THE COMPLETE RESOURCE GUIDE FOR PEOPLE WITH DISABILITIES

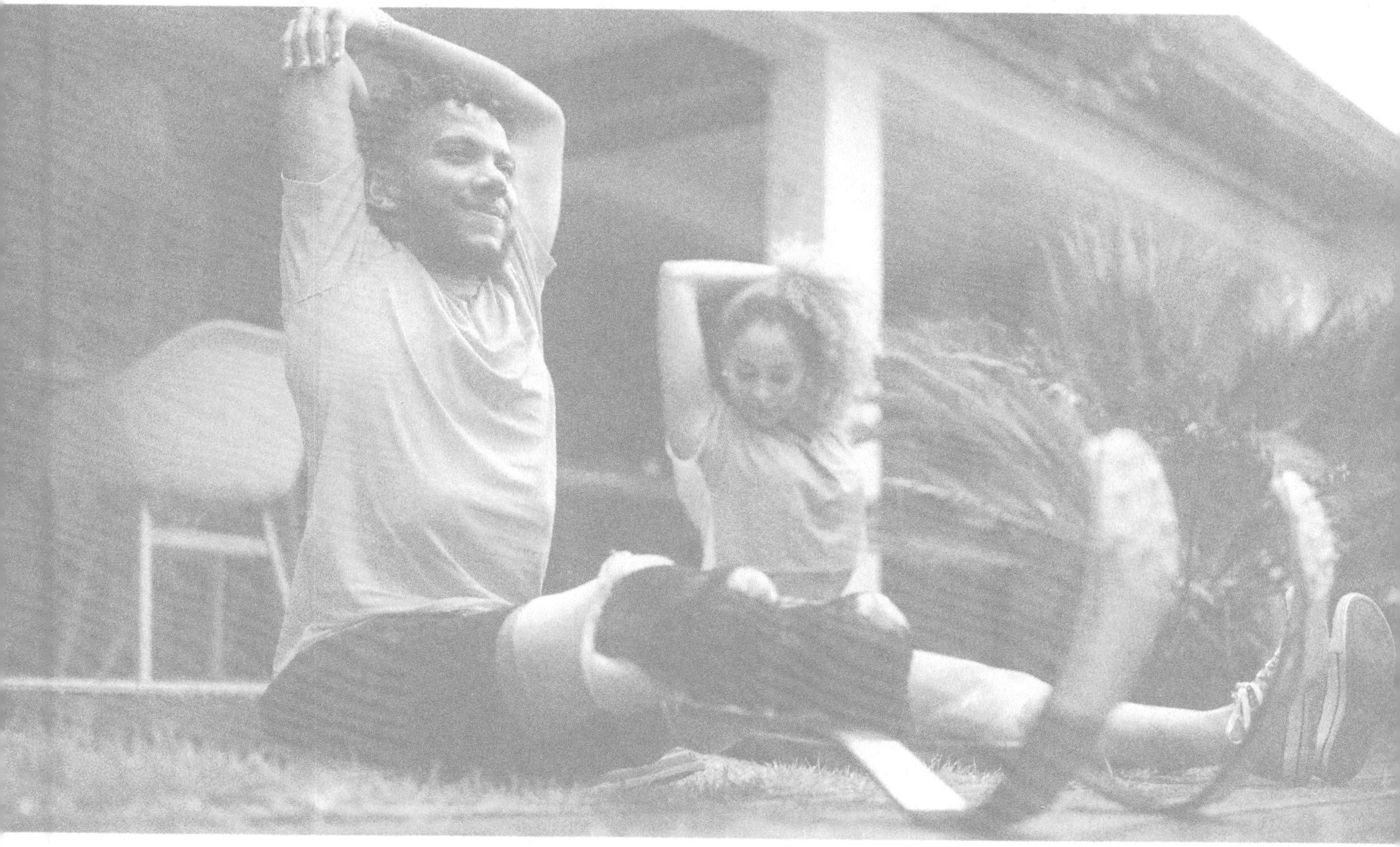

THE COMPLETE RESOURCE GUIDE FOR PEOPLE WITH DISABILITIES

2022
THIRTIETH EDITION

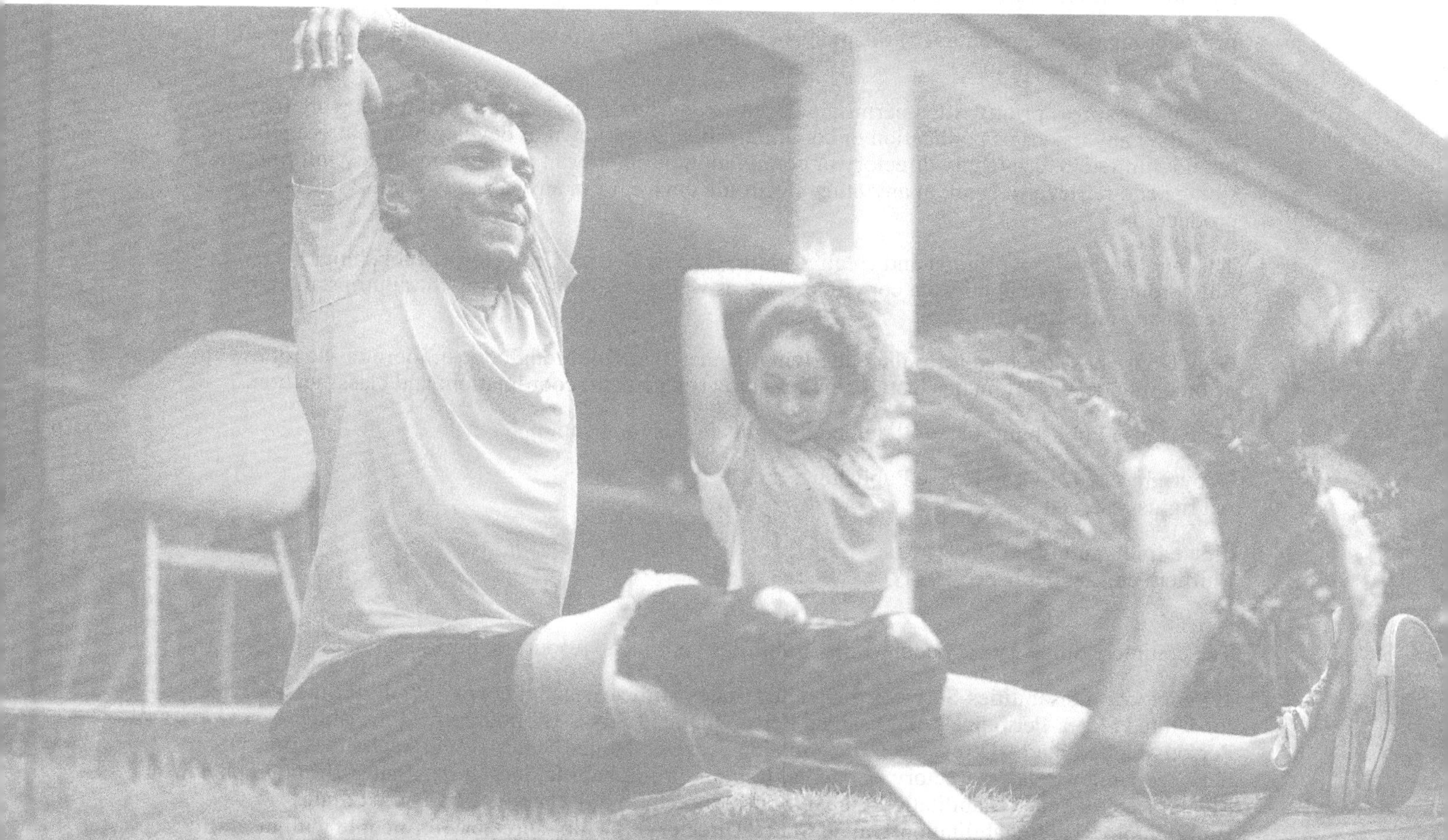

GREY HOUSE PUBLISHING

PUBLISHER: Leslie Mackenzie
EDITORIAL DIRECTOR: Laura Mars
PRODUCTION MANAGER: Kristen Hayes
MARKETING DIRECTOR: Jessica Moody

Grey House Publishing, Inc.
4919 Route 22
Amenia, NY 12501
518.789.8700
Fax: 845.373.6390
www.greyhouse.com
books@greyhouse.com

First edition published 1991
Thirtieth edition published 2021

The complete directory for people with disabilities : products, resources, books, services.-1992-2021

1. People with disabilities-Services for-United States-Directories. 2. People with disabilities-Services for-United States-Periodicals. 3. Disabled Persons-United States-Bibliography. 4. Disabled Persons-United States-Directory. 5. Information Services-United States-Bibliography. 6. Information Services-United States-Directory. 7. Mental Retardation-Rehabilitation-United States-Bibliography. 8. Mental Retardation-Rehabilitation-United States-Directory. 9. Rehabilitation-United States-Bibliography. 10. Rehabilitation-United States-Directory. I. Title: Directory for people with disabilities.

HV1553.C58
362.4/048/02573 92-658843

Printed in the United States

ISBN 13: 9781642658378 Softcover

Table of Contents

Introduction xi
Glossary of Disability-Related Terms xiii
User Guide xix
User Key xxi
2020 Annual Report on People with Disabilities in America xxiii
Disability Impacts Us All lvii
2020 Progress Report on National Disability Policy: Increasing Disability Employment lxiii
A Transition Guide to Postsecondary Education and Employment for Students and Youth with Disabilities lxxxi

General Resources for People with Disabilities

Arts & Entertainment
Resources for the Disabled 1

Assistive Devices
Automobile 8
Bath 12
Bed 14
Communication 15
Chairs 18
Cushions & Wedges 20
Dressing Aids 22
Health Aids 23
Hearing Aids 25
Kitchen & Eating Aids 27
Lifts, Ramps & Elevators 30
Major Catalogs 36
Miscellaneous 41
Office Devices & Workstations 46
Scooters 48
Stationery 51
Visual Aids 52
Walking Aids: Canes, Crutches & Walkers 53
Wheelchairs: Accessories 56
Wheelchairs: General 57
Wheelchairs: Pediatric 60
Wheelchairs: Powered 61
Wheelchairs: Racing 61

Associations
General Disabilities 63

Camps
State Listings 86

Clothing
Clothing 134

Computers
Assistive Devices . . . 139
Braille Products . . . 142
Information Centers & Databases . . . 143
Keyboards, Mouses & Joysticks . . . 148
Scanners . . . 150
Screen Enhancement . . . 150
Speech Synthesizers . . . 151
Software: Math . . . 152
Software: Miscellaneous . . . 154
Software: Professional . . . 164
Software: Reading & Language Arts . . . 165
Software: Vocational . . . 169
Word Processors . . . 170

Conferences & Shows
General . . . 172

Construction & Architecture
Associations . . . 177
Publications & Videos . . . 178

Education
Aids for the Classroom . . . 181
Associations . . . 191
Directories . . . 195
Educational Publishers . . . 197
State Agencies . . . 200
Magazines & Journals . . . 207
Newsletters . . . 213
Professional Texts . . . 217
Testing Resources . . . 250
Treatment & Training . . . 258

Exchange Programs
General . . . 261

Foundations & Funding Resources
State Listings . . . 264
Funding Directories . . . 314

Government Agencies
Federal . . . 318
State Listings . . . 321

Independent Living Centers
State Listings . . . 374

Law
Associations & Referral Agencies . . . 441
Resources for the Disabled . . . 442

Libraries & Research Centers
State Listings . . . 451

Media, Print
Children & Young Adults. 482
Community 483
Employment 484
General Disabilities 485
Parenting: General 504
Parenting: Specific Disabilities 510
Parenting: School 511
Parenting: Spiritual 511
Professional. 512
Specific Disabilities 514
Vocations 515

Media, Electronic
Audio/Visual. 516
Web Sites 524

Toys & Games
General 532

Travel & Transportation
Newsletters & Books 535
Associations & Programs 535
Tours. 536
Vehicle Rentals. 538

Veteran Services
National Administrations 539
State Listings 539

Vocational & Employment Programs
State Listings 563

Rehabilitation Facilities, Acute
State Listings 594

Rehabilitation Facilities, Post-Acute
State Listings 620

Rehabilitation Facilities, Sub-Acute
State Listings 683

Aging
Associations 703
Books 719
Journals. 722
Magazines. 723
Newsletters 731
Support Groups. 733

Blind & Deaf
Audio/Visual. 735
Associations 735
Camps 736
Books 737

Magazines . . . 737
Newsletters . . . 738
Software . . . 739
Sports . . . 739
Support Groups . . . 739

Cognitive
Associations . . . 740
Camps . . . 746
Books . . . 751
Journals . . . 762
Magazines . . . 762
Newsletters . . . 762
Audio/Visual . . . 764
Software . . . 766
Support Groups . . . 766

Dexterity
Associations . . . 767
Books . . . 768
Magazines . . . 768
Newsletters . . . 769

Hearing
Associations . . . 770
Camps . . . 775
Books . . . 777
Journals . . . 787
Magazines . . . 788
Newsletters . . . 788
Audio/Visual . . . 790
Sports . . . 792
Support Groups . . . 792

Mobility
Associations . . . 793
Camps . . . 797
Books . . . 797
Journals . . . 800
Magazines . . . 800
Newsletters . . . 801
Audio/Visual . . . 802
Sports . . . 803
Support Groups . . . 806

General Disorders
Associations . . . 807
Camps . . . 814
Books . . . 826
Journals . . . 845
Magazines . . . 845
Newsletters . . . 846

Sports 849
Support Groups. 849

Speech & Language
Books 853
Associations 853
Camps 856
Books 857
Journals 862
Magazines. 862
Newsletters 862
Audio/Visual. 864
Support Groups. 864

Visual
Associations 866
Camps 873
Books 875
Journals 891
Magazines. 891
Newsletters 892
Audio/Visual. 897
Sports 899
Support Groups. 899

Appendix
2020 Annual Disability Statistics Compendium 901

Indexes
Subject Index 923
Geographic Index. 949
Entry & Publisher Index 965

Introduction

This 30th edition of the award-winning *Complete Resource Guide for People with Disabilities* is invaluable for all those living with a disability, their personal and professional community, and all those committed to empowering these individuals. It offers thousands of ways for people with disabilities to succeed at work, in school, and in their community.

Careful research and compilation of the best data available maintains the reputation of *The Complete Resource Guide for People with Disabilities* among educators, librarians and the disability community. This resource is a repeat recipient of the **National Mature Media Award** and the **National Health Information Award**.

Content

This comprehensive resource opens with valuable front matter, including:

- Glossary of Disability-Related Terms
- 2020 Annual Report on People with Disabilities in America
- "Disability Impacts All of Us" infographic from the CDC
- 2020 Progress Report on National Disability Policy: Increasing Disability Employment
- Transition Guide to Postsecondary Education and Employment for Students and Youth with Disabilities

Coverage continues with subject-specific listing sections (i.e. Arts, Assistive Devices, Camps, Vocational Programs), Rehabilitation Facilities, and disability-specific sections (i.e. Aging, Cognitive, Mobility, Speech). Each disability section includes a range of resources from Associations to Support Groups. The comprehensive Table of Contents guides you through the 33 chapters and more than 100 subchapters contained in this rich resource.

Following the listing chapters is a 2020 Annual Disability Statistics Compendium—a robust section of easy-to-read tables, the first part with numbers of disabled individuals by both state and disability—hearing, vision, cognitive, ambulatory, and self-care and independent-living disabilities—and the second part of individuals who are employed, broken down by the categories listed above.

Sure to save hours of Internet research time, *The Complete Resource Guide for People with Disabilities* provides comprehensive, critical and immediate information in one source that can be accessed quickly and easily. This edition provides 9,367 descriptive listings, 23,933 key contacts, 7,561 fax numbers, 5,894 email addresses, and 8,317 web sites.

Indexes

Three indexes provide quick, easy access to the data.

- **Subject Index** alphabetically organizes listings by relevant topics, i.e. autism, language disorders.
- **Geographic Index** organizes listings alphabetically by state.
- **Entry & Publisher Index** lists all resource guide listings alphabetically.

In addition to the print work, *The Complete Resource Guide for People with Disabilities* is available by subscription on G.O.L.D., Grey House OnLine Databases. This gives you immediate access to the most valuable disability community contacts in the United States, plus offers easy-to-use keyword searches, organization type and subject searches, hotlinks to web sites and emails, and so much more. Call 800-562-2139 for a free trial or visit http://gold.greyhouse.com for more information.

Praise for previous editions:

> *"This comprehensive directory is an excellent starting point...a very useful resource for public, hospital, and consumer-health libraries as well as social-service agencies and nonprofits serving the disabled."*
>
> —Booklist

> *"The strength of this source is in the information referral portion for each entry: the wide range of resources and organizations presented that can assist with additional information and support."*
>
> —ARBA

> *"...thousands of resources...covering a diverse range of services...separate section for specific disabilities...from aging to mobility and from the blind and deaf to speech and language disorders. Libraries...will want to consider..."*
>
> —Against the Grain

We welcome your comments, and look forward to another year of serving the disability community.

Glossary of Disability-Related Terms

Accessible: In the case of a facility, readily usable by a particular individual; in the case of a program or activity, presented or provided in such a way that a particular individual can participate, with or without auxiliary aids(s); in the case of electronic resources, accessible with or without the use of adaptive computer technology.

Access barrier: Any obstruction that prevents people with disabilities from using standard facilities, equipment and resources.

Accessible Web design: Creating World Wide Web pages according to universal design principles to eliminate or reduce barriers, including those that affect people with disabilities.

Accommodation: An adjustment to make a workstation, job, program, facility, or resource accessible to a person with a disability.

Adaptive technology: Hardware or software products that provide access to a computer that is otherwise inaccessible to an individual with a disability.

ALT attribute: HTML code that works in combination with graphical tags to provide alternative text for graphical elements.

Americans with Disabilities Act of 1990 (ADA): A comprehensive Federal law that prohibits discrimination on the basis of disability in employment, telecommunications, public services, public accommodations and services.

American Standard Code for Information Interchange (ASCII): Standard for unformatted text which enables transfer of data between platforms and computer systems.

Assistive technology: Technology used to assist a person with a disability (e.g., a handsplint or computer-related equipment).

Auxiliary aids and services: May include qualified interpreters or other effective methods of making aurally delivered materials available to individuals with hearing impairments; qualified readers, taped texts, or other effective methods of making visually delivered materials available to individuals with visual impairments; acquisition or modification of equipment or devices; and other similar services and actions.

Braille: A system of embossed characters formed by using a Braille cell, a combination of six dots consisting of two vertical columns of three dots each. Each simple Braille character is formed by one or more of these dots and occupies a full cell or space.

Browser: A program that runs on an Internet-connected computer and provides access to the World Wide Web. Web browsers may be text-only, such as Lynx, or graphical, such as Internet Explorer and Netscape Navigator.

Captioned film or videos: Transcription of the verbal portion of films or videos is displayed to make them accessible to people who have hearing impairments.

Closed Circuit TV Magnifier (CCTV): A camera used to magnify books or other materials on a monitor.

Cooperative education: Programs that work with students, faculty, staff, and employers to help students clarify career and academic goals, and expand classroom study by allowing students to participate in paid, practical work experiences.

Compensatory tools: Adaptive computing systems that allow people with disabilities to use computers to complete tasks that would be difficult without a computer (e.g., reading, writing, communicating, accessing information).

Disability: A physical or mental impairment that substantially limits one or more major life activities; a record of such an impairment; or being regarded as having such an impairment (Americans with Disabilities Act of 1990).

Discrimination: The act of treating a person differently in a negative manner based on factors other than individual merit.

Dymo Labeller: A device used to create raised print or Braille labels.

Electronic information: Any digital data for use with computers or computer networks, including disks, CD-ROMs, and World Wide Web resources.

Essential job functions: Those functions of a job or task which must be completed with or without an accommodation.

Facility: All or any portion of a physical complex, including buildings, structures, equipment, grounds, roads, and parking lots.

FM sound amplification system: An electronic amplification system consisting of three components: a microphone/transmitter, monaural FM receiver and a combination charger/carrying case. It provides wireless FM broadcasts from a speaker to a listener who has a hearing impairment.

Frame tags: A means of displaying Web pages. The browser reads the frame tags and produces an output that subdivides output within a browser into discrete windows.

Graphical user interface (GUI): Program interface that presents digital information and software programs in an image-based format as compared to a character-based format.

Hardware: Physical equipment related to computers.

Hearing impairment: Complete or partial loss of the ability to hear, caused by a variety of injuries or diseases, including congenital causes. Limitations, including difficulties in understanding language or other auditory messages and/or in production of understandable speech, are possible.

Independent study: A student works one-on-one with individual faculty members to develop projects for credit.

Informational interview: An activity where students meet with people working in careers to ask questions about their jobs and companies, allowing students to gain personal perspectives on career interests.

Input: Any method by which information is entered into a computer.

Internet: Computer network connecting governmental, educational, commercial, other organizations, and individual computer systems.

Internship: A time-limited, intensive learning experience outside of the typical classroom.

Interpreter: Professional person who assists a person who is deaf in communicating with hearing people.

Job shadowing: A short work-based learning experience where students visit businesses to observe one or more specific jobs to provide them with a realistic view of occupations in a variety of settings.

Keyboard emulation: Uses hardware and/or software in place of a standard keyboard.

Kinesthetic: Refers to touch-based feedback.

Large-print: Most ordinary print is six to ten points in height (about 1/16 to 1/8 of an inch). Large-print type is fourteen to eighteen points (about 1/8 to 1/4 of an inch) and sometimes larger.

Link: a connection between two electronic files or data items.

Lynx: A text-based World Wide Web browser.

Macro: A mini-program that, when run within an application, executes a series of predetermined keystrokes and commands to accomplish a specific task. Macros can automate tedious and often-repeated tasks or create special menus to speed data entry.

Mainstreaming: The inclusion of people with disabilities, with or without special accommodations, in programs, activities, and facilities with non-disabled people.

Major life activities: Functions such as caring for oneself, performing manual tasks, walking, seeing, hearing, speaking, breathing, learning, working, and participating in community activities (Americans with Disabilities Act of 1990).

Multimedia: A computer-based method of presenting information by using more than one medium of communication, such as text, graphics, and sound.

Optical Character Recognition (OCR): Machine recognition of printed or typed text. Using OCR software with a scanner, a printed page can be scanned and the characters converted into text in an electronic format.

Output: Any method of displaying or presenting electronic information to the user through a computer monitor or other device (e.g., speech synthesizer).

Portable Document Format (PDF): The file format for representing documents in a manner that is independent of the original application software, hardware and operating system used to create the documents.

Physical or mental impairment: Any physiological disorder or condition, cosmetic disfigurement, or anatomical loss affecting one or more, but not necessarily limited to, the following body systems: neurological; musculoskeletal; special sense organs; respiratory, including speech organs; cardiovascular; reproductive; digestive; genitourinary; hemic and lymphatic; skin and endocrine; or any mental or psychological disorder, such as mental retardation, organic brain syndrome, emotional or mental illness, and specific learning disabilities (Americans with Disabilities Act of 1990).

Plug-ins: Programs that work within a browser to alter, enhance, or extend the browser,s operation. They are often used for viewing video, animation or listening to audio files.

Proprietary software: Privately owned software based on trade secrets, privately developed technology, or specifications that the owner refuses to divulge, thus preventing others from duplicating a product or program unless an explicit license is purchased. The opposite of proprietary is open (publicly published and available for emulation by others).

Qualified individual with a disability: An individual with a disability who, with or without reasonable modification to rules, policies or practices, the removal of architectural, communication, or transportation barriers, or the provision of auxiliary aids and services, meets the essential eligibility requirements for the receipt of services or participation in programs or activities provided by a public entity (Americans with Disabilities Act of 1990).

Reader: Volunteer or employee of a blind or partially sighted individual who reads printed material in person or records to audiotape.

Relay service: A third-party service (usually free) that allows a hearing person without a TTY/TDD device to communicate over the telephone with a person who has a hearing impairment. The system also allows a person with a hearing impairment who has a TTY/TDD to communicate in voice through a third party, with a hearing person or business.

Screen reader: A text-to-speech system intended for use by computer users who are blind or have low vision that speaks the text content of a computer display using a speech synthesizer.

Service learning: A structured, volunteer work experience where students provide community service in non-paid, volunteer positions to give them opportunities to apply knowledge and skills learned in school while making a contribution to local communities.

Sign language: Manual communication commonly used by people who are deaf. Sign language is not universal; deaf people from different countries speak different sign languages. The gestures or symbols in sign language are organized in a linguistic way. Each individual gesture is called a sign. Each sign has three distinct parts: the hand shape, the position of the hands, and the movement of the hands. American Sign Language (ASL) is the most commonly used sign language in the United States.

Specific learning disability (SLD): A disorder of one or more of the basic psychological processes involved in understanding or in using language, spoken or written, which may manifest itself in difficulties listening, thinking, speaking, reading, writing, spelling, or doing mathematical calculations. Limitations may include hyperactivity, distractibility, emotional instability, visual and/or auditory perception difficulties and/or motor limitations, depending on the type(s) of learning disability.

Speech output system: A system that provides the user with a voice alternative to the text presented on the computer screen.

Speech impairment: A problem in communication and related areas, such as oral motor function, ranging from simple sound substitutions to the inability to understand or use language or use the oral-motor mechanism for functional speech and feeding. Some causes of speech and language disorders include hearing loss; neurological disorders; brain injury; mental retardation; drug abuse; physical impairments, such as cleft lip or palate; and vocal abuse or misuse.

Speech input system: A computer-based system that allows the operator to control the system using his/her voice.

Sticky keys: Enables a computer user to do multiple key combinations on a keyboard using only one finger at a time. The sticky keys function is usually used with the Ctrl, Alt, and Shift keys. Simultaneous keystrokes can be entered sequentially.

Telecommunications Device for the Deaf (TDD) or Teletypewriter (TTY): A device which enables someone who has a speech or hearing impairment to use a telephone when communicating with someone else who has a TDD/TTY. TDD/TTYs can be used with any telephone, and one needs only a basic typing ability to use them.

Trackball: A pointing device consisting of a ball housed in a socket containing sensors to detect the rotation of the ball " like an upside down mouse. The user rolls the ball with his thumb or the palm of his hand to move the pointer.

Traumatic Brain Injury (TBI): An open or closed head injury resulting in impairments in one or more areas, such as cognition; language; memory; attention; reasoning; abstract thinking; judgment; problem-solving; sensory, perceptual, and motor abilities; psychosocial behavior; physical functions; information processing; and speech. The term does not apply to brain injuries that are congenital or degenerative, or brain injuries induced by birth trauma.

Undue hardship: An action that requires significant difficulty or expense in relation to the size of the employer, the resources available, and the nature of the operation (Americans with Disabilities Act of 1990).

Universal design: Designing programs, services, tools, and facilities so that they are usable, without additional modification, by the widest range of users possible, taking into account a variety of abilities and disabilities.

Vocational Rehabilitation Act of 1973: An act prohibiting discrimination on the basis of disability which applies to any program that receives federal financial assistance. Section 504 of the act is aimed at making educational programs and facilities accessible to all people with disabilities. Section 508 of the act requires that electronic office equipment purchased through federal procurement meets disability access guidelines.

Voice input system: A computer-based system that allows the operator to control the system using his/her voice.

Vision impairments: A complete or partial loss of the ability to see, caused by a variety of injuries or diseases including congenital causes. Legal blindness is defined as visual acuity of 20/200 or less in the better eye with correcting lenses, on the widest diameter of the visual field subtending an angular distance no greater than 20 degrees.

World Wide Web (WWW, W3, or Web): Hypertext and multimedia gateway to the Internet.

DO-IT
University of Washington
Box 354842
Seattle, WA 98195-4842
doit@uw.edu
http://www.washington.edu/doit/
206-685-DOIT (3648) (voice/TTY)
888-972-DOIT (3648) (toll free voice/TTY)
206-221-4171 (FAX)
509-328-9331 (voice/TTY) Spokane

Director: Sheryl Burgstahler, Ph.D.

User Guide

Descriptive listings in *The Complete Resource Guide for People with Disabilities* are organized into 33 chapters, by either resource type or disability category type. You will find the following types of listings throughout the book:

- National Agencies & Associations
- State Agencies & Associations
- Camps & Exchanges Programs
- Manufacturers of Assistive Devices, Clothing, Computer Equipment & Supplies
- Print & Electronic Media
- Living Centers & Facilities
- Libraries & Research Centers
- Conferences & Trade Shows

Below is a sample listing illustrating the kind of information that is or might be included in an Association entry. Each numbered item of information is described in the paragraphs on the following page.

---

1 → 1234
2 → **Advocacy Center for Seniors with Disabilities**
3 → 1762 South Major Drive
New Orleans, LA 98087

4 → **800-000-0000**

5 → **058-884-0709**

6 → **Fax: 058-884-0568**

7 → **TDD: 800-000-0001**

8 → **email: info@sadvoc.com**

9 → **www.sadvoc.com**

10 → Barbara Pierce, Executive Director
Diane Watkins, Marketing Director
Robert Goldfarb, Administrative Assistant

11 → The mission of the Center is to advance the dignity, equality, self-determination and choices of senior citizens with disabilities. It provides referrals, publishes information, including a monthly newsletter, offers workshops and consultation on legal, social, travel, and medical issues. The Center works with various local organizations to help seniors with disabilities stay active in their community.

12 → Founded 1964

13 → 18 pages

14 → Monthly

User Key

1 ➔ **Record Number**: Entries are listed alphabetically within each category and numbered sequentially. The entry numbers, rather than page numbers, are used in the indexes to refer to listings.

2 ➔ **Organization Name**: Formal name of company or organization. Where organization names are completely capitalized, the listing will appear at the beginning of the alphabetized section. In the case of publications, the title of the publication will appear first, followed by the publisher.

3 ➔ **Address**: Location or permanent address of the organization.

4 ➔ **Toll Free Number**: This is listed when provided by the organization.

5 ➔ **Phone Number**: The listed phone number is usually for the main office of the organization, but may also be for the sales, marketing, or public relations office as provided by the organization.

6 ➔ **Fax Number**: This is listed when provided by the organization.

7 ➔ **TDD Number**: This is listed when provided. It refers to Telephone Device for the Deaf.

8 ➔ **E-Mail**: This is listed when provided by the organization and is generally the main office e-mail.

9 ➔ **Web Site**: This is also referred to as an URL address. These web sites are accessed through the Internet by typing *http://* before the URL address.

10 ➔ **Key Personnel**: Name and titles of department heads of the organization.

11 ➔ **Organization Description**: This paragraph contains a brief description of the organization and their services.

12 ➔ **Year Founded:** The year in which the organization was established or founded. If the organization has changed its name, the founding date is usually for the earliest name under which it was known.

13 ➔ **Number of Pages**: Number of pages if the listing is a publication.

14 ➔ **Frequency:** The frequency of the listing if it is a publication.

2020

ANNUAL REPORT
ON PEOPLE WITH DISABILITIES IN AMERICA

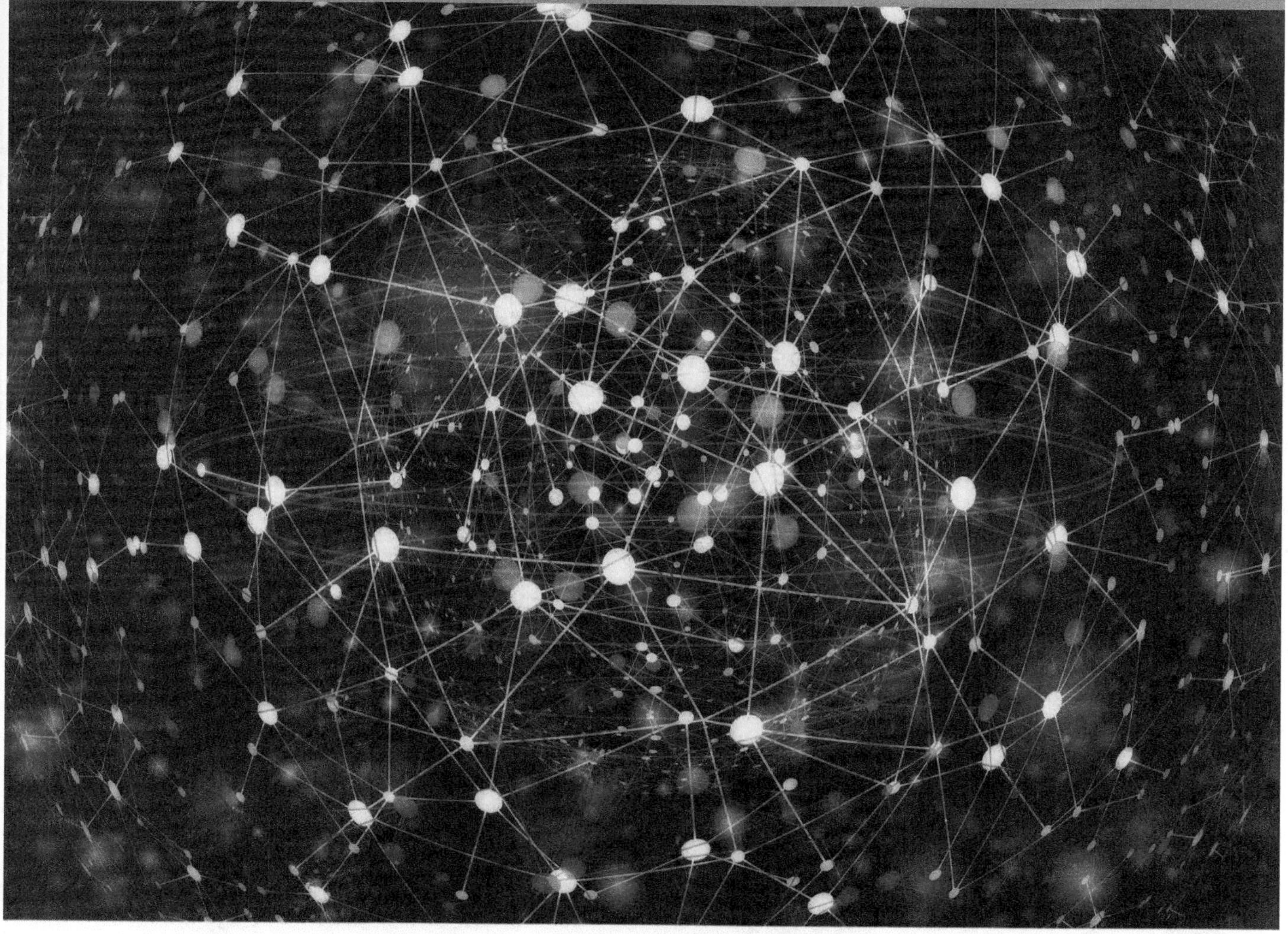

Disability Statistics & Demographics
Rehabilitation Research & Training Center

disabilitycompendium.org

Acknowledgements

Funding for this publication made possible by:

The Rehabilitation Research and Training Center on Disability Statistics and Demographics (StatsRRTC), funded by the U.S. Department of Health and Human Services, Administration for Community, Living National Institute on Disability, Independent Living, and Rehabilitation Research (NIDILRR), grant number 90RTGE0001. The information developed by the StatsRRTC does not necessarily represent the policies of the Department of Health and Human Services, and you should not assume endorsement by the Federal Government (Edgar, 75.620 (b)).

The StatsRRTC is part of the Institute on Disability (IOD) at the University of New Hampshire (UNH). The IOD was established in 1987 to provide a university-based focus for the improvement of knowledge, policies, and practices related to the lives of people with disabilities and their families and is New Hampshire's University Center for Excellence in Disability (UCED). Located within UNH, the IOD is a federally designated center authorized by the Developmental Disabilities Act. Through innovative and interdisciplinary research, academic, service, and dissemination initiatives, the IOD builds local, state, and national capacities to respond to the needs of individuals with disabilities and their families.

Institute on Disability/UCED

University of New Hampshire

10 West Edge Drive, Suite 101 | Durham, NH 03284
603.862.4320 | relay: 711 | contact.iod@unh.edu | https://www.iod.unh.edu

Stay Connected:

This document is available in alternative formats upon request.

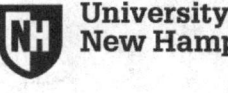

Annual Report on People with Disabilities in America

2020

Rehabilitation Research and Training Center on Disability Statistics and Demographics

A NIDILRR-Funded Center

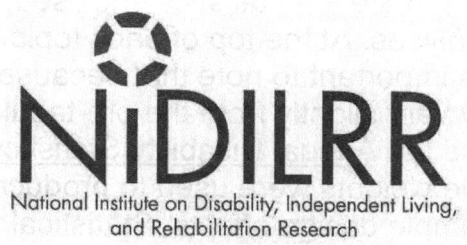

NIDILRR

National Institute on Disability, Independent Living, and Rehabilitation Research

Introduction

Make the Call. Statistics are a powerful tool. The National Bureau of Economic Research tracks changes in the national gross domestic product, a key indicator of economic activity, to "make the call" as to whether the economy is in recession. On the first Friday of each month, the Bureau of Labor Statistics releases the official unemployment rate to monitor the labor market. Each year during the second week of September, the Census Bureau publishes the official poverty rate and whether an increase or decrease in the poverty rate was detected. The Centers of Diseases Control and Prevention's Health People program tracks health indicators over the course of each decade. The goal of the Annual Report on People with Disabilities in America is to track the progress of people with disabilities using key social and economic indicators and each make the call (for each indicator) as to whether an increase or decrease was detected.

Topics. The Annual Report will include many of the key indicators identified in a comprehensive 2008 study, Keeping Track: National Disability Status and Program Performance Indicators, conducted by the National Council on Disability (NCD). This NCD report used a systematic approach of stakeholder input to select indicators based on data availability and ability to address key areas of interest to stakeholders. The resulting indicators were in the following areas of interest: employment, educational attainment, health and health care, financial status and security, leisure recreation, personal relationships, and crime/safety. At the top of each topic the population being studied is noted in parentheses. In the coming years, the Annual Report will add more of the NCD indicators in these areas, as well as indicators for which data has only recently become available.

Methods. The current set of indicators is derived from the American Community Survey (ACS). In future years, other data sources will be used to track other indicators. The ACS is an annual survey conducted by the Census Bureau and is well-suited to track indicators over time due to its large sample size, consistent questionnaire over the years, and multitude of variables to examine. The Public Use Microdata Sample (PUMS) files were used to estimate the statistics enclosed. The PUMS files allow data users to conduct custom analyses. At the top of each topic the population being studied is noted in parentheses. It is important to note that because of this, the estimates presented in this report may vary slightly from the pre-tabulated estimates published in the US Census Bureau's and the Annual Disability Statistics Compendium. Sample weights and replicate sample weights were used to produce nationally representative statistics that account for sample design effects. Statistical significance is based on a one-tail test using a 95 percent level of confidence.

Findings. An important finding – which may help you work your way through the
Ann
"sta ther

words, we are certain (with at least 95 percent confidence) that a given gap exists. It is also important to note that statistical significance is not the same as the term significance or meaningfulness. Whether the magnitude of any gap is meaningful from a social or policy perspective is a matter for further discussion.

Overall, like 2017-2018, it appears that there was not a great deal of change between 2018 to 2019 (the most recent year available) in the indicators track of the Annual Report. The exceptions are

- An increase in the size of the U.S. population with disabilities, percentage-wise,
- A narrowing of the "employment gap,"
- A narrowing of the "recently constructed housing gap," and
- An increase in the "disablement index" (i.e., reporting of independent living difficulty among persons reporting hearing, vision, ambulatory, and cognitive difficulties).

However, many gaps have changed when comparing the gap in 2019 to 2008, the first year the data became available.

Additional Resources. The Annual Report complements the detailed tables of data which can be found in the Annual Disability Statistics Compendium (www.DisabilityCompendium.org). For reasons discussed previously in methods, the statistics reported in the Annual Report might differ from those reported in the Annual Disability Statistics Compendium and Supplement. Help navigating any of the resources described here can be found in the Frequently Asked Questions section at www.DisabilityCompendium.org/faq. Assistance interpreting and locating additional statistics is available via our toll-free number, 886.538.9521, or by email, Disability.Statistics@UNH.edu. For more information about our research project, please visit www.ResearchOnDisability.org.

Suggested Citation. Houtenville, A. and Rafal, M. (2020). *Annual Report on People with Disabilities in America: 2020*. Durham, NH: University of New Hampshire, Institute on Disability.

Population with Disabilities

Focus Population: Civilians, all ages

The size of the population with disabilities—percentage-wise—increased from 2018 to 2019.

When using statistics to track the well-being of people with disabilities and accessibility, it is important to understand the size of the population with disabilities. Table 1 shows that there were 327,011,000 people in the U.S. in 2019. Of these persons, 43,227,000 were people with disabilities. Percentage-wise, people with disabilities comprised 13.2 percent of the U.S. population; i.e., 13.2 percent of the U.S. civilian population were people with disabilities. The size of the population with disabilities—percentage-wise—increased from 13.1 percent in 2018 to 13.2 percent in 2019. (The Appendix contains the questions we used in the American Community Survey to define disability.)

Table 1. Number and Percentage with Disabilities

Year	Total Population	Population with Disabilities	Percentage with Disabilities	
	Estimate (#)	Estimate (#)	Estimate (%)	St. Error (% pts)
2008	302,819,000	38,560,000	12.7‡	0.03
2009	305,701,000	38,583,000	12.6†‡	0.02
2010	308,291,000	38,463,000	12.5†‡	0.02
2011	310,572,000	39,383,000	12.7†‡	0.02
2012	312,873,000	39,710,000	12.7‡	0.02
2013	315,143,000	41,242,000	13.1†‡	0.03
2014	317,861,000	41,827,000	13.2†	0.03
2015	320,399,000	42,050,000	13.1†‡	0.02
2016	322,110,000	42,940,000	13.3†‡	0.02
2017	324,689,000	42,776,000	13.2†	0.02
2018	326,155,000	42,630,000	13.1†‡	0.02
2019	327,011,000	43,227,000	13.2†	0.03

Source: Author's calculation using the data from the 2008-2019 American Community Surveys for civilian respondents of all ages.
† Significantly different from the previous year at the 5 percent level and a one-tailed test.
‡ Significantly different from the 2019 estimate at the 5 percent level and a one-tailed test.

Figure 1. Percentage of People with Disablities

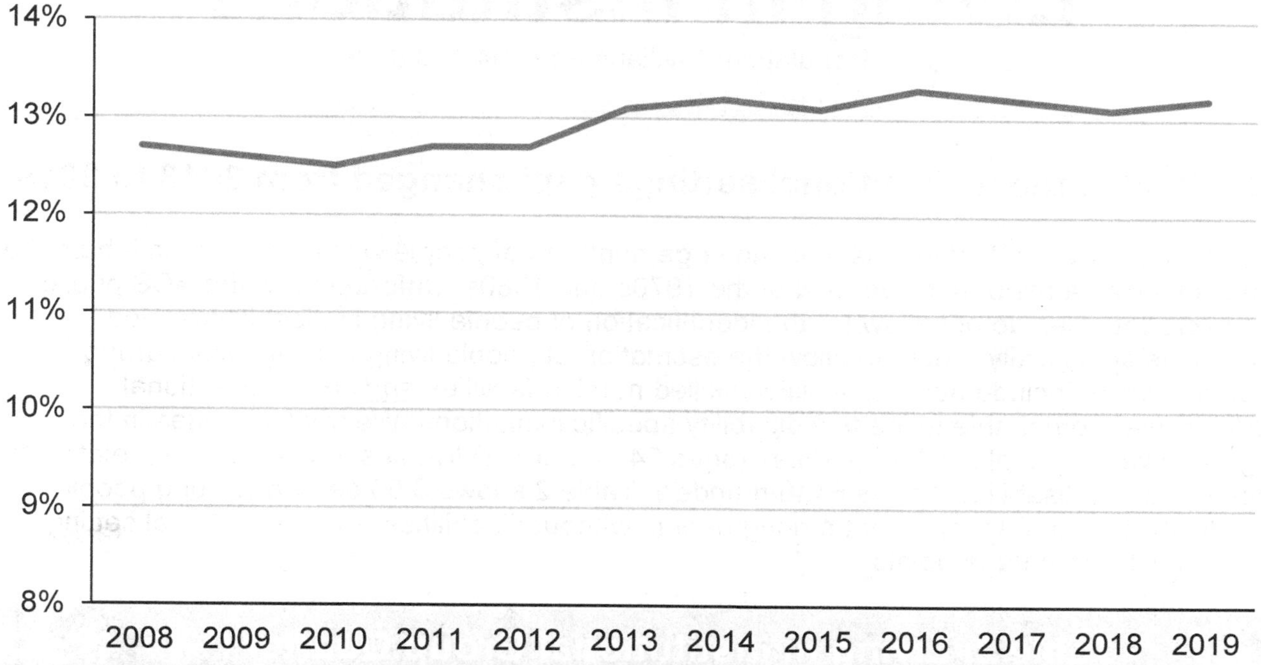

Comparisons & Statistical Significance

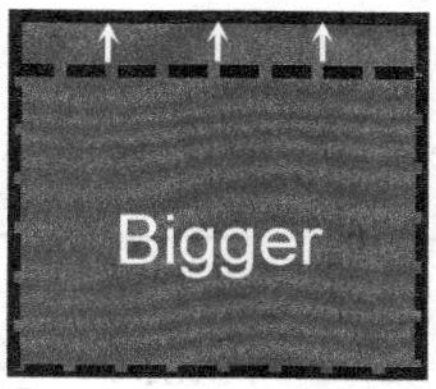

Percentage-wise, did the population with disabilities get larger between 2018 and 2019?
YES. A statistically significant increase in the percentage of the population with disabilities was detected between 2018 and 2019, from 13.1 percent to 13.2 percent.

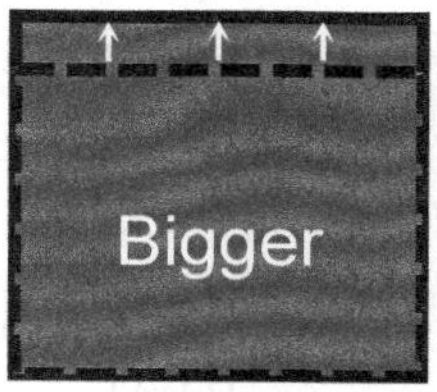

Percentage-wise, did the population with disabilities get larger since the earliest year available, 2008?
YES. A statistically significant increase in the percentage of the population with disabilities was detected between 2008 and 2019, from 12.7 percent in 2008 to 13.2 percent in 2019.

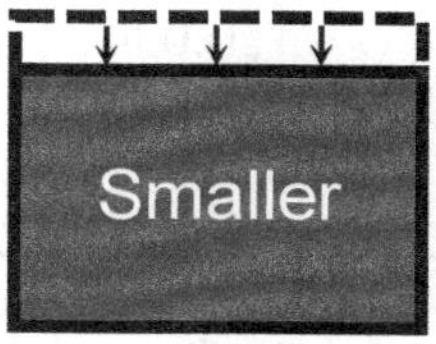

Percentage-wise, did the population with disabilities get larger since its highest level in 2016?
NO. The opposite occurred. A statistically significant decrease in the percentage of the population with disabilities was detected between 2016 and 2019, from 13.3 percent in 2016 to 13.2 percent in 2019.

Living in Institutions

Focus Population: Civilians ages 64 and under

Can't tell if the 'institutional settings gap' changed from 2018 to 2019

The shutting down of institutions housing large numbers of people with disabilities in inhumane conditions was a major achievement of the 1970s and 1980s. Unfortunately, the ACS public use microdata files do not allow for the identification of people living in disability-related institutions specifically. They do allow the estimation of people living in institutional group quarters, which include nursing facilities/skilled nursing facilities _and_ adult correctional facilities, we are not able to identify disability-specific institutions. We track changes in the degree to which people with disabilities (ages 64 and under) live in such institutions, relative to people without disabilities (ages 64 and under). Table 2 shows 3.50 percent among people with disabilities and 0.69 percent among people without disabilities—an "institutional settings gap" of 2.81 percentage points.

Table 2. Living in Institutional Group Quarter (%)

	People with Disabilities		People without Disabilities		Gap (% pts)	
Year	Estimate	St. Error	Estimate	St. Error	Estimate	St. Error
2008	3.97‡	0.048	0.71‡	0.004	3.26*‡	0.048
2009	3.94‡	0.051	0.72†‡	0.003	3.22*‡	0.051
2010	3.75†‡	0.046	0.75†‡	0.004	3.00*†‡	0.046
2011	3.65†‡	0.039	0.75‡	0.004	2.90*‡	0.039
2012	3.75†‡	0.034	0.73†‡	0.003	3.02*†‡	0.034
2013	3.48†	0.035	0.73‡	0.003	2.75*†	0.035
2014	3.64†‡	0.034	0.72†‡	0.003	2.92*†‡	0.034
2015	3.57	0.041	0.71‡	0.004	2.86*	0.041
2016	3.39†‡	0.036	0.71‡	0.003	2.68*†‡	0.036
2017	3.48†	0.034	0.69†	0.003	2.79*†	0.034
2018	3.58†	0.032	0.69	0.003	2.89*†	0.032
2019	3.5	0.037	0.69	0.003	2.81*	0.037

Source: Author's calculation using the data from the 2008-2019 American Community Surveys for civilian respondents ages 64 and under.
* Significant at the 5 percent level and a one-tailed test.
† Significantly different from the previous year at the 5 percent level and a one-tailed test.
‡ Significantly different from the 2019 estimate at the 5 percent level and a one-tailed test.

Figure 2. Percent Living in Institutional Group Quarters

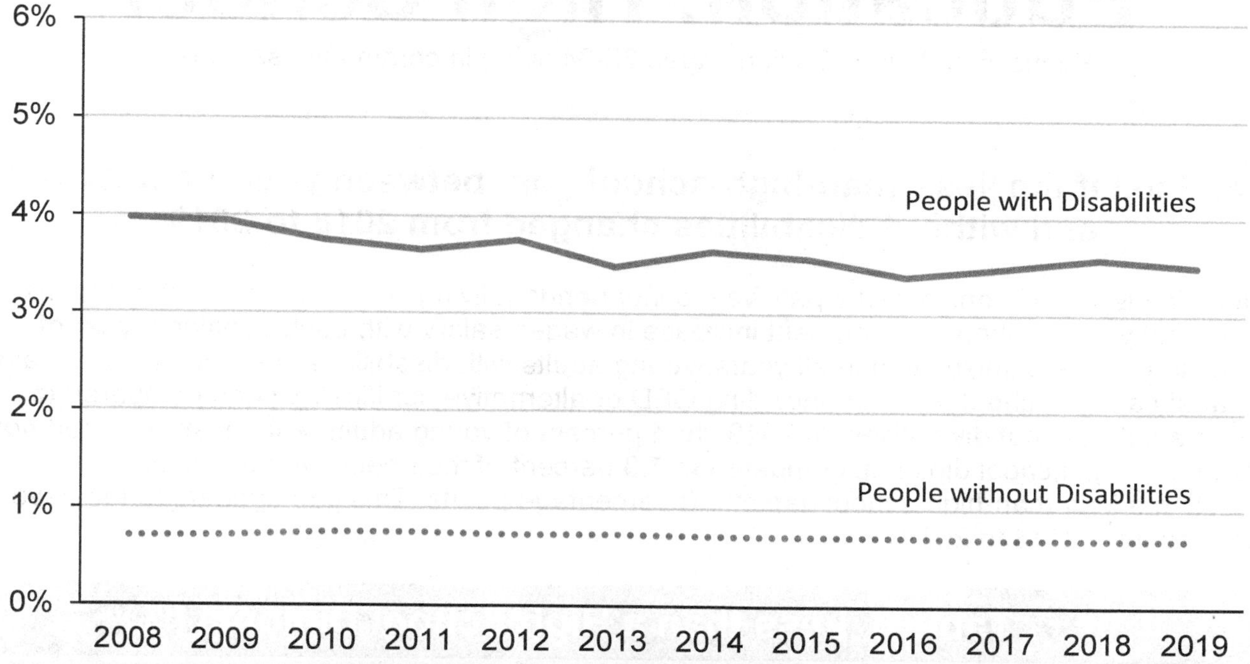

Comparisons & Statistical Significance

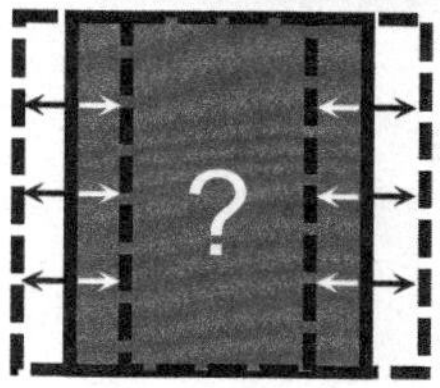

Did the institutional settings gap narrow between 2018 and 2019?

CAN'T TELL. The institutional settings gap appears to narrow from 2.89 percentage points in 2018 to 2.81 percentage points in 2019. However, this narrowing is not statistically significant, meaning that it may be due to the estimates being derived from samples of the U.S. populations.

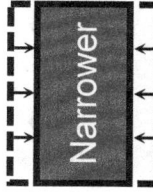

Did the institutional settings gap narrow since the earliest year available, 2008?

YES. A statistically significant narrowing of the institutional settings gap was detected between 2008 and 2019, decreasing from 3.26 percentage points in 2008 to 2.81 percentage points in 2019.

Education: High School

Focus Population: Civilians ages 25-34 living in community settings

Can't tell if the 'less-than-high-school gap' between young adults with and without disabilities changed from 2018 to 2019

Education is widely considered a pathway to independent living. The economics literature has consistently found about a 10 percent increase in wages/salary with each additional year of education. Table 3 shows that in all years, young adults with disabilities are more likely to have *not* attain a high school diploma (including GED or alternative certificate) when compared to young adults without disabilities. In 2019, 16.4 percent of young adults with disabilities had *not* attained a high school diploma, compared to 7.3 percent of their peers without disabilities, reflecting a less-than-high-school gap of 9.0 percentage points. This gap <u>appears</u> not to have changed from 2018 to 2019.

Table 3. Less than a High School Diploma (%)

	People with Disabilities		People without Disabilities		Gap (% pts)	
Year	Estimate	St. Error	Estimate	St. Error	Estimate	St. Error
2008	23.4‡	0.45	12.7‡	0.09	10.7*‡	0.46
2009	24.0‡	0.41	12.0†‡	0.09	12.0*†‡	0.42
2010	22.8†‡	0.32	11.9‡	0.09	10.9*†‡	0.34
2011	22.2‡	0.36	11.1†‡	0.08	11.1*‡	0.37
2012	22.2‡	0.4	10.6†‡	0.08	11.6*‡	0.41
2013	20.6†‡	0.33	10.5‡	0.08	10.1*†‡	0.34
2014	19.8‡	0.3	9.8†‡	0.07	10.0*‡	0.31
2015	19.2‡	0.31	9.4†‡	0.07	9.8*‡	0.32
2016	19.1‡	0.35	8.9†‡	0.07	10.2*‡	0.36
2017	17.3†‡	0.31	8.1†‡	0.07	9.2*†	0.32
2018	16.7	0.29	7.7†	0.07	9.0*	0.29
2019	16.4	0.32	7.3	0.06	9.0*	0.32

Source: Author's calculation using the data from the 2008-2019 American Community Surveys for civilian respondents of ages 25-34 who live in community settings.

* Significant at the 5 percent level and a one-tailed test.

† Significantly different from the previous year at the 5 percent level and a one-tailed test.

‡ Significantly different from the 2018 estimate at the 5 percent level and a one-tailed test.

Figure 3. Percent with Less High School Diploma

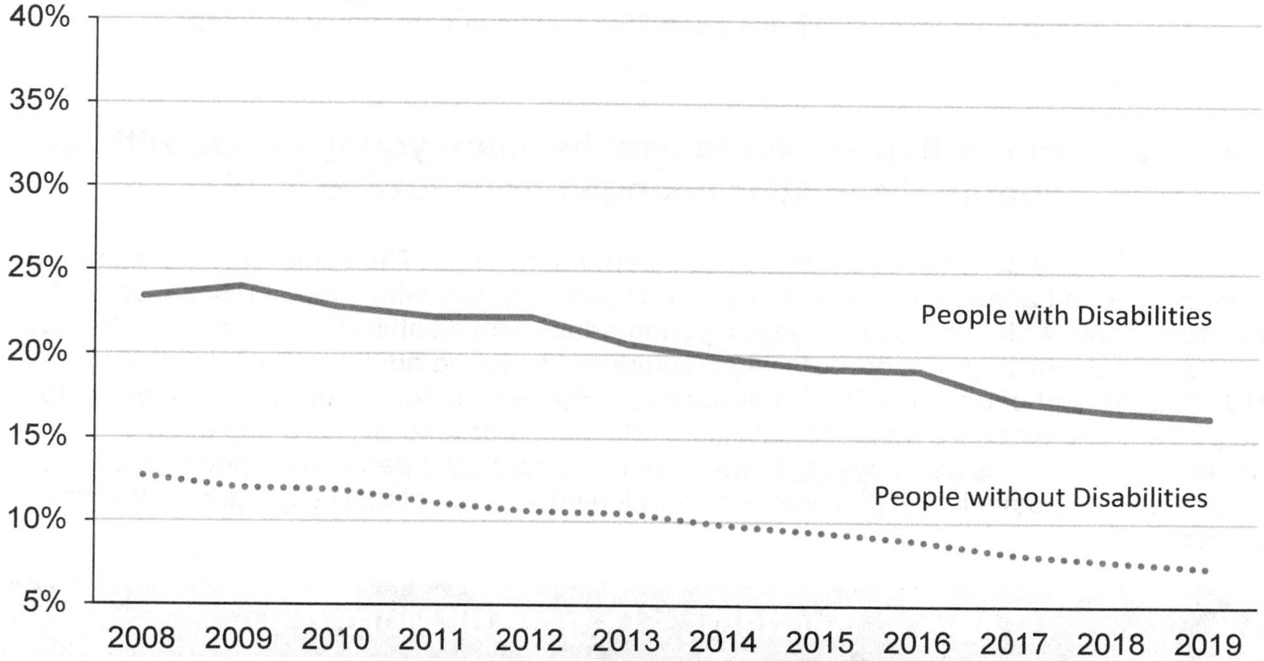

Comparisons & Statistical Significance

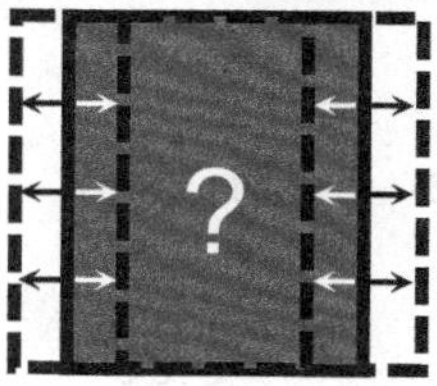

Did the less-than-high-school gap narrow between 2018 and 2019?

NO. The less-than-high-school gap appears to stay the same from 2018 to 2019, at 9.0 percentage points.

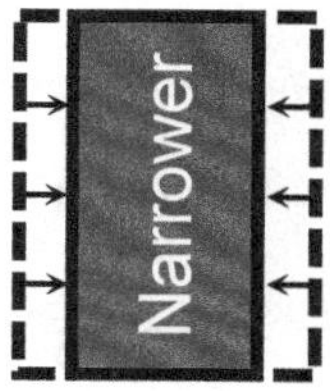

Did the less-than-high-school gap narrow since the earliest year available, 2008?

YES. A statistically significant narrowing of the less-than-high-school gap was detected between 2008 and 2019, decreasing from 10.8 percentage points in 2008 to 9.0 percentage points in 2019. This narrowing was statistically significant, meaning it was not likely due to chance because the estimates are derived from samples of the U.S. populations in 2008 and 2019.

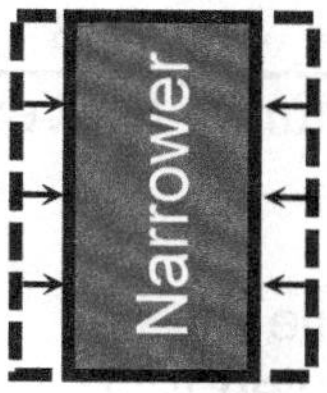

Did the less-than-high-school gap narrow since its widest point?

YES. A statistically significant narrowing of the less-than-high-school gap was detected between its widest point in 2009, decreasing from 12.0 percentage points in 2009 to 9.0 percentage points in 2019.

Education: College

Focus Population: Civilians ages 25-34 living in community settings

Can't tell if the 'college-or-more gap' between young adults with and without disabilities changed from 2018 to 2019

Education is widely considered a pathway to independent living. The economics literature has consistently found about a 10 percent increase in wages/salary with each additional year of education. Table 4 shows that in all years, young adults with disabilities are less likely to have attained a Bachelor's degree or more when compared to young adults without disabilities. In 2019, 16.1 percent of people with disabilities had a Bachelor's degree or more, compared to 39.2 percent of their peers without disabilities, reflecting a college-or-more gap of 23.1 percentage points. This gap appears to have widened from 22.8 percentage points in 2018 to 23.1 percentage points in 2019, however this widening was not statistically significantly greater than zero.

Table 4. Bachelor's Degree or More (%)

	People with Disabilities		People without Disabilities		Gap (% pts)	
Year	Estimate	St. Error	Estimate	St. Error	Estimate	St. Error
2008	9.8‡	0.27	31.3‡	0.13	21.5*‡	0.3
2009	10.0‡	0.26	32.8†‡	0.13	22.8*†	0.29
2010	10.5‡	0.24	33.1‡	0.13	22.6*	0.27
2011	11.0‡	0.3	33.6†‡	0.14	22.6*	0.33
2012	10.7‡	0.27	34.4†‡	0.13	23.7*†	0.3
2013	12.4†‡	0.28	34.8†‡	0.14	22.4*†	0.31
2014	12.8‡	0.3	35.4†‡	0.14	22.6*	0.33
2015	13.5†‡	0.28	36.2†‡	0.13	22.7*	0.31
2016	13.9‡	0.3	37.1†‡	0.14	23.2*	0.33
2017	15.0†‡	0.26	37.7†‡	0.16	22.7*	0.31
2018	15.6	0.3	38.4†	0.14	22.8*	0.33
2019	16.1	0.29	39.2†	0.15	23.1*	0.33

Source: Author's calculation using the data from the 2008-2019 American Community Surveys for civilian respondents of ages 25-34 who live in community settings.
* Significant at the 5 percent level and a one-tailed test.
† Significantly different from the previous year at the 5 percent level and a one-tailed test.
‡ Significantly different from the 2019 estimate at the 5 percent level and a one-tailed test.

Figure 4. Percent with Bachelor's Degree or More

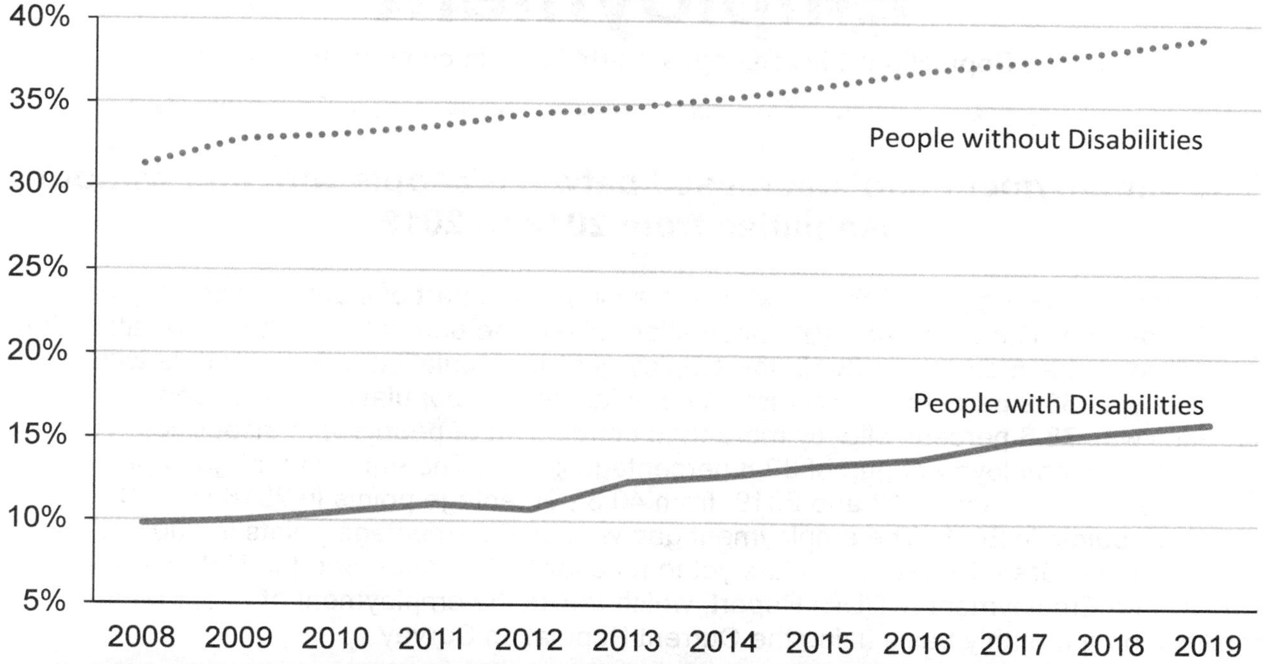

Comparisons & Statistical Significance

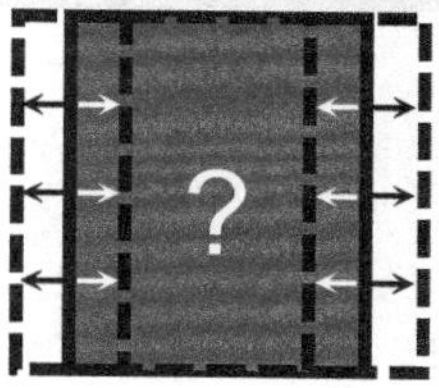

Did the college-or-more gap narrow between 2018 and 2019?
CAN'T TELL. The college-or-more gap appears to widen from 22.8 percentage points in 2018 to 23.1 percentage points in 2019. However, this widening is not statistically significant, meaning that it is not distinguishable (given these data) from zero widening.

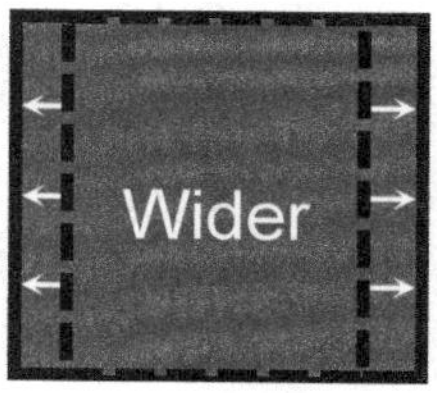

Did the college-or-more gap narrow since the earliest year available, 2008?
NO. The opposite occurred. A statistically significant widening of the college-or-more gap was detected between 2008 and 2019, increasing from 21.5 percentage points to 23.1 percentage points. This widening was statistically significant, meaning it was not likely due to chance because the estimates are derived from samples of the U.S. populations in 2008 and 2019.

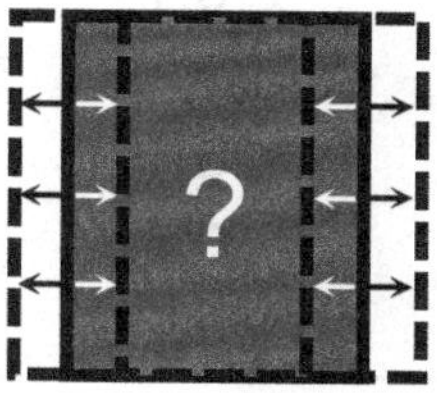

Did the college-or-more gap narrow since its widest point?
CAN'T TELL. The college-or-more gap appears to narrow from its widest point in 2012, decreasing from 23.7 percentage points in 2012 to 23.1 percentage points in 2019. However, this narrowing is not statistically significant, meaning that it is not distinguishable (given these data) from zero widening.

Employment

Focus Population: Civilians ages 18-64 living in community settings

The 'employment gap' decreased between people with and without disabilities from 2018 to 2019

Employment and being part of the workforce is an important part of independent living and social integration. The employment-to-population ratio is the percentage of the population that is employed. Table 5 shows, in 2019, the employment-to-population ratio for people with disabilities was 38.9 percent. In contrast, the employment-to-population ratio of people without disabilities was 78.6 percent, slightly more than double that of people with disabilities. This amounted to an employment gap of 39.8 percentage points. The employment gap appears to have decreased between 2018 and 2019, from 40.3 percentage points in 2018 to 39.8 percentage points in 2018. The employment gap was 38.6 percentage points in 2008 at the beginning of the Great Recession. It has yet to recover to that level. See the National Trends in Disability and Employment (nTIDE) Report, which tracks the employment of people with disabilities on a monthly basis using the Current Population Survey.

Table 5. Employment to Population Ratio (%)

	People with Disabilities		People without Disabilities		Gap (% pts)	
Year	Estimate	St. Error	Estimate	St. Error	Estimate	St. Error
2008	39.1	0.15	77.7‡	0.04	38.6*‡	0.16
2009	35.5†‡	0.15	74.3†‡	0.04	38.9*‡	0.16
2010	33.5†‡	0.12	72.9†‡	0.05	39.4*†‡	0.13
2011	33.0†‡	0.15	73.1†‡	0.05	40.1*†	0.16
2012	33.0‡	0.13	73.8†‡	0.04	40.8*†‡	0.14
2013	34.1†‡	0.12	74.5†‡	0.04	40.4*†‡	0.13
2014	34.2‡	0.14	75.3†‡	0.04	41.1*†‡	0.15
2015	34.9†‡	0.13	76.0†‡	0.04	41.2*‡	0.14
2016	36.0†‡	0.13	76.8†‡	0.05	40.8*†‡	0.14
2017	36.9†‡	0.14	77.2†‡	0.05	40.3*†‡	0.15
2018	37.5†‡	0.12	77.8†	0.05	40.3*‡	0.13
2019	38.9†	0.13	78.6†	0.05	39.8*†	0.14

Source: Author's calculation using the data from the 2008-2019 American Community Surveys for civilian respondents of ages 18-64 who live in community settings.

* Significant at the 5 percent level and a one-tailed test.

† Significantly different from the previous year at the 5 percent level and a one-tailed test.

‡ Significantly different from the 2019 estimate at the 5 percent level and a one-tailed test.

Figure 5. Employment to Population Ratio

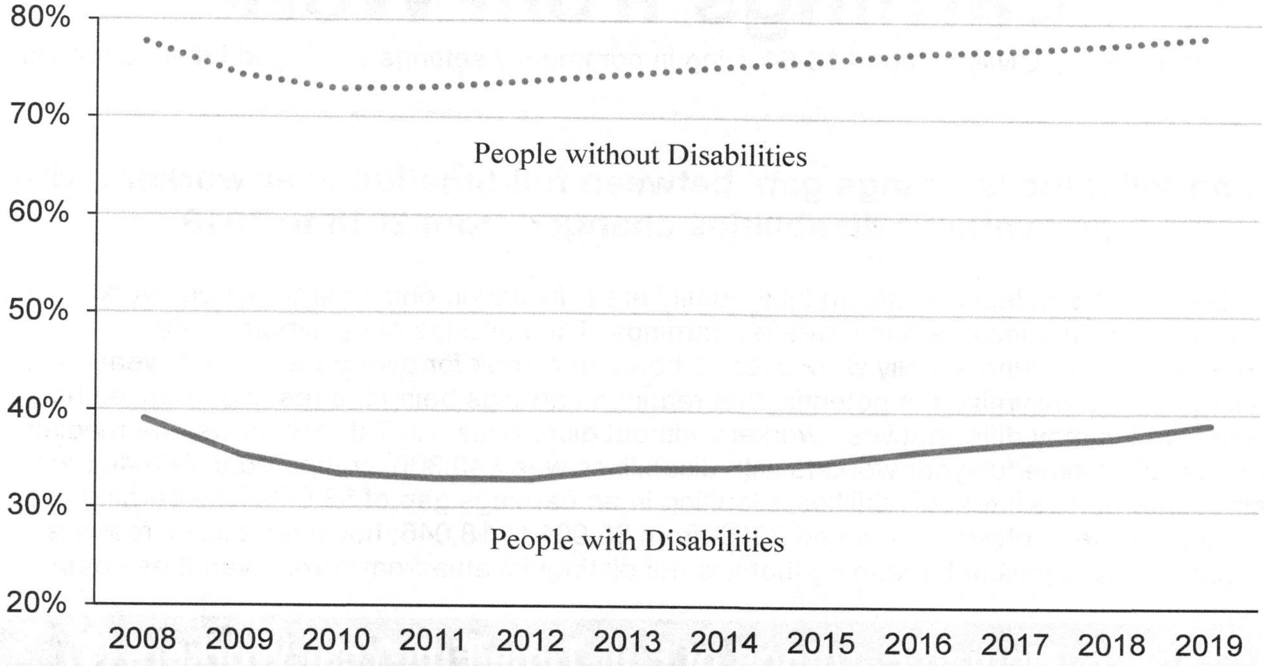

Comparisons & Statistical Significance

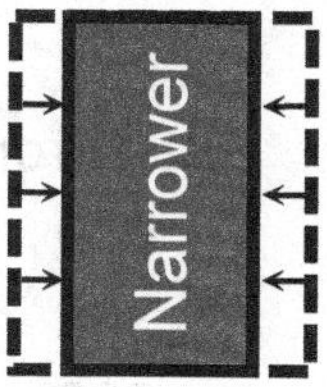

Did the employment gap narrow between 2018 and 2019?
YES. A statistically significant narrowing of the employment gap was detected, decreasing from 40.3 percentage points in 2018 to 39.8 in 2019. This decrease is statistically significant, meaning it is likely not by chance due to the estimates being derived from samples and reflects a non-zero decrease.

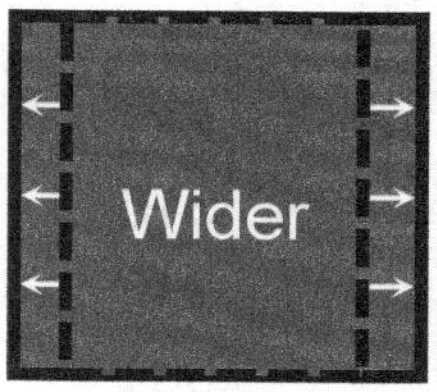

Did the employment gap narrow since the earliest year available, 2008?
NO. The opposite occurred. A statistically significant widening of the employment gap was detected between 2008 and 2019, increasing from 38.6 percentage points to 39.8 percentage points. This widening was statistically significant, meaning it was not likely due to chance because the estimates are derived from samples of the U.S. populations in 2008 and 2019.

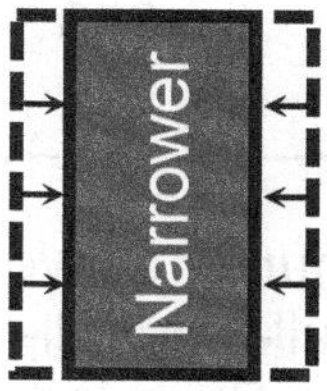

Did the employment gap narrow since its widest point?

YES. A statistically significant narrowing of the employment gap was detected between its widest point in 2015, decreasing from 41.2 percentage points in 2015 to 39.8 percentage points in 2019.

Earnings from Work

Focus Population: Civilians ages 18-64 living in community settings employed full-time/full-year

Can't tell if the 'earnings gap' between full-time/full-year workers with and without disabilities changed from 2018 to 2019

The ability to live independently and job quality are reflected in one's earrings from work; a.k.a., wage/salary income and hereafter earnings. The earnings of full-time/full-year workers—persons who usually work over 35 hours per week for over 50 weeks per year—are tracked in order minimize the potential that reduced earnings being the result of reduced hours worked, which may differ between workers without disabilities. As Table 6 shows, the median earnings of full-time/full-year workers with disabilities was $40,360, compared to $48,406 for their counterparts without disabilities, resulting in an earnings gap of $8,046. The earnings gap appears to widen between 2018 and 2019, from $5,901 to $8,046; however, this increase is not statistically significant, meaning that it is not distinguishable from zero, given these data.

Table 6. Median Earnings of Full-Time/Full-Year Workers ($)

	People with Disabilities		People without Disabilities		Gap	
Year	Estimate	St. Error	Estimate	St. Error	Estimate	St. Error
2008	39,805	348	47,154‡	548	7,394*	649
2009	40,384	289	47,565‡	176	7,181*‡	338
2010	41,234†‡	243	47,194‡	163	5,960*	293
2011	40,444†	374	46,248†‡	206	5,804*	427
2012	39,306†‡	346	44,978†‡	232	5,672*	417
2013	39,796‡	183	44,688‡	155	4,872*	240
2014	40,199	234	45,241†‡	212	5,042*	316
2015	40,512	317	45,336‡	131	4,824*	343
2016	41,776†‡	324	47,144†‡	159	5,368*	361
2017	42,095‡	359	47,404‡	243	5,309*	433
2018	41,187†‡	292	47,808‡	194	5,901*	350
2019	40,360†	282	48,406†	139	8,046*	314

Source: Author's calculation using the data from the 2008-2019 American Community Surveys for civilian respondents of ages 18-64 who live in community settings and work full-time/full-year. All dollar amounts are inflation-adjusted to 2019 dollars using the Consumer Price Index.
* Significant at the 5 percent level and a one-tailed test.
† Significantly different from the previous year at the 5 percent level and a one-tailed test.
‡ Significantly different from the 2019 estimate at the 5 percent level and a one-tailed test.

Figure 6. Median Earnings (thousands, 2019 dollars)

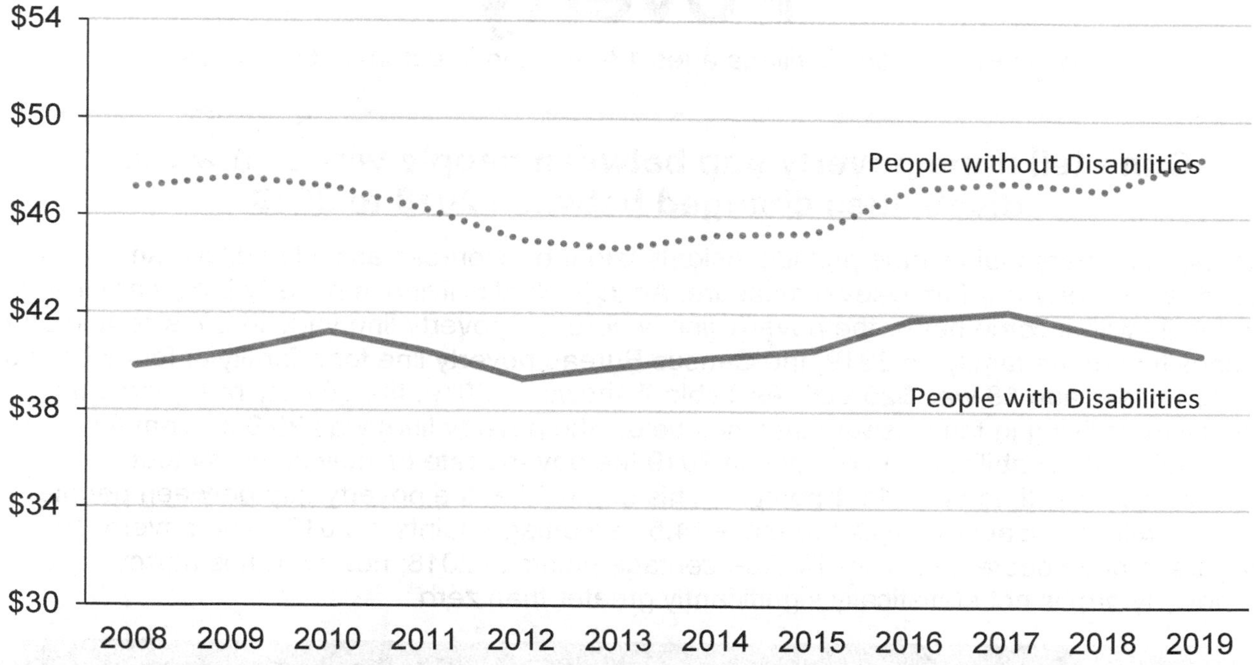

Comparisons & Statistical Significance

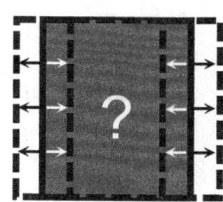

Did the earnings gap narrow between 2018 and 2019?

CAN'T TELL. The earnings gap appears to widen between 2018 and 2019, widening from $5,901 to $8,046. However, this widening is not statistically significant, meaning that it is not distinguishable (given these data) from zero increase. Recall that these estimates are based on full-time, full-year workers, which reduced the sample sizes, making it harder to detect changes.

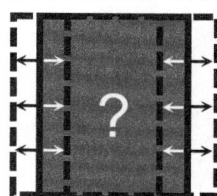

Did the earnings gap narrow since the earliest year available, 2008?

CAN'T TELL. The earnings gap appears to widen between 2008 and 2019, increasing from $7,394 in 2008 to $8,046 in 2019. However, this is not statistically significant meaning it is not distinguishable (given these data) from zero change.

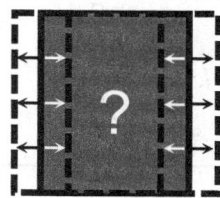

Did the employment gap widen since its narrowest point?

CAN'T TELL. The earnings gap appears to widen from $4,824 in 2015 (its narrowest point) to $8,046 in 2019; however, this widening is not statistically significant.

Poverty

Focus Population: Civilians ages 18-64 living in community settings

Can't tell if the poverty gap between people with and without disabilities changed between 2018 to 2019

Earnings and personal income provide insights into the resources associated with an individual. Poverty is a family-level measure. An individual is living in poverty if they are living in a family with income below the poverty line, where the poverty line varies from size and age composition of the family. In 2019, the Census Bureau poverty line for a family of four with two children under age 18 was $25,926. As Table 7 shows, in 2019, the poverty rate (percentage of individuals living in families with incomes below the poverty line) was 25.9 percent for individuals with disabilities. In contrast, in 2019 the poverty rate of individuals without disabilities was estimated at 11.4 percent. This means that the poverty gap between people with and without disabilities was therefore 14.5 percentage points in 2019. The poverty gap appears to have decreased from 14.7 percentage points in 2018; however, this narrowing of the poverty gap is not statistically significantly greater than zero.

Table 7. Poverty Rate (%)

	People with Disabilities		People without Disabilities		Gap (% pts)	
Year	Estimate Error	St. Error	Estimate	St. Error	Estimate	St. Error
2008	26.2	0.13	11.7‡	0.05	14.4*	0.14
2009	27.2†‡	0.16	12.9†‡	0.05	14.3*	0.17
2010	27.8†‡	0.14	14.1†‡	0.05	13.7*†‡	0.15
2011	28.6†‡	0.12	14.7†‡	0.05	13.9*‡	0.13
2012	29.3†‡	0.14	14.6‡	0.06	14.7*†	0.15
2013	29.2‡	0.15	14.8†‡	0.05	14.4*	0.16
2014	28.8‡	0.14	14.4†‡	0.05	14.4*	0.15
2015	27.7†‡	0.13	13.7†‡	0.05	14.0*†‡	0.14
2016	27.4†‡	0.14	13.1†‡	0.05	14.3*	0.15
2017	26.8†‡	0.15	12.4†‡	0.05	14.4*	0.16
2018	26.9‡	0.15	12.2†	0.05	14.7*	0.15
2019	25.9†	0.13	11.4†	0.05	14.5*	0.14

Source: Author's calculation using the data from the 2008-2019 American Community Surveys for civilian respondents of ages 18-64 who live in community settings.

* Significant at the 5 percent level and a one-tailed test.

† Significantly different from the previous year at the 5 percent level and a one-tailed test.

‡ Significantly different from the 2019 estimate at the 5 percent level and a one-tailed test.

Figure 7. Poverty Rate

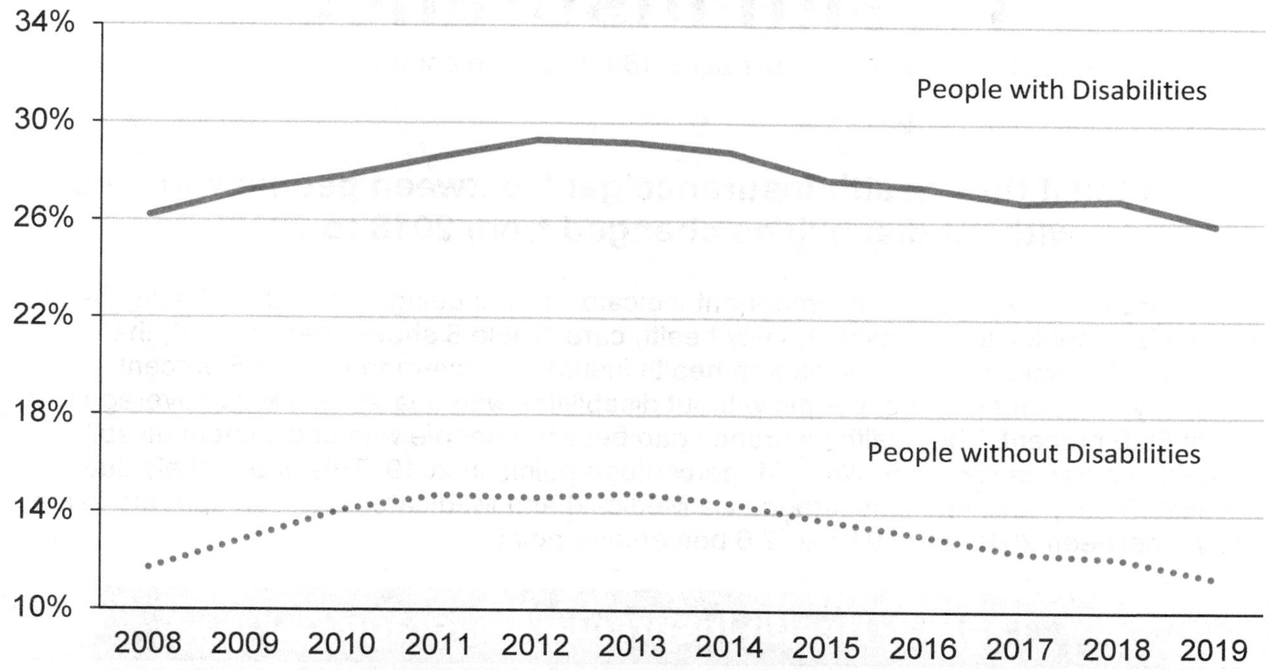

Comparisons & Statistical Significance

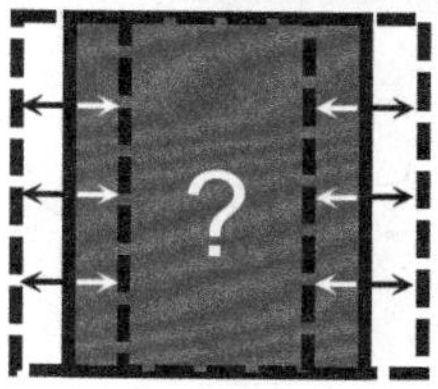

Did the poverty gap narrow between 2018 and 2019?

CAN'T TELL. The poverty gap appears to narrow between 2018 and 2019, decreasing from 14.7 percentage points to 14.5 percentage points; however, this narrowing is not statistically significant, meaning that it is not distinguishable (given these data) from zero change.

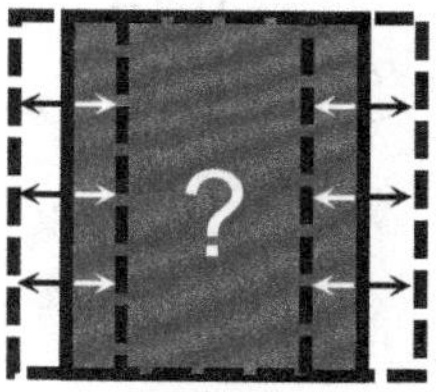

Did the poverty gap narrow since the earliest year available, 2008?

CAN'T TELL. The poverty gap appears to widen between 2008 and 2019, widening from 14.4 percentage points in 2008 to 14.5 percentage points in 2019, but this widening was not statistically significant.

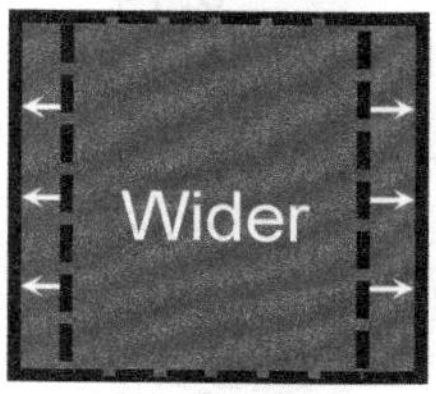

Did the poverty gap widen from its narrowest point in 2010?

YES. A statistically significant widening of the poverty gap was detected between 2010 and 2019, widening from 13.7 percentage points in 2010 to 14.5 percentage points in 2019.

Health Insurance

Focus Population: Civilians ages 18-64 living in community settings

Can't tell if the "health insurance gap" between people with and without disabilities changed from 2018 to 2019

Access to quality health care is an important indicator of well-being. In the U.S., having health insurance is essential to accessing quality health care. Table 8 shows that, in 2019, the percentage of people with disabilities with health insurance coverage was 89.6 percent. Interestingly, the percentage of people without disabilities with health insurance coverage was lower, at 86.9 percent. The health insurance gap between people with and without disabilities with health insurance coverage was -2.6 percentage points in 2019. This gap is likely due to the availability of public health insurance via Medicaid and Medicare. This gap appears to stay the same between 2018 and 2019 at -2.6 percentage points.

Table 8. Health Insurance Coverage (%)

	People with Disabilities		People without Disabilities		Gap (% pts)	
Year	Estimate	St. Error	Estimate	St. Error	Estimate	St. Error
2008	81.6‡	0.12	80.0‡	0.07	-1.6*‡	0.14
2009	82.5†‡	0.11	79.1†‡	0.08	-3.4*†‡	0.14
2010	82.0†‡	0.12	78.3†‡	0.07	-3.7*†‡	0.14
2011	82.4†‡	0.12	78.7†‡	0.08	-3.7*‡	0.14
2012	82.8†‡	0.13	79.0†‡	0.07	-3.8*‡	0.15
2013	83.0‡	0.1	79.3†‡	0.08	-3.7*‡	0.13
2014	86.7†‡	0.12	83.4†‡	0.07	-3.3*†‡	0.14
2015	89.6†	0.1	86.6†‡	0.07	-3.0*‡	0.12
2016	90.3†‡	0.1	87.7†‡	0.06	-2.6*†	0.12
2017	90.2‡	0.1	87.6†‡	0.07	-2.5*	0.12
2018	90.0‡	0.07	87.4†	0.06	-2.6*	0.09
2019	89.6†	0.09	86.9†	0.07	-2.6*	0.12

Source: Author's calculation using the data from the 2008-2019 American Community Surveys for civilian respondents of ages 18-64 who live in community settings.

* Significant at the 5 percent level and a one-tailed test.

† Significantly different from the previous year at the 5 percent level and a one-tailed test.

‡ Significantly different from the 2018 estimate at the 5 percent level and a one-tailed test.

Figure 8. Percent with Health Insurance

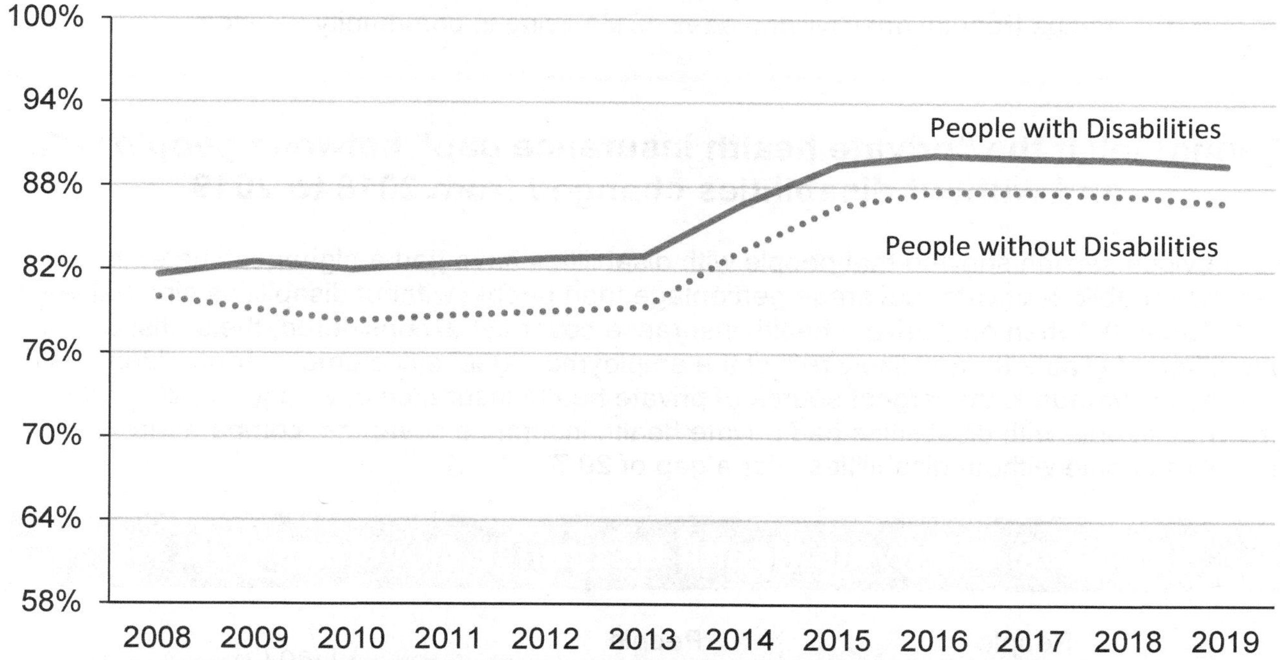

Comparisons & Statistical Significance

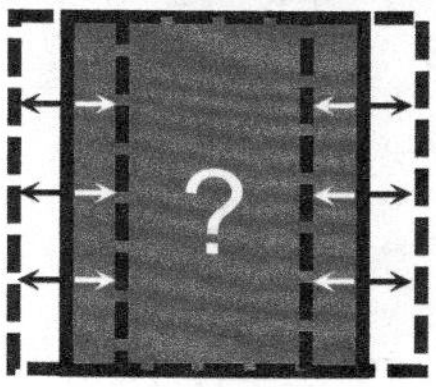

Did the health insurance gap narrow between 2018 and 2019?

NO. The health insurance gap appears to stay the same from 2018 to 2019, at -2.6 percentage points.

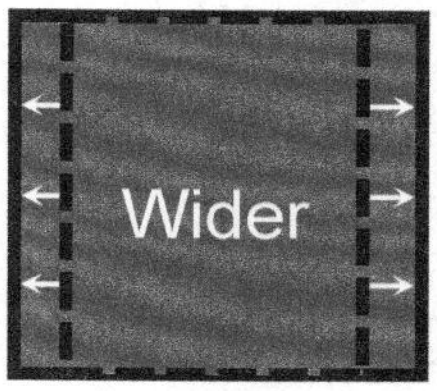

Did the health insurance gap narrow since the earliest year available, 2008?

NO. The opposite occurred. A statically significant widening of the health insurance gap was detected between 2008 and 2019, making it more negative, from -1.6 percentage points in 2008 to -2.6 percentage points in 2019.

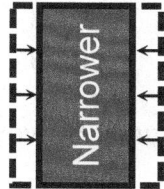

Did the health insurance gap narrow from its widest point in 2012?

YES. A statistically significant narrowing of the health insurance gap was detected between 2012 and 2019, making it less negative, from -3.8 percentage points in 2012 to -2.6 percentage points in 2019.

Private Health Insurance

Focus Population: Civilians ages 18-64 living in community settings

Cannot tell if the "private health insurance gap" between people with and without disabilities changed from 2018 to 2019

The previous section showed that people with disabilities have had a higher estimated health insurance (public & private) coverage percentage than people without disabilities since at least 2008 (Table 8). When only private health insurance coverage is considered, the statistics are quite different (Table 9), and likely reflect the employment gap, since employer provided health insurance coverage is the largest source of private health insurance coverage. In 2019, 46.0 percent of people with disabilities had private health insurance coverage, compared to 75.8 percent of people without disabilities—for a gap of 29.7.

Table 9. Private Health Insurance Coverage (%)

	People with Disabilities		People without Disabilities		Gap (% pts)	
Year	Estimate	St. Error	Estimate	St. Error	Estimate	St. Error
2008	47.0‡	0.17	74.6‡	0.08	27.6*‡	0.19
2009	44.5†‡	0.15	72.5†‡	0.09	28.0*†‡	0.17
2010	43.0†‡	0.15	70.9†‡	0.08	27.9*‡	0.17
2011	42.7‡	0.17	70.9‡	0.08	28.2*‡	0.19
2012	41.8†‡	0.15	71.1†‡	0.08	29.3*†‡	0.17
2013	42.7†‡	0.15	71.2‡	0.09	28.5*†‡	0.17
2014	44.2†‡	0.14	73.6†‡	0.08	29.4*†	0.16
2015	45.3†‡	0.16	75.3†‡	0.08	30.0*†	0.18
2016	46.0†	0.17	76.0†	0.08	30.0*	0.19
2017	45.8	0.18	75.8†	0.09	30.0*	0.2
2018	45.9	0.16	75.9	0.09	30.0*	0.18
2019	46	0.16	75.8	0.09	29.7*	0.19

Source: Author's calculation using the data from the 2008-2019 American Community Surveys for civilian respondents of ages 18-64 who live in community settings.

* Significant at the 5 percent level and a one-tailed test.

† Significantly different from the previous year at the 5 percent level and a one-tailed test.

‡ Significantly different from the 2019 estimate at the 5 percent level and a one-tailed test.

Figure 9. Percent with Private Health Insurance

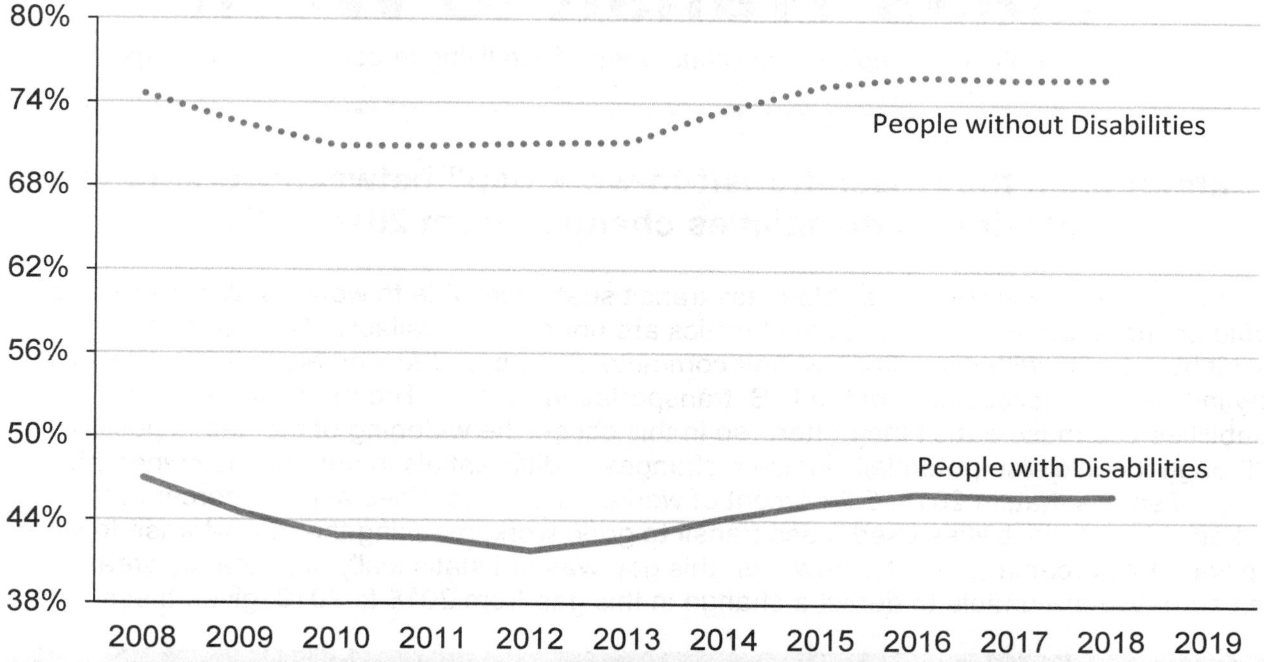

Comparisons & Statistical Significance

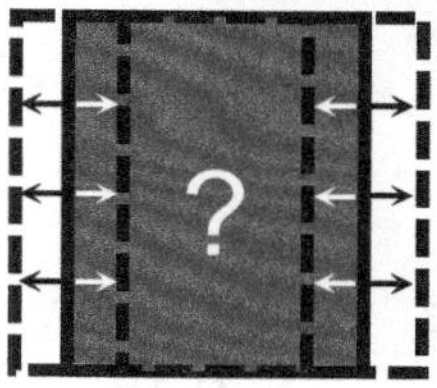

Did the private health insurance gap narrow between 2018 and 2019?

CAN'T TELL. The private health insurance gap appears to narrow from 30.0 percentage points in 2018 to 29.7 in 2019. However, no statistically significant change in the private health insurance gap was detected.

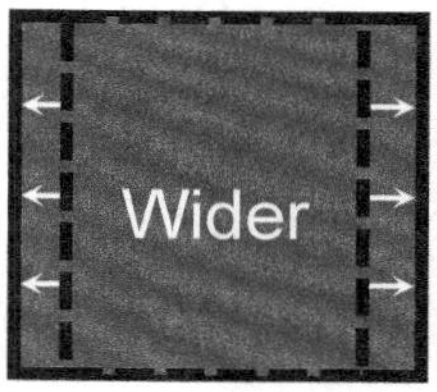

Did the private health insurance gap narrow since the earliest year available, 2008?

NO. The opposite occurred. A statistically significant widening of the private health insurance gap was detected between 2008 and 2019, increasing from 27.6 percentage points in 2008 to 29.7 percentage points in 2019.

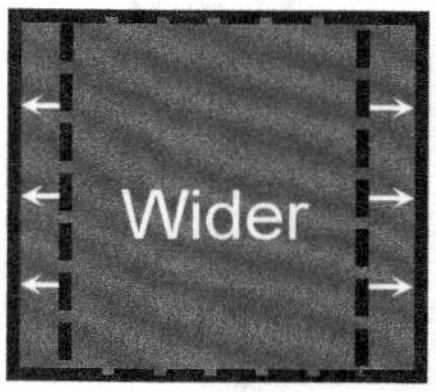

Did the private health insurance gap narrow, when comparing 2019 to the year with the nearest smallest private health insurance gap, 2010?

NO. The opposite occurred. A statistically significant widening of the private health insurance gap was detected between 2010 and 2019, increasing from 27.9 percentage points to 29.7 percentage points in 2019.

Mass Transit to Work

Focus Population: Employed civilians ages 18-64 living in community settings

Cannot tell if the "mass-transit-to-work gap" between workers with and without disabilities changed from 2018 to 2019

Monitoring the number of accessible mass transit seats available to workers with disabilities would be informative; however, such statistics are not readily available. The use of mass transit by workers with disabilities in their commutes, compared to workers without disabilities, may indicate the accessibility of the U.S. transportation system. The more workers with disabilities use mass transit the better—so in this case—the widening of the gap is positive. (Although it could also potentially indicate changes in differentials in automobile ownership.) Table 10 shows that, in 2019, 5.2 percent of workers with disabilities and 5.0 percent of workers without disabilities used mass transit to go to work, meaning the mass-transit-to-work gap was 0.2 percentage points. However, this gap was not statistically significantly greater than zero. We are unable to detect a change in this gap from 2018 to 2019, given these data.

Table 10. Mass Transit to Work (%)

	People with Disabilities		People without Disabilities		Gap (% pts)	
Year	Estimate	St. Error	Estimate	St. Error	Estimate	St. Error
2008	6.1‡	0.13	4.9‡	0.03	1.2*‡	0.13
2009	5.6†‡	0.11	5.0‡	0.03	0.6*†‡	0.11
2010	5.4	0.11	4.9†‡	0.03	0.5*‡	0.11
2011	5.9†‡	0.11	5.0†	0.03	0.9*†‡	0.11
2012	5.9‡	0.12	5.0‡	0.02	0.9*‡	0.12
2013	5.8‡	0.12	5.1†‡	0.02	0.7*‡	0.12
2014	6.1†‡	0.12	5.2‡	0.02	0.9*‡	0.12
2015	5.7†‡	0.12	5.2‡	0.02	0.5*†‡	0.12
2016	5.6‡	0.11	5.1†	0.03	0.5*‡	0.11
2017	5.5‡	0.11	5.0†	0.02	0.5*‡	0.11
2018	5.3	0.11	4.9†	0.02	0.4*	0.11
2019	5.2	0.09	5.0†	0.02	0.2	0.09

Source: Author's calculation using the data from the 2008-2019 American Community Surveys for civilian respondents of ages 18-64 who live in community settings and are employed.
* Significant at the 5 percent level and a one-tailed test.
† Significantly different from the previous year at the 5 percent level and a one-tailed test.
‡ Significantly different from the 2019 estimate at the 5 percent level and a one-tailed test.

Figure 10. Percent of Workers using Mass Transit to Work

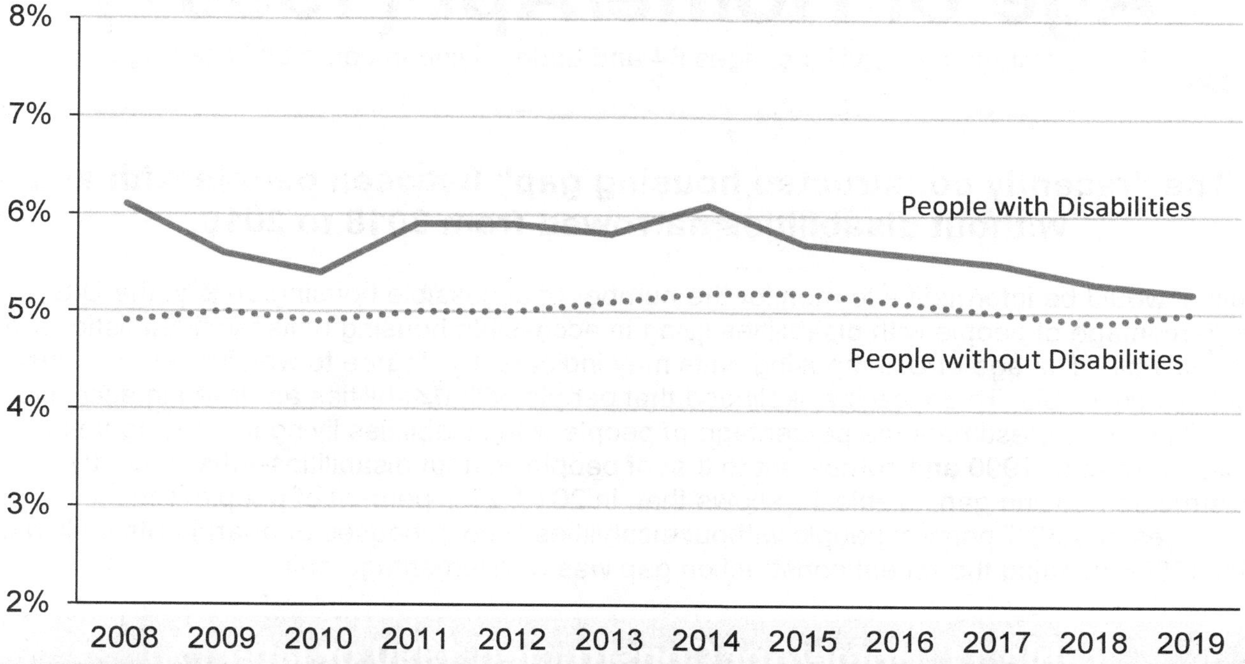

Comparisons & Statistical Significance

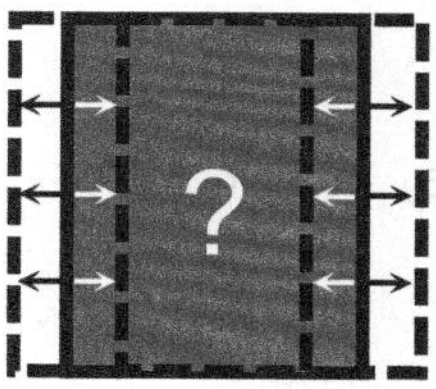

Did the mass-transit-to-work gap widen (a good thing) between 2018 and 2019?

CAN'T TELL. The mass-transit-to-work gap appears to narrow (a bad thing) from 0.4 percentage points in 2018 to 0.2 percentage points in 2019. However, this narrowing is not statistically significant, meaning that it may be due to the estimates being derived from samples of the U.S. populations.

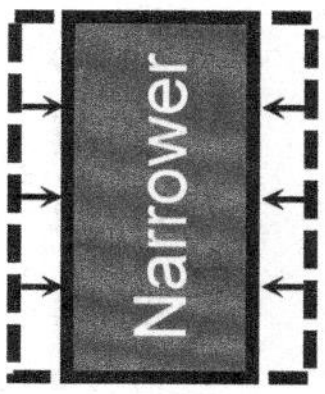

Did the mass-transit-to-work gap widen (a good thing) since the earliest year available, 2008?

NO. The opposite occurred. A statistically significant narrowing (a bad thing) of the mass-transit-to-work gap was detected between 2008 and 2019, decreasing from 1.2 percentage points in 2008 to 0.2 percentage points in 2019.

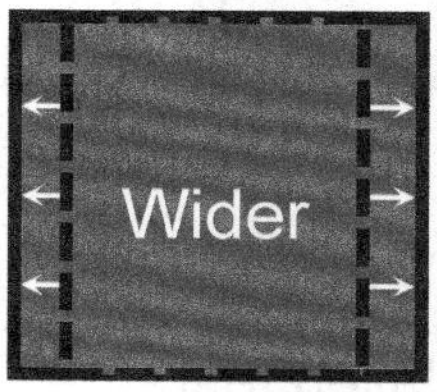

Did the mass-transit-to-work gap ever widen from year to year?

YES. A statistically significant widening (a good thing) occurred between 2010 and 2011, when it increased from 0.5 percentage points to 0.9 percentage points.

Age of Home/Apt (1990+)

Focus Population: Civilians, ages 64 and under, living in community settings

The "recently constructed housing gap" between people with and without disabilities narrowed from 2018 to 2019.

While it would be informative to monitor the number of accessible housing units in the U.S. and the percentage of people with disabilities living in accessible housing units, such statistics are not available. The age of U.S. housing units may indicate the degree to which the U.S. housing stock is accessible. To gauge the likelihood that people with disabilities are living in accessible housing units, we estimate the percentage of people with disabilities living in housing units constructed after 1990 and compare it to that of people without disabilities—the "recently constructed housing gap." Table 11 shows that, in 2019, 27.7 percent of people with disabilities and 33.1 percent people without disabilities lived in houses or apartments built in or after 1990, meaning the recent construction gap was 5.5 percentage points.

Table 11. Home/Apt Constructed 1990 or later (%)

	People with Disabilities		People without Disabilities		Gap (% pts)	
Year	Estimate	St. Error	Estimate	St. Error	Estimate	St. Error
2008	22.1‡	0.12	30.0‡	0.07	7.9*‡	0.14
2009	22.8†‡	0.14	30.7†‡	0.06	7.9*‡	0.15
2010	24.4†‡	0.13	32.1†‡	0.06	7.7*†‡	0.14
2011	24.9†‡	0.16	32.5†‡	0.07	7.6*‡	0.17
2012	25.4†‡	0.14	33.0†‡	0.06	7.6*‡	0.15
2013	26.4†‡	0.13	33.7†‡	0.06	7.3*‡	0.14
2014	26.7‡	0.12	33.9†‡	0.07	7.2*‡	0.14
2015	27.3†‡	0.13	34.5†‡	0.06	7.2*‡	0.14
2016	27.8†	0.12	34.6‡	0.06	6.8*†‡	0.13
2017	27.9	0.14	34.2†‡	0.06	6.3*†‡	0.15
2018	27.7	0.12	33.7†	0.06	6.0*‡	0.13
2019	27.7	0.12	33.1†	0.07	5.5*†	0.14

* Significant at the 5 percent level and a one-tailed test.
† Significantly different from the previous year at the 5 percent level and a one-tailed test.
‡ Significantly different from the 2019 estimate at the 5 percent level and a one-tailed test.

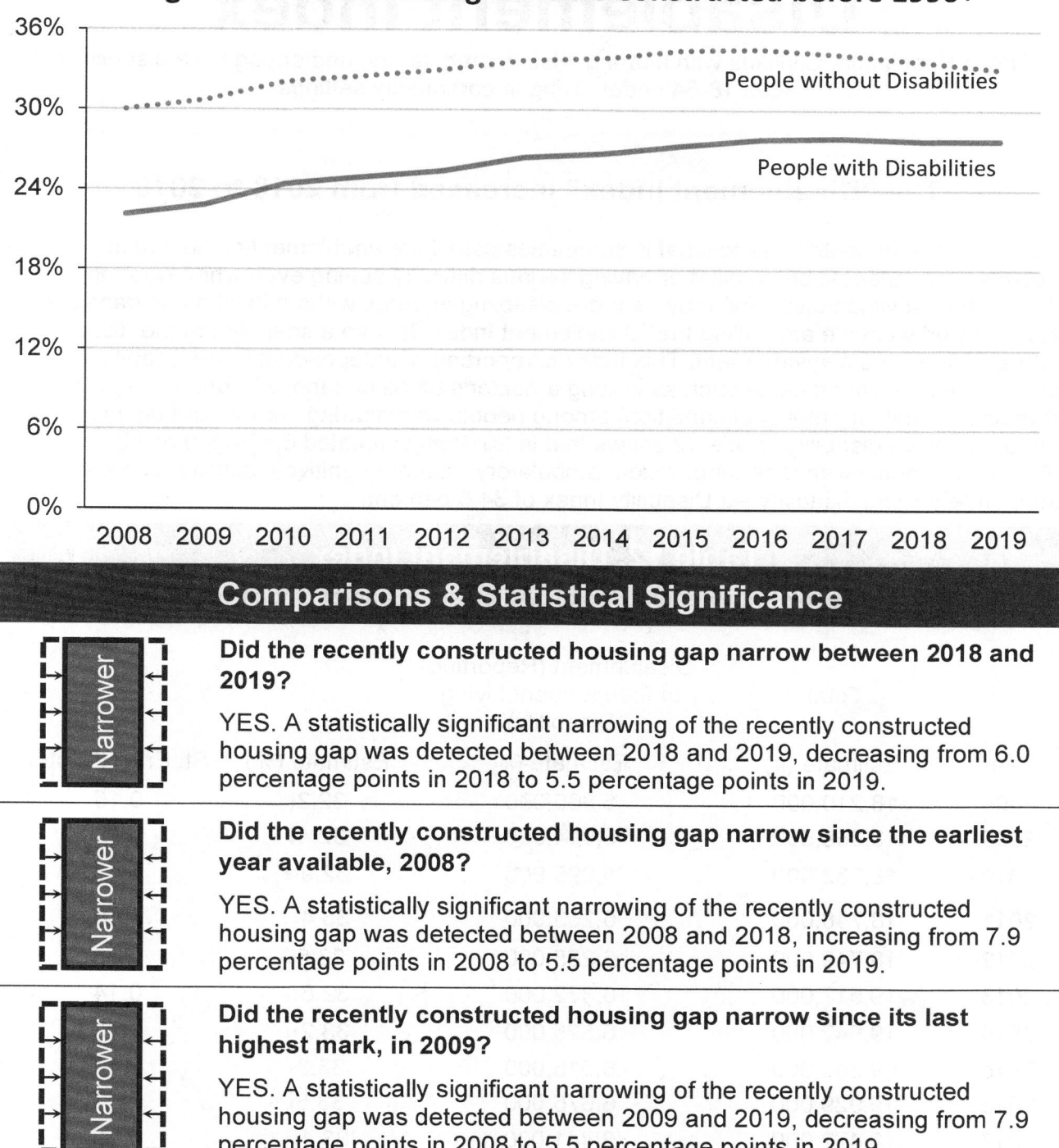

Figure 11. Percent Living in Home Constructed before 1990+

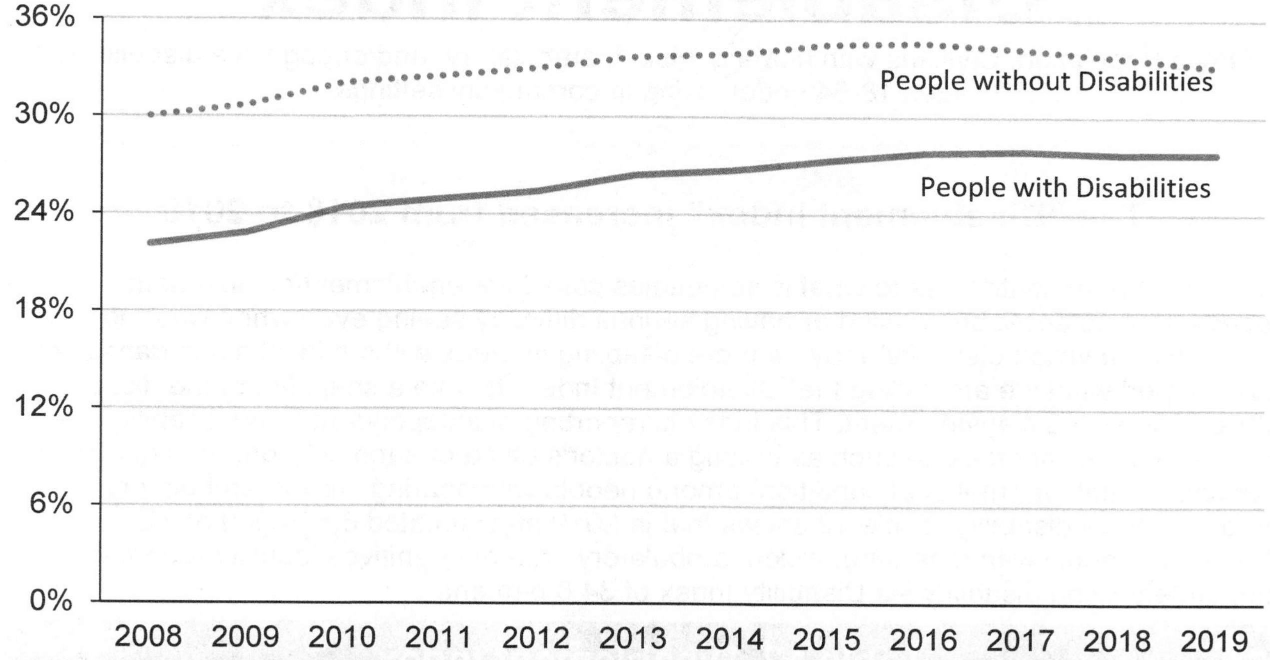

Comparisons & Statistical Significance

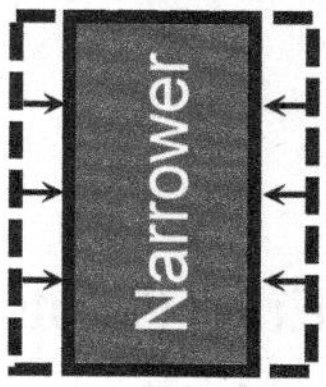

Did the recently constructed housing gap narrow between 2018 and 2019?

YES. A statistically significant narrowing of the recently constructed housing gap was detected between 2018 and 2019, decreasing from 6.0 percentage points in 2018 to 5.5 percentage points in 2019.

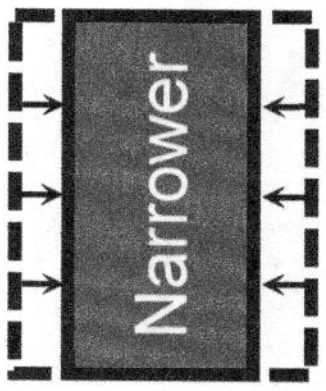

Did the recently constructed housing gap narrow since the earliest year available, 2008?

YES. A statistically significant narrowing of the recently constructed housing gap was detected between 2008 and 2018, increasing from 7.9 percentage points in 2008 to 5.5 percentage points in 2019.

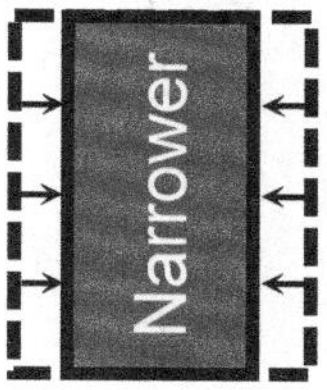

Did the recently constructed housing gap narrow since its last highest mark, in 2009?

YES. A statistically significant narrowing of the recently constructed housing gap was detected between 2009 and 2019, decreasing from 7.9 percentage points in 2008 to 5.5 percentage points in 2019.

Disablement Index

Focus Population: Civilians with hearing, vision, ambulatory, and/or cognitive disabilities, ages 18-64 under, living in community settings

The "Disablement Index" increased from 2018 to 2019

The environment contributes to what is sometimes called the enablement/disablement process. For instance, being blind or having serious difficulty seeing even when wearing glasses (i.e., a vision disability) may be more disabling in areas without local mass transit. We have created what we are calling the "Disablement Index" to take a snapshot at the disabling nature of one's local environment. This Index is reporting of independent living disability (i.e., difficulty doing errands alone such as visiting a doctor's office or shopping, due to a disability physical, mental, or emotional condition) among people with hearing, vision, ambulatory, and/or cognitive disability. Table 12 shows that in 2019 an estimated 6,574,000 of the 19,349,000 people with a hearing, vision, ambulatory, and/or cognitive disability reported independent living disability—a Disability Index of 34.0 percent.

Table 12. Disablement Index

People with Hearing, Vision, Ambulatory, and/or Cognitive Disability

	Total	Disablement (Reporting of Independent Living Disability)		
Year	Estimate (#)	Estimate (#)	Estimate (%)	St. Error (% pts)
2008	18,210,000	5,866,000	32.2‡	0.15
2009	18,268,000	5,914,000	32.4‡	0.16
2010	18,232,000	5,995,000	32.9†‡	0.15
2011	18,748,000	6,263,000	33.4†‡	0.16
2012	18,749,000	6,285,000	33.5‡	0.15
2013	19,517,000	6,372,000	32.6†‡	0.14
2014	19,642,000	6,525,000	33.2†‡	0.15
2015	19,540,000	6,515,000	33.3‡	0.16
2016	19,929,000	6,676,000	33.5‡	0.15
2017	19,472,000	6,441,000	33.1†‡	0.15
2018	19,179,000	6,439,000	33.6†‡	0.14
2019	19,349,000	6,574,000	34.0†	0.16

† Significantly different from the previous year at the 5 percent level and a one-tailed test.
‡ Significantly different from the 2019 estimate at the 5 percent level and a one-tailed test.

Figure 12. Disablement Index

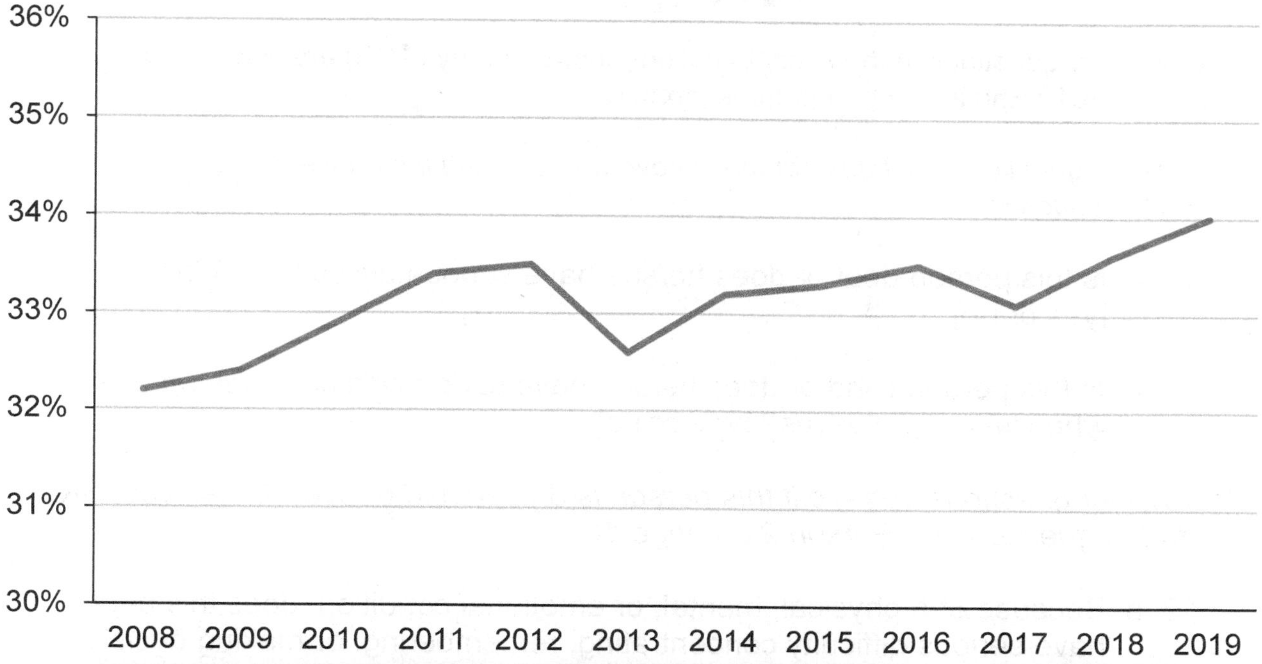

Comparisons & Statistical Significance

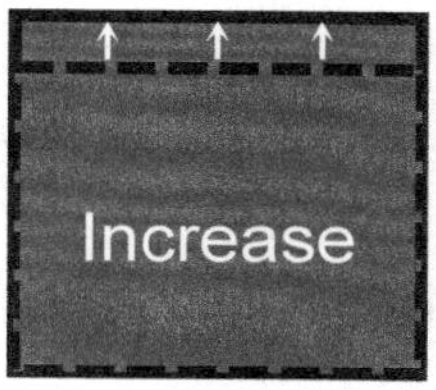

Did the Disablement Index increase between 2018 and 2019?
YES. A statistically significant increase in the percentage of persons with hearing, vision, ambulatory, and/or cognitive disability that reported independent living disability was detected between 2018 and 2019, from 33.6 percent to 34.0 percent. This increase was statistically significant, meaning that it was not likely due to chance because the estimates are derived from samples of the U.S. populations in 2018 and 2019.

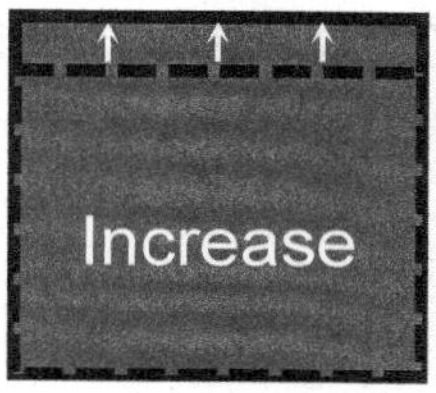

Did the Disablement Index increase since the earliest year available, 2008?
YES. A statistically significant increase in the percentage of persons with hearing, vision, ambulatory, and/or cognitive disability that reported independent living disability was detected between 2008 and 2019, from 32.2 percent to 34.0 percent.

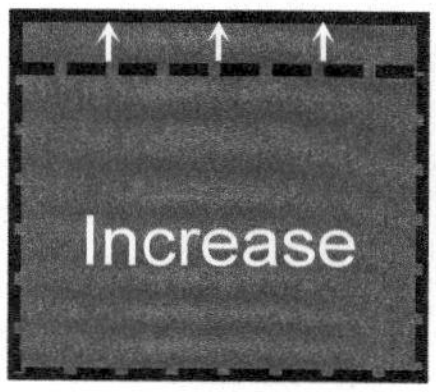

Did the Disablement Index increase above the next highest year, 2016?
YES. The increase—from 33.5 percent in 2016 to 34 percent in 2019—was statistically significant.

Appendix

The six disability questions in the American Community Survey (ACS) are listed below as they appear in the 2019 English language questionnaire:

G. *Answer question 17a if this person is covered by health insurance. Otherwise, SKIP to question 18a.*

18. a. Is this person deaf or does he/she have serious difficulty hearing? [yes or no]

b. Is this person blind or does he/she have serious difficulty seeing even when wearing glasses? [yes or no]

H. *Answer questions 19a – c if this person is 5 years old or over. Otherwise, SKIP to the questions for Person 2 on page 12.*

19. a. Because of a physical, mental, or emotional condition, does this person have serious difficulty concentrating, remembering, or making decisions? [yes or no]

b. Does this person have serious difficulty walking or climbing stairs? [yes or no]

c. Does this person have difficulty dressing or bathing? [yes or no]

I. *Answer question 20 if this person is 15 years old or over. Otherwise, SKIP to the questions for Persons 2 on page 12.*

20. Because of a physical, mental, or emotional condition, does this person have difficulty doing errands alone such as visiting a doctor's office or shopping? [yes or no]

Glossary

American Community Survey (ACS) – The American Community Survey (ACS) is a large, continuous demographic survey conducted by the Census Bureau that will provide accurate and up-to-date profiles of America's communities every year. Annual and multiyear estimates of population and housing data are generated for small areas, including tracts and population subgroups. This information is collected by mailing questionnaires to a sample of addresses. See the Census Bureau website for additional details.

Bachelor's Degree or More – A person has attained a bachelor's degree or more, if the person has received a bachelor's degree (for example, BA and BS), master's degree (for example, MA, MS, MEng, MEd, MSW, MBA), an advanced professional degree (for example, MD, DDS, DVM, LLB, JD), and/or a doctorate degree (for example: PhD, EdD).

Civilian – A person is a civilian, if the person is not in the active-duty military.

Disability – In the ACS, the Census Bureau used responses to six questions to identify whether a person has a disability. These questions ask about difficulties related to vision, hearing, cognition, ambulation, self-care, and independent living. (See Appendix for the wording these six questions.) A person is coded as having a disability, if an affirmative (yes) response is recorded from one or more of these difficulties.

Earnings – Earnings include wages, salary, commissions, bonuses, or tips from all jobs, before deductions for taxes, bonds, dues, or other items. Earnings are reported on an annual basis for the past 12 months reference period. The ACS is fielded over the course of the survey year.

Employed – Individuals were asked a series of questions designed to identify their employment status. Based on the answers, individuals were classified into one of five groups: (1) people who worked at any time during the reference week; (2) people on temporary layoff who were available for work; (3) people who did not work during the reference week but who had jobs or businesses from which they were temporarily absent (excluding layoff); (4) people who did not work during the reference week, but who were looking for work during the last four weeks and were available for work during the reference week; and (5) people not in the labor force.

Gap – The difference between estimates of a given indicator (such as the percentage of people employed) for two different sub-populations, usually people with and without disabilities.

Full-Time, Full-Year – A person is considered to be a full-time, full-year worker, if the person worked 35 hours or more per week for 50 to 52 weeks in the past 12 months.

Health Insurance Coverage – A person is covered by health insurance, if it is indicated that the person is covered by: (a) insurance through a current or former employer or union (of this person or another family member); (b) insurance purchased directly from an insurance company (by this person or another family member); (c) Medicare, for people 65 and older, or people with certain disabilities; (d) Medicaid, Medical Assistance, or any kind of government-assistance plan for those with low incomes or a disability; (e) TRICARE or other military health care; (f) VA (including those who have ever used or enrolled for VA health care); (g) Indian Health Service; and/or (h) Any other type of health insurance or health coverage plan.

Income – The ACS asks for income amounts for the following eight categories: (1) wages, salary, commissions, bonuses, or tips from all jobs (before deductions for taxes, bonds, dues, or other items); (2) self-employment income from own nonfarm businesses or farm businesses, including proprietorships and partnerships (after business expenses); (3) interest, dividends, net rental income, royalty income, or income from estates and trusts; (4) Social Security or Railroad Retirement income; (5) Supplemental Security Income (SSI); (6) any public assistance or welfare payments from the state or local welfare office; (7) retirement, survivor, or disability pensions (not including Social Security); and (8) any other sources of income received regularly such as Veterans' (VA) payments, unemployment compensation, child support or alimony. The sum of these incomes across all persons in a family is used to determine poverty. See the definition of poverty in this glossary.

Less than a High School Diploma – A person has attained less than a high school diploma, if the person has not received a high school diploma, General Equivalency Degree (GED), or alternative credential.

Living in the Community – A person lives in the community, if the person is not living in an institution, such as jail, prison, nursing home, and hospital. A college dormitory is not considered an institution.

No Difference Detected – No difference detected (i.e., statistical insignificance) is a statement, conveying that the *likelihood* of rejecting a null hypothesis, when it is true, is *above* a certain assumed *threshold*, such as 5 percent. For example, in Table 2, no difference was detected between the 2017 employment gap (41.0% pts) and the 2013 employment gap (40.9% pts). In other words, there is a less than a 95 percent chance that we have not detected a difference. Basically, given the data, we can't tell.

Noninstitutionalized Population – Individuals not living in institutions, such as jails, prisons, nursing homes, and hospitals. College dormitories are not considered institutions.

Population Size – The total number of inhabitants in a defined geographic area including all races, classes, and groups.

Poverty – The Office of Management and Budget in Statistical Policy, Directive 14 creates income thresholds (i.e., poverty lines) based on the cost of a standard bundle of goods and services that family needs. Different income thresholds are created based family size and age composition (i.e., number of persons under age 18 and number of persons 65 and older). In the ACS, information about income, household size, and household age composition is used to determine whether a person lives in a family with income below the poverty line of the person's family. See the definition of income in this glossary.

Public Use Microdata Sample (PUMS) Files – The ACS PUMS files contain household- and individual-level data, pertaining to responses to the ACS questionnaire and other variables (such as sample weights). Data are edited to protect anonymity.

Sampling Error – Sampling error occurs when a statistic is estimated using a sample rather than the entire population.

Standard Error – The standard error is a measure of the deviation of a sample estimate from the average of all possible samples. It is a measure of how imprecisely a statistic is measured with respect to sampling error. It typically decreases as sample size increases and decreases as the variation in the phenomenon being measured decreases.

Statistical Significance – Statistical significance is a statement, conveying that the *likelihood* of rejecting a null hypothesis, when it is true, is *below* a certain assumed *threshold*, such as 5 percent. For example, in Table 2, the employment gap in 2017 is statistically significant, because based on the data, there is less than 5 percent chance of rejecting the null hypothesis that the employment gap between people with and without disabilities is greater than zero. In other words, we are 95 percent (or more) confident that we detected a gap between the employment-to-population ratio of people with disabilities and the employment-to-population ratio of people without disabilities.

About the Center

Rehabilitation Research and Training Center on Disability Statistics and Demographics (StatsRRTC)

Policymakers, program administrators, service providers, researchers, advocates for people with disabilities, and people with disabilities and their families need accessible, valid data/statistics to support their decisions related to policy improvements, program administration, service delivery, protection of civil rights, and major life activities. The StatsRRTC supports decision making through a variety of integrated research and outreach activities by (a) improving knowledge about and access to existing data, (b) generating the knowledge needed to improve future disability data collection, and (c) strengthening connections between the data from and regarding respondents, researchers, and decision makers. In this way, the StatsRRTC supports the improvement of service systems that advance the quality of life for people with disabilities.

Led by the University of New Hampshire, the StatsRRTC is a collaborative effort involving the following partners: American Association of People with Disabilities, Center for Essential Management Services, Council of State Administrators of Vocational Rehabilitation, Kessler Foundation, Mathematica Policy Research, and Public Health Institute.

The StatsRRTC is funded by the U.S. Department of Health and Human Services, Administration for Community Living, National Institute on Disability, Independent Living and Rehabilitation Research under grant number 90RTGE00010100, from 2018–2023.

Contact Information

University of New Hampshire, Institute on Disability
10 West Edge Drive, Suite 101
Durham, NH 03824
Toll-Free Telephone/TTY: 866.538.9521
E-mail: Disability.Statistics@unh.edu
https://www.researchondisability.org

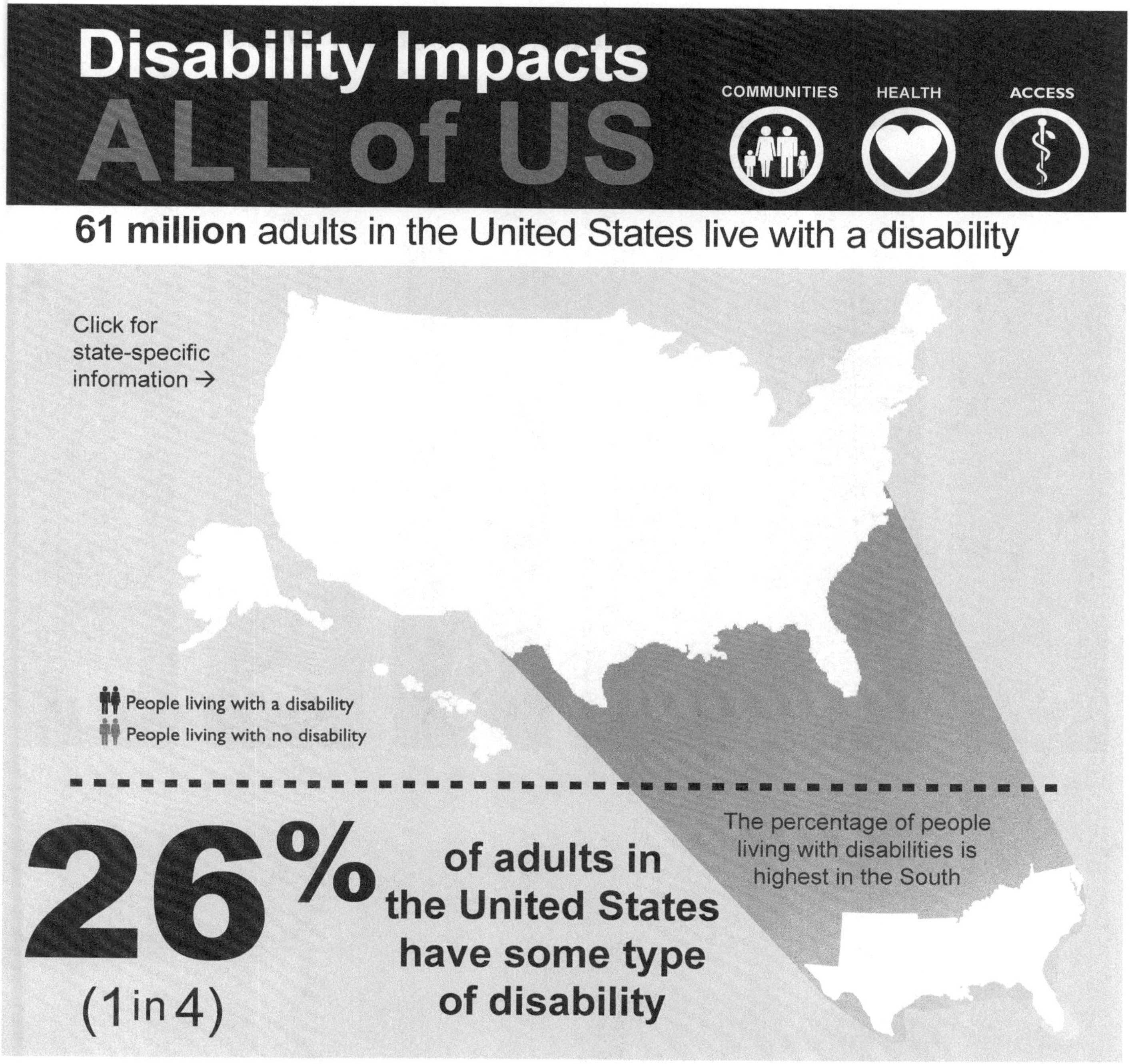
Disability Impacts
ALL of US
COMMUNITIES
HEALTH
ACCESS
61 million adults in the United States live with a disability
Click for state-specific information →
People living with a disability
People living with no disability
26%
(1 in 4)
of adults in the United States have some type of disability
The percentage of people living with disabilities is highest in the South

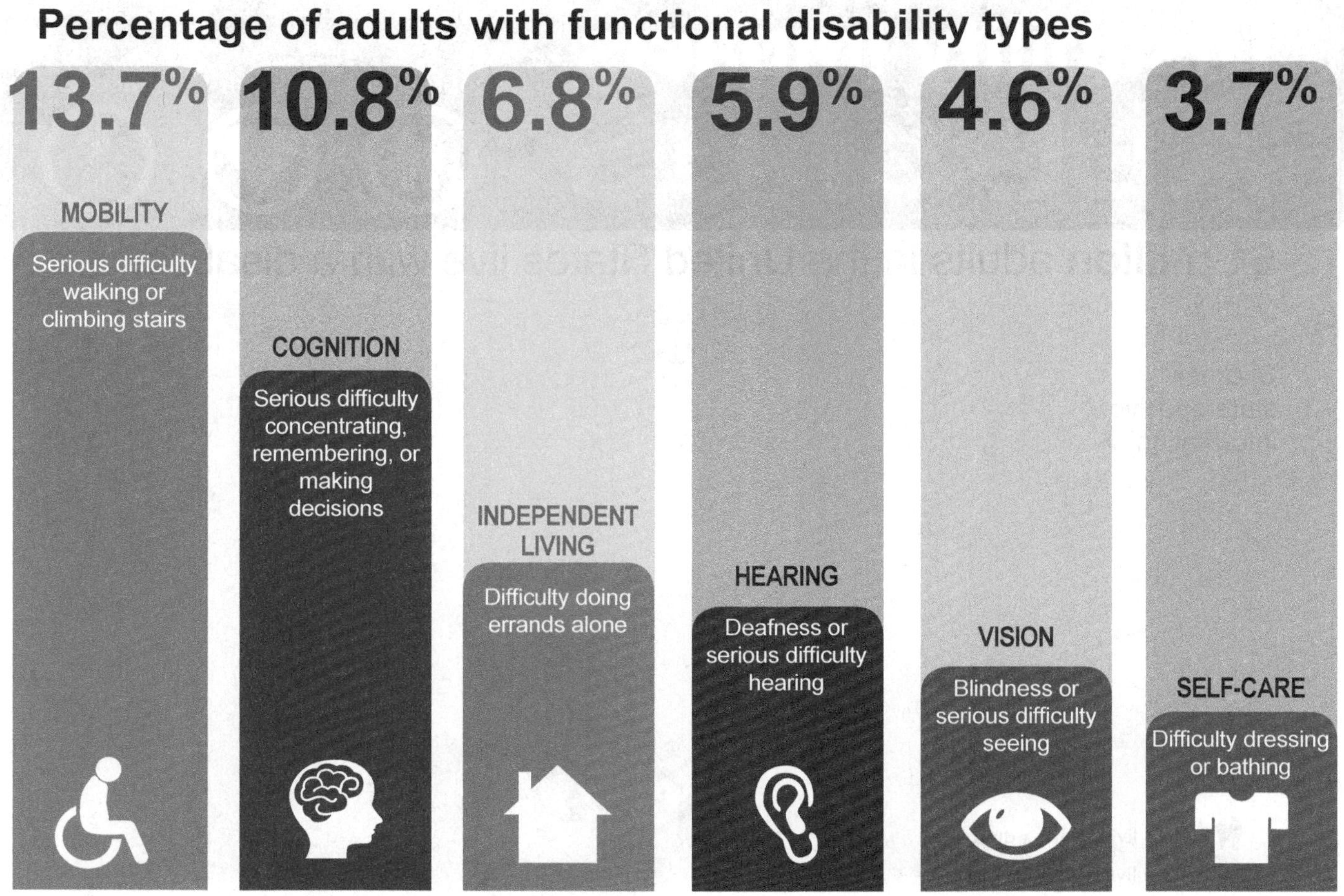
Percentage of adults with functional disability types
13.7%
MOBILITY
Serious difficulty walking or climbing stairs
10.8%
COGNITION
Serious difficulty concentrating, remembering, or making decisions
6.8%
INDEPENDENT LIVING
Difficulty doing errands alone
5.9%
HEARING
Deafness or serious difficulty hearing
4.6%
VISION
Blindness or serious difficulty seeing
3.7%
SELF-CARE
Difficulty dressing or bathing

Disability and COMMUNITIES

Disability is especially common in these groups:

2 in 5 adults age 65 years and older have a disability

1 in 4 women have a disability

2 in 5 Non-Hispanic American Indians/ Alaska Natives have a disability

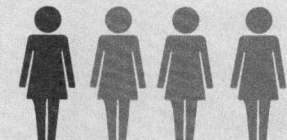

Disability and HEALTH

Adults living with disabilities are more likely to

	With Disabilities	Without Disabilities
HAVE OBESITY	38.2%	26.2%
SMOKE	28.2%	13.4%
HAVE HEART DISEASE	11.5%	3.8%
HAVE DIABETES	16.3%	7.2%

Disability and Healthcare ACCESS

Healthcare access barriers for working-age adults include

1 in 3 adults with disabilities (18-44 years) do not have a **usual healthcare provider**

1 in 3 adults with disabilities (18-44 years) have an **unmet healthcare need because of cost** in the past year

1 in 4 adults with disabilities (45-64 years) did not have a **routine check-up** in the past year

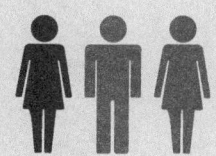

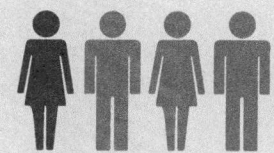

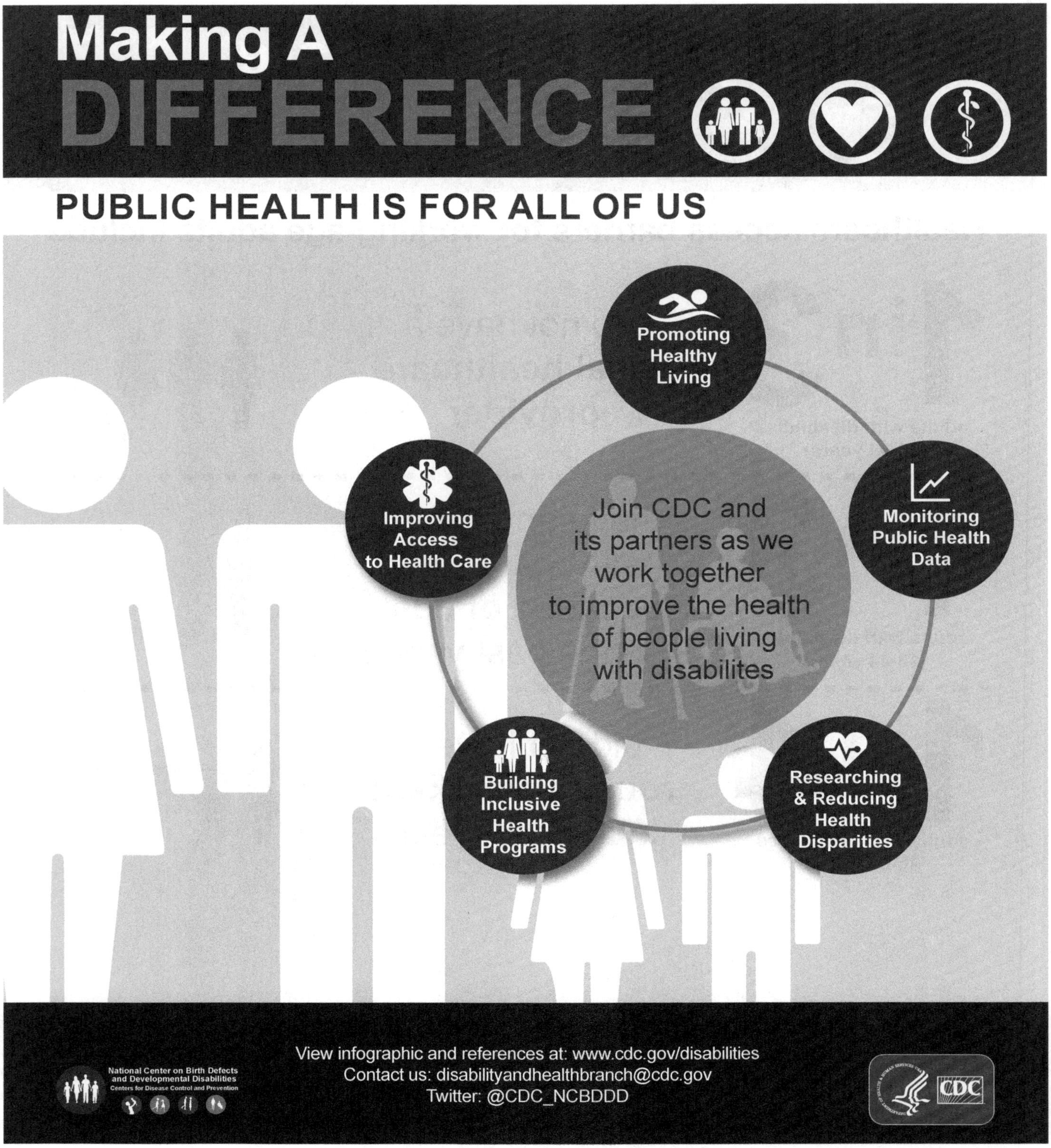
Making A
DIFFERENCE
PUBLIC HEALTH IS FOR ALL OF US
Promoting Healthy Living
Improving Access to Health Care
Join CDC and its partners as we work together to improve the health of people living with disabilites
Monitoring Public Health Data
Building Inclusive Health Programs
Researching & Reducing Health Disparities
National Center on Birth Defects and Developmental Disabilities
Centers for Disease Control and Prevention
View infographic and references at: www.cdc.gov/disabilities
Contact us: disabilityandhealthbranch@cdc.gov
Twitter: @CDC_NCBDDD
CDC

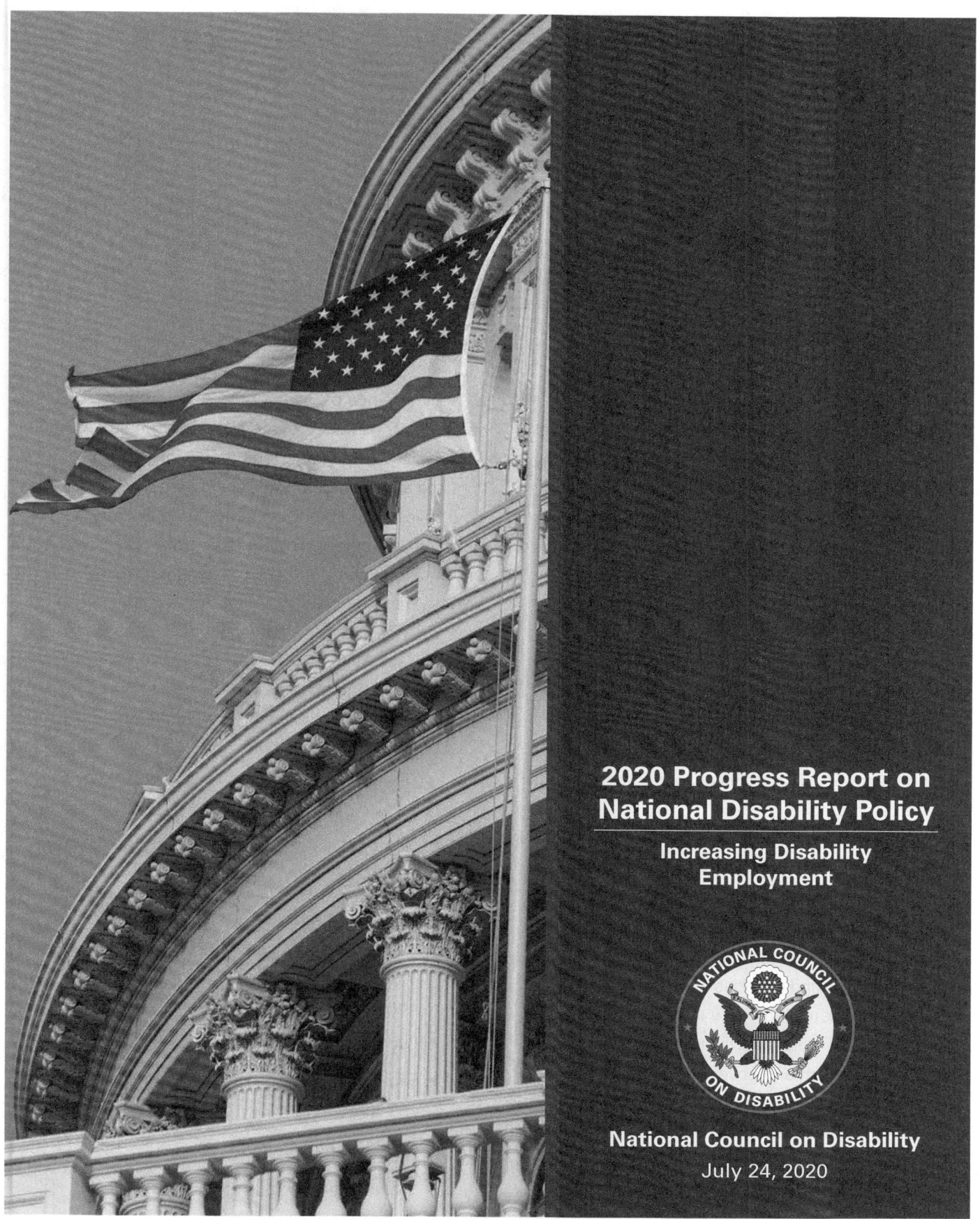

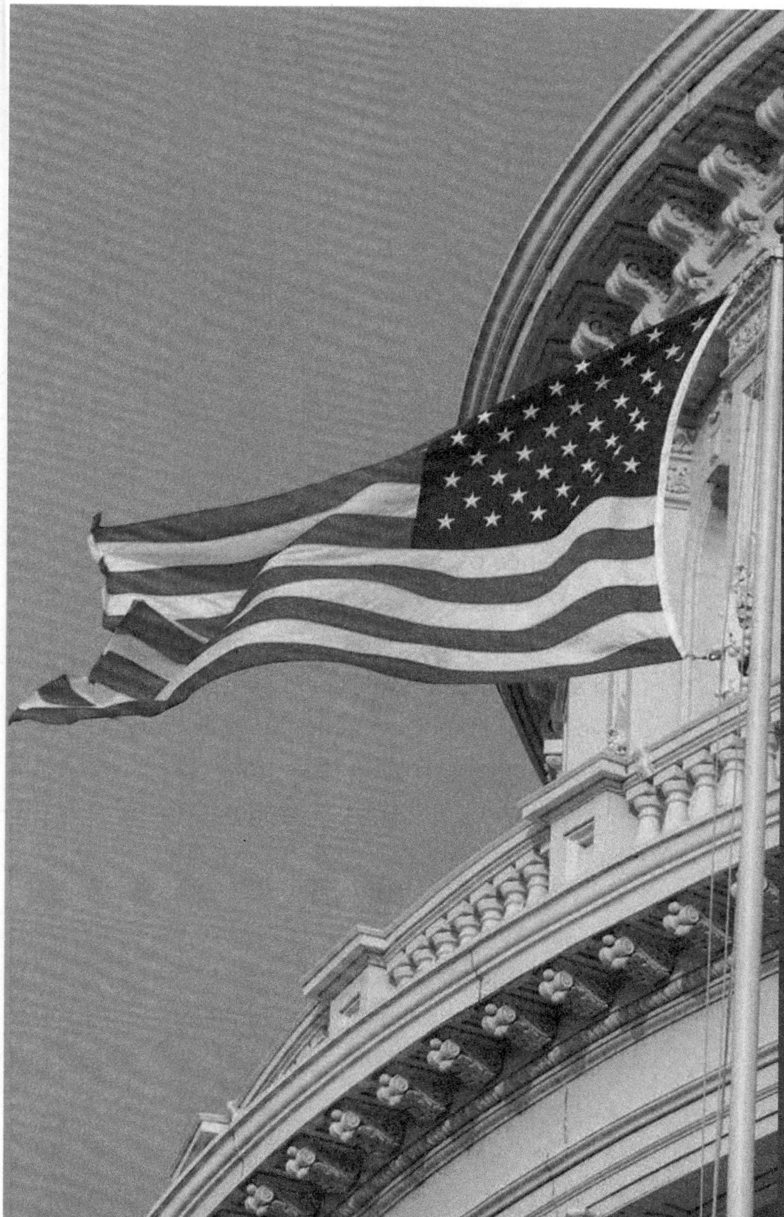

2020 Progress Report on National Disability Policy

Increasing Disability Employment

National Council on Disability

July 24, 2020

Introduction

The National Council on Disability (NCD) is congressionally mandated to advise the President, Congress, and other policymakers on disability policies and practices that enhance equal opportunity for people with disabilities to achieve economic self-sufficiency, independent living, and inclusion and integration into all aspects of society. NCD's 2020 Progress Report fulfills the congressional mandate by advising policymakers on policies and practices that act as barriers to employment and making recommendations for removing these obstacles so that Americans with disabilities can achieve equal opportunity and economic self-sufficiency, and in turn, can achieve and sustain access to independent living, inclusion, and integration in the community.

This Progress Report, issued on the 30th anniversary of the Americans with Disabilities Act (the ADA), focuses on the continuing issues that prevent people with disabilities from obtaining and retaining employment and provides specific, practical recommendations on how to dismantle them. Informed by NCD reports and recommendations on employment and poverty from 1997 to the present, the input of an Advisory Group of six national experts on disability employment, data from five federal agencies, and 23 interviews of stakeholders and Federal Government representatives, it describes the most significant barriers to employment for people with disabilities since passage of the ADA, reviews federal actions taken to improve opportunities for private sector and federal employment, and focuses attention on three areas where federal law, policies, and practices continue to impede or prevent people with disabilities from obtaining and retaining competitive employment. These areas are as follows:

- *Services for transitioning youth*: The need for increased effective coordination, skills training, and employment-related services and supports available to transition-age youth
- *Public benefits*: Long-standing disincentives to work tied to essential health care and other benefits in the Social Security Act and the Medicaid Act

Report Areas of Focus

- Services for transitioning youth
- Public benefits
- Federal employment and support of entrepreneurship
- Employer engagement

- *Federal employment and support of entrepreneurship*: Continued challenges to recruiting and hiring people with targeted disabilities and exclusion from entrepreneurship support

The report also focuses on the topic of *Employer Engagement*: Describing the critical role it plays in increasing employment opportunities for people with disabilities with private sector employers—from the thousands of small businesses across the nation, to major corporations.

As the nation celebrates the 30th anniversary of the enactment of the ADA, the majority of Americans with disabilities are not participants in the nation's workforce—this report provides some of the reasons why and is a call for action. The barriers described can and must be addressed so that people with disabilities who can work, and want to work, can enter or reenter the workforce and achieve financial independence and full inclusion in the economic growth of the nation.

Chapter 1: Employment of People with Disabilities Since Passage of the ADA: A Retrospective of Good and Bad News

The achievement of equal opportunity in employment remains vital to the full inclusion of people with disabilities in the United States nearly 30 years after the enactment of the ADA. Even though the United States has been the leader in the world in advancing the civil and human rights of people with disabilities for the past half century, today Americans with disabilities remain disproportionately poor and unemployed, and they face significant barriers to joining and remaining in the American middle class.

The ADA is indeed an antidiscrimination law, among other things, specifically aimed at ending discrimination in employment.[13] Consequently, it was designed to interrupt the stigma, prejudice, and lack of understanding that accompanied the long history of exclusion of people with disabilities from the American workplace. Yet, even though the ADA was constructed to prevent discriminatory practices, its statutory purpose also conveyed an affirmative vision for employment in America, one of optimism, expansion, and economic freedom. In fact, the statute clearly articulates its purpose "to provide a clear and comprehensive national mandate for the elimination of discrimination against individuals with disabilities . . . the Nation's proper goals regarding individuals with disabilities are to assure equality of opportunity, full participation, independent living, and *economic self-sufficiency* for such individuals" (emphasis added).[14]

[The ADA's] statutory purpose also conveyed an affirmative vision for employment in America, one of optimism, expansion, and economic freedom.

When President George H. W. Bush signed the ADA on the South Lawn of the White House, the following words were among his remarks:

I also want to say a special word to our friends in the business community. You have in your hands the key to the success of this act, for you can unlock a splendid resource of untapped human potential that, when freed, will enrich us all. . . . This act does something important for American business, though—and remember this: You've called for new sources of workers. Well, many of our fellow citizens with disabilities are unemployed. They want to work, and they can work, and this is a tremendous pool of people. And remember, this is a tremendous pool of people who will bring to jobs diversity, loyalty, proven low turnover rate, and only one request: the chance to prove themselves. And when you add together Federal, State, local, and private funds, it costs almost $200 billion annually to support Americans with disabilities—in effect, to keep them dependent. Well, when given the opportunity to be independent, they will move proudly into the economic mainstream of American life, and that's what this legislation is all about.[15] (emphasis added)

That was 30 years ago. This is now. What happened to that "splendid resource of untapped human potential" in the interim? Across all age groups, education, and experience levels, people with disabilities today remain much less likely than workers without disabilities to be employed, or if employed, are more likely to work part-time and in occupations that demand lower wages, offer fewer opportunities for advancement, and lack employer-paid health care and other benefits.[16] This has resulted in additional economic consequences that cascade through the American economy. Among them, people with disabilities have been excluded from savings, asset accumulation, and consumer spending, while the costs of Federal Government programs continue to increase.

Across all age groups, education, and experience levels, people with disabilities today remain much less likely . . . to be employed, or if employed, are more likely to work part-time and in occupations that demand lower wages, offer fewer opportunities for advancement, and lack employer-paid health care and other benefits.

Placed in its proper context, the ADA was a Bill of Rights for Americans with disabilities, one designed to declare an independence that was, in part, *economic*, where economic self-sufficiency was placed on par with equality of opportunity, full participation, and independent living. In this regard, it was one of the explicit purposes of the ADA to address the long history of economic apartheid experienced by people with disabilities, a constituency that had spent the better part of our Nation's history isolated, institutionalized, and removed from what President Bush referred to as "the economic mainstream of American life." It was the ADA that dismantled the long-held assumption, imbued by a medical model of disability, that unemployment and government dependence is an inevitable and irreversible consequence of mental or physical disabilities. Instead, the ADA required an understanding that disability, itself, does not impose a lack of qualification for employment upon people, it is stigma, societal low expectations, and specific environmental barriers in the workplace that so often do. As the World Health Organization has since recognized, "disability exists only in the gap between the person's abilities and capacities and the demands of the environment."[17] In this regard, the ADA codified into law a dramatic shift in societal expectation that a great many people with disabilities can and want to work, and the statute posited that they ought to be given an equal chance to compete when they do so. Even though the ADA has established the right to be free from discrimination in employment, people with disabilities are still vastly underrepresented in workplaces across America, so thus far, we have failed to fulfill the ADA's vision of economic inclusion.

In 2007, at a considerable inflection point for innovation and technological change in the United States,[18] NCD commented on the "good news" and the "bad news" about disability employment: "The bad news is that people with disabilities are currently under-represented in the occupations projected to grow the fastest between 2004 and 2014—they are currently more likely to be in slower-growing service and blue-collar occupations."[19] But the report continued with what was considered then to be grounds for optimism, "The good news is a) growth in computers and new information technologies that help compensate for many types of disabilities and increase the possibilities for productive employment; b) growth in telecommuting and flexible work arrangements, which are appropriate for many people with disabilities; and c) increased attention to issues of diversity in U.S. companies, in which disability is often included as a dimension of diversity." However, despite the occurrence of many of these critical changes to the way work was done over the past 13 years, the changes appear to have done little to disrupt the persistence of the bad news. It raises the important question of why people with disabilities were not included in many of the broadscale changes that the world of work and the U.S. economy experienced over the last several decades.

Indeed, despite both the enactment of the ADA and the rapid pace of innovation infusing disruptive changes into the American workplace—including greater flexibilities, technology, and diversity—the overall picture for Americans with disabilities has remained largely unchanged over the past three decades.

[D]espite both the enactment of the ADA and the rapid pace of innovation infusing disruptive changes into the American workplace—including greater flexibilities, technology, and diversity—the overall picture for Americans with disabilities has remained largely unchanged over the past three decades.

The bird's-eye view of participation of people with disabilities in the labor market is still mostly marked by entrenched poverty and economic exclusion. In 1997, just seven years after the enactment of the ADA, NCD stated, "America's citizens with disabilities want very much to contribute to their country's continued preeminence in the world of nations. They have the talents and the capabilities to do so; and if the proposals presented in this report are enacted, they undoubtedly will."[20] In 2001, 11 years after the enactment of the ADA, NCD lamented the failure to meet the expectations of people with disabilities who can and want to work, stating, "in perhaps no area of public policy has the expectations gap so stubbornly resisted our efforts to achieve equality. Whatever set of statistics one chooses from among the varying estimates of employment rates of

Americans with disabilities, the rate and level of employment for this population remain far too low."[21] In July 2007,17 years after the enactment of the ADA, NCD observed that people with disabilities were nearly three times as likely as people without disabilities to live in poverty—the same ratio as before the passage of the ADA in 1990.[22]

In October 2007, NCD reflected with great optimism upon significant labor shortages caused by the retirement of the Baby Boomer generation, invoking hope that utilizing the untapped resource of workers with disabilities to fill that labor shortage would reverse the disability unemployment trendline.[23] But by the very next fall, the Great Recession took hold, and analysts feared that employers were less likely to take risks on employees with additional support needs, demonstrating concern that bias and discrimination in hiring would take precedence when times were tough. In a 2009 report, NCD remarked:

Today, however, with the ranks of the unemployed growing by hundreds of thousands per month, some may say that unemployment among people with disabilities cannot be a major issue in an environment in which jobs are becoming scarcer for everyone. Such expressions reinforce many of the very stereotypes that explain why, even in periods of rapid economic growth, people with disabilities have not shared in the fruits of the economy.[24]

As predicted, even after the market experienced considerable recovery from the 2008 recession and the nationwide unemployment rate fell dramatically, the employment population ratio for people with disabilities continued at approximately the same level as it had for years.[25]

In 2013, NCD reported, "[e]mployment numbers for Americans with disabilities have not changed much since passage of the ADA, which was intended to increase civil rights protections for millions of Americans with disabilities and to guarantee their equal opportunity in employment. The 40 percent chasm between the employment rates for Americans with and without disabilities is inarguably disparate and unacceptable."[26] The report continued by saying, "[i]t should come as no surprise that the number one topic on the minds of those that NCD interviewed for the 2013 Progress Report was employment and workforce participation."

In 2015, 25 years after the enactment of the ADA and years into the recovery from the Great Recession, the unemployment rate was twice the national average as for people without disabilities, and even when employed, there was a pay gap accounting for average lower wages for workers with disabilities than those without disabilities.[27]

In 2020, now 30 years after the enactment of the ADA, workers with disabilities contend with rising inequality in a job market that is at or near full employment, with a national unemployment rate in February 2020 as low as 3.5 percent.[28] Yet, there remain 22 million working-age Americans with disabilities, with nearly two-thirds of such people left out of the labor market altogether,[29] and for those who are actively looking for work, such people still experience an unemployment rate that is twice that of workers without disabilities.[30] According to the Bureau of Labor Statistics, on average, only approximately 19 percent of people with disabilities were employed during the nine-year period between 2009 and 2018 as compared to approximately more than 65 percent of people without disabilities. See Figures 1 and 2. Significantly, the nearly 40 percentage point gap between the employment population ratio and labor force participation of people with and without disabilities remained steady across the very decade that, as economists have observed, experienced among the greatest disruptions to the way people work and live since the industrial revolution; the same decade that experienced a historic march from recession to recovery to the lowest unemployment rate in decades.[31] The data shows that the technological and social changes that NCD predicted in 2007, and that

According to the Bureau of Labor Statistics, on average, only approximately 19 percent of people with disabilities were employed during the nine-year period between 2009 and 2018 as compared to approximately more than 65 percent of people without disabilities.

Pre-COVID-19 February 2020 national employment

- Job market at or near full employment
- National unemployment rate in February 2020 as low as 3.5 percent.
- Nearly two-thirds of 22 million working-age Americans with disabilities left out of the labor market altogether
- For those people with disabilities actively looking for work, such people still experience an unemployment rate that is twice that of workers without disabilities.

materialized to allow people with disabilities to enter the workforce, had little effect on the overall labor force participation of people with disabilities.

As noted by NCD in its 2018 report, *From the New Deal to the Real Deal*, the nation's economy is increasingly a digital and information-based one, and the physical world is steadily being reimagined and realigned to keep pace with new technologies.[32] Yet, many people with disabilities, in large part, are locked out of these changes and have lacked access to the very kinds of training needed to fill the new demands of the global economy.[33] Secondary school youth transition programs, and the workforce development system, including the Vocational Rehabilitation (VR) program, historically have connected people with disabilities to retail and manual skills training that has become in considerably far less demand than other emerging information, knowledge, and technology-based industries. As a group, people with disabilities continue to be more likely than those without disabilities to work in jobs in the very industries that are most subject to displacement by new technologies.[34]

This is not a new phenomenon, as it has been a persistent theme across time—and since the enactment of the ADA—that people with disabilities are vastly underrepresented in the fastest-growing occupations in the economy and overrepresented in the occupations with

Figure 1. Bureau of Labor Statistics Data Employment-Population Ratios 2009–2018

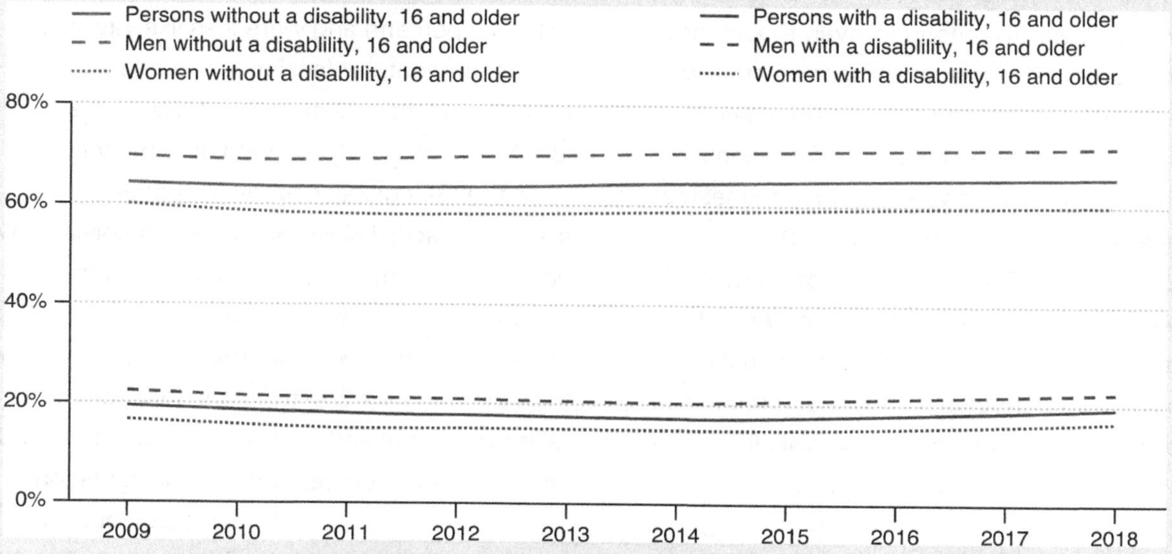

Source: U.S. Bureau of Labor Statistics.

Figure 2. Labor Force Participation Rate of Civilian Population Ages 16–64 Years

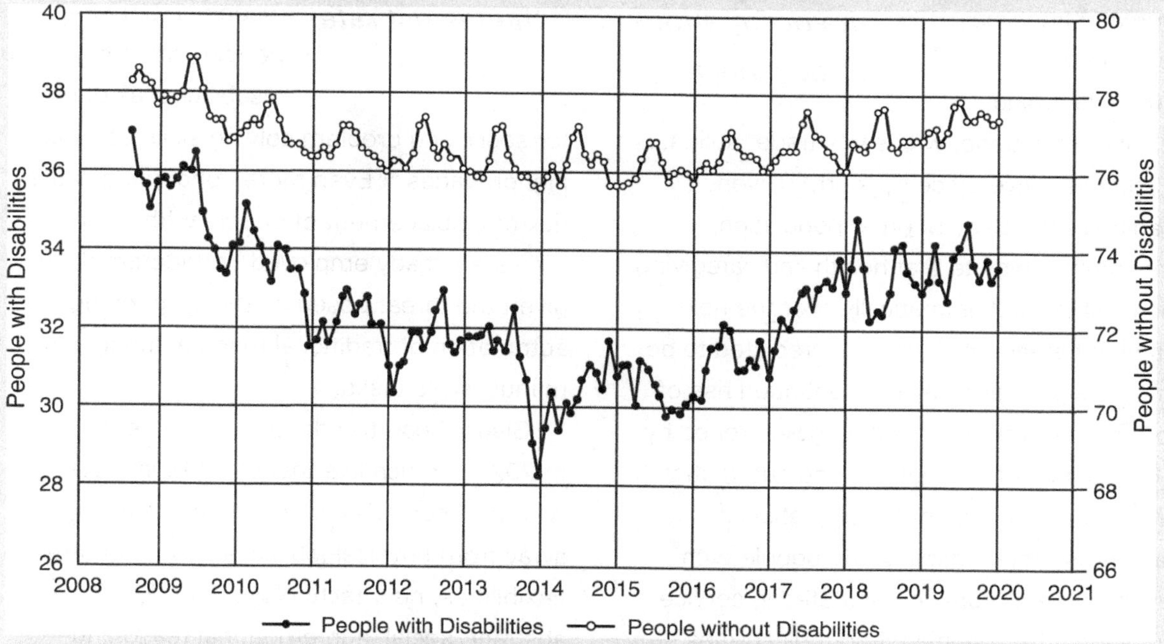

Source: National Trends in Disability and Employment (nTIDE) Report, University of New Hampshire and Kessler Foundation.

the fastest rate of decline. In fact, people with disabilities are most likely to work in jobs that place an unnecessary emphasis on workers' physical limitations, even though new technologies, services, and supports otherwise exist to assist them to enter jobs in a range of new and emerging industries. For example, the sectors projected to experience the fastest annual employment growth from 2018 to 2028 are health care and social assistance, private educational services, computer and mathematical occupations, and construction (including infrastructure projects and renewable energy).[35] The health care and social assistance, private educational assistance, and construction sectors alone are projected to create 4.6 million jobs by 2028.[36] During the same period, the sectors expected to experience the greatest decline in jobs, among others, are manufacturing, sales and retail trade, wholesale trade, utilities, and administrative office support.[37] Given the aging of the Baby Boomer population, demographics dictate that health and caregiving trades will expand dramatically over the next decade, whereas retail jobs are predicted to be disrupted significantly by the continued rise of e-commerce, with manufacturing weakened by the confluence of outsourcing and automation.

[P]eople with disabilities are vastly underrepresented in the fastest-growing occupations in the economy and overrepresented in the occupations with the fastest rate of decline.

Yet, current Bureau of Labor Statistics data demonstrates that in 2018, people with disabilities were more concentrated in service occupations than people without disabilities (19 percent, compared with 17.2 percent).[38] Moreover, workers with disabilities were also more likely than those without disabilities to work in production, transportation, and material moving occupations (13.9 percent, compared with 11.8 percent) and were less likely to work in management, professional, and related occupations than those without disabilities (33.7 percent, compared with 40.3 percent).

In the new global economy, abstract reasoning, social skills, and problem-solving have positive economic returns, while "routine tasks and manual tasks are both negative."[39] A 2013 study found that the tasks that remain resistant to automation are creativity and ideation, tasks related to social and emotional intelligence, and tasks related to perception and manipulation.[40] As one study observed, the fact that people with disabilities are more likely to perform routine or manual tasks may account for the widening wage gap between people with and without disabilities, as demand for social and problem-solving skills command higher wages.[41] Even more concerning is the risk of displacement of people with disabilities who are already employed or underemployed, given the threat posed by the burgeoning automation of traditional manufacturing and manual skills tasks.

Given these trends, the "good news" of 2020 is much like that of 2007, in that—with the market's continued acceleration away from physical job skills toward greater flexibilities, new technology, and demand for abstract, social, and emotional reasoning—the global economy remains ripe for the full inclusion of people with disabilities. The coming decades should give rise to an economy where accommodation is increasingly viewed as an intrinsic part of innovation, rather than something contrary to it. Indeed, we only need to reflect backward in time to understand the dynamism of the present moment and how far we have come. Throughout the 1990s and 2000s, NCD and other commentators focused many of their recommendations about disability employment on the inflexibility of employers in allowing telecommuting and flextime, the cost associated with setting up home offices, and the resistance of large bureaucratic organizations in providing reasonable accommodations; they also criticized the lack of personalized consideration for employees' technology needs.[42]

Today, while there remains more to be accomplished on these fronts, at the very least, workplace flexibility, telecommuting, technology, and workplace modifications have entered the mainstream of successful businesses in the United States. Certainly, workplace policies have become more universally designed for employees with and without disabilities. This makes sense in a market where people can work from anywhere, are connected at all times through smartphones, tablets, and other Internet-connected devices, and enjoy broadband Internet access and cloud computing in the same way that they do other public utilities. Moreover, because of the widespread and common use of technology, the cost of modifications to employers has fallen, making access to accommodation, telecommuting, self-employment, and technology far easier.

More good news is that, over the past 30 years, a new generation of Americans with disabilities has come of age with the ADA well in place, shifting and raising societal expectations and creating demand for meaningful education, job preparation, and experiences in mainstream employment. As the Senate Health, Education, Labor, and Pensions Committee observed in 2012, "we now have a new generation of young adults with disabilities, the 'ADA generation,' who have high expectations for themselves and who are ready, willing and able to pursue a good career in high-growth sectors of our Nation's economy that will allow them to become and stay part of the middle class."[43] Moreover, the desire of not only youth but adults with disabilities to work and achieve economic self-sufficiency and to engage in mainstream employment has been well documented in the years since the passage of the ADA and remains strong.[44]

Additionally, unfounded fears about the high costs of reasonable accommodations have diminished dramatically since the enactment of the ADA, as employers have become accustomed to providing reasonable accommodations at very little cost. In fact, the average accommodations have proven to be less expensive and yield significantly higher returns than critics of the law initially estimated. Survey results from the U.S. Department of Labor's Job Accommodation Network show that, "the benefits employers receive from making workplace accommodations [are documented to] far outweigh the associated costs."[45] Employers reported providing accommodations that resulted in such benefits as "retaining valuable employees, improving productivity and morale, reducing workers' compensation and training costs, and improving company diversity."[46] Employers also reported that "a high percentage

(58 percent) of accommodations cost absolutely nothing to make ($0), while the rest of the accommodations made had a typical cost of only $500."[47]

In addition, companies are engaged in "cutting-edge disability recruitment, hiring, and on-boarding strategies, not as charity or marketing, but because it serves their bottom line."[48] As the executive director of the Marriott Foundation's Bridges from School to Work program told NCD, "there's now a war for talent," and workers with disabilities bring strategic advantage to any employer's position in that war, including by increasing job retention, introducing new efficiencies, and increasing and widening diversity.[49] Companies are increasingly awakening to the economic value and new efficiencies created by hiring people with disabilities.

[C]ompanies are engaged in "cutting-edge disability recruitment, hiring, and on-boarding strategies, not as charity or marketing, but because it serves their bottom line."

A business case for hiring people with disabilities

A 2018 report issued by the consulting giant Accenture that looked at 45 companies that specialized in building disability inclusive policies and practices revealed that those companies achieved, on average, 28 percent higher revenue, double the net income, and 30 percent higher economic profit margins over the four-year period analyzed, compared to other companies in the sample.[50]

In this war for talent, employers now routinely recruit job-ready candidates with disabilities for competitive integrated employment to enhance their bottom line, deeply enrich the skills available within companies, and promote diversity. For example, in 2012, the Federal Home Loan Mortgage Corporation (Freddie Mac) partnered with the Autistic Self Advocacy Network to create an Autism Internship Program to match the needs of its company with the capabilities of autistic people who had college degrees in the fields of computer science, mathematics, and finance.[51] Likewise, companies like JP Morgan, SAP, DXC Technology (formerly Hewlett Packard Enterprise), and Microsoft also have autism hiring programs, built on the idea that such employees have unique skills traits that are especially useful in science, technology, engineering, and mathematics (STEM) industries and that removing barriers to entry for them will allow such companies to access an untapped labor pool. In 2019, JP Morgan Chase reported that employees in its Autism at Work program were 48 percent more accurate and as much as 92 percent more productive than peers in comparable positions.[52]

That was the good news. Unfortunately, there continues to be much bad news. Given the market's strong acceleration toward greater technology, flexibility, and modification, the more people with disabilities are excluded from these important innovations and opportunities, the harder the economic consequences will fall on them, including widening inequality and economic marginalization. It is incumbent upon the public and private sectors to clear the runway for people with disabilities to launch their talents into the twenty-first century global economy, including the necessary education, accessible technology, equipment, advanced skills training, and transportation infrastructure required to compete in it. Even the greatest optimists among us will recognize that the mere presence of technology and training cannot entirely rectify or remove underlying stigma, inattention to the accommodation and accessibility needs of employees, and discriminatory attitudes and stereotypes perpetuated by some employers about the capabilities of employees with disabilities. Consistent work is necessary to build awareness about the good news about disability employment and, most importantly, to convert that knowledge into actual hiring in the coming decades.

Technology and other such disruptive changes at once carry the possibility for transformative inclusion *and* near categorical exclusion of people with disabilities from employment, for instance, "in the past, working as a cashier required a person to have some math skills and the capacity to work a cash register," eliminating some people with intellectual and other disabilities from consideration for the job.[53] "Now, of course, a person just has to scan the bar codes for each product and provide change indicated by the 'point of sale computer' that has replaced cash registers."[54] Alternatively, the authors soberly observed the harsh economic consequences when technology unjustifiably excludes people with disabilities, "if one wants to apply for many jobs in today's employment context, that process begins with filling out a form that is online. If the web browser or computer lacks accessibility, then one cannot complete the form."[55] Certainly the latter scenario applies not just to people who are blind or with intellectual or developmental disabilities, but also to people with disabilities who lack access to a computer or broadband Internet access altogether.

Technology and other such disruptive changes at once carry the possibility for transformative inclusion and *near categorical exclusion of people with disabilities from employment.*

Research has documented the expanding digital divide, as people with disabilities are less likely than those without disabilities to receive computer training or use computers at work or elsewhere, in large part because of resource constraints.

Research has documented the expanding digital divide, as people with disabilities are less likely than those without disabilities to receive computer training or use computers at work or elsewhere, in large part because of resource constraints.[56] At the start of the new millennium, in 2002, the U.S. Department of Commerce documented that people with multiple disabilities aged 25–60 years were almost *half as likely* to have access to the Internet as people without disabilities.[57] However, in the years since, few, if any, government interventions have directly addressed the underlying access to technology issue, let alone as *an employment issue*—including access to basic infrastructure like broadband Internet or mainstream digital computing devices that most businesses now depend on. A 2017 Pew Research survey revealed that the digital divide had expanded exponentially from where it was reported in 2002 to people with disabilities being *three times* as likely not to access the Internet as people without disabilities 15 years later.[58] Instead of directly tackling this digital divide, government systems, in large part, have marshaled resources toward assistive technology (AT), carrying on the narrow mandate to reimburse technology that is definitionally tied to improving deficits caused by disability whether to "increase, maintain, or improve functional capabilities," as defined by the Individuals with Disabilities Education Act (IDEA) and other federal laws.[59] While AT is important, the expansive vision of the ADA toward full economic inclusion is one broader than merely offsetting perceived deficits. It calls for attention to technology as a means to compete and succeed in the open market, not simply to offset deficits to functional capacity.

A study of blind transition-age youth found those with a "high self-perceived level of computer competence" were significantly more likely to have paid jobs than those with "low self-perceived computer competence," when gender, severity of vision loss, and multiple disability status were held constant.[60] The study examined data on 200 in-school youths and 190 out-of-school youths with a primary disability of visual impairment. The data indicated that while the current job market requires computer skills as a threshold matter for most job seekers, computer technologies can also help overcome certain employment barriers specific to visual impairments and blindness. As has been documented by previous studies for years, among other things, technology can overcome access barriers to transportation and mobility, reading print, the lack of job-related information, and difficulties with job applications including accessing and filling out application forms.[61]

Students with intellectual and developmental disabilities (I/DD) often emerge from secondary schools having been trained by special education transition programs in "work readiness" or "prevocational" skills training, a form of vocational training entirely devoid of technology in most instances.

Students with intellectual and developmental disabilities (I/DD) often emerge from secondary schools having been trained by special education transition programs in "work readiness" or "prevocational" skills training, a form of vocational training entirely devoid of technology in most instances.[62] In such programs, students perform manual, often menial, tasks and rote processes in preparation for their transition to postsecondary employment. These programs commonly model and prepare students with I/DD for segregated adult employment programs, including subminimum wage employment in sheltered workshops, rather than competitive integrated employment.[63] The skills training offered in these programs most often consists of such manual tasks, without the use of machines or equipment, as sorting, shredding, folding, recycling, serving food, cleaning, maintaining flower beds, doing laundry, and handling trash.[64] In other words, these programs provide skills training in the industries that will be most subject to decline in the future. Even though computers and personal digital assistants have been documented to improve the performance of people with I/DD in "vocational, transition, and employment skills," most people with I/DD receive skills training that lacks such technology.[65]

Twenty-first century technology is commonplace in employment, and possessing knowledge of information and electronic technology platforms is a requirement for most jobs including those in high-growth industries. Yet many people with disabilities, aside from not receiving training in technology, lack the means to purchase computing devices that fall outside of the narrow definition of AT, or alternatively, for those with the purchasing power, the market has not created technologies universally designed so that they can access and use them. Consequently, the market for job-related and business development technology tailored to people with disabilities has been substantially constrained by the outdated "deficits-based" view of disability. As a result, more research and development pertaining to technology that is individually tailored to people with disabilities' on-the-job needs, and accompanying systematic instruction techniques, is urgently needed.

Likewise, people with disabilities have long faced significant obstacles to employment because they cannot find an accessible or affordable means of transportation to get to work. Some disruptive new technologies are rewriting the rules for transportation. For example, the dawn of ride-sharing apps in 2013 was nearly instantly transformative for some Americans with disabilities who needed a reliable way to get to work. As is the case with new technology, for other people with disabilities, it led to claims of discrimination and exclusion from such services, such as wheelchair users and those travelling with service animals.[66] Nevertheless, the apps were an advancement made possible by a confluence of other technological innovations, including the prevalence of smartphones, effective GPS navigation systems, and cellular networks. The creation of real-time ride-sharing significantly reduced transportation barriers, for instance, for people who are blind; for some, it revolutionized the flexibility of their schedules to work more hours or at alternative times. Likewise, it increased the possibility that other people with disabilities who drive and own vehicles could find work in the gig economy that was flexible and available with low barriers to entry. However, to avail themselves of the new technology, such people still need disposable income to purchase the transportation service, or alternatively own a car to provide the service, and must live somewhat near an urban center where such apps have been mostly deployed. Not to mention that they need smartphones and a cellular connection to even hail their first ride.[67] This explains why only 7 percent of adults with a disability say they have ever used a ride-hailing app, compared with 18 percent of adults who do not have a disability.[68] Similar resource constraints and access issues must be taken into account as governments and the private sector negotiate the future of autonomous vehicles.

In addition, for people with disabilities, perhaps even more so than for people without disabilities, where one lives certainly has direct effects on the likelihood that one will work. According to the 2010 Census, 19 percent of the U.S. population lives in rural areas, but only 6 percent of federal transit funds are allocated to serve rural communities. Moreover, according to the 2014–2018 American Community Survey 5-year estimates, an estimated 9,122,197 noninstitutionalized people with disabilities live in a rural community.[69] This equates to people with disabilities comprising 15.1 percent of people living in rural areas, higher than the national average (12.6 percent).[70] "[T]his means that there is minimal or nonexistent transportation services in many rural areas,"[71] with many Americans with disabilities in rural areas facing limitations in finding *any reliable means of transportation to get to work.* This is partly the result of legal limitations on where paratransit must be provided. By law, paratransit service is only provided within a three-quarter-mile radius of a fixed-route bus stop, to be comparable to existing fixed-route transit (as required by Department of Transportation regulations implementing the ADA's requirements). Moreover, existing paratransit systems often have drawn arbitrary lines between rural jurisdictions, causing interruptions in service between where people live and where they work. Accordingly, the most effective transportation solutions afforded to city-dwellers of the new millennium—including public transportation systems and ride-sharing solutions—may well continue to elude those with disabilities in rural areas or even outer exurbs that lack basic infrastructure, without additional reforms in place.

[T]he most effective transportation solutions afforded to city-dwellers of the new millennium—including public transportation systems and ride-sharing solutions—may well continue to elude those with disabilities in rural areas or even outer exurbs that lack basic infrastructure, without additional reforms in place.

Thus, across various domains—including access to skills training, personal computing devices, business development tools, the Internet and broadband, or transportation—technology and innovation now carry in nearly equal proportion the dramatic potential (1) to include people with disabilities in employment that formerly lacked the kind of supports and accommodations that exist now *or* (2) to resolutely exclude people with disabilities from employment if the means to access these innovations lies out of reach. These two distinct and diametrically opposed possibilities reflect that the future of disability employment balances on a razor's edge. In 2020, it is not an overstatement to suggest that innovations exist that have the potential to fundamentally transform the way people with disabilities work, where they work, how they work, and the impact such work has on the overall economy, but people with disabilities risk not accessing them, sitting curbside as those with low barriers to entry to twenty-first century employment parade by as participants of the new global, information-based, and digital economy. That is only the case, however, if persistent structural barriers to employment and powerful misaligned incentives remain unaddressed. The government has the power to advance new interventions, in partnership with the private sector, that can reverse this course, making the coming decade the beginning of the new century of employment for people with disabilities. In this next decade, the deficits-based view of disability employment can be permanently filed away in the annals of history, and accommodation can become synonymous with innovation and economic potential.

"2020 Progress Report on National Disability Policy: Increasing Disability Employment," p. 17-32. National Council on Disability, July 24, 2020. The full report can be found online at https://ncd.gov/progressreport/2020/2020-progress-report.

A Transition Guide

To Postsecondary Education and Employment
For Students and Youth
With Disabilities

Office of Special Education and Rehabilitative Services

United States Department of Education

Revised August 2020

1. Transition Planning: Opportunities and Programs to Prepare Students with Disabilities for Success

Overview

As a student approaches the time to leave high school, it is important that preparations for adult life are well underway. For early transition planning and active participation in decision making to occur for students with disabilities, members of the planning team need to be well-informed about the student's abilities, needs, and available services. This section highlights educational opportunities, credentials, and employment strategies designed to assist students with disabilities while in school to prepare for a meaningful postsecondary education and/or thriving career.

Transition Planning

"A truly successful transition process is the result of comprehensive team planning that is driven by the dreams, desires and abilities of youth. A transition plan provides the basic structure for preparing an individual to live, work and play in the community, as fully and independently as possible."[1]

Local educational agencies (LEAs) and State Vocational Rehabilitation (VR) agencies participate in planning meetings to assist students and family members to make critical decisions about this stage of the student's life and his or her future post-school goals. During the planning process, schools and VR agencies work together to identify the transition needs of students with disabilities, such as the need for assistive or rehabilitation technology, orientation and mobility services or travel training, and career exploration through vocational assessments or work experience opportunities.

The individualized education program (IEP), developed under the *Individuals with Disabilities Education Act (IDEA),* for each student with a disability must address transition services requirements beginning not later than the first IEP to be in effect when the child turns 16, or younger if determined appropriate by the IEP Team, and must be updated annually thereafter. The IEP must include:

(1) appropriate measurable postsecondary goals based upon age-appropriate transition assessments related to training, education, employment, and, where appropriate, independent living skills; and

(2) the transition services (including courses of study) needed to assist the student with a disability in reaching those goals).

While the *IDEA* statute and regulations refer to courses of study, they are but one example of appropriate transition services. Examples of independent living skills to consider when developing postsecondary goals include self-advocacy, management of the home and personal finances, and the use of public information.

Education and Training Opportunities

There are a number of opportunities and programs available for students preparing to exit secondary school. Many of these education and training opportunities involve formal or informal connections between educational, VR, employment, training, social services, and health services agencies. Specifically, high schools, career centers, community colleges, four-year colleges and universities, and State technical colleges are key partners. These partners offer Federal, State, and local funds to assist a student preparing for postsecondary education.

Further, research suggests that enrollment in more rigorous, academically intense programs (e.g., Advanced Placement (AP), International Baccalaureate (IB), or dual enrollment) in high school prepares students, including those with low achievement levels, to enroll and persist in postsecondary education at higher rates than similar students who pursue less challenging courses of study.[2]

The following are examples of exiting options, programs, and activities that may be available as IEP Teams develop IEPs to prepare the student for the transition to adult life.

Regular High School Diploma

The term "regular high school diploma:"

(A) means the standard high school diploma awarded to the preponderance of students in the State that is fully aligned with State standards, or a higher diploma, except that a regular high school diploma shall not be aligned to the alternate academic achievement standards; and

(B) does not include a recognized equivalent of a diploma, such as a general equivalency diploma, certificate of completion, certificate of attendance, or similar lesser credential.

The vast majority of students with disabilities should have access to the same high-quality academic coursework as all other students in the State that reflects grade-level content for the grade in which the student is enrolled and that enables them to participate in assessments aligned with grade-level achievement standards.

Alternate High School Diploma

Some students with the most significant cognitive disabilities may be awarded a State-defined alternate high school diploma based on alternate academic achievement standards, but that diploma must be standards-based. See the definition of alternate diploma in the **Glossary of Terms** (Glossary).

Working towards an alternate diploma sometimes causes delay or keeps the student from completing the requirements for a regular high school diploma. However, students with the most significant cognitive disabilities who are working towards an alternate diploma must receive instruction that is aligned with the State's challenging academic content standards and that promotes their involvement and progress in the general education curriculum, consistent with the *IDEA*.

Further, States must continue to make a free appropriate public education (FAPE) available to any student with a disability who graduates from high school with a credential other than a regular high school diploma, such as an alternate diploma, General Educational Development (GED), or certificate of completion. While FAPE under the *IDEA* does not include education beyond grade 12, States and school districts are required to continue to offer to develop and implement an IEP for an eligible student with a disability who graduates from high school with a credential other than a regular high school diploma until the student has exceeded the age of eligibility for FAPE under State law. Depending on State law which sets the State's upper age limit for FAPE, the entitlement to FAPE under IDEA of a student with a disability who has not graduated high school with a regular high school diploma could last until the student's 22nd birthday. Note, however, that some State laws may address the provision of educational services to individuals with disabilities beyond their 22nd birthday.

IEPs for students with disabilities could include transition services in the form of coursework at a community college or other postsecondary institution, provided that the State recognizes the coursework as secondary school education under State law. Secondary school education does not include education that is beyond grade 12 and must meet State education standards. See the definition of "secondary school" in the Glossary.

Dual or Concurrent Enrollment Program

Increasingly, States and school districts are permitting students to participate in dual or concurrent enrollment programs while still in high school. The term "dual or concurrent enrollment program" refers to a partnership between a postsecondary education institution and a local school district in which the student who has not yet graduated from high school with a regular high school diploma is able to enroll in one or more postsecondary courses and earn postsecondary credit. The credit(s) can be transferred to the college or university in the partnership and applied toward completion of a degree or recognized educational credential, which the student would earn after leaving high school. Programs are offered both on campuses of colleges or universities, or in high school classrooms. As with all students taking classes at postsecondary institutions, students with disabilities who have IEPs must meet the postsecondary institution's criteria to take the class.

Comprehensive transition programs (CTPs) are a type of postsecondary education. CTPs offered at institutions of higher education (IHEs) provide inclusive, academic, social, and career and technical education programs for individuals with intellectual disabilities seeking a postsecondary or college experience and career path. Participation in a CTP may generate academic credit leading to a postsecondary credential or degree. These programs embrace high expectations and provide valuable opportunities for individuals with intellectual disabilities to gain skills that will maximize their opportunities for achieving employment, including competitive integrated employment. After exiting high school, students can enroll in CTPs on a full-time basis. Additionally, since CTPs are a type of postsecondary education program, students may be able to dually enroll in CTPs while still attending secondary school if the IHE will enroll high school students to take CTP classes. If under State law, attending classes at a postsecondary institution, whether auditing or for credit, is considered secondary school education for students in grade 12 or below and the education provided meets applicable State standards, those services can be designated as transition services on a student's IEP and paid for with *IDEA* Part B funds consistent with the student's entitlement to FAPE.

Dual enrollment can be a helpful option for students in facilitating their transition from secondary school to postsecondary education and the workforce. For further information on dual enrollment and CTPs please see *Increasing Postsecondary Opportunities and Success for Students and Youth with Disabilities* issued by the Department on September 17, 2019, at **https://www2.ed.gov/policy/speced/guid/increasing-postsecondary-opportunities-and-success-09-17-2019.pdf**

Early College High School

The term "early college high school" refers to a partnership between at least one school district and at least one college or university that allows a student to simultaneously complete requirements toward earning a regular high school diploma and earn not less than 12 credits that are transferable to the college or university within the partnership as part of his or her course of study toward a postsecondary degree or credential at no cost to the student or student's family.

Summary of Performance

A summary of performance (SOP) is required for each student with an IEP whose eligibility for services under *IDEA* terminates due to graduation from secondary school with a regular high school diploma or due to exceeding the age of eligibility for FAPE under State law. The school district must provide the student with a summary of the student's academic achievement and functional performance that includes recommendations on how to assist the student in meeting the student's postsecondary goals. This summary of the student's achievement and performance can be used to assist the student in accessing postsecondary education and/or employment services.

Employment Opportunities

Community-Based Work Experiences

Whether the student's next step is employment or entering a postsecondary training or an educational program, it is important for students with disabilities to obtain as much work experience as possible to prepare for adult life. The National Collaborative on Workforce and Disability for Youth (NCWD) reports that the value of a work experience, whether paid or unpaid work:

- Helps students acquire jobs at higher wages after they graduate; and
- Promotes students who participate in occupational education and special education in integrated settings to be competitively employed more than students who have not participated in such activities.

NCWD also recommends that a student with a disability participate in multiple work-based learning experiences and those experiences be directly related to the student's education program.[3]

Community-based work experiences, such as internships, apprenticeships, and other on-the-job training experiences, provide increased opportunities for students to learn a specific job, task, or skill at an integrated employment site, and to transfer the knowledge gained to real-time work experiences. To learn more about the value of community-based work experiences, visit: **http://www.ncwd-youthinfo/.**

VR agencies provide a variety of community-based work experiences and on-the-job training services to students and youth with disabilities on a case-by-case basis under the VR program. The VR counselor and the student or youth with a disability will identify a specific vocational goal to determine whether a community-based work experience is a necessary service for the student or youth with disability to achieve an employment outcome in competitive integrated employment or supported employment. "Competitive integrated employment" is employment with earnings comparable to those paid to individuals without disabilities in a setting that allows them to interact with individuals who do not have disabilities. "Supported employment" is competitive integrated employment or employment in an integrated work setting in which individuals with the most significant disabilities are working on a short-term basis toward competitive integrated employment, while receiving ongoing support services in order to support and maintain those individuals in employment. See the Glossary for more extensive definitions of these terms.

Community-based work experiences allow the student or youth with a disability to explore potential careers related to the specific vocational goal, potential workplace environments and demands, and other aspects of the work. These experiences offer the student opportunities to gain firsthand knowledge of a particular job skill, or to learn the culture of day-to-day employment. These experiences can be offered in lieu of, or to supplement, vocational training or educational programs, or as a stand-alone service. To ensure the success of community-based work experiences, VR agencies are encouraged to develop agreements with employers and the student or youth with a disability that describe the training objectives, services to be provided, timelines, and financial responsibilities necessary for a successful community-based work experience.

The following list describes work-based strategies used to enhance competitive integrated employment opportunities for students and youth with disabilities.

Internships

Internships are formal agreements whereby a student or youth is assigned specific tasks in a workplace over a predetermined period of time. Internships can be paid or unpaid, depending on the nature of the agreement with the company and the nature of the tasks.[4]

Internships are usually temporary on-the-job work experiences. They not only provide individuals, including students and youth with disabilities, actual work experience and the opportunity to develop skills, but also the opportunity to determine if the type of work involved is in keeping with the individuals' career interests, abilities and goals. There is no guarantee that an internship will lead to a permanent employment offer. However, VR counselors refer students or youth with a disability to an internship to increase their employment opportunities. The internship experience is frequently enriched by the provision of services or supports, such as transportation and vocational counseling, as described in an approved individualized plan for employment (IPE) under the VR program (for more information on IPEs, see page 16 of this guide).

Mentorships

A young person with or without a disability may participate in a mentoring relationship to hone his or her occupational skills and work habits. The business community describes mentoring as an employee training system under which a senior or more experienced individual (the mentor) is assigned as an advisor, counselor, or guide to a junior or trainee (mentee). The mentor is responsible for providing support to, and feedback on, the individual in his or her charge. The mentor's area of experience is sought based on his or her career, disability, and history or life experience similar to the mentee or a host of other possibilities. You may learn more about mentoring in the business community at: **http://www.businessdictionary.com/definition/mentoring.html**.

Many schools or existing community organizations, such as the YMCA, Boys and Girls Clubs, and centers for independent living, introduce students and youth to older peer or adult mentors who have achieved success in a particular area that is important for the student and youth (for example, employers, college students, recovering substance abusers).[5] Interaction with successful role models with disabilities enhances the disability-related knowledge and self-confidence of students and youth with disabilities, as well as parents' perceptions of the knowledge and capabilities of their students and youth with disabilities.[6]

Apprenticeships

Apprenticeships are formal, sanctioned work experiences of extended duration in which an apprentice, frequently known as a trainee, learns specific occupational skills related to a standardized trade, such as carpentry, plumbing, or drafting. Many apprenticeships also include paid work components.

In an apprenticeship program, an individual has the opportunity to learn a trade through on-the-job training as well as through related academic knowledge. Often, these programs involve an employer and a community college or university and a trade union. An individual applies for specific training and, once accepted, is able to participate in the apprenticeship program. Employment opportunities are usually offered to an individual who successfully completes the program. VR counselors assist individuals with disabilities to prepare for the apprenticeship application process, develop a plan to gain the pre-requisite knowledge and skills for the trade, and identify support services needed to be successful in the apprenticeship program.

Paid Employment

Paid Employment involves existing standard jobs in a company or customized employment positions that are negotiated with an employer. These jobs always feature a wage paid directly to the student or youth. Such work is scheduled during or after the school day. Paid employment is frequently an integral part of a student's course of study or simply a separate adjunctive experience.[7] Often times, these employment experiences are the first steps towards building a meaningful career for students and youth with disabilities.

Career Pathways[8]

As students and youth with disabilities prepare for their careers, they are counseled to consider and explore a specific career to determine if it meets their career interests, abilities and goals. The Career Pathways model is designed to facilitate an individual's career interest and advancement with multiple entrance and exit points in the individual's career over his or her lifetime. Key program design features of the Career Pathways model include contextualized curricula, integrated basic education and occupational training, career counseling, support services, assessments and credit transfer agreements that ease entry and exit points towards credential attainment.

Career Pathways are also designed as a system strategy for integrating educational instruction, workforce development, and human services, and linking these service delivery systems to labor market trends and employer needs. Career pathways systems use real-time labor market information and active employer involvement to ensure that training and education programs meet the skill and competency needs of local employers. The more the systems are aligned at the State and local levels, the easier it may be to create a level of integration necessary to develop comprehensive programs and ensure an individual's success.

Conclusion: Connections help achieve desired careers

Many of the opportunities, programs, and strategies discussed in this section involve partnerships between high schools, colleges, VR agencies, employers, American Jobs Centers, workforce development boards, social service agencies, students, and their families to identify and secure a career uniquely suited to the student or youth with a disability. It is essential that students and youth with disabilities, along with family members and professional support staff, examine numerous and challenging programs to prepare students and youth with disabilities for their desired post-school goals.

2. Transition Services and Requirements: *IDEA* and the *Rehabilitation Act*

Overview

Both the school system and VR program provide opportunities designed to prepare students and youth with disabilities for postsecondary education and careers in the workforce. This section describes services and key requirements of the *IDEA* and the *Rehabilitation Act* that facilitate the transition from school to post-school activities, including postsecondary education and competitive integrated employment. These requirements are in place for students and youth with disabilities to seamlessly access services and supports to achieve their career goals. Examples of how States implement transition requirements, descriptions of services for youth with disabilities who are no longer in school, and a sample flow chart of key points in the transition process are also presented.

Transition Services

Transition services are integral to FAPE under *IDEA.* A primary purpose of *IDEA* is to ensure that all children with disabilities have available to them a FAPE that emphasizes special education and related services designed to meet their unique needs and prepare them for further education, employment, and independent living. As noted earlier in this guide, *IDEA* contains transition services requirements for students with disabilities, which must be addressed in the first IEP to be in effect when the student turns 16, or younger, if determined appropriate by the IEP Team and updated annually thereafter. The *Rehabilitation Act* authorizes a continuum of services, such as pre-employment transition services for students with disabilities, and transition services, job placement services, other VR services, and supported employment services for students and youth with disabilities, as appropriate, to secure meaningful careers. Implementing regulations for both the schools and the State VR Services program define transition services similarly.

Providing transition services is a shared responsibility between the school and VR agency. The definition of transition services is listed in the Glossary at the end of this guide.

Transition Services for Students under *IDEA*

Schools provide an array of supports and services for *IDEA*-eligible students designed to enable them to be prepared for college or careers. Under *IDEA*, States and school districts must make FAPE available to all eligible children with disabilities in mandatory age ranges. FAPE includes the provision of special education and related services at no cost to the parents in conformity with a properly developed IEP. Each child with a disability must receive FAPE in the least restrictive environment (LRE), and, to the maximum extent appropriate, must be educated with children who do not have disabilities. The LRE requirements apply to transition services, including employment-related transition services, and apply equally to the employment portion of the student's program and placement.[9]

The Individualized Education Program: Postsecondary Goals and Transition Services

The Individualized Education Program

Each student with a disability served under *IDEA,* must have an IEP that is developed, reviewed, or revised at a meeting of the IEP Team that includes:

- The parents of a child with a disability;
- Not fewer than one regular education teacher of such child (if the child is, or may be, participating in the regular education environment);
- Not fewer than one special education teacher or, where appropriate, not fewer than one special education provider of such child;
- A representative of the public agency (generally the local educational agency (LEA)) who is: qualified to provide, or supervise the provision of, specially designed instruction to meet the unique needs of children with disabilities; knowledgeable about the general education curriculum; and knowledgeable about the availability of resources of the LEA;
- An individual who can interpret the instructional implications of evaluation results, who may be a member of the team described above;
- At the discretion of the parent or the agency, other individuals who have knowledge or special expertise regarding the child, including related services personnel as appropriate; and
- Whenever appropriate, the child with a disability.

Parents are an essential source of information in IEP development and play an important role in the IEP Team to establish the student's IEP goals. There are many resources to assist parents through the IEP and transition processes.

Other Agency Representatives at IEP Team Meetings

Representatives of other agencies, such as the VR agency, can be invited to participate at IEP Team meetings in which transition services and postsecondary goals are discussed, if that agency is likely to be responsible for providing or paying for the transition services to be included in the student's IEP. However, *IDEA* requires the consent of the parents or the student who has reached the age of majority under State law to invite other agency representatives to participate in the meeting. See section 4 of this guide for additional information about the age of majority. If a participating agency, other than a public agency, fails to provide the transition services described in the student's IEP, the public agency must reconvene the IEP Team to identify alternative strategies to meet the transition objectives for the student.

To meet *IDEA's* transition services provisions, the IEP must contain the services and supports needed to assist the student to gain the skills and experiences necessary to reach his or her desired post-school goals. In the first IEP to be in effect when the student turns 16, or younger, if determined appropriate by the IEP Team, and updated annually thereafter, the student's IEP must include:

- Appropriate measurable postsecondary goals based upon age-appropriate transition assessments related to training, education, employment, and, where appropriate, independent living skills;
- The transition services (including courses of study) needed to assist the student in reaching those goals; and
- Age-appropriate transition assessments based on the individual needs of the student to be used to determine appropriate measurable postsecondary goals.

States and school districts are in the best position, along with the student and the student's family member or representative, to determine the most appropriate types of transition assessments based upon a student's needs.[10]

As a student gets older, the IEP Team must consider whether the student's needs have changed, taking into account the student's strengths, preferences and interests; and develop measurable goals that are focused on the student's life after high school, specifying the transition services needed to help him or her reach those goals. We strongly encourage parents to recognize that decisions about the specific content of postsecondary goals and transition services are the responsibility of the IEP Team. These decisions are made at IEP Team meetings, which sometimes include additional school personnel with specific knowledge related to the identified goals and services. Nothing in *IDEA* requires a specific service, placement, or course of study to be included in the student's IEP as a transition service. Rather, *IDEA* leaves such decisions to the IEP Team.

Please note that postsecondary goals and transition services are just one component of a student's IEP. It is also important for the student's other annual IEP goals (the student's academic and functional goals) to complement and address the student's transition service needs, as appropriate. IEP Teams assess the relationship of the student's postsecondary goals to the student's needs in developing the student's other annual IEP goals.

School districts, which are responsible for initiating and conducting IEP Team meetings, must:

- Invite the student to an IEP Team meeting if the purpose of the meeting is to discuss the student's postsecondary goals and the transition services needed to assist the student in reaching those goals;
- Take steps to ensure that the student's preferences and interests are considered, if the student does not attend the meeting;
- Take steps to ensure that the parents are present at IEP Team meetings or are afforded the opportunity to participate;

- Notify parents of the meeting early enough to ensure that parents have an opportunity to attend, and specifically inform them if a purpose of the meeting is consideration of postsecondary goals and transition services for the student;
- Schedule the meeting at a mutually convenient time and place;
- Use other methods to ensure parental participation, including individual or conference telephone calls, if neither parent can attend the meeting; and
- Use alternative means of meeting participation, such as videoconferences and conference calls, if agreed to by the parent and the school district.

Parental and student input is also vital in determining postsecondary goals related to postsecondary education and training services needs for post-school activities, including independent living and employment. Students with disabilities and their parents should be knowledgeable about the range of transition services available, and how to access those services at the local level. School districts should encourage both the student and their parents to be fully engaged in discussions regarding the need for and availability of other services, including application and eligibility for VR services and supports to ensure formal connections with agencies and adult services, as appropriate.

For more information about Parent Training and Information Centers, please visit:

https://ww.parentcenterhub.org

https://www2.ed.gov/programs/rsaptp

The participation of a VR agency representative on the IEP Team helps to ensure that the vocational- or employment-related provisions in the IEP provide a bridge from the receipt of services provided by secondary schools to the receipt of services provided by VR agencies. Further, recent amendments to the *Rehabilitation Act* authorize the VR agency, along with the school, to provide or arrange for the early provision of pre-employment transition services for all students with disabilities who are eligible or potentially eligible for VR services and in need of such services. Representation of the VR agency at the IEP meeting fosters the opportunity for pre-employment transition services to be provided early and in keeping with the student's postsecondary goals.

Students with disabilities, including those eligible under IDEA, have rights under Section 504 of the Rehabilitation Act, which prohibits disability discrimination by recipients of Federal financial assistance, including public elementary and secondary schools. Section 504 requires that a free appropriate public education, as defined in the Section 504 regulations, be provided to elementary and secondary students with disabilities through the provision of regular or special education and related aids and services that are designed to meet their individual educational needs as adequately as the needs of nondisabled students are met and that satisfy certain procedural requirements. Section 504 does not specifically require that eligible students receive transition services as defined in IDEA. However, implementation of an IEP developed in accordance with the IDEA is one means of meeting the Section 504 FAPE standard. More information about Section504 is available at: ***https://www.ed.gov/ocr***

Transition Services for Students and Youth with Disabilities under the *Rehabilitation Act*

A Continuum of Services

One of the primary roles of State VR agencies is to empower individuals with disabilities, including students and youth with disabilities, to make informed choices about their careers by providing a continuum of services to achieve employment outcomes in competitive integrated employment or supported employment. Students and youth with disabilities receive a broad range of services under the VR program, in group settings or on an individual basis, as appropriate. The services available will differ from person to person because they are customized for each individual's needs. Furthermore, certain VR services (e.g., pre-employment transition services) are available to students with disabilities, regardless of whether they have applied for VR services, but these same services are not available to youth with disabilities who do not meet the definition of a "student with a disability" under the *Rehabilitation Act*.

Eligibility Requirements for Services Provided under the VR Program

To be eligible for VR services, an individual must meet the following criteria:

- Have a physical or mental impairment that constitutes or results in a substantial impediment to employment; and
- Require VR services to prepare for, secure, retain, advance in, or regain employment.

However, individuals who receive Supplemental Security Income (SSI) and/or Social Security Disability Insurance (SSDI) benefits are presumed to be eligible for VR services, unless there is clear and convincing evidence that they are unable to benefit from VR services. These individuals, including students and youth with disabilities, are determined to be eligible for VR services based on existing documentation indicating that the individual is a recipient of SSI and/or SSDI benefits.

Most notably, section 113 of the *Rehabilitation Act* references "potentially eligible" students with disabilities with respect to the provision of pre-employment transition services. In this regard, all students with disabilities, regardless of whether they have applied for or been determined eligible for VR services, are considered "potentially eligible" for purposes of receiving pre-employment transition services. The term "potentially eligible" is applicable only with respect to the requirements related to pre-employment transition services. Students with disabilities who need other individualized transition services or other VR services beyond the scope of pre-employment transition services must apply and be determined eligible for the VR program and develop an approved IPE with their VR counselor.

Students with disabilities who receive pre-employment transition services before applying for VR services, and are likely to need other VR services, are encouraged to submit an application as early as possible in the transition planning process. A VR agency is required to implement an order of selection for services when it cannot provide the full range of VR services to all eligible individuals with disabilities who apply for services under the State VR services program. If a State has implemented an order of selection due to limited fiscal or staff resources, the assignment to a priority category under the order of selection to be served is based on the date of application for VR services, not the date of referral or receipt of pre-employment transition services.

In other words, a student's position on a VR agency's waitlist for services, in the event the State has implemented an order of selection, is dependent upon applying for VR services. VR agencies that have implemented an order of selection may continue to provide pre-employment transition services to students with disabilities who were receiving these services prior to the determination of eligibility and assignment to a closed priority category.

Distinctions between New Terms

"Student with a Disability" and "Youth with a Disability"

The *Rehabilitation Act*, as amended by Title IV of the *Workforce Innovation and Opportunity Act* (*WIOA*), created distinct definitions for the terms "student with a disability" and "youth with a disability." In general, a "student with a disability" is an individual with a disability who is enrolled in an education program; meets certain age requirements; and is eligible for and receiving special education or related services under *IDEA* or is an individual with a disability for purposes of *Section 504*. Educational programs include: secondary education programs; non-traditional or alternative secondary education programs, including home schooling; postsecondary education programs; and other recognized educational programs, such as those offered through the juvenile justice system. Age requirements for a student with a disability include minimum and maximum age requirements. A student cannot be younger than the earliest age to receive transition services under *IDEA*, unless a State elects to provide pre-employment transition services at an earlier age. A student cannot be older than 21, unless State law for the State provides for a higher maximum age for the receipt of services under *IDEA*, then the student cannot be older than that maximum age. A "youth with a disability" is an individual with a disability who is between the ages of 14 and 24 years of age. There is no requirement that a "youth with a disability" be participating in an educational program. The age range for a "youth with a disability" is broader than that for a "student with a disability" under the *Rehabilitation Act*.

As previously discussed, the continuum of services available through the VR program includes: pre-employment transition services that are available only to VR eligible or potentially eligible students with disabilities; transition services that are available to groups of students or youth with disabilities, or on an individual basis under an approved IPE; and other VR services that are provided to eligible students and youth with disabilities under an approved IPE.

The definitions of "student with a disability" and "youth with a disability" are listed in the Glossary of this guide.

"Pre-Employment Transition Services" and Individualized Transition Services

"Pre-employment transition services" are offered as an early start at job exploration and are designed to help students with disabilities that are eligible or potentially eligible for VR services identify their career interests. These services include:

- Job exploration counseling;
- Work-based learning experiences, which may include in-school or after school opportunities, or experience outside the traditional school setting (including internships) provided in an integrated environment to the maximum extent possible;
- Counseling on opportunities for enrollment in comprehensive transition or postsecondary educational programs at institutions of higher education;
- Workplace readiness training to develop social skills and independent living; and
- Instruction in self-advocacy, (including instruction in person-centered planning), which may include peer mentoring.

As noted earlier, pre-employment transition services are only available to "students with disabilities." For students with disabilities who are not enrolled in an education program administered by an LEA, but who are enrolled in other public programs, VR agencies may coordinate the provision of pre-employment transition services for these students with disabilities with the public entities administering those educational programs. Services arranged or provided by the VR agency should be based upon an individual's need and should enrich, not delay, the transition planning process, application to the VR program, and the continuum of services necessary for movement from school to post-school activities.

Although the five distinct pre-employment transition services discussed above are only available to students with disabilities at the earliest stage of this continuum, either in a group setting or on an individual basis, VR agencies may provide transition services—another set of VR services in the continuum of services—to students and youth with disabilities. Some transition services are provided to groups of students and youth with disabilities prior to or after submitting an application for VR services. While these group services are not individualized or specifically related to the individual needs of the student or an approved IPE, they are beneficial and increase the student's opportunities to participate in activities, such as group tours of universities and vocational training programs; employer site visits to learn about career opportunities; and career fairs coordinated with workforce development and employers.

Individualized transition services or other individualized VR services must be provided to students and youth who have been determined eligible for VR services, and the services are described in an approved IPE. Examples of transition services provided in accordance with an approved IPE include travel expenses, vocational and other training services, employment development activities, job search and placement services, and job coaching.

Transition services are outcome-oriented services designed to facilitate the movement from the receipt of services from schools to the receipt of services from VR agencies, and/or as appropriate, other State agencies. Transition services are also designed to facilitate movement towards post-school activities, including postsecondary education and vocational training that lead to employment outcomes in competitive integrated employment or supported employment.

Individualized VR Services

As noted earlier, if a student or youth with a disability needs individualized VR services, the student or youth must apply and be determined eligible for such services and have an approved IPE in place to receive those services. Individualized VR services are any services described in the IPE necessary to assist an individual with a disability in preparing for, securing, advancing in, retaining, or regaining an employment outcome that is consistent with the strengths, resources, priorities, concerns, abilities, capabilities, interests, and informed choice of the individual.

The VR services provided depend on the student's or youth's individual needs and include, but are not limited to:

- An assessment for determining eligibility and VR needs by qualified personnel, including, if appropriate, an assessment by personnel skilled in rehabilitation technology;
- Counseling and guidance, including information and support services to assist an individual in exercising informed choice consistent with the provisions of section 102(d) of the *Rehabilitation Act*;
- Referral and other services to secure needed services from other agencies through agreements developed, if such services are not available under the VR program;
- Job-related services, including job search and placement assistance, job retention services, follow-up services, and follow-along services;
- Transition services for students with disabilities, that facilitate the transition from school to postsecondary life, such as achievement of an employment outcome in competitive integrated employment, or pre-employment transition services for students;
- Supported employment services for individuals with the most significant disabilities; and
- Services to the family of an individual with a disability necessary to assist the individual to achieve an employment outcome.

The Individualized Plan for Employment Procedures

Once a student or youth is determined eligible for VR services, the student or youth, or his or her representative, develops an IPE. The student or youth, or his or her representative, may seek assistance in the development of the IPE from a qualified VR counselor or another advocate. However, only a qualified VR counselor employed by the VR agency may approve and sign the IPE.

The following IPE requirements facilitate a seamless transition process:

- The IPE is a written document that is agreed to and signed by the eligible individual or the individual's representative;
- The IPE is approved and signed by a qualified VR counselor employed by the VR agency;
- The individual with a disability, including a student or youth, must be given the opportunity to make an informed choice in selecting an employment outcome, needed VR services, providers of those VR services, and related components of the IPE;
- A copy of the IPE must be provided to the individual or individual's representative in writing or appropriate mode of communication;
- The IPE must be reviewed annually by the VR counselor, and amended, as necessary, if there are substantive changes in the components of the IPE; and
- The IPE must be developed no later than 90 days after the date of eligibility determination.

For students with disabilities who receive special education and related services under *IDEA*, the IPE must be developed and approved (i.e., agreed to and signed by the student, or the student's representative, and the VR agency counselor) no later than the time each VR-eligible student leaves the school setting.[11]

Also, the IPE for a student with a disability who receives special education and related services under Part B of *IDEA* or educational services under section 504 must be developed so that it is consistent with and complementary to the student's IEP or plan for section 504 services.

Coordination and Collaboration between State Educational Agency (SEA) and VR Agency

Transition planning and services begin while students are in school. According to program year (PY) 2018 RSA data, of all the individuals with disabilities who applied for VR services between age 14 and 24, 56 percent were referred to VR agencies from elementary and secondary schools. Schools and VR agencies have maintained a longstanding relationship to meet the transition needs of students with disabilities.

A VR agency is required to describe in its VR services portion of the Unified or Combined State Plan, its plans, policies, and procedures for the coordination between VR and education officials to facilitate the transition of students with disabilities from the receipt of educational services in school to the receipt of VR services, including pre-employment transition services. Under *IDEA*, services are provided at no cost to the student or his or her family. Under the *Rehabilitation Act*, VR-eligible individuals may be required to provide financial support towards VR services, such as training and postsecondary education, as outlined in their approved IPE. To ensure effective collaboration and coordination for service delivery, VR agencies and the schools are required to plan and coordinate pre-employment transition services and transition services for students with disabilities, as agreed upon in the State's formal interagency agreement.

The interagency agreements meet the requirement for collaboration between the State education and VR agencies at the State-level and are important because the agreements provide the basis for determining which agency pays for certain services. It is important for students with disabilities and family members to be aware of these agreements, because they serve as the foundation for coordinated services for students with disabilities exiting school and pursuing VR services. In this way, students, family members, and representatives can be more informed participants during the transition planning process and service delivery.

Formal Interagency Agreement

In each State, a formal interagency agreement or other mechanism must be developed between the SEA, the LEA (as appropriate), and the VR agency. This agreement is intended to facilitate a seamless delivery system of services from school to post-school activities.

The formal interagency agreement required under the VR program regulations must include provisions that address, at a minimum, the following:

- Consultation and technical assistance by the State VR agency to assist educational agencies in planning for the transition of students with disabilities from school to post-school activities, including VR services;
- Transition planning by State VR agency and school personnel for students with disabilities that facilitates the development and implementation of their IEPs;
- The roles and responsibilities, including financial responsibilities, of each agency, including provisions for determining State lead agencies and qualified personnel responsible for pre-employment transition services and transition services;
- Procedures for outreach to and identification of students with disabilities who need transition services;
- Coordination necessary to satisfy documentation requirements with regard to students and youth with disabilities who are seeking subminimum wage employment;
- Assurance that neither the SEA nor the LEA will enter into an agreement with an employer holding a section 14(c) certificate under the *Fair Labor Standards Act* for the purpose of operating a program in which students or youth with disabilities are paid subminimum wage; and
- An understanding that nothing in the formal interagency agreement will be construed to reduce the obligation under *IDEA* or the obligation of any other agency to provide or pay for those services that are also considered special education or related services under IDEA and necessary for FAPE.

Additionally, under *IDEA,* these interagency agreements must include:

- An identification of, or method for defining, the financial responsibility of each agency in order to ensure that all services that are needed to ensure a FAPE are provided, provided that the financial responsibility of each public agency, including the State Medicaid agency and other public insurers of youth with disabilities, shall precede the financial responsibility of the LEA (or State agency responsible for developing the child's IEP). The services that are needed to ensure FAPE include, but are not limited to, services described in *IDEA* relating to assistive technology devices and services, related services, supplementary aids and services, and transition services;
- The conditions, terms, and procedures under which a LEA shall be reimbursed by other agencies; and
- Procedures for resolving interagency disputes (including procedures under which LEAs may initiate proceedings) under the agreement or other mechanism to secure reimbursement from other agencies or otherwise implement the provisions of the agreement or mechanism.

It is expected that SEAs, LEAs, and VR agencies will work together to implement the provisions of their respective interagency agreements. Decisions about whether the service is related to an employment outcome or educational attainment, or if it is considered a special education or related service, as well as whether the service is one customarily provided under *IDEA* or the *Rehabilitation Act* are ones that are made at the State and local level by SEA, VR and LEA personnel. For example, work-based learning experiences, such as internships, short-term employment, or on-the-job trainings located in the community may be appropriate pre-employment transition services under the *Rehabilitation Act* or may be considered transition services under *IDEA*, as determined by the IEP Team, in collaboration with the VR counselor, and depending on the student's individualized needs. The mere fact that those services are now authorized under the *Rehabilitation Act* as pre-employment transition services does not mean the school should cease providing them and refer those students to the VR program. If these work-based learning experiences are not customary services provided by an LEA, the VR agencies and LEA are urged to collaborate and coordinate the provision of such services.[12]

Youth with Disabilities No Longer in School

Transition planning is critical for any youth with a disability, whether they are in school or not. A VR counselor can assist youth with disabilities in exploring careers, identifying a career path leading to their vocational goal, and identifying the services and steps to reach that goal. With the exception of pre-employment transition services and transition services provided to groups of individuals with disabilities, VR services are provided only to those individuals with disabilities, including youth with disabilities, who have been determined eligible for services and the services are described in an approved IPE.

Although youth with disabilities who do not meet the definition of a "student with a disability" may not receive pre-employment transition services, they may receive transition services as group transition services, prior to or after applying for VR services, as well as individualized transition or other VR services, after being determined eligible for the VR program and under an approved IPE. Individualized transition services provided under an approved IPE to a youth with a disability eligible for the VR program may consist of, among other things: job exploration counseling, including assessments and vocational guidance and counseling; work adjustment training, vocational/occupational training, or postsecondary education; and job development services, including job search, job placement, and job coaching services.

Coordination of Services

Often, youth with disabilities are not familiar with the community programs and services that are available to them as young adults, especially if they are no longer in school. The VR program is designed to assess, plan, develop, and provide VR services to eligible individuals with disabilities, consistent with their strengths, resources, priorities, concerns, abilities, capabilities, interests, and informed choice. The VR agency assigns a VR counselor to each eligible individual, and the VR counselor can help the youth develop the IPE.

A VR counselor can assist youth in finding and applying for essential daily living services and resources, such as health and housing referrals needed to successfully implement their employment plans. Each community agency sets its criteria for services and, once the youth meets the eligibility criteria, service delivery begins. The VR counselor is available to coordinate VR services with services provided by employment-related programs, such as youth programs funded by the U.S. Department of Labor (DOL) and provided at American Job Centers.

U.S. Department of Labor Youth Programs

Youth programs funded under Title I of *WIOA* include five new program elements: financial literacy instruction; entrepreneurial skills training; provision of local labor market and employment information; activities that help youth transition to postsecondary education and training; and education offered concurrently with workforce preparation activities and training for a specific occupation or occupational cluster.

Two well-known youth programs funded by DOL are the Job Corps and YouthBuild. Each of these programs integrates vocational (including classroom and practical experiences), academic and employability skills training designed to prepare youth for stable, long-term, high-paying employment. Job Corps programs offer career technical training in over 100 career areas. YouthBuild programs focus on the construction trades. Some students are eligible to receive youth services from DOL programs. These youth must be age 14–21, attending school, from a low-income family, and they must meet one or more additional conditions, such as being an English language learner, homeless, an offender, or others.

For more information on these programs, see *Collaboration Opportunities: WIOA Youth and Vocational Rehabilitation Programs* at **https://www2.ed.gov/about/offices/list/osers/rsa/wioa-reauthorization.html**.

Social Security Administration Work Program

The Social Security Administration (SSA) funds the Ticket to Work program to provide career development services to beneficiaries between age 18 to 64 to assist these individuals to become financially independent. SSA issues a letter, referred to as the "Ticket," to eligible beneficiaries that can be used to obtain free employment services from a provider of their choice that is registered with SSA.

Both a single agency and a group of providers are comprised of a consortium of employers referred to as the Employment Network. While pursuing employment, the individual continues to receive SSA benefits and employment-related services to become employed and to maintain that employment. Services include, but are not limited to, vocational counseling, training, education, and job coaching, and are provided based on the individual's needs. More information on this program is located at: **https://choosework.ssa.gov/about/index.html**.

Examples to Consider: States are Coordinating Transition Services

Vocational Rehabilitation Supporting Students with Disabilities

In one State, a community rehabilitation program provides supported employment services and intensive case management services for youth with significant emotional and behavioral disabilities who dropped out of high school or are at risk of dropping out. The program uses work as a means to reach individuals with significant employment challenges. The State VR program works in partnership with the State Department of Justice, Department of Health/Division of Mental Health, and the Department of Children and Families in various sites around this State. Program data report that more than 90 percent of these students were not working when they entered the program; however, after receiving career preparation services and related employment supports and services, approximately three-quarters of the students had paid employment and more than a third of the students achieved an employment outcome.

State Educational Agency and State Vocational Rehabilitation Agency Collaboration

A VR agency partnered with a school district to co-locate a dedicated transition VR counselor and technician in an office with school district transition personnel. Full-time VR agency and school district personnel worked together to secure employment opportunities for eligible students with disabilities. The office space was funded by the school district. The VR agency and school district operated under a signed agreement in which the VR agency provided its own office equipment, clerical supplies, computer, phones, and staff. This collaboration provided an opportunity for VR staff to work side-by-side with school district transition personnel to facilitate improved outcomes.

Conclusion: Coordination is required

Transition services are best delivered within a framework of structured planning, meaningful youth and family engagement, and State agency coordination and accountability.

A Sample Flow Chart of Key Points in the Transition Process[13]

The ultimate purpose of transition planning is to make decisions and assign responsibilities related to the student's desired post-school goals. In this regard, the importance of a common understanding of available services and corresponding activities to receive such services cannot be overstated. All members of the IEP and IPE Teams are encouraged to be active participants, especially students with disabilities, their family members or, as appropriate, representatives.

The following sample flow chart is provided as a quick reference tool for students and their families to have a better understanding of the coordination between IEP and IPE team members with respect to the transition activities in the transition process.

The flow chart begins with activities and services starting while the student is in school, such as participation in IEP meetings, consulting with other State agencies, applying for VR services and moving forward to engage in employment services provided by the VR agency. You may use the following chart to ensure a common understanding among all involved in the transition process.

KEY POINTS IN THE TRANSITION PROCESS

Alignment: IEP and IPE alignment facilitates a seamless service delivery process.

#1	Individualized Education Program	**Participate** in your IEP or child's IEP development to **ensure** that transition services are addressed in your child's IEP by age 16 (or earlier, depending on your State's laws). Students with disabilities and their representative are critical members of the IEP Team and have valuable information that is needed for quality transition planning.
#2	Be Familiar with the Steps to Transition Planning	Schools should: 1. **Invite** student; 2. **Administer** age appropriate transition assessments; 3. **Determine** needs, interests, preferences, and strengths; 4. **Develop** postsecondary goals; 5. **Create** annual goals consistent with postsecondary goals; 6. **Determine** transition services, including course of study needed to assist your student in reaching those goals; 7. **Consult** other agencies, in particular, the VR agency; and 8. **Update** annually.
#3	Implementation of Transition Services	Provide transition services as identified in the IEP. Pre-employment transition services are provided under the *Rehabilitation Act.* Alignment of the IEP and IPE facilitates a seamless service delivery process.
#4	Referral to VR and/or Other Adult Agencies	1. Pre-employment transition services provided under the *Rehabilitation Act*, as appropriate; 2. Familiarize yourself with laws relating to other programs; and 3. Learn about community agencies that provide services to support students, such as travel training and daily living skills.
#5	VR Application Process	1. **Share employment interests** and capabilities during the intake interview. 2. **Focus on assessment(s)** to lead to the student's postsecondary goals.
#6	Individualized Plan for Employment	**Once a student has been determined eligible for VR services**, the IPE must be developed and approved within 90 days, and no later than the time the student leaves the school setting.
#7	Common VR Services Available under the Rehabilitation Act	1. Transition services; 2. Vocational counseling; 3. Vocational training; 4. Postsecondary education; 5. Supported employment services; 6. Career development; and 7. Job placement.
#8	VR Service Record Closure	As a result of the student or youth with disability: 1. Achieving an employment outcome; or 2. No longer pursuing an employment outcome and, therefore, determined ineligible for VR services.

3. Options after Leaving Secondary School: Education and Employment Goals

Overview

Postsecondary education is one of the most important post-school goals; and research has demonstrated that it is the primary goal for most students with disabilities.[14] As students with disabilities transition from secondary school to postsecondary education, training, and employment, it is critical that they are prepared academically and financially. Postsecondary options, with the help of the VR program, include two- and four-year colleges and universities, trade and vocational schools, adult education programs, and employment outcomes in competitive integrated employment or supported employment.

This section will describe specific actions to be taken and available services and supports for students and youth with disabilities. The services described in this section are provided at the secondary and postsecondary levels to help students and youth with disabilities succeed in their post-school goals.

Postsecondary Education and Training Options

Preparing for College

Secondary School

Whether in middle or high school, if an *IDEA*-eligible student is planning to attend college, there are a number of critical steps to be taken to become college-ready. Early in the transition process, a student is encouraged to:

- Take interesting and challenging courses that prepare him or her for college;
- Be involved in school or community-based activities that allow him or her to explore career interests, including work-based learning or internship opportunities;
- Meet with school guidance counselors to discuss career goals, such as vocational and educational goals, programs of study, college requirements, including the admissions process and any standardized tests required for admission; and
- Be an active participant during the IEP meetings.

As noted earlier, the IEP Team is responsible for ensuring that the student's IEP includes the specialized instruction, supports, and services needed to assist the student in preparing for college and/or other postsecondary schools.

Students with disabilities and their families interested in higher education are encouraged to consider the college environment that provides the best educational program and support services to assist students with meeting their needs and career goals.

IDEA-eligible students with disabilities will benefit from discussions with their parents, school guidance counselor, VR counselor (if applicable), and other professional support staff about the services and supports needed to be successful in postsecondary education or training. For *IDEA*-eligible students whose eligibility terminates because the student has graduated from secondary school with a regular high school diploma or the student has exceeded the age of eligibility for FAPE under State law, the school district must provide the student with an SOP that documents the student's academic achievement, functional performance and recommendations on how to assist the student in meeting his or her postsecondary goals.

Paying for College

The Office of Federal Student Aid (FSA) in the U.S. Department of Education plays a central role in the nation's postsecondary education community. Through the FSA, the Department awards about $150 billion a year in grants, work-study funds, and low-interest loans to approximately 13 million students. There are three types of Federal student aid:

Grants and Scholarships: Financial aid that does not have to be repaid, including the Federal Pell grant that can award as much as $6,345 to each low-income student per year;

Work-Study: A program that allows students to earn money for their education; and

Low Interest Loans: Aid that allows students to borrow money for their education; loans must be repaid with interest.

The following website provides information about student aid: **https://studentaid.gov**.

Completing the Free Application for Federal Student Aid (FAFSA®) is the first step toward getting financial aid for college. The FAFSA® not only provides access to the $150 billion in grants, loans, and work-study funds that the Federal government has available, but many States, schools, and private scholarships require students to submit the FAFSA® before they will consider offering any financial aid. That is why it is important that every college-bound student complete the FAFSA®.

Students who participate in comprehensive transition programs (CTPs) are also eligible for Federal student financial aid. Students enrolled in a comprehensive transition and postsecondary program for students with intellectual disabilities who are maintaining satisfactory academic progress in that program may receive Federal student financial aid under the Federal Pell Grant, Federal Supplemental Educational Opportunity Grant, or Federal Work-Study programs.

Choosing the Right College

College is a big investment in time, money, and effort. Therefore, it is important to research and understand the types of schools, tuition and costs, programs available, student enrollment, and a variety of other important factors when choosing the right school.

When researching potential college programs, students and their families are advised to work closely with the Disability Support Services (DSS) office on campus to discuss disability-related concerns and needs, and the disability-related support services available to students at that postsecondary school. Many DSS offices empower, support, and advocate for students with disabilities to achieve their goals by providing access to education and other programs through the coordination of appropriate accommodations and academic adjustments, assistive technology, alternative formats, and other support. These supports and services, including academic adjustments and auxiliary aids, are provided in compliance with Section 504 and the *Americans with Disabilities Act (ADA).* As explained below, Title II of the ADA applies to public postsecondary institutions, and Title III of the ADA applies to certain private postsecondary institutions. Information about the DSS office may be found at the postsecondary school's website. The U.S Department of Education publication "College Scorecard" (**https://collegescorecard.ed.gov**) also provides data on outcomes and affordability to help select the right college.

Rights and Responsibilities in Postsecondary Education and Training

Students with disabilities are encouraged to be well informed about their rights and responsibilities, as well as the responsibilities of postsecondary schools. Being informed about their rights and responsibilities will help ensure that students have full opportunity to enjoy the benefits of the postsecondary education experience without disruption or delay.

A postsecondary student with a disability is *not* entitled to the same services and supports that the student received in high school. While students with disabilities are entitled to comprehensive supports under the FAPE requirements of *IDEA* or Section 504, as applicable, while in high school, they are no longer entitled to FAPE under *IDEA* or Section 504 if they graduate secondary school with a regular high school diploma.

At the postsecondary level, Section 504 prohibits discrimination on the basis of disability by recipients of Federal financial assistance, and Title II prohibits discrimination on the basis of disability by public entities, regardless of receipt of Federal funds.[15] Note that if the postsecondary institution is a private college or university that is not a religious entity, it would be covered by Title III of the *ADA* (Title III). The Department of Education does not enforce the Title III rights of postsecondary students with disabilities. The U.S. Department of Justice enforces Title III.

Section 504 and Title II require that the postsecondary educational institution provide students with disabilities with accommodations, including appropriate academic adjustments and auxiliary aids and services, that are necessary to afford an individual with a disability an equal opportunity to participate in a school's program.[16]

Postsecondary educational institutions are not required to make adjustments or provide aids or services that would result in a fundamental alteration of their academic program or impose an undue financial or administrative burden on the postsecondary institution's programs.[17]

To receive these supports, a student with a disability must inform the college that he or she has a disability and needs one or more accommodations. The college is not required to identify the student as having a disability or assess the student's needs prior to receiving a request for an accommodation. Colleges may set reasonable requirements for documentation that students must provide. While an IEP or Section 504 plan from high school may be helpful in identifying services that have been effective for the student, such a plan will generally not be sufficient documentation by itself.

The IEP Team, VR counselor, or support professionals can provide specific guidance to prepare the student for postsecondary education and training. For example, they may provide an overview of how to self-disclose individual needs or functional limitations in the postsecondary educational setting.

An overview of the rights and responsibilities of students with disabilities who are preparing to attend postsecondary schools, as well as the obligations of a postsecondary school to provide academic adjustments, including auxiliary aids and services, is available on the Department's website. See "Students with Disabilities Preparing for Postsecondary Education: Know Your Rights and Responsibilities" at: **http://www2.ed.gov/about/offices/list/ocr/transition.html**.

Structural Supports and Physical Accessibility

Section 504 and the *ADA* contain requirements related to the physical accessibility of facilities, including those used for higher education purposes. In recent decades, the removal of architectural barriers, such as providing curb cuts, ramps, and elevators, helped make higher education more inclusive for students with disabilities. Structural accommodations involve making buildings accessible to individuals with disabilities. Typical structural accommodations include ramp availability, elevators, convenient parking, doorway and restroom facilities modifications, and architectural barriers removal or modifications. In situations where architectural barriers cannot be removed, some institutions have changed the location of classes or other activities to a site that is accessible.

Vocational Rehabilitation Supports for Postsecondary Education

The VR program assists individuals with disabilities, including students and youth with disabilities, to acquire the knowledge and skills needed to achieve employment that can sustain economic independence. If it is determined to be necessary and is included on the individual's IPE, the VR agencies can provide financial support to eligible individuals to pay for or offset higher education-related expenses, including college expenses not covered by student financial aid, or disability related expenses, such as personal assistants, interpreters, readers, and education support services.

The student's IPE lists the services that the VR agency and other responsible parties will provide. VR financial support commonly listed in an IPE could include the following postsecondary expenses:

- Vocational and other training services;
- Personal and vocational adjustment training; and
- Advanced training in the fields of science, technology, engineering, or mathematics, computer science, medicine, law, or business in an institution of higher education (universities, colleges, vocational schools, technical institutes, hospital schools of nursing or any other postsecondary education institution) books, tools; and other training materials.

Before the VR agency can provide financial support for most VR services, the VR agency and the student must identify other sources of funding. This requirement is frequently referred to as a search for comparable benefits under the VR program. With respect to the provision of training, including postsecondary education at an IHE, both the VR counselor and student or representative, as appropriate, must make every effort to secure grant assistance from other sources to pay for that training prior to the VR agency providing financial support.

Pell grants are identified as grant assistance through the FAFSA® and would be included in a search for comparable benefits. However, scholarships or awards based on merit or student loans do not count as grant assistance, for purposes of searching for comparable benefits, under the VR program. The VR program does not require a student to apply for merit-based scholarships or awards or apply for student loans. If a student accepts a merit-based scholarship that is restricted to specific costs, such as tuition, fees, room and board, the VR program will take that reduction in expenses into consideration when calculating the amount it could pay to assist the student in order to avoid duplication in funding.

Interagency Agreements between State VR Agencies and Public Institutions of Higher Education

To ensure that students with disabilities are able to access services that enable them to fully participate in education, VR agencies must enter into an interagency agreement or other mechanism for interagency coordination with public IHEs in the State. The agreement or mechanism must address the coordination of services, agency financial responsibilities, provision of accommodations and auxiliary aids and services, reimbursement matters, and procedures for resolving interagency disputes. The local VR agency and DSS office can assist students and families with connecting to the support services offered at IHEs.

Postsecondary Education and Training Programs and Opportunities

The following are examples of such programs that are funded through the U.S. Department of Education.

Gallaudet University

Gallaudet University, federally charted in 1864, is a bilingual, diverse, multicultural institution of higher education that ensures the intellectual and professional advancement of deaf and hard of hearing individuals through American Sign Language and English. Deaf and hard-of-hearing undergraduate students can choose from more than 40 majors leading to a Bachelor of Arts or a Bachelor of Science degree. To learn more, you may visit: **https://www.gallaudet.edu/**.

National Technical Institute for the Deaf (NTID)

NTID is one of the nine colleges within Rochester Institute of Technology (RIT), a leading career-oriented, technological university. NTID offers students who are deaf or hard-of-hearing career-focused degree programs, opportunities to participate in the university's cooperative education program, faculty who specialize in educating deaf and hard-of-hearing students, and the opportunity to enroll in RIT's degree programs. For more information, please visit: **https://www.ntid.rit.edu/**.

Model Transition Programs for Students with Intellectual Disabilities (TPSID) into Higher Education

The *Higher Education Opportunity Act* includes provisions to increase access and opportunities for youth and adults with intellectual disabilities who are interested in participating in higher education programs.

The Department's Office of Postsecondary Education (OPE) funded 25 TPSID projects in 2015 to serve students with intellectual disabilities by providing access to academically inclusive college courses, enhancing participation in internships and competitive integrated employment, and encouraging engagement in social and personal development activities. OPE also funds a national coordinating center to provide support, coordination, training, and evaluation services for TPSID grantees and other programs for students with intellectual disabilities nationwide. The national coordinating center is administered by Think College, a project team at the Institute for Community Inclusion at the University of Massachusetts Boston.

For more information about the TPSID program and projects, please visit the Think College website at: **https://thinkcollege.net/about/what-is-think-college/think-college-national-coordinating-center**.

Examples of State and Local Collaboration to Support Postsecondary Options for Individuals with Disabilities

Autism Services

A VR agency, secondary school, and a local community college collaborated in a grant-funded project, which provided comprehensive supports to individuals with autism enrolled at a local community college. At the conclusion of the grant, the VR agency identified a staff person to continue providing supports to 20 students enrolled at three community colleges in the community college system, with some participants transitioning to four-year universities. Supports included faculty trainings, career guidance, self-advocacy instruction, and increased communication with VR counselors, faculty, and family members.

Supported Education

A VR agency collaborated with a community college to develop a supported education program. This initiative provides additional tutoring, study skills training, college life and other training for transition students who enroll in the community college and seek remedial courses before matriculating into a degree or certificate program. The goal is to make community college education and training an option for more transition-age students with disabilities and increase their success rate in college.

A student suffered a stroke at a very young age, and afterwards, was unable to walk, talk, or breathe on his own. However, he did not have any cognitive damage that impacted his intellectual functioning during the stroke. Despite his challenges, he graduated from high school and entered a rigorous four-year college. This student received a bachelor's degree in fine arts. His postsecondary educational success can be largely attributed to his own personal drive, supportive parents, and knowledgeable service providers.

Postsecondary Employment Options

For more than two decades, one of the principal goals of disability policy in the United States, as it influenced special education, vocational rehabilitation, and employment services nationwide, has been to improve employment opportunities for young people with disabilities as they exit secondary education programs.[18] As noted in the *Rehabilitation Act*, as amended by *WIOA*, one of the primary purposes of the *Rehabilitation Act* is to maximize opportunities for individuals with disabilities, including individuals with significant disabilities, for competitive integrated employment.

Preparing for Careers

VR agencies value early engagement with students and youth with disabilities to assist them in preparing for a satisfying career. Early participation in job readiness training can provide the tools and guidance that the student and youth with a disability need to successfully seek, find, advance in, or maintain employment. Job readiness training refers to developing job-seeking skills, such as preparing resumes or completing job applications, practicing interview techniques, honing workplace behaviors, or participating in a job club.

Many models of career development identify stages that are widely accepted as leading to a satisfying and productive career. [19]

These stages include:

Career awareness ► When individuals begin to develop self-awareness and learn about work values and roles in work, usually in elementary school;

Career exploration ► When individuals gather information to explore work interest, skills, abilities, and the requirements of various employment options, usually starting in middle school or early high school; career decision making when individuals begin to select job and career areas that match interests and aptitudes, usually beginning in high school, but often continuing well into adulthood;

Career preparation ► When youth begin to understand their strengths and challenges and make informed choices about preparation activities that will lead to a chosen career area, usually throughout high school and postsecondary school; and

Career placement ► When youth begin to responsibly and productively participate in a job and a career area.

VR counselors have specialized training to assist the youth in developing an IPE. The VR counselor gathers as much information as possible about the youth's work history, education and training, abilities and interests, rehabilitation needs, and possible career goals. In gathering the information, the counselor will first look to existing information to assist in both VR eligibility determination and plan development. VR agencies, SEAs, community rehabilitation programs, and other community partners work together to provide a range of resources to facilitate the objectives and goals of the IPE.

The following work opportunities and options assist students and youth with disabilities to achieve their desired career goals.

On-the-Job Training as a Path to Employment

On-the-job training (OJT) is one type of community-based work experience that is often associated with an existing job opportunity. Through OJT, an individual learns a specific skill taught by an employer in the work environment.

OJT offers an opportunity for the individual to be hired at the conclusion of the training period. A VR counselor and a student or youth with a disability often use the OJT approach as a career exploration opportunity or work experience to obtain entry-level work skills. This training is designed to be short-term and offers a paid or unpaid work experience. VR counselors identify and arrange for the OJT with employers, and frequently provide transportation or other employment related services and supports while the individual is participating in OJT. Additional information about community-based work experiences is discussed in section one of this guide.

Types of Employment Outcomes Authorized under the *Rehabilitation Act*

When developing the IPE, the student or youth with the disability may choose from any employment goal that meets the definition of an "employment outcome" for purposes of the VR program. This means the employment goal must be one in competitive integrated employment (including customized employment and self-employment) or supported employment. Each of these options is discussed in more detail below.

Competitive Integrated Employment

Competitive integrated employment pays a competitive wage in a location where both workers with disabilities and those without disabilities (other than supervisors or individuals supporting the worker with a disability) interact on a daily basis while performing their job. Competitive integrated employment offers the same level of benefits for all employees, including those with disabilities, and offers the same opportunities for advancement for individuals with disabilities and those without disabilities working in similar positions. See the Glossary for the definition of competitive integrated employment.

The *Rehabilitation Act* emphasizes the achievement of competitive integrated employment to ensure that all individuals with disabilities, especially students and youth with disabilities served through the VR program, are provided every opportunity to achieve employment with earnings comparable to those paid to individuals without disabilities, in a setting that allows them to interact with individuals who do not have disabilities. Through the sharing of program information and coordination of joint training, VR program and school staff can explore and identify transition-related services, such as work-based learning, dual enrollment programs, and competitive integrated employment or supported employment opportunities for students exiting school.

WIOA amendments to the *Rehabilitation Act* build on this effort by emphasizing that individuals with disabilities, especially students and youth with disabilities, are given the opportunity to train and work in competitive integrated employment or supported employment. Both school and VR program staff are now responsible for providing documentation of completion of specific services and actions prior to referring a student with a disability to subminimum wage employment. School officials are responsible for providing the VR agency documentation of completion of appropriate transition services under *IDEA*, consistent with the confidentiality requirements of the *Family Educational Rights and Privacy Act*. VR agencies are required to provide the youth with documentation of completion of transition services under *IDEA* in addition to completion of pre-employment transition services and other appropriate services under the VR program. The youth with a disability must obtain this documentation prior to starting a job at subminimum wage with an employer who holds a section 14(c) certificate under the *Fair Labor Standards Act*.

VR agency staff is available to consult with school staff and others to share information that will enable school staff, students, and family members to better understand the medical aspects of disabilities as they relate to employment, the purpose of the VR program, how and when VR staff can best serve the employment needs of the students in the transition process, and how school staff can assist students in their preparation for VR services leading to an employment outcome in competitive integrated employment or supported employment.

Supported Employment

Supported employment refers to competitive integrated employment or employment in an integrated work setting in which individuals are working on a short-term basis toward competitive integrated employment. Supported employment services, including job coaching, are designed for individuals with the most significant disabilities who need ongoing support services because of the nature and severity of their disability in order to perform the work involved. A job coach provides intensive training and on-going support to an individual to learn and perform job tasks at the work site, to teach and reinforce acceptable work behaviors, and to develop positive working relationships with his or her co-workers. As needed, the job coach is able to develop individualized accommodation tools for use on the job, such as picture albums of the sequence of steps in a job or communication aids for individuals with speech or hearing deficits. See the Glossary for the definition of supported employment.

As the student or youth with a disability learns and demonstrates progress in these areas, the job coach decreases the support and time spent with the individual on the job. The job coach makes follow-up or check-in visits on the job site to determine if the individual is performing well on the job and to provide additional job coaching when job tasks change, or the student or youth needs repeated training on a particular task.

Sometimes, the job coach, family member, or youth will identify a co-worker who can provide assistance rather than the job coach. This assistance offers natural support for the individual while working.

A natural support approach refers to enhancing or linking individuals to existing social supports in the work environment that are available either informally (from co-workers and peers on the job) or formally (from supervisors and company-sponsored employment programs). Natural workplace support approaches require more intensive efforts up-front to link the employee to available supports since the approach does not rely on the continuing presence of the job coach.[20]

However, when there is no natural support available and the individual needs ongoing support services, a family member or another agency, such as developmental disabilities, Medicaid, or the VR agencies provides the job coaching or other services. Other services frequently include transportation, daily living, or counseling services relating to attendance or arriving to work on time.

Ongoing support services needed by an individual to maintain a job, such as job placement follow-up, counseling, and training, are considered "extended services." These services are identified on the IPE, along with the service provider that will fund and provide these services. VR agencies may provide extended services to a youth with a most significant disability for a period up to four years or until the youth turns 25 years old. See the Glossary for the definition of extended services.

Customized Employment

While supported employment matches the individual with a position and trains him or her to perform the essential tasks in that position, customized employment designs or tailors job tasks to meet the individual's interests, skills, and capabilities, as well as the needs of the employer. Customized employment is accomplished by using various strategies, including:

- Customizing a job description based on current employer needs or on previously unidentified and unmet employer needs;
- Developing a set of job duties, a work schedule and job arrangement, and specifics of supervision (including performance evaluation and review), and determining a job location;
- Using a professional representative chosen by the individual, or if elected self-representation, to work with an employer to facilitate placement; and
- Providing services and supports at the job location.

Examples of individuals in customized employment across the country are included in "Customized Employment Works Everywhere." You may go to the website to learn more:
https://www.dol.gov/odep/documents/vignette_v3_blue_508_final.pdf

Self-Employment

Self-employment refers to an individual working for him or herself and being responsible for earning his or her own income from a trade or business rather than working for an employer and being paid a salary or wage.

A student or youth with a disability could choose self-employment in a particular business that matches his or her career strengths and interests. Individuals choose self-employment for many reasons, whether it is to work in or out of the home in order to meet family care responsibilities, or to control work schedules or to meet their accessibility needs. The range of occupations for self-employment is vast. For example, individuals with disabilities may choose to be a self-employed certified public accountant, medical billing services provider, comic book artist, or lunch cart operator, among many other options.

VR agencies offer services and guidance to assist a student or youth with a disability to prepare for self-employment, such as training or start-up costs for their business. Typically, the VR counselor will recommend that the individual develop a business plan that includes a market analysis supporting the self-employment venture, the individual's work role in the business, anticipated income based on local market information, identification of the support services needed, and the tools, equipment or supplies needed and their cost. In many cases, the VR counselor refers the student or youth to local community organizations that provide technical assistance to develop the business plan or pay for the development of a business plan. The student or youth and the VR counselor will use the collected information to identify the objectives and goals in their IPE.

Conclusion: Know Your Options to Plan

A range of options is available for students to use in achieving their educational and career aspirations. Students, family members, educators, VR counselors, and other support professionals are encouraged to know about available postsecondary opportunities and services to properly plan and prepare a youth with a disability for adult life.

4. Supporting Student-Made Decisions: Preparation for Adult Life

Overview

Successful post-school transition is most likely to happen when students are actively engaged in their own transition planning. To engage students, families, IEP Teams, VR professionals, and other support professionals should:

- Set high expectations;
- Use a person-centered planning approach;
- Support the student's or youth's social and emotional learning;
- Provide the student or youth with support to make their decisions; and
- Counsel the student and their representative to make informed choices.

This section presents key elements of supported decision-making and describes the practice of informed choice to assist students and youth with disabilities in their decisions for adult life. This section also contains references to resources that will aid students in achieving their life goals.

Setting High Expectations for Secondary School Students with Disabilities

Expectations play a critical role to success in employment and postsecondary educational settings. Low expectations are often cited as significant barriers to academic and career achievement for students with disabilities.[21] For example, the Government Accountability Office (GAO) found that attitudinal barriers of faculty and support service providers in postsecondary educational settings have been shown to inhibit the performance of students with disabilities.[22]

In contrast, setting high expectations for students with disabilities promote successful post-school transition. Research demonstrates that students with disabilities do better when they are held to high expectations and have access to the general education curriculum.[23]

To set high expectations and foster successful post-school outcomes for students with disabilities, all individuals concerned with their education should:

- Establish a school-wide culture of high expectations;
- Provide students with disabilities access to rigorous coursework (see accelerated programs section below);
- Ensure students with disabilities have IEP goals that are aligned with the challenging academic content standards for the grade in which the student is enrolled and ensure that students with disabilities receive the specialized instruction, related services and other supports they need to meaningfully access, be involved, and make progress in the general education curriculum;

- Provide students with disabilities the opportunity to access College and Career Ready Standards and Assessments; and
- Ensure educators have the tools and resources necessary to support success.[24]

Person-Centered Planning

When developing the IEP or the IPE, planning is centered on the interests, strengths, skills, and needs of the student or youth with disability. Person-centered approaches:

- Include in the planning process, individuals who have a deep knowledge of the student's academic and social history;
- View the student as an individual, rather than as a diagnosis or disability;
- Use everyday language in transition planning, rather than "professional jargon;" and
- Ensure that goals are developed based on the student's unique strengths, interests, and capacities.

Addressing Students' Social and Emotional Needs

It is important to address the social and emotional needs of students with disabilities to ensure that they have the skills needed to be successful in a postsecondary educational setting or workplace. Students with disabilities who have well-developed social skills are more likely to be able to successfully navigate employment, community, and postsecondary education settings.[25]

IEP Teams need to take active steps to provide opportunities for students with disabilities to acquire appropriate social skills. Many of these opportunities can be integrated into the student's existing course of study. Specific strategies include:

- **Role-playing**
  Schools can create opportunities for students with disabilities to practice appropriate social skills in a variety of contexts, including school-based, workplace, community, and postsecondary educational settings.
- **Participation in social and emotional learning programs**
  A variety of specific social skill development programs exist that can help students acquire critical social skills.[26]
- **Positive school climate**
  Parents should be aware that a positive school climate is critical to helping students with disabilities develop strong social skills. For example, safe and supportive classrooms build on the students' strengths.[27]

Providing the Student and Youth with Support to Make Their Decisions

Beyond developing social skills, it is crucial for students with disabilities to understand and acquire the skills for self-determination during high school to ensure success in postsecondary education and the workplace.[28] Students with strong self-advocacy skills who understand and fully participate in the development of their IEP and SOP have better transition outcomes.[29]

Key characteristics of self-determination are the ability to:

- Speak for yourself (self-advocacy);
- Solve problems;
- Set goals;
- Make decisions;
- Possess self-awareness; and
- Exhibit independence.[30]

Schools help students develop self-determination skills when they:

- Support students in establishing their own transition goals, including postsecondary education, career, and independent living goals;
- Ensure that students are actively involved in IEP meetings and understand their IEPs, including their specialized instruction and related services, the accommodations they receive for instruction and assessments, if applicable, and supplementary aids and services to facilitate their education in the least restrictive environment;
- Help students develop skills to direct their own learning;
- Use person-centered planning; and
- Create and maintain a system that supports family involvement and empowers families to support the self-determination of their sons and daughters.[31]

Developing self-determination and making informed choices heighten students' knowledge of the transition process and success in post-school settings.

Self-determination activities can be described as activities that result in individuals with developmental disabilities, with appropriate assistance, having the ability, opportunity, authority, and support (including financial support) to:

- Communicate and make personal decisions;
- Communicate choices and exercise control over the type and intensity of services, supports, and other assistance the individual receives;
- Control resources to obtain needed services, supports and other assistance;
- Participate in, and contribute to, their communities; and

- Advocate for themselves and others, develop leadership skills through training in self-advocacy, participate in coalitions, educate policymakers, and play a role in the development of public policies that affect individuals with developmental disabilities.

Making Informed Choices

The VR agency must provide its participants with the opportunity to exercise informed choice throughout the VR process, including making decisions about the following:

- Employment goals;
- Services and service providers;
- Settings for employment and service provision; and
- Methods for procuring services.

The VR agency assists participants by providing information, guidance, and support to make and carry out these decisions. The exercise of informed choice involves communicating clearly, gathering and understanding information, setting goals, making decisions, and following through with decisions. VR counselors provide information through various methods of communication that are helpful to a family in order to assist with identifying opportunities for exercising informed choice from the beginning of the VR process through the achievement of an employment outcome.

Parameters of Informed Choice

While the *Rehabilitation Act* emphasizes the importance of the individual's, including the student's or youth's, ability to exercise informed choice throughout the VR process, the *Rehabilitation Act* requires the VR agencies to ensure that the availability and scope of informed choice is consistent with the VR agencies' responsibilities for the administration of the VR program. Such requirements impose parameters that affect the exercise of informed choice. It is generally the responsibility of the VR counselor to inform the individual about relevant requirements, available options for developing the IPE and for exercising informed choice to assure that the individual understands the options. As appropriate, the VR counselor encourages the participation of family members and others in the VR process.

Parental Consent, Age of Majority, Supported Decision-making and Guardianship

Outreach to parents, family members, caregivers, and representatives plays a critical role in the transition process. For students who receive services under Part B of *IDEA*, States may transfer parental rights to the student when he or she reaches the "age of majority under State law," except for a student who has been determined to be incompetent under State law. The age of majority is the age that a State sets for a minor to become an adult and assume legal responsibility for himself/herself and all decisions that accompany that (e.g., financial, medical, educational).[32] In most States, this is age 18. To learn more about the age of majority, visit: **https://www.parentcenterhub.org/age-of-majority-parentguide**.

At the time a student reaches the age of majority, if parental rights have transferred to the student under State law, the school district must provide any notice required by Part B of IDEA to both the student and the parents. Once parental rights transfer to the student, the student has the right to make his or her own educational, employment, or independent living decisions. VR agencies conduct outreach directly to these students. The consent of the parents or an *IDEA*-eligible student who has reached the age of majority under State law must be obtained before personally identifiable information about the student is released to officials of participating agencies, including VR agencies that are providing or paying for transition services.

As *IDEA*-eligible students with disabilities reach the age of majority, they and their parents are advised to seek information to help them understand their options for making educational decisions. A student need not be placed under guardianship in order for his or her family to remain involved in educational decisions. Guardianship places significant restrictions on the rights of an individual. Students and parents are urged to consider information about less restrictive alternatives.

If State law permits parental rights under the *IDEA* to transfer to a student who has reached the age of majority, that student can become the educational rights holder who invites family members to participate in the IEP meeting. If the adult student does not want to have that role, he or she can execute a power of attorney authorizing a family member to be the educational decision-maker. Alternatively, if a student prefers not to execute a power of attorney, a supported decision-making arrangement can be established consistent with applicable State procedures, in which the parents (or other representatives) assist the student in making decisions.[33] Unlike under guardianship, the student remains an autonomous decision-maker in all aspects of his or her life. To learn more about supported decision-making visit: **http://www.supporteddecisionmaking.org/**.

Families are encouraged to seek services from the Parent Training and Information Centers funded by the Office of Special Education Programs, and Parent Information and Training Programs funded by the Rehabilitation Services Administration.

Conquering Financial Hurdles to Accomplish Goals:

Individuals with disabilities often endure greater expenses than non-disabled individuals. These expenses can create hardships that undermine the careful decision-making processes discussed above and impede the accomplishment of an individual's goals. Fortunately, Congress formally recognized this potential for financial difficulty and passed the Stephen Beck, Jr. Achieving a Better Life Experience ("ABLE") Act of 2014.

What is an ABLE Account?

The ABLE Act amended Section 529 of the IRS Code and authorized States to create tax-advantaged savings programs (ABLE accounts) that individuals with disabilities can establish to help pay for qualified disability expenses. The individual with a disability is considered the ABLE account owner.

Who is eligible for an ABLE Account?

ABLE Accounts can be established for anyone with a disability, at any age, as long as the onset of that disability occurred before age 26. If this age requirement is met and the individual is also already receiving SSI and/or SSDI benefits through the Social Security Administration, then he/she automatically qualifies for an ABLE account. If the individual is not already receiving those benefits, then he/she can still qualify for the account if the individual obtains a letter from a licensed physician. See 26 U.S.C. § 529A(e)(2) for more specific eligibility information.

The individual with a disability who will benefit from the account is the account owner, though other designated individuals may establish the account on the individual's behalf.

How does it work?

Contributions into ABLE accounts are made with post-tax dollars and may not—except in specific circumstances—exceed $15,000 per year in the aggregate. Contributions are not deductible for Federal tax law purposes but may be for State tax law purposes. Any income the account earns will grow tax-free, as long as funds in the account are used solely for qualified disability expenses. Withdrawals from the account will not incur any additional Federal taxes. Most importantly, the ABLE account owner will not lose access to means-tested Federal programs (*e.g.*, Medicare or SSDI), just by having $2,000 or more in the account. The balance of an ABLE account will not impact access to these programs until the account reaches $100,000.

While a majority of States have established ABLE programs, some have not. Individuals with disabilities who reside in States that have not yet established their own programs may enroll in another State's ABLE program. For a current list of State programs and features, please visit: **https://www.ablenrc.org/.**

What expenses may be paid for with an ABLE account?

An ABLE account may be used to pay for all "qualified disability expenses." The Act defines qualified disability expenses as any expenses related to the eligible individual's disability and which are made for the benefit of that individual. The ABLE Act does not list specific costs, but notes that qualifying expenses can be for "education, housing, transportation, employment training and support, assistive technology and personal support services, health prevention and wellness, financial management and administrative services, legal fees, expenses for oversight and monitoring, funeral and burial expenses" but also for "other expenses" consistent with the purpose of the ABLE Act.

For more information about the ABLE Act and ABLE accounts, visit the ABLE National Resource Center website at: **https://www.ablenrc.org**.

Conclusion: Student Empowerment Advances Career Decision-Making

Teaching self-determination and exercising informed choice are not practices limited to the most able youth with disabilities. Schools can help foster self-determination and VR agencies can enhance career decision-making to assist youth with disabilities, including those with the most significant complex or lifelong intellectual or developmental disabilities, to achieve their desired post school goals.

"A Transition Guide to Postsecondary Education and Employment for Students and Youth with Disabilities," p. 1-39. Office of Special Education and Rehabilitative Services, United States Department of Education, revised August 2020. The full report can be found online at https://www2.ed.gov/about/offices/list/osers/transition/products/postsecondary-transition-guide-08-2020.pdf.

Arts & Entertainment

Resources for the Disabled

1 **AbleArts**
P.O. Box 831
Bear, DE 19701
302-368-7477
An organization whose mission is to informthe public of the abilities and talents possessed by individuals with disabilities.

2 **American Art Therapy Association (AATA)**
4875 Eisenhower Ave.
Suite 240
Alexandria, VA 22304
703-548-5860
888-290-0878
Fax: 703-783-8468
info@arttherapy.org
arttherapy.org
Cynthia Woodruff, Executive Director
Barbara Florence, Director, Events & Education
Kat Michel, Senior Manager, Member Services
Clara Keane, Manager, Advocacy & Public Affairs
Not-for-profit organization dedicated to advancing the art therapy profession.

3 **American Council of the Blind**
1703 N Beauregard St
Suite 420
Alexandria, VA 22311
202-467-5081
800-424-8666
Fax: 703-465-5085
info@acb.org
www.acb.org
Eric Bridges, Executive Director
Sharon Lovering, Editor
Tony Stephens, Director, Advocacy and Governmental Affairs
The American Council of the Blind (ACB) is an association working to increase the independence, security, and opportunity for all blind or visually impaired individuals. The Council primarily focuses on developing and maintaining policies to implement the services needed for the blind or visually impaired.

4 **American Dance Therapy Association (ADTA)**
230 Washington Ave.
Suite 101
Albany, NY 12203-3539
518-704-3636
Fax: 518-463-8656
info@adta.org
www.adta.org
Michelle Lavoy, Manager, Operations
Lora Wilson, Continuing Education Administrator
Lauren Hoyt, Office Administrator
Supports the dance and movement therapy profession by promoting education, training, practice and research.

5 **American Music Therapy Association (AMTA)**
8455 Colesville Rd.
Suite 1000
Silver Spring, MD 20910
301-589-3300
Fax: 301-589-5175
info@musictherapy.org
www.musictherapy.org
Adonia Calhoun Coates, Chief Executive Officer
Jane P. Creagan, Director, Professional Programs
Angie K. Elkins, Director, Membership Services & Information Systems
Jennifer McAfee, Director, Communications
AMTA's purpose is the progressive development of the therapeutic use of music in rehabilitation, special education and community settings. Predecessors to the American Music Therapy Association included the National Association for Music Therapy founded in 1950 and the American Association for Music Therapy founded in 1971. AMTA supports the music therapy profession through the advancement of education, training, professional standards, credentialing, and research.

6 **Arena Stage**
The Mead Center for American Theater
1101 Sixth St. SW
Washington, DC 20024
202-554-9066
Fax: 202-488-4056
TTY: 202-484-0247
info@arenastage.org
arenastage.org
Edgar Dobie, Executive Director
Molly Smith, Artistic Director
Joseph Berardelli, CFO
Khady Kamara, Managing Director
Arena Stage has played a pioneering role in providing access to all productions for people with disabilities. Access services and programs include wheelchair accessible seating; infrared assistive listening devices; Braille, large print, audio description and sign interpretation at designated performances.

7 **Art Therapy SourceBook**
McGraw-Hill Company
2 Penn Plaza
New York, NY 10121-101
212-904-2000
www.mhhe.com/hper/physed
Cathy Malchiodi, Author
An overview of the uses of art as a mentally therapeutic tool. *$18.00*
272 pages
ISBN 1-565658-84-1

8 **Art and Disabilities**
Brookline Books
8 Trumbull Rd
Suite B-001
Northampton, MA 01060
413-584-0184
800-666-2665
Fax: 413-584-6184
brbooks@yahoo.com
www.brooklinebooks.com
Florence Ludins-Katz, Author
A step-by-step guide to establishing creative arts centers for people with disabilities. Includes philosophy and making creative arts centers happen.

9 **Art and Healing: Using Expressive Art to Heal Your Body, Mind, and Soul**
Three Rivers Press/Crown Publishing-Random House
1745 Broadway
New York, NY 10019
212-782-9000
crownpublicity@randomhouse.com
www.randomhouse.com/crown/trp.html
Barbara Ganim, Author
Markus Dohle, Chairman & CEO
Melanie Fallon-Houska, Dir., Corporate Contributions
The author believes creating a visual image through any medium can produce physical and emotional benefits for both the creator as well as those who view it. *$17.00*
256 pages
ISBN 0-609803-16-6

10 **Art for All the Children: Approaches to Art Therapy for Children with Disabilities**
Charles C. Thomas
2600 S First St
Springfield, IL 62704-4730
217-789-8980
800-258-8980
Fax: 217-789-9130
books@ccthomas.com
www.ccthomas.com
Frances E Anderson, Author
Sharon Moorman, Editorial Assistant
This second edition is for art therapists in training and for in-service professionals in art therapy, art education and special education who have children with disabilities as a part of their case/class load. *$56.95*
398 pages Paperback
ISBN 0-398060-07-7

11 **Arts Unbound**
542/544 Freeman Street
Orange, NJ 07050
973-675-2787
Fax: 973-678-4408
www.artsunbound.org

Margaret Mikkelsen, Executive Director
Catherine Lazen, Founder and Board Chair
Alan Hirsh, Executive Vice President
Tashea Patterson Carless, Director of Agency Operations

Arts Unbound is a nonprofit organization dedicated to the artistic achievement of youth, adults, and senior citizens with disabilities.

12 **Association of Mouth and Foot Painting Artists (AMPFA)**
2070 Peachtree Court
Suite 101
Atlanta, GA 30341
770-986-7764
877-637- 872
Fax: 770-986-8563
mfpausa@bellsouth.net
www.mfpausa.com

Erich Stegmann, Founder

The AMPF is an international, for-profit association wholly owned and run by disabled artists to help them meet their financial needs. Members paint with brushes held in their mouths or feet as a result of a disability sustained at birth or through an accident or illness that prohibits them from using their hands.

13 **Awakenings Project, The**
PO Box 177
Wheaton, IL 60187
www.awakeningsproject.org

Robert Lundin, Co-Director
Irene O'Neill, President and Co-Director
Mary Lou Lowry, Secretary
John Rakow, Vice President

The Awakenings Project is an organization whose mission is to assist those artists with psychiatric illnesses in developing their talent and finding an outlet for their creative abilities through art in all forms.

14 **Brookline Books**
8 Trumbull Rd
Suite B-001
Northampton, MA 01060
413-584-0184
800-666-2665
Fax: 413-584-6184
brbooks@yahoo.com
www.brooklinebooks.com

15 **Clinical Applications of Music Therapy in Developmental Disability, Pediatrics and Neurolog**
Taylor & Francis
400 Market Street
Suite 400
Philadelphia, PA 19106-4738
215-922-1161
866-416-1078
Fax: 215-922-1474
hello.usa@jkp.com
www.jkp.com

Tony Wigram, Editor
Jessica Kingsley, Chairman, Managing Director
Jemima Kingsley, Director
Octavia Kingsley, Production Director

More and more, music therapy is being practiced as an intervention in medical and special educational settings. This book describes and explains the planning and evaluation of music therapy intervention and how it can be used for assessing complex organic and emotional disabilities. *$34.95*

312 pages
ISBN 1-853027-34-0

16 **Contemporary Art Therapy with Adolescents**
Taylor & Francis
400 Market Street
Suite 400
Philadelphia, PA 19106-4738
215-922-1161
866-416-1078
Fax: 215-922-1474
hello.usa@jkp.com
www.jkp.com

Shirley Riley, Author
Jessica Kingsley, Chairman, Managing Director
Jemima Kingsley, Director
Octavia Kingsley, Production Director

Reviews contemporary theories on adolescent development and therapy and offers solutions to the treatment of young people.
$26.95
285 pages
ISBN 1-853026-37-9

17 **Creative Arts Resources Catalog**
MMB Music
9051 Watson Road
Ste 161
St. Louis, MO 63126
314-531-9635
Fax: 314-531-8384
info@mmbmusic.com
www.mmbmusic.com

Norm Goldberg, Founder & Chair

Publisher and distributor of creative arts therapy materials in the areas of music, dance, art, drama, and poetry. Free catalog contains hundreds of books, recordings, and videos.

18 **Creative Growth Art Center**
355 - 24th St
Oakland, CA 94612
510-836-2340
Fax: 510-836-0769
info@creativegrowth.org
www.creativegrowth.org

Becki Couch-Alvarado, Executive Director
Tom Di Maria, Director
Jennifer Strate O'Neal, Partnerships & Communications Manager

Creative Growth Art Center serves adult artists with developmental, mental and physical disabilities, providing a professional studio environment for artistic development, gallery exhibition and representation and a social atmosphere among peers.

19 **Creativity Explored**
3245 16th St.
San Francisco, CA 94103
415-863-2108
Fax: 415-863-1655
info@creativityexplored.org
www.creativityexplored.org

Linda Johnson, Executive Director

Creativity Explored is a nonprofit visual arts center giving artists with developmental disabilities the means to create and share their work with the community, celebrating the power of art to change lives.

20 **Dancing from the Inside Out**
Fanlight Productions
c/o Icarus Films
32 Court Street, 21st Floor
Brooklyn, NY 11201
718-488-8900
800-876-1710
Fax: 718-488-8642
info@fanlight.com
www.fanlight.com

Ben Achtenberg, Founder

This eloquent video looks at the lives and work of three talented dancers who dance professionally with the acclaimed AXIS Dance Troupe, which includes both disabled and non-disabled dancers. They discuss the process they went through in adapting to their disability and how they came to re-discover physical expression through dance.

21 **Deaf West Theatre**
5114 Lankershim Blvd.
Los Angeles, CA 91601
818-762-2998
Fax: 818-762-2981
info@deafwest.org
deafwest.org

Ed Waterstreet, Founding Artistic Director
David Kurs, Artistic Director
Mark Freund, President

Deaf West Theatre, Inc., was founded in 1991 to directly improve and enrich the cultural lives of the 1.2 million deaf and hard-of-hearing individuals who live in the Los Angeles area. DWT provides exposure and access to professional theatre, filling a void for deaf artists and audiences.

22 **Disability and Social Performance: Using Drama to Achieve Successful Acts**
Brookline Books
8 Trumbull Rd
Suite B-001
Northampton, MA 01060
413-584-0184
800-666-2665
Fax: 413-584-6184
brbooks@yahoo.com
www.brooklinebooks.com

Bernie Warren, Author

This book makes a major contribution to the understanding of disability, people with disabilities and the creative power they possess which can be unleashed through performance. The books name is Disability and Social Performance: Using Drama to Achieve Successful Acts of Being. *$17.95*

23 **Expressive Arts for the Very Disabled and Handicapped of All Ages**
Charles C. Thomas
2600 S First St
Springfield, IL 62704-4730
217-789-8980
800-258-8980
Fax: 217-789-9130
books@ccthomas.com
www.ccthomas.com

Marilyn Wannamaker, Co-Author
Jane G. Cohen, Co-Author

The ideas presented are not only designed to hold the interest of the children and adults, but to meet the needs of professionals and volunteers working with the disabled artists. All crafts are rated on a sliding scale, are of a low difficulty rating, use inexpensive and safe materials, and include explicit instructions. *$49.95*

236 pages Spiral-Paper 1996
ISBN 0-398067-04-5

24 **Fanlight Productions**
c/o Icarus Films
32 Court Street, 21st Floor
Brooklyn, NY 11201
718-488-8900
800-876-1710
Fax: 718-488-8642
info@fanlight.com
www.fanlight.com

Ben Achtenberg, Founder

Fanlight Productions is a leading distributor of innovative film and video works on the social issues of our time, with a special focus on healthcare, mental health, professional ethics, aging and gerontology, disabilities, the workplace, and gender and family issues. Select titles include Acting Blind, Autism: A World Apart, Dancing from the Inside Out, and Able to Laugh.

25 **Fountain House Gallery**
702 Ninth Ave at 48th St
New York, NY 10019
212-262-2756
fountaingallerynyc.com

Ariel Wilmott, Director
Camille Tibaldeo, Communications Director

Fountain House Gallery provides an environment for artists living and working with mental illness to pursue their personal visions and to challenge the stigma that surrounds mental illness.

26 **Friends In Art (FIA)**
4317 Vermont Court
Columbia, MO 65203
573-445-5564
www.friendsinart.com

Peter Altschul, President
Lynn Hedl, Vice President
Don Horn, Corresponding Secretary
Arlo Monthei, Treasurer

Friends in Art is a national organization for blind, visually impaired, and deaf-blind artists, musicians and writers, and art enthusiasts. The organization is dedicated to enhancing the skills and broadening the opportunities of the individuals involved with the organization.

27 **Future Horizons**
721 West Abram Street
Arlington, TX 76013-6995
817-277-0727
800-489-0727
Fax: 817-277-2270
www.fhautism.com

R. Wayne Gilpin, President
Jennifer Gilpin, VP, Foreign Translations
Kelly Gilpin, Editorial Dir.
Teresa Corey, Conference Administration

Founded in 1996, Future Horizons is devoted to supporting and fostering works and programs for those who live and work with autism and asperger's syndrome.

28 **Guide to the Selection of Musical Instruments**
MMB Music
9051 Watson Road
Ste 161
St. Louis, MO 63126
314-531-9635
800-543-3771
Fax: 314-531-8384
info@mmbmusic.com
www.mmbmusic.com

Norm Goldberg, Founder & Chair

A marvelous resource book to aid therapists teaching those who are disabled to play musical instruments. *$7.75*

29 **In-Definite Arts Society**
8038 Fairmount Drive SE
Calgary, AB T2H0Y
403-253-3174
Fax: 403-255-2234
www.indefinitearts.com

Darlene Murphy, Executive Director
Dijana Andric, Client Services Manager
Peter Kelsch, Accountant
Bernice Webb, Facility Coordinator

Promotes opportunities for people with developmental disabilities to express themselves and to grow and develop through their involvement in art.

30 **Infinity Dance Theater**
220 W 93rd St
New York, NY 10025
212-877-3490
info@infinitydance.com
infinitydance.com

Kitty Lunn, RDE, Founder/Artistic Director
Michael A. Fitch, Executive Director

Infinity Dance Theater is a non-traditional dance company committed to expanding the boundaries of dance by featuring dancers with and without disabilities. The company aims to inspire people with and without disabilities, encourage their artistic and other professional aspirations, and empower them through the organization's educational and performance programs.

31 **Instrumental Music for Dyslexics: A Teaching Handbook**
Wiley & Sons
111 River Street
Hoboken, NJ 07030-5774
201-748-6000
Fax: 201-748-6088
info@wiley.com
www.wiley.com

Sheila Oglethorpe, Author
Stephen M. Smith, President and CEO
Ellis E. Cousens, Executive Vice President, Chief Operations Officer
MJ O'Leary, Senior Vice President, Human Resources

Describes dyslexia in layman's terms and explains how the various problems that a dyslexic may have can affect all aspects of learning to play a musical instrument. It alerts the music teacher with a problem pupil to the possibilities of that pupil having some form of dyslexia. It offers suggestions as to how to teach dyslexics, with particular reference to piano teaching, and it suggests ways in which the music teacher may contribute to the welfare of a dyslexic pupil. *$34.95*

200 pages

ISBN 1-861562-91-8

32 **Interact Center for the Visual and Performing Arts**

Interact Center
1860 Minnehaha Ave W
St. Paul, MN 55401
651-209-3575
Fax: 651-209-3579
info@interactcenter.com
interactcenter.com

Jeanne Calvit, Artistic & Executive Director
Shannon Forney, Managing Director
Beth Bowman, Director, Advancement

Creates art in a spirit of radical inclusion; Inspires artists and audiences to explore the full spectrum of human potential; Transforms lives by expanding ideas of what is possible.

33 **Kaleidoscope: Exploring the Experience of Disability through Literature & the Fine Arts**

United Disability Services
701 South Main St
Akron, OH 44311-1019
330-762-9755
Fax: 330-762-0912
kaleidoscope@udsakron.org
www.udsakron.org/services/kaleidoscope

Howard Taylor, President & CEO
Lisa Armstrong, Director of Community Relations & Managing Editor
Gail Willmott, Editor in Chief
Shelley Morris, Chief Financial Officer

Kaleidoscope is a magazine published by United Disability Services. Kaleidoscope challenges and transcends stereotypical, patronizing and sentimental attitudes about disability, looking at the experience of actually living with a disability from a more personal/individual perspective rather than a clinical, sociological or rehabilitative point of view. Included are a variety of articles, fiction, art and poetry relating to issues of disability, literature and the fine arts. *$10.00*

64 pages BiAnnually

34 **Keshet Dance and Center for the Arts**

4121 Cutler Ave NE
Albuquerque, NM 87110
505-224-9808
info@keshetarts.org
keshetarts.org

Shira Greenberg, Artistic Director
Adrian Moore Trask, Director of Business Advancement
Emily Dunkin, Events Director
Carolyn Tobias, Communications Director

Keshet offers youth and adult classes and workshops for individuals with varying levels of physical disabilities and dance experience. Within the Adaptive Dance programming, Keshet pairs dancers with disabilities with able-bodied dancers, which often include siblings, parents, and peers, to create professional-quality dance works.

35 **Learning Disabilities Sourcebook, 3rd Ed.**

Omnigraphics
615 Griswold Street
Suite 520
Detroit, MI 48226
610-461-3548
800-234-1340
Fax: 800-875-1340
contact@omnigraphics.com
www.omnigraphics.com

Peter Ruffner, Co-Founder
Fred Ruffner, Co-Founder

Learning Disabilities Sourcebook, Third Edition provides updated information about specific learning disabilities and other conditions that make learning difficult. These include dyscalculia, dysgraphia, dyslexia, auditory and visual processing, communication disorders, autism spectrum disorders, attention deficit and hyperactivity disorder, hearing and visual impairments, and brain injury. *$84.00*

600 pages Hard cover

ISBN 0-780810-39-6

36 **Manual of Sequential Art Activities for Classified Children and Adolescents**

Charles C. Thomas
2600 S First St
Springfield, IL 62704-4730
217-789-8980
800-258-8980
Fax: 217-789-9130
books@ccthomas.com
www.ccthomas.com

Rocco A L Fugaro, Author

Offers information to the special education professional on art therapy and management. *$41.95*

246 pages Softcover

ISBN 0-39805 -85-6

37 **Mozart Effect: Tapping the Power of Music to Heal the Body, Strengthen the Mind**

Harper Collins Publishers
10 E 53rd St
New York, NY 10022-5244
212-207-7000
www.harpercollins.com

Don Campbell, Author
Brian Murray, President and CEO
Michael Morrison, President and Publisher, U.S. General Books and Canada
Susan Katz, President and Publisher, HarperCollins Children's Books

Offers dramatic accounts of how doctors, shamans, musicians, and others use music to deal with everything from anxiety, cancer, and chronic pain, to dyslexia and mental illness. *$14.95*

352 pages

ISBN 0-060937-20-3

38 **Music Therapy**

Future Horizons, Inc.
721 West Abram St
Arlington, TX 76013-6995
817-277-0727
800-489-0727
Fax: 817-277-2270
www.fhautism.com

Betsey King Brunk, Author
R. Wayne Gilpin, President
Jennifer Gilpin, VP, Foreign Translations
Kelly Gilpin, Editorial Dir.

Music therapy is the use of music to address non-musical goals. Parents and professionals are finding that music can break down barriers for children with autism in areas such as cognition, socialization, and communication. *$19.95*

123 pages

ISBN 1-885477-53-8

39 **Music Therapy and Leisure for Persons with Disabilities**

Sagamore Publishing
1807 N Federal Drive
Urbana, IL 61801
217-359-5940
800-327-5557
Fax: 217-359-5975
books@sagamorepub.com
www.sagamorepub.com

Alicia L. Barksdale, Author
Joseph J. Bannon, Sr., Ph.D., Publisher & CEO
Peter L. Bannon, MBA, President
William Anderson, M.S., Director of Sales and Marketing

Explores the use of musical therapy in order to enhance the development of independent leisure skills with a variety of special populations. Suggestions are provided for alternative avenues through musical experiences enabling individuals to achieve their greatest potential for independence and a high quality of life. *$19.95*

ISBN 1-571675-11-6

40 **Music Therapy for the Developmentally Disabled**
Sage Publications
2455 Teller Road
Thousand Oaks, CA 91320
805-499-9774
800-818-7243
Fax: 800-583-2665
info@sagepub.com
www.sagepub.com

S. Venkatesan, Author

Included are practical guidelines, case samples and step-by-step instructions that enable a music therapist to bring about dramatic improvements in developmentally disabled adults and children. *$40.00*

269 pages Hardcover
ISBN 0-890791-90-2

41 **Music Therapy in Dementia Care**
Jessica Kingsley Publishers
400 Market Street
Suite 400
Philadelphia, PA 19106-4738
215-922-1161
866-416-1078
Fax: 215-922-1474
hello.usa@jkp.com
www.jkp.com

David Aldridge, Editor
Jessica Kingsley, Chairman, Managing Director
Jemima Kingsley, Director
Octavia Kingsley, Production Director

A comprehensive look at music therapy as a means of improving memory, health, and identity in those suffering from dementia, particularly Alzheimer's. For music therapists and those involved in psychogeriatry. *$29.95*

256 pages
ISBN 1-853027-76-6

42 **Music Therapy, Sensory Integration and the Autistic Child**
Jessica Kingsley Publishers
400 Market Street
Suite 400
Philadelphia, PA 19106-4738
215-922-1161
866-416-1078
Fax: 215-922-1474
hello.usa@jkp.com
www.jkp.com

Dorita S. Berger, Author
Jessica Kingsley, Chairman, Managing Director
Jemima Kingsley, Director
Octavia Kingsley, Production Director

Examines the human physiologic function, the brain, information processing, functional adaption, and how that might be affected by music interventions in persons with sensory integration difficulties. *$23.95*

256 pages
ISBN 1-843107-00-7

43 **Music and Dyslexia: A Positive Approach**
Wiley & Sons
111 River Street
Hoboken, NJ 07030-5774
201-748-6000
Fax: 201-748-6088
info@wiley.com
www.wiley.com

John Westcombe, Editor
Stephen M. Smith, President and CEO
Ellis E. Cousens, Executive Vice President, Chief Operations Officer
MJ O'Leary, Senior VP, Human Resources

This book shows how some people who have Dyslexia can be gifted musicians. The main point this books makes is that Dyslexic musicians can succeed provided only that they are given sufficient encouragement and understanding. *$34.95*

200 pages
ISBN 1-861562-05-5

44 **Music for the Hearing Impaired**
MMB Music
9051 Watson Road
Ste 161
St. Louis, MO 63126
314-531-9635
800-543-3771
Fax: 314-531-8384
info@mmbmusic.com
www.mmbmusic.com

Norm Goldberg, Founder & Chair

A resource manual and curriculum guide. It is the product of a four-year developmental music program, placing emphasis on the needs of those with severe and profound losses. *$29.95*

45 **Music: Physician for Times to Come**
Quest Books
P.O. Box 270
Wheaton, IL 60187-270
630-665-0130
800-669-9425
Fax: 630-665-8791
submissions@questbooks.net
www.questbooks.net

Don Campbell, Author

A resource guide for various types of music and their therapeutic outcome.

365 pages
ISBN 0-835607-88-7

46 **NIAD Art Center (Nurturing Independence through Artistic Development)**
551 23rd St.
Richmond, CA 94804-1626
510-620-0290
Fax: 510-620-0326
admin@niadart.org
www.niadart.org

Deborah Dyer, Executive Director

NIAD Art Center) promotes creativity, independence, dignity, and community integration for people with developmental and other disabilities. The visual arts studio supports artists with disabilities by providing materials, space to make art and facilitators to teach skills in drawing, painting, printmaking, ceramics, fiber arts and mixed media. The work that they make is exhibited in the Richmond gallery as well as in other galleries, on-line and other exhibition spaces.

47 **National Arts and Disability Center (NADC)**
Tarjan Center at UCLA
760 Westwood Plaza
Los Angeles, CA 90095-1759
310-825-5054
Fax: 310-794-1143
bstoffmacher@mednet.ucla.edu
www.semel.ucla.edu/nadc

Olivia Raynor, Director
Beth Stoffmacher, Center Coordinator

NADC has a database and website advocating for access to and participation in the arts by people with disabilities.

48 **National Association for Drama Therapy**
1450 Western Avenue
Suite 101
Albany, NY 12203
571-223-6440
888-416-7167
Fax: 518-463-8656
office@nadta.org
www.nadt.org

Nadya Trytan, MA, RDT/BCT, President
Jeremy Segall, MA, RDT, LCAT, Vice President
Jason Butler, RDT/BCT, LCAT, President-Elect
Whitney Sullivan, RDT, LCSW, Secretary

The National Association for Drama Therapy (NADT) was incorporated in 1979 to establish and uphold rigorous standards of professional competence for drama therapists. The NADT promotes drama therapy through information and advocacy.

49 **National Endowment for the Arts: Office for AccessAbility**
1100 Pennsylvania Ave NW
Washington, DC 20506-0001
202-682-5034
Fax: 202-682-5666
TTY: 202-682-5496
webmgr@arts.gov
www.arts.gov/
Jane Chu, Chairman
Beth Bienvenu, Accessibility Director
Wendy Clark, Director of Museums, Visual Arts, and Indemnity
Ayanna N. Hudson, Arts Education Director
The National Endowment for the Arts Office for AccessAbility is the advocacy-technical assistance arm of the Arts Endowment to make the arts accessible for people with disabilities, older adults, veterans, and people living in institutions.

50 **National Library Service for the Blind and Physically Handicapped (NLS)**
1291 Taylor St NW
Washington, DC 20011
202-707-5100
800-424-8567
Fax: 202-707-0712
nls@loc.gov
www.loc.gov/nls
Annual

51 **National Theatre Workshop of the Handicapped (NTWH)**
535 Greenwich Street
New York, NY 10013-1004
212-206-7789
Fax: 212-206-0200
www.ntwh.org
Jason Matthews, Director of Admissions
Rick Curry, President & CEO
John Spalla, General Manager
A non-profit organization that provides individuals within the disabled community with the communication skills and the artistic discipline necessary to pursue a life in professional theatre.

52 **National Theatre of the Deaf**
139 N Main St
West Hartford, CT 06107-1264
860-236-4193
Fax: 860-574-9107
Info@NTD.org
www.ntd.org
Betty Beekman, Executive Director
William C. Martin, Marketing/PR Director
George Ghista, Accountant
Kathy Strauss, Company Interpreter
The mission of the National Theatre of the Deaf is to produce theatrically challenging work of the highest quality, drawing from as wide a range of the world's literature as possible and to perform these original works in a style that links American Sign Language with the spoken word.

53 **New Music Therapist's Handbook, 2nd Ed. Berklee School of Music**
Berklee Press Publications
1140 Boylston Street
Boston, MA 02215
617-747-2146
866-237-5533
www.berkleepress.com
Suzanne B. Hanser, Author
Dr. Hanser's well-respected Music Therapist's Handbook has been revised and thoroughly updated to reflect the latest developments in the field of music therapy. *$29.95*
256 pages
ISBN 0-634006-45-2

54 **No Limits**
9801 Washington Blvd
2nd Fl
Culver City, CA 90232
310-280-0878
Fax: 310-280-0872
michelle@nolimitsfordeafchildren.org
nolimitsfordeafchildren.org
Michelle Christie, Founder & Executive Director
Juliana Scott, Director, Operations & Development
The mission of No Limits is to meet the auditory, speech and language needs of deaf children and enhance their confidence through the theatrical arts and individual therapy as well as provide family support and community awareness on the needs and talents of deaf children who are learning to speak.

55 **Non-Traditional Casting Project**
Ste 1600
1560 Broadway
New York, NY 10036-1518
212-730-4750
Fax: 212-730-4820
TTY: 212-730-4913
www.ntcp.org/
Nancy Kim, Manager
The Non-Traditional Casting Project (NTCP) is a not-for-profit advocacy organization whose purpose is to address and seek solutions to the problems of racism and exclusion in theatre, film and television. NTCP's principal concerns are those of artists of color, female artists, Deaf and hard of hearing artists, and artists with disabilities.

56 **Nuvisions For Disabled Artists, Inc.**
C/O Rose Marcus
1319 Magee Street
Philadelphia, PA 19111
Kaye E Schonbach, Executive Director
Nuvisions was established to enable physically challenged artists to pursue professional and semi-professional artistic opportunities. Nuvisions supports these artists by sponsoring accessible exhibitions, special projects and educational opportunities in Southeastern Pennsylvania and Southern New Jersey.

57 **Open Circle Theatre**
102-500 King Farm Blvd
Rockville, MD 20850
240-683-8934
info@opencircletheatre.org
opencircletheatre.org
Suzanne Richard, Artistic Director
Ian Armstrong, Executive Producer
Open Circle Theatre is a professional theatre dedicated to producing productions that integrate the considerable talents of artists with disabilities. OCT was formed by a group of people with and without disabilities, who possess professional theater experience, love of the theater, and a commitment to full access for all persons in every opportunity our community has to offer.

58 **Pied Piper: Musical Activities to Develop Basic Skills**
Jessica Kingsley Publishers
400 Market Street
Suite 400
Philadelphia, PA 19106-4738
215-922-1161
866-416-1078
Fax: 215-922-1474
hello.usa@jkp.com
www.jkp.com
John Bean, Author
Jessica Kingsley, Chairman, Managing Director
Jemima Kingsley, Director
Octavia Kingsley, Production Director
Describes 78 enjoyable music activities for groups of children or adults who may have learning difficulties. The emphasis is on using music, rather than learning songs or rhythms, so group members do not need any special skills to be able to participate. Full details are given about any equipment required for the games, as well as suggestions for variations or modifications. *$21.95*
96 pages
ISBN 1-853029-94-

59 **Project Onward Gallery**
Bridgeport Art Center
1200 W. 35th St
4th Fl
Chicago, IL 60609
773-940-2992
info@projectonward.org
projectonward.org

60 **Pure Vision Arts**
The Shield Institute
114 W 17th St
3rd Fl
New York, NY 10011
212-366-4263
Fax: 718-269-2059
progers@shield.org
purevisionarts.org

Pamala Rogers, Director
Pure Vision Arts mission is to provide people with autism and developmental disabilities opportunities for artistic expression and to build public awareness of their important creative contributions.

61 **Reaching the Child with Autism Through Art**
Future Horizons, Inc.
721 W Abram St
Arlington, TX 76013-6995
817-277-0727
800-489-0727
Fax: 817-277-2270
www.fhautism.com

Toni Flowers, Author
R. Wayne Gilpin, President
Jennifer Gilpin Yacio, Vice President and Editorial Director
David Reasor, CPA and Administrative Director
This book uncovers how art encourages communication, positive self-image, concept development, spatial relationships, fine-motor skills, and many more facets of health child development.
$19.95
130 pages

62 **Survivors Art Foundation**
PO Box 383
Westhampton, NY 11977
www.survivorsartfoundation.org
Michael Herships, Ph.D, Project Leader & Board President
Candyce Brokaw, Art Director
Candyce M. Brokaw, Executive Director
Margaret Ashe Magistro, Secretary/Treasurer
Dedicated to encourage healing through the arts, committed to empowering Trauma-Survivors with Effective Expressive Outlets via Internet Art Gallery, Outreach Programs, National Exhibitions, Publications and Development of Employment Skills.

63 **Teaching Asperger's Students Social Skills Through Acting**
Future Horizons, Inc.
721 W Abram St
Arlington, TX 76013-6995
817-277-0727
800-489-0727
Fax: 817-277-2270
www.fhautism.com

Amelia Davies, Author
R. Wayne Gilpin, President
Jennifer Gilpin Yacio, Vice President and Editorial Director
David Reasor, CPA and Administrative Director
This book provides the theories and activities needed for setting up acting classes that double as social skills groups for individuals with Asperger's or high-functioning autism. Using these skills, students will be able to develop social understanding through repetition and generalization. *$19.95*
211 pages

64 **Teaching Basic Guitar Skills to Special Learners**
MMB Music
9051 Watson Road
Ste 161
St. Louis, MO 63126
314-531-9635
800-543-3771
Fax: 314-531-8384
info@mmbmusic.com
www.mmbmusic.com

Norm Goldberg, Founder & Chair
The first-of-its-kind guitar book for use with persons who have difficulty learning to play via traditional methods. *$16.00*

65 **The Arts of Life**
2010 W. Carroll Ave
Chicago, IL 60612
312-829-2787
info@artsoflife.org
artsoflife.org

Denise Fisher, Co-Founder & Executive Director
Sara Bemer, Development Coordinator
An organization comprised of people with and without disabilities seeking to promote artistic expression, community building, self-respect, and independence.

66 **Theatre Without Limits**
P.O. Box 4002
Portland, ME 04101
207-607-4016
Fax: 207-761-4740
www.vsartsmaine.org

Kippy Rudy, Executive Director
VSA Maine is a 501 (c) (3) non-profit organization providing educational, arts, and cultural opportunities to children and adults with disabilities in Maine.

67 **VSA - The International Organization on Arts and Disability**
2700 F Street, NW
Washington, DC 20566
202-467-4600
800-444-1324
Fax: 202-429-0868
TTY: 202-737-0645
www.kennedy-center.org/education/vsa/

Ambassador J Kennedy Smith, Founder
David M. Rubenstein, Chair
Michael M. Kaiser, President
Christoph Eschenbach, Music Director, NSO and Kennedy Center
VSA offers a large selection of guides, publications, and other resources dealing with a wide variety of subject matter in education, arts, and disabilities.

68 **VSA arts**
2700 F Street, NW
Washington, DC 20566
202-467-4600
800-444-1324
Fax: 202-429-0868
TTY: 202-737-0645
www.kennedy-center.org/education/vsa/

Ambassador J Kennedy Smith, Founder
David M. Rubenstein, Chair
Michael M. Kaiser, President
Christoph Eschenbach, Music Director, NSO and Kennedy Center
VSA arts is an international, nonprofit organization founded in 1974 by Ambassador Jean Kennedy Smith whose mission is to create a society where all people with disabilities learn through, participate in, and enjoy the arts. Most states offer local programs, such as Arts in Action, that showcases the accomplishments of artists with disabilities and promotes increased access to the arts for people with disabilities.

69 **We Are PHAMALY**
Fanlight Productions
c/o Icarus Films
32 Court Street, 21st Floor
Brooklyn, NY 11201
718-488-8900
800-876-1710
Fax: 718-488-8642
info@fanlight.com
www.fanlight.com

Ben Achtenberg, Owner
Stands for Physically Handicapped Musical Actors League. This dynamic troupe doesn't cut any corners or make any compromises. The musicals they perform are chosen for their appeal to the audience, not because they are easy for the performers, who have a variety of sensory and mobility handicaps. *$199.00*
ISBN 1-572954-08-6

Assistive Devices

Automobile

70 **AUT Secondary Control**
Ace Mobility, LLC
9850 E 30th St.
Indianapolis, IN 46229
317-241-2444
877-223-5301
info@acemobility.us
www.acemobility.us

Doron Mishor, President & CEO
Zvika Amir, Vice President, Marketing & Sales
Controls up to 35 secondary functions.

71 **AUTone**
Ace Mobility, LLC
9850 E 30th St.
Indianapolis, IN 46229
317-241-2444
877-223-5301
info@acemobility.us
www.acemobility.us

Doron Mishor, President & CEO
Zvika Amir, Vice President, Marketing & Sales
Sound-activated signal device that allows drivers to momentarily activate a secondary function by pressing a button, which will play one to eight tones.

72 **Ability Center**
4797 Ruffner St.
San Diego, CA 92111
858-541-0552
833-919-2581
Fax: 858-541-1941
www.abilitycenter.com

Terry Barton, General Manager
Specializes in accessible vehicles and mobility products; the company has more than 100 employees in 14 locations across the western U.S.
1994

73 **Accelerator Shield**
Handicaps, Inc.
4335 S Santa Fe Dr.
Englewood, CO 80110-5417
303-781-2062
800-782-4335
info@handicapsinc.com
www.handicapsinc.com

74 **Accelerator/Brake Foot Control**
Ace Mobility, LLC
9850 E 30th St.
Indianapolis, IN 46229
317-241-2444
877-223-5301
info@acemobility.us
www.acemobility.us

Doron Mishor, President & CEO
Zvika Amir, Vice President, Marketing & Sales
Electronic foot pedals designed for drivers with adaptive driving needs. The pedals can be mounted at any height, spacing, and angle.

75 **Accelerator/Brake Hand Control**
Ace Mobility, LLC
9850 E 30th St.
Indianapolis, IN 46229
317-241-2444
877-223-5301
info@acemobility.us
www.acemobility.us

Doron Mishor, President & CEO
Zvika Amir, Vice President, Marketing & Sales
Hand control device that controls the vehicle's acceleration and brakes. The device can be modified to the needs of the client through the push and pull functions.

76 **Automobile Lifts for Scooters, Wheelchairs and Powerchairs**
Bruno Independent Living Aids, Inc.
1780 Executive Dr.
PO Box 84
Oconomowoc, WI 53066
262-567-4990
800-454-4355
Fax: 262-953-5501
www.bruno.com

Michael R. Bruno, II, President & CEO
Offers automobile lifts for scooters, wheelchairs and power chairs for nearly any car, van, truck or sport utility vehicle that can raise most scooters or wheelchairs under 200 pounds and power chairs up to 300 pounds.

77 **BraunAbility**
645 W Carmel Dr.
Carmel, IN 46032
800-488-0359
888-365-9417
questions@braunability.com
www.braunability.com

Staci Kroon, President & CEO
Manufactures wheelchair lifts and lowered floor minivans as well as many other mobility products.

78 **COM Hand Control**
Ace Mobility, LLC
9850 E 30th St.
Indianapolis, IN 46229
317-241-2444
877-223-5301
info@acemobility.us
www.acemobility.us

Doron Mishor, President & CEO
Zvika Amir, Vice President, Marketing & Sales
A hand control device that integrates Ace Mobility's Hand Control and JoySpinner devices.

79 **Car Cane**
Maxi Aids
42 Executive Blvd.
Farmingdale, NY 11735-4710
631-752-0521
800-522-6294
Fax: 631-752-0689
TTY: 631-752-0738
sales@maxiaids.com
www.maxiaids.com

Elliot Zaretsky, Founder, President & CEO
This device is designed for those who have trouble getting in and out of a car. The portable handle slides into any car door and can be easily stored in the door or glove box. *$15.95*

80 **DW Auto & Home Mobility**
1208 N Garth Ave.
Columbia, MO 65203-4056
573-449-3859
800-568-2271
contactus@dwauto.com
www.dwauto.com

Shawn Bright, Owner
DW manufactures paratransit conversions and personalized conversions for the physically challenged. Products include home elevators and lifts, scooters, and wheelchairs.
1967

81 **Digital Shifter**
Ace Mobility, LLC
9850 E 30th St.
Indianapolis, IN 46229
317-241-2444
877-223-5301
info@acemobility.us
www.acemobility.us

Doron Mishor, President & CEO
Zvika Amir, Vice President, Marketing & Sales
Enables drivers with limited arm strength and range of motion to use buttons to switch between the vehicle's gears. The switch console can be placed at any location to suit the needs of the driver.

82 **Drive Master Company**
37 Daniel Rd. W
Fairfield, NJ 07004-2521
973-808-9709
Fax: 973-808-9713
info@drivemastermobility.com
www.drivemastermobility.com
Peter B. Ruprecht, President
The Drive Master Company offers a full service mobility center, raised tops/doors, drop floors, custom driving equipment. Distributor of name brand devices and systems for full sized and mini vans.

83 **Driving Systems Inc.**
16139 Runnymede St.
Van Nuys, CA 91406-2913
818-782-6793
www.drivingsystems.com

84 **Dual Brake Control**
Kroepke Kontrols
104 Hawkins St.
Bronx, NY 10464
718-885-1100

85 **Entervan**
BraunAbility
645 W Carmel Dr.
Carmel, IN 46032
800-488-0359
888-365-9417
questions@braunability.com
www.braunability.com
Staci Kroon, President & CEO
The Entervan's accessible features include a power sliding door, ramp, and auto-kneel system, allowing for easier entry and exit for wheelchair and scooter users.

86 **Foot Steering Systems**
Drive Master Company
37 Daniel Rd. W
Fairfield, NJ 07004-2521
973-808-9709
Fax: 973-808-9713
info@drivemastermobility.com
www.drivemastermobility.com
Peter B. Ruprecht, President
Custom installed foot steering systems for drivers without the use of their arms.

87 **Four Way Switches**
Gresham Driving Aids
30800 S Wixom Rd.
Wixom, MI 48393-2418
248-624-1533
800-521-8930
Fax: 248-624-6358
www.greshamdrivingaids.com
David Ohrt, General Manager
Craig Wigginton, Sales Consultant
Joyce Martell, Customer Service
Multi-function switches for hand controls. Up to four functions can be added, including left turn signal, right turn signal, horn and dimmer.

88 **Freedom Motors USA, Inc.**
740 Watkins Rd.
Battle Creek, MI 49015
269-244-3497
866-581-7463
Fax: 269-580-8291
www.freedommotors.com
Sieto van Dillen, Chief Executive Officer
Freedom Motors offers van conversions with equipment that is easily installed and accessible for the physically challenged.

89 **Gas and Brake Pedal Guard**
Gresham Driving Aids
30800 S Wixom Rd.
Wixom, MI 48393-2418
248-624-1533
800-521-8930
Fax: 248-624-6358
www.greshamdrivingaids.com
David Ohrt, General Manager
Craig Wigginton, Sales Consultant
Joyce Martell, Customer Service
Designed for drivers who use hand controls, this device guards gas and brake pedals so they do not get accidentally pushed.

90 **Gear Shift Adaptor**
Handicaps, Inc.
4335 S Santa Fe Dr.
Englewood, CO 80110-5417
303-781-2062
800-782-4335
info@handicapsinc.com
www.handicapsinc.com

91 **Gear Shift Extension**
Gresham Driving Aids
30800 S Wixom Rd.
Wixom, MI 48393-2418
248-624-1533
800-521-8930
Fax: 248-624-6358
www.greshamdrivingaids.com
David Ohrt, General Manager
Craig Wigginton, Sales Consultant
Joyce Martell, Customer Service
Allows for easier gear shift operation.

92 **Gresham Driving Aids**
30800 S Wixom Rd.
Wixom, MI 48393-2418
248-624-1533
800-521-8930
Fax: 248-624-6358
www.greshamdrivingaids.com
David Ohrt, General Manager
Craig Wigginton, Sales Consultant
Joyce Martell, Customer Service
Gresham Driving Aids offers mobility solutions to physically challenged individuals including lowered floors, raised roofs and doors and high-quad driver control systems. Dealer for Braun, Ricon, Crow River and Bruno wheelchair lifts.

93 **Hand Brake Control Only**
Kroepke Kontrols
104 Hawkins St.
Bronx, NY 10464
718-885-2100

94 **Hand Control Multi-Function Buttons**
Gresham Driving Aids
30800 S Wixom Rd.
Wixom, MI 48393-2418
248-624-1533
800-521-8930
Fax: 248-624-6358
www.greshamdrivingaids.com
David Ohrt, General Manager
Craig Wigginton, Sales Consultant
Joyce Martell, Customer Service
Enables the driver to operate multiple vehicle controls using only one hand.

95 **Hand Gas & Brake Control**
Kroepke Kontrols
104 Hawkins St.
Bronx, NY 10464
718-885-2100

96 **Hand Parking Brake**
Kroepke Kontrols
104 Hawkins St.
Bronx, NY 10464
718-885-2100

97 **HandBrake**
Ace Mobility, LLC
9850 E 30th St.
Indianapolis, IN 46229
317-241-2444
877-223-5301
info@acemobility.us
www.acemobility.us
Doron Mishor, President & CEO
Zvika Amir, Vice President, Marketing & Sales
Electrical power parking brake aid device for drivers with limited arm or hand strength.

98 **Handicaps, Inc.**
4335 S Santa Fe Dr.
Englewood, CO 80110-5417
303-781-2062
800-782-4335
info@handicapsinc.com
www.handicapsinc.com

99 **Headlight Dimmer Switch**
Kroepke Kontrols
104 Hawkins St.
Bronx, NY 10464 718-885-2100

100 **Horizontal Steering Systems**
Drive Master Company
37 Daniel Rd. W
Fairfield, NJ 07004-2521 973-808-9709
Fax: 973-808-9713
info@drivemastermobility.com
www.drivemastermobility.com
Peter B. Ruprecht, President
The Horizontal Steering System is designed to meet the needs of drivers with spinal cord injuries and other individuals with limited arm strength and range of motion.

101 **Horn Control Switch**
Kroepke Kontrols
104 Hawkins St.
Bronx, NY 10464 718-885-2100

102 **JoySpinner**
Ace Mobility, LLC
9850 E 30th St.
Indianapolis, IN 46229 317-241-2444
877-223-5301
info@acemobility.us
www.acemobility.us
Doron Mishor, President & CEO
Zvika Amir, Vice President, Marketing & Sales
An ergonomic built-in remote-control joystick for secondary driving operations, including turn signals, beams, wipers, and hazard signals.

103 **Kersey Mobility**
6015 160th Ave. E
Sumner, WA 98390 253-863-4744
www.kerseymobility.com
Mike Kersey, Owner
Kersey Mobility is a wheelchair van dealer serving the Pacific Northwest. Also offers a line of mobility products and accessories, including lifts, wheelchair restraints, vehicle transfer seating, and adaptive driving aids.

104 **Kessler Institute for Rehabilitation**
1199 Pleasant Valley Way
West Orange, NJ 07052 973-731-3600
877-322-2580
Fax: 973-243-6819
www.kessler-rehab.com
Sue Kida, President
Driver evaluation training for the physically/mentally challenged. Offers state certified driving instructors. Door-to-door pickup at home, work or rehab centers are available.

105 **Left Foot Gas Pedal**
Kroepke Kontrols
104 Hawkins St.
Bronx, NY 10464 718-885-2100

106 **Left Foot Gas Pedal, The**
Handicaps, Inc.
4335 S Santa Fe Dr.
Englewood, CO 80110-5417 303-781-2062
800-782-4335
info@handicapsinc.com
www.handicapsinc.com

107 **MobilityWorks**
4199 Kinross Lakes Pkwy.
Suite 300
Richfield, OH 44286 877-275-4907
www.mobilityworks.com
Bryan Everett, Chief Executive Officer
Offers a selection of wheelchair accessible vehicles, mobility equipment, adaptive systems, and seating solutions.

108 **Multi-Function Spinner Knobs**
Gresham Driving Aids
30800 S Wixom Rd.
Wixom, MI 48393-2418 248-624-1533
800-521-8930
Fax: 248-624-6358
www.greshamdrivingaids.com
David Ohrt, General Manager
Craig Wigginton, Sales Consultant
Joyce Martell, Customer Service
Spinner knobs that can include up to six vehicle accessory controls.

109 **Park Brake Extension**
Handicaps, Inc.
4335 S Santa Fe Dr.
Englewood, CO 80110-5417 303-781-2062
800-782-4335
info@handicapsinc.com
www.handicapsinc.com

110 **Parking Brake Extension**
Gresham Driving Aids
30800 S Wixom Rd.
Wixom, MI 48393-2418 248-624-1533
800-521-8930
Fax: 248-624-6358
www.greshamdrivingaids.com
David Ohrt, General Manager
Craig Wigginton, Sales Consultant
Joyce Martell, Customer Service
Enables drivers to operate the foot parking/emergency brake by hand.

111 **Portable Hand Controls by Handicaps, Inc.**
Handicaps, Inc.
4335 S Santa Fe Dr.
Englewood, CO 80110-5417 303-781-2062
800-782-4335
info@handicapsinc.com
www.handicapsinc.com

112 **Power Transfer Seat Base (6-Way)**
Ricon
1135 Aviation Pl.
San Fernando, CA 91340 818-267-3000
800-322-2884
Fax: 800-962-1201
ricinsales@wabtec.com
www.riconcorp.com

113 **Push Pull Hand Controls**
Gresham Driving Aids
30800 S Wixom Rd.
Wixom, MI 48393-2418 248-624-1533
800-521-8930
Fax: 248-624-6358
www.greshamdrivingaids.com
David Ohrt, General Manager
Craig Wigginton, Sales Consultant
Joyce Martell, Customer Service
These controls are operated by pushing for brake and pulling back for acceleration.

114 **Push Rock Hand Controls**
Gresham Driving Aids
30800 S Wixom Rd.
Wixom, MI 48393-2418 248-624-1533
800-521-8930
Fax: 248-624-6358
www.greshamdrivingaids.com
David Ohrt, General Manager
Craig Wigginton, Sales Consultant
Joyce Martell, Customer Service
These controls allow the driver to apply the accelerator and brakes by hand.

115 **Rampvan**
BraunAbility
645 W Carmel Dr.
Carmel, IN 46032
800-488-0359
888-365-9417
questions@braunability.com
www.braunability.com
Staci Kroon, President & CEO
Fully accessible minivan conversions with automatic doors and ramps.

116 **Reduced Effort Steering**
Drive Master Company
37 Daniel Rd. W
Fairfield, NJ 07004-2521
973-808-9709
Fax: 973-808-9713
info@drivemastermobility.com
www.drivemastermobility.com
Peter B. Ruprecht, President
Reduced effort steering modifications available for nearly all vehicles. Additional products are pedal extensions which are 1 inch to 4 inch clamp-on aluminum blocks and 6 inch to 12 inch adjustable fold-down pedals.

117 **Right Angle Hand Controls**
Gresham Driving Aids
30800 S Wixom Rd.
Wixom, MI 48393-2418
248-624-1533
800-521-8930
Fax: 248-624-6358
www.greshamdrivingaids.com
David Ohrt, General Manager
Craig Wigginton, Sales Consultant
Joyce Martell, Customer Service
These controls apply the gas and accelerator at a right angle to the brake.

118 **Right Hand Gas and Brake Control**
Gresham Driving Aids
30800 S Wixom Rd.
Wixom, MI 48393-2418
248-624-1533
800-521-8930
Fax: 248-624-6358
www.greshamdrivingaids.com
David Ohrt, General Manager
Craig Wigginton, Sales Consultant
Joyce Martell, Customer Service
Floor-mounted hand control that allows drivers to accelerate and brake using their right hand.

119 **SWAB Steering Wheel**
Ace Mobility, LLC
9850 E 30th St.
Indianapolis, IN 46229
317-241-2444
877-223-5301
info@acemobility.us
www.acemobility.us
Doron Mishor, President & CEO
Zvika Amir, Vice President, Marketing & Sales
The SWAB (Steering Wheel Accelerator-Brake) allows drivers to steer the vehicle and control gas and brake functions with low effort.

120 **Spider Network Systems**
Ace Mobility, LLC
9850 E 30th St.
Indianapolis, IN 46229
317-241-2444
877-223-5301
info@acemobility.us
www.acemobility.us
Doron Mishor, President & CEO
Zvika Amir, Vice President, Marketing & Sales
Modular control network system that allows drivers with disabilities to activate secondary driving functions, including gear-shift, hand-brake, signaling, lights, and more. Also available in touch screen format.

121 **Spinner Knobs**
Ace Mobility, LLC
9850 E 30th St.
Indianapolis, IN 46229
317-241-2444
877-223-5301
info@acemobility.us
www.acemobility.us
Doron Mishor, President & CEO
Zvika Amir, Vice President, Marketing & Sales
Knobs designed to maximize the comfort of drivers with disabilities who have difficulty turning the steering wheel.

122 **Steering Device**
Handicaps, Inc.
4335 S Santa Fe Dr.
Englewood, CO 80110-5417
303-781-2062
800-782-4335
info@handicapsinc.com
www.handicapsinc.com

123 **Steering Wheel Devices**
Drive Master Company
37 Daniel Rd. W
Fairfield, NJ 07004-2521
973-808-9709
Fax: 973-808-9713
info@drivemastermobility.com
www.drivemastermobility.com
Peter B. Ruprecht, President
Steering devices for disabled drivers, including steering knobs, steering cuffs, amputee rings, tri-pins, and grips.

124 **Super Grade IV Hand Controls**
Handicaps, Inc.
4335 S Santa Fe Dr.
Englewood, CO 80110-5417
303-781-2062
800-782-4335
info@handicapsinc.com
www.handicapsinc.com

125 **TapGear**
Ace Mobility, LLC
9850 E 30th St.
Indianapolis, IN 46229
317-241-2444
877-223-5301
info@acemobility.us
www.acemobility.us
Doron Mishor, President & CEO
Zvika Amir, Vice President, Marketing & Sales
Electronic device that allows the driver to control gear positions.

126 **Tim's Trim**
25 Bermar Park
Rochester, NY 14624-1542
585-429-6270
888-468-6784
info@timstrim.com
www.timstrim.com
Tim Miller, Owner
Offers vehicle modifications, drop floors, raised tops/doors, driving equipment, touch pads and lifts.

127 **Transportation Equipment for People with Disabilities**
Gresham Driving Aids
30800 S Wixom Rd.
Wixom, MI 48393-2418
248-624-1533
800-521-8930
Fax: 248-624-6358
www.greshamdrivingaids.com
David Ohrt, General Manager
Craig Wigginton, Sales Consultant
Joyce Martell, Customer Service
Wheelchair lifts and ramps, hand and foot controls, steering and braking modifications, complete van conversions, home modifications, wheelchairs and scooters and wheelchair accessible van rentals.

128 **Turn Signal Cross-Over**
Gresham Driving Aids
30800 S Wixom Rd.
Wixom, MI 48393-2418 248-624-1533
800-521-8930
Fax: 248-624-6358
www.greshamdrivingaids.com
David Ohrt, General Manager
Craig Wigginton, Sales Consultant
Joyce Martell, Customer Service
This device enables the driver to operate the turn signal lever using the right hand.

129 **United Access**
9389 Natural Bridge Rd.
St. Louis, MO 63134 877-578-1962
www.unitedaccess.com
John Beering, President
Various automobile control systems that use hand, foot and steering aids for the disabled, including complete vehicle modifications.

130 **Vantage Mobility International**
5202 S 28th Pl.
Phoenix, AZ 85040 855-864-8267
www.vantagemobility.com
Mark Shaughnessy, Chief Executive Officer
Manufacturer and distributor of accessible vehicles and mobility products.

131 **Vehicle Access Remote Control**
Ace Mobility, LLC
9850 E 30th St.
Indianapolis, IN 46229 317-241-2444
877-223-5301
info@acemobility.us
www.acemobility.us
Doron Mishor, President & CEO
Zvika Amir, Vice President, Marketing & Sales
Universal remote control that opens and closes vehicle doors, raises and lowers hoist and chair elevators, and includes full lift control.

132 **Wheelers Accessible Van Rentals**
6614 W Sweetwater Ave.
Glendale, AZ 85304 623-776-8830
800-456-1371
Fax: 623-776-8930
info@wheelersvanrentals.com
www.wheelersvanrentals.com

Bath

133 **Adjustable Bath Seat**
AliMed, Inc.
297 High Street
Dedham, MA 02026-2852 781-329-2900
800-225-2610
Fax: 781-329-8392
customerservice@alimed.com
www.alimed.com
Julian Cherubini, President
Bath seat that fits easily in any size tub. Easily adjustable to any height for easier maneuverability. *$44.00*

134 **Adjustable Raised Toilet Seat & Guard**
Invacare
1 Invacare Way
Elyria, OH 44035-4190 440-329-6000
800-333-6900
Fax: 877-619-7996
www.invacare.com
Matthew E. Monaghan, Chair, President & CEO
Darcie Karol, Senior Vice President Human Resources
Kathleen P. Leneghan, Senior Vice President & CFO
Anthony C. LePlaca, Senior Vice President, General Counsel & Secretary
The seat features an exclusive pivot locking system so it won't slip or tip and the adjustable guard rail fits all toilets.

135 **ArjoHuntleigh**
ArjoHuntleigh
2349 W Lake St.
Suite 250
Addison, IL 60101 630-785-4490
800-323-1245
Fax: 888-389-2756
us.cc@arjohuntleigh.com
www.arjohuntleigh.us
Joacim Lindoff, CEO and President
Jonas Lindqvist, CFO
ARJO offers a complete line of patient bathing, showering and lift/transport systems, bariatric solutions, and accompanying skin care products for long-term and acute care facilities.

136 **Bath Fixtures**
Fiat Products
41 Cairns Rd.
Mansfield, OH 44904 800-442-1902
www.fiatproducts.com

137 **Bath Products**
R82, Inc.
12801 E Independence Blvd.
P.O. Box 1739
Matthews, NC 28106 Fax: 704-882-0751
information@R82.com
www.r82.com
Kasper Lisby, Controller
Nanneke Dinklo, Marketing Director
Amy Wilson, Product Manager
Nancy Guzman, Product Specialist
Offers a wide range of products to meet the transportation, mobility, seating and bath aid needs for people of all ages. From car seats and standers for children with special needs to versatile wheelchairs that offer adults customized options and the freedom to go anywhere with confidence.

138 **Bath Shower & Commode Chair**
Clark Health Care Products
7830 Steubenville Pike
Oakdale, PA 15071-9226 724-695-2122
888-347-4537
Fax: 724-695-2922
info@clarkehealthcare.com
www.clarkehealthcare.com

139 **Bath and Shower Bench 3301B**
Mada Medical Products
625 Washington Ave.
Carlstadt, NJ 07072-2901 201-460-0454
800-526-6370
Fax: 201-460-3509
saragannon@madamedical.com
www.madamedical.com

140 **Bathroom Transfer Systems**
Inspired By Drive
11724 Willake St.
Santa Fe Springs, CA 90670-5032 800-454-6612
info@inspiredbydrive.com
www.inspiredbydrive.com
Matt Lawrence, Vice President & General Manager
Michael Gipson, Vice President of Sales
Brittany Commodore, Digital Media & Professional Relations Manager
Offers a complete line of bathroom transfer systems, bath lifts, reclining bath chairs, bath/shower/commode chairs, wrap-around bath supports, toilet supports, positioning commodes, premium air, foam and gel seat cushions, giant trainers and positioning restraint car seats that accommodate individuals from 20-130 pounds.

141 **Bathtub Safety Rail**
AliMed, Inc.
297 High Street
Dedham, MA 02026-2852 781-329-2900
800-225-2610
Fax: 781-329-8392
customerservice@alimed.com
www.alimed.com
Julian Cherubini, President

Made of stainless steel, this safety rail fits in any size bathtub and offers safety and independence at bathing time. *$55.00*

142 **Can-Do Products Catalog**
Independent Living Aids
137 Rano Rd.
Buffalo, NY 14207
716-332-2970
800-537-2118
855-746-7452
Fax: 855-937-3906
can-do@independentliving.com
www.independentliving.com

84 pages Quarterly

143 **Clarke Healthcare Products, Inc.**
7830 Steubenville Pike
Oakdale, PA 15071-9226
724-695-2122
888-347-4537
Fax: 724-695-2922
info@clarkehealthcare.com
www.clarkehealthcare.com

144 **Commode**
Maxi Aids
42 Executive Blvd.
Farmingdale, NY 11735-4710
631-752-0521
800-522-6294
Fax: 631-752-0689
TTY: 631-752-0738
sales@maxiaids.com
www.maxiaids.com

Elliot Zaretsky, Founder, President & CEO
Adjustable seat height for patient comfort. Easily assembled, aluminum frame.

145 **Deluxe Bath Bench with Adjustable Legs**
Maxi Aids
42 Executive Blvd.
Farmingdale, NY 11735-4710
631-752-0521
800-522-6294
Fax: 631-752-0689
TTY: 631-752-0738
sales@maxiaids.com
www.maxiaids.com

Elliot Zaretsky, Founder, President & CEO
Bath bench with back support and adjustable legs. *$49.95*

146 **Electric Leg Bag Emptier and Tub Slide Shower Chair**
RD Equipment, Inc.
230 Percival Dr.
West Barnstable, MA 02668-1244
508-362-7498
Fax: 508-362-1458
info@rdequipment.com
www.rdequipment.com

Richard Dagostino, Owner and Founder
Designed for independence, this small, lightweight, battery-operated valve attaches to the bottom of the leg bag. A simple flip of the switch empties the leg bag, allowing the user to take in unlimited amounts of fluids. Tub Slide Shower Chair is a complete bathroom care system. *$200.00*

147 **Freedom Bath**
ArjoHuntleigh
2349 W Lake St.
Suite 250
Addison, IL 60101
630-785-4490
800-323-1245
Fax: 888-389-2756
us.cc@arjohuntleigh.com

Joacim Lindoff, CEO and President
Jonas Lindqvist, CFO
Residents can relax on a semi-reclining seat and enjoy the soothing deluxe whirlpool system. Freedom Bath offers a revolutionary solution with its unique Roll-Door. Includes head cushion and safety belt.

148 **Long Handled Bath Sponges**
Therapro, Inc.
225 Arlington St
Framingham, MA 01702-8723
508-872-9494
800-257-5376
Fax: 508-268-6624
info@therapro.com
www.therapro.com

Karen Conrad Weihrauch, President & Owner
Plastic-handled, 18-inch bath sponge. Handle may be heated and bent for easy reach. *$2.50*

149 **Modular Wall Grab Bars**
Invacare
1 Invacare Way
Elyria, OH 44035-4190
440-329-6000
800-333-6900
Fax: 877-619-7996
www.invacare.com

Matthew E. Monaghan, Chair, President & CEO
Darcie Karol, Senior Vice President Human Resources
Kathleen P. Leneghan, Senior Vice President & CFO
Anthony C. LaPlaca, Senior Vice President, General Counsel & Secretary
Engineered for strength and beauty, these bars can be assembled in various combinations to fit any bath or shower.

150 **P.T. Rail**
Maxi Aids
42 Executive Blvd.
Farmingdale, NY 11735-4710
631-752-0521
800-522-6294
Fax: 631-752-0689
TTY: 631-752-0738
sales@maxiaids.com
www.maxiaids.com

Elliot Zaretsky, Founder, President & CEO
Wall-mounted support rail for safer transfer to and from the toilet. Left side and right side rails available.

151 **Portable Shampoo Bowl**
JK Designs
4004 NE 4th St
Suite 107-456
Renton, WA 98059
206-999-8226
info@portableshampoobowl.com
www.portableshampoobowl.com

152 **Prelude**
ArjoHuntleigh
2349 West Lake Street
Suite 250
Addison, IL 60101
630-785-4490
800-323-1245
Fax: 888-389-2756
usa.info@ArjoHuntleigh.com

Joacim Lindoff, CEO and President
Jonas Lindqvist, CFO
Prelude shower cabinet allows patients to be showered in comfort and privacy, at the same time as protecting staff from excessive splashing.

153 **SLIDER Bathing System**
Assistive Technology
21279 Protecta Dr
Elkhart, IN 46516-9539
574-522-7201
800-478-2363
Fax: 574-293-0202

154 **Shower Bathtub Mat**
Maxi Aids
42 Executive Blvd.
Farmingdale, NY 11735-4710
631-752-0521
800-522-6294
Fax: 631-752-0689
TTY: 631-752-0738
sales@maxiaids.com
www.maxiaids.com

Elliot Zaretsky, Founder, President & CEO
Tub mat provides security against falls in the bath and shower. *$22.95*

155 **Shower and Commode Chair**
Maxi Aids
42 Executive Blvd.
Farmingdale, NY 11735-4710
631-752-0521
800-522-6294
Fax: 631-752-0689
TTY: 631-752-0738
sales@maxiaids.com
www.maxiaids.com

Elliot Zaretsky, Founder, President & CEO
Comes with removable commode bucket and cover, non-skid swivel casters, padded open-front seat, and plastic armrests. Weight limit is 300 lbs. *$169.95*

156 **Suregrip Bathtub Rail**
Invacare
1 Invacare Way
Elyria, OH 44035-4190
440-329-6000
800-333-6900
Fax: 877-619-7996
www.invacare.com

Matthew E. Monaghan, Chair, President & CEO
Darcie Karol, Senior Vice President Human Resources
Kathleen P. Leneghan, Senior Vice President & CFO
Anthony C. LaPlaca, Senior Vice President, General Counsel & Secretary
Compact and versatile, the bars have a soft-touch, contoured, white vinyl gripping area for added safety.

157 **Talking Bathroom Scale**
Independent Living Aids
137 Rano Rd
Buffalo, NY 14207
716-332-2970
800-537-2118
855-746-7452
Fax: 855-937-3906
can-do@independentliving.com
www.independentliving.com

Irwin Schneidmill, President
Michael Gutierrez, Director of Operations
Pamela Strauss, Director of Marketing
Ursula Izurieta, Director of Merchandising
Speaks in a clear voice. Automatically calibrates when stepped on and turns off once weight is announced. Maximum weight of 440lbs. *$59.95*

158 **Terry-Wash Mitt: Medium Size**
Therapro, Inc.
225 Arlington St
Framingham, MA 01702-8723
508-872-9494
800-257-5376
Fax: 508-875-2062
info@therapro.com
www.therapro.com

Karen Conrad Weihrauch, President & Owner
Includes a thumb socket and a palm pocket to hold a bar of soap. *$8.00*

159 **Transfer Tub Bench**
Arista Surgical Supply Company/AliMed
297 High Street
Dedham, MA 02026-2852
781-329-2900
800-225-2610
Fax: 781-329-8392
customerservice@alimed.com
www.alimed.com

Julian Cherubini, President
Curved padded backrest for comfortable support. Backrest also assists patient during lateral transfer. *$64.00*

160 **Tri-Grip Bathtub Rail**
Maxi Aids
42 Executive Blvd.
Farmingdale, NY 11735-4710
631-752-0521
800-522-6294
Fax: 631-752-0689
TTY: 631-752-0738
sales@maxiaids.com
www.maxiaids.com

Elliot Zaretsky, Founder, President & CEO
Two gripping heights for easy bathtub entrance or exit. *$54.95*

161 **Tub Slide Shower Chair**
RD Equipment, Inc.
230 Percival Dr.
West Barnstable, MA 02668-1244
508-362-7498
Fax: 508-362-1458
info@rdequipment.com
www.rdequipment.com

Richard Dagostino, Owner and Founder
The tub slide shower chair was designed for the elderly and disabled to make any bathroom (at home or when travelling) accessible with little or no renovations. *$2000.00*

Bed

162 **ASSISTECH Special Needs**
4801 W Calle Don Miguel
Tucson, AZ 85757-1400
631-752-0521
800-522-6294
Fax: 631-752-0689
TTY: 800-281-3555
www.assistech.com

Oliver Simoes, Owner
ASSISTECH is a division of Maxi-Aids that sells hearing, visual, and mobility aid devices.

163 **Bye-Bye Decubiti Air Mattress Overlay**
Rand-Scot, Inc.
209 Christman Drive
Fort Collins, CO 80525
970-484-7967
800-467-7967
Fax: 970-484-3800
info@randscot.com
www.randscot.com

Joel Lerich, Co-Founder
Barbara Lerich, Co-Founder
Originally designed for hospital beds, the overlay converts any bed into an exceptionally therapeutic, flotation unit when used between the conventional mattress and pad. The complete overlay is comprised of five individually inflatable, 100 percent natural rubber, ventilated sections enclosed within separate pockets of a soft fleece cover. Conforms to any configuration of electric or manual beds. The overlay comes in a kit that includes overlay cover, overlay sections, air pump, and patch kit. *$1588.00*

164 **Dual Security Bed Rail**
Maxi Aids
42 Executive Blvd.
Farmingdale, NY 11735-4710
631-752-0521
800-522-6294
Fax: 631-752-0689
TTY: 631-752-0738
sales@maxiaids.com
www.maxiaids.com

Elliot Zaretsky, Founder, President & CEO
Bed safety rails for the injured or elderly to help getting in and out of bed, and to prevent falling out of bed. The rails are made of steel with a powder coat. *$150.00*

165 **Foam Decubitus Bed Pads**
Profex Medical Products
P.O. Box 140188
Memphis, TN 38114
800-325-0196
Fax: 901-454-9850
customercare@ProfexMed.com
www.profexmed.com

Robert Gates Watel, Founder
Convoluted foam provides extra back support and comfort for wheelchair users.

166 **Global Assistive Devices, Inc.**
5079 N Dixie Highway
Oakland Park, FL 33334
954-806-7796
www.GlobalAssistive.com

167 **Hard Manufacturing Company**
230 Grider Street
Buffalo, NY 14215
800-873-4273
www.hardmfg.com

168 **Hausmann Industries**
130 Union Street
Northvale, NJ 7647-2290
201-767-0255
888-428-7626
Fax: 201-767-1369
info@hausmann.com
hausmann.com

David Hausmann, CEO
George Batchelor, Director Sales & Marketing
Michelle Riley, Mail order Sales
Julie Skoda, Sales and Marketing Adminitrator

Wheelchair acessible exam tables, treatment tables and mat platforms. Hausmann Industries has been in the healthcare sector for 63-plus years.

169 **Home Bed Side Helper**
Maxi Aids
42 Executive Blvd.
Farmingdale, NY 11735-4710
631-752-0521
800-522-6294
Fax: 631-752-0689
TTY: 631-752-0738
sales@maxiaids.com
www.maxiaids.com

Elliot Zaretsky, Founder, President & CEO

The rail attaches to home bed frames and provides support for those who require assistance getting in and out of bed. *$149.95*

170 **SleepSafe Beds**
3629 Reed Creek Drive
Bassett, VA 24055
276-627-0088
866-852-2337
Fax: 276-627-0234
SleepSafeBed@SleepSafeBed.com
www.sleepsafebed.com

Gregg Weinschreider, President
Edward Hettig, Marketing
Rachel Markwood, Publicity/Patient Advocacy
Al Flora, Sales

Perfect for adult home or home care use. SleepSafe offers twin or full size bed frames in classic style. The beds offer an attractive alternative to a hospital bed. SleepSafe beds keeps the user safe during rest and electrically adjusts smoothly for user comfort and caregiver ease of use.

171 **Sonic Alert Bed Shaker**
ASSISTECH
4801 W Calle Don Miguel
Tucson, AZ 85757-1400
631-752-0521
800-522-6294
Fax: 631-752-0689
TTY: 800-281-3555
www.assistech.com

Oliver Simoes, Owner

A vibrator that is put under the pillow or between the mattress and box spring that helps to wake heavy sleepers or individuals who are hard of hearing and/or have hearing impairments. The Sonic Alert Bed Shaker plugs into the Sonic Boom Alarm Clock or remote receiver. *$44.70*

172 **iLuv SmartShaker 2**
ASSISTECH
4801 W Calle Don Miguel
Tucson, AZ 85757-1400
631-752-0521
800-522-6294
Fax: 631-752-0689
TTY: 800-281-3555
www.assistech.com

Oliver Simoes, Owner

The iLuv SmartShaker 2 is a smartphone controlled bed shaker for individuals with hearing loss. The alarm comes with three vibration settings and works with a variety of smartphones. *$29.99*

Communication

173 **Accent 1400**
Prentke Romich Company
1022 Heyl Road
Wooster, OH 44691
330-262-1984
800-262-1984
Fax: 330-263-4829
info@prentrom.com
www.prentrom.com

Dave Hershberger, President & CEO
Barry Romich, Co-Founder

A portable electronic communication device that uses Minspeak so that symbols are used to represent words, sentences, or phrases. Accent 1400 can be accessed by touching the screen or optical/head tracking. Other versions of the Accent are also available. *$7595.00*

174 **Access Control Systems: NHX Nurse Call System**
Aiphone Corporation
535 NJ-38
Suite 340
Cherry Hill, NJ 08002
425-455-0510
800-692-0200
Fax: 800-525-3372
www.aiphone.com

Yusuke Seguchi, President/CEO

AIPHONE manufactures audio and video intercom systems for home or business to help the physically disabled answer doors and communicate through physical barriers; also ADA-compliant emergency call intercom stations for use in public facilities and an Environmental Control System for persons with limited mobility. NHX Nurse Call System provides staff alert in nursing homes, assisted-living facilities, clinics, wards, and hospitals.

175 **Adaptek Systems**
14224 Plank Street
Fort Wayne, IN 46818
260-637-8660
Fax: 260-637-8597
info@adapteksystems.com
www.adapteksystems.com

176 **Amplified Handsets**
HARC Mercantile
5413 S Westnedge Ave.
Suite A
Portage, MI 49002
269-324-1615
800-445-9968
Fax: 269-324-2387
TTY: 269-324-1615
info@harc.com
www.harc.com

Michael Martinson, Owner

Amplified handsets are phones for individuals who are hard of hearing. The phones are louder than other headsets, and can also include extra loud ringers, larger press keypads, and designated speed dial buttons.

177 **Amplified Phones**
HARC Mercantile
5413 S Westnedge Ave.
Suite A
Portage, MI 49002
269-324-1615
800-445-9968
Fax: 269-324-2387
TTY: 269-324-1615
info@harc.com
www.harc.com

Michael Martinson, Owner

Amplified phones are phones for individuals who are hard of hearing. Amplified phones enhance and/or amplify sound, and can have a low frequency ringer, an indicator light, and lighted easy-to-read dial pads.

178 **Amplified Portable Phone**
HARC Mercantile
5413 S Westnedge Ave.
Suite A
Portage, MI 49002
269-324-1615
800-445-9968
Fax: 269-324-2387
TTY: 269-324-1615
info@harc.com
www.harc.com

Michael Martinson, Owner
Cordless phones with amplified or enhanced sound for individuals with hearing loss.

179 **Assistive Technology**
Tobii Dynavox
2100 Wharton Street
Suite 400
Pittsburgh, PA 15203
800-344-1778
Fax: 866-804-1267
www.tobii.com/

Henrik Eskilsson, President/CEO/Co-Founder
John Elvesjo, Deputy CEO/Co-Founder
Marten Skogo, Chief Science Officer/Co-Founder
Johan Wilsby, Chief Financial Officer
A premiere developer of innovative touch and eye tracking technology solutions for people with physical and learning disabilities. Breakthrough products enable people of all ages and abilities to live and learn independently. Supportive material for teachers, clinicians, and those with disabilities.

180 **Big Red Switch**
AbleNet, Inc.
2625 Patton Road
Roseville, MN 55113-1137
651-294-2200
800-322-0956
Fax: 651-294-2259
customerservice@ablenetinc.com
www.ablenetinc.com

Bill Sproull, Chair of the Board
Jennifer Thalhuber, President & CEO
William Mills, Board of Directors
Paul Sugden, CFO & Trustee
Five inches across the top and activates no matter where on its surface it is touched. It is made of shatterproof plastic and contains a cord storage compartment. The Big Red Switch provides auditory, visual, and tactile feedback. Also available in green, yellow, and blue. *$65.00*

181 **Closed Caption Decoder**
HARC Mercantile
5413 S Westnedge Ave.
Suite A
Portage, MI 49002
269-324-1615
800-445-9968
Fax: 269-324-2387
TTY: 269-324-1615
info@harc.com
www.harc.com

Michael Martinson, Owner
Provides closed captions for TV programs, with text displayed as white letters on a black background. *$50.00*

182 **Cornell Communications**
7915 North 81st Street
Milwaukee, WI 53223
414-351-4660
800-558-8957
Fax: 414-351-4657
www.cornell.com

183 **Harc Mercantile, Ltd.**
HARC Mercantile
5413 S Westnedge Ave.
Suite A
Portage, MI 49002
269-324-1615
800-445-9968
Fax: 269-324-2387
TTY: 269-324-1615
info@harc.com
www.harc.com

Michael Martinson, Owner
HARC sells assistive devices for the hard of hearing and deaf, such as amplified telephones, personal amplifiers, personal and large area fm systems, induction hearing loops, signaling systems for wake-up, smoke/fire door and telephone, and hearing aid batteries and supplies.

184 **InfoLoop Induction Receiver**
HARC Mercantile
5413 S Westnedge Ave.
Suite A
Portage, MI 49002
269-324-1615
800-445-9968
Fax: 269-324-2387
TTY: 269-324-1615
info@harc.com
www.harc.com

Michael Martinson, Owner
Sound induction receiver to be used with any loop system (a length of wire around the perimeter of a room and connected to an amplifier). *$99.00*

185 **Large Button Speaker Phone**
HARC Mercantile
5413 S Westnedge Ave.
Suite A
Portage, MI 49002
269-324-1615
800-445-9968
Fax: 269-324-2387
TTY: 269-324-1615
info@harc.com
www.harc.com

Michael Martinson, Owner
HARC Mercantile amplified phones have large, easy-to-read buttons for individuals who have visual impairments. Most phones also have a speakerphone option.

186 **Metropolitan Washington Ear**
12061 Tech Rd.
Silver Spring, MD 20904
301-681-6636
Fax: 301-625-1986
information@washear.org
www.washear.org

Paul W. Schroeder, Chairman
Neely Oplinger, Executive Director
Dr. Margaret R. Pfanstiehl, Founder
Multi-media reading service for the blind and visually impaired. Offering 24 hour audio radio reading, dial-in newspapers and web casting, as well as audio description at theaters, museums and films.

187 **Microloop III Basic**
HARC Mercantile
5413 S Westnedge Ave.
Suite A
Portage, MI 49002
269-324-1615
800-445-9968
Fax: 269-324-2387
TTY: 269-324-1615
info@harc.com
www.harc.com

Michael Martinson, Owner
Home induction loop amplifier for use with hearing aids equipped with T-Coil. Small and compact, the Microloop is also suitable for use in a vehicle. *$198.00*

188 **MyAlert Body Worn Multifunction Receiver**
HARC Mercantile
5413 S Westnedge Ave.
Suite A
Portage, MI 49002
269-324-1615
800-445-9968
Fax: 269-324-2387
TTY: 269-324-1615
info@harc.com
www.harc.com

Michael Martinson, Owner
Composed of a small wireless personal device that receives coded signals and a group of transmitters that send them. Transmitters can send alert signals for telephone, smartphone, door, and window. *$39.00*

189 **PLA240 Room Loop System**
HARC Mercantile
5413 S Westnedge Ave.
Suite A
Portage, MI 49002
269-324-1615
800-445-9968
Fax: 269-324-2387
TTY: 269-324-1615
info@harc.com
www.harc.com
Michael Martinson, Owner
Helps hearing aid users listen to TV or audio equipment via the "T" or "Loop" programs of their hearing aids.

190 **Personal FM Systems**
HARC Mercantile
5413 S Westnedge Ave.
Suite A
Portage, MI 49002
269-324-1615
800-445-9968
Fax: 269-324-2387
TTY: 269-324-1615
info@harc.com
www.harc.com
Michael Martinson, Owner
Wireless FM systems transmit sound via a radio carrier wave.

191 **Phone Ringers**
HARC Mercantile
5413 S Westnedge Ave.
Suite A
Portage, MI 49002
269-324-1615
800-445-9968
Fax: 269-324-2387
TTY: 269-324-1615
info@harc.com
www.harc.com
Michael Martinson, Owner
Uses loud ringers and/or bright flashers to signal phone rings and messages.

192 **Phone Strobe Flasher**
Independent Living Aids
137 Rano Road
Buffalo, NY 14207
516-937-1848
800-537-2118
855-746-7452
Fax: 855-937-3906
can-do@independentliving.com
www.independentliving.com

193 **Pocketalker Personal Amplifier**
HARC Mercantile
5413 S Westnedge Ave.
Suite A
Portage, MI 49002
269-324-1615
800-445-9968
Fax: 269-324-2387
TTY: 269-324-1615
info@harc.com
www.harc.com
Michael Martinson, Owner
Amplifies sounds and voices for better understanding.

194 **Prentke Romich Company**
1022 Heyl Road
Wooster, OH 44691
330-262-1984
800-262-1984
Fax: 330-263-4829
info@prentrom.com
www.prentrom.com
Dave Hershberger, President & CEO
Barry Romich, Co-Founder
The Prentke Romich Company is a full service company offering easy, yet powerful communication aids. The company believes in supporting customers before and after the sale by offering funding assistance, distance learning training, extended warranty, service assistance, and much more.

195 **Silent Call Communications**
5095 Williams Lake Rd.
Waterford, MI 48329
800-572-5227
TTY: 800-572-5227
customerservice@silentcall.com
www.silentcall.com
George J. Elwell, President
Diana Elwell, President
Lisa DeLeuil, Director of Sales & Marketing
Alerting devices such as paging systems and smoke detectors for deaf and deaf-blind people.

196 **Sonic Alert**
Harris Communications
15155 Technology Dr
Eden Prairie, MN 55344-2273
952-906-1180
800-825-6758
Fax: 952-906-1099
TTY: 800-825-9187
info@harriscomm.com
www.harriscomm.com
Robert Harris, Owner & President
Kevin Horsky, Business Director
Randall Moore, Manager
Offers visual alerting devices that provide safety and convenience by turning vital sound into flashing light: telephone ring signalers, doorbell signalers, baby cry signalers, and wake up alarms. Free catalog available.

197 **Speech Adjust-A-Tone Basic**
Maxi Aids
42 Executive Blvd.
Farmingdale, NY 11735-4710
631-752-0521
800-522-6294
Fax: 631-752-0689
TTY: 631-752-0738
sales@maxiaids.com
www.maxiaids.com
Elliot Zaretsky, Founder, President & CEO
Speech Adjust-A-Tone improves speech amplification for use with telephone, TV, radio, tape recorder, or computer sound card. *$155.00*

198 **Step-by-Step Communicator**
AbleNet, Inc.
2625 Patton Road
Roseville, MN 55113-1137
651-294-2200
800-322-0956
Fax: 651-294-2259
customerservice@ablenetinc.com
www.ablenetinc.com
Bill Sproull, Chair of the Board
Jennifer Thalhuber, President & CEO
William Mills, Board of Directors
Paul Sugden, CFO & Trustee
Allows individuals to record a series of messages for later communication. It has a 2 1/2 inches diameter switch surface and is 3 inches at its tallest point. The Step-by-Step Communicator includes 2 minutes of record time, and comes in yellow, green, blue, or red. *$165.00*

199 **TTYs: Telephone Device for the Deaf**
HARC Mercantile
5413 S Westnedge Ave.
Suite A
Portage, MI 49002
269-324-1615
800-445-9968
Fax: 269-324-2387
TTY: 269-324-1615
info@harc.com
www.harc.com
Michael Martinson, Owner
A telecommunications device for individuals who are deaf. The device is a teleprinter that creates text communication over a telephone line. *$239.00*

200 **TalkTrac Wearable Communicator**
AbleNet, Inc.
2625 Patton Road
Roseville, MN 55113-1137
651-294-2200
800-322-0956
Fax: 651-294-2259
customerservice@ablenetinc.com
www.ablenetinc.com

Bill Sproull, Chair of the Board
Jennifer Thalhuber, President & CEO
William Mills, Board of Directors
Paul Sugden, CFO & Trustee

The TalkTrac Wearable Communicator is a personal, portable communication aid that is wearable on the wrist. TalkTrac features simple to use, 80 seconds of recording time, as well as four message locations, rechargeable battery, water resistant coating, and adjustable band. *$145.00*

201 **Talking Calculators**
ASSISTECH
4801 W Calle Don Miguel
Tucson, AZ 85757-1400
631-752-0521
800-522-6294
Fax: 631-752-0689
TTY: 800-281-3555
www.assistech.com

Oliver Simoes, Owner

Calculators for blind and low vision users that announce numbers and calculation results.

202 **Talking Watches**
Maxi Aids
42 Executive Blvd.
Farmingdale, NY 11735-4710
631-752-0521
800-522-6294
Fax: 631-752-0689
TTY: 631-752-0738
sales@maxiaids.com
www.maxiaids.com

Elliot Zaretsky, Founder, President & CEO

Digital display watches that announce the time at the touch of a button.

203 **Unity Language System**
Prentke Romich Company
1022 Heyl Road
Wooster, OH 44691
330-262-1984
800-262-1984
Fax: 330-263-4829
info@prentrom.com
www.prentrom.com

Dave Hershberger, President & CEO
Barry Romich, Co-Founder

A Minspeak application program designed for adolescent and adult individuals with developmental disabilities and associated learning difficulties. The software is used with Prentke Romich Company augmentative communication devices.

204 **Voice Amplified Handsets**
HARC Mercantile
5413 S Westnedge Ave.
Suite A
Portage, MI 49002
269-324-1615
800-445-9968
Fax: 269-324-2387
TTY: 269-324-1615
info@harc.com
www.harc.com

Michael Martinson, Owner

Designed for the person who has a weak speaking voice. Control increases the level of the user's voice and can increase as much as 30%.

Chairs

205 **Adjustable Chair**
Bailey Manufacturing Company
118 Lee Drive
P.O. Box 130
Lodi, OH 44254-0130
330-948-1080
800-321-8372
Fax: 330-948-4439
baileymfg@baileymfg.com
www.baileymfg.com

Larry Strimple, President
Judie Butler, Dealer Contact

The seat and footboard of this versatile chair can be adjusted to accommodate children of various sizes. A classroom-suitable variation of this model is also available.

206 **Adjustable Clear Acrylic Tray**
Bailey Manufacturing Company
118 Lee Drive
P.O. Box 130
Lodi, OH 44254-0130
330-948-1080
800-321-8372
Fax: 330-948-4439
baileymfg@baileymfg.com
www.baileymfg.com

Larry Strimple, President
Judie Butler, Dealer Contact

An clear tray that adjusts for heigh and depth, and is equipped with a spill rim for easy to clean edges.

207 **Adjustable Rigid Chair**
Kuschall USA/Invacare
1 Invacare Way
Elyria, OH 44035-4190
800-333-6900
Fax: 877-619-7996
www.kuschallusa.com/

Matthew E. Monaghan, President/CEO of Invacare

The Champion 3000 is a fully adjustable rigid frame chair weighing only 21 pounds with a new clamping system that adjusts seat height and angle without tools.

208 **Adjustable Tee Stool**
Bailey Manufacturing Company
118 Lee Drive
P.O. Box 130
Lodi, OH 44254-0130
330-948-1080
800-321-8372
Fax: 330-948-4439
baileymfg@baileymfg.com
www.baileymfg.com

Larry Strimple, President
Judie Butler, Dealer Contact

May be used to encourage balance as well as develop integrative and perceptual motor skills. The stool has five adjustable heigt ranges.

209 **BackSaver**
BackSaver Products Company
3000 East Imperial Highway
Lynwood, CA 90262
310-661-3044
800-251-2225
www.backsaver.com

210 **Carendo**
Arjo Inc
2349 West Lake Street
Suite 250
Addison, IL 60101
630-785-4490
800-323-1245
Fax: 630-576-5020
usa.info@ArjoHuntleigh.com
www.arjo.com

Joacim Lindoff, President & CEO
Jonas Lindqvist, CFO
Marion Gullstrand, Executive Vice President, Human Resources & CSR
Katarzyna Bobrow, Executive Vice President, Quality & Regulatory Compliance

The Carendo hygiene chair has been designed for caregivers. The chair is battery powered, and allows for easy access to most parts of the body for sensitive hygiene tasks. Its innovative, ergonomic design makes for better grooming and hygiene routines.

211 **Century Bath System**
Arjo Inc
2349 West Lake Street
Suite 250
Addison, IL 60101
630-785-4490
800-323-1245
Fax: 630-576-5020
usa.info@ArjoHuntleigh.com
www.arjo.com

Joacim Lindoff, President & CEO
Jonas Lindqvist, CFO
Marion Gullstrand, Executive Vice President, Human Resources & CSR
Katarzyna Bobrow, Executive Vice President, Quality & Regulatory Compliance

This bathing system is used with a hygiene lift chair and has a built-in cleaning/disinfectant injection system with adjustable flowmeter. The incorporation of an automatic hot water alarm/shut-off system, and digital temperature monitors, helps to assure resident safety and comfort.

212 **Convert-Able Table**
REAL Design
6332 NY-167
Dolgeville, NY 13329
315-429-3071
800-696-7041
rdesign@twcny.rr.com
www.realdesigninc.com

Sam Camardello, Owner
Kris Wohnsen, Vice President

This table has push button height adjustment and interchangeable tops so it can become a desk, art easel, or a sensory stimulation bowl.

213 **Drive DeVilbiss Healthcare**
99 Seaview Boulevard
Port Washington, NY 11050
877-224-0946
Fax: 516-998-4601
customerSupport@drivemedical.com
www.drivemedical.com

Robert J. Gilligan, CEO
Jeffrey Schwartz, Executive Vice President, Commerical Operations
Amy O'Keefe, Executive Vice President, CFO
Nora Coleman, Executive Vice President, General Counsel

Supplies durable medical equipment, including those dealing with mobility, wheelchairs, beds and sleeping surfaces, personal care products, and electrotherapy devices. Company's goals are to promote independence and improve people's quality of life.

214 **Evac + Chair Emergency Evacuation Chair**
Evac + Chair North America LLC
3000 Marcus Ave.
Suite 3E6
Lake Success, NY 11042-1012
516-502-4240
Fax: 516-327-8220
sales@evac-chair.com
www.evac-chair.com

Richard Perl, VP of Business Development
David Egen, Founder

Gravity driven evaluation chair allows one nondisabled person to smoothly glide a seated passenger down fire stairs and across landings to exit on a combination of wheels and track belts. Pivots in own width for tight landing turns. Features include ability to compactly store on wall mount, a maximum capacity of 400 pounds, and braking features. No installation needed and works on all fire exit stairs.

215 **Golden Technologies**
401 Bridge Sreet
Old Forge, PA 18518
570-451-7477
800-624-6374
Fax: 800-628-5165
www.goldentech.com

Richard Golden, CEO
Robert Golden, Chair
Fred Kiwak, Vice President, Research & Development

The largest facility in the world dedicated to the manufacture of lift chairs, scooters, and power chairs.

216 **High-Low Chair**
REAL Design
6332 NY-167
Dolgeville, NY 13329
315-429-3071
800-696-7041
rdesign@twcny.rr.com
www.realdesigninc.com/

Sam Camardello, President
Kris Wohnsen, Vice President

A high chair and mobile floor sitter in one. The High-Low Chair comes with colorful upholstered wipe clean seat and height adjustable tray. The chair has a single lever adjustment to change the seat height. Lateral and head supports are available as options. *$1720.00*

217 **Ladybug Corner Chair**
REAL Design
6332 NY-167
Dolgeville, NY 13329
315-429-3071
800-696-7041
rdesign@twcny.rr.com
www.realdesigninc.com/

Sam Camardello, President
Kris Wohnsen, Vice President

For children 0-3 years. This chair is adjustable for long leg or conventional sitting positions. The back can also be removed for independent sitting. The Ladybug Chair is upholstered in padded vinyl, and includes an H-strap harness, hip belt, abductor, and removable tray.

218 **Lumex Recliner**
Graham-Field Health Products
2935 Northeast Parkway
Atlanta, GA 30360-2808
770-368-4700
Fax: 770-368-4932
cs@grahamfield.com
www.grahamfield.com

Kenneth Spett, President & CEO
Cherie Antoniazzi, Senior Vice President, Quality, Regulatory & Risk Management
Marc Bernstein, Senior Vice President, Consumer Sales
Lawrence De La Haba, Senior Vice President, Business Development

A recliner designed to improve the mobility of residents in extended care facilities. This chair combines therapeutic benefits of position change with attractive appearance.

219 **Prime Engineering**
Prime Engineering
4202 W Sierra Madre Ave.
Fresno, CA 93722
559-276-0991
800-827-8263
Fax: 800-800-3355
info@primeengineering.com
www.primeengineering.com

Bruce Boegel, CFO
Mary Boegel, President
Mark Allen, Vice President
Dawn Smith Cobb, Customer Service

Prime Engineering is a leading manufacturer of adult and pediatric standing devices and patient transfer equipment. Products include Superstand HLT, Granstand III MSS Standing System, Kidstand III MSS Standing System, Superstand Standing System, Symmetry Youth Standing Systen, UpRite Standing System, and the Symmetry Standing System.

220 **Rifton Equipment**
103 Woodcrest Drive
P.O. Box 260
Rifton, NY 12471-0260
845-658-7750
800-571-8198
Fax: 845-658-7751
sales@rifton.com
www.rifton.com

221 **Roll Chair**
Bailey Manufacturing Company
118 Lee Drive
P.O. Box 130
Lodi, OH 44254-0130
330-948-1080
800-321-8372
Fax: 330-948-4439
baileymfg@baileymfg.com
www.baileymfg.com

Larry Strimple, President
Judie Butler, Dealer Contact
A chair with a padded roll seat that helps maintain proper hip abduction and prevents scissoring of the legs.

222 **Safari Tilt**
Convaid
2830 California Street
Torrance, CA 90503
310-618-0111
888-266-8243
Fax: 310-618-2166
www.convaid.com

Ryan B. Williams, President
A semi-contour seat provides positioning with 5-45 degree tilt adjustment. One step design folds compactly into a lightweight chair.

223 **Spatial Tilt Custom Chair**
Redman Powerchair
1601 South Pantano Road
Suite 107
Tucson, AZ 85710
520-546-6002
800-727-6684
Fax: 520-546-5530
info@redmanpowerchair.com
www.redmanpowerchair.com

Don Redman, CEO
Paula Redman, CFO
Paula Jr. Redman, Vice Executive
Custom chair designed for comfort with a solid seat and back. Modifications available for seat depth, height, or width.

224 **Transfer Bench with Back**
Invacare
1 Invacare Way
Elyria, OH 44035-4190
440-329-6000
800-333-6900
Fax: 877-619-7996
www.invacare.com

Matthew E. Monaghan, Chair, President & CEO
Darcie Karol, Senior Vice President Human Resources
Kathleen P. Leneghan, Senior Vice President & CFO
Anthony C. LaPlaca, Senior Vice President, General Counsel & Secretary
A shower bench with back rest designed to help individuals get in and out of the bathtub. Features a textured seat with drain holes, built-in soap dish, and hand-held shower holder. *$268.84*

Cushions & Wedges

225 **Action Products**
954 Sweeney Dr.
Hagerstown, MD 21740
301-797-1414
800-228-7763
service@actionproducts.com
www.actionproducts.com

Mistie Witt, President
Janet Kaplan, Marketing Director
Wheelchair pads, mattress pads, positioning cushions, and insoles that aid in the prevention and cure of pressure sores by reducing pressure. All products are made of Akton viscoelastic polymer that does not leak, flow, or bottom out. Manufacturer of the Xact line of positioning cushions for patients with high risk of skin breakdown.

226 **Adjustable Wedge**
Bailey Manufacturing Company
118 Lee Drive
P.O. Box 130
Lodi, OH 44254-0130
330-948-1080
800-321-8372
Fax: 330-948-4439
baileymfg@baileymfg.com
www.baileymfg.com

Larry Strimple, President
Judie Butler, Dealer Contact
Orthopedically and neurologically disabled children can freely move arms and hands while lying on this adjustable wedge.

227 **Back-Huggar Pillow**
Bodyline Comfort Systems
3730 Kori Rd.
Jacksonville, FL 32257
904-262-4068
800-874-7715
info@bodyline.com
www.bodyline.com

Dr. John W. Fiore, Owner
Exclusive design makes almost any seat more comfortable by exerting soothing pressure against back muscles and discs. *$32.95*

228 **Bye-Bye Decubiti (BBD)**
Rand-Scot, Inc.
209 Christman Drive
Fort Collins, CO 80525
970-484-7967
800-467-7967
Fax: 970-484-3800
info@randscot.com
www.randscot.com

Joel Lerich, Co-Founder
Barbara Lerich, Co-Founder
The BBD therapeutic wheelchair cushions have been market-proven since 1951 — in the prevention and cure of pressure sores (decubiti). These natural rubber inflatable products have recently been expanded to include pediatric, sports, and double-valve models.

229 **Dynamic Systems, Inc.**
Dynamic Systems, Inc.
104 Morrow Branch Road
Leicester, NC 28748
828-683-3523
855-786-6283
Fax: 844-270-6478
dsi@sunmatecushions.com
www.sunmatecushions.com

Robin W. Yost, President/CEO
Melinda Garrett, Vice President/CFO
Andrew Biebinger, Plant Manager/COO
Susan Yost, Marketing Director
Dynamic Systems, Inc. manufactures high-performance, medical-grade, orthopedic cushion materials for applications where pressure relief, body support, and skin health are critical. Molding seat inserts.

230 **Enhancer Cushion**
ROHO Group
100 North Florida Avenue
Belleville, IL 62221-5429
618-277-9173
800-736-0925
Fax: 888-551-3449
tomb@therohogroup.com
www.therohogroup.com

Tom Borcherding, President
Bobby Graebe, CEO
Tim Richter, Vice President of Finance
Dave McCausland, Senior Vice President of Planning & Government Affairs
Uses AIR IN PLACE progressive positioning for enhanced midline channeling of the femurs, lateral stability, and tissue protection.

231 **Functional Forms**
Consumer Care Products
1446 Pilgrim Rd
Plymouth, WI 53073-4969
920-893-4614
Fax: 800-977-2256

Terry Grall, Owner

These blocks, wedges, rolls, cervical pillows, head and leg supports and barrel rolls in resilient high density foam covered with durable antibacterial, antistatic, flame resistant, nonabsorbent vinyl are used to attain individualized support for the most difficult positioning needs for children and adults. Unique sizes allow fitting for almost any person. Use during exercise, feeding, therapy, recreation and rest at home, school and health care facilities.

232 **Geo-Matt for High Risk Patients**
Span-America Medical Systems
70 Commerce Ctr
Greenville, SC 29615-5814
864-288-8877
800-888-6752
Fax: 864-288-8692
www.spanamerica.com

James D Ferguson, CEO

Provides a line of healthcare products concerned with pressure management and patient positioning, including therapeutic mattress systems, overlay and seat cushions, wound care seating, and skin care. Helps prevent pressure sores in high-risk patients.

233 **High Profile Single Compartment Cushion**
ROHO Group
100 North Florida Avenue
Belleville, IL 62221-5429
618-277-9173
800-736-0925
Fax: 888-551-3449
tomb@therohogroup.com
www.therohogroup.com

Tom Borcherding, President
Bobby Graebe, CEO
Tim Richter, Vice President of Finance
Dave McCausland, Senior Vice President of Planning & Government Affairs

With 4 inch cells, the HIGH PROFILE is the cushion of choice for individuals who suffer from ischemic ulcers (pressure sores) or who have a history of tissue breakdown.

234 **Inflatable Back Pillow**
Corflex Inc.
669 East Industrial Park Dr
Manchester, NH 03109-5625
603-623-3344
800-426-7353
Fax: 603-623-4111
sales@corflex.com
www.corflex.com

Paul Lorenzetti, President & CEO

Corflex specializes in orthopedic rehabilitation products. ReFolds flat to fit into its own carrying case, this inflatable back pillow ensures comfort while at home or traveling.

235 **Jobri**
Jobri
520 North Division Street
Konawa, OK 74849-2223
580-925-3500
800-432-2225
Fax: 580-925-3501
support@jobri.com
www.jobri.com

Brian Gourley, CEO

Jobri manufactures ergonomic back supports, ergonomic chairs, orthopedic soft goods and sleep products.

236 **Lumex Cushions and Mattresses**
Graham-Field Health Products
2935 Northeast Parkway
Atlanta, GA 30360-2808
770-368-4700
Fax: 770-368-4932
cs@grahamfield.com
www.grahamfield.com

Kenneth Spett, President & CEO
Cherie Antoniazzi, Senior Vice President, Quality, Regulatory & Risk Management
Marc Bernstein, Senior Vice President, Consumer Sales
Lawrence De La Haba, Senior Vice President, Business Development

Line of cushions and pillows give comfort and independence to the physically challenged.

237 **Medpro Static Air Chair Cushion**
Medpro
1950 Rutgers Blvd
Lakewood, NJ 08701-4537
732-905-9001
800-257-5145
Fax: 732-905-9899

Jody Gorran, President

Provides a protective layer of air beneath the patient helping prevent and treat pressure ulcers. *$94.95*

238 **Medpro Static Air Mattress Overlay**
Medpro
1950 Rutgers Blvd
Lakewood, NJ 08701-4537
732-905-9001
800-257-5145
Fax: 732-905-9899

Jody Gorran, President

Supports the patient on a cushioned network of air designed to redistribute the patient's weight reducing tissue interface pressure. Medpro's design incorporates a series of 65 air-breather vents that maintain air circulation. Medpro effectively reduces pressure and helps prevent and treat pressure ulcers. *$164.95*

239 **Mini-Max Cushion**
ROHO Group
100 North Florida Avenue
Belleville, IL 62221-5429
618-277-9173
800-736-0925
Fax: 888-551-3449
tomb@therohogroup.com
www.therohogroup.com

Tom Borcherding, President
Bobby Graebe, CEO
Tim Richter, Vice President of Finance
Dave McCausland, Senior Vice President of Planning & Government Affairs

Designed for the active individual with low risk of skin breakdown. The unique air cells of the MINI-MAX provide significant shock and impact absorption, skin protection and stability.

240 **NEXUS Wheelchair Cushioning System**
ROHO Group
100 North Florida Avenue
Belleville, IL 62221-5429
618-277-9173
800-736-0925
Fax: 888-551-3449
tomb@therohogroup.com
www.therohogroup.com

Tom Borcherding, President
Bobby Graebe, CEO
Tim Richter, Vice President of Finance
Dave McCausland, Senior Vice President of Planning & Government Affairs

A unique modular cushion that mates a contoured polyurethane foam base with a dry flotation support pad. It is designed to give the user positioning and stability, while offering maximum protection to the ischia, sacrum and coccyx.

241 **Pediatric Seating System**
ROHO Group
100 North Florida Avenue
Belleville, IL 62221-5429
618-277-9173
800-736-0925
Fax: 888-551-3449
tomb@therohogroup.com
www.therohogroup.com

Tom Borcherding, President
Bobby Graebe, CEO
Tim Richter, Vice President of Finance
Dave McCausland, Senior Vice President of Planning & Government Affairs

ROHO Cushions for kids use individual air cells, creating the most versatile and dynamic cushioning products available. These cushions are designed to specifically fit pediatric wheelchairs.

242 **Quadtro Cushion**
ROHO Group
100 North Florida Avenue
Belleville, IL 62221-5429
618-277-9173
800-736-0925
Fax: 888-551-3449
tomb@therohogroup.com
www.therohogroup.com
Tom Borcherding, President
Bobby Graebe, CEO
Tim Richter, Vice President of Finance
Dave McCausland, Senior Vice President of Planning & Government Affairs
For individuals who require special positioning of the pelvis or thighs and are at risk of skin breakdown, the Quadtro, with 4 inch cell height and air in place, progressive positioning is the cushion of choice.

243 **Silicone Padding**
Spenco Medical Group
P.O. Box 2501
Waco, TX 76702-2501
254-772-6000
800-877-3626
spenco@spenco.com
www.spenco.com
Jeff Antonioli, Vice President of Sales
Ryan Cruthirds, Vice President
For the management of pressure sores, this padding provides a special support system which allows even distribution of pressure and cool, comfortable, well-ventilated support.

244 **Soft-Touch Convertible Flotation Mattress**
Medpro
1950 Rutgers Blvd
Lakewood, NJ 08701-4537
732-905-9001
800-257-5145
Fax: 732-905-9899
Jody Gorran, President
Gives the patient the option to choose between water and gel flotation depending on the needs of the patient. The mattress helps prevent and treat pressure ulcers by spreading the patient's weight over a greater surface area.

245 **Soft-Touch Gel Flotation Cushion**
Medpro
1950 Rutgers Blvd
Lakewood, NJ 08701-4537
732-905-9001
800-257-5145
Fax: 732-905-9899
Jody Gorran, President
Acts like an additional layer of fatty tissue beneath the patient to help prevent and treat pressure sores. *$99.95*

246 **Spenco Medical Group**
Spenco Medical Group
P.O. Box 2501
Waco, TX 76702-2501
254-772-6000
800-877-3626
spenco@spenco.com
www.spenco.com
Jeff Antonioli, Vice President of Sales
Ryan Cruthirds, Vice President
Wheel chair cushions, silicone mattress pads, wound dressings, second skin blister and burn pads, polysorb insoles, elbow, knee and wrist supports and walking shoes.

247 **Stop-Leak Gel Flotation Mattress**
Jefferson Industries
1989 Rutgers Blvd
Lakewood, NJ 08701-4538
732-905-9001
800-257-5145
Fax: 732-905-9899
Charles Landa, General Manager
Protects persons from messy leaks while it protects from pressure ulcers. *$54.00*

248 **Stryker**
2825 Airview Boulevard
Kalamazoo, MI 49002
269-385-2600
Fax: 269-385-1062
www.stryker.com/us/en/about.html
Kevin A. Lobo, Chair & CEO
Glenn S. Boehnlein, Vice President & CFO
Yin C. Becker, Vice President, Communications, Public Affairs & Marketing
Dean H. Bergy, Vice President, Corporate Secretary
Leader in medical technology companies, with the drive to improve healthcare. Provides services and products in Orthopaedics, Medical and Surgical, and Neurotechnology and Spine.

249 **Sun-Mate Seat Cushions**
Dynamic Systems, Inc.
104 Morrow Branch Road
Leicester, NC 28748-5710
828-683-3523
855-786-6283
Fax: 844-270-6478
dsi@sunmatecushions.com
www.sunmatecushions.com
Charles A Yost, CEO
Lewis McCrain, General Manager
Line of cushions, pads and accessory items for personal comfort of the disabled. SunMate Orthopedic foam cushions and sheets that contours slowly to give uniform pressure distribution and soft spring back. Liquid SunMate for Foam-in-Place Seating (FIPS) to make custom molded seat inserts.

250 **Twin-Rest Seat Cushion & Glamour Pillow**
Better Sleep
57 Industrial Road
Berkeley Heights, NJ 07922-1501
908-464-6568
Fax: 908-464-0058
William Emery Jr., President & Founder
Makes any seat more comfortable because it is ingeniously designed to soothe sensitive areas while at work, in the car or at home.

Dressing Aids

251 **Button Aid**
Maxi Aids
42 Executive Blvd.
Farmingdale, NY 11735-4710
631-752-0521
800-522-6294
Fax: 631-752-0689
TTY: 631-752-0738
sales@maxiaids.com
www.maxiaids.com
Elliot Zaretsky, Founder, President & CEO
Makes buttoning possible with the use of only one hand. *$10.95*

252 **Deluxe Sock and Stocking Aid**
Therapro, Inc.
225 Arlington St
Framingham, MA 01702-8723
508-872-9494
800-257-5376
Fax: 508-875-2062
info@therapro.com
www.therapro.com
Karen Conrad Weihrauch, President & Owner
Flexible plastic, lined with blue nylon to reduce friction and outside with beige terry cloth to hold sock firmly until it is on the foot. *$12.95*

253 **Dressing Stick**
Maxi Aids
42 Executive Blvd.
Farmingdale, NY 11735-4710
631-752-0521
800-522-6294
Fax: 631-752-0689
TTY: 631-752-0738
sales@maxiaids.com
www.maxiaids.com
Elliot Zaretsky, Founder, President & CEO
Helps put on coats, sweaters and garments even when arm and shoulder movement is limited. *$16.95*

254 **Elastic Shoelaces**
Therapro, Inc.
225 Arlington St
Framingham, MA 01702-8723
508-872-9494
800-257-5376
Fax: 508-875-2062
info@therapro.com
www.therapro.com

Karen Conrad Weihrauch, President & Owner
The elastic laces allow the wearer to slip tied shoes on and off. *$4.25*

255 **Featherweight Reachers**
Therapro, Inc.
225 Arlington St
Framingham, MA 01702-8723
508-872-9494
800-257-5376
Fax: 508-875-2062
info@therapro.com
www.therapro.com

Karen Conrad Weihrauch, President & Owner
Useful in dressing or retrieving objects. *$17.95*

256 **Mirror Go Lightly**
AbleNet, Inc.
2625 Patton Road
Roseville, MN 55113-1137
651-294-2200
800-322-0956
Fax: 651-294-2259
customerservice@ablenetinc.com
www.ablenetinc.com

Bill Sproull, Chair of the Board
Jennifer Thalhuber, President & CEO
William Mills, Board of Directors
Paul Sugden, CFO & Trustee
Framed in plastic, the mirror can be tilted to provide either a normal or magnified image or to direct its lights at, or away from, the user. *$22.00*

257 **Molded Sock and Stocking Aid**
Therapro, Inc.
225 Arlington St
Framingham, MA 01702-8723
508-872-9494
800-257-5376
Fax: 508-875-2062
info@therapro.com
www.therapro.com

Karen Conrad Weihrauch, President & Owner
Sock or stocking is pulled over the molded plastic and then can be put on more easily. *$13.25*

258 **Say What Clothing Identifier**
Maxi Aids
42 Executive Blvd.
Farmingdale, NY 11735-4710
631-752-0521
800-522-6294
Fax: 631-752-0689
TTY: 631-752-0738
sales@maxiaids.com
www.maxiaids.com

Elliot Zaretsky, Founder, President & CEO
Braille the tag with information that the wearer wants on the tag and place the tag on a hanger. The custom-identification program makes it easier for the user to remember and identify the right clothes. *$4.95*

259 **Shoe Horn and Sock Remover**
Maxi Aids
42 Executive Blvd.
Farmingdale, NY 11735-4710
631-752-0521
800-522-6294
Fax: 631-752-0689
TTY: 631-752-0738
sales@maxiaids.com
www.maxiaids.com

Elliot Zaretsky, Founder, President & CEO
Helps with the removal of socks and shoes. Designed for those with arthritic or weak hands. Easily assembled and taken apart. The handle is 28" (13.75" when disassembled). *$11.95*

Health Aids

260 **AMI**
Aqua Massage International
P.O. Box 808
Groton, CT 06340-808
860-536-3735
800-248-4031
Fax: 860-536-3735
sales@aquamassage.com
www.aquamassage.com

David M. Cote, President
Dow Cote, Vice President Sales
Hilaire Cote, Senior Vice President
Scott Gilbert, Customer Service Manager
The Aqua PT provides the major benefits of Hydrotherapy, Massage Therapy and Dry Heat Therapy. 36 water jets provide continuous full body or localized massage while the user remains clothed and dry. Adjustable water pressure, temperature and pulsation frequency can massage in either a two direction travel mode for musculoskeletal pain management or a one direction mode, flowing water from head to foot for a contrast massage-relax therapy.

261 **American Medical Industries**
EZ Healthcare
Ste 2
330 E 3rd St
Dell Rapids, SD 57022-1918
605-428-5501
801-618-0444
Fax: 605-428-5502
www.ezhealthcare.com

Koby Jackson, Founder
Rick Martin, CEO
Kerina Blauer, VP Client Services
Jim Cannon, SVP Sales and Marketing
Software solutions that allow for healthcare providers to cut back on operational expenses through the automation of office procedures. Tailored to physicians in managing office practices and procedures.

262 **BIPAP S/T Ventilatory Support System**
Respironics
1010 Murry Ridge Ln
Murrysville, PA 15668-8517
724-387-5200
Fax: 724-387-5010
www.respironics.com

John L. Miclot, CEO
Gerald McGinnis, Chair
Daniel Bevevino, Vice President & CFO
Craig Reynolds, Executive Vice President & COO
Respironics, a recognized resource in the medical device market, provides innovative products and unique designs to the health care provider while helping them to grow and manage their business efficiently. As a global leader in the sleep and respiratory fields, Respironics provides innovative products that deal with sleep apnea management, oxygen therapy, noninvasive ventilation, and respiratory drug delivery.

263 **Bed Rails**
Mada Medical Products
625 Washington Ave
Carlstadt, NJ 07072-2901
201-460-0454
800-526-6370
Fax: 201-460-3509
dianelind@mail.madamedical.com
www.madainternational.com

Jeffrey Adam, President
Chrome plated steel rails and crossbars, all welded construction, telescopic side rail length adjustable, and a standard rail height of 16 inches.

264 **Coast to Coast Home Medical**
Coast to Coast Home Medical
Ste 4d
3381 Fairlane Farms Rd
Wellington, FL 33414-8711
561-792-4009
844-877-0707

Keri Suess, Owner
Home-delivered medical supplies for diabetes, respiratory, arthritis and impotence supplies.

265 **Compass Health**
6753 Engle Road
Middleburg Heights, OH 44130
440-572-1962
800-376-7263
Fax: 440-572-4261
corporate@compasshealthbrands.com
www.roscoemedical.com

266 **Drew Karol Industries**
Drew Karol Industries
633 Highway 1 North
P.O. Box 1066
Greenville, MS 38702- 1066
662-378-2188
Fax: 601-378-3188

Andrew K. Hoszowski, Owner
Orally operated toothbrush and dental care system for persons with limited or complete loss of hand or arm use - wheelchair accessible. *$600.00*

267 **Duraline Medical Products Inc.**
Duraline Medical Products Inc.
P.O. Box 67
324 Werner Street
Leipsic, OH 45856-1039
419-943-2044
800-654-3376
Fax: 419-943-3637
duraline@fairpoint.net
www.dmponline.com

Kathy Peck, General Manager
An assortment of quality incontinence products for adults and children.

268 **Duro-Med Industries**
Duro-Med Industries
1931 Norman Drive
Waukegan, IL 60085
800-526-4753
800-622-4714
Fax: 800-479-7968
Service@LiveHealthSmart.com
www.mabisdmi.com

Mike Mazza, President
Tony D'Antonio, Senior Vice President of Sales
Alan Yefsky, Exec Vice President, Sales & Marketing
Manufacturers of a complete line of home health care products. Featured products are patient gowns, back and seat cushions, pillows and a complete line of aids for daily living.

269 **Easy Ply**
BioMedical Life Systems
P.O. Box 1360
Vista, CA 92085-1360
760-579-0801
800-726-8367
Fax: 760-929-9953
information@bmls.com
www.bmls.com

270 **Ekso Bionics**
1414 Harbour Way S.
Suite 1201
Richmond, CA 94804
510-984-1761
customerrelations@eksobionics.com
eksobionics.com

Jack Peurach, President, CEO & Director
Bill Shaw, COO
Chwee Foon Lim, President, APAC
Jack Glenn, CFO
Develops and manufactures exoskeleton solutions to enhance the mobility of users with paralysis. Provides research for the U.S. defense capabilities.

271 **Electronic Amplified Stethoscopes**
HARC Mercantile
5413 S Westnedge Ave.
Suite A
Portage, MI 49002
269-324-1615
800-445-9968
Fax: 269-324-2387
TTY: 269-324-1615
info@harc.com
www.harc.com

Michael Martinson, Owner
A stethoscope designed for hearing aid users. Amplifies heart, breath, and Korotkoff sounds.

272 **Fold-Down 3-in-1 Commode**
Mada Medical Products
625 Washington Ave
Carlstadt, NJ 07072-2901
201-460-0454
800-526-6370
Fax: 201-460-3509
dianelind@mail.madamedical.com
www.madainternational.com

Jeffrey Adam, President
The Fold-Down commode is constructed of heavy duty, 1 inch diameter, steel tubing with X frame, has folding features convenient for storage and transport, easily removable back rest, and full length armrests.

273 **Healing Dressing for Pressure Sores**
Baxter Healthcare Corporation
1 Baxter Pkwy
Deerfield, IL 60015-4625
224-948-1812
800-422-9837
media@baxter.com
www.baxter.com

Robert L. Parkinson Jr., Chair & CEO
Jean-Luc Butel, Corporate Vice President - President, International
Ludwig N. Hantson, Corporate Vice President - President, BioScience
Robert J. Hombach, Corporate Vice President & CFO
A dressing specifically designed to promote healing of pressure sores and other dermal ulcers.

274 **Invacare Corporation**
Invacare
1 Invacare Way
Elyria, OH 44035-4190
440-329-6000
800-333-6900
Fax: 877-619-7996
www.invacare.com

Matthew E. Monaghan, Chair, President & CEO
Darcie Karol, Senior Vice President Human Resources
Kathleen P. Leneghan, Senior Vice President & CFO
Anthony C. LaPlaca, Senior Vice President, General Counsel & Secretary
The world's leading manufacturer and distributor of innovative home and long-term care medical products which promote recovery and active lifestyles.

275 **MADAMIST 50/50 PSI Air Compressor**
Mada Medical Products
625 Washington Ave
Carlstadt, NJ 07072-2901
201-460-0454
800-526-6370
Fax: 201-460-3509
dianelind@mail.madamedical.com
www.madainternational.com

Jeffrey Adam, President
The new compressor rated at 50 PSI is designed to drive humidifiers, nebulizers, mist tents and is ideal to administer pentamidine aerosol therapy.

276 **MedDev Corporation**
MedDev Corporation
730 N Pastoria Ave
Sunnyvale, CA 94085-3522
408-730-9702
800-543-2789
Fax: 408-730-9732
info@meddev-corp.com
www.meddev-corp.com

277 **Medi-Grip**
Therapro, Inc.
225 Arlington St
Framingham, MA 01702-8723
508-872-9494
800-257-5376
Fax: 508-875-2062
info@therapro.com
www.therapro.com

Karen Conrad Weihrauch, President & Owner

Reasonably priced, nonskid material. This nonslip material is available in marine blue, desert sand and burgundy rolls 12 inches x 144 inches. *$11.95*

278 **Osborn Medical Corporation**
Osborn Medical Corporation
7022 S. Revere Pkwy
Suite 240
Centennial, CO 80112
303-223-1800
800-535-5865
Fax: 507-932-5044
info@osbornmedical.com
www.osbornmedical.com

Bill Davis, President and CEO
Keith Walli-Ware, Vice President of Sales and Marketing
Ian MacDonald, COO

Strider allows the user to exercise in most chairs found in at home. No more small, uncomfortable bicycle seats to sit on while exercising. A hands-free exercising experience.

279 **Sivantos US, Inc.**
Sivantos Group
P.O. Box 1397
Piscataway, NJ 08855-1397
800-766-4500
Fax: 732-562-6683
shiconsumerrelations.healthcare@sivantos.com
www.sivantos.com/countrypag e_sivantos_us/

Steve Mahon, CEO
Eric Timm, COO
Tom Strauch, CFO

Sivantos Group is a technological leader and manufacturer of hearing aids, providing the best hearing aids for users. One out of every four hearing aids used throughout the world has been developed and manufacturerd by Sivantos Group.

280 **Standard 3-in-1 Commode**
Mada Medical Products
625 Washington Ave
Carlstadt, NJ 07072-2901
201-460-0454
800-526-6370
Fax: 201-460-3509
dianelind@mail.madamedical.com
www.madainternational.com

Jeffrey Adam, President

The standard commode is constructed of a heavy duty anodized aluminum frame, seat adjustment and an easily removable back rest.

281 **Talking Digital Thermometer**
Maxi Aids
42 Executive Blvd.
Farmingdale, NY 11735-4710
631-752-0521
800-522-6294
Fax: 631-752-0689
TTY: 631-752-0738
sales@maxiaids.com
www.maxiaids.com

Elliot Zaretsky, Founder, President & CEO

Talking and large print thermometer. Announces and displays temperature in Fahrenheit or Celsius. *$15.95*

282 **Talking Thermometers**
Maxi Aids
42 Executive Blvd.
Farmingdale, NY 11735-4710
631-752-0521
800-522-6294
Fax: 631-752-0689
TTY: 631-752-0738
sales@maxiaids.com
www.maxiaids.com

Elliot Zaretsky, Founder, President & CEO

Clearly announces temperature in Fahrenheit or Celsius.

283 **Thinklabs One Stethoscope**
HARC Mercantile
5413 S Westnedge Ave.
Suite A
Portage, MI 49002
269-324-1615
800-445-9968
Fax: 269-324-2387
TTY: 269-324-1615
info@harc.com
www.harc.com

Michael Martinson, Owner

Stethoscope that amplifies sounds by more than 100x. Works with any headphones or hearing aid streamer.

284 **Transfer Bench**
Mada Medical Products
625 Washington Ave
Carlstadt, NJ 07072-2901
201-460-0454
800-526-6370
Fax: 201-460-3509
dianelind@mail.madamedical.com
www.madainternational.com

Jeffrey Adam, President

The transfer bench is a one piece bench with a wide base for stability, 1 inch diameter aluminum framework, corrosion resistant, and an adjustable seat.

Hearing Aids

285 **Auditech: Personal PA Value Pack System**
Auditech
P.O. Box 821105
Vicksburg, MS 39182-1105
800-229-8293
Fax: 800-221-8639
info@auditechusa.com
www.auditechusa.com

286 **Auditech: Pocketalker Pro**
Auditech
P.O. Box 821105
Vicksburg, MS 39182-1105
800-229-8293
Fax: 800-221-8639
www.auditechusa.com

287 **Battery Device Adapter**
AbleNet, Inc.
2625 Patton Road
Roseville, MN 55113-1137
651-294-2200
800-322-0956
Fax: 651-294-2259
customerservice@ablenetinc.com
www.ablenetinc.com

Bill Sproull, Chair of the Board
Jennifer Thalhuber, President & CEO
William Mills, Board of Directors
Paul Sugden, CFO & Trustee

A cable which connects to and adapts battery-operated devices for external switch control. Two sizes are available to adapt devices with either AA or C and D size batteries. *$8.00*

288 **Cochlear**
13059 E. Peakview Avenue
Englewood, CO 80111
303-790-9010
800-523-5798
Fax: 303-792-9025
www.cochlear.com/us/en/home

Dig Howitt, President & CEO
Brent Cubis, CFO
Jennifer Hornery, Senior Vice President, People & Culture
Dr. David N. Cade, Chief Medical Officer

For over three decades, Cochlear has been delivering hearing implant innovation worldwide. Cochlear helps with the communication of implant recipients.

289 **Custom Earmolds**
Lloyd Hearing Aid Corporation
P.O. Box 1645
4435 Manchester Drive
Rockford, IL 61109- 1645
815-964-4191
800-323-4212
Fax: 815-964-8378
info@lloydhearingaid.com
www.lloydhearingaid.com
Andy PalmQuist, President
Hearing aid molds, custom built to the exact fit of the customer.
$29.95

290 **Digital Hearing Aids**
Lloyd Hearing Aid Corporation
P.O. Box 1645
4435 Manchester Drive
Rockford, IL 61109- 1645
815-964-4191
800-323-4212
Fax: 815-964-8378
info@lloydhearingaid.com
www.lloydhearingaid.com
Andy PalmQuist, President
Latest hearing technology. *$7.50*

291 **Duracell & Rayovac Hearing Aid Batteries**
Lloyd Hearing Aid Corporation
P.O. Box 1645
4435 Manchester Drive
Rockford, IL 61109- 1645
815-964-4191
800-323-4212
Fax: 815-964-8378
info@lloydhearingaid.com
www.lloydhearingaid.com
Andy PalmQuist, President
reliable and long lasting, these batteries power the user's hearing aid. Easy to insert into hearing aid.

292 **Harris Communications**
Harris Communications
15155 Technology Dr
Eden Prairie, MN 55344-2273
952-906-1180
800-825-6758
Fax: 952-906-1099
TTY: 800-825-9187
info@harriscomm.com
www.harriscomm.com
Robert Harris, Owner & President
Kevin Horsky, Business Director
Randall Moore, Manager
A national distributor of assistive devices for the deaf and hard-of-hearing with many manufacturers represented. Catalog includes a wide range of assistive devices as well as a variety of books and video tapes related to deaf and hard-of-hearing issues. Products available for children, teachers, hearing professionals, interpreters and anyone interested in deaf culture, hearing loss and sign language.
180 pages Yearly

293 **Hearing Aid Batteries**
HARC Mercantile
5413 S Westnedge Ave.
Suite A
Portage, MI 49002
269-324-1615
800-445-9968
Fax: 269-324-2387
TTY: 269-324-1615
info@harc.com
www.harc.com
Michael Martinson, Owner
Hearing aid batteries in all popular sizes in mercury, zinc air, silver as well as Nicad and Varta and batteries for electrolarynx and infrared systems.

294 **Hearing Aid Battery Testers**
HARC Mercantile
5413 S Westnedge Ave.
Suite A
Portage, MI 49002
269-324-1615
800-445-9968
Fax: 269-324-2387
TTY: 269-324-1615
info@harc.com
www.harc.com
Michael Martinson, Owner
From pocket size to professional type battery testers which test mercury, zinc air, silver, specialty and general usage batteries.
$7.00

295 **Hearing Aid Care Kit**
HARC Mercantile
5413 S Westnedge Ave.
Suite A
Portage, MI 49002
269-324-1615
800-445-9968
Fax: 269-324-2387
TTY: 269-324-1615
info@harc.com
www.harc.com
Michael Martinson, Owner
Includes a hearing aid dehumidifer, stethoset, and cleaning tools.
$40.00

296 **MED-EL Corporation, USA**
2645 Meridian Parkway
Suite 100
Durham, NC 27713
919-572-2222
888-633-3524
Fax: 919-484-9229
www.medel.com/us
Ingeborg Hochmair, CEO
MED-EL is the leader in implantable hearing solutions. In 2017,the company launched the RONDO 2, a revolutionary cochlear implant powered by wireless charging technology.

297 **Micro Audiometrics Corporation**
Micro Audiometrics
655 Keller Road
Murphy, NC 28906-5890
386-888-7878
866-327-7226
Fax: 866-683-4447
sales@microaud.com
www.microaud.com
Jason Keller, President
Manufacturer and distributor of hearing testing instruments, including the complete line of Earscan.

298 **Mushroom Inserts**
Lloyd Hearing Aid Corporation
P.O. Box 1645
4435 Manchester Drive
Rockford, IL 61109- 1645
815-964-4191
800-323-4212
Fax: 815-964-8378
info@lloydhearingaid.com
www.lloydhearingaid.com
Andy PalmQuist, President
A universal earplug useful in wearing behind the ear type hearing instruments. *$2.50*

299 **Oval Window Audio**
33 Wildflower Ct
Nederland, CO 80466
303-447-3607
Fax: 303-447-3607
TTY: 303-447-3607
info@ovalwindowaudio.com
www.ovalwindowaudio.com
Norman Lederman, Director of Research & Development
Paula Hendricks, Educational Director
Manufacturer of induction loop hearing assistance technologies compatible with telecoil-equipped hearing aids used by many hard of hearing people. The company also makes multisensory sound systems for use in speech and music therapy and science classes.

300 **Sonova USA Inc.**
Phonak
4520 Weaver Parkway
Warrenville, IL 60555-3927
800-679-4871
Info@Phonak.com
www.sonova.com/usa/en-us

301 **Starkey Hearing Foundation**
6700 Washington Ave S
Eden Prairie, MN 55344
952-941-6401
866-354-3254
Fax: 952-828-6900
info@starkeyfoundation.org
www.starkeyhearingfoundation.org
Richard S Brown, President
Brady Forseth, Executive Director
Keith Becker, Senior Director of Operations
Bruce Schmaltz, Chief Financial Officer
The Starkey Hearing Foundation works to assist those with hearing impairments by offering hearing aids and aftercare services.
Quarterly

302 **Ultratec**
450 Science Dr
Madison, WI 53711
608-238-5400
800-482-2424
Fax: 608-238-3008
TTY: 800-482-2424
service@ultratec.com
www.ultratec.com
Jackie Morgan, Marketing Director
Amy Mueller, Marketing Communications Specialist
Ultratec works to make telephone access more convenient and reliable for people with hearing loss by providing assistive devices such as amplified phones and text phones.

303 **Widex USA, Inc.**
185 Commerce Drive
Hauppauge, NY 11788
www.widex.com/en-us
Jorgen Jensen, President & CEO
Jan Topholm, Chair & Co-Owner
Julian Topholm, Vice President, Production
Richard Topholm, Director, Neuro Technology
Provider and producer of hearing aids, Widex's design combines technology with functionality and aesthetics.

Kitchen & Eating Aids

304 **Bagel Holder**
Maxi Aids
42 Executive Blvd.
Farmingdale, NY 11735-4710
631-752-0521
800-522-6294
Fax: 631-752-0689
TTY: 631-752-0738
sales@maxiaids.com
www.maxiaids.com
Elliot Zaretsky, Founder, President & CEO
Holds bagels in place for easy slicing. *$4.95*

305 **Big and Bold Low Vision Timer**
Maxi Aids
42 Executive Blvd.
Farmingdale, NY 11735-4710
631-752-0521
800-522-6294
Fax: 631-752-0689
TTY: 631-752-0738
sales@maxiaids.com
www.maxiaids.com
Elliot Zaretsky, Founder, President & CEO
Sixty-minute mechanical timer with large, easy-to-read numbers for the visually impaired. *$14.75*

306 **Box Top Opener**
Performance Health
28100 Torch Parkway
Suite 700
Warrenville, IL 60555-3938
630-393-6000
Fax: 630-393-7600
customersupport@performancehealth.com
www.performancehealth.com
Francis Dirksmeier, CEO
Isabel Afonso, Managing Director & Head of International
Daniel Baumwald, Vice President, North America Retail & eCommerce
Laurie Byrne, Chief Human Resources Officer
This handy device exerts the pressure on those hard-to-open boxes of laundry/dishwasher soap, rice and prepared dinners.
$2.95

307 **Braille Timer**
Maxi Aids
42 Executive Blvd.
Farmingdale, NY 11735-4710
631-752-0521
800-522-6294
Fax: 631-752-0689
TTY: 631-752-0738
sales@maxiaids.com
www.maxiaids.com
Elliot Zaretsky, Founder, President & CEO
Three raised dots at 15, 30 and 45, two raised dots at 0, and one raised dot on all other numbers.

308 **Capscrew**
Access with Ease
P.O. Box 1150
Chino Valley, AZ 86323-1150
928-636-9469
800-531-9479
Fax: 928-636-0292

309 **Cordless Receiver**
AbleNet, Inc.
2625 Patton Road
Roseville, MN 55113-1137
651-294-2200
800-322-0956
Fax: 651-294-2259
customerservice@ablenetinc.com
www.ablenetinc.com
Bill Sproull, Chair of the Board
Jennifer Thalhuber, President & CEO
William Mills, Board of Directors
Paul Sugden, CFO & Trustee
The Cordless Receiver in conjunction with the Cordless Big Red Switch, can be used anywhere a switch is currently used to control battery or electrically-operated toys, games or appliances; augmentative communication systems; and computers (through a computer switch interface). *$79.00*

310 **Deluxe Roller Knife**
Performance Health
28100 Torch Parkway
Suite 700
Warrenville, IL 60555-3938
630-393-6000
Fax: 630-393-7600
customersupport@performancehealth.com
www.performancehealth.com
Francis Dirksmeier, CEO
Isabel Afonso, Managing Director & Head of International
Daniel Baumwald, Vice President, North America Retail & eCommerce
Laurie Byrne, Chief Human Resources Officer
Stainless steel blade rolls smoothly, cutting food cleanly. *$10.95*

311 Dual Brush with Suction Base
Performance Health
28100 Torch Parkway
Suite 700
Warrenville, IL 60555-3938
630-393-6000
Fax: 630-393-7600
customersupport@performancehealth.com
www.performancehealth.com

Francis Dirksmeier, CEO
Isabel Afonso, Managing Director & Head of International
Daniel Baumwald, Vice President, North America Retail & eCommerce
Laurie Byrne, Cheif Human Resources Officer
Two brushes clean the inside and outside of bottles and glasses at the same time using just one hand. *$14.50*

312 Electric Can Opener & Knife Sharpener
Maxi Aids
42 Executive Blvd.
Farmingdale, NY 11735-4710
631-752-0521
800-522-6294
Fax: 631-752-0689
TTY: 631-752-0738
sales@maxiaids.com
www.maxiaids.com

Elliot Zaretsky, Founder, President & CEO
Features include a powerful magnetic lid holder, the ability to open odd-shaped cans, and easy operation for the physically challenged. *$15.99*

313 Folding Pot Stabilizer
Maxi Aids
42 Executive Blvd.
Farmingdale, NY 11735-4710
631-752-0521
800-522-6294
Fax: 631-752-0689
TTY: 631-752-0738
sales@maxiaids.com
www.maxiaids.com

Elliot Zaretsky, Founder, President & CEO
This device holds onto the pot handle and secures the pot in place, allowing for easier use for those with physical challenges. *$27.95*

314 Good Grips Cutlery
Therapro, Inc.
225 Arlington St
Framingham, MA 01702-8723
508-872-9494
800-257-5376
Fax: 508-875-2062
info@therapro.com
www.therapro.com

Karen Conrad Weihrauch, President & Owner
Stainless steel utensils have a special twist built into the metal to facilitate bending of a spoon or fork at any angle for right or left handed people. *$7.50*

315 H.E.L.P. Knife
Maxi Aids
42 Executive Blvd.
Farmingdale, NY 11735-4710
631-752-0521
800-522-6294
Fax: 631-752-0689
TTY: 631-752-0738
sales@maxiaids.com
www.maxiaids.com

Elliot Zaretsky, Founder, President & CEO
Adjustable food slicing system guides the knife for even, uniform slices while protecting the user. *$22.95*

316 Handi Holder
Evio Plastics
P.O. Box 2295
Sandusky, OH 44871-2295
419-621-1105
Fax: 419-626-2183

Doug Didion, Admininstrator Director
Danny Thomas, Owner
Handi Holder is a plastic holder for 1/2 gallon paper cartons of milk or juice. It is used to pour milk or juice without spills by using the handle.

317 Handy-Helper Cutting Board
Maxi Aids
42 Executive Blvd.
Farmingdale, NY 11735-4710
631-752-0521
800-522-6294
Fax: 631-752-0689
TTY: 631-752-0738
sales@maxiaids.com
www.maxiaids.com

Elliot Zaretsky, Founder, President & CEO
Laminated cutting board with unique features to hold food in place with corner ledge for cutting and spreading. *$24.95*

318 Innerlip Plates
Therapro, Inc.
225 Arlington St
Framingham, MA 01702-8723
508-872-9494
800-257-5376
Fax: 508-875-2062
info@therapro.com
www.therapro.com

Karen Conrad Weihrauch, President & Owner
Food may be pushed to the side of the plate, then scooped up with a fork and spoon. Available in beige or blue. *$5.00*

319 Long Oven Mitts
Performance Health
28100 Torch Parkway
Suite 700
Warrenville, IL 60555-3938
630-393-6000
Fax: 630-393-7600
customersupport@performancehealth.com
www.performancehealth.com

Francis Dirksmeier, CEO
Isabel Afonso, Managing Director & Head of International
Daniel Baumwald, Vice President, North America Retail & eCommerce
Laurice Byrne, Chief Human Resources Officer
Protect hands and forearms from heat, flames and oven grates with these practical mitts that allow a longer reach and less bending. *$8.95*

320 Long Ring Low Vision Timers
Maxi Aids
42 Executive Blvd.
Farmingdale, NY 11735-4710
631-752-0521
800-522-6294
Fax: 631-752-0689
TTY: 631-752-0738
sales@maxiaids.com
www.maxiaids.com

Elliot Zaretsky, Founder, President & CEO
Large, bold numerals allows for easy reading at any distance.

321 Nosey Cup
Therapro, Inc.
225 Arlington St
Framingham, MA 01702-8723
508-872-9494
800-257-5376
Fax: 508-875-2062
info@therapro.com
www.therapro.com

Karen Conrad Weihrauch, President & Owner
For those with a stiff neck or persons who can't tip their head back while drinking. *$6.00*

322 Paring Boards
Therapro, Inc.
225 Arlington St
Framingham, MA 01702-8723
508-872-9494
800-257-5376
Fax: 508-875-2062
info@therapro.com
www.therapro.com

Karen Conrad Weihrauch, President & Owner
Suction feet stabilize board and stainless steel prongs hold food in place for easy, one-handed cutting. *$32.50*

323 **Performance Health**
Performance Health
28100 Torch Parkway
Suite 700
Warrenville, IL 60555-3938
630-393-6000
Fax: 630-393-7600
customersupport@performancehealth.com
www.performancehealth.com

Francis Dirksmeier, CEO
Isabel Afonso, Managing Director & Head of International
Daniel Baumwald, Vice President, North America Retail & eCommerce
Laurie Byrne, Chief Human Resources Officer

Performance Health is a leading provider of rehabilitation and assistive devices to help those with disabilities meet daily physical challenges and achieve their greatest level of independence. With one of the industry's largest catalogs, Sammons Preston Rolyan offers a wide range of products available.
Annually

324 **PowerLink 2 Control Unit**
AbleNet, Inc.
2625 Patton Road
Roseville, MN 55113-1137
651-294-2200
800-322-0956
Fax: 651-294-2259
customerservice@ablenetinc.com
www.ablenetinc.com

Bill Sproull, Chair of the Board
Jennifer Thalhuber, President & CEO
William Mills, Board of Directors
Paul Sugden, CFO & Trustee

The PowerLink 2 Control Unit allows switch operation of electrical appliances. It can be used to activate 1 or 2 appliances (up to 1700 watts combined). If 2 appliances are used, they will activate simultaneously. There are four modes of control on the PowerLink 2; direct mode, timed (seconds) mode, timed (minutes) mode and latch mode. Meets safety standards from Underwriters Laboratory (UL) and Canadian Standards Association (CSA) for electrical appliances. *$159.00*

325 **Slicing Aid**
R82, Inc.
12801 E. Independence Blvd.
P.O. Box 1739
Matthews, NC 28106-1739
310-618-0111
844-876-6245
Fax: 704-882-0751
information@r82.com
www.r82.com

Scott Crosswhite, Vice President
Kirk Mackenzie, President
Greg Tilley, Controller
Angela Stegall, Purchasing

The design of these knives allows a better working posture and makes optimal use of strength in the arms and hands.

326 **Small Appliance Receiver**
AbleNet, Inc.
2625 Patton Road
Roseville, MN 55113-1137
651-294-2200
800-322-0956
Fax: 651-294-2259
customerservice@ablenetinc.com
www.ablenetinc.com

Bill Sproull, Chair of the Board
Jennifer Thalhuber, President & CEO
William Mills, Board of Directors
Paul Sugden, CFO & Trustee

The Small Appliance Receiver, in conjunction with the Cordless Big Red Switch, allows you to control small electrical appliances in the environment without a cord. It should only be used with low-wattage appliances (under 500 watts) which have two prong plugs (i.e., radios, fans, lamps, blenders, etc.). It should not be used with heat generating appliances. *$32.00*

327 **Steel Food Bumper**
Maxi Aids
42 Executive Blvd.
Farmingdale, NY 11735-4710
631-752-0521
800-522-6294
Fax: 631-752-0689
TTY: 631-752-0738
sales@maxiaids.com
www.maxiaids.com

Elliot Zaretsky, Founder, President & CEO

Provides stable area to push against while eating. *$16.95*

328 **Stove Knob Turner**
Maxi Aids
42 Executive Blvd.
Farmingdale, NY 11735-4710
631-752-0521
800-522-6294
Fax: 631-752-0689
TTY: 631-752-0738
sales@maxiaids.com
www.maxiaids.com

Elliot Zaretsky, Founder, President & CEO

Lightweight aluminum rod for turning stove knobs. Designed for wheelchair users. *$32.95*

329 **Talking Food Cans**
Maxi Aids
42 Executive Blvd.
Farmingdale, NY 11735-4710
631-752-0521
800-522-6294
Fax: 631-752-0689
TTY: 631-752-0738
sales@maxiaids.com
www.maxiaids.com

Elliot Zaretsky, Founder, President & CEO

Voice recording device for recording descriptions of hard to identify objects, such as food cans, bottles and storage containers. *$24.95*

330 **Thick-n-Easy**
Therapro, Inc.
225 Arlington St
Framingham, MA 01702-8723
508-872-9494
800-257-5376
Fax: 508-875-2062
info@therapro.com
www.therapro.com

Karen Conrad Weihrauch, President & Owner

Instant food thickener that sets in 30 seconds and will not become thicker even after refrigeration. *$6.50*

331 **Thumbs Up Cup**
Therapro, Inc.
225 Arlington St.
Framingham, MA 01702-8723
508-872-9494
800-257-5376
Fax: 508-875-2062
info@therapro.com
www.therapro.com

Karen Conrad Weihrauch, President & Owner

This cup is designed for those with limited strength or coordination or arthritis. The two backward-tilt handles and thumb rests allow finger joints to be used to their greatest mechanical advantage. *$9.50*

332 **Undercounter Lid Opener**
Performance Health
28100 Torch Parkway
Suite 700
Warrenville, IL 60555-3938
630-393-6000
Fax: 630-393-7600
customersupport@performancehealth.com
www.performancehealth.com

Francis Dirksmeier, CEO
Isabel Afonso, Managing Director & Head of International
Daniel Baumwald, Vice President, North America Retail & eCommerce
Laurie Byrne, Chief Human Resources Officer

The gripper of this unit which installs under the counter can help unscrew any cap. *$5.75*

333 **Uni-Turner**
Performance Health
28100 Torch Parkway
Suite 700
Warrenville, IL 60555-3938
630-393-6000
Fax: 630-393-7600
customersupport@performancehealth.com
www.performancehealth.com
Francis Dirksmeier, CEO
Isabel Afonso, Managing Director & Head of International
Daniel Baumwald, Vice President, North America Retail & eCommerce
Laurie Byrne, Chief Human Resources Officer
Odd shaped handles can be turned easily with one-handed, L-shaped Uni-Turner. *$16.50*

334 **Universal Hand Cuff**
Therapro, Inc.
225 Arlington St
Framingham, MA 01702-8723
508-872-9494
800-257-5376
Fax: 508-875-2062
info@therapro.com
www.therapro.com
Karen Conrad Weihrauch, President & Owner
Comfortable cuff with Velcro strap holds utensils, toothbrushes, etc. Washable and adjustable to the user's condition and hand size. *$9.95*

Lifts, Ramps & Elevators

335 **Accessibility Lift**
Inclinator Company of America
601 Gibson Blvd
Harrisburg, PA 17104-3215
717-939-8420
800-343-9007
Fax: 717-939-8075
isales@inclinator.com
www.inclinator.com
Cliff Warner, President & CEO
Mark Crispen, Director of Marketing, Corporate Secretary & Board Member
Brad Rose, Sales Manager
Steve Smith, Sales Manager
An economical lift for restricted usage that provides barrier-free access that can be used by churches, schools, lodging halls and meeting halls to meet compliance requirements, with the dignified convenience and freedom they deserve.

336 **Adjustable Incline Board**
Bailey Manufacturing Company
118 Lee Drive
P.O. Box 130
Lodi, OH 44254-130
330-948-1080
800-321-8372
Fax: 330-948-4439
baileymfg@baileymfg.com
www.baileymfg.com
Larry Strimple, President
Judie Butler, Dealer Contact
Incline board for the physically challenged with a foot board with non-slip tread.

337 **AlumiRamp**
AlumiRamp, Inc.
855 East Chicago Road
Quincy, MI 49082-9450
800-800-3864
Fax: 517-639-4314
sales@alumiramp.com
www.alumiramp.com
Doug Cannon, General Manager
Complete line of modular, aluminum and portable ramps for both home and vehicle use. Welded construction and non-skid extruded surfaces are featured on all our ramps.

338 **Area Access**
Area Access
7131 Gateway Court
Manassas, VA 20109-1015
703-396-4949
800-333-2732
Fax: 703-207-0446
www.areaaccess.com

339 **Back-Saver**
Bruno Independent Living Aids, Inc.
1780 Executive Dr.
PO Box 84
Oconomowoc, WI 53066
262-567-4990
800-454-4355
Fax: 262-953-5501
webinfo@bruno.com
www.bruno.com
Michael R. Bruno, II, President & CEO
Exterior platform lift for transporting manual folding wheelchairs. 100 lb lift capacity.

340 **Basement Motorhome Lift**
Handicaps, Inc.
4335 S Santa Fe Dr.
Englewood, CO 80110-5417
303-781-2062
800-782-4335
info@handicapsinc.com
www.handicapsinc.com

341 **Big Lifter**
Bruno Independent Living Aids, Inc.
1780 Executive Dr.
PO Box 84
Oconomowoc, WI 53066
262-567-4990
800-454-4355
Fax: 262-953-5501
webinfo@bruno.com
www.bruno.com
Michael R. Bruno, II, President & CEO
Hoist-style lift for scooters and power chairs. Can be manually rotated, 400 lb lift capacity.

342 **BraunAbility**
645 W Carmel Dr.
Carmel, IN 46032
800-488-0359
888-365-9417
questions@braunability.com
www.braunability.com
Staci Kroon, President & CEO
Manufactures wheelchair and mobility scooter lifts and ramps for vehicles.

343 **Bruno Independent Living Aids**
Bruno Independent Living Aids, Inc.
1780 Executive Dr.
PO Box 84
Oconomowoc, WI 53066
262-567-4990
800-454-4355
Fax: 262-953-5501
webinfo@bruno.com
www.bruno.com
Michael R. Bruno, II, President & CEO
An ISO 9001 Certified Manufacturer of automotive lifts for scooter, wheelchairs, and power chairs, three and four wheel scooters, and straight and custom curve stairlifts.

344 **Butlers Wheelchair Lifts**
Butler Mobility Products
571 Industrial Drive
Lewisberry, PA 17339
717-938-4253
888-847-0804
Fax: 717-938-4238
www.butlermobility.com
Hal Feinstein, Vice President of Sales & Marketing
Wheelchair lift can be equipped with a ramp and guard. Automatically retractable, it locks firmly into place when the lift is in operation.

345 **Chariot**
Bruno Independent Living Aids, Inc.
1780 Executive Dr.
PO Box 84
Oconomowoc, WI 53066
262-567-4990
800-454-4355
Fax: 262-953-5501
webinfo@bruno.com
www.bruno.com
Michael R. Bruno, II, President & CEO
Exterior lift for transporting scooters and power chairs. The lift includes 360-degree spinning wheels and has a 350 lb lift capacity.

346 **Classique**
Handi-Lift
730 Garden St
Carlstadt, NJ 07072-1625
201-933-0111
800-432-5438
Fax: 201-933-0050
sales@handi-lift.com
www.handi-lift.com
Douglas Boydston, President
The Classique elevator answers access problems in churches, schools and small offices.

347 **Clearway**
Ricon
1135 Aviation Pl.
San Fernando, CA 91340
818-267-3000
800-322-2884
Fax: 800-962-1201
ricinsales@wabtec.com
www.riconcorp.com

348 **Columbus McKinnon Corporation**
Columbus Mckinnon Corporation
205 Crosspoint Parkway
Getzville, NY 14068
716-689-5400
800-888-0985
Fax: 716-689-5644
www.cmworks.com
Timothy T. Tevens, President & CEO
Gregory P. Rustowicz, Vice President & CFO
Charles R. Giesige, Vice President, Corporate Development
Richard A. Steinberg, Vice President, Human Resources
Supplies various lift and transfer systems for independent or attended applications including ceiling mounted or freestanding overhead track lifts and mobile floorbase units for homes, schools and healthcare facilities. Lift Systems for transferring between bed, chair, commode or bath are available with a variety of slings, scales and accessories.

349 **Curb-Sider**
Bruno Independent Living Aids, Inc.
1780 Executive Dr.
PO Box 84
Oconomowoc, WI 53066
262-567-4990
800-454-4355
Fax: 262-953-5501
webinfo@bruno.com
www.bruno.com
Michael R. Bruno, II, President & CEO
A hoist lift that stores fully or partially assembled scooters or power chairs weighing up to 450 pounds in the rear of a van, minivan, SUV, pickup truck, or some station wagon applications.

350 **Curb-Sider Super XL**
Bruno Independent Living Aids, Inc.
1780 Executive Dr.
PO Box 84
Oconomowoc, WI 53066
262-567-4990
800-454-4355
Fax: 262-953-5501
webinfo@bruno.com
www.bruno.com
Michael R. Bruno, II, President & CEO
Provides up to 180 degrees of rotation, allowing for easier raising, lowering, and rotation of fully or partially assembled scooters or power chairs.

351 **Custom Lift Residential Elevators**
Waupaca Elevator Company
1726 N. Ballard Road
Suite 1
Appleton, WI 54911-2444
920-991-9082
800-238-8739
Fax: 920-991-9087
info@waupacaelevator.com
waupacaelevator.com
Bill Mc Michael, Owner
Waupaca Elevator residential elevators and dumbwaiters add value, convenience and reliability to today's homes.

352 **Deluxe Convertible Exercise Staircase**
Performance Health
28100 Torch Parkway
Suite 700
Warrenville, IL 60555-3938
630-393-6000
Fax: 630-393-7600
customersupport@performancehealth.com
www.performancehealth.com
Francis Dirksmeier, CEO
Isabel Afonso, Managing Director & Head of International
Daniel Baumwald, Vice President, North America Retail & eCommerce
Laurie Byrne, Chief Human Resources Officer
An exercise staircase to fit any department configuration. Just reposition a few nuts and bolts to change from a straight to a corner type staircase.

353 **Easy Pivot Transfer Machine**
Rand-Scot, Inc.
209 Christman Drive
Fort Collins, CO 80524-2429
970-484-7967
800-467-7967
Fax: 970-484-3800
info@randscot.com
www.randscot.com
Joel Lerich, Co-Founder
Barbara Lerich, Co-Founder
The Easy Pivot Patient Lifting System allows for strain-free, one-caregiver transfers of the disabled individual.

354 **Easy Stand**
Altimate Medical
262 W. 1st St.
Morton, MN 56270-180
507-697-6393
800-342-8968
Fax: 507-697-6900
info@easystand.com
www.easystand.com
Andrew Gardeen, International Sales Manager
Designed to make standing fast and simple. The easy to operate, hydraulic lift system provides controlled lifting and lowering. With the convenience of simply transferring to the chair and reaching a standing position in seconds with no straps to struggle with.

355 **Economical Liberty**
Handi-Lift
730 Garden St
Carlstadt, NJ 07072-1625
201-933-0111
800-432-5438
Fax: 201-933-0050
sales@handi-lift.com
www.handi-lift.com
Douglas Boydston, President
Installs quickly and easily on most straight stairways. It uses regular household current and mounts over the carpet or directly to the stairs without marring.

356 **Elan Stair Lift**
Bruno Independent Living Aids, Inc.
1780 Executive Dr.
PO Box 84
Oconomowoc, WI 53066
262-567-4990
800-454-4355
Fax: 262-953-5501
webinfo@bruno.com
www.bruno.com
Michael R. Bruno, II, President & CEO

Straight indoor stairlift. Vertical rail design, 300 lb lift capacity.

357 **Elite Curved Stair Lift**
Bruno Independent Living Aids, Inc.
1780 Executive Dr.
PO Box 84
Oconomowoc, WI 53066
262-567-4990
800-454-4355
Fax: 262-953-5501
webinfo@bruno.com
www.bruno.com
Michael R. Bruno, II, President & CEO
Curved stairlift with 400 lb lift capacity. Indoor and outdoor stairlifts available.

358 **Elite Stair Lift**
Bruno Independent Living Aids, Inc.
1780 Executive Dr.
PO Box 84
Oconomowoc, WI 53066
262-567-4990
800-454-4355
Fax: 262-953-5501
webinfo@bruno.com
www.bruno.com
Michael R. Bruno, II, President & CEO
Stairlift with 400 lb lift capacity. Indoor and outdoor stairlifts available.

359 **Freedom Wheels**
Freedom Wheels
580 Tc Jester Blvd
Houston, TX 77007
713-864-1460
888-422-5337
Fax: 713-864-1469
info@freedomwheels.com
www.freedomwheels.com
Carlos Saez, Owner
An assistive technology and mobility equipment provider and is committed to people with disabilities and personal transportation options for an independent lifestyle.

360 **Handi Home Lift**
Handi-Lift
730 Garden St
Carlstadt, NJ 07072-1625
201-933-0111
800-432-5438
Fax: 201-933-0050
sales@handi-lift.com
www.handi-lift.com
Douglas Boydston, President
An outdoor lift designed to provide access over porch stairs or other steps that impede movement.

361 **Handi Lift**
Handi-Lift
730 Garden St
Carlstadt, NJ 07072-1625
201-933-0111
800-432-5438
Fax: 201-933-0050
sales@handi-lift.com
www.handi-lift.com
Douglas Boydston, President
Accessibility with Dignity. Solutions that enable users with mobility impairments to live freely with products like wheelchair lifts and home elevators.

362 **Handi Prolift**
Handi-Lift
730 Garden St
Carlstadt, NJ 07072-1625
201-933-0111
800-432-5438
Fax: 201-933-0050
sales@handi-lift.com
www.handi-lift.com
Douglas Boydston, President
Provides dependable vertical transportation for multi-level buildings.

363 **Handi-Ramp**
Handi-Ramp
510 North Ave
Libertyville, IL 60048-2025
847-680-7700
800-876-7267
Fax: 847-816-7689
info@handiramp.com
www.handiramp.com
Thomas Disch, President & CEO
Alicia C. Johns, Program Manager
Provides a complete line of economical, ADA Compliant access ramping products. Line includes van attachable and wheelchair tie downs; aluminum or expanded metal folding portables; aluminum channels; portable, sectional ramp systems; semi-permanent ramps, platforms and systems. All ramp series are available in varied lengths and widths in combination with platforms and optional hand railing, single or double bar construction with return ends. Special Order ramps and ramp systems.

364 **Homewaiter**
Inclinator Company of America
601 Gibson Blvd
Harrisburg, PA 17104-3215
717-939-8420
800-343-9007
Fax: 717-939-8075
isales@inclinator.com
www.inclinator.com
Cliff Warner, President & CEO
Mark Crispen, Director of Marketing, Corporate Secretary & Board Member
Brad Rose, Sales Manager
Steve Smith, Sales Manager
With its roller truck riding in a specially formed monorail, it is easy to install and highly adaptable to existing conditions. It can travel up to 35 feet, opening on any or all three sides at different stations, whether at counter level or floor level.

365 **Horcher Lifting Systems**
Horcher Medical Systems
324 Cypress Rd
Ocala, FL 34472-3102
352-687-8020
800-582-8732
Fax: 866-378-3318
us-office@horcher.com
www.horcher.com
David Schultz, General Manager
Sharon Harbert, Administrative Assistant
Barrier Free Lifts by Horcher leads the industry for excellence in patient transfers and technology for over 18 years. They offer state of the art ceiling track systems, floor base lifts and bathing systems such as the Unilift, PC-2, Diana, Lexa, and Raisa to achieve greater mobility.

366 **Inclinette**
Inclinator Company of America
601 Gibson Blvd
Harrisburg, PA 17104-3215
717-939-8420
800-343-9007
Fax: 717-939-8075
isales@inclinator.com
www.inclinator.com
Cliff Warner, President & CEO
Mark Crispen, Director of Marketing, Corporate Secretary & Board Member
Brad Rose, Sales Manager
Steve Smith, Sales Manager
Inclinette provides comfort and convenience in providing multi-floor access to persons who have difficulty climbing stairs.

367 **Independent Driving Systems**
Independent Driving Systems
580 T.C. Jester
Houston, TX 77007
713-864-1460
888-422-5337
Fax: 713-864-1469
info@independentdrivingsystems.com
www.independentdrivingsystems.com
Chad Donnelly, Owner
Provides adaptive driving systems for individuals with disabilities with more severe higher levels of injury that require more so-

phisticated types of assistive technology to enable them to drive safely.

368 **Joey Interior Platform Lift**
Bruno Independent Living Aids, Inc.
1780 Executive Dr.
PO Box 84
Oconomowoc, WI 53066
262-567-4990
800-454-4355
Fax: 262-953-5501
webinfo@bruno.com
www.bruno.com

Michael R. Bruno, II, President & CEO
Lifts and stores unoccupied scooters or powerchairs in the back of a minivan at the touch of a button.

369 **KlearVue**
Ricon
1135 Aviation Pl.
San Fernando, CA 91340
818-267-3000
800-322-2884
Fax: 800-962-1201
ricinsales@wabtec.com
www.riconcorp.com

370 **Lectra-Lift**
La-Z-Boy
1284 N Telegraph Rd
Monroe, MI 48162-5138
734-242-1444
800-375-6890
Fax: 734-457-2005
www.lazboy.com

Kurt L. Darrow, CEO
David M. Risley, Senior Vice President & CFO
Patrick H. Norton, Chair
This power recliner has a single motor drive that operates three distinct cycles: lifting, leg elevation and full power recline.

371 **Liberty LT**
Handi-Lift
730 Garden St
Carlstadt, NJ 07072-1625
201-933-0111
800-432-5438
Fax: 201-933-0050
www.handi-lift.com

Douglas Boydston, President
Stair lift with dual armrests that lock into position. The comfortable, contoured seat is designed to swivel and move forward at the bottom or top landings to facilitate transfer.

372 **Lift-All**
Amigo Mobility International
6693 Dixie Highway
Bridgeport, MI 48722-9725
989-777-0910
800-248-9131
Fax: 800-334-7274
info@myamigo.com
www.myamigo.com

Al Thieme, Chair & Founder
Beth Thieme, President & CEO
Sandy Humpert, Sales Representative
Leading manufacturer of electric mobility; Amigo's Lift-All transports your wheelchair easily into the trunk of an automobile and neatly stores it for easy access. *$965.00*

373 **Lifter**
Bruno Independent Living Aids, Inc.
1780 Executive Dr.
PO Box 84
Oconomowoc, WI 53066
262-567-4990
800-454-4355
Fax: 262-953-5501
webinfo@bruno.com
www.bruno.com

Michael R. Bruno, II, President & CEO
Raises and stows folding manual wheelchairs, travel scooters, and travel power chairs. 200 lb lift capacity.

374 **Lifts for Swimming Pools and Spas**
Aquatic Access
1921 Production Dr
Louisville, KY 40299-2110
502-425-5817
800-325-5438
Fax: 502-425-9607
info@AquaticAccess.com
www.aquaticaccess.com

Linda Nolan, President
David Nolan, Vice President & CEO
Aquatic Access manufacturers and sells water-powered lifts providing access to in-ground and above-ground swimming pools, spas, boats and docks. *$2310.00*

375 **Mac's Lift Gate**
Mac's Lift Gate, Inc.
2801 South Street
Long Beach, CA 90805-3751
562-634-5962
800-795-6227
Fax: 562-529-3466
sales@macsliftgate.com
www.macsliftgate.com

Randy Maner, Training Manager
Sales and service of van and truck lifts. Sales and service of wheel chair lifts for vans and automobiles. Sales, installation and service of vertical home lifts, scooter lifts and pool lifts. Sales of scooters.

376 **Mecalift Sling Lifter**
Arjo Inc
2349 West Lake Street
Suite 250
Addison, IL 60101
630-785-4490
800-323-1245
Fax: 630-576-5020
usa.info@ArjoHuntleigh.com
www.arjo.com

Joacim Lindoff, President & CEO
Jonas Lindqvist, CFO
Marion Gullstrand, Executive Vice President, Human Resources & CSR
Katarzyna Bobrow, Executive Vice President, Quality & Regulatory Compliance
Tailored to the mobility level and needs of the resident and patient for the purpose of lifting manoeuvers.

377 **Motorhome Lift**
Handicaps, Inc.
4335 S Santa Fe Dr.
Englewood, CO 80110-5417
303-781-2062
800-782-4335
info@handicapsinc.com
www.handicapsinc.com

378 **One for All Lift All**
Amigo Mobility International
6693 Dixie Highway
Bridgeport, MI 48722-9725
989-777-0910
800-248-9131
Fax: 800-334-7274
info@myamigo.com
www.myamigo.com

Al Thieme, Chair & Founder
Beth Thieme, President & CEO
Sandy Humpert, Sales Representative
Amigo Mobility designs and manufactures a complete line of power operated vehicles and mobility scooters and accessories.

379 **Out-Sider III**
Bruno Independent Living Aids, Inc.
1780 Executive Dr.
PO Box 84
Oconomowoc, WI 53066
262-567-4990
800-454-4355
Fax: 262-953-5501
webinfo@bruno.com
www.bruno.com

Michael R. Bruno, II, President & CEO
Exterior platform lift. Maintains seating and cargo space. Designed specifically for rear-view visibility. Platform folds automatically when not being used. 350 lb lift capacity.

380 **Out-Sider Meridian**
Bruno Independent Living Aids, Inc.
1780 Executive Dr.
PO Box 84
Oconomowoc, WI 53066
262-567-4990
800-454-4355
Fax: 262-953-5501
webinfo@bruno.com
www.bruno.com
Michael R. Bruno, II, President & CEO
Lets the user carry their scooter fully assembled, keeping trunk space available for other possessions.

381 **Parker Bath**
Arjo Inc
2349 West Lake Street
Suite 250
Addison, IL 60101
630-785-4490
800-323-1245
Fax: 630-576-5020
www.arjo.com
Joacim Lindoff, President & CEO
Jonas Lindqvist, CFO
Marion Gullstrand, Executive Vice President, Human Resources & CSR
Katarzyna Bobrow, Executive Vice President, Quality & Regulatory Compliance
This product involves no manual lifting, strain or stress for the caregiver.

382 **Patient Lifting & Injury Prevention**
Arjo Inc
2349 West Lake Street
Suite 250
Addison, IL 60101
630-785-4490
800-323-1245
Fax: 630-576-5020
www.arjo.com
Joacim Lindoff, President & CEO
Jonas Lindqvist, CFO
Marion Gullstrand, Executive Vice President, Human Resources & CSR
Katarzyna Bobrow, Executive Vice President, Quality & Regulatory Compliance
Aids in patient lifting while protecting the caregiver from the risk of backstrain.

383 **Portable Wheelchair Ramp**
Maxi Aids
42 Executive Blvd.
Farmingdale, NY 11735-4710
631-752-0521
800-522-6294
Fax: 631-752-0689
TTY: 631-752-0738
sales@maxiaids.com
www.maxiaids.com
Elliot Zaretsky, Founder, President & CEO
Single-fold ramp designed to help wheelchair or scooter users easily transition from one surface level to another.

384 **Ramplette Telescoping Ramp**
Graham-Field Health Products
2935 Northeast Parkway
Atlanta, GA 30360-2808
770-368-4700
Fax: 770-368-4932
cs@grahamfield.com
www.grahamfield.com
Kenneth Spett, President & CEO
Cherie Antoniazzi, Senior Vice President, Quality, Regulatory & Risk Management
Marc Bernstein, Senior Vice President, Consumer Sales
Lawrence De La Haba, Senior Vice President, Business Development
A multi-functional, easily moved, economical ramp weighing 25 pounds.

385 **Rickshaw Exerciser**
Access to Recreation
8 Sandra Ct
Newbury Park, CA 91320-4302
805-498-7535
800-634-4351
Fax: 805-498-8186
customerservice@accesstr.com
www.accesstr.com
Don Krebs, President & Founder
This Exerciser develops the muscle used most by those in wheelchairs. It develops the strength you need to lift yourself for pressure relief, doing transfers and pushing your wheelchair.

386 **Ricon Classic**
Ricon
1135 Aviation Pl.
San Fernando, CA 91340
818-267-3000
800-322-2884
Fax: 800-962-1201
ricinsales@wabtec.com
www.riconcorp.com

387 **Ricon Corporation**
1135 Aviation Pl.
San Fernando, CA 91340
818-267-3000
800-322-2884
Fax: 800-962-1201
ricinsales@wabtec.com
www.riconcorp.com

388 **Smart Leg**
Invacare
1 Invacare Way
Elyria, OH 44035-4190
440-329-6000
800-333-6900
Fax: 877-619-7996
www.invacare.com
Matthew E. Monaghan, Chair, President & CEO
Darcie Karol, Senior Vice President Human Resources
Kathleen P. Leneghan, Senior Vice President & CFO
Anthony C. LaPlaca, Senior Vice President, General Counsel & Secretary
An ingenious elevating leg rest that automatically extends to correctly fit every outstretched leg.

389 **Smooth Mover**
Dixie EMS
10101 Foster Ave
Brooklyn, NY 11236-3425
718-257-6400
800-347-3494
Fax: 718-257-6401
customerservice@dixieems.com
www.dixieems.com
Eva Silverstein, President
Patient mover is a board designed to transfer patients from bed to stretcher or table with one or two people. Being radio-translucent makes it suitable for x-ray procedures. *$199.95*

390 **Space-Saver**
Bruno Independent Living Aids, Inc.
1780 Executive Dr.
PO Box 84
Oconomowoc, WI 53066
262-567-4990
800-454-4355
Fax: 262-953-5501
webinfo@bruno.com
www.bruno.com
Michael R. Bruno, II, President & CEO
Take-apart hoist-style lift for transporting light mobility devices. 200 lb lift capacity.

391 **SpectraLift**
Inclinator Company of America
601 Gibson Blvd
Harrisburg, PA 17104-3215
717-939-8420
800-343-9007
Fax: 717-939-8075
isales@inclinator.com
www.inclinator.com
Cliff Warner, President & CEO
Mark Crispen, Director of Marketing, Corporate Secretary & Board Member
Brad Rose, Sales Manager
Steve Smith, Sales Manager
A newly designed hydraulic wheelchair lift made of fiberglass construction suitable for commercial and residential use.

392 **Spectrum Products**
Spectrum Aquatics
7100 Spectrum Lane
Missoula, MT 59808-8416
406-542-9781
800-791-8056
Fax: 800-791-8057
info@spectrumproducts.com
www.spectrumproducts.com
Nabil Khaled, Vice President of Sales, Regional Sales Manager
Rob Nelson, Manager of Logistics & Customer Service
Philip Frandsen, Customer Service Representative
Josh Hartley, Business Development Specialist (Southeast Region)
Manufacturers of swimming pool disabled access products such as lifts, ramps, railings, ladders, and stainless steel hydrotherapy tanks for the swimming pool and medical therapy markets.

393 **Spectrum Products Catalog**
Spectrum Aquatics
7100 Spectrum Lane
Missoula, MT 59808-8416
406-542-9781
800-791-8056
Fax: 800-791-8057
info@spectrumproducts.com
www.spectrumproducts.com
Nabil Khaled, Vice President of Sales, Regional Sales Manager
Rob Nelson, Manager of Logistics & Customer Service
Philip Frandsen, Customer Service Representative
Josh Hartley, Business Development Specialist (Southeast Region)
Manufacturers of swimming pool disabled access products such as lifts, ramps, railings, ladders, and stainless steel hydrotherapy tanks for the swimming pool and medical therapy markets.

394 **StairLIFT SC & SL**
Inclinator Company of America
601 Gibson Blvd
Harrisburg, PA 17104-3215
717-939-8420
800-343-9007
Fax: 717-939-8075
isales@inclinator.com
www.inclinator.com
Cliff Warner, President & CEO
Mark Crispen, Director of Marketing, Corporate Secretary & Board Member
Brad Rose, Sales Manager
Steve Smith, Sales Manager
Simple, self-contained and efficient stair units.

395 **Superarm Lift for Vans**
Handicaps, Inc.
4335 S Santa Fe Dr.
Englewood, CO 80110-5417
303-781-2062
800-782-4335
info@handicapsinc.com
www.handicapsinc.com

396 **SureHands Lift & Care Systems**
982 County Route 1
Pine Island, NY 10969-1205
845-258-6500
800-724-5305
Fax: 845-258-6634
info@surehands.com
www.surehands.com
Thomas Herceg, President
Joyce Moraczewski, Marketing Coordinator
Doug Siegel, General Sales Manager
SureHands specializes in lift & care systems for both homecare and professional settings where safety is most important, to assist an individual in overcoming physical and architectural barriers. Some of their products include lifting and body support systems, handi-slides, accessories and bathing equipment.

397 **Thyssen Krupp Access Solutions**
Thyssen Krupp Access Solutions
4001 East 138th Street
Grandview, MO 64030-2837
816-763-3100
800-829-9760
Fax: 816-763-4467
dealerinfo@tkaccess.com
www.tkaccess.com
Mauro Carneiro, CEO
Thyssen Krupp Access provides wheelchair lift, stair lift or elevator solutions to suit any budget and needs. Nationwide network of dealers are in close proximity to the customers.

398 **Vangater, Vangater II, Mini-Vangater**
BraunAbility
645 W Carmel Dr.
Carmel, IN 46032
800-488-0359
888-365-9417
questions@braunability.com
www.braunability.com
Staci Kroon, President & CEO
Tri-fold and fold-in-half lifts for adapted van transportation.

399 **Versatrainer**
Pro- Max/ Division Of Bow- Flex Of America
2200 NE 65th Ave
Vancouver, WA 98661-6978
800-618-8853
800-952-7205
Fax: 360-993-3610
customerservice@bowflex.com
www.bowflex.com

400 **Vestibular Board**
Bailey Manufacturing Company
118 Lee Drive
P.O. Box 130
Lodi, OH 44254-130
330-948-1080
800-321-8372
Fax: 330-948-4439
baileymfg@baileymfg.com
www.baileymfg.com
Larry Strimple, President
Judie Butler, Dealer Contact
Creates tilting in a rolling motion for reclining patients who need help developing balance.

401 **Wheelchair Carrier**
Wheelchair Carrier
7325 Douglas Road
Lambertville, MI 48144-2624
734-568-6084
800-541-3213
Fax: 734-568-6705
admin@WheelChairCarrier.com
wheelchaircarrier.com
David Makulinsky, President
Mike Siler, Engineer
Christina Makulinski, Office Manager
Wheelchair, scooter and powerchair carriers for hitch mount on vehicles, both manual and electric, making it easy and simple to transport the user's mobility device.

402 **Williams Lift Company**
24 S Ave.
Fanwood, NJ 07023
908-325-3648
Fax: 308-322-8020
contact@williamslifts.com
www.williamslifts.com
Barry Williams, Owner
A division of Williams Surgical, Williams Lift Company offers stairlifts, wheelchair ramps, and power lift recliners. Services include installation, repairs, and rentals.

Major Catalogs

403 **Access to Recreation**
Access To Recreation
8 Sandra Ct
Newbury Park, CA 91320-4302
805-498-7535
800-634-4351
Fax: 805-498-8186
customerservice@accesstr.com
www.accesstr.com

Don Krebs, President & Founder

The Access to Recreation catalog is full of recreation and exercise equipment. One can find items such as electric fishing reels and other fishing and hunting equipment for the disabled sportsman. There are also adapted golf clubs, swimming pool lifts, wheelchair gloves and cuffs and bowling equipment. There are devices to help with embroidery, knitting and card playing, videos, books and practical aides such as wheelchair ramps and book.

64 pages Bi-Annually

404 **Achievement Products**
P.O. Box 6013
Carol Stream, IL 60197-6013
800-373-4699
Fax: 800-766-4303
Bids@achievement-products.com
www.specialkidszone.com

Teresa Cardon, Vice President

Offer a wide range of pediatric rehabilitation equipment and special education products including handwriting aids, weighted vests, positioning equipment, sensory integration products and adaptive furniture. Call for your free catalog.

405 **Adaptive Clothing: Adults**
Special Clothes
P.O. Box 333
E Harwich, MA 02645-333
508-385-9171
Fax: 508-430-2410
specialclo@aol.com
www.special-clothes.com

Judith Sweeney, President

Special Clothes produces a catalogue of garments for adults with disabilities and incontinence. Offerings include: undergarments, snap-crotch tee shirts, sleepwear, jumpsuits, bibs and some footwear. Special Clothes produces a catalog of adaptive clothing for children in sizes from toddler through young adults. A full line of clothing is included from undergarments through wheelchair jackets and ponchos.

406 **Adaptive Technology Catalog**
Synapse Adaptive
14 Lynn Ct
San Rafael, CA 94901-5114
415-455-9700
800-317-9611
Fax: 415-455-9801
info@synapse-ada.com
www.synapseadaptive.com

Martin Tibor, President

Adaptive technology for individuals with disabilities, ADA compliant workstations, and ergonomic furniture. Products accommodate blindness, low vision, mobility impairments or learning differences.

407 **Adult Long Jumpsuit with Feet**
Special Clothes
P.O. Box 333
E Harwich, MA 02645-333
508-385-9171
Fax: 508-430-2410
specialclo@aol.com
www.special-clothes.com

Judith Sweeney, President

Line of clothing for people with disabilities. Child and adult catalog available.

408 **Adult Short Jumpsuit**
Special Clothes
P.O. Box 333
E Harwich, MA 02645-333
508-385-9171
Fax: 508-430-2410
specialclo@aol.com
www.special-clothes.com

Judith Sweeney, President

This pull-on jumpsuit provides comfort and full coverage without bulk. Wide leg ribbing ends at mid-thigh, with snaps at the crotch.

409 **AliMed**
Alimed, Inc.
297 High Street
Dedham, MA 02026
781-329-2900
800-225-2610
Fax: 781-329-8392
customerservice@alimed.com
alimed.com

410 **American Discount Medical**
American Discount Medical
459 Main Street
Suite 101-417
Trussville, AL 35173
205-467-6995
800-877-9100
Fax: 205-467-7095
www.americandiscountmed.com

Tom Ruf, General Manager

Medical supply company dedicated to providing medical products of the highest quality. Offers deep discounts for all major brands of medical products.

411 **Apria Healthcare**
Apria Healthcare Group, Inc.
26220 Enterprise Court
Lake Forest, CA 92630
949-639-2000
800-277-4288
contact_us@apria.com
www.apria.com

Dan Starck, CEO
Debra Morris, CFO
Celina M Scally, Senior Vice President
Nichola Denney, Executive Vice President, Revenue Management

Lifts, chairs, bathroom aids, bedroom aids, eating utensils and independent living aids for the physically challenged.

412 **Armstrong Medical**
American Medical Industries, Inc.
575 Knightsbridge Parkway
P.O. Box 700
Lincolnshire, IL 60069-700
847-913-0101
800-323-4220
Fax: 847-913-0138
csr@armstrongmedical.com
www.armstrongmedical.com

Armstrong, CEO
Diane Joseph, Customer Representative
John E. Figel, National Sales Manager

Training aids, anatomical models, medical equipment, pediatrics equipment and rehabilitation equipment.

413 **Assistive Technology Journal**
Technologists, Inc.
1700 N Moore St
Suite 1905
Rosslyn, VA 22209-1905
703-243-1975
Fax: 703-524-6630
email@technologistsinc.com
www.technologistsinc.com

Sayed "Aziz" Azimi, President & CEO

Integrates technical and management in difficult environments. Various disciplines include architecture, engineering, construction management, etc. *$32.50*

Bi-Annually

414 **Assistive Technology Sourcebook**
Special Needs Project
324 State Street
Suite H
Santa Barbara, CA 93101-2364
818-718-9900
800-333-6867
Fax: 818-349-2027
editor@specialneeds.com
www.specialneeds.com

Hod Gray, Owner
Marian Hall, Editor
Provides you with 18 chapters of practical information on all aspects of assistive technology for individuals with functional limitations. *$60.00*
576 pages

415 **Bailey**
Bailey Manufacturing Company
118 Lee Drive
P.O. Box 130
Lodi, OH 44254-130
330-948-1080
800-321-8372
Fax: 330-948-4439
baileymfg@baileymfg.com
www.baileymfg.com

Larry Strimple, President
Judie Butler, Dealer Contact
Ambulation aids, balance aids, benches, chairs, exercise devices, tables, stools, rehabilitation and physical therapy equipment for the physically challenged.
70 pages

416 **Body Suits**
Special Clothes
P.O. Box 333
E Harwich, MA 02645-333
508-385-9171
Fax: 508-430-2410
specialclo@aol.com
www.special-clothes.com

Judith Sweeney, President
Bodysuits, Jumpsuits, back opening garments, incontinence wear, bibs. Features include snap crotches and g-tube pockets.

417 **Cambridge Career Products Catalog**
Cambridge Educational
132 West 31st Street
16th Floor
New York, NY 10001
800-322-8755
800-468-4227
Fax: 800-678-3633
custserv@films.com
cambridge.films.com

Lisa Schmuclei, Marketing Director
A full color catalog featuring hundreds of products designed to aid people in career exploration, selecting specific occupations and obtaining these jobs through resume and interview preparation.
64 pages BiAnnual

418 **Carex Health Brands**
Carex Health Brands
P.O. Box 2526
Sioux Falls, SD 57101-2526
800-526-8051
800-328-2935
Fax: 866-760-8967
customerservice@carex.com
carex.com

Duane Wagner, CEO
The Carex brand provides a full line of home healthCare mobility, bath safety and personal care products that improve quality of life and increase independence. Consistently provides innovative, high-quality, safe and reliable products that exceed customer expectations.

419 **Carolyn's Low Vision Products**
3938 S. Tamiami Trail
Sarasota, FL 34231-3622
941-337-5555
800-648-2266
Fax: 941-957-0933
www.carolynscatalog.com

John Colton, Owner
A trusted leader in low-vision products. Free national mail-order catalog of items for visually impaired and blind people. Well versed in a variety of eye diseases that damage vision and have an expertise in helping customers making product purchasing decisions for their needs.

420 **Communication Aids for Children and Adults**
Crestwood Communication Aids
6589 N
Crestwood Drive
Milwaukee, WI 53209
414-351-0311
crestcomm@aol.com
www.communicationaids.com

Ruth B. Leff, President
A free catalog of communication aids for children and adults with disabilities. Over 300 light and high tech switches and aids, and a large selection of adapted and voice-activated toys. Talking Pictures and Passports communication boards, easy to use and moderately priced talking aids.
32 pages Yearly

421 **Connect Hearing**
Hearing Center
1111 W Centre Ave
Portage, MI 49024
269-324-0301
800-445-9968
888-426-6632
Fax: 269-324-2387
info@connecthearing.com
www.connecthearing.com

Marcello J. Celentano, President & CEO
Specializes in products for the hard of hearing and deaf as required under ADA including visual alerting products for fire, phone, door, wake up, phone amplification, TTY, FM and infrared listening systems. Provides expertise on diagnosing hearing loss.

422 **Danmar Products**
221 Jackson Industrial Dr
Ann Arbor, MI 48103
734-761-1990
800-783-1998
Fax: 734-761-8977
sales@danmarproducts.com
www.danmarproducts.com

Dan Russo, President
Hidie Bowman, Chief Operating Officer
Manufactures adaptive equipment for persons with physical and mental disabilities. Products include seating and positioning equipment, flotation devices, toileting aids, and hard and soft shell helmets.

423 **Dayspring Associates, Inc.**
2111 Foley Road
Havre De Grace, MD 21078-1703
410-939-5900
Fax: 410-939-6252

Benedict Schwartz, Vice President & Director Manager
This publisher provides a directory of 1,000 rehabilitation aids.

424 **Disabilities Sourcebook**
Omnigraphics
615 Griswold Street
Suite 520
Detroit, MI 48226
610-461-3548
800-234-1340
Fax: 800-875-1340
contact@omnigraphics.com
www.omnigraphics.com

Peter Ruffner, Co-Founder
Fred Ruffner, Co-Founder
For people with disabilities and caregivers, this product gives general information concerning birth defects, loss in hearing and vision, speech disorders, learning disorders,intellectual and cognitive disabilities, and other impairments due to illness, injury, and trauma. *$78.00*
616 pages
ISBN 0-780803-89-2

425 **Disability Bookshop Catalog**
P.O. Box 129
Vancouver, WA 98666-129
360-694-2462
800-637-2256
Fax: 360-696-3210

40 pages

426 **Dressing Tips and Clothing Resources for Making Life Easier**
Attainment Company
504 Commerce Parkway
P.O. Box 930160
Verona, WI 53593- 160
608-845-7880
800-327-4269
Fax: 800-942-3865
info@attainmentcompany.com
www.attainmentcompany.com

Autumn Garza, President
Don Bastian, CEO

Offers more than 100 resources specially designed or easy-on/easy-off clothing for men, women, children and wheelchair users. An invaluable resource for people with special dressing needs, people with disabilities, caregivers and healthcare professionals. *$19.00*

144 pages 2000
ISBN 1-578611-19-9

427 **Enrichments Catalog**
Performance Health
28100 Torch Parkway
Suite 700
Warrenville, IL 60555-3938
630-393-6000
Fax: 630-393-7600
customersupport@performancehealth.com
www.performancehealth.com

Francis Dirksmeier, CEO
Isabel Afonso, Managing Director & Head of International
Daniel Baumwald, Vice President, North America Retail & eCommerce
Laurie Byrne, Chief Human Resources Officer

Provides people with physical challenges with the products they need to help live their lives to the fullest. Includes items for everyday tasks and personal care; assistive products for home use; toileting and bathing aids; grooming and dressing devices; kitchen and dining aids. Also items for range of motion, mobility and exercise such as weights, therapy putty and exercise equipment; ergonomic gloves and supports; canes, crutches, walkers and wheelchair accessories. 36-page catalog.

428 **Equipment Shop**
34 Hartford Street
P.O. Box 33
Bedford, MA 01730-33
781-275-7681
800-525-7681
Fax: 781-275-4094
www.equipmentshop.com

Ken Larson, President
Carrie Larson, Manager

Specializing in oral motor therapy equipment, including Flexi Cut Cups, Maroon Spoons, Chewy Tubes, ARK grabbers and z-vibes. Also tricycle foot peal attachments and trike back supports as well as fat wheels.

429 **Essential Medical Supply, Inc.**
6420 Hazeltine National Drive
Orlando, FL 32822
407-770-0710
800-826-8423
Fax: 407-770-0624
essentialmedicalsupply.com

John Hoepner, President
Carol Ann Hoepner, Secretary & Treasurer
Michael J. Hoepner, Vice President & COO
Matthew T. Hoepner, Vice President & Marketing

A broad based supplier of home medical and health related products designed with the needs of the user in mind.

430 **Everest & Jennings**
Division of Graham-Field
2935 Northeast Parkway
Atlanta, GA 30360-2808
770-368-4700
Fax: 770-368-4932
cs@grahamfield.com
www.grahamfield.com

Kenneth Spett, President & CEO
Cherie Antoniazzi, Senior Vice President, Quality, Regulatory & Risk Management
Marc Bernstein, Senior Vice President, Consumer Sales
Lawrence De La Haba, Senior Vice President, Business Development

Manufactures more than 200 items for persons with physical disabilities, including wheelchairs, seat cushions, shower chairs, grab bars and more.

431 **Express Medical Supply**
218 Seebold Spur
Fenton, MO 63026
636-349-8448
800-633-2139
Fax: 800-633-9188
sales@exmed.net
www.exmed.net

Bill Nahm, President

Offers a full line of high quality medical and ostomy supplies to individuals, clinics, and medical institutions.

432 **FlagHouse, Inc.**
601 FLAGHOUSE DRIVE
Hasbrouck Heights, NJ 07604-3116
201-288-7600
800-793-7900
Fax: 800-793-7922
sales@flaghouse.com
www.flaghouse.com

George Carmel, President

Global supplier of products for physical activity, recreation, education and special needs with the mantra of improving the lives of everyone.

Bi-Annually

433 **Freedom Rider**
Freedom Rider
5225 Tudor Court
Naples, FL 34112
603-540-0933
888-253-8811
Fax: 866-522-4708
info@freedomrider.com
www.freedomrider.com

Victoria Surr, President

A catalog of equipment for people with disabilities who ride and drive horses which includes instructional aids, vaulting equipment, and lots of hard to find items. Provides safety in their prod for riders, horses, instructors, and trainers.

434 **Health and Rehabilitation Products**
Luminaud, Inc.
8688 Tyler Blvd
Mentor, OH 44060
440-255-9082
800-255-3408
Fax: 440-255-2250
info@luminaud.com
www.luminaud.com

Thomas M. Lennox, President
Dorothy Lennox, Vice President

Switches for limited capability, stoma and trach covers, shower protectors and thermo-stim oral motor stimulator. Personal voice amplifiers for people with weak voices. Artificial larynges for people with no voices. Small electronic communication boards. Books for laryngectomies and speech pathologists.

435 **HealthCare Solutions**
Blue Chip II
3478 Hauck Road
Cincinnati, OH 45241
513-271-5115
800-417-5115
Fax: 513-527-3686

Michael Leabhart, Manager

Quality rehabilitation equipment sales and rental. Available equipment includes manual and powered mobility, positioning/seating equipment, vehicle modification, environmental controls, augmentative and alternative communication devices, adaptive computer access, ambulance aids and aids for daily living. Equipment provision is carried out through a total team approach. .

436 **Hear You Are**
98 Us Highway 46
Budd Lake, NJ 07828-1818
973-347-7662
Fax: 973-691-0611

Dorinne S Davis, President
A large catalog of various assistive and communication devices for people who are hearing impaired. *$3.00*
42 pages

437 **Hig's Manufacturing**
8375 Sunset Rd Ne
Minneapolis, MN 55418-3238
763-795-9478
Fax: 612-788-1926

Jim Murphy, Owner
Factory direct, lightweight aluminum, portable, 2 & 4-way folding, telescoping tracks, threshold, van, scooter and approach ramps.

438 **Huntleigh Healthcare**
2349 W. Lake Street
Suite 250
Addison, IL 60101
630-785-4490
800-323-1245
Fax: 888-594-2756
www.huntleigh-healthcare.us

439 **Invacare Corporation**
1 Invacare Way
Elyria, OH 44035-4190
440-329-6000
800-333-6900
Fax: 877-619-7996
invacare.com

Matthew E. Monaghan, Chair, President & CEO
Dean Childers, Senior Vice President & General Manager, North America
The global leader in the manufacture and distribution of innovative home and long-term care medical products that promote recovery and active lifestyles.

440 **Kleinert's**
433 Newton St
Elba, AL 36323
800-498-7051
Fax: 305-937-0825
customercare@kleinerts.com
www.kleinerts.com

Michael Brier, President
Offers a complete line of sweat and odor protection products, incontinence products, and skin care products consisting of disposable and reusable panties for women and pants for men. Also disposable liners, diapers, underpads,antiperspirant wipes, deodorants, bedding, underpads, and cleaning solutions.

441 **LS&S**
145 River Rock Drive
Buffalo, NY 14207
716-348-3500
800-468-4789
Fax: 877-498-1482
LSSInfo@LSSproducts.com
www.LSSproducts.com

Melissa Balbach, President
John K. Bace, Executive Vice President
Specializes in products for the blind, visually impaired, hearing impaired, and deaf. A variety of hearing helpers, daily living aids, and vision aids. LS&S aids in the adjustment of alterations in life.

442 **Lighthouse Low Vision Products**
Lighthouse Guild
250 West 64th Street
New York, NY 10023
646-874-8219
800-284-4422
Fax: 212-821-9707
info@lighthouse.org
www.lighthouseguild.org

Alan R. Morse, President & CEO
Lawrence E. Goldschmidt, Deputy Chair & Secretary
Himanshu R. Shah, CFO
Maura J. Sweeney, Senior Vice President, Programs & Services

This organization provides health care services related to vision loss; Career and academic services for people with vision loss; Music instruction and pre K curriculum for visually impaired students.

443 **Luminaud, Inc.**
8688 Tyler Blvd
Mentor, OH 44060-4348
440-255-9082
800-255-3408
Fax: 440-255-2250
info@luminaud.com
www.luminaud.com

Thomas M. Lennox, President
Dorothy Lennox, Vice President
Offers a line of artificial larynx, personal voice amplifiers, special switches, stoma covers and other communication, health and safety items.

444 **MOMS Catalog**
Home Delivery Incontinent Supplies
9385 Dielman Ind Dr
Saint Louis, MO 63132-2214
800-269-4663
Fax: 314-997-0047
custcare@hdis.com
www.hdis.com

Bruce Grench, President
MOMS catalog features high quality, incontinence supplies, mobility products, bath safety products urological products, aids for daily living products, ostomy supplies and many other adaptive items. MOMS offers low prices, excellent customer service and convenient home delivery to your doorstep.
52 pages

445 **Maddak Inc.**
661 Route 23 South
Wayne, NJ 07470
973-628-7600
800-443-4926
Fax: 973-305-0841
custservice@maddak.com
maddak.com

Brian Larkin, President & CEO
Maddak is proud to be a leading manufacturer of home healthcare products for seniors, people with disabilities and people recovering from injuries and illnesses. Marketed under the Ableware brand name, our products make daily living activities easier enabling you to remain active and independent.

446 **Maxi Aids**
Maxi Aids
42 Executive Blvd.
Farmingdale, NY 11735-4710
631-752-0521
800-522-6294
Fax: 631-752-0689
TTY: 631-752-0738
sales@maxiaids.com
www.maxiaids.com

Elliot Zaretsky, Founder, President & CEO
Products specially designed for blind, low vision, visually impaired, deaf, deaf-blind, hard of hearing, arthritic, diabetic, and disabled persons.

447 **New Vision Store**
ASB
919 Walnut Street
Philadelphia, PA 19107-5237
215-627-0600
Fax: 215-922-0692
asbinfo@asb.org
www.asb.org

Karla S. McCaney, President & CEO
Beth Deering, Director, Human Services
Richard Forsythe, Director, Braille Division & Custom Audio
Joyce Robertson, Director, Finance & Information Technology
Catalog for individuals with visual impairments, listing visual aids, magnifiers, large print books and more.
30 pages

448 **Pearson Performance Solutions**
1 North Dearborn
Suite 1150
Chicago, IL 60602
800-922-7343
Fax: 312-242-4403
David Fabianski, Senior Vice President & General Manager
Cindy Hotsky, Finance Director
Julia McClung, Vice President, Talent Management Solutions
Publishes human resource assessment instruments for employment settings. The instruments include job analysis procedures to identify important characteristics for job success and objective assessment procedures to evaluate applicants and employees on these characteristics.

449 **Performance Health**
28100 Torch Parkway
Suite 700
Warrenville, IL 60555-3938
630-393-6000
800-323-5547
Fax: 630-393-7600
customersupport@performancehealth.com
www.performancehealth.com
Francis Dirksmeier, CEO
Isabel Afonso, Managing Director & Head of International
Daniel Baumwald, Vice President, North America Retail & eCommerce
Laurie Byrne, Chief Human Resources Officer
Performance Health is a global provider of rehabilitation, assistive, amd splinting products, working with occupational therapists, physical therapists, long-term care facilities, and clinics.

450 **Performance Health Enrichments Catalog**
Performance Health
28100 Torch Parkway
Suite 700
Warrenville, IL 60555-3938
630-393-6000
Fax: 630-393-7600
customersupport@performancehealth.com
www.performancehealth.com
Francis Dirksmeier, CEO
Isabel Afonso, Managing Director & Head of International
Daniel Baumwald, Vice President, North America Retail & eCommerce
Laurice Byrne, Chief Human Resources Officer
Performance Health Enrichments Catalog offers products that make the tasks and challenges of living at home— bathing, getting dressed, getting around— a little easier. Choose from personal care items to kitchen and dining aids, household helpers to mobility devices, plus a complete selection of pain-reducing products, exercise items, health monitoring equipment and more.
40 pages Yearly

451 **Prentke Romich Company Product Catalog**
1022 Heyl Road
Wooster, OH 44691-9786
330-262-1984
800-262-1984
Fax: 330-263-4829
info@prentrom.com
www.prentrom.com
Dave Hershberger, President & CEO
Barry Romich, Co-Founder
A full line, product catalog containing information on speech-output communication devices, environmental controls and computer access products.

452 **Products for People with Disabilities**
LS&S
145 River Rock Drive
Buffalo, NY 14207
716-348-3500
800-468-4789
Fax: 877-498-1482
LSSInfo@LSSproducts.com
www.LSSproducts.com
Melissa Balbach, President
John K. Bace, Executive Vice President
LS&S, LLC has a free catalog of products for the blind, deaf, visually and hearing impaired including: TTYs, computer adaptive devices, CCTVs, talking blood pressure, blood glucose and talking scales.

453 **Rehabilitation Engineering and AssistiveTechnology Society of North America (RESNA)**
2025 M St. NW
Suite 800
Arlington, VA 20036
202-367-1121
Fax: 202-367-2121
info@resna.org
www.resna.org
Maureen Linden, President
Andrea Van Hook, Interim Executive Director
RESNA improves the potential of people with disabilities to achieve their goals through the use of technology. RESNA promotes research, development, education, advocacy and provision of technology; and by supporting the people engaged in these activities.

454 **Safe Path Products**
Safe Path Products
21 Valley Court
Chico, CA 95973-5011
530-893-1596
800-497-2003
Fax: 530-893-1560
info@safepathproducts.com
www.safepathproducts.com
Tim Vander Heiden, Owner
Lisa Bantum, Sales Administrator
As a ramp manufacturer, Safe Path solves vertical rises with a variety of product solutions. One of the largest online ADA Compliance Catalogs available. Offers everything from innovative barrier removal products to survey equipment, to unique specialty products.

455 **Sportaid**
78 Bay Creek Rd
Loganville, GA 30052
770-554-5033
800-743-7203
Fax: 770-554-5944
stuff@sportaid.com
www.sportaid.com
Stacy Green, Co-Owner
Jimmy Green, Co-Owner
Offers an assortment of wheelchairs (everyday and racing), wheelchair sports equipment, replacement tires, hubs, spokes, pushrims, cushions and more.
68 pages Yearly

456 **Store @ HDSC Product Catalog**
Hearing, Speech & Deafness Center (HDSC)
1625 19th Ave.
Seattle, WA 98122-2848
206-323-5770
888-222-5036
Fax: 206-328-6871
seattle@hsdc.org
www.hsdc.org
Lindsay Klarman, Executive Director
Michelle Coleman, Operations Director
Hearing, Speech & Deaf Center (HSDC) is a nonprofit for clients who are deaf, hard of hearing, or who face other communication barriers such as speech challenges. Their mission is to foster inclusive and accessible communities through communication, advocacy, and education.
32 pages Yearly

457 **Walgreens Home Medical Center**
7173 Cermak Rd
Berwyn, IL 60402-2103
708-795-1295
800-323-2828
Fax: 708-795-1308
www.walgreens.com/store/c/home-medical-suppli
Stan Kozlowski, Manager
Hospital supplies and home medical equipment with nationwide direct mail delivery.

458 **Walton Way Medical**
1225 Walton Way
Augusta, GA 30901-2141
706-722-0276
Fax: 706-722-0279
Michael Bower, President
Offers medical, therapeutic, urological, hygiene and skin care products for disabled persons.

459 **Weitbrecht Communications, Inc. (WCI)**
1500 Olympic Boulevard
Santa Monica, CA 90404
310-656-4924
800-233-9130
Fax: 310-450-9918
TTY: 800-233-9130
www.weitbrecht.com

Robert Weitbrecht, Co-Founder
James C. Marsters, Co-Founder
This catalog offers a variety of products for the deaf and hard of hearing, such as: wake-up devices, alarm clocks, alerting systems, assistive listening devices, signalers, smoke detectors, TTY, captioned telephones and telephone amplifiers. Novelties and educational books and videos are also available.
24 pages

Miscellaneous

460 **Access-USA**
242 James St.
P.O. Box 160
Clayton, NY 13624-160
800-263-2750
Fax: 800-563-1687
info@access-usa.com
www.access-usa.com

Deborah Webster, Manager
Produces Braille business Cards. Access-USA also provides Alternate Format transcription services for documentation, i.e., reports, schedules, menus, statements, brochures, and more. submissions accepted via email or hard copy. AF formats include Braille, Large Print, Accessible Audio as well as Captioning Audio Description. Accessible products are also available for custom projects.

461 **Access-USA: Transcription Services**
242 James St.
P.O. Box 160
Clayton, NY 13624-160
800-263-2750
Fax: 800-563-1687
info@access-usa.com
www.access-usa.com

Deborah Webster, Manager
Access-USA produces Braille business cards as well as offering alternate format services and products to enhance accessibility. Braille, large print, captioning, audio-descriptive forms are available. We help business, government, education, corporations by providing brochures, menus, manuals, books, collateral materials, videos, specialties and promotion items that can be more accessible to more people.

462 **BeOK Key Lever**
Performance Health
28100 Torch Parkway
Suite 700
Warrenville, IL 60555-3938
630-393-6000
Fax: 630-393-7600
customersupport@performancehealth.com
www.performancehealth.com

Francis Dirksmeier, CEO
Isabel Afonso, Managing Director & Head of International
Daniel Baumwald, Vice President, North America Retail & eCommerce
Laurie Byrne, Cheif Human Resources
Handy accessory helps position key to provide maximum leverage enabling the user to work the most stubborn lock. *$11.50*

463 **Big Lamp Switch**
Maxi Aids
42 Executive Blvd.
Farmingdale, NY 11735-4710
631-752-0521
800-522-6294
Fax: 631-752-0689
TTY: 631-752-0738
sales@maxiaids.com
www.maxiaids.com

Elliot Zaretsky, Founder, President & CEO
This three-spoked knob replaces small rotating knobs which are a problem for those with arthritis or other limitations of the fingers.
$10.95

464 **Bookholder: Roberts**
Therapro, Inc.
225 Arlington St
Framingham, MA 01702-8723
508-872-9494
800-257-5376
Fax: 508-875-2062
info@therapro.com
www.therapro.com

Karen Conrad Weihrauch, President & Owner
Gray plastic, ideal for hand free reading, adjusts to all sizes of books and prevents pages from flipping for the physically challenged. *$27.50*

465 **Brandt Industries**
4461 Bronx Blvd.
Bronx, NY 10470-1496
718-994-0800
800-221-8031
Fax: 718-325-7995
brandtequip@yahoo.com
www.brandtind.com

Shaun Semple, President & CEO
Family-owned, Brandt Industries is a provider of Wholesale Medical Equipment desgined for maintaining and operating healthcare facililities. Carries and manufactures medical equipment widely used across the medical industry.

466 **Care Electronics**
3301 W 151 Court
Broomfield, CO 8002
303-444-2273
888-444-8284
Fax: 303-447-3502
tmoody@careelectronics.com
www.medicalshoponline.com

Tom Moody, President
Care Electronics manufactures safety monitoring systems for caregivers, home-health care, and nursing homes. WanderCARE monitors loved ones who tend to wander away from home. Care Deluxe Occupancy systems monitor patients in bed and in wheelchairs to help prevent falls. WetSENSE provides incontinence monitors. Provides FDA Approved Light Therapy for wound care and other injuries, as well as for Dementia, Parkinsons, MS, and other neurological problems.

467 **Child Convertible Balance Beam Set**
Bailey Manufacturing Company
118 Lee Drive
P.O. Box 130
Lodi, OH 44254-130
330-948-1080
800-321-8372
Fax: 330-948-4439
baileymfg@baileymfg.com
www.baileymfg.com

Larry Strimple, President
Judie Butler, Dealer Contact
This convertible set is used to develop balance in two stages.

468 **Child Variable Balance Beam**
Bailey Manufacturing Company
118 Lee Drive
P.O. Box 130
Lodi, OH 44254-130
330-948-1080
800-321-8372
Fax: 330-948-4439
baileymfg@baileymfg.com
www.baileymfg.com

Larry Strimple, President
Judie Butler, Dealer Contact
The four walking beams can be arranged in several different ways for variable balance training.

469 **Child's Mobility Crawler**
Bailey Manufacturing Company
118 Lee Drive
P.O. Box 130
Lodi, OH 44254-130
330-948-1080
800-321-8372
Fax: 330-948-4439
baileymfg@baileymfg.com
www.baileymfg.com

Larry Strimple, President
Judie Butler, Dealer Contact
Neurologically delayed or orthopedically impaired small children can perform crawling and coordination exercises while being comfortably supported by the crawler.

470 **Choice Switch Latch and Timer**
AbleNet, Inc.
2625 Patton Road
Roseville, MN 55113-1137
651-294-2200
800-322-0956
Fax: 651-294-2259
customerservice@ablenetinc.com
www.ablenetinc.com

Bill Sproull, Chair of the Board
Jennifer Thalhuber, President & CEO
William Mills, Board of Directors
Paul Sugden, CFO & Trustee
A Choice Switch Latch and Timer allows one user to learn to make choices. It has two switch inputs and can control two devices. Once one device has been activated, the other will not function until the first one is turned off or completes its timed cycle. *$83.00*

471 **Cordless Big Red Switch**
AbleNet, Inc.
2625 Patton Road
Roseville, MN 55113-1137
651-294-2200
800-322-0956
Fax: 651-294-2259
customerservice@ablenetinc.com
www.ablenetinc.com

Bill Sproull, Chair of the Board
Jennifer Thalhuber, President & CEO
William Mills, Board of Directors
Paul Sugden, CFO & Trustee
The Cordless Big Red Switch, when used in conjunction with either the Cordless Receiver or the Small Appliance Receiver, gives the user cordless control of toys, games, and appliances in one's environment. *$89.00*

472 **DEUCE Environmental Control Unit**
APT Technology
236a N Main St
Shreve, OH 44676
330-567-2001
888-549-2001
Fax: 330-567-3073
www.apt-technology.com

Grace Miller, Office Manager
Allows a severely disabled person to control a variety of useful devices via a dual switch. DEUCE controls phone, 4 AC powered devices such as a radio, 4 switch controlled devices such as a page turner and up to 16 lights and or appliances distributed around the environment.

473 **Dazor Lighting Technology**
2360 Chaffee Drive
St. Louis, MO 63146
314-652-2400
800-345-9103
Fax: 314-652-2069
info@dazor.com
www.dazor.com

Kirk Cressey, Marketing Director
Bob Smith, National Sales Manager
Dazor is a US manufacturer of quality task lighting. Products include fluorescent, incandescent and halogen lighting fixtures. Illuminated magnifiers combine light and magnification to greatly enhance activities such as reading and make hobbies more enjoyable. All lamps come in a variety of mounting options to include desk bases, clamp on, floor stands and wall tracks.

474 **Digi-Flex**
Therapro, Inc.
225 Arlington St
Framingham, MA 01702-8723
508-872-9494
800-257-5376
Fax: 508-875-2062
info@therapro.com
www.therapro.com

Karen Conrad Weihrauch, President & Owner
This is a unique hand and finger exercise unit. Recommended for use of individuation of fingers, web space and general strengthening of work hands. Available in a variety of resistances. *$17.50*

475 **Digital Talking Compass**
Maxi Aids
42 Executive Blvd.
Farmingdale, NY 11735-4710
631-752-0521
800-522-6294
Fax: 631-752-0689
TTY: 631-752-0738
sales@maxiaids.com
www.maxiaids.com

Elliot Zaretsky, Founder, President & CEO
Compass that speaks the direction it is pointed to. Includes eight points for noisy conditions for hard of hearing users. *$74.95*

476 **Door Knock Signaler**
HARC Mercantile
5413 S Westnedge Ave.
Suite A
Portage, MI 49002
269-324-1615
800-445-9968
Fax: 269-324-2387
TTY: 269-324-1615
info@harc.com
www.harc.com

Michael Martinson, Owner
Flashes light to signal a knock on the door. *$31.00*

477 **Doorbell Signalers**
HARC Mercantile
5413 S Westnedge Ave.
Suite A
Portage, MI 49002
269-324-1615
800-445-9968
Fax: 269-324-2387
TTY: 269-324-1615
info@harc.com
www.harc.com

Michael Martinson, Owner
Doorbell signalers to alert with either louder chime or flashing light.

478 **Dormakaba USA Inc.**
1 DORMA Drive, AC Drawer
Reamstown, PA 17567-411
717-336-3881
866-401-6063
Fax: 717-336-2106
archdw@dorma-usa.com
www.dormakaba.com/en

Riet Cadonau, CEO
Bernd Brinker, CFO
Alwin Berninger, COO Access Solutions DACH
Roberto Gaspari, COO Access Solutions EMEA
DORMA provides a complete line of door controls, including barrier-free units that comply with the Americans with Disabilities Act. A wide variety of surface applied and concealed closers, low energy operators, exit devices and electronic access control systems are available to address these equipments.

479 **Dual Switch Latch and Timer**
AbleNet, Inc.
2625 Patton Road
Roseville, MN 55113-1137
651-294-2200
800-322-0956
Fax: 651-294-2259
customerservice@ablenetinc.com
www.ablenetinc.com

Bill Sproull, Chair of the Board
Jennifer Thalhuber, President & CEO
William Mills, Board of Directors
Paul Sugden, CFO & Trustee

A Dual Switch Latch and Timer allows two users to activate two devices at a time in the latch. Timed seconds or timed minutes mode of control. *$88.00*

480 **Enabling Devices**
50 Broadway
Hawthorne, NY 10532-2837
914-747-3070
800-832-8697
Fax: 914-747-3480
sales@enablingdevices.com
www.enablingdevices.com

Seth Kanor, President & CEO

For more than 25 years, Enabling Devices has been dedicated to providing affordable learning and assistive devices for the physically challenged. Products include augmentative communicators, adapted toys, capability switches, training and sensory devices and activity centers.

481 **Foot Inversion Tread**
Bailey Manufacturing Company
118 Lee Drive
P.O. Box 130
Lodi, OH 44254-130
330-948-1080
800-321-8372
Fax: 330-948-4439
baileymfg@baileymfg.com
www.baileymfg.com

Larry Strimple, President
Judie Butler, Dealer Contact

Effective for correcting flat feet. These angled boards require the patient to walk on the outside of the foot instead of the arch.

482 **Foot Placement Ladder**
Bailey Manufacturing Company
118 Lee Drive
P.O. Box 130
Lodi, OH 44254-130
330-948-1080
800-321-8372
Fax: 330-948-4439
baileymfg@baileymfg.com
www.baileymfg.com

Larry Strimple, President
Judie Butler, Dealer Contact

Adjustable cross bars for different length steps. Reinforced metal crosses for easier climbing for the physically-disabled.

483 **HealthCraft SuperPole**
Maxi Aids
42 Executive Blvd.
Farmingdale, NY 11735-4710
631-752-0521
800-522-6294
Fax: 631-752-0689
TTY: 631-752-0738
sales@maxiaids.com
www.maxiaids.com

Elliot Zaretsky, Founder, President & CEO

A floor-to-ceiling grab bar designed for those who require assistance with standing, transferring, or moving. Can be used beside a bed, bath, toilet or chair. *$222.30*

484 **Hocoma AG**
77 Accord Park Drive
Suite D-1
Norwell, MA 02061
877-944-220
Fax: 781-792-0104
service.usa@hocoma.com
www.hocoma.com

Dr. Gery Colombo, President & CEO
Robert McNamara, CFO
Alexander Wallstein, COO
Dr. Patrick Bruno, Chief Sales Officer

Leader in developing, manufacturing and marketing robotic and sensor-based products for functional movement therapy on a global level.

485 **Home Alerting Systems**
HARC Mercantile
5413 S Westnedge Ave.
Suite A
Portage, MI 49002
269-324-1615
800-445-9968
Fax: 269-324-2387
TTY: 269-324-1615
info@harc.com
www.harc.com

Michael Martinson, Owner

Alerting systems featuring bright flasher, loud speaker, and/or bedshaker signals.

486 **Hospital Environmental Control System**
Prentke Romich Company
1022 Heyl Road
Wooster, OH 44691-9786
330-262-1984
800-262-1984
Fax: 330-263-4829
info@prentrom.com
www.prentrom.com

Dave Hershberger, President & CEO
Barry Romich, Co-Founder

Permits the non-ambulatory patient to operate a variety of electrical items in a single room. A large liquid crystal display is mounted in front of the user and they scan through the menu of operations and make a selection using a sip-puff switch. Options include nurse call, standard telephone functions, electric bed control, hospital television operation and electrical appliance on and off. *$3860.00*

487 **Identity Group**
7525 Pennsylvania Ave
Suite 101
Sarasota, FL 34243
941-355-5171
800-237-9447
Fax: 941-351-1787
inquiry@identitygroup.com
www.identitygroup.com

Sam Richardson, President & CEO
Bob Tate, CFO
Lee Brantley, Chief Human Resources Officer
Gary Katz, Chief Marketing Officer

Manufacturer of signs and visual decor for office and personal use.

488 **Labeling Kits**
Maxi Aids
42 Executive Blvd.
Farmingdale, NY 11735-4710
631-752-0521
800-522-6294
Fax: 631-752-0689
TTY: 631-752-0738
sales@maxiaids.com
www.maxiaids.com

Elliot Zaretsky, Founder, President & CEO

Braille and raised letter identification labels for labeling food items, prescriptions, clothing and more. Comes with safety pins and rubber bands for attaching labels.

489 **Leg Elevation Board**
Bailey Manufacturing Company
118 Lee Drive
P.O. Box 130
Lodi, OH 44254-130
330-948-1080
800-321-8372
Fax: 330-948-4439
baileymfg@baileymfg.com
www.baileymfg.com
Larry Strimple, President
Judie Butler, Dealer Contact
Includes seven positions to a 30 degree incline, three pillows with Velcro, easy carry hand slot and a natural finish.

490 **Leveron Door Lever**
Lindustries
21 Shady Hill Rd
Weston, MA 02193-1407
781-237-8177
877-794-9511
Fax: 651-989-2131
www.trademarkia.com/leveron-73486756.html
Willard H. Lind, Owner
Louise T Lind, Vice President
Leveron is a doorknob lever handle for ease of operation. Leveron converts standard doorknobs to lever action without removing existing hardware. No gripping, twisting or pinching when hands are wet, arthritic or arms are full. Leveron provides convenience. ADA access requirements in public and private places. *$16.95*

491 **Longreach Reacher**
Therapro, Inc.
225 Arlington St
Framingham, MA 01702-8723
508-872-9494
800-257-5376
Fax: 508-875-2062
info@therapro.com
www.therapro.com
Karen Conrad Weihrauch, President & Owner
Reacher is useful when reaching, sitting or when standing. Light in weight and easy to control with disabled hands. Operate with one hand or two. Secure grip on any object. *$18.95*

492 **Loop Scissors**
Therapro, Inc.
225 Arlington St
Framingham, MA 01702-8723
508-872-9494
800-257-5376
Fax: 508-875-2062
info@therapro.com
www.therapro.com
Karen Conrad Weihrauch, President & Owner
Pliable, plastic handles that allow for easy and controlled cutting. Extra finger room provides better control when cutting. *$14.25*

493 **Pacific Rehab, Inc.**
36805 N Never Mind Tr.
P.O. Box 5406
Carefree, AZ 85377-5406
888-222-9040
Fax: 480-575-7907
information@pacificrehabinc.com
pacificrehabinc.com

494 **Pedal-in-Place Exerciser**
Thoele Manufacturing
475 County Road 100 N
Montrose, IL 62445-3019
217-924-4553
Fax: 217-924-4553

495 **Pet Partners**
Delta Society National Service Dog Center
875 118th Ave SE
Suite 200
Bellevue, WA 98005-2531
425-679-5550
Fax: 425-379-5539
www.petpartners.org
Annie Peters Magnant, President & CEO
David E. Williams, M.D., Chief Medical Officer
Linda Dicus, Executive Assistant
Chris Calabro, Director of Technology
Pet Partners, formerly Delta Society, is a non-profit organization that helps people live healthier and happier lives by incorporating therapy, service and companion animals into their lives.

496 **Plastic Card Holder**
Therapro, Inc.
225 Arlington St
Framingham, MA 01702-8723
508-872-9494
800-257-5376
Fax: 508-875-2062
info@therapro.com
www.therapro.com
Karen Conrad Weihraucher, President & Owner
For those with reduced finger control. Front extension for pencils and coins. *$4.00*

497 **Power Door**
11240 Gemini Ln
Dallas, TX 75229-4710
800-688-1758
Fax: 972-620-9875
Jim Goldthwaite, National Sales Manager
Power door, low energy door operators. Specialized in the installment and service of automatic doors.

498 **ProtectaCap, ProtectaCap+PLUS, ProtectaChin Guard and ProtectaHip**
Plum Enterprises
P.O. Box 85
Valley Forge, PA 19481-85
610-783-7377
800-321-7586
Fax: 610-783-7577
info@plument.com
www.plument.com
Janice Carrington, Founder & CEO
Plum Enterprises award winning, exquisite, ergonomic protective wear keeps you safe from the dangers of falls. ProtectCap+Plus and ProtectHips are engineered for superior shock-absorption and designed for exquisite simplicity and amazing lightweight comfort.

499 **Quad Commander**
GPK Inc.
535 Floyd Smith Drive
El Cajon, CA 92020-1228
619-593-7381
800-468-8679
Fax: 888-755-5603
www.quadriplegia.com
Rajesh Kanwar, Manager
Joystick for people with quadriplegia.

500 **Real Design Inc.**
187 S. Main Street
Dolgeville, NY 13329
800-696-7041
Fax: 315-429-3071
rdesign@twcny.rr.com
sites.google.com/site/realdesign95/

501 **Rex Bionics, Ltd.**
50 Milk Street
Floor 16
Boston, MA 02109
info@rexbionics.com
www.rexbionics.com
Jon Graham, CEO
Rex Bionics develops and manufactures exoskeletons, capable of performing exercises in multiple positions: upright, backward, sideways, lunge, or ssquat. REX exoskeletons. Permits both at home or gym exercises and stretches for the upper and lower body, accessing different groups of muscles.

502 **Rocker Balance Square**
Bailey Manufacturing Company
118 Lee Drive
P.O. Box 130
Lodi, OH 44254-130
330-948-1080
800-321-8372
Fax: 330-948-4439
baileymfg@baileymfg.com
www.baileymfg.com
Larry Strimple, President
Judie Butler, Dealer Contact
The rocker is used in developing activity, balance control and coordination.

503 **Room Valet Visual-Tactile Alerting System**
HARC Mercantile
5413 S Westnedge Ave.
Suite A
Portage, MI 49002
269-324-1615
800-445-9968
Fax: 269-324-2387
TTY: 269-324-1615
info@harc.com
www.harc.com

Michael Martinson, Owner

ADA compliant built-in visual-tactile alerting system. The Room Valet is fully supervised and has power failure back up. Alerts to in-room smoke, building alarm, door, phone, and alarm clock. Designed for permanent installation.

504 **Series Adapter**
AbleNet, Inc.
2625 Patton Road
Roseville, MN 55113-1137
651-294-2200
800-322-0956
Fax: 651-294-2259
customerservice@ablenetinc.com
www.ablenetinc.com

Bill Sproull, Chair of the Board
Jennifer Thalhuber, President & CEO
William Mills, Board of Directors
Paul Sugden, CFO & Trustee

Allows two-switch operation of any battery-operated device or electrical devices. *$13.00*

505 **Signaling Wake-Up Devices**
HARC Mercantile
5413 S Westnedge Ave.
Suite A
Portage, MI 49002
269-324-1615
800-445-9968
Fax: 269-324-2387
TTY: 269-324-1615
info@harc.com
www.harc.com

Michael Martinson, Owner

Wake up devices. Vibrating alarm clocks, available with flashing lights, louder alarm noises and more.

506 **Smoke Detector with Strobe**
HARC Mercantile
5413 S Westnedge Ave.
Suite A
Portage, MI 49002
269-324-1615
800-445-9968
Fax: 269-324-2387
TTY: 269-324-1615
info@harc.com
www.harc.com

Michael Martinson, Owner

Detects smoke within a radius of 100' and flashes a strobe as a signal.

507 **Spinal Network: The Total Wheelchair Resource Book**
No Limits Communications & New Mobility
75-20 Astoria Blvd.
East Elmhurst, NY 11370-2068
215-675-9133
800-404-2898
888-850-0344
Fax: 215-675-9376
jeff@leonardmedia.com
www.newmobility.com

Jean Dobbs, Publisher & Editorial Director
Josie Byzek, Executive Editor
Tim Gilmer, Editor Emeritus
Ian Ruder, Senior Editor

Nearly 600 pages of profiles, articles and resources on every topic of interest to wheelchair users. Subjects include health, coping, relationships, sexuality, parenthood, computers, sports, recreation, travel, personal assistance services, legal rights, financial strategies, employment, and media images. *$34.95*
400 pages

508 **SteeleVest**
Steele
P.O. Box 7304
Kingston, WA 98346-7304
360-297-4555
888-783-3538
Fax: 360-297-2816
steelevest@gmail.com
www.steelevest.com

Sandra Steele, President

Vest developed by NASA provides an external cooling system. Cooling Vests are tailored to industrial workers while operating in warm environments to keep cool and safe.

509 **Strobe Light Signalers**
HARC Mercantile
5413 S Westnedge Ave.
Suite A
Portage, MI 49002
269-324-1615
800-445-9968
Fax: 269-324-2387
TTY: 269-324-1615
info@harc.com
www.harc.com

Michael Martinson, Owner

Strobe alerts that plug into receivers for signaling systems. A strobe light on the device will flash to alert for calls, visitors, and home alarms.

510 **TV & VCR Remote**
AbleNet, Inc.
2625 Patton Road
Roseville, MN 55113-1137
651-294-2200
800-322-0956
Fax: 651-294-2259
customerservice@ablenetinc.com
www.ablenetinc.com

Bill Sproull, Chair of the Board
Jennifer Thalhuber, President & CEO
William Mills, Board of Directors
Paul Sugden, CFO & Trustee

Controls a TV, a VCR or a TV that is connected through a VCR tuner. It may be programmed to control functions such as on and off, channel up, preprogrammed TV channels and, if desired, other TV functions such as mute and pause. *$82.00*

511 **Tactile Braille Signs**
Maxi Aids
42 Executive Blvd.
Farmingdale, NY 11735-4710
631-752-0521
800-522-6294
Fax: 631-752-0689
TTY: 631-752-0738
sales@maxiaids.com
www.maxiaids.com

Elliot Zaretsky, Founder, President & CEO

Contains raised text and pictograms, Grade 2 Braille, and contrasting colors. Stairs, No Smoking, and various Restroom signs available. *$19.95*

512 **Tactile Thermostat**
ASB
919 Walnut Street
Philadelphia, PA 19107-5237
215-627-0600
Fax: 215-922-0692
asbinfo@asb.org
www.asb.org

Karla S. McCaney, President & CEO
Beth Deering, Director, Human Services
Richard Forsythe, Director, Braille Division & Custom Audio
Joyce Robertson, Director, Finance & Information Technology

Large embossed numbers on cover ring and raised temperature setting knob. *$31.50*

513 **Therapy Putty**
Therapro, Inc.
225 Arlington St
Framingham, MA 01702-8723
508-872-9494
800-257-5376
Fax: 508-875-2062
info@therapro.com
www.therapro.com
Karen Conrad Weihrauch, President & Owner
Designed to exercise and strengthen hands, ranging from soft to firm for developing a stronger grasp. Available in two, four and six ounce sizes. Three ounce putty in unique clear fist shaped container.

514 **Uppertone**
GPK Inc.
535 Floyd Smith Drive
El Cajon, CA 92020-1228
619-593-7381
800-468-8679
Fax: 888-755-5603
www.quadriplegia.com
Rajesh Kanwar, Manager
Unassisted muscle strengthening and conditioning system for quads. *$2495.00*

515 **Window-Ease**
A-Solution
1331 Windridge Drive
Albuquerque, NM 87120
505-856-6632
Fax: 505-856-6652
info@windowease.com
www.windowease.com
Robert Gorrell, President
Jeff Dodd, Sales
Device adapts horizontally and vertically sliding windows to ANSI A117.1 standards. 10:1 mechanical advantage at the crank arm opens a 50lb window with 5lbs force.

Office Devices & Workstations

516 **AdjustaCart**
Infogrip
1899 E. Main Street
Ventura, CA 93001-3411
805-652-0770
800-397-0921
Fax: 805-652-0880
support@infogrip.com
www.infogrip.com
Liza Jacobs, President
Aaron Gaston, Vice President
Sit or stand while working with this easily adjustable desk. With a simple squeeze of a paddle the front surface travel range of 12 3/4. The front surface tilts 9 degrees toward and 15 degrees away from you. Anthro carts are made of 1in thick industrial grade particleboard shelves with high-pressure laminated 16 gauge steel tube legs that safely hold 150 pounds. Spring assisted mechanism. There are holes in 1: increment in the legs so that you can put the shelves and accessories where needed. *$629.00*

517 **BAT Personal Keyboard**
Infogrip
1899 E. Main Street
Ventura, CA 93001-3411
805-652-0770
800-397-0921
Fax: 805-652-0880
support@infogrip.com
www.infogrip.com
Liza Jacobs, President
Aaron Gaston, Vice President
Infogrip has creative computer access solutions for people with all types of disabilities. Alternative keyboards and mice, switches, screen readers, magnifiers and educational software. We also have a retail store, Your Low Vision Store. We have three locations in Southern California offering the best selection of video magnifiers in the industry. *$200.00*

518 **Combination File/Reference Carousel**
Center for Rehabilitation Technology
Ste 118
490 10th St NW
Atlanta, GA 30318-5754
404-712-5667
800-457-9555
Fax: 404-875-9409
TW Gannaway, Executive VP
Anthony Stringer PhD
Offers two reading platforms and file holders joined on one easily rotated carousel. The carousel is easily rotated by head, mouth or handstick. Page retainer adjusts to hold open a variety of books and magazines. *$299.00*

519 **Computer Workstation and Activity Table**
Maxi Aids
42 Executive Blvd.
Farmingdale, NY 11735-4710
631-752-0521
800-522-6294
Fax: 631-752-0689
TTY: 631-752-0738
sales@maxiaids.com
www.maxiaids.com
Elliot Zaretsky, Founder, President & CEO
Height-adjustable wheelchair accessible table. Adjusts with a hand crank. ADA compliant.

520 **Desk-Top Talking Calculator**
Maxi Aids
42 Executive Blvd.
Farmingdale, NY 11735-4710
631-752-0521
800-522-6294
Fax: 631-752-0689
TTY: 631-752-0738
sales@maxiaids.com
www.maxiaids.com
Elliot Zaretsky, Founder, President & CEO
Full-function calculator that announces results in a clear voice. Also features a large 8-digit display. *$13.85*

521 **Don Johnston**
26799 West Commerce Drive
Volo, IL 60073-9675
847-740-0749
800-999-4660
Fax: 847-740-7326
info@donjohnston.com
www.donjohnston.com
Don Johnston, Founder
Ruth Ziolkowski, President
Kevin Johnston, Director of Product Design
Ben Johnston, Director of Marketing
A provider of quality products and services that enable people with special needs to discover their potential and experience success. Products are developed for the areas of Physical Access, Augmentative Communication and for those who struggle with reading and writing.

522 **Extensions for Independence**
360 N. Pacific Coast Highway
Suite 1055
El Segundo, CA 90245
757-416-6575
888-321-4678
Fax: 866-632-7149
support@inmotionhosting.com
Ted Sakis, Director of Operations
Develops, manufactures and markets special vocational equipment for the physically handicapped. Products: mouthsticks, computer mechanical aids: key locks and diskette loaders. Also, turntable desks, wheelchair portable desks, filing trays with slanted sides, telephone adapters, and motorized artist easel. All these products have been designed to solve the functional limitations of people with little or no use of hands and/or arms.

523 **Fairway Spirit Adaptive Golf Car: Model4852**
Fairway Golf Cars
Ste 300
3225 Gateway Rd
Brookfield, WI 53045-5139
262-790-9363
888-320-4850
888-320-4850
Fax: 262-790-9396

524 **Freedom Ryder Handcycles**
Brike International
20589 SW Elk Horn Ct
Tualatin, OR 97062-9518
503-692-1029
800-800-5828
Fax: 970-221-4308
www.freedomryder.com
Mike Lofgren, President & CEO
Brian Stewart, Vice President
The finest handcycle in the world. The cycles incorporate body, lean steering and the finest bicycle components to make this a three-wheeled vehicle without equal. Suitable for both recreation and competition. *$1995.00*

525 **Golf Xpress**
Emotorsports
4400 West M-61
Standish, MI 48658
989-846-6255
Fax: 989-846-6255
www.golfxpress.com

526 **Pencil/Pen Weighted Holders**
Therapro, Inc.
225 Arlington St
Framingham, MA 01702-8723
508-872-9494
800-257-5376
Fax: 508-875-2062
info@therapro.com
www.therapro.com
Karen Conrad Weihrauch, President & Owner
Securely hold any pencil or pen. These weighted holders allow for more control along with proprioceptive feedback to encourage better writing skills.

527 **Perkins Brailler**
Maxi Aids
42 Executive Blvd.
Farmingdale, NY 11735-4710
631-752-0521
800-522-6294
Fax: 631-752-0689
TTY: 631-752-0738
sales@maxiaids.com
www.maxiaids.com
Elliot Zaretsky, Founder, President & CEO
Can emboss 25 lines with 42 cells on an 11 x 11 1/2 sheet. *$775.00*

528 **PhoneMax Amplified Telephone**
Assistech
2738 N Campbell Ave
Tucson, AZ 85719-3141
520-883-8600
866-674-3549
Fax: 520-883-3172
www.assistivedevices.net
Oliver Simoes, Owner

529 **Raised Line Drawing Kit**
Maxi Aids
42 Executive Blvd.
Farmingdale, NY 11735-4710
631-752-0521
800-522-6294
Fax: 631-752-0689
TTY: 631-752-0738
sales@maxiaids.com
www.maxiaids.com
Elliot Zaretsky, Founder, President & CEO
For writing script or drawing graphs by the use of special plastic paper. *$34.95*

530 **Reizen Braille Labeler**
Maxi Aids
42 Executive Blvd.
Farmingdale, NY 11735-4710
631-752-0521
800-522-6294
Fax: 631-752-0689
TTY: 631-752-0738
sales@maxiaids.com
www.maxiaids.com
Elliot Zaretsky, Founder, President & CEO
For labeling in Braille with 3/8 or 1/2 wide labeling tape. *$27.95*

531 **Sharp Calculator with Illuminated Numbers**
Independent Living Aids
137 Rano Rd
Buffalo, NY 14207
716-332-2970
800-537-2118
855-746-7452
Fax: 855-937-3906
can-do@independentliving.com
www.independentliving.com
Irwin Schneidmill, President
Michael Gutierrez, Director of Operations
Pamela Strauss, Director of Marketing
Ursula Izurieta, Director of Merchandising
A trim desktop calculator with large illuminated numbers that can be carried anywhere. *$34.95*

532 **Signature and Address Self-Inking Stamps**
Independent Living Aids
137 Rano Rd
Buffalo, NY 14207
716-332-2970
800-537-2118
855-746-7452
Fax: 516-937-3906
can-do@independentliving.com
www.independentliving.com
Irwin Schneidmill, President
Michael Gutierrez, Director of Operations
Pamela Strauss, Director of Marketing
Ursula Izurieta, Director of Merchandising
Gives thousands of impressions before requiring re-inking. *$11.95*

533 **Steady Write**
Maxi Aids
42 Executive Blvd.
Farmingdale, NY 11735-4710
631-752-0521
800-522-6294
Fax: 631-752-0689
TTY: 631-752-0738
sales@maxiaids.com
www.maxiaids.com
Elliot Zaretsky, Founder, President & CEO
Furnishes the writer with increased holding capacity and stabilizes the hand. *$8.95*

534 **Talking Electronic Organizers**
Independent Living Aids
137 Rano Rd
Buffalo, NY 14207
716-332-2970
800-537-2118
855-746-7452
Fax: 516-937-3906
can-do@independentliving.com
www.independentliving.com
Irwin Schneidmill, President
Michael Gutierrez, Director of Operations
Pamela Strauss, Director of Marketing
Ursula Izurieta, Director of Merchandising
Electronic, portable, personal organizers that talk the user through all the functions and are totally voice interactive. $199.95 and up.

535 **Television Remote Controls with Large Numbers**
Independent Living Aids
137 Rano Rd
Buffalo, NY 14207
716-332-2970
800-537-2118
855-746-7452
Fax: 516-937-3906
can-do@independentliving.com
www.independentliving.com
Irwin Schneidmill, President
Michael Gutierrez, Director of Operations
Pamela Strauss, Director of Marketing
Ursula Izurieta, Director of Merchandising
Large 5 1/2 inch x 8 1/2 inch unit that has easy to see and use buttons. Can be used on nearly every TV, VCR and cable boxes. *$39.95*

536 **Touch-Dots**
Maxi Aids
42 Executive Blvd.
Farmingdale, NY 11735-4710
631-752-0521
800-522-6294
Fax: 631-752-0689
TTY: 631-752-0738
sales@maxiaids.com
www.maxiaids.com
Elliot Zaretsky, Founder, President & CEO
Adhesive-backed dots for identification. Can be used with keyboards, telephones, calculators and more. *$1.95*

Scooters

537 **Ability Center**
4797 Ruffner St.
San Diego, CA 92111
858-541-0552
833-919-2581
Fax: 858-541-1941
www.abilitycenter.com
Terry Barton, General Manager
Specializes in accessible vehicles and mobility products; the company has more than 100 employees in 14 locations across the western U.S.
1994

538 **Aerospace Compadre**
Aerospace America, Inc.
900 Harry Truman Pkwy.
Bay City, MI 48706-4171
989-684-2121
800-237-6414
Fax: 989-684-4486
www.aerospaceamerica.com
Mike Alley, President
Fully customized golf cart type vehicle for the physically impaired person. Fully equipped with hand controls, wheelchair rack, storage racks, head and tail lights and full safety belts.
$2500.00

539 **Alante**
Golden Technologies
401 Bridge Street
Old Forge, PA 18518-2323
570-451-7477
800-624-6374
Fax: 800-628-5165
www.goldentech.com
Richard Golden, President & CEO
Rpbert Golden, Chair
Fred Kiwak, Vice President, Research & Development
Rear-wheel-drive vehicle that represents the best in powered mobility.

540 **Amigo Mobility International**
Amigo Mobility International
6693 Dixie Highway
Bridgeport, MI 48722-9725
989-777-0910
800-248-9131
Fax: 800-334-7274
info@myamigo.com
www.myamigo.com
Al Thieme, Chair & Founder
Beth Thieme, President & CEO
Sandy Humpert, Sales Representative
An industry leader in power operated vehicles and scooters, Amigo provides innovative, durable, and customized mobility solutions for the disabled, injured, and seniors worldwide. Other services include healthcare, travel and transportation services.
$1295.00

541 **Amigo Mobility International Inc.**
6693 Dixie Highway
Bridgeport, MI 48722-9725
989-777-0910
800-248-9131
Fax: 800-334-7274
info@myamigo.com
www.myamigo.com
Al Thieme, Chair & Founder
Beth Thieme, President & CEO
Sandy Humpert, Sales Representative
Amigo Mobility designs and manufactures a complete line of power operated vehicles/mobility scooters and accessories.

542 **Bravo! + Three-Wheel Scooter**
Electro Kinetic Technologies
W194 N11301 McCormick Drive
Germantown, WI 53022
262-250-7740
800-824-1068
Fax: 262-250-7741
info@ek-tech.com
www.ek-tech.com

543 **Cruiser Bus Buggy 4MB**
Convaid
2830 California Street
Torrance, CA 90503
310-618-0111
888-266-8243
Fax: 310-618-2166
www.convaid.com
Ryan B. Williams, President
In sizes from infant through young adult, this positioning buggy is crash-tested.

544 **E-Wheels Electric Senior Mobility Scooter**
Maxi Aids
42 Executive Blvd.
Farmingdale, NY 11735-4710
631-752-0521
800-522-6294
Fax: 631-752-0689
TTY: 631-752-0738
sales@maxiaids.com
www.maxiaids.com
Elliot Zaretsky, Founder, President & CEO
Three-wheel, high-powered scooter for seniors. Travels up to 45 miles on a single charge.

545 **Electric Mobility Corporation**
P.O. Box 156
Sewell, NJ 08080-156
856-468-0083
800-257-7955
Fax: 856-468-3426
www.rascalscooters.com
Linda Autore, CEO
Manufactures Rascal Scooters.

546 **Explorer+ 4-Wheel Scooter**
Electro Kinetic Technologies
W194 N11301 McCormick Drive
Germantown, WI 53022
262-250-7740
800-824-1068
Fax: 262-250-7741
info@ek-tech.com
www.ek-tech.com

547 **Featherlite**
No Boundaries
1 Monster Way
Corona, CA 92879
714-891-5899
800-426-7367
Fax: 714-891-0658
info@hansens.com
www.hansens.com
Hubert Hansen, Founder
Lightweight scooter folds in seconds without tools or bending down for hassle free travel on airplanes, cruise ships, trains, RVs, buses and more. Heaviest component weighs 27 pounds. Fits easily in almost any vehicle trunk.

548 **Invacare Fulfillment Center**
Invacare
1 Invacare Way
Elyria, OH 44035-4190
440-329-6000
800-333-6900
Fax: 877-619-7996
www.invacare.com

Matthew E. Monaghan, Chair, President & CEO
Darcie Karol, Senior Vice President Human Resources
Kathleen P. Leneghan, Senior Vice President & CFO
Anthony C. LaPlaca, Senior Vice President, General Counsel & Secretary

Invacare Corporation is the world's leading manufacturer and distributor of non-acute medical products which promote recovery and active lifestyles for people requiring home and other non-acute health care.

549 **Leisure Lift**
Pace Saver
1800 Merriam Lane
Kansas City, KS 66106-4714
913-722-5658
800-255-0285
Fax: 913-722-2614
www.pacesaver.com

Bill Burke, Founder

Leisure Lift offers light three wheel scooter models and seven power wheelchair models. *$2695.00*

550 **MVP+ 3-Wheel Scooter**
Electro Kinetic Technologies
W194 N11301 McCormick Drive
Germantown, WI 53022
262-250-7740
800-824-1068
Fax: 262-250-7741
info@ek-tech.com
www.ek-tech.com

551 **Moxie**
No Boundaries
1 Monster Way
Corona, CA 92879
714-891-5899
800-426-7367
Fax: 714-891-0658
info@hansens.com
www.hansens.com

Hubert Hansen, Founder

Disassembles into three parts in less than a minute. Heaviest component weighs 41 pounds.

552 **Outdoor Independence**
Palmer Industries
P.O. Box 5707
Endicott, NY 13763-5707
607-754-2957
800-847-1304
Fax: 607-754-1954
palmer@palmerind.com
www.palmerind.com

Jack Palmer, President

The futuristic, one, two and three seater, electric three-wheeler designed to take you almost anywhere.

553 **Pace Saver Plus II**
Pace Saver
1800 Merriam Lane
Kansas City, KS 66106-4714
913-722-5658
800-255-0285
Fax: 913-722-2614
www.pacesaver.com

Bill Burke, Founder

The scooter combines outdoor ruggedness with indoor maneuverability at a low price.

554 **Palmer Independence**
Palmer Industries
P.O. Box 5707
Endicott, NY 13763-5707
607-754-2957
800-847-1304
Fax: 607-754-1954
palmer@palmerind.com
www.palmerind.com

Jack Palmer, President

Futuristic electric outdoor three wheeler designed to take the rider almost anywhere.

555 **Palmer Twosome**
Palmer Industries
P.O. Box 5707
Endicott, NY 13763-5707
607-754-2957
800-847-1304
Fax: 607-754-1954
palmer@palmerind.com
www.palmerind.com

Jack Palmer, President

All electric two seat vehicle for those who can't pedal.

556 **Polaris Trail Blazer**
Polaris Industries
2100 Highway 55
Medina, MN 55340-9770
763-542-0500
888-704-5290
Fax: 763-542-0599
www.polarisindustries.com

Scott Wine, Chair & CEO
Chris Musso, President
Michael W. Malone, Vice President, Finance & Chief Financial Officer
Todd-Michael Balan, Vice President, Corporate Development

A four-wheeler that has many engineered innovations, features such as: full floorboards for full comfort, single lever breaking with auxiliary foot brake, electronic throttle control, parking brake and adjustable handlebars.

557 **Quickie 2**
Sunrise Medical
2842 Business Park Avenue
Fresno, CA 93727
800-333-4000
Fax: 800-300-7502
webmaster@sunmed.com
www.sunrisemedical.com

Thomas Babacan, President & CEO
Adrian Platt, CFO
Bernd Krebs, CTO
Roxane Cromwell, COO

This custom, ultralight, folding, everyday scooter offers portability and performance plus modular flexibility.

558 **Rascal 3-Wheeler**
Mobility Parts and Service
1501 Grandview Avenue
Suite 400
West Deptford, NJ 08066-156
800-257-7955
800-662-4548
info@mobilitypartsandservice.com
mobilitypartsandservice.com

559 **Rascal Convertable**
Mobility Parts and Service
1501 Grandview Avenue
Suite 400
West Deptford, NJ 08066-156
800-257-7955
800-662-4548
info@mobilitypartsandservice.com
mobilitypartsandservice.com

560 **Regent**
Golden Technologies
401 Bridge Street
Old Forge, PA 18518-2323
570-451-7477
800-624-6374
Fax: 800-628-5165
info@goldentech.com
www.goldentech.com

Richard Golden, Presdient & CEO
Robert Golden, Chair
Fred Kiwak, Vice President, Research & Development

Top-rated performance scooter, with extra features and economically priced.

561 **Roadster 20**
ATV Solutions
Unit 4
4700 W 60th Ave
Arvada, CO 80003-6928
303-450-2881
866-777-9727
888-867-1159
Fax: 303-450-2880
sales@atvsolutions.com
www.atvsolutions.com

Andrew Miro, Owner
Great for indoor or outdoor use. The powerful, quiet drive system, independent front suspension and fully reclining high-back seat make for a smooth, quiet ride. The Roadster is loaded with great features at a bargain price.

562 **Safari Scooter**
Ranger All Seasons Corporation
P.O. Box 132
George, IA 51237-132
712-475-2811
800-225-3811
Fax: 712-475-2810
www.rangerallseason.com

Aaron Stegman, National Sales Manager
Ranger all season Corporation is proud to introduce the 'new' auto plug design. Incorporated with our patented take-apart design, it will revolutionize the scooter industry. Ranger is the first company to have this feature on scooters rated with a rider capacity up to 450 lbs.

563 **Scoota Bug**
Golden Technologies
401 Bridge Street
Old Forge, PA 18518-2323
570-451-7477
800-624-6374
Fax: 800-628-5165
www.goldentech.com

Richard Golden, President & CEO
Robert Golden, Chair
Fred Kiwak, Vice President, Research & Development
A lightweight, completely modular scooter, that disassembles and fits into most auto trunks.

564 **Sierra 3000/4000**
Electro Kinetic Technologies
W194 N11301 McCormick Drive
Germantown, WI 53022
262-250-7740
800-824-1068
Fax: 262-250-7741
info@ek-tech.com
www.ek-tech.com

565 **SmartScoot Lightweight Travel Scooter**
Maxi Aids
42 Executive Blvd.
Farmingdale, NY 11735-4710
631-752-0521
800-522-6294
Fax: 631-752-0689
TTY: 631-752-0738
sales@maxiaids.com
www.maxiaids.com

Elliot Zaretsky, Founder, President & CEO
Scooter is lightweight, foldable and adjustable. Airline friendly. Maximum load weight is 300 lb.

566 **Solo Scooter**
Ranger All Seasons Corporation
P.O. Box 132
George, IA 51237-132
712-475-2811
800-225-3811
Fax: 712-475-2810

Aaron Stegman, National Sales Manager
The SOLO is Ranger's flagship model. Introduction of the SOLO 1991 set the standard for easy disassembly of a scooter. The SOLO has a long list of user friendly features including patented take-apart and tiller adjustment mechanisms, non-rusting aluminum frame, comfortable contoured seats as standard, color impregnated-not painted-ABS plastic bodies, charger plug conveniently located on the Accelerator box and many more. Available in ultra-quiet drive and four wheel models.

567 **SoloRider Industries**
Regal Research & Manufacturing Company
1200 East Plano Parkway
Plano, TX 75074
972-422-5324
800-898-3353
Fax: 972-422-8010
info@solorider.com
www.solorider.com

Roger Pretekin, Founder
Manufacturer and distributor of the Solorider Golf Cart. This revolutionary single rider adaptive cart is specifically designed to meet the needs of individuals with mobility impairments.

568 **Sportster 10**
ATV Solutions
Unit 4
4700 W 60th Ave
Arvada, CO 80003-6928
303-450-2881
866-777-9727
888-867-1159
Fax: 303-450-2880
www.atvsolutions.com

Andrew Miro, Owner
Sportster 10 is our most maneuverable scooter, ideal for riders who must operate in tight spaces. Equipped with all of the great features of the Roadster 20, this three-wheeler is an exceptional buy.

569 **Systems 2000**
BioMedical Life Systems
P.O. Box 1360
Vista, CA 92085-1360
760-579-0801
800-726-8367
Fax: 760-929-9953
information@bmls.com
www.bmls.com

570 **Terra-Jet: Utility Vehicle**
TERRA-JET USA
Junction 417 & 419
P.O. Box 918
Innis, LA 70747-918
225-492-2249
800-864-5000
Fax: 225-492-2226
Terra-Jet@Terra-Jet.Com
www.terra-jet.com

Larry Rabalais, President, General Manager & CEO
Shawn Oubre, Sales Manager
TERRA-JET utility vehicles are unique in their ability to traverse many different types of terrain in remote areas otherwise inaccessible. It has a multitude of uses for industry, sportsmen or the whole family. Uniquely designed, industrial duty construction of low maintenance and low fuel consumption.

571 **Terrier Tricycle**
TRIAID
P.O. Box 1364
Cumberland, MD 21501-1364
301-759-3525
800-306-6777
Fax: 301-759-3525
sales@triaid.com
www.triaid.com

572 **Trekker 40**
ATV Solutions
Unit 4
4700 W 60th Ave
Arvada, CO 80003-6928
303-450-2881
866-777-9727
888-867-1159
Fax: 303-450-2880
www.atvsolutions.com

Andrew Miro, Owner
Our biggest, toughest scooter. With a huge 450 pound capacity and five inches of ground clearance, this machine is ideal for the daily outdoor user. The high top speed means you get there fast and the four-wheel suspension makes the ride smooth and comfortable.

573 **Tri-Lo's**
TRIAID
P.O. Box 1364
Cumberland, MD 21501-1364
301-759-3525
800-306-6777
Fax: 301-759-3525
sales@triaid.com
www.triaid.com

574 **Triumph 3000/4000**
Electro Kinetic Technologies
W194 N11301 McCormick Drive
Germantown, WI 53022
262-250-7740
800-824-1068
Fax: 262-250-7741
info@ek-tech.com
www.ek-tech.com

575 **Triumph Scooter**
Electro Kinetic Technologies
W194 N11301 McCormick Drive
Germantown, WI 53022
262-250-7740
800-824-1068
Fax: 262-250-7741
info@ek-tech.com
www.ek-tech.com

Stationery

576 **Access-USA**
242 James St.
P..O Box 160
Clayton, NY 13624-160
800-263-2750
Fax: 800-563-1687
www.access-usa.com

Deborah Webster, Manager
Access-USA provides one-stop alternate format transcription services for almost any type of document-reports, schedules, menus, monthly statements, brochures, reports, etc. Items may be submitted on computer disk, hard copy or email. Alternate formats include Braille, large print, Braille and print, audio recordings, adapted disks as well as video services-open/closed captioning and video descriptions. Accessible products also include Braille Business Cards and ADA signage.

577 **Address Book**
ASB
919 Walnut Street
Philadelphia, PA 19107-5237
215-627-0600
Fax: 215-922-0692
asbinfo@asb.org
www.asb.org

Karla S. McCaney, President & CEO
Beth Deering, Director, Human Services
Richard Forsythe, Director, Braille Division & Custom Audio
Joyce Robertson, Director, Finance & Information Technology
The big print address book is the first personal book to provide enlarged writing spaces, making it easier to write down and retrieve information. *$12.50*

578 **Bold Line Paper**
ASB
919 Walnut Street
Philadelphia, PA 19107-5237
215-627-0600
Fax: 215-922-0692
asbinfo@asb.org
www.asb.org

Karla S. McCaney, President & CEO
Beth Deering, Director, Human Services
Richard Forsythe, Director, Braille Division & Custom Audio
Joyce Robertson, Director, Finance & Information Technology
This pad consists of 100 sheets of paper with bold lines to help guide the writing of an individual with limited vision. *$2.50*

579 **Braille Calendar**
Maxi Aids
42 Executive Blvd.
Farmingdale, NY 11735-4710
631-752-0521
800-522-6294
Fax: 631-752-0689
TTY: 631-752-0738
sales@maxiaids.com
www.maxiaids.com

Elliot Zaretsky, Founder, President & CEO
Calendar with Braille markings for touch reading. *$14.99*

580 **Braille Notebook**
Maxi Aids
42 Executive Blvd.
Farmingdale, NY 11735-4710
631-752-0521
800-522-6294
Fax: 631-752-0689
TTY: 631-752-0738
sales@maxiaids.com
www.maxiaids.com

Elliot Zaretsky, Founder, President & CEO
Made of heavy-duty board, covered with waterproof plastic and contains three rings for binding. *$18.95*

581 **Braille: Greeting Cards**
ASB
919 Walnut Street
Philadelphia, PA 19107-5237
215-627-0600
Fax: 215-922-0692
asbinfo@asb.org
www.asb.org

Karla S. McCaney, President & CEO
Beth Deering, Director, Human Services
Richard Forsythe, Director, Braille Division & Custom Audio
Joyce Robertson, Director, Finance & Information Technology
Birthday, anniversary, get well, sympathy and Christmas cards offering Braille print for the blind. *$.95*

582 **Clip Board Notebook**
ASB
919 Walnut Street
Philadelphia, PA 19107-5237
215-627-0600
Fax: 215-922-0692
asbinfo@asb.org
www.asb.org

Karla S. McCaney, President & CEO
Beth Deering, Director, Human Services
Richard Forsythe, Director, Braille Division & Custom Audio
Joyce Robertson, Director, Finance & Information Technology
Kit includes a pack of Bold Line paper and black ink pen. *$5.95*

583 **Deluxe Signature Guide**
Maxi Aids
42 Executive Blvd.
Farmingdale, NY 11735-4710
631-752-0521
800-522-6294
Fax: 631-752-0689
TTY: 631-752-0738
sales@maxiaids.com
www.maxiaids.com

Elliot Zaretsky, Founder, President & CEO
Consisting of rods supported by two rubber blocks, this device helps to facilitate writing. *$1.95*

584 **Giant Print Address Book**
Maxi Aids
42 Executive Blvd.
Farmingdale, NY 11735-4710
631-752-0521
800-522-6294
Fax: 631-752-0689
TTY: 631-752-0738
sales@maxiaids.com
www.maxiaids.com

Elliot Zaretsky, Founder, President & CEO
Large print address book for storing up to 360 names. Three-ring hardcover binder with removable pages. *$16.95*

585 **Highlighter and Note Tape**
Therapro, Inc.
225 Arlington St
Framingham, MA 01702-8723
508-872-9494
800-257-5376
Fax: 508-875-2062
info@therapro.com
www.therapro.com

Karen Conrad Weihrauch, President & Owner
A great way to highlight and draw attention to words without damaging original. Optimal for people with difficulties in reading and visual processing.

586 **Letter Writing Guide**
Independent Living Aids
137 Rano Rd
Buffalo, NY 14207
716-332-2970
800-537-2118
855-746-7452
Fax: 516-937-3906
can-do@independentliving.com
www.independentliving.com

Irwin Schneidmill, President
Michael Gutierrez, Director of Operations
Pamela Strauss, Director of Marketing
Ursula Izurieta, Director of Merchandising
Sturdy plastic sheet with 13 apertures corresponding to standard line spacing. *$3.49*

587 **Lettering Guide Value Pack**
Independent Living Aids
137 Rano Rd
Buffalo, NY 14207
716-332-2970
800-537-2118
855-746-7452
Fax: 516-937-3906
can-do@independentliving.com
www.independentliving.com

Irwin Schneidmill, President
Michael Gutierrez, Director of Operations
Pamela Strauss, Director of Marketing
Ursula Izurieta, Director of Merchandising
Included in this useful pack are four durable plastic lettering and number guides for tracing letters when the individual is unable to write letters unassisted. *$6.29*

588 **Ottobock**
11501 Alterra Parkway
Suite 600
Austin, TX 78758
800-328-4058
Fax: 800-962-2549
USCustomerService@OttoBock.com
www.ottobockus.com

Visual Aids

589 **Adjustable Folding Support Cane for the Blind**
Maxi Aids
42 Executive Blvd.
Farmingdale, NY 11735-4710
631-752-0521
800-522-6294
Fax: 631-752-0689
TTY: 631-752-0738
sales@maxiaids.com
www.maxiaids.com

Elliot Zaretsky, Founder, President & CEO
Adjustable canes for the visually impaired. *$21.95*

590 **All Terrain Cane**
Maxi Aids
42 Executive Blvd.
Farmingdale, NY 11735-4710
631-752-0521
800-522-6294
Fax: 631-752-0689
TTY: 631-752-0738
sales@maxiaids.com
www.maxiaids.com

Elliot Zaretsky, Founder, President & CEO
A rigid aluminum cane with a curved nylon tip and golf grip with hook handle. Designed to help blind and visually impaired persons navigate unpaved areas. *$49.95*

591 **Audio Book Contractors**
P.O. Box 96
Riverdale, MD 20738-0096
301-439-5830
Fax: 301-439-5830
audiobookcontractors@verizon.net
www.audiobookcontractors.com

Flo Gibson, President
Over 950 titles of unabridged classic books in a variety of genres on audio cassettes in sturdy vinyl covers with picture and spine windows. Discounted prices for disabled patrons.

592 **Beyond Sight, Inc.**
5650 S Windermere St
Littleton, CO 80120-1240
303-795-6455
Fax: 303-795-6425
www.beyondsight.com

Scott Chaplick, Owner & President
Gina Whetzel, Sales & Merchandise Specialist
Products for the blind and visually impaired, including talking clocks, watches and calculators. Beyond Sight, Inc. also carries a large selection of Braille products, magnifiers, reading machines and computer equipment.

593 **Big Number Pocket Sized Calculator**
Independent Living Aids
137 Rano Rd
Buffalo, NY 14207
716-332-2970
800-537-2118
855-746-7452
Fax: 516-937-3906
can-do@independentliving.com
www.independentliving.com

Marvin Sandler, President
A handy pocket size calculator with big numbers that fits easily into purse or pocket. *$14.95*

594 **Braille Elevator Plates**
Maxi Aids
42 Executive Blvd.
Farmingdale, NY 11735-4710
631-752-0521
800-522-6294
Fax: 631-752-0689
TTY: 631-752-0738
sales@maxiaids.com
www.maxiaids.com

Elliot Zaretsky, Founder, President & CEO
The plates have curing type pressure sensitive material applied for metal to metal bonding. *$49.95*

595 **Braille Touch-Time Watches**
Independent Living Aids
137 Rano Rd
Buffalo, NY 14207
716-332-2970
800-537-2118
855-746-7452
Fax: 516-937-3906
can-do@independentliving.com
www.independentliving.com

Marvin Sandler, President
White dial with black numerals and hands makes telling time possible quickly and easily for the visually impaired. *$44.95*

596 **Circline Illuminated Magnifer**
Dazor Lighting Technology
2360 Chaffee Drive
St. Louis, MO 63146
314-652-2400
800-345-9103
Fax: 314-652-2069
info@dazor.com
www.dazor.com

Kirk Cressey, Marketing Director
Bob Smith, National Sales Manager
Provides even, shadow free light under the magnifying lens with a 22-watt circline fluorescent. The magnifier is mounted on a floating arm that allows you to position the light source and lens with the touch of a finger.

597 **Large Display Alarm Clock**
HARC Mercantile
5413 S Westnedge Ave.
Suite A
Portage, MI 49002
269-324-1615
800-445-9968
Fax: 269-324-2387
TTY: 269-324-1615
info@harc.com
www.harc.com

Michael Martinson, Owner

Features a large, easy to read display, as well as an extra loud alarm and bedshaker. *$54.00*

598 **Low Vision Telephones**
2738 N Campbell Ave
Tucson, AZ 85719-3141
520-883-8600
866-674-3549
Fax: 520-883-3172
www.assistivedevices.net

Oliver Simoes, Owner

599 **Low Vision Watches & Clocks**
Maxi Aids
42 Executive Blvd.
Farmingdale, NY 11735-4710
631-752-0521
800-522-6294
Fax: 631-752-0689
TTY: 631-752-0738
sales@maxiaids.com
www.maxiaids.com

Elliot Zaretsky, Founder, President & CEO

Offers a wide range of watches and clocks, including Braille watches, talking watches, and large display clocks.

600 **Magni-Cam & Primer**
Innoventions
9593 Corsair Dr
Conifer, CO 80433-9317
303-797-6554
800-854-6554
Fax: 303-727-4940
www.magnicam.com

Mark Freeman, President

Magni-Cam and Primer are hand-held, light weight, inexpensive auto-focus electronic magnification systems designed to meet the reading and writing needs of those with low vision. The systems present the image in black and white or in color with three different view modes. Connects to any TV monitor in minutes. Systems read any surface with no distortion. A battery powered system is available, providing total portability and flexibility.

601 **Magnifier Bookweight**
Levenger
420 S Congress Ave
Delray Beach, FL 33445-4693
800-544-0880
Fax: 800-544-6910
Cservice@levenger.com
www.levenger.com

Steve Leveen, CEO

The Magnifier Bookweight features an optical quality magnifier and is long enough to enlarge the full width of most book pages while holing the pages open. This magnifier is encased in embossed leather and enlarges approximately four lines of text at a time to twice the original size.

602 **Man's Low-Vision Quartz Watches**
Independent Living Aids
137 Rano Rd
Buffalo, NY 14207
716-332-2970
800-537-2118
855-746-7452
Fax: 516-937-3906
can-do@independentliving.com
www.independentliving.com

Marvin Sandler, President

An inexpensive, easy-to-read watch with chrome case. *$27.95*

603 **MonoMouse Electronic Magnifiers**
Maxi Aids
42 Executive Blvd.
Farmingdale, NY 11735-4710
631-752-0521
800-522-6294
Fax: 631-752-0689
TTY: 631-752-0738
sales@maxiaids.com
www.maxiaids.com

Elliot Zaretsky, Founder, President & CEO

Portable magnifier for people with low vision. Just about the size of a standard computer mouse. Compatible with any desktop or notebook PC. Variable magnification from 3x to 100x.

604 **Stretch-View Wide-View Rectangular Illuminated Magnifier**
Dazor Lighting Technology
2360 Chaffee Drive
St. Louis, MO 63146
314-652-2400
800-345-9103
Fax: 314-652-2069
info@dazor.com
www.dazor.com

Kirk Cressey, Marketing Director
Bob Smith, National Sales Manager

Provides even, shadow free light under the magnifying lens with a 22-watt circline fluorescent. The magnifier is mounted on a floating arm that allows you to position the light source and lens with the touch of a finger.

605 **Timex Easy Reader**
Independent Living Aids
137 Rano Rd
Buffalo, NY 14207
716-332-2970
800-537-2118
855-746-7452
Fax: 516-937-3906
can-do@independentliving.com
www.independentliving.com

Marvin Sandler, President

An easy-to-read large face watch that's water resistant. *$29.95*

606 **Unisex Low Vision Watch**
Independent Living Aids
137 Rano Rd
Buffalo, NY 14207
716-332-2970
800-537-2118
855-746-7452
Fax: 516-937-3906
can-do@independentliving.com
www.independentliving.com

Marvin Sandler, President

Unisex watch with large numbers and wide hands. Gold-toned case with either expansion or leather band. *$31.95*

Walking Aids: Canes, Crutches & Walkers

607 **Aluminum Crutches**
Arista Surgical Supply Company
297 High Street
Dedham, MA 02026-2852
781-329-2900
800-225-2610
Fax: 781-329-8392
customerservice@alimed.com
www.alimed.com

Julian Cherubini, President

Lightweight aluminum crutches with wood underarms and handgrips. Adjusts to custom fit any user. *$25.00*

608 **Aluminum Kiddie Canes**
Maxi Aids
42 Executive Blvd.
Farmingdale, NY 11735-4710
631-752-0521
800-522-6294
Fax: 631-752-0689
TTY: 631-752-0738
sales@maxiaids.com
www.maxiaids.com

Elliot Zaretsky, Founder, President & CEO

Rigid and folding canes for children.

609 **Aluminum Walking Canes**
Maxi Aids
42 Executive Blvd.
Farmingdale, NY 11735-4710
631-752-0521
800-522-6294
Fax: 631-752-0689
TTY: 631-752-0738
sales@maxiaids.com
www.maxiaids.com
Elliot Zaretsky, Founder, President & CEO
Lightweight walking canes made of a heavy gauge aluminum tube with safety locknuts and heavy-duty rubber tips.

610 **Crutches**
Mada Medical Products
625 Washington Ave
Carlstadt, NJ 07072-2901
201-460-0454
800-526-6370
Fax: 201-460-3509
dianelind@mail.madamedical.com
www.madainternational.com
Jeffrey Adam, President
All aluminum construction, underarm crutch with double pushbutton height adjustment.

611 **Deluxe Nova Wheeled Walker & Avant Wheeled Walker**
Performance Health
28100 Torch Parkway
Suite 700
Warrenville, IL 60555-3938
630-393-6000
Fax: 630-393-7600
CustomerSupport@performancehealth.com
www.performancehealth.com
Francis Dirksmeier, CEO
Isabel Afonso, Managing Director & Head of International
Daniel Baumwald, Vice President, North America Retail & eCommerce
Laurie Byrne, Chief Human Resources Officer
Lightweight and simple to handle with an easy-to-operate braking system. *$425.40*

612 **Deluxe Standard Wood Cane**
Arista Surgical Supply Company/AliMed
297 High Street
Dedham, MA 02026-2852
781-329-2900
800-225-2610
Fax: 781-329-8392
info@alimed.com
www.alimed.com
Julian Cherubini, President
A standard old-fashioned wooden cane for the physically challenged. Ideal for those with arthritis. *$10.00*

613 **EasyStand 6000 Glider**
Access To Recreation
8 Sandra Ct
Newbury Park, CA 91320-4302
805-498-7535
800-634-4351
Fax: 805-498-8186
customerservice@accesstr.com
www.accesstr.com
Don Krebs, President & Founder
Provides dynamic leg motion for individuals who are unable to stand upright or walk on their own.

614 **Europa Superior Folding Cane**
Maxi Aids
42 Executive Blvd.
Farmingdale, NY 11735-4710
631-752-0521
800-522-6294
Fax: 631-752-0689
TTY: 631-752-0738
sales@maxiaids.com
www.maxiaids.com
Elliot Zaretsky, Founder, President & CEO
Aluminum folding cane with tapered joints, golf grip with wrist loop, and screw-on glide tip. *$23.95*

615 **Freedom Three Wheel Walker**
Mada Medical Products
625 Washington Ave
Carlstadt, NJ 07072-2901
201-460-0454
800-526-6370
Fax: 201-460-3509
dianelind@mail.madamedical.com
www.madainternational.com
Jeffrey Adam, President
The freedom walker has ultra light touch, locking loop brakes and sure grip hand grips.

616 **Liberty Lightweight Aluminum Stroll Walker**
Mada Medical Products
625 Washington Ave
Carlstadt, NJ 07072-2901
201-460-0454
800-526-6370
Fax: 201-460-3509
dianelind@mail.madamedical.com
www.madainternational.com
Jeffrey Adam, President
The Liberty walker has a spring loaded push down braking system, adjustable handle height with locking system, a 12 inch wide fully padded seat, and a removable shopping basket.

617 **Out-N-About American Walker**
742 Market St
Oregon, WI 53575-1059
608-835-9255
Fax: 608-835-5234
Luann Smith, President
The lightweight Out-N-About is easy to handle. The four wheel design provides greater support and stability than any other walking aids. Its large rubber tires move effortlessly over most surfaces, indoors and out. The small turning radius makes it ideal for getting through confined spaces and narrow doorways. The attractive, burgundy colored, tubular steel frame is extremely durable. The Out-N-About folds flat and stands alone for easy storage. Made in USA.

618 **Patriot Extra Wide Folding Walkers**
Mada Medical Products
625 Washington Ave
Carlstadt, NJ 07072-2901
201-460-0454
800-526-6370
Fax: 201-460-3509
dianelind@mail.madamedical.com
www.madainternational.com
Jeffrey Adam, President
The extra wide walkers have padded foam hand grips, two-stage push button folding mechanism, dual width adjustment, height adjustment, and nonskid tips.

619 **Patriot Folding Walker Series**
Mada Medical Products
625 Washington Ave
Carlstadt, NJ 07072-2901
201-460-0454
800-526-6370
Fax: 201-460-3509
dianelind@mail.madamedical.com
www.madainternational.com
Jeffrey Adam, President
The patriot walker has high density, padded foam hand grips, high strength 1in lightweight, anodized, dull silver aluminum tube construction, adjustable height with push-button lock security, nonskid tips, and a single button folding mechanism.

620 **Patriot Reciprocal Folding Walkers**
Mada Medical Products
625 Washington Ave
Carlstadt, NJ 07072-2901
201-460-0454
800-526-6370
Fax: 201-460-3509
dianelind@mail.madamedical.com
www.madainternational.com
Jeffrey Adam, President
The reciprocal folding walkers have padded foam hand grips, adjustable height with snap-in security, double front cross brace, and nonskid tips.

621 **Prone Support Walker**
Consumer Care Products, LLC
W282 N7109 Main Street
Merton, WI 53056
262-820-2300
info@consumercarellc.com
www.consumercarellc.com

622 **Push-Button Quad Cane**
Arista Surgical Supply Company/AliMed
297 High Street
Dedham, MA 02026-2852
781-329-2900
800-225-2610
Fax: 781-329-8392
info@alimed.com
www.alimed.com

Julian Cherubini, President
A reliable walking cane offering independence to the physically challenged user. *$25.00*

623 **Quad Canes**
Mada Medical Products
625 Washington Ave
Carlstadt, NJ 07072-2901
201-460-0454
800-526-6370
Fax: 201-460-3509
dianelind@mail.madamedical.com
www.madainternational.com

Jeffrey Adam, President
There are large and small base quad canes with high density foam grips.

624 **Rand-Scot**
Rand-Scot, Inc.
209 Christman Drive
Fort Collins, CO 80524-2429
970-484-7967
800-467-7967
Fax: 970-484-3800
info@randscot.com
www.randscot.com

Joel Lerich, Co-Founder
Barbara Lerich, Co-Founder
Manufactures the Easy Pivot patient lift, the BBD wheelchair cushion line and Saratoga Exercise products for the disabled. Offers a line of patient lifts and standers for the disabled. Rand-scot products are designed to help the disabled achieve independence, comfort, and stamina.

625 **Rollators**
Maxi Aids
42 Executive Blvd.
Farmingdale, NY 11735-4710
631-752-0521
800-522-6294
Fax: 631-752-0689
TTY: 631-752-0738
sales@maxiaids.com
www.maxiaids.com

Elliot Zaretsky, Founder, President & CEO
Offers a wide range of rolling walkers.

626 **Secret Agent Walking Stick**
Gold Violin, Inc.
P.O. BOX 126
Jessup, PA 22903
877-648-8400
800-361-3336
customerservice@goldviolin.com
goldviolin.blair.com

Connie Hallquist, CEO
Ian Chaplin, CTO
Kara Carter, Vice President, Business Development
The Secret Agent Walking Stick features a built-in flashlight, a red reflector and a built-in secret pill compartment. This folding aluminum cane is height adjustable and has a derby-style handle and a non-skid rubber tip. A nylon carrying case is included.

627 **StairClimber**
Martin Technology
29 N Main St
Gloversville, NY 12078-3006
518-725-1837
800-800-1410
Fax: 518-725-9522

Michael Lewy, Owner
A walker-capable person can climb and descend stairs with this walker-designed StairClimber.

628 **Standing Aid Frame with Rear Entry**
Consumer Care Products, LLC
W282 N7109 Main Street
Merton, WI 53056
262-820-2300
info@consumercarellc.com
www.consumercarellc.com

629 **Stick Canes**
Mada Medical Products
625 Washington Ave
Carlstadt, NJ 07072-2901
201-460-0454
800-526-6370
Fax: 201-460-3509
www.madainternational.com

Jeffrey Adam, President
Mada's stick canes are adjustable with a locking security system.

630 **TIDI Products, LLC**
570 Enterprise Drive
Neenaha, WI 54956
920-751-4300
800-521-1314
Fax: 920-751-4370
excellence@tidiproducts.com
www.tidiproducts.com

Kevin McNamara, President & CEO
Jeff Hebbard, Vice President & COO
Mike Duski, Vice President & CCO
TIDI Products meets the needs of caregivers for job optimization and providing solutions to other healthcare professionals. Supplies Brand name medical equipment and devices including: POSEY patient safety devices, TIDISHIELD eyewear and devices, C-AMOR drapes, STERILE-Z drapes, GRIP-LOK securement items, and ZERO-GRAVITY radiation protection.

631 **U-Step Walking Stabilizer: Walker**
Maxi Aids
42 Executive Blvd.
Farmingdale, NY 11735-4710
631-752-0521
800-522-6294
Fax: 631-752-0689
TTY: 631-752-0738
sales@maxiaids.com
www.maxiaids.com

Elliot Zaretsky, Founder, President & CEO
Stabilizing walker with braking system, seat and basket. Easily foldable. Weight capacity is 375 lbs. Suitable for users 5'1 to 6'1 tall. *$539.95*

632 **Ventura Enterprises**
4431 S. Eastern Avenue
Las Vegas, NV 89119
702-457-7676
Fax: 317-745-3179
info@venturaenterprises.com
www.venturaenterprises.com

Sam Ventura, President, CEO
Ron Ventura, Vice President of Development
Galit Rozen, Vice President of Acquisitions
Ofir Ventura, ESQ., In House General Council
Manufacturer of everyday living mobility aids. Products include carrying aids for walkers and wheelchairs and also wheelchair cushions.

633 **WCIB Heavy-Duty Folding Cane**
Maxi Aids
42 Executive Blvd.
Farmingdale, NY 11735-4710
631-752-0521
800-522-6294
Fax: 631-752-0689
TTY: 631-752-0738
sales@maxiaids.com
www.maxiaids.com

Elliot Zaretsky, Founder, President & CEO
A four section aluminum folding cane with a golf-type grip handle and flexible wrist loop. *$27.95*

634 **Walker Leg Support**
Performance Health
28100 Torch Parkway
Suite 700
Warrenville, IL 60555-3938
630-393-6000
Fax: 630-393-7600
CustomerSupport@performancehealth.com
www.performancehealth.com
Francis Dirksmeier, CEO
Isabel Afonso, Managing Director & Head of International
Daniel Baumwald, Vice President, North America Retail & eCommerce
Laurie Byrne, Chief Human Resources Officer
For lower extremity trauma. An alternative to crutches that allows safe, stable ambulation and frees hands and arms for daily tasks. *$11.50*

Wheelchairs: Accessories

635 **Advantage Wheelchair & Walker Bags**
Advantage Bag Company
TORRANCE, CA 90505
310-540-8197
800-556-6307
Fax: 310-316-2561
advantagebag@verizon.net
www.advantagebag.com

636 **Automatic Wheelchair Anti-Rollback Device**
Alzheimer's Store
3197 Trout Place Rd
Cumming, GA 30041-8260
678-947-4001
800-752-3238
Fax: 678-947-8411
contact@alzstore.com
www.alzstore.com
Ellen Warner, President & Co-Founder
Mark Warner, Co-Founder
As a wheelchair user transfers to and from the chair, a pair of brake arms grabs the tires to prevent the chair from rolling backwards. Once the individual is seated, the device switches to stand-by mode and the wheelchair returns to standard function.

637 **Battery Operated Cushion**
DA Schulman
3827 Creekside Lane
Holmen, WI 54636
608-782-0031
866-782-9658
Fax: 608-782-0488
aquila@aquilacorp.com
www.aquilacorp.com
Steve Kohlman, Owner & President
Justine Kohlman, Vice President
Battery-operated, dynamic cushion for wheelchairs. The Airpulse PK wheelchair cushion system is Aquila Corporation's most dynamic cushion system. It was designed to be the most advanced solution to help prevent and heal pressure ulcers.

638 **Dual-Mode Charger**
Lester Electrical
625 West A Street
Lincoln, NE 68522-1794
402-477-8988
Fax: 402-474-1769
sales@lesterelectrical.com
www.lesterelectrical.com
Spencer Stock, President & CEO
Fully automatic battery charger.

639 **Equalizer 1000 Series**
Helm Distributing
Deer Park P.O.
PO Box 25105
Red Deer, AB T4R-2M2
403-309-5551
Fax: 403-342-5509
james@equalizerexercise.com
www.equalizerexercise.com

640 **Equalizer 5000 Home Gym**
Helm Distributing
Deer Park P.O.
PO Box 25105
Red Deer, AB T4R-2M2
403-309-5551
Fax: 403-342-5509
james@equalizerexercise.com
www.equalizerexercise.com

641 **Featherspring Shoe Inserts**
Luxis International, Inc.
105 W Lincoln Hwy
DeKalb, IL 60115
815-981-3793
800-628-4693
Fax: 800-261-1164
customerservice@luxis.com
www.luxis.com

642 **Gem Wheelchair & Scooter Service: Mobility & Homecare**
176-39 Union Turnpike
Flushing, NY 11366-1515
718-969-8600
800-943-3578
Fax: 718-969-8300
help@gemwheelchairservice.com
www.gemwheelchairservice.com

643 **MAT Factory, Inc.**
6726 North Figueroa Street
Los Angeles, CA 90042
323-254-6165
800-628-7626
Fax: 323-254-4545
info@matfactoryinc.com
www.matfactoryinc.com

644 **One Thousand FS**
Fortress
P.O. Box 489
Clovis, CA 93613-489
559-322-5437
Fax: 559-323-0299

645 **Pac-All Wheelchair Carrier**
Pac-All Carriers
2321 Carolton Rd
Maitland, FL 32751-3624
407-830-6604
800-628-6672
Fax: 407-339-2847
LE Angel
No more lifting and no more pain wheelchair carrier. VA approved. Made in USA.
$158 - $226.40

646 **Permobil**
300 Duke Drive
Lebanon, TN 37090
800-736-0925
Fax: 800-231-3256
techsupport@permobil.com
www.permobilus.com
Bengt Thorsson, President & CEO
Carl Bandhold, CFO
Jonas Cederhage, Executive Vice President
Peter Jidesjo, Executive Vice President
Develops and manufactures wheelchairs, communication systems, and seating and positioning systems for users with disabilities. Offers a full line of standing wheelchairs for manual operation. Power assisted are fully motorized. *$7000.00*

647 **Safety Deck II**
MAT Factory, Inc.
6726 North Figueroa Street
Los Angeles, CA 90042
323-254-6165
800-628-7626
Fax: 323-254-4545
info@matfactoryinc.com
www.matfactoryinc.com

648 **Scooter & Wheelchair Battery Fuel Gauges and Motor Speed Controllers**
Curtis Instruments, Inc.
200 Kisco Ave
Mount Kisco, NY 10549-1407
914-666-2971
Fax: 914-666-2188
gomezj@curtisinst.com
www.curtisinst.com

Stuart E Marwell, President and CEO
David Matthews, VP Sales Americas
Cheryl Leonaggeo, Customer Service Manager
Richard McFarlane, Customer Support Engineer

Provides a readable, accurate indication of battery in easy to read type of display. Innovative, efficient motor speed controllers for single or dual PM motor vehicles.

649 **Softfoot Ergomatta**
MAT Factory, Inc.
6726 North Figueroa Street
Los Angeles, CA 90042
323-254-6165
800-628-7626
Fax: 323-254-4545
www.matfactoryinc.com

650 **Tilt-N-Table**
Osterguard Enterprises c/o Jim's Shop
3228 W Olive Ave
Fresno, CA 93722-5733
559-275-4695
Jim Ostergaard Ii, Owner

These are lightweight tables for wheelchairs that are angle and height adjustable to your changing needs.

651 **Wheel Life News**
University of Virginia, Rehab Engineering Centers
3363 University Sta
Charlottesville, VA 22903
434-924-5118
www.medicine.virginia.edu
Kristine M. Garza, Ph.D., Executive Director of SACNAS
Steven T. DeKosky, Dean

Features tie downs and other adaptive technology for persons with disabilities.

652 **Wheelchair Accessories**
Diestco Manufacturing Company
P.O. Box 6504
Chico, CA 95927-6504
800-795-2392
info@diestco.com
www.diestco.com

653 **Wheelchair Aide**
Graham-Field
400 Rabro Dr
Hauppauge, NY 11788-4258
631-348-1364

654 **Wheelchair Back Pack and Tote Bag**
Med Covers
320 Roebling Street
Suite 515
Brooklyn, NY 11211
718-302-1923
800-320-7140
Fax: 866-522-6967
info@1800wheelchair.com
www.1800wheelchair.com

655 **Wheelchair Roller**
Access To Recreation
8 Sandra Ct
Newbury Park, CA 91320-4302
805-498-7535
800-634-4351
Fax: 805-498-8186
customerservice@accesstr.com
www.accesstr.com

Don Krebs, President & Founder

The McClain Wheelchair Roller allows you to build strength and stamina in the comfort of your own home.

656 **Wheelchair Work Table**
Bailey Manufacturing Company
118 Lee Drive
P.O. Box 130
Lodi, OH 44254-130
330-948-1080
800-321-8372
Fax: 330-948-4439
baileymfg@baileymfg.com
www.baileymfg.com

Larry Strimple, President
Judie Butler, Dealer Contact

An adjustable height, functional, individual cut-out work table featuring a wood-grain laminate, scratch resistant top with chrome plated steel legs.

Wheelchairs: General

657 **21st Century Scientific, Inc. - Bounder Power Wheelchair**
4931 N Manufacturing Way
Coeur D Alene, ID 83815-8931
208-667-8800
800-448-3680
Fax: 208-667-6600
21st@wheelchairs.com
wheelchairs.com

Ronald E. Prior, Ph.D., President and Founder
RD Davidson, Sales/Marketing Director
Susan Harris, CFO and Webmaster

High performance power chairs for active individuals. Very fast (11+ MPH), OFF-ROAD and Bariatric options available. Power seating options include tilt, recline, 13-inch seat elevator, reverse tilt, leg rests, standing and front load (latitude). 6-drive programmable electronics standard; lights, horn, electric leg bag emptier and many other options available. Customization is our specialty.

658 **Ability Center**
4797 Ruffner St.
San Diego, CA 92111
858-541-0552
833-919-2581
Fax: 858-541-1941
www.abilitycenter.com

Terry Barton, General Manager

Specializes in accessible vehicles and mobility products; the company has more than 100 employees in 14 locations across the western U.S.
1994

659 **Bariatric Wheelchairs Regency FL**
Gendron
520 W. Mulberry St.
Suite 100
Bryan, OH 43506
800-537-2521
Fax: 419-636-9261
www.gendroninc.com

Sebastien Gendron, Co-founder & CEO
Roberta Jacobs, National Sales Manager

Bariatric wheelchairs, for users weighing up to seven hundred pounds. Manual and power styles built to order for specific needs.

660 **Breezy**
Sunrise Medical
2842 Business Park Avenue
Fresno, CA 93727
800-333-4000
Fax: 800-300-7502
webmaster@sunmed.com
www.sunrisemedical.com

Thomas Babacan, President & CEO
Adrian Platt, CFO
Bernd Krebs, CTO
Roxane Cromwell, COO

This lightweight chair is durable, comfortable and flexible enough to meet the needs of a wide range of wheelchair users.

661 **Champion 1000**
Kuschall of America
3601 Rider Trl S
Earth City, MO 63045-1116
314-512-7000
800-654-4768
Fax: 800-542-3567

662 **Champion 2000**
Kuschall of America
3601 Rider Trl S
Earth City, MO 63045-1116
314-512-7000
800-654-4768
Fax: 800-542-3567

663 **Champion 3000**
Kuschall of America
3601 Rider Trl S
Earth City, MO 63045-1116
314-512-7000
800-654-4768
Fax: 800-542-3567

664 **Choosing a Wheelchair: A Guide for Optimal Independence**
Patient-Centered Guides
1005 Gravenstein Hwy N
Sebastopol, CA 95472-3836
707-827-7019
800-889-8969
Fax: 707-824-8268
order@oreilly.com
www.patientcenters.com

Linda Lamb, Series Editor
Shawnde Paull, Marketing
Tim O'Reilly, Publisher
Gary Karp, Author
With the right wheelchair, quality of life increases dramatically and even people with severe disabilities can have a considerable degree of independence and activity. Choosing the wrong chair can indeed the tantamount to confinement. This book describes technology, options, and the selection process to help you identify the chair than can provide you with optimal independence.
$9.95
186 pages Paperback
ISBN 1-565924-11-8

665 **Convaid**
2830 California Street
Torrance, CA 90503
310-618-0111
888-266-8243
Fax: 310-618-2166
www.convaid.com

Ryan B. Williams, President
Five different styles of wheelchairs.

666 **Custom**
Fortress
P.O. Box 489
Clovis, CA 93613-489
559-322-5437
Fax: 559-323-0299

667 **Custom Durable**
21279 Protecta Dr
Elkhart, IN 46516-9539
574-522-7201
800-478-2363
Fax: 574-293-0202

668 **Edge**
Fortress
P.O. Box 489
Clovis, CA 93613-489
559-322-5437
Fax: 559-323-0299

669 **Etac USA: F3 Wheelchair**
Ste J
2325 Parklawn Dr
Waukesha, WI 53186-2938
262-717-9910
800-678-3822
Fax: 262-796-4605
etac1usa@execpc.com

Mark Samolyk, Manager
A Swedish wheelchair designed to provide function, comfort and flexibility. Seat frame and upholstery are adjustable to fit each individual. Swing away, detachable footrests are standard. Available in frame widths from 14, 18 and 20 inch. Numerous accessories are available in order to individualize each chair. Lifetime warranty on frame for original user.

670 **Evacu-Trac**
Garaventa Canada
7505 - 134 A Street, Surrey, BC V3W
Blaine, WA 98231-1769
866-824-8314
productinfo@evacutrac.com

671 **Folding Chair with a Rigid Feel**
Kuschall of America
3601 Rider Trl S
Earth City, MO 63045-1116
314-512-7000
800-654-4768
Fax: 800-542-3567

672 **Formula Series Active Mobility Wheelchairs**
Everest & Jennings
3233 Mission Oaks Blvd
Camarillo, CA 93012-5047
805-389-7450

673 **Freestyle II**
Fortress
P.O. Box 489
Clovis, CA 93613-489
559-322-5437
Fax: 559-323-0299

674 **Gadabout Wheelchairs**
Gadabout Wheelchairs
1165 Portland Ave
Rochester, NY 14621-3945
585-338-2110
800-828-4242
Fax: 585-338-2696

Michael Fonte, Owner
Enjoy independence with the wheelchair that is lightweight, portable, convenient, comfortable and sturdy.

675 **Gem Wheelchair & Scooter Service: Mobility & Homecare**
176-39 Union Turnpike
Flushing, NY 11366-1515
718-969-8600
800-943-3578
Fax: 718-969-8300
help@gemwheelchairservice.com
www.gemwheelchairservice.com

676 **Gendron**
520 W. Mulberry St.
Suite 100
Bryan, OH 43506
419-636-0848
800-537-2521
Fax: 419-636-9261
www.gendroninc.com

Sebastien Gendron, National Sales Manager
Roberta Jacobs, National Sales Manager
Manufacturer of wheelchairs for a variety of other applications, specializing in bariatric mobility products.

677 **HiRider**
Stryker
2825 Airview Boulevard
Kalamazoo, MI 49002
269-385-2600
Fax: 269-385-1062
www.stryker.com/us/en/about.html

Kevin A. Lobo, Chair & CEO
Glenn S. Boehnlein, Vice President & CFO
Yin C. Becker, Vice President, Communications, Public Affairs & Marketing
Dean H. Bergy, Vice President, Corporate Secretary
A wheelchair that provides mobility in both sitting and standing positions.

678 **Innovative Products**
4351 W College Ave
Appleton, WI 54914-3928
920-738-9090
800-424-3369
Fax: 920-738-9050
www.att.com

Fritz H Heerdt, President
Wheelchairs; accessories.

679 **Liberty**
Fortress
P.O. Box 489
Clovis, CA 93613-489
559-322-5437
Fax: 559-323-0299

680 **Lightweight Breezy**
Sunrise Medical
2842 Business Park Avenue
Fresno, CA 93727
800-333-4000
Fax: 800-300-7502
webmaster@sunmed.com
www.sunrisemedical.com

Thomas Babacan, President & CEO
Adrian Platt, CFO
Bernd Krebs, CTO
Roxane Cromwell, COO
A lightweight wheelchair. *$750.00*

681 **Majors Medical Equipment**
415 W Wilshire Blvd.
Suite A
Oklahoma City, OK 73116
405-840-5272
888-444-0122
Fax: 405-840-5274
www.majorsmedicalequipment.com

Pat Metz, Owner
America's largest selection of wheelchairs and homecare medical equipment required safety and mobility needs.

682 **Natural Access**
PO Box 5729
Santa Monica, CA 90409
310-392-9864
800-411-7789
Fax: 310-392-3874
john_egan_2000@yahoo.com

John Egan, Owner
Provides the Landeez all-terrain wheelchair, that can roll easily on sand, gravel and snow for outdoor fun. The entire chair can fit inside a travel bag!

683 **Patient Transport Chair**
Mada Medical Products
625 Washington Ave
Carlstadt, NJ 07072-2901
201-460-0454
800-526-6370
Fax: 201-460-3509
www.madainternational.com

Jeffrey Adam, President
Mada's lightweight design transport chair is constructed of heavy gauge chrome-plated, steel tubing with reinforced cross braces.

684 **Posture-Glide Lounger**
Graham-Field Health Products
2935 Northeast Parkway
Atlanta, GA 30360-2808
770-368-4700
Fax: 770-368-4932
cs@grahamfield.com
www.grahamfield.com

Kenneth Spett, President & CEO
Cherie Antoniazzi, Senior Vice President, Quality, Regulatory & Risk Management
Marc Bernstein, Senior Vice President, Consumer Sales
Lawrence De La Haba, Senior Vice President, Business Development
Provides all day comfort and safe, independent mobilization with feet or hands. The ergonomically engineered seat back provides correct support.

685 **Prairie Cruiser**
Sizewise
8601 Monrovia Street
Lenexa, KS 66215
800-814-9389
info@sizewise.com
www.sizewise.com

686 **Pride Mobility**
182 Susquehanna aaenue
Exter, PA 18643
800-800-4258
info@pridemobility.com
www.pridemobility.com

Scott Meuser, Chair & CEO
Dan Meuser, President
Pride Mobility manufacturers a variety of electric wheelchairs, mobility scooters, and lift chairs for users of all sizes. As a global innovator, Pride Mobility is dedicated to improving the lives of users through mobility solutions.

687 **Redman Apache**
Redman Powerchair
1601 South Pantano Road
Suite 107
Tucson, AZ 85710
520-546-6002
800-727-6684
Fax: 520-546-5530
info@redmanpowerchair.com
www.redmanpowerchair.com

Don Redman, CEO
Paula Redman, CFO
Paula Jr. Redman, Vice Executive
These ultralight, active use wheelchairs offer quick release rear wheels, adjustable arm height and detachable arm swing-away.

688 **Redman Crow Line**
Redman Powerchair
1601 South Pantano Road
Suite 107
Tucson, AZ 85710
520-546-6002
800-727-6684
Fax: 520-546-5530
info@redmanpowerchair.com
www.redmanpowerchair.com

Don Redman, CEO
Paula Redman, CFO
Paula Jr. Redman, Vice Executive
Reclining wheelchair that reclines a full 90 degrees to flat and can be stopped anywhere on the axis.

689 **Rock-King Wheelchair Kit**
Maxi Aids
42 Executive Blvd.
Farmingdale, NY 11735-4710
631-752-0521
800-522-6294
Fax: 631-752-0689
TTY: 631-752-0738
sales@maxiaids.com
www.maxiaids.com

Elliot Zaretsky, Founder, President & CEO
Wheelchair that can turn into a rocking chair with the flip of a lever. The kit includes wheels, footrests, lateral supports, black frame finish, heal-leg strap, cushion and standard head pillow.

690 **Rolls 2000 Series**
Invacare
1 Invacare Way
Elyria, OH 44035-4107
440-329-6000
800-333-6900
Fax: 877-619-7996
www.invacare.com

Matthew E. Monaghan, Chair, President & CEO
Darcie Karol, Senior Vice President Human Resources
Kathleen P. Leneghan, Senior Vice President & CFO
Anthony C. LaPlaca, Senior Vice President, General Counsel & Secretary
The first light-weight wheelchairs designed for rental use. Comes with optional elevating footrests.

691 **Skyway**
Skyway Machine
4451 Caterpillar Rd
Redding, CA 96003-1496
530-243-5151
800-332-3357
Fax: 530-243-5104
sales@skywaywheels.com

Ken Coster, Sales Department
Parrey Cremeans, Sales Department
Rein Stolz, Engineering Department
Patrick McEachen, Customer Service

For over 20 years Skyway has been the world leader in composite wheels. Supplying over 650 different wheel combinations for wheelchairs, lawn and garden products, bicycles and a large assortment of wheeled devices. Wheel sizes range from 4 inch to 24 inch diameter.

692 **Stand-Up Wheelchairs**
Lifestand
P.O. Box 232171
Encinitas, CA 92023-2171
800-782-6324
Fax: 610-586-0847
dallery@msn.com

Jacques A Dallery, President

Offers a complete line of manual, electric and stand-up wheelchairs for the disabled.

693 **Standard Wheelchair**
Mada Medical Products
625 Washington Ave
Carlstadt, NJ 07072-2901
201-460-0454
800-526-6370
Fax: 201-460-3509
www.madainternational.com

Jeffrey Adam, President

Standard wheelchairs designed and built for long-lasting, reliable operation. Each wheelchair is constructed of heavy gauge, chrome plated, steel framework and tube in tube construction at stress points. Mada's state-of-the art engineering uses the most modern components to provide the strength needed while keeping the chair's weight down.

694 **Surf Chair**
2052 S Peninsula Dr
Daytona Beach, FL 32118-5237
386-253-0986
800-841-6610
Fax: 386-253-7600

695 **Vista Wheelchair**
Arista Surgical Supply Company/AliMed
297 High Street
Dedham, MA 02026-2852
781-329-2900
800-225-2610
Fax: 781-329-8392
info@alimed.com
www.alimed.com

Julian Cherubini, President

Vista has a rugged cold-rolled steel frame, durable vinyl upholstery and steel bearings to assure a smooth ride. *$220.00*

696 **Wheelchair with Shock Absorbers**
Iron Horse Productions
3114 Strawberry Ln
Port Huron, MI 48060-1727
810-987-6700
800-426-0354

697 **Wheelchairs and Transport Chairs**
Maxi Aids
42 Executive Blvd.
Farmingdale, NY 11735-4710
631-752-0521
800-522-6294
Fax: 631-752-0689
TTY: 631-752-0738
sales@maxiaids.com
www.maxiaids.com

Elliot Zaretsky, Founder, President & CEO

Offers a wide range of wheelchairs, including lightweight transport chairs, full-reclining wheelchairs, bariatric wheelchairs, and more.

Wheelchairs: Pediatric

698 **Commuter & Kid's Commuter**
Fortress
P.O. Box 489
Clovis, CA 93613-489
559-322-5437
Fax: 559-323-0299

699 **Convaid**
2830 California Street
Torrance, CA 90503-3908
310-618-0111
888-266-8243
Fax: 310-618-2166
www.convaid.com

Ryan B. Williams, President

Convaid manufactures Mobile Positioning Systems for children. The Expedition, Safari Tilt, Cruiser, EZ Rider and Metro offer a non-institutional styling and are lightweight and compact-folding. The steel/aluminum structure is engineered for maximum comfort and durability. The mobile positioning lines come with more than 20 positioning features and a full range of positioning adaptations.

700 **Imp Tricycle**
TRIAID
P.O. Box 1364
Cumberland, MD 21501-1364
301-759-3525
800-306-6777
Fax: 301-759-3525
sales@triaid.com
www.triaid.com

701 **Kid's Custom**
Fortress
P.O. Box 489
Clovis, CA 93613-489
559-322-5437
Fax: 559-323-0299

702 **Kid's Edge**
Fortress
P.O. Box 489
Clovis, CA 93613-489
559-322-5437
Fax: 559-323-0299

703 **Kid's Liberty**
Fortress
P.O. Box 489
Clovis, CA 93613-489
559-322-5437
Fax: 559-323-0299

704 **Kid-Friendly Chairs**
Vector Mobility
5030 E Jensen Ave
Fresno, CA 93725-4010
559-431-3334
800-441-0358
Fax: 559-431-5535

Dave Deatherage, Owner

Manual base offers the lowest available floor to seat height, growth capability, one-third the parts of a conventional chair and no welds to break. The power unit features standard shapes and personality designs from elephants to inch worms and autos to rainbows, lowest seat height, and smallest turning radius on the market.

705 **Koala Miniflex**
Permobil USA
300 Duke Dr
Lebanon, TN 37090
800-736-0925
Fax: 800-231-3256
info@permobilus.com
permobilus.com

706 **Seven Fifty-Five FS**
Fortress
P.O. Box 489
Clovis, CA 93613-489
559-322-5437
Fax: 559-323-0299

707 **TMX Tricycle**
TRIAID
P.O. Box 1364
Cumberland, MD 21501-1364
301-759-3525
800-306-6777
Fax: 301-759-3525
sales@triaid.com
www.triaid.com

Wheelchairs: Powered

708 **Bounder Plus Power Wheelchair**
21st Century Scientific
4931 N Manufacturing Way
Coeur D Alene, ID 83815-8931
208-667-8800
800-448-3680
Fax: 208-667-6600
21st@wheelchairs.com
wheelchairs.com

Ronald E. Prior, Ph.D., President and Founder
RD Davidson, Sales/Marketing Director
Susan Harris, CFO and Webmaster

Available in widths of 16 to 20 inches for users up to 500 pounds with a 2 year warranty on the entire chair. It offers all the standard features of a BOUNDER, plus reinforced rear wheel mounts, reinforced caster barrels, and super duty upholstery (with double liner and web straps under every screw). The BOUNDER Plus also features tandem cross struts, middle vertical support strut, seat rails supported at five points and back upholstery attached with machine screws.

709 **Bounder Power Wheelchair**
21st Century Scientific
4931 N Manufacturing Way
Coeur D Alene, ID 83815-8931
208-667-8800
800-448-3680
Fax: 208-667-6600
21st@wheelchairs.com
wheelchairs.com

Ronald E. Prior, Ph.D., President and Founder
RD Davidson, Sales/Marketing Director
Susan Harris, CFO and Webmaster

Available in a variety of widths from 16 to 18 inches for users up to 250 pounds. The rugged frame is constructed with steel tubing. The standard 12 position Adjustable Front Forks, made of 1/4 inch thick steel, provides impact dampening and seat tilt adjustment. A Dual Group 27 Sliding Battery Box provides extended range and easy battery maintenance. *$8695.00*

710 **Breez 1025**
Electro Kinetic Technologies
W194 N11301 McCormick Dr
Germantown, WI 53022
262-250-7740
800-824-1068
Fax: 262-250-7741
info@ek-tech.com
ek-tech.com

711 **Damaco D90**
Damaco
28918 Hancock Parkway
Valencia, CA 91355
661-775-2020
877-528-2288
Fax: 661-775-2025
www.atbatt.com

712 **Folding Lightweight Power Wheelchair**
Maxi Aids
42 Executive Blvd.
Farmingdale, NY 11735-4710
631-752-0521
800-522-6294
Fax: 631-752-0689
TTY: 631-752-0738
sales@maxiaids.com
www.maxiaids.com

Elliot Zaretsky, Founder, President & CEO

Folding power wheelchair with large foot platform, foam seat design and back seat pocket for storage. Weight capacity is 400 lbs. *$2279.00*

713 **Gem Wheelchair & Scooter Service: Mobility & Homecare**
176-39 Union Turnpike
Flushing, NY 11366-1515
718-969-8600
800-943-3578
Fax: 718-969-8300
help@gemwheelchairservice.com
www.gemwheelchairservice.com

714 **Geronimo**
Redman Powerchair
Ste 202
3840 S Palo Verde Rd
Tucson, AZ 85714-2076
520-294-1466
800-727-6684
Fax: 520-294-1460

Arnie Johnson, Owner

Wheelchair offering direct drive, two year electronic guarantee and micro controls.

715 **One Thousand FS**
Fortress
P.O. Box 489
Clovis, CA 93613-489
559-322-5437
Fax: 559-323-0299

716 **Permobil Max 90**
Permobil
4020 Christopher Way
Plano, TX 75024
877-394-3941
mumu.moorthi@sigmabatteries.com
www.sigmabatteries.com

717 **Permobil Super 90**
Permobil
4020 Christopher Way
Plano, TX 75024
877-394-3941
mumu.moorthi@sigmabatteries.com
www.sigmabatteries.com

718 **Power Wheelchairs**
LaBac Systems
3845 Forest St
Denver, CO 80207-2516
800-370-6808
www.falconrehab.net

Power tilt and recline seating systems for wheelchairs, offering more comfort and dependability for the physically challenged.

719 **Power for Off-Pavement**
Redman Powerchair
1601 South Pantano Road
Suite 107
Tucson, AZ 85710-2076
520-546-6002
800-727-6684
Fax: 520-546-5530
info@redmanpowerchair.com
www.redmanpowerchair.com

Don Redman, CEO
Paula Redman, CFO
Paula Jr. Redman, Vice Executive

Power-drive wheelchair has a solid seat and can handle safely and securely knolls and off-pavement terrain.

Wheelchairs: Racing

720 **Eagle Sportschairs, LLC**
2351 Parkwood Road
Snellville, GA 30039-4003
770-972-0763
800-932-9380
Fax: 770-985-4885
eaglesportschairs@gmail.com
www.eaglesportschairs.com

Barry Ewing, Owner

The Eagle line of custom lightweight performance chairs includes a range of options to fit all racing and sport needs including; track, baseball, quad-rugby, tennis, field events and waterskiing. Also popular for daily use. Ability to customize any chair to accommodate size and disability.

721 **East Penn Manufacturing Company**

East Penn Manufacturing Company
Deka Road P.O. Box 147
Lyon Station, PA 19536-147
610-682-6361
Fax: 610-682-4781
contactus@eastpenn-deka.com
www.eastpenn-deka.com

Daniel Langdon, President & CEO
DeLight Breidegam, Co-Founder & Chair
David Byrne, Director of Finance & Accounting

Specially engineered for demanding deep-cycle applications Gelled electrolyte Deka Dominator Batteries provides maintenance-free operation, longer battery life and hours of reliable performance. Their excellent recharge characteristics provide quick turn around time.

722 **Invacare Top End**

Invacare
1 Invacare Way
Elyria, OH 44035-4107
440-329-6000
800-333-6900
Fax: 877-619-7996
www.invacare.com

Matthew E. Monaghan, Chair, President & CEO
Darcie Karol, Senior Vice President Human Resources
Kathleen P. Leneghan, Senior Vice President & CFO
Anthony C. LaPlaca, Senior Vice President, General Counsel & Secretary

Manufacturers of light weight, rigid, sport-specific wheelchairs, such as the Eliminator line of racing chairs,T-3 tennis and softball chairs, and the Terminator for quad rugby and basketball. The Excelerator, XLT three-wheel hand cycle for adults and juniors.

Associations

General Disabilities

723 **A Loving Spoonful**
1449 Powell St.
Vancouver, BC, Canada V5L-1G8
604-682-6325
Fax: 604-682-6327
info@alovingspoonful.org
alovingspoonful.org
Gerald Regio, President
Quinn Newcomb, Vice President
Ken Channon, Treasurer
Easter Armas, Secretary/Founder
A Loving Spoonful is a volunteer-driven, non-partisan Society that provides free, nutritious meals to people living with HIV/AIDS in Greater Vancouver. Every week volunteers deliver frozen meals and snack packs to men, women, and children who are primarily homebound with AIDS.
1989

724 **ADA National Network**
ADA Knowledge Translation Center
University of Washington
Seattle, WA 98382
800-949-4232
adakt@uw.edu
adata.org

725 **AHF Federation**
AIDS Healthcare Foundation
6255 Sunset Blvd.
21st Floor
Los Angeles, CA 90028
323-860-5200
www.aidshealth.org/about/federation
Michael Weinstein, President
Peter Reis, Senior Vice President
Scott Carruthers, Chief Pharmacy Officer
Michael Wohlfeiler, Chief of Medicine
A consortium of AIDS Service Organizations under the umbrella of the AIDS Healthcare Foundation.

726 **AIDS Healthcare Foundation**
6255 Sunset Blvd.
21st Floor
Los Angeles, CA 90028
323-860-5200
www.aidshealth.org
Michael Weinstein, President
Peter Reis, Senior Vice President
Scott Carruthers, Chief Pharmacy Officer
Michael Wohlfeiler, Chief of Medicine
The Los Angeles-based AIDS Healthcare Foundation (AHF) is a global nonprofit organization providing medicine and advocacy to people all around the world. AHF is currently the largest provider of HIV/AIDS medical care in the U.S.

727 **AIDS Vancouver**
1101 Seymour St.
4th Floor
Vancouver, BC, Canada V6B-0R1
604-893-2201
Fax: 604-893-2205
contact@aidsvancouver.org
aidsvancouver.org
Phillip Banks, Interim Executive Director
Janet Cheng, Finance Director
Adam Reibin, Director, External Relations
Lawrence Chidzambwa, Grocery Program Coordinator
AIDS Vancouver strives to create a community with no new HIV infections while ensuring support for those who are affected through case management services, financial assistance, grocery and nutrition support, and confidential helplines.
1983

728 **Abilities, Inc.**
The Viscardi Center
201 I.U. Willets Rd.
Albertson, NY 11507
516-465-1400
info@viscardicenter.org
viscardicenter.org/services/abilities-inc
John D. Kemp, President & CEO
Sheryl P. Buchel, Executive Vice President & Chief Financial Officer
Michael Caprara, Chief Information Officer
Lauren M. Marzo, Chief Development Officer
The Viscardi Center is a network of nonprofit organizations that provides a lifespan of services for children and adults with disabilities. The Abilities, Inc. program prepares adolescents and adults with disabilities for entering the workforce.

729 **Academy of Integrative Health & Medicine (AIHM)**
6919 La Jolla Blvd.
San Diego, CA 92037
info@aihm.org
aihm.org
Tabatha Parker, Executive Director
Erika Cappelluti, Fellowship Director
April Gruzinsky, Director, Admissions
Bryan Hauf, Associate Director, Online Education
The Academy of Integrative Health & Medicine unites health care professionals from family doctors to psychologists, acupuncturists to nurses, to build bridges between disciplines and offer credible educational and certification programs for licensed health care providers.

730 **Access & Information Network**
2600 N Stemmons Fwy
Suite 151
Dallas, TX 75207
214-943-4444
info@aindallas.org
aindallas.org
Steven Pace, President & CEO
Joni Wysocki, COO
Miranda Grant, Director, Community Relations
Mark Quigley, Director, Development
AIN is a nonprofit organization providing services for individuals with chronic health conditions and prevention programs for at-risk communities.

731 **Accreditation Commission for Acupuncture & Oriental Medicine**
8941 Aztec Dr.
Suite 2
Eden Prairie, MN 55347
952-212-2434
info@acaom.org
acaom.org
Mark McKenzie, Executive Director
Karl Gauby, Director, Regulatory Affairs
Jason Wright, Director, Accreditation Services
Mike Skoglund, Director, Operations & Technology
National accrediting agency of programs in acupuncture and Oriental medicine (AOM), and related institutions.

732 **Accreditation Commission for Midwifery Education (ACME)**
American College of Nurse Midwives
8403 Colesville Rd.
Suite 1230
Silver Spring, MD 20910
240-485-1800
Fax: 240-485-1818
membership@acnm.org
midwife.org/acme
Angela Smith, Executive Director
Kristina Anderson, Accreditation Assistant
Commission of the American College of Nurse Midwives responsible for overseeing all aspects of the accreditation review process.

733 **Advocacy Centre for the Elderly (ACE)**
2 Carlton St.
Suite 701
Toronto, ON, Canada M5B-1J3
416-598-2656
855-598-2656
Fax: 416-598-7924
www.advocacycentreelderly.org
Graham Webb, Executive Director
Susan Bryson, Chair
Alexander Henderson, Vice Chair
Shelley Hobbs, Vice Chair
The Advocacy Centre for the Elderly is a specialty community legal clinic that provides a range of legal services to low-income seniors in Ontario. Legal services include advice and representation to individual and group clients, public legal education, law reform, and community development activities.
1984

734 **Advocates for Children of New York (AFC)**
151 West 30th St.
5th Floor
New York, NY 10001
212-947-9779
Fax: 212-947-9790
info@advocatesforchildren.org
www.advocatesforchildren.org
Kim Sweet, Executive Director
Matthew Lenaghan, Deputy Director
Ivette Greenblatt, Director, Development
Anne Klein, Director, Operations
AFC works on behalf of children from infancy to age 21 who are at risk for school-based discrimination and/or academic failure. These include children with disabilities, ethnic minorities, immigrants, homeless children, foster care children, English language learners, and those living in poverty.

735 **Advocates for Developmental Disabilities**
1225 Lincoln Ave. South
Owatonna, MN 55060
507-451-9769
Molly Tichenal, Director
Advocates for Developmental Disabilities is a local agency that advocates for the dissemination of information regarding developmental disabilities, the enhancement of existing services, and the development of new programs on behalf of individuals with developmental disabilities. Its goal is to develop a better understanding of developmental disabilities by families and others interested in the welfare of individuals with developmental disabilities.

736 **American Academy of Audiology (AAA)**
11480 Commerce Park Dr.
Suite 220
Reston, VA 20191
703-790-8466
Fax: 703-790-8631
infoaud@audiology.org
www.audiology.org
Patrick E. Gallagher, Executive Director
Kathryn Werner, Vice President, Public Affairs
Amy Miedema, Vice President, Communications & Membership
Dina Santucci, Senior Director, Business Development
The American Academy of Audiology is the world's largest professional organization for audiologists. The Academy is dedicated to providing quality hearing care services through professional development, education, research, and increased public awareness of hearing and balance disorders.

737 **American Academy of Environmental Medicine (AAEM)**
PO Box 195
Ashland, MO 65010
316-684-5500
Fax: 888-411-1206
www.aaemonline.org
Jessica Tran, President
Lauren Grohs, Executive Director
William A. Ingram, Secretary
James W. Willoughby, Treasurer
The Academy is an association of physicians and other professionals engaged in investigating and coming up with preventive strategies for medical care relating to environmentally triggered illnesses.

738 **American Academy of Medical Acupuncture**
2512 Artesia Blvd.
Suite 200
Redondo Beach, CA 90278
310-379-8261
info@medicalacupuncture.org
www.medicalacupuncture.org
Kendra Unger, MD, FAAMA, President
Donna Pittman, MD, FAAMA, Vice President
Montiel Rosenthal, MD, FAAMA, Secretary
Joseph Audette, MA, MD, Treasurer
Professional organization for physicians in North America who have incorporated acupuncture into their traditional medical practice.

739 **American Academy of Pain Medicine (AAPM)**
1705 Edgewater Dr.
Suite 7778
Orlando, FL 32804
800-917-1619
Fax: 407-749-0714
info@painmed.org
painmed.org
W. Michael Hooten, President
Vitaly Gordin, Vice President, Scientific Affairs
Farshad M. Ahadian, Treasurer
Steven P. Stanos, Secretary
AAPM is an organization created for physicians practicing the specialty of pain medicine in the United States. AAPM works to provide the most up-to-date information available on the practice of pain medicine, advocate for its members, and bring visibility and credibility to the specialty of pain medicine.

740 **American Academy of Pain Medicine Foundation**
American Academy of Pain Medicine
1705 Edgewater Dr.
Suite 7778
Orlando, FL 32804
800-917-1619
Fax: 407-749-0714
info@painmed.org
painmed.org/aapm-foundation
Charles E. Argoff, President
The Foundation supports AAPM's core purpose to optimize the health of patients in pain and eliminate the major health problem of pain by advancing the practice and the specialty of pain medicine.
1911

741 **American Academy of Pediatrics (AAP)**
345 Park Blvd.
Itasca, IL 60143
800-433-9016
Fax: 847-434-8000
mcc@aap.org
www.aap.org
Mark Del Monte, CEO & Executive Vice President
Christine Bork, Chief Development Officer & Sr. Vice President, Development
Roberta Bosak, Chief Administrative Officer & Sr. Vice President, HR
Vera Tait, Chief Medical Officer
An organization of pediatricians committed to attaining the best physical, mental, and social health and well-being for all infants, children, adolescents, and young adults.

742 **American Acupuncture Council**
1100 W Town & Country Rd.
Suite 1400
Orange, CA 92868
800-838-0383
Fax: 714-571-1863
info@acupuncturecouncil.com
acupuncturecouncil.com
Marilyn Allen, Contact
Provides acupuncture malpractice insurance across the country.

743 **American Association of Acupuncture and Oriental Medicine (AAAOM)**
PO Box 96503
Suite 44114
Washington, DC 20090-6503
admin@aaaomonline.org
www.aaaomonline.org
Carlos Chapa, President
Drea Miller, Vice President
Fotios Sardelis, Treasurer

A national professional organization that is dedicated to the promotion and advancement of high ethical, educational, and professional standards in the practice of acupuncture and Oriental medicine (AOM) in the U.S.

744 **American Association of People with Disabilities (AAPD)**
2013 H St. NW
5th Floor
Washington, DC 20006
202-521-4316
800-840-8844
communications@aapd.com
www.aapd.com

Maria Town, President & CEO
Jasmin Bailey, Manager, Business Operations
Christine Liao, Manager, Programs
Rachita Singh, Coordinator, Public Relations & Communications

Nonprofit cross-disability member organization dedicated to ensuring economic self-sufficiency and political empowerment for Americans with disabilities. AAPD works in coalition with other disability organizations for the full implementation and enforcement of disability nondiscrimination laws, particularly the Americans With Disabilities Act (ADA) of 1990 and the Rehabilitation Act of 1973.

745 **American Association on Health and Disability (AAHD)**
110 N Washington St.
Suite 407
Rockville, MD 20850
301-545-6140
Fax: 301-545-6144
contact@aahd.us
www.aahd.us

Roberta Carlin, Executive Director
Karl Cooper, Director, Public Health Programs
E. Clarke Ross, Director, Public Policy

The American Association on Health and Disability is a cross-disability national nonprofit organization committed to promoting health and wellness initiatives for children and adults with disabilities.

746 **American Association on Intellectual and Developmental Disabilities (AAIDD)**
8403 Colesville Rd.
Suite 900
Silver Spring, MD 20910
202-387-1968
Fax: 202-387-2193
aaidd.org

Margaret A. Nygren, Executive Director & CEO
Paul D. Aitken, Director, Finance & Administration
Ravita Maharaj, Director, Supports Intensity Scale Program
Kathleen McLane, Director, Publications Program

The organization focuses on intellectual and developmental disabilities, advocating for quality of life and rights for individuals with such disabilities.

747 **American Board of Disability Analysts (ABDA)**
4525 Harding Rd.
Second Floor
Nashville, TN 37205
615-327-2984
Fax: 615-327-9235
americanbd@aol.com
www.americandisability.org

Kenneth Anchor, Administrative Officer

Certifies physicians, psychologists, attorneys, and counselors as specialists in disability and personal injury.

748 **American Board of Medical Psychotherapists and Psychodiagnosticians**
American Board of Disability Analysts
4525 Harding Rd.
Second Floor
Nashville, TN 37205
615-327-2984
Fax: 615-327-9235
americanbd@aol.com
www.americandisability.org

Kenneth Anchor, Administrative Officer

Affiliated organization of the American Board of Disability Analysts (ABDA).

749 **American Board of Professional Disability Consultants**
American Board of Disability Analysts
4525 Harding Rd.
Second Floor
Nashville, TN 37205
615-327-2984
Fax: 615-327-9235
americanbd@aol.com
www.americandisability.org

Kenneth Anchor, Administrative Officer

Affiliated organization of the American Board of Disability Analysts (ABDA).

750 **American Botanical Council (ABC)**
6200 Manor Rd.
PO Box 144345
Austin, TX 78714-4345
512-926-4900
800-373-7105
Fax: 512-926-2345
abc@herbalgram.org
herbalgram.org

Mark Blumenthal, Founder & Eexecutive Director
Stefan Gafner, Chief Science Officer
Denise Meikel, Director, Development
Cecelia Thompson, Director, Finance

The American Botanical Council is an independent, nonprofit, international member-based organization providing education using science-based and traditional information to promote the responsible use of herbal medicine.

751 **American Camp Association (ACA)**
5000 State Rd. 67 North
Martinsville, IN 46151-7902
765-342-8456
800-428-2267
Fax: 765-342-2065
www.acacamps.org

Tom Rosenberg, President & CEO
Laurie Browne, Director, Research
Danielle Pinney, Director, Accreditation
Grechen Throop, Director, Membership

The American Camp Association is a community of camp professionals who have joined together to share their knowledge and experience and to ensure the quality of camp programs. Children and adults have the opportunity to engage with a community, developing character building and other skills.

752 **American Chiropractic Association (ACA)**
1701 Clarendon Blvd.
Suite 200
Arlington, VA 22209
703-276-8800
Fax: 703-243-2593
memberinfo@acatoday.org
www.acatoday.org

Michele J. Maiers, President
Kathy A. Boulet, Vice President

The ACA is a professional organization representing chiropractors. Its mission is to preserve, protect, improve, and promote the chiropractic profession. The purpose of the ACA is to provide leadership in health care and a positive vision for the chiropractic profession and its natural approach to health and wellness.

753 **American College of Advancement in Medicine (ACAM)**
380 Ice Center Lane
Suite C
Bozeman, MT 59718
800-532-3688
Fax: 406-587-2451
members@acam.org
www.acam.org

Ahvie Herskowitz, President
Allen Green, Treasurer
Veronica Haynes, Executive Director
Katie VanNatta, Contact, Member Services

The American College for Advancement in Medicine is a nonprofit society dedicated to educating physicians and other health care professionals on the latest findings and emerging procedures in integrative medicine. ACAM's goals are to improve skills, knowledge, and diagnostic procedures as they relate to integrative medicine; to support research; and to develop awareness of alternative methods of medical treatment.

754 **American College of Nurse Midwives (ACNM)**
8403 Colesville Rd.
Suite 1230
Silver Spring, MD 20910
240-485-1800
Fax: 240-485-1818
membership@acnm.org
midwife.org

Katrina Holland, Chief Executive Officer
Marc Rucker, Vice President, Finance & Operations
Amy Kohl, Director, Advocacy & Government Affairs
Hedy Ross, Director, Membership & Communications

The American College of Nurse-Midwives is the oldest women's health care organization in the U.S. ACNM provides research, accredits midwifery education programs, administers and promotes continuing education programs, establishes clinical practice standards, and creates liaisons with state and federal agencies and members of Congress.

755 **American Counseling Association (ACA)**
6101 Stevenson Ave.
Suite 600
Alexandria, VA 22304
703-823-9800
800-347-6647
Fax: 800-473-2329
www.counseling.org

Richard Yep, Chief Executive Officer
Natasha Rankin, Chief Operating Officer
Lynn Linde, Chief Knowledge & Learning Officer
Tiffany Erickson, Chief Communications & Engagement Officer

The American Counseling Association is a not-for-profit, professional and educational organization dedicated to advancing the counseling profession.

756 **American Disabled Golfers Association (ADGA)**
United States Golf Teachers Federation
200 S Indian River Dr.
Suite 206
Fort Pierce, FL 34950
772-888-7483
info@usgtf.com
www.usgtf.com

Brandon Lee, President
Mark Harman, Director, Education

The American Disabled Golfers Association helps create accessibility to golf courses for disabled golfers.

757 **American Disabled for Attendant Programs Today (ADAPT)**
4513 Tyson Ave.
Philadelphia, PA 19135
adapt.org

758 **American Foundation for Suicide Prevention (AFSP)**
199 Water St.
11th Floor
New York, NY 10038
212-363-3500
888-333-2377
Fax: 212-363-6237
info@afsp.org
afsp.org

Robert Gebbia, Chief Executive Officer
Christine Yu Moutier, Chief Medical Officer
Stephanie Rogers, Senior Vice President, Communications & Marketing
Michael F. Lamma, Senior Vice President, Development & Field Management

The American Foundation for Suicide Prevention is a voluntary health organization that gives those affected by suicide a nationwide community empowered by research, education, and advocacy to take action against this disease. AFSP achieves their goal by funding scientific research, educating the public about mental health and suicide prevention, and supporting survivors of suicide loss and all those affected by suicide.

759 **American Herbalists Guild (AHG)**
PO Box 3076
Asheville, NC 28802-3076
617-520-4372
office@americanherbalistsguild.com
www.americanherbalistsguild.com

Bevin Clare, President
Holly Hutton, Vice President
Mimi Hernandez, Executive Director
Heather Lee Compton, Assistant Director

A nonprofit, educational organization that represents the voices of herbalists specializing in the medicinal use of plants. Their mission is to promote a high level of professionalism and education in the study and practice of therapeutic herbalism.
1989

760 **American Massage Therapy Association (AMTA)**
500 Davis St.
Suite 900
Evanston, IL 60201
877-905-2700
info@amtamassage.org
www.amtamassage.org

Steve Albertson, President
Bill Brown, Executive Director
Jeff Flom, Chief Operating Officer

AMTA is a nonprofit professional organization for massage therapists. AMTA works to establish massage therapy as integral to the maintenance of good health and complementary to other therapeutic processes. AMTA aims to advance the profession through ethics and standards, certification, school accreditation, continuing education, professional publications, legislative efforts, public education, and fostering the development of members.

761 **American Occupational Therapy Association (AOTA)**
6116 Executive Blvd.
Suite 200
North Bethesda, MD 20852-4929
301-652-6611
800-729-2682
members@aota.org
www.aota.org

Sherry Keramidas, Executive Director
Neil Harvison, Chief Officer, Knowledge
Matthew Clark, Chief Officer, Innovation & Engagement
Tricia Hopkins, Chief Officer, Finance & Operations

A national professional association that advances the quality, availability, use, and support of occupational therapy through standard setting, advocacy, education, and research on behalf of its members.

762 **American Organization for Bodywork Therapies of Asia (AOBTA)**
391 Wilmington Pike
Suite 3, Box 260
Glen Mills, PA 19342
484-841-6023
office@aobta.org
www.aobta.org

Wayne Mylin, Managing Director
Sarah West, Secretary
Brian Skow, Communications Coordinator
Yolanda Asher, Legislative Consultant

The American Organization for Bodywork Therapies of Asia is a professional membership organizaton that promotes Asian Bodywork Therapy and its practitioners while honoring a diversity of disciplines. AOBTA serves its community of members by supporting appropriate credentialing; defining scope of practice and educational standards; and providing resources for training, professional development, and networking. AOBTA advocates public policy to protect its members.

763 **American Public Health Association (APHA)**
800 I St. NW
Washington, DC 20001
202-777-2742
Fax: 202-777-2534
TTY: 202-777-2500
www.apha.org

Georges C. Benjamin, Executive Director
James Carbo, Chief of Staff
Regina Davis Moss, Associate Executive Director
Kemi Oluwafemi, Chief Financial Officer

The association works to protect all Americans and their communities from preventable, serious health threats. APHA represents a broad array of health officials, educators, environmentalists, policy-makers, and health providers at all levels working both within and outside governmental organizations and educational institutions.
1972

764 **American Red Cross**
431 18th St. NW
Washington, DC 20006
202-303-4498
800-733-2767
www.redcross.org

Bonnie McElveen-Hunter, Chair
Gail J. McGovern, President & CEO
Brian J. Rhoa, Chief Financial Officer
Jennifer L. Hawkins, Corporate Secretary & Chief of Staff

The American Red Cross is an emergency assistance organization offering services in the following areas: disaster relief and recovery; blood donations; health and safety training and education; support for military and veteran families; and international relief and development programs.

765 **American Society for the Alexander Technique (AmSAT)**
11 W Monument Ave.
Suite 510
Dayton, OH 45402-1233
937-586-3732
800-473-0620
info@amsatonline.org
www.amsatonline.org

Matthew Dubroff, Chair
Holly Rocke, Secretary
Rick Carbaugh, Treasurer

The Alexander Technique is a self-help method for improving balance and coordination and increasing movement awareness by eliminating habitual reactions of misuse in every day activities. AmSat, a professional organization of Alexander Technique teachers, aims to define, maintain, and promote the Alexander Technique at its highest standard of professional practice and conduct.

766 **American Society of Clinical Hypnosis (ASCH)**
180 Admiral Cochrane Drive
Suite 370
Annapolis, MD 21401
410-940-6585
Fax: 630-351-8490
info@asch.net
www.asch.net

Eric B. Spiegel, President

The American Society of Clinical Hypnosis is an organization of health and mental health care professionals using clinical hypnosis. ASCH aims to further the knowledge, understanding, and application of hypnosis in health care; to promote the recognition and acceptance of hypnosis as an important tool in clinical health care; and to provide a professional community for clinicians and researchers using hypnosis.

767 **American Therapeutic Recreation Association**
25 Century Blvd.
Suite 505
Nashville, TN 37214
703-234-4140
www.atra-online.com

Brent Wolfe, Executive Director
Brooke Weldon, Director, Operations

Represents the interests and needs of more than 10,000 recreational therapists.

768 **American Tinnitus Association (ATA)**
PO Box 424049
Washington, DC 20042-4049
800-634-8978
ata.org

Torryn Brazell, Chief Executive Officer
Michael Baker, Development Officer
Joy Onozuka, Tinnitus Research & Communications Officer

ATA is an organization dedicated to finding cures for tinnitus and hyperacusis. ATA's research program focuses on providing seed grants for new areas of tinnitus scientific exploration.

769 **Amputee Coalition**
601 Pennsylvania Ave. NW
Suite 600, South Bldg.
Washington, DC 20004
888-267-5669
www.amputee-coalition.org

Mary Richards, President & CEO

The Amputee Coalition is a nonprofit organization dedicated to assisting and empowering people affected by limb loss through education, support groups, and vocal advocacy.

770 **Anxiety and Depression Association of America (ADAA)**
8701 Georgia Ave.
Suite 412
Silver Spring, MD 20910
240-485-1001
Fax: 240-485-1035
information@adaa.org
adaa.org

Susan K. Gurley, Executive Director
Lise Bram, Deputy Executive Director
Vickie Spielman, Associate Director, Membership & Education
Sasha Sicard, Manager, Membership & Education

The Anxiety and Depression Association of America is an international nonprofit organization and a leader in education, training, and research for anxiety, OCD, PTSD, depression, and related disorders. ADAA encourages the advancement of scientific knowledge about the causes and treatment for mental health issues.

771 **Aspies For Freedom (AFF)**
www.aspiesforfreedom.com

Gwen Nelson, Co-Founder
Amy Nelson, Co-Founder

Seeks to change the discourse on autism, including negative treatment in the media. Runs an online chatroom and promotes Autistic Pride Day.

772 **Assistive Technology Industry Association (ATIA)**
330 N Wabash Ave.
Suite 2000
Chicago, IL 60611-4267
312-321-5172
877-687-2842
Fax: 312-673-6659
info@atia.org
www.atia.org

David Dikter, Chief Executive Officer
Caroline Van Howe, Chief Operating Officer
Emily Schmitt, Manager, Marketing

Dedicated to manufacturers, sellers and providers of assistive technology, offering education and research.

773 **Association for Applied Psychophysiology and Biofeedback (AAPB)**
4400 College Blvd.
Suite 220
Overland Park, KS 66211
303-422-8436
800-477-8892
info@aapb.org
www.aapb.org

Ethan Benore, President
Michelle Cunningham, Executive Director
Autumn Menefee, Associate Director

AAPB is a nonprofit organization that aims to advance applied psychophysiology and biofeedback through scientific research, practice, and education.

774 **Association of Assistive Technology Act Programs (ATAP)**
1440 G St. NW
Washington, DC 20005
atapadmin@ataporg.org
www.ataporg.org

Audrey Busch, Executive Director
Dave Scherer, Director, Technical Assistance & Programs
Kim Moccia, Deputy Director
Jamie Anderson, Manager, Membership & Events

The Association of Assistive Technology Act Programs (ATAP) is a national, member-based organization consisting of state Assistive Technology Act Programs funded under the Assistive Technology Act (AT Act). It promotes, represents, and coordinates the state AT Programs at a national level.

775 **Association of Children's Residential Centers (ACRC)**
648 N Plankinton Ave.
Suite 245
Milwaukee, WI 53203
414-403-1565
877-332-2272
info@togetherthevoice.org
togetherthevoice.org

Kari Sisson, Executive Director
Amanda Prange, Training Coordinator
McKenzie Melchoir, Membership Services Specialist
Lisette Burton, Chief Policy & Practice Advisor

The Association of Children's Residential Centers advocates for quality treatment and residential interventions for youth. The organization provides support, training and resources to help members better serve children and families through residential interventions.

776 Association of Educational Therapists (AET)
7044 S 13th St.
Oak Creek, WI 53154
414-908-4949
customercare@aetonline.org
www.aetonline.org

Kaye Ragland, President
Susan Grama, Treasurer
Pamm Scribner, Secretary

AET is a professional association for educational therapists. Educational Therapy offers children and adults with learning disabilities and other learning challenges a wide range of intensive, individualized interventions designed to remediate learning problems.

777 Association of Independent Camps
American Camp Association
5000 State Rd. 67 North
Martinsville, IN 46151-7902
765-342-8456
800-428-2267
Fax: 765-342-2065
www.acacamps.org

Tom Rosenberg, President & CEO, ACA

The Association of Independent Camps is an affiliate of the American Camp Association. Originally founded as a committee in 1954, the AIC has served the independent camp community since 1996. They provide accreditation and public credibility, as well as camper scholarship programs.

778 Association of Medical Professionals with Hearing Losses (AMPHL)
admin@amphl.org
amphl.org

Christopher Moreland, President
Ian DeAndrea-Lazarus, Vice President
Rachel Grosz, Secretary
Zachary Featherstone, Treasurer

The Association of Medical Professionals with Hearing Losses provides information, promotes advocacy and mentorship, and creates a network for individuals with hearing loss interested in or working in health care fields.

779 Association of People Supporting Employment First (APSE)
7361 Calhoun Place
Suite 680
Rockville, MD 20855
301-279-0060
Fax: 301-279-0075
info@apse.org
www.apse.org

Erica Belois-Pacer, Director, Professional Development
Julie Christensen, Director, Policy & Advocacy
Erynn Pawlak, Director, Operations
Christa P. Rainwater, Director, Membership & Chapter Engagement

Through advocacy and education, this nonprofit organization advances employment and self-sufficiency for all people with disabilities.

780 Association of University Centers on Disabilities (AUCD)
1100 Wayne Ave.
Suite 1000
Silver Spring, MD 20910
301-588-8252
Fax: 301-588-2842
aucdinfo@aucd.org
www.aucd.org

John Tschida, Executive Director
Adriane K. Griffen, Senior Director, Public Health & Leadership
Dawn Rudolph, Senior Director, Technical Assistance & Network Engagement
E. Troy Washington, Senior Director, Finance & Grants Administration

AUCD is a membership organization consisting of University Centers for Excellence in Developmental Disabilities (UCEDD), Leadership Education in Neurodevelopmental Disabilities (LEND) Programs, and Intellectual and Developmental Disability Research Centers (IDDRC). AUCD supports its members through advocacy, technical assistance, information dissemination, networking, and leadership.

781 Association on Higher Education & Disability (AHEAD)
8015 West Kenton Circle
Suite 230
Huntersville, NC 28078
704-947-7779
Fax: 704-948-7779
www.ahead.org

Stephan Smith, Executive Director
Carol Funckes, Chief Operations Officer
Oanh Huynh, Chief Financial Officer
Jeremy Jarrell, Director, Innovation and Development

AHEAD is a professional membership organization for individuals involved in the development of policy and in the provision of quality services to meet the needs of persons with disabilities involved in all areas of higher education, promoting full and equal participation.
4,000+ members

782 Bastyr Center for Natural Health
3670 Stone Way N
Seattle, WA 98103
206-834-4100
Fax: 206-834-4131
www.bastyrcenter.org

783 Beacon Tree Foundation
9201 Arboretum Pkwy.
Suite 140
N. Chesterfield, VA 23236
800-414-6427
info@beacontree.org
beacontree.org

Michelle Etheridge, President

Beacon Tree Foundation is dedicated to being an advocate for the family, providing education about treatment and financial resources to help heal children and teens struggling with mental health issues and to provide hope for the future.

784 Birth Defect Research for Children (BDRC)
976 Lake Baldwin Lane
Suite 104
Orlando, FL 32814
407-895-0802
staff@birthdefects.org
www.birthdefects.org

Betty Mekdeci, Executive Director

A nonprofit organization that provides information about birth defects of all kinds to parents and professionals. Offers a library of medical books and files of information on less common categories of birth defects and is involved in research to discover possible links between environmental exposures and birth defects.

785 Bonnie Prudden Myotherapy
4330 E Havasu Rd.
Tucson, AZ 85718
520-529-3979
www.bonnieprudden.com

Enid Whittaker, Managing Director
Sandy Dirks, Treasurer
Lori Drummond, Secretary

Myotherapy is a method for relaxing muscle spasms, improving circulation, and alleviating pain. Pressure is applied using elbows, knuckles or fingers, and held for several seconds to defuse trigger points. The success of this method depends upon the use of specific corrective exercises of the freed muscles.

786 Brain & Behavior Research Foundation
747 Third Ave.
33rd Floor
New York, NY 10017
646-681-4888
800-829-8289
info@bbrfoundation.org
bbrfoundation.org

Jeffrey Borenstein, President & CEO
Louis Innamorato, Vice President, Finance & Chief Financial Officer
Lauren Duran, Vice President, Communications, Marketing & PR
Faith Rothblatt, Vice President, Development

The Brain & Behavior Research Foundation is a nonprofit organization committed to alleviating the suffering caused by mental illness by awarding grants in the field of mental health research.

787 **Brain Injury Association of America (BIAA)**
3057 Nutley St.
Suite 805
Fairfax, VA 22031-1931
703-761-0750
Fax: 703-761-0755
info@biausa.org
www.biausa.org

Susan Connors, President & CEO
Mary S. Reitter, Executive Vice President & COO
Robbie Baker, Vice President & CDO
Marianna Abashian, Director, Professional Services

The Brain Injury Association of America is a national organization serving and representing individuals, families and professionals who are touched by a traumatic brain injury (TBI). Its mission is to improve the quality of life for people affected by brain injury through the advancement of research, treatment, education and awareness.
1980

788 **Burton Blatt Institute (BBI)**
Syracuse University
950 Irving Ave.
Dineen Hall, Suite 446
Syracuse, NY 13244-2130
315-443-2863
315-443-9725
bbi.syr.edu

Peter Blanck, Chair
Michael Morris, Senior Advisor
Jonathan Martinis, Senior Director, Law & Policy
Nanette Goodman, Director, Research

Seeks to advance the full inclusion of people with disabilities through program development, research, and public policy guidance in economic and community participation.

789 **CARF International**
6951 East Southpoint Rd.
Tucson, AZ 85756-9407
520-325-1044
888-281-6531
Fax: 520-318-1129
TTY: 520-495-7077
info@carf.org
carf.org

Brian J. Boon, President & CEO
Leslie Ellis-Lang, Managing Director, Child & Youth Services
Darren M. Lehrfeld, Chief Accreditation Officer
Di Shen, Chief Research Officer

An independent, nonprofit accreditor of human service providers in the areas of aging services, behavioral health, child and youth services, DMEPOS, employment and community services, medical rehabilitation, and opioid treatment programs.

790 **Cambia Health Foundation**
100 SW Market St.
Suite E15B
Portland, OR 97201
503-225-4813
cambiahealthfoundation.org

Peggy Maguire, President & Chair
Kathleen Pitcher Tobey, Director, Operations
Leslie Constans, Director, Digital & Brand Communications
Mary Frances Baldes, Manager, Communications

Cambia Health Foundation is the corporate foundation of Cambia Health Solutions dedicated to transforming the way people experience health care to create a more person-focused and economically sustainable health care system.

791 **Canadian Art Therapy Association (CATA)**
PO Box 658, Stn Main
Parksville, BC, Canada V9P-2G7
admin@canadianarttherapy.org
canadianarttherapy.org

Amanda Gee, President
Nicole Le Bihan, Vice President
Waqas Yousafzai, Treasurer

CATA is a nonprofit organization that works in cooperation with other provincial art therapy associations to promote education and understanding of the value of art therapy, as well as provide ongoing education and professional standards for this field.
1977

792 **Canine Companions for Independence (CCI)**
PO Box 446
Santa Rosa, CA 95402-0446
866-224-3647
800-572-2275
www.canine.org

Paige Mazzoni, Chief Executive Officer
Jack Peirce, Chief Financial Officer & Corporate Treasurer
Barbara Barrow, Chief Development Officer
Sarah Leighton, National Director, Training & Client Services

A nonprofit organization that enhances the lives of people with disabilities by providing highly trained assistance dogs and ongoing support to ensure quality partnerships.

793 **Canine Helpers for the Handicapped**
Canine Helpers for the Handicapped, Inc.
5699 Ridge Rd.
Lockport, NY 14094
716-433-4035
chhdogs@aol.com

Beverly Underwood, Executive Director

A nonprofit organization dedicated to training dogs in order to assist people with disabilities and promote independence.

794 **Case Management Society of America (CMSA)**
5034A Thoroughbred Lane
Brentwood, TN 37027
615-432-0101
800-216-2672
Fax: 615-523-1715
cmsa@cmsa.org
www.cmsa.org

Melanie Prince, President
Patricia Noonan, Treasurer
Janet Coulter, Secretary

The Case Management Society of America is an international, nonprofit organization dedicated to the support and development of the profession of case management through educational forums, networking opportunities, and legislative involvement. Case management workers play a vital role in taking care of patients' health care needs.

795 **Center for Creative Arts Therapy**
4336 Saratoga Ave.
2nd Floor
Downers Grove, IL 60515
847-477-8244
info@c4creativeartstherapy.com
c4creativeartstherapy.com

Azizi Marshall, Founder & CEO
Rachel Wagner-Cantine, Clinical Director
Leslie Kane, Coordinator, Marketing & Outreach

The Center for Creative Arts Therapy offers arts-based psychotherapy services to individuals and their families as a healthy, proactive way to achieve wellness and balance in their lives. Provides art therapy, music therapy, dance therapy and drama therapy, as well as professional counseling.

796 **Center for Disability Resources**
University of South Carolina School of Medicine
Department of Pediatrics
8301 Farrow Rd.
Columbia, SC 29208
803-935-5231
Fax: 803-935-5059
david.rotholz@uscmed.sc.edu
uscm.med.sc.edu/cdrhome

797 **Center for Inclusive Design and Innovation**
512 Means St. NW
Suite 250
Atlanta, GA 30318
404-894-8000
866-279-2964
Fax: 404-894-8323
cidi-support@design.gatech.edu
cidi.gatech.edu

Eric Trevena, Senior Director, Operations
Carolyn Phillips, Director, Services & Learning
Jon Sanford, Professor & Director, RERC TechSAge

CIDI supports individuals with disabilities of any age within the State of Georgia and beyond through expert services, research, design and technological development, information dissemination, and educational programs.

798 **Center for Mind-Body Medicine**
5225 Connecticut Ave. NW
Suite 414
Washington, DC 20015
202-966-7338
Fax: 202-966-2589
www.cmbm.org

James S. Gordon, President
Rosemary L. Murrain, Managing Director
Lynda Richtsmeier, Clinical Director
Tina Fisher, Director, Special Programs
The Center for Mind-Body Medicine is a nonprofit educational organization dedicated to reviving the spirit and transforming the practice of medicine. The Center is working to create a more effective, comprehensive, and compassionate model of health care and education. The Center's model combines the precision of modern science with the best of the world's healing traditions.

799 **Cerebral Palsy Foundation (CPF)**
3 Columbus Circle
15th Floor
New York, NY 10019
212-520-1686
info@yourcpf.org
yourcpf.org

Rachel Byrne, Executive Director
Tracy Pickar, Associate Executive Director
Cynthia Frisina, Senior Vice President, Strategic Partnerships
Debbie Fink, Vice President, Education & Inclusion
The Cerebral Palsy Foundation is dedicated to assisting and empowering people with cerebral palsy through research in both medical breakthroughs and assistive technologies.

800 **Challenged Athletes Foundation (CAF)**
9591 Waples St.
San Diego, CA 92121
858-866-0959
Fax: 858-866-0958
caf@challengedathletes.org
challengedathletes.org

Virginia Tinley, Chief Executive Director
J.D. Douglas, Chief Financial Officer
Kristine Entwistle, Associate Executive Director
Nancy Reynolds, Senior Director, Business Development
The Challenged Athletes Foundation provides opportunities and support to physically challenged persons so they can pursue active lifestyles through physical fitness and competitive athletics.

801 **Change, Inc.**
115 Stoner Ave.
Westminster, MD 21157
410-876-2179
Fax: 410-857-4053
info@penn-mar.org
www.changeinc.cc

Michael F. Shriver, Executive Director
A nonprofit organization that partners with families, caregivers, and advocates to provide opportunities for children with developmental disabilities. A division of Penn-Mar Human Services.

802 **Child and Parent Resource Institute (CPRI)**
600 Sanatorium Rd.
London, ON, Canada N6H-3W7
519-858-2774
877-494-2774
Fax: 519-858-3913
TTY: 519-858-0257
www.cpri.ca

Shannon Bain, Director
Ajit Ninan, Medical Director
Provides highly specialized services to children and youth from 0-18 years of age with complex mental health and/or developmental challenges on a short term inpatient and community basis.

803 **Children's Alliance**
420 Capitol Ave.
Frankfort, KY 40601
502-875-3399
Fax: 502-223-4200
www.childrensallianceky.org

Michelle Sanborn, President
Melissa Muse, Director, Member Services
Kathy Adams, Director, Public Policy
An association of individuals and human services organizations committed to being a voice for at-risk children and families. Interacts with the legislative and executive branches of government and assists members in developing services that most effectively meet the needs of at-risk children and families.

804 **Children's Mental Health Network (CMHN)**
Chapel Hill, NC 27516
information@cmhnetwork.org
www.cmhnetwork.org

Scott Bryant-Comstock, President & CEO
Provides neutral, independent information on children's mental health issues, while sharing ideas on ways to improve the lives of affected children and their families.

805 **Children's National Medical Center**
111 Michigan Ave. NW
Washington, DC 20010
202-476-5000
888-884-2327
childrensnational.org

Kurt Newman, President & CEO
Mark Batshaw, Executive Vice President & Physician-in-Chief
Denice Cora-Bramble, Chief Medical Officer
Aldwin Lindsay, Chief Financial Officer
The Children's National Medical Center provides health care services that enhance the health and well-being of children regionally, nationally, and internationally. Through leadership and innovation, the organization will create solutions to pediatric health care problems.

806 **Clay Tree Society**
838 Old Victoria Rd.
Nanaimo, BC, Canada V9R-6A1
250-753-5322
Fax: 250-753-2749
info@claytree.org
www.claytree.org

Dan Dube, President
Glenys Patmore, Executive Director
Rachel Pearsall, General Manager
Susan Easter, Senior Manager
A nonprofit society providing day programming, assistance and support for people with developmental disabilities.

807 **Coalition for Health Funding**
c/o Cavarocchi Ruscio Dennis Associates, LLC
600 Maryland Ave. SW
Suite 220E
Washington, DC 20024
202-271-8963
Fax: 202-484-1244
emorton@dc-crd.com
www.publichealthfunding.org

Erin Will Morton, Executive Director
Erika Miller, Senior Vice President & Counsel
Katina Pierce, Vice President, Administration & Finance
Lindsey Trischler, Senior Policy Associate
Nonprofit alliance working to preserve and strengthen public health investments via funding for federal agencies and programs.

808 **Communitas Supportive Care Society**
103-2776 Bourquin Cres. W
Abbotsford, BC, Canada V2S-6A4
604-850-6608
800-622-5455
Fax: 604-850-2634
office@communitascare.com
www.communitascare.com

Gary Falk, Chair
Karyn Santiago, Chief Executive Officer
Gillian Viljoen, Chief Program Officer
Kelly Beaulieu, Chief Financial Officer
Communitas Supportive Care Society is a nonprofit, faith-based organization providing care in communities across British Columbia to those living with disabilities. Services include skills-based day programs, residential care, and respite care for families.

809 **Council for Exceptional Children (CEC)**
3100 Clarendon Blvd.
Suite 600
Arlington, VA 22201-5332
888-232-7733
TTY: 866-915-5000
service@exceptionalchildren.org
www.exceptionalchildren.org

Chad Rummel, Executive Director
Laurie VanderPloeg, Associate Executive Director, Professional Affairs
Craig Evans, Chief Financial Officer
Sharon Rodriguez, Director, Governance & Executive Services

The Council for Exceptional Children aims to improve the educational success of individuals with disabilities and/or gifts and talents by advocating for appropriate policies, setting professional standards, and providing resources and professional development for special educators.

810 **Council of Colleges of Acupuncture & Oriental Medicine**
1501 Sulgrave Ave.
Suite 301
Baltimore, MD 21209
410-464-6040
Fax: 410-464-6042
support@ccaom.org
www.ccaom.org

Misti Oxford-Pickeral, President
Kris LaPoint, Vice President
Jennifer Brett, Treasurer
Allyson Wilson, Secretary

The Council seeks to advance the standing of acupuncture and Oriental medicine (AOM) in the U.S. by promoting educational excellence within the field by deepening the knowledge, understanding and skills of the AOM practitioner.

811 **Council of Parent Attorneys and Advocates (COPAA)**
PO Box 6767
Towson, MD 21285
844-426-7224
www.copaa.org

Denise Stile Marshall, Executive Director
Selene A. Almazan, Legal Director
Marcie Hipple, Director, Member Services & Events

Group of attorneys, advocates, parents and related professionals working to protect the rights of students with disabilities and their families, including promoting excellence in education.

812 **Council of State Administrators of Vocational Rehabilitation (CSAVR)**
1 Research Ct.
Suite 450
Rockville, MD 20850
301-519-8023
info@csavr.org
www.csavr.org

Stephen A. Wooderson, Chief Executive Officer
Rita Martin, Deputy Director
Kathy West-Evans, Director, Business Relations
John Connelly, Director, Research & Grants

The Council is made up of the chief administrators of the public rehabilitation agencies that serve people with physical and mental disabilities across the U.S.

813 **Department of Physical Medicine & Rehabilitation at Sinai Hospital**
LifeBridge Health
2401 W Belvedere Ave.
Baltimore, MD 21215-5271
410-601-8823
www.lifebridgehealth.org

Scott E. Brown, Department Chief

Provides health-related services to the people of the Northwest Baltimore region. LifeBridge is dedicated to advancing the health of the community through a variety of health and wellness programs and services. The Department of Physical Medicine & Rehabilitation provides care to individuals with disabling conditions such as traumatic brain injury, spinal cord injury, amputees, and more.

814 **DisAbility LINK**
1901 Montreal Rd.
Suite 102
Tucker, GA 30084
404-687-8890
Fax: 404-687-8298
TTY: 711
www.disabilitylink.org

Kim Gibson, Executive Director
Ken Mitchell, Assistant Director
Joseph Bryant, Director, Finance

disABILITY LINK is an organization committed to promoting the rights of all people with disabilities in allowing them to be independent, achieve goals, have access to their community, and make decisions for themselves.

815 **Disability Funders Network (DFN)**
14241 Midlothian Turnpike
Suite 151
Midlothian, VA 23113-6500
703-795-9646
info@disabilityfunders.org
www.disabilityfunders.org

Kim Hutchinson, President & CEO

Disability Funders Network is a national membership organization dedicated to advocating for equality and rights for disabled individuals and communities.

816 **Disability Research and Dissemination Center**
Arnold School of Public Health, USC
Discovery 1 Bldg.
915 Greene St.
Columbia, SC 29208
info@disabilityresearchcenter.com
www.disabilityresearchcenter.com

Suzanne McDermott, PhD, Research & Administration
Margaret A. Turk, MD, Training & Evaluation
Roberta S. Carlin, MS, JD, Dissemination
Deborah Salzberg Clark, MS, Project Manager

The DRDC was formed in 2012 and is a partnership between the University of South Carolina (USC), the State University of New York Upstate Medical University (SUNY Upstate), and the American Association on Health and Disability (AAHD). Its five core areas are Administration, Research, Research Translation, Evaluation, and Dissemination & Policy.

817 **Disability Rights Bar Association (DBRA)**
c/o Burton Blatt Institute
950 Irving Ave.
Dineen Hall, Suite 446
Syracuse, NY 13244-2130
315-443-2863
Fax: 315-443-9725
drba-law@law.syr.edu
disabilityrights-law.org

Scott LaBarre, Chair
Marc Maurer, Treasurer

The DRBA is an online network of attorneys who specialize in disability civil rights law.

818 **Disability Rights Florida**
2473 Care Dr.
Suite 200
Tallahassee, FL 32308
850-488-9071
800-342-0823
Fax: 850-488-8640
TTY: 800-346-4127
www.disabilityrightsflorida.org

Peter Sleasman, Executive Director
Ann Siegel, Legal Director
Cherie E. Hall, Director, Operations
Tony DePalma, Director, Public Policy

A federally mandated Protection & Advocacy (P&A) organization working to ensure the safety, well-being and success of people with disabilities.
1977

819 **Disability Rights International (DRI)**
1825 K St. NW
Suite 600
Washington, DC 20006 202-296-0800
Fax: 202-697-5422
info@driadvocacy.org
www.driadvocacy.org
Laurie Ahern, President
Eric Rosenthal, Founder & Executive Director
Priscila Rodriguez, Associate Director, Advocacy
Promotes international oversight of disability rights by documenting human rights abuses and publishing reports on enforcement.

820 **Disability Rights Louisiana**
8325 Oak St.
New Orleans, LA 70118 800-960-7705
info@disabilityrightsla.org
disabilityrightsla.org
Christopher Rodriguez, Executive Director
Ron Lospennato, Director, Legal Services
Tory Rocca, Director, Public Policy & Community Engagement
Debra Weinberg, Director, Community Advocacy
Protects and advocates for the rights of seniors and individuals with disabilities in Louisiana.

821 **Disability:IN**
3000 Potomac Ave.
Alexandria, VA 22305 info@disabilityin.org
disabilityin.org
Jill Houghton, President & CEO
Brian Horn, Executive Vice President, Operations
Elizabeth Taub, Executive Vice President, Programs
Philip DeVliegher, Vice President, Supplier Diversity
Nonprofit specializing in disability inclusion in the workplace.

822 **Disabled Athlete Sports Association (DASA)**
1600 Mid Rivers Mall Circle
Suite 2272
St. Peters, MO 63376 dasa@dasasports.org
www.dasasports.org
Kelly Behlmann, Executive Director
Meghan Morgan, Program Director
Brook Matthews, Program Director
Kimi Kemp, Adaptive Training Director
The Disabled Athlete Sports Association is a nonprofit organization specializing in adaptive sport and fitness opportunities. DASA relies heavily upon fundraising events, grants, and individual and corporate donations to sustain its mission.

823 **Disabled Businesspersons Association (DBA)**
6367 Alvarado Crt.
Suite 350
San Diego, CA 92120 619-594-8805
Urban Miyares, Founder
The Disabled Businesspersons Association is a nonprofit public charity and educational organization to help disabled entrepreneurs maximize their potential in the business world, and to encourage the participation and enhance the performance of disabled individuals in the work force.
1991

824 **Disabled Children's Fund (DCF)**
PO Box 4712
Crofton, MD 21114 240-929-4281
Fax: 240-929-4367
helpsomechild@gmail.com
disabled-child.org
Bill Collins, Co-Founder
Erma Collins, Co-Founder
Disabled Children's Fund is a humanitarian organization serving oppressed children and families worldwide. It distributes braces, wheelchairs, crutches, walkers and rehabilitative services globally.
1996

825 **Disabled Drummers Association (DDA)**
18901 NW 19 Ave.
Miami Gardens, FL 33056 305-621-9022
ddafathertime@comcast.net
www.disableddrummers.org

826 **Disabled In Action (DIA)**
PO Box 30954
Port Authority Station
New York, NY 10011- 0109 646-504-4342
Fax: 646-504-4342
TTY: 711
treasurer@disabledinaction.org
www.disabledinaction.org
Jean Ryan, President
Phil Beder, Treasurer
A democratic, nonprofit, membership organization advancing civil rights and seeking to end discrimination for people with disabilities.

827 **Disabled Peoples' International (DPI)**
160 Elgin St.
Place Bell RPO, PO Box 70073
Ottawa, ON, Canada K2P-2M3 dpi.org
Rachel Kachaje, Chair
Jean Luc Simon, Secretary
Shoji Nakanishi, Treasurer
Aims to protect the rights of people with disabilities, while promoting their full and equal role in society.

828 **Disabled and Alone: Life Services for the Handicapped, Inc.**
1440 Broadway
23rd Floor
New York, NY 10018-2326 212-532-6740
800-995-0066
Fax: 212-532-6740
info@disabledandalone.org
www.disabledandalone.org
Leslie D. Park, Chair
Rex L. Davidson, Vice President
Lee Alan Ackerman, Executive Director
William G. Shannon, Treasurer
A national nonprofit humanitarian organization whose primary concern is the well-being of disabled persons, particularly when their families can no longer care for them. The organization helps families do sensible planning for and with their disabled children; provides advocacy and oversight when the parents cannot do so; and advises families, attorneys, and financial planners about life planning for a family with a member with a disability.
1988

829 **Dr. Ida Rolf Institute (DIRI)**
5055 Chaparral Ct.
Suite 103
Boulder, CO 80301 303-449-5903
Fax: 303-449-5978
www.rolf.org
Christina Howe, Executive Director
Mary Contreras, Director, Admissions & Recruitment
Samantha Sherwin, Director, Financial Aid & Compliance
Pat Heckmann, Director, Operations & Systems Management
The Rolf Institute is a nonprofit corporation, dedicated to educating individuals on Rolfing Structural Integration. It is recognized by the US Government as a tax-exempt educational and scientific research organization.
1971

830 **Early Childhood Technical Assistance Center (ETCA)**
CB 8040
Chapel Hill, NC 27599-8040 919-962-2001
Fax: 919-966-7463
ectacenter@unc.edu
ectacenter.org
Christina Kasprzak, Co-Director
Meghan Vinh, Co-Director
Betsy Ayankoya, Associate Director
Katy McCullough, Associate Director
ECTA Center, funded by the Office of Special Education Programs, is a technical assistance center supporting Part C and Section 619 IDEA programs in building quality early intervention and preschool special education service systems, improving and sustaining state systems, and enhancing outcomes for children with disabilities and their families.

831 **Easterseals**
141 W Jackson Blvd.
Suite 1400A
Chicago, IL 60604
312-726-6200
800-221-6827
Fax: 312-726-1494
info@easterseals.com
easterseals.com

Angela F. Williams, President & CEO
Glenda Oakley, Chief Financial Officer
Marcy Traxler, Senior Vice President, Network Advancement
John Osterlund, Senior Vice President, Development

Easterseals provides services, education, outreach and advocacy for people with disabilities, veterans, senior citizens and their families. Programs include early intervention, workforce development, adult day care, autism services, mental health services, and more.

832 **Elwyn**
111 Elwyn Rd.
Media, PA 19063
610-891-2000
info@elwyn.org
elwyn.org

Charles S. McLister, President & CEO
Rex Carney, Chief of Staff
Len Kirby, Chief Operating Officer
Debra Paul, Chief Financial Officer

A nonprofit organization developing programs for children and adults with disabilities and disadvantages.

833 **Employer Assistance and Resource Network on Disability Inclusion (EARN)**
Cornell University, ILR School
201 Dolgen Hall
Ithaca, NY 14853
askearn@cornell.edu
www.askearn.org

834 **Enable America Inc.**
101 E Kennedy Blvd.
Suite 3250
Tampa, FL 33602
877-362-2533
Fax: 813-221-8811
richard.salem@enableamerica.org
www.enableamerica.org

Richard J. Salem, Founder & CEO

Enable America is a nonprofit organization that is dedicated to increasing employment among people with disabilities in the United States.

835 **Esalen Institute**
55000 Highway One
Big Sur, CA 93920
831-667-3000
888-837-2536
info@esalen.org
www.esalen.org

Gordon Wheeler, President
Terry Gilbey, General Manager & CEO
Camille Wright, Chief Financial Officer
Michelle Broderick, Chief Marketing Officer

An alternative education center devoted to East/West philosophies, experiential/didactic workshops, and a steady influx of philosophers, psychologists, artists, and religious thinkers.
1962

836 **Family Resource Center on Disabilities**
11 E Adams St.
Suite 1002
Chicago, IL 60603
312-939-3513
info@frcd.org
www.frcd.org

Michelle Phillips, Executive Director

A not-for-profit advocacy organization dedicated to improving services for all children with disabilities by providing support and services to affected families, informing parents of their rights, and helping parents become advocates for their children. Offers family support services, training, seminars, and information and referral services. Publishes a monthly newsletter.

837 **Family Run Executive Director Leadership Association (FREDLA)**
10632 Patuxent Pkwy.
Suite 234
Columbia, MD 21044
410-707-4547
info@fredla.org
www.fredla.org

Pat Hunt, Executive Director
Millie Sweeney, Deputy Director
Malisa Pearson, Project Coordinator

Aims to strengthen the leadership and organizational capacity of family-run organizations.

838 **Family Voices**
110 Hartwell Ave.
Lexington, MA 02421
781-674-7224
888-835-5669
www.familyvoices.org

Nora Wells, Executive Director
Cara Coleman, Director, Public Poicy & Advocacy
Bev Baker, Associate Director, Operations
Beth Dworetzky, Associate Director, Programs

A not-for-profit organization dedicated to ensuring that children's health issues are addressed as public and private health-care systems undergo change in communities, states, and the nation. They are a national grassroots clearinghouse for information and education in ways to improve health care for children with disabilities and chronic conditions. Family Voices provides materials including pamphlets, a newsletter, and one-page papers on important topics.

839 **Favarh ARC**
225 Commerce Dr.
Canton, CT 06019-2478
860-693-6662
Fax: 860-693-8662
favarh@favarh.org
www.favarh.org

Jerome Chisolm, President
Fay Lenz, Vice President
Tom Smith, Treasurer
Stephen Morris, Executive Director

Favarh ARC provides a variety of programs and services to adults with developmental, physical, or mental disabilities and their families throughout the Farmington Valley communities of Avon, Burlington, and more. Favarh's programs are designed to enhance the personal, social, emotional, vocational, and living capabilities of persons with disabilities.

840 **Fedcap Rehabilitation Services**
633 Third Ave.
6th Floor
New York, NY 10017
212-727-4200
Fax: 212-727-4374
TTY: 646-606-5950
info@fedcap.org
www.fedcap.org

Steve Coons, President
Donald Harreld, Senior Vice President, Education
Aisha Lucas, Vice President, Home Care

Fedcap helps people with barriers achieve economic independence through employment. Through evaluation, vocational and soft-skills training, job placement, job creation, and support programs, each year Fedcap helps thousands of Americans overcome obstacles, rebuild their lives, and find and keep meaningful employment.

841 **Federation for Children with Special Needs**
529 Main St.
Suite 1M3
Boston, MA 02129
617-236-7210
800-331-0688
Fax: 617-241-0330
fcsninfo@fcsn.org
www.fcsn.org

Pam Nourse, Executive Director
Mary Lewis-Pierce, Director, Development
Jacqui Koelsch, Director, Finance
Chetna Putta, Director, Information Technology

The Federation for Children with Special Needs provides information, support, and assistance to parents of children with disabilities, their professional partners, and their communities.

842 Feingold Association of the US
10955 Windjammer Dr. S
Indianapolis, IN 46256
631-369-9340
help@feingold.org
www.feingold.org

Deborah Lehner, Executive Director
An organization of families and professionals, the Feingold Association of the United States is dedicated to helping children and adults apply proven dietary techniques for better behavior, learning, and health.

843 Feldenkrais Guild of North America (FGNA)
401 Edgewater Pl.
Suite 600
Wakefield, MA 01880
781-876-8935
800-775-2118
Fax: 781-645-1322
www.feldenkraisguild.com

Nancy Haller, President
Tom Pappas, Chief Financial Officer
April Veilleux, Manager, Membership
Kayla Chandler, Manager, Events
This organization sets the standards for and certifies all Feldenkrais practitioners in North America. In order to practice, a practitioner must be a graduate of an FGNA accredited program (a minimum of 800 instruction hours over a three to four year period), and agree to follow both the Code of Professional Conduct and the Standards of Practice. FGNA may be contacted for further information about the Feldenkrais Method or for a list of Feldenkrais practitioners sorted by region.

844 Flying Manes Therapeutic Riding, Inc.
PO Box 508
Scarsdale, NY 10583
917-524-6648
info@flyingmanes.org
flyingmanes.org

845 Freedom from Fear
308 Seaview Ave.
Staten Island, NY 10305
718-351-1717
help@freedomfromfear.org
freedomfromfear.org

Mary Guardino, Founder & Executive Director
Freedom From Fear is a national nonprofit mental health advocacy organization whose goal is to better the lives of all those affected by anxiety, depressive, and related disorders through advocacy, education, research, and community support.
1984

846 Genova Diagnostics
63 Zillicoa St.
Asheville, NC 28801
828-253-0621
800-522-4762
info@gdx.net
www.gdx.net

Jeffrey Ledford, Chief Executive Officer
Craig Thiel, Chief Financial Officer
Jeff Ellis, Chief Commercial Officer
Ceco Ivanov, Chief Information Officer
Genova Diagnostics specializes in nutritional, metabolic, and toxicant analyses. Genova is committed to helping health care professionals identify nutritional influences on health and disease, and laboratory procedures in nutritional and biochemical testing.
1984

847 Goodwill Industries International
15810 Indianola Dr.
Rockville, MD 20855
contactus@goodwill.org
www.goodwill.org

Steven C. Preston, President & CEO
Goodwill strives to achieve the full participation in society of disabled persons and other individuals with special needs by expanding their opportunities and occupational capabilities through a network of autonomous, nonprofit, community-based organizations providing services throughout the world in response to local needs.

848 Grand Lodge of the International Association of Machinists and Aerospace Workers
9000 Machinists Pl.
Upper Marlboro, MD 20772-2687
301-967-4500
www.goiam.org

Robert Martinez, Jr., International President
Dora Cervantes, General Secretary-Treasurer
Mark Blondin, General Vice President, Aerospace
Sito Pantoja, General Vice President
Offers placements, programs, and resources for persons with disabilities.

849 HEATH Resource Center at the National Youth Transitions Center
George Washington University
2134 G St. NW
Washington, DC 20052-0001
www.heath.gwu.edu
Joan Kester, Principal Investigator
Christopher Nace, Research Assistant
The HEALTH Resource Center is a national clearinghouse for information about education after high school for people with disabilities. Also serves as an information exchange about educational support services, policies, procedures, adaptations, and opportunities on American campuses, vocational-technical schools, adult education programs, independent living centers, and other training entities after high school.

850 Habilitation Benefits Coalition
c/o Powers Pyles Sutter & Verville PC
1501 M St. NW
7th Floor
Washington, DC 20005
joseph.nahra@powerslaw.com
habcoalition.wordpress.com

Joe Nahra, Contact
The HAB Coalition coordinates, sustains and promotes a unified voice for organizations who are independently active in their support for habilitative services and devices.

851 Haldimand-Norfolk Resource Education and Counseling
101 Nanticoke Creek Pkwy.
Townsend, ON, Canada N0A-1S0
519-587-2441
800-265-8087
Fax: 519-587-4798
info@hnreach.on.ca
www.hnreach.on.ca

Leo Massi, Executive Director
Wendy Carron, Director, Early Childhood Services
Deb Young, Director, Services, Moving on Mental Health
Haldimand-Norfolk REACH is a multi-service agency, providing children's mental health services, developmental services, Autism services, youth justice services, family services, a residential program for transitional-aged youth and several early learning and care services including licensed childcare, Ontario Early Years Centre (s) and Community Action Program for Children.

852 Hanger, Inc.
4534 Westgate Blvd.
Suite 114
Austin, TX 78745
512-614-4612
877-442-6437
Fax: 512-614-4615
hangerclinic.com

Vinit K. Asar, President & CEO
Thomas E. Kiraly, Executive Vice President & Chief Financial Officer
C. Scott Ranson, Executive Vice President & Chief Information Officer
Hanger Clinic specializes in orthotic and prosthetic services with clinic locations across the country.

853 Health Action
5276 Hollister Ave.
Suite 257
Santa Barbara, CA 93111
805-617-3390
www.healthaction.net

Roger Jahnke, Co-Founder & CEO
Rebecca McLean, Co-Founder
Health Action's mission is to foster innovation in health care that will increase health status, customer satisfaction, profitability,

support provider efficiency, enhance clinical outcomes, and encourage consumer self-managed care.

854 **Hearing Health Foundation (HHF)**
575 Eighth Ave.
Suite 1201
New York, NY 10018
212-257-6140
866-454-3924
Fax: 212-257-6139
TTY: 888-435-6104
info@hhf.org
hearinghealthfoundation.org

Timothy Higdon, President & CEO
Noemi Disla, Director, Finance, Operations & Administration
Christopher Geissler, Director, Program & Research Support
Lauren McGrath, Director, Marketing & Communications

Hearing Health Foundation promotes hearing health and advocates for the prevention and cure of hearing loss and tinnitus through research.

855 **High Technology Foundation**
1000 Galliher Dr.
Suite 1000
Fairmont, WV 26554
304-363-5482
877-363-5482
info@wvhtf.org
www.wvhtf.org

Frank W. Blake, Chair
James L. Estep, President & CEO

High Technology Foundation is dedicated to maximizing economic development in West Virginia through the high-technology business sector.

856 **Hogg Foundation for Mental Health**
3001 Lake Austin Blvd.
Austin, TX 78703
512-471-5041
hogg-operations@austin.utexas.edu
hogg.utexas.edu

Octavio N. Martinez Jr., Executive Director
Vicky Coffee, Director, Programs
Colleen Horton, Director, Policy
Crystal Viagran, Director, Finance & Operations

The Hogg Foundation for Mental Health is a nonprofit organization that is dedicated to the advancement of mental wellness for the people of Texas through outreach programs, conferences, seminars, research grants, and more.

857 **Homeopathic Educational Services**
812C Camelia St.
Berkeley, CA 94710
510-649-0294
800-359-9051
email@homeopathic.com
www.homeopathic.com

Dana Ullman, Owner & Director

Resource center for homeopathic products and services including books, tapes, research, medicines, medicine kits, software for the general public and health professionals, and correspondence courses.

858 **Hope Network Neuro Rehabilitation**
3075 Orchard Vista Dr. SE
PO Box 890
Grand Rapids, MI 49546
616-301-8000
800-695-7273
Fax: 616-301-8010
www.hopenetworkrehab.org

Phil Weaver, President & CEO
Tim Becker, Chief Operating Officer
Andre Pierre, Chief Financial Officer
Kiran Taylor, Chief Medical Officer

Neuro Rehabilitation is a service line of Hope Network, helping those with brain or spinal cord injuries or other neurological conditions recover through treatment techniques and person-centered care.

859 **Humanity & Inclusion (HI)**
8757 Georgia Ave.
Suite 420
Silver Spring, MD 20910
301-891-2138
Fax: 301-891-9193
info.usa@hi.org
www.hi-us.org

Jeff Meer, Executive Director
Hannah Deutsch, U.S. Director, Institutional Funding
Mica Bevington, U.S. Director, Development & Communications
Ginette Mballa, U.S. Director, Finance & Administration

International organization promoting disability rights, rehabilitation, and safety in areas of emergency and conflict.

860 **Immune Deficiency Foundation**
110 West Rd.
Suite 300
Towson, MD 21204
800-296-4433
Fax: 410-321-9165
info@primaryimmune.org
primaryimmune.org

Kathryn Stephens, Interim CEO
Sarah Rose, Chief Financial Officer
Katherine Antilla, Vice President, Education
Tammy C. Black, Vice President, Communications

The Immune Deficiency Foundation is the national patient organization dedicated to improving the diagnosis, treatment, and quality of life of persons with primary immunodeficiency diseases through advocacy, education, and research.

861 **Indiana Association for Home and Hospice Care (IAHHC)**
6320-G Rucker Rd.
Indianapolis, IN 46220
317-775-6675
Fax: 317-775-6674
evan@iahhc.org
www.iahhc.org

Evan Reinhardt, Executive Director
Katie Ociepka, Director, Development
Tori Raderstorf, Director, Communications & Events
Michelle Stein-Ordonez, Director, Membership Services

The Indiana Association for Home & Hospice Care represents home nursing services and inpatient hospice care services. The association offers education and resources, advocacy, and a career center to its members.

862 **Institute for Educational Leadership (IEL)**
4301 Connecticut Ave. NW
Suite 100
Washington, DC 20008
202-822-8405
Fax: 202-872-4050
iel@iel.org
iel.org

Jose Munoz, Interim Director
Maame Appiah, Vice President, Finance & Talent
S. Kwesi Rollins, Vice Resident, Leadership & Engagement
Helen Janc Malone, Vice President, Research & Innovation

Assists under-funded communities by preparing children, youth, adults, and families for postsecondary education and training, leading to better career options and greater community engagement.

863 **International Academy of Independent Medical Evaluators**
1061 E Main St.
Suite 300
East Dundee, IL 60118
847-786-0162
Fax: 312-663-1175
iaime@iaime.org
www.iaime.org

Barry Gelinas, Chair
Les Kertay, President
Gayle Whitmer, Executive Director
Sue O'Sullivan, Managing Director

IAIME is an organization serving physicians involved in disability management. Their courses and products cover disability management and evaluations for physicians, health care providers, attorneys, regulators, legislators, and others involved in the care of injured persons.

864 **International Association of Yoga Therapists (IAYT)**
PO Box 251563
Little Rock, AR 72225
928-541-0004
www.iayt.org

Alyssa Wostrel, Executive Director
Beth Whitney-Teeple, Chief of Staff
Nancy Sinton, Manager, Certification
Annette Watson, Manager, Accreditation

IAYT supports research and education in yoga and serves yoga practitioners, teachers, therapists, health care professionals, and researchers worldwide. Its mission is to establish yoga as a recognized and respected therapy in the Western world. IAYT also serves members, the media, and the general public as a comprehensive source of information about contemporary yoga education, research, and statistics.

865 **International Child Amputee Network**
PO Box 13812
Tuscon, AZ 85732
child-amputee.net

866 **International Chiropractors Association (ICA)**
6400 Arlington Blvd.
Suite 650
Falls Church, VA 22042
703-528-5000
Fax: 703-528-5023
info@chiropractic.org
www.chiropractic.org

Beth Clay, Executive Director & CEO
Stephanie Becker, Director, Programs
Sondra J. Thomas, Coordinator, Membership

The Association strives to protect, promote and advance chiropractic throughout the world.
1926

867 **International Clinic of Biological Regeneration (ICBR)**
PO Box 509
Florissant, MO 63032
800-826-5366
Fax: 314-921-8485
icbr@aol.com
www.icbr.com

Judith A. Smith, Co-Founder & Director
William Johnson, Director, Medical Services

The International Clinic of Biological Regeneration is an international cell therapy center dedicated to constantly improving therapeutic results by selecting newer, safer, and more effective treatments.

868 **International Expressive Arts Therapy Association (IEATA)**
PO Box 40707
San Francisco, CA 94140-0707
415-489-0698
info@ieata.org
ieata.org

Christina Hampton, Co-Chair
Janet Rasmussen, Co-Chair
Susan Johnson, Treasurer

The International Expressive Arts Therapy Association is a nonprofit organization dedicated to supporting expressive arts therapists, artists, educators, consultants, and others using creative processes for personal growth and community development.

869 **International League Against Epilepsy (ILAE)**
2221 Justin Rd.
Suite 119-352
Flower Mound, TX 75028
860-586-7547
Fax: 860-201-1111
ilae.org

Samuel Wiebe, President
Alla Guekht, Vice President
Edward H. Bertram, III, Secretary General
J. Helen Cross, Treasurer

ILAE is a nonprofit organization dedicated to the advancement and dissemination of knowledge about epilepsy and to promoting research, education, and training to improve service and care for patients.

870 **International Ventilator Users Network (IVUN)**
50 Crestwood Executive Ctr.
Suite 440
St. Louis, MO 63126-1916
314-534-0475
Fax: 314-534-5070
info@ventusers.org
www.ventnews.org

Saul J. Morse, President & Chair
Daniel J. Wilson, Vice President
Marny K. Eulberg, Secretary
Mike Mrozowicz, Treasurer

To enhance the lives and independence of individuals using ventilators by promoting education, networking and advocacy. IVUN is an affiliate of Post-Polio Health International.

871 **International Women's Health Coalition (IWHC)**
333 Seventh Ave.
6th Floor
New York, NY 10001
212-979-8500
info@iwhc.org
www.iwhc.org

Francoise Girard, President

The Coalition works to generate health and population policies, programs, and funding that promote and protect the rights and health of girls and women worldwide.

872 **Invisible Disabilities Association (IDA)**
PO Box 4067
Parker, CO 80134
invisibledisabilities.org
Wayne Connell, President & CEO
Jess Stainbrook, Executive Director

The Invisible Disabilities Association (IDA) encourages, educates, and connects people and organizations touched by illness, pain, and disability around the globe.

873 **JDRF**
200 Vesey St.
28th Floor
New York, NY 10281
800-533-2873
Fax: 212-785-9595
info@jdrf.org
www.jdrf.org

Timothy Doyle, President & COO
Troy Lindloff, Chief Development Officer
Srinivas Mishra, Chief Data & Technology Officer
Cynthia Rice, Chief Mission Strategy Officer

A nonprofit, nongovernmental diabetes research organization. JDRF's mission is to find a cure for diabetes and its complications through the support of research. JDRF also sponsors international workshops and conferences for biomedical researchers, and individual chapters offer support groups and other activities for families affected by diabetes. JDRF has more than 110 chapters and affiliates worldwide. They publish a quarterly newsletter.
1970

874 **Job Accommodation Network (JAN)**
PO Box 6080
Morgantown, WV 26506-6080
304-293-7186
800-526-7234
Fax: 304-293-5407
TTY: 877-781-9403
jan@askjan.org
askjan.org

Deborah Hendricks, Director
Anne Hirsch, Associate Director

JAN's mission is to facilitate the employment and retention of workers with disabilities by providing employers, employment providers, people with disabilities, their family members, and other interested parties with information on job accommodations, self-employment, and small business opportunities and related subjects.

875 **Joni and Friends (JAF)**
30009 Ladyface Ct.
Agoura Hills, CA 91301
818-707-5664
800-736-4177
Fax: 818-707-2391
www.joniandfriends.org

Joni Eareckson Tada, Founder & CEO
John Nugent, President & COO
Laura Gardner, Executive Vice President & CFO
Greg Hubert, Senior Vice President, Field Services

A nonprofit organization seeking to accelerate Christian ministry with people affected by disabilities. JAF provides resources and training to churches to help create disability-welcoming environments, offers family retreats and mobility programs, and mentors people with disabilities to lead and provide service in their churches and communities.

876 **Lambton County Developmental Services (LCDS)**
339 Centre St.
Petrolia, ON, Canada N0N-1R0
519-882-0933
Fax: 519-882-3386
administration@lcds.on.ca
www.lcdspetrolia.ca

Frank Huybers, President
Barb Frayne, Treasurer
John Douglas, Secretary
Nick Salaris, Executive Director

A network of experts and volunteers working together to provide support services and employment services for people with developmental disabilities.

877 **Laurent Clerc National Deaf Education Center**
800 Florida Ave. NE
Washington, DC 20002
202-651-5855
Fax: 202-651-5857
TTY: 202-250-2856
clerc.center@gallaudet.edu
www.clerccenter.gallaudet.edu

878 **Learning Disabilities Association of America (LDA)**
461 Cochran Rd.
Suite 245
Pittsburgh, PA 15228
412-341-1515
Fax: 412-344-0224
info@ldaamerica.org
www.ldaamerica.org

Cindy Cipoletti, Executive Director
Aaron Goldstein, Director, Federal & State Engagement
Nina DelPrato, Administrative Manager
Lauren Clouser, Coordinator, Marketing & Development

LDA aims to provide opportunities for success and support to individuals with learning disabilities, their parents, teachers, and other professionals. It carries out its mission by supporting research on learning disabilities, advocating for early identification and best practice interventions, and protecting the rights of all persons with learning disabilities.

879 **Learning Disabilities Association of New York State (LDANYS)**
300 Hylan Dr., Suite 6
PO Box 144
Rochester, NY 14623
518-608-8992
Fax: 518-608-8993
www.ldanys.org

Jeffrey Baker, President
Helene Fallon, Vice President
Kathryn Cappella, Treasurer

A nonprofit organization advocating for children and adults with learning disabilities. LDA is a three-tiered organization comprised of a national organization, state affiliates and local chapters. They aim to support and empower individuals with learning disabilities throughout their lives.

880 **Learning Disabilities Worldwide**
179 Bear Hill Rd.
Suite 104
Waltham, MA 02451
help@ldworldwide.org
www.ldworldwide.org

Teresa Allissa Citro, Chief Executive Officer
Mary Laity, Chief Operations Officer
Edwin Masih, Chief Financial Officer

Learning Disabilities Worldwide, Inc. is an international professional organization dedicated to improving the educational, professional, and personal outcomes for individuals with learning disabilities and other related disorders.
1965

881 **LoSeCa Foundation**
215-1 Carnegie Dr.
St. Albert, AB, Canada T8N-5B1
780-460-1400
Fax: 780-459-1380
chorpestad@loseca.ca
www.loseca.ca

Carmen Horpestad, Executive Director
Jules Lefebvre, Director, Operations
Rebecca McLeod, Manager, Human Resources
Patrice Patterson, Administrative Coordinator

A nonprofit organization that provides support services to adults with developmental disabilities.

882 **Mainstream**
300 S Rodney Parham Rd.
Suite 5
Little Rock, AR 72205
501-280-0012
800-371-9026
Fax: 501-280-9267
TTY: 501-280-9262
www.mainstreamilrc.com

Rita Byers, Executive Director

A non-residential, consumer-driven independent living resource center for persons with disabilities. Mainstream operates with the conviction that people with disabilities have the right and responsibility to make choices, to control their lives and to participate fully and equally in the community. Mainstream offers the following services free of charge: Advocacy, Peer Support, Training and Education, Information and Referral, Ramp program, and more.
1988

883 **March of Dimes**
1550 Crystal Dr.
Suite 1300
Arlington, VA 22202
888-663-4637
www.marchofdimes.org

Stacey D. Stewart, President & CEO
Adrian P. Mollo, Senior Vice President, General Counsel & Assistant Secretary
David C. Damond, Senior Vice President, CFO & Assistant Treasurer
Alan Brogdon, Senior Vice President, COO & Officer

The mission of the March of Dimes is to improve the health of babies by preventing birth defects and infant mortality.

884 **McKinnon Body Therapy Center**
2940 Webster St.
Oakland, CA 94609
510-465-3488
info@mckinnonbtc.com
mckinnonbtc.com

1973

885 **Mental Health America (MHA)**
500 Montgomery St.
Suite 820
Alexandria, VA 22314
703-684-7722
800-969-6642
Fax: 703-684-5968
info@mhanational.org
www.mhanational.org

Paul Gionfriddo, President & CEO
Mary Giliberti, Executive Vice President, Policy
Jessica Kennedy, Chief of Staff
Theresa Nguyen, Chief Program Officer & Vice President, Research

A nonprofit organization addressing issues related to mental health and mental illness. MHA works to improve the mental health of all Americans, especially individuals with mental disorders, through advocacy, education, research, and service.

886 **MindFreedom International (MFI)**
454 Willamette, Suite 216
PO Box 11284
Eugene, OR 97440-3484
541-345-9106
877-623-7743
Fax: 480-287-8833
office@mindfreedom.org
mindfreedom.org

Celia Brown, President
Ronald Bassman, Executive Director
Sarah Smith, Office Manager
Nonprofit organization dedicated to winning human rights and alternatives for people with psychiatric disabilities.

887 **Muscular Dystrophy Association USA (MDA)**
161 N Clark
Suite 3550
Chicago, IL 60601
800-572-1717
resourcecenter@mdausa.org
www.mda.org

Donald S. Wood, President & CEO
Kristine Welker, Chief of Staff
Sharon Hesterlee, EVP & Chief Research Officer
Kathy A. Kauffmann, EVP & Chief Strategy Development Officer
MDA provides comprehensive medical services to people with neuromuscular diseases at hospital-affiliated clinics across the country. The Association's worldwide research program, which funds over 400 individual scientific investigations annually, represents the largest single effort to advance knowledge of neuromuscular diseases and to find cures and treatments for them. In addition, MDA conducts far-reaching educational programs for the public and professionals.

888 **National Association for Holistic Aromatherapy (NAHA)**
6000 S 5th Ave.
Pocatello, ID 83204
877-232-5255
Fax: 208-232-4911
info@naha.org
www.naha.org

Annette Davis, President
Jennifer Hochell Pressimone, Vice President
Rose Chard, Secretary
Eric Davis, Treasurer
The NAHA is an educational, nonprofit organization dedicated to enhancing public awareness of the benefits of true aromatherapy. It offers aromatherapy Tele-classes & membership benefits, and acts as a referral service.

889 **National Association of Blind Merchants (NABM)**
National Federation of the Blind
7450 Chapman Hwy.
Suite 319
Knoxville, TN 37920
888-687-6226
blindmerchants.org

Nicky Gacos, President
Harold Wilson, First Vice President
Ed Birmingham, Second Vice President
Pam Schnurr, Treasurer
Serving as an advocacy and support group, NABM is a membership organization of blind persons employed in self-employment work or the Randolph-Sheppard Vending Program. The organization provides information on issues affecting blind merchants, including rehabilitation, social security, and tax.

890 **National Association of City and County health Officials**
1201 Eye St. NW
4th Floor
Washington, DC 20005
202-783-5550
Fax: 202-783-1583
info@naccho.org
naccho.org

Lori Tremmel Freeman, Chief Executive Officer
E. Oscar Alleyne, Chief, Programs & Services
Adriane Casalotti, Chief, Government & Public Affairs
Jerome Chester, Chief Financial Officer
Strengthens and advocates for local health departments to improve the health of communities.

891 **National Association of Councils on Developmental Disabilities (NACDD)**
1825 K St. NW
Suite 600
Washington, DC 20006
202-506-5813
info@nacdd.org
www.nacdd.org

Donna A. Meltzer, Chief Executive Officer
Erin Prangley, Director, Public Policy
Sheryl Matney, Director, Technical Assistance
Robin Troutman, Deputy Director, Operations
NACDD is the national association for the 56 State and Territorial Councils on Developmental Disabilities (DD Councils) which receive federal funding to support programs that promote self-determination, integration, and inclusion for all Americans with developmental disabilities.

892 **National Association of Disability Representatives (NADR)**
1305 W 11th St.
Suite 222
Houston, TX 77008
202-822-2155
800-747-6131
Fax: 972-245-6701
www.nadr.org

C. Greg Cates, President
Michael Wener, Vice President
Cliff Berkley, Secretary
Christopher Mazzulli, Treasurer
NADR is an organization of Professional Social Security Claimants Representatives that focus on issues involving policies to protect the interest of people with disabilities. NADR conducts annual conventions open to members and non-members with educational seminars to keep practitioners up to date on Social Security rulings, regulatory changes, and practice improvements.

893 **National Association of State Directors of Developmental Disabilities Services (NASDDDS)**
301 N Fairfax St.
Suite 101
Alexandria, VA 22314-2633
703-683-4202
www.nasddds.org

Mary P. Sowers, Executive Director
Dan Berland, Director, Federal Policy
Barbara Brent, Director, State Policy
Katherine Snyder, Director, Administrative Services
NASDDDS is the representative for the nation's agencies providing services to people with intellectual and developmental disabilities. They aim to promote the development of effective, efficient service delivery systems for individuals with disabilities.

894 **National Business & Disability Council (NBDC)**
The Viscardi Center
201 I.U. Willets Rd.
Albertson, NY 11507
516-465-1400
info@viscardicenter.org
viscardicenter.org/services/nbdc

John D. Kemp, President & CEO
Sheryl P. Buchel, Executive Vice President & Chief Financial Officer
Michael Caprara, Chief Information Officer
Lauren M. Marzo, Chief Development Officer
The NBDC is a resource for employers seeking to integrate people with disabilities into the workplace and companies seeking to reach them in the consumer marketplace.

895 **National Care Planning Council**
PO Box 1118
Centerville, UT 84014
801-298-8676
800-989-8137
Fax: 801-295-3776
info@longtermcarelink.net
www.longtermcarelink.net

Thomas E. Day, Director
Roxanne Pope, Office Manager
The National Care Planning Council's mission is to help families with long term care planning for seniors. Services include training, eldercare articles, books, workshops and seminars, networking and more.

896 **National Center for College Students with Disabilities (NCCSD)**
8015 West Kenton Circle
Suite 230
Huntersville, NC 28078
844-730-8048
TTY: 651-583-7499
nccsd@ahead.org
www.nccsdonline.org
Wendy Harbour, Center Director
Richard Allegra, Associate Director, Education & Outreach Services
Stephan Smith, Project Director
A federally-funded project under the U.S. Department of Education, housed at the Association on Higher Education And Disability (AHEAD). It provides assistance and information to students, families, educators and more; collects information and conducts research; and reports to the Department of Education.

897 **National Center for Education in Maternal and Child Health (NCEMCH)**
Georgetown University
PO Box 571272
Washington, DC 20057-1272
www.ncemch.org
Rochelle Mayer, Research Professor & Director
John Richards, Executive Director
Provides information on children with special health needs, child health and development, adolescent health, nutrition, violence and injury prevention, and other issues of maternal and child health for health professionals and the public.

898 **National Center for Health, Physical Activity and Disability**
4000 Ridgeway Dr.
Birmingham, AL 35209
800-900-8086
Fax: 205-313-7475
email@nchpad.org
www.nchpad.org
James Rimmer, Principal Investigator
Angela Grant, Business Manager
Jeff Underwood, Program Director
Amy Rauworth, Associate Director
NCHPAD promotes health for people with disability through increased participation in all types of physical and social activities. These include fitness and aquatic activities, recreational and sports programs, adaptive equipment usage, and more.

899 **National Center on Deaf-Blindness (NCDB)**
Hellen Keller National Center
141 Middle Neck Rd.
Sands Point, NY 11050
541-800-0412
support@nationaldb.org
www.nationaldb.org
Sam Morgan, Director
Julie Durando, Evaluation Coordinator
Peggy Malloy, Information Services & Technology Coordinator
Funded by the federal Department of Education, the Center seeks to improve quality of life for children who are deaf-blind and their families.

900 **National Center on Disability and Journalism (NCDJ)**
Walter Cronkite School of Journalism, AZ State U.
555 N Central Ave.
Phoenix, AZ 85004
ncdj.org
Kristin Gilger, Director
Catie Cheshire, Graduate Assistant
Jake Geller, Inaugural Director
Supports journalists as they cover people with disabilities, concerned with accuracy, fairness and diversity in news coverage.

901 **National Certification Commission for Acupuncture and Oriental Medicine**
2001 K St. NW
3rd Floor
Washington, DC 20036
202-381-1140
888-381-1140
Fax: 202-381-1141
info@thenccaom.org
www.nccaom.org
Mina Larson, Chief Executive Officer
Olga Cox, Chief Operations Officer
Irene Basore, Director, Administration & Governance
Jennifer Nemeth, Director, PDA & Education
National organization that provides professional certification for entry-level practitioners of acupuncture and Oriental medicine (AOM), representing 98 percent of the states that regulate acupuncture.

902 **National Collaborative Workforce on Disability (NCWD/Youth)**
c/o Institute for Educational Leadership
4301 Connecticut Ave. NW
Suite 100
Washington, DC 20008-2304
877-871-0744
TTY: 877-871-0665
www.ncwd-youth.info

903 **National Council on Independent Living (NCIL)**
2013 H St. NW
6th Floor
Washington, DC 20006
202-207-0334
844-778-7961
Fax: 202-207-0341
TTY: 202-207-0340
ncil@ncil.org
www.ncil.org
Kelly Buckland, Executive Director
Tim Fuchs, Director, Operations
Cara Liebowitz, Coordinator, Development
Eleanor Canter, Coordinator, Communications
A national cross-disability grassroots organization, NCIL advances independent living and the rights of people with disabilities through consumer-driven advocacy.

904 **National Disability Rights Network (NDRN)**
820 1st St. NE
Suite 740
Washington, DC 20002
202-408-9514
Fax: 202-408-9520
TTY: 202-408-9521
info@ndrn.org
www.ndrn.org
Curtis Decker, Executive Director
Belinda Miller, Deputy Executive Director, Finance & Administration
David Hutt, Deputy Executive Director, Legal Services
Eric Buehlmann, Deputy Executive Director, Public Policy
Voluntary national membership association of protection and advocacy systems and client assistance programs. Promoting and strengthening the role and performance of its members in providing quality legally based advocacy services.

905 **National Federation of Families for Children's Mental Health (NFFCMH)**
15800 Crabbs Branch Way
Suite 300
Rockville, MD 20855
240-403-1901
ffcmh@ffcmh.org
www.ffcmh.org
Lynda Gargan, Executive Director
Michelle Covington, Project Manager
Kelsey Engelbracht, Project Manager
Leann Sherman, Project Coordinator
A national family-run organization serving to provide advocacy at the national level for the rights of children and youth with emotional, behavioral, and mental health challenges and their families. The FFCMH provides leadership and technical assistance to a nation-wide network of family run organizations, and collaborates with organizations to transform mental and substance abuse health care in the U.S.

906 **National Guild of Hypnotists (NGH)**
PO Box 308
Merrimack, NH 03054-0308
603-429-9438
Fax: 603-424-8066
ngh@ngh.net
www.ngh.net

Dr. Dwight Damon, President
Don Mottin, Vice President
Jereme Bachand, Executive Director
Dawn Huard, Membership/Member Services

The National Guild of Hypnotists is a not-for-profit, educational corporation committed to advancing the field of hypnotism.

907 **National Health Council**
1730 M St. NW
Suite 500
Washington, DC 20036-4561
202-785-3910
Fax: 202-785-5923
nationalhealthcouncil.org

Randall L. Rutta, Chief Executive Officer
Eleanor M. Perfetto, EVP, Strategic Initiatives
Susan Gaffney, VP, Membership, Development & Operations
Eric Gascho, VP, Policy & Government Affairs

Seeks to provide a unified voice for people living with chronic diseases and disabilities, and their caregivers.

908 **National Institute on Disability, Independent Living, and Rehabilitation Research (NIDILRR)**
Administration for Community Living
330 C St. SW
Washington, DC 20201
202-401-4634
nidilrr-mailbox@acl.hhs.gov
acl.gov

Anjali Forber-Pratt, Director
Kristi Hill, Deputy Director
Phillip Beatty, Director, Office of Research Sciences
Sarah Ruiz, Associate Director, Office of Research Sciences

NIDILRR, formerly the National Institute on Disability and Rehabilitation Research (NIDRR), aims to promote new research into the abilities of individuals with disabilities, and to use that research to allow those individuals to improve and use those skills within their community. NIDILRR also aims to maximize the full inclusion and integration of individuals with disabilities into society.

909 **National Organization on Disability (NOD)**
77 Water St.
13th Floor
New York, NY 10005
646-505-1191
Fax: 646-505-1184
info@nod.org
www.nod.org

Carol Glazer, President
Moeena Das, Chief of Staff
Priyanka Ghosh, Director, External Affairs
Bernard Blake, Manager, Finance & Administration

The National Organization on Disability is a private, nonprofit organization that promotes the full and equal participation of men, women, and children with disabilities in all aspects of American life.
1982

910 **National Rehabilitation Association (NRA)**
PO Box 150235
Alexandria, VA 22315
703-836-0850
888-258-4295
info@nationalrehab.org
nationalrehab.org

Satinder Atwal, Chief Administrator Officer
James Liin, Coordinator, Membership

NRA members work to eliminate barriers and increase employment opportunities for people with disabilities. They provide opportunities for advocacy and increase awareness of issues through professional development and access to current research topics.

911 **National University of Natural Medicine (NUNM)**
49 South Porter St.
Portland, OR 97201
503-552-1555
reception@nunm.edu
nunm.edu

Melanie Henriksen, Interim President
Gerald Bores, Executive Vice President & Chief Financial Officer
Kathy Stanford, Vice President, Human Resources
Cheryl Miller, Vice President, Institutional Effectiveness

NUNM is an accredited naturopathic medical university, and leads the research on natural medicine. They offer programs in naturopathic medicine, classical Chinese medicine, integrative mental health, global health, massage therapy, and more.
1956

912 **National Vaccine Information Center (NVIC)**
21525 Ridgetop Circle
Suite 100
Sterling, VA 20166
703-938-0342
Fax: 571-313-1268
contactus@nvic.org
www.nvic.org

Barbara Loe Fisher, Co-Founder & President
Kathi Williams, Co-Founder & Vice President
Theresa Wrangham, Executive Director
Paul Arthur, Chief Operations Officer

Provides resources on vaccination and health.

913 **National Women's Health Network (NWHN)**
1413 K St. NW
4th Floor
Washington, DC 20005
202-682-2640
Fax: 202-682-2648
nwhn@nwhn.org
www.nwhn.org

Michelle M. Lockwood, Director, Development
M. Isabelle Chaudry, Senior Policy Manager
Erin Evans, Office Manager

The National Women's Health Network seeks to improve women's health by developing and promoting a critical analysis of health issues in order to affect policy and support consumer decision-making. The Network aspires to a health care system that is guided by social justice and reflects the needs of diverse women.

914 **Native American Disability Law Center**
905 W Apache St.
Farmington, NM 87401
505-566-5880
800-862-7271
Fax: 505-566-5889
info@nativedisabilitylaw.org
www.nativedisabilitylaw.org

Therese Yanan, Executive Director
Laura McClenny, Director, Development

The Native American Disability Law Center is a private nonprofit organization that advocates for the legal rights of Native Americans with disabilities. Through advocacy and education, the center empowers Native people with disabilities to lead independent lives in their own communities.

915 **North Hastings Community Integration Association**
2 Alice St.
PO Box 1508
Bancroft, ON, Canada K0L-1C0
613-332-2090
Fax: 613-332-4762
communityliving@nhcia.ca
www.nhcia.ca

Sandra Phillips, Executive Director
Teena Surma, Manager, Independent Living
Brittany McCaig, Manager, Independent Living
Janet Christie, Manager, Youth & Family Supports

NHCIA offers daily living supports, life planning, community access, dual diagnosis supports, respite services, assistance with funding and resource referral information. The association works closely with many community services, groups, schools, and businesses to offer individualized supports to children, youth and adults with an intellectual disability and their families.

916 **Not Dead Yet**
497 State St.
Rochester, NY 14608
708-420-0539
notdeadyet.org

Diane Coleman, President & CEO
Anita Cameron, Director, Minority Outreach
Disability rights group opposing the legalization of assisted suicide and euthanasia.

917 **PACER Center (Parent Advocacy Coalition for Educational Rights)**
8161 Normandale Blvd.
Bloomington, MN 55437
952-838-9000
800-537-2237
Fax: 952-838-0199
pacer@pacer.org
www.pacer.org

Paula F. Goldberg, Executive Director
Mission is to expand opportunities and enhance the quality of life of children and young adults with disabilities and their families based on the concept of parents helping parents. Offers workshops, individual assistance, and written information for children with disabilities, their parents and families, and professionals working with them. Computer Resource Center/Software Lending Library available.

918 **PEAK Parent Center**
917 East Moreno Ave.
Suite 140
Colorado Springs, CO 80903
719-531-9400
Fax: 719-531-9452
info@peakparent.org
www.peakparent.org

Michele Williers, Executive Director
Pam Christy, Director, Parent Training & Information
PEAK Parent Center is Colorado's federally-designated Parent Training and Information Center (PTI). As a PTI, PEAK supports and empowers parents, providing them with information and strategies to use when advocating for their children with disabilities. PEAK works one-on-one with families and educators helping them realize new possibilities for children with disabilities by expanding knowledge of special education and offering new strategies for success.

919 **Pacific Institute of Aromatherapy**
PO Box 6723
San Rafael, CA 94903
415-479-9120
Fax: 415-479-0614
www.pacificinstituteofaromatherapy.com
Kurt Schnaubelt, Founder & Director
The Pacific Institute on Aromatherapy offers certification courses, seminars, books, and products on aromatherapy treatments and essential oils.

920 **Parent Professional Advocacy League (PPAL)**
77 Rumford Ave.
Waltham, MA 02453
866-815-8122
Fax: 617-542-7832
info@ppal.net
www.ppal.net

Lisa Lambert, Executive Director
Meri Viano, Associate Director
Joel Khattar, Program Manager
A statewide organization focusing on the interests of families with children with mental health needs. PPAL advocates for improved and better access to mental health services for children and their families.

921 **Parents Helping Parents (PHP)**
1400 Parkmoor Ave.
Suite 100
San Jose, CA 95126
408-727-5775
855-727-5775
Fax: 408-286-1116
info@php.com
www.php.com

Maria Daane, Executive Director
Janet Nunez, Director, Programs
Mark Fishler, Director, Development
Virginia Hildebrand, Director, Finance
Dedicated to assisting children with any type of special need: mental, physical, emotional, or learning disability. Mission is to help children with special needs receive love, hope, respect, and services needed to achieve their full potential by strengthening their families and the professionals who serve them. Develops programs and produces educational and support materials, including information packets, brochures, and a newsletter.

922 **Partnership on Employment and Acessible Technology (PEAT)**
info@peatworks.org
www.peatworks.org

923 **Partnership to Improve Patient Care**
100 M St. SE
Suite 750
Washington, DC 20003
www.pipcpatients.org
Sara van Geertruyden, Executive Director
Thayer Surette Roberts, Deputy Director
Promotes a patient-centric healthcare system including comparative effectiveness research, the assessment of treatment value through shared decision-making, and alternate payment models.

924 **People First of Canada**
20-226 Osborne St. North
Winnipeg, MB, Canada R3C-1V4
204-784-7362
Fax: 204-784-7364
info@peoplefirstofcanada.ca
www.peoplefirstofcanada.ca

Shelley Fletcher, Executive Director
Catherine Rodgers, Director, Communications
People First of Canada is the national voice for people who have been labeled with an intellectual disability. People First is a movement of people who want all citizens to live equally in the country.

925 **Peter and Elizabeth C. Tower Foundation**
2351 North Forest Rd.
Suite 106
Getzville, NY 14068-1225
716-689-0370
Fax: 716-689-3716
info@thetowerfoundation.org
thetowerfoundation.org

Tracy A. Sawicki, Executive Director
Donald W. Matteson, Chief Program Officer
Charles E. Colston Jr., Program Officer
Megan T. MacDavey, Program Officer
The Peter and Elizabeth C. Tower Foundation supports community programming that results in children, adolescents, and young adults affected by substance use disorders, learning disabilities, mental illness, and intellectual disabilities achieving their full potential.

926 **Post-Polio Health International**
50 Crestwood Executive Ctr.
Suite 440
St. Louis, MO 63126
314-534-0475
Fax: 314-534-5070
info@post-polio.org
www.post-polio.org

Daniel J. Wilson, President
Mark Mallinger, Vice President
Brian M. Tiburzi, Executive Director
Marny E. Eulberg, Secretary
To enhance the lives and independence of polio survivors, home ventilator users, their caregivers and families, and health professionals through education, networking, and advocacy.

927 **Postpartum Support International (PSI)**
6706 SW 54th Ave.
Portland, OR 97219
503-894-9453
800-944-4773
Fax: 503-894-9452
support@postpartum.net
postpartum.net

Wendy N. Davis, Executive Director
Lianne Swanson, Executive Administrator
Birdie Gunyon Meyer, Certification Director
Jenn Davis, Chapters Manager

The mission of Postpartum Support International is to promote awareness, prevention, and treatment of mental health issues related to childbearing in every country worldwide.

928 **Primary Care Collaborative**
601 13th St. NW
Suite 430N
Washington, DC 20005
202-417-2076
spadre@pcpcc.org
www.pcpcc.org

Ann Grenier, President & CEO
Loren Vandegrift, Director, IT
Stephen Padre, Senior Communications Manager
Evelyn Snyder, Office Manager

Advocates for a health system built on patient-centered primary care. Its four aims are better care, better health, lower costs, and greater joy for clinicians and staff in delivery of care.

929 **Professional Association of Therapeutic Horsemanship International (PATH Intl.)**
PO Box 33150
Denver, CO 80233
303-452-1212
800-369-7433
Fax: 303-252-4610
pathintl@pathintl.org
www.pathintl.org

Kathy Alm, Chief Executive Officer
Carrie Garnett, Director, Membership & Operations
Kaye Marks, Director, Marketing & Communications
Bret Maceyak, Director, Credentialing

A national nonprofit equestrian organization dedicated to serving individuals with disabilities by giving disabled individuals the opportunity to ride horses. Establishes safety standards, provides continuing education, and offers networking opportunities for both its individuals and center members. Produces educational materials including fact sheets, brochures, booklets, audio-visual tapes, a directory, and PATH Intl. magazine Strides.

930 **Raising Deaf Kids**
3440 Market St.
4th Floor
Philadelphia, PA 19104
215-590-7440
Fax: 215-590-1335
TTY: 215-590-6817
info@raisingdeafkids.org
raisingdeafkids.org

Annie Steinberg, Director

This website provides parents/guardians of children with hearing impairments with information and resources. The website is run and funded by the Deafness and Family Communication Center based at the Children's Hospital of Philadelphia.

931 **Rehabilitation International**
866 United Nations Plaza
Office 422
New York, NY 10017
212-420-1500
Fax: 212-505-0871
info@riglobal.org
www.riglobal.org

Teuta Rexhepi, Secretary General
Zhang Haidi, President

RI and its members develop and promote initiatives to protect the rights of people with disabilities and improve rehabilitation and other crucial services for disabled people and their families. RI also works toward increasing international collaboration and advocates for policies and legislation recognizing the rights of people with disabilities and their families, including the establishment of a UN Convention on the Rights and Dignity of Persons with Disabilities.

932 **RespectAbility**
11333 Woodglen Dr.
Suite 102
Rockville, MD 20852
202-517-6272
info@respectability.org
www.respectability.org

Jennifer Laszlo Mizrahi, President
Lauren Appelbaum, Vice President, Communications
Philip Kahn-Pauli, Director, Policy & Practices
Franklin Anderson, Director, Inclusive Philanthropy & Development

Nonprofit, nonpartisan organization providing free educational tools and resources to end stigmas and advance opportunities for people with disabilities and their families.

933 **Ronald McDonald House Charities (RMHC)**
110 N Carpenter St.
Chicago, IL 60607
630-623-7048
info@rmhc.org
www.rmhc.org

Kelly Dolan, President & CEO
Stacey Bifero, Chief Financial Officer
Janet Burton, Chief Operating Officer
Joanna Sabato, Chief Marketing & Development Officer

Ronald McDonald House programs for families with sick children can be found in more than 64 countries around the world. Each house is run by a local nonprofit agency comprised of members of the medical community, McDonald's owners, businesses and civic organizations, and parent volunteers.

934 **Ryan White HIV/AIDS Program**
Health Resources & Services Administration
5600 Fishers Lane
Rockville, MD 20857
301-443-2216
hab.hrsa.gov/about-ryan-white-hivaids-program

Laura Cheever, Associate Administrator
Heather Hauck, Deputy Associate Administrator
Jeanean Willis Marsh, Director, Office of Program Support
Paul Belkin, Director, Office of Operations & Management

The Ryan White HIV/AIDS Program provides a comprehensive system of care that includes primary medical care and essential support services for people living with HIV who are uninsured or underinsured. The Program works with cities, states, and local community-based organizations to provide HIV care and treatment services to more than half a million people each year.

935 **Shirley Ryan AbilityLab**
355 East Erie
Chicago, IL 60611
312-238-1000
844-355-2253
Fax: 312-238-1369
www.sralab.org

Joanne C. Smith, President & CEO
Jonathan Tingstad, Chief Financial Officer
Peggy Kirk, Chief Operating Officer
Betsy Owens, Chief Marketing & Innovation Officer

Shirley Ryan AbilityLab is a research hospital integrating medical and research experts together in real time, applying research and providing patient care in physical medicine and rehabilitation. The AbilityLab has five Innovation Centers, each focusing on an area of biomedical science: Brain; Nerve, Muscle & Bone; Cancer; Spinal Cord; and Pediatric.

936 **Society for Post-Acute and Long-Term Care Medicine (AMDA)**
10500 Little Patuxent Pkwy.
Suite 210
Columbia, MD 21044
410-740-9743
800-876-2632
Fax: 410-740-4572
info@paltc.org
paltc.org

Karl Steinberg, President
Milta Little, Vice President
Swati Gaur, Treasurer
Christopher Laxton, Executive Director

The Society for Post-Acute and Long-Term Care Medicine is a medical society representing medical directors, physicians, nurse practitioners, physician assistants, and other professionals working in post-acute and long-term care settings. The Society's mission is to advance the development of medical practitioners in all post-acute and long-term care settings through professional development, clinical guidance, and advocacy.
1977

937 **Sofia University**
1069 East Meadow Crl.
Palo Alto, CA 94303
888-820-1484
student_services@sofia.edu
sofia.edu
Allan Cahoon, President
Chris Nguyen, Chief Financial Officer & Vice President, Administration
Sofia University is a private, WSCUC-accredited institution focusing on humanistic and transpersonal psychology.

938 **Spartan Stuttering Laboratory**
Michigan State University
1026 Red Cedar Rd.
East Lansing, MI 48824
517-884-2406
stutteringlab.msu.edu
J. Scott Yaruss, Director
The Spartan Stuttering Laboratory is a nonprofit organization that provides specialized assessment and treatment for children, adolescents, and adults who stutter and their families. They also provide education, training, and support for speech-language pathologists who work with people who stutter, and conduct an active program of basic and clinical research on the nature and treatment of stuttering across age groups.

939 **St. Paul Abilities Network**
4637 - 45 Ave.
St. Paul, AB, Canada T0A-3A3
780-645-3441
866-645-3900
Fax: 780-645-1885
www.stpaulabilitiesnetwork.ca
Anthony Opden Dries, Executive Director
Provides support and opportunities to encourage the development of an individual's full potential through education, advocacy, and community partnerships.

940 **Starbridge**
1650 South Ave.
Suite 200
Rochester, NY 14620
585-546-1700
800-650-4967
Fax: 585-224-7100
www.starbridgeinc.org
Colin Garwood, President & CEO
Nikisha Ridgeway, Chief Operating Officer
Terry O'Hare, Chief Financial Officer
Krystyna Staub, Vice President, Philanthropy
A nonprofit organization dedicated to educating, supporting, and advocating for people who have disabilities, their families, and their circles of support.

941 **Student Disability Services (SDS)**
Wayne State University
5155 Gullen Mall
1600 Undergraduate Library
Detroit, MI 48202
313-577-1851
Fax: 313-577-4898
TTY: 313-202-4216
studentdisability@wayne.edu
www.studentdisability.wayne.edu
Cherise Matthews Frost, Interim Director
Their mission is to ensure a university experience in which individuals with disabilities have equitable access to programs and to empower students to self-advocate in order to fulfill their academic goals.

942 **TASH**
1101 15th St. NW
Suite 206
Washington, DC 20005
202-817-3264
Fax: 202-999-4722
info@tash.org
www.tash.org
Michael Brogioli, Executive Director
Linda Metchikoff-Hooker, Director, Special Events
Donald Taylor, Manager, Membership & Operations
Marshall Jones, Office Administrator
Formerly The Association for Persons with Severe Handicaps, it is an international association of people with disabilities, their family members, other advocates, and professionals fighting for a society in which inclusion of all people in all aspects of society is the norm.

943 **The Advocacy Centre**
521 Vernon St.
Nelson, BC, Canada V1L-4E9
250-352-5777
877-352-5777
Fax: 250-352-5723
advocacycentre@nelsoncares.ca
advocacycentre.org

944 **The Cherab Foundation**
PO Box 1771
Jensen Beach, FL 34958
772-335-5135
help@cherab.org
cherabfoundation.org
Lisa Geng, Founder & President
Jolie Abreu, Vice President
The Cherab Foundation is a world-wide nonprofit organization working to improve the communication skills and education of all children with speech and language delays and disorders. The Cherab Foundation is committed to assisting with the development of new therapeutic approaches, preventions, and cures to neurologically-based speech disorders.

945 **The Davis Center**
110 Wesley St.
PO Box 508
Manlius, NY 13104
862-251-4637
Fax: 862-251-4642
ddavis@thedaviscenter.com
www.thedaviscenter.com
Dorinne S. Davis, Director
Offers sound-based therapies supporting positive change in learning, development, and wellness. All ages/all disabilities. Uses The Davis Model of Sound Intervention, an alternative approach.

946 **The Hanen Centre**
1075 Bay St.
Suite 515
Toronto, ON, Canada M5S-2B1
416-921-1073
877-426-3655
Fax: 416-921-1225
info@hanen.org
hanen.org
Elaine Weitzman, Executive Director
The Hanen Centre's mission is to provide parents, caregivers, early childhood educators, and speech-language pathologists with the knowledge and training they need to help young children develop the best possible language, social, and literacy skills. This includes children with or at risk of language delays and those with developmental challenges such as Autism Spectrum Disorder.

947 **The Obesity Medicine Association (OMA)**
7173 S Havana St.
Suite 600-130
Centennial, CO 80112
303-770-2526
Fax: 303-779-4834
info@obesitymedicine.org
obesitymedicine.org
Katrina Crist, Executive Director
Joan Hablutzel, Director, Education
Christin Eriksen, Director, Marketing & Sales
Christian DeSousa, Senior Manager, Membership
The Obesity Medicine Association is an organization of physicians, nurse practitioners, physician assistants, and other health care providers with special interest and experience in the comprehensive treatment of obesity.

948 **The Steve Fund**
PO Box 9070
Providence, RI 02940
401-249-0044
info@stevefund.org
stevefund.org
Laura Sanchez-Parkinson, Director, Partnerships, Programs & Research
Bianca Swift, Director, Operations & Content
The Steve Fund is dedicated to the mental health and emotional well-being of young people of color. It offers programs and ser-

vices designed to assist both institutions of higher education and nonprofits in improving their capacity to support the mental health and emotional well-being of students of color. Programs and services include workshops, webinars, expert speakers, training, and technology innovations.

949 **Therapeutic Touch International Association (TTIA)**
PO Box 130
Delmar, NY 12054
518-325-1185
Fax: 509-693-3537
info@therapeutictouch.org
therapeutictouch.org

Mary Anne Hanley, President
Madonna Pence, Treasurer
Lin Bauer, Contact, Education
Michelle Ferraro, Contact, Membership

This international cooperative network of health care professionals is committed to excellence in healing through Therapeutic Touch. The organization serves as a resource for persons in the field of health care, laypersons, and other organizations interested in information on Therapeutic Touch, and for therapists and teachers searching for teaching and learning materials related to Therapeutic Touch.

950 **Thresholds**
4101 N Ravenswood Ave.
Chicago, IL 60613
773-572-5500
contact@thresholds.org
www.thresholds.org

Mark Ishaug, Chief Executive Officer
Mark Furlong, Chief Operating Officer
Brent Peterson, Chief Development Officer
Al Shoreibah, Chief Financial Officer

Provider of recovery services for persons with mental illnesses and substance abuse disorders in Illinois. It offers 30 programs at more than 75 locations throughout Chicago and surrounding suburbs and counties. Services include case management, housing, employment, education, psychiatry, primary care, substance use treatment, and research.

951 **United States Disabled Golf Association (USDGA)**
598 Dixie Rd.
Clinton, NC 28328
910-214-5983
info@usdga.net
www.usdga.net

Jason Faircloth, Founder

The US Disabled Golf Association provides people with physical, sensory, and mental disabilities an opportunity to play golf at the highest level in the USA.

952 **United States Trager Association**
3755 Attucks Dr.
Powell, OH 43065
440-834-0308
Fax: 888-525-7645
exec@tragerus.org
www.tragerapproach.us

953 **Universal Pediatrics**
10654 Justin Dr.
Urbandale, IA 50322
800-383-0303
www.universalpediatrics.com

Tucker Anderson, Chief Executive Officer

Universal Pediatrics provides high-tech in-home medical care to children and young adults. Emphasis is placed on the provision of services in the rural areas, the ability to service high tech needs, and the promotion of primary nurse concept.

954 **Upledger Institute International (UII)**
11211 Prosperity Farms Rd.
Suite D-325
Palm Beach Gardens, FL 33410
561-622-4334
800-233-5880
Fax: 561-622-4771
upledger@upledger.com
www.upledger.com

Kathy Woll, Chief Operating Officer
Dawn Langnes Shear, Chief Development Officer
Alex Jozefyk, Chief Financial Officer
Jackie Halderman, Director, Marketing

A healthcare resource center focused on comprehensive education programs, advanced treatment options, and outreach initiatives. The Institute has trained more than 125,000 healthcare professionals throughout the globe in the therapeutic approach.

955 **Viability**
60 Brookdale Dr.
Springfield, MA 01104
413-781-5359
viability.org

Francis Fitzgerald, Chair
Jonathon Dean, Vice Chair
Charlene Smolkowicz, Treasurer
Colleen Holmes, President & CEO

Viability's mission is to help individuals with disabilities achieve their full potential. Services include day programs, employment services, and job training and placements.

956 **Volunteers of America (VOA)**
1660 Duke St.
Alexandria, VA 22314
703-341-5000
800-899-0089
info@voa.org
www.voa.org

Michael King, President & CEO
Joseph A. Budzynski, Executive Vice President & CFO
Jatrice Martel Gaiter, Executive Vice President, External Affairs
Sharon Wilson Geno, Executive Vice President, National Services & COO

Volunteers of America is a nonprofit organization serving vulnerable groups, including veterans, at-risk youth, people with disabilities, homeless persons and families, and individuals recovering from addiction. Services include housing, behavioral and mental health services, and community outreach.

957 **WORLD**
389 30th St.
Oakland, CA 94609
510-986-0340
Fax: 510-986-0341
womenhiv.org

958 **Waban Projects**
5 Dunaway Dr.
Sanford, ME 04073
207-324-7955
Fax: 207-324-6050
connect@waban.org
www.waban.org

Jennifer Putnam, Executive Director
Gervaise Flynn, Deputy Director
Ashley Bjornson, Chief Financial Officer
Tiffany Haskell, Director, Clinical Treatment Services

Waban Projects is a nonprofit corporation working to create programs and services for individuals with autism and intellectual, developmental, and other disabilities.

959 **Women to Women Healthcare**
170 US Route 1
Suite 110
Falmouth, ME 04105
207-846-6163
800-540-5906
Fax: 207-846-6167
support@womentowomenhealthcarecenter.com
www.womentowomenhealthcarecente r.com

Marcelle Pick, Co-Founder & Director

Aims to combine alternative and conventional medicine in women's health. Provides integrative care for women and specializes in chronic and difficult cases.

960 **World Federation for Mental Health**
6800 Park Ten Blvd.
Suite 220-N
San Antonio, TX 78213
info@wfmh.global
wfmh.global

Ingrid Daniels, President
Gabriel Ivbijaro, Secretary General & CEO
Henk Parmentier, Treasurer
Tracey Bone, Corporate Secretary

WFMH is an international membership organization that seeks to prevent mental and emotional disorders, advance the proper treatment and care of those with such disorders, and promote mental health.

961 **World Institute on Disability (WID)**
3075 Adeline St.
Suite 155
Berkeley, CA 94703
510-225-6400
Fax: 510-225-0477
wid@wid.org
www.wid.org

Marcie Roth, Executive Director & CEO
Katherine Zigmont, Senior Director, Operations & Deputy Director
Reggie Johnson, Senior Director, Marketing & Communications
Marsha Saxton, Director, Research

The mission of the World Institute on Disability (WID) is to eliminate barriers to full social integration and increase employment, economic security, and health care for persons with disabilities. WID creates innovative programs and tools; conducts research, public education, training, and advocacy campaigns; and provides technical assistance.

962 **YAI: National Institute for People with Disabilities**
220 E 42nd St.
8th Floor
New York, NY 10017
212-273-6100
www.yai.org

George Contos, Chief Executive Officer
Kevin Carey, Chief Financial Officer
Marie Cavallo, Chief Quality, Compliance, & Ethics Officer
Ravi Dahiya, Chief Program Officer

YAI is dedicated to enhancing the lives of people with developmental disabilities and their families. The organization works with individuals, families, government, corporate partners, donors, and foundations to ensure that people with disabilities are recognized for their abilities, achieve the goals that are important to them, and are integrated in the community.

963 **Youth MOVE National**
PO Box 215
Decorah, IA 52101
800-580-6199
youthmovenational.org

Johanna Bergan, Executive Director
Kristin Thorp, Director, Youth Program
Victoria Eckert, Director, Operations
Matt Leavitt, Coordinator, Communications

Aims to strengthen services and systems for issues such as mental health, juvenile justice, education, and child welfare.

964 **Youth as Self Advocates (YASA)**
Family Voices
110 Hartwell Ave.
Lexington, MA 02421
781-674-7224
888-835-5669
bbaker@familyvoices.org
www.familyvoices.org/yasa

Nora Wells, Executive Director, Family Voices
Bev Baker, Associate Director, Operations, Family Voices

National program created by youth with disabilities for other youth, helping them to better advocate for themselves.

Camps

Alabama

965 **Camp Evoked Potential**
Alabama's Special Camp for Children and Adults
PO Box 21
5278 Camp Ascca Dr.
Jacksons Gap, AL 36861
256-825-9226
Fax: 256-269-0714
info@campascca.org
www.campascca.org

Matt Rickman, Camp Director
Amber Cotney, Program Director
Jocelyn Jones, Secretary

Camp Evoked Potential is held one week out of the year for children aged 6-18 with epilepsy at Camp ASCCA. Fully funded by The Epilepsy Foundation, persons wishing to attend the camp must apply. The camp provides a barrier free setting situated on 230 acres of wooded land at Lake Martin. The camp is staffed with medical personnel trained to care for children with all types of disabilities and provides a variety of camp activities.

966 **Camp Seale Harris**
Southeastern Diabetes Education Services
500 Chase Park S.
Ste 104
Birmingham, AL 35244
205-402-0415
Fax: 205-402-0416
info@campsealeharris.org
www.campsealeharris.org

Matthew Munson, Chair
Katie Hester, Vice Chair
Rhonda McDavid, Executive Director
John Latimer, Camp & Community Programs Director

Offering overnight, family, day and community program camps, Camp Seale Harris is a nonprofit organization that offers residential camps for children and teens with diabetes. With multiple programs in Alabama, the volunteer camp counselors are trained adults living with diabetes, to better help the camp attendees gain independence in learning to manage their diabetes. Camp programs run all year round.

967 **Camp Shocco for the Deaf**
216 North St. E
PO Box 602
Talladega, AL 35161
800-264-1225

968 **Camp Smile-A-Mile**
Smile-A-Mile Place
1600 2nd Ave. S.
Birmingham, AL 35233
205-323-8427
Fax: 205-323-6220
info@campsam.org
www.campsam.org

Bruce Hooper, Executive Director
Kellie Reece, Chief Operating Officer
Shannon Rumage, Development Director
Carrie Pomeroy, Camp Director

Camp Smile-A-Mile offers 7 different educational camp opportunities for children and their families who have been affected by childhood cancer in Alabama. The programs run all year long, in a variety of formats.

969 **Camp Smile-A-Mile: Jr./Sr. Camp**
Smile-A-Mile Place
1600 2nd Ave. S.
Birmingham, AL 35233
205-323-8427
Fax: 205-323-6220
info@campsam.org
www.campsam.org

Carrie Pomeroy, Camp Director
Kellie Reece, Chief Operating Officer

Camp Smile-A-Mile's Jr./Sr. Camp is for high school juniors, seniors, and new high school graduates that are both on and off therapy. The weekend camp works to instill independence and responsibility in regards to their diagnosis.

970 **Camp Smile-A-Mile: Off Therapy Family Camp**
Smile-A-Mile Place
1600 2nd Ave. S.
Birmingham, AL 35233
205-323-8427
Fax: 205-323-6220
info@campsam.org
www.campsam.org

Carrie Pomeroy, Camp Director
Kellie Reece, Chief Operating Officer

Camp Smile-A-Mile's Off Therapy Family Camp is a specialized camp for off-therapy patients and their families. Campers up to the age of 18 who are no longer receiving therapy are eligible to attend the camp.

971 **Camp Smile-A-Mile: On Therapy Family Camp**
Smile-A-Mile Place
1600 2nd Ave. S.
Birmingham, AL 35233
205-323-8427
Fax: 205-323-6220
info@campsam.org
www.campsam.org

Carrie Pomeroy, Camp Director
Kellie Reece, Chief Operating Officer

A program of Camp Smile-A-Mile, On Therapy Family Camp is for patients up to 18 years of age, who are currently receiving therapy. The Family Camp is designed to give patients and their immediate families the opportunity to connect outside of an hospital environment.

972 **Camp Smile-A-Mile: Sibling Camp**
Smile-A-Mile Place
1600 2nd Ave. S.
Birmingham, AL 35233
205-323-8427
Fax: 205-323-6220
info@campsam.org
www.campsam.org

Carrie Pomeroy, Camp Director
Kellie Reece, Chief Operating Officer

Camp Smile-A-Mile's Sibling Camp is a specialized camp for the siblings of children and teens with cancer. Campers attending the Sibling Camp range in age from 6-18 and no patients or parents attend the camp.

973 **Camp Smile-A-Mile: Teen Weeklong Camp**
Smile-A-Mile Place
1600 2nd Ave. S.
Birmingham, AL 35233
205-323-8427
Fax: 205-323-6220
info@campsam.org
www.campsam.org

Carrie Pomeroy, Camp Director
Kellie Reece, Chief Operating Officer

A weeklong summer camp session for children, 13 through to the 10th grade, who have cancer. The session is open to those who are and aren't receiving therapy, with campers participating in activities such as swimming, snorkeling, and campfires.

974 **Camp Smile-A-Mile: Young Adult Retreat**
Smile-A-Mile Place
1600 2nd Ave. S.
Birmingham, AL 35233
205-323-8427
Fax: 205-323-6220
info@campsam.org
www.campsam.org

Carrie Pomeroy, Camp Director
Kellie Reece, Chief Operating Officer

A program of Camp Smile-A-Mile, the Young Adult Retreat is for childhood cancer survivors ages 19-30. The retreat is held over a summer weekend and offers educational and camping activities for participants. Those wanting to attend the retreat do not have to be former campers of Camp Smile-A-Mile.

975 **Camp Smile-A-Mile: Youth Weeklong Camp**
Smile-A-Mile Place
1600 2nd Ave. S.
Birmingham, AL 35233
205-323-8427
Fax: 205-323-6220
info@campsam.org
www.campsam.org

Carrie Pomeroy, Camp Director
Kellie Reece, Chief Operating Officer

A weeklong summer camp session for children, ages 6-12, who have cancer. The session is open to those who are and aren't receiving therapy, with campers participating in activities such as arts and crafts, fishing, boating, archery, and canoeing.

976 **Camp WheezeAway**
YMCA Camp Chandler
1240 Jordan Dam Rd
Wetumpka, AL 36092
334-229-0035
Fax: 334-649-7516
jikner@ymcamontgomery.org
ymcamontgomery.org/camp/wheezeaway
Jeff Reynolds, Executive Director
Art Mason, Operations Director
For children ages 8-12 with moderate to severe asthma, Camp WheezeAway offers week long summer camp programs that foster confidence building skills. The camp is free and managed by medical professionals. Those with children wishing to attend must apply to the camp and complete a selection process.

977 **Easterseals Camp ASCCA**
PO Box 21
5278 Camp Ascca Dr.
Jacksons Gap, AL 36861
256-825-9226
Fax: 256-269-0714
info@campascca.org
campascca.org
Matt Rickman, Camp Director
John Stephenson, Administrator
Jocelyn Jones, Secretary
Amber Cotney, Program Director
Easterseals Camp ASCCA is Alabama's Special Camp for Children and Adults, offering therapeutic recreation for children and adults with both physical and intellectual disabilities. The camp is located on 260 acres of barrier free woodland on Lake Martin and campers experience a wide variety of educational and recreational activities, including but not limited to: horseback riding, fishing, tubing, swimming, environmental education, arts, canoeing, and zip-lining. 1 week camp fees are $750.00.

978 **Happy Camp**
Merrimack Hall Performing Arts Center
3320 Triana Blvd SW.
Huntsville, AL 35805
256-534-6455
info@merrimackhall.com
www.merrimackhall.com/happy-headquarters

979 **Rapahope Children's Retreat Foundation**
2701 Airport Blvd
Mobile, AL 36606
251-476-9880
Fax: 251-476-9495
info@rapahope.org
www.rapahope.org
Melissa McNichol, Executive Director
Roz Dorsett, Assistant Director
Rapahope is an organization that offers a one week long summer camp for children who have, or who have had cancer. For children ages 7-17, the camp offers a wide range of summer camp activities, including but not limited to, swimming, kayaking, horseback riding, and arts. The camp is offered at no cost to campers or their families.

Alaska

980 **Adam's Camp: Alaska**
PO Box 242003
Anchorage, AK 99524
907-885-1758
alaska@adamscamp.org
adamscamp.org

981 **Camp Abilities**
Alpine Alternatives
2518 E. Tudor Road
Suite 105
Anchorage, AK 99507-1105
907-561-6655
Fax: 907-563-9232
alpinealternatives@arctic.net
www.alpinealternatives.org

982 **Camp Alpine**
Alpine Alternatives
2518 E. Tudor Road
Suite 105
Anchorage, AK 99507-1105
907-561-6655
Fax: 907-563-9232
alpinealternatives@arctic.net
www.alpinealternatives.org

Arizona

983 **Arizona Camp Sunrise & Sidekicks**
PO Box 27872
Tempe, AZ 85285
www.azcampsunrise.org

984 **Camp AZDA**
American Diabetes Association
5333 N 7th St.
Suite B212
Phoenix, AZ 85014
602-861-4731
Fax: 602-995-1344
ampazda@diabetes.org
www.diabetes.org/adacampazda
Kaylee Gronau, Camp Director
Camp AZDA is the Arizona summer camp program of the American Diabetes Association for children with diabetes. The camp is held at Friendly Pines in Prescott, Arizona with children participating in traditional camp activities while receiving educational information on managing their diabetes.

985 **Camp Abilities Tucson**
8987 East Tanque Verde Rd.
Suite 309-104
Tucson, AZ 85749
campabilitiestucson@gmail.com
www.campabilitiestucson.org
Murry Everson, Camp Director
Maria Lepore-Stevens, Camp Director
Camp Abilities is a privately funded educational sport camp for children and young adults who are blind, deaf-blind or have multiple disabilities including visual impairment. The camp offers sports instruction, with a 1:1 camper to coach ratio, tailored to fit the needs of the individual. The location of camp sessions is the Arizona School for the Deaf and Blind and costs $300.00 per person.

986 **Camp Candlelight**
Epilepsy Foundation Arizona
3620 N 4th Ave.
Suite 228
Phoenix, AZ 85013
602-282-3515
800-332-1000
AZ@EFA.org
epilepsyaz.org/events/campcandlelight
Suzanne Matsumori, Executive Director
Min Skivington, Program Manager
Camp Candlelight provides children ages 8 to 17 a unique camp experience that mixes traditional summer camp with special sessions that teach campers about their seizures and gives them resources to manage the challenges that the seizures represent. Staff inclues a neurologist, several nurses, and a school psychologist, in addition to traditional camp staff who are given specialized training in responding appropriately to the needs of kids with epilepsy.

987 **Camp Civitan**
Civitan Foundation
5008 N Civitan Rd
Williams, AZ 56046
602-953-2944
camp@campcivitan.org
www.civitanfoundationaz.com
Cody Graham, Camp Director
Dawn Trapp, Executive Director
Camp Civitan offers week long summer camp programs, and weekend programs throughout the year, to children with developmental disabilities. The camp is fully wheelchair accessible, is staffed by medical professionals and there is a 2:1 ratio of campers to staff. Camp Civitan offers campers the experience of traditional camp activities including, swimming, adaptive sports, fishing, music, arts and crafts, and talent shows.

988 **Camp H.U.G.**
Arizona Hemophilia Association
826 North 5th Ave
Phoenix, AZ 85003
602-955-3947
888-754-7017
info@arizonahemophilia.org
www.arizonahemophilia.org/camp-programs

Chastity Fermoile, Executive Director
Chelsea Guffy, Business Development Specialist
Yleana Highes, Member Services Supervisor

Camp H.U.G (Hemophilia Uniting Generations) is a weekend camp program of the Arizona Hemophilia Association. The camp is for families who have a member with hemophilia, WWD, and/or other bleeding disorders.

989 **Camp Honor**
Arizona Hemophilia Association
826 North 5th Ave
Phoenix, AZ 85003
602-955-3947
888-754-7017
info@arizonahemophilia.org
www.arizonahemophilia.org/camp-programs

Chastity Fermoile, Executive Director
Chelsea Guffy, Business Development Specialist
Yleana Highes, Member Services Supervisor

Camp Honor offers a week long summer camp to children affected by an inherited bleeding disorders. The cost of the camp is $35 for a single camper and $50 dollars for a family (2 or more campers). Camp Honor offers children the chance to partcipate in outdoor activities and educational opportunities. In order to attend the camp there is an application process.

990 **Camp Not-A-Wheeze**
2689 E Michelle Way
Gilbert, AZ 85234
602-336-6575
Fax: 602-336-6576
info@campnotawheeze.org
campnotawheeze.org

Alan Crawford, Camp Director

Week-long summer camp for children aged 7-14 with moderate to severe asthma living in Arizona. Campers attending Camp Not-A- Wheeze, participate in a wide range of activities such as, horseback riding, hiking, canoeing, and fishing as well as an asthma education class. Those wishing to attend must fill out and send in a camper application.

991 **Camp Rainbow**
Phoenix Childrens Hospital
1919 E Thomas Rd
Phoenix, AZ 85016
602-933-0157
camprainbow@phoenixchildrens.com
www.phoenixchildrens.org

Emilie Jarboe, Camp Director

Camp Rainbow is for children aged 7-17 who have or had cancer or a chronic blood disorder. The camp is offered for one week during the summer, held at camp Friendly Pines in Prescott, Arizona. Campers must be patients of Phoenix Children's Hospital's Center for Cancer and Blood Disorders, with the camp offering participants the opportunity to experience traditional camp activities including but not limited to, horseback riding, canoeing, fishing, swimming, and archery.

992 **Lions Camp Tatiyee**
5283 W White Mountain Blvd
Lakeside, AZ 85929
480-380-4254
pam@camptatiyee.org
camptatiyee.org

Pamela Swanson, Executive Director

Lions Camp Tatiyee is the only organization in Arizona providing a week long summer camp for individuals with special needs. There is no cost for the camp and all of the programs are adaptable. Some activities that campers can participate in are, go-karting, fishing, art, games, cooking, rock wall, swimming, dances and campfires.

993 **Nick & Kelly's Heart Camp**
Nick & Kelly Children's Fund
1321 E Bayview Dr
Tempe, AZ 85283
480-838-1529
contact@nickandkellyfund.org
www.nickandkellyfund.org

Cathy K., Camp Director

Nick & Kelly's Heart Camp is a free camp for children and teens ages 7-17 with congenital heart disease. The camp is held at Friendly Pines in Prescott, Arizona with campers participating in activities such as nature walks, water sports, arts and crafts, and recreational activities.

Arkansas

994 **Camp Aldersgate**
2000 Aldersgate Road
Little Rock, AR 72205
501-225-1444
Fax: 501-225-2019
eballew@campaldersgate.net
www.campaldersgate.net

Sonya S. Murphy, Chief Executive Officer
Ali Miller Berry, Director, Programs
Katie Jenkins, Program Coordinator
Kerri Daniels, Director, Development

Camp Aldersgate is a nonprofit organization, offering summer, weekend camps, and year-round social service programs to children, teens and adults with special needs. The camp promotes outdoor recreation and socialization in a completely accessible environment.

995 **Camp Laughter**
Arkansas Children's Neuroscience Center
1 Children's Way
2nd Floor
Little Rock, AR 72202
501-364-1100
camplaughter@archildrens.org
www.archildrens.org

996 **Camp Quality Arkansas**
PO Box 7754
Little Rock, AR 72217
870-926-3324
arkansas@campqualityusa.org
www.campqualityusa.org/ar

Nick Hankins, Executive Director
Jordan Law, Assistant Director
Audrey Wilkins, Camper Coordinator
Jeana Jucha, Fundraising Coordinator

Camp Quality is an international camping program for children with cancer. The Arkansas Camp Quality is held at Camp Powderfork in Bald Knob, Arkansas and offers children and their siblings summer camps and year round camping opportunities. Volunteer doctors and nurses are at the camp 24 hours a day, and there is a 1:1 staff to camper ratio.

997 **Camp Sunshine**
Burn Program at Arkansas Children's
1 Children's Way
Slot 225
Little Rock, AR 72202
501-364-1635
wilkinsonge@archildrens.org
www.archildrens.org/services/burn-program

Gretta Wilkinson, RN, Camp Director

Camp Sunshine is a 4 day no cost summer camp for children and teens, 4-16, who have experienced burn injuries. Camp Sunshine works to assist campers in the transformation from burn victim to burn survivor. In order to attend the camp, campers must have survived a 10% or greater full thickness burn and/or may have significant scarring, disability or scarring to the hands or face.

998 **Kota Camp**
Junior League Of Little Rock
401 South Scott Street
Little Rock, AR 72201
501-375-5557
info@jllr.org
www.jllr.org

Casey Rockwell, President
Jenna Martin, Vice President, Administrative
Lauren Hall, Treasurer
Betsey Mowery, Vice President, Community

Kota Camp is offered to children aged 6-16 with disabilities or medical conditions. Kota derived from a word used by the Quapaw Native American Tribe indigenous to Arkansas, means friend, and reflects the goals of the camp. Children with a disability bring a sibling or friend without a disability, to create a environment of inclusion, participate in camp activities, and promote an understanding of those with special needs. The camp is held at Camp Aldersgate in Little Rock.

California

999 **Bearskin Meadow Camp**
Diabetic Youth Families
5167 Clayton Rd
Suite F
Concord, CA 94521
925-680-4994
Fax: 925-680-4863
info@dyf.org
www.dyf.org

Kaylor Glassman, Interim Executive Director
Kaylee Gronau, Camp Director
Christi Rossi, Development, Director
Melissa Clarke-Howard, Development Director

Bearskin Meadow Camp, is a camp program offered by the Diabetes Youth Families organization to children (7-13), teens (14-17), and families who are affected by type 1 diabetes. The camp has traditional camp activities as well as educational opportunities for campers.

1000 **Camp Beyond The Scars**
Burn Institute
8825 Aero Drive
Suite 200
San Diego, CA 92123-2269
858-541-2277
Fax: 858-541-7179
ccoppenrath@burninstitute.org
www.burninstitute.org/camp-beyond-the-scar s

Jess Boles Lohmann, Operations Coordinator
Susan Day, Executive Director
Benjamin Hemmings, Director, Operations

Camp Beyond the Scars, is a weeklong sleepaway summer camp for children aged 8-17 who have survived a burn injury. Staffed by adult burn survivors, healthcare professionals, and off-duty firefighters, the camp provides an inclusive environment for burn survivors to participate in activities including, swimming, basketball, volleyball, archery, golf, and arts and crafts. The camp is free of charge, and is hosted at a camp facility in Romano, California.

1001 **Camp Bloomfield**
Wayfinder Family Services
5300 Angeles Vista Blvd.
Malibu, CA 90043
323-295-4555
Fax: 323-296-0424
JLucas@WayfinderFamily.org
www.wayfinderfamily.org

Joshua Lucas, MS, Recreation Programs Manager & Camp Director
Miki Jordan, President & Chief Executive Officer
Veronica Arteaga, Chief Program Officer

Camp Bloomfield is a summer camp with week long sessions for children and youth who are blind, visually impaired or multi-disabled. The 45 acre campground offers campers a variety of activities, specifically designed to meet the needs of the children, with campers attending at no cost.

1002 **Camp Christian Berets**
2508 Oakdale Rd.
Suite 10
Modesto, CA 95355
209-524-7993
Fax: 209-524-7979
www.christianberets.org

Brian Balsbaugh, President
Mark Burns, Vice President
Carletta Evans Steele, Secretary
Kelly Luth, Treasurer

Camp for children, students and adults with special needs.

1003 **Camp Conrad Chinnock**
Diabetes Camping And Educational Services, Inc.
12045 E. Waterfront Dr.
Playa Vista, CA 90094
310-751-3057
Fax: 909-752-5354
info@diabetescamping.org
www.diabetescamping.org

Rocky Wilson, Executive Director
Ryan Martz, Development & Program Director
Dale Lissy, Camp Manager
Melanie Coyne, Director, Camp Operations

Camp Conrad Chinnock offers year round recreational, social, and educational opportunities for children and families with type 1 diabetes.

1004 **Camp Grizzly**
NorCal Services For Deaf & Hard Of Hearing
4044 N Freeway Blvd.
Sacramento, CA 95843
916-349-7500
TTY: 916-349-7500
campgrizzly@norcalcenter.org
www.campgrizzly.org

Molly Bowen, Program Leader
Cheryl Bella, Program Leader

A program of NorCal Services for Deaf & Hard of Hearing, Camp Grizzly is a coed camp for children aged 7-18 who have a hearing impairment. Camp Grizzly takes place at the Camp Lodestar campground facilities and offers sporting activities, performing and creative arts, hiking, swimming, playgrounds and campfires.

1005 **Camp Hollywood HEART**
One Heartland
26001 Heinz Rd.
Willow River, MN 55795
888-216-2028
Fax: 612-824-6303
helpkids@oneheartland.org
www.oneheartland.org

Patrick Kindler, Executive Director
Katie Donlin, Operations Manager
Katie Bartels, Program Director
Stefanie Tywater-Christiansen, Development Director

A program of One Heartland, a nonprofit organization working to provide camping programs for children with serious illnesses or experiencing social isolation. Camp Hollywood HEART is a weeklong summer camp for youths, ages 15-20, who are infected or affected by HIV/AIDS. The camp is held in Malibu, California and is partnership camp between One Heartland and Hollywood Heart.

1006 **Camp Kindle**
Project Kindle
27203 Golden Willow Way
Santa Clarita, CA 91387
877-800-2267
eva@projectkindle.org
www.projectkindle.org

Eva Payne, Founder & CEO
Mandy Nickolite, Vice President

Camp Kindle provides year-round cost free recreational, educational and support services for children with special needs and life challenges.

1007 **Camp Krem**
Camping Unlimited
102 Brook Lane
Boulder Creek, CA 95006 831-338-3210
campkrem@campingunlimited.org
campingunlimited.org
Christina Krem, Camp Director
Kenneth Beebe, Assistant Camp Director
Layla Sharif, Administrator & Mobility Manager
Gail Zigenis, Registrar
Camp Krem - Camping Unlimited offers year-round and summer camping programs for children and adults with developmental disabilities. With a variety of different programs and many facilities on the campground such as a swimming pool, arts and crafts building, amphitheater, music pavilion, and archery range, Camp Krem provides its campers with recreation, education, and adventure opportunities.

1008 **Camp No Limits California**
No Limits Foundation
700 S Wren Dr.
Big Bear Lake, CA 92315 207-569-6411
campnolimits@gmail.com
www.nolimitsfoundation.org
Mary Leighton, Founder & Executive Director
Kelsey Moody, Program Operations Manager
Alix Sandler, Marketing & Development Director
Cheryl Foss, Director, Human Resources
Camp No Limits California, a location of Camp No Limits, is a recreational and educational camp for youth who have experienced limb loss. Camp No Limits, is a program of the nonprofit organization No Limits Foundation. The California camp is held in Big Bear where campers have access to ropes courses, zip lines, and a swimming pool.

1009 **Camp Okizu**
Okizu Foundation
83 Hamilton Dr.
Suite 200
Novato, CA 94949-5755 415-382-9083
Fax: 415-382-8384
info@okizu.org
www.okizu.org
Stuart J. Kaplan, Executive Director
Suzie Randall, Executive Director, Operations
Morgan Santiesteban, Camp Director
Camp Okizu offers a variety of medically supervised, residential camp programs for families who have a child diagnosed with cancer. Programs are offered throughout the year free of charge.

1010 **Camp Okizu: Family Camp**
Okizu Foundation
83 Hamilton Dr.
Suite 200
Novato, CA 94949-5755 415-382-9083
Fax: 415-382-8384
enrollment@okizu.org
www.okizu.org
Stuart J. Kaplan, Executive Director
Suzie Randall, Executive Director, Operations
Morgan Santiesteban, Camp Director
Camp Okizu's Family Camp is no cost camp designed for the families of children, and children who have been diagnosed with cancer. The Family Camp is offered as a weekend program, running on multiple weekends from April to September.

1011 **Camp Okizu: Oncology Camp**
Okizu Foundation
83 Hamilton Dr.
Suite 200
Novato, CA 94949-5755 415-382-9083
Fax: 415-382-8384
enrollment@okizu.org
www.okizu.org
Stuart J. Kaplan, Executive Director
Suzie Randall, Executive Director, Operations
Morgan Santiesteban, Camp Director
A program of Camp Okizu, the Oncology Camp is for children and teens, ages 6-17, who have or have had cancer. The camp is a residential summer camp program and is staffed by pediatric oncology departments from the participating hospitals.

1012 **Camp Okizu: SIBS Camp**
Okizu Foundation
83 Hamilton Dr.
Suite 200
Novato, CA 94949-5755 415-382-9083
Fax: 415-382-8384
enrollment@okizu.org
www.okizu.org
Stuart J. Kaplan, Executive Director
Suzie Randall, Executive Director, Operations
Morgan Santiesteban, Camp Director
SIBS (Special and Important Brothers and Sisters) Camp is for the sibling or siblings, ages 6-17, of a child who has, has had, or has died from cancer. The camp is a no charge, residential summer program, that provides campers the opportunity to learn new skills and get support from others who have experienced having a sibling with cancer.

1013 **Camp Okizu: Teens-N-Twenties Camp**
Okizu Foundation
83 Hamilton Dr.
Suite 200
Novato, CA 94949-5755 415-382-9083
Fax: 415-382-8384
enrollment@okizu.org
www.okizu.org
Stuart J. Kaplan, Executive Director
Suzie Randall, Executive Director, Operations
Morgan Santiesteban, Camp Director
Camp Okizu: Teens-N- Twenties Camp is a weekend recreation and support program that is offered 4 times a year for pediatric oncology patients and their siblings ages 18-25.

1014 **Camp Pacifica**
California Lions Camp
45895 California Hwy 49
Ahwahnee, CA 93601 559-683-4660
deafcamppacifica@gmail.com
www.camppacifica.org
Angelica Martinez, Camp Director
John Martinez, Assistant Director
Camp Pacifica provides a summer camp experience for children, boys and girls, aged 7-15 who have a hearing impairment. The camp is located in the foothills of Sierra on 52 acres of forested woodland. Activities include, but are not limited to, archery, canoeing, ropes course, swimming, horseback riding, and riflery. The camp costs $360.00 plus a registration fee.

1015 **Camp Paivika**
PO Box 3367
Crestline, CA 92325 909-338-1102
Fax: 909-338-2502
camppaivika@abilityfirst.org
www.abilityfirst.org/camp-paivika
Kelly Kunsek, Camp Director
Lauren Wilson, Program Director
Tina Ronning-Fraynd, Coordinator, Camper Services
As a program of AbilityFirst, Camp Paivika offers overnight summer programs for children, teens and adults with developmental and physical disabilities. The camp is completely accessible and the staff is trained to provide any assistance or personal care a camper needs. Located in San Bernardino National Forest, Camp Paivika provides a traditional summer camp experience in a safe and fun environment.

1016 **Camp ReCreation**
9272 Madison Ave.
Orangeville, CA 95662 916-988-6835
camprecreation@outlook.com
www.camprecreation.org
Kathi Barber, Camp Director
Camp ReCreation offers residential summer camps and year round programs for children, teens, and adults with developmental disabilities. The summer camp is held at Camp Ronald McDonald in Lassen National Forest. With a 1:1 staff to camper ratio, Camp ReCreation offers wide variety of camp activities, and campers wishing to participate must fill out a camper application.

1017 **Camp Reach for the Sky**
The Seany Foundation
3530 Camino del Rio N
Suite 101
San Diego, CA 92108 858-551-0922
www.theseanyfoundation.org

Brian Bonert, Camp Advisory Chair
Benji Quintero, Sib Director
Kerry Whittaker, Roc Camp Director
Pauline Kern, Day Camp Director

Previously run by the American Cancer Society, Camp Reach for the Sky (CR4TS) is now run by The Seany Foundation and provides an opportunity for children with cancer and their siblings to attend a free summer camp. Camp Reach for the Sky offers a multiple programs, including a Resident Oncology Camp, a Sibling Camp and Day Camps.

1018 **Camp Ronald McDonald at Eagle Lake**
2555 49th Street
Sacramento, CA 95817 916-734-4230
Fax: 916-734-4238
mdamos@RMHCNC.org
www.campronald.org

Maria Damos, Camp Director

Camp Ronald McDonald at Eagle Lake collaborates with other nonprofit organizations to provide week long summer camp opportunities for children with special medical needs, financial hardship and/or emotional, developmental or physical disabilities. The camp is fully accessible.

1019 **Camp Ronald McDonald for Good Times**
1250 Lyman Place
Los Angeles, CA 90029 310-268-8488
Fax: 310-473-3338
www.campronaldmcdonald.org

Fatima Djelmane Rodriguez, Executive Director
Brian Crater, Associate Executive Director
Chad Edwards, Program Director
Shannon Edwards, Program Associate

Free year-round residential camping for children with cancer and their families.

1020 **Camp Sunburst**
Sunburst Projects United States Headquarters
2143 Hurley Way
Suite 240
Sacramento, CA 95825 916-440-0889
Fax: 916-440-1208
admin@sunburstprojects.org
www.sunburstprojects.org

Geri DeLaRosa, PhD, Founder & Executive Director
Samantha Voelkel, Camp Director

Camp Sunburst is a youth oriented leadership camp that promotes and creates an environment to help youth learn self confidence to change negative social patterns and break cycles of HIV/AIDS infections. Activities campers will participate in include, boating, swimming, art, dance, and sports.

1021 **Camp Sunshine Dreams**
PO Box 28232
Fresno, CA 93729-8232 pam@campsunshinedreams.org
www.campsunshinedreams.com

Stephanie Scharbach, Contact
Pam Aiello, Contact

Camp Sunshine Dreams provides a summer camp experience to children aged 8-15 with cancer and their siblings.

1022 **Camp Taylor**
Camp Taylor, Inc.
8224 West Grayson Rd.
Modesto, CA 95358-9094 209-545-3853
camp@kidsheartcamp.org
www.kidsheartcamp.org

Kimberlie Gamino, Founder & Executive Director

With several programs, Camp Taylor provides youth, teens, and the families of children with heart disease the opportunity to go to a free medically supervised summer sleepaway camp. Campers are able to enjoy activities such as, swimming, snorkeling, horseback riding, rock-wall, skits, archery, and heart education.

1023 **Camp Taylor: Family Camp**
Camp Taylor, Inc.
8224 West Grayson Rd.
Modesto, CA 95358-9094 209-545-3853
camp@kidsheartcamp.org
www.kidsheartcamp.org/familycampca

Kimberlie Gamino, Founder & Executive Director

A program of Camp Taylor, Family Camp is for children of all ages, with congenital heart disease and/or acquired heart disease, and their family including parents and siblings. The camp offers parental heart education and support programs for parents and siblings. Family Camp is geared towards children too young to attend Youth or Teen Camp, or those who are not ready to attend a residential camp.

1024 **Camp Taylor: Leadership Camp**
Camp Taylor, Inc.
8224 West Grayson Rd.
Modesto, CA 95358-9094 209-545-3853
camp@kidsheartcamp.org
www.kidsheartcamp.org/leadershipcamp

Kimberlie Gamino, Founder & Executive Director

Leadership Camp is for teens and youth, ages 16-21, who have previously attended a Camp Taylor California camp program, wishing to be camp mentor for youth, teen, and family camps. Campers wishing to attend this camp should make it known to either a camp counselor or camp director.

1025 **Camp Taylor: Teen Camp**
Camp Taylor, Inc.
8224 West Grayson Rd.
Modesto, CA 95358-9094 209-545-3853
camp@kidsheartcamp.org
www.kidsheartcamp.org/teencamp

Kimberlie Gamino, Founder & Executive Director

The Teen Camp program at Camp Taylor is for teens ages 13-17, with congenital heart disease and/or acquired heart disease. Campers participate in heart education and traditional camp activities. Campers wishing to attend the camp must apply, with campers being accepted on a first come basis.

1026 **Camp Taylor: Young Adult Program**
Camp Taylor, Inc.
8224 West Grayson Rd.
Modesto, CA 95358-9094 209-545-3853
camp@kidsheartcamp.org
www.kidsheartcamp.org/leadershipcamp

Kimberlie Gamino, Founder & Executive Director

The Young Adult Program at Camp Taylor is designed for previous heart campers ages 18-35 with congenital heart disease. The program works to provide support, education, and the opportunities to participate in social events in order to help with the transition to adulthood.

1027 **Camp Taylor: Youth Camp**
Camp Taylor, Inc.
8224 West Grayson Rd.
Modesto, CA 95358-9094 209-545-3853
camp@kidsheartcamp.org
www.kidsheartcamp.org/youthcamp

Kimberlie Gamino, Founder & Executive Director

A program of Camp Taylor, Youth Camp is designed for children, ages 7-12, with congenital heart disease and/or acquired heart disease. Campers participate in heart education and traditional camp activities. Campers wishing to attend the camp must apply, with campers being accepted on a first come basis.

1028 **Camp Tuolumne Trails**
22988 Ferretti Road
Groveland, CA 95321 209-962-7534
info@tuolumnetrails.org
www.tuolumnetrails.org

Jacqui Montero, Program Manager
Jessica Morrison, General Manager

Tuolumne Trails is a camp for individuals with special medical needs. With week long summer camp options, Camp Tuolumne Trails is a completely accessible camp, with a 3:1 staff to camper ratio, that allows campers to participate in camping activities in a safe environment. Campers wishing to attend must complete the application and session assignment process.

1029 **Camp del Corazon**
11615 Hesby St
North Hollywood, CA 91601-3620
818-754-0312
Fax: 818-754-0377
info@campdelcorazon.org
www.campdelcorazon.org

Tiffany Maisonet, Summer Camp Director
Chrissie Endler, Executive Director
Kevin Shannon, MD, President & Medical Director
Kristina Wallace, Director, Development & Operations

Camp del Corazon, is a nonprofit corporation offering a no cost summer camp and other programs to children aged 7-17 living with heart disease. Campers or their guardians must fill out a camp application, with acceptance into the camp dependant upon a nurse review of the parent and cardiology portions of the application.

1030 **Camp-A-Lot and Camp-A-Little**
The Arc of San Diego
3030 Market Street
San Diego, CA 92102
619-685-1175
Fax: 619-234-3759
info@arc-sd.com
www.arc-sd.com

Anthony J. DeSalis, Esq., President & CEO

Programs of The Arc of San Diego, Camp - A - Lot (ages 18 and up) and Camp - A - Little (ages 5-17) offer recreational summer camp opportunities for individuals with physical and developmental disabilities.

1031 **Coelho Epilepsy Youth Summer Camp**
Epilepsy Foundation Of Northern California
1736 Franklin Street
Suite 450
Oakland, CA 94612
510-922-8687
800-632-3532
Fax: 510-922-8659
camp@epilepsynorcal.org
www.epilepsynorcal.org

Carlos Quesada, CEO
Miriam Swanson, Events & Programs Coordinator
Kimberly Bari, Programs Ambassador

Offered to children aged 9-17, Coelho Epilepsy Youth Summer Camp provides a week long sleepaway camp for children with epilepsy. Staffed by medical professional throughout the entire week, campers participate in traditional camp activities. Parents or guardians must fill out an application for a camper and the fee per camper is $150.00.

1032 **Dream Street**
Dream Street Foundation
324 S. Beverly Dr.
Suite 500
Beverly Hills, CA 90212
424-333-1371
Fax: 310-388-0302
www.dreamstreetfoundation.org

Patty Grubman, Founder

Run by The Dream Street Foundation, Dream Street Camps provide camping programs for children (aged 4-14) and young adults (18-24) with chronic and life threatening illnesses. The kids program runs in California, with the young adults program running in Arizona. The programs are free of charge, and campers can participate in different activities such as, swimming, arts and crafts, sports, horseback riding, and archery.

1033 **Easterseals Camp**
Easterseals Southern California
401 S Ivy St.
Escondido, CA 92025
951-264-4855
amanda.showalter@essc.org
www.easterseals.com/southerncal

Mark Whitley, President & CEO
Amanda Showalter, Camp Director

Easterseals Camp is a week long summer camp for children and adults with disabilities. Held at Camp Oakes in the San Bernardino Mountains. Campers participate in activities including, crafts, hayrides, talent shows, dances, swimming, canoeing, archery, hiking, and rope courses. There is a 1:2 counselor to camper ratio. The cost of the camp is $775.00 per camper.

1034 **Easterseals Camp Harmon**
16403 Highway 9
Boulder Creek, CA 95006
831-338-3383
campharmon@es-cc.org
www.campharmon.org

Anna Chambers, Camp Director
Jerardo Pena, Facilities Maintenance Manager

Camp Harmon, the Easterseals Central California camp, offers residential summer camps programs to individuals ages 8-65 with disabilities. Each session at Camp Harmon is designed for a specific age group and offers campers the opportunity to experience traditional summer camp activities. There is a 3:1 counsellor to camper ratio, with camp fees are based on $140.00 a day base.

1035 **Enchanted Hills Camp for the Blind**
Lighthouse for the Blind
1155 Market St.
10th Floor
San Francisco, CA 94103
415-431-1481
afletcher@lighthouse-sf.org
www.lighthouse-sf.org

Tony Fletcher, Director, Enchanted Hills Camp and Retreat
Bryan Bashin, CEO

Enchanted Hills Camp for the Blind is located on 311 acres of land on Mt. Veeder, offering programs for children, teens, adults, deaf-blind, seniors, and families of the blind. The camp gives campers the experience of traditional summer camp but is adapted to meet the needs of the campers.

1036 **Firefighters Kids Camp**
Firefighters Burn Institute
3101 Stockton Blvd.
Sacramento, CA 95820
916-739-8525
info@ffburn.org
www.ffburn.org

Valorie Smart, Camp Contact
Joe Pick, Executive Director
Rachel Crowell, Assistant Director

Firefighters Kids Camp is a program run by the Firefighters Burn Institute for children ages 6-17, who are survivors of burns. With activities such as rocking climbing, bicycling, hiking, kayaking, swimming, and arts and crafts, the ratio of staff to campers is 3:1, with on site 24/7 nurse and physical therapist ensuring a safe and fun environment.

1037 **Lions Wilderness Camp for Deaf Children, Inc.**
Lions Wilderness Camp Headquarters
PO Box 8
Roseville, CA 95661-9998
campdirector@lionswildcamp.org
www.lionswildcamp.org

David Velasquez, Camp Program Director

Lions Wilderness Camp gives deaf children aged 7-15 an outdoor camp experience helping children to learn outdoor skills and enjoy nature.

1038 **Little Heroes Preschool Burn Camp**
Firefighters Burn Institute
3101 Stockton Blvd.
Sacramento, CA 95820
916-739-8525
www.ffburn.org

Valorie Smart, Camp Contact
Joe Pick, Executive Director
Rachel Crowell, Assistant Director

Little Heroes Preschool Burn Camp is a burn recovery program run by the Firefighters Burn Institute. The camp is for children ages 3-6, who are survivors of burns, and their families. The program runs for 3 days, providing support and education for those attending.

1039 **New Horizons Summer Day Camp**
YMCA of Orange County
13821 Newport Ave.
Suite 150
Tustin, CA 92780
714-508-7635
newhorizons@ymcaoc.org
www.ymcaoc.org/new-horizons

1040 **Quest Camp**
907 San Ramon Valley Blvd.
Suite 202
Danville, CA 94526
925-743-2900
800-313-9733
Fax: 925-820-9761
www.questcamps.com
Robert B. Field, PhD., Founder & Executive Director
Debra Forrester-Field, MA, Administrative Director
Aprilyn Artz, MA, Clinical Director
Jodie Knott, Ph.D., Director
Quest Camps are designed using the Quest Camp Therapeutic System developed specifically to help and reduce a campers psychological disability. With locations in San Francisco East Bay, California, Huntington Beach, California, and Pittsburgh, Pennsylvania, camps have a 6:1 camper to staff ratio, with campers receiving sport instruction and participate in physical activity, arts, and games.

1041 **Special Camp For Special Kids**
31641 La Novia Ave
San Juan Capistrano, CA 92675
949-661-0108
Fax: 949-661-8637
lindsay.eres@smes.org
www.specialcamp.org
Lindsay Eres, Executive Director
Stefani Baker, Camp Operations Director
For youths with disabilities, Special Camps for Special Kids, offers day camps with a 1:1 volunteer counselor to camper.

1042 **The Painted Turtle**
1300 4th Street
Suite 300
Santa Monica, CA 90401
310-451-1353
866-451-5367
Fax: 310-451-1357
info@thepaintedturtle.org
www.thepaintedturtle.org
Chris Butler, Chief Executive Officer
Alexis Madrid, Director, Development
Allen McBroom, Chief Operating Officer
April Tani, Director, Camp Programs & Initiatives
The Painted Turtle provides year round camp programs for children, siblings, and families with children who have chronic and life threatening illnesses. The camp is located in Lake Hughes, California.

Colorado

1043 **Adam's Camp**
6767 South Spruce St.
Suite 102
Centennial, CO 80112
303-563-8290
Contact@AdamsCamp.org
www.adamscampcolorado.org
Lindsay Radford, Executive Director
Lesley Pollard, Director, Communications & Events
Kim Kelleher, Therapy Camp Manager
Rob McIntire, Finance Director
Adam's Camp is a nonprofit organization, with multiple locations across the United States, providing therapeutic programs and recreational camps for children, and the families of children with special needs and developmental delays. There is also a location in Northern Ireland.

1044 **Adam's Camp: Colorado**
Adam's Camp
6767 South Spruce St.
Suite 102
Centennial, CO 80112
303-563-8290
Fax: 303-563-8291
Contact@AdamsCamp.org
www.adamscampcolorado.org
Jordan Ficke, Program Driector, Young Adults & Adventure Camp
Karel Horney, Founder
Anne Fiala, Volunteer & Operations Manager
Rob McIntire, Interim Executive Director & Finance Director
Adam's Camp is a nonprofit organization providing therapeutic programs and recreational camps for children and the families of children with special needs. The Colorado location of Adam's Camp, offers both therapy and adventure camps. The adventure camp is held at the YMCA - Snow Mountain Ranch in Granby, Colorado.

1045 **Aspen Camp**
4862 Snowmass Creek Rd.
Snowmass, CO 81654
970-315-0513
TTY: 970-315-0513
hi@aspencamp.org
www.aspencamp.org
Ryan Commerson, President
Karen Immerson, Vice President
Eric Kaika, Treasurer
Open to the deaf community, including family members and friends as well as those who are deaf, deaf blind, hard of hearing, and late deafened, Camp Aspen provides year round programs for youth and adults.

1046 **Breckenridge Outdoor Education Center**
PO Box 697
Breckenridge, CO 80424
970-453-6422
800-383-2632
Fax: 970-453-4676
boec@boec.org
www.boec.org
Sonya Norris, Executive Director
Karen Skruch, Finance Director
Jeff Inouye, Ski Program Director
Jaime Overmyer, Wilderness Program Director
Breckenridge Outdoor Education Center (BOEC) provides year round educational outdoor experiences to individuals with physical and intellectual disabilities. Some programs BOEC offer include, Adaptive Ski and Ride School, Wilderness Programs and adaptive programs for individuals with brain injuries, multiple sclerosis, and Parkinson's Disease.

1047 **Camp Rocky Mountain Village**
Easterseals Colorado
2644 Alvarado Rd.
PO Box 115
Empire, CO 80438
303-569-2333
Fax: 303-569-3857
campinfo@easterseals colorado.org
www.easterseals.com/co
Roman Krafczyk, President & CEO
Tony Garcia, Camp Director
A program of Easterseals Colorado, Rocky Mountain Village in Empire Colorado is a fully accessible camp, with summer camps sessions for children and adults with disabilities. Activities include but are not limited to swimming, fishing, overnight camping, outdoor cooking, arts and crafts, and a zip line.

1048 **Camp Wapiyapi**
191 University Blvd.
PO Box 294
Denver, CO 80206
303-534-0883
Fax: 303-534-0874
Wapiyapi@wapiyapi.org
www.campwapiyapi.org
Darla Dakin, Chief Executive Officer
Rhonda Sheya, Director, Marketing & Development
Megan Blanc, Summer Camp Director
Camp Wapiyapi is a nonprofit organization that fosters friendships, fun and healing outside of the hospital for families facing childhood cancer through a camp experience. For patients ages 6-17. Full-time onsite volunteer medical staff available 24/7.

1049 **Challenge Aspen**
PO Box 6639
Snowmass Village, CO 81615
970-923-0578
Fax: 970-923-7338
info@challengeaspen.org
www.challengeaspen.org
Jeff Hauser, Chief Executive Officer
Anne Adams, Chief Operating Officer
Jenni Petersen, Chief Financial Officer
Challenge Aspen provides recreational, cultural experiences and summer camps for individuals who have cognitive or physical

challenges. Programs are tailored to fit a diversity of needs and interests.

1050 **Champ Camp**
American Lung Association
CO 80481
303-847-0279
www.lung.org/
Bob Doyle, Director
Run by the American Lung Association, Champ Camp is an educational and recreational camp for children ages 7-14 with asthma. Children are able to participate in activities such as canoeing, hiking, and rock climbing. Volunteers and medical staff are on site 24/7 ensuring a safe environment for campers.

1051 **Children's Hospital Burn Camps Program**
13123 E 16th Ave.
PO Box 580
Aurora, CO 80045
720-777-8295
Fax: 720-777-7270
trudy.boulter@childrenscolorado.org
www.noordinarycamps.org
Trudy Boulter, OTH CHT, Program Director
Tim Schuetz, Outreach Coordinator
The Children's Hospital Colorado Burn Camps Program provides rehabilitation and reintegration opportunities for children, teens, adults, and families who have been affected by burn injuries. The Camps Program has partnerships with 7 hospitals across the United States and offers year round programs.

1052 **Children's Hospital Burn Camps Program: England Exchange Program Burn Camp**
13123 E 16th Ave.
PO Box 580
Aurora, CO 80045
720-777-8295
Fax: 720-777-7270
trudy.boulter@childrenscolorado.org
www.noordinarycamps.org
Trudy Boulter, OTH CHT, Program Director
Tim Schuetz, Outreach Coordinator
An international exchange program for campers ages, 13-15, between the Children's Hospital Burn Camps Program and The Manchester Children's Hospital Burns Camp in England. Campers are able to explore a new culture, food, and climate. The camp is located in the Lake District.

1053 **Children's Hospital Burn Camps Program: Family Burn Camp**
13123 E 16th Ave.
PO Box 580
Aurora, CO 80045
720-777-8295
Fax: 720-777-7270
trudy.boulter@childrenscolorado.org
www.noordinarycamps.org
Trudy Boulter, OTH CHT, Program Director
Tim Schuetz, Outreach Coordinator
The Family Burn Camp is for families who have been affected by a burn injury. The camp is designed to give families the opportunity to interact and connect with other families who have had a similar experiences.

1054 **Children's Hospital Burn Camps Program: Summer Burn Camp**
13123 E 16th Ave.
PO Box 580
Aurora, CO 80045
720-777-8295
Fax: 720-777-7270
trudy.boulter@childrenscolorado.org
www.noordinarycamps.org
Trudy Boulter, OTH CHT, Program Director
Tim Schuetz, Outreach Coordinator
The Summer Burn Camp is part of the Children's Hospital Colorado Burn Camps Program, and offers a weeklong summer camp for children and teens, ages 8-18 who have been affected by burn injuries. The camp is held in Estes Park in partnership with Cheley Colorado Camps, and activities include, hiking, mountain biking, challenge courses, horseback riding, mountain climbing, fishing, archery, crafts, riflery, and swimming.

1055 **Children's Hospital Burn Camps Program: Winter Burn Camp**
13123 E 16th Ave.
PO Box 580
Aurora, CO 80045
720-777-8295
Fax: 720-777-7270
trudy.boulter@childrenscolorado.org
www.noordinarycamps.org
Trudy Boulter, OTH CHT, Program Director
Tim Schuetz, Outreach Coordinator
The Winter Burn Camp is for older campers, ages 13-18, who have previously attended the Cheley Children's Hospital Colorado Summer Burn Camp. Held in Steamboat Springs, Colorado at the Steamboat Grand Lodge campers participate in a week of skiing and/or snowboarding.

1056 **Children's Hospital Burn Camps Program: Young Adult Retreat**
13123 E 16th Ave.
PO Box 580
Aurora, CO 80045
720-777-8295
Fax: 720-777-7270
trudy.boulter@childrenscolorado.org
www.noordinarycamps.org
Trudy Boulter, OTH CHT, Program Director
Tim Schuetz, Outreach Coordinator
A program of the Children's Hospital Colorado Burn Camps Program, the Young Adult Retreat is designed to address the specific issues facing burn survivors ages 18-25. The retreat offers a variety of recreational and workshop opportunities working to address the topics of relationships, body image, and goal setting.

1057 **City of Lakewood Recreation and Inclusion Services for Everyone (R.I.S.E.)**
City Of Lakewood
480 S Allison Pkwy
Lakewood, CO 80226
303-987-4867
TTY: 303-987-7057
rise@lakewood.org
www.lakewood.org/rise
Mark Snow, Program Coordinator
The Recreation and Inclusion Services for Everyone (R.I.S.E.) of Lakewood is a therapeutic recreation program for individuals with disabilities, age 6 through senior adult. Some programs offered by R.I.S.E include field trips, social dances, sports and camping.

1058 **Cochlear Implant Camp**
Listen Foundation
6950 E Belleview Ave.
Suite 203
Greenwood Village, CO 80111
303-781-9440
cochlearimplantcamp@gmail.com
www.listenfoundation.org/cicamp
Allison Biever, President
David Kelsall, MD, Medical Director
Held at the YMCA Rockies Estes Park Center, the camp offers a wide range of activities for children from 3-17 years old with cochlear implants. The camp is 4 days and 3 nights, held during the summer and also offers programs for parents and families. The cost is $700 for a family of four.

1059 **Colorado Lions Camp**
28541 Hwy 67 N
PO Box 9043
Woodland Park, CO 80863
719-687-2087
Fax: 719-687-7435
coloradolionscamp@msn.com
www.coloradolionscamp.org
Erin Newport, Camp Director
Michelle Werner, Executive Assistant
Colorado Lions Camp offers summer camp and weekend respite programs for individuals aged 8 and up with special needs. The camp is designed to promote independence and provide an opportunity for campers to discover their potential in a safe environment.

1060 **First Descents**
3001 Brighton Blvd.
Suite 623
Denver, CO 80216
303-945-2490
Fax: 866-592-6911
info@firstdescents.org
www.firstdescents.org

Brad Ludden, Founder
Ryan O'Donoghue, Executive Director
Mackenzie McGrath, Director, Programs
Ray Shedd, Director, Advancement

First Descents offers free outdoor adventure programs for young adults ages 18-39 who have, or who have had cancer. Activities include climbing, paddling and surfing, all offered in a safe environment.

1061 **Roundup River Ranch**
8333 Colorado River Rd.
Gypsum, CO 81637
970-524-2267
Fax: 877-619-0323
info@roundupriverranch.org
www.roundupriverranch.org

Ruth B. Johnson, JD, President & CEO
Sterling Nell Leija, Executive Camp Director
Kendra Perkins, Assustabt Camp Director
Christopher Troxel, Program Coordinator

Roundup River Ranch provides traditional camp experiences for children and their families with chronic and serious illnesses. The Ranch is located in Gypsum, Colorado, with all programs offered free of charge.

Connecticut

1062 **Arthur C. Luf Children's Burn Camp**
Connecticut Burns Care Foundation
601 Boston Post Rd.
Milford, CT 06460
203-878-6744
Fax: 203-878-4044
cbcf@ctburnsfoundation.org
www.ctburnsfoundation.org

Armand J. Cantafio, President
Kathlene Gerrity, Executive Director

The Arthur C. Luf Children's Burn Camp provides a free of charge camp experience for children and teens, ages 8-18, who have survived life altering burn injuries. Camp activities include hiking, fishing, archery, boating, ropes course, and campfires. The volunteer staff is composed of retired firefighters, medical personnel, and burn survivors.

1063 **Camp Discovery**
American Academy of Dermatology
PO Box 1968
Des Plaines, IL 60017
847-240-1280
866-503-7546
888-462-3376
Fax: 847-240-1859
www.campdiscovery.org

1064 **Camp Harkness**
The Arc Eastern Connecticut
125 Sachem St.
Norwich, CT 06360
860-889-4435
Fax: 860-889-4662
info@thearcect.org
thearcect.org/camp-harkness

Kathleen Stauffer, Chief Executive Officer

A week-long summer camp program for individuals with intellectual and developmental disabilities. The camp is held at Camp Harkness in Waterford, CT.

1065 **Camp Horizons**
127 Babcock Hill Rd.
PO Box 323
South Windham, CT 06266
860-456-1032
Fax: 860-456-4721
www.horizonsct.org

Adam Milne, Chair
Chris McNaboe, President & CEO
Kathleen McNaboe, Vice President
L. Sanford Rice, Treasurer

Camp Horizons offers summer camp and weekend camps for children and adults with developmental disabilities.

1066 **Camp Isola Bella**
410 Twin Lakes Rd.
Salisbury, CT 06079
860-824-5558
Fax: 860-824-4276
TTY: 860-596-0110
ibdirector@asd-1817.org
asd-1817.org/programs/camp-isola-bella

David Guardino, Director

Owned and operated by the American School for the Deaf, Camp Isola Bella provides summer camp opportunities for children who are deaf or hard of hearing. Staff is able to communicate with the campers regardless of the mode of communication, including sign language, oral, aural, lipreading or a mix, and activities include, but are not limited to, swimming, ropes course, canoeing, water skiing, archery, hiking, sports, and sailing.

1067 **Camp No Limits Connecticut**
No Limits Foundation
Quinnipiac University
305 Sherman Avenue
Hamden, CT 06518
207-569-6411
campnolimits@gmail.com
www.nolimitsfoundation.org

Mary Leighton, Founder & Executive Director
Kelsey Moody, Program Operations Manager
Alix Sandler, Marketing & Development Director
Cheryl Foss, Director, Human Resources

Camp No Limits Connecticut, a location of Camp No Limits, is a recreational and educational camp for youth who have experienced limb loss. Camp No Limits, is a program of the nonprofit organization No Limits Foundation. The Connecticut camp is hosted at Quinnipiac's York Hill campus and provides campers the opportunity to participate in a variety of different sports, including ice and sled hockey.

1068 **Easterseals Camp Hemlocks**
Easterseals Oak Hill
120 Holcomb St.
Hartford, CT 06112
860-286-3108
jillian.mccarthy@oakhillct.org
www.easterseals.com/oakhill

Barry M. Simon, President & CEO
Jillian McCarthy, Camp Director

A summer camp program of Easterseals Oak Hill, Camp Hemlocks is a completely accessible camp for youth and adults with physical, sensory, intellectual, and developmental disabilities. Activities include swimming, boating, fishing, arts and crafts, and climbing tower.

1069 **SeriousFun Children's Network**
SeriousFun Support Center Office
230 East Ave.
Suite 107
Norwalk, CT 06855
203-562-1203
Fax: 203-341-8707
info@seriousfunnetwork.org
www.seriousfun.org

Blake Maher, Chief Executive Officer
Justin Fusaro, Chief Financial Officer
Tara Fisher, Chief Marketing Officer

The SeriousFun Children's Network is an international organization of camps and programs for children and the families of children with serious illnesses. The Network has 30 camps and programs worldwide.

1070 **The Hole in the Wall Gang Camp**
565 Ashford Center Rd.
Ashford, CT 06278
860-429-3444
info@holeinthewallgang.org
www.holeinthewallgang.org
James H. Canton, Chief Executive Officer
Padraig Barry, Chief Strategy Officer
Kevin Magee, Chief Financial Officer
Hilary Axtmayer, Chief Program Officer
The Hole in the Wall Gang Camp offers summer and weekend camp experiences for children and the siblings of children with serious illnesses. Located in Ashford, Connecticut, campers are able to participate in traditional camp activities in a medically safe environment.

1071 **The Rainbow Club**
The Barton Center for Diabetes Education, Inc.
30 Ennis Rd.
PO Box 356
North Oxford, MA 01537-0356
508-987-2056
Fax: 508-987-2002
info@bartoncenter.org
www.bartoncenter.org
Lynn Butler-Dinunno, Executive Director
Jenna Dufresne, Director, Health Services
Sarah Balko, Director, Camps & Programs
Sadie Vivenzio, Director, Finance
A program of The Barton Center for Diabetes Education, The Rainbow Club is a day camp held in Greenwich, Connecticut for children and teens, ages 5-15 with diabetes. Campers receive diabetes education and participate in games, crafts, and water activities. An adult program designed for parents runs in conjunction with the day camp session.

Delaware

1072 **Camp Manito & Camp Lenape**
United Cerebral Palsy Of Delaware
700A River Rd.
Wilmington, DE 19809
302-764-2400
Fax: 302-764-8713
TTY: 302-764-8708
ucpde@ucpde.org
www.ucpde.org/summer-camps
Moni Edgar, Executive Director
Kim Evans, Director, Camp Program
Camp Manito, located in New Castle County and Camp Lenape, serving Kent and Sussex Counties, are summer camps run by United Cerebral Palsy of Delaware for children and young adults, ages 3-21, with orthopedic disabilities. Both campsites are accessible and activities include swimming, arts and crafts, music, sports, computer education, and outings.

1073 **Children's Beach House**
100 W 10 St.
Suite 411
Wilmington, DE 19801-1674
302-655-4288
Fax: 302-655-4216
www.cbhinc.org
Richard T. Garrett, Executive Director
Patrice Tosi, Vice President, Advancement
Children's Beach House (CBH) is a nonprofit organization providing support and education for children with special needs. CBH offers summer and weekend programs at the Lewes facility on Delaware Bay. Activities are modified for each camper and include, but are not limited to, swimming, sailing, kayaking, arts and crafts, sports, and campfires.

District of Columbia

1074 **Camp Lighthouse**
Columbia Lighthouse for the Blind
1825 K St. NW
Suite 1103
Washington, DC 20006
202-454-6400
Fax: 202-955-6401
info@clb.org
www.clb.org
Tony Cancelosi, President & CEO
Jocelyn Hunter, Senior Director, Communications
Toya Horten, Director, Administrative Operations
Bethany Martin, Manager, Youth & Education Services
Camp Lighthouse is a one week day camp program run by Columbia Lighthouse for the Blind. The camp is for children ages 6-12 with visual impairments.

1075 **Paddy Rossbach Youth Camp**
Amputee Coalition
601 Pennsylvania Ave. NW
Suite 600, South Bldg.
Washington, DC 20004
888-267-5669
www.amputee-coalition.org
Mary Richards, President & CEO
A 6-day camp for youths ages 10-17 who have limb loss or limb difference. Activities include sports, swimming, fishing, arts and crafts. Also offers a Leadership Camp for 18- and 19-year-olds transitioning from high school to college and careers.

Florida

1076 **Camp Amigo**
Children's Burn Camp Of North Florida, Inc.
PO Box 368
Tallahassee, FL 32302
850-509-6200
www.campamigo.com
Rusty Roberts, President
Camp Amigo provides a one week summer camp experience for children ages 6-18 who live in Florida and have survived a burn injury.

1077 **Camp Boggy Creek**
30500 Brantley Branch Rd.
Eustis, FL 32736
352-483-4200
866-462-6449
Fax: 352-483-0589
info@campboggycreek.org
www.boggycreek.org
June Clark, President & CEO
Lisa Hicks, Chief Development Officer
David Mann, Camp Director
Kirstin Cauraugh Youmans, Assistant Camp Director
Part of the SeriousFun Children's Network, Camp Boggy Creek provides year round camping opportunities for children with serious illnesses throughout Florida. The camp has week-long summer camp sessions and retreat weekends.

1078 **Camp No Limits Florida**
No Limits Foundation
Clearwater, FL
207-569-6411
campnolimits@gmail.com
www.nolimitsfoundation.org
Mary Leighton, Founder & Executive Director
Kelsey Moody, Program Operations Manager
Alix Sandler, Marketing & Development Director
Cheryl Foss, Director, Human Resources
Camp No Limits Florida, a location of Camp No Limits, is a recreational and educational camp for youth who have experienced limb loss. Camp No Limits is a program of the nonprofit organization No Limits Foundation. The Florida camp is hosted at the Clearwater Marine Aquarium in Clearwater, Florida.

1079 **Camp Thunderbird**
Quest, Inc.
PO Box 531125
Orlando, FL 32853
407-218-4300
888-807-8378
Fax: 407-218-4301
contact@questinc.org
www.questinc.org/quests-camp-thunderbird
John Gill, President & CEO
Brooke Eakins, Chief Operating Officer
Todd Thrasher, Chief Financial Officer
John Dogaer, Chief Information Officer
A program of Quest, Inc. Camp Thunderbird provides recreational programs for children and adults with developmental disabilities. The camp has six-day overnight sessions with age specific programming. Activities include sports, games, arts and performance, and nature studies.

1080 **Center Academy at Pinellas Park**
6710 86th Ave. N
Pinellas Park, FL 33782
727-541-5716
Fax: 727-544-8186
infopp@centeracademy.com
www.centeracademy.com
Mack R. Hicks, Founder & Chair
Andrew P. Hicks, Chief Executive Officer & Clinical Director
Eric V. Larson, President & Chief Operating Officer
Susan K. Hicks, Vice President
Specifically designed for the learning disabled child and other children with difficulties in concentration, strategy, social skills, impulsivity, distractibility and study strategies. Programs offered include attention training, visual-motor remediation, socialization skills training, relaxation training, and more.

1081 **Dr. Moises Simpser VACC Camp**
Nicklaus Children's Hospital
3200 SW 62nd Ave.
Suite 203
Miami, FL 33155-4076
305-662-8222
Fax: 786-268-1765
bela.florentin@mch.com
www.vacccamp.com
Bela Florentin, Camp Coordinator
Tania Diaz, Camp Clinical Coordinator
VACC Camp is a week-long overnight camp program for ventilation-assisted children and their families. The program includes sailing, swimming, field trips to local attractions, campsite entertainment, structured games, free play, and more. Parents have formal and informal opportunities to network among themselves.

1082 **Dream Oaks Camp**
Foundation For Dreams, Inc.
16110 Dream Oaks Pl.
Bradenton, FL 34212
941-746-5659
www.foundationfordreams.org
Elena Cassella, Executive Director
AnnaMaria Carleton, Director, Children Services
Lauralie Benge, Office Manager
Brynna Shepard, Camp Director
Dream Oaks Camp offers weekend, summer day, summer residential, and specialty camps for children ages 7-17 with special needs and chronic illnesses. The camp is a program of the Foundation for Dreams with a 3:1 staff to camper ratio. Activities include horseback riding, nature programs, sports, games, swimming, talent shows, and arts and crafts.

1083 **Easterseals Camp Challenge**
Easterseals Florida
31600 Camp Challenge Rd.
Sorrento, FL 32776
352-383-4711
camp@fl.easterseals.com
www.easterseals.com/florida
Susan Ventura, President & CEO
Maggie Denk, Camp Director
Located in Sorrento, Florida, Easterseals Camp Challenge provides camp opportunities for children and adults with cognitive and physical disabilities.

1084 **Florida Diabetes Camp**
Florida Camp for Children & Youth with Diabetes
PO Box 14136
Gainesville, FL 32604-2136
352-334-1321
Fax: 352-334-1326
fccydd@floridadiabetescamp.org
www.floridadiabetescamp.org
Gary Cornwell, Executive Director
Chris Stakely, Assistant Director
Janet Silverstein, Medical Director
The Florida Diabetes Camp offers weekend and summer camps for children with type 1 diabetes. The camp combines traditional camp activities and diabetes related educational sessions for campers in order to provide a fun and safe environment.

1085 **Hand Camp**
Hands to Love
3450 Hull Rd., Suite 3341
PO Box 140572
Gainesville, FL 32614-0572
352-273-7382
Fax: 352-273-7388
info@handstolove.org
www.handstolove.org
John Hosman, President
Sean Branch, Vice President
Brian Caslow, Treasurer
Beth Keene, Secretary
A program of Hands to Love, an organization for children and the families of children with upper limb differences, Hand Camp is an annual event held in Starke, Florida at Camp Crystal Lake. Hand Camp offers camp activities, networking and support groups, and special guests.

1086 **Kris' Camp**
Kris' Camp/Therapy Intensive Programs, Inc.
1132 Green Hill Trace
Tallahassee, FL 32317
850-445-4821
kberger62@gmail.com
www.kriscamp.org
Kathy Berger, Director
Kris' Camp provides programs for children with autism and special needs. The camp offers therapy programs led by art, education, music, occupational, physical, and speech therapists.

1087 **Sertoma Camp Endeavor**
1300 Camp Endeavor Blvd.
Dundee, FL 33838
352-422-3435
campendeavorceo@gmail.com
www.campendeavorfl.org
Maureen Tambasco, Camp CEO
Scott Botelho, Camp Assistant Director
Sertoma Camp Endeavor provides camp programs for deaf and hard of hearing youth. Programs are designed to promote social and personal growth, environmental awareness, and independence.

Georgia

1088 **Aerie Experiences**
GA
404-285-0467
mdweneta@aerieexperiences.com
aerieexperiences.com
Matthew Weneta, Owner & Director
Located north of Atlanta, Georgia with summer camp expeditions taking place in Georgia, North Carolina, and Tennessee, Aerie Experiences provides programs for children, families and individuals with special needs. Aerie Experiences is focused on those affected by Aspergers, High Functioning Autism, Learning Disabilities, ADHD, and Neurobiological Disorders.

1089 **Camp Breathe Easy**
American Lung Association
2452 Spring Rd. SE
Smyrna, GA 30080

1090 **Camp Caglewood**
Caglewood, Inc.
5182 Glen Forrest Dr.
Flowery Branch, GA 30542
info@caglewood.org
www.caglewood.org

Paul Freeman, Co-Founder
Jessica Freeman, Co-Founder

A special needs camping program, Camp Caglewood provides active weekend programs for children and adults with developmental disabilities.

1091 **Camp Dream**
Camp Dream Foundation
4355 Cobb Pkwy.
Suite J117
Atlanta, GA 30339
678-367-0040
info@campdreamga.org
www.campdreamga.org

Gary Marshall, Executive Director
Hunter Steng, Operations Director
Amy Blankenship, Medical Director

Camp Dream provides recreational camp programs, Summer Camp and Camp Out, for children and young adults with physical and developmental disabilities.

1092 **Camp Firefly**
The Firefly Foundation
5737 Kanan Rd.
Suite 180
Agoura Hills, CA 91301
campfirefly89@gmail.com
www.campfirefly.com

1093 **Camp Hawkins**
GA Baptist Children's Homes & Family Ministries
800 Rudeseal Rd.
Mount Airy, GA 30563
770-463-3800
georgiachildren.org/camp-hawkins

Kenneth Z. Thompson, President & CEO

Camp Hawkins is a residential summer camp for youth ages 8-21 with developmental disabilities, learning disorders, traumatic brain injury or other special needs. Activities include swimming, canoeing, arts and crafts, games, and Bible study. The camp has locations in Baxley, GA and Mt. Airy, GA.

1094 **Camp Independence**
Camp Twin Lakes
1391 Keencheefoonee Rd.
Rutledge, GA 30663
404-785-0631
campindependence@choa.org
www.choa.org/camps/camp-independence

Donna Hyland, President & CEO, Children's Healthcare of Atlanta

Camp Independence is an overnight, week-long summer camp for children and teens ages 8-18 who have kidney disease, are on dialysis, or have received an organ transplant.

1095 **Camp Juliena**
Georgia Center of the Deaf and Hard of Hearing
2296 Henderson Mill Rd.
Suite 115
Atlanta, GA 30345
404-381-8447
888-297-9461
Fax: 404-297-9465
info@gcdhh.org
www.gcdhh.org/camp-juliena

Jimmy Peterson, Executive Director
Andrea Alston, Coordinator, Community Outreach

A week-long residential summer camp for deaf or hard of hearing youth. Activities help campers develop leadership, team-building, social, and communication skills.

1096 **Camp Kudzu**
Camp Kudzu, Inc.
5885 Glenridge Dr.
Suite 160
Atlanta, GA 30328
833-995-8398
info@campkudzu.org
www.campkudzu.org

Robert G. Shaw, Executive Director
Danielle Holmes, Senior Development Coordinator
Carrie Claiborne, Medical Coordinator
Mandy Conroy, Camp Community Coordinator

Camp Kudzu is a nonprofit organization, offering overnight summer camp, day camp, family camps, and teen programs for individuals and the families of individuals with type 1 diabetes. Programs are held at various locations across Georgia and provide campers with traditional camp experiences and diabetes education.

1097 **Camp Sunshine**
1850 Clairmont Rd.
Decatur, GA 30033
404-325-7979
866-786-2267
Fax: 404-325-7929
info@mycampsunshine.com
www.mycampsunshine.com

Sally Hale, Executive Director
Tenise Newberg, Program Director
Ann Baker, Program Director
Edith Tomasetti, Program Director

Camp Sunshine provides recreational, educational, support, and camp programs for children with cancer and their families.

1098 **Camp Twin Lakes**
1100 Spring St.
Suite 406
Atlanta, GA 30309
404-231-9887
Fax: 404-577-8854
camps@camptwinlakes.org
www.camptwinlakes.org

Jill Morrisey, Chief Executive Officer
Daniel C. Mathews, Chief Operations Officer
Cheryl Belair, Chief Development Officer
Josh Sweat, Chief Program Officer

Camp Twin Lakes provides fully accessible, year round camp programs for children with serious illnesses, disabilities, and other life challenges. Camp Twin Lakes has locations in Rutledge and Winder, Georgia.

1099 **Camp Twin Lakes: Rutledge**
1391 Keencheefoonee Rd.
Rutledge, GA 30663
706-557-9070
Fax: 706-557-9147
camps@camptwinlakes.org
www.camptwinlakes.org

Jill Morrisey, Chief Executive Officer
Daniel C. Mathews, Chief Operations Officer
Cheryl Belair, Chief Development Officer
Josh Sweat, Chief Program Officer

A location of Camp Twin Lakes, which offers camp programs for children with serious illnesses, disabilities, and other life challenges. The Rutledge campus is fully accessible and includes a pool, ropes course, farm, and paddleboat activities.

1100 **Camp Twin Lakes: Will-A-Way**
210 S Broad St.
Unit 5
Winder, GA 30680
770-867-6123
Fax: 770-867-6130
camps@camptwinlakes.org
www.camptwinlakes.org

Jill Morrisey, Chief Executive Officer
Daniel C. Mathews, Chief Operations Officer
Cheryl Belair, Chief Development Officer
Josh Sweat, Chief Program Officer

A location of Camp Twin Lakes, which offers camp programs for children with serious illnesses, disabilities, and other life challenges. The Will-A-Way campus is fully accessible and includes a gymnasium, ropes course, zip line, rock wall, outdoor ampitheater, beachfront, and equestrian program.

1101 **Squirrel Hollow Summer Camp**
The Bedford School
5665 Milam Rd.
Fairburn, GA 30213
770-774-8001
Fax: 770-774-8005
info@thebedfordschool.org
www.thebedfordschool.org

Betsy Box, Admissions Director
Jeff James, Head of School
Allison Day, Associate Head of School

A program of The Bedford School, Squirrel Hollow Summer Camp offers summer sessions for students with academic needs due to a learning disability. Students receive academic instruction in reading, writing, and math through a variety of teaching techniques, with students grouped by age and skill level. The camp also incorporates recreational activities such as swimming, games, and a challenge course.

Hawaii

1102 **Camp Anuenue**
Honolulu, HI
808-349-7325
campanuenue@gmail.com
www.campanuenue.com

B.K. Cannon, President & Director
Alison James, Vice President & Director
Des Medeiros, Medical Director

Camp Anuenue is a nonprofit organization that offers a week long camping experience for children ages 7-18 who have or have had cancer. The camp is held at Camp Mokule'ia on the North Shore of Oahu and accepts children from Hawaii and US territories in the Pacific including Guam, Saipan, Samoa, and Marshall Islands.

1103 **Camp Taylor: Family Camp**
Camp Taylor, Inc.
Hilton Hawaiian Village
2005 Kalia Road
Honolulu, HI 96815
209-545-3853
camp@kidsheartcamp.org
www.kidsheartcamp.org/familycamphi

Kimberlie Gamino, Founder & Executive Director

A program of Camp Taylor, Family Camp is for children of all ages, with congenital heart disease and/or acquired heart disease, and their family including parents and siblings. The camp offers parental heart education and support programs for parents and siblings. The camp is held at the Hilton Hawaiian Village and is open to families from all of the Hawaiian Islands.

Idaho

1104 **Camp Hodia**
Idaho Diabetes Youth Programs, Inc.
5439 W Kendall St.
Boise, ID 83706
208-891-1023
info@hodia.org
www.hodia.org

Lisa Gier, Executive Director
Morgan Coenen, Director, Programs
Ciera Miller, Director, Marketing
Sherilyn Robison, Director, Activities

Camp Hodia offers a variety of educational camp programs for children and teens with type 1 diabetes.

1105 **Camp No Limits Idaho**
No Limits Foundation
Camp Cross Marine Rt.
Coeur d'Alene, ID 83814
207-569-6411
campnolimits@gmail.com
www.nolimitsfoundation.org

Mary Leighton, Founder & Executive Director
Kelsey Moody, Program Operations Manager
Alix Sandler, Marketing & Development Director
Cheryl Foss, Director, Human Resources

Camp No Limits Idaho, a location of Camp No Limits, is a recreational and educational camp for youth who have experienced limb loss. Camp No Limits, is a program of the nonprofit organization No Limits Foundation. The camp is held at Camp Cross on Lake Coeur d'Alene.

1106 **Camp Rainbow Gold**
216 W Jefferson St.
Boise, ID 83702
208-350-6435
info@camprainbowgold.org
www.camprainbowgold.org

Elizabeth Lizberg, Executive Director
Tracy Bryan, Program Director
Christl Holzl, Development Director
KC Covert, Marketing Manager

Camp Rainbow Gold is a independent, nonprofit organization providing year round camp programs, support groups, and scholarships for children, siblings, and the family of children who have been diagnosed with cancer. All camp programs are offered free of charge, with campers participating in activities such as fishing, hiking, campfires, and crafts. The camp is held in the Sawtooth National Forest.

1107 **Cristo Vive International: Idaho Camp**
139 McLean Lane
Kooskia, ID 83539
208-507-1241
www.cristovive.net

Carol McLean, Camp Coordinator

Christian camp with programming for individuals who are blind/deaf, physically or mentally challenged, have multiple disabilities, Down Syndrome, Autism/Asperger's, ADHD/ADD, Cerebral Palsy, and their families and siblings.

Illinois

1108 **ADA Camp GranADA**
American Diabetes Association
55 E Monroe St.
Suite 3420
Chicago, IL 60603
312-346-1805
illinoiscamps@diabetes.org
www.diabetes.org

1109 **ADA Teen Adventure Camp**
American Diabetes Association
55 E Monroe St.
Suite 3420
Chicago, IL 60603
312-346-1805
illinoiscamps@diabetes.org
www.diabetes.org

Paula Williams, Contact

Camping for teenagers with diabetes. Coed, ages 14 to 17. Camp dates are early in August. Located at the YMCA Camp Duncan in Ingleside, Illinois. Featured activities include archery, boating, roller skating, ropes course, and swimming.

1110 **ADA Triangle D Camp**
American Diabetes Association
55 E Monroe St.
Suite 3420
Chicago, IL 60603
312-346-1805
illinoiscamps@diabetes.org
www.diabetes.org

1111 **Camp "I Am Me"**
Illinois Fire Safety Alliance
426 W Northwest Hwy.
Mount Prospect, IL 60056
847-390-0911
Fax: 847-390-0920
ifsa@ifsa.org
www.ifsa.org/programs/camp

Philip Zaleski, Executive Director
Riley Anderson, Program Coordinator
Jenny Tzortzos, Community Outreach Coordinator

Camp I Am Me is a one-week summer camp for children and teens who have experienced burn injuries. The camp is held in Ingleside, Illinois at YMCA Camp Duncan. Activities include archery, games, canoes, kayaks, sailboats, campfires, fishing, ropes course, swimming, and specialized workshops related to burn injuries.

1112 **Camp Callahan**
Camp Callahan, Inc.
PO Box 5253
Quincy, IL 62305
217-883-0137
www.campcallahan.com

Peg Ratliff, Camp Director
Brandy Schlieper, Program Director

Camp Callahan is dedicated to providing a camp experience for youth with disabilities. The camp is held at Saukenauk Scout Reservation.

1113 **Camp Discovery**
American Academy of Dermatology
PO Box 1968
Des Plaines, IL 60017
847-240-1280
866-503-7546
888-462-3376
Fax: 847-240-1859
www.campdiscovery.org

1114 **Camp FRIENDship**
Easterseals Chicagoland & Greater Rockford
1939 W 13th St.
Suite 300
Chicago, IL 60608-1226
312-491-4110
www.easterseals.com/chicago

Sara Ray Stoelinga, President & CEO

A program of Easterseals, Camp FRIENDship is a summer camp program designed to help children ages 5-14 with autism, nonverbal learning disabilities, and intellectual disabilities. The camp promotes the acquiring of social skills in a safe and fun learning environment.

1115 **Camp Little Giant**
Touch of Nature Environmental Center
Southern Illinois University
Mail Code 6888
Carbondale, IL 62901
618-453-3950
Fax: 618-453-1188
jcave@siu.edu
www.ton.siu.edu

Jasmine Cave, Director

A program of the Southern Illinois University and held at the Touch of Nature Environmental Center, Camp Little Giant is a residential camp offering camping opportunities for people with physical, cognitive and developmental disabilities.

1116 **Camp New Hope**
PO Box 764
Mattoon, IL 61938
217-895-2341
Fax: 217-895-3658
officemanager@campnewhopeillinois.org
campnewhopeillinois.org

Paul Semple, Office Manager
Pat Crum, Site Coordinator

Camp New Hope is a year round recreational experience for individuals 8 and up with developmental and physical disabilities. The camp offers summer, weekend respite, and bowling programs. Camp New Hope is situated on 41 acres of land on Lake Mattoon.

1117 **Camp One Step**
Children's Oncology Services Inc.
213 W Institute Pl.
Suite 410
Chicago, IL 60610
312-924-4220
Fax: 312-878-7374
info@camponestep.org
www.camponestep.org

Jeff Infusino, President
Darryl Winston Perkins, Jr., Chief Programs Officer
Katie Weil, Vice President, Philanthropy
Susie Burke, Medical Director

Camp One Step provides 11 different year round camp programs for children and teens ages 7-19 who have been diagnosed with cancer. Camp One Step is open to children and families who live in Illinois, Wisconsin, and the Midwest.

1118 **Camp Quality Illinois**
PO Box 641
Lansing, IL 60438
708-895-8311
illinois@campqualityusa.org
www.campqualityusa.org/il

Mary Lockton, Executive Director
Dawn Winters, Treasurer
Stacy Reynolds, Program Coordinator

Camp Quality is an international camping program for children with cancer. The Illinois Camp Quality is held in Frankfort, Illinois at Camp Manitoqua & Retreat Center and offers children and their siblings summer camps and year round support programs. Volunteer doctors and nurses are at the camp 24 hours a day, and there is a 1:1 staff to camper ratio.

1119 **Camp Red Leaf**
26710 W Nippersink Rd.
Ingleside, IL 60041
847-740-5010
Fax: 847-740-5014
www.campredleaf.org

Ari Strulowitz, Executive Director
Angela McNeal, Camp Director
Tyesha Smith, Business Manager
Lawrence Connealy, Campus Director

Camp Red Leaf provides camp programs for individuals ages 9 and up with developmental disabilities. Programs include youth day and overnight as well as adult overnight and travel camp sessions.

1120 **Illinois Wheelchair Sport Camps**
University of Illinois
1207 S Oak St.
Champaign, IL 61820
217-333-1970
Fax: 217-244-0014
sportscamp@illinois.edu
www.disability.illinois.edu/camps

1121 **MDA Summer Camp**
Muscular Dystrophy Association National Office
161 N Clark
Suite 3550
Chicago, IL 60601
800-572-1717
resourcecenter@mdausa.org
mda.org/summer-camp

Donald S. Wood, President & CEO
Kristine Welker, Chief of Staff
Kathy A. Kauffmann, Executive VP & Chief Strategy Development Officer
Michael J. Kennedy, Executive VP & Chief Financial Officer

MDA Summer Camp is a program of the Muscular Dystrophy Association providing a one-week summer camp for children with muscular dystrophy and related muscle-debilitating diseases.

1122 **Nothern Suburban Special Recreation Association Day Camps**
3105 MacArthur Blvd.
Northbrook, IL 60062
847-509-9400
Fax: 847-509-1177
TTY: 711
info@nssra.org
www.nssra.org/programs/camps

Blair Hill, Recreation Manager, Camps

The Northern Suburban Special Recreation Association (NSSRA) offers year round day camps for children and youth with disabilities.

1123 **Rimland Services for Autistic Citizens**
1265 Hartrey Ave.
Evanston, IL 60202
847-328-4090
Fax: 847-328-8364
TTY: 847-328-4090
www.rimland.org

Lorraine Ganz, President
Barbara Cooper, Secretary

Services include residential living, community day services, and health and wellness programs.

1124 **Shady Oaks Camp**
16300 Parker Rd.
Homer Glen, IL 60491
708-301-0816
Fax: 708-301-5091
soc16300@sbcglobal.net
www.shadyoakscamp.org

Scott Steele, Executive Director
Katie Clark, Camp Director
Gary Schaid, Assistant Director

Shady Oaks is a summer camp for people with disabilities. The camp provides a recreational camp experience with a 1:1 camper to staff ratio.

1125 **Timber Pointe Outdoor Center**
Easterseals Central Illinois
20 Timber Pointe Lane
Hudson, IL 61748
309-365-8021
Fax: 309-365-8934
tpoc@eastersealsci.com
www.easterseals.com/ci

Steve Thompson, President & CEO
Allen McBride, Camp Director

Timber Pointe Outdoor Center (TPOC) is a specialized outdoor recreational center for individuals with disabilities, which is owned and operated by Easterseals Central Illinois and is located on Lake Bloomington. TPOC offers year round programs, including summer and day camps, in a completely accessible environment.

Indiana

1126 **Anderson Woods**
4630 Adyeville Rd.
Bristow, IN 47515
812-639-1079
andersonwoods@psci.net
www.andersonwoods.org

Isaac Gatwood, Executive Co-Director
Megan Gatwood, Executive Co-Director

Anderson Woods is a private, nonprofit organization providing summer camp experiences for children and adults with special needs. The camp typically runs in June and July.

1127 **CHAMP Camp**
494 S Emerson Ave.
Suite H-1
Greenwood, IN 46143
317-679-1860
Fax: 317-245-2291
brittany@champcamp.org
www.champcamp.org

Brittany Sichting, Contact
Emily Miller, Contact

CHAMP Camp is a one week summer camp experience for children and youth ages 6-18 who have tracheostomies or require respiratory assistance. The camp is held at Bradford Woods in Martinsville, Indiana, and activities include fishing, boating, canoeing, arts, swimming, and a 50 foot alpine tower climb.

1128 **Camp About Face**
Riley Hospital For Children, Indiana Univ. Health
705 Riley Hospital Dr.
Indianapolis, IN 46202
317-944-5000
rileychildrens.org/support-services

1129 **Camp Brave Eagle**
Indiana Hemophilia & Thrombosis Center
8326 Naab Rd.
Indianapolis, IN 46260
317-871-0000
www.campbraveeagle.org

Jennifer Maahs, Camp Director

Camp Brave Eagle is a summer camp for children and the siblings of children with bleeding disorders living in the state of Indiana. The camp is supervised by experienced medical staff.

1130 **Camp John Warvel**
American Diabetes Association
8604 Allisonville Rd.
Suite 140
Indianapolis, IN 46250
317-352-9226
campsupport@diabetes.org
www.diabetes.org

1131 **Camp Little Red Door**
Little Red Door Cancer Agency
1801 N Meridian St.
Indianapolis, IN 46202-1411
317-925-5595
Fax: 317-925-5597
camp@littlereddoor.org
www.littlereddoor.org

Fred Duncan, Director & CEO
Mandy Pietrykowski, Chief Advancement Officer
Steve Williams, Chief Financial Officer
Amanda Wolfe, Director, Client Services

Camp Little Red Door is a one week summer camp for children and teens who have or have had cancer. The camp is held at Bradford Woods in Martinsville, Indiana with campers participating in traditional camp activities.

1132 **Camp Millhouse**
25600 Kelly Rd.
South Bend, IN 46614
574-233-2202
Fax: 574-233-2511
campmillhouse@gmail.com
www.campmillhouse.org

Diana Breden, Executive Director
Melissa Swank, Camp Director

Camp Millhouse is a residential summer camp for children and adults with varying disabilities. Ages of campers range from 7 to 75+. The camp offers six week-long summer sessions as well as spring and fall weekend sessions. Activities include arts and crafts, swimming, ropes course, and sports. The camp offers low camper to staff ratios and 24-hour supervision and nursing staff.

1133 **Camp PossAbility**
Camp PossAbility, Inc.
PO Box 370
Huntertown, IN 46748
260-341-5732
info@camppossability.org
www.camppossability.org

Sam Albro, President
Lauren E. Harmison, Founder & Vice President

Camp PossAbility is a one-week summer camp for young adults ages 18-40 with a traumatic spinal cord injury. The camp is held at Bradford Woods in Martinsville, Indiana.

1134 **Camp Quality Kentuckiana**
PO Box 35474
Louisville, KY 40232
502-507-3235
eddie.bobbitt@campqualityusa.org
www.campqualityusa.org/ki

Eddie Bobbitt, Executive Director
Charlie Obranowicz, Camp Director
Heather Barry, Camper Coordinator
Linda Wickliffe, Companion Coordinator

Camp Quality is an international camping program for children with cancer. Camp Quality Kentuckiana, serves Kentucky and Indiana and offers children and their siblings summer camps and year round support programs. Volunteer doctors and nurses are at the camp 24 hours a day, and there is a 1:1 staff to camper ratio.

1135 **Camp Red Cedar**
3900 Hursh Rd.
Fort Wayne, IN 46845
260-637-3608
Fax: 260-637-5483
redcedar@campredcedar.com
www.campredcedar.com

Carrie Perry, Director
Shelly Detcher, Assistant Director
Theresa Prentice, Facilities Manager
Nathan Smith, Camp Program Coordinator

Camp Red Cedar is open to children and adults with or without disabilities. The camp offers summer residental and summer day camps along with year round theraputic and conventional horseback riding. Other activities include fishing, hiking, swimming, and arts and crafts.

1136 **Camp Riley**
Riley's Children Foundation
30 S Meridian St.
Suite 200
Indianapolis, IN 46204-3509
317-634-4474
877-867-4539
Fax: 317-634-4478
riley@rileykids.org
www.rileykids.org/about/camp-riley

Elizabeth Elkas, President & CEO
Meghan Miller, Chief Operations Officer
Karen Spataro, Chief Communications Officer
Katie Askey, Senior Project Manager

Camp Riley is an annual summer camp program for children and teens ages 8-18 with physical disabilities. The program offers camp activities in a safe and accessible environment. The camp is held at Bradford Woods in Martinsville, Indiana.

1137 **Happiness Bag**
Happiness Bag, Inc.
3833 Union Rd.
Terre Haute, IN 47802
812-234-8867
Fax: 812-238-0728
info@happinessbag.org
www.happinessbag.org

1138 **Hillcroft Services**
501 W Air Park Dr.
Muncie, IN 47303
765-284-4166
www.hillcroft.org

Debbie Bennett, President & CEO
Abby Halstead, Chief Financial Officer
Jessica Hammett, Chief Operations Officer
Dan Wolfert, Vice President, Development & Marketing

Offers a summer camp program for children with autism spectrum disorders.

1139 **Hoosier Burn Camp**
PO Box 233
Battle Ground, IN 47920
765-567-0115
Fax: 765-567-0195
info@hoosierburncamp.org
www.hoosierburncamp.org

Mark Koopman, Executive Director
Abby James, Program Manager
Valerie McCain, Administrative Assistant

Hoosier Burn Camp is nonprofit organization that provides an annual summer camp and monthly events for children and teens ages 8-18 who have suffered a burn injury. The camp is held at Camp Tecumseh in Brookston, Indiana.

1140 **Indiana Deaf Camp**
1434 S Wausau St.
Warsaw, IN 46580
260-602-6758
Fax: 317-844-1034
TTY: 574-306-4063
info@indeafcamps.org
www.indeafcamps.org

Barbara Stenacker, Executive Director
Curtis Sigafoose, Director

Indiana Deaf Camp is for children ages 4-17 who have hearing loss or are related to individuals with hearing loss.

Iowa

1141 **Camp Albrecht Acres**
14837 Sherrill Rd.
PO Box 50
Sherrill, IA 52073
563-552-1771
Fax: 563-552-2732
office@albrechtacres.org
www.albrechtacres.org

Eric Veltstra, Executive Director
Cassi Banwarth, Director, Programming

Camp Albrecht Acres is a nonprofit organization offering a residential summer camp program for children and adults with special needs.

1142 **Camp Courageous of Iowa**
12007 190th St.
PO Box 418
Monticello, IA 52310-0418
319-465-5916
Fax: 319-465-5919
info@campcourageous.org
www.campcourageous.org

Charlie Becker, Chief Executive Officer

A year round residential and respite care facility for individuals with special needs and their families. Campers range in age from 1-105 years old. Activities include traditional activities like canoeing, hiking, swimming, and crafts, plus adventure activities like caving and rock climbing.

1143 **Camp Hertko Hollow**
4200 University Ave.
Suite 320
Des Moines, IA 50266
515-471-8523
855-502-8500
Fax: 515-288-2531
www.camphertkohollow.com

Jessica Thornton, Executive Director
Deb Holwegner, Camp Director

Camp Hertko Hollow is an educational and recreational summer camp program for children and teens ages 6-17 with diabetes. Campers participate in traditional camp activities and learn about living with diabetes.

1144 **Camp Sunnyside**
Easterseals Iowa
401 NE 66th Ave.
Des Moines, IA 50313
515-309-2375
campandrespite@eastersealsia.org
www.easterseals.com/ia

Sherri Nielsen, President & CEO

Open to campers age 4 and up, with or without disabilities, Camp Sunnyside is owned and operated by Easterseals Iowa and offers week and day summer camps.

1145 **Camp Tanager**
Tanager Place
1614 W Mount Vernon Rd.
Mount Vernon, IA 52314
319-363-0681
Fax: 319-365-6411
campmail@tanagerplace.org
www.camptanager.org

Donald Pirrie, Camp Director

Camp Tanager offers a wide variety of programs, including medical camps in partnership with local Iowa hospitals. The week long medical programs are for children and teens ages 5-17 with chronic illnesses and disabilities such as hemophilia, diabetes and Tourette's syndrome.

Kansas

1146 **Camp Discovery Kansas**
American Diabetes Association
608 W Douglas Ave.
Wichita, KS 67203
316-684-6091
campsupport@diabetes.org
www.diabetes.org

Lora Furstner, Contact

A program of the American Diabetes Association, Camp Discovery Kansas is for children and teens ages 8-16 with diabetes. Campers participate in traditional camp activities while receiving educational information on diabetes. The camp is held at Rock Springs 4-H Center in Junction City, Kansas.

1147 **Camp Planet D**
American Diabetes Association
608 W Douglas Ave.
Wichita, KS 67203
316-684-6091
campsupport@diabetes.org
www.diabetes.org

Lora Furstner, Contact

A program of the American Diabetes Association, Camp Planet D is for children and teens ages 7-15 with diabetes. Campers participate in traditional camp activities while receiving educational information on diabetes. The camp is held at the Tall Oaks Conference Center in Linwood, Kansas.

1148 **Camp Quality Kansas**
PO Box 781607
Wichita, KS 67278
316-214-4963
shannon.reed@campqualityusa.org
www.campqualityusa.org/ks

Shannon Reed, Executive Director

Camp Quality is an international camping program for children with cancer. Camp Quality Kansas offers children and their siblings summer camps and year round support programs. Volunteer doctors and nurses are at the camp 24 hours a day, and there is a 1:1 staff to camper ratio.

1149 **Camp Sweet Betes**
American Diabetes Association
608 W Douglas Ave.
Wichita, KS 67203
316-684-6091
campsupport@diabetes.org
www.diabetes.org

Lora Furstner, Contact

A program of the American Diabetes Association, Camp Sweet Betes is a day camp for children ages 5-8 with diabetes. Campers learn techniques for managing nutrition, exercise, and medication. The camp is held at Trinity Presbyterian Church in Wichita, Kansas.

Kentucky

1150 **Camp Quality Kentuckiana**
PO Box 35474
Louisville, KY 40232
502-507-3235
eddie.bobbitt@campqualityusa.org
www.campqualityusa.org/ki

Eddie Bobbitt, Executive Director
Charlie Obranowicz, Camp Director
Heather Barry, Camper Coordinator
Linda Wickliffe, Companion Coordinator

Camp Quality is an international camping program for children with cancer. Camp Quality Kentuckiana, serves Kentucky and Indiana and offers children and their siblings summer camps and year round support programs. Volunteer doctors and nurses are at the camp 24 hours a day, and there is a 1:1 staff to camper ratio.

1151 **Kids Cancer Alliance**
611 W Main St., Suite 300
PO Box 24337
Louisville, KY 40224
502-365-1538
info@kidscanceralliance.org
www.kidscanceralliance.org

Shelby Russell, Executive Director
Leah McComb, Program Director
Brandon Padgett, Program Coordinator
Emily Trager, Event Coordinator

The Kids Cancer Alliance is a nonprofit organization that provides summer camps and support programs for children and the families of children with cancer. Camp programs include oncology and sibling camps, as well as teen and and family retreats.

1152 **Lions Camp Crescendo**
1480 Pine Tavern Rd.
PO Box 607
Lebanon Junction, KY 40150
502-264-0120
wibblesb@aol.com
www.lccky.org

Billie J. Flannery, Administrator

Organization dedicated to enhancing quality of life for youths, including those with disabilities, through the delivery of a traditional camping experience.

1153 **The Center for Courageous Kids**
1501 Burnley Rd.
Scottsville, KY 42164
270-618-2900
Fax: 270-618-2902
info@courageouskids.org
www.courageouskids.org

Joanie O'Bryan, President & CEO
Clint Cobb, Chief Operations Officer
Allysa Gooden, Director, Development
Brittany Ransom-Doss, Camp Director

The Center for Courageous Kids is a year round medical camp for children who have chronic or life-threatening illnesses. Offers week-long summer camp sessions and family retreat weekend sessions.

Louisiana

1154 **Camp Bon Coeur**
300 Ridge Rd.
Suite K
Lafayette, LA 70506
337-233-8437
Fax: 337-233-4160
info@heartcamp.com
www.heartcamp.com

Susannah Craig, Executive Director
Chelsea Doyle, Summer Program Coordinator
Jessica Becnel, Family Support Group Coordinator

Camp Bon Coeur is a nonprofit organization offering summer camp sessions for children with congenital heart defects. Also offers weekend family camps, monthly support groups, and outings for individuals with heart defects and their families.

1155 **Camp Challenge**
PO Box 10591
New Orleans, LA 70181
504-347-2267
Fax: 866-295-3803
campdirector@campchallenge.org
www.campchallenge.org

Cathy Allain, Camp Director
R. Tony Ricard, Assistant Camp Director

Camp Challenge is a nonprofit organization offering a week long summer camp for young hematology and oncology patients, including children who have or have had cancer or sickle cell disorders. The camp has an on-site medical team available 24 hours a day. It is held at Louisiana Lions Camp in Leesville, Louisiana.

1156 **Camp Pelican**
PO Box 10235
New Orleans, LA 70181
888-617-1118
Fax: 866-295-3803
camppelican@gmail.com
www.camppelican.org

1157 **Camp Quality Louisiana**
1800 Forsythe Ave.
Suite 2, Box 307
Monroe, LA 71201
315-547-4319
louisiana@campqualityusa.org
www.campqualityusa.org/la

Alan Barth, Executive Director
Gay Nell Barth, Camp Director
Marc Norsworthy, Activities Coordinator
Yolanda Starr, Camper Coordinator

Camp Quality is an international camping program for children with cancer. The Louisiana Camp is held at Kings Camp in Mer Rouge, Louisiana and offers children and their siblings summer camps and year round camping opportunities. Volunteer doctors and nurses are at the camp 24 hours a day, and there is a 1:1 staff to camper ratio.

1158 **Louisiana Lions Camp**
292 L. Beauford Dr.
Anacoco, LA 71403
337-239-6567
Fax: 337-239-9975
lalions@lionscamp.org
www.lionscamp.org

Raymond E. Cecil, Executive Director & Camp Director

Owned and operated by the Louisiana Lions League, Inc. the Louisiana Lions Camp is a no cost residential summer camp for children with intellectual and physical disabilities. Campers are able to experience traditional summer camp activities in a medically safe and fun environment. The Camp is also host to the American Diabetes Association, Camp Victory, and Camp Pelican.

1159 **MedCamps of Louisiana**
102 Thomas Rd.
Suite 615
West Monroe, LA 71291 318-329-8405
Fax: 318-329-8407
info@medcamps.com
www.medcamps.com

Caleb Seney, Executive Director
Kacie Hobson, Camp Director
MedCamps of Louisiana offers week-long residential summer camp programs for children with chronic illnesses and physical or developmental disabilities. Each week during the summer a different camp is held, specifically designed for a particular disability.

Maine

1160 **Camp CaPella**
PO Box 552
Holden, ME 04429 207-843-5104
www.campcapella.org

Deb Breindel, Director
Camp CaPella provides recreational and educational opportunities for children and adults with disabilities. The camp is located on Phillips Lake in Dedham, Maine and offers a variety of programs including day camps, overnight camps, family vacation packages, and travel camp.

1161 **Camp Lawroweld**
288 West Side Rd.
Weld, ME 04285 207-585-2984
bchase@nnec.org
www.camplawroweld.org

Trevor Schlisner, Director
Camp Lawroweld offers several camp programs including a week-long summer camp for individuals who are blind or visually impaired.

1162 **Camp No Limits Maine**
No Limits Foundation
114 Pine Tree Camp Road
Rome, ME 04963 207-569-6411
campnolimits@gmail.com
www.nolimitsfoundation.org

Mary Leighton, Founder & Executive Director
Kelsey Moody, Program Operations Manager
Alix Sandler, Marketing & Development Director
Cheryl Foss, Director, Human Resources
Camp No Limits Maine, a location of Camp No Limits, is a recreational and educational camp for youth who have experienced limb loss. Camp No Limits, is a program of the nonprofit organization No Limits Foundation. The camp is held at Pine Tree Camp in Rome, Maine and is supported by Maine Adaptive Sports & Recreation.

1163 **Camp Sunshine**
35 Acadia Rd.
Casco, ME 04015 207-655-3800
Fax: 207-655-3825
info@campsunshine.org
www.campsunshine.org

Michael Katz, Executive Director
Maureen McAllister, Director, Operations
Michael Smith, Director, Development
Camp Sunshine is a free, year round camp for children and families of children with cancer, hematologic conditions, renal disease, systemic lupus, and solid organ transplantation. The camp also has bereavement programs for families.

1164 **Camp sNOw Maine**
No Limits Foundation
15 South Ridge Road
Newry, ME 04261 207-569-6411
campnolimits@gmail.com
www.nolimitsfoundation.org

Mary Leighton, Founder & Executive Director
Kelsey Moody, Program Operations Manager
Alix Sandler, Marketing & Development Director
Cheryl Foss, Director, Human Resources
Camp sNOw Maine, is a location of Camp No Limits, a recreational and educational camp for youth who have experienced limb loss. Camp No Limits is a program of the nonprofit organization, No Limits Foundation. Partnered with Maine Adaptive Sports & Recreation, the camp is weekend of winter activities including, skiing and snowboarding. The camp takes place in March.

1165 **Pine Tree Camp**
Pine Tree Society
114 Pine Tree Camp Rd.
Rome, ME 04963 207-386-5990
Fax: 207-397-5324
ptcamp@pinetreesociety.org
www.pinetreesociety.org

Dawn Willard-Robinson, Camp Director
Mary Schafhauser, Assistant Camp Director
Lori Chesley, Coordinator, Camp Relations
Offering day camps, overnight camps, retreats, and specialized programs, Pine Tree Camp provides children and adults with disabilities the opportunity to participate in recreational activities, such as swimming, fishing, kayak, hiking, and boating. The camp is located in North Pond in Rome, Maine.

Maryland

1166 **Camp Great Rock**
Brainy Camps, Children's National
1 Inventa Pl.
4th Floor West
Silver Spring, MD 20910 202-476-5142
brainycamps@childrensnational.org
www.brainycamps.com/camps/camp-great-rock

Sandra Cushner-Weinstein, Director, Brainy Camps
Camp Great Rock is a one-week overnight summer camp for children and teens ages 7-17 with epilepsy. Campers participate in a variety of activities and receive educational information regarding epilepsy.

1167 **Camp Littlefoot**
The Treatment and Learning Centers
2092 Gaither Rd.
Suite 100
Rockville, MD 20850 301-424-5200
Fax: 301-424-8063
TTY: 301-424-5203
info@ttlc.org
www.ttlc.org

Patricia Ritter, Executive Director
Camp Littlefoot offers a variety of programs for children requiring speech-language and/or occupational therapy.

1168 **Camp No Limits Maryland**
No Limits Foundation
11 Horseshoe Point Lane
North East, MD 21901 207-569-6411
campnolimits@gmail.com
www.nolimitsfoundation.org

Mary Leighton, Founder & Executive Director
Kelsey Moody, Program Operations Manager
Alix Sandler, Marketing & Development Director
Cheryl Foss, Director, Human Resources
Camp No Limits Maryland, a location of Camp No Limits, is a recreational and educational camp for youth who have experienced limb loss. Camp No Limits, is a program of the nonprofit organization No Limits Foundation.

1169 **Camp SunSibs**
Johns Hopkins Children's Center
1800 Orleans St.
Baltimore, MD 21287 www.hopkinsmedicine.org
Joe Young, Director
A weekend camp for children ages 5-16 who have siblings diagnosed with cancer.

1170 **Camp Sunrise**
Johns Hopkins Children's Center
1800 Orleans St.
Baltimore, MD 21287 campsunriseappliations@gmail.com
www.hopkinsmedicine.org
Ashley Richards, Camp Director
Lauren Murphy, Camper Coordinator
Camp Sunshine is a week-long summer camp open to children and teens ages 4-18 who are currently being treated for cancer or who have undergone bone marrow transplants at Johns Hopkins Hospital.

1171 **Deaf Camps, Inc.**
Manidokan Outdoor Ministry Center
1600 Harpers Ferry Rd.
Knoxville, MD 21758 deafcampsinc@gmail.com
deafcampsinc.org
Louise Rollins, President
Erin Krug, Vice President
David Shepard, Secretary
Kathy MacMillan, Treasurer
Deaf Camps, Inc. is a volunteer-run nonprofit organization dedicated to providing camp experiences for deaf and hard of hearing children and children learning American Sign Language.

1172 **Easterseals Camp Fairlee**
Easterseals Delaware & Maryland's Eastern Shore
22242 Bay Shore Rd.
Chestertown, MD 21620 410-778-0566
Fax: 410-778-0567
fairlee@esdel.org
www.easterseals.com/de
Kenan J. Sklenar, President & CEO
Sallie Price, Camp Director
Easterseals Camp Fairlee provides year-round recreation and respite to children and adults with all types of disabilities. Best known for week long summer camp sessions June-August. Camp Fairlee was rebuilt in 2015 with new cabins, activity, center, health center and dining hall. Activities include, but are not limited to, swimming, wall climbing, zip lining, canoeing, kayaking, arts and crafts, indoor and outdoor games. Accredited by the American Camp Association.

1173 **League at Camp Greentop**
The League for People with Disabilities, Inc.
1111 E Cold Spring Lane
Baltimore, MD 21239 410-323-0500
info@leagueforpeople.org
www.leagueforpeople.org
David Greenberg, President & CEO
Margy Ryan, Senior Vice President, Finance
Shiketa Jenkins, Vice President, Workforce, Community & Youth Programs
Lauren Yankolonis, Vice President, Development
A traditional sleepaway summer camp for youth and adults with disabilities. The League at Camp Greentop is located in Thurmont, Maryland, and has youth and all ages sessions, with campers participating in activities such as swimming, arts and crafts, sports, and games.

1174 **Lions Camp Merrick**
PO Box 56
Nanjemoy, MD 20662 301-870-5858
Fax: 301-246-9108
info@lionscampmerrick.org
www.lionscampmerrick.org
Heidi A. Fick, Executive Director
Donna Wadsworth, Office Administrator
A recreational camp for children ages 6-16 who are deaf, blind, or have type 1 diabetes. Camp activities include archery, canoeing, ropes courses, swimming, fishing, and games.

Massachusetts

1175 **Camp Howe**
557 East St.
PO Box 326
Goshen, MA 01032 413-268-7635
Fax: 413-268-8206
office@camphowe.com
www.camphowe.com
Terrie Campbell, Executive Director
Camp Howe provides camp programs for youth ages 7 to 17. The camp's ECHO Program offers one-week and two-week sessions for youth with physical and developmental disabilities.

1176 **Camp Jabberwocky**
200 Greenwood Ave. Ext.
PO Box 1357
Vineyard Haven, MA 02568 508-693-2339
info@campjabberwocky.org
www.campjabberwocky.org
Liza Gallagher, Executive Director
Kelsey Grousbeck, Director, Outreach
Camp Jabberwocky offers summer camp and family camp programs for individuals with physical and intellectual disabilities. The camp is located in Martha's Vineyard with campers usually staying between 1 and 4 weeks. Camp activities include day trips, horseback riding, barbecues, boating, biking, and spending time at the beach.

1177 **Camp Starfish**
636 Great Rd.
Suite 2
Stow, MA 01775 978-637-2617
Fax: 978-637-2617
info@campstarfish.org
www.campstarfish.org
Emily Golinsky, Interim Executive Director
Jamie Mahnken, Camp Director
Laura Petersen, Director, Staff Experience
Em Adolphsen, Director, Operations
Camp Starfish provides summer camps, day camps, and year round respite programs for children with emotional, behavioral, and learning disabilities. Camp Starfish has a 1:1 staff to camper ratio at all times.

1178 **Eagle Hill School: Summer Program**
Eagle Hill School
242 Old Petersham Rd.
PO Box 116
Hardwick, MA 01037 413-477-6000
Fax: 413-477-6837
www.eaglehill.school
PJ McDonald, Head of School
Michael Riendeau, Assistant Head of School, Academic Affairs
Kristyl Kelly, Assistant Head of School, Student Life
Erin Wynne, Assistant Head of School, Institutional Advancement
A program of Eagle Hill School, a school for students diagnosed with learning disabilities including ADHA. The Eagle Hill Summer session is a five week summer camp for students ages 10-16 with learning disabilities. The summer session incorporates education and recreation to address the specific academic and social skills of the student.

1179 **Kamp for Kids at Camp Togowauk**
Behavioral Health Network Inc.
417 Liberty St.
Springfield, MA 01104 413-246-9675
www.bhninc.org
Steve Winn, President & CEO
Anne Benoit, Program Manager
Kamp for Kids at Camp Togowauk is an integrated summer camp for youth with or without disabilities.

1180 **Open Hearts Camp**
The Edward J. Madden Open Hearts Camp
250 Monument Valley Rd.
Great Barrington, MA 01230 413-528-2229
hearts@openheartscamp.org
www.openheartscamp.org
David Zaleon, Executive Director

The Open Hearts Camp is a summer camp program divided into four age-specific sessions for children and teens who have had open heart surgery. Campers must be in stable health and the program blends sports, recreation, arts and crafts and rest periods into a camper's day.

1181 **Summer@Carroll**
Carroll School
25 Baker Bridge Rd.
Lincoln, MA 01773
781-259-8342
summeradmissions@carrollschool.org
www.carrollschool.org

Kristin Curry, Director
Donna Brown, Assistant Director

A program of the Carroll School, an independent day school for elementary and high school students diagnosed with learning disabilities, Summer@Carroll is a 5 week day camp incorporating education and recreation for children with learning disabilities. Students participate in academic classes in the morning, splitting into smaller groups during the afternoon for recreational activities. Campers attending the day camp do not have to be students of the school during the regular school year.

1182 **The Barton Center**
The Barton Center for Diabetes Education, Inc.
30 Ennis Rd.
PO Box 356
North Oxford, MA 01537-0356
508-987-2056
Fax: 508-987-2002
info@bartoncenter.org
www.bartoncenter.org

Lynn Butler-Dinunno, Executive Director
Jenna Dufresne, Director, Health Services
Sarah Balko, Director, Camps & Programs
Sadie Vivenzio, Director, Finance

The Barton Center for Diabetes Education is a year round camp, retreat and conference center offering education, recreation, and support programs for children and teens with diabetes and their families. The center offers a variety of programs in Massachusetts, Connecticut, and New York.

1183 **The Barton Center Camp Joslin**
The Barton Center for Diabetes Education, Inc.
30 Ennis Rd.
PO Box 356
North Oxford, MA 01537-0356
508-987-2056
Fax: 508-987-2002
info@bartoncenter.org
www.bartoncenter.org

Lynn Butler-Dinunno, Executive Director
Jenna Dufresne, Director, Health Services
Sarah Balko, Director, Camps & Programs
Sadie Vivenzio, Director, Finance

A summer camp program of The Barton Center for Diabetes Education, Camp Joslin provides boys ages 6-16 with diabetes a traditional summer camp experience combined with diabetes education. Activities include sports, swimming, kayaking, canoeing, fishing, hiking, arts and crafts, and campfires.

1184 **The Barton Center Clara Barton Camp**
The Barton Center for Diabetes Education, Inc.
30 Ennis Rd.
PO Box 356
North Oxford, MA 01537-0356
508-987-2056
Fax: 508-987-2002
info@bartoncenter.org
www.bartoncenter.org

Lynn Butler-Dinunno, Executive Director
Jenna Dufresne, Director, Health Services
Sarah Balko, Director, Camps & Programs
Sadie Vivenzio, Director, Finance

A summer camp program of the Barton Center for Diabetes Education, Clara Barton Camp provides girls ages 6-16 with diabetes a traditional summer camp experience combined with diabetes education. Activities include sports, swimming, kayaking, canoeing, fishing, hiking, arts and crafts, and campfires.

1185 **The Barton Center Danvers Day Camp**
The Barton Center for Diabetes Education, Inc.
30 Ennis Rd.
PO Box 356
North Oxford, MA 01537-0356
508-987-2056
Fax: 508-987-2002
info@bartoncenter.org
www.bartoncenter.org

Lynn Butler-Dinunno, Executive Director
Jenna Dufresne, Director, Health Services
Sarah Balko, Director, Camps & Programs
Sadie Vivenzio, Director, Finance

A coed day camp for children and teens, ages 5-15, with type 1 diabetes. The camp is held in Danvers, Massachusetts at the St. John's Preparatory School. Campers get the opportunity to explore the 175-acre facility, play games, and construct art pieces.

1186 **The Barton Center Family Camp**
The Barton Center for Diabetes Education, Inc.
30 Ennis Rd.
PO Box 356
North Oxford, MA 01537-0356
508-987-2056
Fax: 508-987-2002
info@bartoncenter.org
www.bartoncenter.org

Lynn Butler-Dinunno, Executive Director
Jenna Dufresne, Director, Health Services
Sarah Balko, Director, Camps & Programs
Sadie Vivenzio, Director, Finance

The Barton Center Family Camp is offered for the families of youth with diabetes. Families participate in traditional camp activities and diabetes education sessions.

1187 **The Barton Center Worcester Day Camp**
The Barton Center for Diabetes Education, Inc.
30 Ennis Rd.
PO Box 356
North Oxford, MA 01537-0356
508-987-2056
Fax: 508-987-2002
info@bartoncenter.org
www.bartoncenter.org

Lynn Butler-Dinunno, Executive Director
Jenna Dufresne, Director, Health Services
Sarah Balko, Director, Camps & Programs
Sadie Vivenzio, Director, Finance

A coed day camp for children and teens ages 5-15 with diabetes. The camp is held in North Oxford, Massachusetts at the Clara Barton Birthplace Museum. Campers experience boating, canoeing, arts and crafts, and camp games.

1188 **The Bridge Center**
470 Pine St.
Bridgewater, MA 02324
508-697-7557
info@thebridgectr.org
www.thebridgectr.org

Karen Ellis, Finance Coordinator
Abby Ross, Year Round & Summer Camp Program Coordinator
Peggy O'Neill, Coordinator, Volunteers

A therapeutic recreational facility in Bridgewater, Massachusetts offering after-school programs, special events, school vacation full-week and summer day camp programs for individuals with disabilities.

Michigan

1189 **Camp Barefoot**
The Fowler Center for Outdoor Learning
2315 Harmon Lake Rd.
Mayville, MI 48744
989-673-2050
Fax: 989-673-6355
info@thefowlercenter.org
www.thefowlercenter.org

Lynn M. Seeloff, Camp Director
Lillia Sheline, Program Director

Offered to adults 18 or older with traumatic brain injuries/closed head injuries. A wide variety of activities are offered. The participants in Camp Barefoot request their week's activities, allowing each participant to design their own activity schedule.

1190 **Camp Catch-A-Rainbow**
YMCA Storer Camps
6941 Stony Lake Rd.
Jackson, MI 49201
517-536-8607
Fax: 517-536-4922
ccar@ymcastorercamps.org
www.ymcastorercamps.org

Katie Wilson, Camp Catch-A-Rainbow Coordinator

Camp Catch-A-Rainbow is a free camp for cancer survivors ages 4-17. The camp is held at YMCA Storer Camps in Jackson, Michigan.

1191 **Camp Chris Williams**
MI Coalition for Deaf & Hard of Hearing People
PO Box 16234
Lansing, MI 48901-6234
586-932-6090
campchris@michdhh.org
www.michdhh.org/camp-chris-williams

Val Boyer, Camp Director

A program of the Michigan Coalition for Deaf and Hard of Hearing, Camp Chris Williams is a one week summer camp for youths ages 11-17 who are deaf or hard of hearing. Sessions are normally held the first full week of August each year. Registration is online only.

1192 **Camp Grace Bentley**
8250 Lakeshore Rd.
Burtchville Township, MI 48059
313-962-8242
campgracebentley@gmail.com
campgracebentley.org

1193 **Camp Midicha**
American Diabetes Association
20700 Civic Center Dr.
Suite 100
Southfield, MI 48076
248-433-3830
campsupport@diabetes.org
www.diabetes.org

1194 **Camp Quality North Michigan**
PO Box 345
Boyne City, MI 49712
231-582-2471
mioffice@campqualityusa.org
www.campqualityusa.org/MI

Jean McDonough, Executive Director
Amy Smitter, Development Director

Camp Quality is an international camping program for children with cancer. The Michigan Camp Quality is held in Lake Ann, Michigan and offers children and their siblings summer camps and year round camping opportunities. Volunteer doctors and nurses are at the camp 24 hours a day, and there is a 1:1 staff to camper ratio.

1195 **Camp Quality South Michigan**
PO Box 345
Boyne City, MI 49712
231-582-2471
mioffice@campqualityusa.org
www.campqualityusa.org/MI

Jean McDonough, Executive Director
Amy Smitter, Development Director

Camp Quality is an international camping program for children with cancer. The South Michigan Camp Quality is held in Fenton, Michigan and offers children and their siblings summer camps and year round camping opportunities. Volunteer doctors and nurses are at the camp 24 hours a day, and there is a 1:1 staff to camper ratio.

1196 **Echo Grove Camp**
Salvation Army
1101 Camp Rd.
Leonard, MI 48367
248-628-3108
Fax: 248-628-7055
shayna.stubblefield@usc.salvationarmy.org
www.echogrove.org

Shayna Stubblefield, Program Director

The Salvation Army's Echo Grove Camp offers a structured camping program for children, adults and seniors referred through Corps Community Centers. In addition to outdoor recreation, camps may include religious, musical and skill-building instruction.

1197 **Indian Trails Camp**
IKUS Life Enrichment Services
O-1859 Lake Michigan Dr. NW
Grand Rapids, MI 49534
616-677-5251
Fax: 616-677-2955
info@ikuslife.org
www.ikuslife.org

Scott Blakeney, Executive Director
Amy DeMott, Director, Programs & Services
Nikki Outhier, Director, Development
Sarah Streng, Camp Director & Respite Coordinator

The Indian Trails Camp is a program of IKUS Life Enrichment Services. The camp offers summer, day, and weekend respite programs for individuals of all ages with disabilities. Campers are able to participate in adaptive recreation opportunities in a barrier-free environment.

1198 **St. Francis Camp On The Lake**
10120 Murrey Rd.
Jerome, MI 49249
517-688-9212
Fax: 517-688-9298
director@saintfranciscamp.org
www.saintfranciscamp.org

Victoria Petty, Camp Director

St. Francis Camp on the Lake offers residential summer camps, day camps, and respite care for children and adults with developmental and intellectual disabilities.

1199 **Trail's Edge Camp**
c/o Mott Respiratory Care, 8-714
1540 E Hospital Dr. SPC 4208
Ann Arbor, MI 48109-4208
director.trailsedgecamp@gmail.com
www.trailsedgecamp.org

Jeff Cain, Director
Betsy Howell, Activities Coordinator

Trail's Edge Camp is a one-week summer camp for children and teens ages 5-18 who are ventilator dependent. Campers are able to participate in camp activities such as games, horseback riding, and fishing. The camp is limited to 32 campers and campers must be able to communicate with other children through speech or sign language.

Minnesota

1200 **AuSM Summer Camp**
Autism Society of Minnesota
2380 Wycliff St.
Suite 102
St. Paul, MN 55114
651-647-1083
Fax: 651-642-1230
camp@ausm.org
www.ausm.org

Ellie Wilson, Executive Director
Dawn Brasch, Senior Director, Finance & Operations
Kelly Thomalla, Senior Director, Integration & Advancement
Eric Ringgenberg, Director, Education Programs

A program of the Autism Society of Minnesota (AuSM), the Summer Camps are offered to children, teens, and adults with autism, ages 6 and up, in a variety of formats including day and residential summer camp. The camp offers the following programs: Camp Hand in Hand, for ages 9+, held at Camp Knutson in Crosslake, Minnesota; Camp Discovery, for ages 10+, held at True Friends/Courage North in Lake George, Minnesota; and Wahode Day Camps, for ages 6-12, held at Camp Butwin in Eagan, Minnesota.

1201 **Camp Buckskin**
PO Box 389
Ely, MN 55731
763-432-9177
info@campbuckskin.com
www.campbuckskin.com

Tom Bauer, Camp Co-Director
Mary Bauer, Camp Co-Director

Camp Buckskin is for campers ages 6-18 with underdeveloped social skills who may struggle to interact with others and make friends. The camp is also open to children who have been diagnosed with AD/HD, Aspergers, and/or a learning disability.

1202 **Camp Confidence**
Confidence Learning Center
1620 Mary Fawcett Memorial Dr.
East Gull Lake, MN 56401
218-828-2344
info@confidencelearningcenter.org
www.campconfidence.com
Jeff Olson, Executive Director
Bob Slaybaugh, Camp Director
Camp Confidence works to promote self-confidence and self-esteem for individuals with developmental and cognitive disabilities. Programs run year round with campers participating in hands on activities and outdoor recreation experiences.

1203 **Camp Courage**
True Friends
8046 83rd St. NW
Maple Lake, MN 55358
952-852-0101
800-450-8376
Fax: 952-852-0123
info@truefriends.org
www.truefriends.org
John Leblanc, President & CEO
Conor McGrath, Senior Director, Camp & Operations
Jon Salmon, Director, Programs
Camp is located in Maple Lake, Minnesota. Summer sessions for campers with a variety of disabilities. Camp Courage is owned and operated by True Friends.

1204 **Camp Courage North**
True Friends
37569 Courage North Dr.
Lake George, MN 56458
952-852-0101
800-450-8376
Fax: 952-852-0123
info@truefriends.org
www.truefriends.org
John Leblanc, President & CEO
Conor McGrath, Senior Director, Camp & Operations
Jon Salmon, Director, Programs
Camp is located in Lake George, Minnesota. Summer camp programs for individuals with disabilities. Camp Courage North is owned and operated by True Friends.

1205 **Camp Eden Wood**
True Friends
6350 Indian Chief Rd.
Eden Prairie, MN 55346
952-852-0101
800-450-8376
Fax: 952-852-0123
info@truefriends.org
www.truefriends.org
John Leblanc, President & CEO
Conor McGrath, Senior Director, Camp & Operations
Jon Salmon, Director, Programs
Offers resident camp programs for children, teenagers and adults with developmental, physical or multiple disabilities.

1206 **Camp Heartland**
One Heartland
26001 Heinz Rd.
Willow River, MN 55795
888-216-2028
Fax: 612-824-6303
helpkids@oneheartland.org
www.oneheartland.org
Patrick Kindler, Executive Director
Katie Donlin, Operations Manager
Katie Bartels, Program Director
Stefanie Tywater-Christiansen, Development Director
A program of One Heartland, a nonprofit organization working to provide camping programs for children with serious illnesses or experiencing social isolation, Camp Heartland is a weeklong summer camp for children, ages 7-15, who are infected or affected by HIV/AIDS. The camp is held in Willow River, Minnesota.

1207 **Camp Knutson**
11148 Manhattan Pt. Blvd.
Crosslake, MN 56442
218-543-4232
camp.knutson@lssmn.org
www.lssmn.org/campknutson
Jared Griffin, Senior Camp Director
Caitlin Malin, Program Director
Camp Knutson is an accessible camp that hosts a variety of different programs for children with special needs such as skin disease, autism, down syndrome, heart disease, and children who have HIV/AIDS.

1208 **Camp Odayin**
Camp Odayin
3503 High Point Dr. N
Suite 250
Oakdale, MN 55128
651-351-9185
Fax: 651-351-9187
info@campodayin.org
www.campodayin.org
Sara Meslow, Executive Director
Alison Boerner, Assistant Director
Matt Olson, Finance Director
Brooke Hohag, Program Director
Camp Odayin provides camping experiences for youth and the families of youth with heart disease. Camp Odayin offers a variety of programs including residential, day, family, and winter camps as well as retreats.

1209 **Camp Odayin Family Camp**
Camp Odayin
3503 High Point Dr. N
Suite 250
Oakdale, MN 55128
651-351-9185
Fax: 651-351-9187
info@campodayin.org
www.campodayin.org
Sara Meslow, Executive Director
Alison Boerner, Assistant Director
Matt Olson, Finance Director
Brooke Hohag, Program Director
Camp Odayin's Family Camp is a two-night program for families with a child who has heart disease.

1210 **Camp Odayin Residential Camp**
Camp Odayin
3503 High Point Dr. N
Suite 250
Oakdale, MN 55128
651-351-9185
Fax: 651-351-9187
info@campodayin.org
www.campodayin.org
Sara Meslow, Executive Director
Alison Boerner, Assistant Director
Matt Olson, Finance Director
Brooke Hohag, Program Director
A program of Camp Odayin, the Residential Camp is for children in grades 1-11 with heart disease. Camps are hosted at Camp Lutherdale in Elkhorn, WI and Camp Knutson in Crosslake, MN.

1211 **Camp Odayin Summer Camp**
Camp Odayin
3503 High Point Dr. N
Suite 250
Oakdale, MN 55128
651-351-9185
Fax: 651-351-9187
info@campodayin.org
www.campodayin.org
Sara Meslow, Executive Director
Alison Boerner, Assistant Director
Matt Olson, Finance Director
Brooke Hohag, Program Director
Camp Odayin offers a variety of summer camp programs for children in grades 1-11 with heart disease. Camper eligibility is determined upon the recommendation of a pediatric cardiologist and the camp's medical director.

1212 **Camp Odayin Winter Camp**
Camp Odayin
3503 High Point Dr. N
Suite 250
Oakdale, MN 55128
651-351-9185
Fax: 651-351-9187
info@campodayin.org
www.campodayin.org

Sara Meslow, Executive Director
Alison Boerner, Assistant Director
Matt Olson, Finance Director
Brooke Hohag, Program Director

A winter camp program for youth in grades 1-12 with heart disease.

1213 **Cristo Vive International: Minnesota Camp**
Ironwood Springs Christian Ranch
7291 County 6 Rd. SW
Stewartville, MN 55976
218-910-8151
cvimncamp@gmail.com
www.cristovive.net

Kristin Munoz, Camp Coordinator

Christian camp with programming for individuals who are blind/deaf, physically or mentally challenged, have multiple disabilities, Down Syndrome, Autism/Asperger's, ADHD/ADD, Cerebral Palsy, and their families and siblings.

1214 **Down Syndrome Camp**
Down Syndrome Foundation
17186 Daniel Lane
Eden Prairie, MN 55346
651-321-2267
www.downsyndromefoundation.org

Angie Kniss, President & Founder
Nick Engbloom, Secretary
Ellie Wilson, Counselor Coordinator

A week-long coed summer camp for youth ages 10-21 who have Down Syndrome. The camp is held at Camp Knutson in Crosslake, Minnesota. The camp is fully accessible and activities include swimming, boating, fishing, tubing, paddleboarding, horseback riding, arts and crafts, and campfires. The camp's staff is trained to work with children and adults with special needs.

1215 **True Friends**
10509 108th St. NW
Annandale, MN 55302
952-852-0101
800-450-8376
Fax: 952-852-0123
info@truefriends.org
www.truefriends.org

John Leblanc, President & CEO
Conor McGrath, Senior Director, Camp & Operations
Jon Salmon, Director, Programs

True Friends provides camp experiences for children and adults with disabilities. Programs are held at five locations: Camp Courage in Maple Lake, MN; Camp Eden Wood in Eden Prairie, MN; Camp Friendship in Annandale, MN; Camp Courage North in Lake George, MN; and True Friends' office in Plymouth, MN.

Mississippi

1216 **Camp Dream Street**
3863 Morrison Rd.
Utica, MS 39175
601-885-3793
info@dreamstreetms.org
www.dreamstreetms.org

Aimee Adler, Director
Ashley Rubinsky, Assistant Director

Dream Street is a five-day camp program for children ages 8-14 with physical disabilities. The camp offers activities such as swimming, arts and crafts, horseback riding and more.

Missouri

1217 **Camp Barnabas**
PO Box 3200
Spingfield, MO 65808
417-476-2565
info@campbarnabas.org
www.campbarnabas.org

John Tillack, Chief Executive Officer
Krystal Simon, Chief Operations Officer
Mike Mrosko, Camp Director
Debbie Weathermon, Director, Development

Camp Barnabas is a Christian camp for children, the siblings of children, and adults with special needs. The camp serves children and adults ages 7 and up.

1218 **Camp Encourage**
4025 Central St.
Kansas City, MO 64111
816-830-7171
Fax: 816-301-6228
info@campencourage.org
www.campencourage.org

Kelly Lee, Executive Director
Aimee Gorrow, Program Coordinator

Provides overnight and summer camp sessions for children and youth with autism spectrum disorders.

1219 **Camp Hickory Hill**
PO Box 1942
Columbia, MO 65205
573-445-9146
camphickoryhill@gmail.com
www.camphickoryhill.com

Jessica Bernhardt, Camp Director

Camp Hickory Hill is a residential summer camp for children ages 7-17 with diabetes. Campers participate in traditional summer camp activities as well as educational programs.

1220 **Camp MITIOG**
7615 N Platte Purchase Dr.
Suite 116
Kansas City, MO 64118
www.campmitiog.org

1221 **Camp No Limits Missouri**
No Limits Foundation
13528 State Route AA
Potosi, MO 63664
207-569-6411
campnolimits@gmail.com
www.nolimitsfoundation.org

Mary Leighton, Founder & Executive Director
Kelsey Moody, Program Operations Manager
Alix Sandler, Marketing & Development Director
Cheryl Foss, Director, Human Resources

Camp No Limits Missouri, is a location of Camp No Limits, a recreational and educational camp for youth who have experienced limb loss. Camp No Limits, is a program of the nonprofit organization No Limits Foundation.

1222 **Camp Quality Central Missouri**
PO Box 953
Jefferson City, MO 65012
636-795-7229
cmo@campqualityusa.org
www.campqualityusa.org/cmo

Casey Bucher, Co-Director
Erin Carl, Co-Director

Camp Quality is an international camping program for children with cancer. The Central Missouri Camp is held in St.Clair, Missouri and offers children and their siblings summer camps and year round camping opportunities. Volunteer doctors and nurses are at the camp 24 hours a day, and there is a 1:1 staff to camper ratio.

1223 **Camp Quality Greater Kansas City**
3111 SE 3rd Terr.
Lee's Summit, MO 64063
816-809-8600
crystal.davison@campqualityusa.org
www.campqualityusa.org/gkc

Crystal Davison, Executive Director
Jacinda Farmer, Camp Director
Taylor Edgar, Volunteer Coordinator

Camp Quality Greater Kansas City is a local chapter of a nationwide nonprofit dedicated to serving children with cancer and their families. They host a signature week-long summer camping experience for children with cancer and their siblings in addition to programs and support throughout the year for the entire family. Their mission is to promote hope while fostering life skills. Hosted at the Lake Maurer Retreat Center, each camper is paired 1:1 with a companion volunteer during camp.

1224 **Camp Quality Northwest Missouri**
1325 Village Dr.
St. Joseph, MO 64506 816-232-2267
erikka.dunn@campqualityusa.org
www.campqualityusa.org/nwmo
Lynette Bingaman, Office Manager
Kandi LaMar, Regional Director
Camp Quality is an international camping program for children with cancer. The Northwest Missouri Camp is held in Stewartsville, Missouri and offers children and their siblings summer camps and year round camping opportunities. Volunteer doctors and nurses are at the camp 24 hours a day, and there is a 1:1 staff to camper ratio.

1225 **Camp Quality Ozarks**
PO Box 302
Joplin, MO 64802 ozarks@campqualityusa.org
www.campqualityusa.org/oz
Kristin Patterson, Executive Director
Camp Quality is an international camping program for children with cancer. The Missouri Ozarks Camp is held in Neosho, Missouri and offers children and their siblings summer camps and year round camping opportunities. Volunteer doctors and nurses are at the camp 24 hours a day, and there is a 1:1 staff to camper ratio.

1226 **Sunnyhill Adventures**
6555 Sunlit Way
Dittmer, MO 63023 636-274-9044
sunnyhilladventures.org
Rob Darroch, Director
Summer camps and year-round programs are offered for youth and adults of all abilities.

1227 **Wonderland Camp**
18591 Miller Circle
Rocky Mount, MO 65072 573-392-1000
info@wonderlandcamp.org
www.wonderlandcamp.org
Jill Wilke, Executive Director
Stephanie Dehner, Director, Administration
Mike Clayton, Director, Fund Development & Communication
Wonderland Camp provides residential summer camps and year round weekend camps for children, teens, and adults with disabilities.

Montana

1228 **Big Sky Kids Cancer Camps**
Eagle Mount Bozeman
6901 Goldenstein Lane
Bozeman, MT 59715 406-586-1781
Fax: 406-586-5794
bigskykids@eaglemount.org
www.eaglemount.org
Kevin Sylvester, Executive Director
Shannon Stober, Senior Director, Programs
Trevor Olson, Director, Operations
Provides recreational opportunities for kids and young adults ages 5-23 with cancer. Big Sky offers skiing, swimming, fishing, ice skating, golf, cycling, and other outdoor activities.

1229 **Camp Mak-A-Dream**
PO Box 1450
Missoula, MT 59806 406-549-5987
Fax: 406-549-5933
info@campdream.org
www.campdream.org
Kim McKearnan, Executive Director
Jennifer Benton, Program Director
Camp Mak-A-Dream provides a cost-free summer camp experience to children, teens, young adults, women and families affected by cancer. Participants experience regular camp activities such as swimming and zip lining, as well as the chance to interact with ranch staff.

1230 **Charles Campbell Childrens Camp**
PO Box 23342
Billings, MT 59102 406-670-2496
campbellcamp@msn.com
billingslions.org/clubnews/campbell-camp
Doug Hanson, Director
Sue Hanson, Director
Camp is open to young adults with physical disabilities that include sight or hearing impairment, spina bifida, cerebral palsy, gross motor skill impairments and other disabilities. Campers enjoy hiking, swimming, fishing, dances, campfires and much more.

Nebraska

1231 **Camp Floyd Rogers**
PO Box 541058
Omaha, NE 68154 402-885-9022
director@campfloydrogers.com
www.campfloydrogers.com
Dylan Helberg, Camp Director
Carrie Busing, Operations Director
A camp for children ages 8-18 with diabetes. While at the camp, campers enjoy activities, participate in special events, engage in evening programs, and meet other children their own age with diabetes.

1232 **Camp Kindle**
Project Kindle
PO Box 81147
Lincoln, NE 68501 877-800-2267
eva@projectkindle.org
www.campkindle.org
Eva Payne, Founder & President
Mandy Nickolite, Vice President & Camp Director
Camp Kindle provides educational and recreational camp programs for children and youth with a chronic or life-threatening illness, disability, or life challenge.

1233 **Camp Quality Heartland**
PO Box 24322
Omaha, NE 68124 402-450-1674
heartland@campqualityusa.org
www.campqualityusa.org/htl
Laura Peitzmeier, Executive Director
Camp Quality is for children with cancer and their siblings. The camp offers a stress-free environment that offers exciting activities and fosters new friendships, while helping to give the children courage, motivation and emotional strength.

1234 **Easterseals Nebraska Camp**
Easterseals Nebraska
12565 West Center Rd.
Omaha, NE 68144 402-930-4053
Fax: 888-611-6396
campesn@ne.easterseals.com
www.easterseals.com/ne
James C. Summerfelt, President & CEO
Jami Biodrowski, Director, Camp & Respite
Offers a variety of camp and recreational programs to help people with disabilities gain independence in a safe and adapted environment.

1235 **Kamp Kaleo**
46872 Willow Springs Rd.
Burwell, NE 68823 308-346-5083
kampkaleo@gmail.com
www.kampkaleo.com
David Butz, Camp Administrator
Offers an overnight summer camp for individuals with developmental disabilities. Participants can expect to experience outdoor recreational activities such as canoeing, fishing, and swimming, and there is a strong focus on religious education.

1236 **National Camps for Blind Children**
Christian Record Services
5900 S 58th St.
Suite M
Lincoln, NE 68516
402-488-0981
Fax: 402-488-7582
info@christianrecord.org
www.christianrecord.org

Diane Thurber, President
Lonnie Kreiter, Vice President, Finance
National Camps for Blind Children is a program of Christian Record Services offering summer camps for individuals who are considered legally blind.

Nevada

1237 **Camp Buck**
Nevada Diabetes Association
18 Stewart St.
Reno, NV 89501
775-856-3839
800-379-3839
Fax: 775-348-7591
camp@diabetesnv.org
www.diabetesnv.org

Sarah Gleich, Executive Director
Nate Gibson, Director, Camps
Dakota Ostrenger, Director, Marketing
Tara Winkelman, Director, Programs
Co-ed summer camp for children ages 7-17 with diabetes. Campers participate in recreational and athletic activities as well as diabetes education.

1238 **Camp Lotsafun**
Amplify Life
480 Galletti Way
Bldg. 2
Sparks, NV 89431
775-827-3866
Fax: 775-827-0334
info@amplifylife.org
www.amplifylife.org

Jessica Daum, Executive Director
Luis Chavez Torres, Program Coordinator
Cindy Oesterle-Prescott, Office Manager
Provides therapeutic, educational, and recreational opportunities for individuals with developmental disabilities. Camp activities include swimming, kayaking, pet therapy, arts and crafts, drama and music. The camp is held at Eagle Lake, California.

1239 **CampCare**
PO Box 12155
Reno, NV 89510-2155
775-323-3737
cmoore@campcarenevada.org
www.campcarenevada.org

Carol Moore, Camp Director
The camp provides programs for individuals with special needs such as ADHD, autism and cerebral palsy.

1240 **Discovery Day Camp**
Nevada Blind Children's Foundation
95 S Arroyo Grande Blvd.
Henderson, NV 89012
702-735-6223
info@nvblindchildren.org
nvblindchildren.org/programs/day-camp

Emily Smith, Chief Executive Officer
Maribel Garcia, Director, Programs
Paula Farrell, Director, Finances & Facilities
A summer day camp program for children in grades K-12 who are visually impaired. Discovery Day Camp provides traditional camp activities that have been adapted to meet the needs of children with visual impairments.

New Hampshire

1241 **Adam's Camp: New England**
26 Shaker Rd.
Concord, NH 03301
508-901-9610
NewEngland@AdamsCamp.org
www.adamscampnewengland.org

Adrienne Evans, Executive Director
Offers both therapy and adventure camps for children and the families of children with special needs and developmental delays. Camps are available in New Hampshire and Massachusetts.

1242 **Camp Allen**
56 Camp Allen Rd.
Bedford, NH 03110
603-622-8471
Fax: 603-626-4295
michael@campallennh.org
www.campallennh.org

Michael Constance, Executive Director
Stephen Daley, Camp Director
Debra Schulte, Office Manager
A residential summer camp for individuals with disabilities. All of the activities are conducted by individual coordinators under the supervision of the Program Director. Activities include aquatics, arts, crafts, games and nature programs. All camp events, special events, evening programs, and field trips are scheduled throughout the summer and are structured to meet the individual abilities and needs of each camper.

1243 **Camp Carefree**
American Diabetes Association
Lions Camp Pride
154 Camp Pride Way
New Durham, NH 03855
campsupport@diabetes.org
www.diabetes.org

Phyllis Woestemeyer, Director
The camp is located at Lions Camp Pride in New Durham, New Hampshire. Camp Carefree is a American Diabetes Association summer camp for children with diabetes.

1244 **Camp Connect**
Easterseals New Hampshire
555 Auburn St.
Manchester, NH 03103
603-623-8863
www.easterseals.com/nh

Maureen Beauregard, President & CEO
A summer day camp for children in grades K-12 with Asperger Syndrome, Autism, Nonverbal Learning Disorder, and other social communication disorders. The camp has a large focus on continuing to address academic needs of the campers, but also incorporates music, drama, and arts and crafts.

1245 **Camp Inter-Actions**
Inter-Actions
170 West Rd.
Suite 6-B
Portsmouth, NH 03801
603-319-6120
campinfo@inter-actions.org
inter-actions.org

Debbie Gross, Camp Director
Camp Inter-Actions is a summer camp for children ages 8-15 who are blind or visually impaired. The camp is located in Kingston, New Hampshire and runs one, two, and three week sessions. Activities include swimming, fishing, adapted sports/games, woodworking, pottery, and more.

1246 **Camp Sno Mo**
Easterseals New Hampshire
Hidden Valley Reservation
260 Griswold Ln.
Gilmanton Iron Works, NH 03837
603-364-5818
cellis@eastersealsnh.org
www.easterseals.com/nh

Maureen Beauregard, President & CEO
Chris Ellis, Camp Director
Camp Slo Mo is is a camp program for children with disabilities. Activities include water sports, team sports, hiking, archery, arts and crafts, and more offered in an accessible setting.

1247 **Camp Wediko**
Wediko Children's Services, New Hampshire Campus
11 Bobcat Blvd.
Windsor, NH 03244
603-478-5236
Fax: 603-478-2049
www.wediko.org
Edward Zadravec, Interim Executive Director
This program is a six-week residential program for youth ages 8-19 with social, emotional, and behavior challenges. This program serves children with disabilities such as ADHD, autism, mood disorders, and more.

1248 **Camp Yavneh: Yedidut Program**
Summer Office
18 Lucas Pond Rd.
Northwood, NH 03261
603-942-5593
info@campyavneh.org
www.campyavneh.org/yedidut
Bil Zarch, Executive Director
Miriam Loren, Director, Camper Care & Yedidut
Michelle Rosenhek Zelermyer, Director, Summer Camp
Netanel Spiegel, Director, Operations
A residential Jewish summer camp program for children with disabilities. Traditional camp activities with a strong focus on Judaism and Jewish education.

New Jersey

1249 **Camp Chatterbox**
Children's Specialized Hospital
200 Somerset St.
New Brunswick, NJ 08901
908-301-5548
campchatterbox@childrens-specialized.org
csh.recdesk.com
Sara Barnhill, Clinical Coordinator
Camp Chatterbox is an overnight camp for people ages 5-22 who use augmentative communication devices. The camp offers recreational activities such as swimming, arts, and sports.

1250 **Camp Deeny Riback**
208 Flanders Netcong Rd.
Flanders, NJ 07836
973-929-2901
Fax: 973-463-3998
camps@jccmetrowest.org
cdr.jccmetrowest.org
Dana Gottfried, Director
Debra Scher, Assistant Director
Todd Seideman, Assistant Director
A Jewish summer camp for children of all ages. The camp integrates children with special needs through their Camp Friends program. The camp provide traditional outdoor camp activities.

1251 **Camp Dream Street**
Kaplen JCC on the Palisades
411 East Clinton Ave.
Tenafly, NJ 07670
201-569-7900
Fax: 201-569-7448
info@jccotp.org
www.jccotp.org
Jordan Shenker, Chief Executive Officer
Miriam Chilton, Chief Operating Officer
Kevin Cunningham, Chief Financial Officer
Dream Street is a camp program for children with cancer and other blood disorders. Activities include swimming, arts and crafts, horseback riding and more.

1252 **Camp Jaycee**
Camp Jaycee Administrative Office
985 Livingston Ave.
North Brunswick, NJ 08902
732-737-8279
Fax: 732-737-8279
info@campjaycee.org
www.campjaycee.org
Maureen Brennan, Camp Director
Nicole Goodwin, Coordinator, Camping Services
Camp Jaycee offers residential summer camp programs for adults with developmental and intellectual disabilities. The campsite is located in Effort, PA.

1253 **Camp Jotoni**
51 Old Stirling Rd.
Warren, NJ 07059
908-753-4244
www.campjotoni.org
Josh Burke, Director
Sponsored by the Arc of Somerset County, Camp Jotoni is a day and residential camp for children and adults with developmental disabilities. Campers are ages 5-21.

1254 **Camp Merry Heart**
Easterseals New Jersey
21 O'Brien Rd.
Hackettstown, NJ 07840
908-852-3896
Fax: 908-852-9263
camp@nj.easterseals.com
www.easterseals.com/nj
Brian Fitzgerald, President & CEO
An organized program of swimming, arts and crafts, boating, nature study and travel offered to campers with a variety of disabilities.

1255 **Camp Nejeda**
Camp Nejeda Foundation
910 Saddleback Rd.
PO Box 156
Stillwater, NJ 07875
973-383-2611
Fax: 973-383-9891
info@campnejeda.org
www.campnejeda.org
Bill Vierbuchen, Executive Director
Ginnie Ramberger, Registrar & Staff Coordinator
Jim Daschbach, Camp Director
Victoria Benyo, Program Director
For children with diabetes, ages 7-16. Provides an active and safe camping experience which enables the children to learn about and understand diabetes. Activities include boating, swimming, fishing, archery, and camping skills.

1256 **Camp Quality New Jersey**
PO Box 264
Adelphia, NJ 07710
908-770-2105
newjersey@campqualityusa.org
www.campqualityusa.org/nj
Al Passy, Executive Director
Kaitlin DeGennaro, Camp Director
Camp Quality is for children with cancer and their siblings. The camp offers a stress-free environment that offers exciting activities and fosters new friendships, while helping to give the children courage, motivation and emotional strength.

1257 **Camp Sun'N Fun**
The Arc Gloucester
1555 Gateway Blvd.
West Deptford, NJ 08096
856-629-4502
camp@thearcgloucester.org
www.thearcgloucester.org
Lisa Conley, Chief Executive Officer
Camp is located in Williamstown, New Jersey. Summer sessions for campers with developmental disabilities. Coed, ages 5+. Activities include swimming, arts and crafts, sports, games, music, dance and drama.

1258 **Explorer's Club Camp**
New Behavioural Network
2 Pin Oak Lane
Suite 250
Cherry Hill, NJ 08003
856-874-1616
Fax: 856-424-7660
nbh@nbngroup.com
www.newbehavioralnetwork.com/summer-camp

1259 **Happiness Is Camping**
62 Sunset Lake Rd.
Hardwick, NJ 07825
908-362-6733
Fax: 908-362-5197
rich@happinessiscamping.org
www.happinessiscamping.org
Laura San Miguel, President
Julie McMahon, Secretary
Beth Fuchs, Treasurer

Located in Hardwick, New Jersey, Happiness is Camping is a week-long camp for kids with cancer and their siblings, ages 6-16. The camp is free for all attendees, and campers participate in a variety of traditional outdoor activities, including caneoing, fishing, swimming, archery, and more.

1260 **Harbor Haven Summer Program**
4 Hanover Rd.
Unit C3
Florham Park, NJ 07932
908-964-5411
Fax: 908-964-0511
info@harborhaven.com
www.harborhaven.com

Robyn Tanne, Director
Kim Van Woeart, Associate Director
Ryan Cox, Assistant Director

A seven-week summer program for children ages 3-15 with mild special needs. Harbor Haven offers traditional outdoor recreation activities and a daily academic period which reinforces math, reading, and language arts.

1261 **Mane Stream**
83 Old Turnpike Rd.
PO Box 305
Oldwick, NJ 08858
908-439-9636
Fax: 908-439-2338
info@manestreamnj.org
www.manestreamnj.org

Trish Hegeman, Executive Director
Jane Banta, Camp Director
Louisa Bartok, Manager, Marketing & Communications

A summer day camp for children with physical and cognitive challenges, their siblings, and non-disabled children. The camp is primarily focused on horsemanship lessons, with activities such as riding lessons, grooming, tacking, leading, basic horse care, and more. Eight week-long sessions available.

1262 **Rising Treetops at Oakhurst**
111 Monmouth Rd.
Oakhurst, NJ 07755
732-531-0215
Fax: 732-531-0292
info@risingtreetops.org
www.risingtreetops.org

Robert Pacenza, Executive Director
Charles Sutherland, Camp Director
Lori Schenck, Assistant Director, Services

A summer and day camp for adults and children with special needs, including autism and physical and intellectual disabilities. Campers experience traditional camp activities while gaining skills for greater independence.

1263 **Round Lake Camp**
NJY Camps
21 Plymouth St.
Fairfield, NJ 07004
973-575-3333
Fax: 973-575-4188
rlc@njycamps.org
www.roundlakecamp.org

Aryn Barer, Director

Round Lake Camp is for children ages 7-17 with learning differences and social communication disorders. Campers enjoy swimming, boating, sailing, mountain biking, and arts and crafts. The camp is located in Milford, PA.

New Mexico

1264 **ADA Camp 180**
American Diabetes Association
Fort Lone Tree Camp
307 Fort Lone Tree Rd.
Capitan, NM 88316
602-861-4731
campsupport@diabetes.org
www.diabetes.org

1265 **Camp Enchantment**
Rio Grande Community Development Corporation
318 Isleta Blvd. SW
Albuquerque, NM 87105
info@campenchantment.org
www.campenchantment.org

Shayna Rosenblum, Camp Director

A summer camp for children and teens ages 7-17 who have been diagnosed with cancer. The camp is held at Manzano Mountain Retreat in Torreon, NM. Activities include swimming, kayaking, dancing, archery, and more. The camping session is seven days.

1266 **Camp Rising Sun**
Center for Development and Disability
2300 Menaul Blvd. NE
Albuquerque, NM 87107
505-272-3000
800-270-1861
Fax: 505-272-5896
hsc.unm.edu/cdd

Paul Brouse, Camp Director

Held at the Manzano Mountain Retreat southeast of Albuquerque, Camp Rising sun is a summer camp designed specifically for children and teens with Autism Spectrum Disorder and their peers, ages 8-17. Activities include hiking, sports, photography, kayaking, campouts, and other nature activities.

New York

1267 **ADA Camp Aspire**
American Diabetes Association
809 Five Points Rd.
Rush, NY 14543
585-458-3040
www.diabetes.org

1268 **Autism Summer Respite Program**
Commonpoint Queens
58-20 Little Neck Pkwy.
Little Neck, NY 11362
718-225-6750
larmband@commonpointqueens.org
www.commonpointqueens.org/summercamp

Lisa Armband, Contact

An afternoon camping program for children, teens, and young adults ages 5-21 with Autism and similar disabilities. Located at Sam Field Center.

1269 **AutismUp: YMCA Summer Social Skills Program**
AutismUp
50 Science Pkwy.
Rochester, NY 14620
585-248-9011
Fax: 585-248-9159
contact@autismup.org
autismup.org

Sarah Milko, Executive Director
Christina Hilton, Director, Finance & Operations
Lisa Ponticello, Director, Marketing & Development
Rachel Rosner, Director, Education & Support

This program is a collaboration between AutismUp and the Greater Rochester YMCA. The Summer Social Skills Program is a day camp held at Camp Arrowhead for children, 4-16, with Autism Spectrum Disorders. Half day and full day sessions available, and campers are integrated into regular camp activities.

1270 **Camp Abilities Brockport**
The College at Brockport, State Univ of New York
350 New Campus Drive
Brockport, NY 14420
585-395-5361
campabilitiesbrockport01@gmail.com
www.campabilitiesbrockport.org

Lauren Lieberman, PhD, Camp Director
Alex Stribing, Assistant Director
Emily Gilbert, Aquatics Director

A one-week sports camp for children who are visually impaired, blind or deaf blind. Children learn to be more physically active, which in turn improves their health and well being.

1271 **Camp Adventure**
KiDS NEED MoRE
PO Box 305
Copiague, NY 11726
631-608-3135
Fax: 631-532-4944
info@kidsneedmore.org
kidsneedmore.org

Melissa Firmes, President
John Ray, Treasurer
Jacqueline Lorenz, Secretary

Camp Adventure is a one-week sleep away camp for children and teens ages 6-18 dealing with cancer and other life threatening illnesses. The camp takes place on Shelter Island at Quinipet Camp and Retreat Center.

1272 **Camp Anne**
AHRC New York City
228 Four Corners Lane
Ancramdale, NY 12503
518-329-5649
Fax: 518-329-5689
michael.rose@ahrcnyc.org
camping.ahrcnyc.org

Michael Rose, Camp Director

A day summer camp program for children and adults with intellectual and developmental disabilities. The camp offers activities such as cooking, crafts, nature, sports, swimming, and more. Camp Anne offers three 11-day sessions for adults ages 21-59, and two 11-day sessions for childres ages 5-20. Each session can accommodate 100 campers.

1274 **Camp EAGR**
Empowering People's Independence (EPI)
2 Townline Circle
Rochester, NY 14623
585-442-4430
Fax: 585-442-6964
info@epiny.org
www.epiny.org

Michael Radell, Camp Director

Camp EAGR is a summer sleep-away camp for children with epilepsy and their siblings. Activities include swimming, horseback riding, and rock climbing.

1275 **Camp Good Days and Special Times**
1332 Pitsford-Mendon Rd.
PO Box 665
Mendon, NY 14506
585-624-5555
800-785-2135
Fax: 585-624-5799
info@campgooddays.org
www.campgooddays.org

Wendy Bleier-Mervis, Executive Director
Sheri Watkins, CFO & Director, Administration

The camp is dedicated to improving the quality of life for children and adults affected by cancer or other life challenges. The camp offers week-long sessions that are free of charge.

1276 **Camp High Hopes**
82 Pixley Rd.
Chenango Forks, NY 13746
607-226-5474
joe@camphighhopes.org
www.camphighhopes.org

Joe Brennan, Director
Hope Woodcock-Ross, Health Director

A week-long summer camp program for boys with hemophilia. The camp has a 24-hour physician and nursing staff. Ages 7-17, boys only.

1277 **Camp Huntington**
56 Bruceville Rd.
High Falls, NY 12440-5100
845-687-7840
855-707-2267
Fax: 855-707-2267
www.camphuntington.com

Daniel Falk, Executive Director
Dylan Sloan, Program Director
Margaret Short, Health Director

A co-ed residential summer camp specifically designed to focus on adaptive and therapeutic recreation. Campers include those with learning and developmental disabilities, ADD/HD, Autism Spectrum Disorders, Asperger's, PDD, and other special needs. Programs focus on recreation and social skills, independence, and participation.

1278 **Camp Kehilla**
Henry Kaufmann Campgrounds
75 Colonial Springs Rd.
Wheatley Heights, NY 11798
516-484-1545
jwasserman@sjjcc.org
www.campkehilla.org

Joe Wasserman, Camp Director
Victoria Granatelli, Assistant Camp Director

A year-round camp for children, teens, and young adults with developmental disabilities and other neurodevelopmental conditions. Ages 5-21.

1279 **Camp Little Oak**
Aldersgate Camp & Retreat Center
7955 Brantingham Rd.
Greig, NY 13345
425-770-1801
camplittleoak.org

Hannah Russell, Camp Director

A non-profit, week-long summer camp for girls diagnosed with a bleeding disorder. The camp is held at Aldersgate Camp in Greig, New York. Camp Little Oak runs traditional summer camp activities such as swimming, canoeing, and archery, as well as provides education about blood disorders and conducts community service projects.

1280 **Camp Mark Seven**
Mark Seven Deaf Foundation
144 Mohawk Hotel Rd.
Old Forge, NY 13420
315-207-5706
TTY: 315-357-6089
registrar@campmark7.org
www.campmark7.org

Dave Staehle, Camp Director

A camp program for hard-of-hearing, deaf and hearing people. Coed, open to all ages. The camp is located on the Fourth Lake in the Adirondack Mountains.

1281 **Camp Pa-Qua-Tuck**
2 Chet Swezey Rd.
Center Moriches, NY 11934
631-878-1070
www.camppaquatuck.com

Alyssa Pecorino, Executive Director
Melissa Locrotondo, Chief of Programming
Tommy Ryan, Director, Respite Camp
Johneen Feehan, Office Manager

Camp Pa-Qua-Tuck is a residential camp for individuals with physical and developmental disabilities. The camp also offers Respite Camp, a weekend camp program for ages 6-40.

1282 **Camp Ramapo**
Ramapo for Children
Rt. 52/Salisbury Turnpike
PO Box 266
Rhinebeck, NY 12572
845-876-8403
Fax: 845-876-8414
office@ramapoforchildren.org
www.ramapoforchildren.org

Matthew McKnight, Camp Director
Lenora Sealey, Associate Camp Director

A residential summer camp for youth ages 6-16 with social, emotional, or learning challenges.

1283 **Camp Reece**
1782 S Johnsburg Rd.
Johnsburg, NY 12843-1909
212-289-4872
info@campreece.org
www.campreece.org

Duncan Lester, Executive Director
Octavia Man, Camp Director
Kiersten Twitchell, Camp Director

A sleep-away camp for children ages 10-17 with special needs. The camp is located at Skidmore College and offers activities such as photography, rafting, biking, sports, and more. The camp serves boys and girls with disabilities such as ADD/ADHD, learning disabilities, and high-functioning autism. There are two 3-week sessions or the full 6-week session available.

1284 **Camp Sisol**
Jewish Community Center of Greater Rochester/JCC
1200 Edgewood Ave.
Rochester, NY 14618
585-461-2000
Fax: 585-461-0805
bettertogether@jccrochester.org
www.jccrochester.org
Josh Weinstein, Chief Executive Officer
Coed, ages 5-16. Camp Sisol accommodates children with special needs.

1285 **Camp Tova**
92nd Street Y
1395 Lexington Ave.
New York, NY 10128
212-415-5573
www.92y.org
Seth Pinsky, Chief Executive Officer
Alyse Myers, President
Lauren Wexler, Director, Camps
Camp Tova is a program for children with developmental disabilities. Campers participate in sports, arts, and outdoor activities and develop their creative, social, and physical skills.

1286 **Camp Venture, Inc.**
25 Smith St.
Suite 510
Nanuet, NY 10954
845-624-3860
www.campventure.org
Matthew Shelley, Chief Executive Officer
Celia Solomita, Chief Financial Officer
Marie Pardi, Chief Program Officer
Camp Venture is a day camp for children ages 5-12 with and without developmental disabilities. Located in Stony Point, the camp also offers a young adult group for teens ages 13-21 with developmental disabilities. Children will experience regular camp activities while benefitting from group engagement.

1287 **Camp Whitman on Seneca Lake**
PO Box 24393
Rochester, NY 14624
315-201-0193
Fax: 315-531-4002
camp@campwhitman.org
www.campwhitman.org
Lea Kone, Camp Director
Provides camp opportunities for individuals with developmental disabilities. Campers are encouraged to participate in a full range of activities including games, sports, swimming, singing, and dancing.

1288 **Clover Patch Camp**
Center for Disability Services
55 Helping Hand Lane
Glenville, NY 12302
518-384-3042
Fax: 518-384-3001
cloverpatchcamp@cfdsny.org
www.cloverpatchcamp.org
Cindy Francis, Camp Director
Jackie Richards, Director, Residential Services
Clover Patch Camp is operated by the Center for Disability Services and is located in Glenville, New York. The camp is for individuals with a variety of disabilities. For ages 5+.

1289 **Double H Ranch**
97 Hidden Valley Rd.
Lake Luzerne, NY 12846
518-696-5676
Fax: 518-696-4528
myurenda@doublehranch.org
www.doublehranch.org
Max Yurenda, CEO & Executive Director
Kate Walsh, Camp Director
Alex Griffen, Assistant Camp Director, Programs
Chris Pezzulo, Assistant Camp Director, Residential Life
Summer residential camp and winter sports programs for children and young adults ages 6-16 who have cancer and other life threatening illnesses. The programs are free of charge and some of the recreational activities include bead making, arts and crafts, tennis, soccer, and volleyball.

1290 **Friendship Circle Day Camp**
Friendship Circle Upper East Side
419 E 77th St.
New York, NY 10075
office@friendshipcirclenyc.org
www.friendshipcirclenyc.org
Shlomo Gutnick, Executive Director
Sara Gutnick, Program Director
Dassy Chein, Program Coordinator
Rochel Greisman, Office Administrator
The Friendship Circle Day Camp allows children with special needs the opportunity to have a full camp experience. Campers participate in activities such as field trips, music, arts and crafts, and performances.

1291 **Gow School Summer Programs**
2491 Emery Rd.
South Wales, NY 14139
716-687-2004
Fax: 716-687-2003
summer@gow.org
www.gow.org
Matthew Fisher, Director
Co-ed summer programs for students ages 8-16 with dyslexia or similar learning disabilities. Offers a blend of morning academics, afternoon/evening traditional camp activities and weekend overnights.

1292 **Kamp Kiwanis**
New York District Kiwanis Foundation
9020 Kiwanis Rd.
Taberg, NY 13471
315-336-4568
Fax: 315-336-3845
kamp@kampkiwanis.org
www.kampkiwanis.org
Rebecca Lopez Clemence, Executive Director
Luke Clemence, Camp Director
Dori Gross, Assistant Camp Director
Kamp Kiwanis is a mainstream camp for underprivileged youth with and without special needs. Twenty campers with disabilities are integrated into weekly sessions. Programs are offered for children, teens, and adults.

1293 **Katy Isaacson Elaine Gordon Lodge**
AHRC New York City
653 Colgate Rd.
Box 37
East Jewett, NY 12424
518-589-6000
Fax: 518-589-6583
matthew.hatcher@ahrcnyc.org
camping.ahrcnyc.org
Matt Hatcher, Camp Director
An alternative and traditional summer day camp for adults and teens with intellectual and developmental disabilities. The lodge offers five 11-day sessions for adults ages 18-29, and one session for teens ages 13-17. Activities include boating, swimming, pony rides, sports, and more.

1294 **Lisa Beth Gerstman Camp**
Lisa Beth Gerstman Foundation
439 Oak St.
Suite 1
Garden City, NY 11530
516-594-4400
Fax: 516-594-7085
info@lisabethgerstman.org
www.lisabethgerstman.org
Harvey Gerstman, Co-Founder
Carol Gerstman, Co-Founder
Linda Gerstman, Co-Founder
Dan Gerstman, Co-Founder
A summer day camp for children with special needs. Activities include swimming, sports, and arts and crafts. Camps are located across the New York Metropolitan Area.

1295 **Maplebrook School**
5142 Route 22
Amenia, NY 12501
845-373-9511
Fax: 845-373-7029
admissions@maplebrookschool.org
www.maplebrookschool.org

Donna Konkolics, Head of School
Roger Fazzone, President
Jennifer Scully, Assistant Head, Postsecondary Studies
Lori Hale, Executive Director

A coeducational boarding school which offers a six week camp for children with learning differences and ADD.

1296 **Marist Brothers Mid-Hudson Valley Camp**
1455 Broadway
PO Box 197
Esopus, NY 12429
845-384-6620
info@maristbrotherscenter.org
www.maristbrotherscenter.org

Jim Sheldon, Camp Director
Timothy Hagan, Director, Operations
Donnell Neary, Assistant Director

The camp provides week-long summer sessions for children who have a variety of special needs and illnesses, including cancer and physical, developmental, and mental disabilities. Each session is specific to the special need or illness.

1297 **Mosholu Day Camp**
Mosholu Montefiore Community Center
3450 Dekalb Ave.
New York, NY 10467
718-882-4000
frontdesk@mmcc.org
www.mmcc.org/camp

Rita Santelia, Chief Executive Officer
Shakil M. Khan, Chief Financial Officer
Jackina Farshtey, Chief of Staff
Ivan Diaz, Director, Facilities & Operations

A day camp program for children in grades 1-10. The day camp offers specific programs for children and teens who are developmentally disabled. Camp Sunshine is for children ages 5-12, and Camp Elan is for children ages 12-16.

1298 **Southampton Fresh Air Home**
36 Barkers Island Rd.
Southampton, NY 11968
631-283-1594
Fax: 631-283-7596
www.sfah.org

Thomas Naro, Executive Director
David Billingham, Camp Director
Nathan Unwin, Assistant Camp Director

A residential camp facility accommodating physically challenged children. The Special Needs Summer Camp is for children and teens ages 8-18. One or three week sessions available, as well as day camp. The SFAH provides adapted programs and activities that allow campers to develop physically, emotionally, and psychologically.

1299 **Special Services Summer Day Camp**
Commonpoint Queens
58-20 Little Neck Pkwy.
Little Neck, NY 11362
718-225-6750
larmband@commonpointqueens.org
www.commonpointqueens.org/summercamp

Lisa Armband, Contact

A day camp program for children and youth ages 5-21 with developmental disabilities. Activities include dancing, swimming, arts and crafts, and community-based field trips. The program is held at the Henry Kaufmann Campgrounds.

1300 **Summit Camp**
55 W 38th St.
4th Floor
New York, NY 10018
570-253-4381
info@summitcamp.com
www.summitcamp.com

Shepherd Baum, Director
Leah Love, Assistant Director
Thea Mullis, Travel Director
Maryann Santoro, Admissions Director

The camp is located in Honesdale, Pennsylvania, and is for children ages 8-19 who have a variety of developmental, social, or learning challenges. In addition to traditional camp activities, Summit Camp has a strong focus on social skills development and interpersonal growth.

1301 **Sunshine Campus**
809 Five Points Rd.
Rush, NY 14543
585-533-2080
www.sunshinecamp.org

Tracey Dreisbach, Executive Director
Brandi Koch, Camp Director
Jarod Alexander, Facility Director
Princeton Jones, Maintenance Manager

The camp is located in Rush, New York. Camping sessions for children and young adults with a variety of disabilities. Ages 7-21. Campers experience a variety of traditional summer camp activities, including climbing wall, swimming, boating, hiking, and sports.

1302 **VISIONS Vacation Camp for the Blind (VCB)**
VISIONS Center on Blindness
111 Summit Park Rd.
Spring Valley, NY 10977
845-354-3003
888-245-8333
info@visionsvcb.org
www.visionsvcb.org

Krystal Findley-Jones, Director

A nonprofit agency that promotes the independence of people of all ages who are blind or visually impaired. Camp offers Braille classes, computers with large print and voice output, support groups, discussions, cooking classes, personal and home management training, and large print and Braille books.

1303 **Wagon Road Camp**
Children's Aid Society
117 W 124th St.
3rd Floor
New York, NY 10027
212-949-4800
www.childrensaidnyc.org

Phoebe Boyer, President & CEO
Vince Canziani, Camp Director

Wagon Road Day Camp is a co-ed program for children ages 6-13 with a variety of disabilities held in Chappaqua, New York. Activities include athletics, horsemanship, theater arts, nature studies, and arts and crafts.

1304 **West Hills Day Camp**
21 Sweet Hollow Rd.
Huntington, NY 11743
631-427-6700
Fax: 631-427-6504
info@westhillscamp.com
westhillsdaycamp.com

Susan Diamond, Director
Kimberly Doxey, Director

A summer day camp program for children with autism spectrum disorders an other related neurobiological disorders. Located on Long Island, activities include swimming, climbing/ropes course, photography, arts and crafts, and more.

1305 **YMCA Camp Chingachgook on Lake George**
Capital District YMCA
1872 Pilot Knob Rd.
Kattskill Bay, NY 12844
518-656-9462
Fax: 518-656-9362
chingachgook@cdymca.org
www.lakegeorgecamp.org

Jine Andreozzi, Executive Director
Mike Obermayer, Director, Summer Program
Carol Lewis, Office Manager

Offers sailing programs for people with disabilities.

North Carolina

1306 **Camp Carefree**
275 Carefree Lane
Stokesdale, NC 27357
336-427-0966
directors@campcarefree.org
www.campcarefree.org

Diane Samelak, Executive Director
Tony McCallum, Program Director
JeNai Davis, Program Director
A free, one-week camp for children with chronic illnesses. The camp also offers programs for siblings of ill children and children with a sick parent.

1307 **Camp Carolina Trails**
American Diabetes Association
1300 Baxter St.
Suite 150
Charlotte, NC 28204
704-373-9111
campsupport@diabetes.org
www.diabetes.org

1308 **Camp Dogwood**
7062 Camp Dogwood Dr.
PO Box 39
Sherrills Ford, NC 28673
828-478-2135
tammy@nclionsinc.org
nclionscampdogwood.org

Tammy Thomas, Camp Administrator
A recreational facility on Lake Norman offering 10 week-long sessions for adults who are blind and visually impaired. Ages 18 and up. Activities include swimming, tubing, local field trips, bowling, and more. Service dogs welcome.

1309 **Camp New Hope**
PO Box 154
Glendale Springs, NC 28629
336-982-3797
campnewhopenc.com

Randy Brown, Executive Director
Camp New Hope is a privately owned facility for children with life-threatening medical conditions and their families. Families are able to enjoy fishing, canoeing, tubing, swimming, and more at their leisure.

1310 **Camp Royall**
250 Bill Ash Rd.
Moncure, NC 27559
919-542-1033
Fax: 919-533-5324
camproyall@autismsociety-nc.org
www.autismsociety-nc.org/camp-royall

Sara Gage, Director
A week-long overnight and day camp for children and adults with autism. Campers participate in traditional camp activities such as swimming, boating, hiking, and arts and crafts. Counselor-to-camper ratio is 1:1 or 1:2, depending on the campers' needs.

1311 **Camp Sertoma**
Millstone 4-H Center
1296 Mallard Dr.
Ellerbe, NC 28338
sertomadeafcamp@gmail.com
www.campsertomaclub.org

Sandy Waterman, Contact
Keith Russell, Camp Director, Millstone 4-H Center
Camp Sertoma is a camp program for deaf and hard of hearing youth. Activities include swimming, canoeing, fishing, hiking, hayrides, campfires, and games. Coed, ages 8-16.

1312 **Camp Tekoa**
United Methodist Camp Tekoa
PO Box 1793
Flat Rock, NC 28731-1793
828-692-6516
Fax: 828-697-3288
www.camptekoa.org

John Isley, Executive Director
Dave Bollen, Assistant Director
Karen Rohrer, Business Manager
Melisa Coates, Administrative Assistant
Offers special needs camp programs for individuals with developmental disabilities.

1313 **SOAR Summer Adventures**
226 SOAR Lane
PO Box 388
Balsam, NC 28707
828-456-3435
Fax: 801-820-3050
admissions@soarnc.org
www.soarnc.org

John Willson, Executive Director
A nonprofit adventure program working with disadvantaged youth diagnosed with learning disabilities in an outdoor, challenge-based environment. Focuses on esteem building and social skills development through rock climbing, backpacking, whitewater rafting, mountaineering, sailing, snorkeling, and more. Offers two week, one month, and semester programs. Locations include North Carolina, Florida, Wyoming, California, New York, Belize, Costa Rica, and the Caribbean.

1314 **Talisman Summer Camp**
64 Gap Creek Rd.
Zirconia, NC 28790
828-697-6313
info@talismancamps.com
www.talismancamps.com

Linda Tatsapaugh, Operations Director & Owner
Robiyn Mims, Admissions Director & Owner
Cory Greene, Camp Director
Talisman Summer Camp is located 40 minutes south of Asheville, North Carolina. Offers a program of hiking, rafting, climbing, and caving for young people with autism, ADHD and learning disabilities. Coed, ages 6-22.

1315 **Victory Junction**
4500 Adam's Way
Randleman, NC 27317
336-498-9055
info@victoryjunction.org
www.victoryjunction.org

Chad Coltrane, President & CEO
Lisa Weber, Chief Financial Officer
Frances Beasley, Chief Development Officer
Jonathan Lemmon, Chief Operating Officer
The camp serves children with a variety of chronic medical conditions or serious illnesses, including Autism, Cancer, Craniofacial Anomalies, Diabetes, Sickle Cell, Spina Bifida and more. Victory Junction provides traditional camp activities and also includes a NASCAR themed area.

North Dakota

1316 **Camp Sioux**
American Diabetes Association
106 Solid Rock Circle
Park River, ND 58270
763-593-5333
campsupport@diabetes.org
www.diabetes.org

Ohio

1317 **Camp Arye**
Jewish Community Center of Greater Columbus
1125 College Ave.
Columbus, OH 43209
614-231-2731
Fax: 614-231-8222
www.columbusjcc.org

Raeann Cronebach, Director
Ariana Solomon, Inclusion Coordinator
A Jewish summer camp for children and young adults with developmental, physical, emotional, mental and learning disabilities. Camp Arye is co-ed and for children in grades 1-7.

1318 **Camp Cheerful**
Achievement Centers For Children
15000 Cheerful Lane
Strongsville, OH 44136-5420
440-238-6200
Fax: 440-238-1858
www.achievementcenters.org

Sally Farwell, President & CEO
Scott Peplin, Executive Vice President & CFO
Deborah Osgood, Vice President, Development & Marketing
Maureen Davis, Program Contact

Camp Cheerful provides a number of day and overnight camping options for children and adults who have disabilities. The camp hosts traditional camp activities as well as year-round therapeutic horseback riding sessions and an accessible high ropes challenge course during the summer. The focus of activities is to increase the quality of life while encouraging confidence and independence.

1319 **Camp Christopher: SumFun Day Camp**
Catholic Charities Disability Services
Camp Christopher
930 N Hametown Rd.
Akron, OH 44333
330-376-2267
800-296-2267
campchristopher@ccdocle.org
ccdocle.org/programs/sumfun-day-camp

Tess Flannery, Contact

A multi-week summer day camp for children, teens, and young adults ages 5-21 with developmental disabilities. Campers participate in regular camp activities while building confidence and social skills.

1320 **Camp Echoing Hills**
36272 County Rd. 79
Warsaw, OH 43844
740-327-2311
www.ehvi.org

Lauren Unger, Camp Administrator

Summer camp for children and adults with physical, intellectual and developmental disabilities. The camp focuses on religion, social interaction, and skill development.

1321 **Camp Emanuel**
PO Box 752343
Dayton, OH 45475
937-477-5504
crawford@campemanuel.org
www.campemanuel.weebly.com

Brian Demarke, President
Stephanie Ackner, Vice President
Mary Foreman, Secretary
Nan Crawford, Executive Director

Camp Emanuel is a camp for hearing impaired and hearing youth. There are day sessions for children 5-14 and overnight resident sessions for children and teens 9-17. The camp aims to promote descision making, self-esteem, and acceptance by integrating non-hearing children with hearing children.

1322 **Camp Hamwi**
LifeCare Alliance - Central Ohio Diabetes Assoc.
1699 West Mound St.
Columbus, OH 43223
614-278-3130
amyer@lifecarealliance.org
www.lifecarealliance.org

Anthony Myer, Director, Youth & Family Program

A summer camp for kids with diabetes, ages 7-17. Sessions are divided by age group, with a Junior Challenge Week for ages 7-12 and a Senior Challenged week for ages 13-17. Activities include horseback riding, sports, swimming, and other outdoor activities.

1323 **Camp Happiness**
Catholic Charities Disability Services
7911 Detroit Ave.
Cleveland, OH 44102
216-334-2900
Fax: 216-334-2905
ccdocle.org/programs/camp-happiness

Marilyn Scott, Director
Lauren Mailey, Program Administrator

Camp Happiness welcomes children and young adults ages 5-21 with intellectual and developmental disabilities. In addition to recreational services, Camp Happiness also provides educational and social services to help participants continue to practice and develop skills throughout the year.

1324 **Camp Ho Mita Koda**
14040 Auburn Rd.
Newbury, OH 44065
440-739-4095
info@camphomitakoda.org
www.camphomitakoda.org

Ian Roberts, Executive Director
Eric Brown, Camp Director

Camp Ho Mita Koda is a summer camp for children with type 1 diabetes. The camp aims to provide outdoor activities while also educating and building life skills for children with diabetes. Offers overnight camp, family camp, specialty camp, and leadership development programs.

1325 **Camp Joy**
10117 Old 3C Hwy.
PO Box 157
Clarksville, OH 45113
937-289-2031
info@camp-joy.org
camp-joy.org

Jen Eismeier, Executive Director
Casey Miller, Director, Operations
Jen Alvis, Director, Business Operations
Erin Policinski, Camp Director

A summer camp organization for children and teens with a variety of disabilities. Sessions for children, teens and young adults with asthma, HIV/AIDS, spina bifida, limb loss, cancer, blood diseases, and immune disorders.

1326 **Camp Ko-Man-She**
Diabetes Dayton
2555 S Dixie Dr.
Suite 112
Dayton, OH 45409
937-220-6611
Fax: 937-224-0240
admin@diabetesdayton.org
www.diabetesdaytoncamp.com

Susan McGovern, Executive Director

Camp Ko-Man-She is located in Bellefontaine, Ohio, and is held annually for children with diabetes. The camp's goal is for children to socialize with other children who also have diabetes and to have fun outdoors in a medically supervised setting. Co-ed, ages 8-17.

1327 **Camp Korelitz**
American Diabetes Association
Camp Joy
10117 Old 3C Hwy.
Clarksville, OH 45113
513-759-9330
campsupport@diabetes.org
www.diabetes.org

1328 **Camp Nuhop**
1077 Township Rd. 2916
Perrysville, OH 44864
419-938-7151
www.nuhop.org

Trevor Dunlap, Executive Director & CEO
Chris Clyde, Associate Director
Matt Poland, Director, Outdoor Education
Katelyn Seroka, Director, Summer Camp & Respite Programs

A summer residential program for youth ages 6-18 with learning disabilities, behavioral disorders, or other neuroatypical disorders. Activities include outdoor education and team-building workshops. The staff-to-camper ratio is 3:7 or 3:8.

1329 **Camp Oty'Okwa**
24799 Purcell Rd.
South Bloomingville, OH 43152-9740
740-385-5279
rperkins@bbbscentralohio.org
campotyokwa.org

Rick Perkins, Camp Director
Matt Smith, Youth Camp Director
Emily Kridel, Environmental Education Director
Rachel Gratz, Life Skills Director

Owned and operated by Big Brothers Big Sisters of Central Ohio, this summer camp accommodates children with disabilities such as ADD/ADHD, autism, learning disabilities, and behavioral or mood disorders.

1330 **Camp Paradise**
SHC, The Arc of Medina County
4283 Paradise Rd.
Seville, OH 44273
330-722-1900
shc@shc-medina.org
shc-medina.org/camp-paradise
Melanie Kasten-Krause, Executive Director
Shelly Wharton, Associate Executive Director
Michael Beh, Director, Finance
Jennifer Roman Anzalone, Director, Development & Community Relations
Camp Paradise is a summer camp for adults with developmental disabilities. The camp offers five weeks of themed programs. Day and residential camp available. Activities include music, art therapy, sports, swimming, bonfires, and more.

1331 **Camp Quality Ohio**
PO Box 358
Uniontown, OH 44685
234-738-2073
ohio@campqualityusa.org
www.campqualityusa.org/oh
Sarah Givens, Executive Director
Brian Krebs, Camp Director
Kelly Krebs, Camper Registrar
Katelyn Koppelberger, Program Coordinator
Camp Quality is for children with cancer and their siblings. The camp offers a stress-free environment that offers exciting activities and fosters new friendships, while helping to give the children courage, motivation and emotional strength.

1332 **Camp Stepping Stone**
Stepping Stones Inc. - Given Campus
5650 Given Rd.
Cincinnati, OH 45243
513-831-4660
Fax: 513-831-5918
steppingstonesohio.org
Chris Adams, Executive Director
Sam Allen, Director, Programs & Operations
Chris Brockman, Director, Facilities
Kelly Crow, Director, Development
A summer day camp program for youth with disabilities, ages 5-22. Activities include swimming, fishing, art, and music. Three separate three-week sessions are available. The camp is located at the Stepping Stones Given Campus in Cincinnati, Ohio.

1333 **Camp Tiponi**
Diabetes Dayton
2555 S Dixie Dr.
Suite 112
Dayton, OH 45409
937-220-6611
Fax: 937-224-0240
admin@diabetesdayton.org
www.diabetesdaytoncamp.com
Susan McGovern, Executive Director
A summer camp for youth with type 2 diabetes, prediabetes, or metabolic disorders. Campers participate in activities such as swimming, archery, hiking, and sports while gaining education and skills needed to maintain a healthy lifestyle. The camp is located at Camp Willson in Bellefontaine, Ohio.

1334 **Courageous Acres**
Courageous Community Services
12701 Waterville Swanton Rd.
Whitehouse, OH 43571
419-875-6828
Fax: 419-875-5598
info@ccsohio.org
www.ccsohio.org
Laura Kuhlenbeck, Executive Director
Courageous Acres is an accessible summer camp for children, teens, and adults with disabilities. Open to individuals ages 4+ in Northwest Ohio and Southeast Michigan.

1335 **Flying Horse Farms**
5260 State Route 95
Mt. Gilead, OH 43338
419-751-7077
Fax: 419-751-7010
info@flyinghorsefarms.org
flyinghorsefarms.org
Nichole E. Dunn, President & CEO
Rachel Escusa, Chief Advancement Officer
Stacey Kyser, Director, Development
Susan Murray, Director, Finance
Flying Horse Farms is a camp for children with serious illnesses, ages 7-15, and their families. The camp serves campers diagnosed with cancer, heart conditions, asthma, blood disorders, and more. Activities include swimming, fishing, and other traditional camp activities.

1336 **Highbrook Lodge**
Cleveland Sight Center
1909 E 101st St.
Cleveland, OH 44106
216-791-8118
Fax: 216-791-1101
TTY: 216-791-8119
info@clevelandsightcenter.org
www.clevelandsightcenter.org
Larry Benders, President & CEO
Kevin Krencisz, Chief Financial & Administrative Officer
Jassen Tawil, Director, Business Development & Customer Success
Ali Thomas, Director, Human Resources
Camp is located in Chardon, Ohio. Summer sessions for children, adults and families who are blind or have low vision. Sessions include a wide range of outdoor camp activities. Camp activities focus on gaining independent skills, mobility, orientation and self-confidence in an accessible and traditional camp setting.

1337 **Insight Horse Camp**
Marmon Valley
7754 State Route 292 S
Zanesfield, OH 43360
937-593-8000
Fax: 937-593-6900
info@marmonvalley.com
marmonvalley.com
Matt Wiley, Executive Director
A coed resident camp program for children who are blind or visually impaired. The main focus of camp is on learning basic horsemanship skills. Campers also participate in traditional camp activities and Bible study discussions.

1338 **Recreation Unlimited: Day Camp**
Recreation Unlimited Foundation
7700 Piper Rd.
Ashley, OH 43003
740-548-7006
Fax: 740-747-2640
info@recreationunlimited.org
www.recreationunlimited.org
Paul L. Huttlin, Executive Director & CEO
Sarah Kelley, Camps Director
Camping sessions for children and teens, ages 5-22, with physical or developmental disabilities and their siblings. The camp provides a full day of traditional camp activities and aims to create an inclusive experience for all participants.

1339 **Recreation Unlimited: Residential Camp**
Recreation Unlimited Foundation
7700 Piper Rd.
Ashley, OH 43003
740-548-7006
Fax: 740-747-2640
info@recreationunlimited.org
www.recreationunlimited.org
Paul L. Huttlin, Executive Director & CEO
Sarah Kelley, Camps Director
Camping sessions for children and adults with a variety of physical and developmental disabilities. Two week long sessions for ages 8-22, one week long session for ages 18-35, and four week long sessions for ages 23 and up. The camp provides traditional outdoor recreation such as fishing, archery, exploration, campfires and more. A week long winter camp is offered for ages 18 and up.

1340 **Recreation Unlimited: Respite Weekend Camp**
Recreation Unlimited Foundation
7700 Piper Rd.
Ashley, OH 43003
740-548-7006
Fax: 740-747-2640
info@recreationunlimited.org
www.recreationunlimited.org

Paul L. Huttlin, Executive Director & CEO
Sarah Kelley, Camps Director

Camping sessions for children and adults with a variety of physical and developmental disabilities. There are seven weekend camps for youth ages 8-22 and eight weekend camps for adults ages 23 and up. Traditional outdoor activities are provided, along with lodging, meals, site nursing, and more.

1341 **Recreation Unlimited: Specialty Camp**
Recreation Unlimited Foundation
7700 Piper Rd.
Ashley, OH 43003
740-548-7006
Fax: 740-747-2640
info@recreationunlimited.org
www.recreationunlimited.org

Paul L. Huttlin, Executive Director & CEO
Sarah Kelley, Camps Director

Weekend and week-long camping sessions for youth and adults. The camps are dedicated to a specific disability or health concern and designed to meet the needs of certain groups.

1342 **Rotary Camp**
Rotary Club of Akron
4460 Rex Lake Dr.
Akron, OH 44319
330-644-4512
Fax: 330-644-1013
danr@akronymca.org
www.akronrotary.org

Dan Reynolds, Camp Director

Offers camping experiences for children and adults with disabilities. Rotary Camp provides traditional camping experiences while focusing on socialization and independence.

1343 **St. Augustine Rainbow Camp**
Disability Ministries at St. Augustine Parish
2486 W 14th St.
Cleveland, OH 44113
216-781-5530
Fax: 216-781-1124
TTY: 216-302-2375
augustine.rainbow.camp@gmail.com
www.staugustinecleveland.org

Rev. William O'Donnell, Administrator

Day camp for disabled and non-disabled youth ages 5-13. The camp serves youth from the deaf, hard-of-hearing, blind, and developmentally disabled communities of Greater Cleveland, as well as youth from the Tremont area.

1344 **Stepping Stones: Camp Allyn**
Stepping Stones Inc. - Allyn Campus
1414 Lake Allyn Rd.
Batavia, OH 45103
513-831-4660
Fax: 513-831-5918
steppingstonesohio.org

Chris Adams, Executive Director
Sam Allen, Director, Programs & Operations
Chris Brockman, Director, Facilities
Kelly Crow, Director, Development

An overnight residential camp for children and adults with disabilities. Coed, ages 16-65. Campers participate in crafts, swimming, hiking, and sports activities. The camp session lasts five days and is located at the Stepping Stones Allyn Campus in Batavia, Ohio.

1345 **YMCA Outdoor Center Campbell Gard**
4803 Augspurger Rd.
Hamilton, OH 45011
513-867-0600
Fax: 513-867-0127
campoffice@gmvymca.org
www.ccgymca.org

Pete Fasano, Executive Director

The camp is located in Hamilton, Ohio. Offers camp programs for youth with developmental disabilities. Runs overnight and day sessions for ages 7-22 and families.

Oklahoma

1346 **Camp CANOE**
Camp Fire Heart of Oklahoma
3309 E Hefner Rd.
Oklahoma City, OK 73131
405-478-5646
info@campfirehok.org
www.campfirehok.org

Penn Henthorn, Director, Programs & Camps

Camp CANOE is a summer day camp for children with autism and Down Syndrome. Camp CANOE focuses on skills such as self-reliance, confidence, communication, social skills, problem-solving, and more.

1347 **Camp ClapHans**
J.D. McCarty Center
2002 E Robinson St.
Norman, OK 73071
405-307-2865
camp@jdmc.org
www.campclaphans.com

Bobbie Hunter, Camp Director

A summer camp for children, teens, and young adults ages 8-18 with developmental disabilities. Activities include archery, arts and crafts, scavenger hunts, stargazing, and more. Sessions are four days and three nights, and are limited to 12 campers per session (6 boys and 6 girls).

1348 **Camp Endres**
Diabetes Solutions of Oklahoma, Inc.
3333 NW 63rd
Suite 100
Oklahoma City, OK 73116
405-843-4386
Fax: 888-665-2741
natalie@dsok.net
dsok.net/programs/camp-endres-day-camp

Kim Boaz-Wilson, Executive Director
Natalie Bayne, Camp Director

Camp Endres is a summer camp for individuals with diabetes. Programs include Day Camp (ages 4-10), Junior (ages 7-13), Senior (ages 14-18), Adult (ages 21+), and Family Camp sessions.

1349 **Camp Lo-Be-Gon**
American Diabetes Association
5401 S Harvard
Suite 120
Tulsa, OK 74135
918-492-3839
Fax: 918-492-4262
campsupport@diabetes.org
www.diabetes.org

1350 **Camp Loughridge**
4900 W 71st St.
Tulsa, OK 74131
918-446-4194
registrar@camploughridge.org
camploughridge.org

Jacob McIntosh, Executive Director
Loren Pirtle, Program Director

Camp Loughridge is a Christian summer day camp for children ages 6-10. The camp offers an Autism Inclusion program for children diagnosed with austism. Space is limited to two campers with autism per session.

1351 **Camp Perfect Wings**
Baptist General Convention of Oklahoma
3800 N May Ave.
Oklahoma City, OK 73112
405-942-3800
www.oklahomabaptists.org

Becka Johnson, Camp Director

Camp program for children and adults with special needs, ages 8 and up. Activities include canoeing, pool games, low ropes challenges, and crafts. Held in spring/early summer.

Oregon

1352 **Adventures Without Limits**
1341 Pacific Ave.
Forest Grove, OR 97116
503-359-2568
Fax: 503-359-4671
info@awloutdoors.org
awloutdoors.com
Brad Bafaro, Founder & Executive Director
Jennifer Wilde, Director, Outreach & Development
Carrie Morton, Program Director
Adventures Without Limits facilitates inclusive outdoor adventures for people of all ages and ability levels. Trip activities include hiking, rafting, caving, rock climbing, kayaking, snowshoeing, and more.

1353 **B'nai B'rith Camp: Kehila Program**
6443 SW Beaverton-Hillsdale Hwy.
Suite 234
Portland, OR 97221
503-496-7444
Fax: 503-452-0750
info@bbcamp.org
bbcamp.org
Michelle Koplan, Chief Executive Officer
Ben Charlton, Chief Program Officer
Bette Amir-Brownstein, Camp Director
Rikki Nouri, Director, Community Care & Inclusion
The Kehila Program at B'nai B'rith Camp is a Jewish summer camp program for children with special needs. This program is run during the camp's Maccabee session.

1354 **Camp Magruder**
17450 Old Pacific Hwy.
Rockaway Beach, OR 97136
503-355-2310
Fax: 503-355-8701
troy@campmagruder.org
www.campmagruder.org
Troy Taylor, Camp Director
Hope Montgomery, Program Director
Rik Gutzke, Facilities Manager
Camp is located in Rockaway Beach, Oregon. Sessions for teens and adults with developmental disabilities through Camp Hope.

1355 **Camp Meadowood Springs**
77650 Meadowood Rd.
Weston, OR 97886
541-276-2752
Fax: 541-276-7227
camp@meadowoodsprings.org
www.meadowoodsprings.org
Michelle Nelson, Camp Director
This camp is designed to help children with communication disorders and learning differences. A full range of activities in recreational and clinical areas is available.

1356 **Camp Millennium**
2880 NW Stewart Pkwy.
Suite 200
Roseburg, OR 97471
541-677-0600
campmoregon@gmail.com
campmillennium.org
Mindy Bean, Camp Director
Steve Maine, Program Director
A week-long residential summer camp for children diagnosed with cancer, ages 5-16. The camp is free to attend, and activities include hiking, archery, horeseback riding, and more.

1357 **Camp Starlight**
PO Box 13107
Portland, OR 97213
503-964-1516
info@camp-starlight.org
camp-starlight.org
Melanie Smith-Wilusz, Camp Director
Kit Noble, Operations Director
Spike Huntington-Kline, Program Director
Jessica Retan, Mental Health Director
Camp Starlight is a week-long sleep-away summer camp for children in Oregon and Washington whose lives are affected by HIV/AIDS. There is a 1:1 staff-to-camper ratio. Activities include swimming, hiking, arts and crafts, archery, sports, and games. The camp is free to attend.

1358 **Camp Taloali**
15934 N Santiam Hwy. SE
PO Box 32
Stayton, OR 97383
503-400-6547
campadmin@taloali.org
www.taloali.org
Randall Smith, Camp Administrator
Summer sessions for children who are deaf, hard of hearing, or have a hearing impairment. Camp Taloali emphasizes communication, leadership, and social development.

1359 **Camp Ukandu**
601 SW 2nd Ave.
Suite 2300
Portland, OR 97204
503-276-2178
info@ukandu.org
www.ukandu.org
Jason Hickox, Executive Director
Ashley Light, Development Director
Kendra Gish, Program Director
Sage Nicholson, Development Coordinator
Camp Ukandu is a summer camp for children and teens with cancer, ages 8-18, and their siblings. Activities include campfires, horseback riding, rock walls, and more. The camp is free to attend.

1360 **Creating Memories**
Creating Memories for Disabled Children
59895 Pollock Rd.
Joseph, OR 97846
541-398-0169
cmfdc777@yahoo.com
creatingmemoriesfordisabledchildren.com
Ken Coreson, Founder
Creating Memories for Disabled Children is a camp for children and adults with disabilities. The camp's goal is to connect individuals with disabilities to nature. The camp offers a variety of outdoor activities, including hiking and fishing. Attendance is free.

1361 **Easterseals Oregon Summer Camp**
Easterseals Oregon
7300 SW Hunziker St.
Suite 103
Portland, OR 97223
503-228-5108
Fax: 503-228-1352
www.easterseals.com/oregon
Carol Salter, President & CEO
A camp program for children with disabilities. Activities include boating and fishing, swimming, horseback riding, arts and crafts, archery, sports and recreation, outdoor education, and campfires.

1362 **Gales Creek Diabetes Camp**
Gales Creek Camp Foundation
6950 SW Hampton St.
Suite 242
Tigard, OR 97223
503-968-2267
Fax: 503-992-6785
office@galescreekcamp.org
www.galescreekcamp.org
Robert Dailey, Executive Director
Maddie Ehl, Office & Programming Manager
Camp is located in Gales Creek, Oregon. Summer sessions for children with Type 1 diabetes. Coed and family and pre-school family camps also available. Gales Creek also helps teach campers about testing themselves, giving injections, and how to manage their own bodies.

1363 **Hull Park and Retreat Center**
Oral Hull Foundation for the Blind
43233 SE Oral Hull Rd.
PO Box 157
Sandy, OR 97055
503-668-6195
oralhull@gmail.com
oralhull.org
Kerith Vance, Executive Director
The Oral Hull Foundation for the Blind provides recreational, educational, and social activities programs designed to fit the needs of guests with vision loss. Programs include week-long summer and winter retreats and three-night getaways for adults with vision impairments.

1364 **Mt Hood Kiwanis Camp**
10725 SW Barbur Blvd.
Suite 50
Portland, OR 97219
503-452-7416
info@mhkc.org
www.mhkc.org

Dave McDonald, Executive Director
Allan Cushing, Director, Operations
Skye Burns, Director, Development & Communications
Kayla Plessinger, Director, Programs
Camp is located in Government Camp, Oregon. Summer sessions for children and adults with a variety of disabilities. Coed, ages 12 and up. Family and off-site adventure programs available.

1365 **Strength for the Journey**
Oregon-Idaho Conference UMC - Camp Registrar
1505 SW 18th Ave.
Portland, OR 97201
503-802-9214
registrar@gocamping.org
suttlelake.gocamping.org

Daniel Petke, Co-Director, Suttle Lake Camp
Jane Petke, Co-Director, Suttle Lake Camp
Camp is located near Sisters, Oregon at Suttle Lake Camp. Strength for the Journey is a program for adults living with HIV/AIDS.

1366 **Suttle Lake Camp**
29551 Suttle Lake Rd.
Sisters, OR 97759
541-595-6663
suttlelake@gocamping.org
suttlelake.gocamping.org

Daniel Petke, Co-Director
Jane Petke, Co-Director
Offers a variety of camp programs, including sessions for individuals with HIV/AIDS.

1367 **Upward Bound Camp**
40151 Gates School Rd.
Gates, OR 97346
503-897-2447
Fax: 503-897-4116
camp@upwardboundcamp.org
www.upwardboundcamp.org

Diane Turnbull, Executive Director
Upward Bound Camp is a Christian camp for children and adults with a variety of disabilities, ages 12 and up.

Pennsylvania

1368 **Aces Adventure Weekend**
Camp Hebron
957 Camp Hebron Rd.
Halifax, PA 17032
412-281-7244
www.easterseals.com/wcpenna

James G. Bennett, President & CEO
A weekend respite program for youth with high-functioning Austism, ages 11-22. Activities include canoeing, rock climbing, and cooking. The camp takes place at Camp Hebron in Halifax, Pennsylvania.

1369 **Camp AIM**
YMCA of Greater Pittsburgh
680 Andersen Dr.
Suite 400
Pittsburgh, PA 15220
412-227-3800
campaiminfo@gmail.com
www.ycamps.org/camp-aim

Kevin Bolding, President & CEO
Angela Schuettler, Chief Financial Officer
Carolyn Grady, Chief Development Officer
Greg Swetoha, Chief Operating Officer
Camp AIM is a 6-week summer program for children, teens, and young adults with physical, cognitive, social/communication, and emotional/behavioral disabilities. The program combines life skills and social and recreational activities with music, art, physical education, and more. Ages 3-21.

1370 **Camp Achieva**
711 Bingham St.
Pittsburgh, PA 15203
412-995-5000
888-272-7229
Fax: 412-995-5001
cscuilli@achieva.info
www.achieva.info

Stephen H. Suroviec, President & CEO
Cathy Scuilli, Camp Director
Achieva provides life-long services such as early intervention therapies, in-home support, older adult protective services, and more, to individuals with disabilities. Offers summer day camp programs for youth up to age 21 with intellectual disabilities. The camp is located in Monaca, Pennsylvania.

1371 **Camp Akeela**
Camp Akeela Winter Address
314 Bryn Mawr Ave.
Bala Cynwyd, PA 19004
866-680-4744
Fax: 866-462-2828
www.campakeela.com

Eric Sasson, Camp Director
Debbie Sasson, Camp Director
Ben Jerez, Staffing Director
Rob Glyn-Jones, Assistant Director
Camp Akeela is a co-ed, overnight camp for children and young adults ages 9-17 who have been diagnosed with Asperger's Syndrome or a non-verbal learning disability. The camp is located in Thetford Center, Vermont.

1372 **Camp Amp**
Easterseals Western & Central Pennsylvania, York
2550 Kingston Rd.
Suite 219
York, PA 17402
717-741-3891
Fax: 717-741-5359
www.easterseals.com/wcpenna

James G. Bennett, President & CEO
Dane Schick, Director, Camping & Recreation
Camp Amp is an overnight summer camp for children ages 7-17 with any disability or special need. The camp offers a mini session and a full week session. Activities include talent shows, sports, swimming, ropes course, hiking, and more. Camp Amp's goal is to foster independence and encourage socialization.

1373 **Camp Can Do**
Administrative Office
3 Unami Trail
Chalfont, PA 18914
717-273-6525
campcandoforever.org

Tom Prader, Director, Patient Camp
Stephanie Cole, Director, Patient Camp
Caitlyn McLarnon, Director, Sibling Camp
Camp Can Do is for children ages 8-17 who have been diagnosed with cancer in the last five years. The camp also offers a session for siblings of children with cancer.

1374 **Camp Courage**
American Diabetes Association
YMCA Camp Soles
134 Camp Soles Ln.
Rockwood, PA 15557
412-824-1181
campsupport@diabetes.org
www.diabetes.org

1375 **Camp Discovery**
American Academy of Dermatology
PO Box 1968
Des Plaines, IL 60017
847-240-1280
866-503-7546
888-462-3376
Fax: 847-240-1859
www.campdiscovery.org

1376 **Camp Freedom**
American Diabetes Association
150 Monument Rd.
Suite 100
Bala Cynwyd, PA 19004
610-828-5003
campsupport@diabetes.org
www.diabetes.org

1377 **Camp Hot-to-Clot**
National Hemophilia Foundation - Western PA
20411 Route 19
Unit 14
Cranberry Township, PA 16066-7512
724-741-6160
Fax: 724-741-6167
www.hemophilia.org

Brittani Spencer, President
Kara Dornish, Executive Director

Camp Hot-to-Clot is a summer camp for children ages 7-17 with bleeding disorders and their siblings. The camp is held at Camp Kon-O-Kwee in Fombell, PA. Activities include rock climbing, arts and crafts, field games, and more.

1378 **Camp Lee Mar**
Winter Address
805 Redgate Rd.
Dresher, PA 19025
215-658-1708
Fax: 215-658-1710
ari@leemar.com
www.leemar.com

Ari Segal, Director
Lynsey Trohoske, Assistant Director
Laura Leibowitz, Assistant Director

Seven week summer camp for children and young adults ages 7-21 with developmental, learning, communication, and other disabilities. The camp incorporates an Academic and Speech program with traditional camp activities.

1379 **Camp Lily Lehigh Valley**
Easterseals Eastern Pennsylvania
1501 Lehigh St.
Suite 201
Allentown, PA 18103
610-289-0114
camp@esep.org
www.easterseals.com/esep

Nancy Knoebel, President & CEO
Janine Noel, Camp Director

Camp Lily is a week-long day camp for children and young adults with a variety of disabilities. Coed, ages 8-21. The camp offers a variety of traditional camp activities and field trips so that campers can enhance their social skills and increase their independence. The camp takes place on the campus of Cedar Crest College.

1380 **Camp Orchard Hill**
640 Orange Rd.
Dallas, PA 18612
570-333-4098
Fax: 570-333-4058
office@camporchardhill.com
www.camporchardhill.com

Jim Payne, Executive Director
Derek Hodne, Program Director
Matt Chase, Facilities Director
Lauren Hodne, Office Manager

Camp Orchard Hill provides day and overnight summer camps for ages 4-17. The camp is inclusive to children with mild to moderate special needs. Special needs campers participate alongside non-disabled campers in a multitude of outdoor activities.

1381 **Camp Ramah in the Poconos**
2100 Arch St.
Philadelphia, PA 19103
215-885-8556
Fax: 215-885-8905
info@ramahpoconos.org
www.ramahpoconos.org

Rabbi Joel Seltzer, Executive Director
Rachel Dobbs Schwartz, Camp Director
Bruce I. Lipton, Director, Finance & Operations
Leah Schatz, Program Director

Camp Ramah is a Jewish summer camp that runs three separate programs for children with various disabilities and their families. There are two residential programs and one family program, the Tikvah Family Camp.

1382 **Camp STAR**
2504 Atlas St.
Pittsburgh, PA 15235
412-370-5481
www.chp.edu

Cindy McCue, Camp Director

A week-long summer camp for children and teens ages 8-18 who are amputees. The camp is held at the YMCA Camp Kon-O-Kwee in Fombell, Pennsylvania. Activities include arts and crafts, zip lining, canoeing, rock climbing, and more. Campers are also able to learn about prosthetics, physical and recreational therapy, and limb care.

1383 **Camp Setebaid**
Setebaid Services, Inc.
PO Box 196
Winfield, PA 17889-0196
570-524-9090
Fax: 570-523-0769
info@setebaidservices.org
www.setebaidservices.org

Mark Moyer, Executive Director

Camping sessions for children with diabetes. The camp also hosts a family day for children with diabetes and their families.

1384 **Camp Spencer Superstars**
YMCA Camp Kon-O-Kwee
126 Nagel Rd.
Fombell, PA 16123
724-758-6238
Fax: 724-758-2705
campkon-o-kwee@ymcapgh.org
www.ycampkok.org

Charlie Deer, Camp Director

An overnight respite camp for adults, ages 18 and up, with special needs. The camp is fully inclusive and aims to encourage campers to develop social and life skills. Campers have access to all activities and programs, such as canoeing, bonfires, swimming, and more.

1385 **Camp Victory**
58 Camp Victory Rd.
PO Box 810
Millville, PA 17846
570-458-6530
www.campvictory.org

Jamie Huntley, Executive Director
Kate Stepnick, Camp Director

Camp Victory provides camping opportunities for children with chronic health problems or physical or mental challenges.

1386 **Camp Wesley Woods: Exceptional Persons Camp**
1001 Fiddlersgreen Rd.
Grand Valley, PA 16420
814-436-7802
info@wesleywoods.com
www.wesleywoods.com

Emily Reed, Chair

The Exceptional Persons Camp is a camp program for individuals with disabilities. Activities include swimming, games, sports, crafts, and Bible study.

1387 **Camp Woodlands**
The Woodlands Foundation
134 Shenot Rd.
Wexford, PA 15090
724-935-6533
www.woodlandsfoundation.org

Samantha Ellwood, Executive Director
Denise Balkovec, Deputy Director, Advancement & Operations
Clarissa Amond, Program Manager
Rachel Clark, Administrative Manager

Camp Woodlands is a camp for youth, teens, and adults with varying disabilities and chronic illness. The camp runs a number of programs for children, teens, adults, and seniors.

1388 **Dragonfly Forest Summer Camp**
YMCA Camp Speers
143 Nichecronk Rd.
Dingmans Ferry, PA 18328
570-828-2329
Fax: 570-828-2984
campspeers@philaymca.org
www.dragonflyforest.org

1389 **Handi Camp**
Handi Vangelism Ministries International
PO Box 122
Akron, PA 17501-0122
717-859-4777
Fax: 717-721-7662
info@hvmi.org
www.hvmi.org

Tim Sheetz, Founder
Mark Amey, Assistant Director, Handi Camp
Brian Robinson, Office Manager, Handi Camp

Christian overnight camping program for people with disabilities, ages 9-50, in Eastern Pennsylvania. Sponsored by Handi Vangelism Ministries International.

1390 **Innabah Camps**
United Methodist Church: Eastern Pennsylvania
712 Pughtown Rd.
Spring City, PA 19475
610-469-6111
Fax: 610-469-0330
www.innabah.org

Michael Hyde, Director
Samantha Wagaman, Assistant Director
Gina James, Office Manager
Innabah Camps runs a number of sessions for children, teens, and adults with developmental disabilities. The Challenge camps are for ages 12 and up.

1391 **Mainstay Life Services Summer Program**
Mainstay Life Services
200 Roessler Rd.
Pittsburgh, PA 15220
412-344-3640
Fax: 412-344-5486
info@mainstaylifeservices.org
mainstaylifeservices.org

Kim Sonafelt, Chief Executive Officer
Barbara Dyer, Coordinator, Community Services
Mainstay Life Services' summer respite and recreation program offers one or two week sessions on a college campus in Pittsburgh, Pennsylvania. The program is open to adults age 18 and over who live with families and caregivers.

1392 **Outside In School Of Experiential Education, Inc.**
PO Box 639
Greensburg, PA 15601
724-837-1518
Fax: 724-837-0801
www.myoutsidein.org

Michael C. Henkel, Executive Director
Camp programs primarily focus on substance abuse, but some services are available for special needs related to school/work. Programs are for boys ages 13-18.

1393 **Phelps School Academic Support Program**
583 Sugartown Rd.
Malvern, PA 19355
610-644-1754
Fax: 610-540-0156
admis@thephelpsschool.org
www.thephelpsschool.org

Charles A. McGeorge, Head of School
The Phelps School is a college preparatory day and boarding school dedicated to the individual boy. They serve students in grades 6 through 12/PG in a supportive and structured environment. Their supplemental Academic Support Program offers small (4:1) courses in reading, writing, and mathematics, as well as introductions to history and science, for young men with diagnosed learning differences. Also features a dedicated Executive Functioning Skill resource center.

1394 **Sequanota Lutheran Conference Center and Camp**
PO Box 245
Jennerstown, PA 15547
814-629-6627
contact@sequanota.com
www.sequanota.com

Rev. Nathan Pile, Executive Director
Angie Pile, Director, Business Management
Ann Ferry, Director, Hospitality
Ron Druist, Director, Facilities
Runs Camp Bethesda, a summer camp for adults with developmental and intellectual disabilities. For ages 18 and up.

1395 **Variety Club Camp and Developmental Center**
2950 Potshop Rd.
PO Box 609
Worcester, PA 19490
610-584-4366
Fax: 610-584-5586
www.varietyphila.org

Dominique Bernardo, Chief Executive Officer
Nicholas Larcinese, Director, Programming
Kristin Podwojski, Director, Operations
Year-round camping and recreation facility for children with special needs and their families. Includes summer camping, aquatics, weekend retreats and other specialty programs. Coed, ages 5-21.

1396 **West Penn Burn Camp**
Allegheny Health Network
120 Fifth Ave.
Suite 2900
Pittsburgh, PA 15222
412-578-5295
www.ahn.org

Christine Perlick, Outreach Coordinator
Founded in 1986, West Penn Burn camp is a week-long overnight camp for children and teens, ages 7-17, who have burn injuries. The camp provides traditional camp activities as well as therapeutic services through the support and guidance of camp counselors. The camp is held at the YMCA Camp Kon-O-Kwee in Fombell, Pennsylvania.

1397 **YMCA Camp Fitch**
12600 Abels Rd.
North Springfield, PA 16430
814-922-3219
877-863-4824
Fax: 814-922-7000
registrar@campfitchymca.org
campfitchymca.org

Tom Parker, Executive Director
Joe Wolnik, Summer Camp Director
Brandy Duda, Outdoor Education Director
Hannah Kight, Office Manager
Camp is located in North Springfield, Pennsylvania. Camp programs include sessions for children with diabetes or epilepsy.

Rhode Island

1398 **Camp Mauchatea**
Rhode Island Lions Sight Foundation, Inc.
PO Box 19671
Johnston, RI 02919-0671
www.lions4sight.org
Robert P. Andrade, President
Earle U. Schahrff III, First Vice President
Steve Krohn, Secretary
Lisa M. Bartoshevich, Treasurer
Camp serving those who are blind/visually impaired. Campers enjoy developing and maintaining friendships with fellow campers. Some of the activities include boating and other water sports, as well as hiking and nature studies.

1399 **Camp Ruggles**
PO Box 353
Chepachet, RI 02814
401-567-8914
campruggles@gmail.com
www.campruggles.org

Jim Field, Executive Director
Ethan Roe, Assistant Director
Camp Ruggles is located in Glocester, RI and is a summer day camp for children with emotional and behavioral disabilities. The camp offers 240 hours of supervised therapeutic care for children ages 6-12.

1400 **Canonicus Camp & Conference Center**
54 Exeter Rd.
Exeter, RI 02822
401-294-6318
Fax: 401-294-7780
www.canonicus.org

Kathy Black, Director, Conferencing
Amanda Hosley, Director, Camping Ministries
Matt Black, Facilities Manager
Carolyn Lynch, Camp Registrar
Canonicus Camp offers camp and conference programs and facilities for children, adults, and groups with special needs. The camp is owned by the American Baptist Churches of Rhode Island.

1401 **Hasbro Children's Hospital Asthma Camp**
593 Eddy St.
Providence, RI 02903
401-444-8340
malsina@lifespan.org
www.hasbrochildrenshospital.org

Miosotis Alsina, Administrative Director
Camp for children with asthma, hosted by Canonicus Camp and Conference Center. Children learn about asthma and asthma management through interactive and educational activities. The camp

also offers activities such as swimming, canoeing, and arts and crafts. Coed, ages 9-13.

South Carolina

1402 **Burnt Gin Camp**
SC Department of Health and Environmental Control
2100 Bull St.
Columbia, SC 29201
803-898-0784
Fax: 803-898-0613
campburntgin@dhec.sc.gov
www.scdhec.gov
Marie Aimone, Camp Director
A residential camp for youth who have physical disabilities and/or chronic illnesses. Camp Burnt Gun runs four six-day sessions for children ages 7-15; two six-day sessions for teenagers ages 16-20; and one four-day session for young adults ages 21-25. The camp is held in Wedgefield, South Carolina.

1403 **Camp Adam Fisher**
PO Box 2543
Columbia, SC 29202-2543
campadamfisher@gmail.com
www.campadamfisher.com
Scott McFarland, Camp Director
Maria McGregor Mullendore, Assistant Camp Director
Katherine Lewis, Medical Director
A week-long overnight camp for children with diabetes and their siblings, ages 6-17. Campers enjoy swimming, horseback riding, tubing, basketball, volleyball, and arts and crafts, while also learning how to manage their diabetes so they can live longer, healthier lives.

1404 **Camp Courage**
Prisma Health Children's Hospital
900 W Faris Rd.
2nd Floor
Greenville, SC 29605
864-455-8898
Fax: 864-455-5164
www.ghschildrens.org/programs
Ericka Turner, Camp Director
Camp Courage is a non-profit organization that provides a summer camp experience for children and teens with cancer or blood disorders. Programs include week-long summer camps for children, weekend camp for siblings, fall carnival for patients and families, counselor training sessions, evening and weekend retreats, and monthly support groups. The camp is held at Pleasant Ridge Camp and Retreat Center.

1405 **Camp Debbie Lou**
726 Lucky Run
Latta, SC 29565
843-845-2617
Dean Richardson, Camp Director
For children between the ages of 4-14 who have been diagnosed with cancer and their families.

1406 **Camp Luv-A-Lung**
Prisma Health Children's Hospital
900 W Faris Rd.
2nd Floor
Greenville, SC 29605
864-455-8898
Fax: 864-455-5164
www.ghschildrens.org/programs
Jessica Herron, Contact
A summer camp for children ages 6-12 who have respiratory problems. The camp takes place at Pleasant Ridge Camp and Retreat Center in Marietta, South Carolina. Activities include swimming, archery, campfires, arts and crafts, and more.

1407 **Camp Spearhead**
Greenville County Recreation District
4806 Old Spartanburg Rd.
Taylors, SC 29687
864-467-3398
Fax: 864-288-6499
campspearhead@greenvillecounty.org
www.greenvillerec.com
Randy Murr, Therapeutic Recreation Manager
Camp for children with disabilities ages 8 and up. The camp is held at Pleasant Ridge Camp and Retreat Center in Marietta, South Carolina. Activities include canoeing, kayaking, swimming, archery, sports, and games.

South Dakota

1408 **Camp Friendship**
PO Box 1986
Rapid City, SD 57709-1986
www.campfriendshipsd.org

1409 **Camp Gilbert**
Camp Gilbert, Inc.
PO Box 89406
Sioux Falls, SD 57109-9406
605-610-8775
campgilbertinfo@gmail.com
www.campgilbert.com
Laura Parish, Camp Director
For children ages 8-18 with diabetes. Campers can enjoy a week of canoeing, swimming, sing-a-longs, crafts, and games, while also attending educational programs covering nutrition, exercise and lifestyle management.

1410 **NeSoDak**
Lutherans Outdoors in South Dakota
2001 S Summit Ave.
Sioux Falls, SD 57197
605-947-4440
800-888-1464
nesodak@losd.org
www.losd.org/nesodak
Vicki Foss, Director
Camp is located in Waubay, South Dakota. Hosts Camp Gilbert, a summer camp program for children with diabetes. Coed, ages 8-18.

Tennessee

1411 **ACM Lifting Lives Music Camp**
Vanderbilt Kennedy Center
110 Magnolia Circle
Nashville, TN 37203
615-322-8240
vkc.vumc.org
Jeffrey Neul, Director, IDDRC
Erik Carter, Co-Director, UCEDD
Elise McMillan, Co-Director, UCEDD
Zachary E. Warren, Executive Director, TRIAD
A camp for individuals with developmental disabilities where they can come to celebrate music by participating in songwriting workshops, recording sessions and live performances. For ages 18 and up. The program is specifically designed for people with Williams syndrome.

1412 **All Days Are Happy Days Summer Camp**
UTHSC Center on Developmental Disabilities
920 Madison Ave.
Suite 939
Memphis, TN 38103
901-448-6511
888-572-2249
Fax: 901-448-3844
TTY: 901-448-4677
www.uthsc.edu/cdd
Bruce Keisling, Executive Director
Week long camp for children ages 6-11 years of age who have been diagnosed with ADHD. The goal of the camp is to provide activities specifically designed for children with ADHD and to educate children and their parents on the treatment and management of ADHD and related behaviours.

1413 **Bill Rice Ranch**
627 Bill Rice Ranch Rd.
Murfreesboro, TN 37128
615-893-2767
800-253-7423
Fax: 615-898-0656
info@billriceranch.org
www.billriceranch.org
Wil Rice IV, President
Troy Carlson, Vice President
Matt Downs, Camp Director

Camping for hearing impaired children and youth ages 9-19. Also runs camps and retreats for deaf or hearing impaired adults.

1414 Camp Conquest
3934 West Union Rd.
Millington, TN 38053 901-545-2267
info@campconquest.com
www.campconquest.com
Becca Bryant, Camp Director
Camp Conquest is a Christian camp that provides life-changing experiences for children and adults with special needs, chronic illnesses, and disabilities. Activities include horseback riding, canoeing, ropes course, rock climbing wall, zip line, lake slide, swimming pool, and more.

1415 Camp Discovery
Tennessee Jaycees and Tennessee Jaycee Foundation
400 Camp Discovery Lane
Gainesboro, TN 38562 931-268-0239
director@jayceecamp.org
www.jayceecamp.org
Chester Lowe, Vice President
Serves children, teens, and adults ages 7 and up with disabilities. The camp is a project of the Tennessee Jaycees and the Tennessee Jaycee Foundation.

1416 Camp Joy
Lakeshore Camp and Retreat Center
1458 Pilot Knob Rd.
Eva, TN 38333 731-584-6102
Fax: 731-584-2267
office@lakeshorecamp.org
lakeshorecamp.org/summer-camp
Rev. Gary D. Lawson, Sr., Executive Director
Allison Doyle, Program Director
Katlyn White, Director, Communications
Vickie Lawson, Office Manager
A summer camp for adults ages 31 and up with disabilities. The camp takes place at Lakeshore Camp and Retreat Center and runs regular camp activities such as swimming, arts and crafts, and other outdoor activities.

1417 Camp Koinonia
Koinonia Foundation of Tennessee
244 N Peters Rd.
Suite 211
Knoxville, TN 37923 865-888-7365
info@kftn.org
www.kftn.org/campkoinonia
Jacqui Pearl, Executive Director
Camp program for children and young adults ages 7-21 with disabilities. The camp offers recreational activities such as canoeing, music and games. The camp is operated by the Koinonia Foundation and the University of Tennessee's Therapeutic Recreation Program.

1418 Camp Oginali
Koinonia Foundation of Tennessee
244 N Peters Rd.
Suite 211
Knoxville, TN 37923 865-888-7365
info@kftn.org
www.kftn.org/campkoinonia
Jacqui Pearl, Executive Director
A weekend retreat for individuals ages 7 and up with Down syndrome. The camp is held every fall at Camp Montvale. Activities include fishing, low ropes courses, cooking, arts and crafts, and more.

1419 Camp Okawehna
Dialysis Clinic, Inc.
1633 Church St.
Suite 500
Nashville, TN 37203 615-327-3061
Fax: 605-341-8814
campo@dciinc.org
www.dciinc.org/camps
Andy Parker, Camp Director
Week-long summer camp for children ages 6-18 with kidney disease. Children who have had kidney transplants as well as children on hemodialysis and peritoneal dialysis are welcome.

1420 Camp Sugar Falls
American Diabetes Association
220 Great Circle Rd.
Nashville, TN 37228 615-298-3066
campsupport@diabetes.org
www.diabetes.org

1421 Camp Wonder
Lakeshore Camp and Retreat Center
1458 Pilot Knob Rd.
Eva, TN 38333 731-584-6102
Fax: 731-584-2267
office@lakeshorecamp.org
lakeshorecamp.org/summer-camp
Rev. Gary D. Lawson, Sr., Executive Director
Allison Doyle, Program Director
Katlyn White, Director, Communications
Vickie Lawson, Office Manager
A summer camp for children and adults ages 14-30 with disabilities. The camp takes place at Lakeshore Camp and Retreat Center. Activities include swimming, crafts, games, and more traditional camp activities.

1422 Easterseals Tennessee Camping Program
Easterseals Tennessee
500 Wilson Pike Cir.
Suite 228
Brentwood, TN 37027 615-292-6640
Fax: 615-251-0994
www.easterseals.com/tennessee
Tim Ryerson, President & CEO
Offers overnight, day, and weekend programs for youths ages 7-16 and adults ages 16 and up with disabilities or traumatic brain injuries. The camps are held at the YMCA's Camp Widjiwagan.

1423 LeBonheur Cardiac Kids Camp
LeBonheur Children's Hospital
848 Adams Ave.
Memphis, TN 38103 866-870-5570
cardiac@lebonheur.org
www.lebonheur.org
Christopher Knott-Craig, MD, Co-Director, Heart Institute
Jeffrey Towbin, MD, Co-Director, Heart Institute
Camp for LeBonheur patients ages 10-17 who are being treated for a congenital heart condition or have a pacemaker. The camp provides recreational and educational activities while promoting healthy lifestyles.

Texas

1424 Camp Ailihpomeh
Texas Bleeding Disorders Camp Foundation
20212 Champion Forest Dr.
Suite 700-312
Spring, TX 77379 info@camp-ailihpomeh.org
www.camp-ailihpomeh.org
Grant Spikes, Camp Director
Amanda Wolgamott, Camp Administrator
A six-day overnight camp for boys ages 7-17 who have a bleeding disorder. The camp takes place at Camp John Marc and provides recreational and educational activities.

1425 Camp Aranzazu
5420 Loop 1781
Rockport, TX 78382 361-727-0800
Fax: 361-727-0818
info@camparanzazu.org
www.camparanzazu.org
Virginia Calton Ballard, Executive Director, Camp Aranzazu Foundation
Amelia Halsam, Camp Director
Lillian Anfosso, Finance & Administrative Director
Kate Plouvier, Development Director
A summer camp program for children with a variety of special needs and chronic illnesses, such as cancer, autism, asthma, cerebral palsy, Down Syndrome, epilepsy, and more. Activities center around emphasizing spiritual awareness, environmental awareness, team building and sports, the arts, and social skills.

1426 **Camp Be An Angel**
2003 Aldine Bender Rd.
Houston, TX 77032
281-219-3313
angel@beanangel.org
www.beanangel.org/camp

Marti Boone, Executive Director
Margaret Adsit, Development Director
Russ Massey, Program Director
Larry Blanton, Office Manager

Camp Be An Angel is a summer camp program for children with special needs under the age of 22 and their immediate families.

1427 **Camp Blessing**
7227 Camp Blessing Lane
Brenham, TX 77833
281-259-5789
info@campblessing.org
campblessing.org

Greg Anderson, Executive Director
Rachel Landon, Programs Coordinator
Dean Forland, Facilities Manager
Debbie Forland, Guest Services Manager

A Christian summer camp for children and adults with special needs and their siblings. The camp serves individuals ages 7 and up with a physical, developmental, or intellectual disability. Camp Blessing offers traditional summer camp activities for campers of all levels of ability.

1428 **Camp CAMP**
Children's Association for Maximum Potential
PO Box 27086
San Antonio, TX 78227
210-671-5411
Fax: 210-671-5225
campmail@campcamp.org
www.campcamp.org

Susan Osborne, Chief Executive Officer
Brandon G. Briery, Chief Program Officer & Executive Camp Director
Sarah Coulombe, Chief Administrative Officer
Dianna Hopkins, Chief Development Officer

Camping for children, teens, and adults ages 5-50 with a variety of disabilities and their siblings. The camp is held in Center Point, Texas. Activities are modified to include each camper's physical or developmental needs.

1429 **Camp CPals**
5501A Balcones
Suite 160
Austin, TX 78731
866-742-7284
info@cpathtexas.com
www.cpathtexas.com

Victoria Polega, President
Marielle Deckard, Secretary
Jamie Eppele, Director, Development

Camp CPals is an overnight weekend camp for campers of all ages with cerebral palsy. The camp's goal is to allow campers to gain confidence, independence, learn new skills, and meet other people with cerebral palsy. The camp is held in Burton, Texas.

1430 **Camp Can-Do**
YMCA Camp Carter
6200 Sand Springs Rd.
Fort Worth, TX 76114
817-738-9241
camper@ymcafw.org
www.ymcacampcarter.org

Holly Martin, Executive Camp Director

A week-long summer camp designed specifically for blind/visually impaired children, ages 6-12. The camp is held at the YMCA Camp Carter, and activities include hiking, canoeing, skeet shooting, and more.

1431 **Camp Discovery**
American Academy of Dermatology
PO Box 1968
Des Plaines, IL 60017
847-240-1280
866-503-7546
888-462-3376
Fax: 847-240-1859
www.campdiscovery.org

1432 **Camp John Marc**
4925 Greenville Ave.
Suite 400
Dallas, TX 75206
214-360-0056
mail@campjohnmarc.org
www.campjohnmarc.org

Kevin Randles, Executive Director
Megan White, Camp Director
Bre Loveless, Operations Manager

Year-round camping for children with a variety of chronic medical and physical challenges. Campers can participate in a number of traditional camp activities.

1433 **Camp Neuron**
Epilepsy Foundation Texas
2401 Fountain View Dr.
Suite 900
Houston, TX 77057
713-789-6295
888-548-9716
Fax: 713-789-5628
info@eftx.org
eftx.org

Donna Stahlhut, Chief Executive Officer

Camp Neuron offers an overnight camping experience for children and teens ages 8-14 with epilepsy or a diagnosed seizure disorder. There is no cost to attend the camp, and the camp is located at the Texas Lions Camp in Kerrville, Texas.

1434 **Camp New Horizons North**
American Diabetes Association
4100 Alpha Rd.
Dallas, TX 75244
972-392-1181
campsupport@diabetes.org
www.diabetes.org

Sherry Hill, Contact

A week-long summer camp program of the American Diabetes Association for children ages 5-12 and teens ages 13-17 with diabetes. The camp is held at Cross Creek Ranch in Parker, Texas.

1435 **Camp New Horizons South**
American Diabetes Association
4100 Alpha Rd.
Dallas, TX 75244
972-392-1181
campsupport@diabetes.org
www.diabetes.org

Sherry Hill, Contact

A summer camp program of the American Diabetes Association for children ages 5-12 and teens ages 13-17 with diabetes. The camp is held at Southern Creek Ranch in Dallas, Texas.

1436 **Camp No Limits Texas**
No Limits Foundation
6301 Rehburg Rd
Burton, TX 77835
207-569-6411
campnolimits@gmail.com
www.nolimitsfoundation.org

Mary Leighton, Founder & Executive Director
Kelsey Moody, Program Oprations Manager
Alix Sandler, Marketing & Development Director
Cheryl Foss, Director, Human Resources

Camp No Limits Texas, is a location of Camp No Limits, a recreational and educational camp for youth who have experienced limb loss. Camp No Limits, is a program of the nonprofit organization No Limits Foundation. The weeklong camp is for children ages 5 and up, with campers participating in a variety of activities such as archery, kayaking, and fishing. The camp is held at Camp For All in Burton, Texas.

1437 **Camp NoLoHi**
American Diabetes Association
4100 Alpha Rd.
Dallas, TX 75244
972-392-1181
campsupport@diabetes.org
www.diabetes.org

Sherry Hill, Contact

A summer camp program for children ages 5-13 and teens ages 14-17 with diabetes. The camp is held in Lubbock, Texas. Activities include swimming, fishing, outdoor games, and arts and crafts.

1438 **Camp Quality Texas**
18035 Melissa Springs Dr.
Tomball, TX 77375
713-553-7872
texas@campqualityusa.org
www.campqualityusa.org/TX

Falyne Kirkpatrick, Executive Director
Eric Pitts, Co-Camp Director
Lyndsey Gerhart, Co-Camp Director
Alban Rector, Camper Coordinator

Camp Quality is for children with cancer and their siblings. The camp offers a stress-free environment that offers exciting activities and fosters new friendships, while helping to give the children courage, motivation and emotional strength.

1439 **Camp Rainbow**
American Diabetes Association
4100 Alpha Rd.
Dallas, TX 75244
972-392-1181
campsupport@diabetes.org
www.diabetes.org

1440 **Camp Sandcastle**
American Diabetes Association
4100 Alpha Rd.
Dallas, TX 75244
972-392-1181
campsupport@diabetes.org
www.diabetes.org

1441 **Camp Spike 'n' Wave**
Epilepsy Foundation Texas
2401 Fountain View Dr.
Suite 900
Houston, TX 77057
713-789-6295
888-548-9716
Fax: 713-789-5628
info@eftx.org
eftx.org

Donna Stahlhut, Chief Executive Officer

Camp Spike 'n' Wave is a residential camp for children and teens ages 8-14 with epilepsy or a seizure disorder. The camp is located at Camp For All in Burton, Texas, and runs activities such as swimming, boating, and sports. There is no cost to attend the camp.

1442 **Camp Summit**
17210 Campbell Rd.
Suite 180-W
Dallas, TX 75252
972-484-8900
Fax: 972-620-1945
camp@campsummittx.org
www.campsummittx.org

Carla R. Weiland, President & CEO
Lisa Braziel, Director, Camp Operations & Strategy
Amanda Davis, Camp Director
Zoe Galtelli, Assistant Camp Director

Camp Summit offers camping for children and adults with a variety of disabilities. The program is coed, for ages 6-99.

1443 **Camp Sweeney**
PO Box 918
Gainesville, TX 76241
940-665-2011
Fax: 940-665-9467
info@campsweeney.org
www.campsweeney.org

Ernie Fernandez, Camp Director
Bob Cannon, Program Director
Billie Hood, Business Manager
Kelley King, Registrar

Camp Sweeney teaches self-care and self-reliance to children ages 5-18 with type 1 diabetes. Campers participate in activities such as swimming, fishing, horseback riding and arts and crafts while learning how to self manage their diabetes.

1444 **Camp for All**
6301 Rehburg Rd.
Burton, TX 77835
979-289-3752
Fax: 979-289-5046
bdeans@campforall.org
www.campforall.org

Pat Prior Sorrells, President & CEO
Mary Beth Mosley, Development Director
April McIntosh, Human Resource & Finance Director
Kurt R. Podeszwa, Camp Director

Camp For All is a fully accessible year-round camp facility located in Burton, Texas. The camp is for children and adults with a variety of disabilities. Some disabilities that the camp serves include autism, muscular dystrophy, spinal cord injuries, and more.

1445 **Charis Hills Camp**
498 Faulkner Rd.
Sunset, TX 76270
940-964-2145
Fax: 940-964-2147
info@charishills.org
www.charishills.org

Rand Southard, Co-Director
Colleen Southard, Co-Director
Cara Krueger, Program Director
Liz Austin, Registrar

A Christian summer camp for children with learning disabilities, such as ADD/ADHD, Autism, Asperger's, and more. Campers will participate in traditional camp activities while also learning about Christ and improving social skills, self-esteem and confidence.

1446 **Cristo Vive International: Texas Camp Conroe**
702 Barbara Lane
Conroe, TX 77301
832-703-3733
www.cristovive.net

Rachel Larson, Camp Coordinator

Christian camp with programming for individuals who are blind/deaf, physically or mentally challenged, have multiple disabilities, Down Syndrome, Autism/Asperger's, ADHD/ADD, Cerebral Palsy, and their families and siblings.

1447 **Cristo Vive International: Texas Camp Rio Grande Valley**
4300 S US Highway 281
Edinburg, TX 78539
956-532-8033
www.cristovive.net

Mayra Green, Camp Coordinator

Christian camp with programming for individuals who are blind/deaf, physically or mentally challenged, have multiple disabilities, Down Syndrome, Autism/Asperger's, ADHD/ADD, Cerebral Palsy, and their families and siblings.

1448 **Dallas Academy**
950 Tiffany Way
Dallas, TX 75218
214-324-1481
Fax: 214-327-8537
www.dallas-academy.com

Elizabeth Murski, Head of School

Dallas Academy is a school for children with diagnosed learning differences such as autism, ADD/ADHD, dyslexia, and more. The academy offers a number of summer camps and programs.

1449 **Hill School of Fort Worth**
4817 Odessa Ave.
Fort Worth, TX 76133
817-923-9482
Fax: 817-923-4894
hillschool@hillschool.org
www.hillschool.org

Roxann Breyer, Head of School
Matt Errico, Dean, Student Success
Jimmy Cessna, Registrar

Provides an alternative learning environment for students with learning differences. Hill School caters to individuals with disabilities by offering smaller class sizes and individualized learning programs. Offers an academic summer program during the month of June.

1450 Kamp Kaleidoscope
Epilepsy Foundation Texas
2401 Fountain View Dr.
Suite 900
Houston, TX 77057
713-789-6295
888-548-9716
Fax: 713-789-5628
info@eftx.org
eftx.org

Donna Stahlhut, Chief Executive Officer

Kamp Kaleidoscope is a residential camp for teens ages 15-19 with epilepsy or a seizure disorder. The camp takes place at the YMCA Collin County Adventure Camp in Anna, Texas, and is provided at no cost.

1451 Texas Lions Camp
PO Box 290247
Kerrville, TX 78029
830-896-8500
Fax: 830-896-3666
tlc@lionscamp.com
www.lionscamp.com

Stephen S. Mabry, President & CEO
Karen-Anne King, Vice President, Summer Camps
Milton Dare, Director, Development
Joan Dixon, Director, Finance

Texas Lions Camp is a camp dedicated to serving children ages 7-16 in Texas with physical disabilities. While at camp, campers will participate in a variety of activities and be encouraged to become more independent and self-confident.

Utah

1452 Action X-Treme Camp
National Ability Center
1000 Ability Way
Park City, UT 84060
435-649-3991
Fax: 435-658-3992
info@discovernac.org
www.discovernac.org

Dan Glasser, Chief Executive Officer

Week-long overnight camp for teens with physical and visual disabilities. Activities include skiing, snowboarding, rock climbing, and more.

1453 Camp Giddy-Up
National Ability Center
1000 Ability Way
Park City, UT 84060
435-649-3991
Fax: 435-658-3992
info@discovernac.org
www.discovernac.org

Dan Glasser, Chief Executive Officer

Camp Giddy Up is a horsemanship camp, ages 8-18, for campers with and without disabilities. Campers will be participating in all activities related to horseback riding, including grooming, riding, and barn activities.

1454 Camp Hobe
PO Box 520755
Salt Lake City, UT 84152-0755
801-631-2742
www.camphobekids.org

Christina Beckwith, Executive Director
Ashley Clinger, Deputy Director
Nicole Bailey, Program Director
Laura James, Program Director

A summer camp for children with cancer (and similarly-treated disorders) and their siblings. The camp's goal is to allow kids to take part in a normal aspect of childhood in a safe and medically supervised environment. Camp Hob, offers a two-day session for ages 4-7, one five-day session for ages 7-12, and one five-day session for ages 12-19.

1455 Camp ICANDO
American Diabetes Association
Holladay, UT
campsupport@diabetes.org
www.diabetes.org

1456 Camp Kostopulos
Kostopulos Dream Foundation
4180 E Emigration Canyon Rd.
Salt Lake City, UT 84108
801-582-0700
Fax: 801-583-5176
kdf@campk.org
www.campk.org

Mircea Divricean, President & CEO
Michael Divricean, Chief Operating Officer
Natalie Norris, Administrative Manager

Summer camping for children and adults ages 7 and up with disabilities. There are four types of summer camp programs offered: Day Camp, Residential Camp, Travel Trip Camp, and Partner Day Camps. There is also year round recreation on site and community based activities. Programs are designed to foster independence, confidence, physical fitness, and social and communication skills.

1457 Camp Nah-Nah-Mah
University of Utah Health Care Burn Camp Programs
50 N Medical Dr.
Salt Lake City, UT 84132
801-585-2847
healthcare.utah.edu/burncenter

Kristen Quinn, Camp Director

For children ages 6-13 who are burn survivors. Some of the activities include canoeing, rock climbing and archery. The camp takes place in Millcreek Canyon and is a five-day overnight camp.

1458 Discovery Camp
National Ability Center
1000 Ability Way
Park City, UT 84060
435-649-3991
Fax: 435-658-3992
info@discovernac.org
www.discovernac.org

Dan Glasser, Chief Executive Officer

Summer and winter camps for children ages 8-18 with and without physical and developmental disabilities. Also offers overnight camps for adults.

1459 FCYD Camp Utada
Foundation for Children and Youth with Diabetes
1995 W 9000 S
West Jordan, UT 84088
801-566-6913
www.fcydcamputada.org

Dave Okubo, MD, Co-Founder & Trustee
Elizabeth Elmer, Co-Founder & Trustee
Nathan Gedge, Co-Founder & Trustee

Camp Utada is a summer camp for children with diabetes. Coed, ages 1-18 and families.

1460 Kids Rock The World Day Camp
National Ability Center
1000 Ability Way
Park City, UT 84060
435-649-3991
Fax: 435-658-3992
info@discovernac.org
www.discovernac.org

Dan Glasser, Chief Executive Officer

A day camp program for children and teens ages 11-16 with diabetes. Activities include cycling, indoor climbing, arts and crafts, and more.

1461 Overnight Camps
National Ability Center
1000 Ability Way
Park City, UT 84060
435-649-3991
Fax: 435-658-3992
info@discovernac.org
www.discovernac.org

Dan Glasser, Chief Executive Officer

Overnight Camps are available for teens and young adults ages 15-24. Campers participate in traditional camp activities during the day. During the evenings, campers may attend campfires and sometimes sleep in tents.

1462 **Pathfinders Camp**
National Ability Center
1000 Ability Way
Park City, UT 84060
435-649-3991
Fax: 435-658-3992
info@discovernac.org
www.discovernac.org

Dan Glasser, Chief Executive Officer

Outdoor camp for children ages 8-14 with physical disabilities and their siblings and friends. Activities include adaptive cycling, rock climbing, paddle boarding, and more.

Vermont

1463 **Camp Thorpe**
PO Box 82
Brandon, VT 05733
802-247-6611
director@campthorpe.org
www.campthorpe.org

Heather Moore, Executive Director
Lyllie Harvey, Director, Operations
Karen Davidson, Assistant Director
Jessica Houck, Assistant Director

Camp Thorpe is a residential summer camp for children, teens and adults with a range of social, behavioral, mental, and developmental disabilities. The camp offers two programs: Mountain Reach (ages 12-20) and Pine Haven (ages 21 and up).

1464 **Silver Towers Camp**
PO Box 166
Ripton, VT 05766
802-388-6446
Fax: 802-388-0219
www.vtelks.org/programs/silver-towers

Carolyn Ravenna, Camp Director

Two-week residential camp for individuals ages 6-75 with physical or mental disabilities. Activities include swimming, horseback riding, music, sing-a-longs, dancing, nature studies and more.

1465 **Vermont Overnight Camp**
The Barton Center for Diabetes Education, Inc.
30 Ennis Rd.
PO Box 356
North Oxford, MA 01537-0356
508-987-2056
Fax: 508-987-2002
info@bartoncenter.org
www.bartoncenter.org

Lynn Butler-Dinunno, Executive Director
Jenna Dufresne, Director, Health Services
Sarah Balko, Director, Camps & Programs
Sadie Vivenzio, Director, Finance

The Vermont Overnight Camp provides children and teens ages 6-16 with diabetes a traditional summer camp experience combined with diabetes education. Activities include sports, swimming, kayaking, canoeing, fishing, hiking, arts and crafts, and campfires. The camp is held at Camp Ta-Kum-Ta in South Hero, Vermont.

Virginia

1466 **Camp Dickenson**
Holston Conference of United Methodist Church
801 Camp Dickenson Lane
Fries, VA 24330
276-744-7241
office@campdickenson.com
www.campdickenson.com

Anthony Gomez, Camp Director

Camp Dickenson's Celebration Camp is a four-day camp for youth and adults with mild to moderate developmental disabilities. Activities include archery, hiking, swimming, and games.

1467 **Camp Easterseals UCP**
Easterseals UCP North Carolina & Virginia
900 Camp Easter Seals Rd.
New Castle, VA 24127
540-864-5750
camp@eastersealsucp.com
www.easterseals.com/ncva

Luanne Welch, President & CEO
Alex Barge, Camp Director

Summer camp, weekend respite, and family camp sessions for children and adults with disabilities and special needs. Therapeutic recreation activities including swimming, fishing, sports, horseback riding, rock climbing, and more.

1468 **Camp Holiday Trails**
400 Holiday Trails Lane
Charlottesville, VA 22903
434-977-3781
Fax: 866-342-7850
info@campholidaytrails.org
www.campholidaytrails.org

Tina LaRoche, Executive Director
McKenzie Markham, Program Director
Katrina Beitz, Director, Communications
Ina Stephens, Medical & Education Director

Private, nonprofit camp for children with special health needs and various chronic illnesses. Coed, ages 7-17. Activities include canoeing, swimming, horseback riding, arts and crafts, drama, ropes course, etc. 24-hour medical supervision by doctor and nursing staff.

1469 **Camp Jordan**
Camp Hanover
3163 Parsleys Mill Rd.
Mechanicsville, VA 23111
804-779-2811
info@camphanover.org
www.camphanover.org

Doug Walters, Executive Director
Harry Zweckbronner, Associate Director, Programs
Lisa VanderPloeg, Office Manager
Larry Covington, Facilities Manager

Camp Jordan is a sleepover camp session for children with diabetes in grades 6-12. The camp is a part of Camp Hanover, and activities include hiking, archery, campfires, paddle boards, and more.

1470 **Camp Loud And Clear**
Holiday Lake 4-H Educational Center
1267 4-H Camp Rd.
Appomattox, VA 24522
434-248-5444
Fax: 434-248-6749
info@holidaylake4h.com
holidaylake4h.com

Preston Willson, President & CEO
Heather Benninghove, Center Director
Levi Callahan, Program Director
Cindy Morris, Marketing Director

Camp Loud And Clear is a summer camp for youth ages 9-18 who are deaf or have hearing loss. Activities include swimming, archery, Bible study, and more.

1471 **Camps for Children & Teens with Diabetes**
American Diabetes Association
2451 Crystal Dr.
Suite 900
Arlington, VA 22202
800-342-2383
campsupport@diabetes.org
www.diabetes.org

Tracey D. Brown, Chief Executive Officer
Charlotte Carter, Chief Financial Officer
Charles Henderson, Chief Development Officer
Kathy Nesbitt, Chief Operating & Strategy Officer

The American Diabetes Association sponsors day camps, family camps and resident camps for children and teens. These camps provide an opportunity for children with diabetes to go to camp, meet other children and gain a better understanding of their diabetes. Camps are located all across the country.

1472 **Civitan Acres**
Eggleston Services
1161 Ingleside Rd.
Suite A
Norfolk, VA 23502
757-625-2044
info@egglestonservices.org
www.egglestonservices.org

Paul J. Atkinson, President & CEO
Ron Fritch, Chief Financial Officer
Tasha Jones, Vice President, Rehabilitation Services
Chris Hoagland, Vice President, Federal Contracts

Offers a summer camp for adults and children with disabilities. Sessions run for one week and aim to help campers improve their emotional, intellectual, and physical dimensions of life.

1473 **Loudoun County Adaptive Recreation Camps**
Loudoun County Parks, Recreation & Community Svcs
PO Box 7800
Leesburg, VA 20177-7800
703-777-0343
Fax: 703-771-5354
prcs@loudoun.gov
www.loudoun.gov

Steve Torpy, Director

Loudoun County's Adaptive Recreation Camps offer and promote integration opportunities for individuals with disabilities. All camps are designed to meet the individual needs of the participants and aim to provide traditional summer camp experiences.

1474 **Oakland School & Camp**
128 Oakland Farm Way
Troy, VA 22974
434-293-9059
Fax: 434-296-8930
information@oaklandschool.net
www.oaklandschool.net

Carol Williams, Head of School

A highly individualized program that stresses improving reading ability. Subjects taught are reading, English composition, math and word analysis. Recreational activities include horseback riding, sports, swimming, tennis, crafts, archery and camping. For girls and boys, ages 7-13. Students who attend the summer camp often have a variety of learning disabilities, such as ADHD, dyslexia, visual/auditory processing disorders, and more.

Washington

1475 **Camp Beausite NW**
PO Box 1227
Port Hadlock, WA 98339
360-732-7222
campbeausitenw.org

Raina Baker, Executive Director

The camp is located in Chimacum, Washington. Campers range from 7-65 in age and includes those with developmental disabilities, cerebral palsy, autism, Down syndrome, and other physical or mental disabilities. The camp offers five week-long overnight summer camp sessions for adults and children.

1476 **Camp Goodtimes**
The Goodtimes Project
7400 Sand Point Way NE
Suite 101S
Seattle, WA 98115
206-556-3489
Fax: 206-877-4437
info@thegoodtimesproject.org
www.thegoodtimesproject.org

Bridget K. Dolan, Executive Director
Tanya Krohn, Director, Programming
Becky Felak, Program & Event Manager

A week-long residential summer camp for children ages 8-17 diagnosed with cancer and their siblings. The Goodtimes Project also runs Kayak Adventure Camp for childhood cancer survivors, aged 18-25.

1477 **Camp Killoqua**
15207 E Lake Goodwin Rd.
Stanwood, WA 98292
360-652-6250
killoqua@campfiresnoco.org
www.campkilloqua.org

Cassie Anderson, Camp Director, Outdoor Education & Operations
Pearl Verbon, Camp Director, Summer Camp, Rentals & Retreats

Camp Killoqua offers Inclusion Programs for all of its traditional camp programs. The inclusion program allows campers ages 7-21 with mild to moderate developmental disabilities the chance to participate in any Camp Killoqua session.

1478 **Camp Korey**
3616 Colby Ave.
PMB 247
Everett, WA 98201
425-440-0850
Fax: 425-404-2158
info@campkorey.org
campkorey.org

Chris McReynolds, Co-President
Tim Rose, Co-President
Sue Colbourne, Vice President
Claudia Campanile, Secretary

A summer camp for children with life-altering medical conditions and their families. The camp is free of charge and aims to allow children to experience camp in a safe environment with specialized medical support.

1479 **Camp Sealth**
14500 SW Camp Sealth Rd.
Vashon, WA 98070-8222
206-463-3174
Fax: 206-463-6936
info@campfireseattle.org
campfireseattle.org

Rick Taylor, Executive Director
Kristen Cook, Marketing & Development Director
Carrie Kishline, Summer Camp Director
Meaghan Baumgartner, Summer Camp Program Manager

Camp Sealth is a camp program for youth ages 5-17. The camp is open to children with a variety of abilities and special needs.

1480 **Easterseals Camp Stand by Me**
Easterseals Washington
17809 S Vaughn Rd. NW
PO Box 289
Vaughn, WA 98394
253-884-2722
campadmin@wa.easterseals.com
www.easterseals.com/washington

Cathy Bisaillon, President & CEO
Angela Cox, Camp Director

Camp Stand by Me is a camp program for children and adults with disabilities. Offers week-long summer sessions and weekend respite in the fall, winter, and spring.

1481 **Prime Time, Inc.**
6 S. 2nd St.
Suite 815
Yakima, WA 98901
509-248-2854
Fax: 509-248-5505
office@campprimetime.org
www.campprimetime.org

Bill Schorzman, Camp Manager
Merita Sletten, Office Manager

Camp Prime Time serves children with developmental disabilities or serious or terminal illnesses and their families.

1482 **STIX Diabetes Programs**
PO Box 8308
Spokane, WA 99203
509-484-1366
Fax: 509-955-1329
stix@stixdiabetes.org
www.stixdiabetes.org

Tonya Kobluk, Director, Administration & Camps
Cindy Schneider, Director, Community Outreach
Jill Strom, Director, Development

STIX Diabetes Programs is a non-profit organization providing camp experiences for children and teens with diabetes. STIX offers a three-day non-residential day camp for children ages 6-8; a week-long residential camp for youth ages 9-16; and an excursion-based Adventure Camp for teens ages 16-19.

West Virginia

1483 **Mountaineer Spina Bifida Camp**
534 New Goff Mountain Rd.
Charleston, WV 25313
info@drewsday.org
www.drewsday.org

Suzie Humphreys, Contact
A summer camp for individuals with spina bifida. Campers can participate in activities such as swimming, wheelchair hockey, baseball, and more.

Wisconsin

1484 **Camp Daypoint**
American Diabetes Association
375 Bishops Way
Brookfield, WI 53005
414-778-5500
campsupport@diabetes.org
www.diabetes.org

Becky Barnett, Camp Director
Camp Daypoint is a day camp for children ages 5-9 with diabetes. Activities include swimming, crafts, hikes, games, and more. The camp is held at YMCA Camp St. Croix in Hudson, Wisconsin.

1485 **Camp Kee-B-Waw**
Easterseals Wisconsin
1450 State Hwy. 13
Wisconsin Dells, WI 53965
608-254-8319
800-422-2324
Fax: 608-277-8333
TTY: 608-277-8031
camp@easterseals wisconsin.com
camp.easterseals wisconsin.com

Paul Leverenz, President & CEO
Carissa Peterson, Vice President, Camp & Respite Services
Stevie Thomas, Director, Camp Operations
Alex Peters, Camp Wawbeek Director
Located at Camp Wawbeek, Camp Kee-B-Waw is a day camp for children ages 6-13 from Wisconsin Dells and surrounding communities.

1486 **Camp Klotty Pine**
Great Lakes Hemophilia Foundation
638 N 18th St.
Milwaukee, WI 53233
414-937-6782
888-797-4543
Fax: 414-257-1225
info@glhf.org
glhf.org

Karin Koppen, Camp Director
An overnight summer camp for children ages 7-15 who have been diagnosed with a bleeding disorder. The camp is held at Camp Lakotah in Wautoma, Wisconsin. The camp runs recreational camp activities such as archery, canoeing, and campfires, as well as education about their disorder and self-infusion instruction.

1487 **Camp Needlepoint**
American Diabetes Association
375 Bishops Way
Brookfield, WI 53005
414-778-5500
campsupport@diabetes.org
www.diabetes.org

Becky Barnett, Camp Director
Camp Needlepoint is a summer camp for children who have type 1 diabetes. Coed, ages 8-16. The camp takes place at the YMCA Camp St. Croix in Hudson, Wisconsin.

1488 **Easter Seal Camp Wawbeek**
Easterseals Wisconsin
1450 State Hwy. 13
Wisconsin Dells, WI 53965
608-254-8319
800-422-2324
Fax: 608-277-8333
TTY: 608-277-8031
camp@easterseals wisconsin.com
camp.easterseals wisconsin.com

Paul Leverenz, President & CEO
Carissa Peterson, Vice President, Camp & Respite Services
Stevie Thomas, Director, Camp Operations
Alex Peters, Camp Wawbeek Director
Camp Wawbeek is a summer camp for children and adults with physical disabilities. Coed, ages 7 and up. During the summer, the camp runs six-day youth and teen sessions; six-day adult, young adult, and transition sessions; and weekend sessions from September to May.

1489 **Lutherdale Bible Camp**
Lutherdale Ministries
N7891 US Hwy. 12
Elkhorn, WI 53121
262-742-2352
Fax: 888-248-4551
info@lutherdale.org
www.lutherdale.org

Jeff Bluhm, Executive Director
David Box, Associate Director
Paul Degner, Operations & Facilities Manager
Kathy Dittner, Registrar
Lutherdale Bible Camp currently offers Team USA, a summer camp program for adults with developmental disabilities. Activities include talent show, parade, and campfires.

1490 **Phantom Lake YMCA Camp**
S110W30240 YMCA Camp Rd.
Mukwonago, WI 53149
262-363-4386
office@phantomlakeymca.org
www.phantomlakeymca.org

Karin Mulrooney, Chair
Sara Hacker, Secretary
Bill Canfield, Treasurer
Phantom Lake Camp offers day and residential camping sessions for children ages 3-17. All programs are open to individuals with disabilities.

1491 **Timbertop Camp for Youth with Learning Disabilities**
PO Box 423
Plover, WI 54467
715-869-6262
info@timbertopcamp.org
www.timbertopcamp.org

Pete Matthai, Camp Director
Timbertop Camp is a seven-day outdoor camp for children and youth with learning disabilities. Campers participate in traditional camp activities as well as activities that focus on enhancing cooperative abilities, interpersonal relationships, and self-esteem. The program includes nature exploration, canoeing, arts and crafts, archery, fishing, games, reading instruction, and campfires.

1492 **Wisconsin Badger Camp**
1250 US-151 BUS
PO Box 723
Platteville, WI 53818
608-348-9689
Fax: 608-348-9737
wiscbadgercamp@badgercamp.org
www.badgercamp.org

Brent Bowers, Executive Director
Austin Rist, Program Director
Steve Van Kooten, Camp Director
Morgan Heidenreich, Public Relations Director
Wisconsin Badger Camp, established in 1966, is a summer camp that serves individuals with developmental disabilities. Badger Camp offers eight one-week sessions and one two-week session, with one week for children ages 3-13, one week for teens ages 14-21, and eight weeks for adults.

1493 **Wisconsin Elks/Easterseals Respite Camp**
Easterseals Wisconsin
1550 Waubeek Rd.
Wisconsin Dells, WI 53965
608-254-2502
800-422-2324
Fax: 608-277-8333
TTY: 608-277-8031
camp@eastersealswisconsin.com
camp.eastersealswisconsin.com

Paul Leverenz, President & CEO
Carissa Peterson, Vice President, Camp & Respite Services
Stevie Thomas, Director, Camp Operations
Jamie Lloyd, Respite Camp Director

The Wisconsin Elks/Easterseals Respite Camp is a year-round camp for individuals with disabilities, including those with severe or multiple disabilities. Activities include arts and crafts, sports, games, high ropes course, and local field trips.

1494 **Wisconsin Lions Camp**
Wisconsin Lions Foundation
3834 County Rd. A
Rosholt, WI 54473
715-677-4969
877-463-6953
Fax: 715-677-4527
info@wisconsinlionscamp.com
www.wisconsinlionscamp.com

Evett Hartvig, Executive Director
Andrea Yenter, Camp Director
Phillip Potter, Assistant Camp Director
Peter Rekowski, Facility Director

Provides camp programs for youth and adults in Wisconsin with disabilities, including autism, intellectual disabilities, diabetes, epilepsy, visual impairments, and hearing impairments. ACA accredited, located in central Wisconsin, near Stevens Point.

Wyoming

1495 **Camp Hope**
3920 W 45th St.
Casper, WY 82604
307-259-3327
Fax: 307-472-5008
camphopewyoming@gmail.com
www.camphopewy.net

Steve Johnson, Director
Nancy Johnson, Director

Camp Hope is a camp for children and young adults with diabetes. Activities include hiking, swimming, sports and games.

1496 **Eagle View Ranch**
SOAR
184 Uphill Rd.
PO Box 584
Dubois, WY 82513
307-455-3084
Fax: 801-820-3050
admissions@soarnc.org
www.soarnc.org

John Willson, Executive Director
Jeremy Neidens, Director, Eagle View Ranch

Camp for youth with ADHD and learning disabilities. Campers participate in a broad range of wilderness adventure experiences that help them to overcome challenges and develop problem-solving skills, effective communication strategies, and social skills.

Clothing

Clothing

1497 Adaptations by Adrian
PO Box 7
San Marcos, CA 92079-0007
760-744-3565
888-214-8372
Fax: 760-471-7560
adrians1@sbcglobal.net
www.adaptationsbyadrian.com

1498 Adaptive Clothing: Adults
Special Clothes
P.O. Box 333
E Harwich, MA 02645-333
508-385-9171
Fax: 508-430-2410
specialclo@aol.com
www.special-clothes.com

Judith Sweeney, President

Special Clothes produces a catalogue of garments for adults with disabilities and incontinence. Offerings include: undergarments, snap-crotch tee shirts, jumpsuits, and denim travel cath. The catalogue is available without charge. Comparable to department store prices. Special Clothes produces a catalog of adaptive clothing for children in sizes from toddler through young adults. A full line of clothing is included from undergarments through wheelchair jackets and ponchos.

1499 Adult Absorbent Briefs
Special Clothes
P.O. Box 333
E Harwich, MA 02645-333
508-385-9171
Fax: 508-430-2410
specialclo@aol.com
www.special-clothes.com

Judith Sweeney, President

Soft, comfortable, 100% cotton knit brief is seven layers thick at the crotch. Sides of the brief are a non-bulky single layer. The waistband elastic is enclosed in a soft cotton knit casing and does not touch the skin. Comfortable cotton rib knit bands circle the leg. This brief will not replace a diaper, but provides absorbency for light incontinence. *$18.50*

1500 Adult Lap Shoulder Bodysuit
Special Clothes
P.O. Box 333
E Harwich, MA 02645-333
508-385-9171
Fax: 508-430-2410
specialclo@aol.com
www.special-clothes.com

Judith Sweeney, President

Bodysuit styles fasten at the crotch with sturdy snaps to stay neatly tucked. All are made of soft, absorbent 100% cotton knit for maximum comfort. They are cut wide at the hip and seat for full coverage, and will accomodate a diaper if necessary. Soft knit rib circles the neck and leg. Deep armholes are banded with rib knit.

1501 Adult Short Jumpsuit
Special Clothes
P.O. Box 333
E Harwich, MA 02645-333
508-385-9171
Fax: 508-430-2410
specialclo@aol.com
www.special-clothes.com

Judith Sweeney, President

This pull-on jumpsuit provides comfort and full coverage without bulk. Wide leg ribbing ends at mid-thigh, with snaps at the crotch.

1502 Adult Sleeveless Bodysuit
Special Clothes
P.O. Box 333
E Harwich, MA 02645-333
508-385-9171
Fax: 508-430-2410
specialclo@aol.com
www.special-clothes.com

Judith Sweeney, President

Bodysuit styles fasten at the crotch with sturdy snaps to stay neatly tucked. All are made of soft, absorbent 100% cotton knit for maximum comfort. They are cut wide at the hip and seat for full coverage, and will accomodate a diaper if necessary. Soft knit rib circles the neck and leg. Deep armholes are banded with rib knit.

1503 Adult Swim Diaper
Special Clothes
P.O. Box 333
E Harwich, MA 02645-333
508-385-9171
Fax: 508-430-2410
specialclo@aol.com
www.special-clothes.com

Judith Sweeney, President

This pant is made of soft, silent, light-weight, impermeable fabric- waterproof and secure. It is a containment brief, designed to be used in the pool in place of cloth or disposable diapers, which can become waterlogged or disintegrate in the water. Waist and legbands should be snug for proper fit, so please consult sizing chart before ordering. Darlex with lining of 100% cotton knit. *$40.00*

1504 Adult Tee Shoulder Bodysuit
Special Clothes
P.O. Box 333
E Harwich, MA 02645-333
508-385-9171
Fax: 508-430-2410
specialclo@aol.com
www.special-clothes.com

Judith Sweeney, President

Styles fasten at the crotch with sturdy snaps to stay neatly tucked. All are made of soft, absorbent 100% cotton knit for maximum comfot. They are cut wide at the hip and seat for full coverage, and will accommodate a diaper if necessary. Soft knit rib circles the neck and leg. This bodysuit looks like a regular tee shirt, but snaps at the crotch.

1505 Adult Waterproof Overpant
Special Clothes
P.O. Box 333
E Harwich, MA 02645-333
508-385-9171
Fax: 508-430-2410
specialclo@aol.com
www.special-clothes.com

Judith Sweeney, President

Overpants are made of a soft, silent, lightweight fabric which is waterproof and very secure. It is designed to be used over our Adult Absorbent Brief, or cloth diapers. It is completely latex-free and is an excellent non-allergenic substitute for rubber or vinyl pants. Waist and legbands snug to minimize leakage. Lycra waist and legbands. *$40.00*

1506 Basic Rear Closure Sweat Top
Buck & Buck
3111 27th Ave S
Seattle, WA 98144-6502
206-722-4196
800-458-0600
Fax: 800-317-2182
info@buckandbuck.com
www.buckandbuck.com

Julie Buck, Owner

Top opens completely down the back for ease of dressing with snaps. *$19.00*

1507 Body Suits
Special Clothes
P.O. Box 333
E Harwich, MA 02645-333
508-385-9171
Fax: 508-430-2410
specialclo@aol.com
www.special-clothes.com

Judith Sweeney, President

These are one piece garments that can be used to protect skin under braces, to add warmth and to shield incisions.

1508 **Booties with Non-Skid Soles**
Buck & Buck
3111 27th Ave S
Seattle, WA 98144-6502
206-722-4196
800-458-0600
Fax: 800-317-2182
info@buckandbuck.com
www.buckandbuck.com
Julie Buck, Owner
Acrylic knit or quilted cotton/poly and shearling inner. *$17.00*

1509 **Briefs**
Special Clothes
P.O. Box 333
E Harwich, MA 02645
508-385-9171
Fax: 508-430-2410
specialclo@aol.com
www.special-clothes.com
Judith Sweeney, President
A variety of unique brief styles available for easy access and practicality.

1510 **Buck and Buck Clothing**
3111 27th Ave S
Seattle, WA 98144-6502
206-722-4196
800-458-0600
Fax: 800-317-2182
info@buckandbuck.com
www.buckandbuck.com
Julie Buck, Owner
Clothing for the disabled and elderly.
88 pages Yearly

1511 **Budget Cotton/Poly Open Back Gown**
Buck & Buck
3111 27th Ave S
Seattle, WA 98144-6502
206-722-4196
800-458-0600
Fax: 800-317-2182
info@buckandbuck.com
www.buckandbuck.com
Julie Buck, Owner
Short raglan sleeves, lace at neck and bodice over lapping snapback closure. *$14.00*

1512 **Budget Flannel Open Back Gown**
Buck & Buck
3111 27th Ave S
Seattle, WA 98144-6502
206-722-4196
800-458-0600
info@buckandbuck.com
www.buckandbuck.com
Julie Buck, Owner
3/4 raglan sleeve, lace at neck and bodice. *$17.00*

1513 **Carolyn's Low Vision Products**
3938 S. Tamiami Trail
Sarasota, FL 34231-3622
941-337-5555
800-648-2266
Fax: 941-957-0933
www.carolynscatalog.com
John Colton, Owner
A trusted leader in low-vision products. Free national mail-order catalog of items for visually impaired and blind people. Well versed in a variety of eye diseases that damage vision and have an expertise in helping customers making product purchasing decisions for their needs.

1514 **Cotton Full-Back Vest**
Buck & Buck
3111 27th Ave S
Seattle, WA 98144-6502
206-722-4196
800-458-0600
Fax: 800-317-2182
info@buckandbuck.com
www.buckandbuck.com
Julie Buck, Owner
Wide shoulder straps that don't slide off shoulders. *$5.00*

1515 **Cotton/Poly House Dress**
Buck & Buck
3111 27th Ave S
Seattle, WA 98144-6502
206-722-4196
800-458-0600
info@buckandbuck.com
www.buckandbuck.com
Julie Buck, Owner
Comes in short and long sleeves, assorted florals and plaids. *$36.00*

1516 **Creative Designs**
3704 Carlisle Ct
Modesto, CA 95356-924
209-523-3166
800-335-4852
robes4you@aol.com
www.robes4you.com
Barbara Arnold, Owner
Designer of the original Change-A-Robe and the new Handi-Robe, which allows the wearer to put it on without having to stand up. Robes are designed especially for physically challenged, disabled individuals, and wheelchair users. *$69.95*

1517 **Dusters**
Buck & Buck
3111 27th Ave S
Seattle, WA 98144-6502
206-722-4196
800-458-0600
info@buckandbuck.com
www.buckandbuck.com
Julie Buck, Owner
Three types: Floral, Budget Better. Snap front styles and gathered yokes, flannel $16.00-$24.00. *$36.00*

1518 **Dutch Neck T-Shirt**
Buck & Buck
3111 27th Ave S
Seattle, WA 98144-6502
206-722-4196
800-458-0600
Fax: 800-317-2182
info@buckandbuck.com
www.buckandbuck.com
Julie Buck, Owner
Stretchy neck makes it easy to get over the head. *$5.50*

1519 **Exquisite Egronomic Protective Wear**
Plum Enterprises
P.O. Box 85
Valley Forge, PA 19481-85
610-783-7377
800-321-7586
Fax: 610-783-7577
info@plument.com
www.plument.com
Janice Carrington, President/CEO
Egronomic Protective Wear; ProtectaCap custom-fitting headgear has earned an unparalleled reputation for quality, safety, and comfort. ProtectaCap+Plus technologically-advanced protective headgear closes the gap between hard and soft helmets. Comes with optional ProtectaChin Guard and new sporty design. Protectahip protective undergarment is the intelligent, innovative solution to the problem of hip injuries for both men and women.

1520 **Flannel Gowns**
Buck & Buck
3111 27th Ave S
Seattle, WA 98144-6502
206-722-4196
800-458-0600
info@buckandbuck.com
www.buckandbuck.com
Julie Buck, Owner
Comes in long or short with a deep button-front opening for ease of slipping on. Shorter long length. *$21.00*

1521 **Flannel Pajamas**
Buck & Buck
3111 27th Ave S
Seattle, WA 98144-6502
206-722-4196
800-458-0600
Fax: 800-317-2182
info@buckandbuck.com
www.buckandbuck.com

Julie Buck, Owner
$25.00

1522 **Float Dress**
Buck & Buck
3111 27th Ave S
Seattle, WA 98144-6502
206-722-4196
800-458-0600
info@buckandbuck.com
www.buckandbuck.com

Julie Buck, Owner
A safe bet for everyone from a size medium to a 3X. Gathered yoke front and back and literally yards of fabric for fullness. Comes in cotton or polyester. *$32.00*

1523 **Foot Snugglers**
Buck & Buck
3111 27th Ave S
Seattle, WA 98144-6502
206-722-4196
800-458-0600
Fax: 800-317-2182
info@buckandbuck.com
www.buckandbuck.com

Julie Buck, Owner
Quilted poly/cotton outers lined with plush shearling pile, provide a thick, comfortable cushion which helps minimize the pressure points on tender areas. *$.30*

1524 **Headliner Hats**
Designs for Comfort
PO Box 671044
Marietta, GA 30066-2429
770-565-8246
800-443-9226
Fax: 770-565-8425
headliner@mindspring.com
www.headlinerhats.com

Curt Maurer, President
A patented cap and hairpiece combination, the Headliner is both a quick, stylish coverup and an upbeat wig alternative for women experiencing hair care problems or hair loss. Ideal for social gatherings and outdoor activities as well as for sleeping and hospital stays. *$25.00*

1525 **His & Hers**
Wishing Wells Collection
Ste 965
11684 Ventura Blvd
Studio City, CA 91604-2699
818-840-6919
Fax: 818-760-3878
www.dawnwells.com

Dawn Wells, Owner
This sleep shirt is designed for him or her. *$21.99*

1526 **Jumpsuits**
Special Clothes
P.O. Box 333
E Harwich, MA 02645-333
508-385-9171
Fax: 508-430-2410
specialclo@aol.com
www.special-clothes.com

Judith Sweeney, President
Several styles of one-piece garments are available for dressing ease. Front opening styles are designed for easy access. *$55.00*

1527 **Knee Socks**
Buck & Buck
3111 27th Ave S
Seattle, WA 98144-6502
206-722-4196
800-458-0600
Fax: 800-317-2182
info@buckandbuck.com
www.buckandbuck.com

Julie Buck, Owner
Comes in regular and large size. $3.00 - $8.00

1528 **M&M Health Care Apparel Company**
Fashion Collection
1541 60th St
Brooklyn, NY 11219-5023
718-871-8188
800-221-8929
Fax: 718-436-2067
info@fashionease.com
www.fashionease.com

Abraham Klein, Owner
Specialized clothing for disabled people.

1529 **Muu Muu**
Buck & Buck
3111 27th Ave S
Seattle, WA 98144-6502
206-722-4196
800-458-0600
info@buckandbuck.com
www.buckandbuck.com

Julie Buck, Owner
Comes in long and short styles, assorted bright floral prints. $20.00-$22.00. *$31.00*

1530 **Nightshirts**
Buck & Buck
3111 27th Ave S
Seattle, WA 98144-6502
206-722-4196
800-458-0600
Fax: 800-317-2182
info@buckandbuck.com
www.buckandbuck.com

Julie Buck, Owner
Come in flannel or cotton patterns and prints in sizes S/M, 4XL, 2XL/3XL *$29.00*

1531 **Open Back Nightgowns**
Buck & Buck
3111 27th Ave S
Seattle, WA 98144-6502
206-722-4196
800-458-0600
Fax: 800-317-2182
info@buckandbuck.com
www.buckandbuck.com

Julie Buck, Owner
Come in cotton (sizes S-4X) or flannel (sizes S-3X). *$20.00*

1532 **Panties**
Buck & Buck
3111 27th Ave S
Seattle, WA 98144-6502
206-722-4196
800-458-0600
Fax: 800-317-2182
info@buckandbuck.com
www.buckandbuck.com

Julie Buck, Owner
Come in nylon or cotton, band leg for comfort. *$5.00*

1533 **Polyester House Dress**
Buck & Buck
3111 27th Ave S
Seattle, WA 98144-6502
206-722-4196
800-458-0600
info@buckandbuck.com
www.buckandbuck.com

Julie Buck, Owner
Comes in short and long sleeves, assorted florals. *$36.00*

1534 **Printed Rear Closure Sweat Top**
Buck & Buck
3111 27th Ave S
Seattle, WA 98144-6502
206-722-4196
800-458-0600
Fax: 800-317-2182
info@buckandbuck.com
www.buckandbuck.com

Julie Buck, Owner
Comes in assorted colors, plain or with animal motifs and snaps all the way down the back. *$28.00*

1535 **Professional Fit Clothing**
Ste 1
831 N Lake St
Burbank, CA 91502-1600
818-563-1975
800-422-2348
Fax: 818-563-1834
sales@professionalfit.com
www.professionalfit.com
Kurt Rieback, Owner
Professional fit clothing caters to homes that care for people with developmental disabilities and individuals who are physically challenged. Our clothing is fashionable, affordable and can be adapted to each person's special needs.

1536 **Propet Leather Walking Shoes**
Buck & Buck
3111 27th Ave S
Seattle, WA 98144-6502
206-722-4196
800-458-0600
Fax: 800-317-2182
info@buckandbuck.com
www.buckandbuck.com
Julie Buck, Owner
Two velcro straps, leather upper, shock-absorbing sole. *$58.00*

1537 **Rear Closure Shirts**
Buck & Buck
3111 27th Ave S
Seattle, WA 98144-6502
206-722-4196
800-458-0600
Fax: 206-722-1144
info@buckandbuck.com
www.buckandbuck.com
Julie Buck, Owner
Snaps down the back on T-shirts and dress shirts. *$33.00*

1538 **Rear Closure T-Shirt**
Buck & Buck
3111 27th Ave S
Seattle, WA 98144-6502
206-722-4196
800-458-0600
Fax: 800-317-2182
info@buckandbuck.com
www.buckandbuck.com
Julie Buck, Owner
Closes down the back with velcro snaps. *$10.00*

1539 **Seersucker Shower Robe**
Buck & Buck
3111 27th Ave S
Seattle, WA 98144-6502
206-722-4196
800-458-0600
Fax: 800-317-2182
info@buckandbuck.com
www.buckandbuck.com
Julie Buck, Owner
Totally covers a man or woman being wheeled to and from the shower or bath. A crisp, light weight shower robe. *$34.00*

1540 **Side Velcro Slacks**
Buck & Buck
3111 27th Ave S
Seattle, WA 98144-6502
206-722-4196
800-458-0600
Fax: 800-317-2182
info@buckandbuck.com
www.buckandbuck.com
Julie Buck, Owner
Slacks open down both sides from waist to hip with snap closures at sides. *$36.00*

1541 **Side-Zip Sweat Pants**
Buck & Buck
3111 27th Ave S
Seattle, WA 98144-6502
206-722-4196
800-458-0600
Fax: 800-317-2182
info@buckandbuck.com
www.buckandbuck.com
Julie Buck, Owner
Out-seam zippers un-zip 22-inch zippers down both sides to enable dressing a resident with severe leg contractures. *$25.00*

1542 **Spec-L Clothing Solutions**
849 Performance Drive
Stockton, CA 95206
714-427-0781
800-445-1981
Fax: 800-683-6510
www.clothingsolutions.com
Jim Lechner, Owner
The nation's leading designer and manufacturer of assistive clothing for men and women. Free 56 page catalog available.

1543 **Special Clothes Adult Catalogue**
Special Clothes
P.O. Box 333
E Harwich, MA 02645-333
508-385-9171
Fax: 508-430-2410
specialclo@aol.com
www.special-clothes.com
Judith Sweeney, President
Produces a catalogue of adaptive clothing for adults with disabilities. Offers include undergarments, casual bottoms, jumpsuits, swimwear, footwear and bibs. Prices are comparable to deparment store prices.

1544 **Special Clothes for Special Children**
Special Clothes
P.O. Box 333
E Harwich, MA 02645-333
508-385-9171
Fax: 508-430-2410
specialclo@aol.com
www.special-clothes.com
Judith Sweeney, President
All special adaptations, such as velcro closures, snap crotches, bib fronts and G-tube access openings. Every item is fully washable. Offering optional features to customize each item to meet the needs of the user's child.

1545 **Specialty Care Shoppe**
16126 E 161st St S
Bixby, OK 74008-7325
918-366-2901
Fax: 918-366-9445
www.specialtycareshoppe.com
K J Marshall, Owner
Catalog of attractive, affordable clothing and accessories for adults with special needs. Includes items for edema, incontinence, alzheimers, limited mobility, and hand impairment.

1546 **Super Stretch Socks**
Buck & Buck
3111 27th Ave S
Seattle, WA 98144-6502
206-722-4196
800-458-0600
Fax: 800-317-2182
info@buckandbuck.com
www.buckandbuck.com
Julie Buck, Owner
This sock has been improved to stretch laterally throughout the foot area as well as at the top. *$3.75*

1547 **Support Plus**
5581 Hudson Industrial Parkway
PO Box 2599
Hudson, OH 44236-0099
508-359-2910
866-229-2910
Fax: 800-950-9569
www.supportplus.com
Ed Janos, President
Offers a selection of support undergarments, braces and shoes for the physically challenged and medical professionals.

1548 **TRU-Mold Shoes**
42 Breckenridge St
Buffalo, NY 14213-1555
716-881-4484
800-843-6653
Fax: 716-881-0406
www.trumold.com
Husain Syed, Production Manager
Custom made, fully molded shoes, relieve pressure in sensitive areas by taking all of the weight off the painful areas.

1549 **Thigh-Hi Nylon Stockings**
Buck & Buck
3111 27th Ave S
Seattle, WA 98144-6502
206-722-4196
800-458-0600
Fax: 800-317-2182
info@buckandbuck.com
www.buckandbuck.com
Julie Buck, Owner
A sheer, full length stocking. *$4.50*

1550 **Trunks**
Buck & Buck
3111 27th Ave S
Seattle, WA 98144-6502
206-722-4196
800-458-0600
Fax: 800-317-2118
info@buckandbuck.com
www.buckandbuck.com
Julie Buck, Owner
Come in cotton or nylon, flare leg, full cut. *$5.00*

1551 **Velcro Booties**
Buck & Buck
3111 27th Ave S
Seattle, WA 98144-6502
206-722-4196
800-458-0600
Fax: 800-317-2182
info@buckandbuck.com
www.buckandbuck.com
Julie Buck, Owner
The high-domed toe, and extra-wide, non-skid sole design accommodates virtually every foot related problem. *$20.00*

1552 **Washable Shoes**
Buck & Buck
3111 27th Ave S
Seattle, WA 98144-6502
206-722-4196
800-458-0600
Fax: 800-317-2182
info@buckandbuck.com
www.buckandbuck.com
Julie Buck, Owner
Vinyl upper with velcro closure, nonskid sole. *$20.00*

1553 **Waterproof Bib**
Buck & Buck
3111 27th Ave S
Seattle, WA 98144-6502
206-722-4196
800-458-0600
Fax: 800-317-2182
info@buckandbuck.com
www.buckandbuck.com
Julie Buck, Owner
Made with 3 layers of fabric including waterproof backing, these attractive bibs will not soak through like most others, protecting clothing from stains. *$18.00*

1554 **Wishing Wells Collection**
Ste 965
11684 Ventura Blvd
Studio City, CA 91604-2699
818-840-6919
Fax: 818-760-3878
www.dawnwells.com
Dawn Wells, Owner
Lorraine Parker, General Manager
Features designs full of back overlap construction and all velcro closures clothing.

Computers

Assistive Devices

1555 **Ability Research**
PO Box 1721
Minnetonka, MN 55345-721
952-939-0121
Fax: 952-227-5809
info@abilityresearch.net
www.abilityresearch.net

Suzanne Severson, Administrator
Manufacturers and marketers of assistive technology equipment.

1556 **Academic Software Inc**
3504 Tates Creek Rd
Lexington, KY 40517-2601
859-552-1020
Fax: 253-799-4012
asistaff@acsw.com
www.acsw.com

Warren E Lacefield PhD, President
Penelope Ellis, Marketing Director
Sylvia P Lacefield, Graphic Artist
Employs a unique, goal-oriented approach to aid individuals in identifying adaptive devices with potential to support various physical limitations. Devices are categorized in seven databases: Existence, Travel, In-situ Motion, Environmental Adaptation, Communication, and Sports & recreation. ADLS provides its users with device descriptions, pictures and lists of sources for locating products and product information.

1557 **Adaptivation**
Ste 100
2225 W 50th St
Sioux Falls, SD 57105-6536
605-335-4445
800-723-2783
Fax: 605-335-4446
info@adaptivation.com
www.adaptivation.com

Jonathan Eckrich, President
Manufacturers of switches, voice output devices and enviromental controls.

1558 **Analog Switch Pad**
Academic Software
331 W 2nd St
Lexington, KY 40507-1113
859-233-2332
800-842-2357
Fax: 859-231-0725

Warren E Lacefield PhD, President
Penelope Ellis, Marketing Director
A touch-activated, force-adjustable, low-voltage DC, electronic switch designed to control battery-operated toys, environmental controls, and computer access interfaces. This device features a large activation area that is soft and compliant to the touch. Force sensitivity is adjusted by a small dial from approximately 1 ounce to 32 ounces activation pressure, applied over an area ranging from the size of a fingertip to the size of the entire switch surface.

1559 **Arkenstone: The Benetech Initiative**
480 S California Ave
Palo Alto, CA 94306-1609
650-644-3400
Fax: 650-475-1066
www.hrdag.org

Jim Fruthterman, CEO
Roberta G Brosnaha, General Manager/VP
Patrick Ball, Executive Director
Offers various models of ready-to-read personal computers for the disabled.

1560 **Augmentative Communication Systems (AAC)**
ZYGO-USA
48834 Kato Road
Suite 101A
Freemont, CA 94538
510-249-9660
800-234-6006
Fax: 510-770-4930
www.zygo-usa.com

Lawrence Weiss, President
Full range of AAC systems and assistive technology including computer-based systems and computer access programs and devices.

1561 **Away We Ride IntelliKeys Overlay**
Soft Touch Inc
12301 Central Ave NE
Ste 205
Blaine, NE 55434
763-755-1402
888-755-1402
sales@marblesoft.com
www.softtouch.com

Joyce Meyer, President
Four full color preprinted overlays to use with Away We Ride. Just put them on an IntelliKeys keyboard and you are ready to go.

1562 **BIGmack Communication Aid**
AbleNet, Inc.
2625 Patton Road
Roseville, MN 55113-1137
651-294-2200
800-322-0956
Fax: 651-294-2259
customerservice@ablenetinc.com
www.ablenetinc.com

Bill Sproull, Chair of the Board
Jennifer Thalhuber, President & CEO
William Mills, Board of Directors
Paul Sugden, CFO & Trustee
A single message communication aid, BIGmack has 2 minutes of memory and has a 5 inches in diameter switch surface. *$86.00*

1563 **Close-Up 6.5**
Norton- Lambert Corporation
PO Box 4085
Santa Barbara, CA 93140-4085
805-964-6767
www.norton-lambert.com

Jeannie Vesely, Marketing Coordinator
Remotely controls PC's via modem. Telecommute from your home or laptop PC to your office PC. Run applications, update spreadsheets, print documents remotely and access networks on remote PCs. Features: fast screen and file transfers, synchronize files, unattended transfers, multi-level security, transaction logs, automated installation. *$99.95*

1564 **Concepts on the Move Advanced Overlay CD**
Soft Touch Inc
12301 Central Ave NE
Ste 205
Blaine, MN 55434
763-755-1402
888-755-1402
Fax: 763-862-2920
sales@marblesoft.com
www.softtouch.com

Joyce Myer, President
Use this overlay CD with Concepts on the Move Advanced Preacademics. Overlays match the concepts and graphics in the program. Includes standard overlays with all the choices and SoftTouch's changeable format overlays. Print and laminate the blank templates. Then print and laminate the picture keys in all three sizes - small, medium and large. Includes Overlay Printer by IntelliTools for easy printing. *$115.00*

1565 **Concepts on the Move Basic Overlay CD**
Soft Touch Inc
12301 Central Ave NE
Ste 205
Blaine, MN 55434
763-755-1402
888-755-1403
Fax: 763-862-2920
sales@marblesoft.com
www.softtouch.com

Joyce Meyer, President
Use this Overlay CD with Concepts on the Move Basic Preacademics. Overlays match the conepts and graphics in the program. Includes standard overlays with all the choices and SoftTouch's changeable format overlays. Print and laminate the blank templates. Then print and laminate the picture keys in all three sizes - small, medium and large. It is easy and fast to place the images on the blank templates. *$115.00*

1566 **Darci Too**
WesTest Engineering Corporation
810 Shepard Ln
Farmington, UT 84025-3846
801-451-9191
Fax: 801-451-9393
larryk@westest.com
westest.com
Robert Lessmann, President
A universal device which allows people with physical disabilities to replace the keyboard and mouse on a personal computer with a device that matches their physical capabilities. DARCI TOO works with almost any personal computer and provides access to all computer functions. *$995.00*

1567 **Eyegaze Computer System**
LC Technologies Inc
10363A Democracy Lane
Fairfax, VA 22030
703-385-7133
800-393-4293
Fax: 703-385-7137
www.eyegaze.com
Nancy Cleveland, Medical Coordinator
Enables people with physical disabilities to do many things with their eyes that they would otherwise do with their hands.

1568 **Five Green & Speckled Frogs IntelliKeys Overlay**
Soft Touch Inc
12301 Central Ave NE
Ste 205
Blaine, MN 55434
763-755-1402
888-755-1403
Fax: 763-862-2920
sales@marblesoft.com
www.softtouch.com
Joyce Meyer, President
Seven full color preprinted overlays to use with Five Green and Speckled Frogs. Just put them on an IntelliKeys keyboard and you are ready to go. *$49.00*

1569 **GW Micro**
725 Airport North Office Park
Fort Wayne, IN 46825-6707
260-489-3671
Fax: 260-489-2608
www.gwmicro.com
Dan Weirich, Sales Executive
Marty Hord, Sales Manager
Computer hardware and software products for people with disabilities.

1570 **InvoTek, Inc.**
1026 Riverview Dr
Alma, AR 72921
479-632-4166
Fax: 479-632-6457
invotek.org
Thomas Jakobs, President
Diane Jakobs, Vice President, Operations
John Riggins, Chief Marketing Officer
InvoTek, Inc. is a research and development company that improves the quality of life for people who find it difficult or impossible to use their hands by giving them new, efficient ways to access computers.

1571 **Jelly Bean Switch**
AbleNet, Inc.
2625 Patton Road
Roseville, MN 55113-1137
651-294-2200
800-322-0956
Fax: 651-294-2259
customerservice@ablenetinc.com
www.ablenetinc.com
Bill Sproull, Chair of the Board
Jennifer Thalhuber, President & CEO
William Mills, Board of Directors
Paul Sugden, CFO & Trustee
A momentary touch switch made of shatterproof plastic, small and sensitive to 2-3 ounces of pressure, this switch is provided audible feedback when activated and is a compact version of the Big Red Switch. Choice of colors: red, blue, green and yellow.

1572 **Large Print Keyboard Labels**
Hooleon Corp
P.O. Box 589
Melrose, NM 88124-589
575-253-4503
800-937-1337
Fax: 928-634-4620
sales@hooleon.com
www.hooleon.com
Shannen Aikman, Admin Manager/Sales
Joan Crozier, President/Sales
Pressure sensitive labels for computer keyboards.

1573 **MessageMate**
Words+ Inc
42505 10th Street W
Lancaster, CA 93534-7059
661-723-6523
800-869-8521
Fax: 661-723-2114
www.words-plus.com
Jeff Dahlan, President
Ginger Woltosz, General Manager
Lightweight, hand-held communicator providing high-quality analog recording capability using either direct select keyboards or 1 to 2 switch access. Price ranges from $549.00 to $999.00. *$1550.00*

1574 **Mouthsticks**
Performance Health
28100 Torch Parkway
Suite 700
Warrenville, IL 60555-3938
630-393-6000
Fax: 630-393-7600
customsupport@performancehealth.com
www.performancehealth.com
Francis Dirksmeier, CEO
Isabel Afonso, Managing Director & Head of International
Daniel Baumwald, Vice President, North America Retail & eCommerce
Laurie Byrne, Chief Human Resources Officer
Wide offering of mouthsticks: BK 5380, 5381, 5383, 5385, 6002, or BK 5370 series). Designed for typing and page turning. Suitable for both personal and professional use.

1575 **Old MacDonald's Farm IntelliKeys Overlay**
Soft Touch Inc
12301 Central Ave NE
Ste 205
Blaine, MN 55434
763-755-1402
888-755-1403
Fax: 763-862-2920
sales@marblesoft.com
www.softtouch.com
Joyce Meyer, President
Extend your students' learning with more than 45 pre-made overlays that support all of the skills learned at the farm. Use with the IntelliKeys keyboard. Simply print and use. Print an extra set to make off computer activities, too. Note: Requires Overlay Maker or Overlay Printer by IntelliTools.

1576 **Origin Instruments Corporation**
854 Greenview Dr
Grand Prairie, TX 75050
972-606-8740
Fax: 972-606-8741
support@orin.com
www.orin.com

1577 **Perfect Solutions**
2685 Treanor Ter
Wellington, FL 33414-6460
561-790-1070
800-726-7086
Fax: 561-790-0108
perfect@gate.net
www.perfectsolutions.com
Andrew Kramer, President
A computer for every student and it speaks! Wireless laptop computers starting at $299.00 are ideal for students to carry with them all day. Text-to-speech and web browsing are available. *$299.00*

1578 **Phillip Roy, Inc.**
P.O. Box 130
Indian Rocks Beach, FL 33785-130
727-593-2700
800-255-9085
Fax: 877-595-2685
info@philliproy.com
www.philliproy.com

Ruth Bragman, PhD, President
Phil Padol, Consultant

Offers multimedia materials appropriate for use with individuals with disabilities. Programs range from preschool through the adult level. Many of the programs are high interest topics/low vocabulary, ideal for transition and employability skills. Materials are also available which focus on social and personal development. Lesson Plans, teacher's guides, pre/post assessment, and other support materials are provided at no additional cost.

1579 **SS-Access Single Switch Interface for PC'swith MS-DOS**
Academic Software
3504 Tates Creek Road
Lexington, KY 40517-2601
859-552-1020
800-842-2357
Fax: 253-799-4012
asistaff@acsw.com
www.acsw.com

Warren E Lacefield PhD, President
Penelope Ellis, Marketing Director

A general purpose single switch hardware and software interface for DOS and the IBM and compatible PC family. It is designed to be easy to install, simple to use, and compatible with the widest possible range of computers and application software programs. SS-ACCESS! connects to one of the PC serial ports and provides a jack to connect an external switch. The DOS version of the software works by sending a user defined keystroke to the PC keyboard buffer whenever the switch is pressed. *$90.00*

1580 **Simplicity**
Words+
42505 10th Street W
Lancaster, CA 93534-7059
661-723-6523
800-869-8521
Fax: 661-723-2114
info@words-plus.com
www.words-plus.com

Jeff Dahlan, President
Ginger Wolosz, General Manager

Swing-down mount for portable computers and other devices is made from high-quality aircraft aluminum. Simplicity contains very few moving parts and installs in minutes, providing a positive, secure support for computer/device in both the stored and overlap position. *$1199.00*

1581 **Slim Armstrong Mounting System**
AbleNet, Inc.
2625 Patton Road
Roseville, MN 55113-1137
651-294-2200
800-322-0956
Fax: 651-294-2259
customerservice@ablenetinc.com
www.ablenetinc.com

Bill Sproull, Chair of the Board
Jennifer Thalhuber, President & CEO
William Mills, Board of Directors
Paul Sugden, CFO & Trustee

Slim Armstrong is a mounting system strong enough to hold up to five pounds in any position. Mix and match parts to create the system length you desire. *$188.00*

1582 **Songs I Sing at Preschool IntelliKeys Overlay**
Soft Touch
12301 Central Ave NE
Ste 205
Blaine, MN 55434
763-755-1402
888-755-1403
Fax: 763-862-2920
sales@marblesoft.com
www.softtouch.com

Joyce Meyer, President

Pre-made overlays for use with Songs I Sing at Preschool. Simply print and use with an IntelliKeys keyboard. Print an extra set to make off computer activities, too.

1583 **Switch Basics IntelliKeys Overlay**
Soft Touch
12301 Central Ave NE
Ste 205
Blaine, MN 55434
763-755-1402
888-755-1403
Fax: 763-862-2920
sales@marblesoft.com
www.softtouch.com

Joyce Meyer, President

Four preprinted overlays to use with Switch Basics. Just put them on an IntelliKeys keyboard and you're ready to go.

1584 **Teach Me Phonemics Blends Overlay CD**
SoftTouch Inc.
12301 Central Ave NE
Ste 205
Blaine, MN 55434
763-755-1402
888-755-1403
Fax: 763-862-2920
sales@marblesoft.com
wwww.softtouch.com

Roxanne Butterfield, Marketing
Joyce Meyer, President

Teach Me Phonemics Blends Overlay CD contains over 40 IntelliKeys overlays for use with Teach Me Phonemics - Blends program. Choose either 4-item or 9-item layout to match the presentation you use in the program. Print extra copies of the overlays for off computer activites, too.

1585 **Teach Me Phonemics Medial Overlay CD**
SoftTouch Incorporated
Ste C
17117 Oak Dr
Omaha, NE 68130-2193
402-330-1301
877-763-8868
Fax: 402-334-8478
support@softtouch.com
www.softtouch.com

Kip Fisher, Manager
Roxanne Butterfield, Marketing

Teach Me Phonemics Medial Overlay CD contains over 40 IntelliKeys overlays for use with Teach Me Phonemics - Medial program. Choose either 4-item or 9-item layout to match the presentation you use in the program. Print extra copies of the overlays for off computer activites, too.

1586 **Teach Me Phonemics Overlay Series Bundle**
SoftTouch
Ste 401
4300 Stine Rd
Bakersfield, CA 93313-2352
661-396-8676
877-763-8868
Fax: 661-396-8760
www.softtouch.com

Roxanne Butterfield, Marketing
Joyce Meyer, President

Teach Me Phonemics Overlay Series Bundle includes one copy of each Teach Me Phonemics Overlay CD - Initial, Medial, Final and - four CD's in all.

1587 **Teach Me to Talk Overlay CD**
Soft Touch
12301 Central Ave NE
Ste 205
Blaine, MN 55434
763-755-1402
888-755-1403
Fax: 763-862-2920
sales@marblesoft.com
www.softtouch.com

Joyce Meyer, President

For older version of Teach Me to Talk. Mac only version with red label and PC only version with yellow label. More than 48 pre-made overlays that match the activities on Teach Me to Talk. Simply print and use with an IntelliKeys keyboard. Print an extra set to make off computer activities, too.

1588 **Teach Me to Talk: USB-Overlay CD**
Soft Touch
12301 Central Ave NE
Ste 205
Blaine, MN 55434
763-755-1402
888-755-1403
Fax: 763-862-2920
sales@marblesoft.com
www.softtouch.com
Joyce Meyer, President
Revised version of Teach Me to Talk Overlays for the newest version that is USB IntelliKeys compatible. This CD contains more than 48 overlays that match the activities and updated graphics of Teach Me to Talk. Includes Overlay Printer by IntelliTools for easy printing.

1589 **Teen Tunes Plus IntelliKeys Overlay**
Soft Touch
12301 Central Ave NE
Ste 205
Blaine, MN 55434
763-755-1402
888-755-1403
Fax: 763-862-2920
sales@marblesoft.com
www.softtouch.com
Joyce Meyer, President
Seven full color, preprinted overlays to use with Teen Tunes Plus. Just put them on an IntelliKeys keyboard and you're ready to go. *$49.00*

1590 **U-Control III**
Words+
42505 10th St W
Lancaster, CA 93534-7059
575-253-4503
800-869-8521
Fax: 661-723-2114
www.words-plus.com
Jeff Dahlen, President
Ginger Wolosz, General Manager
Works with the Words+ system (EX Keys, Morse WSKE, Scanning WSKE, Talking Screen) to provide wireless, portable control of items which are already infrared-controlled such as a TV, VCR, CD player, etc. *$499.00*

1591 **Universal Switch Mounting System**
AbleNet, Inc.
2625 Patton Road
Roseville, MN 55113-1137
651-294-2200
800-322-0956
Fax: 651-294-2259
customerservice@ablenetinc.com
www.ablenetinc.com
Bill Sproull, Chair of the Board
Jennifer Thalhuber, President & CEO
William Mills, Board of Directors
Paul Sugden, CFO & Trustee
Mounting system that allows switch placement in any position. A single lever locks all joints securely in place. Extends to 20 1/2 inches and holds up to five pounds. A mounting system for quick and easy positioning. *$210.00*

1592 **WinSCAN: The Single Switch Interface for PC's with Windows**
Academic Software
3504 Tates Creek Rd
Lexington, KY 40517-2601
859-522-1020
Fax: 253-799-4012
asistaff@acsw.com
www.acsw.com
Warren E Lacefield, President
Penelope Ellis, Marketing Director/COO
A general purpose single-switch control interface for Windows. It provides single-switch users independent control access to educational and productivity software, multimedia programs, and recreational activities that run under Windows 3.1 and higher versions on IBM and compatible PC's. The user can navigate through Windows; choose program icons and run programs, games, and CD's; even surf the Internet with WinSCAN and his or her adaptive switch. *$349.00*

1593 **Words+ IST (Infrared, Sound, Touch)**
Words+
42505 10th St W
Lancaster, CA 93534-7059
575-253-4503
800-869-8521
Fax: 661-723-2114
www.words-plus.com
Jeff Dahlan, President
Ginger Wolosz, General Manager
A unique switch that is activated by slight movement or faint sound. The switch provides user control when connected to a device driven by a single switch. Individuals are currently accessing a wide variety of communication and computer systems with movement using the IST switch. *$395.00*

Braille Products

1594 **Braille Keyboard Labels**
Hooleon Corporation
PO Box 589
Melrose, NM 88124-589
928-634-7515
800-937-1337
Fax: 928-634-4620
sales@hooleon.com
www.hooleon.com
Barry Green, Sales Manager
Joan Crozier, President/Sales
Also large print keyboard labels and large print with Braille.

1595 **Braille Paper**
Maxi Aids
42 Executive Blvd.
Farmingdale, NY 11735-4710
631-752-0521
800-522-6294
Fax: 631-752-0689
TTY: 631-752-0738
sales@maxiaids.com
www.maxiaids.com
Elliot Zaretsky, Founder, President & CEO
Paper for Braille embossing. Sizes include 8.5 by 11 inch and 11 by 11.5 inch.

1596 **Brailon Plastic Sheets**
Maxi Aids
42 Executive Blvd.
Farmingdale, NY 11735-4710
631-752-0521
800-522-6294
Fax: 631-752-0689
TTY: 631-752-0738
sales@maxiaids.com
www.maxiaids.com
Elliot Zaretsky, Founder, President & CEO
Brailon plastic sheets used with Thermoform machines to copy Braille text and graphics.

1597 **Brailon Thermoform Duplicator**
American Thermoform Corporation
1758 Brackett St
La Verne, CA 91750-5855
909-593-6711
800-331-3676
Fax: 909-593-8001
pnunnelly@americanthermoform.com
www.americanthermoform.com
Patrick Nunnelly, VP
Gary Nunnelly, Owner
This copy machine, for producing tactile images, copies any Brailled or embossed original, by a vacuum forming process. This model is for the reproduction of teaching aids and mobility maps.

1598 **Duxbury Braille Translator**
Duxbury Systems
Ste 6
270 Littleton Rd
Westford, MA 01886-3523
978-692-3000
Fax: 978-692-7912
info@duxsys.com
www.duxburysystems.com
Joe Sullivan, President

A complete line of easy to use word processing and Braille translation software available for Windows (including 64 bit windows. Applications for anyone wanting to produce or communicate with Braille; signs, note cards, textbooks, business communications and forms, telephone bills, etc. Simple to use, FREE technical support. Free one year upgrades. DBT is for producing Braille in English, Spanish, French, Portuguese, Italian, Latin, Greek, German and 125 other languages. *$600.00*

1599 **Enabling Technologies Company**
1601 NE Braille Pl
Jensen Beach, FL 34957-5345
772-225-3687
800-777-3687
Fax: 772-225-3299
info@Brailler.com
www.Brailler.com

Tony Schenk, President
Kate Schenk, Product Manager Western US
Greg Schenk, Sales & Marketing

Manufactures the most complete line of American made Braille embossers, including desktop or portable models capable of producing high quality single sided or interpoint Braille. Also carries a complete line of adaptive technology aids for the blind community at affordable prices.

1600 **Freedom Scientific Blind/Low Vision Group**
11800 31st Ct N
St Petersburg, FL 33716-1805
727-803-8000
800-444-4443
Fax: 727-803-8001
info@freedomscientific.com
www.freedomscientific.com

Brad Davis, VP Hardware Product Management
Dr Lee Hamilton, President/CEO

Developer and manufacturer of assistive technology products for people who are blind or who have low vision. Innovative blindness products include: JAWS® screen reading software; the PAC Mate Omni™, an accessible Pocket PC; the SARA™ scanning and reading appliance; OpenBook™ scanning and reading software; FSReader™ DAISY player; FaceToFace™ deaf-blind communications solution; and PAC Mate and Focus Braille Displays. *$16.95*

1601 **Hooleon Corporation**
PO Box 589
Melrose, NM 88124-589
928-634-7515
800-937-1337
Fax: 928-634-4620
sales@hooleon.com
www.hooleon.com

Kim Green, Manager
Joan Crozier, President/Sales

Large print and combination Braille adhesive keytop labels for computer keyboards. Helps visually impaired computer users access correct key strokes either by sight or by touch. Raised Braille meets ADA specifications and large print fills key top surface.

1602 **Humanware**
1 UPS Way
P.O. Box 800
Champlain, NY 12919
800-722-3393
Fax: 888-871-4828
info@humanware.com
humanware.com

Gilles Pepin, CEO

Humanware manufactures electronics to provide solutions that empower the visually impaired.

1603 **Large Print/Braille Keyboard Labels**
Infogrip
1899 E. Main Street
Ventura, CA 93001-3411
805-652-0770
800-397-0921
Fax: 805-652-0880
support@infogrip.com
www.infogrip.com

Liza Jacobs, President
Aaron Gaston, Vice President

Makes a standard keyboard more accessible for visually impaired individuals with large print or Braille keyboard labels. Characters on the large print labels are .5 by .25 inches, about 3 times larger than standard keyboard characters. Braille labels are available as clear labels with Braille dots or large print with Braille. Each set includes all the keys used on a standard Windows keyboard. *$29.00*

1604 **Raised Dot Computing**
Duxbury Systems Incorporated
270 Littleton Rd.
Unit 6
Westford, MA 01886-3523
978-692-3000
Fax: 978-692-7912
info@duxsys.com
www.duxburysystems.com

Joe Sullivan, President
Peter Sullivan, VP of Software Development
Genevieve Sullivan, Treasurer
Dana Winikates, Software Engineer

Software for the visually impaired.

1605 **Touchdown Keytop/Keyfront Kits**
Hooleon Corporation
P.O. Box 589
304 West Denby Ave
Melrose, NM 88124
575-253-4503
800-937-1337
Fax: 575-253-4299
Sales@Hooleon.com
www.hooleon.com

Bob Crozier, Founder
Joan Crozier, President
Barry Green, Sales Manager

These kits enlarge the key legends of a computer and include Braille for easy recognition.

Information Centers & Databases

1606 **ATTAIN**
Division of Disability Aging & Rehab Services
Ste 1400
32 E Washington St
Indianapolis, IN 46204-3552
317-232-1147
800-528-8246
Fax: 317-486-8809

Gary R Hand, Executive Director
Peter Bisbecos, Manager

Nonprofit organization that creates system change by expanding the availability of community-based technology-related activities, outreach services, empowerment and advocacy activities through the development of a comprehensive, consumer-responsive, statewide program to serve individuals with disabilities, of all ages and all disabilities, their families, caregivers, educators and service providers. Provides training, information and referrals, system change and assessments for equipment needs.

1607 **AbleData**
103 W Broad St
Suite 400
Falls Church, VA 22046
301-608-8998
800-227-0216
Fax: 301-608-8958
TTY: 301-608-8912
abledata@neweditions.net
www.abledata.com

Katherine Belknap, Director
David Johnson, Publications Director

AbleData is an electronic database containing information on assistive technology and rehabilitation equipment products for children and adults with physical, cognitive and sensory disabilities. AbleData staff can perform database searches or the database can be searched via the website, informed consumer guides or fact sheets.

1608 **Aloha Special Technology Access Center**
710 Green St
Honolulu, HI 96813-2119
808-523-5547
Fax: 808-536-3765
astachi@yahoo.com

Ali Silvert, President
Ms. Jacquely Brand, Founder

Computer technology center.

1609 **Birmingham Alliance for Technology Access Center**
Birmingham Independent Living Center
206 13th St S.
Birmingham, AL 35233-1317
205-251-2223
Fax: 205-251-0605
TTY: 205-251-2223
www.drradvocates.org

Kathy Lovell, President
Phil Klebine, Vice President
Daniel Kessler, Executive Director
Judy Roy, Programs Coordinator
Computer technology center.

1610 **Bluegrass Technology Center**
409 Southland Drive
Lexington, KY 40503
859-294-4343
800-209-7767
Fax: 866-576-9625

Debbie Sharon, Acting Executive Director
Linnie Lee, Assistive Technology Specialist
Jean Isaacs, Assistive Technology Consultant
Linda Gassaway, PhD, Assistive Technology Consultant
Provides assistive technology information, consulting and training for education, health professionals, consumers and parents of consumers. Maintains extensive lending library of assistive devices and adapted toys. Statewide training such as; AAC, how to obtain funding for assistive technology, augmentative and alternate communication, equipment implementation strategies, specific to hardware and software, etc.

1611 **CITE: Lighthouse for Central Florida**
215 East New Hampshire Street
Orlando, FL 32804
407-898-2483
Fax: 407-898-0236
csacca@lcf-fl.org
www.lighthousecentralflorida.org/Default.asp

Lee Nasehi, MSW, President/CEO
Donna Esbensen CPA,MBA, VP/CFO
Jeff Whitehead, MPA, MS, Director of Program Services
Casey Mathews, Access Technology Specialist
CITE promotes the independence of adults and children with blindness, low vision and other disabilities through technology, education, support and advocacy.

1612 **Carolina Computer Access Center**
P.O. Box 247
Cramerton, NC 28032
704-342-3004
Fax: 704-342-1513

Linda Schilling, Executive Director
Nonprofit, community-based technology resource center for people with disabilities, providing information about and demonstration of the technology tools that enable individuals with disabilities to control and direct their own lives. Services and programs include: assessments, demonstrations, resource information, lending library, workshops and outreach.

1613 **Center for Accessible Technology**
3075 Adeline
Suite 220
Berkeley, CA 94703
510-841-3224
Fax: 510-841-7956
info@cforat.org
www.cforat.org

Dmitri Belser, Executive Director
Eric Smith, Associate Director
A consumer-based technology resource and demonstration center for adults and children with disabilities, families, teachers, and professionals. The primary focus is on assistive technology for computer access. Seen by appointment only.

1614 **Center for Applied Special Technology**
40 Harvard Mills Square
Suite 3
Wakefield, MA 01880-3233
781-245-2212
Fax: 781-245-5212
cast@cast.org
www.cast.org/

Anne Meyer, Founder
David H. Rose, Founder
Lisa Poller, Co-President
Gabrielle Rappolt-Schlichtmann, Co-President
Expands opportunities for individuals with special needs through innovative use of computers and related technology. We pursue this mission through research and product development that further universal design for learning.

1615 **Center for Assistive Technology & Inclusive Education Studies**
2000 Pennington Rd.
P.O. Box 7718
Ewing, NJ 08628-0718
609-771-3016
Fax: 609-637-5179
caties@tcnj.edu
caties.pages.tcnj.edu

Amanda Norvell, President
Matt Bender, VP
Regina Morin, Parliamentarian
Laurie Wanat, Secretary
Computer technology center offering resource time, workshops, technology, training and evaluations.

1616 **Center on Evaluation of Assistive Technology**
National Rehabilitation Hospital
102 Irving St NW
Washington, DC 20010
202-877-1000
TTY: 202-726-3996
justin.m.carter@medstar.net
www.medstarhealth.org

Kenneth A. Samet, FACHE, President, CEO
Michael J. Curran, EVP, Chief Administrative and Financial Officer
Christine Swearingen, EVP, Planning, Marketing and Community Relations
Stephen R.T. Evans, MD, EVP, Medical Affairs and Chief Medical Officer
The center develops ways of collecting, producing and distributing information to help users, prescribers and third-party payers make intelligent selections of devices.

1617 **Compuserve: Handicapped Users' Database**
5000 Arlington Centre Blvd
Columbus, OH 43220-2913
614-326-1002
800-848-8990
Fax: 614-538-4023
webcenters.netscape.compuserve.com

1618 **Computer Access Center**
P.O. Box 12464
Albuquerque, NM 87195
505-242-9588
info@cac.org
www.cac.org

Richard Barlow, Board of Director
Richard Rohr, Board of Director
Michael Poffenberger, Board of Director
Damien Faughnan, Board of Director
Computer technology center.

1619 **Computer Center for Visually Impaired People: Division of Continuing Studies**
Baruch College
1 Bernard Baruch Way
Box H-648
New York, NY 10010
646-312-1420
Fax: 646-312-5101
www.baruch.cuny.edu/ccvip

Karen Gourgey, Director
Judith Gerber, Operations Manager
Lynette Tatum, Training Specialist
William Reed, Assistant Director
Offers courses, tutors, equipment and assistance.

1620 **Computer Resources for People with Disabilities**
Hunter House Publishers, Inc
424 Church Street
Suite 2240
Nashville, TN 37219
615-255-BOOK
info@turnerpublishing.com
www.hunterhouse.com

Kiran Rana, Publisher
Chris Alexander, Author
Sheila Alson, Author
Peter Axt, Author

Part One describes conventional and assistive technologies and gives strategies for accessing the Internet. Part Two features easy-to-use charts organized by key access concerns, and provides detailed descriptions of software, hardware, and communication aids. Part Three is a gold mine of Web resources, publications, support organizations, government programs, and technology vendors.

1621 **Computer-Enabling Drafting for People with Physical Disabilities**
County College of Morris
214 Center Grove Road
Randolph, NJ 07869-2086
973-328-5000
888-226-8001
Fax: 973-328-5067
www.ccm.edu

Edward J Yaw, President
Dr. Dwight Smith, Vice President of Academic Affairs
Karen VanDerhoof, Vice President for Business and Finance
Dr. Bette M. Simmons, VP of Student Development & Enrollment Management

Since they opened in 1968, more than 40,000 graduates have passed through their halls. Many have become teachers, nurses, police officers, doctors and engineers. CCM has also been a community resource for those seeking to enhance their careers through additional education. They drafted a newsletter on Computer-Enabling Drafting for People with Physical Disabilities

1622 **DIRLINE**
National Library of Medicine
8600 Rockville Pike
Bethesda, MD 20894
301-594-5983
888-346-3656
Fax: 301-402-1384
TTY: 800-735-2258
www.nlm.nih.gov/

Dr. Donald A B. Lindberg, Director
Milton Corn, Deputy Director
Betsy Humphreys, Deputy Director
Todd Danielson, Office of Administration

18,000 listings of organizations that serve as information resources, including libraries, professional associations and government agencies.

1623 **Developmental Disabilities Council**
626 Main Street, Suite A
P.O. Box 3455
Baton Rouge, LA 70821-3455
225-342-6804
800-450-8108
Fax: 225-342-1970
shawn.fleming@la.gov
www.laddc.org

Sandee Winchell, Executive Director
Shawn Fleming, Deputy Director
Derek White, Program Manager
Robbie Gray, Program Monitor

The Louisiana Developmental Disabilities Council is made up of people from every region of the state who are appointed by the governor to develop and implement a five year plan to address the needs of persons with disabilities. Membership includes persons with developmental disabilities, parents, advocates, professionals, and representatives from public and private agencies.

1624 **Employment Resources Program**
330 South Grand Avenue West
Springfield, IL 62704
217-523-2587
800-447-4221
Fax: 217-523-0427
TTY: 217-523-2587
scil@scil.org
www.scil.org

Pete Roberts, Executive Director
Susanne Cooper, Program Director
Robin Ashton- Hale, Reintegration Coordinator
Kathryn Cline, Business Manager

An information and referral service that encourages inquiries from professionals, individuals with disabilities, family members, organizations or anyone requesting information pertaining to disabilities. The staff at DRN uses both computer listings and in-house library files to provide the programs services. The DRN program is funded by a grant from the Illinois Department of Rehabilitation Services.

1625 **Functional Skills Screening Inventory**
Functional Resources
3905 Huntington Dr
Amarillo, TX 79019-4047
806-353-1114
Fax: 806-353-1114
www.winfssi.com

Ed Hammer, Owner
Heather Becker PhD, Owner

Assesses the individual's level of functional skills and identifies supports needed by educational, rehabilitation and residential programs serving moderately and severely disabled persons. Includes environmental assessments as well as profiles of jobs and training sites.

1626 **High Tech Center**
Sacremento State
6000 J Street
Sacramento, CA 95819
916-278-6011
sswd@csus.edu
www.csus.edu

Alexander Gonzalez, President
Judy Dean, Co-Director
Melissa Repa, Co-Director
Terry Gomez, Office Manager

The Center offers assessment and training in adaptive hardware/software for eligible students with disabilities at Sacramento State upon referral from the Office of Services to Students with Disabilities.

1627 **Idaho Assistive Technology Project**
121 W 3rd St
Moscow, ID 83843-2268
208-885-3557
Fax: 208-885-3628
www.idahoat.org

Ron Seiler, Project Director
Sue House, Information Specialist

A federally funded program managed by the center on disabilities and human development at the university of Idaho. The goal of the IATP is to increase the availability of assistive technology devices and services for Idahoans with disabilities. The IATP offers free trainings and technical assistance, a low-interest loan program, assistive technology assessments for children and agriculture workers, and free informational materials.

1628 **Increasing Capabilities Access Network**
525 W.Capitol
Little Rock, AR 72201
501-666-8868
800-828-2799
Fax: 501-666-5319
TTY: 501-666-8868
nfo@ar-ican.org
www.arkansas-ican.org

Bryen Ayres, Member of Advisory Council
Billy Altom, Member of Advisory Council
Adrienne Brown, Member of Advisory Council
Carolyn Boyles, Member of Advisory Council

A consumer responsive statewide systems change program promoting assistive technology for persons of all ages with disabilities. The program provides information on new and existing technology and maintains an equipment exchange free of charge. Training on assistive technology is also provided.

1629 International Center for the Disabled
340 E 24th St
New York, NY 10010-4019
212-585-6000
Fax: 212-585-6161
info@icdnyc.org
www.icdnyc.org

Jill Bowman, Manager
Les Halpert, CEO

The ICD is a comprehensive outpatient rehabilitation facility, providing medical rehabilitation, behavioral health and vocational services to children and adults with a broad range of physical, communication, emotional and cognitive disabilities.

1630 Kentucky Assistive Technology Service Network
200 Juneau Dr.
Suite 200
Louisville, KY 40243
502-429-4484
800-327-5287
Fax: 502-429-7114
www.katsnet.org

Derrick Cox, Manager

Statewide network of four regional assistive technology centers with a central coordinating office in Louisville and two regional centers in eastern Kentucky. Network services include but are not limited to assistive technology of services, loan of assistive devices, funding information and referral, assessment and evaluations, consultations on appropriate technologies, training, and technical assistance.

1631 Learning Independence Through Computers
2301 Argonne Drive
Baltimore, MD 21218
410-554-9134
Fax: 410-261-2907
info@linc.org
www.linc.org

Theo Pinette, Executive Director
Sandy Fishman, Office and Computer Center Coordinator
Angela Tyler, Volunteer Services Manager
Christy Wooden, AT Learning Specialist

V-LINC creates technological solutions to improve the independence and quality of life for individuals of all ages with disabilities in Maryland. We do this through a mix of off-the-shelf computer software and equipment, and one-of-a-kind, customized assistive technology.

1632 MEDLINE
Dialog Corporation
2250 Perimeter Park Drive
Suite 300
Morrisville, NC 27560
800-334-2564
919-804-6400
Fax: 919-804-6410
www.dialog.com

Tim Wahlberg, Genral Manager
Morten Nicholaisen, VP Global Sales and Account Mana
Libby Trudell, VP Strategic Initiatives
Tim Hall, Director Integration and Busines

Bibliographic citations to biomedical literature.

1633 Maine CITE
University of Maine at Augusta
46 University Avenue
Augusta, ME 04330
207-621-3195
Fax: 207-629-5429
TTY: 877-475-4800
iweb@mainecite.org
www.mainecite.org

Robert McPhee, Member of Advisory Council
Deborah Gardner, Member of Advisory Council
Anita Dunham, Member of Advisory Council
Sandra Jaeger, Member of Advisory Council

Computer technology center.

1634 Maryland Technology Assistance Program
Maryland Department of Disabilities
2301 Argonne Drive
Rm T-17
Baltimore, MD 21218
410-554-9361
800-832-4827
Fax: 410-554-9237
TTY: 866-881-7488
www.mdtap.org

James McCarthy, Executive Director
Denise Schuler, Assistive Technology Specialist
Tanya Goodman, Loan Program Assistant Director
Lori Markland, Director of Communications, Outreach &Program Development

Assistive technology center. Information and referral, equipment display loans and demonstration, funding sources, alternative media, training, workshops and seminars. Rural outreach for individuals with disability in Maryland.

1635 Minnesota STAR Program
358 Centennial Office Building 658
Saint Paul, MN 55155- 1402
651-201-2640
800-627-3529
888-234-1267
Fax: 651-282-6671
star.program@state.mn.us

Chuck Rassbach, Program Director
Jennis Delisi, Program Staff
Jaoan Gillum, Program Staff
Kim Moccia, Program Staff

STAR's mission is to help all Minnesotans with disabilities gain access to and acquire the assistive technology they need to live, learn, work and lay. The Minnesota STAR program is federally funded by the Rehabilitation Services Administration.

1636 Mississippi Project START
2550 Peachtree Street
Jackson, MS 39216
601-987-4872
800-852-8328
Fax: 601-364-2349
pgaltelli@mdrs.ms.gov
www.msprojectstart.org

Patsy Galtelli, Executive Director
Dorothy Young, Project Director
Nekeba Simmons, Administrative Assistant
Jason Mac McMaster, Repair Specialist

Project START is a Tech Act project established to bring about systems change in the field of assistive technology in the State of Mississippi. Activities include providing training opportunities for consumers and service providers on subjects such as state-of-the-art AT devices, their application and funding resources; referral information on AT evaluation centers; technical assistance to AT users; establishment of an AT equipment loan program and an Information and Referral Service.

1637 National Technology Database
American Foundation for the Blind/ AF B Press
2 Penn Plaza
Suite 1102
New York, NY 10121
212-502-7600
800-232-5463
Fax: 888-545-8331
afbinfo@afb.net
www.afb.org

Carl.R Augusto, President and CEO
Robin Vogel, Vice President, Resource Development
Kelly Bleach, Chief Administrative Officer
Rick Bozeman, Chief Financial Officer

This database includes resources for visually impaired persons.
$99.00

1638 New Jersey Department of Labor & Workforce Development
Office of the Commissioner
1 John Fitch Plaza
P.O. Box 110
Trenton, NJ 08625-0110
609-292-7060
Fax: 609-633-1359
www.state.nj.us/labor

Harold J. Wirths, Commissioner
Aaron R. Fichtner, Ph.D., Deputy Commissioner
Frederick J. Zavaglia, Chief of Staff
David Ramsay, Director

Oversees various federal and state vocational rehabilitation services including sheltered workshops and independent living centers; adjudication of permanent disability claims filed with the Social Security Administration; oversees New Jersey's temporary disability program covering non-work related illnesses and injuries

1639 New Mexico Technology Assistance Program
625 Silver Ave SW
Suite 100 B
Albuquerque, NM 87102
505-841-4464
877-696-1470
Fax: 505-841-4467
www.tap.gcd.state.nm.us

Tracy Agiovlasitis, Program Manager

Examines and works to eliminate barriers to obtaining assistive technology in New Mexico. Has established a statewide program for coordinating assistive technology services; is designed to assist people with disabilities to locate, secure, and maintain assistive technology.

1640 Northern Illinois Center for Adaptive Technology
3615 Louisiana Rd
Rockford, IL 61108
815-229-2163
Dave Grass, President

Computer technology center.

1641 OCCK
1710 W. Schilling Road
Salina, KS 67402-1160
785-827-9383
800-526-9731
Fax: 785-823-2015
TTY: 785-827-9383
occk@occk.com
www.occk.com

Shelia Nelson Stout, President, CEO
Carolee Miner, CEO

Computer technology center; training center for employment and independent living for people with disabilities; family support center. Kansas AgrAbility program coordinator, Kansas equipment exchange site.

1642 Options, Resource Center for Independent Living
318 3rd St. NW
East Grand Forks, MN 56721
218-773-6100
800-726-3692
Fax: 218-773-7119
options@myoptions.info
www.rcil.com

Burt Danovitz, Executive Director

The RCIL aggressively advocates for and defends the rights of persons with disabilities. RCIL believes in integration adn assisting people to reach their full potential, encouraging a culture of risk-taking, creativity and innovation through our programs and services. They monitor and assess the current legal climate around rights for persons with disabilities on an ongoing bases and are committed and deliberate in speaking about the problems and obstacles faced by persons with disabilities.

1643 Parents, Let's Unite for Kids
516 N 32nd St
Billings, MT 59101-6003
406-255-0540
800-222-7585
Fax: 406-255-0523
TTY: 406-657-2055
info@pluk.org

Roger Holt, Executive Director

Computer technology center. Parents, Let's Unite for Kids offers an assistive technology lab that is open to people of all ages. The lab is a computer and assistive technology demonstration site. There is no charge for services.

1644 Pennsylvania's Initiative on Assistive Technology
Temple University
1755 N. 13th St.
Student Center, Room 411 South
Philadelphia, PA 19122-6024
215-204-1356
800-204-7428
Fax: 215-204-6336
TTY: 866-268-0579
ATinfo@temple.edu
www.disabilities.temple.edu

Kim Singleton, Director

Pennsylvania's Initiative on Assistive Technology (PIAT) offers information and referral about assistive Technology (AT), device demonstrations, and awareness-level presentations. PIAT also operates Pennsylvania's AT Lending Library, a free, state-supported program that loans AT devices to Pennsylvanians of all ages.

1645 Rehabilitation Engineering and AssistiveTechnology Society of North America (RESNA)
2025 M St. NW
Suite 800
Arlington, VA 20036
202-367-1121
Fax: 202-367-2121
info@resna.org
www.resna.org

Maureen Linden, President
Andrea Van Hook, Interim Executive Director

RESNA improves the potential of people with disabilities to achieve their goals through the use of technology. RESNA promotes research, development, education, advocacy and provision of technology; and by supporting the people engaged in these activities.

1646 SACC Assistive Technology Center
P.O. Box 1325
Simi Valley, CA 93062-1325
805-582-1881
www.semel.ucla.edu

Debi Schultze, CEO

SACC connects children, adults and seniors with special needs to computers, technologies and resources. We provide information and referral, assessments, tutoring, presentations and outreach awareness.

1647 South Dakota Department of Human Services: Computer Technology Services
Properties Plaza
500 East Capitol Avenue
Pierre, SD 57501
605-773-5990
800-265-9684
Fax: 605-773-5483
TTY: 605-773-6412
infodhs@state.sd.us
dhs.sd.gov

Dan Lusk, Division Director
Ted Williams, Director
Eric Weiss, Director
Gaye Mattke, Director

Computer technology center.

1648 Star Center
1119 Old Humboldt Rd
Jackson, TN 38305-1752
731-668-3888
888-398-5619
Fax: 731-668-1666
TTY: 731-668-9664
information@starcenter.tn.org
www.starcenter.tn.org

John Borden, CEO

Nation's largest assistive technology center dedicated to helping children and adults with disabilities achieve their goals for competitive employment, effective learning, returning to or starting school and independent living. Programs include: high-tech training, music therapy, art therapy, low vision evaluation, orientation and mobility evaluation and training, augmentative communication evaluation, vocational evaluations, assistive technology, job placement services and job skills training.

1649 **Students with Disabilities Office**
University of Texas at Austin
100 West Dean Keeton A5800
Austin, TX 78712-1100 512-471-5017
Fax: 512-471-7833
deanofstudents@austin.utexas.edu
deanofstudents.utexas.edu
Soncia Reagins-Lilly, Ed.D., Senior Associate VP for Student Affairs & Dean of Students
Douglas Garrard, Ed.D., Senior Associate Dean of Students
Wanda Brune, Administrative Associate
Sara LeStrange, Manager of Communications

1650 **TASK Team of Advocates for Special Kids**
100 W Cerritos Ave
Anaheim, CA 92805 714-533-8275
866-828-8275
Fax: 714-533-2533
task@taskca.org
www.taskca.org
Marta Anchondo, Executive Director
Tom Bratkovich, Treasurer
Leana Way, Director
Computer technology center.

1651 **Tech Connection**
35 Haddon Avenue
Shrewsbury, NJ 07702 732-747-5310
Fax: 732-747-1896
info@frainc.org
www.frainc.org
Bill Sheeser, President
Nancy Phalanukom, Executive Director
Sue Levine, Program Administrator
Vicky Butler, EI Program Coordinator
Offers a noncommercial center to examine and try computers, adapted equipment, alternative input devices, and a variety of software. Program of Family Resource Associates and a member of the Alliance for Technology Access (ATA), a growing national coalition of computer resource centers, professionals, technology developers and vendors, interacting with new technology to enrich the lives of people with disabilities. Tech Connection offers evaluations, for computer technology.

1652 **Tech-Able**
1451 Klondike Road, Suite D
Conyers, GA 30094 770-922-6768
Fax: 770-922-6769
Cassandra Baker, Executive Director
Pat Hanus, Program Assistant
Erika Ruffin-Mosley, Assistive Technology Trainer
Jason Chadwell, AT & Blind / Low Vision Trainer
Provide assistive technology to individuals with disabilities, toy-lending and software libraries, product demonstration, access to technology devices and fabrication of keyguards for keyboards. Low vision consultant on Thursdays; computer training for persons with disabilities.

1653 **Technology Access Center of Tucson**
P.O. Box 13178
Tucson, AZ 85732-3178 520-638-2733
Fax: 520-519-7954
tact1@qwestoffice.net
http://www.uacoe.arizona.edu/tact/

1654 **Technology Assistance for Special Consumers**
1856 Keats Dr NW.
Huntsville, AL 35810 256-859-8300
Fax: 256-859-4332
ucphuntsville.org/what-we-do/t-a-s-c/
Cheryl Smith, Chief Executive Officer
T.A.S.C. is a computer resource center with 10 computers, which are equipped with special adaptations for those who are blind, visually impaired, or severely physically disabled. The staff demonstrates and trains individuals on this equipment so that they can become more independent at home, school, and work. Over 2,500 pieces of educational software are available.

1655 **Tidewater Center for Technology Access Special Education Annex**
1415 Laskin Rd
Virginia Beach, VA 23451 757-424-2672
Fax: 757-263-2801
www.tcta.access.org
Pat Mc Gee, Manager
Myra Jessie Flint, Designee
Nonprofit organization providing persons with disabilities access, support, and knowledge—re: technology; organization contracts for consultations, workshops and training, or conventional and assistive technologies including computers, augmented communication devices and software; resources: extensive lending library of educational software; books and videotape library; yearly individual membership and corporate membership fees; working/presentation and evaluation fees available upon request.

1656 **Vermont Assistive Technology Project: Department of Aging & Disabilities**
Agency of Human Services
103 South Main Street
Weeks Building
Waterbury, VT 05671-2305 802-871-3353
800-750-6355
Fax: 802-871-3048
TTY: 802-241-1464
atp.vermont.gov
Amber Fulcher, Program Director
Sharon Alderman, Assistive Technology Reuse Coordinator
Emma Cobb, Assistive Technology Services Coordinator
Increase the awareness and change policies to insure assistive technology is available to all Vermonters with disabilities.

Keyboards, Mouses & Joysticks

1657 **A4 Tech (USA) Corporation**
5585 Brooks St
Montclair, CA 91763-4547 909-988-9633
www.a4tech.com
Robert C
Manufacturers of a cordless mouse, trackballs and joysticks that emulate mouse controls, flatbed scanners, modified keyboards, and other specialty mouses.

1658 **Abacus**
3150 Patterson Ave SE
Grand Rapids, MI 49512 616-698-0330
800-451-4319
Fax: 616-698-0325
www.abacuspub.com
Arnie Lee, President
Designs a mouse software program that permits programs written for one computer to be run on another computer.

1659 **Ability Center of Greater Toledo**
5605 Monroe St.
Sylvania, OH 43560 419-885-5733
Fax: 419-882-4813
www.abilitycenter.org
Tim Harrington, Executive Director
Ash Lemons, Associate Director
Debbie Andriette, Director, Human Resources
Jack Perion, Director, Finance & Operations
Manufactures keyboard wrist supports to help prevent repetitive motion disorders.

1660 **Dreamer**
TS Micro Tech
17109 Gale Ave
City of Industry, CA 91745-1810 626-939-8998
Fax: 626-839-8516
Steve Heung, Owner
An intelligent, add-on function keyboard providing single-keystroke access to multiple-keystroke functions.

1661 **FlexShield Keyboard Protectors**
Hooleon Corporation
P.O. Box 589
Melrose, NM 88124-589
928-634-7515
800-937-1337
Fax: 928-634-4620

Barry Green, Sales Manager
Joan Crozier, President

Transparent keyboard protectors allowing instant recognition of keytop legends. They have a matte finish to reduce glare. Also available are large print and Braille keyboard labels and large print/Braille combo labels.

1662 **IntelliKeys**
Intelli Tools
1720 Corporate Circle
Petaluma, CA 94954
707-773-2000
800-899-6687
Fax: 707-773-2001
info@intellitools.com
www.intellitools.com

Dayton Johnson, VP, Sales
Arjan Khalsa, CEO

Alternative, touch-sensitive keyboards; plugs into any Macintosh or Windows computer. *$395.00*

1663 **IntelliKeys USB**
Intelli Tools
1720 Corporate Circle
Petaluma, CA 94954
707-773-2000
800-899-6687
Fax: 707-773-2001
info@intellitools.com
www.intellitools.com

Dayton Johnson, VP, Sales
Arjan Khalsa, CEO

IntelliKeys alternative keyboard for USB computers and Windows 2000, Mac OSX. *$69.95*

1664 **Key Tronic KB 5153 Touch Pad Keyboard**
KeyTronic
N. 4424 Sullivan Road
Spokane Valley, WA 99216
509-928-8000
Fax: 509-927-5555
EMSsales@keytronicems.com
www.keytronic.com

Craig.D Gates, President/CEO
Ronald.F Klawitter, EVP of Administration and Chief Financial Officer
Douglas G. Burkhardt, Executive Vice President of Worldwide Operations
Philip S. Hochberg, Executive Vice President of Business Development

Integrates a regular full-function keyboard, a numeric keypad with a cursor key capability and a touch pad into one unit.

1665 **King Keyboard**
Infogrip
1899 E. Main Street
Ventura, CA 93001-3411
805-652-0770
800-397-0921
Fax: 805-652-0880
support@infogrip.com
www.infogrip.com

Liza Jacobs, President
Aaron Gaston, Vice President

Giant alternative keyboard that plugs directly into a computer—no special interface is required. The keys are 1.25 inches in diameter, slightly recessed, and provide both tactile and auditory feedback. The King has a built-in keyboard so that you can rest on its surface without activating keys. This keyboard allows you to control both keyboard and mouse functions, making it great for people who have difficulty maneuvering a standard mouse. *$130.00*

1666 **Large Print Keyboard**
Infogrip
1899 E. Main Street
Ventura, CA 93001-3411
805-652-0770
800-397-0921
Fax: 805-652-0880
support@infogrip.com
www.infogrip.com

Liza Jacobs, President
Aaron Gaston, Vice President

Standard Windows keyboard with large print keys. The keyboard and its keys are the same size as a standard keyboard; however, the print has been enhanced. The characters measure .5 by .25 inches, about 3 times larger than standard keyboard characters. *$130.00*

1667 **Magic Wand Keyboard**
In Touch Systems
11 Westview Road
Spring Valley, NY 10977
845-354-7431
800-332-6244
sc@magicwandkeyboard.com
www.magicwandkeyboard.com

Jerry Crouch, President
Susan Crouch, VP

The magic wand keyboard allows your child to use a keyboard and mouse easily-no light beams, microphones, or sensors to wear of position. This miniature computer keyboard has zero-force keys that work with the slightest touch of a wand (hand-held of mouthstick). No strength required.

1668 **McKey Mouse**
In Touch Systems
11 Westview Road
Spring Valley, NY 10977
845-354-7431
800-332-6244
sc@magicwandkeyboard.com
www.magicwandkeyboard.com

Jerry Crouch, President
Susan Crouch, VP

Microsoft compatible mouse for persons with little or no hand/arm movement; it's an option for the Magic Wand Keyboard and adds full mouse function without adding any extra devices.

1669 **OnScreen**
Infogrip
1899 E. Main Street
Ventura, CA 93001-3411
805-652-0770
800-397-0921
Fax: 805-652-0880
support@infogrip.com
www.infogrip.com

Liza Jacobs, President
Aaron Gaston, Vice President

OnScreen features word prediction/completion (with an editable dictionary), Key Dwell Timer (a timer that selects a key under the cursor), integrated Verbal Keys Feedback, Show and Hide Keys (turns on/off keys to prevent access and minimize confusion) a Smart Window (automatically re-positions the keyboard or panels off of the area in use). On Screen also offers edit, numeric, macro, calculator and Windows enhancement capabilities. *$200.00*

1670 **PortaPower Plus**
Words+
42505 10th Street West
Lancaster, CA 93534-7059
661-723-7723
800-869-8521
Fax: 661-723-5524
info@simulations-plus.com
www.simulations-plus.com

Walter S Woltosz, M.S., M.A.S., President, CEO
John A. DiBella, Vice President, Marketing & Sales
John R. Kneisel, Chief Financial Officer
Robert D. Clark, Ph.D., Director, Life Sciences

Rechargeable battery pack designed to give longer life and remote usage time to laptop computers and other portable battery-operated devices and accessories. Requires a 12 volt auto adapter. *$149.00*

1671 Unicorn Keyboards
Intelli Tools
1720 Corporate Circle
Petaluma, CA 94954
707-773-2000
800-899-6687
Fax: 707-773-2001
info@intellitools.com
www.intellitools.com

Dayton Johnson, VP, Sales
Arjan Khalsa, CEO
Alternative keyboards with membrane surface and large, user-defined keys. Large and small sizes are available. *$250.00*

Scanners

1672 Scanning WSKE
Words+
42505 10th Street West
Lancaster, CA 93534-7059
661-723-7723
888-266-9294
Fax: 661-723-5524
info@simulations-plus.com
www.simulations-plus.com

Walter S Woltosz, M.S., M.A.S., President, CEO
John A. DiBella, Vice President, Marketing & Sales
John R. Kneisel, Chief Financial Officer
Robert D. Clark, Ph.D., Director, Life Sciences
A software and a hardware product designed to operate on an IBM compatible PC. The software provides dual word prediction, abbreviation expansion, five different methods of voice output, and access to commercial software applications.

1673 System 2000/Versa
Words+
42505 10th Street West
Lancaster, CA 93534-7059
661-723-7723
800-869-8521
Fax: 661-723-5524
info@simulations-plus.com
www.simulations-plus.com

Walter S Woltosz, M.S., M.A.S., President, CEO
John A. DiBella, Vice President, Marketing & Sales
John R. Kneisel, Chief Financial Officer
Robert D. Clark, Ph.D., Director, Life Sciences
Provides all of the strategies currently being used in AAC, from dynamic display color pictographic language, to dual-word prediction text language, in a single system.

1674 Zygo-Usa
SVC Corporation
48834 Kato Road Suite 101-A
Fremont, CA 94538
510-249-9660
800-234-6006
Fax: 510-770-4930
www.zygo-usa.com

Adam Weiss, Vp Sales & Marketing
ZYGO-USA has been involved in manufacturing and distributing assistive technologies since 1974. They specialize in augmentative and alternative computer access. They offer a wide range of technology products to our clients so they can achieve a greater independence and to enhance the quality of their lives. These soloutins improve and individual's ability to learn, work, and interact with family and friends.

Screen Enhancement

1675 Boxlight
Boxlight Corporation
151 State Highway 300, Suite A
P.O. Box 2609
Belfair, WA 98528
360-464-2119
866-972-1549
sales@boxlight.com
www.boxlight.com

Herb Myers, CEO/Founder
Sloan Myers, Founder
Hank Nance, President
BOXLIGHT is a global presentation solutions partner for trainers, educators and professional speakers. Solutions include projector sales, national rental service, technical support, repair, and presentation peripherals. For more information visit us online.

1676 FDR Series of Low Vision Reading Aids
Optelec U S
Breslau 4
Barendrecht, LT 92081-8358
886-783-444
800-826-4200
Fax: 886-783-400
info@optelec.com
in.optelec.com

Stephan Terwolbeck, President
Michiel van Schaik, VP
Janet Lennex, Director of Customer Excellence
Jade Arbelo, Director of Human Resources
The Low Vision Reading Aids features; high resolution, positive and negative display, a high-quality zoom lens, versatile swivel and a 12 inch or 19 inch high-resolution monitor, color or black and white, computer compatible, or portable.

1677 InFocus
AI Squared
130 Taconic Business Park Road
Manchester Center, VT 05255
802-362-3612
800-859-0270
Fax: 802-362-1670
sales@aisquared.com
www.aisquared.com

David Wu, CEO
Jost Eckhardt, VP of Engineering
Scott Moore, VP of Marketing
Shawn Warren, VP of Product Support
A memory-resident program that magnifies text and graphics - the entire screen, a single line or a portion of the screen.

1678 Portable Large Print Computer
Human Ware
1800, Michaud street
Drummondville, CA 94520-1213
819-471-4818
888-723-7273
Fax: 925-681-4630
ca.info@humanware.com
www.humanware.com/en-australia/home

Real Goulet, Chairman
Gilles Pepin, CEO
Michel Cote, Corporate Director
Georges Morin, Corporate Director
A portable large print computer which magnifies up to 64 times. It is linked to a PC and has a hand-held camera.

1679 ZoomText
A I Squared
130 Taconic Business Park Road
Manchester Center, VT 05255
802-362-3612
800-859-0270
Fax: 802-362-1670
sales@aisquared.com
www.aisquared.com

David Wu, CEO
Jost Eckhardt, VP of Engineering
Scott Moore, VP of Marketing
Shawn Warren, VP of Product Support
A RAM-resident program that enlarges screen characters up to eight times. It runs on IBM PC, XT, AT and PS/2.

Speech Synthesizers

1680 **Artic Business Vision (for DOS) and Artic WinVision (for Windows 95)**
Artic Technologies
3456 Rodchester Road
Troy, MI 48083
248-689-9883
Fax: 248-588-2650
info@ablezone.com

Dale McDaniel, Founder
Kathy Gargagliano, Founder

A speech processor for blind computer users featuring true interactive speech with spread sheets, word processors, database managers, etc. Now available with both Windows 3.1 and Windows 95 access. *$495.00*

1681 **Computerized Speech Lab**
Kay Elemetrics Corporation
3 Paragon Drive
Montvalle, NJ 07645
973-628-6200
800-289-5297
Fax: 201-391-2063
www.kaypentax.com

John Crump, President

Hardware/software for the acquisition, analysis/display, playback and storage of speech signals.

1682 **DynaVox Technologies Speech Communication Devices**
Dyna Vox Technologies
2100 Wharton St
Suite 400
Pittsburgh, PA 15203-1945
412-381-4883
866-396-2869
Fax: 412-381-5241
www.dynavoxtech.com

Ed Donnelly, CEO
Michelle Heying, President and COO
Kenneth Misch, CFO
Ray Merk, VP Finance

Develops and manufactures speech communication devices that help individuals who are unable to speak due to speech, language and/or learning disabilities to communicate quickly and easily.

1683 **Electronic Speech Assistance Devices**
Luminaud, Inc.
8688 Tyler Blvd
Mentor, OH 44060-4348
440-255-9082
800-255-3408
Fax: 440-255-2250
info@luminaud.com
www.luminaud.com

Thomas M. Lennox, President
Dorothy Lennox, Vice President

Offers a full line of speech aids, voice amplifiers, mini-vox amplifiers, laryngectomee products.

1684 **Keywi**
Hoffmann + Krippner Inc.
200 Westpark Drive
Suite 270
Peachtree City, GA 30269
770-487-1950
Fax: 770-487-1945
www.keywi-usa.com

1685 **Little Mack Communicator**
AbleNet, Inc.
2625 Patton Road
Roseville, MN 55113-1137
651-294-2200
800-322-0956
Fax: 651-294-2259
customerservice@ablenetinc.com
www.ablenetinc.com

Bill Sproull, Chair of the Board
Jennifer Thalhuber, President & CEO
William Mills, Board of Directors
Paul Sugden, CFO & Trustee

The Little Mack Communicator has 2 minutes of memory and has an angled switch surface making it easy to see and access. The switch surface is 2 1/2 inches in diameter. Detachable mounting base makes it easy to position a single unit in a variety of locations. *$129.00*

1686 **Mega Wolf Communication Device**
Wayne County Regional Educational Service Agency
33500 Van Born Rd
Wayne, MI 48184-2474
734-334-1300
Fax: 734-334-1620
www.resa.net

Lynda S. Jackson, President
Kenneth E. Berlinn, Vice President
James Petrie, Secretary
Mary E. Blackmon, Treasurer

A low cost voice output communication device which is primarily intended to provide the power of speech to those individuals who are most severely challenged mentally and/or physically. The WOLF device is User programmable and uses the Texas Instruments' Touch and Tell case and touch panel; ADAMLAB electronics with synthesized (robotic) voice. For users able to point with approximately 6 ounces of pressure. *$400.00*

1687 **Talking Screen**
Words+
42505 10th St W
Lancaster, CA 93534-7059
661-723-7723
888-266-9294
Fax: 661-723-5524
info@simulations-plus.com
www.simulations-plus.com

Walter S Woltosz, M.S., M.A.S., Chairman, President and Chief Ex
John R. Kneisel, Chief Financial Officer
John DiBella, Vice President, Marketing and Sales
Robert D. Clark, Ph.D, Director, Life Sciences

An augmentative communication program that allows the user to select graphic symbols on the display to produce speech output. Symbols can be used either singly or in sequence as picture abbreviations. *$1395.00*

1688 **Turnkey Computer Systems for the Visually, Physically, and Hearing Impaired**
E VA S
39 Canal St P.O. Box 371
Westerly, RI 02891-1511
401-596-3155
800-872-3827
Fax: 401-596-3979
TTY: 401-596-3500
contact@evas.com
www.evas.com

Gerald Swerdlick, Owner
Jerry Swerdlick, CEO

Offers clear speech with pleasant inflection and tonal quality as well as variable pitch, intonation and voices.

1689 **Voice-It**
V XI Corporation Incorporated
271 Locust Street
Denver, NH 03820
603-742-2888
800-742-8588
Fax: 603-742-5065
info@vxicorp.com
www.vxicorp.com

Michael Ferguson, President
Tom Manero, Chief Financial Officer
Phil Pane, Vice President Operations
Brian Cole, Vice President Engineering

Adds voice to popular spreadsheet and word processing applications on IBM PCs and compatibles, turning spreadsheets and word processing documents into talking documents.

1690 **Window-Eyes**
G W Micro
725 Airport North Office Park
Fort Wayne, IN 46825
260-489-3671
Fax: 260-489-2608
www.gwmicro.com

Dan Weirich, Owner/Vice President of Sales an
Doug Geoffray, Owner

Provides access to available software automatically reading information important to the user while ignoring the rest. A screen reader for the windows operative system.

Software: Math

1691 **AIMS Multimedia**
Discovery Education
8145 Holton Dr
Florence, KY 41042-3009
859-342-7200
Fax: 877-324-6830

Mike Wright, Director
Lynn Fassett, Administrative Assistant
Cindy Vogt, Human Resources Executive
AIMS Multimedia is a leader in the production and distribution of training and educational programs for the business and K-12 communities via YHS, interactive CD-ROM, DVD and Internet streaming video.

1692 **Basic Math: Detecting Special Needs**
Allyn & Bacon
One Liberty Square
Suite 1200
Boston, MA 02109-3988
617-261-0040
800-852-8024
Fax: 617-944-7273
samplingdept@pearson.com
www.greenellp.com

Thomas M Greene, Attorney at Law
Michael Tabb, Attorney at Law
Describes special mathematics needs of special learners.
180 pages
ISBN 0-205116-35-3

1693 **Campaign Math**
Mindplay
4400 E. Broadway Blvd
Suite 400
Tucson, AZ 85711-1726
520-888-1800
800-221-7911
Fax: 520-888-7904
mail@mindplay.com
www.mindplay.com

Judith Bliss, CEO
Brian Williams, Development Manager
Lisa Garcia, Director of Educational Services
Chris Coleman, Vice President of Business Development
A complete program on the electoral process as well as a math package which teaches ratios, fractions and percentages.

1694 **Educational Activities Software**
5600 W 83rd Street
Suite 300, 8200 Tower
Bloomington, MN 55437
866-243-8464
Fax: 239-225-9299
jwest@orchardlng.com
www.edmentum.com

Vin Riera, President & Chief Executive Officer
Rob Rueckl, Chief Financial Officer
Dave Adams, Chief Academic Officer
Paul Johansen, Chief Technology Officer
Comprehensive MATH SKILLS software tutorials teach concepts ranging from rounding and tables to measuring area. MAC/WIN compatible. *$369.00*
Per Unit

1695 **Fraction Factory**
Queue
80 Hathaway Drive
Stratford, CT 06615
800-232-2224
Fax: 800-775-2729
jdk@queueinc.com
qworkbooks.com

Anna Christopoulos, General Manager
Peter Uhrynowski, Comptroller
Steve Pernett, Director of Printing and Graphic
Ann Pleszko, Shipping Manager
In 1980, Jonathan Kantrowitz started Queue, Inc. as an educational software company. After twenty thriving years publishing and distributing high-quality software to educators, Queue began transitioning from software to workbooks, focusing on state-specific test preparation.

1696 **Information & Referral Services**
Information + Referral Services
2590 N. Alvernon Way
Tucson, AZ 85712
520-323-1708
Fax: 520-325-8841
www.azinfo.org

Patti Caldwell, Executive Director
Chuck Palm, Treasurer
Ben Rensvold, Vice President
Tom DeSollar, President
Provides information about health and human services for people in Arizona over the telephone. Information specialists help callers clarify their needs, and provide referrals to the appropriate service agency.

1697 **King's Rule**
WINGS for Learning
1600 Green Hills Rd
Scotts Valley, CA 95066-4981
831-426-2228
Fax: 831-464-3600

Ani Stocks, Owner
A software mathematical problem solving game. Students discover mathematical rules as they work their way through a castle and generate and test a working hypothesis by asking questions.

1698 **Learning About Numbers**
C&C Software
5713 Kentford Cir
Wichita, KS 67220-3131
316-683-6056
800-752-2086

Carol Clark, President
Three programs use the power of computer graphics to provide young children with a variety of experiences in working with numbers. *$50.00*

1699 **Math Rabbit**
Learning Company
Ste 1900
100 Pine St
San Francisco, CA 94111-5205
415-659-2000
800-825-4420
Fax: 415-659-2020
thelearningco@hmhpub.com
www.hmhco.com

Linda K. Zecher, President, Chief Executive Officer and Director
Eric Shuman, Chief Financial Officer
William Bayers, Executive Vice President and General Counsel
Dr. Tim Cannon, Executive Vice President,
Teaches early math concepts by matching objects to numbers, then adding and subtracting up to 18.

1700 **Math for Everyday Living**
Educational Activities Software
5600 W 83rd Street
Suite 300, 8200 Tower
Bloomington, MN 55437
866-243-8464
Fax: 239-225-9299
jwest@orchardlng.com
www.edmentum.com

Vin Riera, President & Chief Executive Officer
Rob Rueckl, Chief Financial Officer
Dave Adams, Chief Academic Officer
Paul Johansen, Chief Technology Officer
Real life math skills are taught with this tutorial and practice software program. Examples include Paying for a Meal (addition and subtraction), Working with Sales Slips (multiplication), Unit Pricing (division), Sales Tax (percent), Earning with Overtime (fractions) plus more. Software: CD-ROM, Windows, MAC, and DOS. *$159.00*

1701 **Math for Successful Living**
Siboney Learning Group
5600 W 83rd Street
Suite 300, 8200 Tower
Bloomington, MN 55437
866-243-8464
Fax: 239-225-9299
jwest@orchardlng.com
www.edmentum.com

Vin Riera, President & Chief Executive Officer
Rob Rueckl, Chief Financial Officer
Dave Adams, Chief Academic Officer
Paul Johansen, Chief Technology Officer

These programs include managing a checking account, budgeting, shopping strategies and buying on credit.

1702 **Piece of Cake Math**
Queue Inc
80 Hathaway Drive
Stratford, CT 06615
800-232-2224
Fax: 800-775-2729
jdk@queueinc.com
www.qworkbooks.com

Anna Christopoulos, General Manager
Peter Uhrynowski, Comptroller
Steve Pernett, Director of Printing and Graphic
Ann Pleszko, Shipping Manager

In 1980, Jonathan Kantrowitz started Queue, Inc. as an educational software company. After twenty thriving years publishing and distributing high-quality software to educators, Queue began transitioning from software to workbooks, focusing on state-specific test preparation.

1703 **Puzzle Tanks**
WINGS for Learning
1600 Green Hills Rd
Scotts Valley, CA 95066-4981
831-426-2228
Fax: 831-464-3600

Ani Stocks, Owner

A mathematical problem solving game that involves multi-step problems.

1704 **Right Turn**
WINGS for Learning
1600 Green Hills Rd
Scotts Valley, CA 95066-4981
831-426-2228
Fax: 831-464-3600

Ani Stocks, Owner

Requires students to predict, experiment and learn about the mathematical concepts of rotation and transformation.

1705 **RoboMath**
4400 E. Broadway Blvd
Suite 400
Tucson, AZ 85711-1726
520-888-1800
800-221-7911
Fax: 520-888-7904
mail@mindplay.com
www.mindplay.com

Judith Bliss, CEO
Brian Williams, Development Manager
Lisa Garcia, Director of Educational Services
Chris Coleman, Vice President of Business Development

A complete program on the electoral process as well as a math package which teaches ratios, fractions and percentages.

1706 **Stickybear Math I Deluxe**
Optimum Resource
1 Mathews Drive
Suite 107
Hilton Head Island, SC 29926- 3689
843-689-8000
Fax: 843-689-8008
info@stickybear.com
www.stickybear.com

Richard Hefter, President

Sharpen basic addition and subtraction skills with this captivating series of math exercises. Grades Pre-K to 2. Available in as single edition with sizing up to 30 users at a site. English/Spanish. *$59.95*

1707 **Stickybear Math II Deluxe**
Optimum Resource
1 Mathews Drive
Suite 107
Hilton Head Island, SC 29926- 3689
843-689-8000
Fax: 843-689-8008
info@stickybear.com
www.stickybear.com

Richard Hefter, President

Multiplication and division, beginning with the elementary problems and developing into the more complex problems with regrouping. Grades 2-4. Available for single user through the 30 user site package. English/Spanish. *$59.95*

1708 **Stickybear Math Splash**
Optimum Resource
1 Mathews Drive
Suite 107
Hilton Head Island, SC 29926- 3689
843-689-8000
Fax: 843-689-8008
info@stickybear.com
www.stickybear.com

Richard Hefter, President

Unique multiple activities keep the learning level high while children acquire skills in addition, subtraction, multiplication and division. K-5th grade. Available as single edition up to 30 user site package. English/Spanish. *$59.95*

1709 **Stickybear Math Word Problems**
Optimum Resource
1 Mathews Drive
Suite 107
Hilton Head Island, SC 29926- 3689
843-689-8000
Fax: 843-689-8008
info@stickybear.com
www.stickybear.com

Richard Hefter, President

Hundreds of different word problems make it easy for students to practice basic math skills around analyzing and solving word problems. Grades 1-5. Available as single edition up to 30 user site package. English/Spanish. *$59.95*

1710 **Stickybear Money**
Optimum Resource
1 Mathews Drive
Suite 107
Hilton Head Island, SC 29926- 3667
843-689-8000
Fax: 843-689-8008
info@stickybear.com
www.stickybear.com

Chris Gintz, President

Teaches children to recognize US coins and paper money and introduces simple counting. K to 3rd grade. Bilingual. *$59.95*

1711 **Stickybear Numbers Deluxe**
Optimum Resource
1 Mathews Drive
Suite 107
Hilton Head Island, SC 29926- 3689
843-689-8000
Fax: 843-689-8008
info@stickybear.com
www.stickybear.com

Richard Hefter, President

Counting and number recognition are as easy as 1-2-3 with this award-winning program. Teaches number recognition of numbers 0-9 and 0-30. Pre-K to 2nd grade. Available as single edition up to 30 user site package. *$59.95*

1712 **Tomorrow's Promise: Mathematics**
Compass Learning
203 Colorado Street
Austin, TX 78701
512-478-9600
800-678-1412
866-586-7387
www.compasslearning.com

Eric Loeffel, President
Trey Chambers, Chief Financial Officer
Arthur Vanderveen, Vice President, Business Strategy and Development
Chipp Walters, Chief Designer Officer

By integrating interdisciplinary content and real-world application of skills, this product emphasizes the practical value of fundamental math skills. It helps your students develop a problem-solving aptitude for ongoing mathematics achievement.

Software: Miscellaneous

1713 **Adventures in Musicland**
Electronic Courseware Systems
1713 S State St
Champaign, IL 61820-7258
217-359-7099
800-832-4965
Fax: 217-359-6578
support@ecsmedia.com
http://ecsmedia.com.np/

G Peters, President
Jodie Varner, Marketing Manager
This unique set of music games features characters from Lewis Carroll's, Alice in Wonderland. Players learn through pictures, sounds, and animation which help develop understanding of musical tones, composers, and musical symbols. Games include MusicMatch, Melody Mixup, Picture Perfect and Sound Concentration. *$49.95*

1714 **Ai Squared**
130 Taconic Business Park Road
Manchester Center, VT 05255-669
802-362-3612
800-859-0270
Fax: 802-362-1670
sales@aisquared.com
http://www.aisquared.com

David Wu, CEO
Jost Eckhardt, VP of Engineering
Scott Moore, VP of Marketing
Shawn Warren, VP of Product Support
Developers of software for the visually impaired.

1715 **All About You: Appropriate Special Interactions and Self-Esteem**
P CI Educational Publishing
P.O. Box 34270
San Antonio, TX 78265-4270
210-377-1999
800-594-4263
800-471-3000
Fax: 888-259-8284

Lee Wilson, President and CEO
Randy Pennington, Executive VP
Jeff McLane, Founder
David Keith, Vice President of IT
This game offers parents and game players a new line of communication when discussing various issues such as learning to be thoughtful, respecting the rights and feelings of others, how to make and keep friends and more. *$49.95*

1716 **All Star Review**
Tom Snyder Productions
100 Talcott Ave
Watertown, MA 02472-5703
800-342-0236
www.tomsnyder.com

Rick Abrams, Manager
Tom Synder, Founder
Bridget Dalton, Ed.D., Author
Peggy Healy Stearns, Ph.D., Author
This package turns group review into a baseball game for small and large groups.

1717 **Attainment Company**
I ET Resources
504 Commerce Parkway
P.O. Box 930160
Verona, WI 53593- 0160
608-845-7880
800-327-4269
Fax: 800-942-3865
info@attainmentcompany.com
www.attainmentcompany.com

Autumn Garza, President
Don Bastian, CEO
Augmentative and alternative communication, software, videos, print and hands-on functional life skills and basic acdemics materials for developmental and cognitive disabilities.

1718 **Attention Getter**
Soft Touch
12301 Central Ave NE Ste 205
4300 Stine Rd
Blaine, MN 55434
763-755-1402
888-755-1402
Fax: 763-862-2920
support@marblesoft.com
www.softtouch.com

Joyce Meyer, President
The whimsical photos morph to another photo and then to a third photo in categories. Paired with interesting sounds and music, the photo animations are so engaging that the student is motivated to activate the computer to see and hear the next one. This is a perfect vehicle to achieve goals aimed at attention getting, activating a switch or intentionally. Compatible with USB IntelliKeys keyboards.

1719 **Attention Teens**
Soft Touch
12301 Central Ave NE Ste 205
Blaine, MN 55434
763-755-1403
888-755-1403
Fax: 763-862-2921
support@marblesoft.com
www.softtouch.com

Joyce Meyer, President
Attention Teens (formerly known as Loony Teens) is a program for teens with disabilities who need powerful input to get their attention. Attention Teens is a computer program to do just this. Paired with interesting sounds and music, the photo animations are so engaging that the student is motivated to activate the computer to see and hear the next one. Compatible with USB IntelliKeys keyboards.

1720 **Away We Ride**
Soft Touch
12301 Central Ave NE Ste 205
4300 Stine Rd
Blaine, MN 55434
763-755-1404
888-755-1404
Fax: 763-862-2922
support@marblesoft.com
www.softtouch.com

Joyce Meyer, President
Software for children and teens. For Macintosh and PC.

1721 **Battenberg & Associates**
11135 Rolling Springs Dr
Carmel, IN 46033-3629
317-843-2208
Jan Battenberg, Owner
Offers various software programs that develop the user's visual memory, sequencing skills, word recognition, hand-eye coordination and more.

1722 **Behavior Skills: Learning How People Should Act**
PCI Education Publishing
P.O. Box 34270
San Antonio, TX 78265-4270
210-377-1999
800-471-3000
Fax: 888-828-
www.pcieducation.com

Jeff Clain, CEO
Erin Kinard, VP Product Development/Publisher
Helps players learn what behavior is acceptable and what behavior is not acceptable in the real world. *$49.95*

1723 **Blocks in Motion**
Don Johnston
26799 West Commerce Drive
Volo, IL 60073-9675
847-740-0749
800-999-4660
Fax: 847-740-7326
info@donjohnston.com
www.donjohnston.com

Don Johnston, Founder
Ruth Ziolkowski, President
Kevin Johnston, Director of Product Design
Ben Johnston, Director of Marketing

This unique art and motion program makes drawing, creating and animating fun and educational for all users. Based on the Piagetian Theory for motor-sensory development, this program promotes the concept that the process is as educational and as much fun as the end result. *$79.00*

1724 **Car Builder Deluxe**
Optimum Resource
1 Mathews Drive
Suite 107
Hilton Head Island, SC 29926- 3689
843-689-8000
Fax: 843-689-8008
info@stickybear.com
www.stickybear.com

Richard Hefter, President

As design engineers, users build cars on screen, specifying chassis length, wheelbase, engine type, transmission, fuel tank size, suspension, steering, tires and brakes. All functional choices are interrelated and will affect the performance of the final design. Grades 3 & up. *$59.99*

1725 **Center for Best Practices in Early Childhood**
Horrabin Hall 32
Macomb, IL 61455
309-298-1634
Fax: 309-298-2305
jk-johanson@wiu.edu
www.wiu.edu/thecenter/

Linda Robinson, Assistant Director

The Center, part of the College of Education and Human Services at Western Illinois University, provides products, training materials, and information related to best practices for educators and families of young children with disabilities.

1726 **Clock**
Compass Learning
203 Colorado Street
Austin, TX 78701-3922
512-478-9600
800-678-1412
866-586-7387
www.compasslearning.com

Eric Loeffel, President
Trey Chambers, Chief Financial Officer
Arthur Vanderveen, Vice President, Business Strategy and Development
Chipp Walters, Chief Designer Officer

An extremely simple, easy-to-use program for children who are learning how to read the time of day from clocks and digital displays. Apple and MS-DOS and Mac available. *$39.95*

1727 **Community Skills: Learning to Function in Your Neighborhood**
Programming Concepts
8700 Shoal Creek Boulevard
Austin, TX 78757-6897
210-377-1999
800-594-4263
800-471-3000
Fax: 888-259-8284
www.proedinc.com

Lee Wilson, President and CEO
Randy Pennington, Executive VP
Jeff McLane, Founder
David Keith, Vice President of IT

Offers parents and educators a functional way to teach community life skills. *$49.95*

1728 **Companion Activities**
Soft Touch
12301 Central Ave NE Ste 205
4300 Stine Rd
Blaine, MN 55434
763-755-1404
888-755-1404
Fax: 763-862-2922
support@marblesoft.com
www.softouch.com

Joyce Meyer, President

Print your own books, worksheets, flash cards, board games, matching games, bingo games, card games and many more. This CD offers numerous companion activities to different SoftTouch software titles. Activities range from very easy to difficult. Companion activities are great tools to reinforce learning. Use the work sheets - black and white and color - in the inclusion class for students with special needs.

1729 **Concepts on the Move Advanced Preacademics**
Soft Touch
12301 Central Ave NE Ste 205
P.O. Box 490215
Blaine, MN 55449
763-862-2920
888-755-1402
Fax: 763-862-2922
support@marblesoft.com
www.marblesoft.com

Joyce Meyer, President

Choose from five concepts groups: categories, occupations, functions, goes with and prepositions. Use our Steps to Learning Design to choose how many concepts to present at one time and where to place each one in the scan array, on screen keyboard or IntelliKeys keyboard. Watch and listen as the concept morphs or changes and music plays. The words are also shown to reinforce emerging literacy skills. Compatible with USB IntelliKeys.

1730 **Cooking Class: Learning About Food Preparation**
Programming Concepts
8700 Shoal Creek Boulevard
Austin, TX 78757-6897
512-451-3246
800-897-3202
800-471-3000
Fax: 800-397-7633
general@proedinc.com
www.proedinc.com

Jeff McLane, Founder
Lee Wilson, President and CEO
Randy Pennington, Executive VP
David Keith, Vice President of IT

This game offers parents and educators a new way to teach basic preparation skills. Kitchen safety and sanitation are stressed throughout the game. *$49.95*

1731 **Dilemma**
Educational Activities Software
5600 West 83rd Street
Suite 300, 8200 Tower
Bloomington, MN 55437
800-447-5286
Fax: 239-225-9299
info@edmentum.com
www.edmentum.com

Vin Riera, President/CEO
Dan Juckniess, SVP, Sales & Professional Services
Stacey Herteux, VP, Human Resources
Rob Rueckl, Chief Financial Officer

Realistic stories with a choice of different gripping endings, color graphics, a built-in dictionary and a user controlled reading rate make these computer programs compelling enough to interest all students. Comprehension and vocabulary questions follow each story. *$159.00*

1732 **Dino-Games**
Academic Software
3504 Tates Creek Road
Lexington, KY 40517-2601
859-552-1020
859-552-1040
Fax: 253-799-4012
asistaff@acsw.com
www.acsw.com

Dr. Warren E Lacefield PhD, President
Penelope D. Ellis, COO, Sales & Marketing Director
Sylvia B. Lacefield, Graphic Artist
Cindy L George, Author

Dino-Games are single switch software programs for early switch practice. Dinosaur games provide practice in pattern recognition, cause and effect demonstration, directionality training, number concepts and problem solving. They are compatible with most popular switch interfaces and alternate keyboards. For Macintosh, IBM and compatibles. DINO-LINK is a matching game; DINO-MAZE is a series of maze games; DINO-FIND is a game of concentration; and DINO-DOT is a collection of dot-to-dot games.
$39.95 per game

1733 **Directions: Technology in Special Education**
DREAMMS for Kids
273 Ringwood Road
Freeville, NY 13068-5606
607-539-3027
Fax: 607-539-9930
janet@dreamms.org
www.dreamms.org

Janet P. Hosmer, Editor/Publisher
Chester D. Hosmer, Jr., Technical Editor
Susan Lait, Regular Contributor
Lorianne Hoenninger, Regular Contributor

A CD containing all of 'Directions' past articles and information gathered from their newsletter which lists resources for assistive and adaptive computer ethnologies in the home, school and community. *$24.95*

1734 **ESI Master Resource Guide**
Educational Software Institute
4213 S 94th St
Omaha, NE 68127-1223
402-592-3300
800-955-5570
Fax: 402-592-2017

Lee Myers, President
Kathy Cavanaugh, Catalog Manager

Educational Software Institute (ESI) provides a one-stop shop to purchase software titles by all of the best publishers. The ESI Master Gold Book catalog and CD-ROM represents more than 400 software publishers, with information on more than 8,000 software titles. Take the confusion out of software selection by calling ESI for all of your software needs - including competitive prices, software previews, knowledgeable assistance, and the largest selection available all in one place.
Yearly

1735 **EZ Keys**
Words+
42505 10th Street West
Suite 109
Lancaster, CA 93534- 7059
661-723-7723
888-266-9294
Fax: 661-723-5524
info@simulations-plus.com
www.simulations-plus.com

Walter S Woltosz, M.S., M.A.S., Chairman, President and Chief Executive Officer
John A. Dibella, VP, Marketing & Sales
Virginia E. Woltosz. M.B.A., Secretary & Treasurer
John R. Kneisel, Chief Financial Officer

A software and hardware product designed to operate on an IBM compatible PC. The software provides dual word prediction, abbreviation expansion, five different methods of voice output and access to commercial software applications. *$1395.00*

1736 **Early Games for Young Children**
Queue Incorporated
80 Hathaway Drive
Stratford, CT 06615
800-232-2224
Fax: 800-775-2729
jdk@queueinc.com
www.qworkbooks.com

Anna Christopoulos, General Manager
Peter Uhrynowski, Comptroller
Steve Perrett, Director of Printing and Graphics
Ann Pleszko, Shipping Manager

Software that includes nine activities that entertain preschoolers in honing basic math and language skills.

1737 **Early Music Skills**
Electronic Courseware Systems
1713 S State St
Champaign, IL 61820-7258
217-359-7099
800-832-4965
Fax: 217-359-6578
support@ecsmedia.com
www.ecsmedia.com

G Peters, President
Jodie Varner, Marketing Manager

A tutorial and drill program designed for the beginning music student. It covers four basic music reading skills: recognition of line and space notes; comprehension of the numbering system for the musical staff; visual and aural identification of notes moving up and down; and recognition of notes stepping and skipping up and down. *$39.95*

1738 **Eating Skills: Learning Basic Table Manners**
PCI Education Publishing
P.O. Box 34270
San Antonio, TX 78265-4270
210-377-1999
800-594-4263
Fax: 210-377-1121

Erin Kinard, VP Product Development/Publisher
Jeff Clain, CEO

Offers parents and educators a functional way to teach and reinforce basic table manners. *$49.95*

1739 **Electronic Courseware Systems**
1713 S State St
Champaign, IL 61820-7258
217-359-7099
800-832-4965
Fax: 217-359-6578
support@ecsmedia.com
www.ecsmedia.com

Jodie Varner, Manager
G Peters, President

Offers a complete library of instructional software for music, math, science and social studies.

1740 **Fall Fun**
Soft Touch
12301 Central Ave NE Ste 205
P.O. Box 490215
Blaine, MN 55449
763-862-2920
888-755-1402
Fax: 763-862-2922
support@marblesoft.com
www.marblesoft.com

Joyce Meyer, President

Your students can begin their day with the Pledge of Allegiance, Pumpkins, Owls, and Cats. Witches adorn Five Pumpkins Sitting on the Gate. Five Fat Turkeys out smart the pilgrims with song and antics. The owl and cat have songs of their own. A variety of activities reinforce concepts such as short, tall, first, second, third, same and different. Fall Fun includes cause and effect and easy to more difficult levels. Eight songs in all.

1741 **Five Green & Speckled Frogs**

Soft Touch
12301 Central Ave NE Ste 205
P.O. Box 490215
Blaine, MN 55449
763-862-2920
888-755-1402
Fax: 763-862-2922
support@marblesoft.com
www.marblesoft.com

Joyce Meyer, President

Laugh, learn and sing with Five Humorous Frogs. Activities start with cause and effect and progress to teach directionality and simple subtraction. This classic song makes learning numbers and number worlds easy. Selections can be set to 2, 3, 4, 5, or 6 on-screen choices. Two games are included. One teaches direction on a number line. If the child moves the frog in the correct direction, the frog gets a point. The other game teaches beginning subtraction.

1742 **Free and User Supported Software for the IBM PC: A Resource Guide**

McFarland & Company
960 NC Highway 88 W
P.O. Box 611
Jefferson, NC 28640-8813
336-246-4460
800-253-2187
Fax: 336-246-5018
info@mcfarlandpub.com
www.mcfarlandpub.com

Robert McFarland Franklin, Founder
Kenneth.J Ansley, Author
Victor.D Lopez, Author

A selection of word processing, database management, spreadsheets, and graphics programs are described and evaluated. Describes how the program works and its strengths and weaknesses. Rating charts cover such aspects as ease of use, ease of learning, documentation, and general utility. *$27.50*

224 pages Paperback
ISBN 0-89950 -99-0

1743 **GoalView: Special Education and RTI Student Management Information System**

Learning Tools International
2391 Circadian Way
Santa Rosa, CA 95407-5439
707-521-3530
800-333-9954

Cathy Zier, President/CEO
Natalie Sipes, VP
Michael R. Paul, Director of IT/Senior Web Engine

A Web Based information system for students, educators and parents that enables accountability and achievement tracking; prepares IDEA compliant IEP's in minutes; provides over 250,000 education standards and special education goals and objectives in English and Spanish; generates Federal compliance reports; and creates IDEA GoalCard progress reports for students, schools and districts for every reporting period.

1744 **HELP**

V OR T Corporation
P.O. Box G (George)
Menlo Park, CA 94026
650-322-8282
888-757-8678
Fax: 650-327-0747
custserv@vort.com
vort.com

Tom Holt, Owner

A software version of HELP, covers over 650 skills in 6 developmental areas; cognitive, motor skills, language, gross motor, social and self-help.

1745 **Handbook of Adaptive Switches and Augmentative Communication Devices**

Academic Software
3504 Tates Creek Road
Lexington, KY 40517-2601
859-552-1020
859-552-1040
Fax: 253-799-4012
asistaff@acsw.com
www.acsw.com

Dr. Warren E Lacefield PhD, President
Penelope D. Ellis, COO, Sales & Marketing Director
Cindy L George, Author
Sylvia B. Lacefield, Graphic Artist

This second edition contains physical descriptions and laboratory test data for a variety of commercially available pressure switches and augmentative communication devices and chapters on physical interaction, seating and positioning, and control access. It is an essential tool for assistive technology professionals and therapists who make decisions concerning physical access. *$60.00*

300 pages Hardcover

1746 **HandiWARE**

Microsystems Software
600 Worcester Rd
Framingham, MA 01702-5303
508-626-8511
800-828-2600
Fax: 508-879-1069
infor@microsys.com
www.handiware.com

Terri McGrath, Sales/Marketing
Bill Kilroy, Product Manager

Adapted access software, assists persons with physical, hearing and visual impairments in accessing computers running DOS and Windows. HandiWARE is a suite of 8 software programs which provide users with screen magnification, alternate keyboard access, word prediction, augmentative communication, hands free telephone access, a visual beep. $20.00-$595.00.

1747 **How to Write for Everyday Living**

Educational Activities Software
5600 West 83rd Street
Suite 300, 8200 Tower
Bloomington, MN 55437-585
800-447-5286
Fax: 239-225-9299
info@edmentum.com
www.edmentum.com

Vin Riera, President/CEO
Dan Juckniess, SVP, Sales & Professional Services
Stacey Herteux, VP, Human Resources
Rob Rueckl, Chief Financial Officer

An individualized Life Skills WRITING Software program emphasizing the reading, writing, communication and reference skills needed for real-life tasks: preparing a resume, an employment form, a business letter and envelope, a learner's permit, a social security application and banking forms. *$159.00*

1748 **I KNOW American History**

Soft Touch
12301 Central Ave NE Ste 205
P.O. Box 490215
Blaine, MN 55449-2352
763-862-2920
888-755-1402
Fax: 763-862-2922
support@marblesoft.com
www.marblesoft.com

Joyce Meyer, President

The new I KNOW programs is the way students practice attending, choice making and turn-taking while uncovering learning puzzles. Each press reveals more of the image while the narrator reads the text on the screen. Offers three levels of language: short phrases, short sentences and longer sentences to match the student's learning level. Choose from the five topic areas: American Symbols, Westward Movement, Early Colonial Americans, Industrial Revolution and Biographies.

1749 I KNOW American History Overlay CD
Soft Touch
12301 Central Ave NE Ste 205
P.O. Box 490215
Blaine, MN 55449-2352
763-862-2920
888-755-1402
Fax: 763-862-2922
support@marblesoft.com
www.marblesoft.com

Joyce Meyer, President
Use this Overlay CD with I KNOW American History program. Includes standard overlays and SoftTouch's changeable overlays. Includes Overlay Printer by IntelliTools. Use Overlay Maker by IntelliTools (not included) to modify the overlays or to make additional learning materials.

1750 Incite Learning Series
Don Johnston
26799 West Commerce Drive
Volo, IL 60073-9675
847-740-0749
800-999-4660
Fax: 847-740-7326
info@donjohnston.com
www.donjohnston.com

Don Johnston, Founder
Ruth Ziolkowski, President
Kevin Johnston, Director of Product Design
Ben Johnston, Director of Marketing
A collection of original short films and a thought-provoking instruction model to engage every student in the critical thinking and feeling process. This research-based program was developed around the science of how students learn best using the theory of 'anchored instruction' and 'front-loading' standards-based curriculum. *$79.00*

1751 Innovation Management Group
179 Niblick Rd
Ste 454
Paso Robles, CA 93446
818-701-1579
800-889-0987
Fax: 818-936-0200
cs@imgpresents.com
www.imgpresents.com

Jerry Hussong, VP of Marketing
Publisher of the Assistive Technology Suite. The ultimate set of general purpose, adaptive computer access available today. Site License includes ALL computers and ALL active students and teachers at a single or multi-site location.

1752 IntelliPics Studio 3
Intelli Tools
1720 Corporate Cir
Petaluma, CA 94954-6924
707-773-2000
800-547-6747
Fax: 707-773-2001

Arjan Khalsa, CEO
Multimedia authoring tool for both students and teachers to create activities, games, quizzes, slide shows, reports and presentations. *$395.00*

1753 KIDS (Keyboard Introductory Development Series)
Electronic Courseware Systems
1713 S State St
Champaign, IL 61820-7258
217-359-7099
800-832-4965
Fax: 217-359-6578
support@ecsmedia.com
www.ecsmedia.com

G Peters, President
Jodie Varner, Marketing Manager
A four disk series for the very young. Zoo Puppet Theater reinforces learning correct finger numbers for piano playing; Race Car Keys teaches keyboard geography by recognizing syllables or note names; Dinosaurs Lunch teaches placement of the notes on the treble staff; and Follow Me asks the student to play notes that have been presented aurally. *$49.95*

1754 Keyboard Tutor, Music Software
Electronic Courseware Systems
1713 S State St
Champaign, IL 61820-7258
217-359-7099
800-832-4965
Fax: 217-359-6578
support@ecsmedia.com
www.ecsmedia.com

G Peters, President
Jodie Varner, Marketing Manager
Presents exercises for learning elementary keyboard skills including knowledge of names of the keys, piano keys matched to notes, notes matched to piano keys, whole steps and half steps. Each lesson allows unlimited practice of the skills. The program may be used with or without a midi keyboard attached to the computer. *$39.95*

1755 Keyboarding by Ability
Teachers Institute for Special Education
9933 NW 45th St
Sunrise, FL 33351-4744
954-235-7940
Fax: 866-843-0765
Support@Special-Education-Soft.com
www.special-education-soft.com

Gary Byowitz, President
Allows the learning disabled or dyslexic student to acquire keyboarding skills through visually cued alphabetical approach designed and tested to meet the specific learning style needs of this unique population at every grade level. Package contains: IBM software, a set of lesson plans and instructional goals; supplemental graded data input exercises. *$369.00*

1756 Keyboarding for the Physically Handicapped
Teachers Institute for Special Education
9933 NW 45th Street
Sunrise, FL 33351
954-235-7940
Fax: 866-843-0765
Support@Special-Education-Soft.com
www.special-education-soft.com

Jack Heller, Director/Owner
Gary Byowitz, President
Custom designed touch typing programs for any student. A person needs order by the number of usable fingers on each hand (not counting the thumb), and whether or not a one finger or a head-pointer edition is wanted. Package includes IBM software; a complete set of lesson plans and instructional goals. *$149.95*

1757 Keyboarding with One Hand
Teachers Institute for Special Education
P.O. Box 2300
Wantagh, NY 11793-140
Fax: 516-781-4070
jackheller@aol.com

Jack Heller, Director
This 22 lesson tutorial developed through 25 years of research, testing and teaching allows a student with one hand to acquire employable keyboarding skills using a touch system designed for the standard IBM PC keyboard. *$79.95*

1758 LPDOS Deluxe
Optelec U S
3030 Enterprise Court
STE C
Vista, CA 92081-8358
800-826-4200
Fax: 800-368-4111
info@optelec.com
us.optelec.com

Stephan Terwolbeck, President
Michiel van Schaik, VP
Janet Lennex, Director of Customer Excellence
Jade Arbelo, Director of Human Resources
Large print software programs. *$595.00*

1759 **Large Print DOS**
Optelec U S
3030 Enterprise Court
STE C
Vista, CA 92081-8358
800-826-4200
Fax: 800-368-4111
info@optelec.com
us.optelec.com

Stephan Terwolbeck, President
Michiel van Schaik, VP
Janet Lennex, Director of Customer Excellence
Jade Arbelo, Director of Human Resources

1760 **Laureate Learning Systems**
110 E Spring St
Winooski, VT 05404-1898
802-655-4755
800-562-6801
Fax: 802-655-4757
www.laureatelearning.com

Mary Wilson, Owner
Kathy Hollandsworth, Office Manager

Laureate publishes award-winning talking software for children and adults with disabilities. Programs cover cause and effect, language development, cognitive processing, and reading. High-quality speech, colorful graphics and amusing animation make learning fun. Accessible with touchscreen, single switch, keyboard and mouse. No reading required. Available on a hybrid CD-ROM for Windows and Macintosh. Visit our website for more information or call for a free catalog.

1761 **Learning Company**
Ste 400
222 3rd Ave SE
Cedar Rapids, IA 52401-1542
319-395-9626
888-242-6747
Fax: 319-395-0217
info@riverdeep.net
http://web.riverdeep.net

Barry O'Callaghan, Executive Chairman & Chief Executive Officer
Tony Mulderry, Executive Vice President, Corporate Development
Ciara Smyth, Executive Vice President, Global Business Operations
Scott Campbell, Executive Vice President, Strategic Sales

Software for children. For Macintosh or Windows (3.1 DOS or Windows 95, Windows 98 required). The Learning Company has been added to Riverdeep.

1762 **Little Red Hen**
Compass Learning
203 Colorado Street
Austin, TX 78701
512-478-9600
800-678-1412
866-586-7387
Fax: 619-622-7873
support@compasslearning.com
www.compasslearning.com

Eric Loeffel, President, CEO
Tammy Deal, VP, Human Resources
Eric Wasser, VP, Sales
Eileen Shihadeh, VP, Marketing

Children learn about the rewards of hard work when they discover who the Little Red Hen's friends miss out on freshly baked bread. Puzzles, rhymes, story writing and other interactive exercises enhance the creative learning process. *$34.95*

1763 **Looking Good: Learning to Improve Your Appearance**
Programming Concepts
8700 Shoal Creek Boulevard
Austin, TX 78757-6897
512-451-3246
800-897-3202
800-471-3000
Fax: 800-397-7633
general@proedinc.com
www.proedinc.com

Jeff McLane, Founder
Lee Wilson, President and CEO
Randy Pennington, Executive VP
David Keith, Vice President of IT

This game offers a creative way to discuss all areas of grooming. *$49.95*

1764 **Monkeys Jumping on the Bed**
Soft Touch
12301 Central Ave NE Ste 205
P.O. Box 490215
Blaine, MN 55449-2352
763-862-2920
888-755-1402
Fax: 763-862-2922
support@marblesoft.com
www.marblesoft.com

Joyce Meyer, President

This program combines a favorite preschool song with number and color activities. Children and adults will enjoy engaging music and delightful animation. Students with cognitive delays respond to upbeat music and interesting sounds. Large graphics help learners focus on the action. Several important concepts are presented in enjoyable activity formats. Students learn cause and effect in Let's Play and Just for Fun.

1765 **Morse Code WSKE**
Words+
42505 10th Street West
Suite 109
Lancaster, CA 93534- 7059
661-723-7723
888-266-9294
Fax: 661-723-5524
info@simulations-plus.com
www.simulations-plus.com

Walter S Woltosz, M.S., M.A.S., Chairman, President and Chief Executive Officer
John A. Dibella, VP, Marketing & Sales
Virginia E. Woltosz. M.B.A., Secretary & Treasurer
John R. Kneisel, Chief Financial Officer

A software and hardware product designed to operate on an IBM compatible PC.

1766 **Multi-Scan Single Switch Activity Center**
Academic Software
3504 Tates Creek Road
Lexington, KY 40517-2601
859-552-1020
859-552-1040
Fax: 253-799-4012
asistaff@acsw.com
www.acsw.com

Dr. Warren E Lacefield PhD, President
Penelope D. Ellis, COO, Sales & Marketing Director
Cindy L George, Author
Sylvia B. Lacefield, Graphic Artist

A single switch activity center containing four educational games: Match, Maze, Dot-to-Dot, and Concentration, along with six graphics libraries; Dinosaurs, Sports, Animals, Independent Living, Vocations, and Cosmetology. MULTI-SCAN allows you to select a graphic library, choose games for each user, and adjust the difficulty level and other settings for each game. Other features allow you to save the game setups under each user's name and print out individual performance reports after sessions. *$154.00*

1767 **Muppet Learning Keys**
WINGS for Learning
1600 Green Hills Rd
Scotts Valley, CA 95066-4981
831-426-2228
Fax: 831-464-3600

Ani Stocks, Owner

Designed to introduce children to the world of the computer as they become familiar with letters, numbers and colors.

1768 **My Own Pain**
Soft Touch
12301 Central Ave NE Ste 205
P.O. Box 490215
Blaine, MN 55449-2352
763-862-2920
888-755-1402
Fax: 763-862-2922
support@marblesoft.com
www.marblesoft.com

Joyce Meyer, President

Three activities - three levels. Press the switch and the paint brush chooses the color and paints the vehicle. Music reinforces the sounds when the picture is complete. A second activity allows the student to choose the color and paint the vehicle parts any color he or she wants. The third activity is a blueprint. Print the color that matches the one in the wire drawing. Color the drawing to complete the picture.

1769 **NanoPac**
4823 S Sheridan Rd
Suite 302
Tulsa, OK 74145-5717
918-665-0329
800-580-6086
Fax: 918-665-0361
TTY: 918-665-2310
www.nanopac.com

Silvio Cianfrone, President
NanoPac offers assistive technology for those with low vision, blindness and reading disabilities. Some of their products include voice recognition, environmental controls, text to speech, magnifiers and door openers.

1770 **Old MacDonald's Farm Deluxe**
Soft Touch
12301 Central Ave NE Ste 205
P.O. Box 490215
Blaine, MN 55449-2352
763-862-2920
888-755-1402
Fax: 763-862-2922
support@marblesoft.com
www.marblesoft.com

Joyce Meyer, President
Toddlers, preschoolers and early elementary students will be entertained and captivated by the six major activities and animations in the delightful program. Includes 18 real animation images or 9 cartoon like characters. The teacher or child can choose which animals they want to sing about. Some activities are designed for children within the normal population, others are designed for students with moderate and severe disabilities.

1771 **Optimum Resource Educational Software**
Optimum Resource
1 Mathews Drive
Suite 107
Hilton Head Island, SC 29926
843-689-8000
Fax: 843-689-8008
info@stickybear.com
www.stickybear.com

Richard Hefter, President
A complete topical curriculum of reading, math, keyboard skills and science programs that are age and skill specific. Programs include: Early Learning for Pre-K to 1st grade with introductions to numbers, language, shapes, and time; Language Arts from Pre-K to 12; Math for Pre-K to 12; two distinct Science programs; Tools for Educators provides Spelling and Math generators; and Bilingual programs for Pre-K through 9th grade. All are available as single user up to 30 user site packages.

1772 **Optimum Resources/Stickybear Software**
1 Mathews Drive
Suite 107
Hilton Head Island, SC 29926
843-689-8000
Fax: 843-689-8008
info@stickybear.com
www.stickybear.com

Richard Hefter, President
Publisher of award-winning educational software for thirty years. Programs in use by millions of students nationwide.
$59.95

1773 **Please Understand Me: Software Program and Books**
Cambridge Educational
132 West 31st Street
17th Floor
New York, NY 10001
800-322-8755
Fax: 800-678-3633
custserv@films.com
www.films.com

209 pages BiAnnual
ISBN 0-927368-56-x

1774 **Pond**
WINGS for Learning
1600 Green Hills Rd
Scotts Valley, CA 95066-4981
831-426-2228
Fax: 831-464-3600

Ani Stocks, Owner
Software game that teaches pattern recognition and encourages observation, trial and error and the interpretation of data.

1775 **Print, Play & Learn #1 Old Mac's Farm**
Soft Touch Incorporated
12301 Central Ave NE Ste 205
P.O. Box 490215
Blaine, MN 55449-2352
763-862-2920
888-755-1402
Fax: 763-862-2922
support@marblesoft.com
www.marblesoft.com

Joyce Meyer, President
Once your students have completed Old Mac's Farm, let them use the fun off-computer activities to continue learning. Over 25 activities with 250 sheets you print. Board games, dot-to-dot drawings, word puzzles, make a scene, flash cards. Concentration, sentence strips, worksheets and much more are available for teachers to expand their teaching goals. This CD is full of activities to print and use.

1776 **Print, Play & Learn #7: Sampler**
Soft Touch
12301 Central Ave NE Ste 205
P.O. Box 490215
Blaine, MN 55449-2352
763-862-2920
888-755-1402
Fax: 763-862-2922
support@marblesoft.com
www.marblesoft.com

Joyce Meyer, President
Print, Play and Learn Sampler gives you over 200 activities organized by training, easy, medium and hard levels so you can ready to help your student advance. Activities cover a wide range of basic knowledge, including colors, shapes, numbers, letters and much, much more. Note: Requires Overlay Maker or Overlay Printer by IntelliTools and a color printer.

1777 **Puzzle Power: Sampler**
Soft Touch
12301 Central Ave NE Ste 205
P.O. Box 490215
Blaine, MN 55449-2352
763-862-2920
888-755-1402
Fax: 763-862-2922
support@marblesoft.com
www.marblesoft.com

Joyce Meyer, President
Puzzle Power - Sampler offers a variety of puzzles in different themes. Each theme puzzle is followed by a puzzle of one item in this category. For example, first solve a puzzle for occupations. Then, solve a puzzle that is a baker. The pictures are large, clear and easily identifiable.

1778 **Puzzle Power: Zoo & School Days**
Soft Touch
12301 Central Ave NE Ste 205
P.O. Box 490215
Blaine, MN 55449-2352
763-862-2920
888-755-1402
Fax: 763-862-2922
support@marblesoft.com
www.marblesoft.com

Joyce Meyer, President
Here is a program for all of our students who need puzzle skills, but cannot access commercial puzzles. Puzzle Power puzzles start with just two pieces and progress to 16 pieces. The pictures are large, clear and easily identifiable. Four different activities enable all students to be successful. Automatic Placement: the student just presses the switch or keyboard to place the pieces. Magnet Mouse: all the student needs to do is move the mouse and it drops into place.

1779 **Rodeo**
Soft Touch
12301 Central Ave NE Ste 205
P.O. Box 490215
Blaine, MN 55449-2352
763-862-2920
888-755-1402
Fax: 763-862-2922
support@marblesoft.com
www.marblesoft.com

Joyce Meyer, President

Rodeo action and familiar tunes for teens and preteens. Four activities invite students to learn, laugh, and sing as they go to the rodeo with up to six age-peer friends. Age-appropriate graphics with surprising animations reinforce the learning. The graphics are large and colorful, the melodies familiar, and the words descriptive of the action on the screen.

1780 **Shop Til You Drop**
Soft Touch
12301 Central Ave NE Ste 205
P.O. Box 490215
Blaine, MN 55449-2352
763-862-2920
888-755-1402
Fax: 763-862-2922
support@marblesoft.com
www.marblesoft.com

Joyce Meyer, President

Designed specifically for preteens and teens with moderate and severe disabilities, this program will become a staple for the classroom. The student goes shopping and can choose which outfits to put together. They may choose to purchase the outfit - of course, with mom's credit card. Another activity is a video arcade game about money. Shop 'Til You Drop can be adjusted from a single switch cause-and-effect program to row-and-column scanning to direct choice.

1781 **Songs I Sing at Preschool**
Soft Touch
12301 Central Ave NE Ste 205
P.O. Box 490215
Blaine, MN 55449-2352
763-862-2920
888-755-1402
Fax: 763-862-2922
support@marblesoft.com
www.marblesoft.com

Joyce Meyer, President

Songs I Sing at Preschool offers many options for the teacher and the student. Over the years, our software has used music because our students really respond to the sounds and rhythms of songs. Teachers select which songs to present, how many to present at one time and where to place each song on the overlay, keyboard or scan array.

1782 **Stickybear Early Learning Activities**
Optimum Resource
1 Mathews Drive
Suite 107
Hilton Head Island, SC 29926
843-689-8000
Fax: 843-689-8008
info@stickybear.com
www.stickybear.com

Richard Hefter, President

Two modes of play allow youngsters to learn through prompted direction or by the discovery method. Lively animation and sound keep attention levels high as children learn writing, counting, shapes, opposites and colors. Stickybear Early Learning Activities is bilingual, so youngsters can build skills in both English and Spanish. Pre-K to 1st grade. *$59.95*

1783 **Stickybear Kindergarden Activities**
Optimum Resource
1 Mathews Drive
Suite 107
Hilton Head Island, SC 29926
843-689-8000
Fax: 843-689-8008
info@stickybear.com
www.stickybear.com

Richard Hefter, President

This dynamic new multifaceted program covers a wide range of preschool skills that go far beyond the strictly academic. At Stickybear's house, children discover the alphabet, numbers, shapes, colors, plus - social skills, important safety messages and delightful off-screen activities that foster creativity. Over three hours of original music can be composed by a child and saved for future use. *$59.95*

1784 **Stickybear Science Fair Light**
Optimum Resource
1 Mathews Drive
Suite 107
Hilton Head Island, SC 29926
843-689-8000
Fax: 843-689-8008
info@stickybear.com
www.stickybear.com

Richard Hefter, President

The first in the new series of science-based programs Stickybear Science Fair Light presents a content rich environment which allows students in grades 7-12 to explore, experiment with and understand light and it's properties. The program presents experiments, both structured and free-form, which allow users to work with prisms, lenses, color mixing, optical illusions and more. *$59.95*

1785 **Stickybear Town Builder**
Optimum Resource
1 Mathews Drive
Suite 107
Hilton Head Island, SC 29926
843-689-8000
Fax: 843-689-8008
info@stickybear.com
www.stickybear.com

Richard Hefter, President

Children learn to read maps, build towns, take trips and use a compass in this simulation program. *$59.95*

1786 **Stickybear Typing**
Optimum Resource
1 Mathews Drive
Suite 107
Hilton Head Island, SC 29926
843-689-8000
Fax: 843-689-8008
info@stickybear.com
www.stickybear.com

Richard Hefter, President

Sharpen typing skills with three challenging activities: Stickybear Keypress, Stickybear Thump and Stickybear Stories. Pre-K to 5th. *$59.95*

1787 **Storybook Maker Deluxe**
Compass Learning
203 Colorado Street
Austin, TX 78701
512-478-9600
800-678-1412
866-586-7387
Fax: 619-622-7873
support@compasslearning.com
www.compasslearning.com

Eric Loeffel, President, CEO
Tammy Deal, VP, Human Resources
Eric Wasser, VP, Sales
Eileen Shihadeh, VP, Marketing

Using Storybook Maker Deluxe and their imaginations, students can create and publish stories filled with exciting graphics. Students can write stories and watch as the text appears in the setting they've chosen. Engaging sounds and music, plus lively animations, provide positive learning reinforcement throughout the program. *$44.95*

1788 **Super Challenger**
Electronic Courseware Systems
1713 S State St
Champaign, IL 61820-7258
217-359-7099
800-832-4965
Fax: 217-359-6578
www.ecsmedia.com

Jodie Varner, Manager
G Peters, President

An aural-visual musical game that increases the player's ability to remember a series of pitches as they are played by the computer. The game is based on a 12-note chromatic scale, a major scale, and a minor scale. Each pitch is reinforced visually with a color representation of a keyboard on the display screen. Computer/software. *$39.95*

1789 Switch Basics
Soft Touch
12301 Central Ave NE Ste 205
P.O. Box 490215
Blaine, MN 55449-2352
763-862-2920
888-755-1402
Fax: 763-862-2922
support@marblesoft.com
www.marblesoft.com
Joyce Meyer, President

Discover whimsical animations and real life pictures while learning switch operations. Intriguing and humorous, nine different programs offer a multitude of learning experiences for all ages. Program options include: cause and effect, scanning, step scanning, row and column activities for one or two players. Watch the clouds roll away revealing African animals; visit the beauty salon or barber shop; work two to sixteen piece puzzles; or add swimming fish to a huge aquarium.

1790 Switch Interface Pro 5.0
Don Johnston
26799 West Commerce Drive
Volo, IL 60073-9675
847-740-0749
800-999-4660
Fax: 847-740-7326
info@donjohnston.com
www.donjohnston.com
Don Johnston, Founder
Ruth Ziolkowski, President
Kevin Johnston, Director of Product Design
Ben Johnston, Director of Marketing

Allows individuals with physical disabilities to access the computer. Five ports accommodate multiple switches and emulate everything from a single-click to a return. Consequently, individuals gain access to the widest variety of switch-accessible software available. It requires no software and can be used with both Windows and Macintosh computers. *$79.00*

1791 Teach Me Phonemics Series Bundle
SoftTouch
Ste 401
4300 Stine Rd
Bakersfield, CA 93313-2352
661-396-8676
877-763-8868
Fax: 661-396-8760
support@softtouch.com
www.funsoftware.com
Joyce Meyer, President
Roxanne Butterfield, Marketing

The Teach Me Phonemics Series Bundle includes one copy of each Teach Me Phonemics program - Initial, Medial, Final and Blends - four CD's in all.

1792 Teach Me Phonemics Super Bundle
SoftTouch
Ste 401
4300 Stine Rd
Bakersfield, CA 93313-2352
661-396-8676
877-763-8868
Fax: 661-396-8760
www.funsoftware.com
Roxanne Butterfield, Marketing
Joyce Meyer, President

Teach Me Phonemics Super Bundle includes all 4 Teach Me Phonemics programs and all 4 Teach Me Phonemics overlay CD's - eight CD's in all.

1793 Teach Me Phonemics: Blends
SoftTouch
Ste 401
4300 Stine Rd
Bakersfield, CA 93313-2352
661-396-8676
877-763-8868
Fax: 661-396-8760
Roxanne Butterfield, Marketing
Joyce Meyer, President

Teach Me Phonemics - Blends helps students explore words and hear the initial blend sounds. It features musical interludes and movement to engage the student. Teachers select the best combination options to motivate and engage the student. Options turn off and on the fly so you can quickly make changes to keep the student engaged.

1794 Teach Me Phonemics: Final
SoftTouch
Ste 401
4300 Stine Rd
Bakersfield, CA 93313-2352
661-396-8676
877-763-8868
Fax: 661-396-8760
Roxanne Butterfield
Joyce Meyer, President

Teach me Phonemics - Final helps students explore words and hear the final sounds. It features musical interludes and movement to engage the student. Options turn off and on the fly so you can quickly make changes to keep the student engaged.

1795 Teach Me Phonemics: Initial
SoftTouch
12301 Central Ave NE
Ste 205
Blaine, MN 55434
763-755-1402
888-755-1403
Fax: 763-862-2920
sales@marblesoft.com
www.softtouch.com
Roxanne Butterfield, Marketing
Joyce Meyer, President

Teach Me Phonemics - Initial helps students explore the words and hear the initial sounds. It features musical interludes and movement to engage the student. Teachers select the best combination options to motivate and engage the student. Options turn off and on the fly so you can quickly make changes to keep the student engaged.

1796 Teach Me Phonemics: Medial
SoftTouch
12301 Central Ave NE
Ste 205
Blaine, MN 55434
763-755-1402
888-755-1403
Fax: 763-862-2920
sales@marblesoft.com
www.softtouch.com
Roxanne Butterfield, Marketing
Joyce Meyer, President

Teach Me Phonemics - Medial helps students explore the words and hear the medial sounds. It features musical interludes and movement to engage the student. Teachers select the best combination options to motivate and engage the student. Options turn off and on the fly so you can quickly make changes to keep the student engaged.

1797 Teach Me to Talk
Soft Touch
12301 Central Ave NE Ste 205
P.O. Box 490215
Blaine, MN 55449-2352
763-862-2920
888-755-1402
Fax: 763-862-2922
support@marblesoft.com
www.marblesoft.com
Joyce Meyer, President

The first activity Teach Me to Talk is used as a springboard for the student to learn to speak the word. There are 150 real pictures. When a picture is chosen, it appears on a clear background with musical interludes, movement, written word and spoken word. It culminates by morphing to the corresponding black and white Mayer-Johnson symbol. The second activity Story Time, takes some of these nouns and puts them in four line poetry. This helps students hear the word in the midst of a sentence.

1798 **Teen Tunes Plus**

Soft Touch
12301 Central Ave NE Ste 205
P.O. Box 490215
Blaine, MN 55449-2352
763-862-2920
888-755-1402
Fax: 763-862-2922
support@marblesoft.com
www.marblesoft.com

Joyce Meyer, President

Introduce switch use to older students with disabilities. Large interesting graphics, a variety of musical interludes, and surprising animations are combined with calm soothing music and beautiful pictures in the software specifically designed for preteens and teens with severe cognitive delays and/or physical disabilities, and older students learning to use a switch.

1799 **There are Tyrannosaurs Trying on Pants in My Bedroom**

Compass Learning
203 Colorado Street
Austin, TX 78701-3922
512-478-9600
800-678-1412
866-586-7387
Fax: 619-622-7873
support@compasslearning.com
www.compasslearning.com

Eric Loeffel, President, CEO
Tammy Deal, VP, Human Resources
Eric Wasser, VP, Sales
Eileen Shihadeh, VP, Marketing

In this popular story, Saturday chores turn into fun-filled frolicking when dinosaurs come for a visit. Sounds, music and animation make learning about phonics and vocabulary dyno-mite. *$34.95*

1800 **Three Billy Goats Gruff**

Compass Learning
203 Colorado Street
Austin, TX 78701-3922
512-478-9600
800-678-1412
866-586-7387
Fax: 619-622-7873
support@compasslearning.com
www.compasslearning.com

Eric Loeffel, President, CEO
Tammy Deal, VP, Human Resources
Eric Wasser, VP, Sales
Eileen Shihadeh, VP, Marketing

Motivating exercises and creative activities provide hours of learning fun while young students follow the adventure of The Three Billy Goats Gruff in this animated version of the timeless tale. *$34.95*

1801 **Three Little Pigs**

Compass Learning
203 Colorado Street
Austin, TX 78701-3922
512-478-9600
800-678-1412
866-586-7387
Fax: 619-622-7873
support@compasslearning.com
www.compasslearning.com

Eric Loeffel, President, CEO
Tammy Deal, VP, Human Resources
Eric Wasser, VP, Sales
Eileen Shihadeh, VP, Marketing

Help young students build reading comprehension and writing skills with this interactive version of the children's classic, The Three Little Pigs. Animated storytelling and creative activities inspire children to read, write and rhyme. *$34.95*

1802 **TouchCorders**

Soft Touch
12301 Central Ave NE Ste 205
P.O. Box 490215
Blaine, MN 55449-2352
763-862-2920
888-755-1402
Fax: 763-862-2922
support@marblesoft.com
www.marblesoft.com

Joyce Meyer, President

TouchCorders are the flexible and easy-to-use communicator designed by Jo Meyer and Linda Bidabe for reach classroom use. TouchCorders are sensitive to touch at every angle and give the student kinesthetic feedback. With the unique Add 'n Touch system, Jo connects the puzzles bases of 2 or more TouchCorders on the fly to present vocabulary, sequencing, story telling, social stories, concepts and other curriculum and communication opportunities.

1803 **TouchWindow Touch Screen**

Riverdeep Incorporated
100 Pine Street
Suite 1900
San Francisco, CA 94111
415-659-2000
800-542-4222
Fax: 415-659-2020
info@riverdeep.net
www.riverdeep.net

Barry O'Callaghan, Executive Chairman & Chief Executive Officer
Tony Mulderry, Executive Vice President, Corporate Development
Ciara Smyth, Executive Vice President, Global Business Operations
Scott Campbell, Executive Vice President, Strategic Sales

Software for children. *$335.00*

1804 **Turtle Teasers**

Soft Touch
12301 Central Ave NE Ste 205
P.O. Box 490215
Blaine, MN 55449-2352
763-862-2920
888-755-1402
Fax: 763-862-2922
support@marblesoft.com
www.marblesoft.com

Joyce Meyer, President

Three Games, Three Levels from Easy, Medium to Hard. The Shell Game - easy: Watch one of the three turtles get the tomato. Then watch carefully as they switch positions and pop shut. Choose incorrectly and the frog disappears until the correct one is displayed. The Pond - medium: Watch the tomato disappear somewhere in the pond scene. Tomato Dump - hard: Hit the shell and it turns into the tomato, giving a score. There are different difficulty levels to equalize all students.

1805 **What Was That!**

Compass Learning
203 Colorado Street
Austin, TX 78701-3922
512-478-9600
800-678-1412
866-586-7387
Fax: 619-622-7873
support@compasslearning.com
www.compasslearning.com

Eric Loeffel, President, CEO
Tammy Deal, VP, Human Resources
Eric Wasser, VP, Sales
Eileen Shihadeh, VP, Marketing

In this bedtime story, noises in the night send three brother bears scurrying out of bed. Thoughtful questions test young readers' comprehension, while games, voice recording, writing practice and other playful activities stimulate their creativity.

1806 **Wivik 3**

Prentke Romich Company
1022 Heyl Road
Wooster, OH 44691
330-262-1984
800-262-1984
Fax: 330-263-4829
info@prentrom.com
www.prentrom.com

Dave Hershberger, President & CEO
Barry Romich, Co-Founder

On-screen keyboard provides access to any application in the latest Windows operating systems. Selections are made by clicking, dwelling or switch scanning. Enhancements include word prediction and abbreviation expansion.

1807 **WordMaker**
Don Johnston
26799 West Commerce Drive
Volo, IL 60073-9675
847-740-0749
800-999-4660
Fax: 847-740-7326
info@donjohnston.com
www.donjohnston.com

Don Johnston, Founder
Ruth Ziolkowski, President
Kevin Johnston, Director of Product Design
Ben Johnston, Director of Marketing

The computer version of Dr Patricia Cunningham's book 'Systematic Sequential Phonics They Use.' The program systematically builds spelling and word decoding skills for struggling readers and writers. *$79.00*

1808 **Write: Out Loud**
Don Johnston
26799 West Commerce Drive
Volo, IL 60073-9675
847-740-0749
800-999-4660
Fax: 847-740-7326
info@donjohnston.com
www.donjohnston.com

Don Johnston, Founder
Ruth Ziolkowski, President
Kevin Johnston, Director of Product Design
Ben Johnston, Director of Marketing

Write: Out Loud is an easy-to-use talking word processor that uses text-to-speech and revision and editing supports to help students write more effectively, more often and with more enthusiasm as they share creative thoughts on paper. *$79.00*

1809 **You Tell Me: Learning Basic Information**
Programming Concepts
8700 Shoal Creek Boulevard
Austin, TX 78757-6897
512-451-3246
800-897-3202
800-471-3000
Fax: 800-397-7633
general@proedinc.com
www.proedinc.com

Jeff McLane, Founder
Lee Wilson, President and CEO
Randy Pennington, Executive VP
David Keith, Vice President of IT

This game teaches and reinforces basic information all individuals need to know. Questions asked in this game help prepare people to communicate personal identification information important to community survival. *$49.95*

Software: Professional

1810 **Acrontech International**
5500 Main St
Williamsville, NY 14221-6755
Fax: 716-854-4014

1811 **DPS with BCP**
V OR T Corporation
P.O. Box G (George)
Menlo Park, CA 94026
650-322-8282
888-757-8678
Fax: 650-327-0747
custserv@vort.com
vort.com

Tom Holt, Owner

This program uses unique DPS branching techniques to access goals and objectives.

1812 **Descriptive Language Arts Development**
Educational Activities Software
5600 West 83rd Street
Suite 300, 8200 Tower
Bloomington, MN 55437
888-351-4199
800-447-5286
Fax: 239-225-9299
info@edmentum.com
www.edmentum.com

Vin Riera, President/CEO
Dan Juckniess, SVP, Sales & Professional Services
Stacey Herteux, VP, Human Resources
Rob Rueckl, Chief Financial Officer

This multimedia language arts development program provides instruction and application of fundamental English skills and concepts. *$395.00*

1813 **Diagnostic Report Writer**
Parrot Software
P.O. Box 250755
West Bloomfield, MI 48325
248-788-3223
800-727-7681
Fax: 248-788-3224
support@parrotsoftware.com
www.parrotsoftware.com

Dr. Frederic Weiner, Ph. D., CCC-SP, President, Owner

Creates a three page single-spaced diagnostic report for a child with a communication disorder from a list of questions; sections of the report include developmental and background history, oral peripheral exam, speech and language analysis, summary and recommendations.

1814 **Draft: Builder**
Don Johnston
26799 West Commerce Drive
Volo, IL 60073-9675
847-740-0749
800-999-4660
Fax: 847-740-7326
info@donjohnston.com
www.donjohnston.com

Don Johnston, Founder
Ruth Ziolkowski, President
Kevin Johnston, Director of Product Design
Ben Johnston, Director of Marketing

A software-based graphic organizer that breaks down the writing process into manageable chunks to structure planning, organizing, and draft-writing. *$79.00*

1815 **EZ Dot**
CAPCO Capability Corporation
3910 S. Union Court
Spokane Valley, WA 99206-6345
509-927-8195
800-827-2182
Fax: 800-827-2182
info@skilltran.com
www.skilltran.com

Jeff Truthan, President

A critical software tool used in vocational counseling, job restructuring, recruitment and placement, better utilization of workers, and safety issues. This software offers occupational data by title, code, industry, GEO, DPT, or OGA. *$295.00*

1816 **EZ Keys for Windows**
Words+
Ste 109
42505 10th St W
Lancaster, CA 93534-7059
661-723-6523
800-869-8521
Fax: 661-723-2114
info@words-plus.com

Jean Dobbs, Editorial Director
Tim Gilmer, Editor
Josie Byzek, Managing Editor
Doug Lathrop, Senior Correspondent

A software and hardware product designed to operate on an IBM compatible PC. The software provides dual word prediction, abbreviation expansion, five different methods of voice output and access to commercial software applications. *$1395.00*

1817 **Goals and Objectives**
JE Stewart Teaching Tools
P.O. Box 15308
Seattle, WA 98115-308
206-262-9538
Fax: 206-262-9538

Jeff Stewart, Owner
Goals and Objectives software helps teachers make student plans including IEP's, IPP's and IHP's. The system provides curricula for all students and programs to develop and evaluate plans, print reports and make data forms. Systems are available for Windows and Macintosh for $139.

1818 **Goals and Objectives IEP Program Curriculum Associates LLC**
153 Rangeway Road
P.O. Box 2001
North Billerica, MA 01862-0901
978-667-8000
800-225-0248
Fax: 800-366-1158
www.curriculumassociates.com

Frank E. Ferguson, Chairman
Renee Foster, President & Publisher
Woody Palk, Senior Vice President, Sales
Robert Waldron, CEO
BRIGANCE CIBS-R standardized scoring conversion software, is a teacher's tool that prints goal and objective pages of the IEP. In less than two minutes per student, a teacher types student data into the computer.

1819 **Nasometer**
Kay Elemetrics Corporation
3 Paragon Drive
Montvale, NJ 07645
973-628-6200
800-289-5297
Fax: 201-391-2063
sales@kaypentax.com
www.kaypentax.com

John Crump, President
Steve Crump, Direct Sales
Measures the ratio of acoustic energy for the nasal and real-time visual cueing during therapy. Used clinically in the areas of cleft palate, motor speech disorders, hearing impairment and palatal prosthetic fittings.

1820 **PSS CogRehab Software**
Psychological Software Services
3304 W 75th St
Indianapolis, IN 46268-1664
317-257-9672
Fax: 317-257-9674
www.neuroscience.cnter.com

Odie L Bracy, Executive Director
PSS CogRehab Software is a comprehensive and easy-to-use multimedia cognitive rehabilitation software available, for clinical and educational use with head injury, stroke LD/ADD and other brain compromises. The packages include 64 computerized therapy tasks which contain modifiable parameters that will accommodate most requirements. Exercises include attention and executive skills, multiple modalities of visuosatial and memory skills, simple, complex, problem-solving skills.
$260 - $2500

1821 **Parrot Easy Language Simple Anaylsis**
Parrot Software
P.O. Box 250755
West Bloomfield, MI 48325
248-788-3223
800-727-7681
Fax: 248-788-3224
support@parrotsoftware.com
www.parrotsoftware.com

Dr. Frederic Weiner, Ph. D., CCC-SP, President, Owner
Designed for grammatical analysis of language samples. The user types and translates language samples of up to 100 utterances.

1822 **SOLO Literacy Suite**
Don Johnston
26799 West Commerce Drive
Volo, IL 60073-9675
847-740-0749
800-999-4660
Fax: 847-740-7326
info@donjohnston.com
www.donjohnston.com

Don Johnston, Founder
Ruth Ziolkowski, President
Kevin Johnston, Director of Product Design
Ben Johnston, Director of Marketing
Places all of the right tools, and a wide-range of embedded learning supports, at their fingertips. SOLO includes word prediction, a text reader, graphic organizer and talking word processor, putting students in charge of their own learning and accommodations. Students of varying ages and abilities have access to, and make progress in, the general education curriculum. *$79.00*

1823 **TOVA**
Universal Attention Disorders
3321 Cerritos Avenue
Los Alamitos, CA 90720
562-594-7700
800-729-2886
Fax: 800-452-6919
info@tovatest.com
www.tovatest.com

Lawrence M. Greenberg, MD
A computerized assessment which, in conjunction with classroom behavior ratings, is a highly effective screening tool for ADD. TOVA includes software, complete instructions, and supporting data including norms.

1824 **Visi-Pitch III**
Kayelemetrics Corporation
3 Paragon Drive
Montvale, NJ 07645
973-628-6200
800-289-5297
Fax: 201-391-2063
sales@kaypentax.com

John Crump, President
Steve Crump, Direct Sales
Assists the speech/voice clinician in assessment and treatment tasks across an expansive range of disorders.

Software: Reading & Language Arts

1825 **Choices, Choices 5.0**
Tom Snyder Productions
100 Talcott Avenue
Watertown, MA 02472-5703
800-342-0236
www.tomsnyder.com

Tom Snyder, Founder
Bridget Dalton, Ed.D, Author
Peggy Healy Stearns, Ph.D., Author
David Dockterman, Ed.D., Author
Teaches students to take responsibility for their behavior. Helps students develop the skills and awareness they need to make wise choices and to think through the consequences of their actions.

1826 **Co: Writer**
Don Johnston
26799 West Commerce Drive
Volo, IL 60073-9675
847-740-0749
800-999-4660
Fax: 847-740-7326
info@donjohnston.com
www.donjohnston.com

Don Johnston, Founder
Ruth Ziolkowski, President
Kevin Johnston, Director of Product Design
Ben Johnston, Director of Marketing
A software-based writing assistant that uses word prediction to cut through writing barriers and improve written expression. It is intended for students who struggle to write because of difficulty with spelling, syntax, and translating thoughts into writing. As students type, Co: Writer learns the context of the sentence and

accurately 'predicts' words even when spelled phonetically or inventively. *$79.00*

1827 **Community Exploration**
Compass Learning
203 Colorado Street
Austin, TX 78701-3922
512-478-9600
800-678-1412
866-586-7387
Fax: 619-622-7873
support@compasslearning.com
www.compasslearning.com

Eric Loeffel, President, CEO
Tammy Deal, VP, Human Resources
Eric Wasser, VP, Sales
Eileen Shihadeh, VP, Marketing

An award-winning learning adventure takes students who are learning English as a second language on a field trip to the make-believe town of Cornerstone. More than 50 community locations come to life with sound and animation. While exploring places in this typical American community where people live, work and play, students also enhance important English language skills. Offers an exciting approach for any age student who needs to improve their English language proficiency. 4-12. *$19.95*

1828 **Conversations**
Educational Activities Software
5600 West 83rd Street
Suite 300, 8200 Tower
Bloomington, MN 55437
888-351-4199
800-447-5286
Fax: 239-225-9299
info@edmentum.com
www.edmentum.com

Vin Riera, President/CEO
Dan Juckniess, SVP, Sales & Professional Services
Stacey Herteux, VP, Human Resources
Rob Rueckl, Chief Financial Officer

Using American digitized voices, CONVERSATIONS provides 14 different dialogues in which the student can participate. The topics offer learners important information about American culture and the workplace. Available for DOS. *$195.00*

1829 **Core-Reading and Vocabulary Development**
Educational Activities
P.O. Box 87
Baldwin, NY 11510
516-223-4666
800-797-3223
Fax: 516-623-9282
www.edact.com

Alfred Harris, President
Carol Stern, VP

Students begin with 36 basic words and progress to more than 200. Reading and writing activities are coordinated and integrated throughout the program for more substantial permanent learning. Five units covering readability levels from pre-primer to grade three.
Full Program

1830 **Friday Afternoon**
203 Colorado Street
Austin, TX 78701-3922
512-478-9600
800-678-1412
866-586-7387
Fax: 619-622-7873
support@compasslearning.com
www.compasslearning.com

Eric Loeffel, President, CEO
Tammy Deal, VP, Human Resources
Eric Wasser, VP, Sales
Eileen Shihadeh, VP, Marketing

Save hours of preparation time and dazzle your students with interesting new activities to supplement their classroom learning. With Friday afternoon, you'll produce flash cards, word puzzles, even customized bingo cards and more, all at the click of a mouse. MacIntosh diskette. *$99.95*

1831 **How to Read for Everyday Living**
Educational Activities Software
5600 West 83rd Street
Suite 300, 8200 Tower
Bloomington, MN 55437
888-351-4199
800-447-5286
Fax: 239-225-9299
info@edmentum.com
www.edmentum.com

Vin Riera, President/CEO
Dan Juckniess, SVP, Sales & Professional Services
Stacey Herteux, VP, Human Resources
Rob Rueckl, Chief Financial Officer

Basic vocabulary and key words are taught and, when need, retaught using alternative teaching strategies. Passages that students read help put the vocabulary into context. Each lesson is followed by crossword and other puzzles check comprehension.

1832 **Learning English: Primary**
203 Colorado Street
Austin, TX 78701-3922
512-478-9600
800-678-1412
866-586-7387
Fax: 619-622-7873
support@compasslearning.com
www.compasslearning.com

Eric Loeffel, President, CEO
Tammy Deal, VP, Human Resources
Eric Wasser, VP, Sales
Eileen Shihadeh, VP, Marketing

Four stories and rhymes help students familiarize themselves with essential English language concepts, recognize patterns in language and associate words with objects. *$49.95*

1833 **Learning English: Rhyme Time**
Compass Learning
203 Colorado Street
Austin, TX 78701-3922
512-478-9600
800-678-1412
866-586-7387
Fax: 619-622-7873
www.compasslearning.com

Eric Loeffel, President, CEO
Tammy Deal, VP, Human Resources
Eric Wasser, VP, Sales
Eileen Shihadeh, VP, Marketing

Using classic children's rhymes in an animated multimedia program, students work on language skills, vocabulary and comprehension.

1834 **Lexia I, II and III Reading Series**
Lexia Learning Systems
200 Baker Ave Ext.
Concord, MA 01742
978-405-6200
800-435-3942
800-507-2772
Fax: 978-287-0062
info@lexialearning.com
www.lexialearning.com

Nick Gaehde, President and CEO
Paul More, Vice President, Finance
Collin Earnst, Vice President of Marketing
Peter Koso, Vice President of Operations

Lexia's software helps children and adults with learning disabilities master their core reading skills. Based on the Orton Gillingham method, Lexia Early Reading, Phonics Based Reading and SOS (Strategies for Older Students) apply phonics principles to help students learn essential sound-symbol correspondence and decoding skills. The Quick Reading Tests generate detailed skill reports in only 5-8 minutes per student to provide data for further instruction. Price: $40-400 per workstation.

1835 **Memory Castle**
WINGS for Learning
1600 Green Hills Rd
Scotts Valley, CA 95066-4981
831-426-2228
Fax: 831-464-3600

Ani Stocks, Owner

Introduces a strategy to increase memory skills via an adventure Q198game. Set in a castle, the game requires memory, reading, spelling skills and more to win.

1836 On a Green Bus: A UKanDu Little Book
Don Johnston
26799 West Commerce Drive
Volo, IL 60073-9675
847-740-0749
800-999-4660
Fax: 847-740-7326
info@donjohnston.com
www.donjohnston.com

Don Johnston, Founder
Ruth Ziolkowski, President
Kevin Johnston, Director of Product Design
Ben Johnston, Director of Marketing

This early literacy program that consists of several create-your-own 4-page animated stories that help build language experience on each page and then watch the page come alive with animation and sound. After completing the story, students can print it out to make a book which can be read over and over again. Because there are no wrong answers, all children can have a successful literacy experience. *$45.00*

1837 Open Book
Freedom Scientific
11800 31st Court North
St Petersburg, FL 33716
727-803-8000
800-444-4443
Fax: 727-803-8001
info@freedomscientific.com
www.freedomscientific.com

Lee Hamilton, President, CEO, and Chairman of
Mike Self, Sales Representative (Alabama)
Joseph McDaniel, Sales Representative (Alaska and
Bobby Lakey, Sales Representative (Arkansas)

Software that reads scanned text allowed and includes other features that aid the vision-impaired. *$995.00*

1838 Optimum Resource Software
1 Mathews Drive
Suite 107
Hilton Head Island, SC 29926
843-689-8000
Fax: 843-689-8008
info@stickybear.com
www.stickybear.com

Richard Hefter, President

Optimum Resource publishes over 100 K-12 education curriculum software titles under its varietal brands, StickyBear, MiddleWare, High School and Tools for Teachers. Most programs are available in Bilingual English/Spanish, and are offered with options for the single user through 30 users.

1839 Parts of Speech
Optimum Resource
1 Mathews Drive
Suite 107
Hilton Head Island, SC 29926
843-689-8000
Fax: 843-689-8008
info@stickybear.com
www.stickybear.com

Richard Hefter, President

Designed to help students build grammar and vocabulary as they strengthen reading and writing ability. Grades 3 to 9. *$59.95*

1840 Programs for Aphasia and Cognitive Disorders
Parrot Software
P.O. Box 250755
West Bloomfield, MI 48325
248-788-3223
800-727-7681
Fax: 248-788-3224
support@parrotsoftware.com
www.parrotsoftware.com

Dr. Frederic Weiner, Ph. D., CCC-SP, President, Owner

Over 50 different computer programs that facilitate language, memory and attention training. Programs are available for MS DOS, WINDOWS and Apple II.

1841 Punctuation Rules
Optimum Resource
1 Mathews Drive
Suite 107
Hilton Head Island, SC 29926
843-689-8000
Fax: 843-689-8008
info@stickybear.com
www.stickybear.com

Richard Hefter, President

Punctuation Rules is designed to help students improve their punctuation skills. Students work with appropriate level sentences which follow common rules of punctuation. The program covers material ranging from categories of sentences to forming possessives and allows students to gain strength in their ability to correctly use periods, commas, apostrophes, question marks, colons, hyphens, quotation marks, exclamation points and more. Grades 3-9. Bilingual. *$59.95*

1842 Quick Reading Test, Phonics Based Reading, Reading SOS (Strategies for Older Students)
Lexia Learning Systems
200 Baker Ave Ext.
Concord, MA 01742
978-405-6200
800-435-3942
800-507-2772
Fax: 978-287-0062
info@lexialearning.com
www.lexialearning.com

Nick Gaehde, President and CEO
Paul More, Vice President, Finance
Collin Earnst, Vice President of Marketing
Peter Koso, Vice President of Operations

Lexia's software helps children and adults with learning disabilities master their core reading skills. Based on the Orton Gillingham method, Phonics Based Reading and S.O.S. (Strategies for the Older Student) apply phonics principles to help students learn essential sound-symbol correspondence and decoding skills. The Quick Reading Tests generate detailed phonemic skills reports in only 5-8 minutes per student to provide teachers with accurate data to focus their instruction. Price: $67-$500.

1843 Quick Talk
Educational Activities Software
5600 West 83rd Street
Suite 300, 8200 Tower
Bloomington, MN 55437
888-351-4199
800-447-5286
Fax: 239-225-9299
info@edmentum.com
www.edmentum.com

Vin Riera, President/CEO
Dan Juckniess, SVP, Sales & Professional Services
Stacey Herteux, VP, Human Resources
Rob Rueckl, Chief Financial Officer

Students will learn and use new vocabulary immediately: high-frequency, everyday vocabulary words are introduced and used contextually using human speech, graphics and text. Voice-interactive program (MS-DOS). *$65.00*

1844 Race the Clock
Mindplay
4400 E. Broadway Blvd
Suite 400
Tucson, AZ 85711
520-888-1800
800-221-7911
Fax: 520-888-7904
mail@mindplay.com
www.mindplay.com

Dan Figurski, Senior Vice President of Business
Chris Coleman, VP, Business Development
Judith Bliss, CEO
Brian Williams, Development Manager

A matching game, uses the animation capabilities to teach verbs. The player chooses a matching game from a menu.

1845 **Read: Out Loud**
Don Johnston
26799 West Commerce Drive
Volo, IL 60073-9675
847-740-0749
800-999-4660
Fax: 847-740-7326
info@donjohnston.com
www.donjohnston.com

Don Johnston, Founder
Ruth Ziolkowski, President
Kevin Johnston, Director of Product Design
Ben Johnston, Director of Marketing

An accessible text reader that provides access to the curriculum. It features high-quality text to speech and study tools that help students read with comprehension. *$79.00*

1846 **Reader Rabbit**
Learning Company
Ste 1900
100 Pine St
San Francisco, CA 94111-5205
415-659-2000
800-825-4420
Fax: 415-659-2020
thelearningco@hmhpub.com
www.thelearningcompany.com

Linda K. Zecher, President and CEO
Eric Shuman, Chief Financial Officer
John K. Dragoon, Executive Vice President and Chi
William Bayers, Executive Vice President and Gen

Supports young students in building fundamental reading readiness skills in a playful, multi-sensory environment.

1847 **Reading Comprehension Series**
Optimum Resource
1 Mathews Drive
Suite 107
Hilton Head Island, SC 29926- 3765
843-689-8000
Fax: 843-689-8008
info@stickybear.com
www.stickybear.com

Richard Hefter, President

The Reading Comprehension Series, includes seven volumes packed with intriguing multi-level stories. Each volume will capture the interest of children ages 8-14 while teaching them crucial reading comprehension skills. These open-ended programs are versatile and easy to use, and Bilingual. *$59.95*

1848 **Simon SIO**
Don Johnston
26799 West Commerce Drive
Volo, IL 60073-9675
847-740-0749
800-999-4660
Fax: 847-740-7326
info@donjohnston.com
www.donjohnston.com

Don Johnston, Founder
Ruth Ziolkowski, President
Kevin Johnston, Director of Product Design
Ben Johnston, Director of Marketing

A researched and widely field-tested phonics program for beginning readers, developed in collaboration with Dr. Ted Hasselbring of Vanderbilt University. The program uses a personal tutor to deliver individualized instruction and corrective feedback. *$79.00*

1849 **Sound Sentences**
Educational Activities Software
5600 West 83rd Street
Suite 300, 8200 Tower
Bloomington, MN 55437
888-351-4199
800-447-5286
Fax: 239-225-9299
info@edmentum.com
www.edmentum.com

Vin Riera, President/CEO
Dan Juckniess, SVP, Sales & Professional Services
Stacey Herteux, VP, Human Resources
Rob Rueckl, Chief Financial Officer

This sound-interactive program breaks away from traditional language instruction. Instead of formal concentration on verb and basic vocabulary, students meet everyday English with colloquialisms they will hear in real life situations. They reinforce their knowledge of sentence structure while acquiring the ability to communicate in daily settings. (For MAC, MS-DOS and Windows). *$65.00*

1850 **Spelling Rules**
Optimum Resource
1 Mathews Drive
Suite 107
Hilton Head Island, SC 29926- 3765
843-689-8000
Fax: 843-689-8008
info@stickybear.com
www.stickybear.com

Richard Hefter, President

A curriculum based, easy-to-use program that provides students with the practice they need to build strong spelling skills. Concepts discussed include plurals, compounds, i-before-e, capitalization, and more. Grades 3 to 9. Bilingual. *$59.95*

1851 **Start-to-Finish Library**
Don Johnston
26799 West Commerce Drive
Volo, IL 60073-9675
847-740-0749
800-999-4660
Fax: 847-740-7326
info@donjohnston.com
www.donjohnston.com

Don Johnston, Founder
Ruth Ziolkowski, President
Kevin Johnston, Director of Product Design
Ben Johnston, Director of Marketing

Offers struggling readers a wide selection of engaging narrative chapter books written at two readability levels (2-3rd and 4-5th grade) and delivered in three media formats. Professionally-narrated audio and computer supports help scaffold reading to ensure success. *$79.00*

1852 **Start-to-Finish Literacy Starters**
Don Johnston
26799 West Commerce Drive
Volo, IL 60073-9675
847-740-0749
800-999-4660
Fax: 847-740-7326
info@donjohnston.com
www.donjohnston.com

Don Johnston, Founder
Ruth Ziolkowski, President
Kevin Johnston, Director of Product Design
Ben Johnston, Director of Marketing

A reading series intended for students with multiple disabilities who are in 3-12th grade, but reading at a beginning level. Dr. Karen Erickson developed this series, which combines switch-accessible software with three types of text. *$79.00*

1853 **Stickybear Reading Comprehension**
Optimum Resource
1 Mathews Drive
Suite 107
Hilton Head Island, SC 29926- 3765
843-689-8000
Fax: 843-689-8008
info@stickybear.com
www.stickybear.com

Richard Hefter, President

This multi-level reading comprehension program helps children improve reading skills with 30 high-interest stories and question sets created by the Weekly Reader editors. Children learn to recognize main ideas, define sequence, using context to identify words, and more. Grades 2 to 4. Bilingual. *$59.95*

1854 **Stickybear Reading Fun Park**
Optimum Resource
1 Mathews Drive
Suite 107
Hilton Head Island, SC 29926- 3765
843-689-8000
Fax: 843-689-8008
info@stickybear.com
www.stickybear.com

Richard Hefter, President

Children discover and practice critical reading skills as the Stickybear family guides users through unique, action-packed activities, each with multiple levels of difficulty and skills that address both the auditory and visual needs of budding readers. Pre-K through 3rd grade. *$59.95*

1855 **Stickybear Reading Room Deluxe**
Optimum Resource
1 Mathews Drive
Suite 107
Hilton Head Island, SC 29926- 3765
843-689-8000
Fax: 843-689-8008
www.stickybear.com
Richard Hefter, President
Children build vocabulary and reading comprehension skills using hundreds of word/picture sets and thousands of put-together sentence parts. K-3rd grade. Bilingual, English/Spanish. *$59.95*

1856 **Stickybear Spelling**
Optimum Resource
1 Mathews Drive
Suite 107
Hilton Head Island, SC 29926- 3765
843-689-8000
Fax: 843-689-8008
www.stickybear.com
Richard Hefter, President
Children discover and practice critical spelling skills as they work with three unique action-packed activities, each with four graded levels of difficulty. The program is open-ended and teachers may add, change and modify the word lists for each individual. Stickybear Spelling contains more than 2000 recorded words. Levels may be set to allow students of different ages or abilities to compete effectively. Grades 2 through 4. *$59.95*

1857 **Tomorrow's Promise: Language Arts**
Compass Learning
13500 Evening Creek Drive North
Suite 600
San Diego, CA 92128
858-668-2586
866-475-0317
Fax: 858-408-2903
info@bridgepointeducation.com
www.bridgepointeducation.com
Andrew S. Clark, Founder, Chief Executive Officer
Diane Thompson, SVP, General Counsel
Charlene Dackerman, SVP, Human Resources
Daniel J. Devine, Executive Vice President & CFO
You'll strengthen students' grammar, usage and vocabulary skills and promote higher order thinking skills with this comprehensive Language Arts curriculum. It utilizes cross-curricular, thematic instruction engaging multimedia learning exercises that encourage writing, speaking and listening proficiency. Promotes higher order thinking skills. *$279.95*

1858 **Tomorrow's Promise: Reading**
Compass Learning
203 Colorado Street
Austin, TX 78701-3922
512-478-9600
800-678-1412
866-586-7387
Fax: 619-622-7873
www.compasslearning.com
Eric Loeffel, President, CEO
Tammy Deal, VP, Human Resources
Eric Wasser, VP, Sales
Eileen Shihadeh, VP, Marketing
This multimedia curriculum balances thematic, interactive exploration with core skills development, increasing your students' early reading proficiency, building a solid literacy foundation and fostering a lifelong love for reading. *$279.95*

1859 **Tomorrow's Promise: Spelling**
Compass Learning
203 Colorado Street
Austin, TX 78701-3922
512-478-9600
800-678-1412
866-586-7387
Fax: 619-622-7873
www.compasslearning.com
Eric Loeffel, President, CEO
Tammy Deal, VP, Human Resources
Eric Wasser, VP, Sales
Eileen Shihadeh, VP, Marketing
Lovable characters and engaging multimedia effects put young students on a fast-track to early spelling proficiency with fourteen activities and three games. A full year's instruction on each CD includes 30 world lists per grade, in story context, or create word lists to suit your needs. This program addresses students' multiple learning styles and rewards students as they progress through each stage of spelling skill acquisition. *$99.95*

1860 **Vocabulary Development**
Optimum Resource
1 Mathews Drive
Suite 107
Hilton Head Island, SC 29926- 3765
843-689-8000
Fax: 843-689-8008
www.stickybear.com
Richard Hefter, President
A featured program in the middle school series. Vocabulary Development is designed to help students increase vocabulary as they strengthen reading skills. Students relate their current knowledge of vocabulary to the context in which they discover an unfamiliar word. Utilizing a variety of contextual aids, this program illustrates synonyms, antonyms, prefixes, suffixes, homophones, multiple meanings and context clues, allowing students to apply experience and context. *$59.95*

1861 **Whoops**
Cornucopia Software
P.O. Box 6111
Albany, CA 94706
510-528-7000
supportstaff@practicemagic.com
www.practicemagic.com
Christina Morua, Manager
Checks spelling three ways. It checks words as they are typed, it checks an entire screen and highlights the errors and it reads ASCII text files from a disk and lists errors.

Software: Vocational

1862 **Films Media Group**
Infobase Publishing
132 W 31st St, 17th Floor
New York, NY 10001
800-322-8755
Fax: 800-678-3633
custserv@factsonfile.com
www.infobaselearning.com
Melinda Gallo, Senior Account Executive
Educational publisher of DVD programming for schools and libraries. *$64.86*
ISBN 0-927368-59-5

1863 **Functional Literacy System**
Conover Company
4 Brookwood Court
Appleton, WI 54914
920-231-4667
800-933-1933
Fax: 800-933-1943
support@conovercompany.com
www.conovercompany.com
Terry Schmitz, Founder and Owner
Mike, Vice President of Operations
Art Janowiak, Vice President of Sales
Assessment and skill building for basic functional literacy. This multimedia software program is adult in format and uses live action video taken in actual community settings to help learners become more capable of functioning independently. Twenty different programs are currently available. *$99.00*

1864 **Learning Activity Packets**
4 Brookwood Court
Appleton, WI 54914
920-231-4667
800-933-1933
Fax: 800-933-1943
support@conovercompany.com
www.conovercompany.com
Terry Schmitz, Founder and Owner
Mike, Vice President of Operations
Art Janowiak, Vice President of Sales
Demonstrates how basic academic skills relate to 30 major career areas. LAPs provide valuable diagnostics in applied academic ap-

plications and demonstrates to users the importance of academics as they relate to the workplace. Software. *$99.00*

1865 **Microcomputer Evaluation of Careers & Academics (MECA)**
Conover Company
4 Brookwood Court
Appleton, WI 54914
920-231-4667
800-933-1933
Fax: 800-933-1943
support@conovercompany.com
www.conovercompany.com

Terry Schmitz, Founder and Owner
Mike, Vice President of Operations
Art Janowiak, Vice President of Sales

A cost-effective, technology-based, career development system which provides users with opportunities to get their hands dirty. The MECA system utilizes work simulations and is built around common occupational clusters. Each cluster, or career area, consists of hands-on WORK SAMPLES which provide a variety of career exploration and assessment experiences, linked to LEARNING ACTIVITY PACKETS, which integrate basic academic skills into the career planning and placement process. $580-$1,070.

1866 **OASYS**
Vertek
12835 Bellevue-Redmond Road
Suite 310
Bellevue, WA 98005
425-455-9921
800-220-4409
Fax: 425-454-7264

Debra Callahan, Sales Representative, Northern California
Tim Whitney, Sales Representative, Ohio, Michigan
Beverly Duncan, Sales Representative, Florida
Debbie Gordon, Sales Representative, Illinois

A software system that matches a person's skills and abilities to occupations and employers.

1867 **Reading in the Workplace**
Educational Activities Software
5600 West 83rd Street
Suite 300, 8200 Tower
Bloomington, MN 55437-585
888-351-4199
800-447-5286
Fax: 239-225-9299
info@edmentum.com
www.edmentum.com

Vin Riera, President/CEO
Dan Juckniess, SVP, Sales & Professional Services
Stacey Herteux, VP, Human Resources
Rob Rueckl, Chief Financial Officer

A job-based, reading software program using real-life problems and solutions to capture students' attention and improve their vocabulary and comprehension skills. Units include: automotive, clerical, health care and construction. *$295.00*

1868 **Stickybear Typing**
Optimum Resource
1 Mathews Drive
Suite 107
Hilton Head Island, SC 29926- 3765
843-689-8000
Fax: 843-689-8008
www.stickybear.com

Richard Hefter, President

The award winning Stickybear Typing program allows users to sharpen typing skills and achieve keyboard mastery with three engaging and amusing multi-level activities. *$59.95*

1869 **Work-Related Vocational Assessment Systems: Computer Based**
Valpar International
P.O. Box 5767
Tucson, AZ 85703-767
262-797-0840
800-633-3321
Fax: 262-797-8488
sales@valparint.com
www.valparint.com

Neal Gunderson, President

Criterion-referenced to Department of Labor standards. Evaluate academic levels for reading, spelling, math and language, interests, personalities, cognitive and physical aptitudes.

1870 **Workplace Skills: Learning How to Function on the Job**
Programming Concepts
8700 Shoal Creek Boulevard
Austin, TX 78757-6897
512-451-3246
800-897-3202
Fax: 800-397-7633
general@proedinc.com
www.proedinc.com

Jeff McLane, Founder
Lee Wilson, President and CEO
Randy Pennington, Executive VP
David Keith, Vice President of IT

Offers parents and educators a functional means by which to discuss all aspects of finding and keeping a job. *$49.95*

Word Processors

1871 **DARCI**
Wes Test Engineering Corporation
810 Shepard Lane
Farmington, UT 84025
801-451-9191
Fax: 801-451-9393
westest.com

Robert Lessmann, President
James Lynds

Provides transparent access to all computer functions by replacing the computer's keyboard with a smart joystick. *$975.00*

1872 **Eye Relief Word Processing Software**
SkiSoft Publishing Corporation
P.O. Box 364
Lexington, MA 02420-4
781-863-1876
www.skisoft.com

Ken Skier, President
Cynthia Skier, CFO

Large-type word processing program for visually-impaired PC users. *$295.00*

1873 **IntelliTalk**
Intelli Tools
24 Prime Parkway
Natick, MA 01760
707-773-2000
800-547-6747
Fax: 707-773-2001
customerservice@cambiumtech.com

Beth Davis, Director Sales Operations
Lori Castle, Supervisor
Arjan Khalsa, CEO

Talking word-processing program available for MacIntosh, Apple IIe, IBM compatible and Windows computers. *$39.95*

1874 **Large Type**
P.O. Box T
Hewitt, NJ 07421-2088
973-853-6585
800-736-2216
Fax: 928-832-2894
http://www.angelfire.com

Don Selwyn, Vice President
Rev. Tom Schwanda, President & Chairman
Robt. Fondiller, Ph.D., P.E, Vice President
Everett G. Ball, Treasurer

Display enlargement programs for visually impaired users. Consist of a variety of programs for different needs, ranging from basic to full-featured.

1875 **Pegasus LITE**
Words+
Ste 109
42505 10th St W
Lancaster, CA 93534-7059
661-723-6523
800-869-8521
Fax: 661-723-2114
info@words-plus.com

Phil Lawrence, VP

Provides all of the strategies currently being used in AAC, from dynamic display color pictographic language, to dual-word prediction text language, in a single system. *$6995.00*

1876 **Up and Running**

Intelli Tools
24 Prime Parkway
Natick, MA 01760
707-773-2000
800-547-6747
Fax: 707-773-2001
customerservice@cambiumtech.com

Beth Davis, Director Sales Operations
Lori Castle, Supervisor
Arjan Khalsa, CEO

Instantly use hundreds of popular commercial software programs with this custom collection of setups and overlays. *$69.95*

1877 **Write: OutLoud**

Don Johnston
26799 West Commerce Drive
Volo, IL 60073-9675
847-740-0749
800-999-4660
Fax: 847-740-7326
info@donjohnston.com
www.donjohnston.com

Don Johnston, Founder
Ruth Ziolkowski, President
Kevin Johnston, Director of Product Design
Ben Johnston, Director of Marketing

The award-winning feasible and user friendly talking word processor with talking spell checker. Text-to-speech technology provides multi-sensory learning and positive reinforcements for writers of all ages and ability levels. *$99.00*

Conferences & Shows

General

1878 **AACRC Annual Conference**
Association of Children's Residential Centers
648 N Plankinton Ave.
Suite 245
Milwaukee, WI 53203
414-403-1565
877-332-2272
info@togetherthevoice.org
togetherthevoice.org
Kari Sisson, Executive Director
Amanda Prange, Training Coordinator
McKenzie Melchoir, Membership Services Specialist
Lisette Burton, Chief Policy & Practice Advisor
August

1879 **AADB National Conference**
American Association of the Deaf-Blind
248 Rainbow Drive
Suite 14864
Livingston, TX 77399-2048
aadb-info@aadb.org
www.aadb.org
Rene Pellerin, President
A week of general meetings, workshops, tours and evening recreational activities.

1880 **AAIDD Annual Meeting**
American Assn on Intellecutal/Devel. Disabilities
8403 Colesville Rd.
Suite 900
Silver Spring, MD 20910
202-387-1968
Fax: 202-387-2193
maria@aaidd.org
aaidd.org
Maria Alfaro, Manager, Meetings & Website
This annual meeting offers workshops, symposia, multiperspective sessions, and social events over four days.
May/June

1881 **AAO Annual Meeting**
American Academy Of Opthamology
655 Beach St.
San Francisco, CA 94109-1336
415-561-8500
Fax: 415-561-8533
www.aao.org/annual-meeting
David W. Parke II, Chief Executive Officer
Debra Rosencrance, VP, Meetings & Events
Offers the most comprehensive program with more than 2000 scientific presentations and six subspecialty day programs.
October/November

1882 **ACA Annual Conference**
American Counseling Association
6101 Stevenson Ave.
Suite 600
Alexandria, VA 22304
703-823-9800
800-347-6647
Fax: 800-473-2329
www.counseling.org/conference
Richard Yep, Chief Executive Officer
Theresa Holmes, Director, Conference Planning & Events
Promotes the development of professional counselors, advances the counseling profession, and uses the profession and practice of counseling to promote respect for human dignity and diversity.
March/April

1883 **ADA Annual Scientific Sessions**
American Diabetes Association
2451 Crystal Dr.
Suite 900
Arlington, VA 22201
800-342-2383
askada@diabetes.org
www.diabetes.org
Tracey D. Brown, Chief Executive Officer
Linda Cann, SVP, Professional Services
Brings together physicians, scientists and other health care professionals from around the world to learn about the latest advances in basic and clinical science for diabetes.

1884 **AER Annual International Conference**
Assoc. for Educ. & Rehab of the Blind/Vis. Imp.
5680 King Centre Dr.
Suite 600
Alexandria, VA 22315
703-671-4500
Fax: 703-671-6391
conference@aerbvi.org
www.aerbvi.org
Neva Fairchild, President
Dedicated to rendering support and assistance to the professionals who work in all phases of education and rehabilitation of blind and visually impaired children and adults.
July

1885 **AG Bell Global Listening and Spoken Language Symposium**
Alexander Graham Bell Association
3417 Volta Pl., NW
Washington, DC 20007
202-337-5220
Fax: 202-337-8314
TTY: 202-337-5221
info@agbell.org
agbellsymposium.com
Emilio Alonso-Mendoza, Chief Executive Officer
A meeting of professionals who serve those who are deaf and hard of hearing.
June/July

1886 **APSE National Conference**
APSE
7361 Calhoun Place
Suite 680
Rockville, MD 20855
301-279-0060
Fax: 301-279-0075
info@apse.org
www.apse.org
Erica Belois-Pacer, Director, Professional Development
Julie Christensen, Director, Policy & Advocacy
Erynn Pawlak, Director, Operations
Christa P. Rainwater, Director, Membership & Chapter Engagement
A major conference on Supported Employment. The conference includes sessions presented by nationally recognized leaders in the field. Conference attendees come from all 50 states, Canada and several foreign countries and include professionals in supported employment, occupational therapy, rehabilitation technology and other related fields.
July

1887 **ASHA Convention**
American Speech-Language-Hearing Association
2200 Research Blvd.
Rockville, MD 20850-3289
301-296-5700
800-638-8255
Fax: 301-296-8580
convention@asha.org
convention.asha.org
Arlene A. Pietranton, Chief Executive Officer
Craig E. Coleman, VP, Planning
Exhibits by companies specializing in alternative and augmentative communication products, publishers, software and hardware companies, and hearing aid testing equipment manufacturers. Speech-Language Pathologists are professionals who identify, assess, and treat speech and language problems. Audiologists are hearing health care professionals who specialize in preventing, identifying and assessing hearing disorders as well as providing audiologic treatment including hearing aids and more.
November

1888 **ASIA Annual Scientific Meeting**
American Spinal Injury Association
9702 Gayton Rd.
Suite 306
Richmond, VA 23238
877-274-2724
asia.office@asia-spinalinjury.org
www.asia-spinalinjury.org

Patty Duncan, Executive Director
Carolyn Moffatt, Association Manager
Kim Ruff, Administrative Assistant

Professional association for physicans and other health professionals working in all aspects of spinal cord injury. Also holds an annual scientific that surveys the latest advancements in the field.
May

1889 **ATIA Conference**
Assistive Technology Industry Association
330 N Wabash Ave.
Suite 2000
Chicago, IL 60611-4267
312-321-5172
877-687-2842
Fax: 312-673-6659
info@atia.org
www.atia.org

David Dikter, Chief Executive Officer
Caroline Van Howe, Chief Operating Officer
Emily Schmitt, Manager, Marketing
Katie Isdonas, Registration Senior Associate

The ATIA Conference is the largest international conference showcasing excellence in assistive technology.

1890 **Abilities Expo**
299 N Euclid Ave.
2nd Floor
Pasadena, CA 91101
323-363-2099
info@abilities.com
abilities.com

David Korse, President & CEO
Caryn Bates, Director, Operations

Abilities Expo is a national event for people with disabilities, their families, caregivers, and healthcare professionals. Meets in Phoenix, Dallas, Chicago, Los Angeles, Miami, Houston, New York, and Toronto.

1891 **American Academy for Cerebral Palsy and Developmental Medicine Annual Conference**
555 East Wells
Suite 1100
Milwaukee, WI 53202
414-918-3014
Fax: 414-276-2146
info@aacpdm.org
www.aacpdm.org

Tamara Wagester, Executive Director
Erin Trimmer, Senior Meetings Manager

The Annual Meeting is a 3-day event, held in the Fall, designed to provide targeted opportunities for dissemination of information in the basic sciences, prevention, diagnosis, treatment, and technical advances as applied to persons with cerebral palsy and development disorders.
September

1892 **American Academy of Audiology Conference**
American Academy of Audiology
11480 Commerce Park Dr.
Suite 220
Reston, VA 20191
703-790-8466
Fax: 703-790-8631
infoaud@audiology.org
www.audiology.org

Patrick E. Gallagher, Executive Director
Kathryn Werner, Vice President, Public Affairs
Amy Miedema, Vice President, Communications & Membership
Dina Santucci, Senior Director, Business Development

The American Academy of Audiology is the world's largest professional organization for audiologists. The Academy is dedicated to providing quality hearing care services through professional development, education, research, and increased public awareness of hearing and balance disorders.
March-April

1893 **American Academy of Environmental Medicine Annual Conference**
PO Box 195
Ashland, MO 65010
316-684-5500
Fax: 888-411-1206
aaemonline.org

Jessica Tran, President
Lauren Grohs, Executive Director
William A. Ingram, Secretary
James W. Willoughby, Treasurer

The Academy is an association of physicians and other professionals engaged in investigating and coming up with preventive strategies for medical ccare relating to environmentally triggered illnesses.

1894 **American Board of Disability Analysts Annual Conference**
4525 Harding Rd.
Second Floor
Nashville, TN 37205
americanbd@aol.com
www.americandisability.org

Kenneth Anchor, Administrative Officer

Bi-annual conference held for members to meet and discuss current events and attend seminars.

1895 **Annual Conference on Dyslexia and Related Learning Disabilities**
New York Branch International Dyslexia Association
1550 Deer Park Ave.
Suite C
Long Island, NY 11729
631-261-7441
www.lidyslexia.org

Concetta Russo, President
Caryl Deiches, Vice President
Carolyn McIntyre, Secretary
Julia Bunyatov, Treasurer

The International Dyslexia Association (IDA) is an organization focused on the complex issues of dyslexia and related language-based learning disabilities which make it difficult to learn to read and write.
March

1896 **Annual TASH Conference**
TASH
1101 15th St. NW
Suite 206
Washington, DC 20005
202-817-3264
Fax: 202-999-4722
info@tash.org
www.tash.org/conferences

Michael Brogioli, Executive Director
Linda Metchikoff-Hooker, Director, Special Events
Donald Taylor, Manager, Membership & Operations
Marshall Jones, Office Administrator

Each year, the TASH Conference connects attendees to information and resources, facilitates connections between stakeholders within the disability movement, and helps attendees reignite their passion for an inclusive world.
December

1897 **Arc National Convention, The**
The Arc
1825 K St., NW
Suite 1200
Washington, DC 20006
202-534-3700
800-433-5255
Fax: 202-534-3731
convention.thearc.org

Peter Berns, Chief Executive Officer
Tanisha Forte, Director, Conference & Events

Experts and professionals gather from all over the world share best practices, struggles, successes and hopes for the future, and continue the conversation about protecting and promoting the human and civil rights for individuals with intellectual and developmental disabilities.
October

1898 Attention Deficit Disorders Association, Southern Region: Annual Conference
12345 Jones Rd.
Suite 287-7
Houston, TX 77070
281-897-0982
Fax: 281-894-6883
addaoffice@sbcglobal.net
www.adda-sr.org

Carlye Read, President
Barbara Beard, Vice President
Judy German, Treasurer
The Attention Deficit Disorders Association provides a resource network, supports individuals impacted by ADHHD and related condition and to advocate for the development of community resources.
February

1899 Blind Children's Center Annual Meeting
Blind Children's Center
4120 Marathon St.
Los Angeles, CA 90029-3584
323-664-2153
info@blindchildrenscenter.org
www.blindchildrenscenter.org

Sarah E. Orth, CEO
Fernanda Armenta-Schmitt, Director, Education & Family Services
A family-centered agency which serves children with visual impairments from birth to school-age. The center-based and home-based services help the children to acquire skills and build their independence. The Center utilizes its expertise and experience to serve families and professionals worldwide through support services, education and research.
September

1900 Blinded Veterans Association National Convention
Blinded Veterans Association
1101 King St.
Suite 300
Alexandria, VA 22314
800-669-7079
bva@bva.org
www.bva.org

Donald D. Overton, Jr., Executive Director
The convention has three functions: to serve as a platform for Association business, to educate blinded veterans about the resources available to them, and to provide a means whereby blinded veterans can support one another.
August

1901 CQL Accreditation
Council on Quality and Leadership
100 West Rd.
Suite 300
Towson, MD 21204
410-275-0488
info@thecouncil.org
www.c-q-l.org/accreditation

Mary Kay Rizzolo, President & CEO
Katherine Dunbar, VP, Accreditation
CQL Accreditation is a leader in working with human service organizations and systems to continuously define, measure and improve quality of life and quality of services.

1902 Centers of Excellence Leadership Conference
National Parkinson Foundation
200 SE 1st St.
Suite 800
Miami, FL 33131
800-473-4636
contact@parkinson.org
parkinson.org

John L. Lehr, CEO
James Beck, VP & Chief Scientific Officer
Yashnahia Cortorreal, VP & Chief Human Resources & Administration Pfficer
Curt DeGreff, SVP & CFO
The mission of the National Parkinson Foundation is to make life better for people affected by Parkinson's through expert care, research, and education. The goal of the conference is to convene the medical directors, center coordinators and other leaders from the Centers of Excellence to discuss the latest research and best practices in care delivery and to highlight NPF's programs.
July/August

1903 Closing the Gap's Annual Conference
P.O. Box 68
Henderson, MN 56044
507-248-3294
Fax: 507-248-3810
www.closingthegap.com

Dolores Hagen, Co-Founder
Budd Hagen, Co-Founder
Topics cover a broad spectrum of technology as it is being applied to all disabilities and age groups in education, rehabilitation, vocation and independent living. People with disabilities, special educators, rehabilitation professionals, administrators, service/care providers, personnel managers, government officials, and hardware/software developers share their experiences and insights at this significant networking experience.
October/November

1904 Conference of the Association on Higher Education & Disability (AHEAD)
8015 West Kenton Circle
Suite 230
Huntersville, NC 28078
704-947-7779
Fax: 704-948-7779
www.ahead.org

Stephan Smith, Executive Director
Carol Funckes, Chief Operations Officer
Howard Kramer, Conference Director
Jeremy Jarrell, Director, Innovation and Development
An annual conference focused on aiding and meeting the needs of persons with disabilities attending higher education institutions.

1905 Council for Exceptional Children Annual Convention and Expo
3100 Clarendon Blvd.
Suite 600
Arlington, VA 22201-5332
888-232-7733
TTY: 866-915-5000
service@cec.sped.org
cecconvention.org

Chad Rummel, Executive Director
Sharon Rodriguez, Governance & Executive Services Coordinator
Works to improve the educational success of children with disabilities and/or gifts and talents.
March/April

1906 Disability Matters
Springboard Consulting
4740 S Ocean Blvd.
Suite 505
Highland Beach, FL 33487
973-813-7260
Fax: 973-813-7261
info@consultspringboard.com
www.consultspringboard.com

Nadine Vogel, Chief Executive Officer
Elizabeth Ladu, Chief Financial Officer
Ivette Lopez, Chief of Staff
Susan Hamilton, Legal Counsel
Features outstanding content as delivered by leading disability experts from corporations, academia, national non-profits and governments across North America. Conferences also take place in Europe and Asia-Pacific.

1907 Eye Bank Association of America Annual Meeting
Eye Bank Association of America
1101 17th St., NW
Suite 400
Washington, DC 20036
202-775-4999
Fax: 202-429-6036
www.restoresight.org

Kevin Corcoran, CAE, President & CEO
Genevieve Casaceli, Education & Programs Manager
Bernie Dellario, Director, Finance
Jennifer DeMatteo, Director, Regulations & Standards
A four day program, which includes a series of presentations in administrative, hospital development, scientific and technical fields that are relative to eye banking.
June

1908 **IDF National Conference**
Immune Deficiency Foundation
110 West Rd.
Suite 300
Towson, MD 21204
800-296-4433
Fax: 410-321-9165
info@primaryimmune.org
primaryimmune.org

Kathryn Stephens, Interim CEO
Sarah Rose, Chief Financial Officer
Katherine Antilla, Vice President, Education
Tammy C. Black, Vice President, Communications

The four-day conference brings together primary immunodeficiency patients, caregivers and clinicians to participate in youth programs, panel discussions, educational sessions and networking opportunities.
June

1909 **Lowe Syndrome Conference**
Lowe Syndrome Association
P.O. Box 417
Chicago Ridge, IL 60415
216-630-7723
www.lowesyndrome.org

Lisa Waldbaum, President
Jane Gallery, Treasurer
Tiffany Johnson, Director, Medical & Scientific Affairs

An international conference held approximately every two years where family, friends, medical and other professionals gather to exchange ideas and information.
June

1910 **NACDD Annual Conference**
1825 K St. NW
Suite 600
Washington, DC 20006
202-506-5813
info@nacdd.org
www.nacdd.org

Donna A. Meltzer, Chief Executive Officer
Erin Prangley, Director, Public Policy

NACDD is the national association for the 56 State and Territorial Councils on Developmental Disabilities (DD Councils) which receive federal funding to support programs that promote self-determination, integration, and inclusion for all Americans with developmental disabilities.
July

1911 **NADR Conference**
National Association of Disability Representatives
1305 W 11th St.
Suite 222
Houston, TX 77008
202-822-2155
800-747-6131
Fax: 972-245-6701
www.nadr.org

C. Greg Cates, President
Michael Wener, Vice President
Cliff Berkley, Secretary
Christopher Mazzulli, Treasurer

NADR is an organization of Professional Social Security Claimants Representatives that focus on issues involving policies to protect the interest of people with disabilities. NADR conducts annual conventions open to members and non-members with educational seminars to keep practitioners up to date on Social Security rulings, regulatory changes, and practice improvements.

1912 **NASW-NYS Chapter**
NASW
188 Washington Ave.
Albany, NY 12210
518-463-4741
800-724-6279
Fax: 518-463-6446
info.naswnys@socialworkers.org
www.naswnys.org

Samantha Fletcher, Executive Director
Marcia Schwartzman Levy, President

Workshops, keynote speakers, and presentations offered at this event will develop and enhance practice skills and knowledge in the provision of quality mental health and community services.
March

1913 **NEXT Conference & Exposition**
American Physical Therapy Association
1111 North Fairfax St.
Alexandria, VA 22314-1488
703-684-2782
800-999-2782
Fax: 703-706-8536
consumer@apta.org
apta.org

Sharon L. Dunn, President
Matthew R. Hyland, Vice President
Kip Schick, Secretary
Jeanine Gunn, Treasurer

The American Physical Therapy Association is a national professional organization sponsors this annual conference. The goal is to foster advancements in physical therapy practice, research, and education.

1914 **National Association for the Dually Diagnosed Conferences**
12 Hurley Ave.
Kingston, NY 12401
845-331-4336
info@thenadd.org
www.thenadd.org

Jeanne M. Farr, CEO
Michelle Jordan, Office Manager
Jeffrey Schmunk, Operations Manager
Edward Seliger, Project Coordinator

NADD is a non-for-profit membership organization designed to promote awareness of, and services for, individuals who have co-occuring intellectual disability and mental illness. NADD provides training, consultation services, and publishes journals and books. it also offers two conferences per year.

1915 **National Council on the Aging Conference**
251 18th St. S.
Suite 500
Arlington, VA 22202
571-527-3900
membership@ncoa.org
www.ncoa.org

James Knickman, Interim President & CEO
Donna Whitt, Senior Vice President, Chief Financial Officer
Kristin Kiefer, Chief Administrative Officer
Josh Hodges, Chief Customer Officer

Offers ideas and programs to increase program and administrative skills through NCOA's professional development tracks and offering of continuing education units.
May

1916 **PVA Summit & Expo**
Paralyzed Veterans of America
801 18th St. NW
Washington, DC 20006-3517
800-424-8200
TTY: 800-795-4327
summit@pva.org
summitpva.org

David Zurfluh, National President
Charles Brown, National Senior Vice President
Carl Blake, Executive Director
Shaun Castle, Deputy Executive Director

The annual 3-day medical conference brings together leaders from medicine, health care, policy, and government to explore and implement holistic strategies to strengthen the continuum of care for patients with spinal cord injuries or related diseases.

1917 **PWSA (USA) Conference**
Prader-Willi Alliance Of New York
244 5th Ave.
Suite D-110
New York, NY 10001
800-442-1655
alliance@prader-willi.org
www.prader-willi.org/conference

Amy McDougall, President
Barbara McManus, Treasurer
Brian Burgin, 1st Vice President
Rachel Johnson, Executive Director

Through conferences, publications, electronic communication and networking (parent-to-parent, parent-to professional, and professional-to-professional), the Prader-Willi Alliance pro-

vides a valuable resource for individuals and families sharing the same concerns.
July

1918 **Pacific Rim International Conference on Disability And Diversity**
Center on Disability Studies
1410 Lower Campus Rd.
Unit 171F
Honolulu, HI 96822
808-956-8816
prinfo@hawaii.edu
pacrim.coe.hawaii.edu
Patricia Morrissey, Director of the Center on Disability
The Pacific Rim International Conference on Disability and Diversity encourages and respects voices from diverse perspective across numerous areas including voices from persons representing all disability areas, and experiences of family members and supporters across all disability and diversity areas.

1919 **RESNA Annual Conference**
Rehab Engineering & Assistive Tech. North America
2025 M St. NW
Suite 800
Arlington, VA 20036
202-367-1121
Fax: 202-367-2121
info@resna.org
www.resna.org
Maureen Linden, President
James Lenker, Treasurer
Meghan Donahue, Secretary
Sponsored by a multidisciplinary association for the advancement of rehabilitation and assistive technologies, this annual conference brings together a large number of rehabilitation professionals, products and services from around the world and has something to offer for both professionals and consumers. The conference provides an informative and thought provoking forum for anyone with interests in rehabilitation technology.
June

1920 **Rehabilitation International World Congress**
866 United Nations Plaza
Office 422
New York, NY 10017
212-420-1500
Fax: 212-505-0871
info@riglobal.org
www.riglobal.org
Teuta Rexhepi, Secretary General
Zhang Haidi, President
RI is a global network of people with disabilities, service providers, researchers, government agencies, and advocates protecting and promoting the rights and inclusion of people with disabilities.
Quadrennial

1921 **Southwest Conference On Disability**
University of New Mexico
2300 Menaul Blvd., NE
Albuquerque, NM 87107
505-272-3000
Fax: 505-272-2014
HSC-swdisabilityconference@salud.unm.edu
www.cdd.unm.edu/apps/SWConf/pre sentation

1922 **Tourette Association of America National Education Conference**
42-40 Bell Blvd.
Suite 205
Bayside, NY 11361
888-486-8738
support@tourette.org
tourette.org
Amanda Talty, President & CEO
This is a biannual conference that includes members of the TS community and their families, educators, TS advocates, physicians, researchers, allied professionals, and TSA staff members. Attendees interact, socialize, share ideas, discuss issues of concern, and learn from experts.
1972

1923 **Young Onset Parkinson Conference**
National Parkinson Foundation & ADPF
200 SE 1st St.
Suite 800
Miami, FL 33131
800-473-4636
Fax: 305-537-9901
contact@parkinson.org
www.parkinson.org
John L. Lehr, President and CEO
James Beck, Vice President, Chief Scientific Officer
Yasnahia Cortorreal, Vice President, Human Resources & Administration
Curt DeGreff, Vice President, Chief Development Officer
Purpose is to find the cause and cure for Parkinson's Disease and related neurodegenerative disorders through research, education and dissemination of current information to patients, care-givers and families.
Annual

Construction & Architecture

Associations

1924 **Adaptive Environments Center**
200 Portland Street
Suite 1
Boston, MA 02114
617-695-1225
Fax: 617-482-8099
info@HumanCenteredDesign.org
www.humancentereddesign.org

Ralph Jackson, FAIA, President
Chris Pilkington, Vice President
Nancy Jenner, Treasurer
Valerie Fletcher, Executive Director

Develops educational programs and materials on universal design, Americans with Disabilities Act, home adaptation, and more. Central Adaptive Environments publication list also available.

1925 **American Institute of Architects**
1735 New York Ave. NW
Washington, DC 20006-5292
800-242-3837
memberservices@aia.org
www.aia.org

Robert A. Ivy, FAIA, EVP/Chief Executive Officer
Abigail Warnecke Gorman, Chief of Staff
Sarah Dodge, SVP, Advocacy & Relationships
Terri S. Stewart, AIA, CAE, SVP, Knowledge & Practice

The organization, with 200 chapters worldwide and 95,000 members, advocates for the value of architecture and ethical standards in the profession.

1926 **American Society of Landscape Architects**
636 Eye St. NW
Washington, DC 20001-3736
202-898-2444
888-999-2752
Fax: 202-898-1185
info@asla.org
www.asla.org

Roxanne Blackwell, Co-Interim EVP & CEO
Curt Millay, Co-Interim EVP & CEO
Susan Cahill-Aylward, Director, Information & Professional Practice
Kevin Fry, Director, Public Relations & Communications

Professional organization for landscape architects in the U.S., with 15,000 members.

1927 **Building Owners and Managers Association International**
1101 15th St., NW
Suite 800
Washington, DC 20005
202-326-6300
Fax: 202-326-6377
info@boma.org
www.boma.org

Henry Chamberlain, President & COO
Patricia Areno, Senior Vice President
Luci Vallejo, Director, Executive Services
Lisa Prats, Managing Director, Standards & International Affairs

Conducts seminars nationwide and publishes resource guidebooks for building owners and managers on ADA requirements for commercial facilities and places of public accommodation.

1928 **Department of Insurance/OSFM**
North Carolina Department of Insurance
325 N. Salisbury St.
Raleigh, NC 27603
919-647-0014
Fax: 919-715-0067
tara.barthelmess@ncdoi.gov

Tara Barthelmess, Chief Accessibility Code Consultant

The Chief Accessibility Code Consultant interprets building code accessibility requirements for new and existing buildings undergoing construction or alteration. The position also receives and initiates investigation of accessibility-related complaints within the State of North Carolina whenever possible.

1929 **Institute for Human Centered Design**
Formerly Adaptive Environments
200 Portland St
Ste 1
Boston, MA 02214
617-695-1225
Fax: 617-482-8099
TTY: 617-695-1225
info@humancentereddesign.org
humancentereddesign.org

Valerie Fletcher, Executive Director
Gabriela Bonome-Sims, Director, Administration & Finance

Formerly known as Adaptive Environments, the Insititute focuses on collaborating and working with citizens to design communal places to be accessible for all, including those with disabilities.

1930 **Mark Elmore Associates Architects**
Ste 104
42 East St
Crystal Lake, IL 60014-4400
815-455-7260
800-801-7766
Fax: 815-455-2238
www.elmore-architects.com

Mark A Elmore, Owner

Architectural designs for accessible residential and commercial buildings. ADA compliance reviews.

1931 **National Conference on Building Codes and Standards**
505 Huntmar Park Drive
Suite 210
Herndon, VA 20170
703-437-0100
Fax: 703-481-3596
www.ncsbcs.org

Cynthia Wilk, President
Robert C. Wible, Executive Director
Debbie Becker, Administrative Assistant
Kevin Egilmez, Project Manager

Serves as a forum in the interchange of information and provides technical services, education and training to our members to enhance the public's social and economic well being through safe, durable, affordable, accessible and efficient buildings.

1932 **National Council of Architectural Registration Boards (NCARB)**
1401 H Street NW
Suite 500
Washington, DC 20006
202-879-0520
ncarb.org

Michael J. Armstrong, Chief Executive Officer
Mary S. de Sousa, Chief Operating Officer
Guillermo Ortiz de Zarate, Chief Innovation & Information Officer

Research service in print and online information. Large collection of books and periodicals on the building/architectural environments.

1933 **National Institute of Building Sciences**
1090 Vermont Ave. NW
Suite 700
Washington, DC 20005
202-289-7800
Fax: 202-289-1092
nibs@nibs.org
www.nibs.org

Lakisha Ann Woods, President & CEO
Rebecca Liko, Vice President, Finance & Controller
Sarah Swango, Senior Director, Business Development
Kristen Petersen, Managing Director, Marketing & Communications

The organization supports advances in building science and technology to improve the built environment. The U.S. Congress established it in the the Housing and Community Development Act of 1974.

1934 **Overcoming Mobility Barriers International**
1022 S 4st St
Omaha, NE 68105
402-342-5731
Fax: 402-342-5731

Kay Neil, Executive Director

Members are government officials, service consumers and providers, and other persons interested in removing mobility barriers for elderly, handicapped and disadvantaged persons. Advises and works in conjunction with other groups and government agencies to establish safety standards for special equipment used in retrofitting vehicles and works to retrain drivers in the use of nonconventional driving controls.

1935 **PVA Architecture**
Paralyzed Veterans of America
801 18th St. NW
Washington, DC 20006-3517
202-416-7645
800-424-8200
TTY: 800-795-4327
pvaarchitecture@pva.org
www.pva.org

David Zurfluh, National President
Charles Brown, National Senior Vice President
Carl Blake, Executive Director
Shaun Castle, Deputy Executive Director
Provides architectural consulting services related to accessible designs. Experience includes product design and building codes and standards.

1936 **United States Access Board**
Ste 1000
1331 F St NW
Washington, DC 20004-1111
202-272-0080
800-872-2253
Fax: 202-272-0081
TTY: 800-993-2822
info@access-board.gov
www.access-board.gov

Lance Robertson, Chair
Gregory S. Fehribach, Vice Chair
Offers information and technical assistance to the public on accessible design under the Americans with Disabilities Act and other laws. Guidance and publications are available free that address access to facilities, transit vehicles and information technology.

Publications & Videos

1937 **Access Currents**
United States Access Board
1331 F Street, NW
Suite 1000
Washington, DC 20004-1111
202-272-0080
800-872-2253
Fax: 202-272-0081
TTY: 800-993-2822
info@access-board.gov
www.access-board.gov

Lance Robertson, Chair
Gregory S. Fehribach, Vice Chair
Offers information and referrals on architectural accessibility for architects, designers, government agencies, building owners and consumers. A list of free publications is available on request.
bi-monthly

1938 **Access Equals Opportunity**
Council of B BB s Foundation
3033 Wilson Blvd
Suite 600
Arlington, VA 22201
703-276-0100
www.bbb.org

Beverly Baskin, Senior VP, Chief Mission Officer
Genie Barton, Vice President and Director, Onl
Rodney L. Davis, Senior VP Enterprise Programs
Joseph E. Dillon, VP and CFO
These six Title III compliance guides for existing small businesses offer creative cheap and easy suggestions for complying with the public accommodations section of the ADA. Each guide is industry specific for: retail stores, car sales/service, restaurants/bars, medical offices and fun/fitness centers. They include suggestions for readily achievable removal of architectural barriers; effective communication; and guidance for nondiscriminatory policies or procedures. *$2.50*

1939 **Access for All**
Hospital Audiences
548 Broadway
3rd Floor
New York, NY 10012
212-575-7676
Fax: 212-575-7669

David Sweeny, Executive Director
Jane Kleinsinger, Director of Operations
Jill Bernard, Marketing & Outreach Manager
JoAnne Brockways, Chief Financial Officer
Provides physical and program accessibility information for people with disabilities to New York City cultural institutions including theaters, museums, galleries, etc.

1940 **Accessible Home of Your Own**
Accent Special Publications
Bloomington, IL 61702-700
Raymond C Cheever, Publisher
Betty Garee, Editor
This guide includes 14 articles on the popular subject of how to make a disabled persons home more accessible. *$7.99*
52 pages Paperback 1990
ISBN 0-915708-29-9

1941 **Adaptable Housing: A Technical Manual for Implementing Adaptable Dwelling**
H UD U SE R
P.O. Box 23268
Washington, DC 20026-3268
202-708-3178
800-245-2691
Fax: 202-708-9981
TTY: 800-927-7589
helpdesk@huduser.org
www.huduser.org

Patrick J. Tewey, Director, Budget, Contracts, and Program Control Division
Jacqueline D Buford, Director, Management and Administrative Services Division
Jean Lin Pao, General Deputy Assistant Secretary
Katherine M. O'Regan, Assistant Secretary for Policy Development and Research
An illustrated manual describing methods for implementing adaptability in housing. *$3.00*

1942 **Architect Magazine**
Hanley Wood Media Inc.
One Thomas Circle NW
Washington, DC 20003
202-452-0800
etters@architectmagazine.com
www.architectmagazine.com

Ned Cramer, Editor-in-Chief
Grieg O'Brien, Managing Editor
Official journal of the American Institute of Architects

1943 **BOMA Magazine**
Building Owners & Managers Association
1101 15th St., NW
Suite 800
Washington, DC 20005
202-326-6300
Fax: 202-326-6377
info@boma.org
www.boma.org

Henry Chamberlain, President & COO
Courtney McKay, Vice President, Communications & Marketing
Official magazine of the Building Owners & Managers Association.

1944 **Consumer's Guide to Home Adaptation**
Institute for Human Centered Design
200 Portland Street
Suite 1
Boston, MA 02114
617-695-1225
Fax: 617-482-8099
TTY: 617-695-1225
info@HumanCenteredDesign.org
www.humancentereddesign.org

Valerie Fletcher, Executive Director
Tzesika Iliovits, Project Manager, Inclusive Design Projects

A workbook that enables people with disabilities to plan the modifications necessary to adapt their homes. Describes how to widen doorways, lower countertops, etc. *$12.00*

52 pages Paperback

ISBN 0-970835-80-9

1945 **Design for Acessibility**

National Endowment for the Arts Office
400 7th Street, SW
Washington, DC 20506-0001
202-682-5400
Fax: 202-682-5715
webmgr@arts.gov
arts.gov

Jane Chu, Chairman
Joan Shigekawa, Senior Deputy Chairman
Mike Burke, Chief Information Officer
Joseph Smith, Deputy Chief Information Officer

A handbook for compliance with Section 504 of the Rehabilitation Act of 1973 and the Americans with Disabilities Act of 1990 including technical assistance on making arts programs accessible to staff, performers and audience.

101 pages

ISBN 0-160042-83-6

1946 **Directory of Accessible Building Products**

N AH B Research Center
400 Prince George's Blvd
Upper Marlboro, MD 20774
301-249-4000
800-638-8556
Fax: 301-430-6180
www.homeinnovation.com

Michael Luzier, CEO & President
Michelle Desiderio, Vice President of Innovation Services
Tom Kenney, P.E, Vice President of Engineering & Research
Phil Davis, Senior Economist & Analyst

Contains descriptions of more than 200 commercially available products designed for use by people with disabilities and age-related limitations. Paperback. *$5.00*

104 pages Yearly

1947 **Do-Able Renewable Home**

AARP Fulfillment
601 E Street NW
Washington, DC 20049
202-434-3525
888-687-2277
877-342-2277
Fax: 202-434-3443
member@aarp.org
www.aarp.org

John Wider, President, CEO, AARP Services Inc.
Lisa M. Ryerson, President, AARP Foundation
Robert R. Hagans, Jr., Executive Vice President & Chief Financial Officer
Hollis Terry Bradwell III, Executive Vice President & Chief Information Officer

Describes how individuals with disabilities can modify their homes for independent living. Room-by-room modifications are accompanied by illustrations.

1948 **ECHO Housing: Recommended Construction and Installation Standards**

601 E Street NW
Washington, DC 20049
202-434-3525
888-687-2277
877-342-2277
Fax: 202-434-3443
member@aarp.org
www.aarp.org

John Wider, President, CEO, AARP Services Inc.
Lisa M. Ryerson, President, AARP Foundation
Robert R. Hagans, Jr., Executive Vice President & Chief Financial Officer
Hollis Terry Bradwell III, Executive Vice President & Chief Information Officer

Illustrated design, construction, and installation standards for temporary dwelling units for elderly people on single family residential property.

1949 **Electronic House: Enhanced Lifestyles with Electronics**

Electronic House
111 Speen Street, Suite 200
P.O. Box 989
Framingham, MA 01701-2000
508-663-1500
800-375-8015
Fax: 508-663-1599
eheditorial@ehpub.com
electronichouse.com

Kenneth D. Moyes, President
Karen Bligh, Marketing Director
John Brillon, Web Creative Director
Guy Caiola, Director of Internet Operations

Dedicated to home automation. Featuring both extravagant and affordable smart homes that can be controlled with one touch. EH covers electronic systems that give homeowners more security, entertainment, convenience, and fun. Articles cover whole house control and subsystems like residential lighting, security, home theater, energy management and telecommunications. *$23.95*

84 pages BiMonthly

ISSN 0886-66 3

1950 **Fair Housing Design Guide for Accessibility**

National Council on Multifamily Housing Industry
1201 15th Street NW
Washington, DC 20005
202-266-8200
800-368-5242
Fax: 202-266-8400
www.nahb.com

Kevin Kelly, Chairman of the Board
Tom Woods, First Vice Chairman of the Board
Ed Brady, Second Vice Chairman of the Board
Gerald M. Howard, CEO

Specifically tailored to address the needs of architects and builders. The book includes a detailed technical analysis of the legislation's impact on multifamily design, highlights potential construction problems, and identifies possible solutions. *$29.95*

1951 **Ideas for Making Your Home Accessible**

Accent Books & Products
P.O. Box 700
Bloomington, IL 61702-0700
309-378-2961
800-787-8444
Fax: 309-378-4420
acmtlvng@aol.com
www.accentonliving.com

Raymond C Cheever, Publisher
Betty Garee, Editor

Offers over 100 pages of tips and ideas to help build or remodel a home. Includes many special devices and where to get them. *$7.50*

94 pages Paperback

ISBN 0-91570 -08-6

1952 **Landscape Architecture Magazine**

American Society of Landscape Architects
636 Eye St. NW
Washington, DC 20001-3736
202-898-2444
888-999-2752
Fax: 202-898-1185
landscapearchitecturemagazine.org

Bradford McKee, Editor
Michael D. O'Brien, Publisher

Official publication of the American Society of Landscape Architects.

1953 **National Institute of Building Sciences**

1090 Vermont Ave. NW
Suite 700
Washington, DC 20005
202-289-7800
Fax: 202-289-1092
nibs@nibs.org
www.nibs.org

Lakisha Ann Woods, President & CEO
Rebecca Liko, Vice President, Finance & Controller
Sarah Swango, Senior Director, Business Development
Kristen Petersen, Managing Director, Marketing & Communications

The organization supports advances in building science and technology to improve the built environment. The U.S. Congress established it in the the Housing and Community Development Act of 1974.

1954 **Removing the Barriers: Accessibility Guidelines and Specifications**

A PP A
1643 Prince Street
Alexandria, VA 22314
703-684-1446
Fax: 703-549-2772
webmaster@appa.org
www.appa.org

John F. Bernhards, Associate Vice President
E. Lander Medlin, Executive VP
Steve Glazner, Director of Knowledge Management
Suzanne M. Healy, Director of Professional Development

Offers site accessibility, building entrances, doors, interior circulation, restrooms and bathing facilities, drinking fountains and additional resources. *$45.00*

125 pages
ISBN 0-91335 -59-9

1955 **Smart Kitchen/How to Design a Comfortable, Safe & Friendly Workplace**

Ceres Press
P.O. Box 87
Woodstock, NY 12498-87
845-679-5573
Fax: 845-679-5573
cem620@aol.com
healthyhighways.com

David Goldbeck, Owner

This book provides information about designing kitchens that may be helpful to people with disabilities as well as safe and energy efficient. *$16.95*

132 pages Paperback

1956 **United Spinal Association**

75-20 Astoria Blvd
Suite 120
East Elmhurst, NY 11370- 1177
718-803-3782
800-444-0120
Fax: 718-803-0414
mkurtz@unitedspinal.org
www.unitedspinal.org

Paul Tobin, President
Maria Kurtz, Executive Assistant

Information on spinal cord injury and laws and regulations concerning people with disabilities, including veterans.

Monthly

1957 **Whole Building Design Guide**

National Institute of Building Sciences
1090 Vermont Ave. NW
Suite 700
Washington, DC 20005
202-289-7800
Fax: 202-289-1092
nibs@nibs.org
www.wbdg.org

Lakisha Ann Woods, President & CEO
Kristen Petersen, Managing Director, Marketing & Communications

Online portal with access to published materials on integrated whole-building design techniques and technologies, with an emphasis on integrated design and team efforts during planning and programming.

Education

Aids for the Classroom

1958 ACT Assessment Test Preparation Reference Manual

American College Testing Program
P.O. Box 414
Iowa City, IA 52243-0414
319-337-1270
act.org

Marten Roorda, Chief Executive Officer
Suzana Delanghe, Chief Commercial Officer
Lucas Kuhlmann, Chief Technology Officer
Janet Goodwin, Chief Operating Officer

This reference manual was developed as a resource for high school teachers and counselors in assisting students with test preparation. Offers accommodation for individuals with disabilities.

1959 AEPS Child Progress Record: For Children Ages Three to Six

Brookes Publishing
PO Box 10624
Baltimore, MD 21285-624
410-337-9580
800-638-3775
Fax: 800-638-3775
custserv@brookespublishing.com
www.brookespublishing.com

Paul Brooks, President
Melissa Behm, Executive VP
George Stamathis, VP and Publisher

This chart helps monitor change by visually displaying current abilities, intervention targets, and child progress. In packages of 30. *$21.00*

8 pages Gate-fold
ISBN 1-557662-51-7

1960 AEPS Curriculum for Three to Six Years

Brookes Publishing
PO Box 10624
Baltimore, MD 21285-0624
410-337-9580
800-638-3775
Fax: 410-337-8539
webmaster@brookespublishing.com
www.brookespublishing.com

Paul H. Brookes, Chairman of the Board
Jeffrey D. Brookes, President
George S. Stamathis, VP/Publisher
Melissa A. Behn, Executive Vice President

Used after the AEPS® Test is completed and scored, this developmentally sequenced curriculum allows professionals to match the child's IFSP/IEP goals and objectives with activity-based interventions — beginning with simple skills and moving on to more advanced skills. *$65.00*

304 pages Spiral-bound
ISBN 1-557665-65-6

1961 AEPS Data Recording Forms: For Children Ages Three to Six

Brookes Publishing
PO Box 10624
Baltimore, MD 21285-624
410-337-9580
800-638-3775
Fax: 800-638-3775
custserv@brookespublishing.com
www.readplaylearn.com

Paul Brooks, President

These forms can be used by child development professionals on four separate occasions to pinpoint and then monitor a child's strengths and needs in the six key areas of skill development measured by the AEPS Test. Packages of 10. *$24.00*

36 pages Saddle-stiched
ISBN 1-557662-49-5

1962 AEPS Family Interest Survey

Brookes Publishing
PO Box 10624
Baltimore, MD 21285-624
410-337-9580
800-638-3775
Fax: 800-638-3775
custserv@brookespublishing.com
www.brookespublishing.com

Paul Brooks, President
Tracy Gracy, Educational Sales Manager

This is a 30-item checklist that helps families to identify interests and concerns to address in a child's IEP/IFSP. Comes in packages of 30. *$15.00*

8 pages Saddle-stiched
ISBN 1-557660-98-0

1963 Adaptivemall.com

15 South Second Street
Dolgeville, NY 13329
315-429-7112
800-371-2778
Fax: 315-429-8862
info@adaptivemall.com
www.adaptivemall.com

Katie Bergeron Peglow,PT,MS, COO

Adaptivemall.comr help families find the best equipment to support their children at their highest functioning level.

1964 Advanced Language Tool Kit

School Specialty
625 Mt. Auburn Street, 3rd Floor
PO Box 9031
Cambridge, MA 02139-9031
617-547-6706
800-225-5750
Fax: 888-440-2665
Feedback.EPS@schoolspecialty.com
eps.schoolspecialty.com

Rick Holden, President, EPS
Jean S Osman, Co-Author
Paula D Rome, Author

Provides an overview o the structure, organization, and sound units that are needed to develop skills for advanced reading and spelling. The kit contains a teacher's manual and 3 pack of cards, with features similar to the cards in the Language Tool Kit. *$60.00*

ISBN 0-838885-48-9

1965 All Kinds of Minds

School Specialty
625 Mt. Auburn Street, 3rd Floor
PO Box 9031
Cambridge, MA 02139-9031
617-547-6706
800-225-5750
Fax: 888-440-2665
Feedback.EPS@schoolspecialty.com
eps.schoolspecialty.com

Rick Holden, President, EPS
Melvin D Levine, Author

A fictitious account of five different students who have learning disabilities. *$33.00*

296 pages
ISBN 0-838820-90-5

1966 American Sign Language Handshape Cards

T J Publishers, Distributor
Ste 206
817 Silver Spring Ave
Silver Spring, MD 20910- 4617
301-585-4440
800-999-1168
Fax: 301-585-5930
tjpubinc@aol.com

Angela K Thames, President
Jerald A Murphy, VP

Durable flashcards illustrate basic handshapes, classifiers and the American manual alphabet. An instructional booklet describes games for differing skill levels to improve vocabulary, increase hand and eye coordination, sign recognition and usage. *$16.95*

1967 **Asthma Action Cards: Child Care Asthma/Allergy Action Card**
Asthma and Allergy Foundation of America
8201 Corporate Drive
Suite 1000
Landover, MD 20785
202-466-7643
800-727-8462
Fax: 202-466-8940
info@aafa.org
www.aafa.org

Tom Flanigan, Chariman
William Mclin, President and CEO
Yolanda Miller, VP and CFO

Includes necessary information a provider needs to care for a young child who has asthma and allergies. The card includes a medication plan, a list of the child's specific signs and symptoms that indicate the child is having trouble breathing, and steps on how to handle an emergency situation.

1968 **Asthma Action Cards: Student Asthma Action Card**
Asthma and Allergy Foundation of America
1233 20th St NW
Suite 610
Washington, DC 20036-2330
202-833-1700
800-727-8462
Fax: 202-833-2351
info@aafa.org
www.swmlaw.com

Bill Mc Lin, Executive Director
Ben C Hadden, VP Finance & Treasurer
Bill Lin, Executive Director

Tool for communicating school aged children's and teen's asthma managment plan to school personnel. Includes sections for asthma triggers, daily medications, and emergency directions.

1969 **Auditech: Classroom Amplification System Focus CFM802**
Auditech
PO Box 821105
Vicksburg, MS 39182-1105
800-229-8293
Fax: 800-221-8639
www.auditechusa.com

1970 **Auditech: Personal FM Educational System**
Auditech
PO Box 821105
Vicksburg, MS 39182-1105
800-229-8293
Fax: 800-221-8639
www.auditechusa.com

1971 **Auditory-Verbal Therapy for Parents and Professionals**
Alexander Graham Bell Association
3417 Volta Place, NW
Washington, DC 20007
202-337-5220
Fax: 202-337-8314
TTY: 202-337-5221
info@agbell.org
www.listeningandspokenlanguage.org

Meredith K. Sugar, Esq. (OH), President
Donald M. Goldberg, Immediate Past President
Ted A. Meyer, M.D., Ph.D. (SC, President-Elect, Secretary, Treasurer
Emilio Alonso Mendoza (DC), Chief Executive Officer

A must-have for hearing health professionals, students entering hearing health fields and parents who want to explore the theory and practices of auditory-verbal therapy. *$54.95*
313 pages Paperback

1972 **Autism Community Store**
7800 E. Iliff Ave.
Suite J
Denver, CO 80231
303-309-3647
866-709-4344
Fax: 303-756-2311
support@autismcommunitystore.com
www.autismcommunitystore.com

Shannon Sullivan, Co-Founder

The Autism Community Store is a parent-owned autism and special needs resource, a special little shop helping families, teachers and therapists get hard-to-find products for kids with ASD, PDD-NOS, Aspergers, SPD, ADHD and other special needs at reasonable prices.

1973 **Autism-Products.com**
8776 E. Shea Blvd.
Suite 106-552
Scottsdale, AZ 85260
Fax: 815-550-1819
Kelly@Autism-Products.com
www.autism-products.com

1974 **Beginning Reasoning and Reading**
School Specialty
625 Mt. Auburn Street, 3rd Floor
PO Box 9031
Cambridge, MA 02139-9031
617-547-6706
800-225-5750
Fax: 888-440-2665
Feedback.EPS@schoolspecialty.com
eps.schoolspecialty.com

Rick Holden, President, EPS
Joanne Carlisle, Author

This workbook develops basic language and thinking skills that build the foundation for reading comprehension. Workbook exercises reinforce reading as a critical reasoning activity. *$10.45*
ISBN 0-838830-01-3

1975 **Blue Skies: A Complete Multi-Media Curriculum on the Cloud**
Phillip Roy, Inc.
P.O. Box 130
Indian Rocks Beach, FL 33785
727-593-2700
800-255-9085
Fax: 877-595-2685
info@philliproy.com
www.philliproy.com

Ruth Bragman, PhD, President
Phil Roy Padol, Consultant

A complete PDF duplicatable curriculum that indlues Life Skills Curriculum, Academic Curriculum, Vocational Curriculum, Special Educational Curriculum, and Parenting/Early Learning Curriculum. This curriculum was designed for students to learn to be successful. Lesson plans, teacher's guides, pre/post assessments, and other support materials provided. *$495.00*
ISBN 1-568184-12-8

1976 **Buy!**
JE Stewart Teaching Tools
PO Box 15308
Seattle, WA 98115-308
206-262-9538
Fax: 206-262-9538

Jeff Stewart, Owner

Teaches 50 words as they appear in commercial and community situations such as clinic, sale, receipt, price and cleaner. These words are functional at school, on the job and shopping. *$32.50*
116 pages
ISBN 1-877866-05-9

1977 **Catalog for Teaching Life Skills to Persons with Development Disability**
PCI Education Publishing
PO Box 34270
San Antonio, TX 78265-4270
210-377-1999
800-594-4263
Fax: 888-259-8284

Lee Wilson, President/CEO
Erin Kinard, VP Product Development/Publisher
Randy Pennington, VP, Sales & Marketing

Over 200 educational products that help individuals learn and maintain the life skills they need to succeed in an inclusive society.

1978 **Classroom GOALS: Guide for Optimizing Auditory Learning Skills**
Alexander Graham Bell Association
3417 Volta Pl. NW
Washington, DC 20007
202-337-5220
Fax: 202-337-8314
TTY: 202-337-5221
info@agbell.org
www.agbell.org

Emilio Alonso-Mendoza, Chief Executive Officer

This reader-friendly teacher's guide filled with tips, source materials and sample charts and plans is designed for educators who have yearned for a resource that explains how to incorporate auditory goals into academic learning for students with different degrees of hearing loss. *$34.95*
Paperback

1979 **Classroom Notetaker: How to Organize a Program Serving Students with Hearing Impairments**
Alexander Graham Bell Association
3417 Volta Pl. NW
Washington, DC 20007
202-337-5220
Fax: 202-337-8314
TTY: 202-337-5221
info@agbell.org
www.agbell.org
Emilio Alonso-Mendoza, Chief Executive Officer
This detailed manual for instructors, administrators and staff notetakers promotes classroom notetaking within long-term educational programs as absolutely vital for students who are deaf and hard of hearing from elementary school to college. *$24.95*
127 pages Paperback

1980 **Community Services for the Blind and Partially Sighted Store: Sight Connection**
9709 Third Ave NE
Ste 100
Seattle, WA 98115-2027
206-525-5556
800-458-4888
Fax: 206-525-0422
info@sightconnection.org
www.sightconnection.org
Miles Otoupal, Chair
Jonathan Avedovech, Vice Chair
David McBride, Treasurer
Mary Lewis, Secretary
Over 400 products specifically designed to make life easier for people with vision loss.

1981 **Community Signs**
JE Stewart Teaching Tools
P.O. Box 15308
Seattle, WA 98115-308
206-262-9538
Fax: 206-262-9538
Jeff Stewart, Owner
Teaches 50 words like go, fire, rest room, men, women, danger and walk needed to successfully navigate our environment. *$32.50*

1982 **Comprehensive Assessment of Spoken Language (CASL)**
AGS
PO Box 99
Circle Pines, MN 55014-99
800-328-2560
Fax: 800-471-8457
agsmail@agsnet.com
www.agsnet.com
Kevin Brueggeman, President
Robert Zaske, Market Manager
CASL is an individually and orally administered research-based, theory-drive oral language assessment battery for ages 3 through 21. Fifteen tests measure language processing skills - comprehension, expression, and retrieval - in four language structure categories: lexical/semantic, syntactic, supralinguistic and pragmatic. *$299.95*

1983 **Creative Arts Therapy Catalogs**
MMB Music
9051 Watson Road
Suite 161
Saint Louis, MO 63126-1019
314-531-9635
800-543-3771
Fax: 314-531-8384
info@mmbmusic.com
www.mmbmusic.com
Marcia Goldberg, President
Catalogs of books, videos, recordings for the creative arts and wellness (music, art, dance, poetry, drama, therapies, photography).

1984 **Cursive Writing Skills**
School Specialty
625 Mt. Auburn Street, 3rd Floor
PO Box 9031
Cambridge, MA 02139-9031
617-547-6706
800-225-5750
Fax: 888-440-2665
Feedback.EPS@schoolspecialty.com
eps.schoolspecialty.com
Rick Holden, President, EPS
Diana Hanbury King, Author
Boosts writing achievement through handwriting skills. Handwriting instruction helps students become fluent writers, allowing them to focus on their thoughts and ideas rather than on letter and word formation. *$12.00*

1985 **Different Roads to Learning**
37 East 18th Street
10th Floor
New York, NY 10003
212-604-9637
800-853-1057
Fax: 212-206-9329
info@difflearn.com
www.difflearn.com
Julie Azuma, Founder
Its product line supports the social, academic and communicative development of children on the autism spectrum through Applied Behavior Analysis (ABA) and Verbal Behavior interventions

1986 **Discount School Supply**
PO Box 6013
Carol Stream, IL 60197-6013
800-627-2829
Fax: 800-879-3753
customerservice@discountschoolsupply.com
www.discountschoolsupply.com
Ron Elliott, Founder
Kelly Crampton, Chief Executive Officer
Discount School Supply offers the highest quality educational products at the lowest possible prices, supported by an extraordinary level of service.

1987 **Do2learn**
3204 Churchill Road
Raleigh, NC 27607
919-755-1809
Fax: 919-420-1978
www.do2learn.com

1988 **Don Johnston**
26799 West Commerce Drive
Volo, IL 60073-9675
847-740-0749
800-999-4660
Fax: 847-740-7326
info@donjohnston.com
www.donjohnston.com
Don Johnston, Founder
Ruth Ziolkowski, President
Kevin Johnston, Director of Product Design
Ben Johnston, Director of Marketing
A provider of quality products and services that enable people with special needs to discover their potential and experience success. Products are developed for the areas of Physical Access, Augmentative Communication and for those who struggle with reading and writing.

1989 **Dyslexia Training Program**
School Specialty
625 Mt. Auburn Street, 3rd Floor
PO Box 9031
Cambridge, MA 02139-9031
617-547-6706
800-225-5750
Fax: 888-440-2665
Feedback.EPS@schoolspecialty.com
eps.schoolspecialty.com
Rick Holden, President, EPS
This 2-year, cumulative series of daily 1-hour video lessons and accompanying Student's Books and Teacher's Guides is a structured, multisensory sequence of alphabet, reading, spelling, cursive handwriting, listening, language history, and review activities. Written by the Texas Scottish Rite Hospital for Children.

1990 **ESpecial Needs**
11704 Lackland Industrial Drive
St. Louis, MO 63146
314-692-2424
877-664-4565
Fax: 314-692-2428
www.especialneeds.com

1991 **Encyclopedia of Basic Employment and Daily Living Skills**
Phillip Roy, Inc.
13064 Indian Rocks Rd.
P.O. Box 130
Indian Rocks Beach, FL 33785
727-593-2700
800-255-9085
Fax: 877-595-2685
info@phillipr oy.com
www.PhillipRoy.com

Ruth Bragman, PhD, President
Phil Roy Padol, Consultant
Contains developmental skills for special education students. Contains lessons in 6 curriculum areas covering 80 objects with 541 lessons. Also includes objectives, instructional strategies, and assessment tasks. Curriculum is in PDF format and unlimited duplication is allowed after purchase. *$300.00*
ISBN 1-568184-15-8

1992 **Exceptional Teaching Inc**
Exceptional Teaching Inc
3994 Oleander Way
PO Box 2330
Castro Valley, CA 94546
510-889-7282
800-549-6999
Fax: 510-889-7382
info@exceptionalteaching.com
www.exceptionalteaching.com

Helene Holman, Owner/manager
Providing educational products for those with special needs via catalog and online store.

1993 **Explode the Code**
School Specialty
625 Mt. Auburn Street, 3rd Floor
PO Box 9031
Cambridge, MA 02139-9031
617-547-6706
800-225-5750
Fax: 888-440-2665
Feedback.EPS@schoolspecialty.com
eps.schoolspecialty.com

Rick Holden, President, EPS
Nancy M Hall, Author
Helps students build the essential literacy skills needed for reading success: phonological awareness, decoding, vocabulary, comprehension, fluency and spelling. *$6.20*
Grades K-4, 1-3

1994 **Food!**
JE Stewart Teaching Tools
PO Box 15308
Seattle, WA 98115-308
206-262-9538
Fax: 206-262-9538

Jeff Stewart, Owner
Teaches 50 words like salt, pepper, hamburger, fruit, milk and soup, seen commonly on menus, packages and in directions used at home and at play. *$32.50*

1995 **Fun for Everyone**
AbleNet, Inc.
2625 Patton Road
Roseville, MN 55113-1137
651-294-2200
800-322-0956
Fax: 651-294-2259
customerservice@ablenetinc.com
www.ablenetinc.com

Bill Sproull, Chair of the Board
Jennifer Thalhuber, President & CEO
William Mills, Board of Directors
Paul Sugden, CFO & Trustee
Today, simple technology allows children and adults with disabilities to participate in leisure activities they were limited or excluded from in the past. *$20.00*

1996 **Fundamentals of Autism**
Slosson Educational Publications Inc.
538 Buffalo Road
East Aurora, NY 14052-280
716-652-0930
800-655-3840
888-756-7760
Fax: 716-655-3840
slossonprep@gmail.com
www.slosson.com

Steven Slosson, President
John Slosson, VP
David Slosson, VP
The Fundamentals of Autism handbook provides a quick, user friendly, effective and accurate approach to help in identifying and developing educationally related program objectives for children diagnosed as autistic. These materials have been designed to be easily and functionally used by teachers, therapists, special education/learning disability resource specialists, psychologists and others who work with children diagnosed as autistic. *$56.00*
72 pages

1997 **GO-MO Articulation Cards- Second Edition**
Sage Publications
2455 Teller Road
Thousand Oaks, CA 91320
805-499-9774
800-818-7243
Fax: 800-583-2665
info@sagepub.com
www.sagepub.com

Blaise R Simqu, President & CEO
Tracey Ozmina, VP and COO
Chris Hickok, Senior VP and CFO
Stephen Barr, Managing Director
The most popular system used for remedying defective speech articulation in children and adults. This popular card set was the first and is still the best therapy tool of its kind, as it continues to produce results and maintains the interest of students of all ages.

1998 **Gillingham Manaual**
School Specialty
625 Mt. Auburn Street, 3rd Floor
PO Box 9031
Cambridge, MA 02139-9031
617-547-6706
800-225-5750
Fax: 888-440-2665
Feedback.EPS@schoolspecialty.com
eps.schoolspecialty.com

Rick Holden, President, EPS
Anna Gillingham, Author
Bessie W Stillman, Co-Author
Remedial training for children with specific disability in reading, spelling, and penmanship.
352 pages 69.95
ISBN 0-83880 -00-

1999 **Guide to Teaching Phonics**
School Specialty
625 Mt. Auburn Street, 3rd Floor
PO Box 9031
Cambridge, MA 02139-9031
617-547-6706
800-225-5750
Fax: 888-440-2665
Feedback.EPS@schoolspecialty.com
eps.schoolspecialty.com

Rick Holden, President, EPS
June Lyday Orton, Author
This flexible teacher's guide presents multisensory procedures developed in association with the late Dr. Samuel Orton. They consist of 100 phonograms for teaching phonetic elements and their sequences in words for reading, writing and spelling. Also contains coordinated Phonics Cards. *$19.25*
96 pages
ISBN 0-838802-41-9

2000 **Homemade Battery-Powered Toys**
Special Needs Project
324 State Street
Suite H
Santa Barbara, CA 93101-2364
818-718-9900
800-333-6867
Fax: 818-349-2027
editor@specialneeds.com
www.specialneeds.com
Hod Gray, Owner
Laraine Gray, Coordinator
Describes how to make simple switches and educational devices for severely handicapped children. *$7.50*

2001 **Idaho Assistive Technology Project**
University of Idaho
PO Box 444061
Moscow, ID 83844-4061
208-885-6097
800-432-8324
Fax: 208-885-6145
janicec@uidaho.edu
www.idahoat.org
Janice Carson, Project Director
Sue House, Information/Referral Specialst
A federally funded program managed by the Center on Disabilities and Human Development at the University of Idaho. The goal is to increase the availability of assistive technology devices and services for Idahoans with disabilities. *$15.00*

2002 **If It Is To Be, It Is Up To Me To Do It!**
AVKO Educational Research Foundation
3084 Willard Road
Birch Run, MI 48415-9404
810-686-9283
866-285-6612
Fax: 810-686-1101
webmaster@avko.org
www.avko.org
Don McCabe, President, Research Director Emeritus, Birch Run, Michigan
Linda Heck, VP, Clio, Michigan
Michael Lane, Treasurer, Clio, Michigan
Amy Messer, Board Member, Flint, Michigan
A student and tutor's text, for use on dyslexics and non-dyslexics, by parents, spouses, or friends. *$29.95*
206 pages
ISBN 1-564007-42-1

2003 **Inclusive Play People**
Educational Equity Concepts
Fl 8
100 5th Ave
New York, NY 10011-6903
212-243-1110
Fax: 212-627-0407
TTY: 212-725-1803
www.iconcapital.com
Jacqueline Johnson, Manager
Six sturdy multiracial wooden figures that provide a unique variety of nonstereotyped work and family roles and are inclusive of disabled and nondisabled people of various ages. For block building and dramatic play. *$25.00*

2004 **Individualized Keyboarding**
AVKO Educational Research Foundation
3084 Willard Road
Birch Run, MI 48415-9404
810-686-9283
866-285-6612
Fax: 810-686-1101
webmaster@avko.org
www.avko.org
Don McCabe, President, Research Director Emeritus, Birch Run, Michigan
Linda Heck, VP, Clio, Michigan
Michael Lane, Treasurer, Clio, Michigan
Amy Messer, Board Member, Flint, Michigan
Utilizes a multi-sensory approach to teach typing skills. It not only teaches typing skills, it also reinforces the reading patterns that are necessary for typing proficiency. *$14.95*
96 pages
ISBN 1-654004-01-5

2005 **Instruction of Persons with Severe Handicaps**
McGraw-Hill School Publishing
PO Box 182604
Columbus, OH 43272
877-833-5524
Fax: 614-759-3749
customer.service@mcgraw-hill.com
www.mcgraw-hill.com
Harold McGraw, President and CEO
Jack Callahan, Executive VP
John Berisford, Executive VP of HR
A complete introduction to the status of education as it pertains to people with severe handicaps.

2006 **Kaplan Early Learning Company**
1310 Lewisville Clemmons Rd
Lewisville, NC 27023
336-766-7374
800-334-2014
Fax: 800-452-7526
info@kaplanco.com
www.kaplanco.com
Hal Kaplan, President & CEO
Kaplan Early Learning Company is a international provider of products and services that enhance children's learning.

2007 **Keeping Ahead in School**
Educators Publishing Service
PO Box 9031
Cambridge, MA 2139-9031
617-547-6706
800-225-5750
Fax: 888-440-2665
feedback@epsbooks.com
www.epsbooks.com
Charles H Heinle, VP
Alexandra S Bigelow, Author
Gunnar Voltz, President
This book helps students not only understand their own strengths and weaknesses but also more fully appreciate their individuality. He suggests specific ways to approach work, bypass or overcome learning disorders, and manage other struggles that may beset students in school. *$24.75*
320 pages Paperback
ISBN 0-838820-69-7

2008 **KeyMath Teach and Practice**
AGS
P.O. Box 99
Circle Pines, MN 55014-99
800-328-2560
Fax: 800-471-8457
agsmail@agsnet.com
www.agsnet.com
Kevin Brueggeman, President
Robert Zaske, Market Manager
This set of materials provides all the tools needed to assess students' math skills...and the strategies to deal with problem areas. Three sets are available: Basic Concepts Package; Operations Package; and Applications Package. $219.95 each or $599.95 for whole set.

2009 **Lakeshore Learning Materials**
2695 E. Dominguez Street
Carson, CA 90895
310-537-8600
800-421-5354
Fax: 800-537-5403
lakeshore@lakeshorelearning.com
www.lakeshorelearning.com
Bo Kaplan, President/CEO
Josh Kaplan, VP Merchandising
Mat, Vice President of Operations
Offers books, resources, testing materials, assessment information and special education materials for the professional in the field of special education.
190 pages

2010 **Language Parts Catalog**
School Specialty
625 Mt. Auburn Street, 3rd Floor
PO Box 9031
Cambridge, MA 02139-9031
617-547-6706
800-225-5750
Fax: 888-440-2665
Feedback.EPS@schoolspecialty.com
eps.schoolspecialty.com

Rick Holden, President, EPS
Melvin D Levine, Author
Offers a humorous and informative explanation of the various aspects of language and how they operate. Laid out in the form of a catalog, the book presents various parts that can help students improve their language abilities. *$12.65*
ISBN 0-838819-80-X

2011 **Language Tool Kit**
School Specialty
625 Mt. Auburn Street, 3rd Floor
PO Box 9031
Cambridge, MA 02139-9031
617-547-6706
800-225-5750
Fax: 888-440-2665
Feedback.EPS@schoolspecialty.com
eps.schoolspecialty.com

Rick Holden, President, EPS
Paula D Rome, Author
Jean S Osman, Co-Author
Designed for use by a teacher or parents, teaches reading and spelling to students with specific language disability. *$43.25*
32 pages English Edition
ISBN 0-838885-20-3

2012 **Language, Speech and Hearing Services in School**
American Speech-Language-Hearing Association
10801 Rockville Pike
Rockville, MD 20852-3226
301-296-5700
800-638-8255
Fax: 301-296-8580
actioncenter@asha.org
www.asha.org

Paul Rao, President
Robert Augustine, VP of Finance
Arlene Pietranton, Executive Director
Professional journal for clinicians, audiologists and speech-language pathologists. *$30.00*

2013 **Learning American Sign Language**
Harris Communications
15155 Technology Dr
Eden Prairie, MN 55344-2273
952-906-1180
800-825-6758
Fax: 952-906-1099
TTY: 800-825-9187
info@harriscomm.com
www.harriscomm.com

Robert Harris, Owner & President
Kevin Horsky, Business Director
Randall Moore, Manager
Offers over 700 titles on ASL including books, videotapes, CDs & DVDs. Free catalog available. *$78.95*
350 pages Video & Book

2014 **Learning Resources**
380 N. Fairway Drive
Vernon Hills, IL 60061
800-333-8281
Fax: 888-892-8731
info@learningresources.com
www.learningresources.com

2015 **Learning to Sign in My Neighborhood**
T J Publishers
2544 Tarpley Rd
Suite 108
Carrollton, TX 75006-2288
972-416-0800
800-999-1168
Fax: 301-585-5930
tjpubinc@aol.com

Angela K Thames, President
Jerald A Murphy, VP
Beautifully illustrated coloring book lets children learn signs from kids just like themselves! Recommended for ages 4 and up, let children have fun while they learn signs for words typically used in day-to-day activities. *$3.50*
32 pages Softcover
ISBN 0-93266 -36-1

2016 **Literacy Program**
School Specialty
625 Mt. Auburn Street, 3rd Floor
PO Box 9031
Cambridge, MA 02139-9031
617-547-6706
800-225-5750
Fax: 888-440-2665
Feedback.EPS@schoolspecialty.com
eps.schoolspecialty.com

Rick Holden, President, EPS
Paula D Rome, Author
Jean S Osman, Co-Author
Written by the Texas Scottish Rite Hospital for Children. A one-year course that consists of 160 one-hour videotaped lessons accompanied by student workbooks, designed for high school students and adults who read below sixth grade level.

2017 **Literature Based Reading**
Oryx Press
4041 N Central Ave
Phoenix, AZ 85012-3330
602-265-2651
800-279-6799
Fax: 800-279-4663

2018 **Living an Idea: Empowerment and the Evolution of an Alternative School**
Brookline Books
8 Trumbull Rd, Suite B-001
Northampton, MA 1060-4533
413-584-0184
800-666-2665
Fax: 413-584-6184
brbooks@yahoo.com
www.brooklinebooks.com

William H Walters, Author
Esther Wilder, Co-Author
This book is about the creation and 14 year evolution of a public alternative inner-city high school. The school lived an idea - empowerment. Students were encouraged to participate in shaping many aspects of their education, teachers were responsible for running the school, and parents invited to help govern. *$27.95*
ISBN 0-91479 -68-9

2019 **Low Tech Assistive Devices: A Handbook for the School Setting**
Therapro, Inc.
225 Arlington Street
Framingham, MA 02139-8723
508-872-9494
800-257-5376
Fax: 508-875-2062
info@therapro.com
www.therapro.com

Karen Conrad Weihrauch, President & Owner
A how-to book with step by step directions and detailed illustrations for fabrication of frequently requested low-tech assistive devices. *$45.00*
320 pages Paperback

2020 **MTA Readers**
Educators Publishing Service
625 Mt. Auburn Street, 3rd Floor
PO Box 9031
Cambridge, MA 02139-9031
617-547-6706
800-225-5750
Fax: 888-440-2665
Feedback.EPS@schoolspecialty.com
www.epsbooks.com

Rick Holden, President, EPS
Illustrated readers for grades 1-3 that accompany the MTA Reading and Spelling Program (Multisensory Teaching Approach). Phonetic elements in a structured, but entertaining context.
48+ pages $4.65 - $11.65
ISBN 0-83882 -33-3

2021 **Making School Inclusion Work: A Guide to Everyday Practice**
Brookline Books
8 Trumbull Rd, Suite B-001
Northampton, MA 2445-4533
413-584-0184
800-666-2665
Fax: 413-584-6184
brbooks@yahoo.com
www.brooklinebooks.com
William H Walters, Author
Esther Wilder, Co-Author
This book tells the reader how to conduct a truly inclusive program, regardless of ethnic or racial background, economic level and physical or cognitive ability. *$24.95*
254 pages
ISBN 0-914791-96-4

2022 **Making the Writing Process Work: Strategies for Composition and Self-Regulation**
Brookline Books
8 Trumbull Rd, Suite B-001
Northampton, MA 2445-4533
413-584-0184
800-666-2665
Fax: 413-584-6184
brbooks@yahoo.com
www.brooklinebooks.com
William H Walters, Author
Esther Wilder, Co-Author
This book is geared toward students who have difficulty organizing their thoughts and developing their writing. The specific stategies teach students how to approach, organize, and produce a final written product.. *$24.95*
240 pages Paperback
ISBN 1-571290-10-9

2023 **Manual Alphabet Poster**
TJ Publishers
Ste 108
2544 Tarpley Rd
Carrollton, TX 75006-2288
972-416-0800
800-999-1168
Fax: 972-416-0944
TJPubinc@aol.com
www.TJpublishers.com
Pat O'Rourke, President
Poster presents the manual alphabet. *$4.50*

2024 **Many Faces of Dyslexia**
International Dyslexia Association
40 York Rd.
4th Floor
Baltimore, MD 21204-5243
410-296-0232
Fax: 410-321-5069
info@dyslexiaida.org
dyslexiaida.org
Margaret Byrd Rawson, Author
Provides information on the teaching and rehabilitation techniques for people with dyslexia. *$20.00*
269 pages Paperback

2025 **Match-Sort-Assemble Job Cards**
Exceptional Education
PO Box 15308
Seattle, WA 98115-308
206-262-9538
Jeff Stewart, Owner
Teaches workers to use a series of symbolic cues to control their own production cycles. *$565.00*
Class Set

2026 **Match-Sort-Assemble Pictures**
Exceptional Education
PO Box 15308
Seattle, WA 98115-308
206-262-9538
Jeff Stewart, Owner
People with profound, severe and moderate developmental disabilities have immediate access with MSA Pictures. Students work with pictures (and if necessary a template) to match, sort, assemble and disassemble parts that vary in shape, length and diameter. *$426.00*
Class Set

2027 **Match-Sort-Assemble SCHEMATICS**
Exceptional Education
PO Box 15308
Seattle, WA 98115-308
206-262-9538
Jeff Stewart, Owner
Students with moderate and mild developmental disabilities and those who have completed MSA Pictures are ready for MSA Schematics. It increases abstraction and displacement of instruction from the work clearly and simply. *$495.00*
Class Set

2028 **Match-Sort-Assemble TOOLS**
Exceptional Education
PO Box 15308
Seattle, WA 98115-308
206-262-9538
Fax: 475-486-4510
Jeff Stewart, Owner
Students and clients learn to use the tools required for many jobs in light industry. Mastery of the production cycle with independence, endurance and the ability to learn new tasks through pictures and schematics and basic hand functions will help clients acquire and maintain employment in a competitive field. *$595.00*
Class Set

2029 **Meeting-in-a-Box**
Asthma and Allergy Foundation of America
1233 20th St NW
Suite 610
Washington, DC 20036-7322
202-833-1700
800-7AS-THMA
Fax: 202-833-2351
info@aafa.org
Bill McLin, Executive Director
A series of self-contained, comprehensive kits that contain all the necessary components for a successful asthma presentation.

2030 **More Food!**
JE Stewart Teaching Tools
PO Box 15308
Seattle, WA 98115-308
206-262-9538
Fax: 206-262-9538
Jeff Stewart, Owner
Teaches 50 more words found in restaurants, grocery stores, cookbooks such as pizza, carrot, tacos, oysters and pineapple. These words are functional at home, going shopping and during leisure. *$32.50*

2031 **More Work!**
J E Stewart Teaching Tools
PO Box 15308
Seattle, WA 98115-308
206-262-9538
Fax: 206-262-9538
Jeff Stewart, Owner
Teaches 50 words as they appear on parts, tools, job instructions, signs and labels, such as fill, grasp, release, lock, search, position and select. These words are functional in school and on-the-job. *$32.50*

2032 **Multisensory Teaching Approach**
Educators Publishing Service
PO Box 9031
Cambridge, MA 2139-9031
617-367-2700
800-225-5750
Fax: 617-547-0412
www.epsbooks.com
$110 - $140
ISBN 0-83888 -10-9

2033 **National Autism Resources**
6240 Goodyear Rd.
Benicia, CA 94510
707-745-3308
877-249-2393
Fax: 877-259-9419
customerservice@nationalautismresources.com
www.nationalautismresources. com

2034 **Peabody Articulation Decks**
AGS
PO Box 99
Circle Pines, MN 55014-99
651-287-7220
800-328-2560
Fax: 763-786-9007
agsmail@agsnet.com
www.agsnet.com

Keith Powel, Special Education Transition Coo
Robert Zaske, Marketing Manager
Complete kit of playing-card sized PAD decks let students focus on the 18 most commonly misarticulated English consonants and blends. *$115.95*
ISBN 0-88671 -75-4

2035 **Phonemic Awareness in Young Children: A Classroom Curriculum**
Brookes Publishing
PO Box 10624
Baltimore, MD 21285-624
410-337-9580
custserv@brookespublishing.com
www.brookespublishing.com

Clary Creighton, Exhibits Coordinator
Tracy Gray, Educational Sales Manager
Paul Brooks, Owner
This is a supplemental, whole-class curriculum for improving pre-literacy listening skills. It contains activities that are fun, easy to use, and proven to work in any kindergarten classroom - general, bilingual, inclusive, or special education. This program takes only 15-20 minutes a day. *$24.95*
208 pages Spiral-bound
ISBN 1-557663-21-1

2036 **Phonics for Thought**
Educators Publishing Service
PO Box 9031
Cambridge, MA 2139-9031
617-367-2700
800-225-5750
Fax: 617-547-0412
www.epsbooks.com

Paperback

2037 **Phonological Awareness Training for Reading**
Sage Publications
2455 Teller Road
Thousand Oaks, CA 91320
805-499-9774
800-818-7243
Fax: 800-583-2665
info@sagepub.com
www.sagepub.com

Blaise R Simqu, President & CEO
Tracey Ozmina, Executive VP
Chris Hickok, Executive VP and CFO
Stephen Barr, Managing Director
Designed to increase the level of phonological awareness in young children. Can be taught individually or in small groups and takes about 12 to 14 weeks to complete if children are taught in short sessions three or four times a week. *$129.00*

2038 **Play!**
JE Stewart Teaching Tools
PO Box 15308
Seattle, WA 98115-308
206-262-9538
Fax: 206-262-9538

Jeff Stewart, Owner
Teaches 50 more words as they appear at recreation sites, on signs and labels and in newspapers and magazines, such as movie, visitor, ticket, gallery and zoo. These words are functional in school and at leisure. *$32.50*

2039 **Power Breathing Program**
Asthma and Allergy Foundation of America
8201 Corporate Drive
Suite 1000
Landover, MD 20785
202-466-7643
800-727-8462
Fax: 202-466-8940
info@aafa.org
www.aafa.org

Bill McLin, Executive Director
Devoloped the only asthma education program specifically designed for and pre-tested with teens. Teens with asthma have special challenges. This interactive program covers everything from the basics of asthma to dealing with their asthma in social situations, in college, and on the job. Includes everything you need to present this three-four session program. *$295.00*

2040 **Primary Phonics**
School Specialty
625 Mt. Auburn Street, 3rd Floor
PO Box 9031
Cambridge, MA 02139-9031
617-547-6706
800-225-5750
Fax: 888-440-2665
Feedback.EPS@schoolspecialty.com
eps.schoolspecialty.com

Rick Holden, President, EPS
Barbara W Makar, Author
A program of storybooks and coordinated workbooks that teaches reading for grades K-2. A structured phonetic approach. Contains 8 student workbooks, with 8 sets of 10 coordinated storybooks; consonant workbooks; initial consonant blend workbooks; picture dictionary, and coloring book.
ISSN 0838-83 0

2041 **Reading for Content**
School Specialty
625 Mt. Auburn Street, 3rd Floor
PO Box 9031
Cambridge, MA 02139-9031
617-547-6706
800-225-5750
Fax: 888-440-2665
Feedback.EPS@schoolspecialty.com
eps.schoolspecialty.com

Rick Holden, President, EPS
Carol Einstein, Author
A series of 4 books designed to help students improve their reading comprehension skills. Each book contains 43 reading passages followed by 4 questions. Two questions as for a recall of main ideas, and two ask the student to draw conclusions from what they have read. *$11.45*
96 pages

2042 **Reading from Scratch**
Educators Publishing Service
P.O. Box 9031
Cambridge, MA 2139-9031
617-367-2700
800-225-5750
Fax: 617-547-0412
www.epsbooks.com

$6.25 - $49.30
ISBN 0-83888 -75-5

2043 **Recipe for Reading**
School Specialty
625 Mt. Auburn Street, 3rd Floor
PO Box 9031
Cambridge, MA 02139-9031
617-367-2700
800-225-5750
Fax: 888-440-2665
Feedback.EPS@schoolspecialty.com
eps.schoolspecialty.com

Rick Holden, President, EPS
Nina Traub, Author
Frances Bloom, Co-Author
Contains comprehensive, multisensory, phonics-based reading program presents a skill sequence and lesson structured designed for beginning, at-risk, or struggling readers.

2044 **Rewarding Speech**
Speech Bin
PO Box 1579
Appleton, WI 54912-1579
772-770-0007
888-388-3224
Fax: 888-388-6344
customercare@schoolspecialty.com
www.speechbin.com

Jan J Binney, Senior Editor
Reproducible reward certificates for children. *$12.95*
32 pages

2045 SAYdee Posters
Speech Bin
PO Box 1579
Appleton, WI 54912-1579
772-770-0007
888-388-3224
Fax: 888-388-6344
customercare@schoolspecialty.com
www.speechbin.com

Jan J Binney, Senior Editor
Colorful speech and language posters. *$20.00*
24 pages
ISBN 0-93785 -47-5

2046 Sensation Products
74 Cotton Mill Hill
Unit A-350
Brattleboro, VT 5301
802-254-4480
Fax: 802-254-4481
www.sensationproducts.com

2047 Sensory University Toy Company, The
4992 Bristol Industrial Hwy
Buford, GA 30518
888-831-4701
Fax: 770-904-6418
sales@sensoryuniversity.com
sensoryuniversity.com

2048 Sequential Spelling: 1-7 with 7 Student Response Books
AVKO Educational Research Foundation
3084 Willard Rd
Birch Run, MI 48415-9404
810-686-9283
866-285-6612
Fax: 810-686-1101
webmaster@avko.org
www.avko.org

Deborah Wolf, President
Aaron Miller, Vice President
Sequential Spelling uses immediate student self-correction. It builds from easier words of a word family such as all and then builds on them to teach; all, tall, stall, install, call, fall, ball, and their inflected forms such as: stalls, stalled, stalling, installing, installment. *$89.95*
72 pages $8.95 each
ISBN 1-56400 -11-6

2049 Signing Naturally Curriculum
Harris Communications
15155 Technology Dr
Eden Prairie, MN 55344-2273
952-906-1180
800-825-6758
Fax: 952-906-1099
TTY: 800-825-9187
info@harriscomm.com
www.harriscomm.com

Robert Harris, Owner & President
Kevin Horsky, Business Director
Randall Moore, Manager
A series based on the functional approach that is the most popular and widely used sign language curriculum designed for teaching American Sign Language. Book and videotape set for level 1 & 2. Teacher's curriculum is also available. *$59.95*

2050 Small Wonder
AGS
PO Box 99
Circle Pines, MN 55014-99
651-287-7220
800-328-2560
Fax: 763-786-9007
agsmail@agsnet.com
www.agsnet.com

Kevin Brueggeman, President
Robert Zaske, Marketing Manager
This infant through toddler program offers a delightful array of activities to teach babies about themselves, others, their surroundings and the world outside. Level One - zero to 18 months; Level Two 18-36 months. Discount price of $389.95 when both levels ordered. *$229.95*
ISBN 0-91347 -62-5

2051 Solving Language Difficulties
School Specialty
625 Mt. Auburn Street, 3rd Floor
PO Box 9031
Cambridge, MA 02139-9031
617-547-6706
800-225-5750
Fax: 888-440-2665
Feedback.EPS@schoolspecialty.com
eps.schoolspecialty.com

Rick Holden, President, EPS
Amey Steere, Author
Caroline Z Peck, Co-Author
This basic workbook can be used in any corrective reading program. It deals extensively with syllables, syllable division, prefixes, suffixes and accent. *$9.75*
176 pages
ISBN 0-838803-26-1

2052 Speech Bin
Abilitations
PO Box 1579
Appleton, WI 54912-1579
772-770-0007
800-513-2465
Fax: 80- 51- 246
onlinehelp@schoolspecialty.com
www.speechbin.com

Jan J Binney, Senior Editor
Activities, worksheets and games to encourage practice of speech and language skills. *$25.00*
128 pages
ISBN 0-93785 -42-4

2053 Speech-Language Delights
1965 25th Ave
Vero Beach, FL 32960-3062
772-770-0007

2054 Spell of Words
School Specialty
625 Mt. Auburn Street, 3rd Floor
PO Box 9031
Cambridge, MA 02139-9031
617-547-6706
800-225-5750
Fax: 888-440-2665
Feedback.EPS@schoolspecialty.com
eps.schoolspecialty.com

Rick Holden, President, EPS
Elsie T Rak, Author
Covers syllabication, word building along with prefixes, phonograms, word patterns, suffixes, plurals, and possessives. *$14.70*
128 pages Grades 7-Adult

2055 Spellbound
School Specialty
625 Mt. Auburn Street, 3rd Floor
PO Box 9031
Cambridge, MA 02139-9031
617-547-6706
800-225-5750
Fax: 888-440-2665
Feedback.EPS@schoolspecialty.com
eps.schoolspecialty.com

Rick Holden, President, EPS
Elsie T Rak, Author
This workbook begins with teaching simple, consistent rules and then moves on to those that are more difficult. By an inductive process, students use their own observations to confirm the spelling rules they learn. Each portion of the text is followed by exercises for drill and kinesthetic reinforcement. *$12.85*
144 pages Grades 7-Adult
ISBN 0-838801-65-X

2056 **Spelling Dictionary**
School Specialty
625 Mt. Auburn Street, 3rd Floor
PO Box 9031
Cambridge, MA 02139-9031
617-547-6706
800-225-5750
Fax: 888-440-2665
Feedback.EPS@schoolspecialty.com
eps.schoolspecialty.com

Rick Holden, President, EPS
Gregory Hurray, Author
Contains the most frequently used and misspelled words for students at these grade levels. Designed to be useable and reliable, to build research and writing skills, and to help teachers promote independent learning in a classroom setting *$6.35*
ISBN 0-838820-56-5

2057 **Starting Over**
School Specialty
625 Mt. Auburn Street, 3rd Floor
PO Box 9031
Cambridge, MA 02139-9031
617-547-6706
800-225-5750
Fax: 888-440-2665
Feedback.EPS@schoolspecialty.com
eps.schoolspecialty.com

Rick Holden, President, EPS
Joan Knight, Author
For students who are ready to try to learn to read again, or for those who are learning English as a second language. *$38.40*
ISBN 0-838881-65-5

2058 **Studio 49 Catalog**
MMB Music
9051 Watson Road
Suite 161
Saint Louis, MO 63126-1019
314-531-9635
800-543-3771
Fax: 314-531-8384
info@mmbmusic.com
www.mmbmusic.com

Marcia Goldberg, President
Michelle Greenlaw, VP
Percussion instruments for school, therapy, church and family.

2059 **Syracuse Community-Referenced Curriculum Guide for Students with Disabilties**
Brookes Publishing
PO Box 10624
Baltimore, MD 21285-624
410-337-9580
800-638-3775
Fax: 410-337-8539
custserv@brookespublishing.com
www.readplaylearn.com

Paul Brooks, President
Serving learners from kindergarten through age 21, this field-tested curriculum is a for professionals and parents devoted to directly preparing a student to function in the world. it examines the role of community living domains, functional academics, and embedded skills and includes practical implementation strategies and information for preparing students whose learning needs go beyond the scope of traditional academic programs. *$54.95*
416 pages Spiral-bound
ISBN 1-557660-27-1

2060 **Teaching Individuals with Physical and Multiple Disabilities**
McGraw-Hill, School Publishing
PO Box 182604
Columbus, OH 43272
877-833-5524
Fax: 614-759-3749
www.mcgraw-hill.com

Harold McGraw, President and CEO
Jack Callahan, Executive VP
John Berisford, Executive VP of HR
Focuses on the functional needs of the handicapped and the teaching skills of background teachers that they need to help them reach the highest possible level of self-sufficiency.
410 pages

2061 **Teaching Students Ways to Remember**
Brookline Books
8 Trumbull Rd, Suite B-001
Northampton, MA 1060
60- 66- 703
800-666-2665
Fax: 413-584-6184
brbooks@yahoo.com
www.brooklinebooks.com

ISBN 0-914797-67-0

2062 **Teaching Test-Taking Skills: Helping Students Show What They Know**
Brookline Books
8 Trumbull Rd, Suite B-001
Northampton, MA 1060
60- 66- 703
800-666-2665
Fax: 414-584-6184
brbooks@yahoo.com
www.brooklinebooks.com

ISBN 0-914797-76-X

2063 **Therapy Shoppe**
P.O. Box 8875
Grand Rapids, MI 49518
616-696-7441
800-261-5590
Fax: 616-696-7471
info@therapyshoppe.com
www.therapyshoppe.com

2064 **To Teach a Dyslexic**
AVKO Educational Research Foundation
3084 Willard Rd
Birch Run, MI 48415-9404
810-686-9283
866-686-9283
Fax: 810-686-1101
webmaster@avko.org
www.avko.org

Deborah Wolf, President
Aaron Miller, Vice President
A video available in DVD or video CD that shows Don McCabe working with a dyslexic teenager. The video helps teachers learn more about dyslexia and how to go about teaching a dyslexic student using the AVKO methodology and philosophy. This is a free video.
288 pages Paperback

2065 **Tools for Transition**
AGS
PO Box 99
Circle Pines, MN 55014-99
651-287-7220
800-328-2560
Fax: 763-786-9007
agsmail@agsnet.com
www.agsnet.com

Kevin Brueggeman, President
Robert Zaske, Marketing Manager
This program prepares students with learning disabilities for postsecondary education. *$129.95*

2066 **United Art and Education**
PO Box 9219
Fort Wayne, IN 46899-9219
260-478-1121
800-322-3247
Fax: 800-858-3247
www.unitednow.com

2067 **VAK Tasks Workbook: Visual, Auditory and Kinesthetic**
Educational Tutorial Consortium
4400 S 44th St
Lincoln, NE 68516-1109
402-489-8133
Fax: 402-489-8160

T Elli Cross, Owner
A workbook emphasizing the multisensory approach to teaching vocabulary and spelling. It is intended for middle-grade and older students working with prefixes, roots, suffixes, homonyms, and the spelling of easily confused endings. Includes spelling posters. *$7.00*
96 pages Paperback

2068 Volunteer Transcribing Services
Ste 200
205 E 3rd Ave
San Mateo, CA 94401-4028
650-357-1571
Fax: 650-632-3510

Alanah Hoffman, Coordinator
VTS is a nonprofit California corporation that produces large print school books for visually impaired students in grades K-12.

2069 Wordly Wise 3000
School Specialty
625 Mt. Auburn Street, 3rd Floor
PO Box 9031
Cambridge, MA 02139-9031
617-547-6706
800-225-5750
Fax: 888-440-2665
Feedback.EPS@schoolspecialty.com
eps.schoolspecialty.com

Rick Holden, President, EPS
Kenneth Hodkinson, Author
Sandra Adams, Co-Author
Cheryl Dressler, Co-Author
Begins with a word list of 8-12 words, followed by clear, brief definitions and sentences that illustrate the meaning of the word. Books B and C often present more than one meaning of a word. Throughout all three books, drawings illustrate the meanings.
ISSN 0838-84 8

2070 Work!
JE Stewart Teaching Tools
PO Box 15308
Seattle, WA 98115-308
206-328-7664
Fax: 206-262-9538

Jan Gleason, Executive Director
Teaches 50 words as they appear on parts, tools, job instructions, signs, labels such as: hard hat, assembly, clamp, cut, drill, package and schedule. These words are functional in school and on-the-job. *$32.50*

2071 Working Together & Taking Part
A GS
PO Box 99
Circle Pines, MN 55014-99
651-287-7220
800-328-2560
Fax: 763-786-9007
agsmail@agsnet.com
www.agsnet.com

Kevin Brueggeman, President
Robert Zaske, Market Manager
Two programs to build children's social skills in grades 3-6 through folk literature. Has 31 activity-rich lessons, teaching skills like: following rules, accepting differences, speaking assertively and helping others. Discount price of $279.00 when ordering both. *$149.95*

Associations

2072 AVKO Educational Research Foundation
3084 Willard Rd
Birch Run, MI 48415-9404
810-686-9283
Fax: 810-686-1101
webmaster@avko.org
www.avko.org

Don McCabe, President
Linda Heck, Vice President
Comprised of individuals interested in helping others learn to read and spell. Develops and sells materials for teaching dyslexics or others with learning disabilities using a method involving audio, visual, kinesthetic and oral (multi-sensory) techniques.

2073 Academy of Rehabilitative Audiology
PO Box 2323
Albany, NY 12220-0323
ara@audrehab.org
www.audrehab.org

Karen Doherty, Ph.D, President
Brittney Carlson, Au.D, Ph.D, Treasurer
Ali Marinelli, Au.D, Ph.D, Secretary
Anne D. Olsen, JARA Editor
The Academy of Rehabilitative Audiology provides professional education, research and programs for hearing handicapped persons. The primary purpose of the ARA is to promote excellence in hearing care through the provision of comprehensive rehabilitative and habilitative services.

2074 Alternative Work Concepts
PO Box 11452
Eugene, OR 97440
541-345-3043
Fax: 541-345-9669
www.alternativeworkconcepts.org

Liz Fox, Executive Director
To promote individualized, integrated, and meaningful employment opportunities in the community for adults with multiple disabilities; to improve the quality of life and provide continuous opportunities for personal growth for these individuals; and to assist businesses with workforce diversification.

2075 American Migraine Foundation
19 Mantua Rd.
Mount Royal, NJ 08061
856-423-0043
Fax: 856-423-0082
amf@talley.com
www.achenet.org

Lawrence C. Newman, MD, FAHS, Chair
Christine Lay, MD, FAHS, Vice-Chair
Nim Lalvani, MPH, Executive Director
Nonprofit, patient-health, professional partnership dedicated to advancing the treatment and management of headaches and to raising the public awareness of headache as valid, biologically based illness.

2076 American School Counselor Association
American Counselling Association
1101 King St.
Suite 310
Alexandria, VA 22314-2957
703-683-2722
800-306-4722
Fax: 703-997-7572
asca@schoolcounselor.org
www.schoolcounselor.org

Richard Wong, Executive Director
Kathleen Rakestraw, Director of Communications
Jennifer Walsh, Director of Education and Training
ASCA focuses on providing professional devleopment, enhancing school counseling programs, and research effective school counseling practices. Mission is to promote excellence in professional school counseling and the development of all students.

2077 Association for Driver Rehabilitation Specialists
200 First Ave. NW
Suite 505
Hickory, NC 28601
866-672-9466
Fax: 828-855-1672
info@aded.net
www.aded.net

Elizabeth Green, Executive Director
Adrienne Segundo, Credentialing Specialist
Keith Segundo, Director, Education
The Association for Driver Rehabilitation Specialists was established to support professionals working in the field of driver education and driver training and transportation equipment modifications for persons with disabilities through education and information dissemination.

2078 Association on Higher Education & Disability (AHEAD)
8015 West Kenton Circle
Suite 230
Huntersville, NC 28078
704-947-7779
Fax: 704-948-7779
www.ahead.org

Stephan Smith, Executive Director
Carol Funckes, Chief Operations Officer
Oanh Huynh, Chief Financial Officer
Jeremy Jarrell, Director, Innovation and Development
AHEAD is a professional membership organization for individuals involved in the development of policy and in the provision of quality services to meet the needs of persons with disabilities involved in all areas of higher education, promoting full and equal participation.
4,000+ members

2079 **CARF International**
6951 East Southpoint Rd.
Tucson, AZ 85756-9407
520-325-1044
888-281-6531
Fax: 520-318-1129
TTY: 520-495-7077
info@carf.org
carf.org

Brian J. Boon, President & CEO
Leslie Ellis-Lang, Managing Director, Child & Youth Services
Darren M. Lehrfeld, Chief Accreditation Officer
Di Shen, Chief Research Officer

An independent, nonprofit accreditor of human service providers in the areas of aging services, behavioral health, child and youth services, DMEPOS, employment and community services, medical rehabilitation, and opioid treatment programs.

2080 **CEC Pioneers Division (CEC-PD)**
Council for Exceptional Children (CEC)
3100 Clarendon Blvd.
Suite 600
Arlington, VA 22201-5332
888-232-7733
TTY: 866-915-5000
cecpioneers@gmail.com
cecpioneers.exceptionalchildren.org

Chad Rummel, Executive Director, CEC

Exists to support the programs and activities of the Council for Exceptional Children.

2081 **Center for Inclusive Design and Innovation**
512 Means St. NW
Suite 250
Atlanta, GA 30318
404-894-8000
866-279-2964
Fax: 404-894-8323
cidi-support@design.gatech.edu
cidi.gatech.edu

Eric Trevena, Senior Director, Operations
Carolyn Phillips, Director, Services & Learning
Jon Sanford, Professor & Director, RERC TechSAge

CIDI supports individuals with disabilities of any age within the State of Georgia and beyond through expert services, research, design and technological development, information dissemination, and educational programs.

2082 **Council for Children with Behavioral Disorders (CCBD)**
Council for Exceptional Children (CEC)
3100 Clarendon Blvd.
Suite 600
Arlington, VA 22201-5332
888-232-7733
TTY: 866-915-5000
service@cec.sped.org
www.ccbd.net

Chad Rummel, Executive Director, CEC

Advocates for the education and welfare of youth with behavioral and emotional disorders.

2083 **Council for Educational Diagnostic Services (CEDS)**
Council for Exceptional Children (CEC)
3100 Clarendon Blvd.
Suite 600
Arlington, VA 22201-5332
888-232-7733
TTY: 866-915-5000
cedscec@gmail.com
ceds.exceptionalchildren.org

Chad Rummel, Executive Director, CEC

Focused on diagnostic and prescriptive procedures involving the education of gifted persons or those with disabilities.

2084 **Council for Exceptional Children (CEC)**
3100 Clarendon Blvd.
Suite 600
Arlington, VA 22201-5332
888-232-7733
TTY: 866-915-5000
service@exceptionalchildren.org
www.exceptionalchildren.org

Chad Rummel, Executive Director
Laurie VanderPloeg, Associate Executive Director, Professional Affairs
Craig Evans, Chief Financial Officer
Sharon Rodriguez, Director, Governance & Executive Services

The Council for Exceptional Children aims to improve the educational success of individuals with disabilities and/or gifts and talents by advocating for appropriate policies, setting professional standards, and providing resources and professional development for special educators.

2085 **Council of Administrators of Special Education (CASE)**
Osigian Office Center
101 Katelyn Circle
Suite E
Warner Robins, GA 31088
478-333-6892
Fax: 478-333-2453
lpurcell@casecec.org
www.casecec.org

Luann Purcell, Executive Director

Provides professional leadership and personal and professional development for special education administrators.

2086 **Disability Research and Dissemination Center**
Arnold School of Public Health, USC
Discovery 1 Bldg.
915 Greene St.
Columbia, SC 29208
info@disabilityresearchcenter.com
www.disabilityresearchcenter.com

Suzanne McDermott, PhD, Research & Administration
Margaret A. Turk, MD, Training & Evaluation
Roberta S. Carlin, MS, JD, Dissemination
Deborah Salzberg Clark, MS, Project Manager

The DRDC was formed in 2012 and is a partnership between the University of South Carolina (USC), the State University of New York Upstate Medical University (SUNY Upstate), and the American Association on Health and Disability (AAHD). Its five core areas are Administration, Research, Research Translation, Evaluation, and Dissemination & Policy.

2087 **Division for Communication, Language, and Deaf/Hard of Hearing (DCD)**
Council for Exceptional Children (CEC)
3100 Clarendon Blvd.
Suite 600
Arlington, VA 22201-5332
888-232-7733
TTY: 866-915-5000
service@cec.sped.org
dcdcec.org

Chad Rummel, Executive Director, CEC

Dedicated to improving education for deaf/hard of hearing students, and those with communicative disabilities.

2088 **Division for Culturally and Linguistically Diverse Exceptional Learners (DDEL)**
Council for Exceptional Children (CEC)
3100 Clarendon Blvd.
Suite 600
Arlington, VA 22201-5332
888-232-7733
TTY: 866-915-5000
ddel.exceptionalchildren@gmail.com
ddel.exceptionalchildren.org

Chad Rummel, Executive Director, CEC

Serves culturally and linguistically diverse students with disabilities.

2089 **Division for Early Childhood (DEC)**
PO Box 662089
Los Angeles, CA 90066
310-428-7209
Fax: 855-678-1989
dec@dec-sped.org
www.dec-sped.org

Peggy Kemp, Executive Director
Diana Stanfill, Associate Director
Brittany Clark, Operations Manager

Serves educators who work with children with special needs from birth through age 8.

2090 **Division for Early Childhood of the Council for Exceptional Children**
Council for Exceptional Children
3100 Clarendon Blvd.
Suite 600
Arlington, VA 22201-5332
888-232-7733
TTY: 866-915-5000
service@cec.sped.org
www.dec-sped.org

Peggy Kemp, Executive Director
Diana Stanfill, Associate Director
Brittany Clark, Operations Coordinator

Promotes policies and advances evidence-based practices that support families and enhance the optimal development of young children who have or are at risk for developmental delays and disabilities.

2091 **Division for Learning Disabilities (DLD)**
Council for Exceptional Children (CEC)
3100 Clarendon Blvd.
Suite 600
Arlington, VA 22201-5332
888-232-7733
TTY: 866-915-5000
service@cec.sped.org
www.teachingld.org

Chad Rummel, Executive Director, CEC

Seeks to enhance services, research, and legislation for persons with learning disabilities.

2092 **Division for Physical, Health & Multiple Disabilities: Complex and Chronic Conditions**
Council for Exceptional Children (CEC)
3100 Clarendon Blvd.
Suite 600
Arlington, VA 22201-5332
888-232-7733
TTY: 866-915-5000
cecdphmd@gmail.com
ccc.exceptionalchildren.org

Chad Rummel, Executive Director, CEC

Dedicated to quality education for all individuals with physical disabilities, multiple disabilities, and special health care needs.

2093 **Division for Research (CEC-DR)**
Council for Exceptional Children (CEC)
3100 Clarendon Blvd.
Suite 600
Arlington, VA 22201-5332
888-232-7733
TTY: 866-915-5000
service@cec.sped.org
www.cecdr.org

Chad Rummel, Executive Director, CEC

Seeks to advance research into education for the gifted and/or disabled.

2094 **Division of International Special Education and Services (DISES)**
Council for Exceptional Children (CEC)
3100 Clarendon Blvd.
Suite 600
Arlington, VA 22201-5332
888-232-7733
TTY: 866-915-5000
info@dises-cec.org
dises-cec.org

Chad Rummel, Executive Director, CEC

Dedicated to special education programs in other countries.

2095 **Division of Visual and Performing Arts Education (DARTS)**
Council for Exceptional Children (CEC)
3100 Clarendon Blvd.
Suite 600
Arlington, VA 22201-5332
888-232-7733
TTY: 866-915-5000
cecdartswebmaster@gmail.com
darts.exceptionalchildren.org

Chad Rummel, Executive Director, CEC

Promotes art, music, drama, and dance for students with disabilities.

2096 **Division on Autism and Developmental Disabilities (DADD)**
Council for Exceptional Children (CEC)
3100 Clarendon Blvd.
Suite 600
Arlington, VA 22201-5332
888-232-7733
TTY: 866-915-5000
service@cec.sped.org
www.daddcec.com

Chad Rummel, Executive Director, CEC

Seeks to improve quality of life for individuals with autism and other intellectual disabilities, especially youth.

2097 **Division on Career Development and Transition (DCDT)**
Council for Exceptional Children (CEC)
3100 Clarendon Blvd.
Suite 600
Arlington, VA 22201-5332
888-232-7733
TTY: 866-915-5000
jrazeghi@gmu.edu
www.exceptionalchildren.org

Jane Razeghi, Executive Director

Dedicated to assisting disabled students with their transition from school to adult life.

2098 **Division on Visual Impairments and Deafblindness (DVIDB)**
Council for Exceptional Children (CEC)
3100 Clarendon Blvd.
Suite 600
Arlington, VA 22201-5332
888-232-7733
TTY: 866-915-5000
dvidbwebmaster@gmail.com
dvidb.exceptionalchildren.org

Chad Rummel, Executive Director, CEC

Dedicated to assisting students with visual impairments or deafblindness.

2099 **Filomen M. D'Agostino Greenberg Music School**
111 E 59th St.
New York, NY 10022
315-842-4489
music@fmdgmusicschool.org
fmdgmusicschool.org

Leslie Jones, Executive Director
Dalia Sakas, Director, Music Studies
Amanda Wheeler, Director, Administration

Formerly affiliated with the Lighthouse Guild, the Filomen M. D'Agostino Greenberg Music School is the only community music school in the US for people who are blind or visually impaired, offering instruction and an accessible music technology center.

2100 **HEAL: Health Education AIDS Liaison**
New York, NY
347-867-4497
michaelellner2@gmail.com
www.healaids.com

Michael Ellner, President
Barnett J. Weiss, Board Member
Roberto Giraldo, Board Member

Nonprofit, community-based educational organization providing information, hope, and support to people who are HIV positive or living with AIDS. The men and women at HEAL are health professionals, people living with life threatening diseases, and volunteers.

2101 **Incight**
111 SW Columbia St
Suite 940
Portland, OR 97201
971-244-0305
scott@incight.org
incight.org

Scott Hatley, Executive Director
Vail Horton, Director, Results
Hannah Rankin, Director, Results

Incight in a non-profit organization that supports people with disabilities in the areas of education, employment, and independent living. Incight offers programs that address workplace descrimination, college application process and recreational needs of those they serve.

2102 **Innovations in Special Education Technology Division (ISET)**
Council for Exceptional Children (CEC)
3100 Clarendon Blvd.
Suite 600
Arlington, VA 22201-5332
888-232-7733
TTY: 866-915-5000
service@cec.sped.org
www.isetcec.org
Chad Rummel, Executive Director, CEC
Advocates for technology and media to assist gifted persons and those with disabilities.

2103 **International Childbirth Education Association**
110 Horizon Dr.
Suite 210
Raleigh, NC 27615
919-674-4183
Fax: 919-459-2075
info@icea.org
www.icea.org
Katesha Phillips, Executive Director
Jenna Westheimer, Membership & Certification Coordinator
Allison Winter, Marketing Coordinator
The Association offers teaching certificates, seminars, continuing education workshops, and mail order center.

2104 **International Dyslexia Association**
40 York Rd.
4th Floor
Baltimore, MD 21204
410-296-0232
Fax: 410-321-5069
info@dyslexiaida.org
dyslexiaida.org
Sonja Banks, Chief Executive Officer
David Holste, Chief Financial Officer
Jason Marshall, Interim Chief Communications & Engagement Officer
Regina Gooden, Chair, Accreditation
Provides free information and referral services for diagnosis and tutoring for parents, educators, physicians, and individuals with dyslexia. Membership includes yearly journal and quarterly newsletter, and Pennsylvania newsletter; discounts to conferences and events.

2105 **Job Accommodation Network**
PO Box 6080
Morgantown, WV 26506-6080
304-293-7186
800-526-7234
Fax: 304-293-5407
TTY: 877-781-9403
jan@askjan.org
askjan.org
Deborah Hendricks, Director
Anne Hirsch, Associate Director
JAN's mission is to facilitate the employment and retention of workers with disabilities by providing employers, employment providers, people with disabilities, their family members, and other interested parties with information on job accommodations, self-employment, and small business opportunities and related subjects.

2106 **LD Online**
2775 S. Quincy St.
Arlington, VA 22206
Fax: 703-998-2060
ldonline@weta.org
ldonline.org
Noel Gunther, Executive Director
Christian Lindstrom, Director, Learning Media
Lydia Breiseth, Director, Colorin Colorado
Tina Chovanec, Director, Reading Rockets
LD OnLine seeks to help children and adults reach their full potential by providing accurate and up-to-date information and advice about learning disabilities and ADHD. The site features hundreds of helpful articles, multimedia, monthly columns by noted experts, first person essays, children's writing and artwork, a comprehensive resource guide, very active forums, and a Yellow Pages referral directory of professionals, schools, and products.

2107 **Lighthouse Guild**
250 W 64th St.
New York, NY 10023
212-769-6200
800-284-4422
www.lighthouseguild.org
Calvin W. Roberts, President & CEO
Paul D. Misiti, Chief of Staff
Himanshu R. Shah, Chief Financial Officer
Maura J. Sweeney, Chief Program Officer
Lighthouse Guild is a not-for-profit vision & healthcare organization, addressing the needs of people who are blind or visually impaired, including those with multiple disabilities or chronic medical conditions.

2108 **Michigan Psychological Association**
124 W Allegan St.
Suite 1900
Lansing, MI 48933
517-347-1885
Fax: 517-484-4442
www.michiganpsychologicalassociation.org
Antu Segal, President
Valencia Montgomery, Treasurer
Cynthia S. Rodriguez, Secretary
LaVone Swanson, Executive Director
Nonprofit organization of over 1000 psychologists, working to advance psychology as a science and a profession and to promote the public welfare by encouraging the highest professional standards, offering public education and providing a public service, and by participating in the public policy process on behalf of the profession and health care consumers.

2109 **National Association for Adults with Special Learning Needs**
P.O. Box 716
Bryn Mawr, PA 19010
naasln.org
Richard Cooper, Co-President
Joan Hudson-Miller, Co-President
Frances A. Holthaus, Vice President
Jeanne Brunette-Tregoning, Treasurer
NAASLN is an association for those who serve adults with special learning needs. NAASLN members include educators, trainers, employers and human service providers.

2110 **National Association of Colleges and Employers**
62 Highland Ave.
Bethlehem, PA 18017
610-868-1421
admin@naceweb.org
naceweb.org
Jennifer Lasater, President
Shawn Vanderziel, Executive Director
A national association with services for career planning, placement and recruitment professionals.

2111 **National Association of Parents with Children in Special Education**
3642 E Sunnydale Dr.
Chandler Heights, AZ 85142
800-754-4421
Fax: 800-424-0371
contact@napcse.org
www.napcse.org
George Giuliani, President
NAPCSEis a national membership organization dedicated to rendering all possible support and assistance to parents whose children receive special education services, both in and outside of school.

2112 **National Association of State Directors of Special Education**
1000 Diagonal Rd.
Suite 600
Alexandria, VA 22314
703-519-3800
Fax: 703-519-3808
www.nasdse.org
John Eisenberg, Executive Director
Valerie Williams, Director, Government Relations
Joanne Cashman, Member Services
NASDSE focuses on improving educational services and outcomes for children and youth with disabilities throughout the United States, the Department of Defense, the federated territo-

ries and the Freely Associated States of Palau, Micronesia and the Marshall Islands.

2113 **National Center for Homeopathy**
1120 Route 73
Suite 200
Mount Laurel, NJ 08054
856-437-4752
Fax: 856-439-0525
www.homeopathycenter.org

Deb Dupnik, Executive Director
Natascha Williams, Meeting Manager
Steve Clark, Membership Coordinator
Christina DeRose, Industry Relations

The National Center for Homeopathy (NCH) is a non-profit organization dedicated to promoting health through homeopathy by advancing the use and practice of homeopathy.

2114 **National Council on Rehabilitation Education (NCRE)**
1099 E. Champlain Dr.
Suite A-137
Fresno, CA 93720
559-906-0787
info@ncre.org
ncre.org

David A. Rosenthal, Ph.D, CRC, President
Mona Robinson, Ph.D, CRC, First Vice President
Allison Fleming, Ph.D, CRC, Second Vice President

Members include academic institutions and organizations, professional educators, researchers, and students. Assists in the documentation of the effect of education in improving services to persons with disabilities; determines the skills and training necessary for effective rehabilitation services; develops role models, standards and uniform licensure and certification requirements for rehabilitation personnel.

2115 **National Education Association of the United States**
1201 16th St. NW
Washington, DC 20036-3290
202-833-4000
Fax: 202-822-7974
www.nea.org

Lily Eskelsen Garcia, President
Becky Pringle, Vice President
Princess R. Moss, Secretary/Treasurer
Kim Anderson, Executive Director

The National Education Association (NEA) is committed to advancing the cause of public education.

2116 **National Society for Experiential Education**
19 Mantua Rd.
Mount Royal, NJ 08061
856-423-3427
Fax: 856-423-3420
nsee@talley.com
www.nsee.org

Haley Burst, Executive Director
Wendy Stevens, Meeting Manager
Arianna B., Program Manager
Denise Smith, Exhibits & Membership Services Manager

National nonprofit organization which advocates experiential learning and works with college administrators and high school and college internship programs.

2117 **Servcies for Students with Disabilities (SSD)**
College Board
P.O. Box 7504
London, KY 40742-7504
212-713-8333
844-255-7728
Fax: 866-360-0114
ssd@info.collegeboard.org
www.collegeboard.com

David Coleman, Chief Executive Officer
Jeremy Singer, President
Tracy MacMahon, Senior Vice President, Operations

National, nonprofit association dedicated to preparing, inspiring and connecting students to college and opportunity. Provide the accomodations students with disabilities need to complete test and other evaluations.

2118 **Society for Disability Studies**
P.O. Box 5570
Eureka, CA 95502
510-206-5767
sds@disstudies.org
www.disstudies.org

Devva Kasnitz, Ph.D, Interim Executive Director

SDS is a scholarly association of more than 400 artists, scholars and activists who promote Disability Studies, recognizing disability as a complex and valuable aspect of human experience.

2119 **Teacher Education Division (TED)**
Council for Exceptional Children (CEC)
3100 Clarendon Blvd.
Suite 600
Arlington, VA 22201-5332
888-232-7733
TTY: 866-915-5000
service@cec.sped.org
tedcec.org

Chad Rummel, Executive Director, CEC
Sharon Rodriguez, Governance & Executive Services Coordinator

Advocates for continual professional development of professionals in special education and related fields.

2120 **The AG Academy for Listening and Spoken Language**
Alexander Graham Bell Association
3417 Volta Pl. NW
Washington, DC 20007
202-337-5220
Fax: 202-337-8314
TTY: 202-337-5221
academy@agbell.org
agbellacademy.org

Jenna Voss, Chair
Emilio Alonso-Mendoza, Chief Executive Officer

Listening and Spoken Language Specialsts (LSLST) work with infants and children who are deaf or hard of hearing and their families seeking a listening and spoken language outcome in a variety of settings: home-based intervention, public schools, independent schools, private therapy, clinical centers for the deaf and hard of hearing, audiological and cochlear implant centers.

2121 **The Association for the Gifted (TAG)**
Council for Exceptional Children (CEC)
3100 Clarendon Blvd.
Suite 600
Arlington, VA 22201-5332
888-232-7733
TTY: 866-915-5000
tag.cec@gmail.com
cectag.com

Chad Rummel, Executive Director, CEC
Sharon Rodriguez, Governance & Executive Services Coordinator

Serves parents and professionals working with gifted and talented children.

2122 **United Cerebral Palsy**
1825 K St. NW
Suite 600
Washington, DC 20006-5638
202-776-0406
www.ucp.org

Armando Contreras, President & CEO
Anita Porco, Vice President, Affiliate Network
Michael Ludgardo, Manager, Development

United Cerebral Palsy (UCP) educates, advocates and provides support services to ensure a life without limits for people with a spectrum of disabilities. UCP and its nearly 68+ affiliates have a mission to advance the independence, productivity and full citizenship of people with a broad range of disabilities by providing services and support to children and adults.

Directories

2123 **ADDitude Directory**
108 West 39th St.
Suite 805
New York, NY 10018
646-366-0830
Fax: 646-366-0842
customerservice@additudemag.com
directory.additudemag.com

2124 BOSC: Directory of Facilities for People with Learning Disabilities
Books on Special Children
PO Box 3378
Amherst, MA 1004-3378 413-256-8164
Fax: 413-256-8896
Michael Young, President
Directory of schools, independent living programs, clinics and centers, colleges and vocational programs, agencies and commercial products. Five sections in special post binder that can be updated annually. Hardcover. *$70.00*
300+ pages Yearly
ISSN 0961-3888

2125 Community Resource Directory
5300 Hiatus Road
Sunrise, FL 33351 954-745-9779
800-963-5337
webmaster@adrcbroward.org
www.adrcbroward.org

2126 Complete Learning Disabilities Resource Guide
Grey House Publishing
4919 Route 22
P.O. Box 56
Amenia, NY 12501 518-789-8700
800-562-2139
Fax: 518-789-0556
books@greyhouse.com
www.greyhouse.com
Leslie Mackenzie, Publisher
Laura Mars, Editorial Director
Jessica Moody, Vice President, Marketing
A comprehensive educational guide offering over 6,000 listings on associations and organizations, schools, government agencies, testing materials, camps, products, books, newsletters, legal information, classroom materials and more. Includes separate chapters on ADD and Literacy, as well as informative articles. *$165.00*
800 pages Annual

2127 Complete Mental Health Resource Guide
Sedgwick Press/Grey House Publishing
4919 Route 22
P.O. Box 56
Amenia, NY 12501 518-789-8700
800-562-2139
Fax: 518-789-0556
books@greyhouse.com
www.greyhouse.com
Leslie Mackenzie, Publisher
Laura Mars, Editorial Director
Jessica Moody, Vice President, Marketing
This directory offers comprehensive information covering the field of behavioral health, with critical information for both the layman and the mental health professional. It covers, in depth, 22 specific mental disorders, and includes informative descriptions and a complete list of resources. *$165.00*
800 pages Annual

2128 Complete Resource Guide for Pediatric Disorders
Sedgwick Press/Grey House Publishing
4919 Route 22
P.O. Box 56
Amenia, NY 12501 518-789-8700
800-562-2139
Fax: 518-789-0556
books@greyhouse.com
www.greyhouse.com
Leslie Mackenzie, Publisher
Laura Mars, Editorial Director
Jessica Moody, Vice President, Marketing
An annual directory for professionals, parents and caregivers. Provides valuable information on more than 200 pediatric conditions, disorders, diseases and disabilities, including informative descriptions and a wide variety of resources, from associations to publications. *$165.00*
1000 pages Annual

2129 Complete Resource Guide for People with Chronic Illness
Grey House Publishing
4919 Route 22
P.O. Box 56
Amenia, NY 12501 518-789-8700
800-562-2139
Fax: 518-789-0556
books@greyhouse.com
www.greyhouse.com
Leslie Mackenzie, Publisher
Laura Mars, Editorial Director
Jessica Moody, Vice President, Marketing
This directory is structured around the 80 most prevalent chronic illnesses. Each chronic illness chapter includes an informative description, plus a comprehensive listing of resources and support services available for people diagnosed with chronic illness and their network of supportive individuals. *$165.00*
1000 pages Annual

2130 Directory Of Services For People With Disabilities
117 W. Duval St.
Suite 205
Jacksonville, FL 32202-4111 904-630-4940
Fax: 904-630-3476
TTY: 904-630-4933
disabledservices@coj.net
www.coj.net

2131 Directory for Exceptional Children
Prorter Sargent
2 LAN Drive
Suite 100
Westford, MA 01886 978-692-5092
800-342-7470
Fax: 978-692-4714
info@carnegiecomm.com
www.carnegiecomm.com
Joe Moore, President, CEO
Mark Cunningham, SVP, Enrollment Marketing
Melissa Rekos, SVP, Digital Services
Gary Allen Williams, VP, Special Projects
Supports parents and professionals seeking the optimal educational, therapeutic or clinical environment for special-needs youth. *$75.00*
1120 pages Trienniel
ISBN 0-875581-50-1

2132 Educators Resource Guide
Grey House Publishing
4919 Route 22
PO Box 55
Amenia, NY 12501 518-789-8700
800-562-2139
Fax: 845-373-6390
books@greyhouse.com
www.greyhouse.com
Leslie Mackenzie, Publisher
Laura Mars, Editorial Director
Jessica Moody, Vice President, Marketing
Gives education professionals immediate access to Associations and Organizations, Conferences and Trade Shows, Educational Research Centers, Employment Opportunities and Teaching Abroad, School Library Services, Scholarships, Financial Resources and much more. *$145.00*
650 pages Annual

2133 Greater Milwaukee Area Health Care Guide for Older Adults
PO Box 285
Germantown, WI 53022 262-253-0901
Fax: 262-253-0903
info@seniorresourcesonline.com
www.seniorresourcesonline.com
Gary Knippen, President
This directory is designed for older adults, family members and professionals looking for health care options in Milwaukee, Ozaukee, Washington and Waukesha counties. The directory is comprehensive with all providers included at no charge.

2134 **Greater Milwaukee Area Senior Housing Options**
PO Box 285
Germantown, WI 53022 262-253-0901
Fax: 262-253-0903
info@seniorresourcesonline.com
www.seniorresourcesonline.com

Gary Knippen, President
This directory is designed for older adults, family members and professionals looking for senior housing options in Milwaukee, Ozaukee, Washington and Waukesha counties. The directory is comprehensive with all providers included at no charge.

2135 **Indiana Directory of Disability Resources**
225 S. University Street
ABE Bldg.
West Lafayette, IN 47907-2093 765-494-5013
800-825-4264
bng@ecn.purdue.edu
engineering.purdue.edu/~bng/IDDR/

2136 **Nevada's Care Connection**
3416 Goni Road
Suite D-132
Carson City, NV 89706 702-486-3600
cpasquale@adsd.nv.gov
www.nevadaadrc.com

Cheyenne Pasquale, ADRC Project Manager
Nevada's Care Connection: Aging and Disability Resource Center (ADRC) program provides information and access to programs and services that benefit Nevada's seniors, people with disabilities and caregivers.

2137 **Northeast Wisconsin Directory of Servicesfor Older Adults**
PO Box 285
Germantown, WI 53022 262-253-0901
Fax: 262-253-0903
info@seniorresourcesonline.com
www.seniorresourcesonline.com

Gary Knippen, President
This directory is designed for older adults, family members and professionals looking for housing and health care options in Brown, Calumet, Door, Fond du Lac, Green Lake, Kewaunee, Manitowoc, Marinette, Marquette, Oconto, Outagamie, Shawano, Sheboygan, Waupaca, Waushara and Winnebago counties.

2138 **ODHH Directory of Resources and Services**
1521 N. 6th Street
Harrisburg, PA 17102 717-783-4912
TTY: 717-783-4912
RA-LI-OVR-ODHH@pa.gov

2139 **Responding to Crime Victims with Disabilities**
2000 M Street NW
Suite 480
Washington, DC 20036 202-467-8700
Fax: 202-467-8701
www.victimsofcrime.org

Philip M. Gerson, Chair
G. Morris Gurley, Vice-Chair
Mai Fernandez, Executive Director
Jeffrey R. Dion, Deputy Executive Director
The mission of the National Center for Victims of Crime is to forge a national commitment to help victims of crime rebuild their lives. It is dedicated to serving individuals, families, and communities harmed by crime.

2140 **Selective Placement Program Coordinator Directory**
1900 E Street, NW
Washington, DC 20415-1000 202-606-1800
www.opm.gov

2141 **South Central Wisconsin Directory of Services for Older Adults**
PO Box 285
Germantown, WI 53022 262-253-0901
www.seniorresourcesonline.com

Gary Knippen, President
This directory is designed for older adults, family members and professionals looking for housing and health care options in Columbia, Dane, Dodge, Grant, Green, Iowa, Jefferson, Juneau, Lafayette, Richland, Rock, Sauk, and Walworth counties.

2142 **Southeast Wisconsin Directory of Servicesfor Older Adults**
PO Box 285
Germantown, WI 53022 262-253-0901
www.seniorresourcesonline.com

Gary Knippen, President
This directory is designed for older adults, family members and professionals looking for housing and health care options in Kenosha, Racine and Walworth counties.

2143 **Teaching Special Students in Mainstream**
Books on Special Children
P.O. Box 305
Congers, NY 10920-305 845-638-1236
Fax: 845-638-0847

515 pages Softcover

Educational Publishers

2144 **AFB Press**
American Foundation for the Blind / AFB Press
2 Penn Plaza
Suite 1102
New York, NY 10121 212-502-7600
Fax: 888-545-8331
afbinfo@afb.net
www.afb.org

Carl R. Augusto, President and CEO
Paul Schroeder, Vice President, Programs and Policy
Rick Bozeman, Chief Financial Officer
Kelly Bleach, Chief Administrative Officer
Develops, publishes, and sells a wide variety of informative books, pamphlets, periodicals, and videos for students, professionals, and researchers in the blindness and visual impairment fields, for people professionally involved in making the mainstream community accessible, and for blind and visually impaired people and their families; publication and video orders.

2145 **Academic Therapy Publications**
Academic Therapy Publications / High Noon Books
20 Leveroni Ct.
Novato, CA 94949-5746 415-883-3314
800-422-7249
Fax: 888-287-9975
sales@academictherapy.com
www.academictherapy.com

Jim Arena, President
Stacy Frauwirth, Assessment Project Manager
Holly Melton, Head Writer & Senior Project Manager
Academic Therapy Publications produces and distributes psychological and educational tests used by professionals involved in special education and learning differences in the K-12 school system as well as adult services.

2146 **AccessText Network**
512 Means St. NW
Suite 250
Atlanta, GA 30318 866-271-4968
membership@accesstext.org
www.accesstext.org

Dawn Evans, AccessText Network Coordinator
AccessText is a conduit between the publishing world and colleges and universities across the country, with a shared mission to ensure students with disabilities have equal access to their textbooks in an accessible format and in a timely manner.

2147 **American Counseling Association (ACA)**
6101 Stevenson Ave.
Suite 600
Alexandria, VA 22304 703-823-9800
800-347-6647
Fax: 800-473-2329
www.counseling.org

Richard Yep, Chief Executive Officer
Carolyn Baker, Associate Publisher
Offers tools and books for counseling professionals.

2148 **Association of University Centers on Disabilities (AUCD)**
AUCD
1100 Wayne Ave.
Suite 1000
Silver Spring, MD 20910
301-588-8252
Fax: 301-588-2842
aucdinfo@aucd.org
www.aucd.org

John Tschida, Executive Director
Adriane K. Griffen, Senior Director, Public Health & Leadership
Dawn Rudolph, Senior Director, Technical Assistance & Network Engagement
E. Troy Washington, Senior Director, Finance & Grants Administration

AUCD is a membership organization consisting of University Centers for Excellence in Developmental Disabilities (UCEDD), Leadership Education in Neurodevelopmental Disabilities (LEND) Programs, and Intellectual and Developmental Disability Research Centers (IDDRC). AUCD supports its members through advocacy, technical assistance, information dissemination, networking, and leadership.

2149 **Brookes Publishing Company**
PO Box 10624
Baltimore, MD 21285-0624
410-337-9580
800-638-3775
Fax: 410-337-8539
webmaster@brookespublishing.com
www.brookespublishing.com

Paul H. Brookes, Chairman of the Board
Jeffrey D. Brookes, President
George S. Stamathis, VP/Publisher
Melissa A. Behn, Executive Vice President

Publishes highly respected resources in early childhood, early intervention, inclusive and special education, developmental disabilities, learning disabilities, communication and language, behavior and mental health.

2150 **Brookline Books**
8 Trumbull Rd
B-001
Northampton, MA 01060
413-584-0184
800-666-2665
Fax: 413-584-6184
brbooks@yahoo.com
www.brooklinebks.com

2151 **Brooks/Cole Publishing Company**
511 Forest Lodge Rd
Pacific Grove, CA 93950-5040
831-373-0728
800-354-9706
Fax: 831-375-6414

2152 **BurnsBooks Publishing**
680 Ridge Road
Middletown, CT 6457
860-344-0233
Fax: 860-344-0233
burnsbookspub@aol.com
www.burnsbookspublishing.com

2153 **Charles C Thomas Publisher LTD**
2600 S 1st Street
Springfield, IL 62704-4730
217-789-8980
800-258-8980
Fax: 217-789-9130
books@ccthomas.com
www.ccthomas.com

Michael P. Thomas, President

Publishes specialty titles and textbooks in medicine, dentistry, nursing, and veterinary medicine, as well as a complete line in the behavioral sciences, criminal justice, education, special education, and rehabilitation. Aims to accommodate the current needs for information.

2154 **DisabilityAdvisor.com**
37 North Orange Ave.
Suite 500
Orlando, FL 32801
321-332-7800
888-393-1010
Fax: 888-985-6060
www.disabilityadvisor.com

Joseph E. Ram, Publisher
Kay Derochie, Editor
Jackie Booth, Ph.D., Editor

DisabilityAdvisor.com provides free information on federal and state disability benefits programs and other resources for readers and their families. This includes disabled children and students, military veterans, injured workers and disabled seniors. Readers are encouraged to submit their questions and comments online. The website also offers information on managing finances, education, parenting, relationships and other issues of interest to the disabled and their friends and families.

2155 **Dolphin Computer Access**
231 Clarksville Road
Suite 7
Princeton Junction, NJ 8550
866-797-5921
Fax: 609-799-0475
info@dolphinusa.com
www.yourdolphin.com

Noel Duffy, Managing Director

Dolphin helps vision and print impairments

2156 **Gallaudet University Press**
800 Florida Avenue, NE
Washington, DC 20002-3695
202-651-5488
Fax: 202-651-5489
gupress@gallaudet.edu
gupress.gallaudet.edu

David F Armstrong, Executive Director

Publishes scholarly trade books and journals about deaf people and their language, history, and culture for deaf people, parents of deaf children, professionals, educators and the general public. Produces spring and fall catalogs.

2157 **Greenwood Publishing Group**
88 Post Rd W
Westport, CT 06880-4208
203-226-3571
Fax: 203-222-1502
webmaster@greenwood.com
greenwood.com

Wayne Smith, President
Kirstin Olsen, Author

ABC-CLIO and Greenwood Press are recognized as industry-leading providers of the highest-quality reference materials. These imprints offer authoritative reference scholarship and innovative coverage of history and humanities topics across the secondary and higher education curriculum.

2158 **Grey House Publishing**
4919 Route 22
P.O. Box 56
Amenia, NY 12501
518-789-8700
800-562-2139
Fax: 518-789-0556
books@greyhouse.com
www.greyhouse.com

Leslie Mackenzie, Publisher
Laura Mars, Editorial Director
Jessica Moody, Vice President, Marketing
Kristen Hayes, Production Manager

Grey House Publishing publishes directories, handbooks and reference works for public, high school and academic libraries and the business and health communities. Most titles are available as online databases.

2159 **Hammill Institute on Disabilities**
8700 Shoal Creek Blvd.
Austin, TX 78757-6897
512-451-3521
Fax: 512-451-3728
info@hammill-institute.org
hammill-institute.org

2160 **Harbor House Law Press**
PO Box 480
Hartfield, VA 23071
804-758-8400
Fax: 202-318-3239
webmaster@wrightslaw.com
www.harborhouselaw.com

2161 **High Noon Books**
Academic Therapy Publications / High Noon Books
20 Leveroni Ct
Novato, CA 94949-5746
800-422-7249
888-287-9975
products@academictherapy.com
www.highnoonbooks.com

Jim Arena, President
Holly Melton, Head Writer & Senior Project Manager
High Noon Books produces and distributes a variety of phonic-based and high-interest/low level chapter books, ebooks, and audio for beginning, at-risk, and struggling readers.

2162 **Information from HEATH Resource Center**
National Clearinghouse on Postsecondary Education
2134 G Street, N.W.
Washington, DC 20052
202-939-9320
800-544-3284
Fax: 202-833-5696
www.HEATH-resource-center.org

2163 **Lynne Rienner Publishers**
1800 30th St.
Ste. 314
Boulder, CO 80301
303-444-6684
Fax: 303-444-0824
www.rienner.com

2164 **MAPCON Technologies**
8191 Birchwood Court
Suite A
Johnston, IA 50131-2930
515-331-3358
800-223-4791
Fax: 515-331-3373
www.mapcon.com

Joel Tesdall, President/CEO
Diane Wiand, Client Solutions Advocate
Lora Whicker, Accounting
Bailey Merritt, Administrative Assistant
MAPCON is a computerized maintainance management software.

2165 **McGraw-Hill Company**
PO Box 182605
Columbus, OH 43218
800-338-3987
Fax: 609-308-4480
customer.service@mheducation.com
www.mcgraw-hill.com

David Levin, President, CEO
Ellen Haley, President, CTB
Peter Cohen, President, School Education
Mark Dorman, President, International
Offers a catalog of testing resources and materials for the special educator.

2166 **National Association of School Psychologists**
4340 East West Hwy.
Suite 402
Bethesda, MD 20814
301-657-0270
866-331-6277
Fax: 301-657-0275
TTY: 301-657-4155
www.nasponline.org

Kathleen Minke, Executive Director
Laura Benson, Chief Operating Officer
Represents over 25,000 school psychologists and related professionals. It serves its members and society by advancing the profession of school psychology and advocating for the rights, welfare, education and mental health of children, youth and their families.

2167 **National Center for Learning Disabilities**
32 Laight St
2nd Floor
New York, NY 10013
212-545-7510
888-575-7373
Fax: 212-545-9665
info@ncld.org
www.ncld.org

Frederic M Poses, Chairman
Mimi Corcoran, President & CEO
Rashonda Ambrose, Director of Strategic Partnerships
Michele Aweeky, Manager of Communications & Content
Contains features, articles, human interest news and other practical material to benefit children and adults with learning disabilities and their families, as well as educators and other helping professionals. The center also offers online forums and other resources on their website.
Quarterly

2168 **PEAK Parent Center**
917 East Moreno Ave.
Suite 140
Colorado Springs, CO 80903
719-531-9400
Fax: 719-531-9452
info@peakparent.org
www.peakparent.org

Michele Williers, Executive Director
Pam Christy, Director, Parent Training & Information
PEAK Parent Center is Colorado's federally-designated Parent Training and Information Center (PTI). As a PTI, PEAK supports and empowers parents, providing them with information and strategies to use when advocating for their children with disabilities. PEAK works one-on-one with families and educators helping them realize new possibilities for children with disabilities by expanding knowledge of special education and offering new strategies for success.

2169 **PRO-ED**
8700 Shoal Creek Boulevard
Austin, TX 78757-6897
512-451-3246
800-897-3202
Fax: 512-451-8542
info@proedinc.com
www.proedinc.com

2170 **Peytral Publications**
P.O. Box 1162
Minnetonka, MN 55345
952-949-8707
TTY: 952-906-9777
www.peytral.com

2171 **Prufrock Press**
PO Box 8813
Waco, TX 76714
254-756-3337
800-998-2208
Fax: 800-240-0333
jmcintosh@prufrock.com
www.prufrock.com

Joel McIntosh, Publisher
Lacy Compton, Senior Editor
Rachel Taliaferro, Editor
Raquel Trevino, Graphic Designer and Production Coordinator
Publishes books, textbooks, teaching materials supporting the education of gifted, advanced, and twice-exceptional learners.

2172 **Research Press**
P.O. Box 7886
Champaign, IL 61826
217-352-3273
800-519-2707
Fax: 217-352-1221
orders@researchpress.com
www.researchpress.com

Robert W. Parkinson, Founder
Dr Richard M Foxx, Author
Jeffrey S. Allen, Author
Bryce Alvord, Author
Research Press is an independent, family-owned business founded in 1968 by Robert W. Parkinson (1920-2001). During the past 40 years, the company has earned a solid reputation for publishing practical and effective educational and mental health resources. Authors from the early years include well-known names

in the field of psychology, such as B.F. Skinner, Albert Ellis, Gerald Patterson, Wesley Becker, John Guttmann, Richard Foxx, Arnold Lazarus, and Joseph Cautela.

2173 **Research Press Company**
2612 N. Mattis Ave.
Champaign, IL 61822
217-352-3273
800-519-2707
Fax: 217-352-1221
www.researchpress.com

2174 **Sage Publications**
2455 Teller Road
Thousand Oaks, CA 91320
805-499-0721
800-818-7243
Fax: 800-583-2665
info@sagepub.com
www.sagepub.com
Sara Miller McCune, Founder, Publisher & Executive Chairman
Blaise R Simqu, President/CEO
Chris Hickok, Senior Vice President & Chief Financial Officer
Stephen Barr, Managing Director/SAGE London, President of SAGE Internation
Publishes books, text books, journals, reference books, and databases mainly related to psychology, special education and speech, language and hearing.

2175 **Special Needs Project**
Special Needs Project
324 State Street
Suite H
Santa Barbara, CA 93101-2364
818-718-9900
800-333-6867
Fax: 818-349-2027
editor@specialneeds.com
www.specialneeds.com
Hod Gray, Owner
Publishes child development textbooks, books about aspergers syndrome, autism, and other disabilities.

2176 **Supporting Success for Children with Hearing Loss**
15619 Premiere Drive
Suite 101
Tampa, FL 33624
850-363-9909
Fax: 480-393-4331
accounting@successforkidswithhearingloss.com
successforkidswithhearinglo ss.com
Karen Anderson, PhD, Director
Improving the Outcomes of Children with Hearing Loss

2177 **Woodbine House**
6510 Bells Mill Road
Bethesda, MD 20817
800-843-7323
info@woodbinehouse.com
www.woodbinehouse.com

State Agencies: Alabama

2178 **Alabama Department of Education: Division of Special Education Services**
50 North Ripley St
P.O. Box 302101
Montgomery, AL 36104
334-242-9700
Fax: 334-262-2677
www.alsde.edu
Crystal Richardson, Program Coordinator
Provides technical assistance to all education agencies serving Alabama's gifted children as well as children with disabilities.

State Agencies: Alaska

2179 **Alaska Department of Education: Special Education**
State of Alaska
801 West 10th St
Ste 200, P.O. Box 110500
Juneau, AK 99811-0500
907-465-8693
Fax: 907-465-2806
TTY: 907-465-2815
sped@alaska.gov
www.education.alaska.gov/TLS/SPED
Dr. Susan McCauley, Division Director
Paul Prussing, Deputy Director
Cassidy Jones, Special Education Programs Manager
Administers special educational programs to the disabled residents of Alaska, through the Division of Teaching & Learning Support.

State Agencies: Arkansas

2180 **Arkansas Department of Special Education**
1401 West Capitol Ave, Victory Bldg
Suite 450
Little Rock, AR 72201
501-682-4221
Fax: 501-682-3456
TTY: 501-682-4222
spedsupport@arkansas.gov
arksped.k12.ar.us
Tom Hicks, Interim Associate Director
Ella Albert, Management Project Analyst
Howie Knoff, Director
Tony Boaz, Director
Provides oversight of all educational programs for children and youth with disabilities, ages 3 to 21. Provides technical assistance to all public agencies providing educational services to this population.

State Agencies: California

2181 **California Department of Education: Special Education Division**
1430 N Street
Sacramento, CA 95814-5901
916-319-0800
Fax: 916-327-3516
scheduler@cde.ca.gov
www.cde.ca.gov
Tom Torlakson, State Superintendent of Public Instruction and Director of E
Fred Balcom, Director
Gordon Jackson, Director
Phyllis Bramson, Director
Information and resources to serve the unique needs of persons with disabilities so that each person will meet or exceed high standards of achievement in academic and nonacademic skills.

State Agencies: Colorado

2182 **Colorado Department of Education: Special Education Service Unit**
Colorado Department of Education
201 E Colfax Ave
Denver, CO 80203-1704
303-866-6600
Fax: 303-830-0793
www.cde.state.co.us
Ed Steinberg, Commissioner
Provides consultation on materials and educational services for visually handicapped children, supervises volunteer services, transcribes textbooks for visually handicapped students.

State Agencies: Connecticut

2183 **Connecticut Department of Education: Bureau of Special Education**
165 Capitol Avenue
Hartford, CT 06106
860-713-6543
Fax: 860-713-7014
www.sde.ct.gov

Anne Louise Thompson, Bureau Chief
Lisa Spooner, Administrative Assistant
Regina Gaunichaux, Secretary
Carol Leddy, Secretary, Due Process Unit
The State Board of Education believes each student is unique and needs an educational environment that provides for, and accommodates, his or her strengths and areas of needed improvement.

2184 **Department of Rehabilitation Services & Bureau of Education And Services for the Blind**
State of Connecticut Agency
184 Windsor Ave
Windsor, CT 06095-4536
860-602-4000
800-842-4510
Fax: 860-602-4020
TTY: 860-602-4221
brian.sigman@ct.gov
www.ct.gov/besb

State Agencies: Delaware

2185 **Department of Public Instruction: Exceptional Children & Special Programs Division**
Department of Education
Ste 2
401 Federal St
Dover, DE 19901-3639
302-739-5471
Fax: 302-739-2388
www.doe.k12.de.us

Martha Toomey, Executive Director

State Agencies: DC

2186 **Administration for Community Living**
330 C St. NW
Washington, DC 20001
202-401-4634
800-677-1116
aclinfo@acl.hhs.gov
www.acl.gov

Alison Barkoff, Acting Administrator
Rick Nicholls, Chief of Staff
ACL's mission is to maximize the independence and well-being of people with disabilities so that they can participate fully in society. ACL achieves its goals by funding services provided by community-based organizations and investing in research, education and innovation.

2187 **District of Columbia Public Schools: Special Education Division**
1200 First Street, NE
Washington, DC 20002-4210
202-442-5885
202-442-5517
Fax: 202-442-5026
www.dcps.dc.gov

Paul L Vance MD, Superintendent
Committed to providing a continuum of services that offers students with disabilities the opportunity to actively participate in the learning environment of their neighborhood school.

2188 **Federal Emergency Management Agency**
500 C Street S.W.
Washington, DC 20472
202-646-2500
800-621-3362
TTY: 800-427-5593
www.fema.gov

W. Craig Fugate, Administrator
Michael Coen, Jr., Chief of Staff
Joseph Nimmich, Deputy Administrator
Alyson Vert, Director
FEMA's mission is to support the citizens and first responders to ensure that as a nation we work together to build, sustain and improve our capability to prepare for, protect against, respond to, recover from and mitigate all hazards.

2189 **Lab School of Washington**
4759 Reservoir Rd NW
Washington, DC 20007-1921
202-965-6600
www.labschool.org

Mimi W. Dawson, Chair
Mac Bernstein, Vice Chair
Mike Tongour, Secretary
Bill Tennis, Treasurer
The Lab School six week summer session includes individualized reading, spelling, writing, study skills and math programs. A multisensory approach addresses the needs of bright learning disabled children. Related services such as speech/language therapy and occupational therapy are integrated into the curriculum. Elementary/Intermediate; Junior High/High School.

2190 **National Clearinghouse on Family Support and Children's Mental Health**
Ste 800
1 Dupont Cir NW
Washington, DC 20036-1149
202-939-9320
800-544-3284
Fax: 202-833-4760
ncfy.acf.hhs.gov/

State Agencies: Florida

2191 **Florida Department of Education: Bureau of Exceptional Education And Student Services**
325 West Gaines Street
Turlington Building, Suite 1514
Tallahassee, FL 32399
850-245-0505
Fax: 850-245-9667
Monica.Verra-Tirado@fldoe.org
www.fldoe.org/ese

Monica Verra-Tirado, Ed.D., Bureau Chief
Gerard Robinson, Commissioner
Randy Hanna, Chancellor
Pam Stewart, Chancellor
Administers programs for students with disabilities and for gifted students. Coordinates student services throughout the state and participates in multiple inter-agency efforts designed to strengthen the quality and variety of services to students with special needs.

2192 **Florida State College at Jacksonville Services for Students with Disabilities**
501 W State St
Jacksonville, FL 32202
904-633-8100
888-873-1145
Fax: 904-633-5955
info@fscj.edu
fscj.edu

Randle P DeFoor, Chair
Cynthia A Bioteau, President
Richard Turner, Associate Vice President of Enrollment Management
Sarah Ashbrook, Project Coordinator
Florida State College ensures acessibility of its services, activities, facilities and academic programs to students with disabilities. Special accmmodations are provided to anyone with a physical, mental or learning disability.

State Agencies: Hawaii

2193 **Hawaii Department of Education: Special Needs**
Hawaii Department of Education
3430 Leahi Ave
Honolulu, HI 96815-4246
808-941-3894
Fax: 808-941-3894

Margaret Donovan MD, State Administrator
Provides consultation on educational services for local schools, offers psychological testing and evaluation, maintains resource rooms in district schools and more for the blind and handicapped throughout the state.

State Agencies: Illinois

2194 **Illinois State Board of Education: Department of Special Education**
100 N 1st St
Springfield, IL 62777
217-782-5589
Fax: 217-782-0372
www.isbe.net

Elizabeth Hanselman, Asst Superintendent Special Ed.
Mission is to advance the human and civil rights of people with disabilities in Illinois. Statewide advocacy organization providing self-advocacy assistance, legal services, education and public policy initiatives. Designated to implement the federal protection and advocacy system; has broad statutory power to enforce the rights of people with physical and mental disabilities, including developmental disabilities and mental illnesses.

State Agencies: Indiana

2195 **Indiana Department of Education: Special Education Division**
Indiana Department of Education
South Tower, Suite 600
115 W. Washington Street
Indianapolis, IN 46204-2731
317- 23- 661
877-851-4106
Fax: 317- 23- 800
webmaster@doe.in.gov
www.doe.in.gov/

Robert A Marra, Manager
Tony Bennett, Chair
Provides consultation on educational services for local schools, offers psychological testing and evaluation, maintains resource rooms in district schools and more for the blind and handicapped throughout the state.

State Agencies: Iowa

2196 **Iowa Department of Public Instruction: Bureau of Special Education**
400 E 14th St
Des Moines, IA 50319-9000
515-457-2000
Fax: 515-242-6019
www.educateiowa.gov/

Tom Kuehl, CEO
Jason Glass, Director
Jeff Berger, Administrative Services

State Agencies: Kansas

2197 **Kansas State Board of Education: Special Education Services**
900 SW Jackson Street
Topeka, KS 66612-1212
785-296-3201
800-203-9462
Fax: 785-296-7933
TTY: 785-296-6338
contact@ksde.org
www.ksde.org

Ethan Erickson, Director
Kathy Gosa, Director
Denise Kahler, Director
Scott Myers, Director
Provides leadership and support for exceptional learners receiving special education services throughout Kansas schools and communities.

State Agencies: Kentucky

2198 **Kentucky Department of Education: Divisionof Exceptional Children's Services**
500 Mero St
Capital Tower Plaza
Frankfort, KY 40601
502-564-4770
Fax: 502-564-7749
www.education.ky.gov

Darlene Jesse, Director
Provides consultation on educational services for local schools, offers psychological testing and evaluation, maintains resource rooms in district schools and more for the blind and handicapped throughout the state.

State Agencies: Louisiana

2199 **Louisiana Department of Education: Office of Special Education Services**
Louisiana Department of Education
1201 North Third Street
Baton Rouge, LA 70802
225-342-0090
877-453-2721
Fax: 225-342-0193
www.doe.state.la.us

David Elder, Manager
Kim Fitch, Director Human Resources
George Nelson, President

State Agencies: Massachusetts

2200 **Getting Ready for the Outside World (G.R.O.W.)**
Riverview School
551 Route 6A East Sandwich
Cape Cod, MA 2537-1448
508-888-0489
Fax: 508-833-7001
admissions@riverviewschool.org
www.riverviewschool.org

Janice James, Vice Chairman
Deborah Cowan, Vice Chair
James Shallcross, Treasurer
Kathleen Yazbak, Secretary
Riverview School's G.R.O.W. Program is a unique ten month transitional prgoram (1-3 years) for young adults with complex language, learning and cognitive disabilities. This post secondary program is designed to further develop academic, vocational and independent living skills, to enable students to function as independently as possible.

2201 **Massachusetts Department of Education: Program Quality Assurance**
Massachusetts Department of Education
75 Pleasant Street
Malden, MA 2148-4906
781-388-3300
Fax: 617-388-3476
boe@doe.mass.edu
www.doe.mass.edu/pqa/

Pamela Kaufamann, Administrator

State Agencies: Maryland

2202 **Agency for Healthcare Research and Quality**
540 Gaither Road
Rockville, MD 20850
301-427-1364
www.ahrq.gov

Richard G. Kronick, PhD, Director, Director
Sharon B. Arnold, PhD, Deputy Director

The Agency for Healthcare Research and Quality's (AHRQ) mission is to produce evidence to make health care safer, higher quality, more accessible, equitable, and affordable, and to work within the U.S. Department of Health and Human Services and with other partners to make sure that the evidence is understood and used.

2203 **Center for Mental Health Services**
5600 Fishers Lane
Rockville, MD 20857
240-276-1310
Fax: 240-276-1320
www.samhsa.gov

Anita Everett, Director

The Center for Mental Health Services leads federal efforts to promote the prevention and treatment of mental disorders.

2204 **Centers for Medicare & Medicaid Services**
7500 Security Boulevard
Baltimore, MD 21244
410-786-3000
877-267-2323
TTY: 866-226-1819
www.cms.gov

Dr. Mandy Cohen, M.D., MPH, Chief of Staff
Deborah Taylor, Acting Chief Operating Officer
Andy Slavitt, Acting Administrator
Patrick Conway, MD, MSc, Acting Principal Deputy Admin

US federal agency which administers Medicare, Medicaid, and the State Children's Health Insurance Program.

2205 **Maryland State Department of Education: Division of Special Education**
200 West Baltimore Street
Baltimore, MD 21201-2595
410-767-0100
888-246-0016
Fax: 410-333-8165
www.marylandpublicschools.org

Nancy S Grasmick, State Supertintendent
Dr. Lillian Lowery, Superintendent of Schools
James V. Foran, Assistant State Superintendent
Katharine Oliver, Assistant State Superintendent

Collaborates with families, local early intervention systems, and local school systems to ensure that all children and youth with disabilities have access to appropriate services and educational opportunities to which they are entitled under federal and state laws.

2206 **National Human Genome Research Institute**
National Institutes of Health
Building 31, Room 4B09
31 Center Drive, MSC 2152
Bethesda, MD 20892-2152
301-402-0911
Fax: 301-402-2218
lbrody@mail.nih.gov
www.genome.gov

Eric D. Green, M.D., Ph.D., Director
Lawrence Brody, Ph.D., Director
Bettie Graham, Ph.D., Director
Ellen Rolfes, M.A., Director, Division of Management

The National Human Genome Research Institute began as the National Center for Human Genome Research (NCHGR), which was established in 1989 to carry out the role of the National Institutes of Health (NIH) in the International Human Genome Project (HGP).

2207 **National Institute of General Medical Sciences**
45 Center Drive MSC 6200
Bethesda, MD 20892-6200
301-496-7301
info@nigms.nih.gov
www.nigms.nih.gov

Jon R. Lorsch, Ph.D., Director
Judith H. Greenberg, Ph.D., Deputy Director
Ann Hagan, Ph.D., Associate Director
Sally Lee, Executive Officer

The National Institute of General Medical Sciences (NIGMS) supports basic research that increases understanding of biological processes and lays the foundation for advances in disease diagnosis, treatment and prevention.

State Agencies: Michigan

2208 **Michigan Department of Education: Special Education Services**
608 W. Allegan Street
PO Box 30008
Lansing, MI 48909
517-373-3324
Fax: 517-373-7504
DHS-OCS-PEP@michigan.gov
www.michigan.gov/mde

John C. Austin, President
Kathleen N. Straus, President of the State Board
Michelle Fecteau, Executive Director
Daniel Varner, Chief Executive Officer of Excellent Schools Detroit

Oversees the administrative funding of education and early intervention programs and services for young children and students with disabilities.

2209 **Services for Students with Disabilities**
University of Michigan
G-664 Haven Hall
505 South State St.
Ann Arbor, MI 48109-1045
734-763-3000
Fax: 734-936-3947
TTY: 734-615-4461
ssdoffice@umich.edu
www.ssd.umich.edu

Stuart Segal, Director

Offers information to students of the University of Michigan and their parents.

State Agencies: Minnesota

2210 **Community Supports for People with Disabilities (CSP)**
South Central Technical College (SCTC)
1920 Lee Blvd
North Mankato, MN 56003-2504
507-389-7200
800-722-9359
online@southcentral.edu
www.southcentral.edu

Christensen Tami, Executive Director
Keith Stover, President

Human services program available as a physical or online program, designed for those wanting to earn a certificate, diploma or associate degree as a Direct Support Professional for use in the health and human services industries. The program comprises eight courses relating to professional services and support for people with disabilities.

2211 **Professional Development Programs**
6303 Osgood Ave. N.
Ste 104
Stillwater, MN 55082
651-439-8865
877-439-8865
Fax: 877-259-5906
www.pdppro.com

Cindy Lacosse, VP
Lori Lacrosse, President

Sponsors cutting edge and popular continuing education workshops and symposia of interest to professionals who provide services to children and adults with special needs.

State Agencies: Missouri

2212 **Missouri Department of Elementary and Secondary Education: Special Education Programs**
205 Jefferson St
PO Box 480
Jefferson City, MO 65102 573-751-5739
Fax: 573-526-4404
TTY: 800-735-2966
Stephen Barr, Assistant Commissioner
The Office of Special Education administers state and federal funds to support services for students and adults with disabilities.

State Agencies: Mississippi

2213 **Mississippi Department of Education: Office of Special Services**
359 North West Street
P.O. Box 771
Jackson, MS 39201 601-359-3513
Fax: 601-987-3892
Dr Tom Burnham, Superintendent
Key priorities are: reading, early literacy, student achievement, teachers/teaching, leadership/principals, safe and orderly schools, parent relations/community involvement, and technology.

State Agencies: Montana

2214 **Department of Public Health Human Services**
PO Box 4210
Helena, MT 59604-4210 406-444-5622
Fax: 406-444-1970
www.dphhs.mt.gov
Anna Whitin Sorrell, Director
Bernie Jacobs, Chief Legal Counsel
Deb Sloat, Human Resources Office
Jon Ebelt, Public Information Office
Provides consultation on educational services for local schools, offers psychological testing and evaluation, maintains resource rooms in district schools and more for the blind and handicapped throughout the state.

State Agencies: North Carolina

2215 **National Institute of Environmental Health Sciences**
111 T.W. Alexander Drive
Research Triangle Park, NC 27709 919-541-4580
birnbaumls@niehs.nih.gov
www.niehs.nih.gov
Linda S. Birnbaum, Ph.D., Director
Richard Woychik, Ph.D., Deputy Director
Sheila A. Newton, Ph.D., Policy, Planning, and Evaluation
Ericka Reid, Ph.D., Science Education & Diversity
The mission of the NIEHS is to discover how the environment affects people in order to promote healthier lives.

2216 **North Carolina Department of Public Instruction: Exceptional Children Division**
301 N Wilmington St
Raleigh, NC 27601 919-807-3300
Fax: 919-715-1569
www.ncpublicschools.org
June St. Clair Atkinson, Ed.D, State Superintendent of Public Instruction
Mike McLaughlin, Senior Policy Advisor to the State Superintendent
Rachel Beaulieu, Legislative & Community Affairs Director
Jeani Allen, Director of Internal Auditing
The mission is to assure that students with disabilities develop mentally, physically, emotionally, and vocationally through the provision of an appropriate individualized education in the least restrictive environment.

State Agencies: North Dakota

2217 **North Dakota Department of Education: Special Education**
600 E. Boulevard Avenue, Dept. 201
Floors 9, 10, and 11
Bismarck, ND 58505-0440 701-328-2260
866-741-3519
Fax: 701-328-2461
TTY: 701-328-4920
mdanderson@nd.gov
www.dpi.state.nd.us
Kirsten Baesler, State Superintendent
Jerry Coleman, Director, School Finance & Organization
Linda Schloer, Child Nutrition & Food Distribution, Director
Gerry Teevens, Director, Special Education
Provides consultation on educational services for local schools, offers psychological testing and evaluation, maintains resource rooms in district schools and more for the blind and handicapped throughout the state.

State Agencies: Nebraska

2218 **Nebraska Department of Education: Special Populations Office**
1200 N Street, Suite 400
PO Box 98922
Lincoln, NE 68509 402-471-2186
877-253-2603
Fax: 402-471-2909
NDEQ.moreinfo@Nebraska.gov
deq.ne.gov
Rod Gangwish Shelton, Council Member
Douglas Anderson Aurora, Council Member
Mark Whitehead Lincoln, Council Member
Mark Czaplewski Grand Islan, Council Member
Assists school districts in establishing and maintaining effective special education programs for children with disabilities (date of diagnosis through the school year when a child reaches 21). Major function: provide technical assistance to school districts and to parents of children with disabilities, assist programs in meeting state and federal special education regulations. Also responsible for assuring that the rights of children with disabilities and their parents are protected.

State Agencies: New Hampshire

2219 **Institute on Disability**
University of New Hampshire
10 West Edge Drive
Suite 101
Durham, NH 03824
603-862-4320
Fax: 603-862-0555
contact.iod@unh.edu
www.iod.unh.edu

Charles E. Drum, Director & Professor
Andrew Houtenville, Director of Research
Matthew Gianino, Director of Communications
Mary Schuh, Director of Development and Consumer Affairs
Provides coherent university-based focus for the improvement of knowledge, policies, and practices related to the lives of persons with disabilities and their families.

2220 **New Hampshire Department of Education: Bureau for Special Education Services**
101 Pleasant Street
Concord, NH 03301-3860
603-271-3494
Fax: 603-271-1953
Lori.Temple@doe.nh.gov
www.education.nh.gov

Santina Thibedeau, Administrator
Virginia Barry, Commissioner
Linda Breden, Secretary
Traci Biron, Secretary
The mission of Special Education is to improve educational outcomes for children and youth with disabilities by providing and promoting leadership, technical assistance and collaboration statewide. Provides oversight and implementation of federal and state laws that ensure a free appropriate public education for all children and youth with disabilities in New Hampshire.

State Agencies: New Jersey

2221 **New Jersey Department of Education: Office of Special Education Program**
New Jersey Department of Education
PO Box 500
Trenton, NJ 8625-500
609-292-0147
Fax: 609-984-8422
www.nj.gov/education/specialed/info/

Barbara Gantwerk, Director
Alfred Murray, Executive Director

2222 **New Jersey Speech-Language-Hearing Association**
174 Nassau St
Suite 337
Princeton, NJ 08542
888-906-5742
Fax: 888-729-3489
info@njsha.org
njsha.org

Mary Faella, President
Robynne Kratchman, Vice President
Joan Warner, Treasurer
Kristie Soriano, Secretary
The New Jersey Speech-Language-Hearing Association offers services to audiologists, speech-language pathologists, and scientists studying in these fields. Services include resources, advocacy, information and programs to help foster professional development.

2223 **The Arc of New Jersey**
985 Livingston Ave
North Brunswick, NJ 08902
732-246-2525
Fax: 732-214-1834
info@arcnj.org
arcnj.org

Joanne Bergin, President
Thomas Baffuto, Executive Director
Celine Fortin, Associate Executive Director
Anna Scruggs, Coordinator, Financial Services
The Arc of New Jersey is committed to enhancing the quality of life of children and adults with intellectual and developmental disabilities and their families, through advocacy, empowerment, education and prevention.

State Agencies: New Mexico

2224 **New Mexico State Department of Education**
300 Don Gaspar Ave
Santa Fe, NM 87501-2744
505-827-6508
Fax: 505-827-6696
www.sde.state.nm.us

Bill Trant, Assistant Director
Judy Parks, Assistant Director
Provides consultation on educational services for local schools, offers psychological testing and evaluation, maintains resource rooms in district schools and more for the blind and handicapped throughout the state.

State Agencies: Nevada

2225 **Nevada Department of Education: Special Eduction Branch**
700 E Fifth St
Carson City, NV 89701-5096
775-687-9800
Fax: 775-687-9101
www.doe.nv.gov

Nick Gakalatos, Manager
The Office of Special Ed and School Improvement Program of the Nevada State Department of Education is responsible for management of state and federal programs providing educational opportunities for students with diverse learning needs. Included are such programs as: special education/disabled (IDEA); disadvantaged/at-risk programs (Title I/IASA); early childhood programs (Title I/ESEA); early childhood programs; migrant education; English language learners; NRS 395 student placement program.

State Agencies: New York

2226 **New York State Education Department**
1606 One Commerce Plz
Albany, NY 12234
518-474-5930
Fax: 518-486-6880
www.nysed.gov

Bernard Margolis, Manager
Provides vocational rehabilitation and educational services for eligible individuals with disabilities throughout New York State. Services include evaluation, counseling, job placement, and referral to other agencies.

State Agencies: Ohio

2227 **Ohio Department of Education: Division of Special Education**
Ohio Department of Education
25 S Front St
Columbus, OH 43215-4183
614-995-1545
877-644-6338
Fax: 614-728-1097
TTY: 888-886-0181
www.ode.state.oh.us

Mike Armstrong, Manager
Provides technical assistance to educational agencies for the development and implementation of educational services to meet the needs of students with disabilities and/or those who are gifted. Provides information to parents. Administers state and federal funds allocated to educational agencies for the provision of services to students with disabilities and/or those who are gifted.

2228 **The Arc of Allen County**
546 S Collett St
Lima, OH 45805
419-225-6285
Fax: 419-228-7770
info@thearcofohio.org
www.arcallencounty.org

Brad Perrott, Executive Director
Vicki Alves, Day Service Manager
Lisa Hengstler, Office Assistant
Elaine Copeland, Day Care Aide
Offers services to people with intellectual and developmental disabilities. Some programs include day care, educational training, human rights advocacy, and information and referral.

State Agencies: Oklahoma

2229 **Oklahoma State Department of Education**
2500 N Lincoln Blvd
Oklahoma City, OK 73105-4599
405-521-3301
Fax: 405-521-6205

Misty Kimbrough, Manager
Sandy Garrett, Administrator
Janet Barresi, State Superintendent
Provides consultation on educational services for local schools, offers psychological testing and evaluation, maintains resource rooms in district schools and more for the blind and handicapped throughout the state.

State Agencies: Oregon

2230 **Oregon Department of Education: Office of Special Education**
Oregon Department of Education:
255 Capitol St NE
Salem, OR 97310-1300
503-945-5600
Fax: 503-378-2897
www.dpeducation.com

Bruce Goldberg, Manager
Heidi Cockrell, Executive Assistant
Katy Coba, Executive Director
State agency ensuring provision of special education services to children with disabilities from birth to age 21.

State Agencies: Pennsylvania

2231 **Pennsylvania Department of Education: Bureau of Special Education**
333 Market St
Harrisburg, PA 17126-333
717-783-6788
Fax: 717-783-6139
TTY: 717-783-8445
00specialed@psupen.psu.edu
www.pde.state.pa.us

Linda Rhen, Administrator
John Tommasini, Assistant Director
Provides effective and efficient administration of the Commonwealth of Pennsylvania's resources dedicated to enabling school districts to maintain high standards in the delivery of special education services and programs for all exceptional students.

State Agencies: Rhode Island

2232 **Rhode Island Department of Education: Office of Special Needs**
255 Westminster St
Providence, RI 2903
401-222-4600
Fax: 401-784-9513
www.ride.ri.gov

Al Moscola, Manager
Alfred Moscola, Manager

Provides consultation on educational services for local schools, offers psychological testing and evaluation, maintains resource rooms in district schools and more for the blind and handicapped throughout the state.

State Agencies: South Carolina

2233 **South Carolina Assistive Technology Program (SCATP)**
Center for Disability Resources
8301 Farrow Rd
Columbia, SC 29208-3245
803-935-5263
800-915-4522
Fax: 800-935-5342
www.sc.edu/scatp

Carol Page, Program Director
Mary Bechter, Program Coordinator
SCATP is a federally funded project concerned with getting technology into th hands of people with disabilities so that they might live, work, learn and be a more independent part of the community.

2234 **South Carolina Department of Education: Office of Exceptional Children**
1429 Senate St
Suite 808
Columbia, SC 29201-3730
803-734-8224
Fax: 803-734-4824
sdeservicedesk@sde.ok.gov
www.scschools.com

Susan Durant, State Director
Provides consultation on educational services for local schools, offers psychological testing and evaluation, maintains resource rooms in district schools and more for the blind and handicapped throughout the state.

State Agencies: South Dakota

2235 **South Dakota Department of Education & Cultural Affairs: Office of Special Education**
700 Governors Dr
Pierre, SD 57501-2291
605-773-3804
Fax: 605-773-6041

Chelle Somsen, Manager
Dorothy Liegl, Manager

State Agencies: Tennessee

2236 **Tennessee Department of Education**
710 James Robertson Pkwy
Nashville, TN 37243-1219
615-741-2731
888-212-3162
Fax: 615-741-1791

Ruth S Letson, Manager
Kevin Huffman, Commissioner
Provides consultation on educational services for local schools, offers psychological testing and evaluation, maintains resource rooms in district schools and more for the blind and handicapped throughout the state.

State Agencies: Texas

2237 **Texas Education Agency**
1701 N Congress Ave
Austin, TX 78701-1494
512-463-8532
Fax: 512-463-8057
www.tealighthouse.org

Shirley J Neeley, Commissioner of Education
Provides consultation on educational services for local schools, offers psychological testing and evaluation, maintains resource rooms in district schools and more for the blind and handicapped throughout the state.

2238 **Texas Education Agency: Special Education Unit**
1701 Congress Ave
PO Box 420637
Austin, TX 77242-637
512-463-8532
Fax: 512-463-8057
info@tdea.org
www.tdea.org
Gene Lenz, Deputy Associate Commissioner
Shirley Neeley, Administrator

2239 **Texas School of the Deaf**
1102 S Congress Ave
Austin, TX 78704-1791
512-462-5353
800-332-3873
Fax: 512-462-5424
ercod@tsd.state.tx.us
tsd.state.tx.us
Claire Bugen, Superintendent
Russell West, Residential Services Director
Gary Bego, Business and Operations Director
Brenda Fraenkel, Special Education Director
Ensures that students excel in an environment where they learn, grow and belong. Supports deaf students, families and professionals in Texas by providing resources through outreach services.

State Agencies: Utah

2240 **Utah State Office of Education: At-Risk and Special Education Service Unit**
Utah State Office of Education
250 East 500 South
P.O. Box 144200
Salt Lake City, UT 84114-4200
801-538-7500
Fax: 801-538-7521
webmaster@schools.utah.gov
schools.utah.gov
Sandra Cox, Financial Analyst
Mark Peterson, Director
Glenna Gallo, State Director of Special Educat
Rebecca Donovan, Administrative Secretary
Provides consultation on educational services for local schools, offers psychological testing and evaluation, maintains resource rooms in district schools and more for the blind and handicapped throughout the state.

State Agencies: Virginia

2241 **National Science Foundation**
4201 Wilson Blvd
Arlington, VA 22230
703-292-5111
TTY: 703-292-5090
info@nsf.gov
www.nsf.gov
France A. C¢rdova, Director
Richard O. Buckius, Chief Operating Officer
Michael Van Woert, Executive Officer/Director
Dr. James L. Olds, Assistant Director
NSF is the only federal agency whose mission includes support for all fields of fundamental science and engineering, except for medical sciences.

2242 **Virginia Department of Education: Divisionof Pre & Early Adolescent Education**
Virginia Department Of Education
James Monroe Building, 101, N. 14th
P.O. Box 2120
Richmond, VA 23219
804-236-3631
Fax: 804-236-3635
webmaster@doe.virginia.gov
www.pen.k12.va.us
Dr. Steven R Staples, Superintendent of Public Instruction
Kent Dickey, Deputy Superintendent, Finance & Operations
Chris Sorensen, Director, Budget
Becky Marable, Director, Human Resources
Provides consultation on educational services for local schools, offers psychological testing and evaluation, maintains resource rooms in district schools and more for the blind and handicapped throughout the state.

State Agencies: Washington

2243 **Superintendent of Public Instruction: Special Education Section**
Old Capitol Building, 600 Washingto
P.O. Box 47200
Olympia, WA 98504-7200
360-725-6000
Fax: 360-586-0247
TTY: 360-664-3631
www.k12.wa.us
Randy I. Dorn, State Superintendent of Public I
Alan Burke, Deputy Superintendent
Robert Butts, Assistant Superintendent
Bob Harmon, Assistant Superintendent
Provides leadership, service and support for the development and implementation of research-based curriculum to assure that all learners achieve at all levels.

State Agencies: West Virginia

2244 **West Virginia Department of Education: Office of Special Education**
Rm 6
1900 Kanawha Blvd E
Charleston, WV 25305-0001
304-558-3660
Fax: 304-558-3741
wvde.state.wv.us
Liza Cordeiro, Executive Director
Mary Nunn, Assistant Director
Marshall Patton, Executive Director
Brenda Williams, Executive Director
Provides consultation on educational services for local schools, offers psychological testing and evaluation, maintains resource rooms in district schools and more for the blind and handicapped throughout the state.

State Agencies: Wyoming

2245 **Wyoming Department of Education**
2300 Capitol Avenue
Hathaway Building, 2nd Floor
Cheyenne, WY 82002-2060
307-777-7690
Fax: 307-777-6234
edu.wyoming.gov
Cindy Hill, WDE Superintendent
Deb Lindsey, Division Administrator, Assessment
Teri Wigert, Division Administrator, Support Systems & Resources
Dianne Bailey, Division Administrator, Finance & Data
Mission is to lead, model, and support continuous improvement of education for everyone in Wyoming.

Magazines & Journals

2246 **Adapted Physical Activity Programs**
Human Kinetics
1607 N. Market Street
P.O. Box 5076
Champaign, IL 61820
800-747-4457
Fax: 217-351-1549
info@hkusa.com
www.humankinetics.com
Patty Lehn, Publicity Manager
Lori Cooper, Marketing Manager
Bill Dobrik, Sales Associate
Dan Stebel, Sales Associate

Human Kinetics produces a variety of resources for adapted physical education practitioners, including books on activities, a research journal and higher education references. *$24.00*
Quarterly
ISSN 0736-58 9

2247 **Advance for Providers of Post-Acute Care**
Merion Publications
2900 Horizon Drive
King of Prussia, PA 19406 610-278-1400
800-355-5627
Fax: 610-278-1421
webmaster@advanceweb.com
advanceweb.com
Timothy Baum, MS, CRNP, Author
A free magazine for providers of post-acute care.

2248 **American Journal of Occupational Therapy (AJOT)**
American Occupational Therapy Association
6116 Executive Blvd.
Suite 200
North Bethesda, MD 20852-4929 301-652-6611
800-729-2682
members@aota.org
ajot.aota.org
Sherry Keramidas, Executive Director
Neil Harvison, Chief Officer, Knowledge
Matthew Clark, Chief Officer, Innovation & Engagement
Tricia Hopkins, Chief Officer, Finance & Operations
Official peer-reviewed publication of the American Occupational Therapy Association.
6 issues/year

2249 **American Journal on Intellectual and Developmental Disabilities (AJIDD)**
AAIDD
8403 Colesville Rd.
Suite 900
Silver Spring, MD 20910 202-387-1968
Fax: 202-387-2193
books@aaidd.org
aaidd.org
Frank Symons, PhD, Editor
American Journal on Intellectual and Developmental Disabilities (AJIDD)is a scientific, scholarly, and archival multidisciplinary journal for reporting original contributions to knowledge of intellectual disability, its causes, treatment, and prevention.
Bimonthly

2250 **Behavioral Disorders**
Council for Exceptional Children
3100 Clarendon Blvd.
Suite 600
Arlington, VA 22201-5332 888-232-7733
TTY: 866-915-5000
services@exceptionalchildren.org
www.exceptionalchildren.org
Daniel M. Maggin, Editor
Provides professionals with a means to exchange information and share ideas related to research, empirically tested educational innovations and issues and concerns relevant to students with behavioral disorders.
Quarterly

2251 **CEC Catalog**
Council for Exceptional Children
3100 Clarendon Blvd.
Suite 600
Arlington, VA 22201-5332 888-232-7733
TTY: 866-915-5000
service@exceptionalchildren.org
www.exceptionalchildren.org/store
Chad Rummel, Executive Director
Laurie VanderPloeg, Associate Executive Director, Professional Affairs
Craig Evans, Chief Financial Officer
Sharon Rodriguez, Director, Governance & Executive Services
Catalog from the Council for Exceptional Children offering books, guides, materials, and specialty items for special educators.

2252 **Career Development and Transition for Exceptional Individuals**
2455 Teller Road
Thousand Oaks, CA 91320 800-818-7243
Fax: 800-583-2665
journals@sagepub.com
cde.sagepub.com
Blaise R. Simqu, President/ CEO
Tracey A. Ozmina, EVP/ COO
Chris Hickok, SVP/ CFO
Phil Denvir, Global Chief Information Officer
Career Development and Transition for Exceptional Individuals (CDTEI) specializes in the fields of secondary education, transition, and career development for persons with documented disabilities and special needs.

2253 **Case Manager Magazine**
Elsevier Health
3251 Riverport Lane
Maryland Heights, MO 63043 314-447-8070
800-222-9570
textbook@elsevier.com
Thomas Reller, Vice President Global Corporate
Harald Boersma, Senior Manager Corporate Relatio
Ylann Schemm, Corporate Relations Manager
Sacha Boucherie, Press Officer
This national magazine is for medical case managers, social workers, counselors and home health professionals who work with people with serious injury or illness. It is a membership benefit of CMSA, the national association for case managers. *$55.00*
84 pages BiMonthly

2254 **Catalyst**
The Catalyst
Ste 275
1259 El Camino Real
Menlo Park, CA 94025-4208 800-647-0314
Sue Swezey, Editor
Digest of news and information on the use of computers in special education. *$15.00*
20 pages Quarterly

2255 **Challenge Magazine**
451 Hungerford Drive
Suite 100
Rockville, MD 20850 301-217-0960
Fax: 301-217-0968
Info@dsusa.org
www.disabledsportsusa.org
Kirk Bauer, Executive Director
Claire Duffy, Program Coordinator
Orlando Gill, Field Representative
Huarya Gomez-Garcia, Program Manager
Challenge Magazine is a publication of Disabled Sports USA, providing adaptive sports information to adults and children with disabilities, including those who are visually impaired, amputees, spinal cord injured (paraplegic and quadriplegic), and those who have multiple sclerosis, head injury, cerebral palsy, autism and other related intellectual disabilities.

2256 **Clinical Connection**
American Advertising Dist of Northern Virginia
708 Pendleton St
Alexandria, VA 22314-1819 703-549-5126
Fax: 703-548-5563
Kathie Harrington, M.A., CCC, Author
Covers speech language pathology.

2257 **College and University**
AACRAO
One Dupont Circle NW
Suite 520
Washington, DC 20036 202-293-9161
Fax: 202-872-8857
reillym@aacrao.org
aacrao.org
Brad Myers, President
Dan Garcia, President Elect
Adrienne McDay, Past President
Stan DeMerritt, VP, Finance

Scholarly research journal. American Association of Collegiate Registrars and Admissions Offers (AACRAO) is a nonprofit, voluntary, professional, educational association of degree-granting, postsecondary institutions, government agencies, private educational organizations and education-oriented businesses in the United States and abroad. $80 per year US; $90 per year international.

30 pages Quarterly
ISSN 0010-0889

2258 **Communication Disorders Quarterly**
2455 Teller Road
Thousand Oaks, CA 91320
800-818-7243
Fax: 800-583-2665
journals@sagepub.com
cde.sagepub.com

Blaise R. Simqu, President/ CEO
Tracey A. Ozmina, EVP/ COO
Chris Hickok, SVP/ CFO
Phil Denvir, Global Chief Information Officer

Communication Disorders Quarterly (CDQ) presents cutting edge information on typical and atypical communication — from oral language development to literacy.

2259 **Continuing Care**
Stevens Publishing Corporation
14901 Quorum Dr,
Suite 425
Dallas, TX 75254
972-687-6700
Fax: 972-687-6750
info@1105media.com
1105media.com

Neal Vitale, President & Chief Executive Officer
Richard Vitale, Senior Vice President & Chief Financial Officer
Mike Valenti, Executive Vice President
Jeff Klein, Non-Executive Chairman of the Board

A national magazine for case management and discharge planning professionals published monthly except for December. *$119.00*

34 pages Monthly

2260 **Counseling & Values**
American Counseling Association
6101 Stevenson Ave.
Suite 600
Alexandria, VA 22304
703-823-9800
800-347-6647
Fax: 800-473-2329
ahconley@vcu.edu
www.counseling.org

Richard Yep, Chief Executive Officer
Abigail H. Conley, Editor

Counseling and Values is the official journal of the Association for Spiritual, Ethical, and Religious Values in Counseling (ASERVIC), a member association of the American Counseling Association. Counseling and Values is a professional journal of theory, research, and informed opinion concerned with the relationships among psychology, philosophy, religion, social values, and counseling. *$20.00*

Bi-annual

2261 **Counseling Psychologist**
American Psychological Association
2455 Teller Road
Thousand Oaks, CA 91320
805-499-0721
800-818-7243
Fax: 800-583-2665
info@sagepub.com
www.sagepub.com

Sara Miller McCune, Founder, Publisher & Executive Chairman
Blaise R Simqu, President/CEO
Chris Hickok, Senior Vice President & Chief Financial Officer
Stephen Barr, Managing Director/SAGE London

Thematic issues in the theory, research and practice of counseling psychology. *$78.00*

Bi-Monthly

2262 **Counselor Education & Supervision**
American Counseling Association
6101 Stevenson Ave.
Suite 600
Alexandria, VA 22304
703-823-9800
800-347-6647
Fax: 800-473-2329
acesjournal@gmail.com
www.counseling.org

Richard Yep, Chief Executive Officer
James S. Korcuska, Editor

Dedicated to the growth and development of the counseling profession and those who are served. *$14.00*

Quarterly

2263 **Disability & Society**
711 3rd Avenue
8th Floor
New York, NY 10017
212-216-7800
800-634-7064
Fax: 212-564-7854
www.routledge.com

Len Barton, Author

The study of disability has traditionally been influenced mainly by medical and psychological models. The aim of this new text, Disability and Society, is to open up the debate by introducing alternative perspectives reflecting the increasing sociological interest in this important topic.

2264 **Disability Studies Quarterly**
552 Park Hall
Buffalo, NY 14260-4130
marembis@buffalo.edu
dsq-sds.org

Michael Rembis, Interim Editor-in-Chief
Tanja Aho, Interim Managing Editor

Disability Studies Quarterly (DSQ) is the journal of the Society for Disability Studies (SDS). It is a multidisciplinary and international journal of interest to social scientists, scholars in the humanities, disability rights advocates, creative writers, and others concerned with the issues of people with disabilities.

2265 **Disability and Health Journal**
American Association on Health and Disabiity
110 N Washington St.
Suite 407
Rockville, MD 20850
301-545-6140
Fax: 301-545-6144
contact@aahd.us
www.aahd.us/disability-and-health-journal

Monika Mitra, Editor
Margaret A. Turk, Editor

Disability and Health Journal is a scientific, scholarly and multidisciplinary journal for reporting original contributions that advance knowledge in disability and health.

2266 **Early Intervention**
Early Childhood Intervention Clearinghouse
51 Gerty Drive
Room 20
Champaign, IL 61820-7469
217-333-1386
877-275-3227
Fax: 217-244-7732
Illinois-eic@illinois.edu
www.eiclearinghouse.org

Susan Fowler, Director

Features articles, conference calendar, material reviews and news concerning early childhood intervention and disability.

4 pages Quarterly

2267 **Emerging Horizon**
PO Box 278
Ripon, CA 95366-0278
209-599-9409
emerginghorizons.com

2268 **Exceptional Children (EC)**
Council for Exceptional Children
3100 Clarendon Blvd.
Suite 600
Arlington, VA 22201-5332
888-232-7733
TTY: 866-915-5000
service@exceptionalchildren.org
www.exceptionalchildren.org
John Wills Lloyd, Editor
William Therrien, Editor
Peer-reviewed journal with articles including research, literature surveys and position papers concerning exceptional children, special education and mainstreaming.
Quarterly

2269 **Focus on Autism and Other Developmental Disabilities**
Sage Publications
2455 Teller Road
Thousand Oaks, CA 91320
805-499-0721
800-818-7243
Fax: 800-583-2665
info@sagepub.com
www.sagepub.com
Sara Miller McCune, Founder, Publisher & Executive Chairman
Blaise R. Simqu, President & CEO
Chris Hickok, Senior Vice President & Chief Financial Officer
Stephen Barr, Managing Director/SAGE London
Practical management, treatment and planning strategies; a must for persons working with individuals with autism and other developmental disabilities. *$43.00*
64 pages Quarterly

2270 **Focus on Exceptional Children**
Love Publishing Company
9101 East Kenyon Avenue
Suite 2200
Denver, CO 80237
303-221-7333
Fax: 303-221-7444
lpc@lovepublishing.com
www.lovepublishing.com
Steve Graham, Consulting Editor
Ron Nelson, Consulting Editor
Eva Horn, Consulting Editor
Contains research and theory-based articles on special education topics, with an emphasis on application and intervention, of interest to teachers, professors and administrators. *$36.00*
Monthly

2271 **HerbalGram**
American Botanical Council
6200 Manor Rd.
PO Box 144345
Austin, TX 78714-4345
512-926-4900
800-373-7105
Fax: 512-926-2345
abc@herbalgram.org
herbalgram.org
Mark Blumenthal, Founder, Executive Director & Editor
Tyler Smith, Editor
Hannah Bauman, Assistant Editor
Connor Yearsley, Assistant Editor
Official quarterly journal of the American Botanical Council.

2272 **HomeCare Magazine**
Cahaba Media Group
1900-28th Ave S.
Ste 200
Birmingham, AL 35209
205-212-9402
cahabamedia.com
Wally Evans, Publisher
Greg Meineke, Vice President, Sales
Stephanie Gibson Lepore, Editor
The business magazine of the home medical equipment industry offering information on legislation and regulations affecting the homecare industry, monthly profiles of suppliers, operational tips, newest products in the industry, advice on sales, government regulations. *$65.00*
120 pages Monthly

2273 **I Wonder Who Else Can Help**
AARP
601 E Street NW
Washington, DC 20049
202-434-3525
888-687-2277
877-342-2277
Fax: 202-434-3443
member@aarp.org
www.aarp.org
John Wider, President, CEO, AARP Services Inc.
Lisa M. Ryerson, President, AARP Foundation
Robert R. Hagans, Jr., Executive Vice President & Chief Financial Officer
Hollis Terry Bradwell III, Executive Vice President & Chief Information Officer
Contains information about crisis counseling, needs and resources, written in lay terms.

2274 **Inclusion**
AAIDD
8403 Colesville Rd.
Suite 900
Silver Spring, MD 20910
202-387-1968
Fax: 202-387-2193
books@aaidd.org
aaidd.org
Colleen Thoma, PhD, Co-Editor
LaRon Scott, PhD, Co-Editor
Inclusionis an open submission ejournal. Inclusion is published quarterly in an online-only format, enabling timely dissemination of emerging and promising research, policy, and practices.
Quarterly

2275 **Intellectual and Developmental Disabilities (IDD)**
AAIDD
8403 Colesville Rd.
Suite 900
Silver Spring, MD 20910
202-387-1968
Fax: 202-387-2193
books@aaidd.org
aaidd.org
James R. Thompson, PhD, Editor
Intellectual and Developmental Disabilities (IDD) is a peer reviewed multidisciplinary journal disseminating information on policies, practices, and concepts relating to intellectual and developmental disabilities.
Bimonthly

2276 **Intervention in School and Clinic**
Sage Publications
2455 Teller Road
Thousand Oaks, CA 91320
805-499-0721
800-818-7243
Fax: 800-583-2665
info@sagepub.com
www.sagepub.com
Sara Miller McCune, Founder, Publisher & Executive Chairman
Blaise R. Simqu, President & CEO
Chris Hickok, Senior Vice President & Chief Financial Officer
Stephen Barr, Managing Director/SAGE London
A hands-on, how-to resource for teachers and clinicians working with students for whom minor curriculum and environmental modifications are ineffective. *$35.00*
64 pages

2277 **Journal of Addictions & Offender Counseling**
American Counseling Association
6101 Stevenson Ave.
Suite 600
Alexandria, VA 22304
703-823-9800
800-347-6647
Fax: 800-473-2329
jaoc.iaaoc@utoledo.edu
www.counseling.org
Richard Yep, Chief Executive Officer
John M. Laux, Editor
Official journal of the International Association of Addictions and Offender Counselors, a member association of the American

Counseling Association. Contains information on programs, theory, and research into addictions and offender counseling. *$25.00*
Bi-annual

2278 **Journal of Applied School Psychology**
Haworth Press
711 Third Avenue
New York, NY 10017
212-216-7800
800-354-1420
Fax: 212-244-1563
subscriptions@tandf.co.uk
www.haworthpress.com
BiAnnually

2279 **Journal of Counseling & Development**
American Counseling Association
6101 Stevenson Ave.
Suite 600
Alexandria, VA 22304
703-823-9800
800-347-6647
Fax: 800-473-2329
jcd@unt.edu
www.counseling.org
Richard Yep, Chief Executive Officer
Matthew Lemberger-Truelove, Editor
Publishes practice, theory, and research articles across 18 different counseling and development specialty areas. Sections include research, assessment and diagnosis, theory and practice, and trends. *$35.00*
128 pages Quarterly

2280 **Journal of Disability Policy Studies**
2455 Teller Road
Thousand Oaks, CA 91320
800-818-7243
Fax: 800-583-2665
journals@sagepub.com
cde.sagepub.com
Blaise R. Simqu, President/ CEO
Tracey A. Ozmina, EVP/ COO
Chris Hickok, SVP/ CFO
Phil Denvir, Global Chief Information Officer
Journal of Disability Policy Studies (DPS) addresses compelling variable issues in ethics, policy and law related to individuals with disabilities.

2281 **Journal of Emotional and Behavioral Disorders**
Sage Publications
2455 Teller Road
Thousand Oaks, CA 91320
805-499-0721
800-818-7243
Fax: 800-583-2665
info@sagepub.com
www.sagepub.com
Sara Miller McCune, Founder, Publisher & Executive Chairman
Blaise R. Simqu, President & CEO
Chris Hickok, Senior Vice President & Chief Financial Officer
Stephen Barr, Managing Director/SAGE London
An international, multidisciplinary journal featuring articles on research, practice and theory related to individuals with emotional and behavioral disorders and to the professionals who serve them. *$39.00*
64 pages Quarterly

2282 **Journal of Learning Disabilities**
Sage Publications
2455 Teller Road
Thousand Oaks, CA 91320
805-499-0721
800-818-7243
Fax: 800-583-2665
info@sagepub.com
www.sagepub.com
Sara Miller McCune, Founder, Publisher & Executive Chairman
Blaise R. Simqu, President & CEO
Chris Hickok, Senior Vice President & Chief Financial Officer
Stephen Barr, Managing Director/SAGE London
An international, multidisciplinary publication containing articles on practice, research and theory related to learning disabilities. Published bi-monthly. *$49.00*
Magazine

2283 **Journal of Midwifery & Women's Health (JMWH)**
American College of Nurse Midwives
8403 Colesville Rd.
Suite 1230
Silver Spring, MD 20910
240-485-1800
Fax: 240-485-1818
membership@acnm.org
midwife.org
Frances Likis, Editor-in-Chief
Brittany Swett, Managing Editor
Tekoa King, Deputy Editor
Patricia Murphy, Deputy Editor
Official journal of the American College of Nurse Midwives.

2284 **Journal of Motor Behavior**
Heldref Publications
325 Chestnut Street
Suite 800
Philadelphia, PA 19106
215-625-8900
800-354-1420
Fax: 215-625-2940
customer.service@taylorandfrancis.com
www.heldref.org
Emilli Pawlowsky, Marketing Manager
Laura Rosse, Assistant Marketing Manager
Douglas Kirkpatrick, Publisher
A professional journal aimed at psychologists, therapists and educators who work in the areas of motor behavior, psychology, neurophysiology, kinesiology, and biomechanics. Offers up-to-date information on the latest techniques, theories and developments concerning motor control. Titles previously published by Heldref Publications will be joining the T&F portfolio. *$77.00*
115 pages Quarterly

2285 **Journal of Musculoskeletal Pain**
Haworth Press
711 Third Avenue
New York, NY 10017
212-216-7800
800-354-1420
Fax: 212-244-1563
subscriptions@tandf.co.uk
www.haworthpress.com
110 pages Quarterly

2286 **Journal of Positive Behavior Interventions**
2455 Teller Road
Thousand Oaks, CA 91320
800-818-7243
Fax: 800-583-2665
journals@sagepub.com
cde.sagepub.com
Blaise R. Simqu, President/ CEO
Tracey A. Ozmina, EVP/ COO
Chris Hickok, SVP/ CFO
Phil Denvir, Global Chief Information Officer
Journal of Positive Behavior Interventions (PBI) offers sound, research-based principles of positive behavior support for use in school, home and community settings with people with challenges in behavioral adaptation.

2287 **Journal of Postsecondary Education & Disability (JPED)**
AHEAD
8015 West Kenton Circle
Suite 230
Huntersville, NC 28078
704-947-7779
Fax: 704-948-7779
jped@ahead.org
www.ahead.org
Stephan Smith, Executive Director
Ezekiel Kimball, Executive Editor
Ryan Wells, Executive Editor
An annual publication dedicated to the advancement of full participation in higher education for persons with disabilities. The journal focuses on a variety of related topics that emphasize research, issues, and trends related to the theory and practice of postsecondary disability services.
Quarterly

2288 Journal of Prosthetics and Orthotics
330 John Carlyle Street
Suite 210
Alexandria, VA 22314
703-836-7114
Fax: 703-836-0838
info@abcop.org
www.abcop.org
Catherine Carter, Executive Director
Debbie Ayres, Director, Marketing & Public Relations
Stephen Fletcher, CPO, LPO, Director, Clinical Resources
Heather Harris, Director, Continuing Education Programs
Provides the latest research and clinical thinking in orthotics and prosthetics, including information on new devices, fitting techniques and patient management experiences. Each issue contains research-based information and articles reviewed and approved by a highly qualified editorial board. *$60.00*
64 pages Quarterly
ISSN 1040-88 0

2289 Journal of Reading, Writing and Learning Disabled International
Hemisphere Publishing Corporation
7625 Empire Drive
Florence, KY 41042-2919
800-634-7064
Fax: 800-248-4724
orders@taylorandfrancis.com
www.taylorandfrancis.com

2290 Journal of Rehabilitation
National Rehabilitation Association (NRA)
PO Box 150235
Alexandria, VA 22315
703-836-0850
888-258-4295
journalofrehab@email.arizona.edu
nationalrehab.org/journal-of-rehabilitation
Wendy Parent-Johnson, Editor
Official journal of the National Rehabilitation Association.
Quarterly

2291 Journal of School Health Association
Suite 403
4340 East West Highway
Bethesda, MD 20814
301-652-8072
Fax: 301-652-8077
info@ashaweb.org
ashaweb.org
Jeffrey K. Clark, President
Stephen Conley, Executive Director
Julie Greenfield, Marketing and Conferences Direct
Beverly Samek, Chair of Advocacy
This is a monthly journal which offers information to professionals and parents on school health. Membership dues, $95.00.

2292 Journal of Special Education
Sage Publications
2455 Teller Road
Thousand Oaks, CA 91320
805-499-0721
800-818-7243
Fax: 800-583-2665
info@sagepub.com
www.sagepub.com
Sara Miller McCune, Founder, Publisher & Executive Chairman
Blaise R. Simqu, President & CEO
Chris Hickok, Senior Vice President & Chief Financial Officer
Stephen Barr, Managing Director/SAGE London
Internationally known as the prime research journal in special education. JSE provides research articles of special education for individuals with disabilities, ranging from mild to severe. Published quarterly. *$39.00*
Magazine

2293 Journal of Vocational Behavior
Academic Press, Journals Division

2294 Learning Disabilities: A Contemporary Journal
179 Bear Hill Rd.
Suite 104
Waltham, MA 02451
978-897-5399
Fax: 978-897-5355
help@ldworldwide.org
www.ldw-ldcj.org
Matthias Grunke, Editor
Teresa Allissa Citro, Editor
Marco G. P. Hessels, Associate Editor
Erin K. Washburn, Associate Editor
Learning Disabilities: A Contemporary Journal (LDCJ) is a peer-reviewed forum for research, practice, and opinion regarding learning disabilities (LD) and associated disorders.

2295 Learning Disabilities: A Multidisciplinary Journal
Learning Disabilities Association of America
461 Cochran Rd.
Suite 245
Pittsburgh, PA 15228
412-341-1515
Fax: 412-344-0224
info@ldaamerica.org
www.ldaamerica.org
Cindy Cipoletti, Executive Director
The journal is a vehicle for disseminating the most current thinking on learning disabilities and to provide information on research, practice, theory, issues, and trends regarding learning disabilities from the perspectives of varied disciplines involved in broadening the understanding of learning disabilities.

2296 Learning Disability Quarterly
2455 Teller Road
Thousand Oaks, CA 91320
800-818-7243
Fax: 800-583-2665
journals@sagepub.com
ldq.sagepub.com
Blaise R. Simqu, President/ CEO
Tracey A. Ozmina, EVP/ COO
Chris Hickok, SVP/ CFO
Phil Denvir, Global Chief Information Officer
Learning Disability Quarterly (LDQ) publishes high-quality research and scholarship concerning children, youth, and adults with learning disabilities.

2297 MDA/ALS Newsmagazine
Muscular Dystrophy Association
161 N Clark
Suite 3550
Chicago, IL 60601
800-572-1717
alsn.mda.org
Lynn O'Connor Vos, President & CEO
Presents news related to muscular dystrophy and other neuromuscular diseases including research, personal profiles, fundraising activities and patient services.

2298 Movement Disorders
555 East Wells Street
Suite 1100
Milwaukee, WI 53202- 3823
414-276-2145
Fax: 414-276-3349
info@movementdisorders.org
www.movementdisorders.org
Matthew B. Stern, President
Oscar S. Gershanik, President-Elect
Francisco Cardoso, Secretary
Christopher Goetz, Treasurer
Movement Disorders, the official Journal of the International Parkinson and Movement Disorder Society (MDS), is a highly read and referenced journal covering all topics of the field - both clinical and basic science.

2299 People & Families
PO Box 700
Trenton, NJ 8625-700
609-292-345
800-792-8858
Fax: 609-292-7114
TTY: 609-777-3238
njcdd@njcdd.org
www.njcdd.org
Kevin T. Jonathan, Waller
Editor

People & Families, the NJCDD's nationally recognized magazine, focuses on issues of importance to the developmental disabilities community in New Jersey.

2300 **Psychiatric Staffing Crisis in Community Mental Health**
Nat l Council for Community Behavioral Healthcare
76 Ninth Avenue
New York, NY 10011
201-559-3882
800-THE-BOOK
amilevoj@bn.com
www.barnesandnoble.com
Andy Milevoj, Vice President, Investor Relations
Mary Ellen Keating, SVP, Corporate Communications & Public Affairs
Carolyn Brown, Director of Corporate Communications
Find out some of the simple, low-cost ways you can increase workplace satisfaction among staff psychiatrists and compete successfully for their talents. *$20.00*

2301 **Quest Magazine**
Muscular Dystrophy Association
161 N Clark
Suite 3550
Chicago, IL 60601
800-572-1717
ResourceCenter@mdausa.org
www.mda.org/quest
Lynn O'Connor Vos, President & CEO
Magazine of the Muscular Dystrophy Association.

2302 **Readings: A Journal of Reviews and Commentary in Mental Health**
American Orthopsychiatric Association
3524 Washington Avenue
P.O. Box 1048
Sheboygan, WI 53081-1048
920-457-5051
800-558-7687
Fax: 920-457-1485
info@americanortho.com
www.americanortho.com
Michael Bogenschuetz, President
Randy Benz, Chief Executive Officer
Charles Achter, Assistant Controller
Deb Schmidt, Administrative Manager
Reviews of recent books in mental health and allied disciplines. Includes essay reviews and brief reviews. *$25.00*
32 pages Quarterly

2303 **Rehab Pro**
1926 Waukegan Rd
Suite 1
Glenview, IL 60025-1770
847-657-6964
Fax: 847-657-6963
carlw@tcag.com
www.rehabpro.org
Carl Wangman, Executive Director
The magazine is to promote the profession and to inform the public about the activities of the national organization, its state chapter affiliates, and the work of its special interest sections.
38 pages BiMonthly

2304 **Remedial and Special Education**
Sage Publications
2455 Teller Road
Thousand Oaks, CA 91320
805-499-0721
800-818-7243
Fax: 800-583-2665
info@sagepub.com
www.sagepub.com
Sara Miller McCune, Founder, Publisher & Executive Chairman
Blaise R. Simqu, President & CEO
Chris Hickok, Senior Vice President & Chief Financial Officer
Stephen Barr, Managing Director/SAGE London
A professional journal that bridges the gap between theory and practice. Emphasis is on topical reviews, syntheses of research, field evaluation studies and recommendations for the practice of remedial and special education. Published six times a year. *$39.00*
64 pages

2305 **Structural Integration: The Journal of the Rolf Institute**
5055 Chaparral Ct.
Suite 103
Boulder, CO 80301
303-449-5903
Fax: 303-449-5978
www.rolf.org
Christina Howe, Executive Director
Mary Contreras, Director, Admissions & Recruitment
Samantha Sherwin, Director, Financial Aid & Compliance
Pat Heckmann, Director, Operations & Systems Management
Professional journal consisting of articles on research, practice building, faculty perspectives, reviews, and other topics relating to the field of Rolfing Structural Integration.

2306 **Teaching Exceptional Children (TEC)**
Council for Exceptional Children
3100 Clarendon Blvd.
Suite 600
Arlington, VA 22201-5332
888-232-7733
TTY: 866-915-5000
service@exceptionalchildren.org
www.exceptionalchildren.org
Dawn Rowe, Ph.D, Academic Editor
Journal designed for teachers of gifted students and students with disabilities, featuring practical methods and materials for classroom use.
61 pages BiMonthly

Newsletters

2307 **APA Access**
750 First Street, NE
Washington, DC 20002-4242
202-336-5500
800-374-2721
rllowman@gmail.com
www.apa.org
Rodney L. Lowman, PhD, Chair
Barry Anton, PhD, President
Bonnie Markham, PhD, PsyD, Treasurer
Norman Anderson, PhD, CEO, EVP
Exclusively for APA members, APA Access provides a helpful insider's view of the latest APA news. Each monthly issue highlights an array of current topics, such as advocacy updates, continuing education opportunities, press releases, previews of Monitor on Psychology articles, APA publishing news, new APA products and a calendar of events.

2308 **Alert**
Association on Handicapped Student Service Program
P.O. Box 21192
Columbus, OH 43221
614-365-5216
Fax: 614-365-6718

2309 **Children's Mental Health and EBD E-news**
PACER Center
8161 Normandale Blvd.
Bloomington, MN 55437
952-838-9000
800-537-2237
Fax: 952-838-0199
pacer@pacer.org
www.pacer.org
Paula F. Goldberg, Executive Director
Newsletter providing resources for parents with children affected by mental health and emotional or behavioral issues.

2310 **Counseling Today**
American Counseling Association
6101 Stevenson Ave.
Suite 600
Alexandria, VA 22304
703-823-9800
800-347-6647
Fax: 800-473-2329
ct.counseling.org
Richard Yep, Chief Executive Officer
Aims to serve individuals active in professional counseling, as well as other citizens, community leaders and policy makers who appreciate the importance of the role of professional counselors in today's society. The publication features news and articles on

professional counseling developments, resources, strategies, regulations, and more.
Monthly

2311 **Disability Compliance for Higher Education**
LRP Publications
P.O. Box 24668
West Palm Beach, FL 33416-4668
561-622-2423
800-341-7874
Fax: 561-622-1375
custserve@lrp.com
lrp.com
Kenneth F. Kahn, Owner and President
Ed Chase, Vice President
The only newsletter that is dedicated to the exclusive coverage of disability issues that affect colleges and universities. *$195.00*
8 pages Monthly

2312 **Disability Pride Newsletter**
900 Rebecca Avenue
Pittsburgh, PA 15221
800-633-4588
Fax: 412-371-9430
lgray@trcil.org
Rachel Rogan, CEO
Gregory Daigle, Chief Financial Officer
Lisa Wilson, HR Program Manager
Victoria Johnson, Human Resources Assistant
Three Rivers Center for Independent Living (TRCIL) is a non-residential, non-profit, community-based human service organization. There purpose is to assist people with disabilities to lead self-directed and productive lives within the community.

2313 **Disability Resources Monthly**
Disability Resources
4 Glatter Ln
South Setauket, NY 11720-1032
631-585-0290
Fax: 631-585-0290
Avery Klauber, Executive Director
A newsletter that monitors, reviews and reports on resources for independent living. A monthly newsletter that features short topical articles, news items and reviews of books, pamphlets, periodicals, videotapes, on-line services, organizations and other resources for and about people with disabilities. It is intended primarily for librarians, social workers, educators, rehabilitation specialists, disability advocates, ADA coordinators and other health and social service professionals. *$33.00*
4 pages Monthly
ISSN 1070-72 0

2314 **Early Childhood Reporter**
LRP Publications
P.O. Box 24668
West Palm Beach, FL 33416-4668
561-622-2423
800-341-7874
Fax: 561-622-1375
custserve@lrp.com
www.lrp.com
Kenneth F. Kahn, Owner and President
Ed Chase, Vice President
Monthly reports with information on federal, state, and local legislation affecting the implementation of early intervention and preschool programs for children with disabilities. *$145.00*
12-16 pages $10 shipping

2315 **FYI**
AAIDD
8403 Colesville Rd.
Suite 900
Silver Spring, MD 20910
202-387-1968
Fax: 202-387-2193
aaidd.org
Margaret A. Nygren, Executive Director & CEO
Kathleen McLane, Director, Publications Program
A monthly newsletter that provides news about AAIDD resources, educational opportunities, and activities.

2316 **Family Engagement**
PACER Center
8161 Normandale Blvd.
Bloomington, MN 55437
952-838-9000
800-537-2237
Fax: 952-838-0199
pacer@pacer.org
www.pacer.org
Paula F. Goldberg, Executive Director
E-newsletter providing parents and professionals with resources for supporting family engagement with schools.

2317 **Fellow Insider**
AAIDD
8403 Colesville Rd.
Suite 900
Silver Spring, MD 20910
202-387-1968
Fax: 202-387-2193
aaidd.org
Margaret A. Nygren, Executive Director & CEO
Kathleen McLane, Director, Publications Program
Quarterly newsletter for Fellows of the American Association on Intellectual and Developmental Disabilities.

2318 **Field Notes**
AAIDD
8403 Colesville Rd.
Suite 900
Silver Spring, MD 20910
202-387-1968
Fax: 202-387-2193
aaidd.org
Margaret A. Nygren, Executive Director & CEO
Kathleen McLane, Director, Publicatons Program
A monthly newsletter providing summaries of studies published in peer reviewed journals, along with links to the original articles.

2319 **Gram Newsletter, The**
PO Box 1114
Claremont, CA 91711
909-621-1494
Arline Krieger, President
Pam Hamilton, 1st Vice-President
EunMi Cho, 3rd Vice-President
William McKinley, Treasurer
The Learning Disabilities Association of California's (LDA-CA's) quarterly newsletter, The GRAM, provides LDA-CA members with timely information.

2320 **Growing Readers**
LD Online
2775 S. Quincy St.
Arlington, VA
Fax: 703-998-2060
ldonline@weta.org
www.ldonline.org
Noel Gunther, Executive Director
Christian Lindstrom, Director, Learning Media
Monthly tips for raising strong readers and writers, written especially for parents. Used by schools and PTAs in parent newsletters, and by libraries and community literacy organizations.

2321 **Healthline**
CV Mosby Company
1600 John F. Kennedy Boulevard
Suite 1800
Philadelphia, PA 19103-2822
215-239-3900
800-523-1649
Fax: 215-239-3990
www.us.elsevierhealth.com
Monthly

2322 **Help Newsletter**
Learning Disabilities Association of Arkansas
P.O. Box 23514
Little Rock, AR 72221
501-666-8777
Fax: 501-666-8777
www.ldaarkansas.org
Nathan Green, President
Rebecca Walker, VP
Becca Green, Past President, Treasurer
Doris Pierce, Secretary

Information on how to overcome obstacles and to achieve in spite of learning disabilities. *$30.00*
8 pages Quarterly

2323 **HerbalEGram**
American Botanical Council
6200 Manor Rd.
PO Box 144345
Austin, TX 78714-4345
512-926-4900
800-373-7105
Fax: 512-926-2345
abc@herbalgram.org
herbalgram.org
Mark Blumenthal, Founder, Executive Director & Editor
Hannah Bauman, Assistant Editor
Electronic newsletter of the American Botanical Council, with current editions available to members only.

2324 **Insights**
135 Parkinson Avenue
Staten Island, NY 10305
800-223-2732
Fax: 718-981-4399
apda@apdaparkinson.org
www.apdaparkinson.org
Fred Greene, Chairman
Patrick McDermott, 1st Vice Chairman
Jerry Wells, Esq., Secretary
Elena Imperato, Treasurer
APDA was founded in 1961 with the dual purpose to Ease the Burden - Find the Cure for Parkinson's disease.

2325 **Inspiring Possibilities**
PACER Center
8161 Normandale Blvd.
Bloomington, MN 55437
952-838-9000
800-537-2237
Fax: 952-838-0199
pacer@pacer.org
www.pacer.org
Paula F. Goldberg, Executive Director
From PACER's National Parent Center on Transition and Employment, the e-newsletter provides news and updates for youth with disabilities transitioning from school to the workforce.

2326 **LD Monthly Report**
LD Online
2775 S. Quincy St.
Arlington, VA
Fax: 703-998-2060
ldonline@weta.org
www.ldonline.org
Noel Gunther, Executive Director
Christian Lindstrom, Director, Learning Media
LD OnLine seeks to help children and adults reach their full potential by providing accurate and up-to-date information and advice about learning disabilities and ADHD.

2327 **MA Report**
National Allergy and Asthma Network
Ste 200
3554 Chain Bridge Rd
Fairfax, VA 22030-2709
703-385-4403
Fax: 703-352-4354
Monthly

2328 **Member Update**
AAIDD
8403 Colesville Rd.
Suite 900
Silver Spring, MD 20910
202-387-1968
Fax: 202-387-2193
aaidd.org
Margaret A. Nygren, Executive Director & CEO
Kathleen McLane, Director, Publications Program
A weekly newsletter providing updates on professional development opportunities, including conferences and webinars, job postings, calls for papers, and opportunities to join advisory committees and provide comments on federal initiatives.

2329 **National Bullying Prevention Center Newsletter**
PACER Center
8161 Normandale Blvd.
Bloomington, MN 55437
952-838-9000
800-537-2237
Fax: 952-838-0199
pacer@pacer.org
www.pacer.org
Paula F. Goldberg, Executive Director
Provides resources from PACER's National Bullying Prevention Center (NBPC). Publishes information on bullying prevention as well as news on anti-bullying events. Published quarterly and during National Bullying Prevention Month in October.

2330 **O&P Almanac**
American Orthotic & Prosthetic Association
330 John Carlyle Street
Suite 200
Alexandria, VA 22314
571-431-0876
Fax: 571-431-0899
info@aopanet.org
www.aopanet.org
Anita Liberman-Lampear, MA, President
Charles H. Dankmeyer, Jr, CPO, President-Elect
James Campbell, CO, Ph.D., Vice President
Jim Weber, MBA, Treasurer
Offers in-depth coverage on orthotics and prosthetics to current professional, government, business and reimbursement activities affecting the orthotics and prosthetics industry. *$59.00*
80 pages Monthly

2331 **Occupational Therapy in Health Care**
Haworth Press
711 Third Avenue
New York, NY 10017
212-216-7800
800-354-1420
Fax: 212-244-1563
subscriptions@tandf.co.uk
www.haworthpress.com

2332 **Ohio Coalition for the Education of Children with Disabilities**
165 W Center St, 3rd Floor, Chase B
Suite 302
Marion, OH 43302
740-382-5452
800-374-2806
Fax: 740-383-6421
ocecd@ocecd.org
www.ocecd.org
Martha Lause, Manager
Lee Ann Derugen, Co-Director
Margaret Burley, Executive Director
Lee Ann Derugen, Co-Director
Forum is a newsletter reporting on educational, legislative and other developments affecting persons with disabilities.
8 pages

2333 **PACER E-News**
PACER Center
8161 Normandale Blvd.
Bloomington, MN 55437
952-838-9000
800-537-2237
Fax: 952-838-0199
pacer@pacer.org
www.pacer.org
Paula F. Goldberg, Executive Director
E-newsletter providing information on special events and other news. Published monthly.

2334 **PACER Partners**
PACER Center
8161 Normandale Blvd.
Bloomington, MN 55437
952-838-9000
800-537-2237
Fax: 952-838-0199
pacer@pacer.org
www.pacer.org
Paula F. Goldberg, Executive Director
Published by PACER's Development Office, the newsletter connects families, friends, donors, and the staff of PACER.

2335 PACESETTER
PACER Center
8161 Normandale Blvd.
Bloomington, MN 55437
952-838-9000
800-537-2237
Fax: 952-838-0199
pacer@pacer.org
www.pacer.org
Paula F. Goldberg, Executive Director
Provides resources and information on special education and PACER programs. PACER's main newsletter.

2336 SAMHSA News
US Department of Health and Human Services
5600 Fishers Lane
Rockville, MD 20857
877-726-4727
TTY: 800-487-4889
samhsainfo@samhsa.hhs.gov
www.samhsa.gov
Tom Coderre, Acting Assistant Secretary
Sonia Chessen, Chief of Staff
This quarterly agency newsletter reports on information on substance abuse, mental health treatment and prevention programs of the Substance Abuse and Mental Health Services Administration.
Quarterly

2337 Sibling Information Network Newsletter
AJ Pappanikou Center
270 Farmington Avenue
Suite 181
Farmington, CT 06030
860-679-1500
866-623-1315
Fax: 860-679-1571
TTY: 860-679-1502
contact.us.ucedd@uchc.edu
www.uconnucedd.org
Mary Beth Bruder, PhD, UCEDD/LEND Director
Gerarda Hanna, J.D., M.Ed., Associate UCEDD Director
Gabriela Freyre-Calish, MSW, Coordinator, Director, Cultural Diversity
Linda Procko, Program Coordinator
Contains information aimed at the varying interested of our membership. Program descriptions, requests for assistance, conference announcements, literature summaries and research reports.
$8.50

2338 Sibpage
AJ Pappanikou Center
270 Farmington Avenue
Suite 181
Farmington, CT 06030
860-679-1500
866-623-1315
Fax: 860-679-1571
TTY: 860-679-1502
contact.us.ucedd@uchc.edu
www.uconnucedd.org
Mary Beth Bruder, PhD, UCEDD/LEND Director
Gerarda Hanna, J.D., M.Ed., Associate UCEDD Director
Gabriela Freyre-Calish, MSW, Coordinator, Director, Cultural Diversity
Linda Procko, Program Coordinator
Developed specifically for children containing games, recipes, pen pals, and articles written by siblings relating to developmental disabilities.
4 pages

2339 Special Edge
Resources in Special Education
Fl 4
1107 9th St
Sacramento, CA 95814-3616
916-492-9999
877-493-7833
Fax: 916-492-4004
Virigina Reynolds, President
Provides education news, collaborative programs, amendments to the laws, tools for accommodations, resource information, a calendar of events, and more.
BiMonthly

2340 Special Education Report
LRP Publications
360 Hiatt Dr
Dept. 150F
Palm BeachGardens, FL 33418
800-341-7874
Fax: 561-622-2423
custserve@lrp.com
lrp.com
Current, pertinent information about federal legislation, regulations, programs and funding for educating children with disabilities. Covers federal and state litigation on the Individuals with Disabilities Education Act and other relevant laws. Looks at innovations and research in the field.

2341 Topics in Early Childhood Special Education
Sage Publications
2455 Teller Road
Thousand Oaks, CA 91320
805-499-0721
800-818-7243
Fax: 800-583-2665
info@sagepub.com
www.sagepub.com
Sara Miller McCune, Founder, Publisher & Executive Chairman
Blaise R. Simqu, President & CEO
Chris Hickok, Senior Vice President & Chief Financial Officer
Stephen Barr, Managing Director/SAGE London
Designed for professionals helping young children with special needs in areas such as assessment, special programs, social policies and developmental aids. *$43.00*
Quarterly

2342 Treatment Review
AIDS Treatment Data Network
57 Willoughby St.
2nd Floor
Brooklyn, NY 11201
347-473-7400
800-734-7104
TTY: 212-925-9560
info@housingworks.org
www.housingworks.org
Charles King, Chair
Linney Smith, Vice Chair
Earl Ward, Vice Chair
Andrew Coarney, Secretary
Individual members receive treatment education, counseling, referrals and case management support. Services are available in both English and Spanish. The Treatment Review newsletter includes descriptions of approved, alternative and experimental treatments, as well as announcements of seminars and forums on treatments and clinical trials.
Quarterly

2343 VIP Newsletter
Blind Children's Fund
6761 West US 12
P.O. Box 363
Three Oaks, MI 49128
989-779-9966
Fax: 269-756-3133
www.blindchildrensfund.org
Karla B. Kwast, Executive Director
Jeremy Murphy, President
Robert R. Storrer Jr., Vice President
Carrie L. Owens, Director
Provides parents and professionals with information, materials and resources that help them successfully teach and nurture blind, visually and multi-impaired infants and preschoolers. *$10.00*

Professional Texts

2344 7 Steps for Success
Council for Exceptional Children
3100 Clarendon Blvd.
Suite 600
Arlington, VA 22201-5332
888-232-7733
TTY: 866-915-5000
service@exceptionalchildren.org
www.exceptionalchildren.org

Elizabeth C. Hamblet, Author

A book helping young adults with disabilities transitioning from high school to college.

2345 A Guide to Teaching Students With Autism Spectrum Disorders
Council for Exceptional Children
3100 Clarendon Blvd.
Suite 600
Arlington, VA 22201-5332
888-232-7733
TTY: 866-915-5000
service@exceptionalchildren.org
www.exceptionalchildren.org

Monica E. Delano, Co-Author
Darlene E. Perner, Co-Author

This book is a resource for all special educators and general educators who work with students with autism spectrum disorders (ASD). The underlying premise is that students with ASD should be explicitly taught a full range of social, self-help, language, reading, writing and math skills, as are their typically developing classmates.

2346 A Teacher's Guide to Isovaleric Acidemia
150 North 18th Avenue
Phoenix, AZ 85007
602-542-1025
Fax: 602-542-0883
www.azdhs.gov

Will Humble, Director
Thomas Salow, Manager

Resource book for preschool teachers and school staff on isovaleric academia basics and classroom activities. *$2.50*

2347 A Teacher's Guide to Methylmalonic Acidemia
Arizona State Department of Health Services
150 North 18th Avenue
Phoenix, AZ 85007
602-542-1025
Fax: 602-542-0883
www.azdhs.gov

Will Humble, Director
Thomas Salow, Manager

Resource book for preschool teachers and school staff on methylmalonic academia basics and classroom activities. *$2.50*

2348 A Teacher's Guide to PKU
Arizona Department of Health Services
150 North 18th Avenue
Phoenix, AZ 85007
602-542-1025
Fax: 602-542-0883
www.azdhs.gov

Will Humble, Director
Thomas Salow, Manager

Resource book for preschool teachers and school staff on PKU basics, NutraSweet warning, and classroom activities. *$2.50*
13 pages

2349 AD/HD and the College Student: The Everything Guide to Your Most Urgent Questions
750 First Street, NE
Washington, DC 20002-4242
202-336-5500
800-374-2721
rllowman@gmail.com
www.apa.org

Patricia O. Quinn, MD, Author

Whether you are looking for information or facing an urgent situation,AD/HD and the College Studentprovides answers to your most pressing questions. Organized in a question-and-answer format, this guide is loaded with helpful information, practical tips, and resources.

2350 ADD Challenge: A Practical Guide for Teachers
2612 N. Mattis Ave.
P.O. Box 7886
Champaign, IL 61822
217-352-3273
800-519-2707
Fax: 217-352-1221
orders@researchpress.com
www.researchpress.com

Robert W. Parkinson, Founder
Steven B. Gordon, Author
Dr Richard M Foxx, Author
Michael J. Asher, Author

Research Press is an independent, family-owned business founded in 1968 by Robert W. Parkinson (1920-2001).

2351 ADHD Coaching: A Guide for Mental Health Professionals
750 First Street, NE
Washington, DC 20002-4242
202-336-5500
800-374-2721
rllowman@gmail.com
www.apa.org

Frances Prevatt, PhD, Co-Author
Abigail Levrini, PhD, Co-Author

This book describes the underlying principles as well as the nuts and bolts of ADHD coaching. Step-by-step details for gathering information, conducting the intake, establishing goals and objectives, and working through all stages of coaching are included, along with helpful forms and a detailed list of additional resources.

2352 ADHD in the Classroom: Strategies for Teachers
Guilford Publication
72 Spring Street
New York, NY 10012
212-431-9800
800-365-7006
Fax: 212-966-6708
info@guilford.com
www.guilford.com

Bob Matloff, President
Seymour Weingarten, Editor-in-Chief
Russell A. Barkley, Author
Gary Stoner, Author

Designed specifically to help teachers with their ADHD students, thereby providing a better learning environment for the entire class. *$95.00*
ISBN 0-898629-85-3

2353 ADHD in the Schools: Assessment and Intervention Strategies
72 Spring Street
New York, NY 10012
212-431-9800
800-365-7006
Fax: 212-966-6708
info@guilford.com
www.guilford.com

Bob Matloff, President
Seymour Weingarten, Editor-in-Chief
George J. DuPaul, Author
Gary Stoner, Author

The landmark volume emphasizes the need for a team effort among parents, community-based professionals, and educators. Provides practical information for educators that is based on empirical findings. Chapters Focus on how to identify and assess students who might have ADHD, the relationship between ADHD and learning disabilities; how to develop and supplement classroom-based programs. Communication strategies to assist physicians and the need for community-based treatments *$36.00*
269 pages Paperback
ISBN 0-898622-45-X

2354 AEPS Curriculum for Birth to Three Years
Brookes Publishing
P.O. Box 10624
Baltimore, MD 21285-0624
410-337-9580
800-638-3775
Fax: 410-337-8539
custserv@brookespublishing.com
readplaylearn.com

496 pages
ISBN 1-557660-96-4

2355 Access to Health Care
World Institute on Disability
3075 Adeline St.
Suite 155
Berkeley, CA 94703
510-225-6400
Fax: 510-225-0477
wid@wid.org
www.wid.org

Marcie Roth, Executive Director & CEO
Katherine Zigmont, Senior Director, Operations & Deputy Director
Reggie Johnson, Senior Director, Marketing & Communications
Marsha Saxton, Director, Research

Policy bulletins focusing on the capacity of the private and public health insurance systems to respond to the health care needs of persons with disabilities or chronic illness.

2356 Activity-Based Approach to Early Intervention, 2nd Edition
Brookes Publishing
P.O. Box 10624
Baltimore, MD 21285-0624
410-337-9580
800-638-3775
Fax: 410-337-8539
webmaster@brookespublishing.com
www.brookespublishing.com

Paul H. Brookes, Chairman of the Board
Jeffrey D. Brookes, President
George S. Stamathis, VP/Publisher
Melissa A. Behn, Executive Vice President

Activity-based intervention shows how to use natural and relevant events to teach infants and young children, of all abilities, effectively and efficiently. *$24.00*
240 pages
ISBN 1-55766 -87-5

2357 Adapted Physical Education for Students with Autism
Charles C. Thomas
2600 S First St
Springfield, IL 62704-4730
217-789-8980
800-258-8980
Fax: 217-789-9130
books@ccthomas.com
www.ccthomas.com

Kimberly Davis, Author

Focuses on the physical education needs and curriculum for autistic children. Available in cloth, paperback and hardcover. *$27.95*
142 pages Paper
ISBN 0-398060-85-1

2358 Adapting Early Childhood Curricula for Children with Special Needs (9th Edition)
Pearson Higher Education
330 Hudson St
New York, NY 10013
212-641-2400
www.pearsonhighered.com

Ruth E. Cook, Author
M. Diane Klein, Author
Deborah Chen, Author

This highly readable, well researched, and current resource uses a developmental focus, rather than a disability orientation, to discuss typical and atypical child development and curricular adaptations, and encourage the treatment of students as children first, without regard to their learning differences. *$102.67*
528 pages Loose-Leaf or Access Code Card 1915
ISBN 0-134019-41-3

2359 Adapting Instruction for the Mainstream: A Sequential Approach to Teaching
McGraw-Hill School Publishing
P.O. Box 182605
Columbus, OH 43218
800-338-3987
Fax: 609-308-4480
customer.service@mheducation.com
mcgraw-hill.com

David Levin, President, CEO
Ellen Haley, President, CTB
Peter Cohen, President, School Education
Mark Dorman, President, International

This text gives both regular and special education teachers everything they need to help mildly handicapped students succeed in the mainstream.
226 pages

2360 Adaptive Education Strategies Building on Diversity
Brookes Publishing Company
P.O. Box 10624
Baltimore, MD 21285-0624
410-337-9580
800-638-3775
Fax: 410-337-8539
webmaster@brookespublishing.com
www.brookespublishing.com

Paul H. Brookes, Chairman of the Board
Jeffrey D. Brookes, President
George S. Stamathis, VP/Publisher
Melissa A. Behn, Executive Vice President

Based on more than two decades of systematic research, this comprehensive manual provides a road map to the effective implementation of adaptive education. *$35.00*
304 pages Paperback
ISBN 1-557880-84-0

2361 Adolescents and Adults with Learning Disabilities and ADHD
370 Seventh Avenue
Suite 1200
New York, NY 10001-1020
800-365-7006
Fax: 212-966-6708
info@guilford.com
www.guilford.com

No%l Gregg, PhD, Author

Most of the literature on learning disabilities and attention-deficit/hyperactivity disorder (ADHD) focuses on the needs of elementary school-age children, but older students with these conditions also require significant support.

2362 Advanced Sign Language Vocabulary: A Resource Text for Educators
Charles C. Thomas
2600 S First St
Springfield, IL 62704-4730
217-789-8980
800-258-8980
Fax: 217-789-9130
books@ccthomas.com
www.ccthomas.com

Elizabeth E. Wolf, Author
Janet R. Coleman, Author

This book is a collection of advanced sign language vocabulary for use by educators, interpreters, parents or anyone wishing to enlarge their sign vocabulary. *$53.95*
202 pages Spiralbound
ISBN 0-398057-22-2

2363 Advances in Cardiac and Pulmonary Rehabilitation
Haworth Press
711 Third Avenue
New York, NY 10017
212-216-7800
800-354-1420
Fax: 212-244-1563
subscriptions@tandf.co.uk
www.haworthpress.com

74 pages Hardcover
ISBN 0-866869-86-3

2364 Aging Brain
Taylor & Francis Group
Ste 800
325 Chestnut St
Philadelphia, PA 19106-2608
215-625-8900
800-354-1420
Fax: 215-625-2940
www.taylorandfrancisgroup.com

225 pages Paperback
ISBN 0-85066 -78-0

2365 Aging and Disability: Crossing Network Lines
Springer Publishing
11 West 42nd Street
15th Floor
New York, NY 10036
212-431-4370
877-687-7476
Fax: 212-941-7842
marketing@springerpub.com
springerpub.com

Theodore C. Nardin, CEO/Publisher
Jason Roth, VP/Marketing Director
Annette Imperati, Marketing/Sales Director
Stephanie Drew, Acquisitions Editor,Social Work

Michelle Putnam has set forth this volume to reflect the current research, facilitate collaboration across service networks, and encourage movement toward more effective service policies. Professional stakeholders evaluate the bridges and barriers to crossing network lines, and chapter on current websites, agencies, and coalitions provides the much needed tools to bring collaboration into practice.

2366 Aging and Rehabilitation II: The State ofthe Practice
Springer Publishing Company
11 W 42nd St
15th Fl
New York, NY 10036-8002
212-431-4370
877-687-7476
Fax: 212-941-7842
cs@springerpub.com
www.springerpub.com

Ted Nardin, chief Executive Officer
Jason Roth, Vice President, Marketing & Sales
Kathy Weiss, Senior Sales Director
Annette Imperati, Sales Director, Corporate, Government, & Associations

Current, multidisciplinary investigations of various practice issues. Leading experts in the field use a practical perspective to provide specific comments on interventions. The scope of this work encompasses the autonomy of elderly disabled, mobility, mental health and value issues, as well as basic aspects in rehabilitation of the elderly. *$8.95*

348 pages Hardcover 1990
ISBN 0-826170-80-3

2367 Alphabetic Phonics Curriculum
Educators Publishing Service
625 Mount Auburn Street
3rd Floor
Cambridge, MA 02138- 3039
617-547-6706
800-225-5750
Feedback.EPS@schoolspecialty.com
www.epsbooks.com

Rick Holden, President, EPS

Ungraded multisensory curriculum for teaching phonics and the structure of language. Uses Orton-Gillingham approach to teach handwriting, spelling, reading, reading comprehension, and oral and written expression. program includes basic manual, workbooks, tests, teachers' guides, drill cards and all cards. *$28.15*

ISSN 8388-42

2368 Alternative Educational Delivery Systems
National Association of School Psychologists
4340 East West Highway
Suite 402
Bethesda, MD 20814
301-657-0270
866-331-NASP
Fax: 301-657-0275
TTY: 301-657-4155
webmaster@naspweb.org
nasponline.org

Stephen E. Brock, President
Todd A. Savage, President-Elect
Laura Benson, Chief Operating Officer
Susan Gorin, Executive Director

A book offering information to the professional on how to enhance educational options for all students.

2369 Alternative Teaching Strategies
Special Needs Project
324 State Street
Suite H
Santa Barbara, CA 93101-2364
818-718-9900
800-333-6867
Fax: 818-349-2027
editor@specialneeds.com
www.specialneeds.com

Hod Gray, Owner

Offers help for teachers who teach behaviorally troubled students.

2370 Antecedent Control: Innovative Approaches to Behavioral Support
Brookes Publishing
P.O. Box 10624
Baltimore, MD 21285-0624
410-337-9580
800-638-3775
Fax: 410-337-8539
webmaster@brookespublishing.com
www.brookespublishing.com

Paul H. Brookes, Chairman of the Board
Jeffrey D. Brookes, President
George S. Stamathis, VP/Publisher
Melissa A. Behn, Executive Vice President

This book explains the theory and methodology of antecedent control. The treatment techniques in this book are effective for both children and adults.

416 pages Paperback
ISBN 1-55766 -34-3

2371 Anxiety-Free Kids: An Interactive Guide for Parents and Children
Prufrock Press
PO Box 8813
Waco, TX 76714-8813
800-998-2208
Fax: 800-240-0333
info@prufrock.com
www.prufrock.com

Joel McIntosh, Publisher & Marketing Director
Lacy Compton, Senior Editor
Rachel Taliaferro, Editor
Raquel Trevino, Graphic Designer and Production Coordinator

Offers parents strategies that help children happy and worry-free, methods that relieve a child's excessive anxieties and phobias, and tools for fostering interaction and family-oriented solutions. *$19.95*

280 pages Paperback
ISBN 1-593633-43-1

2372 **Applied Rehabilitation Counseling (Springer Series on Rehabilitation)**
Springer Publishing Company
11 W 42nd St
15th Fl
New York, NY 10036-8002
212-431-4370
877-687-7476
Fax: 212-941-7842
cs@springerpub.com
www.springerpub.com

Ted Nardin, Chief Executive Officer
Jason Roth, Vice President, Marketing & Sales
Kathy Weiss, Senior Sales Director
Annette Imperati, Sales Director, Corporate, Government, & Associations

This comprehensive text describes current theories, techniques, and their applications to specific disabled populations. Perspectives on varying counseling approaches such as psychodynamic, existential, gestalt, behavioral and psychoeducational orientations are systematically outlined in an easy-to-follow format. Practical applications for counseling are emphasized with attention given to strategies, goal-setting and on-going evaluations. *$43.95*
404 pages Paperback 1986
ISBN 0-826153-71-2

2373 **Art-Centered Education and Therapy for Children with Disabilities**
Charles C. Thomas
2600 S First St
Springfield, IL 62704-4730
217-789-8980
800-258-8980
Fax: 217-789-9130
books@ccthomas.com
www.ccthomas.com

Frances E. Anderson, Author

This book has been written to help both the regular education, and art and special education teachers, both pre- and in-service, better understand some of the issues and realities of providing education and remediation to children with disabilities. The book is also offered as model concept that has govern the author's personal and professional career of over thirty years. *$41.95*
284 pages Paperback
ISBN 0-398060-06-1

2374 **Assessing the Handicaps/Needs of Children**
Books on Special Children
P.O. Box 3378
Amherst, MA 01004-3378
413-256-8164
Fax: 413-256-8896

260 pages Hardcover
ISBN 0-12218 -02-0

2375 **Assessment & Management of Mainstreamed Hearing-Impaired Children**
Sage Publications
2455 Teller Road
Thousand Oaks, CA 91320
805-499-0721
800-818-7243
Fax: 800-583-2665
info@sagepub.com
www.sagepub.com

Sara Miller McCune, Founder, Publisher & Executive Chairman
Blaise R. Simqu, President & CEO
Chris Hickok, Senior Vice President & Chief Financial Officer
Stephen Barr, Managing Director/SAGE London

The theoretical and practical considerations of developing appropriate programming for hearing-impaired children who are being educated in mainstream educational settings are presented in this book.

2376 **Assessment Log & Developmental Progress Charts for the Carolina Curriculum**
Brookes Publishing
P.O. Box 10624
Baltimore, MD 21285-0624
410-337-9580
800-638-3775
Fax: 410-337-8539
webmaster@brookespublishing.com
www.brookespublishing.com

Paul H. Brookes, Chairman of the Board
Jeffrey D. Brookes, President
George S. Stamathis, VP/Publisher
Melissa A. Behn, Executive Vice President

This 28-page booklet allows the progress of children with skills in the 12-36 month development range to be easily recorded. Available in packages of 10. *$23.00*
28 pages Saddle-stiched
ISBN 1-557662-21-5

2377 **Assessment and Remediation of Articulatoryand Phonological Disorders**
McGraw-Hill School Publishing
PO Box 182604
Columbus, OH 43218
877-833-5524
800-338-3987
Fax: 609-308-4480
customer.service@mheducation.com
www.mcgraw-hill.com

David Levin, President/Chief Executive Officer
David Stafford, Senior Vice President/General Counsel
Maryellen Valaitis, Senior Vice President Human Resources
Patrick Milano, Chief Financial Officer/Chief Administrative Officer

Offers comprehensive coverage of articulation disorders.

2378 **Assessment in Mental Handicap: A Guide to Assessment Practices & Tests**
Brookline Books
8 Trumbull Rd
Suite B-001
Northampton, MA 01060
413-584-0184
800-666-2665
Fax: 413-584-6184
brbooks@yahoo.com
www.brooklinebooks.com

Esther Wilder, Co-Author

Helps professionals understand the rationale and uses for assessment practices, and provides details of appropriate instruments within each type: adaptive behavior scales, assessment of behavioral disturbances, early development and Plagetian tests. *$20.00*
Hardcover
ISBN 0-91479 -31-X

2379 **Assessment of Children and Youth**
Longman Education/Addison Wesley
1185 Avenue of the Americas
New York, NY 10036-2601
212-997-8500
866-203-6215
TTY: 800-231-5469
www.hess.com

Dr. Mark R. Williams, Chairman of the Board
Gregory P. Hill, President/COO
John B. Hess, Chief Executive Officer
Gary Boubel, Senior Vice President-Developments

Introductory text for preservice and in-service special educators on assessment, based on the principle that every child is unique. Comprehensive coverage of both formal and informal assessment instruments. *$50.00*
640 pages Paperback
ISBN 0-80131 -02-5

2380 **Assessment of Individuals with Severe Disabilities**
Brookes Publishing Company
PO Box 10624
Baltimore, MD 21285-0624
410-337-9580
800-638-3775
Fax: 410-337-8539
custserv@brookespublishing.com
www.brookespublishing.com
Paul H. Brookes, Chairman
Jeffrey D. Brookes, President
Melissa A. Behm, ExecutiveVice President
George S. Stamathis, Vice President & Publisher
This expanded text offers instructors guidelines to design a comprehensive educational assessment for individuals with severe disabilities. *$34.00*
432 pages Paperback
ISBN 1-557660-67-0

2381 **Assessment of the Technology Needs of Vending Facilitiy Managers In Tennessee**
Mississippi State University
108 Herbert - South
Room 150/PO Drawer 6189
Mississippi State Univers, MS 39762-6189
662-325-2001
800-675-7782
Fax: 662-325-8989
TTY: 662-325-2694
nrtc@colled.msstate.edu
www.blind.msstate.edu
Jacqui Bybee, Research and Training Coordinato
Michele Capella McDonnall, Ph.D., Research Professor/Interim Director
Jessica Thornton, Business Manager
Marty Giesen, Ph.D., Senior Research Scientist
This report summarizes the results and recommendations of a survey conducted of vending facility managers throughout the state of Tennessee who participate in the Randolph-Sheppard program. *$15.00*
39 pages Paperback

2382 **Assessment: The Special Educator's Role**
Brookes Publishing Company
PO Box 10624
Baltimore, MD 21285-0624
410-337-9580
800-638-3775
Fax: 410-337-8539
custserv@brookespublishing.com
www.brookespublishing.com
Paul H. Brooks, Chairman
Jeffrey D. Brookes, President
Melissa A. Behm, ExecutiveVice President
George S. Stamathis, Vice President & Publisher
Aimed at students with little or no classroom experience in assessment, the book focuses on the integration of dynamic, curriculum-based and norm-referenced data for diagnostic decisions and program planning.
580 pages Casebound
ISBN 0-53421 -32-1

2383 **Assistive Technology in the Schools: A Guide for Idaho Educators**
Idaho Assistive Technology Project
University of Idaho
1187 Alturas Dr.
Moscow, ID 83843- 8331
205-885-3557
800-432-8324
Fax: 208-885-6102
idahoat@uidaho.edu
www.idahoat.org
LaRhae Rhoads, Author
Ron Seiler, Author
Michelle Doty, Author
This manual is designed to provide educators, parents, students with disabilities and related service providers with assistance in identifying, selecting, and acquiring assistive technology (AT) devices and services.

2384 **Asthma Management and Education**
Asthma and Allergy Foundation of America
8201 Corporate Drive
Suite 1000
Landover, MD 20785
202-466-7643
800-727-8462
info@aafa.org
www.aafa.org
Lynn Hanessian, Chair
Mitchell Grayson, MD, Chair, Research
Barbara Corn, Chair, Governance
Calvin Anderson, Chair/Finance/Treasurer
One session, two hour program developed to educate allied health professionals about up-to-date asthma care and patient education, information and materials. Includes hands on experience with peak flow meters and demonstrations of medical devices.

2385 **Aston-Patterning**
PO Box 3568
Incline Village, NV 89450-3568
775-831-8228
Fax: 775-831-8955
office@astonkinetics.com
www.astonkinetics.com
J Aston, Owner
Angelina Calafiore, Office Manager
Integrated system of movement education, body assessment, environmental modification and fitness training.

2386 **Attention Deficit Disorder in Children**
Charles C. Thomas
2600 S First St
Springfield, IL 62704-4730
217-789-8980
800-258-8980
Fax: 217-789-9130
books@ccthomas.com
www.ccthomas.com

2387 **Aural Habilitation**
Alexander Graham Bell Association
3417 Volta Pl NW
Washington, DC 20007-2737
202-337-5220
Fax: 202-337-8314
TTY: 202-337-5221
info@agbell.org
www.listeningandspokenlanguage.org
Meredith K. Sugar, Esq. (OH), President
Ted A. Meyer, M.D., Ph.D, President-Elect/Secretary-Treasurer
Emilio Alonso-Mendoza, Chief Executive Officer
Susan Boswell, Director of Communications and Marketing
This classic text for professionals, educators and parents discusses verbal learning and aural habilitation of young children with hearing losses to ensure that each child is educated in the best setting. It discusses communication, normal development of spoken language, speech audiologic assessment, hearing aids and use of residual hearing, and program designs for individualized needs, including the assessment and planning of IEPs. *$26.95*
324 pages

2388 **Behavior Analysis in Education: Focus on Measurably Superior Instruction**
Brookes Publishing Company
PO Box 10624
Baltimore, MD 21285-0624
410-337-9580
800-638-3775
Fax: 410-337-8539
custserv@brookespublishing.com
www.brookespublishing.com
Paul H. Brookes, Chairman
Jeffrey D. Brookes, President
Melissa A. Behm, ExecutiveVice President
George S. Stamathis, Vice President & Publisher
Designed to disseminate measurably superior instructional strategies to those interested in advancing sound, pedagogically effective, field-tested educational practices, this book is intended for graduate-level courses and seminars in special education and/or psychology focusing on behavior analysis and instruction.
512 pages Casebound
ISBN 0-53422 -60-9

2389 **Behavior Modification**
Sage Publications
2455 Teller Rd
Thousand Oaks, CA 91320-2218
805-499-0721
800-818-7243
Fax: 800-583-2665
info@sagepub.com
www.sagepub.com
Sara Miller McCune, Founder, Publisher and Executive Chairman
Blaise R. Simqu, President & CEO
Chris Hickok, Senior Vice President & Chief Financial Officer
Stephen Barr, Managing Director/SAGE London
Describes in detail for replication purposes assessment and modification techniques for problems in psychiatric, clinical, educational and rehabilitation settings. *$53.00*
640 pages Quarterly

2390 **Behind Special Education**
Love Publishing Company
9101 E Kenyon Ave
Suite 2200
Denver, CO 80237-1854
303-221-7333
Fax: 303-221-7444
lpc@lovepublishing.com
www.lovepublishing.com
ISBN 0-89108 -17-4

2391 **Biomedical Concerns in Persons with Down's Syndrome**
Paul H Brookes Publishing Company
PO Box 10624
Baltimore, MD 21285-0624
410-337-9580
800-638-3775
Fax: 410-337-8539
custserv@brookespublishing.com
www.brookespublishing.com
Paul H. Brookes, Chairman
Jeffrey D. Brookes, President
Melissa A. Behm, ExecutiveVice President
George S. Stamathis, Vice President & Publisher
Written by leading authorities and spanning many disciplines and specialties, this comprehensive resource provides vital information on biomedical issues concerning individuals with Down's Syndrome. *$45.00*
336 pages Hardcover
ISBN 1-557660-89-1

2392 **Breaking Barriers**
AbleNet, Inc.
2625 Patton Road
Roseville, MN 55113-1137
651-294-2200
800-322-0956
Fax: 651-294-2259
customerservice@ablenetinc.com
www.ablenetinc.com
Bill Sproull, Chair of the Board
Jennifer Thalhuber, President & CEO
William Mills, Board of Directors
Paul Sugden, CFO & Trustee
A practical resource for parents, caregivers, teachers and therapists. *$15.00*

2393 **Building Skills for Independence in the Mainstream**
15619 Premiere Drive
Suite 101
Tampa, FL 33624
850-363-9909
Fax: 480-393-4331
accounting@successforkidswithhearingloss.com
successforkidswithhearinglo ss.com
Karen L. Anderson, Director/ Co-Author
Gale Wright, Co-Author
Building Skills for Independence in the Mainstream was developed as a Guide for DHH professionals to support their work with classroom teachers and with students to develop the skills needed for independence with hearing aids and self-advocacy.

2394 **Building Skills for Success in the Fast-Paced Classroom**
15619 Premiere Drive
Suite 101
Tampa, FL 33624
850-363-9909
Fax: 480-393-4331
accounting@successforkidswithhearingloss.com
successforkidswithhearinglo ss.com
Karen L. Anderson, PhD, Co-Author
Kathleen A. Arnoldi, MA
The purpose of this book is to provide resources that will assist these students in optimizing their achievement through improved access and self-advocacy. The information contained in this book targets the expanded core curriculum, or those skills that must be mastered in order to benefit from the core curriculum. This book is meant to be a practical ready-to-go resource for professionals who work with school-age children with hearing loss.

2395 **Building the Healing Partnership: Parents, Professionals and Children with Chronic Illnesses**
Brookline Books
8 Trumbull Rd
Ste B-001
Northampton, MA 01060
413-584-0184
800-666-2665
Fax: 413-584-6184
brbooks@yahoo.com
www.brooklinebks.com
Patricia Tanner Leff, Author
Elaine H. Walizer, Author
Successful programs understand that the disabled child's needs must be considered in the context of a family. This book was specifically written for practitioner's who must work with families but who have insufficient training in family systems assessment and intervention. It is a valuable blend of theory and practice with pointers for applying the principles. *$24.95*
312 pages Paperback 1992
ISBN 0-914797-60-3

2396 **CAI, Career Assessment Inventories for the Learning Disabled**
Academic Therapy Publications
20 Leveroni Crt
Novato, CA 94949-5746
415-883-3314
800-422-7249
Fax: 888-287-9975
sales@academictherapy.com
www.academictherapy.com
Carol Weller, Author
Mary Buchanan, Author
Takes personality, ability and interest into account in pointing learning disabled students of all ages toward intelligent and realistic career choices. Contains binder with paperback teaching guide plus 50 interest inventories and 50 abilities inventories.
64 pages 1983
ISBN 0-878793-50-X

2397 **Caring for Children with Chronic Illness**
11 W 42nd St
15th Floor
New York, NY 10036-8002
212-431-4370
877-687-7476
Fax: 212-941-7842
cs@springerpub.com
www.springerpub.com
Ursula Springer, President
Theodore C. Nardin, CEO/Publisher
Jason Roth, VP/Marketing Director
James C. Costello, Vice President, Journal Publishing
A critical look at the current medical, social, and psychological framework for providing care to children with chronic illnesses. Emphasizing the need to create integrated, interdisciplinary approaches, it discusses issues such as the roles of families, professionals, and institutions in providing health care, the impact of a child's illness on various family structures, financing care, the special problems of chronically ill children as they become adolescents and more. *$36.95*
320 pages Hardcover
ISBN 0-82615 -00-1

2398 Carolina Curriculum for Infants and Toddlers with Special Needs (3rd Edition)

Brookes Publishing
P.O. Box 10624
Baltimore, MD 21285-0624
410-337-9580
800-638-3775
Fax: 410-337-8539
custserv@brookespublishing.com
www.brookespublishing.com

Nancy M. Johnson-Martin, Author
Susan M. Attermeier, Author
Bonnie J. Hacker, Author

This book includes detailed assessment and intervention sequences, daily routine integration strategies, sensorimotor adaptations, and a sample 24-page assessment log that shows readers how to chart a child's individual progress.

504 pages Spiral-bound

2399 Carolina Curriculum for Preschoolers with Special Needs

Brookes Publishing
PO Box 10624
Baltimore, MD 21285-0624
410-337-9580
800-638-3775
Fax: 410-337-8539
custserv@brookespublishing.com
www.brookespublishing.com

Paul H. Brookes, Chairman
Jeffrey D. Brookes, President
Melissa A. Behm, ExecutiveVice President
George S. Stamathis, Vice President & Publisher

This curriculum provides detailed teaching and assessment techniques, plus a sample 28-page assessment log that shows readers how to chart a child's individual progress. This guide is for children between 2 and 5 in their developmental stages who are considered at risk for developmental delay or who exhibit special needs. *$34.00*

352 pages Spiral-bound
ISBN 1-55766 -32-8

2400 Challenge of Educating Together Deaf and Hearing Youth: Making Manistreaming Work

Charles C. Thomas
2600 S First St
Springfield, IL 62704-4730
217-789-8980
800-258-8980
Fax: 217-789-9130
books@ccthomas.com
www.ccthomas.com

198 pages Hardcover
ISBN 0-398063-91-5

2401 Challenged Scientists: Disabilities and the Triumph of Excellence

Greenwood Publishing Group
130 Cremona Drive
Santa Barbara, CA 93117
805-968-1911
800-368-6868
Fax: 866-270-3856
CustomerService@abc-clio.com
www.abc-clio.com

208 pages
ISBN 0-275938-73-5

2402 Child Care and the ADA: A Handbook for Inclusive Programs

Brookes Publishing
PO Box 10624
Baltimore, MD 21285-0624
410-337-9580
800-638-3775
Fax: 410-337-8539
custserv@brookespublishing.com
www.brookespublishing.com

Paul H. Brookes, Chairman
Jeffrey D. Brookes, President
Melissa A. Behm, ExecutiveVice President
George S. Stamathis, Vice President & Publisher

This book is designed for educators and administrators in child care settings. It offers a straightforward discussion of the Americans with Disabilities Act including children with disabilities in community programs. *$25.95*

240 pages Paperback
ISBN 1-55766 -85-5

2403 Child with Disabling Illness

Lippincott, Williams & Wilkins
16522 Hunters Green Pkwy
Hagerstown, MD 21740
301-223-2300
800-638-3030
Fax: 301-223-2400
orders@lww.com
www.lww.com

700 pages

2404 Childhood Behavior Disorders: Applied Research & Educational Practice

Sage Publications
2455 Teller Road
Thousand Oaks, CA 91320-2218
805-499-0721
800-818-7243
Fax: 800-583-2665
info@sagepub.com
www.sagepub.com

Sara Miller McCune, Founder, Publisher, Chairperson
Blaise R. Simqu, President/CEO
Chris Hickok, Senior Vice President & Chief Fi
Stephen Barr, Managing Director/SAGE London, P

The only comprehensive overview of childhood behavior disorders. This book gives you the how and why for helping children with behavior disorders.

2405 Childhood Disablity and Family Systems (Routledge Library Editions) (Volume 5)

Routledge (Taylor & Francis Group)
711 Third Ave
New York, NY 10017
212-216-7800
800-634-7064
Fax: 202-564-7854
enquiries@taylorandfrancis.com
www.routledge.com

Michael Ferrari, Editor
Marvin B. Sussman, Editor

Focuses on what the presence of a disabled child means to a family. Those professionals involved in teaching, research, and direct care with families having disabled children will value the coverage of such topics as the contemporary context of disability, ethical issues, family effects, and care systems. First published in 1987 by Haworth Press, the book is now published under Routledge. *$140.00*

256 pages Hardcover 1916
ISBN 1-138101-55-9

2406 Children and Youth Assisted by Medical Technology in Educational Settings, 2nd Edition

Brookes Publishing
PO Box 10624
Baltimore, MD 21285-0624
410-337-9580
800-638-3775
Fax: 410-337-8539
custserv@brookespublishing.com
www.brookespublishing.com

Paul H. Brookes, Chairman
Jeffrey D. Brookes, President
Melissa A. Behm, ExecutiveVice President
George S. Stamathis, Vice President & Publisher

Contains detailed daily care guidelines and emergency-response techniques, including information on working with a range of students who have the HIV infection, that rely on ventilators, that utilize tube feeding, or require catheterization. Also covers every aspect of planning for inclusive classrooms, including information on personnel training, entrance planning and transition, legal requirements, and transportation issues. *$52.00*

432 pages Spiral-bound
ISBN 1-55766 -36-3

2407 Children's Needs Psychological Perspective
National Association of School Psychologists
4340 East West Hwy.
Suite 402
Bethesda, MD 20814
301-657-0270
866-331-6277
Fax: 301-657-0275
TTY: 301-657-4155
www.nasponline.org
Kathleen Minke, Executive Director
Laura Benson, Chief Operating Officer
This monograph was developed with the recognition that many factors beyond the classroom and the child's own personal characteristics influence school success.
637 pages

2408 Choices: A Guide to Sex Counseling with Physically Disabled Adults
Krieger Publishing Company
1725 Krieger Dr
Malabar, FL 32950
321-724-9542
800-724-0025
Fax: 321-951-3671
info@krieger-publishing.com
www.krieger-publishing.com
Maureen E. Neistadt, Author
Provides rehabilitation professionals with the basic information necessary for limited sexuality counseling of physically disabled adults. *$20.90*
132 pages
ISBN 0-898749-03-4

2409 Choosing Options and Accommodations for Children
Brookes Publishing
PO Box 10624
Baltimore, MD 21285-0624
410-337-9580
800-638-3775
Fax: 410-337-8539
custserv@brookespublishing.com
www.brookespublishing.com
192 pages
ISBN 1-55766 -06-5

2410 Cirriculum Development for Students with Mild Disabilities
Charles C. Thomas
2600 S First St
Springfield, IL 62704-4730
217-789-8980
800-258-8980
Fax: 217-789-9130
books@ccthomas.com
www.ccthomas.com
Carroll J. Jones, Author
This book was designed to provide the foundation from which to write cirrocumuli that will provide academic and social skills for Individual Education Programs (IEPs). *$38.95*
258 pages Spiral-Paper
ISBN 0-398070-18-2

2411 Clinical Alzheimer Rehabilitation
Springer Publishing
11 W 42nd St
15th Floor
New York, NY 10036-8002
212-431-4370
877-687-7476
Fax: 212-941-7842
cs@springerpub.com
www.springerpub.com
Theodore C. Nardin, CEO/Publisher
Jason Roth, VP/Marketing Director
Annette Imperati, Marketing/Sales Director
James C. Costello, Vice President, Journal Publishing
This comprehensive and easy-to-read guidebook contains the latest research on dementia and AD in the elderly population, including the causes and risk factors of AD, diagnosis information, and symptoms and progressions of the disease. Significant emphasis is given to the physical, mental, and verbal rehabilitation challenges of patients with AD. The authors outline specific rehabilitation goals for the physical therapist, speech-language pathologist, and general caregiver.

2412 Clinical Management of Childhood Stuttering, 2nd Edition
Sage Publications
2455 Teller Road
Thousand Oaks, CA 91320-2218
805-499-0721
800-818-7243
Fax: 800-583-2665
info@sagepub.com
www.sagepub.com
Sara Miller McCune, Founder, Publisher, Chairperson
Blaise R. Simqu, President/CEO
Chris Hickok, Senior Vice President/CFO
Stephen Barr, Managing Director/SAGE London
Updates and integrates recent findings in childhood stuttering into a broad range of therapeutic strategies for assessing and treating the young dysfluent child. *$38.00*
336 pages

2413 Cognitive Approaches to Learning Disabilities
Sage Publications
2455 Teller Road
Thousand Oaks, CA 91320-2218
805-499-0721
800-818-7243
Fax: 800-583-2665
info@sagepub.com
www.sagepub.com
Sara Miller McCune, Founder, Publisher, Chairperson
Blaise R. Simqu, President/CEO
Chris Hickok, Senior Vice President/CFO
Stephen Barr, Managing Director/SAGE London
The first to bridge the gap between cognitive psychology and information processing theory in understanding learning disabilities. *$39.00*
495 pages Hardcover

2414 Cognitive Strategy Instruction That Really Improves Children's Academic Skills
Brookline Books
8 Trumbull Rd
Suite B-001
Northampton, MA 01060
413-584-0184
800-666-2665
Fax: 413-584-6184
brbooks@yahoo.com
www.brooklinebooks.com
Esther Isabe Wilder, Author
A concise and focused work that summarily presents the few procedures for teaching strategies that aid academic subject matter learning: decoding reading comprehension, vocabulary, math, spelling and writing. Learning unrelated facts and science. Completely revised in 1995. *$27.95*
Paperback
ISBN 1-571290-07-9

2415 Collaborating for Comprehensive Services for Young Children and Families
Brookes Publishing Company
PO Box 10624
Baltimore, MD 21285-0624
410-337-9580
800-638-3775
Fax: 410-337-8539
custserv@brookespublishing.com
www.brookespublishing.com
Paul H. Brookes, Chairman
Jeffrey D. Brookes, President
Melissa A. Behm, ExecutiveVice President
George S. Stamathis, Vice President & Publisher
Taking collaboration a step beyond basic implementation, this useful book shows agency and school leaders how to coordinate their efforts to stretch human services dollars while still providing quality programs. Provides the building blocks needed to establish a local interagency coordinating council. *$37.00*
272 pages
ISBN 1-557661-03-0

2416 Collaborative Teams for Students with Severe Disabilities

Brookes Publishing
PO Box 10624
Baltimore, MD 21285-0624
410-337-9580
800-638-3775
Fax: 410-337-8539
custserv@brookespublishing.com
www.brookespublishing.com

Paul H. Brookes, Chairman
Jeffrey D. Brookes, President
Melissa A. Behm, ExecutiveVice President
George S. Stamathis, Vice President & Publisher

How can educators, parents and therapists work together to ensure the best possible educational experience for students with severe disabilities? This resource describes how a collaborative team can successfully create exciting learning opportunities for students, while teaching them to participate fully at home, school, work and play. *$30.00*

304 pages
ISBN 1-55766 -88-3

2417 Communicating with Parents of Exceptional Children

Love Publishing Company
9101 E Kenyon Ave
Suite 2200
Denver, CO 80237-1854
303-221-7333
Fax: 303-221-7444
lpc@lovepublishing.com
www.lovepublishing.com

Roger L. Kroth, Author
Denzil Denzil Edge, Author

This book shows how teachers can facilitate parent involvement with children's education. It presents the mirror model of parent involvement, family, dynamics, how to listen actively to parents, values and perceptions, problem-solving, parent conferences and training groups. *$19.95*

ISBN 0-89108 -67-4

2418 Communication & Language Acquisition: Discoveries from Atypical Development

Brookes Publishing
PO Box 10624
Baltimore, MD 21285-0624
410-337-9580
800-638-3775
Fax: 410-337-8539
custserv@brookespublishing.com
www.brookespublishing.com

Paul H. Brookes, Chairman
Jeffrey D. Brookes, President
Melissa A. Behm, ExecutiveVice President
George S. Stamathis, Vice President & Publisher

This text demonstrates how the study of language acquisition in children with atypical development promotes advances in basic theory. *$44.00*

352 pages Hardcover
ISBN 1-557662-79-7

2419 Communication Skills for Working with Elders

Springer Publishing Company
11 W 42nd St
15th Floor
New York, NY 10036-8002
212-431-4370
877-687-7476
Fax: 212-941-7842
cs@springerpub.com
www.springerpub.com

Ursula Springer, President
Theodore C. Nardin, CEO/Publisher
Jason Roth, VP/Marketing Director
James C. Costello, Vice President, Journal Publishing

How aging and illness affects communication. *$17.95*

160 pages Softcover
ISBN 0-82615 -20-7

2420 Communication Unbound

Teachers College Press
Ste 2115
14781 Memorial Dr
Houston, TX 77079-5210
415-738-4323
Fax: 415-738-4329
tcc.orders@aidcvt.com
www.pearsonhighered.com

240 pages Paperback
ISBN 0-087737-21-4

2421 Complete Handbook of Children's Reading Disorders: You Can Prevent or Correct LDs

Gallery Bookshop
319 Kasten Street
PO Box 270
Mendocino, CA 95460-270
707-937-2215
Fax: 707-937-3737
info@gallerybookshop.com
www.gallerybooks.com

Tony Miksak, Owner

The complete handbook of children's reading disorders. *$34.95*

732 pages Paperback
ISBN 0-80772 -83-3

2422 Computer Access/Computer Learning

Special Needs Project
324 State Street
Suite H
Santa Barbara, CA 93101-2364
818-718-9900
800-333-6867
Fax: 818-349-2027
editor@specialneeds.com
www.specialneeds.com

Mark Darrow, Founder,The Prolotherapy Institu

A resource manual in adaptive technology and computer training. *$22.50*

2423 Consulting Psychologists Press

1055 Joaquin Rd
Suite. 200
Mountain View, CA 94043-1243
650-969-8901
800-624-1765
Fax: 650-969-8608
custserv@cpp.com

Carl E. Thoresen, Chairman
Jeffrey Hayes, President and Chief Executive Officer
Andrew Bell, Vice President of International
Catey DeBalko, Vice President of Marketing

Catalog offering job assessment software, career development reports, educational assessment information and books for the professional.

2424 Counseling Persons with Communication Disorders and Their Families

Sage Publications
2455 Teller Road
Thousand Oaks, CA 91320-2218
805-499-0721
800-818-7243
Fax: 800-583-2665
info@sagepub.com
www.sagepub.com

Sara Miller McCune, Founder, Publisher, Chairperson
Blaise R. Simqu, President & CEO
Chris Hickok, Senior Vice President & Chief Fi
Stephen Barr, Managing Director/SAGE London, P

A learning manual for speech-language pathologists and audiologists on how to deal with the emotional issues facing them in their work with clients with communication disorders and their families. *$29.00*

187 pages

2425 **Counseling in the Rehabilitation Process**
Charles C. Thomas
2600 S First St
Springfield, IL 62704-4730
217-789-8980
800-258-8980
Fax: 217-789-9130
books@ccthomas.com
www.ccthomas.com
Gerald L. Gandy, Author
E. Davis Martin Jr, Author
Richard E. Hardy, Author
This text provides the reader with a comprehensive overview and introduction to the field of rehabilitation counseling and services, and also has applicability in the growing field of community counseling. *$51.95*
358 pages paper 1999
ISBN 0-398069-70-4

2426 **Creating Positive Classroom Environments: Strategies for Behavior Management**
Brooks / Cole Publishing Company
511 Forest Lodge Rd
Pacific Grove, CA 93950-5040
831-373-0728
800-354-9706
Fax: 831-375-6414
bc-info@brookscole.com
www.cengage.com
448 pages Paperbound
ISBN 0-53422 -54-4

2427 **Cristine M. Trahms Program for Phenylketonuria**
University of Washington
PO Box 357920
Seattle, WA 98195
206-598-1800
877-685-3015
Fax: 206-598-1915
pku@u.washington.edu
www.depts.washington.edu/pku
C. Ronald Scott, MD, Professor, Pediatrics, Division
Clinical program for children and adults with phenylketonuria.

2428 **Critical Voices on Special Education: Problems & Progress Concerning the Mildly Handicapped**
State University of New York Press
22 Corporate Woods Boulevard
3rd Floor
Albany, NY 12211-2504
518-472-5000
866-430-7869
Fax: 518-472-5038
info@sunypress.edu
www.sunypress.edu
James Peltz, Associate Director
Janice Vunk, Assistant to the Director
Scott B Sigmon, Editor
Problems and progress concerning the mildly handicapped. *$24.95*
265 pages Paperback 1990
ISBN 0-79140 -20-3

2429 **Cultural Diversity, Families and the Special Education System**
Teachers College Press
1234 Amsterdam Ave
New York, NY 10027-6602
212-678-3929
800-575-6566
Fax: 212-678-4149
tcpress@tc.columbia.edu
www.teacherscollegepress.com
Beth Harry, Author
This timely and thought-provoking book explores the quadruple disadvantage faced by the parents of poor, minority, handicapped children whose first language is not that of the school they attend. *$22.95*
296 pages Paperback
ISBN 0-807731-19-6

2430 **Curriculum Decision Making for Students with Severe Handicaps**
Teachers College Press
1234 Amsterdam Ave
New York, NY 10027-6602
212-678-3929
800-575-6566
Fax: 212-678-4149
www.teacherscollegepress.com
192 pages Paperback
ISBN 0-807728-61-6

2431 **Deciphering the System: A Guide for Families of Young Disabled Children**
Brookline Books
8 Trumbull Rd
Ste B-001
Northampton, MA 01060
413-584-0184
800-666-2665
Fax: 413-584-6184
brbooks@yahoo.com
www.brooklinebks.com
Paula Beckman, Author
This book informs parents of disabled children (0-5) of their rights and the service system, e.g., ways to manage the cumulating information, tips on IEP and IFSP meetings and the educational assessment process, and how parents can work with multiple service providers. It includes contributions from both parents and professionals who have experience with the service system. *$21.95*
208 pages Paperback 1999
ISBN 0-914797-87-5

2432 **Defining Rehabilitation Agency Types**
Mississippi State University
108 Herbert - South
Room 150 Industrial Education Depar
Mississippi State, MS 39762-6189
662-325-2001
800-675-7782
Fax: 662-325-8989
TTY: 662-325-2694
nrtc@colled.msstate.edu
www.blind.msstate.edu
Jacqui Bybee, Research Associate II
Michele Capella McDonnall, Ph.D., Research Professor/Interim Director
Jessica Thornton, Business Manager
Marty Giesen, Ph.D., Senior Research Scientist
Relationships of participant selection and cost factors of service delivery across rehabilitation agency types. A national survey of state agencies for the blind was conducted to examine factors that define the characteristics of different agencies; similar programs were grouped together. Classification criteria were developed to distinguish agencies into logical groups based on line of authority, funding and operating procedures. *$10.00*
15 pages Paperback

2433 **Designing and Using Assistive Technology: The Human Perspective**
Brookes Publishing
PO Box 10624
Baltimore, MD 21285-0624
410-337-9580
800-638-3775
Fax: 410-337-8539
custserv@brookespublishing.com
www.brookespublishing.com
Paul H. Brookes, Chairman
Jeffrey D. Brookes, President
Melissa A. Behm, ExecutiveVice President
George S. Stamathis, Vice President & Publisher
Presented here is a holistic perspective on how and why people choose and use AT. Features personal insights and the latest research on design and development. *$31.00*
352 pages Paperback
ISBN 1-55766 -14-9

2434 **Developing Cross-Cultural Competence:Guideto Working with Young Children & Their Families**
Brookes Publishing
PO Box 10624
Baltimore, MD 21285-0624
410-337-9580
800-638-3775
Fax: 410-337-8539
custserv@brookespublishing.com
www.brookespublishing.com
Paul H. Brookes, Chairman
Jeffrey D. Brookes, President
Melissa A. Behm, ExecutiveVice President
George S. Stamathis, Vice President & Publisher
This enlightening book perceptively and sensitively explores cultural, ethnic, and language diversity in human services. For those who work with families whose infants and young children may have or be at risk for a disability or chronic illness. (Second Edition) *$32.00*
448 pages Paperback
ISBN 1-55766 -31-9

2435 **Developing Individualized Family Support Plans: A Training Manual**
Brookline Books
Suite B-001
8 Trumbull Rd
Northampton, MA 01060
413-584-0184
800-666-2665
Fax: 413-584-6184
brbooks@yahoo.com
www.brooklinebooks.com
Esther Wilder, Co-Author
This manual provides in-service training coordinators, administrators, supervisors and university personnel with a compact package of functional and practical methods to train professionals about implementing family-centered individualized family support plans (IFSP'S). Also, case studies provide concrete examples to aid in learning to write IFSP's. *$24.95*
ISBN 0-914797-69-7

2436 **Developing Staff Competencies for Supporting People with Disabilities**
Brookes Publishing
PO Box 10624
Baltimore, MD 21285-0624
410-337-9580
800-638-3775
Fax: 410-337-8539
custserv@brookespublishing.com
www.brookespublishing.com
Paul H. Brookes, Chairman
Jeffrey D. Brookes, President
Melissa A. Behm, ExecutiveVice President
George S. Stamathis, Vice President & Publisher
This timely second edition, now in a new easier to read format, gives service providers helpful strategies for increasing effectiveness and maintaining well-being while working in the rewarding yet challenging field of human services. *$34.00*
480 pages Paperback
ISBN 1-55766 -07-3

2437 **Development of Language**
McGraw-Hill, School Publishing
220 E Danieldale Rd
Desoto, TX 75115-2490
800-648-2970
Fax: 800-593-4418
www.mhschool.com
464 pages

2438 **Developmental Disabilities of Learning**
Gallery Bookshop
319 Kasten Street
PO Box 270
Mendocino, CA 95460-270
707-937-2215
Fax: 707-937-3737
info@gallerybookshop.com
www.gallerybooks.com
Tony Miksak, Owner
Manual for professionals on developmental and learning disabilities in the growing child. *$25.00*
224 pages Illustrated

2439 **Developmental Disabilities: A Handbook for Occupational Therapists**
Haworth Press
711 Third Avenue
New York, NY 10017
212-216-7800
800-354-1420
Fax: 212-244-1563
subscriptions@tandf.co.uk
www.haworthpress.com
268 pages Hardcover
ISBN 0-866569-59-6

2440 **Developmental Disabilities: A Handbook for Interdisciplinary Practice**
Brookline Books
8 Trumbull Rd
Suite B-001
Northampton, MA 01060
413-584-0184
800-666-2665
Fax: 413-584-6184
brbooks@yahoo.com
www.brooklinebooks.com
Esther Wilder, Co-Author
Successful interdisciplinary team practice for persons with developmental disabilities that require each team member to understand and respect the contributions of the others. This handbook explains the professions most often represented on interdisciplinary teams: their natures, concerns and roles in the interdisciplinary context. *$29.95*
256 pages
ISBN 1-571290-03-6

2441 **Developmental Variation and Learning Disorders**
Educators Publishing Service
PO Box 9031
Cambridge, MA 02139-9031
617-367-2700
800-225-5750
Fax: 617-547-0412
eps@schoolspecialty.com
www.epsbooks.com
Rick Holden, President
Discusses seven major areas of development and four major areas of academic proficiency and then ties this information together by examining factors that predispose a child to dysfunction and disability, offering guidelines to assessment and management, and analyzing long-range outcomes and factors that promote resiliency for parents, educators and clinicians. *$69.00*
640 pages Cloth
ISBN 0-838819-92-3

2442 **Digest of Neurology and Psychiatry**
Institute of Living: Hartford Hospital
80 Seymour Street
Hartford, CT 06106-3309
860-545-5000
800-673-2411
Fax: 860-545-5066
www.harthosp.org
Douglas Elliot, Chair of the Board
Stuart K. Markowitz, MD, FACR, President/SVP
Gerald J. Boisvert, HHC Regional Vice President / Chief Financial Officer,
Peter Q. Fraser, Regional Vice President Human Resources
Abstracts and reviews of selected current literature in psychiatry, neurology and related fields.

2443 **Disability Funding News**
8204 Fenton St
Silver Spring, MD 20910-4502
301-588-6380
800-666-6380
Fax: 301-588-6385
www.cdpublications.com
Mike Gerecht, Publisher

2444 Disability Studies and the Inclusive Classroom
711 3rd Avenue
8th Floor
New York, NY 10017
212-216-7800
800-634-7064
Fax: 212-564-7854
www.routledge.com

Susan Baglieri, Co-Author
Arthur Shapiro, Co-Author
This book's mission is to integrate knowledge and practice from the fields ofdisability studiesandspecial education. Parts I & II focus on the broad, foundational topics that comprise disability studies (culture, language, and history) and Parts III & IV move into practical topics (curriculum, co-teaching, collaboration, classroom organization, disability-specific teaching strategies, etc.) associated with inclusive education.

2445 Disability and Rehabilitation
Taylor & Francis
7625 Empire Dr
Florence, KY 41042-2919
800-634-7064
Fax: 800-248-4724
orders@taylorandfrancis.com
www.taylorandfrancis.com

Monthly
ISSN 0963-82 8

2446 Disability, Sport and Society
711 3rd Avenue
8th Floor
New York, NY 10017
212-216-7800
800-634-7064
Fax: 212-564-7854
www.routledge.com

Nigel Thomas, Co-Author
Andy Smith, Co-Author
Disability sport is a relatively recent phenomenon, yet it is also one that, particularly in the context of social inclusion, is attracting increasing political and academic interest. The purpose of this important new text - the first of its kind - is to introduce the reader to key concepts in disability and disability sport and to examine the complex relationships between modern sport, disability and other aspects of wider society.

2447 Disabled Rights: American Disability Policy and the Fight for Equality
3240 Prospect Street, NW
Suite 250
Washington, DC 20007
202-687-5889
Fax: 202-687-6340
gupress@georgetown.edu
press.georgetown.edu/

Jacqueline Vaughn Switzer, Author
Disabled Rights explains how people with disabilities have been treated from a social, legal, and political perspective in the United States.

2448 Divided Legacy: A History of the Schism in Medical Thought, The Bacteriological Era
North Atlantic Books
2526 Martin Luther King Jr. Way
Berkeley, CA 94704
510-549-4270
800-337-2665
Fax: 510-549-4276
orders@northatlanticbooks.com
www.northatlanticbooks.com

Alla Spector, Director of Finance & Office Operations
Doug Reil, Executive Director/Associate Publisher
Ed Angel, Director of Office Administration
Janet Levin, Senior Director of Sales & Distribution
Concluding volume of Coulter's history of medical philosophy, from ancient times to today. Covers the origins of bacteriology and immunology in world medicine; describes the clash between orthodox and alternative medicine.

2449 Dual Relationships in Counseling
American Counseling Association
6101 Stevenson Ave.
Suite 600
Alexandria, VA 22304
703-823-9800
800-347-6647
Fax: 800-473-2329
www.counseling.org

Richard Yep, Chief Executive Officer
Discusses issues involving dual relationships in counseling.

2450 Early Communication Skills for Children with Down Syndrome
Woodbine House
6510 Bells Mill Rd
Bethesda, MD 20817-1636
301-897-3570
800-843-7323
Fax: 301-897-5838
info@woodbinehouse.com
www.woodbinehouse.com

Nancy Gray Paul, Acquisitions Editor
Libby Kumin, Author
An expert shares her knowledge of speech and language development in young children with Down syndrome. Intelligibility, hearing loss, apraxia and other factors that affect communications are discussed. It also covers speech-language assessments and alternative communication options and literacy. *$19.95*
368 pages
ISBN 1-890627-27-5

2451 Early Intervention: Implementing Child & Family Services for At-Risk Infants and Toddlers
PRO-ED Inc.
8700 Shoal Creek Blvd
Austin, TX 78757-6897
512-451-3246
800-897-3202
Fax: 800-397-7633
general@proedinc.com
www.proedinc.com

Marci J. Hanson, Author
Eleanor W. Lynch, Author
New directions and recent legislation have produced a need for this guide which is designed for professionals facing the challenge of program development for disabled and at-risk infants, toddlers and their families. *$68.20*
394 pages Paperback 1995
ISBN 0-890796-21-1

2452 Ecology of Troubled Children
Brookline Books Publications
8 Trumbull Rd
Suite B-001
Northampton, MA 01060
413-584-0184
800-666-2665
Fax: 413-584-6184
brbooks@yahoo.com
www.brooklinebooks.com

Esther Isabe Wilder, Author
Designed for frontline mental health clinicians working with children with serious emotional disturbances; shows how to make children's' worlds more supportive by changing the places, activities and people in their lives. *$15.95*
256 pages
ISBN 1-571290-57-5

2453 Educating Children with Disabilities: A Transdisciplinary Approach
Brookes Publishing
PO Box 10624
Baltimore, MD 21285-0624
410-337-9580
800-638-3775
Fax: 410-337-8539
custserv@brookespublishing.com
www.brookespublishing.com

Paul H. Brookes, Chairman
Jeffrey D. Brookes, President
Melissa A. Behm, ExecutiveVice President
George S. Stamathis, Vice President & Publisher
Widely respected textbook presents you with the strategies you need for developing an inclusive curriculum, integrating health

care and educational programs and addressing needs and concerns. *$38.00*
512 pages
ISBN 1-557662-46-0

2454 **Educating Children with Multiple Disabilities: A Transdisciplinary Approach**
Brookes Publishing
PO Box 10624
Baltimore, MD 21285-0624
410-337-9580
800-638-3775
Fax: 410-337-8539
custserv@brookespublishing.com
www.brookespublishing.com
Paul H. Brookes, Chairman
Jeffrey D. Brookes, President
Melissa A. Behm, ExecutiveVice President
George S. Stamathis, Vice President & Publisher
Emphasizing transdisciplinary cooperation between teachers, therapists, nurses and parents, this book describes a general model and specific techniques for effectively educating children with multiple disabilities. *$29.00*
496 pages Paperback
ISBN 1-557662-46-0

2455 **Educating Individuals with Disabilities: IDEIA 2004 and Beyond (1st Edition)**
Springer Publishing Company
11 W 42nd St
15th Fl
New York, NY 10036-8002
212-431-4370
877-687-7476
Fax: 212-941-7842
cs@springerpub.com
www.springerpub.com
Ted Nardin, Chief Executive Officer
Jason Roth, Vice President, Marketing & Sales
Kathy Weiss, Director, Sales
Elena L. Grigorenko, Editor
Discusses how learning-disabled students are identified and assessed today, in light of the 2004 Individuals with Disabilities Education Improvement Act. Grigorenko's interdisciplinary collection is the first to comprehensively review the IDEIA 2004 Act and distill the changes professionals working with learning-disabled students face. The text takes an overarching perspective, first discussing the IDEIA in its historical, political, and legal context. *$100.00*
512 pages Hardcover 1908
ISBN 0-826103-56-1

2456 **Educating Students Who Have Visual Impairments with Other Disabilities**
Brookes Publishing
PO Box 10624
Baltimore, MD 21285-0624
410-337-9580
800-638-3775
Fax: 410-337-8539
custserv@brookespublishing.com
www.brookespublishing.com
Paul H. Brookes, Chairman
Jeffrey D. Brookes, President
Melissa A. Behm, ExecutiveVice President
George S. Stamathis, Vice President & Publisher
This introductory text provides techniques for facilitating functional learning in students with a wide range of visual impairments and multiple disabilities. With a concentration on educational needs and learning styles, the authors of this multidisciplinary volume demonstrate functional assessment and teaching adaptations that will improve students' inclusive learning experiences. *$49.95*
552 pages Paperback
ISBN 1-557662-80-0

2457 **Educating all Students in the Mainstream**
Brookes Publishing Company
PO Box 10624
Baltimore, MD 21285-0624
410-337-9580
800-638-3775
Fax: 410-337-8539
custserv@brookespublishing.com
Paul H. Brookes, Chairman
Jeff Brookes, President
Melissa A. Behm, ExecutiveVice President
Cary Gold, Educational Sales Representative
Incorporating the research and viewpoints of both regular and special educators, this textbook provides an effective approach for modifying, expanding, and adjusting regular education to meet the needs of all students. *$34.00*
304 pages
ISBN 1-557660-22-0

2458 **Educational Audiology for the Limited Hearing Infant and Preschooler**
Charles C. Thomas
2600 S First St
Springfield, IL 62704-4730
217-789-8980
800-258-8980
Fax: 217-789-9130
books@ccthomas.com
www.ccthomas.com
Donald Goldberg, Author
Nancy Coleffe-Schenck, Author
Doreen Pollack, Author
Offers information on current concepts and practices in audio-logic screening and evaluation, development of the listening function, development of speech, development of language, the role of parents, parent education, mainstreaming of the limited-hearing child, and program modifications for the severely learning disabled child. Also includes information on auditory assessment, sensory aides, cochlear implants, acoupedics and auditory verbal programs. *$79.95*
430 pages Paperback
ISBN 0-398067-51-1

2459 **Educational Care**
Educators Publishing Service
625 Mount Auburn St
3rd Floor
Cambridge, MA 02138-3039
617-547-6706
800-225-5750
Feedback.EPS@schoolspecialty.com
www.eps.schoolspecialty.com
Paula Fabbro, Sales Consultant
Leo Micale, Sales Consultant
Kristen Colson, Sales Consultant
Flora Francis, Sales Consultant
This book, written for both parents and teachers, is based on the view that education should be a system of care that is able to look after the specific needs of individual students. Using case studies, it analyzes various types of learning disorders and then suggests ways to help students with these problems. *$31.50*
325 pages
ISBN 0-838819-87-7

2460 **Educational Intervention for the Student**
Charles C. Thomas
2600 S First St
Springfield, IL 62704-4730
217-789-8980
800-258-8980
Fax: 217-789-9130
books@ccthomas.com
www.ccthomas.com

2461 **Educational Prescriptions**
Educators Publishing Service
625 Mount Auburn St
3RD Floor
Cambridge, MA 02138-3039
617-547-6706
800-225-5750
Feedback.EPS@schoolspecialty.com
Paula Fabbro, Sales Consultant
Leo Micale, Sales Consultant
Kristen Colson, Sales Consultant
Flora Francis, Sales Consultant
This book provides specific recommendations for the classroom management of students who are experiencing subtle developmental and/or learning difficulties. Intended for regular classroom teachers, specific examples of accommodations teachers can make are provided for grades 1-3 and 4-6. *$13.50*
64 pages
ISBN 0-838819-90-7

2462 **Effective Instruction for Special Education**
Sage Publications
2455 Teller Road
Thousand Oaks, CA 91320-2218
805-499-0721
800-818-7243
Fax: 800-583-2665
info@sagepub.com
www.sagepub.com
Sara Miller McCune, Founder, Publisher, Chairperson
Blaise R. Simqu, President/CEO
Chris Hickok, Senior Vice President/CFO
Stephen Barr, Managing Director/SAGE London, P
This exciting and wide-ranging book provides special educators with effective methods for teaching students with mild and moderate learning and behavioral problems, as well as for teaching remedial students in general. *$37.00*
419 pages Paperback

2463 **Effectively Educating Handicapped Students**
Longman Publishing Group
9th Fl
Upper Saddle River, NJ 07458-1813
201-236-3281
800-922-0579
Fax: 201-236-3290
www.pearsoned.com
468 pages Paperback
ISBN 0-801303-17-6

2464 **Emotional Problems of Childhood and Adolescence**
McGraw-Hill School Publishing
PO Box 182604
Columbus, OH 43218
877-833-5524
800-338-3987
Fax: 609-308-4480
customer.service@mheducation.com
www.mcgraw-hill.com
David Levin, President/Chief Ex
David Stafford, Senior Vice President/General Counsel
Maryellen Valaitis, Senior Vice President Human Resources
Patrick Milano, Chief Financial Officer Chief Administrative Officer
For future special educators, psychologists and others who work with emotionally disturbed children and adolescents.

2465 **Enabling & Empowering Families: Principles & Guidelines for Practice**
Brookline Books
8 Trumbull Rd
Suite B-001
Northampton, MA 01060
413-584-0184
800-666-2665
Fax: 413-584-6184
brbooks@yahoo.com
www.brooklinebooks.com
Esther Wilder, Co-Author
This book was written for practitioners who must work with families but who have insufficient training in family systems assessment and intervention. The authors' system enables professionals to help the family identify its needs, locate the formal and informal resources to meet these needs and develop the abilities to effectively access these resources. *$24.95*
220 pages
ISBN 0-914797-59-X

2466 **Evaluation and Educational Programming of Students with Deafblindness & Severe Disabilities**
Charles C. Thomas
2600 S First St
Springfield, IL 62704-4730
217-789-8980
800-258-8980
Fax: 217-789-9130
books@ccthomas.com
www.ccthomas.com
Carroll J. Jones, Author
Subtitle: Sensorimotor Stage. This second edition offers a very complete package of information on the special education of deaf-blind students; including detailed diagnostic information to assist the instructor in evaluating the physical, social, mental status of the student, as well as the educational progress. *$50.95*
265 pages Spiral-Paper 2001
ISBN 0-398072-16-2

2467 **Evaluation and Treatment of the Psychogeriatric Patient**
Haworth Press
711 Third Avenue
New York, NY 10017
212-216-7800
800-354-1420
Fax: 212-244-1563
subscriptions@tandf.co.uk
www.haworthpress.com
111 pages Hardcover
ISBN 1-560240-52-0

2468 **Exceptional Children in Focus**
McGraw-Hill School Publishing
PO Box 182604
Columbus, OH 43218
877-833-5524
800-338-3987
Fax: 609-308-4480
customer.service@mheducation.com
www.mcgraw-hill.com
David Levin, President/Chief Ex
David Stafford, Senior Vice President/General Counsel
Maryellen Valaitis, Senior Vice President Human Resources
Patrick Milano, Chief Financial Officer Chief Administrative Officer
Combines a light, personal look at the problems of special educators experiences with the basic facts of exceptionality.
288 pages

2469 **Exceptional Lives: Special Education in Today's Schools, 4th Edition**
Pearson Education
1 Lake St
Upper Saddle River, NJ 07458-1813
201-236-3281
800-922-0579
Fax: 201-236-3290
www.pearsoned.com
592 pages
ISBN 0-131126-00-8

2470 **Facilitating Self-Care Practices in the Elderly**
Haworth Press
711 Third Avenue
New York, NY 10017
212-216-7800
800-354-1420
Fax: 212-244-1563
subscriptions@tandf.co.uk
www.haworthpress.com
185 pages Hardcover
ISBN 1-560240-13-X

2471 **Family-Centered Early Intervention with Infants and Toddlers**

Brookes Publishing
PO Box 10624
Baltimore, MD 21285-0624
410-337-9580
800-638-3775
Fax: 410-337-8539
custserv@brookespublishing.com
www.brookespublishing.com

Paul H. Brookes, Chairman
Jeffrey D. Brookes, President
Melissa A. Behm, ExecutiveVice President
George S. Stamathis, Vice President & Publisher

This informative text provides professionals with insight and practical guidelines to help fulfill the federal requirements for provision of early intervention services. *$37.00*

368 pages Hardcover
ISBN 1-557661-24-3

2472 **Feeding Children with Special Needs**

Arizona Department of Health Services
150 North 18th Avenue
Phoenix, AZ 85007-2607
602-542-1025
Fax: 602-542-0883
www.azdhs.gov

Will Humble, Director
Jeff Bloomberg, J.D., Manager
Robert Lane, Esq., Administrative Counsel
Lynn Golder, Esq., Administrative Counsel & HIPAA Privacy Officer

Guide designed to help develop a greater awareness of the special challenges involved in the nutrition and feeding concerns for children with special health care needs, and ways to approach the issues. *$5.00*

2473 **Focal Group Psychotherapy**

New Harbinger Publications
5674 Shattuck Ave
Oakland, CA 94609-1662
510-652-0215
800-748-6273
Fax: 800-652-1613
customerservice@newharbinger.com
www.newharbinger.com

Matthew McKay, Founder
Patrick Fanning, Co-Founder/Writer

Guide to leading brief, theme-based groups. This book offers an extensive week-by-week description of the basic concepts and interventions for 14 theme or focal groups for: codependency, rape victims, shyness, survivors of incest, agoraphobia, survivors of toxic parents, depression, child molesters, anger control, domestic violence offenders, assertiveness, alcohol and drug abuse, eating disorders, and parent training. *$59.95*

544 pages Cloth
ISBN 1-879237-18-0

2474 **Free Hand: Enfranchising the Education of Deaf Children**

TJ Publishers

Margaret Walworth, Author
Donald F. Moores, Author
Terrence J. O'Rourke, Author

A select group of nationally prominent educators, linguists and researchers met at Hofstra University to consider the most vital and controversial question in education of the deaf: what role should ASL play in the classroom? Become part of that discussion with A Free Hand. *$16.95*

204 pages Softcover
ISBN 0-93266 -40-X

2475 **Friendship 101**

Council for Exceptional Children
3100 Clarendon Blvd.
Suite 600
Arlington, VA 22201-5332
888-232-7733
TTY: 866-915-5000
service@exceptionalchildren.org
www.exceptionalchildren.org

Juliet E. Hart Barnett, Co-Author & Editor
Kelly J. Whalon, Co-Author & Editor

Book and webinar for general special educators who work with children with autism spectrum disorder (ASD). Presents evidence-based practices shown to enhance social competence in children with ASD.

2476 **Functional Assessment Inventory Manual**

Stout Vocational Rehab Institute
655 15th St. NW
Suite 800
Washington, DC 20005
715-232-1411
800-538-3742
Fax: 715-232-2356
botterbuschd@uwstout.edu
www2.epa.gov

Gina McCarthy, Administrator
Gwen Keyes Fleming, Chief of Staff
Bob Perciasepe, Deputy Administrator
Craig E. Hooks, Office of Administration and Resource Management (OARM)

The Functional Assessment is a systematic enumeration of a client's vocactionally relevant strengths and limitations. *$12.00*

96 pages Paperback
ISBN 0-916671-53-4

2477 **Get Ready for Jetty!: My Journal About ADHD and Me**

750 First Street, NE
Washington, DC 20002-4242
202-336-5500
800-374-2721
rllowman@gmail.com
www.apa.org

Jeanne Kraus, Author

Jetty writes about these things as well as her recent ADHD diagnosis in her journal.

2478 **Getting Around Town**

Council for Exceptional Children
3100 Clarendon Blvd.
Suite 600
Arlington, VA 22201-5332
888-232-7733
TTY: 866-915-5000
service@exceptionalchildren.org
www.exceptionalchildren.org

M. Sherril Moon, Co-Author
Emily M. Luedtke, Co-Author
Elizabeth Halloran-Tornquist, Co-Author

This bookprovides examples of possible IEP goals and field-tested lesson plans for individual students or entire classes across all age and grade levels. *$34.95*

2479 **Global Perspectives on Disability: A Curriculum**

Mobility International USA
132 E Broadway
Suite 343
Eugene, OR 97401
541-343-1284
Fax: 541-343-6812
TTY: 541-343-1284
clearinghouse@miusa.org
www.miusa.org

Susan Sygall, Chief Executive Officer
Cindy Lewis, Director, Programs

Designed for secondary and higher education instructors. Includes five lesson plans covering disability awareness, disability rights and international perspectives on disability. Available in alternative formats.

2480 **Glossary of Terminology for Vocational Assessment/Evaluation/Work**

Rehabilitation Resource University
University of Wisconsin-Stou
Menomonie, WI 54751
715-232-2236
Fax: 715-232-2356
gundlachj@uwstout.edu

Ronald Fry, Manager
Jennifer Gundlach Klatt, Program Assistant

This glossary contains 254 terms and their definitions. Primary focus is on the terminology related to the practice and professionals of vocational assessment, vocational evaluation and work adjustment. *$9.50*

40 pages Softcover

2481 Graduate Technological Education and the Human Experience of Disability
Haworth Press
711 Third Avenue
New York, NY 10017
212-216-7800
800-354-1420
Fax: 212-244-1563
subscriptions@tandf.co.uk
www.haworthpress.com

115 pages Hardcover
ISBN 0-789060-08-6

2482 HIV Infection and Developmental Disabilities
Brookes Publishing
PO Box 10624
Baltimore, MD 21285-0624
410-337-9580
800-638-3775
Fax: 410-337-8539
custserv@brookespublishing.com
www.brookespublishing.com

Paul H. Brookes, Chairman
Jeffrey D. Brookes, President
Melissa A. Behm, ExecutiveVice President
George S. Stamathis, Vice President & Publisher

A resource for service providers pinpointing the most crucial medical, legal and educational issues to control HIV infection. *$47.00*
320 pages
ISBN 1-557660-83-2

2483 Handbook for Implementing Workshops for Siblings of Special Children
Special Needs Project
324 State Street
Suite H
Santa Barbara, CA 93101-2364
818-718-9900
800-333-6867
Fax: 818-349-2027
editor@specialneeds.com
www.specialneeds.com

Mark Darrow, Founder,The Prolotherapy Institu

Based on three years of professional experience, this handbook provides guidelines and techniques for those who wish to start and conduct workshops for siblings. *$40.00*

2484 Handbook for Speech Therapy
Psychological & Educational Publications
PO Box 520
Hydesville, CA 95547
800-523-5775
Fax: 800-447-0907
psych-edpublications@suddenlink.net

143 pages paperback

2485 Handbook for the Special Education Administrator
Edwin Mellen Press
PO Box 450
Lewiston, NY 14092-1205
716-754-2266
Fax: 716-754-4056
jrupnow@mellenpress.com
www.mellenpress.com

Arthur R. Crowell, Author
Bonnie Crogan, Marketing
Irene Miller, Accounting
Patricia Schultz, Production

Organization and procedures for special education. *$49.95*
96 pages Hardcover
ISBN 0-88946 -22-9

2486 Handbook of Acoustic Accessibility
15619 Premiere Drive
Suite 101
Tampa, FL 33624
850-363-9909
Fax: 480-393-4331
accounting@successforkidswithhearingloss.com
successforkidswithhearinglo ss.com

Joseph J. Smaldino, Co-Author
Carol Flexer, Co-Author

Most students with hearing loss are educated in mainstream education classrooms the majority of each school day.Communication - between peers and with teachers - is the coin of education and upon which a wealth of knowledge is built.Unfortunately for students with hearing loss, the typical classroom environment is hazardous for listening and interferes with access to all classroom communication.

2487 Handbook of Developmental Education
Greenwood Publishing Group
130 Cremona Drive
Santa Barbara, CA 93117
805-968-1911
800-368-6868
Fax: 866-270-3856
CustomerService@abc-clio.com
www.abc-clio.com

This comprehensive handbook has brought together the leading practitioners and researchers in the field of developmental education to focus on the developmental learning agenda. Hardcover.
400 pages $65 - $75
ISBN 0-275932-97-4

2488 Handbook on Supported Education for Peoplewith Mental Illness
Brookes Publishing
PO Box 10624
Baltimore, MD 21285-0624
410-337-9580
800-638-3775
Fax: 410-337-8539
custserv@brookespublishing.com
www.brookespublishing.com

Paul H. Brookes, Chairman
Jeffrey D. Brookes, President
Melissa A. Behm, ExecutiveVice President
George S. Stamathis, Vice President & Publisher

Here you will find all necessary information that mental health professionals need in order to provide supported education services. There are specific suggestions on how to help people with mental illness return to or remain in college, trade school, or GED programs. Also addressed are funding and legal issues, accommodations, and specific interventions.
208 pages Paperback
ISBN 1-55766 -52-1

2489 Head Injury Rehabilitation: Children
Taylor & Francis
47 Runway Dr
Ste G
Levittown, PA 19057-4738
267-580-2622
Fax: 215-785-5515

460 pages Cloth
ISBN 0-85066 -67-1

2490 Health Care Management in Physical Therapy
Charles C. Thomas
2600 S First St
Springfield, IL 62704-4730
217-789-8980
800-258-8980
Fax: 217-789-9130
books@ccthomas.com
www.ccthomas.com

2491 Health Care for Students with Disabilities
Brookes Publishing Company
PO Box 10624
Baltimore, MD 21285-0624
410-337-9580
800-638-3775
Fax: 410-337-8539
custserv@brookespublishing.com
www.brookespublishing.com

Paul H. Brookes, Chairman
Jeffrey D. Brookes, President
Melissa A. Behm, ExecutiveVice President
George S. Stamathis, Vice President & Publisher

This practical guidebook provides detailed descriptions of the 16 health-related procedures most likely to be needed in the classroom by students with disabilities. *$25.00*
304 pages Paperback
ISBN 1-557660-37-9

2492 **Helping Learning- Disabled Gifted Children Learn Through Compensatory Active Play**
Charles C. Thomas
2600 S First St
Springfield, IL 62704-4730
217-789-8980
800-258-8980
Fax: 217-789-9130
books@ccthomas.com
www.ccthomas.com

James Harry Humphrey, Author
$36.95
156 pages Hardcover 1990
ISBN 0-398056-95-1

2493 **Helping Students Grow**
American College Testing Program
500 ACT Drive
PO Box 168
Iowa City, IA 52243-0168
319-337-1000
info@keytrain.com
www.act.org

Jon Whitmore, Chief Executive Officer
Tom J. Goedken, Chief Financial Officer/Senior Vice President
Patricia C. Steinbrech, Chief Information Officer
Janet E. Godwin, Chief of Staff/Accountability Officer
Designed to assist counselors in using the wealth of information generated by the ACT Assessment.

2494 **Home Health Care Provider: A Guide to Essential Skills**
Springer Publishing
11 W 42nd St
15th Floor
New York, NY 10036-8002
212-431-4370
877-687-7476
Fax: 212-941-7842
cs@springerpub.com
www.springerpub.com

Theodore C. Nardin, CEO/Publisher
Jason Roth, VP/Marketing Director
Annette Imperati, Marketing/Sales Director
James C. Costello, Vice President, Journal Publishing
This book is designed to foster quality care to home care recipients. Prieto provides information, tips, and techniques on personal care routines as well as additional responsibilities, including home safety and maintenance, meal planning, errand running, caring for couples, and making use of recreational time. The book focuses on the psycho-social needs of home care recipients, stressing the need to maintainthe house as a home, and sustaining the recipient's way of life throughout caregiving.

2495 **How to Teach Spelling/How to Spell**
Educators Publishing Service
625 Mount Auburn St
3rd Floor
Cambridge, MA 02138-3039
617-547-6706
800-225-5750
Feedback.EPS@schoolspecialty.com

Paula Fabbro, Sales Consultant
Leo Micale, Sales Consultant
Kristen Colson, Sales Consultant
Flora Francis, Sales Consultant
This is a comprehensive resource manual based on the Orton-Gillingham approach to reading and spelling. It recommends what and how much to teach at each grade level at the beginning of each lesson or section. There are four student manuals that accompany this. *$22.50*
Teachers Manual
ISBN 0-838818-47-1

2496 **Human Exceptionality: School, Community,and Family (12th Edition)**
Cengage Learning
20 Channel Center St
Boston, MA 02210
617-289-7700
617-289-7844
www.cengage.com/us

Michael L. Hardman, Author
M. Winston Egan, Author
Clifford J. Drew, Author
An evidence-based testament to the critical role of cross-professional collaboration in enhancing the lives of exceptional individuals and their families. This text's unique lifespan approach combines powerful research, evidence-based practices, and inspiring stories, engendering passion and empathy and enhancing the lives of individuals with exceptionalities.
544 pages Hardcover

2497 **I Can't Hear You in the Dark: How to Lean and Teach Lipreading**
Charles C. Thomas
2600 S First St
Springfield, IL 62704-4730
217-789-8980
800-258-8980
Fax: 217-789-9130
books@ccthomas.com
www.ccthomas.com

Betty Woerner Carter, Author
The goal of this text is to improve communication and strengthen relationships with others. *$40.95*
226 pages Spiral-Paper 1997
ISBN 0-398067-89-2

2498 **I Heard That!**
3417 Volta Pl NW
Washington, DC 20007-2737
202-337-5220
Fax: 202-337-8314
TTY: 202-337-5221
info@agbell.org
www.listeningandspokenlanguage.org

Meredith K. Sugar, Esq. (OH), President
Ted A. Meyer, M.D., Ph.D, President-Elect/Secretary-Treasurer
Emilio Alonso-Mendoza, Chief Executive Officer
Susan Boswell, Director of Communications and Marketing
Provides a framework for teachers, clinicians and parents when writing objectives and designing activities to develop listening skills in children with hearing loss from newborn to 3 years. *$7.95*
36 pages

2499 **I Heard That!2**
Alexander Graham Bell Association
3417 Volta Pl NW
Washington, DC 20007-2737
202-337-5220
Fax: 202-337-8314
TTY: 202-337-5221
info@agbell.org
www.listeningandspokenlanguage.org

Meredith K. Sugar, Esq. (OH), President
Ted A. Meyer, M.D., Ph.D, President-Elect/Secretary-Treasurer
Emilio Alonso-Mendoza, Chief Executive Officer
Susan Boswell, Director of Communications and Marketing
Provides a framework for teachers, clinicians and parents when writing objectives and designing activities to develop listening skills in children who are deaf or hard of hearing. *$7.95*
36 pages

2500 **If It Is To Be, It Is Up To Us To Help!**
AVKO Educational Research Foundation
3084 Willard Rd
Ste W
Birch Run, MI 48415-9404
810-686-9283
866-285-6612
Fax: 810-686-1101
www.avko.org

Don Mc Cabe, President
Ted A. Meyer, M.D., Ph.D, Vice-President
Michael Lane, Treasurer
Birch Run, Research Director Emeritus
A book of lesson plans for an Adult Community Education Course for Volunteer Tutors. Contains information on how to go about establishing such a course and how to secure cooperation from local and national organizations. Free as an e-book for Foundation members. *$14.95*
ISBN 1-56400 -42-1

2501 Images of the Disabled, Disabling Images
ABC-CLIO
130 Cremona Dr
Santa Barbara, CA 93117 805-968-1911
800-368-6868
Fax: 866-270-3856
customerservice@abc-clio.com
www.abc-clio.com

Alan Gartner, Author
Combines an examination of the presentation of persons with disabilities in literature, film and the media with an analysis of the ways in which these images are expressed in public policy concerning the disabled. *$84.00*
227 pages Hardcover 1986
ISBN 0-275921-78-6

2502 Implementing Family-Centered Services in Early Intervention
Brookline Books
8 Trumbull Rd
Suite B-001
Northampton, MA 01060 413-584-0184
800-666-2665
Fax: 413-584-6184
brbooks@yahoo.com
www.brooklinebooks.com

180 pages Paperback
ISBN 0-91479 -62-

2503 Including All of Us: An Early Childhood Curriculum About Disability
Educational Equity Concepts
381 Park Ave South
Suite 701
New York, NY 10016 212-243-1110
Fax: 212-367-4640
lcolon@fhi360.org
www.fhi360.org

Frank Schneiger, President
Antonia Cottrell Martin, Founder and President
Merle Froschl, Director, Educational Equity
Barbara Sprung, Co-director
The first nonsexist, multicultural, mainstreamed curriculum. Step-by-step activities incorporate disability into three curriculum areas: Same/Different (hearing impairment), Body Parts (visual impairment), and Transportation (mobility impairment). *$14.95*
144 pages
ISBN 0-93162 -00-4

2504 Including Students with Severe and Multiple Disabilites in Typical Classrooms
Brookes Publishing
PO Box 10624
Baltimore, MD 21285-0624 410-337-9580
800-638-3775
Fax: 410-337-8539
custserv@brookespublishing.com
www.brookespublishing.com

Paul H. Brookes, Chairman
Jeffrey D. Brookes, President
Melissa A. Behm, ExecutiveVice President
George S. Stamathis, Vice President & Publisher
This straightforward and jargon free resource gives instructors the guidance needed to educate learners who have one or more sensory impairments in addition to cognitive and physical disabilities. *$32.95*
224 pages Paperback
ISBN 1-55766 -39-8

2505 Including Students with Special Needs: A Practical Guide for Classroom Teachers
Allyn & Bacon
75 Arlington St
Suite 300
Boston, MA 02116-3988 ab_webmaster@abacon.com
www.pearson.com/us/higher-education.html

544 pages
ISBN 0-20528 -85-4

2506 Inclusive & Heterogeneous Schooling: Assessment, Curriculum, and Instruction
Brookes Publishing
PO Box 10624
Baltimore, MD 21285-0624 410-337-9580
800-638-3775
Fax: 410-337-8539
custserv@brookespublishing.com
www.brookespublishing.com

Paul H. Brookes, Chairman
Jeff Brookes, President
Melissa A. Behm, ExecutiveVice President
Cary Gold, Educational Sales Representative
Presents methods for successfully restructuring classrooms to enable all students, particularly those with disabilities, to flourish. Provides specific strategies for assessment, collaboration, classroom management, and age-specific instruction. *$34.95*
448 pages Paperback
ISBN 1-55766 -02-9

2507 Independent Living Approach to Disability Policy Studies
World Institute on Disability
3075 Adeline St.
Suite 155
Berkeley, CA 94703 510-225-6400
Fax: 510-225-0477
wid@wid.org
www.wid.org

Marcie Roth, Executive Director & CEO
Katherine Zigmont, Senior Director, Operations & Deputy Director
Reggie Johnson, Senior Director, Marketing & Communications
Marsha Saxton, Director, Research
A collection of essays and bibliographies aiming to build a framework for understanding how the relationship between public policy, disability studies and disability policy studies will impact the future.

2508 Information & Referral Center
Mississippi State University
108 Herbert - South
Room 150/PO Drawer 6189
Mississippi State Univers, MS 39762-6189 662-325-2001
800-675-7782
Fax: 662-325-8989
TTY: 662-325-2694
nrtc@colled.msstate.edu
www.blind.msstate.edu

Jacqui Bybee, Research and Training Coordinato
Michele Capella McDonnall, Ph.D., Research Professor/Interim Director
Jessica Thornton, Business Manager
Marty Giesen, Ph.D., Senior Research Scientist
A comprehensive website that includes information about client assistance programs, vocational rehabilitation agencies, low vision clinics and information about blindness and low vision. *$25.00*
150 pages

2509 Instructional Methods for Students
Allyn & Bacon
75 Arlington St
Suite 300
Boston, MA 02116-3988 ab_webmaster@abacon.com
www.home.pearsonhighered.com

450 pages
ISBN 0-205087-35-3

2510 Interactions: Collaboration Skills for School Professionals
Longman Education/Addison Wesley
75 Arlington St
Suite 300
Boston, MA 02116-3988 ab_webmaster@abacon.com

270 pages Paperback
ISBN 0-80131 -21-2

2511 International Journal of Arts Medicine
MMB Music
9051 Watson Road
Suite 161
Saint Louis, MO 63126
314-531-9635
800-543-3771
Fax: 314-531-8384
info@mmbmusic.com
www.mmbmusic.com
Norm Goldberg, Founder/chairman
Exploration of the creative arts and healing. Presents peer-reviewed articles clearly written by educators in the creative arts, as well as internationally prominent physicians, therapists and health care professionals.

2512 Interpreting Disability: A Qualitative Reader
Teachers College Press
1234 Amsterdam Avenue
New York, NY 10027
212-678-3929
800-575-6566
Fax: 212-678-4149
tcpress@tc.columbia.edu
www.tcpress.com
Brian Ellerbeck, Executive Acquisitions Editor
Marie Ellen Larcada, Senior Acquisitions Editor
Emily Spangler, Acquisitions Editor
Meg Hartmann, Acquisitions Assistant
This book offers a collection of exemplary qualitative research affecting people with disabilities and their families. Instead of focusing upon methodological details, the chapters illustrate the variety of styles and formats that interpretive research can adopt in reporting its results. *$24.95*
328 pages Paperback
ISBN 0-807731-21-8

2513 Intervention Research in Learning Disabilities
Gallery Bookshop
319 Kasten Street
PO Box 270
Mendocino, CA 95460-270
707-937-2215
Fax: 707-937-3737
info@gallerybookshop.com
www.gallerybooks.com
Tony Miksak, Owner
Based on the Symposium on Intervention Research, this volume presents 12 papers addressing issues in intervention research, academic interventions, social and behavioral interventions, and postsecondary interventions. *$30.00*
347 pages

2514 Introduction to Learning Disabilities
Allyn & Bacon
75 Arlington St
Suite 300
Boston, MA 02116-3988
www.pearsonhighered.com
608 pages
ISBN 0-20529 -43-4

2515 Introduction to Special Education: Teaching in an Age of Challenge, 4th Edition
Allyn & Bacon
75 Arlington St
Suite 300
Boston, MA 02116-3988
www.pearsonhighered.com
640 pages cloth
ISBN 0-20526 -94-4

2516 Introduction to the Profession of Counseling
McGraw-Hill School Publishing
PO Box 182604
Columbus, OH 43218
877-833-5524
800-338-3987
Fax: 609-308-4480
customer.service@mheducation.com
www.mcgraw-hill.com
David Levin, President/Chief Executive Officer
David Stafford, Senior Vice President/General Counsel
Maryellen Valaitis, Senior Vice President Human Resources
Patrick Milano, Chief Financial Officer/Chief Administrative Officer
Offers information, theories and techniques for counseling numerous cases from drug addiction to special populations.
464 pages

2517 Issues and Research in Special Education
Teachers College Press
PO Box 20
Williston, VT 05495-0020
800-575-6566
Fax: 802-664-7626
tcp.orders@aidcvt.com
www.teacherscollegepress.com
264 pages Hardcover
ISBN 0-807731-95-1

2518 Kendall Demonstration Elementary School Curriculum Guides
Gallaudet University Bookstore
800 Florida Ave NE
Washington, DC 20002-3695
202-651-5488
800-621-2736
Fax: 202-651-5489
TTY: 888-630-9347
gupress@gallaudet.edu
www.gupress.gallaudet.edu
Dr. T Alan Hurwitz, President
Edward Bosso, Vice President for Administration
Dr. Lynne Murray, Vice President for Development
Donald Beil, Chief of Staff
KDES is a day school serving students from birth through age 15, beginning with the Parent-Infant Program and ending in grade 8. Students come from the Washington, D.C., metropolitan area.

2519 Language Arts: Detecting Special Needs
Allyn & Bacon
75 Arlington St
Suite 300
Boston, MA 02116-3988
617-848-7500
800-852-8024
Fax: 617-944-7273
www.home.pearsonhighered.com
Bill Barke, Chairman/CEO
Nancy Forfyth, President
Kevin Stone, Vice President, National Sales M
Thomas A. Rakes, Author
Describes special language arts needs of special learners.
180 pages paperback
ISBN 0-205116-36-1

2520 Language Learning Practices with Deaf Children
Sage Publications
2455 Teller Road
Thousand Oaks, CA 91320
805-499-9774
800-818-7243
Fax: 800-583-2665
books.claim@sagepub.com
www.sagepub.com
Sara Miller McCune, Founder, Publisher, Chairperson
Stephen P. Quigley, Co-Author
Susan Rose, Co-Author
Patricia L. McAnally, Co-Author
This new edition describes the variety of language-development theories and practices used with deaf children without advocating anyone. *$38.00*
321 pages Hardcover

2521 Language and Communication Disorders in Children
McGraw-Hill School Publishn
PO Box 182604
Columbus, OH 43218
877-833-5524
800-338-3987
Fax: 609-308-4480
customer.service@mheducation.com
www.mcgraw-hill.com
David Levin, President/Chief Executive Officer
David Stafford, Senior Vice President/General Counsel
Maryellen Valaitis, Senior Vice President Human Resources
Patrick Milano, Chief Financial Officer/Chief Administrative Officer

Comprehensive coverage encompassing all aspects of children's language disorders.
512 pages

2522 Learning Disabilities, Literacy, and Adult Education
Brookes Publishing
PO Box 10624
Baltimore, MD 21285-0624
410-337-9580
800-638-3775
Fax: 410-337-8539
custserv@brookespublishing.com
www.brookespublishing.com
Paul H. Brookes, Chairman
Jeffrey D. Brookes, President
Melissa A. Behm, ExecutiveVice President
George S. Stamathis, Vice President & Publisher
This book focuses on adults with severe learning disabilities and the educators who work with them. Described are the characteristics, demographics, and educational and employment status of adults with LD and the laws that protect them in the workplace and in educational settings.
450 pages Paperback
ISBN 1-55766 -47-5

2523 Learning Disabilities: Concepts and Characteristics
McGraw-Hill School Publishing
220 E Danieldale Rd
Desoto, TX 75115-2490
972-224-4772
800-442-9685
Fax: 972-228-1982
Harold McGraw III, Chairman/ President/ Chief Ex
Jack F. Callahan, Executive Vice President, Chief
James A. McLoughlin, Co-Author
Gerald Wallace, Co-Author
Covers the conceptual basis of learning disabilities, identification, etiology and diagnosis.
448 pages

2524 Learning Disability: Social Class and the Cons of Inequality In American Education
Greenwood Publishing Group
130 Cremona Drive
Santa Barbara, CA 93117
805-968-1911
800-368-6868
Fax: 866-270-3856
CustomerService@abc-clio.com
www.abc-clio.com
James Carrier, Author
Presents a detailed historical description of the social and educational assumptions integral to the idea of learning disability.
167 pages $43.95 - $47.95
ISBN 0-313253-96-X

2525 Learning and Individual Differences
National Association of School Psychologists
4340 East West Hwy.
Suite 402
Bethesda, MD 20814
301-657-0270
866-331-6277
Fax: 301-657-0275
TTY: 301-657-4155
www.nasponline.org
Kathleen Minke, Executive Director
Laura Benson, Chief Operating Officer

2526 Learning to Feel Good and Stay Cool: Emotional Regulation Tools for Kids With AD/HD
750 First Street, NE
Washington, DC 20002-4242
202-336-5500
800-374-2721
rllowman@gmail.com
www.apa.org
Judith M. Glasser, PhD, Co-Author
Kathleen G. Nadeau, PhD, Co-Author
Packed with practical advice and fun activities, this book will show you how to Understand your emotions, Practice healthy habits to stay in your Feel Good Zone, Feel better when you get upset, Know the warning signs that you are heading into your Upset Zone, Problem-solve so upsets come less often

2527 Learning to See: American Sign Language asa Second Language
Gallaudet University Press
800 Florida Ave NE
Washington, DC 20002-3695
202-651-5206
800-621-2736
Fax: 800-621-8476
TTY: 888-630-9347
clerc.center@gallaudet.edu
www.gupress.gallaudet.edu
Dr. T Alan Hurwitz, President
Edward Bosso, Vice President for Administration
Phyliss Wilcox, Co-Author
Sherman Wilcox, Co-Author
This important book has been updated to help teachers teach American Sign Language as a second language, including information on Deaf culture, the history and structure of ASL, teaching methods and issues facing educators. *$19.95*
160 pages Softcover

2528 Let's Write Right: Teacher's Edition
AVKO Educational Research Foundation
3084 Willard Rd
Ste W
Birch Run, MI 48415-9404
810-686-9283
866-285-6612
Fax: 810-686-1101
Barry Chute, President
Julie Guyette, Vice President
Don Mc Cabe, Research Director
Clifford Schroeder, Treasurer
A manuscript and cursive writing program designed not only to teach handwriting but help with reading and spelling patterns as well. Teaches students to learn to read cursive as manuscript is being taught and ease the transition to cursive by using a D'Nealian-like script. Exercises involve phoically consistent patterns to help reinforce fluency with spelling and handwriting. *$39.95*
164 pages

2529 Library Manager's Guide to Hiring and Serving Disabled Persons
McFarland & Company
960 NC Hwy 88 W
Jefferson, NC 28640
336-246-4460
800-253-2187
Fax: 336-246-5018
infoinso@mcfarlandpub.com
www.mcfarlandbooks.com
Kieth C. Wright, Author
Judith F. Davie, Author
Information for library staff on hiring and serving disabled persons. *$27.50*
171 pages Library binding 1990
ISBN 0-899505-16-3

2530 Life-Span Approach to Nursing Care for Individuals with Developmental Disabilities
Brookes Publishing
PO Box 10624
Baltimore, MD 21285-0624
410-337-9580
800-638-3775
Fax: 410-337-8539
custserv@brookespublishing.com
www.brookespublishing.com
Paul H. Brookes, Chairman
Jeffrey D. Brookes, President
Melissa A. Behm, ExecutiveVice President
George S. Stamathis, Vice President & Publisher
This reference book was written by and for nurses. This guide addresses fundamental nursing issues such as health promotion, infection control, seizure management, adaptive and assistive technology, and sexuality. Also offered are in-depth case studies, helpful charts and tables, and problem-solving strategies. *$49.95*
464 pages Hardcover
ISBN 1-557661-51-0

2531 **Mainstreaming Deaf and Hard of Hearing Students: Questions and Answers**
Gallaudet University Bookstore
800 Florida Ave NE
Washington, DC 20002-3600
202-651-5000
800-451-1073
Fax: 202-651-5489
TTY: 888-630-9347
clerc.center@gallaudet.edu
www.gupress.gallaudet.edu
Dr. T Alan Hurwitz, President
Debra S. Lipkey, University Budget Director
Donald Beil, Chief of Staff
Edward Bosso, Vice President for Administratio
This booklet presents mainstreaming as one educational option and suggests some considerations for parents, teachers and administrators. *$6.00*
40 pages

2532 **Mainstreaming Exceptional Students: A Guide for Classroom Teachers**
Allyn & Bacon
75 Arlington St
Suite 300
Boston, MA 02116-3988
617-848-7500
800-852-8024
Fax: 617-944-7273
www.home.pearsonhighered.com
Nancy Forfyth, President
Bill Barke, CEO
Jane B. Schulz, Co-Author
C. Dale Carpenter, Co-Author
Covers the various categories of exceptional students and discusses educational strategies and classroom management.
464 pages paperback
ISBN 0-20515 -24-6

2533 **Mainstreaming: A Practical Approach for Teachers**
McGraw-Hill School Publishing
PO Box 182604
Columbus, OH 43218
877-833-5524
800-338-3987
Fax: 609-308-4480
customer.service@mheducation.com
www.mcgraw-hill.com
David Levin, President/Chief Executive Officer
David Stafford, Senior Vice President/General Counsel
Maryellen Valaitis, Senior Vice President Human Resources
Patrick Milano, Chief Financial Officer/Chief Administrative Officer
Provides teachers, administrators and school psychologists with the background, techniques and strategies they need to offer appropriate services for mildly handicapped students in the mainstream classroom.

2534 **Managing Diagnostic Tool of Visual Perception**
Gallery Bookshop
319 Kasten Street
PO Box 270
Mendocino, CA 95460-270
707-937-2215
Fax: 707-937-3737
info@gallerybookshop.com
www.gallerybooks.com
Constantine Mangina, Author
For diagnosing specific perceptual learning abilities and disabilities. *$14.00*
ISBN 0-80580 -83-4

2535 **Medical Rehabilitation**
Lippincott, Williams & Wilkins
227 S 6th St
Suite 227
Philadelphia, PA 19106-3713
215-545-5630
800-777-2295
Fax: 215-732-9988
www.lpub.com
Cheryl Murkey, Manager
Information for the professional on new techniques and treatments in the medical rehabilitation fields. *$80.50*
368 pages Illustrated
ISBN 0-88167 -85-5

2536 **Meeting the ADD Challenge: A Practical Guide for Teachers**
Research Press
PO Box 7886
Champaign, IL 61826-9177
217-352-3273
800-519-2707
Fax: 217-352-1221
rp@researchpress.com
www.researchpress.com
Robert W. Parkinson, Founder
Dr. Michael Asher, Co-Author
Dr. Steven B Gordon, Co-Author
$24.95
ISBN 0-878223-45-9

2537 **Mental & Physical Disability Law Digest**
A BA Commission on Mental and Physical Disability
1050 Connecticut Ave. N.W.
Suite 400
Washington, DC 20036-1019
202-662-1000
800-285-2221
Fax: 202-442-3439
cmpdl@abanet.org
www.americanbar.org
Robert M. Carlson, Chair, House of Delegates:
James R. Silkenat, President
William C. Hubbard, President-Elect
Cara Lee, Secretary
Provides comprehensive, summary and analysis of federal and state disability and state disability laws from mental disability law and disability discrimination law perspectives. *$60.00*
376 pages
ISBN 1-590310-05-5

2538 **Mental Health Concepts and Techniques for the Occupational Therapy Assistant**
Lippincott, Williams & Wilkins
227 S 6th St
Suite 227
Philadelphia, PA 19106-3713
215-521-8300
800-777-2295
Fax: 301-824-7390
www.lpub.com
J Lippincott, CEO
This text offers clear and easily understood explanations of the various theoretical and practiced health models. *$36.00*
344 pages
ISBN 0-88167 -53-X

2539 **Mental Health and Mental Illness**
Lippincott, Williams & Wilkins
227 S 6th St
Suite 227
Philadelphia, PA 19106-3713
215-592-5400
800-777-2295
Fax: 301-824-7390
www.lpub.com
Kathy Sykes, Manager
Concise, comprehensive and completely up to date, this book presents the most current theory in mental health nursing for the student and the new practitioner. *$28.95*
480 pages
ISBN 0-39755 -73-7

2540 **Mentally Ill Individuals**
Mainstream
Ste 830
3 Bethesda Metro Ctr
Bethesda, MD 20814-6301
301-961-9299
800-247-1380
Fax: 301-654-6714
Charles Moster
Mainstreaming mentally ill individuals into the workplace. *$2.50*
12 pages

2541 Midland Treatment Furniture
Performance Health
28100 Torch Parkway
Suite 700
Warrenville, IL 60555-3938 630-393-6000
Fax: 630-393-7600
customersupport@performancehealth.com
www.performancehealth.com
Francis Dirksmeier, CEO
Isabel Afonso, Managing Director & Head of International
Daniel Baumwald, Vice President, North America Retail & eCommerce
Laurie Byrne, Chief Human Resources Officer
This catalog has the biggest selection of OT/PT products anywhere. Whether you deal with larger or smaller caseloads, you need treatment furniture you can count on. Midland Treatment Furniture from SPR is designed and built to stand up to the heaviest use. From tilt tables and traction packages to mat platforms and parallel bars, you'll find the complete line of Midland Treatment Furniture inside this brochure. All products are assembled from premium materials and carefully crafted.
Free

2542 Multisensory Teaching of Basic Language Skills: Theory and Practice
Brookes Publishing
PO Box 10624
Baltimore, MD 21285-0624 410-337-9580
800-638-3775
Fax: 410-337-8539
custserv@brookespublishing.com
www.brookespublishing.com
Paul H. Brookes, Chairman
Jeffrey D. Brookes, President
Melissa A. Behm, ExecutiveVice President
George S. Stamathis, Vice President & Publisher
This book presents specific multisensory methods for helping students who are having trouble learning to read due to dyslexia or other learning disabilities. Recommended techniques are offered for teaching alphabet skills, composition, comprehension, handwriting, math, organization and study skills, phonological awareness, reading and spelling. *$59.00*
608 pages Hardcover
ISBN 1-557663-49-1

2543 Music, Disability, and Society
1852 North 10th Street
Philadelphia, PA 19122 215-926-2140
800-621-2736
www.temple.edu/tempress
Alex Lubet, Author
In Music, Disability, and Society, Alex Lubet challenges the rigid view of technical skill and writes about music in relation to disability studies. He addresses the ways in which people with disabilities are denied the opportunity to participate in music.

2544 Occupational Therapy Across Cultural Boundaries
Haworth Press
711 Third Avenue
New York, NY 10017 212-216-7800
800-354-1420
Fax: 212-244-1563
subscriptions@tandf.co.uk
www.taylorandfrancisgroup.com
Derek Mapp, Non-Executive Chairman
Roger Horton, CEO
Emma Blaney, Group HR Director - Head of Corporate Responsibility
Isobel Peck, Group Chief Marketing Officer
Examines the concept of culture from a unique perspective, that of individual occupational therapists who have worked in environments very different from those in which they were educated or had worked previously. Journal publications formerly published by Haworth Press are now listed on the Taylor & Francis Journals website. *$74.95*
107 pages Hardcover
ISBN 1-560242-23-X

2545 Occupational Therapy Approaches to Traumatic Brain Injury
Routledge (Taylor & Francis Group)
711 Third Ave
New York, NY 10017 212-216-7800
800-634-7064
Fax: 212-564-7854
enquiries@taylorandfrancis.com
www.routledge.com
Laura H. Krefting, Author
Jerry A. Johnson, Author
Focusing on the disabled individual, the family, and the societal responses to the injured, this comprehensive book covers the spectrum of available services from intensive care to transitional and community living. Formerly published by Haworth Press, titles are now listed on Routledge/Taylor Francis Group. *$140.00*
137 pages Hardcover
ISBN 1-560240-64-4

2546 Overcoming Dyslexia in Children, Adolescents and Adults
Sage Publications
2455 Teller Road
Thousand Oaks, CA 91320 805-499-9774
800-818-7243
Fax: 800-583-2665
books.claim@sagepub.com
www.sagepub.com
Sara Miller McCune, Founder, Publisher, Chairperson
Blaise R Simqu, President/CEO
Tracey A. Ozmina, Executive Vice President & Chief
Dale R. Jordan, Author
This book describes some forms of dyslexia in detail and then relates those problems to the social, emotional and personal development of dyslexic individuals. *$34.00*
350 pages Paperback

2547 Oxford Textbook of Geriatric Medicine
Oxford University Press
198 Madison Ave
New York, NY 10016-4308 212-726-6000
800-445-9714
Fax: 919-677-1303
custserv.us@oup.com
global.oup.com
Rebecca Seger, Director, Institutional Sales, Americas
Lesa Moran Owen, Library Sales Operations Manager
Lenny Allen, Director, Institutional Accounts
Nancy Roy, Library Sales Manager
This comprehensive text brings together extensive experience in clinical geriatrics with a strong scientific base in research. *$125.00*
784 pages

2548 Pain Centers: A Revolution in Health Care
Lippincott Williams And Wilkins
227
227 S 6th St
Philadelphia, PA 19106-3713 215-521-8300
800-777-2295
Fax: 301-824-7390
www.lpub.com
J Lippincott, CEO
$103.00
280 pages

2549 Parental Concerns in College Student Mental Health
Haworth Press
711 Third Avenue
New York, NY 10017 212-216-7800
800-354-1420
Fax: 212-244-1563
subscriptions@tandf.co.uk
www.taylorandfrancisgroup.com
Derek Mapp, Non-Executive Chairman
Roger Horton, CEO
Emma Blaney, Group HR Director - Head of Corporate Responsibility
Isobel Peck, Group Chief Marketing Officer

An instructive guide for parents and mental health professionals regarding the most important issues about psychological development in college students. Journal publications formerly published by Haworth Press are now listed on the Taylor & Francis Journals website. *$74.95*

204 pages Hardcover

ISBN 0-866567-20-8

2550 **Parents and Teachers**

Alexander Graham Bell Association
3417 Volta Pl NW
Washington, DC 20007-2737 202-337-5220
866-337-5220
Fax: 202-337-8314
TTY: 202-337-5221
info@agbell.org
www.listeningandspokenlanguage.org

Kathleen S. Treni, M.Ed., M.A., President
Meredith K. Knueve, Esq., Secretary-Treasurer
Alexander T. Graham, Executive Director/CEO
Corrine Altman, Director

This excellent book offers in-depth guidance to parents and teachers whose partnership can foster language in school-aged children with hearing impairments. The first section examines roles of parents, teachers, professionals and children in language acquisition, residual hearing and audiological management, language development stages and readying children for preschool. The second portion of the book presents specific objectives and teaching strategies to use at school and at home. *$27.95*

386 pages

2551 **Patient and Family Education**

Springer Publishing Company
11 W 42nd St
15th Floor
New York, NY 10036-8002 212-431-4370
877-687-7476
Fax: 212-941-7842
cs@springerpub.com
www.springerpub.com

Dr. Ursula Springer, President
Ted Nardin, CEO
James C. Costello, Vice President, Journal Publishi
James C. Costello, Vice President, Journal Publishing

This guide outlines the actual clinical content needed to develop, implement and maintain patient education programs. Conveniently arranged in one-hour long lesson plans, each disease or condition is organized in an easy-to-follow format. *$26.95*

272 pages Softcover

ISBN 0-82615 -41-7

2552 **Person to Person: Guide for Professionals Working with the Disabled**

Paul H Brookes Publishing Company
PO Box 10624
Baltimore, MD 21285-0624 410-337-9580
800-638-3775
Fax: 410-337-8539
custserv@brookespublishing.com
www.brookespublishing.com

Paul H. Brookes, Chairman
Jeffrey D. Brookes, President
Melissa A. Behm, ExecutiveVice President
George S. Stamathis, Vice President & Publisher

This second edition of an already-popular book helps professionals approach interactions with a people-first, disability second attitude. *$29.00*

288 pages Paperback

ISBN 1-557661-00-6

2553 **Personality and Emotional Disturbance**

Taylor & Francis
Ste G
47 Runway Dr
Levittown, PA 19057-4738 267-580-2622
Fax: 215-785-5515

Richard Roberts, CEO

The brain injured person has unique needs. Recent findings have highlighted that it is the personality, behavioral and emotional problems which most prohibit a return to work, create the greatest burden for the long-term care and rehabilitation of physical and cognitive functions. *$72.00*

260 pages Cloth

ISBN 0-85066 -71-3

2554 **Phenomenology of Depressive Illness**

Human Sciences Press
233 Spring St
New York, NY 10013-1522 212-229-2859
877-283-3229
Fax: 212-463-0742
ainy@aveda.com
www.aveda.edu

263 pages Cloth

ISBN 0-89885 -69-9

2555 **Physical Disabilities and Health Impairments: An Introduction**

McGraw-Hill School Publishing
PO Box 182604
Columbus, OH 43218 877-833-5524
800-338-3987
Fax: 609-308-4480
customer.service@mheducation.com
www.mcgraw-hill.com

David Levin, President/Chief Executive Officer
David Stafford, Senior Vice President/General Counsel
Maryellen Valaitis, Senior Vice President Human Resources
Patrick Milano, Chief Financial Officer/Chief Administrative Officer

A comprehensive text which presents a wealth of up-to-date medical information for teachers.

2556 **Physical Education and Sports for Exceptional Students**

McGraw-Hill Company
2460 Kerper Blvd
Dubuque, IA 52001-2224 800-338-3987
Fax: 614-755-5654
www.mhhe.com/hper/physed

Michael Horvat, Author
Harold McGraw III, Chairman, President and Chief Ex
Jack F. Callahan, Executive Vice President, Chief
John Berisford, Executive Vice President, Human

Physical education for exceptional students and teaching students with learning and behavior exceptionalities.

Cloth

2557 **Physical Management of Multiple Handicaps: A Professional's Guide**

Brookes Publishing Company
PO Box 10624
Baltimore, MD 21285-0624 410-337-9580
800-638-3775
Fax: 410-337-8539
custserv@brookespublishing.com
www.brookespublishing.com

Paul H. Brookes, Chairman
Jeffrey D. Brookes, President
Melissa A. Behm, ExecutiveVice President
George S. Stamathis, Vice President & Publisher

Comprehensive guide, takes a transdisciplinary approach to therapeutic/technological management of persons with multiple handicaps. *$36.00*

352 pages Hardcover

ISBN 1-557660-47-6

2558 **Physically Handicapped in Society**

Ayer Company Publishers
Ste 322
400 Bedford St
Manchester, NH 03101-1195 603-669-9307
888-267-7323
Fax: 603-669-7945
www.ayerpub.com

Kathy Train, Office Manager
Ellie Phipps, Customer Service

A group of 39 books. Biographies that offer studies on attitudes, sociological and psychological. Please write or call for catalog. *$965.00*
Hardcover
ISBN 0-40513 -00-3

2559 Practicing Rehabilitation with Geriatric Clients
Springer Publishing Company
11 W 42nd St
15th Floor
New York, NY 10036-8002 212-431-4370
877-687-7476
Fax: 212-941-7842
cs@springerpub.com
www.springerpub.com
Dr. Ursula Springer, President
Ted Nardin, CEO
James C. Costello, Vice President, Journal Publishi
James C. Costello, Vice President, Journal Publishing
Physical therapy in the geriatric client, psychological and psychiatric considerations in the rehabilitation of the elderly. *$32.95*
256 pages Hardcover
ISBN 0-82616 -80-5

2560 Pragmatic Approach
Educators Publishing Service
625 Mount Auburn St
3RD Floor
Cambridge, MA 02138-3039 617-547-6706
800-225-5750
Fax: 617-547-0285
Paula Fabbro, Sales Consultant
Leo Micale, Sales Consultant
Kristen Colson, Sales Consultant
Flora Francis, Sales Consultant
Monograph on evaluation of children's performances on Slingerland Pre-Reading Screening Procedures to Identify First Grade Academic Needs. *$6.00*
56 pages
ISBN 0-838816-85-1

2561 Preschoolers with Special Needs: Children At-Risk, Children with Disabilities
Allyn & Bacon
75 Arlington St
Suite 300
Boston, MA 02116-3988 617-848-7500
800-852-8024
Fax: 617-944-7273
www.home.pearsonhighered.com
Bill Barke, CEO
Janet W. Lerner, Co-Author
Barbara Lowenthal, Co-Author
Rosemary W. Egan, Co-Author
Explores ways of providing preschool children with special needs and their families with a learning environment that will help them develop and learn. Emphasizes the needs of preschoolers age three to six and provides information to teachers and others who work with young children in all settings. Current models of curricula, which incorporate new features from research and practical expreiences with children who have special needs, are described and discussed. *$59.00*
336 pages cloth
ISBN 0-205358-79-9

2562 Preventing Academic Failure - Teachers Handbook
Educators Publishing Service
625 Mount Auburn St
3rd Fl
Cambridge, MA 02138-3039 617-547-6706
800-225-5750
Fax: 617-547-0285
eps.schoolspecialty.com
Paperback
ISBN 0-838852-71-8

2563 Preventing School Dropouts
Sage Publications
2455 Teller Road
Thousand Oaks, CA 91320 805-499-9774
800-818-7243
Fax: 800-583-2665
books.claim@sagepub.com
www.sagepub.com
Sara Miller McCune, Founder, Publisher, Chairperson
Blaise R Simqu, President/ CEO
Tracey A. Ozmina, Executive Vice President & Chief
Thomas C. Lovitt, Author
For secondary teachers, special education and regular, who have difficulty teaching youth in their classes. Presented are 120 tactics, specific instructional techniques, for helping adolescents to stay in school. Each tactic is written in a format that includes five sections. *$38.00*
509 pages

2564 Prevocational Assessment
Exceptional Education
P.O. Box 15308
Seattle, WA 98115-308 206-262-9538
Fax: 475-486-4510
Jeff Stewart, Owner
Use the PACG to assess your students in nine areas (attendance and endurance, learning and behavior, communication skills, social skills, grooming and eating and toileting) covering 46 specific workshop experiences. *$12.00*
16 pages Complete Set
ISBN 1-87786 -23-7

2565 Primary Special Needs and the National Curriculum
7625 Empire Drive
Florence, KN 41042-2919 800-634-4724
orders@taylorandfrancis.com
Ann Lewis, Author
This new edition of Ann Lewis's widely acclaimed text has been substantially revised and updated to take into account the recent revisions to the National Curriculum and the guidance of the Code of Practice.

2566 Progress Without Punishment: Approaches for Learners with Behavior Problems
Teachers College Press
1234 Amsterdam Ave
New York, NY 10027-6602 212-678-3929
800-575-6566
Fax: 212-678-4149
tcpress@tc.columbia.edu
www.teacherscollegepress.com
Anne M. Donnellan, Author
In this volume, the authors argue against the use of punishment, and instead advocate the use of alternative intervention procedures. *$17.95*
184 pages Paperback
ISBN 0-807729-11-6

2567 Promoting Postsecondary Education for Students with Learning Disabilities
Sage Publications
2455 Teller Road
Thousand Oaks, CA 91320 805-499-9774
800-818-7243
Fax: 800-583-2665
books.claim@sagepub.com
www.sagepub.com
Sara Miller McCune, Founder, Publisher, Chairperson
Stan F. Shaw, Co-Author
Joan M. McGuire, Co-Author
Loring Cowles Brinckerhoff, Co-Author
Primarily designed for postsecondary service providers who are responsible for serving college students with learning disabilities. *$41.00*
440 pages

2568 **Psychiatric Mental Health Nursing**
Lippincott, Williams & Wilkins
227 S 6th St
Suite 227
Philadelphia, PA 19106-3713
215-521-8300
800-777-2295
Fax: 301-824-7390
J Lippincott, CEO
This text emphasizes and contrasts the roles of the generalist nurse and the psychiatric nurse specialist. *$52.00*
1120 pages Illustrated

2569 **Psychoeducational Assessment of Visually Impaired and Blind Students**
Sage Publications
2455 Teller Road
Thousand Oaks, CA 91320
805-499-9774
800-818-7243
Fax: 800-583-2665
books.claim@sagepub.com
www.sagepub.com
Sara Miller McCune, Founder, Publisher, Chairperson
Blaise R Simqu, President/CEO
Tracey A. Ozmina, Executive Vice President & Chief
Sharon Bradley-Johnson, Author
Professional reference book that addresses the problems specific to assessment of visually impaired and blind children. Of particular value to the practitioner are the extensive reviews of available tests, including ways to adapt those not designed for use with the visually handicapped. *$29.00*
140 pages Paperback
ISBN 0-890791-08-2

2570 **Psychological and Social Impact of Illness and Disability**
Springer Publishing
11 W 42nd St
15th Floor
New York, NY 10036-8002
212-431-4370
877-687-7476
Fax: 212-941-7842
cs@springerpub.com
www.springerpub.com
Dr. Ursula Springer, President
Ted Nardin, CEO
Ph.D. Orto Arthur E. Dell, Editor
James C. Costello, Vice President, Journal Publishing
The newest edition of Psychological and Social Impact of Illness and Disability continues the tradition of presenting a realistic perspective on life with disabilies and then improves upon its predecessors with the inclusion of illness as a major influence on client care needs. Further broadening the scope of this edition is the inclusion of personal perspectives and stories from those living with illness or disabilities. These stories offer a look into what it is like to cope with these issues.

2571 **Reading and Deafness**
Sage Publications
2455 Teller Road
Thousand Oaks, CA 91320
805-499-9774
800-818-7243
Fax: 800-583-2665
books.claim@sagepub.com
www.sagepub.com
Sara Miller McCune, Founder, Publisher, Chairperson
Beverly J Trezek, Co-Author
Peter V. Paul, Co-Author
Ye Wang, Co-Author
Three areas are looked at in this book: deaf children's prereading development of real-world knowledge, cognitive abilities and linguistic skills. *$39.00*
422 pages

2572 **Readings on Research in Stuttering**
Longman Publishing Group
1 Penn Plaza
Suite 2222
New York, NY 10119
646-556-8401
Fax: 646-556-8415
coffee@rothfos.com
www.rothfos.com
Dan Dwyer, CEO
Thomas Minogue, CFO
Maria Tanpinco-Queyquep, Traffic Manager
Joseph P. Thomas, Traffic Coordinator
Collection of the key journal articles published on stuttering over the past decade, addressing trends in recent research in the field.
231 pages Paperback
ISBN 0-801304-10-5

2573 **Recreation Activities for the Elderly**
Springer Publishing Company
11 W 42nd St
15th Floor
New York, NY 10036-8002
212-431-4370
877-687-7476
Fax: 212-941-7842
cs@springerpub.com
www.springerpub.com
Dr. Ursula Springer, President
Ted Nardin, CEO
James C. Costello, Vice President, Journal Publishi
James C. Costello, Vice President, Journal Publishing
Included in this volume are simple crafts that utilize easily obtainable, inexpensive materials, hobbies focusing on collections, nature, and the arts' and games emphasizing both mental and physical activity. *$23.95*
240 pages Softcover
ISBN 0-82616 -30-1

2574 **Reference Manual for Communicative Sciences and Disorders**
Pro- Ed Publications
8700 Shoal Creek Blvd
Austin, TX 78757-6897
512-451-3246
800-897-3202
Fax: 512-451-8542
info@proedinc.com
www.proedinc.com
Raymond D. Kent, Author
An indispensable guide to standards and values essential in the assessment of communication disorders. *$54.00*
393 pages

2575 **Rehabilitation Interventions for the Institutionalized Elderly**
Haworth Press
711 Third Avenue
Floor 8th
New York, NY 10017
212-216-7800
800-354-1420
Fax: 212-564-7854
subscriptions@tandf.co.uk
Derek Mapp, Non-Executive Chairman
Roger Horton, CEO
Emma Blaney, Group HR Director - Head of Corporate Responsibility
Isobel Peck, Group Chief Marketing Officer
Gerontology professionals offer suggestions to enrich the quality of rehabilitation services offered to the institutionalized elderly. This volume examines up to the minute ideas, some that would have been unlikely even a few years ago, that focus exclusively on rehabilitation services for the institutionalized elderly. Journal publications formerly published by Haworth Press are now listed on the Taylor & Franc *$44.95*
77 pages Hardcover
ISBN 0-866568-33-6

2576 Rehabilitation Nursing for the Neurological Patient
Springer Publishing Company
11 W 42nd St
15th Fl
New York, NY 10036-8002
212-431-4370
877-687-7476
Fax: 212-941-7842
cs@springerpub.com
www.springerpub.com

Ted Nardin, Chief Executive Officer
Jason Roth, Vice President, Sales & Marketing
Kathy Weiss, Director, Sales
Marcia Hanak, Author

Reviews the physiology, pathophysiology, & nursing management of problems frequently encountered in neuro- rehabilitation and reviews the pathphysiology of specific disabilities & the related nursing interventions. *$32.95*
229 pages Hardcover 1992
ISBN 0-826176-60-7

2577 Rehabilitation Resource Manual: VISION
Resources for Rehabilitation
22 Bonad Rd
Winchester, MA 01890-1302
781-368-9094
Fax: 781-368-9096
info@rfr.org
www.rfr.org

Marshall E. Flax, MS, Author

A desk reference that enables service providers, librarians and others to make effective referrals. Includes guidelines on establishing self-help groups, information on research and service organizations, and chapters on assistive technology, for special population groups and by eye condition. *$44.95*
Biennial

2578 Rehabilitation Technology
CRC Press
6000 Broken Sound Pkwy NW
Ste 300
Boca Raton, FL 33487
800-634-7064
Fax: 800-374-3401
orders@crcpress.com
www.crcpress.com

Glenn E. Hedman, Author

Learn how the use of technological devices can enhance the lives of disabled children. Informs physical therapists, occupational therapists, and rehabilitation technologists about the devices that are available today and provides important background information on these devices. CRC Press is part of the Taylor & Francis Group. *$39.95*
173 pages Hardcover 1990
ISBN 1-560240-33-4

2579 Report Writing in Assessment and Evaluation
Stout Vocational Rehab Institute
University of Wisconsin-Stout
712 South Broadway
Menomonie, WI 54751
715-232-1478
Fax: 715-232-2356
giffordj@uwstout.edu
www.uwstout.edu

Charles W. Sorensen, Chancellor
Judy Gifford, Director
Stephen W. Thomas, Author
Linda Vanderloop, CFSC Office

This examines questions of who are you writing for and what does the referral source want. Defines characteristics of good reports, common problems, writing in different settings, types of reports, getting ready to write, and writing prescriptive recommendations. *$17.75*
188 pages Softcover

2580 Resource Room, The
State University of New York Press
22 Corporate Woods Boulevard
3rd Floor
Albany, NY 12210-2314
518-472-5000
866-430-7869
Fax: 518-472-5038
info@sunypress.edu
www.sunypress.edu

Barry Edwards McNamara, Author

Provides teachers and administrators with helpful, practical information and explores the role of the resource room teacher as it relates to three major functions: assessment, instruction and consultation. It will also assist supervisors and administrators in evaluating their resource programs. *$28.95*
148 pages Paperback
ISBN 0-887069-84-0

2581 Resources for Rehabilitation
22 Bonad Rd
Winchester, MA 01890-1302
781-368-9094
Fax: 781-368-9096
info@rfr.org
www.rfr.org

2582 Restructuring High Schools for All Students: Taking Inclusion to the Next Level
Brookes Publishing
PO Box 10624
Baltimore, MD 21285-0624
410-337-9580
800-638-3775
Fax: 410-337-8539
custserv@brookespublishing.com
www.brookespublishing.com

Paul H. Brookes, Chairman
Jeffrey D. Brookes, President
Melissa A. Behm, ExecutiveVice President
George S. Stamathis, Vice President & Publisher

Details the process of creating an inclusive, collaborate community of learners and teachers at the secondary level. *$29.95*
304 pages Paperback
ISBN 1-557663-13-0

2583 Restructuring for Caring and Effective Education: Administrative Guide
Brookes Publishing
PO Box 10624
Baltimore, MD 21285-0624
410-337-9580
800-638-3775
Fax: 410-337-8539
custserv@brookespublishing.com
www.brookespublishing.com

Paul H. Brookes, Chairman
Jeffrey D. Brookes, President
Melissa A. Behm, ExecutiveVice President
George S. Stamathis, Vice President & Publisher

In this empowering book, leading general and special education schools reform experts synthesize the major school restructuring initiatives and describe the processes and rationale for changing the organizational structure and instructional practices of schools. *$29.00*
384 pages Paperback
ISBN 1-55766 -91-3

2584 Scoffolding Student Learning
Brookline Books
8 Trumbull Rd
Suite B-001
Northampton, MA 01060
413-584-0184
800-666-2665
Fax: 413-584-6184
brbooks@yahoo.com
www.brooklinebooks.com

Paul H. Brookes, Chairman
Jeffrey D. Brookes, President
Melissa A. Behm, ExecutiveVice President
George S. Stamathis, Vice President & Publisher

Collection of papers on the theory and practice of scoffolding—an interactive style of instructions that helps students develop more powerful thinking tools. *$21.95*
180 pages Paperback
ISBN 1-571290-36-2

2585 Selective Nontreatment of Handicapped
Oxford University Press
2001 Evans Rd
Cary, NC 27513-2009
919-677-0977
800-445-9714
Fax: 919-677-1303
custserv.us@oup.com
www.global.oup.com
Lesa Moran Owen, Library Sales Operations Manager
Rebecca Seger, Director, Institutional Sales, Americas
Lenny Allen, Director, Institutional Accounts
Nancy Roy, Library Sales Manager
Information on selective nontreatment of handicapped newborns, moral dilemmas in neonatal medicine. *$17.95*
304 pages Paperback

2586 Semiotics and Dis/ability: Interogating Categories of Difference
State University of New York Press
22 Corporate Woods Boulevard
3rd Floor
Albany, NY 12210-2314
518-472-5000
866-430-7869
Fax: 518-472-5038
info@sunypress.edu
www.sunypress.edu
James Peltz, Associate Director
Linda Rogers, Editor
Beth Blue Swadener, Editor
Examines the ways the words disability and difference and socially and culturally constructed. *$25.95*
265 pages Paperback 1990
ISBN 0-791449-06-6

2587 Service Coordination for Early Intervention: Parents and Friends
Brookline Books
8 Trumbull Rd
Suite B-001
Northampton, MA 01060
413-584-0184
800-666-2665
Fax: 413-584-6184
brbooks@yahoo.com
www.brooklinebooks.com
Deborah D. Hatton, Co-Author
R. A. McWilliam, Co-Author
P. J. Winton, Co-Author
This book helps administrators and professionals to structure early intervention and ongoing services so that professionals work collaboratively with parents to promote the health, well being and development of children with special needs. *$19.95*
110 pages Paperback
ISBN 0-91479 -91-3

2588 Services for the Seriously Mentally Ill: A Survey of Mental Health Centers
Nat'l Council for Community Behavioral Healthcare
12300 Twinbrook Pkwy
Ste 320
Rockville, MD 20852-1606
301-984-6200
Fax: 301-881-7159
Linda Rosenberg, CEO
Dale K Klatzker, Board Chair
This ground-breaking report documents what administrators and practitioners have maintained for many years: community mental health organizations devote a significant percentage of the human and financial resources to serving the seriously mentally ill. *$30.00*

2589 Sexuality and Disability
Springer Publishing
11 W 42nd St
15th Fl
New York, NY 10036-8002
212-431-4370
Fax: 212-460-1575
www.springer.com
Sigmund Hough, Editor-in-Chief
A journal devoted to the psychological and medical aspects of sexuality in rehabilitation and community settings. The journal features original scholarly articles that address the psychological and medical aspects of sexuality in the field of rehabilitation, case studies, clinical practice reports, and guidelines for clinical practice.
Quarterly

2590 Shop Talk
PO Box 7886
Champaign, IL 61826-9177
217-352-3273
800-519-2707
Fax: 217-352-1221
rp@researchpress.com
www.researchpress.com
Robert W. Parkinson, Founder
Philip Roth, Author

2591 Signed English Schoolbook
Gallaudet University Press
800 Florida Ave NE
Washington, DC 20002-3600
202-651-5488
800-451-1073
Fax: 202-651-5489
TTY: 888-630-9347
clerc.center@gallaudet.edu
www.gupress.gallaudet.edu
Harry Bornstein, Co-Author
Karen L. Saulnier, Co-Author
Dr. T Alan Hurwitz, President
Edward Bosso, Vice President for Administratio
The Signed English Schoolbook provides vocabulary for teachers and others who serve school-age children and adolescents and covers the full range of school activities. *$13.95*
184 pages Softcover

2592 Social Skills for Students With Autism Spectrum Disorders and Other Developmental Disorders
Council for Exceptional Children
3100 Clarendon Blvd.
Suite 600
Arlington, VA 22201-5332
888-232-7733
TTY: 866-915-5000
service@exceptionalchildren.org
www.exceptionalchildren.org
Laurence R. Sargent, Co-Author
Toni Cook, Co-Author
Darlene E. Perner, Co-Author
A book teaching children to understand their own behaviours. *$24.95*

2593 Social Studies: Detecting and Correcting Special Needs
Allyn & Bacon
75 Arlington St
Suite 300
Boston, MA 02116-3988
617-848-7500
800-852-8024
Fax: 617-944-7273
www.home.pearsonhighered.com
Harry Bornst Barke, CEO
Nancy Forfyth, President
Lana J. Smith, Co-Author
Dennie L. Smith, Co-Author
Describes social studies and special needs for special learners.
180 pages
ISBN 0-205121-51-9

2594 **Social and Emotional Development of Exceptional Students: Handicapped**
Charles C. Thomas
2600 S First St
Springfield, IL 62704-4730
217-789-8980
800-258-8980
Fax: 217-789-9130
books@ccthomas.com
www.ccthomas.com
Michael P. Thomas, President
Carroll J. Jones, Author
Sixteen years after the passage of P.L. 94-142, the dream of special educators to educate the handicapped and nonhandicapped children and youth together resulting in increased academic gains and age-appropriate school skills for handicapped children and youth has not yet materialized. This book helps eliminate an existing void by providing teachers with understandable information regarding the social and emotional development of exceptional students. Also in cloth at $41.95 (ISBN# 0-398-05781-8) *$29.95*
218 pages Softcover
ISBN 0-398061-94-7

2595 **Special Education Today**
LifeWay Christian Resources Southern Baptist Conv.
One LifeWay Plaza
Nashville, TN 37234
615-251-2000
800-458-2772
Fax: 615-532-9412
www.lifeway.com
Thom S. Rainer, President/CEO
Brad Waggoner, Executive Vice President
Eric Geiger, Vice President, Church Resources Division
Tim Hill, Vice President/Chief Information Officer
This unique quarterly publications ministers to people with special education needs and to their families, the church, and other caregivers. It offers a variety of helps and encouragement, including: What's working in churches, Suggestions for adapting teaching techniques, inspirational stories about people who have disabilities, Parenting and family issues, Ideas for reaching, witnessing, worship, and recreation. *$4.25*
36 pages Quarterly

2596 **Special Education for Today**
Allyn & Bacon
75 Arlington St
Suite 300
Boston, MA 02116-3988
617-848-7500
800-852-8024
Fax: 617-944-7273
www.home.pearsonhighered.com
See search r Barke, CEO
Michael S. Rosenberg, Co-Author
David L. Westling, Co-Author
James McLeskey, Co-Author
An undergraduate introduction to special education covering all major areas of exceptionality. Contains pedagogical features designed to make the book accessible to the undergraduate.
576 pages hardcover
ISBN 0-138264-53-8

2597 **Speech and the Hearing-Impaired Child**
Alexander Graham Bell Association
3417 Volta Pl NW
Washington, DC 20007-2737
202-337-5220
866-337-5220
Fax: 202-337-8314
TTY: 202-337-5221
info@agbell.org
www.listeningandspokenlanguage.org
Meredith K. Sugar, Esq. (OH), President
Ted A. Meyer, M.D., Ph.D, President-Elect/Secretary-Treasurer
Emilio Alonso-Mendoza, Chief Executive Officer
Susan Boswell, Director of Communications and Marketing
This textbook for professionals deals with basic theoretical issues in the acquisition of speech and the form of language (phonetics and phonology) in children with hearing losses. It provides a systematic framework to develop and evaluate speech target behaviors and their underlying subskills. *$29.95*
402 pages Paperback

2598 **Speech-Language Pathology and Audiology: An Introduction**
McGraw-Hill School Publishing
PO Box 182604
Columbus, OH 43218
877-833-5524
800-338-3987
Fax: 609-308-4480
customer.service@mheducation.com
www.mcgraw-hill.com
David Levin, President/Chief Executive Officer
David Stafford, Senior Vice President/General Counsel
Maryellen Valaitis, Senior Vice President Human Resources
Patrick Milano, Chief Financial Officer & Chief Administrative Officer
Offers classroom-tested coverage of clinical objectives and functioning.
301 pages

2599 **Spinal Cord Dysfunction**
Oxford University Press
2001 Evans Rd
Cary, NC 27513-2009
919-677-0977
800-451-7556
Fax: 919-677-1303
humanres@oup-usa.org
Lesa Moran Owen, Library Sales Operations Manager
Rebecca Seger, Director, Institutional Sales, Americas
Lenny Allen, Director, Institutional Accounts
Nancy Roy, Library Sales Manager
Offers information on restoration of function after spinal cord damage as seen from the point of view of identification of impaired or absent function in the nerve cells and processes which survive after the initial insult, intact but with impaired functions.
$95.00
368 pages

2600 **Steps to Success: Scope & Sequence for Skill Development**
15619 Premiere Drive
Suite 101
Tampa, FL 33624
850-363-9909
Fax: 480-393-4331
accounting@successforkidswithhearingloss.com
successforkidswithhearinglo ss.com
Lynne H. Price, Author
Steps to Success is a curriculum for students who are deaf or hard of hearing in grades kindergarten through 12.

2601 **Strategies for Teaching Learners with Special Needs**
McGraw-Hill School Publishing
PO Box 182604
Columbus, OH 43218
877-833-5524
800-338-3987
Fax: 609-308-4480
customer.service@mheducation.com
www.mcgraw-hill.com
David Levin, President/Chief Executive Officer
David Stafford, Senior Vice President/General Counsel
Maryellen Valaitis, Senior Vice President Human Resources
Patrick Milano, Chief Financial Officer & Chief Administrative Officer
This is a text that helps special educators develop the full range of teaching competencies needed to be effective.
560 pages

2602 **Strategies for Teaching Students with Learning and Behavior Problems**
Allyn & Bacon
75 Arlington St
Suite 300
Boston, MA 02116-3988
617-848-7500
800-852-8024
Fax: 617-944-7273
www.home.pearsonhighered.com
Bill Barke, CEO
Nancy Forfyth, President
Sharon R. Vaughn, Co-Author
Candace S. Bos, Co-Author
Provides descriptions of methods and strategies for teaching students with learning and behavior problems, managing profes-

sional roles, and collaborating with families, professionals, and paraprofessionals.
544 pages
ISBN 0-205113-89-3

2603 **Students with Acquired Brain Injury: The School's Response**
Brookes Publishing
PO Box 10624
Baltimore, MD 21285-0624
410-337-9580
800-638-3775
Fax: 410-337-8539
custserv@brookespublishing.com
www.brookespublishing.com
Ann Glang, Editor
Bonnie Todis, Editor
Paul H. Brooks, Chairman of the Board
Cary Gold, Educational Sales Representative
This book is designed for school professionals and describes a range of issues that this population faces and presents proven means of addressing them in ways that benefit all students. Included topics are hospital-to-school transitions, effective assessment strategies, model programs in public schools, interventions to assist classroom teachers, and ways to involve family members in the educational program. *$29.95*
424 pages Paperback
ISBN 1-55766 -85-1

2604 **Students with Mild Disabilities in the Secondary School**
Longman Group
75 Arlington St
Suite 300
New York, NY 10036-2601
212-782-3300
800-852-8024
www.home.pearsonhighered.com
William Hitchings, Co-Author
Michael Horvath, Co-Author
Bonnie Schmalle, Co-Author
Paul Retish, Co-Author, Editor
Provides methods and strategies for curriculum delivery to students with mild disabilities at the secondary school level.
2313G pages Paperback
ISBN 0-801301-66-1

2605 **Supporting and Strengthening Families**
Brookline Books
8 Trumbull Rd
Suite B-001
Northampton, MA 01060
413-584-0184
800-666-2665
Fax: 413-584-6184
brbooks@yahoo.com
www.brooklinebooks.com
Carl J Dunst, Author
A collection of papers addressing the theory, methods, strategies, and practices involved in adopting an empowerment and family-centered resources approach to supporting families and strengthening individual and family functioning. *$30.00*
252 pages Paperback
ISBN 0-91479 -94-8

2606 **TESTS**
Slosson Educational Publications
538 Buffalo rd
PO Box 280
East Aurora, NY 14052
716-652-0930
888-756-7766
Fax: 800-665-3840
slossonprep@gmail.com
www.slosson.com
Steven W. Slosson, President
Dr. Georgina Moynihan, Office Personnel
Slosson Educational Publications, Inc. offers educators an extensive selection of testing products, along with books on autism. ADED and other special needs materials. Our catalog includes 30 pages of speech-language testing and language rehabilitation products. The behavioral conduct. Special needs section includes checklist and scales on aberrant/disruptive behavior, tapes on ADD, as well as products for dyslexia and remediation of reversals.

2607 **Teacher's Guide to Including Students with Disabilities in Regular Physical Education**
Brookes Publishing
PO Box 10624
Baltimore, MD 21285-0624
410-337-9580
800-638-3775
Fax: 410-337-8539
custserv@brookespublishing.com
www.brookespublishing.com
Martin E. Block, Author
Melissa A. Behm, Executive Vice President
Paul H. Brooks, Chairman of the Board
Cary Gold, Educational Sales Representative
Provides simple and creative strategies for meaningfully including children with disabilities in regular physical education programs. *$39.00*
288 pages Paperback
ISBN 1-557661-56-1

2608 **Teachers Working Together**
Brookline Books
8 Trumbull Rd
Suite B-001
Northampton, MA 01060
413-584-0184
800-666-2665
Fax: 413-584-6184
brbooks@yahoo.com
www.brooklinebooks.com
Carol Davis, Co-Author
Alice Yang, Co-Author
This collection of papers describes collaborative efforts for such classroom settings as preschools, elementary, middle and high schools, for content area teaching and into the transition to work. Each chapter describes actual practice and analyzes what is required to accomplish this collaboration. *$19.95*
Paperback
ISBN 1-57139 -66-4

2609 **Teachig Students with Special Needs in Inclusive Classrooms**
SAGE Publications
2455 Teller Rd
Thousand Oaks, CA 91320
800-818-7243
Fax: 800-583-2665
orders@sagepub.com
us.sagepub.com
Diane P. Bryant, Author
Brian P. Bryant, Author
Deborah D. Smith, Author
Using the research-validated ADAPT framework, Teaching Students with Special Needs in Inclusive Classrooms helps future teachers determine how, when, and with whom to use proven academic and behavioral interventions to obtain the best outcomes for students with disabilities. This book will provide the skills and inspiration that teachers need to make a positive difference in the educational lives of struggling learners.

2610 **Teaching Adults with Learning Disabilities**
Krieger Publishing Company
1725 Krieger Drive
Malabar, FL 32902
321-724-9542
800-724-0025
Fax: 321-951-3671
info@krieger-publishing.com
www.krieger-publishing.com
Dale R. Jordan, Author
R Krieger, Owner
Designed to teach literacy providers and classroom instructors how to recognize specific learning disability (LD) patterns and block reading, spelling, writing and arithmetic skills in students of all ages. One of the major problems faced by literary providers is keeping low-skill adults involved in basic education programs long enough to increase their literacy skills to the level of success. Shows instructors in adult education how to modify teaching strategies. *$25.50*
160 pages
ISBN 0-894649-10-8

2611 Teaching Children With Autism in the General Classroom
Prufrock Press
PO Box 8813
Waco, TX 76714-8813
254-756-3337
800-998-2208
Fax: 254-756-3339
gbates@prufrock.com
www.prufrock.com
Joel McIntosh, Publisher & Marketing Director
Ginny Bates, Customer Service and Office Manager
Lacy Compton, Senior Editor
Rachel Taliaferro, Editor
Provides an introduction to inclusionary practices that serve children with autism, giving teachers the practical advice they need to ensure each students receives the quality education he or she deserves. *$39.95*
350 pages Paperback
ISBN 1-593633-64-6

2612 Teaching Disturbed and Disturbing Students: An Integrative Approach
Sage Publications
2455 Teller Road
Thousand Oaks, CA 91320
805-499-9774
800-818-7243
Fax: 800-583-2665
books.claim@sagepub.com
www.sagepub.com
Sara Miller McCune, Founder, Publisher, Chairperson
Blaise R Simqu, President & CEO
Tracey A. Ozmina, Executive Vice President & Chief
Paul Zionts, Author
Using an integrative approach, this text provides teachers with step-by-step details of how to implement and use the methods and theories discussed in each chapter. *$37.00*
465 pages

2613 Teaching Every Child Every Day: Integrated Learning in Diverse Classrooms
Brookline Books
8 Trumbull Rd
Suite B-001
Northampton, MA 01060
413-584-0184
800-666-2665
Fax: 413-584-6184
brbooks@yahoo.com
www.brooklinebooks.com
Karen R. Harris, Editor
Steve Graham, Editor
Don Deshler, Editor
Collection of articles addressing various issues in teaching to diverse classrooms—varied in need for special educational services, English proficiency, and socioeconomic and racial backgrounds. *$19.95*
224 pages Paperback
ISBN 0-57129 -40-0

2614 Teaching Infants and Preschoolers with Handicaps
Mc Graw- Hill, School Publishing
PO Box 182604
Columbus, OH 43218
877-833-5524
800-338-3987
Fax: 609-308-4480
customer.service@mheducation.com
www.mcgraw-hill.com
David Levin, President/Chief Executive Officer
David Stafford, Senior Vice President/General Counsel
Maryellen Valaitis, Senior Vice President Human Resources
Patrick Milano, Chief Financial Officer & Chief Administrative Officer
Builds a solid background in early childhood special education.
380 pages

2615 Teaching Language-Disabled Children: A Communication/Games Intervention
Brookline Books
8 Trumbull Rd
Ste B-001
Northampton, MA 01060
413-584-0184
800-666-2665
Fax: 413-584-6184
brbooks@yahoo.com
www.brooklinebks.com
Susan Conant, Author
Offers practitioners specific teaching methods for helping students play communication games. *$22.95*
185 pages Hardcover 1983
ISBN 0-914797-38-7

2616 Teaching Learners with Mild Disabilities: Integrating Research and Practice
Brooke Publishing
PO Box 10624
Baltimore, MD 21285-0624
410-337-9580
800-638-3775
Fax: 410-337-8539
custserv@brookespublishing.com
www.brookespublishing.com
Ruth Lyn Meese, Author
Melissa A. Behm, Executive Vice President
Paul H. Brooks, Chairman of the Board
Cary Gold, Educational Sales Representative
The authors illustrate interactions among regular teachers, special education teachers and students with mild disabilities through the use of hypothetical case studies of students and teachers.
496 pages Paperbound
ISBN 0-53421 -02-0

2617 Teaching Mathematics to Students with Learning Disabilities
Sage Publications
2455 Teller Road
Thousand Oaks, CA 91320
805-499-9774
800-818-7243
Fax: 800-583-2665
www.sagepub.com
Sara Miller McCune, Founder, Publisher, Chairperson
Blaise R Simqu, President & CEO
Nancy S. Bley, Co-Author
Carol A. Thornton, Co-Author
New trends in school mathematics have surfaced in the teaching world. Problem-solving, estimation and the use of computers are receiving considerably greater emphasis than in the past and these areas are included in the new text. *$38.00*
486 pages Paperback

2618 Teaching Mildly and Moderately Handicapped Students
Allyn & Bacon
75 Arlington St
Suite 300
Boston, MA 02116-3988
617-848-7500
800-852-8024
Fax: 617-944-7273
www.home.pearsonhighered.com
Bill Barke, CEO
Nancy Forfyth, President
B. R. Gearheart, Author
Kevin Stone, Vice President, National Sales M
A cross-categorical text providing teaching ideas and techniques. Focuses on the theme of learning as a constructive process in which the learner interacts with the environment, constructing new systems of knowledge, Behavioral techniques and research are also presented.
hardcover
ISBN 0-138939-00-4

2619 **Teaching Reading to Children with Down Syndrome: A Guide for Parents and Teachers**
Woodbine House
6510 Bells Mill Rd
Bethesda, MD 20817-1636
301-897-3570
800-843-7323
Fax: 301-897-5838
info@woodbinehouse.com
www.woodbinehouse.com
Irvin Shapell, Publisher
Patricia Logan Oelwein, Author
Beth Binns, Special Marketing Manage
Fran Marinaccio, Marketing Manager
Guide includes lessons customized to meet the unique interests and learning style of each child. *$16.95*
371 pages Paperback
ISBN 0-933149-55-7

2620 **Teaching Reading to Disabled and Handicapped Learners**
Charles C. Thomas
2600 S First St
Springfield, IL 62704-4730
217-789-8980
800-258-8980
Fax: 217-789-9130
books@ccthomas.com
www.ccthomas.com
Michael P. Thomas, President
Freddie W. Litton, Author
Harold D. Love, Author
Designed as a text for undergraduate and graduate students, this resource aims to help the many children, adolescents, and adults who encounter difficulty with reading. It guides prospective and present special education teachers in assisting and teaching handicapped learners to read. The text integrates traditional methods with newer perspectives to provide and effective reading program in special education. *$43.95*
252 pages Paperback 1996
ISBN 0-398062-48-X

2621 **Teaching Reading to Handicapped Children**
Love Publishing Company
9101 E Kenyon Ave
Suite 2200
Denver, CO 80237-1854
303-221-7333
Fax: 303-221-7444
lpc@lovepublishing.com
www.lovepublishing.com
Charles H. Hargis, Author
The author covers skills teaching through letter sound association, word identification, synthetic and analytic methods and others, plus testing and assessment. *$24.95*
ISBN 0-89108 -13-5

2622 **Teaching Self-Determination to Students with Disabilities**
Brookes Publishing
PO Box 10624
Baltimore, MD 21285-0624
410-337-9580
800-638-3775
Fax: 410-337-8539
custserv@brookespublishing.com
www.brookespublishing.com
Michael L. Wehmeyer, Co-Author
Martin Agran, Co-Author
Paul H. Brooks, Chairman of the Board
Cary Gold, Educational Sales Representative
Basic skills for successful transition. This teacher-friendly source will help educators prepare students with disabilities with the specific skills they need for a satisfactory, self-directed life once they leave school. *$34.95*
384 pages Paperback
ISBN 1-55766 -02-5

2623 **Teaching Students with Learning Problems**
McGraw-Hill School Publishing
PO Box 182604
Columbus, OH 43218
877-833-5524
800-338-3987
Fax: 609-308-4480
customer.service@mheducation.com
www.mcgraw-hill.com
David Levin, President/Chief Executive Officer
David Stafford, Senior Vice President/General Counsel
Maryellen Valaitis, Senior Vice President Human Resources
Patrick Milano, Chief Financial Officer & Chief Administrative Officer
Expanded coverage of learning strategies, generalization training, self-monitoring techniques, and techniques for increasing the time students spend on academic tasks.
608 pages

2624 **Teaching Students with Learning and Behavior Problems**
Sage Publications
2455 Teller Road
Thousand Oaks, CA 91320
805-499-9774
800-818-7243
Fax: 800-583-2665
www.sagepub.com
Sara Miller McCune, Founder, Publisher, Chairperson
Blaise R Simqu, President & CEO
Sharon R. Vaughn, Co-Author
Candace S. Bos, Co-Author
$65.00
444 pages Paperback
ISBN 0-890799-28-4

2625 **Teaching Students with Mild and Moderate Learning Problems**
Allyn & Bacon Longman College Faculty
75 Arlington St
Suite 300
Boston, MA 02116-3988
617-367-0025
800-852-8024
Fax: 617-367-2155
www.home.pearsonhighered.com
Bill Barke, CEO
John Langone, Author
Kevin Stone, Vice President, National Sales M
Kevin Stone, Vice President, National Sales M
Provides teachers with skills for assisting students with mild to moderate handicaps in making successful transitions in school and community environments.
496 pages
ISBN 0-205123-62-7

2626 **Teaching Students with Moderate/Severe Disabilities, Including Autism**
Charles C. Thomas
2600 S First St
Springfield, IL 62704-4730
217-789-8980
800-258-8980
Fax: 217-789-9130
books@ccthomas.com
www.ccthomas.com
Michael P. Thomas, President
Elva Duran, Author
This resource and guide was written to help teachers, parents, and other caregivers provide the best educational opportunities for their students with moderate and severe disabilities. The author addresses functional language and other language intervention strategies, vocational training, community based instruction, transition and postsecondary programming, the adolescent student with autism, students with multiple disabilities, parent and family issues, and legal concerns. *$58.95*
416 pages Paperback
ISBN 0-398067-01-5

2627 Teaching Students with Special Needs in Inclusive Settings
Allyn & Bacon
75 Arlington St
Suite 300
Boston, MA 02116-3988
617-848-7500
800-852-8024
Fax: 617-944-7273

Tom E.C. Smith, Co-Author
Edward A. Polloway, Co-Author
James Patton, Co-Author
Carol A. Dowdy, Co-Author

This text is intended to be a survey text providing practical guidance to general education teachers. It will help them to meet the diverse needs of students with disabilities.
544 pages
ISBN 0-20527 -16-6

2628 Teaching Young Children to Read
Brookline Books
8 Trumbull Rd
Suite B-001
Northampton, MA 01060
413-584-0184
800-666-2665
Fax: 413-584-6184
brbooks@yahoo.com
www.brooklinebooks.com

Dolores Durkin, Author
John P.

Detailed instructions on teaching reading to preschoolers. Gradually develops full fluency. *$16.95*
192 pages Paperback
ISBN 0-57129 -48-6

2629 Teaching the Bilingual Special Education Student
Ablex Publishing Corporation
P.O. Box 811
Stamford, CT 06904-811
Fax: 201-767-6717
ISBN 0-89391 -23-4

2630 Teaching the Learning Disabled Adolescent: Strategies and Methods
Love Publishing Company
9101 E Kenyon Ave
Ste 2200
Denver, CO 80237-1813
303-221-7333
Fax: 303-221-7444
lpc@lovepublishing.com
www.lovepublishing.com

Gordon R. Alley, Author

This book gives expert strategies and methods for teaching learning disabled adolescents how, rather than what, to learn. *$39.95*
360 pages Hardcover 1979
ISBN 0-891080-94-5

2631 Technology and Handicapped People
Springer Publishing Company
11 W 42nd St
15th Floor
New York, NY 10036-8002
212-431-4370
877-687-7476
Fax: 212-941-7842
cs@springerpub.com
www.springerpub.com

Dr. Ursula Springer, President
Ted Nardin, CEO
James C. Costello, Vice President, Journal Publishi
James C. Costello, Vice President, Journal Publishing

Important information for concerned professionals about new rehabilitation techniques and treatments for handicapped people. *$29.95*
224 pages Hardcover
ISBN 0-82614 -10-8

2632 Textbooks and the Student Who Can't Read Them: A Guide for Teaching Content
Brookline Books
8 Trumbull Rd
Suite B-001
Northampton, MA 01060
413-584-0184
800-666-2665
Fax: 413-584-6184
brbooks@yahoo.com
www.brooklinebooks.com

Paperback
ISBN 0-91479 -57-3

2633 The Education of Children with Acquired Brain Injury
David Fulton Publishers (Routledge)
711 Third Ave
New York, NY 10017
212-216-7800
Fax: 212-564-7854
orders@taylorandfrancis.com
www.routledge.com

Sue Walker, Author
Beth Wicks, Author

Teachers have to be aware of their pupils' special educational needs. Find out what an acquired brain injury is and how to maximize learning opportunities for those with the condition with this book.
128 pages

2634 The Fundamentals of Special Education: A Practical Guide for Every Teacher
Corwin Press Inc.
2455 Teller Rd
Thousand Oaks, CA 91320
805-499-9734
800-233-9936
Fax: 805-499-5323
order@corwin.com
us.corwin.com

Bob Algozzine, Author
Jim Ysseldyke, Author

This guide highlights major concepts in special education-from disability categories, identification issues, and IEPs to appropriate learning environments and the roles general and special educators play.
104 pages

2635 The K&W Guide to Colleges for Studentswith Learning Disabilties (13th Edition)
The Princeton Review - Penguin Random House
1745 Broadway
New York, NY 10019
212-782-9000
customerservice@penguinrandomhouse.com
www.penguinrandomhouse.com

848 pages Paperback 1916
ISBN 1-101920-38-6

2636 There's a Hearing Impaired Child in My Class
Gallaudet University Bookstore
800 Florida Ave NE
Washington, DC 20002-3600
202-651-5000
800-451-1073
Fax: 202-651-5489
TTY: 888-630-9347
clerc.center@gallaudet.edu

Debra Nussbaum, Author
Dr. T Alan Hurwitz, President
Edward Bosso, Vice President for Administratio
Donald Beil, Chief of Staff

This complete package provides basic facts about deafness, practical strategies for teaching hearing impaired children, and the question-and-answer information for all students. *$16.95*
44 pages

2637 Toward Effective Public School Program for Deaf Students
Teachers College Press
525 W 120th St
New York, NY 10027-6605
212-678-3000
800-575-6566
Fax: 212-678-4149
webcomments@tc.columbia.edu
www.tc.columbia.edu
Susan H. Fuhrman, Ph.D., President of the College
Harvey Spector, Vice President for Finance and Administration
Suzanne M. Murphy, Vice President for Development and External Affairs
Janice S. Robinson, Vice President for Diversity and Community Affairs
This book translates research and data into useable recommendations and possible courses of action for organizing effective public school programs for deaf students. *$22.95*
272 pages Paperback
ISBN 0-807731-59-5

2638 Treating Adults with Physical Disabilities: Access and Communication
World Institute on Disability
3075 Adeline St.
Suite 155
Berkeley, CA 94703
510-225-6400
Fax: 510-225-0477
wid@wid.org
www.wid.org
Marcie Roth, Executive Director & CEO
Katherine Zigmont, Senior Director, Operations & Deputy Director
Reggie Johnson, Senior Director, Marketing & Communications
Marsha Saxton, Director, Research
A training curriculum for medical professionals who want to improve the quality of care for people with disabilities and chronic illnesses. Also covers architectural, communication, attitudinal and economic policy barriers to quality health care and specific skills to increase good communication and rapport.

2639 Treating Cerebral Palsy for Clinicians by Clinicians
Sage Publications
2455 Teller Road
Thousand Oaks, CA 91320
805-499-9774
800-818-7243
Fax: 800-583-2665
www.sagepub.com
Sara Miller McCune, Founder, Publisher, Chairperson
Blaise R Simqu, President & CEO
Tracey A. Ozmina, Executive Vice President & Chief
Eugene T. McDonald, Editor
A clinical manual for professionals beginning to work with persons who have cerebral palsy. *$31.00*
312 pages

2640 Treating Disordered Speech Motor Control
Sage Publications
2455 Teller Road
Thousand Oaks, CA 91320
805-499-9774
800-818-7243
Fax: 800-583-2665
www.sagepub.com
Sara Miller McCune, Founder, Publisher, Chairperson
Blaise R Simqu, President & CEO
Deanie Vogel, Author
Michael Cannito, Editor
This book about neuromotor disturbances of speech production is aimed at practicing professionals and advanced graduate students interested in the neuropathologies of communication. *$36.00*
410 pages

2641 Treating Families of Brain Injury Survivors
Springer Publishing Company
11 W 42nd St
15th Floor
New York, NY 10036-8002
212-431-4370
877-687-7476
Fax: 212-941-7842
cs@springerpub.com
www.springerpub.com
Dr. Ursula Springer, President
Ted Nardin, CEO
James C. Costello, Vice President, Journal Publishi
James C. Costello, Vice President, Journal Publishing
Provides the mental health practitioner with a comprehensive program for helping families of head injury survivors cope with the change in their lives. Includes background on medical aspects of head injury, family structure functioning and special needs of various family members.
220 pages
ISBN 0-82616 -20-1

2642 Understanding and Teaching Emotionally Disturbed Children & Adolescents
Sage Publications
2455 Teller Road
Thousand Oaks, CA 91320
805-499-9774
800-818-7243
Fax: 800-583-2665
www.sagepub.com
Sara Miller McCune, Founder, Publisher, Chairperson
Blaise R Simqu, President & CEO
Tracey A. Ozmina, Executive Vice President & Chief
Phyllis L. Newcomer, Author
The teacher's handbook provides information that will change misconceptions about children who are frequently labeled as emotionally disturbed. It also gives information about a wide variety of intervention methods and approaches for use in educational settings. *$41.00*
620 pages Hardover

2643 Using the Dictionary of Occupational Titles in Career Decision Making
Stout Vocational Rehab Institute
University of Wisconsin Stou
Menomonie, WI 54751
715-232-2470
Fax: 715-232-5008
luij@uwstout.edu
John Lui, Contact Person
This is a self-study manual for learning how to use the 1991 U.S. Department of Labor's Dictionary of Occupational Titles. It gives the DOT user a tool to understand the DOT and then put its information to work. Shows how to quickly obtain information about the work performed in 12,741 occupations listed and described in the DOT and the worker requirements for those occupations. *$24.00*
142 pages Softcover

2644 VBS Special Education Teaching Guide
Life Way Christian Resources Southern Baptist Conv
1 Lifeway Plz
Nashville, TN 37234-1001
615-251-2000
www.lifeway.com
Tom Hellam, VP of Executive Communications a
Thom Rainer, President & CEO
This book contains teaching plans for five bible study sessions with reproducible handouts for learners. The plans use multisensory, experiential-based learning activities designed for adults and older youth who have developmental disabilities. Suggestions for Bible learning, crafts, recreation, snacks and theme interpretation are included. Designed primarily for Vacation Bible School, but may be used in camp/retreat settings. *$9.95*
56 pages Yearly

2645 **Vermont Interdependent Services Team Approach (VISTA)**
Brookes Publishing
PO Box 10624
Baltimore, MD 21285-624
410-337-9580
800-638-3775
Fax: 410-337-8539
custserv@brookespublishing.com
www.brookespublishing.com
Paul Kelly, National Textbook Sales Manager
Tracy Gray, Educational Sales Manager
Paul Brooks, President
A guide to coordinating educational support services. This manual enables IEP team members to fulfill the related services provisions of IDEA as they make effective support services decisions using a collaborative team approach. *$27.95*
176 pages Spiral bound
ISBN 1-55766 -30-4

2646 **What School Counselors Need to Know**
Council for Exceptional Children
3100 Clarendon Blvd.
Suite 600
Arlington, VA 22201-5332
888-232-7733
TTY: 866-915-5000
service@exceptionalchildren.org
www.exceptionalchildren.org
Barbara E. Baditoi, Co-Author
Pamelia E. Brott, Co-Author
This book provides counselors (and school administrators) with essential information to make the most of their participation in providing special education services. *$25.95*

2647 **When You Have a Visually Impaired Student in Your Classroom: A Guide for Teachers**
American Foundation for the Blind
2 Penn Plaza
Suite1102
New York, NY 10121
212-502-7600
800-232-5463
Fax: 888-545-8331
afbinfo@afb.net
afb.org
Carl Augusto, President
This guide provides information on students' abilities and needs, resources and educational team members, federal special education requirements, and technology materials used by students. *$9.95*
84 pages
ISBN 0-891283-93-5

2648 **Working Bibliography on Behavioral and Emotional Disorders**
Natl. Clearinghouse for Alcohol & Drug Information
1 Choke Cherry Road
Rockville, MD 20857
301-468-2600
877-SAM-SA 7
Fax: 301-468-6433
Lizabeth J Foster, Librarian/Info. Resource Manager
Pamela S. Hyde, Administrator
NCADI is a service of the U.S. Substance Abuse and Mental Health Services Administration. As the national focal point for information on alcohol and other drugs, NCADI collects, prepares, classifies, and distributes information about alcohol, tobacco and other drugs, prevention strategies and materials, research, treatment, etc.
40 pages

2649 **Working Together with Children and Families: Case Studies**
Brookes Publishing Company
PO Box 10624
Baltimore, MD 21285-624
410-337-9580
800-638-3775
Fax: 410-337-8539
custerv@brookespublishing.com
www.brookespublishing.com
Paul Kelly, National Textbook Sales Manager
Tracy Gray, Educational Sales Manager
Paul Brooks, Owner
Early interventionists will be able to bridge the gap between theory and practice with this edited collection of case studies. *$23.00*
336 pages
ISBN 1-557661-23-5

2650 **Working with Visually Impaired Young Students: A Curriculum Guide for 3 to 5 Year Olds**
Charles C. Thomas
2600 S First St
Springfield, IL 62704-4730
217-789-8980
800-258-8980
Fax: 217-789-9130
books@ccthomas.com
www.ccthomas.com
Michael P. Thomas, President
Ellen Trief, Editor
The first step in the education process of a visually impaired child is the early identification and treatment by an eye care specialist. This book is geared to the age of birth through 3-years. Available in cloth, paperback and hardcover. *$42.95*
194 pages Paperback
ISBN 0-398068-75-2

Testing Resources

2651 **ADD-SOI Center, The**
2007 Cedar Avenue
Manhattan Beach, CA 90266
310-546-6500
Fax: 310-546-9068
ADDSOI@aol.com
www.addsoi.com

2652 **AEPS Child Progress Report: For Children Ages Birth to Three**
Brookes Publishing
PO Box 10624
Baltimore, MD 21285-624
410-337-9580
800-638-3775
Fax: 410-337-8539
custserv@brookespublishing.com
www.brookespublishing.com
Paul Kelly, National Textbook Sales Manager
Tracy Gray, Educational Sales Manager
Paul Brooks, Owner
This chart helps monitor change by visually displaying current abilities, intervention targets, and child progress. In packages of 30. *$18.00*
6 pages Gate-fold
ISBN 1-55766 -65-0

2653 **AEPS Data Recording Forms: For Children Ages Birth to Three**
Brookes Publishing
PO Box 10624
Baltimore, MD 21285-624
410-337-9580
800-638-3775
Fax: 410-337-8539
custserv@brookespublishing.com
readplaylearn.com
Paul Brooks, Owner
Melissa Behm, Executive Vice President
These forms can be used by child development professionals on four separate occasions to pinpoint and then monitor a child's strengths and needs in the six key areas of skill development measured by the AEPS Test. Packages of 10. *$23.00*
36 pages Saddle-stiched
ISBN 1-55766 -97-2

2654 **AEPS Measurement for Birth to Three Years**
Brookes Publishing
PO Box 10624
Baltimore, MD 21285-624 410-337-9580
800-638-3775
Fax: 410-337-8539
custserv@brookespublishing.com
www.brookespublishing.com
Paul Kelly, National Textbook Sales Manager
Tracy Gray, Educational Sales Manager
Paul Brooks, Owner
This dynamic volume explains the Assessment, Evaluation and Programming System, provides the complete AEPS Test and parallel assessment/evaluation tools for families and includes the forms and plans needed for implementation. *$39.00*
352 pages

2655 **AEPS Measurement for Three to Six Years**
Brookes Publishing
PO Box 10624
Baltimore, MD 21285-624 410-337-9580
800-638-3775
Fax: 410-337-8539
custserv@brookespublishing.com
www.brookespublishing.com
Paul Kelly, National Textbook Sales Manager
Tracy Gray, Educational Sales Manager
Paul Brooks, Owner
Resources in early childhood, early intervention, inclusive and special education, developmental disabilities, learning disabilities, communication and language, behavior, and mental health. *$57.00*
400 pages Spiral-bound
ISBN 1-55766 -87-1

2656 **AIR: Assessment of Interpersonal Relations**
Sage Publications
2455 Teller Road
Thousand Oaks, CA 91320 805-499-0721
800-818-7243
Fax: 800-583-2665
info@sagepub.com
www.sagepub.com
Sara Miller McCune, Founder, Publisher, Chairperson
Blaise R Simqu, President & CEO
A thoroughly researched and standardized clinical instrument assessing the quality of adolescents' interpersonal relationships in a hierarchical fashion, including global relationship quality and relationship quality with three domains: Family, Social and Academic. *$89.00*

2657 **ALST: Adolescent Language Screening Test**
Sage Publications
2455 Teller Road
Thousand Oaks, CA 91320 805-499-0721
800-818-7243
Fax: 800-583-2665
info@sagepub.com
www.sagepub.com
Sara Miller McCune, Founder, Publisher, Chairperson
Blaise R Simqu, President & CEO
Provides speech/language pathologists and other interested professionals with a rapid thorough method for screening adolescents (ages 11-17). *$119.00*

2658 **Adaptive Mainstreaming: A Primer for Teachers and Principals, 3rd Edition**
Longman Publishing Group
1330 Avenue of the Americas
New York, NY 10019 212-641-2400
800-745-8489
www.pearson.com
Glen Moreno, Chairman
Marjorie Scardino, Chief Executive Officer
An introduction to education for handicapped and gifted students. Presents research-based rationales for teaching exceptional students in the least restrictive environment. Provides historical perspectives, offers realistic descriptions of prevailing practices in the field, and reviews trends and new directions.
366 pages Paperback
ISBN 0-582285-04-6

2659 **Ages & Stages Questionnaires**
Brookes Publishing
PO Box 10624
Baltimore, MD 21285-624 410-337-9580
800-638-3775
Fax: 410-337-8539
custserv@brookespublishing.com
www.brookespublishing.com
Paul Kelly, National Textbook Sales Manager
Tracy Gray, Educational Sales Manager
Paul Brooks, Owner
ASQ is an economical and field-tested system for identifying whether infants and young children may require further developmental evaluation and offers a screening and tracking program that helps early intervention professionals, service coordinators, and administrators maximize financial resources while promoting the health and growth of the children they serve. Set includes 11 color-coded, reproducible questionnaires, 11 reproducible, age appropriate scoring sheets. *$135.00*

2660 **American College Testing Program**
500 Act Drive
PO Box 168
Iowa City, IA 52243-168 319-337-1000
Fax: 319-339-3021
act.org
John Whitmore, CEO
Mark D Musik, President Emeritus
An independent, nonprofit organization that provides a variety of educational services to students and their parents, to high schools and colleges, and to professional associations and government agencies.

2661 **Assessing Students with Special Needs**
Longman Publishing Group
10 Bank Street
9th Floor
White Plains, NY 10606-1933 914-993-5000
www.ablongman.com
Joanne Dresner, President
Step-by-step guide to informal, classroom assessment of students with special needs.
174 pages Paperback
ISBN 0-801301-77-7

2662 **Assessment Log & Developmental Progress Charts for the CCPSN**
Brookes Publishing
P.O. Box 10624
Baltimore, MD 21285-624 410-337-9580
800-638-3775
Fax: 410-337-8539
custserv@brookespublishing.com
www.brookespublishing.com
Paul Kelly, National Textbook Sales Manager
Tracy Gray, Educational Sales Manager
Paul Brooks, Owner
This 28-page booklet allows readers to actually chart the ongoing progress of each preschool child. Available in packages of 10. *$22.00*
28 pages Saddle-stiched
ISBN 1-55766 -39-5

2663 **Assessment of Learners with Special Needs**
Allyn & Bacon
75 Arlinton Street
Ste 300
Boston, MA 2116-3988 617-848-7500
800-852-8024
Fax: 617-944-7273
www.ablongman.com
Bill Barke, CEO
Thomas Longman, Founder
The central goal of this book is to help teachers become sophisticated, informed test consumers in terms of choosing, using and

interpreting commercially prepared tests for their special needs students.
508 pages Casebound
ISBN 0-205227-33-3

2664 **Benchmark Measures**
Educators Publishing Service
PO Box 9031
Cambridge, MA 2139
617-547-6706
800-225-5750
Fax: 888-440-2665
feedback@epsbooks.com
www.epsbooks.com
Charles H Heinle, VP
Alexandra S Bigelow, Author
Gunnar Voltz, President
Ungraded test containing three sequential levels that assess alphabet and dictionary skills, reading, handwriting and spelling, and correspond to the first three schedules of the Alphabetic Phonics curriculum. The tests can be used at any level to measure a student's general knowledge of phonics. *$64.40*
Kit

2665 **Brain Clinic, The**
19 West 34th Street
Penthouse
New York, NY 10001
212-268-8900
nurosvcs@aol.com
thebrainclinic.com
Dr. James Lawrence Thomas, Director
The brain clinic offers diagnosis and Treatment of ADD, Learning Disabilities, Migraines, and Traumatic Brain Injury.

2666 **CREVT: Comprehensive Receptive and Expressive Vocabulary Test**
Sage Publications
2455 Teller Road
Thousand Oaks, CA 91320
805-499-0721
800-818-7243
Fax: 800-583-2665
info@sagepub.com
www.sagepub.com
Sara Miller McCune, Founder, Publisher, Chairperson
Blaise R Simqu, President & CEO
A new, innovative, efficient measure of both receptive and expressive oral vocabulary. The CREVT has two subtests and is based on the most current theories of vocabulary development, suitable for ages 4 through 17. *$174.00*
Complete Kit

2667 **Carolina Curriculum for Preschoolers with Special Needs**
Brookes Publishing
P.O. Box 10624
Baltimore, MD 21285-624
410-337-9580
800-638-3775
Fax: 410-337-8539
custserv@brookespublishing.com
www.brookespublishing.com
Paul Kelly, National Textbook Sales Manager
Tracy Gray, Educational Sales Manager
Paul Brooks, Owner
This curriculum provides detailed teaching and assessment techniques, plus a sample 28-page Assessment Log that shows readers how to chart a child's individual progress. This guide is for children between 2 and 5 in their developmental stages who are considered at risk for developmental delay or who exhibit special needs. *$35.95*
352 pages Spiral-bound
ISBN 1-557660-32-8

2668 **Center For Personal Development**
405 North Wabash Ave.
Suite 208 & 1114
Chicago, IL 60611
312-755-7000
Fax: 312-755-7001
info@chicagotherapist.com
www.chicagotherapist.com
Steven Nakisher, Licensed Clinical Psychologist
Cara McCanse, Licensed Clinical Psychologist
Sarah Krcmarik, Staff Psychotherapist
Amy Zurawic, Staff Psychotherapist
The Center for Personal Development was founded in 1998 to provide a diverse range of high-quality mental health services.

2669 **Center for Human Potential**
525 East 100 South
Suite 120
Salt Lake City, UT 84102
801-483-2447
801-486-8705
www.c4hp.com
C. Brendan Hallett Psy.D., Clinical Director
Michael DeCaria, Ph.D., Licensed Clinical Psychologist
Annice Julian, Psy.D., Licensed Clinical Psychologist
Stephanie Voigt, Psy.D., Licensed Clinical Psychologist
Center for Human Potentialis a human services company that helps individuals, businesses and organizations reach their potential by achieving balance in the fundamental areas of life: Emotional, Physical, Mental, Spiritual and Financial. We offer individual, couples, and family counseling to help with a number of issues.

2670 **Center for Neuropsychology, Learning & Development**
1955 Pauline Blvd
Suite 100A
Ann Arbor, MI 48103
734-994-9466
Fax: 734-994-9465
www.cnld.org
Roger E. Lauer, Clinical Director
Jodene Goldenring Fine, Ph.D., Licensed Psychologist
CNLD was founded over 20 years ago to serve Southeast Michigan and the greater Ann Arbor community by providing quality mental health care for children, adolescents, adults and families.

2671 **Center for Student Health and Counseling**
1825 SW Broadway
Portland, OR 97201
503-725-3000
800-547-8887
Fax: 503-725-4882
askadm@pdx.edu
www.pdx.edu/shac/ldadhd

2672 **Children's Assessment Center, The**
2500 Bolsover St.
Houston, TX 77005
713-986-3300
Fax: 713-986-3553
info@cac.hctx.net
cachouston.org
Brady E. Crosswell, Chairman
Gail Prather, President
Elaine Stolte, Executive Director
Mark Anderson, Treasurer
The Children's Assessment Center (CAC)provides a safe haven to sexually abused children and their families.

2673 **Cognitive Solutions Learning Center**
2409 N. Clybourn Ave.
Chicago, IL 60614
773-755-1775
Fax: 773-439-5499
info@helpforld.com
www.helpforld.com/index.php/about-us/
Dr. Ari Goldstein, Founder
Jason Almodovar, M.S.Ed., Office Manager
Cognitive Solution offers a broad range of services, including learning disability and attention deficit disorder assessment and remediation, executive functions training, and the latest neurofeedback technologies.

2674 **DAYS: Depression and Anxiety in Youth Scale**
Sage Publications
2455 Teller Road
Thousand Oaks, CA 91320
805-499-0721
800-818-7243
Fax: 805-376-9443
info@sagepub.com
www.sagepub.com
Sara Miller McCune, Founder, Publisher, Chairperson
Blaise R Simqu, President & CEO
A unique battery of three norm-references scales useful in identifying major depressive disorder and overanxious disorders in children and adolescents. *$129.00*
Complete Kit

2675 **DOCS: Developmental Observation Checklist System**
Pro- Ed Publications
8700 Shoal Creek Blvd
Austin, TX 78757-6897
512-451-3246
800-897-3202
Fax: 800-397-7633
general@proedinc.com
www.proedinc.com
Donald D Hammill, Owner
Courtney King, Marketing Coordinator
A three-part system for the assessment of very young children with respect to general development, adjustment behavior and parent stress and support. *$124.00*

2676 **Dennis Developmental Center**
1 Children's Way
Little Rock, AR 72202-3591
501-364-1100
TTY: 501-364-1184
www.archildrens.org

2677 **Developmental Services Center**
Therapeutic Nursery Program
4525 Lee St NE
Washington, DC 20019
202-388-3216
Fax: 202-576-8799
Alice Anderson
Offers assessment information and evaluation for developmentally delayed students.

2678 **Frames of Reference for the Assessment of Learning Disabilities**
Brookes Publishing
P.O. Box 10624
Baltimore, MD 21285-624
410-337-9580
800-638-3775
Fax: 410-337-8539
custserv@brookespublishing.com
www.brookespublishing.com
Paul Kelly, National Textbook Sales Manager
Tracy Gray, Educational Sales Manager
Paul Brooks, Owner
New views on measurement issues. Here you'll find an in=depth look at the fundamental concerns facing those who work with children with learning disabilities - assessment and identification. *$55.00*
672 pages Hardcover
ISBN 1-55766 -38-3

2679 **How to Conduct an Assessment**
FSSI
3905 Huntington Dr
Amarillo, TX 79109-4047
806-353-1114
Fax: 806-353-1114
Ed Hammer, Owner
The Functional Skills Screening Inventory,this behavioral checklist allows for parents and professionals to observe critical behaviors in individuals with multiple disabilities (7 years to adult years).

2680 **Inclusive & Heterogeneous Schooling: Assessment, Curriculum, and Instruction**
Brookes Publishing
P.O. Box 10624
Baltimore, MD 21285-624
410-337-9580
800-638-3775
Fax: 410-337-8539
custserv@brookespublishing.com
www.brookespublishing.com
Paul Kelly, National Textbook Sales Manager
Tracy Gray, Educational Sales Manager
Paul Brooks, Owner
Presents methods for successfully restructuring classrooms to enable all students, particularly those with disabilities, to flourish. Provides specific strategies for assessment, collaboration, classroom management, and age-specific instruction. *$34.95*
448 pages Paperback
ISBN 1-557662-02-9

2681 **Infant & Toddler Convection of Fairfield: Falls Church**
Joseph Willard Health Center
3750 Old Lee Hwy
Fairfax, VA 22030-1806
703-246-7180
Fax: 703-246-7307
Susan Sigler, Program Coordinator
Allan Phillips, Director Early Intervention
Offers assessments, evaluations and educational/therapeutic infant programs for parents infants and toddlers birth to age 3.
Sliding Scale

2682 **K-BIT: Kaufman Brief Intelligence Test**
AGS
Ste 1000
5910 Rice Creek Pkwy
Shoreview, MN 55126-5023
651-287-7220
800-328-2560
Fax: 800-471-8457
agsmail@agsnet.com
www.agsnet.com
Kevin Brueggeman, President
Robert Zaske, Market Manager
Quick and easy-to-use, KBIT assesses verbal and non-verbal abilities through two reliable subtests - vocabulary and matricies.
$124.95
Ages 4-90

2683 **K-FAST: Kaufman Functional Academic Skills Test**
AGS
Ste 1000
5910 Rice Creek Pkwy
Shoreview, MN 55126-5023
651-287-7220
800-328-2560
Fax: 800-471-8457
agsmail@agsnet.com
www.agsnet.com
Robert Zaske, Market Manager
Helps assess a person's capacity to function effectively in society regarding functional reading and math skills. *$99.95*
Ages 15-85+

2684 **K-SEALS: Kaufman Survey of Early Academic and Language Skills**
AGS
5910 Rice Creek Pkwy
Shoreview, MN 55126-5025
651-287-7220
800-328-2560
Fax: 800-471-8457
agsmail@agsnet.com
www.agsnet.com
Kevin Brueggeman, President
Robert Zaske, Market Manager
An individually administered test of children's of both expressive and receptive skills, pre-academic skills and articulation. K-SEALS offers reliable scores usually in less than 25 minutes.
$179.95
Ages 3-0; 6-11

2685 KLST-2: Kindergarten Language Screening Test Edition, 2nd Edition
Sage Publications
2455 Teller Road
Thousand Oaks, CA 91320
805-499-9774
800-818-7243
Fax: 800-583-2665
info@sagepub.com
www.sagepub.com
Paul Kelly, National Textbook Sales Manager
Blaise R Simqu, President & CEO
Identifies children who need further diagnostic testing to determine whether or not they have language deficits that will accelerate academic failure. *$94.00*

2686 Kaufman Test of Educational Achievement (K-TEA)
AGS
PO Box 99
Circle Pines, MN 55014-99
800-328-2560
Fax: 800-471-8457
agsmail@agsnet.com
www.agsnet.com
Robert Zaske, Marketing Manager
Kevin Brueggeman, President
K-TEA is an individually administered diagnostic battery that measures reading, mathematics, and spelling skills. Setting the standards in achievement testing today, K-TEA Comprehensive provides the complete diagnostic information you need for educational assessment and program planning. The Brief Forum is indispensable for school and clinical psychologists, special education teachers when a quick a measure of achievement is needed. *$249.95*

2687 Learning House
264 Church Street
Guilford, CT 6437
203-453-3691
Susan Santora, Founder and Director
Learning House is a professional community committed to enhancing the lives of individuals with dyslexia and other learning disabilities in safe and supportive surroundings.

2688 LearningRx
5085 List Drive
Suite 200
Colorado Springs, CO 80919
719-264-8808
www.learningrx.com
Dr. Ken Gibson, Founder
LearningRx is a brain training program.

2689 Life Centered Career Education: A Contemporary Based Approach
Council for Exceptional Children
3100 Clarendon Blvd.
Suite 600
Arlington, VA 22201-5332
888-232-7733
TTY: 866-915-5000
service@exceptionalchildren.org
www.exceptionalchildren.org
Chad Rummel, Executive Director
Laurie VanderPloeg, Associate Executive Director, Professional Affairs
Craig Evans, Chief Financial Officer
Sharon Rodriguez, Director, Governance & Executive Services
Provides a framework for building 97 functional skill competencies appropriate for preparing for adult life and special education students. *$28.00*
175 pages

2690 Measure of Cognitive-Linguistic Abilities (MCLA)
Speech Bin
PO Box 1579
Appleton, VA 54912-1579
772-770-0007
888-388-3224
Fax: 888-388-6344
onlinehelp@schoolspecialty.com
www.speechbin.com
Jan J Binney, Senior Editor
A diagnostic test of cognitive-linguistic abilities of adolescents and adults with traumatically induced brain injuries. High level. Normed. *$89.00*
100 pages
ISBN 0-93785 -72-

2691 Miriam
501 Bacon Avenue
St. Louis, MO 63119-1512
314-968-3893
Fax: 314-962-0482
athorp@miriamstl.org
www.miriamstl.org/learning-center
Andrew Thorp, Executive Director
Sarah Scott, Development Director
Carol Faust, Business Manager
Tam Nguyen, Facilities Manager
Miriam improves the quality of life for children with learning disabilities and their families through innovative and comprehensive programs.

2692 Neuropsychology Assessment Center
One University Place
Chester, PA 19013
610-499-4273
www.widenernac.org
Mary F. Lazar, PsyD, Director
Wendy M. Sarkisian, PsyD, Assistant Director
Located in the Philadelphia area, the Neuropsychology Assessment Center (NAC) specializes in neuropsychological evaluations for the investigation of a variety of psychological conditions.

2693 ONLINE
West Virginia Research and Training Center
P.O. Box 1004
Institute, WV 25112-1004
304-766-9495
800-624-8284
Fax: 304-766-2689
www.icdi.wvu.edu
Clifford Lantz, President
A quarterly newsletter offering information about hardware technology, software (commercial and home grown); applications that work and bonuses such as an exchange program for copyright-free software. *$25.00*
Quarterly

2694 OWLS: Oral and Written Language Scales LC/OE & WE
AGS
P.O. Box 99
Circle Pines, MN 55014-99
800-328-2560
Fax: 800-471-8457
www.agsnet.com
Kevin Brueggeman, President
Robert Zaske, Market Manager
One kit provides an assessment of listening comprehension while the other assesses oral expression tasks: semantic, syntactic, pragmatic, and supralinguistic aspects of language. Written Expression may be administered individually or in small groups. *$249.95*

2695 PAT-3: Photo Articulation Test
Sage Publications
2455 Teller Road
Thousand Oaks, CA 91320
805-499-9774
800-818-7243
Fax: 800-583-2665
info@sagepub.com
www.sagepub.com
Paul Kelly, National Textbook Sales Manager
Blaise R Simqu, President & CEO
This test consists of 72 color photographs. The first 69 photos test consonants and all but one vowel and one diphthong. The remaining pictures test connected speech and the remaining vowel and diphthong. *$144.00*
Complete Kit

2696 **Peabody Early Experiences Kit (PEEK)**
AGS
P.O. Box 99
Circle Pines, MN 55014-99
800-328-2560
Fax: 800-471-8457
www.agsnet.com

Kevin Brueggeman, President
Robert Zaske, Market Manager
1,000 activities and all the materials you need to build youngsters' cognitive, social and language skills. Manuals, puppets, manipulatives, picture card deck, picture mini decks and more to teach early development concepts. *$789.95*

2697 **Peabody Individual Achievement Test-Revised Normative Update (PIAT-R-NU)**
AGS
P.O. Box 99
Circle Pines, MN 55014-99
800-328-2560
Fax: 800-471-8457
www.agsnet.com

Kevin Brueggeman, President
Robert Zaske, Market Manager
PIAT-R-NU is an efficient individual measure of academic achievement. Reading, mathematics, and spelling are assessed in a simple, non-threatening format that requires only a pointing response for most items. This multiple choice format makes the PIAT-R ideal for assessing individuals who hesitate to give a spoken response, or have limited expressive abilities. *$289.98*

2698 **Peabody Language Development Kits (PLDK)**
AGS
P.O. Box 99
Circle Pines, MN 55014-99
800-328-2560
Fax: 800-471-8457
www.agsnet.com

Kevin Brueggeman, President
Robert Zaske, Market Manager
The main goals of the Peabody Kit language program are to stimulate overall language skills in Standard English and, for each level of the program, advance children's cognitive skills about a year. *$649.95*
Level P
ISBN 0-88671 -25-1

2699 **Pediatric Early Elementary (PEEX II) Examination**
Educators Publishing Service
625 Mount Auburn Street
3rd Floor
Cambridge, MA 2138- 3039
617-547-6706
800-225-5750
Fax: 888-440-2665
feedback@epsbooks.com
www.epsbooks.com

Charles H Heinle, VP
Alexandra S Bigelow, Author
Gunnar Voltz, President
Assesses the second-fourth grade child's performance on thirty-two tasks in six specific areas of development: fine-motor function, language, gross-motor function, memory, visual processing, and delayed recall. At three points during the exam, the child is rated on selective attention and behavior and effect.
$15.40 - $93
ISBN 0-83888 -80-6

2700 **Pediatric Exam of Educational-PEERAMID Readiness at Middle Childhood**
Educators Publishing Service
625 Mount Auburn Street
3rd Floor
Cambridge, MA 2138- 3039
617-547-6706
800-225-5750
Fax: 888-440-2665
feedback@epsbooks.com
www.epsbooks.com

Charles H Heinle, VP
Alexandra S Bigelow, Author
Gunnar Voltz, President
Assesses the 4th-10th grade child's performance on thirty-one tasks in six specific areas: minor neurological indicators, fine-motor function, language, gross-motor function, temporal-sequential organization, and visual processing. Complete set.
$15.40 - $109
ISBN 0-83888 -99-3

2701 **Pediatric Examination of Educational Readiness**
Educators Publishing Service
625 Mount Auburn Street
3rd Floor
Cambridge, MA 2139- 3039
617-547-6706
800-225-5750
Fax: 888-440-2665
feedback@epsbooks.com
www.epsbooks.com

Charles H Heinle, VP
Alexandra S Bigelow, Author
Gunnar Voltz, President
Assesses the Pre-1st grade child's performance on twenty-nine tasks in six specific areas of development: orientation, gross-motor, visual-fine motor, sequential, linguistic and preacademic learning. The child is rated on ten dimensions of selective attention/activity processing efficiency and adaptation. Complete set.
$12.85 - $86.40
ISBN 0-83888 -80-1

2702 **Pediatric Extended Examination at-PEET Three**
Educators Publishing Service
625 Mount Auburn Street
3rd Floor
Cambridge, MA 2138- 3039
617-547-6706
800-225-5750
Fax: 888-440-2665
feedback@epsbooks.com
www.epsbooks.com

Charles H Heinle, VP
Alexandra S Bigelow, Author
Gunnar Volta, President
Assesses the preschool-age child's performance on twenty-eight tasks in five basic areas of development: gross-motor, language, visual-fine motor, memory, and intersensory integration. Complete set.
$13.75 - $126
ISBN 0-83888 -79-4

2703 **Pre-Reading Screening Procedures**
Educators Publishing Service
625 Mount Auburn Street
3rd Floor
Cambridge, MA 2138- 3039
617-547-6706
800-225-5750
Fax: 888-440-2665
feedback@epsbooks.com
www.epsbooks.com

Charles H Heinle, VP
Alexandra S Bigelow, Author
Gunnar Voltz, President
This revised group test, for grades K-1, evaluates auditory, visual and kinesthetic strengths in order to identify children who may have some form of dyslexia or specific language disability. *$18.00*
Grades K-1
ISBN 0-83885 -23-4

2704 **Preparing for ACT Assessment**
American College Testing Program
500 Act Drive
PO Box 168
Iowa City, IA 52243-168
319-337-1000
Fax: 319-339-3021
act.org

Richard L Ferguson, CEO
Designed to help high school students ready themselves for the ACT Assessment's subject area tests, explains the purposes of the four tests, describes their content and format, provides tips and exercises to improve student's test-taking skills and includes a complete sample text with scoring key.

2705 **Psycho-Educational Assessment of Preschool Children**
National Association of School Psychologists
Ste 105
4340 East West Hwy
Bethesda, MD 20814-4468
301-657-0270
866-331-NASP
Fax: 301-657-0275
ADMIN@SOELIN.COM
soelin.com
Susan Gorin, Executive Director
This is a contributed text on assessing specific skills of preschool children.
592 pages

2706 **RULES: Revised**
Speech Bin
PO Box 1579
Appleton, VA 54912-1579
772-770-0007
888-388-3224
Fax: 888-388-6344
customercare@schoolspecialty.com
www.speechbin.com
Jan J Binney, Senior Editor
Treatment program for young children who have phonological disorders. *$43.95*
280 pages
ISBN 0-93785 -51-3

2707 **Receptive-Expressive Emergent-REEL-2 Language Test, 2nd Edition**
Sage Publications
2455 Teller Road
Thousand Oaks, CA 91320
805-499-9774
800-818-7243
Fax: 800-583-2665
info@sagepub.com
www.sagepub.com
Paul Kelly, National Textbook Sales Manager
Blaise R Simqu, President & CEO
A revision of the popular scale used for the multidimensional analysis of emergent language. The REEL-2 is specifically designed for use with a broad range of at risk infants and toddlers in the new multidisciplinary programs developing under P.L. 99-457. *$79.00*

2708 **Regents' Center for Learning Disorders**
103 Hooper Street
Athens, GA 30602
706-542-4589
Fax: 706-583-0001
rcld@uga.edu
rcld.uga.edu
Tasha Falkingham, Office Manage
Karen Myers, Budget Analyst
Trish Foels, Staff Clinician, Psychologist
Lisa McLain, Staff Clinician
Provide assessment, training, research, andresources related to students who have learning disorders (e.g., Attention-Deficit/Hyperactivity Disorder, Autism Spectrum Disorders, Learning Disabilities, Emotional Disorders, and Traumatic Brain Injury) that impact their functioning in the academic environment.

2709 **Schmieding Developmental Center**
519 Latham Drive
Lowell, AR 72745
479-750-0125
Fax: 479-750-0323
www.archildrens.org
Mary Ann Scott, PhD, Program Director
Damon Lipinski, PhD, Program Director
Jerie Beth Karkos, MD, Medical Director
Arkansas Children's Hospital (ACH) is the a pediatric medical center in Arkansas.

2710 **Slingerland Screening Tests**
Educators Publishing Service
625 Mount Auburn Street
3rd Floor
Cambridge, MA 2138- 3039
617-547-6706
800-435-7728
Fax: 888-440-2665
feedback@epsbooks.com
www.epsbooks.com
Charles H Heinle, VP
Alexandra S Bigelow, Author
Gunnar Voltz, President
These tests, by Beth Slingerland, for individuals or groups of children, grades 1-6, identify children who show indications of having specific language disability in reading, handwriting, spelling or speaking. Form D evaluates personal orientation in time and space as well as the ability to express ideas in writing.
$14.80 - $27.45
ISBN 0-83882 -02-2

2711 **Special Needs Advocacy Resource Book**
Prufrock Press
PO Box 8813
Waco, TX 76714-8813
800-998-2208
Fax: 800-240-0333
info@prufrock.com
www.prufrock.com
Joel McIntosh, Publisher & Marketing Director
Rich Weinfield, Author
Michelle Davis, Author
Subtitle: What You Can Do Now to Advocate for Your Exceptional Child's Education. This is a unique hadnbook that teaches parents how to work with schools to achieve optimal learning situations and accommodations for their child's needs. *$19.95*
328 pages
ISBN 1-593633-09-7

2712 **Speech Bin**
PO Box 1579
Appleton, VA 54912-1579
772-770-0007
888-388-3224
Fax: 888-388-6344
customercare@schoolspecialty.com
www.speechbin.com
Jan J Binney, Senior Editor
Catalog offering test materials, assessment information, books and special education resources for speech-language pathologists, occupational and physical therapists, audiologists, and other rehabilitation professionals in schools, hospitals, clinics and private practices.
ISSN 4773-324

2713 **Stuttering Severity Instrument for Children and Adults**
Psychological & Educational Publications
P.O. Box 520
Hydesville, CA 95547-520
707-768-1807
800-523-5775
Fax: 800-447-0907
Morrison Gardner, President
With this tool teachers can determine whether to schedule a child for therapy or to evaluate the effects of treatment.

2714 **TLC Speech-Language/Occupational TherapyCamps**
2092 Gaither Rd.
Suite 100
Rockville, MD 20850
301-424-5200
Fax: 301-424-8063
TTY: 301-424-5203
info@ttlc.org
www.ttlc.org
Patricia Ritter, Executive Director
TLC provides small group summer programs for children with special needs. Offers speech-language and occupational therapy summer camps for children ages 3-7.

2715 **Taking Part: Introducing Social Skills to Young Children**
AGS
P.O. Box 99
Circle Pines, MN 55014-99
800-328-2560
Fax: 800-471-8457
www.agsnet.com

Kevin Brueggeman, President
Robert Zaske, Market Manager
The first social skills curriculum to be linked directly to an assessment tool. More than 30 lessons correlate with the skills assessed by the Social Skills Rating System, a multirater approach to assessing prosocial and problem behaviors. *$149.95*

2716 **Teaching of Reading: A Continuum from Kindergarten through College, The**
AVKO Educational Research Foundation
3084 Willard Rd
Birch Run, MI 48415-9404
810-686-9283
866-285-6612
Fax: 810-686-1101
avko.org

Don Mc Cabe, Executive Director
A textbook for teaching teachers how to teach language arts with lessons about dyslexia, phonics, learning to write, the connection between reading and spelling, and diagnostic and prescriptive tests. Free as an e-book for Foundation members. *$49.95*
364 pages

2717 **Test Critiques: Volumes I-X**
Sage Publications
2455 Teller Road
Thousand Oaks, CA 91320
805-499-9774
800-818-7243
Fax: 800-583-2665
info@sagepub.com
www.sagepub.com

Paul Kelly, National Textbook Sales Manager
Blaise R Simqu, President & CEO
Provides the professional and nonprofessional with in-depth, evaluative studies of more than 800 of the most widely used of these assessment instruments. *$649.00*

2718 **Test of Early Reading Ability Deaf or Hard of Hearing**
Pro- Ed Publications
8700 Shoal Creek Blvd
Austin, TX 78757-6816
512-451-3246
800-897-3202
Fax: 800-397-7633
general@proedinc.com
www.proedinc.com

Donald D Hammill, Owner
Courtney King, Marketing Coordinator
This adaptation of the TERA-2 for simultaneous communication of American Sign Language is the ONLY individually administered test of reading designed for children with moderate to profound sensory hearing loss. *$169.00*
Complete Kit

2719 **Test of Language Development: Primary**
Sage Publications
2455 Teller Road
Thousand Oaks, CA 91320
805-499-9774
800-818-7243
Fax: 800-583-2665
info@sagepub.com
www.sagepub.com

Paul Kelly, National Textbook Sales Manager
Blaise R Simqu, President & CEO
TOLD P:2 and TOLD 1:2 are the most popular tests of spoken language used by clinicians today. They are used to identify children who have language disorders and to isolate the particular types of disorders they have. Primary Edition for ages 1-4 to 8-11: Intermediate Edition for ages 8-6 to 12-11.

2720 **Test of Mathematical Abilities, 2nd Edition**
Sage Publications
2455 Teller Road
Thousand Oaks, CA 91320
805-499-9774
800-818-7243
Fax: 800-583-2665
info@sagepub.com
www.sagepub.com

Paul Kelly, National Textbook Sales Manager
Blaise R Simqu, President & CEO
The latest version was developed for use in grades 3 through 12. It measures math performance on the two traditional major skill areas in math as well as attitude, vocabulary and general application of math concepts in real life. *$84.00*

2721 **Test of Nonverbal Intelligence, 3rd Edition**
Sage Publications
2455 Teller Road
Thousand Oaks, CA 91320
805-499-9774
800-818-7243
Fax: 800-583-2665
info@sagepub.com
www.sagepub.com

Paul Kelly, National Textbook Sales Manager
Blaise R Simqu, President & CEO
A language-free measure of intelligence, aptitude and reasoning. The administration of the test requires no reading, writing, speaking or listening on the part of the test subject. The items included in this test are problem-solving tasks that increase in difficulty. Each item presents a set of figures in which one or more components is missing. The test items include one or more of the characteristics of shape, position, direction, rotation, contiguity, shading, size, movement or pattern. *$229.00*
Complete Kit

2722 **Test of Phonological Awareness**
Sage Publications
2455 Teller Road
Thousand Oaks, CA 91320
805-499-9774
800-818-7243
Fax: 800-583-2665
info@sagepub.com
www.sagepub.com

Paul Kelly, National Textbook Sales Manager
Blaise R Simqu, President & CEO
Measures young children's awareness of the individual sounds in words. Children who are sensitive to the phonological structure of words in oral language have a much easier time learning to read than children who are not. *$143.00*

2723 **Test of Written Spelling, 3rd Edition**
Pro- Ed Publications
8700 Shoal Creek Blvd
Austin, TX 78757-6897
512-451-3246
800-897-3202
Fax: 800-397-7633
general@proedinc.com
www.proedinc.com

Donald D Hammill, Owner
Courtney King, Marketing Coordinator
This revised edition assesses the student's ability to spell words whose spellings are readily predictable in sound-letter patterns, words whose spellings are less predictable and both types of words considered together. *$74.00*

2724 **Texas Scottish Rite Hospital for Children**
2222 Welborn Street
Dallas, TX 75219
214-559-5000
Fax: 800-421-1121
tsrhdv@tsrh.org
www.tsrhc.org

Robert L. Walker, President/ CEO
Mark G. Bateman, SVP, Public Relations
Leslie A. Clonch, Jr., Vice President/ CIO
Stephanie Brigger, Vice President, Development
TSRHC treats children with orthopedic conditions, such as scoliosis, clubfoot, hand disorders, hip disorders and limb length differences, as well as certain related neurological disorders and learning disorders, such as dyslexia.

2725 **Woodcock Reading Mastery Tests**
Pearson
5601 Green Valley Dr
Bloomington, MN 55437-1099
800-627-7271
Fax: 800-232-1223
pearsonassessments@pearson.com
www.pearsonassessments.com
Christine Carlson, Product Manager
Doug Kubach, President & CEO
The Woodcock Reading Mastery Tests - Revised provides an interpretive system and age range to help you assess reading skills of children and adults. Two forms, G and II, make it easy to test and retest, or you can combine the results of both forms for a more comprehensive assessment. Revised with recent updates.
$329.95

2726 **Young Children with Special Needs: A Developmentally Appropriate Approach**
Allyn & Bacon
75 Arlington Street
Ste 300
Boston, MA 2116-3988
617-848-7500
800-852-8024
Fax: 617-944-7273
www.ablongman.com
Bill Barke, CEO
Thomas Longman, Founder
This book is designed to prepare students in making curriculum decisions in order to care for and foster the development of young children with special needs in normal early childhood settings.
270 pages
ISBN 0-20518 -94-X

Treatment & Training

2727 **ABLE Program MCC-Longview**
3200 Broadway
Kansas City, MO 64111-2105
816-604-1000
Fax: 816-672-2719
joan.bergstrom@mcckc.edu
mcckc.edu/ABLE
Joan Bergstrom, Director
Kay Owens, Administrative Assistant
Intensive support services program for post secondary students with neurological disabilities. The ABLE Program can be reached at http://mcckc.edu/ABLE

2728 **Academy for Guided Imagery**
30765 Pacific Coast Hwy
Ste 355
Malibu, CA 90265-3643
800-726-2070
Fax: 800-727-2070
info@acadgi.com
www.acadgi.com
David E Bresler, President
The Academy aims to teach people to access and use the power of the mind/body connection for healing, and to further understanding of the imagery process in human life and development. They provide systematic training and guidance to health professionals who are interested in the use of Guided Imagery in their practice. The Academy's Imagery Store offers guided imagery CDs, DVDs and books for self-healing.

2729 **Adventist HealthCare**
820 West Diamond Avenue
Suite 600
Gaithersburg, MD 20878
301-315-3030
Fax: 301-315-3000
www.adventisthealthcare.com
David E. Weigley, M.B.A., Chairman
Robert T. Vandeman, Vice-Chair
Terry Forde, Secretary
dventist HealthCare, based in Gaithersburg, Md., is a not-for-profit organization of dedicated professionals who work together to provide excellent wellness, disease management and health-care services to the community.

2730 **Asthma & Allergy Education for Worksite Clinicians**
Asthma and Allergy Foundation of America
8201 Corporate Drive
Suite 1000
Landover, VA 20785
202-466-7643
800-727-8462
Fax: 202-466-8940
info@aafa.org
aafa.org
Bill Mc Lin, President & CEO
Helen Taylor, Information Specialist
Developed to teach health professionals in the worksite about asthma and allergies and ultimately improve the health of the employees who have theses de\iseases. The program gives worksite clinicians the knowledge and tools they need to give employees guidance on how to control environmental factors both in the home and in the workplace, self-manage thier asthma and/or allergies and to determaine if ti is necessary for employees to see an allergist if symptoms persist.

2731 **Asthma & Allergy Essentials for Children's Care Provider**
Asthma and Allergy Foundation of America
8201 Corporate Drive
Suite 1000
Landover, VA 20785
202-466-7643
800-727-8462
Fax: 202-466-8940
info@aafa.org
aafa.org
Bill Mc Lin, President & CEO
Helen Taylor, Information Specialist
Course gives child care providers the tools and knowledge they need to care for children with asthma and allergies. During the interactive, three hour program, a trained health professional teaches providers how to recognize the signs and symptoms of an asthma or allergy episode, how to institute environmental control measures to prevent these episodes, and how to properly use medication and the tools for asthma management. In areas of the country serviced by AAFA's 14 chapters.

2732 **Asthma Care Training for Kids (ACT)**
Asthma and Allergy Foundation of America
8201 Corporate Drive
Suite 1000
Landover, VA 20785
202-466-7643
Fax: 202-466-8940
info@aafa.org
www.aafa.org
Bill Mc Lin, President & CEO
Helen Taylor, Information Specialist
Interactive program for children ages seven to 12 and their families. Children and their families attend three group sessions seperately to learn their own unique styles and then come together at the end of each session to share their knowledge.

2733 **Ayurvedic Institute**
PO Box 23445
Albuquerque, NM 87292-1445
505-291-9698
800-863-7721
Fax: 505-294-7572
ayurveda.com
Wynn Werner, Administrator
Directed by Dr. Vasant Lad, trains people in Ayurveda.

2734 **Brooks Rehabilitation Hospital**
3599 University Blvd S
Jacksonville, FL 32216
904-345-7600
Fax: 904-345-7619
www.brookshealth.org
Gary W. Sneed, Chairman
Michael Spigel, President/ COO
Douglas M. Baer, Chief Executive Officer
Bruce M. Johnson, Vice-Chair
Brooks Rehabilitation provides the most advanced therapy and medical care.

2735 **Center for Parent Information and Resources**
35 Halsey St
4th Floor
Newark, NJ 07102 973-642-8100
www.parentcenterhub.org
Debra A. Jennings, Director
Myriam Alizo, Project Assistant
Lisa K□pper, Product Development Coordinator
Jessica Wilson, Communications Director
The Center for Parent Information and Resources (CPIR) serves as a central resource of information and products to the community of Parent Training Information (PTI) Centers and the Community Parent Resource Centers (CPRCs), so that they can focus their efforts on serving families of children with disabilities.

2736 **Center for Spinal Cord Injury Recovery**
261 Mack
Detroit, MI 48201 866-724-2368
Fax: 313-745-9064
krodgers@dmc.org
www.centerforscirecovery.org
Krystal Rodgers, Administrative Assistant
The Center for SCI Recoveryr (CSCIR)provides long-term, high intensity, non-traditional, activity based therapy to maximize recovery.

2737 **Cottage Rehabilitation Hospital**
400 W. Pueblo Street
Santa Barbara, CA 93105 805-682-7111
mzate@sbch.org
www.cottagehealth.org

2738 **Courage Kenny Rehabilitation Institute**
Allina Health
800 E 28th St.
Minneapolis, MN 55407 612-863-4495
www.allinahealth.org

2739 **Harriet & Robert Heilbrunn Guild School**
JGB Audio Library for the Blind
15 W 65th St
New York, NY 10023-6601 212-769-6200
800-284-4422
Fax: 212-769-6266
www.JGB.org
Allen R Morse, JD, PhD, President & CEO
Ken Stanley, Manager
A Jewish Guild for the blind.

2740 **Howard School, The**
1192 Foster St NW
Atlanta, GA 30318-4329 404-377-7436
Fax: 404-377-0884
admissions@howardschool.org
howardschool.org
Marifred Cilella, Head Of School
The Howard School educates students 5 years old through 12th grade with language learning disabilities and learning differences. Small student/teacher ratios allow for instruction that is personalized to complement the individual learning styles and to help each student understand his/her learning process. Students gain the tools and strategies needed to become independent, life-long learners.

2741 **Kennedy Krieger Institute**
707 North Broadway
Baltimore, MD 21205 443-923-9200
800-873-3377
888-554-2080
www.kennedykrieger.org
Jennifer Accardo, M.D., Neurologist
Adrianna Amari, Ph.D., Training & Research Coordinator
Roberta L. Babbitt, Ph.D, Program Director
Amy J. Bastian, Ph.D., P.T., Chief Science Officer
Kennedy Krieger Institute is an internationally recognized institution dedicated to improving the lives of children and young adults with pediatric developmental disabilities and disorders of the brain, spinal cord and musculoskeletal system, through patient care, special education, research, and professional training.

2742 **Kessler Institute for Rehabilitation**
1199 Pleasant Valley Way
West Orange, NJ 07052 973-731-3600
877-322-2580
Fax: 973-243-6819
www.kessler-rehab.com
Sue Kida, President
Provides physical medicine and rehabilitation through the integration of highly specialized care, treatment, technology, education, research, and advocacy.

2743 **Lake Michigan Academy**
West Michigan Learning Disabilities Foundation
2428 Burton St SE
Grand Rapids, MI 49546-4806 616-464-3330
Fax: 616-285-1935
Amy Barto, Executive Director
Is a private day school for children with learning disabilities.

2744 **Levinson Medical Center**
98 Cutter Mill Road
Suite 90
Great Neck, NY 11021 516-482-2888
800-334-7323
Fax: 516-482-2480
drlevinson@aol.com
www.dyslexiaonline.com
Dr. Harold Levinson, Psychiatrist, Neurologist
Carolyn Malman, Office Manager
Lisa Danziger, Patient Coordinator
Dr. Margaret, Neurological Test & Evaluations
Medical center groundbreaking medical treatment offers rapid and often dramatic help to suffering dyslexic/ADHD children and adults

2745 **Mad Hatters: Theatre That Makes a World of Difference**
P.O. Box 50002
Kalamazoo, MI 49005-2 Fax: 269-385-5868
Bobbe A Luce, Executive Director
A nationally-known theater which has presented effective and innovative programs to more than 175,000 people in over 1,150 performances in the past 15 years. Our presentations and training programs are a proven method of changing attitudes and behaviors. The Mad Hatters is a leader in the field of sensitivity training to build community and foster the inclusion of all people in society. Fees: $500-$4000 per program, depending on topic and audience.

2746 **MedStar National Rehabilitation Network**
102 Irving Street NW
Washington, DC 20010 202-877-1000
www.medstarnrh.org

2747 **Missouri Rehabilitation Center**
One Hospital Drive
Columbia, MO 65212 573-882-4141
www.muhealth.org

2748 **Neuroxcel**
401 Northlake Blvd.
North Palm Beach, FL 33048 866-391-6247
www.neuroxcel.com

2749 **Ramapo Training**
Ramapo for Children
Rt. 52/Salisbury Turnpike
PO Box 266
Rhinebeck, NY 12572 845-876-8403
Fax: 845-876-8414
office@ramapoforchildren.org
www.ramapoforchildren.org
Adam Weiss, Chief Executive Officer
Bruce Kuziola, Chief Financial & Administrative Officer
Adam St. Bernard Jacobs, Director, Development & Communications
Kazz A. Pinkard, Deputy Director, Ramapo Training
Ramapo Training was established to provide staff training and program support for educational and recreational programs, especially those that serve children-at-risk and those with special needs.

2750 **Sandhills School**
1500 Hallbrook Dr
Columbia, SC 29209-4021
803-695-1400
Fax: 803-695-1214
info@sandhillsschool.org
www.sandhillsschool.org

Anne Vickers, Head of School
Erika Senneseth, Asst Head of School
Angela Daniel, Director of Development
Carmen Kennedy, Business Manager

Exists to provide educational programs and intellectual development for average to above average students, six to 15, who learn differently and to promote the development of self-awareness, joy in learning and a vision of themselves as life-long learners.

2751 **Senior Program for Teens and Young Adults with Special Needs**
Camp J CC
6125 Montrose Rd
Rockville, MD 20852-4860
301-881-0100
Fax: 301-881-6549
jcccamp@jccgw.org
www.jccgw.org

Scott Cohen, President
Mindy Burger, Vice President for Development

The senior Program is a transitional program for teens and young adults with severe learning disabilities and multiple disabilities. Socialization, recreation and independent living skills are enhanced in a fun enviroment. Activities include art, music, recreational swim and more.

2752 **Spinal Cord Injury Center**
132 S. 10th Street
375 Main Building
Philadelphia, PA 19107
215-955-6579
Fax: 215-955-5152

Marilyn P. Owens, RN, BSN, Project Coordinator
Brittany Hayes, Research Coordinator
Jacqueline Robinson, Administrative Assistant
Susan Sakers Sammartino, BS, Data Coordinator

SCI provides medical care for their injuries, along with emotional, social, vocational and psychological rehabilitation to cope with the changes in their bodies and in their lifestyles that often result from the injury.

2753 **Stanford Health Care**
300 Pasteur Drive
Stanford, CA 94304
650-498-3333
800-756-9000
stanfordhealthcare.org

Amir Dan Rubin, President and CEO
Raj Behal, MD, Chief Quality Officer
James Hereford, Chief Operating Officer
Daniel J. Morissette, Chief Financial Officer

Stanford Health Care provides patients with the very best in diagnosis and treatment.

2754 **Teacher of Students with Visual Impairments**
3635 Coal Mountain Rd.
Cumming, GA 30028
c.willings@teachingvisuallyimpaired.com
www.teachingvisuallyimpaired.com

2755 **The Glenholme School**
Devereux Advanced Behavioral Health Connecticut
81 Sabbaday Ln.
Washington, CT 06793
860-868-7377
Fax: 860-868-7894
info@theglenholmeschool.org
www.theglenholmeschool.org

2756 **UAB Spain Rehabilitation Center**
1720 2nd Ave South
Birmingham, AL 35294
205-934-4011
TTY: 205-934-4642
www.uab.edu

Ray L. Watts, M.D., President
G. Allen Bolton Jr., VP, Financial Affairs

UAB's missionis to be a research university and academic health center that discovers, teaches and applies knowledge for the intellectual, cultural, social and economic benefit of Birmingham, the state and beyond.

2757 **University of Maryland Rehabilitation and Orthopaedic Institute**
Uni of MD Rehab & Ortho Institute
2200 Kernan Drive
Baltimore, MD 21207
410-448-2500
888-453-7626
TTY: 800-735-2258
www.umrehabortho.org

Cynthia A. Kelleher, MPH, MBA, Interim President and CEO
John P. Straumanis, VP, Medical Affairs
W. Walter Augustin, III, CPA, VP of Financial Services
Cheryl D. Lee, RN, MSN, CRRN, VP, Patient Care Services

University of Maryland Rehabilitation & Orthopaedic Institute (formerly Kernan Hospital), a committed provider of orthopaedic surgery and the largest inpatient rehabilitation hospital and provider of rehabilitation services in the state of Maryland, has been serving the Baltimore community for over 100 years.

2758 **Vanguard School, The**
Valley Forge Specialized Educational Services
1777 N Valley Rd
Paoli, PA 19301
610-296-6700
Fax: 610-640-0132
www.vanguardschool-pa.org

Tim Lanshe, Director of Education
James Kirkpatrick, CFO
Peg Osborne, Admissions Director

An Approved Private School (APS) for students aged 4-21 years with exceptionalities including autism spectrum disorder, mild emotional disturbances and/or neurological impairments.

2759 **Worthmore Academy**
3535 Kessler Boulevard East Dr
Indianapolis, IN 46220-5154
317-902-9896
877-700-6516
Fax: 317-251-6516
bjackson@worthmoreacademy.org
www.worthmoreacademy.org

Brenda Jackson, Director
Alyssa Blaire Cook, Assistant Director

A place where children with learning disabilities receive individualized instruction to help remediate his or her condition. The most common learning disabilities we work with are Dyslexic, A.D.D, A.D.H.D, Autism Spectrum (including Asperger's Syndrome), and communication disorders.

Exchange Programs

General

2760 A Guide to International Educational Exchange
Mobility International USA
132 E Broadway
Suite 343
Eugene, OR 97401
541-343-1284
Fax: 541-343-6812
TTY: 541-343-1284
clearinghouse@miusa.org
www.miusa.org

Susan Sygall, Chief Executive Officer
Cindy Lewis, Director, Programs
A Guide to International Educational Exchange, Community Service and Travel for People with Disabilities includes information travel and international programs, as well as personal experience stories from people with disabilities who have had successful international experiences.
600 pages

2761 American Institute for Foreign Study
River Plaza 9 W Broad St
Stamford, CT 6902-3788
203-399-5000
866-906-2437
Fax: 203-399-5590
info@aifs.com
www.aifs.com

William L Gertz, CEO
Organizes cultural exchange programs throughout the world for more than 50,000 students each year and arranges insurance coverage for our own participants as well as participants of other organizations. Also provides summer travel programs overseas and in the US ranging from one week to a full academic year.

2762 American Universities International Programs
307 S College Ave
Fort Collins, CO 80524-2801
970-495-0084
888-730-2847
Fax: 970-495-0114
info@auip.com
www.auip.com

Laurie Klith, Executive Director
Study abroad organization sending students to universities in Australia and New Zealand.

2763 American-Scandinavian Foundation
58 Park Ave
38 Street
New York, NY 10016-3007
212-779-3587
Fax: 212-686-1157
info@amscan.org
scandinaviahouse.org

Edward Gallagher, President
Promotes international understanding through educational and cultural exchange between the United States and Denmark, Finland, Iceland, Norway and Sweden.

2764 Antioch College
One Morgan Place
Yellow Springs, OH 45387-1635
937-319-6082
Fax: 937-319-6085

Mark Roosevelt, President
Thomas Brookley, CFO & COO
Gariot Louima, Chief Communications Officer
Education abroad offers numerous programs which can be included in undergraduate and graduate study programs.

2765 Army and Air Force Exchange Services
PO Box 660202
Dallas, TX 75266-202
214-312-2011
800-527-2345
Fax: 800-446-0163
TTY: 800-423-2011
www.aafes.com

James Moore, Senior VP
MG Bruce Casella, Commander/CEO
Brings a tradition of value, service, and support to its 11.5 million authorized customers at military installations in the United States, Europe and in the Pacific.

2766 Association for International Practical Training
10400 Little Patuxent Pkwy
Suite 250
Columbia, MD 21044-3519
410-997-2200
Fax: 410-992-3924
aipt@aipt.org
aipt.org

Elizabeth Chazottes, CEO
Nonprofit organization dedicated to encouraging and facilitating the exchange of qualified individuals between the US and other countries so they may gain practical work experience and improve international understanding.

2767 Basic Facts on Study Abroad
International Education
809 United Nations Plz
New York, NY 10017-3503
212-883-8200
Fax: 212-984-5452
publications@un.org
iie.org

Allen E Goodman, CEO
Peggy Blumenthal, Executive Vice President
Information book including foreign study planning, educational choices, finances and study abroad programs. *$35.00*
30 pages

2768 Beaver College
Arcadia University
450 S Easton Rd
Glenside, PA 19038-3215
215-572-2901
888-232-8379
Fax: 215-572-2174

Lorna Stern, Deputy Director
One of the largest college-based study abroad programs in the country. Prices from $8000.00 semester to $22000.00 a year.

2769 Buffalo State (SUNY)
1300 Elmwood Ave
South Wing 410
Buffalo, NY 14222-1095
716-878-4620
Fax: 716-878-3054
intleduc@buffalostate.edu

Lee Ann Grace, Asst Dean Int'l/Exchange Program
Provides international educational exchange opportunities for students of university age and older through its Office of International Education.

2770 Building Bridges: Including People with Disabilities in International Programs
Mobility International USA
132 E Broadway
Suite 343
Eugene, OR 97401
541-343-1284
Fax: 541-343-6812
TTY: 541-343-1284
clearinghouse@miusa.org
www.miusa.org

Susan Sygall, Chief Executive Officer
Cindy Lewis, Director, Programs
Empowers people with disabilities around the world through international exhange and international development to achieve their human rights. The international exchange programs usually last two-four weeks and are held throughout the year in the US and abroad. Activities include living with homestay families, leadership seminars, disability rights workshops, cross cultural learning and teambuilding activities such as river rafting and challenging courses.

2771 Davidson College, Office of Study Abroad
Davidson College
PO Box 7171
Davidson, NC 28035-7171
704-894-2000
Fax: 704-894-2005
kocampbell@davidson.edu
www3.davidson.edu

Carol Quillen, President

Recognizes the value of study abroad for both the devlopment of worl understanding and the development of the student as a broadminded, objective and mature individual.

2772 High School Students Guide to Study, Travel, and Adventure Abroad
300 Fore Street
Portland, ME 4101
207-553-4000
Fax: 207-553-4299
contact@ciee.org
www.ciee.org

Robert E. Fallon, CEO & President
Kenton Keith, Senior Vice President for Progra
This guide provides high school students with all the information they need for a successful trip abroad. Included are sections to help students find out if they're ready for a trip abroad, make the necessary preparations and get the most from their experience. Over 200 programs are described including language study, summer camps, homestays, study tours and work camps. The program descriptions include information for people with disabilities.
ISSN 0312-11

2773 IPSL Institute of Global Learning
4110 SE Hawthorne Blvd.
Suite 200
Portland, OR 97214
503-395-4775
Fax: 503-954-1881
info@ipsl.org
ipsl.org

Thomas Morgan, President
Arianne Newton, Director, Programs
IPSL is an educational organization servicing students, colleges, universities, service agencies and related organizations around the world by fostering programs that link volunteer service and academic study. IPSL is a registered Social Benefit Corporation that is committed to its mission and dedicated to promoting an ethic of service. They invest over 83% of our revenues directly back into the communities where they serve.

2774 International Christian Youth Exchange
134 W 26th St
New York, NY 10001-6803
212-206-7307
Fax: 212-633-9085

Ed Gragert
Offers participants a unique experience to learn about another culture and make friends from different countries.

2775 International Student Exchange Programs (I SEP)
1655 N Fort Myer Drive
Suite 400
Arlington, VA 22209
703-504-9960
Fax: 703-243-8070
info@isep.org
www.isep.org

Dr. Thomas Hochstettler, Chair
Dr. Tony Atwater, President
ISEP is a network of 275 post-secondary institutions in the United States and 38 other countries cooperating to provide affordable international educational experiences for a diverse student population.

2776 International University Partnerships
University of Pennsylvania
1011 South Dr
Indiana, PA 15705-1046
724-357-2100
Fax: 724-357-6213
iup.edu

David Werner, President
Offers a variety of international educational exchange programs to students who wish to study overseas.

2777 Lake Erie College
391 W. Washington St.
Painesville, OH 44077
440-296-1856
800-533-4996
Fax: 440-375-7005
admissions@lec.edu
www.lec.edu

Michael Victor, President
Michael Keresman lll, Director
Sends students abroad for a term or longer to develop intellectual awareness and individual maturity.

2778 Lane Community College
4000 E 30th Ave
Eugene, OR 97405
541-463-3100
Fax: 541-463-5201
asklane@lanecc.edu
www.lanecc.edu

Margaret Hamilton, Ph.D, President
Lane Community College offers a wide variety of instructional programs including transfer credit programs, career and technical degree and certificate programs, continuing education noncredit courses, ESL, GED programs, and customized training for local businesses. The college offers support services for those with disabilities through their Center for Accessible Resources.

2779 Lions Clubs International
300 W 22nd St
Oak Brook, IL 60523-8842
630-571-5466
Fax: 630-571-8890
www.lionsclubs.org

Joe Preston, International President
Jitsuhiro Yamada, First Vice President
Robert E. Corlew, Second Vice President
Eric R. Carter, First Year Directors
Over 46,000 individual clubs in over 194 countries and geographical areas which provide community service and promote better international relations. Clubs work with local communities to provide needed and useful programs for sight, diabetes and hearing, and aid in study abroad.

2780 Lisle
900 County Road 269
Leander, TX 78641-1633
512-259-4404
Barbara E Bratton, Owner
Educational organization which works toward world peace and better quality of human life through increased understanding between persons of similar and different cultures.

2781 National 4-H Council
7100 Connecticut Ave
Chevy Chase, MD 20815-4934
301-961-2800
Fax: 301-961-2894
www.4-h.org

Donald Floyd, President
Jennifer Sirangelo, Executive Vice President
4-H opened the door for young people to learn leadership skills and explore ways to give back. 4-H revolutionized how youth connected to practical, hands-on learning experiences while outside of the classroom.

2782 New Directions for People with Disabilities
5276 Hollister Ave.
Suite 207
Santa Barbara, CA 93111
805-967-2841
888-967-2841
Fax: 805-964-7344
hello@newdirectionstravel.org
www.newdirectionstravel.org

Dee Duncan, Executive Director
A nonprofit organization providing local, national, and international travel vacations and holiday programs for people with mild to moderate developmental disabilities.

2783 People to People International
911 Main Street
Suite 2110
Kansas City, MO 64105-2246
816-531-4701
Fax: 816-561-7502
ptpi@ptpi.org
www.ptpi.org

Mary Eisenhower, CEO
Roseanne Rosen, Senior Vice President of Operati
Brian Hueben, Senior Director, Administration
Stacey Chance, Director, Publications
Exchanges international understanding and friendship through educational, cultural and humantarian activities involving the exchange of ideas and experiences directly among people of different countries and diverse cultures. Is also dedicated to enhancing

cross cultural communication within each communityand across communities and nations.

2784 **Rotary Youth Exchange**
Rotary International
1560 Sherman Ave
Evanston, IL 60201-4818
847-866-3000
866-976-8279
Fax: 847-328-4101
youthexchange@rotary.org
www.rotary.org

Kalyan Banerjee, International President
Noel A Bajat, Vice President
Kenneth R Boyd, Director
Elizabeth Demaray, Director

This worldwide organization of business and professional leaders provides humanitarian service, encourages high ethical standards in all vocations, and helps build goodwill and peace in the world. Approximately 1.2 million Rotarians belong to more than 31,000 Rotary clubs located in 167 countries for exchange opportunities.

2785 **Scandinavian Exchange**
24 Dickinson Street
Amherst, MA 1002
413-253-9737
Fax: 413-253-5282
howery@scandinavianseminar.org
www.scandinavianseminar.org

Jacqueline D Waldman, CEO
William Kaufmann, Chair

Student exchange program founded in 1949.

2786 **Sister Cities International**
915 15th Street, NW
4th Floor
Washington, DC 20005
202-347-8630
Fax: 202-393-6524
info@sister-cities.org
sister-cities.org

Patrick Madden, President
Jim Doumas, Executive Vice President, & Inte

A non profit citizen diplomacy network creating and strengthening partnerships between US and international communities in an effort to increase global cooperation at the municipal level, to promote cultural understnading and to stimulate economic development. Encourages local community development and volunteer action by motivating and empowering private citizens, municipal officials and business leaders to conduct long term programs of mutual benefits including exchange situations.

2787 **State University of New York**
1400 Washington Ave
Albany, NY 12222-100
518-442-3300
Fax: 518-442-5383
ugadmissions@albany.edu
www.albany.edu

George Philip, President
Alain Kaloyeros, Senior Vice President & CEO
Susan Phillips, Provost & VP for Academic Affai
James Dias, VP for Research

Offers over 150 international educational exchange programs in 37 different countries. Broad mission of excellence in undergraduate and graduate education, research and public service engages 17,000 diverse students in nine schools and colleges across three campuses.

2788 **University of Minnesota at Crookston**
2900 University Ave
Crookston, MN 56716-5000
218-281-6510
800-862-6466
Fax: 218-281-8050
UMCinfo@umn.edu
www.crk.umn.edu

Charles Casey, CEO
Eric Kaler, President

The University of Minnesota, Crookston (UMC) is a public, baccalaureate, coeducational institution and a coordinate campus of the University of Minnesota

2789 **University of Oregon**
5000 N Willamette Blvd
Portland, OR 97203-5798
503-943-8000
Fax: 503-725-3067
webmaster@up.edu
up.edu

Patricia Esley, Manager
Rev.E.Willia Beauchamp, President
James Lyons, VP University Relations
Jim Ravelli, VP for University Research

Study/cultural experience is available in Tokyo and other Japanese cities as part of the Japan Studies Program at the University.

2790 **Western Washington University**
516 High St
Bellingham, WA 98225-5996
360-650-3000
Fax: 360-650-3022
www.wwu.edu

Bruce Shepard, President
Paul Dunn, Senior Executive Asst. to the Pr
Barbara Stoneberg, Assistant to the President
Mary Lacher, Receptionist, President & Provis

2791 **World Experience Teenage Exchange Program**
2440 S Hacienda Blvd
Suite 116
Hacienda Heights, CA 91745-4763
626-330-5719
800-633-6653
Fax: 626-333-4914

Kerry Gonzales, President
Marge Archaumbault, President

Offers a quality and affordable program for over two decades and continues to provide students and host families a youth exchange program based on individual attention, with the help of an international network of overseas directors and USA coordinators.

2792 **World of Options**
Mobility International USA
132 E Broadway
Suite 343
Eugene, OR 97401
541-343-1284
Fax: 541-343-6812
TTY: 541-343-1284
clearinghouse@miusa.org
www.miusa.org

Susan Sygall, Chief Executive Officer
Cindy Lewis, Director, Programs

Empowering people with disabilities around the world through international exchange and international development to achieve their human rights.
338 pages

2793 **Youth for Understanding International Exchange**
6400 Goldsboro Road
Suite 100
Bethesda, MD 20817-5841
240-235-2100
800-833-6243
Fax: 240-352-2104
admissions@yfu.org
yfu.org

Rachel Andreson, Founder
Samantha Brizzolara, Chair

Youth for Understanding (YFU) International Exchange, an educational, nonprofit organization, prepares young people for the opportunities and responsabilities in a changing, independent world. With YFU, students can choose a year, semenster, or summer program in one or more than 35 countries worldwide. More than 200,000 young people from more than 50 nations in Asia, Europe, North and South America, Africa and the Pacific have participated in YFU exchanges.

Foundations & Funding Resources

Alabama

2794 **Alabama Power Foundation**
PO Box 2641
Birmingham, AL 35203
205-257-2508
powerofgood.com
Myla Calhoun, President
Hallie Bradley, Manager, Community Initiatives
Brandon Glover, Manager, Strategic Initiatives
Honoring its mission to strengthen the communities the company serves, the foundation focuses its efforts on organizations that support education, civic activities, health services, the environment and the arts. By supporting the state's educational system from pre-K to universities, the foundation is investing in Alabama's future and the well-being of its residents.

2795 **Andalusia Health Services**
700 River Falls Street
PO Box 667
Andalusia, AL 36420
334-222-2030
Fax: 334-222-7844
chrissie@andalusiachamber.com
www.andalusiachamber.com
Janna McGlamory, President
Debbie Marcum, Vice President
Ashley Eiland, Executive Vice President
Gail Hayes, Treasurer
Only offers grants to the residents of Covington County in Alabama who are pursuing a degree in a medical field.

2796 **Arc Of Alabama, The**
557 S Lawrence St
Montgomery, AL 36104-4611
334-262-7688
866-243-9557
Fax: 334-834-9737
www.thearcofal.org/#!contact/c1d94
Larry Bailey, President
Sherron Culpepper, 1st Vice President
Bruce Koppenhoeffer, 2nd Vice President
Jack Knight, Treasurer
The Arc of Alabama, Inc. is a volunteer-based membership organization made up of individuals with intellectual, developmental and other disabilities, their families, friends, interested citizens, and professionals in the disability field.

2797 **Rapahope Children's Retreat Foundation**
2701 Airport Blvd
Mobile, AL 36606
251-476-9880
Fax: 251-476-9495
info@rapahope.org
www.rapahope.org
Melissa McNichol, Executive Director
Roz Dorsett, Assistant Director
Rapahope is an organization that offers a one week long summer camp for children who have, or who have had cancer. For children ages 7-17, the camp offers a wide range of summer camp activities, including but not limited to, swimming, kayaking, horseback riding, and arts. The camp is offered at no cost to campers or their families.

Alaska

2798 **Arc of Alaska**
The Arc of Anchorage
2211 Arca Dr
Anchorage, AK 99508-3462
907-277-6677
800-258-2232
Fax: 907-272-2161
TTY: 907-277-0735
info@thearcofanchorage.org
Rod Shipley, President
Dave Falsey, Vice President
Meredith Parham, Secretary
Sharon Purkis, Treasurer
The Arc helps Alaskans who experience developmental disabilities, behavioral health concerns or deafness achieve lives of dignity and independence as valued members of our community.

2799 **Rasmuson Foundation**
301 West Northern Lights Blvd.
Suite 400
Anchorage, AK 99503
907-297-2700
877-366-2700
Fax: 907-297-2770
www.rasmuson.org
Edward B. Rasmuson, Chairman
Cathryn Rasmuson, Vice Chair
Diane Kaplan, President & CEO
Chris Perez, Program Officer
The Rasmuson Foundation invests both in individuals and well managed organizations dedicated to improving the quality of life for Alaskans.

Arizona

2800 **American Foundation Corporation**
4518 North 32nd Street
Phoenix, AZ 85018
602-955-4770
Fax: 602-955-4700
www.americanfoundation.org
Ben L. Schaub, Founder and CEO
The American Foundation can be your sponsor, and help your company set up a corporate foundation in a public charity or support organization format.

2801 **Arizona Autism Resources**
The Arc of Arizona
PO Box 90714
Phoenix, AZ 85066
602-234-2721
800-433-5255
Fax: 602-234-5959
arc@arcarizona.org
www.arcarizona.org
Robert Snyder, President
Michael Leyva, Vice President
Jon Meyers, Executive Director
Kim Dorshaw, Secretary
The Arc is committed to securing for all people with developmental disabilities the opportunity to choose and realize their goals in regard to where they live, learn, work and play.

2802 **Arizona Community Foundation**
2201 E Camelback Road
Suite 405B
Phoenix, AZ 85016
602-381-1400
800-222-8221
Fax: 602-381-1575
info@azfoundation.org
www.azfoundation.org
Ron Butler, Chair
Shelly Cohn, Vice Chair
Steven G. Seleznow, President & CEO
John Gogolak, Treasurer
The mission of the Arizona Community Foundation is to empower and align philanthropic interests with community needs and build a legacy of living.

2803 **Arizona Instructional Resource Center for Students who are Blind or Visually Impaired, The**
Foundation For Blind Children
1235 E. Harmont Drive
Phoenix, AZ 85020
602-678-5800
800-322-4870
Fax: 602-678-5819
mashton@SeeItOurWay.org
www.seeitourway.org
Dee Nortman, CFO
Marc Ashton, Chief Executive Officer
Barbra Smith, Chief of Staff
Alexander Pushman, Director, Mark & Dev
The Foundation for Blind Children contracts with the Arizona Department of Education to provide statewide media services for students between pre-kindergarten and 12th grade who have a vi-

sual impairment or are blind andEneed their instructional materials in a specialized medium such as Braille, large print, or electronic files as well as adaptive equipment.

2804 Civitan Foundation
12635 N 42nd St.
Phoenix, AZ 85032 602-953-2944
www.civitanfoundationaz.com
Dawn Trapp, Executive Director
Mike Prochelo, Chief Administrative Officer
Jeanne Anastasopoulos, Director, Program Services & HR
Sophia Campbell, Director, Mission Advancement
The foundation aims to enhance the quality of life for children and adults with developmental disabilities through programs such as camp, employment opportunities, adult learning, respite, and summer programs for teens.

2805 Margaret T Morris Foundation
PO Box 592
Prescott, AZ 86302-592 928-445-6633
Fax: 928-445-6633
Susan Rheem, Executive Director

Arkansas

2806 Arc of Arkansas
2004 Main St
Little Rock, AR 72206-1526 501-375-7770
Fax: 501-372-4621
www.arcark.org
Willie Jones, President
Steve Hitt, Chief Executive Officer
Roger Williams, Chief Financial Officer
Cynthia Stone, Chief Operating Officer
Serving people with disabilites and their families for over fourty years.

2807 Winthrop Rockefeller Foundation
225 East Markham Street
Suite 200
Little Rock, AR 72201 501-376-6854
Fax: 501-374-4797
webfeedback@wrfoundation.org
www.wrfoundation.org
Phillip N. Baldwin, Chair
David Rainey, Ed.D., Vice chair
Sherece Y. West-Scantlebury, Ph.D, President & CEO
Andrea M. Dobson, CPA, COO & CFO
Mission is to improve the quality of life in Arkansas. It focuses its grantmaking efforts in three areas: education, economic development and civic affairs. Education projects funded in the past have included grants to schools that are working to involve teachers and parents in making decisions about what happens at their schools, projects that work to remove prejudice from the educational process and more. Major grants are made to support the development of new programs.

California

2808 AIDS Healthcare Foundation
6255 Sunset Blvd.
21st Floor
Los Angeles, CA 90028 323-860-5200
www.aidshealth.org
Michael Weinstein, President
Peter Reis, Senior Vice President
Scott Carruthers, Chief Pharmacy Officer
Michael Wohlfeiler, Chief of Medicine
The Los Angeles-based AIDS Healthcare Foundation (AHF) is a global nonprofit organization providing medicine and advocacy to people all around the world. AHF is currently the largest provider of HIV/AIDS medical care in the U.S.

2809 Ahmanson Foundation
9215 Wilshire Blvd
Beverly Hills, CA 90210 310-278-0770
info@theahmansonfoundation.org
www.theahmansonfoundation.org
William H. Ahmanson, President
Karen Ahmanson Hoffman, Managing Director & Secretary
Kristen K. O'Connor, CFO & Treasurer
Jennie H. Chin, Senior Accountant
The Foundation primarily gives in Southern California with major emphasis in Los Angeles County. The Foundation focuses on the arts and humanities, education, mental health and support for a broad range of social welfare programs.

2810 Alice Tweed Touhy Foundation
205 E Carrillo Street
Suite 219
Santa Barbara, CA 93101-7186 805-962-6430
Jeanne Mc Kay, Manager
Rehabilitation, recreation and building funds are given to organizations only within the Santa Barbara area.

2811 Alternating Hemiplegia of Childhood Foundation
2000 Town Center
Suite 1900
Southfield, MI 48075 313-663-7772
Fax: 313-733-8987
sharon@ahckids.org
ahckids.org
Lynn Egan, President
Joshua Marszalek, Vice President
Gene M Andrasco, Treasurer
Vicky Platt, Secretary
Non-profit organization dedicated to promoting professional and public awareness of Alternating Hemiplegia of Childhood (AHC) and providing current information to affected individuals and their families. The foundation also supports ongoing medical research into the cause, treatment and potential cure of AHC and maintains a registry of families, affected chidren and physicians who are familiar with AHC.

2812 Arc of California
1225 8th Street
Suite 350
Sacramento, CA 95815 916-552-6619
800-698-6619
Fax: 916-441-3494
www.thearcca.org
Tony Anderson, Executive Director
Richard Fitzmaurice, President
Betsy Katz, Secretary
Bruce MacKenzie, Treasurer
Advocates for people with intellectual and all developmental disabilities since 1953. The ARC of California is committed to securing for all people with developmental disabilities, in partnership with thier families, legal guardians or conservators the opportunity to choose and realize their goals of where and how they learn, live, work and play.

2813 Atkinson Foundation
1660 Bush Street
Suite 300
San Mateo, CA 94109 415-561-6540
Fax: 650-357-1101
sangeles@pfs-llc.net
www.atkinsonfdn.org
Elizabeth Curtis, Administrator
Stacey Angels, Grants Manager
The Foundation focuses and awards grants to community service and civic organizations serving the residents of San Mateo County, California through programs that benefit children, youth, seniors, the disadvantaged and those in need of rehabilitation. Grants are also made to local churches and schools, and overseas for sustainable development, health education and family planning. No grants to individuals or for research, travel, special events, annual campaigns, media and publications.

2814 Baker Commodities Corporate Giving Program
4020 Bandini Blvd
Vernon, CA 90058
323-268-2801
Fax: 323-268-5166
info@bakercommodities.com
Jim Andreoli, President
Baker Commodities has been one of the nation's leading providers of rendering, and grease removal services. Baker Commodities, Inc. is a completely sustainable company, recycling animal by-products and kitchen waste into valuable products that can be used to feed livestock, power vehicles, and act as a base for everyday items.

2815 Bank of America Foundation
315 Montgomery St
Fl 8
San Francisco, CA 94104-1803
415-622-8248
888-488-9802
Fax: 704-386-6444
www.bankamerica.com/foundation
Ilana Orin, Manager
The Foundation will consider grants in four categories including: Health & Human Services, which provides support to health & human service organizations primarily through grants to the United Way campaigns; Education, with the focus on preparing people to become productive employees and participating citizens; Conservation & Environment, the improvement of California communities for the benefit of their citizens; and Culture & The Arts, supporting the leading performing and visual arts groups.

2816 Blind Babies Foundation
1814 Franklin Street
Suite 300
Oakland, CA 94612
510-446-2229
Fax: 510-446-2262
www.blindbabies.org
Dottie Bridge, President
Sharon Sacks, PhD, 1st Vice President
Clare Friedman, PhD, 2nd Vice President
Deborah Orel-Bixler, PhD, OD, Secretary
Founded in 1949, the foundation provides home-based early intervention services to families with young children with vision impairment in the Northern and Central regions of California.

2817 Bothin Foundation
1660 Bush Street
Suite 300
San Francisco, CA 94109
415-561-6540
Fax: 415-561-6477
ccasey@pfs-llc.net
Lyman H. Casey, President
A. Michael Casey, Vice President & Treasurer
Devon Laycox, Vice President
Charlie Casey, Program Officer
The Bothin Foundation makes grants for capital, building, and equipment needs to organizations providing direct services to low-income, at risk children, youth and families, the elderly, and the disabled in San Francisco, Marin, Sonoma, and San Mateo counties.

2818 Briggs Foundation
1969 Lancewood Ln
Carlsbad, CA 92009-6826
760-704-6481
Fax: 760-704-6483
Blaine A Briggs, President
Private non-operating foundation.

2819 Burns-Dunphy Foundation
5 3rd Street
Suite 528
San Francisco, CA 94103-3213
415-421-6995
Fax: 415-882-7774
Walter Gleason
Cressey Nakagawa
Grants are given to promote wellness for the visually impaired, physically and mentally disabled and to promote research in these areas.

2820 California Community Foundation
221 S. Figueroa Street
Suite 400
Los Angeles, CA 90012
213-413-4130
Fax: 213-383-2046
info@ccf-la.org
www.calfund.org
Cynthia A. Telles, Chairman
Antonia Hernandez, President & CEO
John E. Kobara, EVP & COO
Stephen J. Cobb, VP & CFO
Areas of funding priority include grants for the disabled, child welfare, rehabilitation, developmentally disabled, employment projects, research and computer projects. Giving is limited to the greater Los Angeles area.

2821 California Endowment
1000 N Alameda St
Los Angeles, CA 90012
213-628-1001
800-449-4149
Fax: 213-703-4193
questions@calendow.org
Zac Guevara, Vice Chair
Robert Ross, President & CEO
Martha Jimenez, EVP/ Counsel
Anthony Iton, SVP
California Endowment's mission is to expand access to affordable, quality health care for underserved individuals and communities, and to promote fundamental improvements in the health status of all Californians.

2822 Carrie Estelle Doheny Foundation
707 Wilshire Boulevard
Suite 4960
Los Angeles, CA 90017
213-488-1122
Fax: 213-488-1544
doheny@dohenyfoundation.org
www.dohenyfoundation.org
Robert A. Smith,III, President
Nina Shepherd, CAO/ CFO
Pam Thomas, Grants Administrator
Lisa Rogers, Grants Administrator
The Foundation primarily funds local, not-for-profit organizations endeavoring to advance education, medicine and religion, to improve the health and welfare of the sick, aged, incapacitated, and to aid the needy.

2823 Coeta and Donald Barker Foundation
3740 Cahuenga Blvd
Studio City, CA 91604
760-340-1162
818-980-3630
Fax: 818-980-2709
info@scga.org
www.scga.org
Nancy Harris, President
Kevin Heaney, Executive Director
Andrea Fredlin, Admin Asst., Club Services
Evan Belfi, Asst. Director, Marketing
It is an independent organization that gives its attention to organizations that are charitable or nonprofit under the laws of the state of Oregon or California.

2824 Conrad N Hilton Foundation
30440 Agoura Road
Agoura Hills, CA 91301
818-851-3700
Fax: 310-694-9051
cnhf@hiltonfoundation.org
hiltonfoundation.org
Steven M. Hilton, Chairman, President & CEO
Barron Hilton, Chairman Emeritus
Donald H Hubbs, Director Emeritus
Katherine Miller, Facilities and Office Services M
Our grant-making style is to initiate and develop major long-term projects and then seek out the organizations to implement them. As a consequence of this proactive approach, the Foundation does not generally consider unsolicited proposals. Our major projects currently include: blindness prevention and treatment, support the work of the Catholic Sisters, drug abuse prevention among youth, support of the Conrad N. Hilton College of Hotel and Restaurant Management, and much more.

2825 **Crescent Porter Hale Foundation**
1660 Bush Street
Suite 300
San Francisco, CA 94109
415-561-6540
Fax: 415-561-5477
evalentine@pfs-llc.net
www.crescentporterhale.org

E. William Swanson, President
Sr. Estela Morales, MSW, Vice President
Eunice Valentine, Executive Director
Patricia Fata, Secretary/Treasurer

Serves organizations in the San Francisco Bay Area who are involved in the following areas of concern: education in the fields of art and music; private elementary, high school and university education; capital funding; and other worthwhile programs which can be demonstrated as serving broad community purposes, leading toward the improvement of the quality of life.

2826 **David and Lucile Packard Foundation**
343 Second Street
Los Altos, CA 94022
650-917-7142
Fax: 650-948-5793
communications@packard.org
www.packard.org

Susan Packard Orr, Chairman
Julie E. Packard, Vice Chairman
Nancy Packard Burnett, Vice Chairman
Carol S Larson, President & CEO

This foundation provides grants to nonprofit organizations in the following areas: conservation; population; science; children, familes, and communities; arts and organizational effectiveness; and philanthropy. It provides national and international grants and also has a special focus on the Northern California Counties.

2827 **Deutsch Foundation**
5454 Beethoven St
Los Angeles, CA 90066
310-862-3000
877-340-7700
Fax: 310-862-3100
deutschinc.com

Linda Sawyer, Chairman
Kim Getty, President, North America
Val Difebo, CEO, Deutsch NY
Mike Sheldon, CEO, North America

Learning disabled, visually impaired, mental health, eye research, child welfare, speech and hearing impaired, physically disabled and independence projects are funded through this Foundation. Giving is limited to California.

2828 **Dream Street Foundation**
324 S. Beverly Dr.
Suite 500
Beverly Hills, CA 90212
424-333-1371
Fax: 310-388-0302
www.dreamstreetfoundation.org

Patty Grubman, Founder

Provides nationwide camping programs for children and young adults with cancer, chronic and life threatening illnesses.

2829 **East Bay Community Foundation**
De Domenico Building
200 Frank H Ogawa Plaza
Oakland, CA 94612
510-836-3223
Fax: 510-836-7418
jwhead@eastbaycf.org
www.ebcf.org

Sherry M. Hirota, Chair
Ingrid Lamirault, Vice Chair
Peter Garcia, Vice Chair
James W. Head, President & CEO

A collection of funds created by many people, organizations and businesses, the Foundation helps those people and groups to support effective nonprofit organizations to the East Bay and beyond.

2830 **Evelyn and Walter Hans Jr**
114 Sansome Street
Suite 600
San Francisco, CA 94104
415-856-1400
Fax: 415-856-1500
www.haasjr.org

Walter J. Haas, Chair
Ira S. Hirschfield, President & Trustee
Michael Blake, VP of Finance
Robert D. Haas, Treasurer

A private foundation interested in programs which assist people who are hungry, homeless, or at risk of homelessness; enable older adults to maintain independent lives in the community and support Hispanic community development in San Francisco's Mission District. The Foundation also encourages proposals for corporate social responsibility efforts within the business community.

2831 **Family Caregiver Alliance**
785 Market St.
Suite 750
San Francisco, CA 94103
415-434-3388
800-445-8106
Fax: 415-434-3508
info@caregiver.org
www.caregiver.org

Ping Hao, MBA, President
Jacquelyn Kung, Vice President
Kathleen Kelly,MPA, Executive Director
Deborah Wolter, Secetary

To improve the quality of life for caregivers and those they care for through information, services, and advocacy.

2832 **Financial Aid for the Disabled and Their Families**
Reference Service Press
2310 Homestead Rd.
Suite C1 #219
Los Altos, CA 94024
650-861-3170
Fax: 650-861-3171
info@rspfunding.com
www.rspfunding.com

Gail Schlachter, President
R David Weber, Editor-in-Chief
Mike Fields, Database and Website Manager
Sandy Perez, Online and Print Sales

This directory, which Children's Bookwatch calls invaluable describes more than 1,100 financial aid opportunities available to support persons with disabilities and members of their families. Updated ever 2 years. *$39.50*

300 pages
ISBN 1-588410-31-5

2833 **Firemans Fund Foundation**
Firemans Fund Insurance Companies
777 San Marin Dr
Novato, CA 94998
415-899-2000
800-227-1700
Fax: 415-899-3600

Lori Dickerson Fouche, President & CEO
Jill Paterson, Chief Financial Officer
Eleanor Barnard, Chief Distribution & Sales
Sally Narey, Chief Counsel, Corp. Secretary

Provides discretionary grants to the disabled only in Marin and Sonoma counties in the San Francisco Bay area.

2834 **Fred Gellert Foundation**
1038 Redwood Highway
Building B, Suite 2
Mill Valley, CA 94941
415-381-7575
Fax: 415-381-8526
foundationcenter.org/grantmaker/fredgellert/

Fred Gellert, Founder
Patty Oday, Administrator

Focuses on organizations and programs serving residents of San Mateo and San Francisco and Marin counties in California, with the exception of environmentally concerned organizations.

2835 Gallo Foundation
P.O. Box 1130
Modesto, CA 95353-1130
209-579-3204
877-687-9463
Fax: 209-341-3307
www.ejgallo.com
John Gallo, Senior VP Operations
Physically and mentally disabled, child welfare, Special Olympics, United Cerebral Palsy and Easter Seal Society are among the grants provided by this foundation.

2836 Glaucoma Research Foundation
251 Post Street
Suite 600
San Francisco, CA 94108
415-986-3162
800-826-6693
Fax: 415-986-3763
question@glaucoma.org
www.glaucoma.org
Andrew Iwach, MD, Board Chair
Robert L. Stamper, MD, Vice Chair
Thomas M. Brunner, President/CEO
Fred H. Brinkmann, Treasurer
A national organization dedicated to protecting the sight of people with glaucoma through research and education. The Foundation conducts and supports research that contributes to improved patient care and a better understanding of the disease process. Provides education, advocacy and emotional support to patients and their families.

2837 Harden Foundation
1636 Ercia Street
Salinas, CA 93906
831-442-3005
Fax: 831-443-1429
joe@hardenfoundation.org
www.hardenfoundation.org
Patricia Tynan Chapman, President
C. Bill Elliott, Vice President/Treasurer
Joseph C. Grainger, Executive Director
Linda Taylor, Secretary
Founded to assist charitable organizations in the Salinas Valley.

2838 Henry J Kaiser Family Foundation
2400 Sand Hill Rd
Menlo Park, CA 94025-6941
650-854-9400
Fax: 650-854-4800
www.kff.org
Drew Altman, President/CEO
Gary Claxton, Vice President
Esther Dicks, Vice President
Mollyann Brodie, SVP for Executive Operations
A non-profit, private operating foundation focusing on the major health care issues facing the US, with a growing role in global health. Kaiser develops and runs its own research and communications programs, sometimes in partnership with other non-profit research organizations or major media companies.

2839 Henry W Bull Foundation
Santa Barbara Bank & Trust
P.O. Box 2340
Santa Barbara, CA 93120
202-720-7871
Fax: 805-884-1404
info@coreprojects.com
www.activistfacts.com/about/
Janice Gibbons, VP/Senior Trust Officer
Grant given to a wide range of organizations that include those which provide services for the disabled; arts, education, services for elderly and youth grants awarded two times a year. Grant size ranges from $500 to $5,000. Proposal deadlines April 1, Sept 1.

2840 Irvine Health Foundation
18301 Von Karman Avenue
Suite 440
Irvine, CA 92612-0120
949-253-2959
Fax: 949-253-2962
info@ihf.org
www.ihf.org
Timothy L. Strader, Sr., Chairman
Carol Mentor McDermott, Vice Chairman
Edward B. Kacic, President
Ptricia A. Meredith, VP, Administration & Programs
Mission is to improve the physical, mental and emotional well-being of all Orange County residents.

2841 Joseph Drown Foundation
1999 Avenue of the Stars
Suite 2330
Los Angeles, CA 90067
310-277-4488
Fax: 310-277-4573
staff@jdrown.org
www.jdrown.org
Norman C Obrow, President
Giving is focused primarily in California. No support for religious purposes or to individuals. Goal is to assist individuals in becoming successful, self-sustaining, contributing citizens.

2842 Kenneth T and Eileen L Norris Foundation
11 Golden Shore
Suite 450
Long Beach, CA 90802
562-435-8444
Fax: 562-436-0584
grants@ktn.org
www.norrisfoundation.org
Lisa D Hanson, Chairman
Ronald R Barnes, Executive Director & Trustee
Walter J Zanino, Controller
William G Corey, Medical Advisor
The Foundation is primarily focused on medicine and education. To a lesser extent the foundation contributes to community programs including visually impaired, autism, mentally and physically disabled, deaf and mental health in the Southern California area. Average grant size in this area is $5,000-$10,000. Grants are also given in the area of culture and youth.

2843 Koret Foundation
33 New Montgomery Street
Suite 1090
San Francisco, CA 94105-4526
415-882-7740
Fax: 415-882-7775
info@koretfoundation.org
www.koretfoundation.org
Susan Koret, Board Chair
Anita L. Friedman, President
Michael J. Boskin, President
Jeffery A. Farber, CEO
Koret seeks to fund outstanding examples of innovative approaches to community challenges and opportunities.

2844 LA84 Foundation
2141 W Adams Blvd
Los Angeles, CA 90018
323-730-4600
Fax: 323-730-9637
info@la84.org
www.la84.org
Frank M. Sanchez, Chair
Anita L. DeFrantz, President
F. Patrick Escobar, VP, Grants & Programs
Robert Wagner, Vice President, Partnerships
The LA84 Foundation was established to manage Southern California's share of the surplus from the highly successful 1984 Olympic Games in Los Angeles and offers sports programs, a premier sports library and meeting facilities. The foundation currently serves two million youth in eight Southern California counties.

2845 LJ Skaggs and Mary C Skaggs Foundation
1221 Broadway
21st Floor
Oakland, CA 94612-1837
510-451-3300
Fax: 510-451-1527
skaggs@fablaw.com
Philip M Jelley, President
Jayne C Davis, Vice President
Robert N Janopaul, Director
Joseph W Martin, Jr., Secretary, Treasurer
The Foundation presently makes grants under four program categories: performing arts, social concerns, projects of historic interest and special projects.

2846 **Legler Benbough Foundation**
2550 Fifth Avenue
Suite 132
San Diego, CA 92103
619-235-8099
Fax: 619-235-8077
peter@benboughfoundation.org

Peter K. Elsworth, President
John G. Rebelo, Jr., Treasurer
Nbob Kelly, Director
Peter K. Ellsworth, Director

The mission of the foundation is to improve the quality of life of the people of San Diego. The foundation focuses on three target areas for funding, one in the area of providing economic opportunity, one in the area of enhancing cultural opportunity, and one that provides focus for health, education and welfare funding.

2847 **Levi Strauss Foundation**
1155 Battery St
San Francisco, CA 94111-1264
415-501-7208
800-872-5384
Fax: 415-544-3490
www.levistrauss.com/levi-strauss-foundation

Chip Bergh, President & CEO
Roy Bagattini, EVP/President
Lisa Collier, EVP/President
James Curleigh, EVP/President

Has a funding initiative to support organizations which provide services for people with AIDS, and/or educational programs which help prevent the further spread of the HIV virus. The Foundation will assist in the development and enhancement of such services only in those communities where Levi Strauss & Co. has plants and distribution centers.

2848 **Louis R Lurie Foundation**
555 California Street
Suite 5100
San Francisco, CA 94104-1707
415-392-2470
Fax: 415-421-8669
www.foundationcenter.org/grantmaker/lurie

Nancy Terry, Foundation Administrator

Visually impaired, hard-of-hearing and physically disabled in the San Francisco Bay Area and Metropolitan Chicago areas only.

2849 **Luke B Hancock Foundation**
360 Bryant St
Palo Alto, CA 94301-1409
650-321-5536
Fax: 650-321-0697

Ruth Ramel, Director

Has concentrated its resources over the past year on programs which provide job training and employment for at-risk youth. Consortium funding with other foundations in areas where there is unmet need; emergency and transitional funding; and selected funding for music education. .

2850 **Marin Community Foundation**
5 Hamilton Landing
Suite 200
Novato, CA 94949
415-464-2500
Fax: 415-464-2555
info@marincf.org
www.marincf.org

Cleveland Justis, Chair
Thomas Peters, Ph.D., President & CEO
Sid Hartman, CFO/COO
Aileen Sweeney, VP Of Finance

Mission is to encourage and apply philanthropic contributions to help improve the human condition, embrace diversity, promote a humane and democratic society, and enhance the communities quality of life, now and for future generations.

2851 **Mary A Crocker Trust**
57 Post Street
Suite 610
San Francisco, CA 94104-5023
650-576-3384
Fax: 415-982-0141
staff@mactrust.org
www.mactrust.org

2852 **MedicAlert Foundation International**
5226 Pirrone Crt
Salida, CA 95368
800-432-5378
customer_service@medicalert.org
www.medicalert.org

Barton G. Tretheway, CAE, Chairt
David Leslie, President & CEO
Melody Howard, Vice President Of Call Center Operations

A trusted emergency support network dedicated to educating emergency responders and medical personnel for facing everyday emergency situations, as well as providing emergency care services for members.

2853 **National Center on Caregiving at Family Caregiver Alliance (FCA)**
785 Market Street
Suite 750
San Francisco, CA 94103
415-434-3388
800-445-8106
Fax: 415-434-3508
info@caregiver.org
www.caregiver.org

Ping Hao, MBA, President
Jacquelyn Kung, Vice President
Kathleen Kelly, MPA, Executive Director
Jeff Kumataka, CPA, MBA, Treasurer

FCA offers programs at national, state and local levels to support and sustain caregivers. The National Center on Caregiving (NCC) program works to advance the development of high-quality, cost-effective policies and programs for caregivers in every state of the country. Uniting research, public policy and services, the NCC serves as a central source of information on caregiving and long term care issues for policy makers, service providers, media, funders and family caregivers.

2854 **National Foundation of Wheelchair Tennis**
940 Calle Amanecer
Suite B
San Clemente, CA 92673-6218
714-361-3663
Fax: 714-361-6603
www.nfwt.org

Bill Butler

Founded in January of 1980, the intention of this foundation is to assist the newly physically disabled individual to realize his full potential in society by enhancing his esteem, independence productivity and physical capabilities regardless of age, sex, creed or disability extent.

2855 **Parker Foundation**
2604-B El Camino Real
Suite 244
Carlsbad, CA 92008
760-720-0630
Fax: 760-720-1239
mail@theparkerfoundation.org
www.theparkerfoundation.org

Judy McDonald, President
Gordon Swanson, Vice President
Ann Davies, Secretary
Raymond Ellis, Treasurer

The assets are directed to projects which will contribute to the betterment of any aspect of the people of San Diego County, California and solely to entities which, among other things, are organized exclusively for charitable purposes and are operating in San Diego County, California.

2856 **Pasadena Foundation**
301 East Colorado Boulevard
Suite 810
Pasadena, CA 91101-2824
626-796-2097
Fax: 626-583-4738
pcfstaff@pasadenacf.org
www.pasadenacf.org

David M. Davis, Chair
Judy Gain, Vice Chair
Jennifer Fleming DeVoll, Executive Director
Mariver Copeland, Director of Finance

The mission of the Pasadena Foundation is to improve the quality of life for citizens of the Pasadena area through support of nonprofit organizations that provide services beneficial to the community.

2857 RC Baker Foundation
P.O. Box 6150
Orange, CA 92863-6150 714-750-8987
F L Scott, Manager
Established in 1952, for general philanthropic purposes. The bulk of assistance and support has been to religious, scientific, educational institutions and youth organizations.

2858 Ralph M Parsons Foundation
888 West Sixth Street
Suite 700
Los Angeles, CA 90017 213-362-7600
Fax: 213-482-8878
www.rmpf.org
James A. Thomas, Chairman
Elizabeth Lowe, Vice Chairman
Wendy Garen, President & CEO
Astra Anderson Galang, CFO
The Foundation is concerned with the encouragement and support of projects and programs deemed beneficial to mankind in several major areas of interest such as: education; social impact; civic and cultural; health and special products. Only funds in Los Angeles County.

2859 Robert Ellis Simon Foundation
312 S Canyon View Drive
Los Angeles, CA 90049-3812 310-275-7335
Joan Willens
Mental health and visually impaired grants are the main concerns of this organization.

2860 San Francisco Foundation
One Embarcadero Cente
Suite 1400
San Francisco, CA 94111 415-733-8500
Fax: 415-477-2783
info@sff.org
www.sff.org
Sandra R Hernandez, CEO
Nick Hodges, VP for Philanthropic Services
Bobbie Chapman, Director of Business Development
Shona Carter, Donor Relations Officer
The Foundation's purpose is to improve life, promote greater equality of opportunity and assist those in need or at risk in the San Francisco Bay Area. The Foundation strives to protect and enhance the unique resources of the Bay Area, committed to equality of opportunity for all and the elimination of any injustice, seeks to enhance human dignity and seeks to establish mutual trust, respect and communication among the Foundation.

2861 Santa Barbara Foundation
1111 Chapala Street
Suite 200
Santa Barbara, CA 93101 805-963-1873
Fax: 805-966-2345
info@sbfoundation.org
www.sbfoundation.org
Eileen Sheridan, Chair
James Morouse, Vice Chair
Ronald Gallo, President & CEO
Maria Caudillo, Exec. Asst. to President & CEO
The Foundations mission is to enrich the lives of the people of Santa Barbara County through philanthropy. The Foundation awards grants to nonprofits within the County in the areas of education, health, human services, personal development, cluture, recreation, community enhancement and environment. No support is given to individuals except through student aid.

2862 Seany Foundation
3530 Camino del Rio N
Suite 101
San Diego, CA 92108 858-551-0922
www.theseanyfoundation.org
Paula Lutzky, CFO
Emily Brody, Director, Marketing & Media
Tiana LaCerva, Director, Special Events
Funds programs dedicated to bringing joy to children with cancer and their families.

2863 Sidney Stern Memorial Trust
860 Via de la Paz
PO Box 457
Pacific Palisades, CA 90272 310-459-2117
info@sidneysternmemorialtrust.org
www.sidneysternmemorialtrust.org
Betty Hoffenberg, Director
A Southern California-based foundation providing grants to non-profit organizations for various projects. The foundation gives priority to the following areas of interest: education, health and science, community service projects, youth, services to the mentally and emotionally disabled, the arts, organizations and activities serving California. The Board prefers to make contributions to organizations that use the funds directly in the furtherance of their charitable and public purposes.

2864 Sierra Health Foundation
1321 Garden Hwy
Sacramento, CA 95833 916-922-4755
Fax: 916-922-4024
info@sierrahealth.org
www.sierrahealth.org
Jose Hermocillo, Chair
David W. Gordon, Vice Chair
Chet P. Hewitt, President & CEO
Gil Alvarado, VP of Administration/CFO
The Foundation strives to establish a collaborative relationship with its grantees, and with other funders and foundations, through an open dialogue. The Foundation approaches each grant as a partnership, with opportunities for the grantee and grantor to work cooperatively to enhance the effectiveness of the grant project.

2865 Silicon Valley Community Foundation
2400 West El Camino Real
Suite 300
Mountain View, CA 94040-1498 650-450-5400
Fax: 650-450-5401
info@siliconvalleycf.org
www.siliconvalleycf.org
C.S. Parker, Chair
Samuel Johnson,Jr., Vice Chair
Emmitt D. Carson, Ph.D, President & CEO
George Dallas, Administrative Asst.
Serving all of San Mateo & Santa Clara counties, Silicon Valley Foundation has more than $1.5B in assets under management and 1500 philanthropic funds. The community provides grants through donor advised and corporate funds in addition to its own Community Endowment Fund. In addition, the community foundation serves as a regional center for philanthropy, providing donors simple and effective ways to give locally & globally.

2866 Sonora Area Foundation
362 S Stewart Street
Sonora, CA 95370 209-533-2596
Fax: 209-533-2412
www.sonora-area.org
Jim Johnson, President SAF
Roger Francis, Vice President
Edward B. Wyllie, Executive Director
Lin Freer, Program Manager
The Sonora Area Foundation strengthens its community through assisting donors, making grants, and providing leadership.

2867 Stella B Gross Charitable Trust C/O Bank of The West Trust Department
PO Box 1121
San Jose, CA 95108-1121 408-947-5203
Gabe Padilla, Trust Admin
Organization must be federal and state tax-exempt and reside within the bounds of Santa Clara County, California to be eligible.

2868 Teichert Foundation
3500 American River Dr
Sacramento, CA 95864 916-484-3011
Fax: 916-484-6506
www.teichert.com
Frederick Teichert, LHD, Executive Director
Awards grants to community organizations and provides employee matching grants. Teichert Foundation expresses the

companie's commitment to build and preserve a healthy and prosperous region.

2869 **WM Keck Foundation**
550 South Hope Street
Suite 2500
Los Angeles, CA 90071- 2617
213-680-3833
Fax: 213-614-0934
info@wmkeck.org
www.wmkeck.org

Allison Keller, Executive Director & CFO
Maria Pellegrini, Ph.D, Executive Director of Programs
Thomas Everhart, Ph.D, Senior Scientific Advisor
Matesh Varma, Ph.D, Senior Program Director

Created to support accredited colleges and universities with particular emphasis on the sciences, engineering and medical research. The Foundation also maintains a Southern California Grant Program that provides support for non-profit organizations in the field of civic and community services, health care, precollegiate education and the arts.

2870 **Wayfinder Family Services**
5300 Angeles Vista Blvd
Los Angeles, CA 90043
323-295-4555
800-352-2290
Fax: 323-296-0424
info@wayfinderfamily.org
www.wayfinderfamily.org

Miki Jordan, President & CEO
Jay Allen, EVP & COO
Karen Alvord, EVP & Chief Impact Officer
Veronica Arteaga, Chief Program Officer

Formerly Junior Blind of America, Wayfinder provides programs and services for children and adults who are blind or visually impaired and their families to achieve independence and self-esteem. Programs include; Camp Bloomfield, Visions: Adventures in Learning, Infant-Family Program, Early Childhood Program, Special Education School, Children's Residential Program, Davidson Program for Independence, and Student Transition and Enrichment Program, Vision Screening and After School enrichment.

2871 **Whittier Trust**
Whittier Trust Company
1600 Huntington Dr
South Pasadena, CA 91030
626-441-5111
Fax: 626-441-0420
hrdept@whittiertrust.com
www.whittiertrust.com

Michael J Casey, Chairman
David A Dahl, President & CEO
Brian H Flynn, Senior Vice President, Business Development
Sandip A Bhagat, Chief Investment Officer

Whittier Trust offers financial services and expertise in the area of family wealth management. Some of their other areas of consultation include philanthropic advising, investment management, legal services and real estate.

2872 **Willam G Gilmore Foundation**
1660 Bush Street
Suite 300
San Francisco, CA 94109
415-561-0650
Fax: 415-561-5477

William N Hancock, Owner

Colorado

2873 **AV Hunter Trust**
650 South Cherry Street
Suite 535
Glendale, CO 80246- 1897
303-399-5450
Fax: 303-399-5499
afreeman@pfs-llc.net
www.avhuntertrust.org

Mary K. Anstine, President
George C. Gibson, Vice President
Barbara L. Howie, Executive Director
Jessica Sutton, Grants Manager

Donated nearly $50 million to nonprofit organizations serving those who captured Mr. Hunter's attention and sparked his compassion. Trust gives aid, comfort, support, or assistance to children or aged people or indigent adults.

2874 **Adolph Coors Foundation**
215 St. Paul Street
Suite 300
Denver, CO 80206
303-388-1636
Fax: 303-388-1684
www.coorsfoundation.org

John W. Jackson, Executive Director
Jeanne L. Bistranin, Senior Program Officer
Carrie C. Tynan, Program Officer
Carol S. Strathman, Financial/Special Projects Coord

Applicant organizations must be classified as 501 and must operate within the United States. The areas covered by the Foundation are health, education, youth, community services, civic and cultural and public affairs.

2875 **Arc of Colorado**
1580 Logan Street
Suite 730
Denver, CO 80203
303-864-9334
800-333-7690
Fax: 303-864-9330
mrymer@thearcofco.org
www.thearcofco.org

Randy Patrick, President
Tonna Kelly, Vice President
Marijo Rymer, Executive Director
Lynnelle Zackroff, Secretary

A private not-for-profit, membership-based, grassroots association. The Arc of Colorado is the state office whith local units located in various areas throughout the state.

2876 **Bonfils-Stanton Foundation**
Daniels and Fisher Tower
1601 Arapahoe St.
Suite 500
Denver, CO 80202
303-825-3774
Fax: 303-825-0802
webinfo@bonfils-stanton.org
bonfils-stantonfoundation.org

Gary P. Steuer, President/CEO
Gina A. Ferrari, Director, Grants Program
Ann M. Hovland, CFO/Treasurer
Monique M. Loseke, Executive Assistant

Grants limited to Colorado 501 (c) (3) organizations and are evaluatied based on alignment with these Foundation objectives: 1) The Bonfils-Stanton Foundation supports cultural organizations that consistently demonstrate artistic excellence, visionary leadership, and adaptive capacity; and 2) They idenitfy and nurture grassroots innovative organizations and initiative that enhance the values, spirit, and diversity of Denver's cultural community.

2877 **Comprecare Foundation**
PO Box 740610
Arvada, CO 80006
303-432-2808
Fax: 303-432-2808
www.comprecarefoundation.org

Milton W. Bollman, Chairman of the Board
Dr. Ellen Mangione, MD, MPH, Vice Chairman
James R. Gilsdorf, Executive Director
Dennis E. Baldwin, Secretar/Treasurer

The purpose of the Comprecare Foundation is to encourage, aid or assist specific health related programs and to make grants to support the activities of organizations which are designed to advance and promote health care education, the delivery of health care services, and the improvement of community health and welfare.

2878 **Denver Foundation**
55 Madison Street
8th Floor
Denver, CO 80206
303-300-1790
Fax: 303-300-6547
information@denverfoundation.org
www.denverfoundation.org

Sandra Shreve, Chair
Ginny Bayless, Vice Chair and Chair-Elect
David M Miller, President & CEO
Sarah Bock, Secretary

Neighbors helping neighbors, that's what the foundation is for. As Denver's only community foundation we've been accepting charitable donations since 1925. Those funds have been given back to the community in ongoing grants to nonprofit organizations - organizations that touch nearly every meaningful artistic, cultural, civic, health and human services interest of metro Denver's citizens.

2879 **El Pomar Foundation**
10 Lake Circle
Colorado Springs, CO 80906
719-633-7733
800-554-7711
Fax: 719-577-5702
grants@elpomar.org
www.elpomar.org

William J. Hybl, Chairman/CEO
William Ward, Vice Chair
R. Thayer Tutt, Jr., President/CIO
Kyle Hybl, COO/General Counsel

Mission of El Pomar is to enhance, encourage and promote the current and future well being of the people of Colorado through grantmaking and community stewardship.

2880 **Helen K and Arthur E Johnson Foundation**
1700 Broadway
Suite 1100
Denver, CO 80290-1718
303-861-4127
800-232-9931
Fax: 303-861-0607
www.johnsonfoundation.org

Ms. Lynn H. Campion, Chairman
Ms. Berit K. Campion, Vice Chair
John H Alexander Jr, President
Jacque Beaty, Finance Director

A nonprofit, grantmaking private foundation incorporated under the laws of the State of Colorado in 1948. The Foundation is a general purpose foundation whose grant program consists of a wide variety of creative efforts to solve problems and to enrich the quality of life. The areas of interest are: education, youth, health, community services, civic and culture and senior citizens. Grants limited to the state of Colorado.

2881 **Listen Foundation**
6950 E Belleview Ave.
Suite 203
Greenwood Village, CO 80111
303-781-9440
info@listenfoundation.org
www.listenfoundation.org

Allison Biever, President
David Kelsall, MD, Medical Director

The Listen Foundation provides access to Listening and Spoken Language Therapy (LSL) for children are deaf and hard of hearing.

Connecticut

2882 **Aetna Foundation**
151 Farmington Ave
Hartford, CT 06156
860-273-0123
800-872-3862
www.aetnahealthinsurance.com

Mark T Bertolini, Chairman/CEO
Karen S. Rohan, President
William J. Casazza, EVP & General Counsel
Richard di Benedetto, EVP, Aetna International

The Aetna Foundation is the independent charitable and philanthropic arm of Aetna Inc. The Foundation helps build healthy communities by promoting volunteerism, forming partnerships and funding initiatives that improve the quality of life where our employees and customers live and work.

2883 **Arc of Connecticut**
43 Woodland Street
Suite 260
Hartford, CT 6105-2300
860-246-6400
Fax: 860-246-6406
arcct@aol.com
www.arcct.com

Leslie Simoes, Interim Executive Director

The Arc of Connecticut is an advocacy organization committed to protecting the rights of people with intellectual, cognitive, and developmental disabilities and to promoting opportunities for their full inclusion in the life of thier communities.

2884 **Community Foundation of Southeastern Connecticut**
68 FederalStreet
PO Box 769
New London, CT 06320
860-442-3572
877-442-3572
Fax: 860-442-0584
maryam@cfect.org
www.cfect.org

Susan Pochal, Chair
Dianne E. Williams, Vice Chair
Maryam Elahi, President & CEO
Alison Woods, Vice President & COO

Provides donors with an easy and convenient way to give back to our community with joy and impact. We make grants to nonprofit organizations and support their efforts to strengthen our community.

2885 **Connecticut Mutual Life Foundation**
140 Garden St
Hartford, CT 6154
860-727-3000

Astrida Olds, Executive Director

Distinguished throughout its long history by unusual commitment to high principles of corporate purpose and business ethics. That commitment has been reflected not only in the firm belief that normal business functions must be carried out with a sense of responsibility beyond that required by the marketplace. Maintains an ongoing program of corporate contributions, a nationwide matching gifts plan for all employees on behalf of private and public education, skills training programs, and more.

2886 **Cornelia de Lange Syndrome Foundation**
302 West Main Street
#100
Avon, CT 06001
860-676-8166
800-753-2357
Fax: 860-676-8337
info@cdlsusa.org
www.cdlsusa.org

Robert Boneberg, Esq., President
Richard Haaland, Ph.D., Vice President
David Harvey, Vice President
Wendy Miller, Esq., Secretary

Provides information about birth defects caused by Cornelia de Lange Syndrome.

2887 **Fidelco Guide Dog Foundation**
103 Vision Way
Bloomfield, CT 06002
860-243-5200
Fax: 860-769-0567
admissions@fidelco.org
www.fidelco.org

Karen C. Tripp, Chair
G. Kenneth Bernhard, Esq., Vice Chair
Gregg Barratt, Chief of Staff
Julie Unwin, Chief Operating Officer

The Fidelco Guide Dog Foundation creates increased freedom and independence for men and women who are blind by providing them with guide dogs.

2888 **GE Foundation**
General Electric Company
3135 Easton Tpke
Fairfield, CT 6828
203-373-3216
Fax: 203-373-3029
gefoundation@ge.com
www.ge.com

Jeffrey R. Immelt, Chairman/ CEO
Daniel C. Heintzelman, Vice Chair
Jeffrey S. Bornstein, SVP & CFO, GE
Shane Fitzsimons, SVP Global Operations

Believes that our greatest national resource is the work force. If we are to successfully compete in the global arena, then we become involved in improving the education of all of our citizens. The Foundation sets examples for others to emulate helping people with their international grant program to higher education and to health care for children in developing countries.

2889 **Hartford Foundation for Public Giving**
10 Columbus Blvd
8th Floor
Hartford, CT 06106
860-548-1888
Fax: 860-524-8346
lindakelly@hfpg.org
www.hfpg.org

Yvette Melendez, Chair
Bonnie J. Malley, Vice Chair
Linda J. Kelly, President
Julie Feidner, Exec. Asst. to the President

Developmentally disabled, housing, deaf, recreation and education grants.

2890 **Hartford Insurance Group**
1 Hartford Plz
Hartford, CT 6155-1708
860-547-5000
www.thehartford.com

Christopher Swift, Chairman/ CEO
Doug Elliot, President
Beth Bombara, Chief Financial Officer
Kathy Bromage, Chief Marketing Officer

Giving is primarily in the Hartford, CT area and in communities where the company has a regional office. No support is available for political or religious purposes. Grants are given in the areas of education, health and United Way organizations.

2891 **Henry Nias Foundation**
20 Carmen Rd
Milford, CT 6460-7508
203-874-2787
Charles D Fleischman, President

Giving limited to NY metropolitan area. Arts, cultural programs, medical school/education, and children and youth.

2892 **Jane Coffin Childs Memorial Fund for Medical Research**
333 Cedar St, SHM
L300
New Haven, CT 6510-3206
203-785-4612
Fax: 203-785-3301
www.jccfund.org

Dr Randy Schekman, Director

The Fund awards fellowships to suitably qualified individuals for full time postdoctoral studies in the medical and related sciences bearing on cancer.

2893 **John H and Ethel G Nobel Charitable Trust**
Bankers Trust Company
1 Fawcett Pl
PO Box 1297
New York, NY 1008-1297
203-629-7120
Fax: 203-629-7170

Paul J Bisset, VP

2894 **Scheuer Associates Foundation**
960 Lake Ave
Greenwich, CT 6831-3032
203-622-5002
Fax: 203-622-5002

Thomas Scheuer, President

2895 **Swindells Charitable Foundation Trust**
Shawmut Bank
1221SW YamhillStreet
Suite 100
Portland, OR 97205-2303
503-222-0689
Fax: 503-222-0726
dwecker@swindellstrust.org
www.swindellstrust.org

Maggie Willard, President

Grants made to charitable organizations or societies incorporated for the relief of sick and suffering poor children and/or the relief of sick suffering and indigent aged men and women and/or the support of public charitable hospitals. Geographic area includes Hartford, CT area primarily. Application is required, deadlines are Feb. 1 and Aug. 1.

Delaware

2896 **Arc of Delaware**
2 S Augustine Street
Suite B
Wilmington, DE 19804-2504
302-996-9400
Fax: 302-996-0683
TTY: 800-232-5460
eraign@arcde.org
www.thearcofdelaware.org

Bill Seufert, President
Becky Hill, Vice President
Merry Jones, Vice President
Barbara Robeleto, Vice President

The Arc of Delaware is a non-profit organization of volunteers and staff who work together to improve the quality of life for people with disabilitiesand their families. We strive to include all children and adults with cognitive, intellectual and developmental disabilities in every community.

2897 **Longwood Foundation**
100 W 10th St
Suite 1109
Wilmington, DE 19801-1694
302-683-8200
Fax: 302-654-2323
www.longwoodfoundation.com

ThŠre du Pont, President
Peter Morrow, Executive Director

Offers grants to the mentally and physically disabled - capital, program, education and housing grants in the state of Delaware.

District of Columbia

2898 **Alexander and Margaret Stewart Trust**
Brawner Building
888 17th Street NW
Suite 1250
Washington, DC 20006-3321
202-333-1277
Fax: 202-333-3128
aplatt@projectsinternational.com
www.projectsinternational.com

Chas W. Freeman, Chairman
Peter J.C, Young, President
Imtiaz T. Ladak, Chief Financial Officer
Landon K. Thorne, Managing Director

Grants are given only to the Washington, DC area organizations providing care or treatment to cancer patients or those with childhood afflictions.

2899 **American Hotel and Lodging Association Foundation**
1201 Eye St. NW.
Suite 1100
Washington, DC 20005
202-289-3100
Fax: 202-289-3199
ahleffoundation@ahla.com
www.ahlafoundation.org

Rosanna Maietta, President
Shelly Weir, Senior VP, Career Development
Kara Filer, VP, Donor Relations & Development
Abigail Kang, Director, Impact

Programs include apprenticeship, community-based initiatives for youth, hospitality certification, funding for employee education, and a career center.

2900 Arc of the District of Columbia
415 Michigan Avenue, NE
Suite 150
Washington, DC 20017- 2144
202-636-2950
Fax: 202-635-7086
www.arcdc.net

Robert A. Anderson, President
Mary Lou Meccariello, Executive Director
Michael Gonzales, Chief Operating Officer
Ed Cabatic, Director of Finance

Advocating for and providing services to persons with developmental disabilities.

2901 Eugene and Agnes E Meyer Foundation
The Meyer Foundation
1250 Connecticut Ave NW
Suite 800
Washington, DC 20036- 2620
202-483-8294
Fax: 202-328-6850
meyer@meyerfdn.org
www.meyerfoundation.org

Joshua Bernstein, Chair
Deborah Ratner Salzberg, Vice Chair
Nicky Goren, President & CEO
Barbara Lang, Secretary-Treasurer

Awards grants to projects dealing with the learning disabled, blind, mental health and vocational training in the Washington metropolitan area.

2902 Federal Student Aid Information Center
US Department of Education
400 Maryland Ave SW
Washington, DC 20202
202-275-5446
800-872-5327
www.ed.gov

Arne Duncan, Secretary of Education
Tony Miller, Deputy Secretary
Martha Kanter, Under Secretary

Answers questions about Federal student aid from students, parents and Members of Congress, as well as financial aid administrators.

2903 GEICO Philanthropic Foundation
1 Geico Plz
Washington, DC 20076
301-986-3000
800-841-3000
Fax: 301-986-2851
www.geico.com

Tony M Nicely, CEO

Hospitals, physically disabled and Special Olympics.

2904 Jacob and Charlotte Lehrman Foundation
1836 Columbia Rd NW
Washington, DC 20009-2002
202-328-8400
Fax: 202-338-8405
www.lehrmanfoundation.org

Elizabeth Berry, Director
Robert Lehrman, Trustee
Samuel Lehrman, Trustee
Barbara Ferguson, Administrative/Program assistant

The Jacob & Charlotte Lehrman Foundation supports and seeks to enrich Jewish life in Washington DC, Israel and around the world. It is committed to making Washington a better place for all people and supports the arts, education and undeserved children, the environment, and healthcare.

2905 John Edward Fowler Memorial Foundation
79 Fifth Avenue
16th Street
New York, NY 10003-3076
212-620-4230
800-424-9836
Fax: 212-807-3677
www.foundationcenter.org

Bradforth K. Smith, President
Lisa Philp, Vice President
Lawrence T. McGill, Vice President
Jen Bokoff, Director

Although not a program priority, the foundation does offer grants to the physically disabled in the Washington, DC area only.

2906 Joseph P Kennedy Jr Foundation
1133 19th Street NW
12th Floor
Washington, DC 20036-3604
202-393-1250
Fax: 202-824-0351

Rebecca Salon, President
Steven Eidelman, Executive Director

Has two firm objectives: to seek the prevention of developmental disabilities, and to improve the way society deals with its citizens who are already affected. The Foundation uses its funds in areas where a multiplier effect can be achieved through development of innovative models for the prevention and amelioration, through provision of seed money that encourages new researchers, and thorough use of the Foundation's influence to promote public awareness.

2907 Kiplinger Foundation
1100 13th Street, NW
Suite 750
Washington, DC 20005-3938
202-887-6400
800-544-0155
Fax: 202-778-8976
www.kiplinger.com

Knight Kiplinger, VP

Limited to the greater Washington, DC area, the grants focus primarily on education, social welfare, cultural activities and community programs. Matching grants to eligible secondary or higher education institutions are provided on behalf of employees and retirees of Kiplinger Washington Editors, Inc. The Foundation does not fund scholarships.

2908 Morris and Gwendolyn Cafritz Foundation
1825 K St NW
Ste 1400
Washington, DC 20006-1271
202-223-3100
800-544-0155
Fax: 202-296-7567
info@cafritzfoundation.org
www.cafritzfoundation.org

Calvin Cafritz, Chairman/President/ CEO
John E. Chapoton, Vice Chairman and Treasurer
Ed McGeogh, Vice President - Asset Managemen
Rohan Rodrigo, Vice President - Finance

Grants are awarded to only 501 (c) (3) organizations that are in the DC area. Grants are not awarded for capitol purposes, special events, endowments, or to individuals.

2909 Paul and Annetta Himmelfarb Foundation
4545 42nd St NW
Ste 203
Washington, DC 20016-4623
202-966-3796

M Preston, Executive Director

Primary areas of interest include health, children, human need, and Israel.

2910 Public Welfare Foundation
1200 U St NW
Washington, DC 20009-4443
202-965-1800
info@publicwelfare.org
www.publicwelfare.org

Lydia M. Marshall, Chair
Mary E. McClymont, President
Phillipa Taylor, Chief Financial and Administrati
Alyssa Piccirilli, Manager of Administration

The foundation's funding is specifically targeted to economically disadvantaged populations. Proposals must fall within one of the following categories: criminal justice, disadvantaged elderly, disadvantaged youth, environment, health and population and reproductive health, human rights and global security, and community economic developmental and participation. Proposals should be addressed to the Review Committee.

Florida

2911 Able Trust
3320 Thomasville Road
Suite 200
Tallahassee, FL 32308
850-224-4493
Fax: 850-224-4496
TTY: 850-224-4493
info@abletrust.org
www.abletrust.org

Susanne Homant, President
Guenevere Crum, Senior Vice President
Kathryn McManus, MA, Chief Development Director
Allison Chase, MS, State Director, Florida High Sch

The Able Trust is a non-profit, public/private partnership that supports non-profit vocational rehabilitation programs throughout Florida with fundraising, grant making and public awareness of disability issues.

2912 American Academy of Pain Medicine Foundation
American Academy of Pain Medicine
1705 Edgewater Dr.
Suite 7778
Orlando, FL 32804
800-917-1619
Fax: 407-749-0714
info@painmed.org
painmed.org/aapm-foundation

Charles E. Argoff, President

The Foundation supports AAPM's core purpose to optimize the health of patients in pain and eliminate the major health problem of pain by advancing the practice and the specialty of pain medicine.
1911

2913 Arc of Florida
2898 Mahan Dr
Ste 1
Tallahassee, FL 32308-5462
850-921-0460
800-226-1155
info@arcflorida.org
www.arcflorida.org

Pat Young, President
Dick Bradley, Vice President Administration
Linda Bloom, Vice President Advocacy
Greg Roe, Treasurer

Advocates for all people with developmental disablilities, through education, awareness, research, advocacy and the support of families, friends and community.

2914 Bank of America Client Foundation
50 Central Avenue
Suite 750
Sarasota, FL 34236-5900
941-951-4103
maryann.l.smith@ustrust.com
www.fdnweb.org/boacf/

Maryann L. Smith, Vice President, Senior Trust Off

Committed to creating meaningful change in the communities we serve through our philanthropic efforts, associate volunteerism, community development activities and investing, support of arts and culture programming and environmental initiatives.

2915 Barron Collier Jr Foundation
2600 Golden Gate Pkwy
Naples, FL 34105-3227
239-262-2600
Fax: 239-262-1840
ContactUs@BarronCollier.com
www.barroncollier.com

Karen V. Triplett, Director of Property Management
Jose Medina, Facilities Manager

Barron Collier Companies - dedicated to the responsible development, management and stewardship of its extensive land holdings and other assets in the businesses of agriculture, real estate, and mineral management.

2916 Camiccia-Arnautou Charitable Foundation
Ste 402
980 N Federal Hwy
Boca Raton, FL 33432-2712
561-368-5757
Fax: 561-368-8505

Ronda Gluck, President

2917 Chatlos Foundation
PO Box 915048
Longwood, FL 32791-5048
407-862-5077
info@chatlos.org
www.chatlos.org

Bill Chatlos, Trustee

Funds nonprofit organizations in the USA and around the globe. Funding is provided in the following areas of giving: Bible Colleges/Seminaries, Religious Causes, Medical Concerns, Liberal Arts Colleges and Social Concerns. Category of placement is determined by the organizations overall mission rather than the project under consideration. The Foundation does not make scholarship grants directly to individuals but rather to educational institutions which in turn select recipients.

2918 Edyth Bush Charitable Foundation
199 E Welbourne Ave
Ste 100
Winter Park, FL 32789-4365
407-647-4322
888-647-4322
Fax: 407-647-7716
dodahowski@edythbush.org
www.edythbush.org

Gerald F. Hilbrich, Chairman
Herbert W. Holm, Vice Chairman
David A. Odahowski, President/CEO
Mary Ellen Hutcheson, Vice-President/Treasurer

Funding is resrticted to 501c3 nonprofit organizations located and operating in Orange, Osceola, Seminole and Lake Counties, Florida. Visit www.edythbush.org for a list of funding policies.

2919 FPL Group Foundation
700 Universe Blvd
Juno Beach, FL 33408-2657
561-694-4000
888-488-7703
Fax: 561-694-4620
PoweringFlorida@FPL.com
www.fpl.com

Maria V. Fogarty, Senior Vice President, Internal
James L. Robo, President and Chief Operating Of
Joseph T. Kelliher, Executive Vice President, Federa
Antonio Rodriguez, Executive Vice President, Power

The company consistently outperforms national averages for service reliability while customer bills are below the national average. A clean energy leader, FPL has one of the lowest emissions profiles and one of the leading energy efficiency programs among utilities nationwide. FPL is a subsidiary of Juno Beach, Fla.-based NextEra Energy, Inc.

2920 Jefferson Lee Ford III Memorial Foundation
9600 Collins Ave
Bal Harbour, FL 33154-2202
305-868-2609
Fax: 305-868-2640

Sanford L King, Director
Yvonne Quatrale, President

Disabled children, hearing and speech center. Grants are only given to tax exempt organizations, no individual grants are offered.

2921 Jessie Ball duPont Fund
40 East Adams Street
Ste 300
Jacksonville, FL 32202-3302
904-353-0890
800-252-3452
Fax: 904-353-3870
contactus@dupontfund.org
www.dupontfund.org

Sherry P. Magill, President
Mark D. Constantine, Vice President for Strategy, Pol
Barbara Roole, Senior Program Officer
Katie Ensign, Senior Program Officer

Established under the terms of the will of the late Jessie Ball duPont. The fund is a national foundation having a special though not exclusive interest in issues affecting the South. The Fund works with the approximately 325 individual institutions to which Mrs. duPont personally contributed during the five-year period, 1960 through 1964.

2922 **Lost Tree Village Charitable Foundation**
8 Church Lane
North Palm Beach, FL 33408-2908 561-622-3780
Fax: 561-841-6773
info@losttreefoundation.org
www.losttreefoundation.org

Pam Rue, Executive Director
Teresa Elu, Executive Assistant
Bob Heon, Controller

The Lost Tree Village Charitable Foundation is dedicated to building a stronger community and improving the quality of life for all local residents. Grants are awarded annually to local non-profit health and human service organizations providing information, expertise and assistance to those in need. Applications are only accepted from organizations located in Palm Beach and Southern Martin Counties. Visit the website for guidelines and further information.

2923 **Miami Foundation, The**
40 NW 3rd Street
Suite 405
Miami, FL 33128 305-371-2711
Fax: 305-371-5342
info@miamifoundation.org
www.miamifoundation.com

Javier Alberto Soto, President and CEO
Rebecca Mandelman, VP for Strategy and Engagement

The Foundation approaches all of its program activities with a focus on building the community. We conduct acticvities and support efforts that build community assets and relationships among individuals, organizations, and communities that connect people with resources and opportunities to improve their quality of life.

2924 **Mount Sinai Medical Center**
4300 Alton Road
Miami Beach, FL 33140-6574 305-674-2121
305-674-2777
www.msmc.com/foundation

Wayne Chaplin, Chairman
Steven D. Sonenreich, President & CEO
Jason Loeb, Foundation President
Kenneth L. Davis, MD, Chief Executive Officer and Pres
Autism Research

2925 **National Parkinson Foundation**
200 SE 1st Street
Suite 800
Miami, FL 33131-1494 800-473-4636
contact@parkinson.org
www.parkinson.org

John L. Lehr, President & CEO
James Beck, SVP & Chief Scientific Officer
Yasnahia Cortorreal, VP & chief Human Resources & Administration Officer
Curt De Graff, SVP & CFO

The mission of the NPF is to improve the quality of care for people with Parkinson's disease through research, education, and outreach.

2926 **Publix Super Markets Charities**
Publix Super Market Corporation Office
PO Box 407
Lakeland, FL 33802-0407 800-242-1227
www.publix.com

Gino DiGrazia, Vice President of Finance
Maria Brous, Director of Media & Community R
Kimberly Reynolds, Media & Community Relations

In addition to giving to thousands of local projects, Publix annually supports five organizations in companywide campaigns: Special Olympics, March of Dimes, Children's Miracle Network, United Way and Food for All

2927 **The Cherab Foundation**
PO Box 1771
Jensen Beach, FL 34958 772-335-5135
help@cherab.org
cherabfoundation.org

Lisa Geng, Founder & President
Jolie Abreu, Vice President

The Cherab Foundation is a world-wide nonprofit organization working to improve the communication skills and education of all children with speech and language delays and disorders. The Cherab Foundation is committed to assisting with the development of new therapeutic approaches, preventions, and cures to neurologically-based speech disorders.

Georgia

2928 **Arc Of Georgia**
100 Edgewood Ave NE
Ste 1675
Atlanta, GA 30303-3068 678-733-8969
888-401-1581
Fax: 678-733-8970
info@thearcofgeorgia.org
www.thearcofgeorgia.org

Torin Togut, President
David Glass, Vice President
Julie Lee, Secretary
Will Hudson, Treasurer

The Arc of Georgia advocates for the rights and full participation of all children and adults with intellectual and developmental disabilities. Together with our network of members and other local Chapters, we improve systems of supports and services, connect families, inspire communities, and influence public policy.

2929 **Community Foundation for Greater Atlanta**
50 Hurt Plz SE
Ste 449
Atlanta, GA 30303-2915 404-688-5525
Fax: 404-688-3060
info@cfgreateratlanta.org
www.cfgreateratlanta.org

Suzanne Boas, Board Chair
Alicia Philipp, President
Robert Smulian, Vice President of Philanthropic
Lesley Grady, Senior Vice President of Communi

The Community Foundation for Greater Atlanta is a creative, cost-effective and tax-efficient way for people to invest in our community. We help donors and their families meet their charitable goals by educating them or critical issues and by matching them with organizations that serve their interests. By working with donors and the community, we improve the quality of life for residents in our region.

2930 **Florence C and Harry L English Memorial Fund**
Sun Trust Bank Atlanta
PO Box 4418
Mail Code 041
Atlanta, GA 30302 404-588-8250
Fax: 404-724-3082

Anil T. Cheriyan, Chief Information Officer
Kenneth J. Carrig, Chief Human Resources Officer
Rilla S. Delorier, Chief Marketing and Client Exper
Thomas E. Freeman, Chief Risk Officer

Grants only made to Metro Atlanta non-profit organizations; no grants to churches or individuals.

2931 **Georgia Power**
96 Annex
Atlanta, GA 30308-3374 404-506-6526
888-655-5888
www.georgiapower.com

W. Paul Bowers, Chairman/ President/ CEO
John L. Pemberton, Senior VP/SPO,

Georgia Power is an investor-owned, tax-paying utility that serves 2.25 million customers in all but four of Georgia's 159 counties.

2932 **Grayson Foundation**
1701 Willa Place Drive
Kernersville, NC 2728 336-650-9914
graysonfoundation@gmail.com
www.graysonfoundation.net

Donna Sherrell, Finance- Public Relations
Tricia Gladstone, Behavior Analyst-Finance Public
Roger Sherrell, Information Technology-Web Manag
Bob Sherrell, Finance

Grayson Foundation enhances the quality of public educationfor the students of the Grayson cluster of schools by providing funds which enrich and extend educational oppurtunities.

2933 **Harriet McDaniel Marshall Trust in Memory of Sanders McDaniel**
Sun Trust Bank Atlanta
96 Annex
PO Box 4418
Atlanta, GA 30396
404-588-8250
888-891-0938
Fax: 404-724-3082

Anil T. Cheriyan, Chief Information Officer
Kenneth J. Carrig, Chief Human Resources Officer
Rilla S. Delorier, Chief Marketing and Client Exper
Thomas E. Freeman, Chief Risk Officer

Grants only made to Metro Atlanta non-profit organizations, no grants to churches or individuals.

2934 **IBM Corporation**
1 New Orchard Rd
Armonk, NY 10504-1772
914-499-1900
800-425-3333
TTY: 804-068-4225
response@in.ibm.com
www.ibm.com

Samuel J Palmisano, Chairman
Virginia M. Rometty, President and Chief Executive Of
Rodney C. Adkins, Senior Vice President
Michael E. Daniels, Senior Vice President and Group

Manages disability programs (which leverage IBM resources through partnerships) designed to train persons with disabilities and assist them in gaining employment. Also, disseminates information regarding products and resources for persons with disabilities with those of other companies and organizations.

2935 **John H and Wilhelmina D Harland Charitable Foundation**
3565 Piedmont Road, NE
Two Piedmont Center, Suite 710
Atlanta, GA 30305-1502
404-264-9912
Fax: 404-266-8834
info@harlandfoundation.org
www.harlandfoundation.org

Margaret C. Reiser, President
Winifred S. Davis, Vice President/Treasurer
Robert E. Reiser, Secretary
Jane G. Hardesty, Executive Director

The Harland Charitable Foundation was established in 1972 by John H. and Wilhelmina D. Harland to support worthy local causes in Atlanta, with a particular interest in improving the welfare of children and youth as well as support of community services and arts and culture.

2936 **Lettie Pate Whitehead Foundation**
191 Peachtree Street NE
Suite 3540
Atlanta, GA 30303- 2951
404-522-6755
Fax: 404-522-7026
fdns@woodruff.org
www.woodruff.org

James B. Williams, Chairman
James M. Sibley, Vice Chairman
Lawrence L. Gellerstedt, President /CEO
J. Lee Tribble, Treasurer

Non-profit organization dedicated to the support of needy women in nine southeastern states.

2937 **Rich Foundation**
222 Summer Street
Stamford, CT 06901
203-359-2900
Fax: 203-328-7980
info@fdrich.com
www.fdrich.com

2938 **SunTrust Bank, Atlanta Foundation**
Sun Trust Bank Atlanta
PO Box 4418
Mail Code 041
Atlanta, GA 30302
404-588-8250
Fax: 404-724-3082
www.suntrust.com

Anil T. Cheriyan, Chief Information Officer
Kenneth J. Carrig, Chief Human Resources Officer
Rilla S. Delorier, Chief Marketing and Client Exper
Thomas E. Freeman, Chief Risk Officer

Hawaii

2939 **Arc of Hawaii**
3989 Diamond Head Rd
Honolulu, HI 96816-4413
808-737-7995
Fax: 808-732-9531
info@thearcinhawaii.org
www.thearcinhawaii.org

Thomas Huber, President
Lee Moriwaki, Vice President
Duane Bartholomew, Secretary
Kevin Dooley, Treasurer

The Arc is a national, grassroots organization of and for people with intellectual and related developmental disabilities. With more then 140,000 members in 1000 local and state chapters. The Arc is the largest volunteer organization devoted soley to working on behalf of people with intellectual disabilities.

2940 **Atherton Family Foundation**
827 Fort Street Mall
Honolulu, HI 96813-2817
808-566-5524
888-731-3863
Fax: 808-521-6286
foundations@hcf-hawaii.org

Patricia R. Giles, Vice President
Judith M. Dawson, President
Frank C. Atherton, Vice President and Treasurer
Paul F. Morgan, Vice President

Supports educational projects, programs and institutions as the highest priority, with the enterprises of a religious nature and those concerned with health and social services given careful attention. The Foundation is one of the largest private resources in the State devoted exclusively to the support of activities of a charitable nature.

2941 **GN Wilcox Trust**
Bank of Hawaii
PO Box 3170
Honolulu, HI 96802-3170
808-649-8580
800-272-7262
Fax: 808-538-4006
stafford.kiguchi@boh.com
www.boh.com

Paul Boyce, AVP and Grants Administrator
Elaine Moniz, Trust Specialist
William L. Carpenter, Senior Vice President
Diane W. Murakami, Senior Vice President

Benefits the people of Hawaii by funding programs that support social services, education, culture, the arts, youth services, religion, health and rehabilitation.

2942 **Hawaii Community Foundation**
827 Fort Street Mall
Honolulu, HI 96813-2817
808-537-6333
888-731-3863
Fax: 808-521-6286
info@hcf-hawaii.org
www.hawaiicommunityfoundation.org

Kelvin Taketa, President/CEO
Chris van Bergeijk, Vice President/Chief Operating O
Joseph Martyak, Vice President of Communications
Tom Kelly, Vice President for Knowledge, Ev

The Hawaii Community Foundation is a public, statewide, charitable services and grantmaking organization supported by donor contributions for the benefit of Hawaii's people.

2943 **McInerny Foundation Bank Of Hawaii, Corporate Trustee**
PO Box 3170
Honolulu, HI 96802-3170
808-649-8580
800-272-7262
Fax: 808-538-4006
stafford.kiguchi@boh.com
www.boh.com

Paula Boyce, Avp And Grants Administrator
Elaine Moniz, Trust Specialist
William L. Carpenter, Senior Vice President
Diane W. Murakami, Senior Vice President

Although the Trust is broad-purposed, it does not make grants to churches or individuals, nor for endowments, reserve purposes, deficit financing, or for the purchase of real estate.

2944 **Sophie Russell Testamentary Trust Bank Of Hawaii**
PO Box 3170
Honolulu, HI 96802-3170
808-649-8580
800-272-7262
Fax: 808-538-4006
stafford.kiguchi@boh.com
www.boh.com

Paula Boyce, Asst. Vice President
Elaine Moniz, Trust Specialist
William L. Carpenter, Senior Vice President
Diane W. Murakami, Senior Vice President

Supports qualified tax-exempt charitable organizations, in the State of Hawaii only. Offers grants to the Humane Society and institutions giving nursing care and serving the physically and mentally handicapped.

Illinois

2945 **Alzheimer's Association**
225 N Michigan Ave
Fl 17
Chicago, IL 60601-7633
312-335-8700
800-272-3900
Fax: 866-699-1246
TTY: 312-335-5886
info@alz.org
www.alz.org

Stewart Putnam, Chair
Christopher Binkley, Vice Chair
Harry Johns, President /CEO
Deborah Jones, Secretary

Mission is to eliminate Alzheimer's disease through the advancement of research, to provide and enhance care and support for all affected, and to reduce the risk of dementia through the promotion of brain health.

2946 **American National Bank and Trust Company**
33 N La Salle St
PO Box 191
Danville, VA 24543-0191
312-661-6000
800-240-8190
Fax: 815-961-7745
www.amnb.com

Charles H. Majors, Chairman/ CEO
Jeffrey V. Haley, President
Charles T. Canaday, Jr., Senior Vice President
R. Helm Dobbins, Senior Vice President

Supports the endeavors of organizations working to meet the critical needs of the city and its surrounding communities. Success is greatly affected by the well-being of the communities the company serves, thus the foundation seeks to fulfill the social obligations both through financial funding and human resources. The Foundation funding categories include organizations and programs involved in economic development, education, community and social services, healthcare and culture and the arts.

2947 **Amerock Corporation**
P.O. Box 7018
Rockford, IL 61125-7018
815-963-9631
800-435-6959
Fax: 800-618-6733
www.amerock.com

Robert Bailey, President

Grants are given to organizations promoting wellness, health and rehabilitation of the visually impaired and physically disabled.

2948 **Arc of Illinois**
The Illinois Life Span Project
20901 S La Grange Rd
Ste 209
Frankfort, IL 60423-3213
815-464-1832
800-588-7002
Fax: 815-464-5292
www.thearcofil.org

Brain Rubin, President
Therese Devine, Vice President
Tony Paulauski, Executive Director
Janet Donahue, Director of Development

The Arc of Illinois is committed to empowering persons with disabilities to achieve full participation in community life thru informed choices.

2949 **Benjamin Benedict Green-Field Foundation**
18313 Greenleaf Ct
Tinley Park, IL 60487-2176
708-444-4241
Fax: 708-614-0496
www.greenfieldfoundation.org

Colin Fisher, Chairman of the Board
Kathryn Groenendal, President
Dan Jarke, Vice President
Sheldon K. Rachman, Secretary

A privately endowed grantmaking organization trying to improve the qaulity of life for children and the elderly in the city of chicago.

2950 **Blowitz-Ridgeway Foundation**
1701 E Woodfield Rd
Suite 201
Schaumburg, IL 60173-5127
847-330-1020
Fax: 847-330-1028
laura@blowitzridgeway.org
www.blowitzridgeway.org

Daniel L Kline, President
Pierre R. LeBreton, Ph.D., Vice-President
Thomas P. Fitzgibbon, Treasurer
Sandra Swantek, M.D., Secretary

Provides limited program, capital and research grants to organizations aiding the physically and mentally disabled, and agencies serving children and youth. Grants generally limited to Illinois.

2951 **Chaddick Institute for Metropolitan Development**
2352 N. Clifton Ave.
Suite 130
Chicago, IL 60614-2302
773-325-7310
Fax: 312-362-5506
lasadvising@depaul.edu
las.depaul.edu

Joseph P Scwieterman PhD, Director
Marisa Schulz, LEED AP, Assistant Director
Justin Kohls, Program Manager
Susan Aaron, Civic Program Design

Advances the principals of effective land use, transportation, and community planning. Offers planners, attorneys, developers, and entrepreneurs a forum to share expertise on difficult land-use issues through workshops, conferences, and policy studies.

2952 **Chicago Community Trust**
225 North Michigan Avenue
Suite 2200
Chicago, IL 60601- 4501
312-616-8000
Fax: 312-616-7955
www.cct.org

Frank M. Clark, Chairman
Terry Mazany, President /CEO
Jamie Phillippe, Vice President-Development and D
Chae Dawning, Sr. Director of Human Resources

A community foundation established in 1915, which receives gifts and bequests from individuals, families or organizations interested in providing through the community foundation, financial support for the charitable agencies or institutions which serve the residents of metropolitan Chicago.

2953 **Chicago Community Trust and Affiliates**
225 North Michigan Avenue
Suite 2200
Chicago, IL 60601- 4501
312-616-8000
Fax: 312-616-7955
TTY: 312-853-0394
www.cct.org

Frank M. Clark, Chairman
Terry Mazany, President /CEO
Jamie Phillippe, Vice President-Development and D
Chae Dawning, Sr. Director of Human Resources
Provides critical charitable resources in the arts, community and economic development, education, health and wellness, hunger and homeless alleviation, legal services, programs for youth, the elderly, and people with disabilities, and services to assure that basic human needs are met for all members of our community.

2954 **Community Foundation of Champaign County**
307 W University Ave
Champaign, IL 61820-3411
217-359-0125
Fax: 217-352-6494
www.cfeci.org

Brooke Didier Starks, Chair
Tom Costello, Vice-Chair
Joan M. Dixon, President /CEO
Bradley Uken, Treasurer
A network of cultural resource providers and educational organizations who collaborate in the creation, coordination, and promotion of cultural resource programs for Champaign County Schools.

2955 **Dr Scholl Foundation**
1033 Skokie Blvd
Ste 230
Northbrook, IL 60062-4109
847-559-7430
www.drschollfoundation.com

Pamela Scholl, President
The Foundation is dedicated to providing financial assistance to organizations committed to improving our world. Grants are made annually after an executive review by the staff and all the directors.

2956 **Duchossois Foundation**
Chamberlain Group
845 N Larch Ave
Elmhurst, IL 60126-1114
630-279-3600
Fax: 630-530-6091
employment@duch.com
www.duch.com

Richard L. Duchossois, Chairman
Robert L. Fealy, President /COO
Craig J. Duchossois, Chief Executive Officer
Michael E. Flannery, Executive Vice President/Chief F
Established in 1984, the foundation returns dollars to the communities supporting its facilities and employees. Within these following areas, organizations are carefully selected on the basis of community needs and the organization's value and performance. Areas aimed at include: medical research, children/youth programs and cultural institutions.

2957 **Evenston Community Foundation**
1560 Sherman Ave
Suite 535
Evanston, IL 60201-5910
847-492-0990
Fax: 847-492-0904
info@evanstonforever.org
www.evanstonforever.org

Sara Schastok, Phd., President and CEO
Gwen Jessen, Vice President for Philanthropy
Marybeth Schroeder, Vice President for Programs
Jan Fischer, Chief Financial Officer
The Foundation is a publicly supported plilanthropic organization dedicated to enriching Evanston and the lives of its people, now and in the future. The Foundation builds and manages its own and other community endowments, addresses Evanston's changing needs through grant making, and provides leadership on important community needs.

2958 **Field Foundation of Illinois**
200 S Wacker Dr
Ste 3860
Chicago, IL 60606-5848
312-831-0910
Fax: 312-831-0961
byoung@fieldfoundation.org
www.fieldfoundation.org

Lyle Logan, Board Chair
Aurie A. Pennick, Executive Director and Treasurer
Sarah M. Linsley, Secretary
Mark C. Murray, Program Director
The Field Foundation seeks to provide support for community, civic and cultural organizations in the Chicago area, enabling both new and established programs to test innovations, to expand proven strengths or to address specific, time-limited operational needs.

2959 **Francis Beidler Charitable Trust**
53 W Jackson Blvd
Ste 530
Chicago, IL 60604-3422
312-922-3792
Fax: 312-922-3799

Francis Beidler, Owner
Children/youth, services. Community development, business promotion, crime and violence prevention. Federated giving programs, higher education, human services and family planning.

2960 **Fred J Brunner Foundation**
9300 King St
Franklin Park, IL 60131-2114
847-678-3232
Fax: 847-678-0642

Fred J Brunner, CEO
General disability grants.

2961 **George M Eisenberg Foundation for Charities**
Ste 480
2340 S Arlington Heights Rd
Arlington Heights, IL 60005-4507
847-981-0545
Fax: 847-941-0548

James Marousis, Manager

2962 **Grover Hermann Foundation**
233 S Wacker Dr
Suite 6600
Chicago, IL 60606-6473
312-258-5500
Fax: 312-258-5600
rsafer@schiffhardin.com
www.schiffhardin.com

Ronald S. Safer, Managing Partner, Executive Comm
Provides funds for educational, health, public policy, community and religious organizations throughout the United States. Its major interests are in higher education and health.

2963 **John D and Catherine T MacArthur Foundation**
Office of Grants Management
140 S Dearborn St
Chicago, IL 60603-5285
312-726-8000
Fax: 312-920-6258
TTY: 312-920-6285
4answers@macfound.org
www.macfound.org

Marjorie M. Scardino, Chair
Julia Statch, Interim President
Cecilia A. Conrad, Vice President-MacArthur Fellows
Susan E. Manske, Vice President/Chief Investment
The Foundation supports creative people and effective institutions committed to building a more just, verdant, and peaceful world. In addition, we work to defend human rights, advance global conservation, & security, make cities better places, and understand how technology is affecting children and society.

2964 **Les Turne Amyotrophic Lateral Sclerosis Foundation**
5550 Touhy Ave
Ste 302
Skokie, IL 60077-3254
847-679-3311
888-257-1107
Fax: 847-679-9109
info@lesturnerals.org
www.lesturnerals.org

Ken Hoffman, President
Andrea Paul Backman, Executive Director
Shari Diamond, RN, BSN, Director of Patient Services
Kim McIver, Director

Voluntary health organization dedicated to raising funds for ALS research, patient services and public awareness. Provides educational materials for affected individuals and family members, health care professionals, and the general public. Program services include referrals and counseling; audio-visual aids and periodic newsletters. Offers support groups and patient networking to affected individuals, family members, and caregivers.

2965 **Little City Foundation**
1760 W Algonquin Rd
Palatine, IL 60067-4799
847-358-5510
Fax: 847-358-3291
info@littlecity.org
www.littlecity.org

Matthew B. Schubert, President
B. Timothy Desmond, Executive Vice President
David Rose, Vice President
Douglas A. Wilson, Vice President

We offer innovative and personalized programs to fully assist and empower children & adults with autism and other intellectual and developmental disabilities. With a commitment to attaining a greater quality of life for Illinois most vulnerable citizens, we actively promote choice, person-centered planning and a holistic approach to health and wellness. 'ChildBridge' services include in-home personal & family supports, clinical behavior intervention, 24/7 residential services and much more.

2966 **MAGIC Foundation for Children's Growth**
6645 North Ave
Oak Park, IL 60302-1057
708-383-0808
800-362-4423
Fax: 708-383-0899
ContactUs@magicfoundation.org
www.magicfoundation.org

Rich Buckley, Chairman
Ken Dickard, Vice Chairman
Mary Andrews, CEO and Co-Founder
Dianne Kremidas, Executive Director

This is a national nonprofit organization providing support and education regarding growth disorders in children and related adult disorders, including adult GHD. Dedicated to helping children whose physical growth is affected by a medical problem by assisting families of afflicted children through local support groups, public education/awareness, newsletters, specialty divisions and programs for the children.

2967 **McDonald's Corporation Contributions Program**
2111 McDonalds Dr
Oak Brook, IL 60523-5500
630-623-3000
800-244-6227
Fax: 630-623-5700
www.mcdonalds.com

Don Thompson, President and Chief Executive Of
Tim Fenton, Chief Operating Officer
Peter J. Bensen, Executive Vice President and Chi
Jose Armario, Corporate Executive Vice Preside

2968 **Michael Reese Health Trust**
150 N Wacker Dr
Ste 2320
Chicago, IL 60606-1608
312-726-1008
Fax: 312-726-2797
www.healthtrust.net

Herbert S. Wander, Chairman
The Hon. How Carroll, Vice Chairman
Walter R. Nathan, Secretary
Gregory S. Gross, EdD, President

The trust seeks to improve the health of people in Chicago's metropolitan communities through effective grantmaking in health care, health education, and health research.

2969 **National Eye Research Foundation**
910 Skokie Blvd
Ste 207a
Northbrook, IL 60062-4033
847-564-9400
800-621-2258
Fax: 847-564-0807
info@nerf.org
www.subway.com

Joel Tenner, Manager

Dedicated to improving eye care for the public and meeting the professional needs of eye care practitioners; sponsors eye research projects on contact lens applications and eye care problems. Special study sections in such fields as orthokertology, primary eyecare, pediatrics, and through continuing education programs. Provides eye care information for the public and professionals. Educational materials including pamphlets. Program activities include education and referrals.

2970 **National Foundation for Ectodermal Dysplasias**
6 Executive Dr
Suite 2
Fairview Heights, IL 62208-1360
618-566-2020
Fax: 618-566-4718
info@nfed.org
www.nfed.org

Anil Vora, President
George Barbar, Vice President
Mary Fete, Executive Director
Kelley Atchison, Director

To empower and connect people touched by ectodermal dysplasias through education, support, and research.

2971 **National Headache Foundation**
820 N Orleans St
Ste 411
Chicago, IL 60610-3131
312-274-2650
888-643-5552
Fax: 312-640-9049
info@headaches.org
www.headaches.org

Seymour Diamond, M.D., Executive Chairman
Roger K. Cady, M.D., Associate Executive Chairman
Arthur H. Elkind, M.D., President
Vincent Martin, M.D., Vice President

Foundation exists to enhance the healthcare of headache sufferers. It is a source of help to sufferers' families, physicians who treat headache sufferers, allied healthcare professionals and to the public.

2972 **OMRON Foundation OMRON Electronics**
1 Commerce Dr
Schaumburg, IL 60173-5330
847-843-7900
800-556-6766
Fax: 847-884-1866
aoisales@omron.com
www.omron247.com

Tastu Goto, CEO

Supports local community projects through direct donations and matching employee-directed contributions.

2973 **Parkinson's Disease Foundation**
1359 Broadway
Suite 1509
New York, NY 10018-2331
212-923-4700
800-457-667
Fax: 212-923-4778
info@pdf.org
www.pdf.org

Howard D. Morgan, Chair
Constance Woodruff Atwell, Ph.D., Vice Chair
Robin Anthony Elliott, President
James Beck, Ph.D., Vice President

International voluntary not-for-profit organization dedicated to patient services; education of affected individuals, family members, and healthcare professionals; and promotion and support of research for Parkinson's Disease and related disorders. Offers an extensive referral service to guide affected individuals to proper

diagnosis and clinical care. Provides referrals to genetic counseling and support groups; promotes patient advocacy; and offers a variety of educational and support materials
Quarterly

2974 **Peoria Area Community Foundation**
331 Fulton St
Ste 310
Peoria, IL 61602-1449
309-674-8730
Fax: 309-674-8754
jim@communityfoundationci.org
www.communityfoundationci.org
Donna Maracci, Chair
David Wynn, Vice Chair
Mark Roberts, CEO
Jessica Dillon, Program Manager
Established to meet a wide variety of social, cultural, educational and other charitable needs throughout Central Illinois.

2975 **Polk Brothers Foundation**
20 W Kinzie St
Ste 1110
Chicago, IL 60654-5815
312-527-4684
Fax: 312-527-4681
questions@polkbrosfdn.org
www.polkbrosfdn.org
Sandra P. Guthman, Chair
Raymond F. Simon, Vice Chair
Gordon S. Prussian, Secretary
Gillian Darlow, CEO
The Polk Brothers Foundation seeks to improve the quality of life for the people of Chicago. We partner with local nonprofit organizations that work to reduce the impact of poverty and provide area residents with better access to quality education, preventive health care and basic human services.

2976 **Retirement Research Foundation**
8765 W Higgins Rd
Ste 430
Chicago, IL 60631-4170
773-714-8080
Fax: 773-714-8089
info@rrf.org
www.rrf.org
Nathaniel P. McParland, M.D., Chairman
Ruth Ann Watkins, Secretary
Downey R. Varey, Treasurer
Irene Frye, Executive Director
A private philanthropy with primary interest in improving the quality of life of older persons in the United States.

2977 **Sears-Roebuck Foundation**
3333 Beverly Rd
Hoffman Estates, IL 60179
847-286-2500
800-932-3188
Fax: 800-326-0485
www.sears.com
W Bruce Johnson, CEO
Has a special interest in projects that address women, families, and diversity, but awards most of its funding to disease-specific charities and United Way in the Chicago area.

2978 **Siragusa Foundation**
1 E Wacker Dr
Ste 2910
Chicago, IL 60601-1912
312-755-0064
Fax: 312-755-0069
www.siragusa.org
John E. Hicks, Chair & President
Ross D. Siragusa, Vice Chair
John R. Siragusa, Treasurer
Sharmila Rao Thakkar, Executive Director
The Siragusa Foundation, is a private family foundation that is committed to honoring its founder by sustaining and developing Chicago's extraordinary nonprofit resources.

2979 **Square D Foundation**
1415 S Roselle Rd
Palatine, IL 60067-7337
847-397-2600
Fax: 847-925-7500
www.schneider-electric.com

2980 **WP and HB White Foundation**
540 W Frontage Rd
Ste 3240
Northfield, IL 60093-1232
847-446-1441
Margaret Blandford, Executive Director
The Foundation's funds are allocated on a continuing basis within the metropolitan area of Chicago where our founder's business prospered. The Foundation helps organizations specializing in the visually impaired, mental health, youth and recreation.

2981 **Washington Square Health Foundation**
875 N Michigan Ave
Ste 3516
Chicago, IL 60611-1957
312-664-6488
Fax: 312-664-7787
washington@wshf.org
www.wshf.org
William N. Werner, MD, MPH, Board Chair
Howard Nochumson, Executive Director/President
William B. Friedeman, Secretary
James M. Snyder, Treasurer
Grants funds in order to promote and maintain access to adequate healthcare for all people in the Chicagoland area regardless of race, sex, creed or financial need.

2982 **Wheat Ridge Ministries**
1 Pierce Pl
Ste 250 E
Itasca, IL 60143-2634
630-766-9066
800-762-6748
Fax: 630-766-9622
www.wheatridge.org
Kevin Boettcher, Chair
Richard Herman, President
Brain Becker, Senior Vice President
Holly Harrison Fiala, Vice President of Advancement
Weat Ridge supports more then 100 new health-related ministries each year through a variety of grant programs

Indiana

2983 **Arc of Indiana**
107 N Pennsylvania St
Suite 800
Indianapolis, IN 46204- 2423
317-977-2375
800-382-9100
Fax: 317-977-2385
thearc@arcind.org
www.arcind.org
Kerry Fletcher, President
Marlene Lu, Vice President
Mike Foddrill, Treasurer
Erika Steuterman, Secretary
Arc of Indiana is commited to people with cognitive and developmental disabilities realizing their goals of learning, living, working, and playing in the community.

2984 **Ball Brothers Foundation**
222 S Mulberry St
Muncie, IN 47305-2802
765-741-5500
Fax: 765-741-5518
info@ballfdn.org
www.ballfdn.org
James A. Fisher, Chairman/ CEO
Jud Fisher, President/Chief Operating Office
Frank B. Petty, Vice Chairman
Tammy Phillips, Treasurer, ex-officio
The Ball Brothers Foundation is dedicated to the stewardship legacy of the Ball brothers and to the pursuit of improving the quality of the Muncie, Delaware County, east Central Indiana and Indiana, through philanthropy and leadership.

2985 **Community Foundation of Boone County**
102 N. Lebanon
Suite 200
Lebanon, IN 46052
317-873-0210
Fax: 317-873-0219
info@communityfoundationbc.org
www.communityfoundationbc.org
Marc Applegate, Chairman of the Board
Ray Ingham, Vice Chair
Mike Harlos, Treasurer
Suzy Rich, Secretary
The Community Foundation of Boone County provides pathways for connecting people who care with causes that matter for now and in the future.

2986 **John W Anderson Foundation**
402 Wall St
Valparaiso, IN 46383-2562
219-462-4611
Fax: 219-531-8954
andersonfnd@aol.com
Bruce Wargo, Manager
Physically and mentally disabled, recreation and youth agencies in Northwest Indiana area.

Iowa

2987 **Arc of Iowa**
114 S. 11th Street
Ste 302
West Des Moines, IA 50265- 3259
515-402-1618
800-362-2927
Fax: 515-330-2195
casey@thearcofiowa.org
www.thearcofiowa.org
Casey Westhoff, Executive Director
The Arc of Iowa exists to ensure that people with intellectual disabilities and developmental disabilities receive the services, supports and opportunities necessary to fully realize their right to live, work and enjoy life in the community without discrimination.

2988 **Hall-Perrine Foundation**
115 3rd St SE
Ste 803
Cedar Rapids, IA 52401-1222
319-362-9079
Fax: 319-362-7220
www.hallperrine.org
William Whipple, Chairman
Jack Evans, President
Darrel Morf, Vice President
Iris Muchmore, Secretary
This foundation is dedicated tio improving the quality of life for peole in Linn County, IA by responding to the changing social, economic, and cultural needs of the community.

2989 **Mid-Iowa Health Foundation**
3900 Ingersoll Ave
Ste 104
Des Moines, IA 50312-3535
515-277-6411
Fax: 515-271-7579
info@midiowahealth.org
www.midiowahealth.org
Becky Miles-Polka, Chairman
Rob Hayes, Vice Chair
Suzanne Mineck, President
Cheryl Harding, Secretary/Treasurer
Mission is to serve as a partner and catalyst for improving the health of vulnerable people in greater Des Moines.

2990 **Principal Financial Group Foundation**
711 High St
Des Moines, IA 50392
515-247-5111
800-986-3343
Fax: 515-235-5724
Larry Zimpleman, Chairman/ President/ CEO
Daniel J. Houston, President - Retirement, Insuranc
James P. McCaughan, President - Principal Global Inv
Luis Valdes, President - Principal Internatio
The Principal Financial Group is a leading global financial company offering businesses, individuals and industrial clients a wide range of financial products and services.

2991 **Siouxland Community Foundation**
505 5th St
Suite 412
Sioux City, IA 51101-1507
712-293-3303
Fax: 712-293-3303
office@siouxlandcommunityfoundation.org
www.siouxlandcommunityfoundation .org
Richard J. Dehner, President
Robert F. Meis, Vice President
Marilyn J. Hagberg, Secretary
Mary E. Anderson, Treasurer
The Siouxland Community Foundation strives to enhance the quality of life in the greater Siouxland tri-state area by seeking charitable gifts to build permanent endowments as charitable capital for the community, providing a flexable vehicle to receive and distribute gifts of any size, making grants in response to community needs, and providing services that will help shape the well-being of Siouxland.

Kansas

2992 **Arc of Kansas**
2701 SW Randolph Ave
Topeka, KS 66611-1536
785-232-0597
Fax: 785-232-3770
info@tarcinc.org
www.tarcinc.org
Barbara Duncan, President
Matthew Bergman, Vice President
Travis Stryker, Secretary
Kim Savage, Treasurer
Organzation works to ensure that the estimated 7.2 million Americans with intellectual and developmental disabilities have the services and supports they need to grow, develop, and live in communities across the nation.

2993 **Hutchinson Community Foundation**
1 North Main, Suite 501
PO Box 298
Hutchinson, KS 67504-0298
620-663-5293
Fax: 620-663-9277
info@hutchcf.org
www.hutchcf.org
Aubrey Abbot Patterson, President and Executive Director
Terri L. Eisiminger, Vice President of Administration
Janet Hamilton, Community Investment Officer
Maria G. Kicklighter, Finance Assistant
Connects donors to community needs and opportunities, increases philanthropy and provides community leadership.

2994 **Richard W Higgins Charitable Foundation**
Marshall & Ilsley Trust of Florida
2520 South Iowa
Ste 100
Lawrence, KS 66046-2713
877-202-9234
www.applebees.com
Ken Krei, President
Jessica James, Executive Chef
Patrick Humphrey, Executive Chef
Michael Slavin, Executive Chef
Gives primarily for medical research with geographical focus on New York and Florida.

Kentucky

2995 Arc of Kentucky
706 E. Main Street
Suite A
Frankfort, KY 40601-2408
502-875-5225
800-281-1272
Fax: 502-875-5226
arcofky@aol.com
arcofky.org

James Cheely, President
Patty Dempsey, Executive Director
Ellen Nicholson, Secretary
Bob Gray, Treasurer

The Arc of Kentucky works to ensure a quality of life for children and adults with intellectual and developmental disabilities to help in securing a positive future. The Arc values services and supports that enhance the quality of life through independence, friendship, choice and respect for individuals with intellectual and developmental disabilities.

Louisiana

2996 Arc of Louisiana
606 Colonial Dr
Ste G
Baton Rouge, LA 70714-6535
225-383-1033
866-966-6260
Fax: 225-383-1092
info@thearcla.org
www.thearcla.org

Larry Pete, President
Henry Friloux, Vice President
Kelly Serrett, Executive Director
Ashley Courville, Project Director

The Arc of Louisiana advocates for and with individuals with intellectual and developmental disabilities and their families that they shall live to their fullest potential.

2997 Baton Rouge Area Foundation
402 N 4th St
Baton Rouge, LA 70802-5506
225-387-6126
877-387-6126
Fax: 225-387-6153
mverma@braf.org
www.braf.org

C. Kris Kirkpatrick, Chair
S. Dennis Blunt, Vice Chair
John G. Davies, President/CEO
Annette D. Barton, Secretary

The Foundation provides grants to nonprofits to make lives better in the region. It also takes on projects, often with parters, to remake Baton Rouge.

2998 Community Foundation of Shreveport-Bossier
401 Edwards St
Ste 105
Shreveport, LA 71101-5551
318-221-0582
Fax: 318-221-7463
info@cfnla.org
www.cfnla.org

Janie D. Richardson, Chairman
Thomas H. Murphy, Vice Chairman
Terry C. Davis, Ph.D, Secretary
Rand Falbaum, Treasurer

Provides a variety of charitable funds and gift options to help our partners achieve their vision for a stronger, more vibrant community. By bringing together fund donors, their financial advisors and non profit agencies, the Foundation is a powerful catalyst for building charitable giving and effecting positive change in our area

Maine

2999 BCR Foundation
83 Mussey Rd.
Scarborough, ME 04074
207-883-8000
800-227-6111
Fax: 207-883-0100
solutions@bcr.net

3000 No Limits Foundation
265 Centre Dr.
Wales, ME 04280
207-569-6411
info@nolimitsfoundation.org
www.nolimitsfoundation.org

Mary Leighton, Founder & Executive Director
Kelsey Moody, Program Operations Manager
Alix Sandler, Marketing & Development Director
Cheryl Foss, Director, Human Resources

Non-profit organization offering camps for children with limb loss and differences.

3001 UNUM Charitable Foundation
Maine Association of Non Profits
565 Congress St
Ste 301
Portland, ME 04101-3308
207-871-1885
Fax: 207-780-0346
Manp@NonprofitMaine.org
www.nonprofitmaine.org

Doug Woodbury, Board President
Ted Scontras, Board Vice President
Joan Smith, Board Treasurer
Stephanie Eglinton, Board Secretary

The Foundation encourages projects that: stimulate others in the private or public sector to participate in problem solving; advance innovative and cost-effective approaches for addressing defined, recognized needs; and demonstrate ability to obtain future project funding, if needed. The foundation generally limits its consideration of capital campaign requests to the Greater Portland, Maine area.

Maryland

3002 ACNM Foundation, Inc.
American College of Nurse Midwives
8403 Colesville Rd.
Suite 1230
Silver Spring, MD 20910
240-485-1800
Fax: 240-485-1818
membership@acnm.org
midwife.org

Holly Kennedy, President
Lisa Paine, Chief Executive Officer

Charitable foundation of the American College of Nurse Midwives.

3003 American Health Assistance Foundation
22512 Gateway Center Dr
Clarksburg, MD 20871-2005
301-948-3244
800-437-2423
Fax: 301-258-9454
info@brightfocus.org
www.brightfocus.org

Stacy Pagos Haller, President / CEO
Donna Callison, Vice President of Development
Michael Buckley, Vice President of Public Affairs
Guy Eakin, Ph.D., Vice President of Scientific Aff

The American Health Assistance Foundation (AHAF) is a registered non-profit organization that funds research into cures for Alzheimer's disease, macular degeneration and glaucoma, and provides the public with informantion about risk factors, preventative lifestyles, availiable treatments and coping strategies.

3004 **American Occupational Therapy Foundation**
4720 Montgomery Lane
Suite 202
Bethesda, MD 20814-3449
240-292-1079
Fax: 240-396-6188
aotf@aotf.org
aotf.org

Diana L. Ramsay, Chair
Wendy J. Coster, Vice Chair
Scott Campbell, CEO
Emily Kringle, President

AOFT provides advanced research, education and public awareness for occupational therapy, so that all people may participate fully in life regardless of their physical, social, mental or developmental circumstances.

3005 **Arc of Maryland**
121 Cathedral St, 2B
PO Box 1747
Annapolis, MD 21401- 1747
410-571-9320
888-272-3449
Fax: 410-974-6021
info@thearcmd.org
www.thearcmd.org

Richard Dean, President
Aileen O'Hare, Vice President
Annette Hinkle, Treasurer
Adam Vanderhook, Secretary

The Arc of Maryland works to create a world where children and adults with cognitive and developmental disabilities have and enjoy equal rights and opportunities.

3006 **Baltimore Community Foundation**
2 E Read Street
Floor 9
Baltimore, MD 21202-6903
410-332-4171
Fax: 410-837-4701
questions@bcf.org
www.bcf.org

Raymond L. Bank, Chair
Tedd Alexander, Vice Chair
Laura L. Gamble, Vice Chair
Thomas E. Wilcox, President

Makes grants in Baltimore City and Baltimore County; see website for how to apply. BCF is governed by a 30-member board of trustees, made up of a cross section of Baltimore.

3007 **Candlelighters Childhood Cancer Foundation**
10920 Connecticut Ave.
PO Box 498
Kensington, MD 20895- 0498
301-962-3520
855-858-2226
Fax: 301-962-3521
staff@acco.org
www.acco.org

Naomi Bartley, President
Janine Lynne, Vice President
Ken Phillips, Treasurer
Judy Mendoza, Secretary

An international organization providing information and support, and advocacy to parents of children with cancer and survivors of childhood cancer.Health and Education professionals also welcome as members.Network of local support groups. Information on disabilities related to treatment of childhood cancer. Publications.

3008 **Children's Fresh Air Society Fund**
Baltimore Community Foundation
2 E Read St
Baltimore, MD 21202-2470
410-332-4171
Fax: 410-837-4701
grants@bcf.org
bcf.org

Tom E. Wilcox, President
Danista Hunte, Vice President, Community Invest
Ralph M. Serpe, CFRE, Vice President, Development
Amy T. Seto, CPA, Vice President, Finance and Admi

Makes grants to nonprofit camps to provide tuition for disadvantaged and disabled Maryland children to attend summer camp. See website for how to apply.

3009 **Clark-Winchcole Foundation**
3 Bethesda Metro Ctr
Suite 550
Bethesda, MD 20814-5358
301-654-3607

Laura Phillips, President

Supported tax-exempt charitable organizations operating in the metropolitan area of Washington, DC in the following areas: deaf, higher education and physically disabled.

3010 **Columbia Foundation**
10630 Little Patuxent Parkway
Century Plaza, Suite 315
Columbia, MD 21044
410-730-7840
Fax: 410-997-6021
www.cfhoco.org

Bruce Harvey, Chair
Joseph Maranto, Vice Chair
Barb Van Winkle, Secretary
Lynne Schaefer, Treasurer

The Columbia Foundation serves as a catalyst for building a more caring, creative and effective community in Howard County by promoting and creating opportunities for personal and corporate philanthropy, managing endowments, anticipating and responding to community needs, and strategically granting funds.

3011 **Corporate Giving Program**
Ryland Group
11000 Broken Land Pkwy
Columbia, MD 21044
410-715-7022
800-267-0998
Fax: 410-715-7909

Bruce N Haas, President

Contributions of equipment, volunteers and financial support to organizations working to meet the challenges and needs of modern society.

3012 **Cystic Fibrosis Foundation**
6931 Arlington Rd
2nd floor
Bethesda, MD 20814-5200
301-951-4422
800-344-4823
Fax: 301-951-6378
info@cff.org
www.cff.org

Catherine C. McLoud, Board Chair
Robert J. Beall, Ph.D., President/Chief Executive Office
C. Richard Mattingly, Executive Vice President/Chief O
Preston W. Campbell, III, M.D., Executive Vice President for Med

The mission of the Cystic Fibrosis Foundation, a nonprofit donor-supported organization is to assure the development of the means to cure and control cystic fibrosis and to improve the quality of life for those with the disease.

3013 **Foundation Fighting Blindness**
7168 Columbia Gateway Dr.
Suite 100
Columbia, MD 21046
410-423-0600
800-683-5555
TTY: 410363713951
info@FightBlindness.org
www.blindness.org

William T. Schmidt, Chief Executive Officer
Valerie Navy-Daniels, Chief Development Officer
Stephen M. Rose, PhD, Chief Research Officer

The Foundation Fighting Blindness (FFB) works to promote research in order to prevent, treat and restore vision. FFB is currently the world's leading private funder of retinal disease research, funding over 100 research grants and 150 researchers.

3014 **George Wasserman Family Foundation**
Grossberg Company
6707 Democracy Blvd
Suite 300
Bethesda, MD 20817-1176
301-571-4977
Fax: 301-571-6250

Helen Salud, Manager
Anthony Cpa, Partner

3015 **Giant Food Foundation**
8301 Professional Pl
Ste 115
Landover, MD 20785-2351
301-341-4100
888-469-4426
jmiller@giantfood.com
www.giantfood.com

Anthony Hucker, President
Brian Beatty, Md. Director of Marketing and Ex
Stefanie Cain, Md. District Director
Bob Haas, Md. District Director

Offers grants in the areas of mental health, recreation, community and cultural programs, art, and educational programs for the health and prosperity of the greater Washington area.

3016 **Harry and Jeanette Weinberg Foundation**
7 Park Center Ct
Owings Mills, MD 21117-4200
410-654-8500
Fax: 410-654-4900
cdemchak@hjweinberg.org
hjweinbergfoundation.org

Ellen M. Heller, Chair
Barry I. Schloss, Treasurer
Alvin Awaya, Vice-President
Rachel Garbow Monroe, President and Chief Executive Of

The Harry & Jeanette Weinberg Foundation, Inc. is dedicated to assisting the poor, primarily through operating and capital grants to direct service organizations located in Baltimore, Hawaii, Northeastern Pennsylvania, New York, Israel and the Former Soviet Union. These grants are focused on meeting basic needs such as shelter, nutrition, health & socialization & on enhancing an individual's ability to meet those needs. Within that focus, emphasis is placed on the elderly & Jewish community.

3017 **Immune Deficiency Foundation**
110 West Rd.
Suite 300
Towson, MD 21204
800-296-4433
Fax: 410-321-9165
info@primaryimmune.org
primaryimmune.org

Kathryn Stephens, Interim CEO
Sarah Rose, Chief Financial Officer
Katherine Antilla, Vice President, Education
Tammy C. Black, Vice President, Communications

The Immune Deficiency Foundation is the national patient organization dedicated to improving the diagnosis, treatment, and quality of life of persons with primary immunodeficiency diseases through advocacy, education, and research.

3018 **Kennedy Krieger Institute**
707 North Broadway
Baltimore, MD 21205
443-923-9200
800-873-3377
888-554-9400
TTY: 443-923-2645
findaspecialist@kennedykrieger.org
www.kennedykrieger.org

Gary W. Goldstein, MD

Internationally recognized for improving the lives of children and adolescents with disorders and injuries of the brain, spinal cord and musculoskeletal system, the Kennedy Krieger Institute serves more than 20,000 individuals each year through inpatient and outpatient clincs, home and community services and school-based programs. Kennedy Krieger provides a wide range of services for children and young adults with developmental concerns mid to severe, and is home to a team of investigators.

3019 **Miracle-Ear Children's Foundation**
5000 Cheshire Ln N
Minneapolis, MN 55446-3706
763-268-4000
800-464-8002
Fax: 763-268-4365
www.miracle-ear.com/en-us/

3020 **National Federation of the Blind**
200 E Wells St.
Baltimore, MD 21230
410-659-9314
Fax: 410-685-5653
nfb@nfb.org
nfb.org

Mark Riccobono, President
John Berggren, Executive Director, Operations
Anil Lewis, Executive Director, Blindness Initiatives
John G. Pare, Jr., Executive Director, Advocacy & Policy

The National Federation of the Blind (NFB) works to help blind people achieve self-confidence, self-respect and self-determination and to achieve complete integration into society on a basis of equality. The Federation provides public educations, information and referral services, scholarships, literature and publications, adaptive equipment, advocacy services, legal services, employment assistance and more.

3021 **Optometric Extension Program Foundation**
2300 York Road
Suite 113
Timonium, MD 21093
410-561-3791
Fax: 949-250-8157
Kelin.Kushin@oep.org
www.oepf.org

Paul A. Harris, OD, President
Robin Lewis, OD, Vice President
Kelin Kushin, Executive Director
Eric Ikeda, Secretary-Treasurer

Vision care for learning disabilities and head trauma patients.

3022 **Sjogren's Syndrome Foundation**
6707 Democracy Blvd
Suite 325
Bethesda, MD 20817-1164
301-530-4420
800-475-6473
Fax: 301-530-4415
tms@sjogrens.org
www.sjogrens.org

Kenneth Economou, Chairman of the Board
Stephen Cohen, OD, Chairman-Elect
Vidya Sankar, DMD, MHS, Treasurer
Janet Ee. Church, Secretary

Provides patients practical information and coping strategies that minimize the effects of Sjogren's syndrome. In addition, the Foundation is the clearinghouse for medical information and is the recognized national advocate for Sjogren's syndrome. *$25.00 Monthly*

Massachusetts

3023 **Abbot and Dorothy H Stevens Foundation**
P.O. Box 111
North Andover, MA 01845
978-688-7211
Fax: 978-686-1620

Josh Miner, Executive Director

Established in 1953, Purpose is giving primarily to the arts, education, conservation, and health and human services.

3024 **Arc of Massachusetts, The**
217 South St
Waltham, MA 02453-2710
781-891-6270
Fax: 781-891-6271
arcmass@arcmass.org
www.arcmass.org

Leo Sarkissian, Executive Director
Joshua Komyerox, Government Affairs Director
Brenda Asis, Development Director

Quarterly newsletter for The Arc of Massachusetts is Advocate.

3025 **Arc of Northern Bristol County**
141 Park St
Attleboro, MA 02703-3020
508-226-1445
888-343-3301
Fax: 508-226-1476
info@arcnbc.org
arcnbc.org

Richard Harwood, Chairperson
Valerie Zagami, Vice Chairperson
Paul Oliveira, Treasurer
D. Randall Hays, III, Secretary/Clerk

Mission is to strive for the right of all people with developmental disabilities to be valued as individuals, to experience choice, and to be fully included in all aspects of community life

3026 **Boston Foundation**
75 Arlington St
10th Fl
Boston, MA 02116-3992
617-338-1700
Fax: 617-338-1604
tbf.org

Michael Keating, Esq., Chair
Catherine D'Amato, Vice Chair
Paul S. Grogan, President & CEO
Alfred F. Van Ranst, Jr., CFO and Treasurer

The Foundation's grantmaking, special initiatives and civic leadership promote innovation across a broad range of compelling community issues, from educational excellence to affordable housing to workforce development and the arts.

3027 **Boston Globe Foundation**
P.O. Box 55819
Boston, MA 02205-5819
617-929-2000
bostonglobe.com

Mary Jacobus, President

The mission of the Boston Globe Foundation is to empower community-based organizations to effect real change in the ares of greatest need, where the Globe is uniquely postioned to add the most value. Priority focus areas: strengthen the reading, writing and critical thinking of young people, while fostering their inherent love of learning. Strengthen the roads that link people to culture. Strengthen the civic fabric of the city. Be responsive to the needs of our immediate community.

3028 **Bushrod H Campbell and Ada F Hall Charity Fund**
Palmer & Dodge
111 Huntington Ave
Boston, MA 02199-7610
617-239-0540
Fax: 617-227-4420

Brenda Taylor, Foundation Administrator

The fund's areas of interest include organizations and/or their projects supporting aid to the elderly, healthcare and population control. Medical research grants are administered through the Medical Foundation. No grants are awarded to individuals and the geographical area of support is limited to organizations located in Massachusetts within the area of Boston and Route 128.

3029 **Clipper Ship Foundation**
77 Summer St
8th Floor
Boston, MA 02110-1006
617-391-3088
Fax: 617-426-7087
hblaisdell@gmafoundations.com
clippershipfoundation.org

Ron Ancrum, President

Makes grants to federally tax-qualified non-profit organizations offering human services to individuals living in Greater Boston and the cities of Lawrence and Brockton.

3030 **Community Foundation of Western Massachusetts**
1500 Main Street, Suite 2300
P.O. Box 15769
Springfield, MA 01115-5769
413-732-2858
Fax: 413-733-8565
wmass@communityfoundation.org
www.communityfoundation.org

Katie Allan Zobel, President and CEO
Nancy Reiche, M.S.W., Vice President for Programs
Donna Roseman David, Chief Financial Officer/Chief Ad
Kristin Leutz, Vice President of Philanthropic

Provides a simple way to achieve the charitable objectives of donors most effectively; supports nonprofit organizations that offer programs in the arts, education, human services, healthcare, housing, and the environment; and works to improve the quality of life in our region.

3031 **Frank R and Elizabeth Simoni Foundation**
1401 Boston Providence Tpke
Norwood, MA 02062-5053
781-762-3449
Fax: 781-769-6166

Matthew Mac Donald, President
Ann Mac Donald, Secretary
Robert Mac Donald, Clerk

3032 **Friendly Ice Cream Corp Contributions Program**
1855 Boston Rd
Wilbraham, MA 01095-1002
413-543-3544
800-966-9970
Fax: 413-731-4467
friendlys.com

John Maguire, Chief Financial Officer
Steve Weigel, EVP, Chief Operating Officer
Pat Hickey, EVP, Chief Financial Officer
Tim Hopkins, EVP, Retail and Manufacturing

3033 **Greater Worcester Community Foundation**
370 Main St
Ste 650
Worcester, MA 01608-1738
508-755-0980
Fax: 508-755-3406
info@greaterworcester.org
greaterworcester.org

Gerald Gaudette III, Chair
Warner S. Fletcher, Vice Chair
Thomas J. Bartholomew, Treasurer
Carolyn Stempler, Clerk

By focusing on the entire community rather then on any specific issue, the community foundation is able to address matters of greater importance to the people of the region. The Foundation has built a permanent, flexable endowment and has distributed grants and awards to a broad range of organizations and people throughout the region.

3034 **Hyams Foundation**
50 Federal St
9th Floor
Boston, MA 02110
617-426-5600
Fax: 617-426-5696
info@hyamsfoundation.org
hyamsfoundation.org

Martella Wilson-Taylor, Chair
Angela Brown, Director of Programs
Mike Givens, Communications Manager
Jocelyn V Sargent, Executive Director

The mission of the foundation is to increase economic and social stregnth within low-income communities in Boston and Chelsea, Massachusetts. Some areas they provide funding to include community identified issues, racial justice and transitional funding.

3035 **Raytheon Company Contributions Program**
870 Winter St
Waltham, MA 02451-1449
781-522-3000
Fax: 781-860-2172
raytheon.com

Thomas A. Kennedy, Chief Financial Officer
David C. Wajsgras, Senior Vice President and Chief
Keith J. Peden, Senior Vice President - Human Re
Jay B. Stephens, Senior Vice President - General

Industry leader in defense and government electronics, space, information technology, technical services, and business aviation and special mission aircraft.

3036 **TJX Foundation**
TJX Companies
770 Cochituate Rd
Framingham, MA 01701-4666
508-390-1000
Fax: 508-390-2091
www.tjx.com

Carol Meyrowitz, CEO

The purpose of the TJX Foundation's Giving Program is to support qualified, tax-exempt nonprofit organizations that provide services which promote and improve the quality of life for children, women and families in need.

3037 **The Beveridge Family Foundation, Inc.**
3 Upland Ln.
West Newbury, MA 01985
800-229-9667
administrator@beveridge.org
www.beveridge.org

Ward Slocum Caswell, President
Philip Caswell, Chairman and Vice President
Ruth S. DuPont, Treasurer
Leah Beveridge Richardson, Clerk

The mission of The Frank Stanley Beveridge Foundation, Inc. is to preserve and enhance the quality of life by embracing and perpetuating Frank Stanley Beveridge's philanthropic vision through grantmaking initiatives in support of The Stanley Park of Westfield, Inc. and programs in youth development, health, education, religion, art, and environment primarily in Hampden and Hampshire Counties, Massachusetts.

3038 **Vision Foundation**
8901 Strafford Cir
Knoxville, TN 37923-1500
865-357-4603
Fax: 865-690-9322

Gordon Adams, President

Offers counseling, support groups, seminars and transportation for the blind providing 600 members.

Michigan

3039 **Ann Arbor Area Community Foundation**
301 N Main St
Ste 300
Ann Arbor, MI 48104-1296
734-663-0401
Fax: 734-663-3514
info@aaacf.org
aaacf.org

Michelle Crumm, Chair
Tim Wadhams, Vice Chair
Neel Hajra, President & CEO
Shelley Strickland, Vice President

Interested in funding projects which will improve the quality of life for citizens of the Ann Arbor area. Eligible projects generally fall within these categories: education, culture, social service, community development, environmental awareness and health and wellness. The Foundation aims to support creative approaches to community needs and problems by making grants which will benefit the widest possible range of people.

3040 **Arc of Michigan**
State of Michigan
1325 S Washington Ave
Lansing, MI 48910-1652
517-487-5426
800-292-7851
Fax: 517-487-0303
dhoyle@arcmi.org
arcmi.org

Shari Fitzpatrick, President
Kim Brown, Vice President
Bob Altizer, Secretary
Laurel Robb, Treasurer

The Arc Michigan empowers local chapters to assure that citizens with disabilities are valued and that they and their families participate fully in and contribute to the life of their community.

3041 **Berrien Community Foundation**
2900 S State St
Ste 2e
Saint Joseph, MI 49085-2467
269-983-3304
Fax: 269-983-4939
bcf@BerrienCommunity.org
berriencommunity.org

Hillary Bubb, Chair
Mabel Mayfield, Vice Chair
Lisa Cripps-Downey, President
Sandra Tardi, Finance Director

The Foundation is a union of numerous gifts, bequests and other contributions that form permanent endowments and other funds.

3042 **Blind Children's Fund**
P.O. Box 187
Grand Ledge, MI 48837
517-488-4887
www.blindchildrensfund.org

Carrie L Owens, Board President
Diana Popp, Executive Director

Provides parents and professionals information materials and resources to help them teach and nurture blind and visually impaired children so they may reach their potential.

3043 **Community Foundation of Monroe County**
P.O. Box 627
28 S. Macomb St.
Monroe, MI 48161-627
734-242-1976
Fax: 734-242-1234
info@cfmonroe.org
cfmonroe.org

Kathleen Russeau, MBA, Executive Director
Michele Sandiefer, Office Manager
Julie Rhinehart, YAC Coordinator
Doug Redding, Project Manager

The mission of the Community Foundation of Monroe County is to encourage and facilitate philanthropy in Monroe County.

3044 **Cowan Slavin Foundation**
7881 Dell Rd
Saline, MI 48176-9744
734-944-1439
Fax: 734-944-3529

David Bovee, Owner

3045 **Daimler Chrysler**
Automobility Program
P.O. Box 5080
Troy, MI 48007-5080
800-255-9877
Fax: 855-409-0475
rebates@chrysler.com

3046 **Frank & Mollie S VanDervoort Memorial Foundation**
4646 Okemos Rd
Okemos, MI 48864-1795
517-349-7232
Ann L Gessert, Secretary

3047 **Fremont Area Community Foundation**
4424 W. 48th Street
PO Box B
Fremont, MI 49412-176
231-924-5350
Fax: 231-924-5351
tfacf.org

Robert Zeldenrust, Chair
William Johnson, Vice Chair
Carla Roberts, President & CEO
Cathy Kissinger, Secretary

A local nonprofit organization serving the residence of Newaygo County. We connect the needs of the community with those who have the conviction to make a lasting impact. Our mission is to improve the quality of life for the people of Newaygo County.Zeldenrust

3048 **Grand Rapids Foundation**
185 Oakes St SW
Grand Rapids, MI 49503-4008
616-454-1751
Fax: 616-454-6455
grfound@grfoundation.org
grfoundation.org

Paul M. Keep, Chair
Laurie Finney Beard, Vice Chair
Diana R. Sieger, President
Ren Guttrich, Executive Assistant

Grand Rapids Community Foundation leads the community in making positive, sustainable change. Through our grantmaking and leadership initiatives we help foster academic achievement, build economic prosperity, achieve healthy ecosystems, encourage healthy people, support social enrichment, and create vibrant neighborhoods.

3049 **Granger Foundation**
6267 Aurelius Rd
Lansing, MI 48911-2187
517-393-1670
Fax: 517-393-1382
grangerconstruction.com

Alton Granger, Chairman
Glenn D. Granger, President & CEO

The primary purpose of the Granger Foundation is to enhance the quality of life within the Greater Lansing, Michigan Area. Our mission is to support Christ-centered activities. We also support efforts that enhance the lives of youth in our community.

3050 **Harvey Randall Wickes Foundation**
4800 Fashion Square Blvd
Suite 472
Saginaw, MI 48604- 2677 989-799-1850
Fax: 989-799-3327
www.tgci.com

James Finkbeiner
Grants for rehabilitation.

3051 **Havirmill Foundation**
3505 Greenleaf Blvd
Ste 203
Kalamazoo, MI 49008-2580 269-375-1193
millenniumrestaurants.com

Ken Miller, CEO, Principal Partner
Matthew Burian, President
Bob Lewis, Operating Partner
Shelly Pastor, Operating Partner

3052 **Kelly Services Foundation**
999 W Big Beaver Rd
Troy, MI 48084-4782 248-362-4444
Fax: 248-244-4588
kfirst@kellyservices.com
kellyservices.com

George S. Corona, Chief Operating Officer
Carl T. Camden, President & CEO
Terence E. Adderley, Executive Chairman
Olivier Thirot, Acting Chief Financial Officer

3053 **Kent County Arc**
2922 Fuller Ave. NE
Ste 201
Grand Rapids, MI 49505 616-459-3339
Fax: 401-737-8907
info@arckent.org
www.arckent.org

Pam Cross, President
Tim Lundgren, Vice-President
Tammy Finn, Executive Director
Maggie Kolk, Advocate/WIPA Benefits Counselor
Providing individuals with disabilties meaningful opportunities throughout their communities.

3054 **Kresge Foundation**
3215 W Big Beaver Rd
Troy, MI 48084-2818 248-643-9630
Fax: 248-643-0588
info@kresge.org
kresge.org

Rip Rapson, President and CEO
Amy B. Coleman, VP/ CFO
Ariel H. Simon, Vice President, Chief Program
Marcus L. McGrew, Director of Grants Management
This foundation offers challenge grants for capital projects, most often for construction or renovation of buildings, but also for the purchase of major equipment and real estate. As challenge grants, they are intended to stimulate new, private gifts in the midst of an organized fund raising effort. Offers special opportunities to build capacity, both in providing enhanced facilities in which to present programs and in generating private support. Only charitable organizations may apply.

3055 **Lanting Foundation**
1575 S Shore Dr
Holland, MI 49423-4436 616-335-2033
Arlyn Lanting, Partner

3056 **Rollin M Gerstacker Foundation**
PO Box 1945
Midland, MI 48641-1945 989-631-6097
www.gerstackerfoundation.org

Gail E. Lanphear, Chairperson
Lisa J. Gerstacker, President
E. N. Brandt, Vice President /Secretary
Alan W Ott, Vice President /Treasurer
The Rollin M. Gerstacker Foundation was founded by Mrs. Eda U. Gerstacker in 1957, in memory of her husband. Its primary purpose is to carry on, indefinitely, financial aid to charities of all types supported by Mr. and Mrs. R.M. Gerstacker during their lifetimes. These charities are concentrated in the states of Michigan and Ohio.

3057 **Steelcase Foundation**
PO Box 1967
GH-4E
Grand Rapids, MI 49501-1967 616-246-4695
Fax: 616-475-2200
foundation@Steelcase.com
steelcase.com

Julie Ridenour, President
The Foundation focuses on the areas of human service, health, education, community development, the arts and the environment; giving particular concern to people who are disadvantaged, disabled, young and elderly as they attempt to improve the quality of their lives.
1951

Minnesota

3058 **Arc of Minnesota**
800 Transfer Road
Suite 7A
St. Paul, MN 55114 651-523-0823
800-582-5256
Fax: 651-523-0829
mail@arcmn.org
www.arcmn.org

John Rentschler, President
Lisa Schoneman, Vice President
Amy Hewitt, Secretary
Rob Wolf, Treasurer
Your membership in The Arc of Minnesotta benefits persons with developmental disabilities and their families as they live, learn, work and play. Please join today!

3059 **Burnett Foundation**
P.O. Box 633
Northfield, MN 55057-6881 817-877-3344
tomburnettfamilyfoundation@msn.com
www.tomburnettfoundation.org

V Neils Agather, Executive Director

3060 **Deluxe Corporation Foundation**
Deluxe Corporation
3680 Victoria St N
Shoreview, MN 55126-2966 651-483-7111
800-328-0304
Fax: 651-483-7270
feedback@deluxe.com
ww.deluxe.com

Lee J Schram, CEO
Terry D. Peterson, CFO /Senior VP
Malcolm J. McRoberts, Senior Vice President, Small Bus
John D. Filby, Senior Vice President, Financial
Funds programs such as schools, museums, programs for the disadvantaged. We believe programs and services like these represent the heart and soul of our communities.

3061 **General Mills Foundation**
P.O. Box 9452
Minneapolis, MN 55440-9452 800-248-7310
Fax: 763-764-8330
corporate.response@genmills.com
generalmills.com

Kendall J. Powell, Chairman / CEO
Ann W.H. Simonds, Senior Vice President/ Chief Mar
Keith A Woodward, Vice President, Treasurer
Gary Chu, Senior Vice President

3062 **Hugh J Andersen Foundation**
342 5th Ave N
Suite 200
Bayport, MN 55003-4502
651-439-1557
888-439-9508
Fax: 651-439-9480
contact@srinc.biz
www.srinc.biz
Brad Kruse, Program Director
Established in 1962, this fund is a nonprofit charitable corporation classified as a private foundation. The Foundation was established as a general charitable fund, but now identifies projects that build individual and community capacity to be a priority. Giving is focused primarily in the counties of Washington, Minnesota, & St, Croix, Polk and Pierce of WI. Grants are given in the areas of human services, health, education, arts and culture, community services and the environment.

3063 **James R Thorpe Foundation**
5866 Oakland Avenue
Minneapolis, MN 55417-5418
763-250-9304
info@jamesrthorpefoundation.org
www.jamesrthorpefoundation.org
Tim Thorpe, President
Robert C. Cote, Treasurer
Kerrie Blevins, Foundation Manager
S. Ruggles Cote, Board Member
Foundation based on values of respect and compassion, and is dedicated to making the greater Minneapolis area better for all its citizens.

3064 **Jay and Rose Phillips Family Foundation**
615 First Ave. NE
Ste. 330
Minneapolis, MN 55413
612-623-1654
Fax: 612-623-1653
info@phillipsfamilyfoundationmn.org
Patrick Troska, Executive Director
Joel Luedtke, Senior Program Officer
Tracy Lamparty, Grants and Operations Manager
Salena Acox, Vista Program Manager

3065 **Minneapolis Foundation**
80 S 8th St
800 IDS Center
Minneapolis, MN 55402-2100
612-672-3878
866-305-0543
Fax: 612-672-3846
email@mplsfoundation.org
www.mplsfoundation.org
Sandra L. Vargus, President and CEO
Jean M. Adams, Chief Operating Officer/Chief Fi
Teresa Morrow, Vice President, External Relatio
Luz Maria Frias, Vice President, Community Impact
Provides a variety of charitable fund and gift options to help Minnesotans make a difference.

3066 **Ordean Foundation**
424 W Superior St
Duluth, MN 55802-1591
218-726-4785
Steve Mangan, Executive Director
Grants are given for a variety of purposes including: treatment and rehabilitation for persons who are chronically or temporarily mentally ill, persons whose physical capacity is impaired by injury or illness, promotes mental and physical health of the elderly, provides for youth guidance programs designed to avoid delinquency, and provides relief, aid and charity to people with no or low incomes. Grants are only offered to certain cities and townships near and around St. Louis County/Duluth.

3067 **Otto Bremer Foundation**
445 Minnesota St
Ste 2250
Saint Paul, MN 55101-2161
651-227-8036
888-291-1123
Fax: 651-312-3665
obf@ottobremer.org
www.ottobremer.org
Kari Suzuki, Director of Operations
Diane Benjamin, Executive Director
Danielle Cheslog, Grants Manager
Rose Carr, Program Officer
Mission is to assist people in achieving full economic, civic and social participation in and for the betterment of their communities.

3068 **Rochester Area Foundation**
400 South Broadway
Suite 300
Rochester, MN 55904
507-282-0203
Fax: 507-282-4938
info@rochesterarea.org
rochesterarea.org
JoAnn Stormer, President
Max Evans, Administration/Communications
Ann Fahy-Gust, Grants and Impact Officer
Paul Harkess, Development Officer
The mission of the Rochester Area Foundation is to strengthen community philanthropy by promoting responsible and informed giving and to assist donors in meeting their charitable objectives.

Mississippi

3069 **Arc of Mississippi**
704 North President Street
Jackson, MS 39202
601-355-0220
800-717-1180
Fax: 601-355-0221
info@arcms.org
www.arcms.org
Kim Duffy, President
Ronnie Raggio, Senior Vice-President
Shirley Miller, Secretary
Cherri Hedglin, Treasurer
The Arc is Committed to securing for all people with developmental disabilities the opportunity to choose and realize their goals of where and how they learn live work and play.

Missouri

3070 **Allen P & Josephine B Green Foundation**
1055 Broadway
Suite 130
Kansas City, MO 64105
816-627-3420
Fax: 816-268-3420
greenfoundation@gkccf.org
www.greenfdn.org
Matthew Fuller, Manager of Community Investment
While the Foundation makes grants in a variety of fields, in the past its major support was in the field of medical research. During a 20-year period, 1951-71, it contributed over $900,000 to research in Parkinson's and related diseases of the nervous system; $600,000 for research in pediatric neurology and lesser amounts in other areas of medical research, but the board is now trending in other directions. Grants are limited to Missouri and none are offered to individuals.

3071 **Anheuser-Busch**
1 Busch Pl
Saint Louis, MO 63118-1852
314-577-2000
800-342-5283
Fax: 314-577-2900
anheuser-busch.com
August A Busch Iv, President

Supports education, helped fund health and human services organizations, provided disaster relief, and worked to preserve the environment.

3072 Arc of the US Missouri Chapter
PO Box 7823
Columbia, MO 65205
573-552-7648
www.arcofmissouri.org

3073 Greater Kansas City Community Foundation & Affiliated Trusts
1055 Broadway Blvd
Suite 130
Kansas City, MO 64105-1595
816-842-0944
866-719-7886
Fax: 816-842-8079
info@gkccf.org
www.growyourgiving.org

William S. Berkley, Past Chair
Dr. Jim Hinson, Vice Chair
William H. Coughlin, President
Mary Bloch, Community Volunteer

Mission is to improve the quality of life in Greater Kansas City by increasing charitable giving, connecting donors to community needs they care about, and providing leadership on critical community issues.

3074 Greater St Louis Community Foundation
319 N 4th St
Ste 300
Saint Louis, MO 63102-1906
314-588-8200
Fax: 314-588-8088

Stephen J. Rafferty, Chair
Thomas R. Collins, Vice Chair & Secretary
Amelia A.J. Bond, President & CEO
Mara Mitch Meyers, Treasurer

To improve the quality of life across the region by helping individuals, families and businesses make a difference through charitable giving.

3075 H&R Block Foundation
1 H and R Block Way
Kansas City, MO 64105-1905
816-854-4363
Fax: 816-854-8025
foundation@hrblock.com
www.blockfoundation.org

Henry W. Bloch, Chairman/ Treasurer/ Director
Thomas M. Bloch, Vice Chairman & Director
David P. Miles, President
Carey Wilker Looney, Vice President and Secretary

A charitable organization under the not-for-profit corporation law of the state of Missouri. Grants are made only to organizations which are tax exempt from Federal Income taxation and which are not classified as private foundations. Major emphasis is placed in the metropolitan areas of Kansas City, Missouri: and Columbus, Ohio. The goal is to provide proportionately significant support of relatively few activities, as opposed to minor support for a great many.

3076 James S McDonnell Foundation
1034 S Brentwood Blvd
Suite 1850
Saint Louis, MO 63117- 1284
314-721-1532
Fax: 314-721-7421
info@jsmf.org
jsmf.org

Susan M Fitzpatrick, President
John T. Bruer, President Emeritus
Cheryl A. Washington, Grants Manager
M. Brent Dolezalek, Senior Program Associate

The Foundation supports scientific, educational, and charitable causes locally, nationally and internationally.

3077 Lutheran Charities Foundation of St Louis
8860 Ladue Road
Suite 200
Saint Louis, MO 63124
314-231-2244
Fax: 314-727-7688
info@lutheranfoundation.org
www.lutheranfoundation.org

Karl A. Dunajcik, Chairperson of the Board
Ann L. Vazquez, President/ CEO
Melinda K. McAliney, Program Director
Donna Luker, Office/Grants Manager

Seeks the improved care of people in the greater St. Louis metropolitan region. Lutheran Foundation of St. Louis manages the endowment established upon the sale of the Lutheran Medical Center and provides grant awards for health, human care, Lutheran congregations' community service programs, and Lutheran education.

3078 RA Bloch Cancer Foundation
1 H and R Block Way
Kansas City, MO 64105-1905
816-854-5050
800-433-0464
Fax: 816-854-8024
hotline@blochcancer.org
www.blochcancer.org

Vangie Rich, Executive Director
Rosanne Wickman, Hotline Director

Provides a hotline that matches newly diagnosed cancer patients with someone who has survived the same kind of cancer. Offers free infomration, resources and support groups, and distributes lists of multidisciplinary second opinion centers. Also supplies three books at no charge: Fighting Cancer; Cancer... There's Hope; and A Guide for Cancer Supporters. All services and books are free of charge.

3079 Victor E Speas Foundation
10434 Indiana Ave
Kansas City, MO 64137-1532
816-868-9300
mo.grantmaking@ustrust.com
www.bankofamerica.com

Latricia Scott Adams, President

VCC is a membership-based organization that brings together area volunteer managers and others interested in volunteerism for mutual support, exchange of ideas and information, and educational programs of timely interest.

Nebraska

3080 Arc of Nebraska
215 Centennial Mall South
Suite 508
Lincoln, NE 68508
402-475-4407
888-519-6524
Fax: 402-475-0214
info@arc-nebraska.org
www.arc-nebraska.org

Debbie Salomon, President
David Rowe, 1st Vice President
Kadi Holmberg, 2nd Vice President
Michael Chittenden, Executive Director

Arc of Nebraska is commited to helping children and adults with disabilities secure the oppurtunity to choose and realize their goals of where and how they learn, live, work, and play.

3081 Cooper Foundation
1248 O St
Suite 870
Lincoln, NE 68508-1493
402-476-7571
Fax: 402-476-2356
info@cooperfoundation.org
cooperfoundation.org

Jack Campbell, Chair
Brad Korell, VP Business Development
Art Thompson, President
Robert Nefsky, Attorney & Partner

Serves only Nebraska with the primary interest in education, arts and humanities and the human services area.

3082 **Mosaic**
4980 S 118th St
Omaha, NE 68137-2200
402-896-9988
877-366-7242
Fax: 402-896-1511
info@mosaicinfo.org
www.mosaicinfo.org

Linda Timmons, President / CEO
Cindy Schroeder, Chief Financial Officer
Raul Saldivar, Chief Operating Officer
Scott Hoffman, Senior Vice President of Finance

Headquarters for the faith-based organization providing services to people with disabilities in communities nationwide, and in conjunction with international partners. Mosaic was born of a merger of these two Lutheran organizations: Bethpage and Martin Luther Homes Society.

3083 **Slosburg Family Charitable Trust**
10040 Regency Cir
Ste 200
Omaha, NE 68114-3734
402-391-7900
Fax: 402-391-2991
richdale.com

David Slosburg, Owner

3084 **Union Pacific Foundation**
1400 Douglas Street
Omaha, NE 68179
402-544-5000
888-870-8777
888-877-7267
Fax: 402-501-0021
www.up.com

John J. Koraleski, Executive Chairman
Lance M. Fritz, President & COO of Union Pacific
Eric L. Butler, EVP, Marketing and Sales
Diane K. Duren, EVP/ Corporate Secretary

The Union Pacific Foundation is the philanthropic arm of the Union Pacific Corporation and Union Pacific Railroad. Union Pacific believes that the quality of life in the commuinities in which its employees live and work is an integral part of its own success.

Nevada

3085 **EL Wiegand Foundation**
165 W Liberty St
Suite 200
Reno, NV 89501-1955
775-333-0310
Fax: 775-333-0314
www.thewiegandfoundationinc.com

Kristen A Avansino, President/Executive Director

3086 **Nell J Redfield Foundation**
PO Box 61
Reno, NV 89504-0061
775-323-1373
Fax: 775-323-4476
redfieldfoundation@yahoo.com

Jerry Smith, Manager
Gerald C. Smith, V.P. and Secy

3087 **William N Pennington Foundation**
441 W Plumb Ln
Reno, NV 89509-3766
775-333-9100
Fax: 775-333-9111

William Pennington, Owner

New Hampshire

3088 **Agnes M Lindsay Trust**
660 Chestnut St
Manchester, NH 03104-3550
603-669-1366
866-669-1366
Fax: 603-665-8114
admin@lindsaytrust.org
lindsaytrust.org

Susan E. Bouchard, Administrative Director
Ernest E. Dion, CPA, Trustee
Alan G. Lampert, Esq., Trustee
Michael S. Delucia, Esq., Trustee

Funding for health and wefare organizations, special needs, mental health, blind, deaf and cultural programs to organizations, specifically for capital needs, not operating funds, located in the New England states of Maine, Massachusetts, New Hampshire and Vermont. We highly recommend you visit our web site.

3089 **Foundation for Seacoast Health**
100 Campus Dr
Ste 1
Portsmouth, NH 03801-5892
603-422-8200
Fax: 603-422-8206
ffsh@communitycampus.org
ffsh.org

Debra S. Grabowski, Executive Director
Kathleen Taylor, Finance Director
Eligio Santana, Facility Manager
Noreen Hodgdon, Executive Assistant

Giving limited to Portsmouth, Rye, New Castle, Greenland, Newington, North Hampton, NH; and Kittery, Eliot, and York, ME.

New Jersey

3090 **American Migraine Foundation**
19 Mantua Rd.
Mount Royal, NJ 08061
856-423-0043
Fax: 856-423-0082
amf@talley.com
www.achenet.org

Lawrence C. Newman, MD, FAHS, Chair
Christine Lay, MD, FAHS, Vice-Chair
Nim Lalvani, MPH, Executive Director

Nonprofit, patient-health, professional partnership dedicated to advancing the treatment and management of headaches and to raising the public awareness of headache as valid, biologically based illness.

3091 **Arc of New Jersey**
985 Livingston Ave
N Brunswick, NJ 08902-1843
732-246-2525
Fax: 732-214-1834
arcnj.org

Robert Hage, President
Joanne Bergin, First Vice President
Kevin Sturges, Second Vice President
Elspeth Moore, Secretary

The Arc of New Jersey is committed to enhancing the quality of life of children and adults with intellectual and developmental disabilities and their families, through advocacy, empowerment, education and prevention.

3092 **Arnold A Schwartz Foundation**
15 Mountain Blvd
Warren, NJ 7059-5611
908-757-7800
Fax: 908-757-8039

Steven A Kunzman, President

3093 **Campbell Soup Foundation**
1 Campbell Pl
Camden, NJ 08103-1701
800-257-8443
media@campbellsoup.com
campbellsoup.com

Denise M. Morrison, President/ CEO
Anthony P. DiSilvestro, Senior Vice President and Chief
Mark Alexander, President
Carlos J. Barraso, Senior Vice President - Global R

Goal of this foundation is to match the company's assets with community needs in order to help forge solutions to community challenges. The Foundation believes that involvement at the community level can play a catalytic role in improving the quality of life. Giving is located in the areas of education, nutrition and health, cultural and youth related programs. The major focus of the foundation is on nutrition and health related matters, and places a high priority on Camden, New Jersey areas.

3094 **Children's Hopes & Dreams Wish Fulfillment Foundation**
280 US Highway 46
Dover, NJ 07801-2084 — 706-482-2248
Fax: 706-482-2289

3095 **Community Foundation of New Jersey**
35 Knox Hill Road Morristown
PO Box 338
Morristown, NJ 07963-0388 — 973-267-5533
800-659-5533
Fax: 973-267-2903
info@cfnj.org
www.cfnj.org

Hans Dekker, President
Madeline Rivera, Program Officer
Susan I. Soldivieri, Chief Financial Officer
Faith Krueger, Chief Operating Officer

The Community Foundation of New Jersey is an alliance of families, businesses, and foundations that work together to create lasting differences in lives and communities today and tomorrow.

3096 **FM Kirby Foundation**
17 DeHart Street
PO Box 151
Morristown, NJ 07963-0151 — 973-538-4800
www.fdncenter.org/grantmaker/kirby

S. Dillard Kirby, President and Director
Jefferson W Kirby, Vice President and Director
Alice Kirby Horton, Assistant Secretary and Director
Walker D. Kirby, Director

Family foundation, grants made to a wide range of nonprofit organizations in education, health and medicine, the arts and humanities, civic and public affairs, as well as religious, welfare and youth organizations.

3097 **Fannie E Rippel Foundation**
14 Maple Avenue
Suite 200
Morristown, NJ 07960 — 973-540-0101
Fax: 973-540-0404
info@rippelfoundation.org
www.rippelfoundation.org

Laura K Landy, President/ CEO
Chana Fitton, Chief Operating Officer
John D. Campbell, Chairman
Elizabeth G. Christopherson, Secretary

Core purposes: research and treatment related to cancer and heart disease, the health of women and the elderly, and the quality of our nation's hospitals.

3098 **Fund for New Jersey**
One Palmer Square East
Suite 303
Princeton, NJ 08542 — 609-356-0421
fundfornj.org

Kiki Jamieson, President
Lucy Vandenberg, Senior Program Officer
Laura Mandell, Office Manager
Ami Kachalia, Program Associate

Our grants promote projects that share a high purpose of furthering effective democracy through a range of methods encompassing education, advocacy, public policy analysis, and community problem-solving.

3099 **Merck Company Foundation**
2000 Galloping Hill Road
Kenilworth, NJ 07033 — 908-740-4000
merck.com

Kenneth C. Frazier, Chairman
Robert M. Davis, Executive Vice President and Chi
Willie A. Deese, EVP and President, Merck Manufac
Clark Golestani, Executive Vice President and Chi

Mission of the foundation is to support organizations and innovative programs in alignment with four strategic profiles: Improving access to quality health care and the appropriate use of medicines and vaccines,building capacity in the biomedical and health sciences, promoting environments that support innovation, economic growth and development in and ethical and fair context, and supporting communities where Merck employees work and live.

3100 **Nabisco Foundation**
7 Campus Dr
Parsippany, NJ 07054-4413 — 973-682-7096
Fax: 973-503-3018

Henry Sandbach, Director

3101 **Ostberg Foundation**
PO Box 1098
Alpine, NJ 07620-1098 — 201-569-6800
Fax: 201-767-8006

3102 **Prudential Foundation**
Prudential Financial
751 Broad St
15th Floor
Newark, NJ 07102-3714 — 973-802-6000
Fax: 973-802-7486
community.resources@prudential.com
prudential.com

John R Strangfeld, Chairman and CEO
Mark B. Grier, Vice Chairman
Charles Lowrey, Executive Vice President, Chief
Sharon C. Taylor, Senior Vice President, Corporate

Gives priority to national programs that further our objectives and programs serving areas where The Prudential has a substantial employee presence. Places special emphasis on the home state of New Jersey and the headquarters city, Newark.

3103 **Robert Wood Johnson Foundation**
Route 1 and College Road East
P.O. Box 2316
Princeton, NJ 08543-2316 — 609-452-8701
877-843-7953
Fax: 888-727-1966
mail@rwjf.org
rwjf.org

Roger S. Fine, Chairman
Risa Lavizzo-Mourey, President and CEO
Robin E. Mockenhaupt, Chief of Staff
Joan F. McKay, Executive Assistant, Executive O

Our mission is to assure that all Americans have access to basic health care at reasonable cost, improve care and support for people with chronic health conditions, promote healthy communities and lifestyles and also, reduce the personal, social and economic harm caused by substance abuse.

3104 **Victoria Foundation**
31 Mulberry Street
5th Floor
Newark, NJ 07102-1397 — 973-792-9200
Fax: 973-792-1300
info@victoriafoundation.org
www.victoriafoundation.org

Frank Alvarez, President
Margaret H. Parker, Vice President
Gary M. Wingens, Treasurer
Irene Cooper-Basch, Executive Officer

Desire is to help individuals in need reach their potential remains. Provides emergency coal for needy families and treated rheumatic fever in children.

New Mexico

3105 **Arc of New Mexico**
3655 Carlisle NE
Albuquerque, NM 87110-1644
505-883-4630
800-358-6493
Fax: 505-883-5564
rcostales@arcnm.org
arcnm.org

John Hall, President
Dolores Harden, Senior Vice President
Elaine Palma, Secretary
Randy Costales, Executive Director

Our mission is to improve the quality of life for individuals with developmental disabilities of all ages by advocating for equal opportunities and choices in where and how they learn, live, work, play and socialize. The Arc of New Mexico promotes self-determination, healthy families, effective community support systems and partnerships.

3106 **Frost Foundation**
511 Armijo St
Suite A
Santa Fe, NM 87501-2899
505-986-0208
info@frostfound.org
frostfound.org

Mary Amelia Whited-Howell, President
Philip B. Howell, Executive Vice President
Taylor F. Moore, Secretary/Treasurer
Ann Rogers Gerber, Board Member

The Frost Foundation was created to be operated excusively for educational, charitable, and religious purposes.

3107 **McCune Charitable Foundation**
345 E Alameda St
Santa Fe, NM 87501-2229
505-983-8300
Fax: 505-983-7887
mccune@nmmccune.org
nmmccune.org

Sarah McCune Losinger, Chair
Wendy Lewis, Executive Director
Henry Rael, Program Officer
Carla Romero, Administrative Director

Dedicated to enriching the health, education, environment, and cultural and spiritual life of New Mexicans.

3108 **Santa Fe Community Foundation**
501 Halona Street
Santa Fe, NM 87505
505-988-9715
Fax: 505-988-1829
foundation@santafecf.org
www.santafecf.org

Suzanne Ortega Cisneros, Chair
Barry Herskowitz, Vice Chair
Kenneth Romero, Secretary
Stephen G. Gaber, Treasurer

New York

3109 **AFB Center on Vision Loss**
American Foundation for the Blind
2 Penn Plaza
Suite 1102
New York, NY 10121-4524
212-502-7600
Fax: 888-545-8331
afbinfo@afb.net
afb.org

Carl R Augusto, President & CEO
Kelly Bleach, Chief Administrative Officer
Rick Bozeman, Chief Financial Officer
Paul Schroeder, Vice President

National nonprofit organization that expands possibilities for people with vision loss.

3110 **AT&T Foundation**
32 Avenue of the Americas
24th Floor
New York, NY 10013-2473
212-226-2216
Fax: 212-387-5097
info@att.com
www.att.com

Randall L Stephenson, Chairman, Chief Executive Office
John T. Stanky, Group President and Chief Strate
Wayne Watts, Senior Executive Vice President
John Stephens, Senior Executive Vice President

Committed to advancing education, strengthening communities and improving lives.

3111 **Altman Foundation**
521 5th Ave
Fl 35
New York, NY 10175-3500
212-682-0970
Fax: 212-682-1648
info@altman.org
altmanfoundation.org

Karen L. Rosa, President
Jeremy Tennenbaum, Chief Financial Officer
Ann E. Maldonado, Office Manager
Megan McAllister, Program Officer

For the benefit of such charitable and educational institutions in the City of New York as said directors shall approve. Foundation grants support programs and institutions that enrich the quality of life in the city, with a particular focus on initiatives that help individuals, families and communities benefit from the services and opportunities that will enable them to achieve their full potential.

3112 **Ambrose Monell Foundation**
1 Rockefeller Plz
Suite 301
New York, NY 10020-2002
212-586-0700
Fax: 212-245-1863
www.monellvetlesen.org

Ambrose K. Monell, President and Treasurer
Eugene P. Grisanti, Vice-President
George Rowe, Vice-President
Kristen G. Pemberton, Secretary

Voluntary aiding and contributing to religious, charitable, scientific, literary, and educational uses and purposes, in New York, elsewhere in the US and throughout the world.

3113 **American Chai Trust**
41 Madison Ave
Suite 400
New York, NY 10010-2202
212-889-0575
Fax: 212-743-8120
info@perlmanandperlman.com
www.perlmanandperlman.com

3114 **American Foundation for Suicide Prevention (AFSP)**
199 Water St.
11th Floor
New York, NY 10038
212-363-3500
888-333-2377
Fax: 212-363-6237
info@afsp.org
afsp.org

Robert Gebbia, Chief Executive Officer
Christine Yu Moutier, Chief Medical Officer
Stephanie Rogers, Senior Vice President, Communications & Marketing
Michael F. Lamma, Senior Vice President, Development & Field Management

The American Foundation for Suicide Prevention is a voluntary health organization that gives those affected by suicide a nationwide community empowered by research, education, and advocacy to take action against this disease. AFSP achieves their goal by funding scientific research, educating the public about mental health and suicide prevention, and supporting survivors of suicide loss and all those affected by suicide.

3115 **American Foundation for the Blind**
2 Penn Plaza
Suite 1102
New York, NY 10121
800-232-5463
www.afb.org

Kirk Adams, President & CEO
Darren M. Davis, Executive Administrator Executive Office

The American Foundation for the Blind (AFB) is a national nonprofit that is dedicated to removing barriers, creating solutions, and expanding possibilities for the blind and visually impaired. The AFB is focused on spreading access to technology, elevating the quality of information and tools for professional who serve people with vision loss, and the promotion of independent living for those with vision loss.

3116 **Arthur Ross Foundation**
20 E 74th St
Ste 4c
New York, NY 10021-2654
212-737-7311
Fax: 212-650-0332

Arthur Ross, President

3117 **Artists Fellowship**
47 5th Ave
New York, NY 10003-4303
212-255-7740
info@artistsfellowship.org
www.artistsfellowship.org

Babette Bloch, President

Private, charitable foundation that assists professional fine arts and their families in times of emergency, disability, or bereavement.

3118 **Bodman Foundation**
767 3rd Ave
4th Floor
New York, NY 10017-2023
212-644-0322
Fax: 212-759-6510

John N. Irwin III, Chairman
Russell P. Pennoyer, President
Peter Frelinghuysen, Vice President
John B. Krieger, Executive Director

Foundation concentrates their grant programs in New York City, but foundation also makes some grants in Northern New Jersey. Funding is concentrated in six program areas: Arts & Culture, Education, Employment, Health, Public Policy and Youth and Families.

3119 **Brain & Behavior Research Foundation**
747 Third Ave.
33rd Floor
New York, NY 10017
646-681-4888
800-829-8289
info@bbrfoundation.org
bbrfoundation.org

Jeffrey Borenstein, President & CEO
Louis Innamorato, Vice President, Finance & Chief Financial Officer
Lauren Duran, Vice President, Communications, Marketing & PR
Faith Rothblatt, Vice President, Development

The Brain & Behavior Research Foundation is a nonprofit organization committed to alleviating the suffering caused by mental illness by awarding grants in the field of mental health research.

3120 **Brooklyn Home for Aged Men**
P.O. Box 280062
Brooklyn, NY 11228
718-745-1638
Fax: 718-745-0813
www.brooklynhome.org

Catherine M. Birdseye, Co-President
William E. Spaulding, Co-President
Andelusia Wheeler, Co-President
Edwin A. Ames, Co-President

The Brooklyn Home For Aged Men has served the community for more than one hundred years. Although originally set up as a residence for men, it later accepted women and couples as well.

3121 **Cancer Care**
275 7th Avenue
22nd Floor
New York, NY 10001-6754
212-712-8400
800-813-4673
Fax: 212-712-8495
info@cancercare.org
www.cancercare.org

Patricia J. Goldsmith, Chief Executive Officer
John Rutigliano, Chief Operating Officer
Sue Lee, Senior Director of Development
Ann Navarria, Director of Human Resources

A national non-profit organization that provides free, professional support services to anyone affected by cancer: people with cancer, caregivers, children, loved ones, and the bereaved.

3122 **Children's Tumor Foundation**
120 Wall Street
16th Floor
New York, NY 10005-3904
212-344-6633
800-323-7938
Fax: 212-747-0004
info@ctf.org
ctf.org

Linda Halliday Martin, Chairperson
Colin Bryar, Vice Chairperson
Annette Bakker, PhD, President and Chief Scientific Officer
Tracy Galloway, Secretary

A nonprofit 501 (c) (3) medical foundation, dedicated to improving the health and well-being of individuals and families affected by neurofibromatosis. The Foundation sponsors medical research, clinical services, public education programs and patient support services. It is the central source for up-to-date and accurate information about NF. It also assists patients and families with referrals to NF clinics and healthcare professionals specializing in NF. The goal is to find a cure for NF.

3123 **Commonwealth Fund**
1 E 75th St
New York, NY 10021-2692
212-606-3800
Fax: 212-606-3500
info@cmwf.org
www.commonwealthfund.org

Benjamin K. Chu, Chairman
Cristine Russell, Vice Chairman
Donald Moulds, Executive Vice President for Pro
Barry Scholl, Senior Vice President for Commun

A private foundation with the broad charge to enhance the common good. Carries out this mandate by supporting efforts that help people live healthy and productive lives, and by assisting certain groups with serious and neglected problems. Supports independent research on health and social issues and makes grants to improve heathcare practice and policy.

3124 **Community Foundation for Greater Buffalo**
726 Exchange Street,
Suite 525
Buffalo, NY 14210
716-852-2857
Fax: 716-852-2861
mail@cfgb.org
cfgb.org

Marsha Joy Sullivan, Chair
William Joyce, Vice Chair
Gary L. Mucci, Secretary
Ross Eckert, Treasurer

Mission is connecting people, ideas, and resources to improve lives in Western New York

3125 **Community Foundation of Herkimer & Oneida Counties**
2608 Genesee Street
Utica, NY 13502-4728
315-735-8212
Fax: 315-735-9363
info@foundationhoc.org
foundationhoc.org

Alicia Dicks, President/CEO
Gilles Lauzon, Director of Finance
Elayne Johnson, Director of Fund Administration
Laura Cohen, Program Officer

Mission of the foundation is to improve the lives of the residents of Herkimer and Oneida Counties.

3126 **Community Foundation of the Capitol Region**
Six Tower Place
Albany, NY 12203-3749
518-446-9638
Fax: 518-446-9708
info@cfgcr.org
www.cfgcr.org

Karen Bilowith, President/CEO
Mindy Derosia, Development Officer
Shelly Connolly, Program Assistant
Jackie Mahoney, Vice President of Programs
Mission is to strengthen our community by attracting charitable endowments both large and small, maximizing benefits to donors, making effective gtants, and providing leadership to address community needs.

3127 **Comsearch: Broad Topics**
Foundation Center
79 5th Ave
New York, NY 10003-3034
212-620-4230
800-424-9836
Fax: 212-807-3677
communications@foundationcenter.org
www.fdncenter.org

Bradford K. Smith, President
Lisa Philip, Vice President for Strategic Phi
Jen Bokoff, Director of GrantCraft
Steven Lawrence, Director of Research
Subset publications of The Foundation Grants Index, are printouts of actual foundation grants, covering 26 key areas of grantmaking. This tool is designed for fundraisers who wish to examine grantmaking activities in a broad field of interest.
$55.00

3128 **DE French Foundation**
Ste 503
120 Genesee St
Auburn, NY 13021-3672
315-252-3634
Walter Lowe, Owner

3129 **Dana Foundation**
Dana Alliance for Brain Initiatives
505 Fifth Avenue
6th floor
New York, NY 10017
212-223-4040
Fax: 212-317-8721
danainfo@dana.org
www.dana.org

Edward F Rover, President /Chairman
Burton M. Mirsky, Executive Vice President, Financ
Barbara Rich, Ed.D., EVP, Communications; Assistant S
Barbara E Gill, Executive Vice President
A private philanthropy with principal interests in brain science, immunology, and arts education.

3130 **David J Green Foundation**
Ste 12
599 Lexington Ave
New York, NY 10022-6030
212-317-8820
Fax: 212-371-5099

Valerie Ventolora, Manager
Michael Greene, Manager

3131 **Easterseals New York**
633 3rd Ave.
New York, NY 10017
212-943-4364
www.easterseals.com/newyork
Marianne Gribbon, Senior Director, Childhood Services
Robert Lambert, Director, Workforce & Veterans Services
Offers resources and expertise that allow children and adults with disabilities to live with dignity and independence. Provides programs and solutions that enhance the lives of people with disabilities, while heightening community awareness and acceptance.

3132 **Edna McConnel Clark Foundation**
415 Madison Ave
Tenth Floor
New York, NY 10017-7949
212-551-9100
Fax: 212-421-9325
info@emcf.org
emcf.org

Nancy Roob, President
Woodrow C. McCutchen, Vice President, Senior Portfolio
Kelly Fitzsimmons, Vice President, Chief Program an
Charles Harris, Portfolio Manager
Helps young people, ages 9-24, from low-income backgrounds become independent, productive adults.

3133 **Edward John Noble Foundation**
Fl 19
32 E 57th St
New York, NY 10022-8562
212-759-4212
Fax: 212-888-4531

June Noble Larkin, Owner
June Larkin, Owner

3134 **Epilepsy Foundation of Long Island**
1500 Hempstead Turnpike
East Meadow, NY 11554
516-739-7733
888-672-7154
Fax: 516-739-1860
efli.org

Thomas Hopkins, President & CEO
Paul Giotis, Chief Operating Officer
Lawrence Boord, Chief Financial Officer
Gladys Brown, Director of Intake Coordination
Provides education, counseling and residential care to Long Island residents with epilepsy and related conditions.

3135 **Episcopal Charities**
1047 Amsterdam Avenue
New York, NY 10025-1747
212-316-7575
episcopalcharities@dioceseny.org
episcopalcharities-newyork.org

John Talty, President
Lorraine A. LaHuta, Vice President
Evan A. Davis, Secretary
John P Banning, Treasurer
Provides funding and support to a broad range of community-based human service programs throughout the Diocese of New York. These programs, sponsored by Episcopal congregations, serve disadvantaged individuals, youth and families on a non-sectarian basis.

3136 **Esther A & Joseph Klingenstein Fund**
125 Park Ave.
Suite 1700
New York, NY 10017
212-492-6181
www.klingfund.org

3137 **Fay J Lindner Foundation**
189 Wheatley Road
Brookville, NY 11545
516-686-4440
www.fayjlindnercenter.org

Terrence Ullrich, President
Dr. Robert Steinberger, Vice President
Thomas F. Moore, Treasurer
Frederick Sterbenz, Secretary

3138 **Ford Foundation**
320 E 43rd St
New York, NY 10017-4890
212-573-5000
Fax: 212-351-3677
office-of-communications@fordfoundation.org
www.fordfound.org

Darren Walker, President
Kenneth T Monterio, Vice President, Secretary and Ge
Alfred Ironside, Vice President/Communications
Nicholas M. Gabriel, Vice President, Treasurer and Ch
A resource for innovative people and institutions worldwide. Goals are to: strenghthen democratic values; reduce poverty and injustice; promote international cooperation; and advance human achievement. While not specific to disabilities, the Ford Foundation operates on several levels that indirectly assist and support those with disabilities through human and civil rights issues, so-

cial justice support, economic fairness and opportunity, and access to education involvements.

3139 **Fortis Foundation**
28 Liberty Street
New York, NY 10005-1401
212-859-7197
Fax: 212-859-7010
ir.assurant.com
Elaine D. Rosen, Chair
Howard L. Carver, Director
Melissa Kivett, Senior Vice President, Investor
Suzanne Shepherd, Director, Investor Relations

3140 **Foundation Center**
79 5th Ave
16th Street
New York, NY 10003-3076
212-620-4230
800-424-9836
Fax: 212-807-3677
communications@foundationcenter.org
foundationcenter.org
Bradford K Smith, President
Lisa Philip, VP, Strategic Philanthropy
Jen Bokoff, Director of GrantCraft
Steven Lawrence, Director of Research
The Foundation Center publishes Foundation Directory Online, with key facts on the US grantmakers and their grants.

3141 **Foundation Center Library Services**
Foundation Center
79 5th Ave
16th Street
New York, NY 10003-3076
212-620-4230
800-424-9836
Fax: 212-807-3677
communications@foundationcenter.org
foundationcenter.org
Bradford K Smith, President
Lisa Philip, VP, Strategic Philanthropy
Jen Bokoff, Director of GrantCraft
Steven Lawrence, Director of Research
The Center disseminates current information on foundation and corporate giving through our national collections in New York City and Washington D.C., our field offices in San Francisco and our network of over 180 cooperating libraries in all 50 states and abroad.

3142 **Foundation for Advancement in Cancer Therapy**
PO Box 1242
Old Chelsea Station
New York, NY 10113-1242
212-675-6349
info@rethinkingcancer.org
www.rethinkingcancer.org
Ruth Sackman, Founder
A clearinghouse for information regarding alternative cancer therapies, emphasizing nutritional and metabolic approaches.

3143 **Gebbie Foundation**
215 Cherry St
Jamestown, NY 14701-5207
716-487-1062
Fax: 716-484-6401
info@gebbie.org
www.gebbie.org
Gregory J Edwards, CEO
Daniel Kathman, President
Jonathan Taber, Vice President
Nancy Gleason, Secretary
Giving in Chautauqua County, and secondly, in neighboring areas of western New York. Giving is offered in other areas only when the project is consonant with program objectives that cannot be developed locally.

3144 **Gladys Brooks Foundation**
1055 Franklin Avenue
Suite 208
Garden City, NY 11530
www.gladysbrooksfoundation.org
Jessica L Rutledge, Director
The purpose of this Foundation is to provide for the intellectual, moral and physical welfare of the people of this country by establishing and supporting nonprofit libraries, educational institutions, hospitals and clinics. The Foundation will make grants only to private, publicly supported, nonprofit, tax-exempt organizations.

3145 **Glickenhaus Foundation**
546 5th Ave
New York, NY 10036-5000
212-953-7800
info@glickenhaus.com
Seth M. Glickenhaus, Senior Partner and Chief Investm

3146 **Guide Dog Foundation for the Blind**
371 East Jericho Turnpike
Smithtown, NY 11787-2976
631-930-9000
800-548-4337
Fax: 631-930-9009
info@guidedog.org
www.guidedog.org
James C. Bingham, Chair
Alphonce J. Brown, Vice Chair
Barbara J. Kelly, Secretary
Donald Dea, Treasurer
Providing mobility through the use of trained guide or service dogs to individuals who are blind or with other special needs.

3147 **Hearing Health Foundation (HHF)**
575 Eighth Ave.
Suite 1201
New York, NY 10018
212-257-6140
866-454-3924
Fax: 212-257-6139
TTY: 888-435-6104
info@hhf.org
hearinghealthfoundation.org
Timothy Higdon, President & CEO
Noemi Disla, Director, Finance, Operations & Administration
Christopher Geissler, Director, Program & Research Support
Lauren McGrath, Director, Marketing & Communications
Hearing Health Foundation promotes hearing health and advocates for the prevention and cure of hearing loss and tinnitus through research.

3148 **Hearst Foundations**
300 W 57th St
Fl 26
New York, NY 10019-3741
212-649-2000
Fax: 212-887-6855
hearst.com
Steven R. Swartz, President and Chief Executive Of
National philanthropic resources for organziations and institutions working in the fields of education, health, culture and social services. Our goal is to ensure that people of all backgrounds have the opportunity to build healthy, productive and inspiring lives.

3149 **Henry and Lucy Moses Fund**
405 Lexington Ave
New York, NY 10174-1299
212-554-7800
Fax: 212-554-7700
www.mosessinger.com
Irving Sitnick, President
Provides legal services to many prominent industries, individuals and families in the New York City area.

3150 **Herman Goldman Foundation**
Fl 18
61 Broadway
New York, NY 10006-2708
212-797-9090
Alan Nisselson, President
A private nonoperating foundation.

3151 **Kenneth & Evelyn Lipper Foundation**
Fl 6
101 Park Ave
New York, NY 10178
212-883-6333
Kenneth Lipper, Director

3152 **Long Island Alzheimer's Foundation**
5 Channel Drive
Port Washington, NY 11050-2216
516-767-6856
Fax: 516-767-6864
www.liaf.org

Paul Eibeler, Chairman
Fred Jenny, Executive Director
Sean Phillips, Director of Development
Tiffany Ewald, Program Assistant

3153 **Louis and Anne Abrons Foundation**
First Manhattan Company
399 Park Avenue
New York, NY 10022-7001
212-756-3300
Fax: 212-223-4175
firstmanhattan.com

David Manischewitz, CEO
Sam Colin, Senior Managing Director
Allan Glick, Senior Managing Director
Neal Sterns, Senior Managing Director

3154 **Margaret L Wendt Foundation**
Ste 277
40 Fountain Plz
Buffalo, NY 14202-2200
716-855-2146
Fax: 716-855-2149

Robert J Kresse, Manager

3155 **Merrill Lynch & Company Foundation**
250 Vesey St
New York, NY 10080
212-449-1000
800-637-7455
Fax: 212-449-7969
ml.com

Brian T Moynihan, CEO
John Theil, Head
Andy M Sieg, Managing Director
John Hogarty, Chief Operating Officer

Ongoing support for the arts, health, human services, and civic issues. Merrill Lynch's philanthropic priority is a sustained investment in education. Q992

3156 **Metzger-Price Fund**
Ste 2300
230 Park Ave
New York, NY 10169
212-867-9500
Fax: 212-599-1759

Isaac A Saufer, Secretary/Treasurer

3157 **Milbank Foundation for Rehabilitation**
116 Village Boulevard
Suite 200
New York, NY 08540
609-951-2283
Fax: 609-951-2281
fdnweb.org/milbank

Jeremiah M. Bogert, Chairman & Secretary
Jeremiah Milbank III, President and Treasurer
Carl Helstrom, Executive Director
Carmel Mazzola, Administrative Assistant

Awarding grants from trust funds based on a competitive selection process or the preferences of the foundation managers and granters. The foundations mission is to integrate people with disabilities into all aspects of american life. Current priorities include, but are not limited to: consumer-focused initiatives that enable people with disablities to lead fulfilling,independent lives; innovative policy research and education on market-based approaches to health care and rehabilitation...

3158 **Morgan Stanley Foundation**
1585 Broadway
New York, NY 10036-8293
212-761-4000
Fax: 212-761-0086
mediainquiries@morganstanley.com
morganstanley.com

James P. Gorman, Chairman and Chief Executive Off
Thomas Nides, Vice Chairman
Jeff Brodsky, Chief Human Resources Officer
Jim Rosenthal, Chief Operating Officer

Our overachieving mission is threefold: build the potential of individuals and families, encourage and support our employees charitable efforts, and strengthen relationships with our communities.

3159 **National Foundation for Facial Reconstruction**
333 East 30th St.
Lobby Office
New York, NY 10016-4974
212-263-6656
Fax: 212-263-7534
info@myface.org
myface.org

Barbara H. Zuckerberg, President
John R. Gordon, Chairman
Sondra Neuschotz, Secretary
Jeremiah M. Bogert, Treasurer

A nonprofit organization whose major purposes are to provide facilities for the treatment and assistance of individuals who are unable to afford private reconstructive surgical care, to train and educate professionals in this surgery, to encourage research in the field and to carry on public education.

3160 **National Hemophilia Foundation**
7 Penn Plaza
Suite 1204
New York, NY 10001
212-328-3700
888-463-6643
Fax: 212-328-3777
info@hemophilia.org
www.hemophilia.org

Leonard Valentino, President & CEO
Dawn Rotellini, Chief Operating Officer
Kevin Mills, Chief Scientific Officer
Michelle Rice, Chief External Affairs Officer

Dedicated to finding better treatments and cures for bleeding and clotting disorders and to preventing the complications of these disorders through education, advocacy and research.

3161 **Neisloss Family Foundation**
Ste 7
1737 Veterans Hwy
Central Islip, NY 11749-1533
631-234-1600
Fax: 631-234-1066

Stanley Neisloss, President/Owner

3162 **New York Community Trust**
909 3rd Ave
22nd Floor
New York, NY 10022-4752
212-686-0010
Fax: 212-532-8528
aw@nyct-cfi.org
nycommunitytrust.org

Lorie A Slutsky, President
Carolyn M Weiss, CFO
Mary Z. Greenebaum, Chief Investment Officer
Eileen Casey, Director of Investment Reporting

Our goal is to out charitable money to work, making grants to the city's nonprofit community and building an endowment to tackle future problems.

3163 **New York Foundation**
10 E 34th St
10th Floor
New York, NY 10016-4327
212-594-8009
info@nyf.org
nyf.org

Marlene Provizer, Chair
Roger Schwed, Vice Chair
Sue A Kaplan, Secretary
Gail Gordon, Treasurer

Grants are given that involve New York City or a particular neighborhood of the city. Emphasize advocacy and community organizing. Address a critical need or disadvantaged population, particularly youth or the elderly. Are strongly identified with a particular community. Require an amount of funding to which a Foundation grant would make a substantial contribution. And can show a clear role for the Foundation's funds.

3164 Northern New York Community Foundation
120 Washington St
Suite 400
Watertown, NY 13601-3376
315-782-7110
Fax: 315-782-0047
info@nnycf.org
www.nnycf.org

Joseph W. Russell, President
Linda S. Merrell, Vice President
Jacquelyn A. Schell, Secretary
Rande S. Richardson, Executive Director

Raises, manages and administers an endowment and collection of funds for the benefit of the community

3165 Parkinson's Disease Foundation
1359 Broadway
Room 1509
New York, NY 10018-7867
212-923-4700
800-457-6676
Fax: 212-923-4778
info@pdf.org
www.pdf.org

Howard D Morgan, Chair
Constance Atwell, Vice Chair
Isobel Konecky, Secretary
Stephen Ackerman, Treasurer

The Parkinson's Disease Foundation is a leading national presence in Parkinson's disease research, education and public advocacy. We are working for the nearly one million people in the US who live with Parkinson's by funding promising scientific research to find the causes of and a cure for Parkinson's while supporting people with Parkinson's, their families and caregivers through educational programs and support services.

3166 Peter and Elizabeth C. Tower Foundation
2351 North Forest Rd.
Suite 106
Getzville, NY 14068-1225
716-689-0370
Fax: 716-689-3716
info@thetowerfoundation.org
thetowerfoundation.org

Tracy A. Sawicki, Executive Director
Donald W. Matteson, Chief Program Officer
Charles E. Colston Jr., Program Officer
Megan T. MacDavey, Program Officer

The Peter and Elizabeth C. Tower Foundation supports community programming that results in children, adolescents, and young adults affected by substance use disorders, learning disabilities, mental illness, and intellectual disabilities achieving their full potential.

3167 Reader's Digest Foundation
Readers Digest Association
Readers Digest Rd
Pleasantville, NY 10570
914-238-1000
Fax: 914-238-4559
letters@rd.com
rd.com

Mary G Berner, CEO

Dedicated to creating opportunities and promoting efforts that encourage individuals to make a positive difference in their communities, and to supporting programs designed to help young people learn, grow and enrich their lives.

3168 Research to Prevent Blindness
645 Madison Ave
Floor 21
New York, NY 10022-1010
212-752-4333
800-621-0026
Fax: 212-688-6231
www.rpbusa.org

Diane S. Swift, Chair
Brian F. Hofland PhD, President
David H Brenner, Vice President and Secretary
Richard E. Baker, Treasurer and Assistant Secretar

National voluntary health foundation supported by foundations, corporations and voluntary gifts and bequests from individuals. Established to stimulate basic and applied research into the causes, prevention and treatment of blinding eye diseases.

3169 Rita J and Stanley H Kaplan Foundation
Rm 306
866 United Nations Plz
New York, NY 10017-1822
212-688-1047
Fax: 212-688-6907
www.kaplanfoundation.org

Nancy Kaplan Belsky, President
Susan B. Kaplan, Vice President
Scott Kaplan Belsky, Secretary & Treasurer
Rebecca Tobin, Executive Director

3170 Robert Sterling Clark Foundation
135 E 64th St
New York, NY 10065-7045
212-288-8900
Fax: 212-288-1033
rscf@rsclark.org
rsclark.org

James Allen Smith, Chairman
Vincent McGee, President
Clara Miller, Treasurer
Julie Muraco, Secretary

Giving primarily in New York with emphasis on advocacy, research, and public education aimed at informing New York City of state policies.

3171 Skadden Fellowship Foundation
4 Times Sq
New York, NY 10036-6518
212-735-3000
Fax: 212-735-2000
info@skadden.com
www.skadden.com

Alan C Myers, Director
William Schumann, Legal Assistant

The aim of the Foundation is to give Fellows the freedom to pursue public intrest work, thus the Fellows create their own projects at public interest organizations with at least 2 lawyers on staff before they apply.

3172 St George's Society of New York
216 E 45th St
Suite 901
New York, NY 10017-3304
212-682-6110
Fax: 212-682-3465
info@stgeorgessociety.org
stgeorgessociety.org

John Shannon, Almoner
Anna Titley, Director of Operations and Commu
Samantha Hamilton, Director of Development and Memb
Daisy Rowan, Operations Executive

St George's Society provides monthly stipends to the elderly and the handicapped.

3173 Stanley W Metcalf Foundation
Ste 503
120 Genesee St
Auburn, NY 13021-3672
315-252-3634
Walter Lowe, Owner

3174 Stonewall Community Foundation
446 West 33rd Street
New York, NY 10001-1913
212-367-1155
Fax: 212-367-1157
stonewall@stonewallfoundation.org
www.stonewallfoundation.org

Dante Mastri, President
Neill Coleman, Vice President
Chris Davis, Secretary
Tina Salandra, Treasurer

Mission is to promote the well being of lesbian, gay, bisexual, and transgender (LGBT) individuals and strengthen the LGBT community. We do this by increasing resources; targeting those resources strategically to areas of greatest need; and by serving as a catalyst and clearinghouse for ideas and solutions. Through grant-making donor-advised funds, endowment funds and charitable education, Stonewall supports LGBT organizations and helps donors realize their philanthropic goals.

3175 **Surdna Foundation**
330 Madison Ave
30th Floor
New York, NY 10017-5016
212-557-0010
grants@surdna.org
surdna.org

Jocelyn Downie, Chairperson
Peter B Benedict, Vice Chairperson
Lawrence S.C Griffth, Secretary & Treasurer
Jonathan Goldberg, Director of Grants Management, L

The Foundation makes grants in the areas of environment, community revitalization, effective citizenry, the arts and the non-profit sector.

3176 **The Adaptive Sports Foundation**
100 Silverman Way
PO Box 266
Windham, NY 12496
518-734-5070
Fax: 518-734-6740
info@adaptivesportsfoundation.org
www.adaptivesportsfoundation.org

Robert W Stubbs, Chair
Todd Munn, Executive Director
Pam Greene, Program Director
Ginny Scahill, Administrative Director

The Adaptive Sports Foundation is a non-profit organization providing programs for children and adults with physical and cognitive disabilities. Programs center around outdoor physical activities and sports, including skiing and snowboarding, canoeing and cycling.

3177 **Tisch Foundation**
Fl 19
655 Madison Ave
New York, NY 10065-8043
212-521-2930
Fax: 212-521-2983

Mark J Krinsky, VP

3178 **Van Ameringen Foundation**
509 Madison Avenue
New York, NY 10022-5501
212-758-6221
Fax: 212-688-2105
info@vanamfound.org
www.vanamfound.org

Kenneth A. Kind, President / Treasurer
Steadman Westergaard, Vice President and Secretary
Eleanor Sypher, Executive Director
Helaine Williams, Office Manager

From its beginning the Foundation has sought to stimulate prevention, education, and direct care in the mental health field with an emphasis on those individuals and populations having an impoverished background and few opportunities, for whom appropriate intervention would produce positive change.

3179 **Verizon Foundation**
1 Verizon Way
Basking Ridge, NJ 07920-1097
866-247-2687
Fax: 908-630-2660
www.verizon.com

Lowell C McAdam, Chairman & CEO
Roy H Chestnutt, Executive Vice President
James J Gerace, Chief Communications Officer
Craig Silliman, Executive Vice President

Mission is to improve education, literacy, family safety and healthcare by supporting Verizon's commitment to deliver technology that touches life. We focus our philanthropic efforts on 3 areas: Education, Safety and Health. & Volunteerism.

3180 **Western New York Foundation**
11 Summer St
Third Floor
Buffalo, NY 14209-2256
716-839-4225
Fax: 716-883-1107
bgosch@wnyfoundation.org
www.wnyfoundation.org

Jennifer S. Johnson, Chairman
James A. W. McLeod, President
John N. W. Walsh III, Vice President
Theodore V. Buerger, Treasurer

The Western New York Foundation makes grants in the seven counties of Western New York State: Erie, Niagra, Genesee, Wyoming, Allegany, Cattaraugus and Chautauqua

3181 **William T Grant Foundation**
570 Lexington Avenue
18th Floor
New York, NY 10022-6837
212-752-0071
Fax: 212-752-1398
info@wtgrantfdn.org
wtgrantfoundation.org

Adam Gamoran, President
Vivian Tseng, Vice President, Program
Deborah McGinn, Vice President, Finance and Admi
Vivian Louie, Program Officer

Purpose is to further the understanding of human behavior through research. The mission focuses on improving the lives of youth ages 8 to 25 in the United States.

North Carolina

3182 **Arc of North Carolina**
343 East Six Forks Rd.
Suite 320
Raleigh, NC 27609
919-782-4632
800-662-8706
Fax: 919-782-4634
info@arcnc.org
www.arcnc.org

Adonis Brown, President
Robert Rusty Bradstock, Senior Vice President
Rhonda Schandevel, Secretary
Ed McShane, Treasurer

Committed to securing for all people with developmental disabilities the opportunity to choose and realize their goals of where and how they learn, live, work, and play.

3183 **Bob & Kay Timberlake Foundation**
1660 E Center Street Ext
Lexington, NC 27292-1309
336-243-7777
800-776-0822
Fax: 336-249-2469
bobtimberlake.com

Daniel Timberlake, President

3184 **Duke Endowment**
800 East Morehead Street
Charlotte, NC 28202-4012
704-376-0291
Fax: 704-376-9336
dukeendowment.org

Eugene W. Cochrane Jr., President
Arthur E. Morehead IV, Vice President/General Counsel
Susan L. McConnell, Director of Higher Education
Terri W. Honeycutt, Corporate Secretary

Mission is to serve the people of North Carolina and South Carolina by supporting selected programs of higher education, health care, children's welfare, and spiritual life.

3185 **First Union Foundation**
301 S College St
Charlotte, NC 28288
704-383-0525
Fax: 704-374-2484

Judy Allison, Director

3186 **Foundation for the Carolinas**
220 N. Tryon Street
Charlotte, NC 28202
704-973-4500
800-973-7244
Fax: 704-973-4599
mmarsicano@fftc.org
fftc.org

Michael Marsicano, Ph.D., President & CEO
Brian Collier, Executive Vice President
Debra S. Watt, SVP, Information Technology
Laura Smith, Executive Vice President

Giving primarily to organizations serving the citizens of North and South Carolina.

3187 **Kate B Reynolds Charitable Trust**
128 Reynolda Village
Winston Salem, NC 27106-5123
336-397-5500
800-485-9080
Fax: 336-723-7765
kbr.org

Karen McNeil-Miller, President
Lori Fuller, Director, Evaluation and Learnin
Joel Beeson, Director, Operations
Nora Ferrell, Director, Communications
Mission is to improve the quality of life and quality of health for the financially needy of North Carolina. Grants resricted to the state of North Carolina only.

3188 **Mary Reynolds Babcock Foundation**
2920 Reynolda Rd
Winston Salem, NC 27106-3016
336-748-9222
Fax: 336-777-0095
info@mrbf.org
mrbf.org

Jennifer Barksdale, Finance Officer
Toshawia Bruner, Office Assistant
Lavastian Glenn, Network Officer
Justin Maxson, Executive Director
For 1994, this foundation is committed to an extensive educational and planning process to better understand the Southeast and to articulate the role the foundation seeks to play in the region into the twenty-first century.

3189 **Triangle Community Foundation**
324 Blackwell St
Suite 1220
Durham, NC 27701-3690
919-474-8370
Fax: 919-941-9208
info@trianglecf.org
trianglecf.org

Lacy M. Presnell, Chair
Pat Nathan, Secretary
C. Perry Colwell, Assistant Secretary
James A. Stewart, Treasurer
Triangle Community Foundation connects philanthropic resources with community needs, creates opportunity for enlightned change and encourages philanthropy as a way of life.

North Dakota

3190 **Alex Stern Family Foundation**
4141 28th South Avenue
Suite 102
Fargo, ND 58104-8403
701-271-0263
Fax: 701-271-0408
alexsternfamilyfoundation.org

Don Scott, Executive Director
Rondi McGovern, Trustee
Dan Carey, Trustee
The Foundation supports the arts, social welfare/human services, education, youth recreation, civic projects and health issues for the benefit of the greater Fargo-Moorhead area.

3191 **Arc of North Dakota**
2500 DeMers Avenue
Grand Forks, ND 58201-2420
701-772-6191
877-250-2022
Fax: 701-772-2195
thearc@arcuv.com
www.thearcuppervalley.com

Peggy Johnson, President
Joan Karpenko, First Vice President
Ruth Jenny, Secretary
Pam Heyd, Treasurer
Mission is to work in partnership with our constituents, members and affiliated chapters to ensure that children and adults with intellectual and developmental disabilities have the supports, benefits, and services they need, and are accepted, respected and fully included in their communities.

3192 **North Dakota Community Foundation**
309 N Mandan Street
309 N Mandan Street, Suite 2
P.O. Box 387
Bismarck, ND 58502-0387
701-222-8349
kdvorak@ndcf.net
www.ndcf.net

Kevin J Dvorak, CFP, President & CEO
Amy N. Warnke, CFRE, Development Director East
Kara L. Geiger, Development Director West
Cynthia Kaip, Accountant/Administrator
The mission of the North Dakota Community Foundation is to improve the quality of life for North Dakota's citizens through charitable giving and promothing philanthropy.

Ohio

3193 **Akron Community Foundation**
345 W Cedar St
Akron, OH 44307-2407
330-376-8522
Fax: 330-376-0202
jpetures@akroncf.org

Mark Alio, Chair
Steven Cox, Vice Chair
Dr. Sandra Selby, Secretary
Paul Belair, Treasurer
Mission is to improve the quality of life in the Greater Akron area by building permanent endowments, and providing philanthropic leadership that enables donors to make lasting investments in the community.

3194 **Albert G and Olive H Schlink Foundation**
49 Benedict Avenue, Suite C
Norwalk, OH 44857
curtis@hwak.com
www.schlinkfoundation.org

3195 **Arc of Ohio**
1335 Dublin Rd
Suite 100-A
Columbus, OH 43215-7037
614-487-4720
800-875-2723
Fax: 614-487-4725
info@thearcofohio.org
thearcofohio.org

Gary Tonks, Executive Director
John Hannah, President
Connie Calhoun, Vice President
Josh Ebling, Treasurer
The mission of The Arc of Ohio is to advocate for human rights, personal dignity and community participation of individuals with developmental disabilities, through legislative and social action, information and education, local chapter support and family involvement.

3196 **Bahmann Foundation**
8041 Hosbrook Rd
Suite 210
Cincinnati, OH 45236-2909
513-891-3799
Fax: 513-891-3722
info@bahmann.org
www.bahmann.org

John Gatch, Executive Director
The mission of the Bahmann Foundation is to reduce isolation of low-income older adults through technology.

3197 **Cleveland Foundation**
1422 Euclid Ave
Suite 1300
Cleveland, OH 44115-2063
216-861-3810
Fax: 216-861-1729
Hello@CleveFdn.org
clevelandfoundation.org

James A. Ratner, Chairman
Paul J. Dolan, Vice Chairman
Ronald B. Richard, President and CEO
Robert E. Eckardt, Executive Vice President
In general, grants are made in (but not restriced to) the areas of arts and culture, community development, economic development, education, environment, health and human services.

3198 **Columbus Foundation and Affiliated Organizations**
1234 E Broad St
Columbus, OH 43205-1453
614-251-4000
Fax: 614-251-4009
info@columbusfoundation.org
columbusfoundation.org
Doug F. Kridler, President & CEO
Raymond J. Biddiscombe, CPA, Senior Vice President - Finance
Lisa Schweitzer Courtice, P, EVP - Community Research and Gra
Alicia Szempruch, Scholarship Manager
The Columbus Foundation offers a range of charitable fund types that can be used for individuals, families and businesses.

3199 **Eleanora CU Alms Trust**
Fifth Third Bank
Department 00864
9990 Montgomery Rd
Cincinnati, OH 45263
513-793-2200
Robert W Laclair, President
Giving is limited to Cincinnati, OH.

3200 **Eva L And Joseph M Bruening Foundation**
Foundation Management Services
1422 Euclid Ave
Suite 966
Cleveland, OH 44115-1952
216-621-2901
Fax: 216-621-8198
www.fmscleveland.com
Janet E. Narten, Founder
Cristin N. Slesh, President
Valerie Schramm, Operations Assistant
Kara L. McCullough, Manager, Grants and Office Opera
Charitable foundation providing grants to noprofit organizations located inCuyahoga county Ohio. No grant are awarded to inviduals.

3201 **Fred & Lillian Deeks Memorial Foundation**
P.O. Box 1118
Cincinnati, OH 45201-1118
937-339-2329
Fax: 937-339-1861

3202 **GAR Foundation**
277 East Mill Street
Akron, OH 44308
330-576-2926
Fax: 330-294-5315
info@garfdn.org
Christine Amer Mayer, President
Kirstin S. Toth, Senior Vice President
Candace Campbell Jackson, Consulting Program Officer
Brittany G. Zaehringer, Senior Program Officer
The mission of the Foundation is to strengthen communities in our region through discerning and creative support of worthy organizations.

3203 **George Gund Foundation**
1845 Guildhall Building
45 Prospect Avenue, West
Cleveland, OH 44115-1008
216-241-3114
Fax: 216-241-6560
info@gundfdn.org
gundfoundation.org
Geoffrey Gund, President & Treasurer
Ann L. Gund, Vice President
David T. Abbott, Executive Director
Catherine Gund, Secretary
The George Gund Foundation was established in 1952 as a private, nonprofit institution with the sole purpose of contributing to human well-being and the progress of society.

3204 **Greater Cincinnati Foundation**
200 West Fourth St.
Cincinnati, OH 45202-2775
513-241-2880
Fax: 513-852-6886
info@gcfdn.org
www.gcfdn.org
Kathryn e. Merchant, President/CEO
Terri Masur, Executive Assistant
Elizabeth Reiter Benson, APR, Vice President for Communic
Shiloh Turner, Vice President for Community Inv
Offers a wide variety of giving tools to help people achieve their charitable goals and create lasting good work in their communities.

3205 **HCR Manor Care Foundation**
333 N. Summit St.
P.O. Box 10086
Toledo, OH 43699-0086
419-252-5500
Fax: 419-252-6404
foundation@hcr-manorcare.com
hcr-manorcare.com
Paul A Ormond, Chairman, President and CEO
An independent, not-for-profit corporation that provides funding for organizations and programs that address the needs of the elderly and individuals requiring post-acute care services.

3206 **HWH Foundation**
Canton, OH
330-818-1300
contacthwh@hwhfoundation.org
www.hwhfoundation.org
Elizabeth Lacey Hoover, Chairman
Colton Hoover Chase, Vice Chairman
Mark Butterworth, Executive Director
Caiti Pomerance, Esq, Program & Outreach Director
The Herbert W Hoover Foundation funds unique opportunities that provide solutions to issues related to the Community, Education and the Environment.

3207 **Harry C Moores Foundation**
100 South Third Street
Columbus, OH 43215-4291
614-227-2300
Fax: 614-227-2390
info@bricker.com
bricker.com
Kurtis A Tunnell, Managing Partner
Ahmad Sino, Chief Information Officer
Steve P Odum, Chief Financial Officer
Angela M Gelst, Chief Human Resources Officer

3208 **Helen Steiner Rice Foundation**
1301 Western Ave.
Cincinnati, OH 45203
513-287-7022
800-877-2665
helensteinerrice.com
Virginia J. Ruehlmann, Creative Consultant
Dorothy C. Lingg, Office Manager
Willis D. Gradison, Jr., Board of Trustee
Gregory Ionna, Board of Trustee
Non-profit corporation whose purpose is to award grants to worthy charitable programs that aid the poor, the needy, and the elderly.

3209 **Nationwide Foundation**
One Nationwide Plaza
Columbus, OH 43215-2220
614-249-7111
800-882-2822
Fax: 614-249-5721
www.nationwide.com
Kirt A. Walker, President and COO Nationwide Fin
Mark A. Pizzi, President and Chief Operating Of
Stephen S. Rasmussen, Chief Executive Officer, Nationw
W. Kim Austen, President and COO, Allied Group,
The Nationwide Foundation is an independent corporation funded by Nationwide Companies to help positively impact the quality of life in communities where our associates, agents and their families live and work.

3210 **Nordson Corporate Giving Program**
28601 Clemens Rd
Westlake, OH 44145-1148
440-892-1580
Fax: 440-892-9507
kladiner@nordson.com
nordson.com
Michael F. Hilton, President and Chief Executive O
Gregory A. Thaxton, Senior Vice President, Chief Fin
John J. Keane, Senior Vice President, Advanced
Gregory P. Merk, Senior Vice President, Adhesive
Nordson Corporation encourages individual financial support of nonprofit organizations, colleges, and universities

3211 **Parker-Hannifin Foundation**
6035 Parkland Blvd
Cleveland, OH 44124-4141
216-896-3000
800-272-7537
Fax: 216-896-4000
parker.com
Donald E. Washkewicz, Chairman, Chief Executive Office
Lee C. Banks, Executive Vice President and Ope
Robert P. Barker, Executive Vice President, Operat
Jon P. Marten, Executive Vice President - Finan
To be a leading worldwide manufacturer of components and systems for the builders and users of durable goods.

3212 **Reinberger Foundation**
30000 Chagrin Blvd.
Suite 300
Cleveland, OH 44124-4439
216-292-2790
Fax: 216-292-4466
info@reinbergerfoundation.org
www.reinbergerfoundation.org
Karen R. Hooser, President
Sally R. Dyer, Trustee
Richard H. Oman, Trustee
William C. Reinberger, Trustee
Committed to enhancing the quality of life for individuals from all walks of life. To achieve this goal, proposals in the areas of the arts, education, healthcare, and social service are favored.

3213 **Robert Campeau Family Foundation**
7 West Seventh Street
Cincinnati, OH 45202-2424
513-579-7000
Fax: 513-579-7555
Terry J Lundgren, Chairman and Chief Executive Officer

3214 **Sisler McFawn Foundation**
P.O. Box 149
Akron, OH 44309
330-849-8887
Fax: 330-996-6215
Charlotte M Stanley, Grants Manager
Our trust restricts giving to certain programs and types of organizations. You can see recent giving has been by referring to the list of grants approved and paid during the past year. Call foundation office to request a guidelines brochure and list.

3215 **Stark Community Foundation**
400 Market Ave North
Suite 200
Canton, OH 44702-1557
330-454-3426
Fax: 330-454-5855
info@starkcf.org
www.starkcommunityfoundation.org
Mark Samolczyk, President
Patricia Quick, VP/ CFO
Chris Decker, Finance and Systems Officer
Bridgette Neisel, Vice President of Advancement
Stark Community Foundation is dedicated to promoting the betterment of Stark County and enhancing the quality of life of all its citizens.

3216 **Stocker Foundation**
201 Burns Road
Elyria, OH 44035
440-366-4884
Fax: 440-366-4656
contact@stockerfoundation.org
stockerfoundation.org
Brenda Norton, President
Dawn Dobras, Treasurer
Patricia O'Brien, Executive Director
Melanie R Wilson, Office Manager
The Stocker Foundation seeks creative ideas and projects that are catalysts for constructive change in the community through arts and culture, community needs, education, health social services and women's issues.

3217 **Toledo Community Foundation**
300 Madison Avenue
Suite 1300
Toledo, OH 43604-1583
419-241-5049
Fax: 419-242-5549
toledocf@toledocf.org
www.toledocf.org
David F. Waterman, Chair
Dr. Anthony Armstrong, Vice Chair
Rita N.A. Mansour, Secretary
Scott A Estes, Treasurer
The Toledo Community Foundation is a public, charitable foundation which exists to improve the quality of life in the region.

3218 **William J and Dorothy K O'Neill Foundation**
7575 Northcliff Ave.
Suite 205
Cleveland, OH 44144
216-831-4134
Fax: 216-378-0594
info@oneill-foundation.org
www.oneillfdn.org
Leah S Gary, President & CEO
Symone R McClain, Manager of Grants & Office Opera
Timothy M. McCue, MPH, Senior Program Officer

3219 **Youngstown Foundation**
100 Federal Plaza East, Suite 101
P.O. Box 1162
Youngstown, OH 44503-1162
330-744-0320
Fax: 330-744-0344
Jan@youngstownfoundation.org
www.youngstownfoundation.org
Jan Strasfeld, Executive Director
Crissi Jenkins, Program Coordinator
Rena Colarossi, Admin. Assistant
Funds proposals that provide direct services to children with medically diagnosed disabilities. Grants are awarded to Ohio non-profit agencies that are qualified under the Internal Revenue Service Code 501 (c) (3) for the care of such children in the greater Youngstown Area.

Oklahoma

3220 **Anne and Henry Zarrow Foundation**
401 S Boston Ave
Suite 900
Tulsa, OK 74103-4012
918-295-8004
Fax: 918-295-8049
bmajor@zarrow.com
www.zarrow.com

3221 **Sarkeys Foundation**
530 East Main St
Norman, OK 73071-5823
405-364-3703
Fax: 405-364-8191
angela@sarkeys.org
sarkeys.org
Kim Henry, Executive Director
Lori Sutton, Facilities Manager
Angella Holladay, Director of Grants Management
Susan C. Frantz, Senior Program Officer
Improves the quality of life in Oklahoma. Offers contributions in the areas of social services, arts and cultural programs, educational funding and health care and medical research. Funding only in agencies in the state of Oklahoma.

Oregon

3222 **Arc of Oregon**
2405 Front Street NE
Suite 120
Salem, OR 97301-4342
503-581-2726
877-581-2726
Fax: 503-363-7168
www.thearcoregon.org
Marcie Ingledue, Executive Director
Tiffany Tombleson, Administrative Assistant
Paula Boga, OSNT Program Director
Cici Gaynor, OSNT Administrative Assistant
Guardianship, Advocacy and Planning Services. Oregon special needs trust; information and referral.

3223 **Cambia Health Foundation**
100 SW Market St.
Suite E15B
Portland, OR 97201
503-225-4813
cambiahealthfoundation.org
Peggy Maguire, President & Chair
Kathleen Pitcher Tobey, Director, Operations
Leslie Constans, Director, Digital & Brand Communications
Mary Frances Baldes, Manager, Communications
Cambia Health Foundation is the corporate foundation of Cambia Health Solutions dedicated to transforming the way people experience health care to create a more person-focused and economically sustainable health care system.

3224 **Chiles Foundation**
1614 Mahan Center Boulevard
Suite 104
Tallahassee, Fl 32308
805-385-7800
Fax: 805-385-7808
kchiles@lawtonchiles.org
chilesfoundation.org
Kitty Chiles, Executive Director
Bud Chiles, President
Dr. Wil J. Blechman, Board Member
Todd Abernethy, Chief Financial Officer
Giving in Oregon, with emphasis on Portland, and the Pacific Northwest.

3225 **Jackson Foundation**
P.O. Box 3168
Portland, OR 97208-3168
503-275-4414
march.voyles@usbank.com
www.thejacksonfoundation.com
Robert H Depew, Vice President & Senior Trust Of
Libby Voyles, Trust Relationship Associate
Purpose is to respond to the requests deemed appropriate to promote the welfare of the public of the city of Portland or the State of Oregon or both.

3226 **Leslie G Ehmann Trust**
P.O. Box 3168
Portland, OR 97208-3168
503-275-5929
800-522-9100
Fax: 503-275-4117
William Dolan, Trustee

Pennsylvania

3227 **Air Products Foundation**
7201 Hamilton Blvd
Allentown, PA 18195-9642
610-481-4911
Fax: 610-481-5900
gigmrktg@airproducts.com
www.airproducts.com
Seifi Ghasemi, Chairman & CEO
M. Scott Crocco, Senior Vice President and Chief
Guillermo Novo, Senior Vice President
Corning F. Painter, Executive Vice President
Giving primarily in areas of company operations throughout the US.

3228 **Arc of Pennsylvania**
301 Chestnut Street
Suite 403
Harrisburg, PA 17101-2535
717-234-2621
800-692-7258
Fax: 717-234-2622
info@thearcpa.org
thearcpa.org
Maureen Cronin, Executive Director
Pam Klipa, Government Relations Director
Gwen Adams, Operations Director
Ashlinn Masland-Sarani, Policy and Development Director
The Arc's mission is to work to include all children and adults with cognitive, intellectual, and developmental disabilities in every community. We promote active citizenship and inclusion in every community.

3229 **Arcadia Foundation**
105 E Logan St
Norristown, PA 19401-3058
202-747-0876
Marilyn L Steinbright, President
Robert Carmona-Borjas, Founder

3230 **Brachial Plexus Palsy Foundation**
210 Springhaven Cir
Royersford, PA 19468-1178
www.brachialplexuspalsyfoundation.org

3231 **Columbia Gas of Pennsylvania Corporate Giving**
650 Washington Rd
Pittsburgh, PA 15228-2702
412-572-7104
Fax: 412-572-7140
www.columbiagaspamd.com/html/
Rosemary Martinelli, Manager Corporation

3232 **Connelly Foundation**
100 Front Street,
Suite 1450
West Conshohocken, PA 19428-2873
610-834-3222
Fax: 610-834-0866
info@connellyfdn.org
connellyfdn.org
Josephine C. Mandeville, Chair & President
Emily C Riley, Executive Vice President
Lewis W Bluemle, Senior Vice President
Carol L. Cromie, Executive Assistant
Seeks to foster learning and to improve the quality of life in the Greater Philadelphia area. The Foundation supports local non-profit organizations in the fields of education, health and human services, arts and culture and civic enterprise.

3233 **Dolfinger-McMahon Foundation**
30 South 17th Street
Philadelphia, PA 19103-4196
215-979-1768
www.dolfingermcmahonfoundation.org
Sheldon M. Bonovitz, Trustee
David E. Loder, Trustee
Frank G. Cooper, Counsel
Sharon M. Renz, Executive Secretary

3234 **Heinz Endowments**
Howard Heinz Endowment
625 Liberty Ave
30 Dominion Tower
Pittsburgh, PA 15222- 3115
412-281-5777
Fax: 412-281-5788
bobbyvagt@heinz.org
heinz.org
Grant Oliphant, President
Edward Kolano, Vice President Finance and Admin
Ann C. Plunkett, Director, Human Resources
Donna Evans Sebastian, Executive Assistant
Mission is to help our region thrive as a whole community-economically, ecologically, educationaly, and culturaly while advancing the state of knowledge and practice in the fields in which we work.

3235 **Henry L Hillman Foundation**
310 Grant Street
Suite 2000
Pittsburgh, PA 15219 412-338-3466
foundation@hillmanfo.com
hillmanfamilyfoundations.org
David K Roger, President
Lisa R Johns, Treasurer and Senior Program Off
Lauri K. Fink, Senior Program Officer
D.Tyler Gourley, Program Officer
Established with a broad purpose to improve the quality of life in Pittsburgh and southwestern Pennsylvania.

3236 **Jewish Healthcare Foundation of Pittsburgh**
650 Smithfield Street
Suite 2400
Pittsburgh, PA 15222- 3915 412-594-2550
Fax: 412-232-6240
info@jhf.org
jhf.org
Karen Wolk Feinstein, PhD, President and Chief Executive Of
Carla Barricella, Communications Director
Lindsey Kirstatter Hartle, Accounting Manager
Millie Greene, Executive Assistant
The mission of the JHF is to support and foster the provision of healthcare services, healthcare education, and, when appropriate, medical and scientific research, and to respond to the health-related needs of elderly, underprivileged, indigent, and undeserved persons in both the Jewish and general community throughout Western Pennsylvania. .

3237 **Juliet L Hillman Simonds Foundation**
310 Grant Street
Suite 2000
Pittsburgh, PA 15219 412-338-3466
Fax: 412-338-3520
foundation@hillmanfo.com
hillmanfamilyfoundations.org
David K. Roger, President
Lisa R. Johns, Treasurer and Senior Program Off
Lauri K. Fink, Senior Program Officer
D.Tyler Gourley, Program Officer

3238 **Oberkotter Foundation**
1600 Market St
Suite 3600
Philadelphia, PA 19103-7212 215-751-2601
Fax: 215-751-2678
info@oberkotterfoundation.org
oberkotterfoundation.org
George H Nofer, Executive Director
Mildred L. Oberkotter, M.S.W., Trustee
Bruce A. Rosenfield, J.D., Trustee
David A. Pierson, Ph.D., Trustee
The Oberkotter Foundation focuses its efforts on supporting families who have chosen listening and spoken language for their child and on opportunities for children learning listening and spoken language to develop their social, emotional, language and educational skills.

3239 **PECO Energy Company Contributions Program**
Fl 7toorh
2301 Market St
Philadelphia, PA 19103-1338 215-841-4000
800-494-4000
Fax: 215-841-6830
www.peco.com
Denis P O'Brien, SVP/ CEO
Michael A. Innocenzo, SVP/ COO
Phillip S. Barnett, SVP/ CFO/ Treasurer
Scott A. Bailey, VP/ Controller

3240 **PNC Bank Foundation**
249 5th Ave
Pittsburgh, PA 15222-2707 412-762-2000
Fax: 412-762-7829
marianna.hallett@pnc.com
www.pncbank.com
Samuel R Patterson, Senior VP
The PNC Foundation's priority is to form partnerships with community-based nonprofit organizations within the markets PNC serves in order to enhance educational opportunities for children, particularly underserved pre-K children though our signature, PNC Grow Uo Great Program, and to promote the growth of targeted communities through economic development initiatives.

3241 **Philadelphia Foundation**
1234 Market St
Suite 1800
Philadelphia, PA 19107-3704 215-563-6417
Fax: 215-563-6882
philafound.org
R Andrew Swinney, President
Pat Meller, Vice President for Finance & Adm
Andrea Congo, Executive Assistant
Betsy Anderson, Communications Director
The Philadelphia Foundation improves our community by advancing change, leading on issues of importance, forging meaningful relationships and providing knowledge, resources and stewardship.

3242 **Pittsburgh Foundation**
Five PPG Place
Suite 250
Pittsburgh, PA 15222-5405 412-391-5122
Fax: 412-391-7259
oliphantg@pghfdn.org
pittsburghfoundation.org
Maxwell King, President and CEO
Jonathan Brelsford, Vice President of Investments
Jay Donato, Senior Investment Analyst
Marianne Cola, Special Assistant
The Pittsburgh Foundation works to improve the quality of life in the Pittsburgh region by evaluating and addressing community issues, promoting responsible philanthropy, and connecting donors to the critical needs of the community.

3243 **Shenango Valley Foundation**
7 West State Street
Suite 301
Sharon, PA 16146-2713 724-981-5882
866-901-7204
Fax: 724-983-9044
comm-foundation.org
Lawrence E. Haynes, Executive Director
Amy Atkinson, Associate Director
Shelly Mason, Chief Financial Officer
Tristan Rice, Development Coordinator
Mission is to promote the betterment of our region and enhancement of the quality of life for all of its citizens.

3244 **Staunton Farm Foundation**
650 Smithfield Street
Suite 210
Pittsburgh, PA 15222- 3907 412-281-8020
Fax: 844-281-8020
office@stauntonfarm.org
stauntonfarm.org
Joni S. Schwager, Executive Director
Bethany Hemingway, Program Officer
Jason Fate, Office Manager
Robert Musca, Financial Manager
Dedicated to improving the lives of people who live with mental illness.

3245 **Stewart Huston Charitable Trust**
50 South First Avenue
Coatesville, PA 19320-3418 610-384-2666
Fax: 610-384-3396
admin@stewarthuston.org
stewarthuston.org
Scott G. Huston, Executive Director
Charles L. Huston III, Trustee
Shelton P Sanford, Trustee
Elinor Lashley, Trustee
The purpose of the Trust is to provide funds, technical assistance and collaboration on behalf of non-profit organizations engaged exclusively in religious, charitable or educational work; to extend opportunities to deserving needs persons and, in general, to promote any of the above causes.

3246 **Teleflex Foundation**
155 S Limerick Rd
Limerick, PA 19468-1603
610-948-5100
Fax: 610-948-5101
teleflex.com
Jeffrey P Black, CEO
The Teleflex Foundation strives to create an impact on the quality of life in Teleflex communities and build supportive relationships among our stakeholders. The Foundation places a priority on progrmas that have the commitmenet and volunteer involvement of Teleflex communities.

3247 **USX Foundation**
600 Grant St
Pittsburgh, PA 15219-2702
412-433-1121
Fax: 412-433-6847
www.ussteel.com
CD Mallick, General Manager
Patricia Funaro, Program Manager
Giving primarily in areas of company operations located within the United States.

3248 **William B Dietrich Foundation**
Duane Morrs Llt
30 S 17th St
Philadelphia, PA 19103-4001
215-979-1000
Fax: 215-979-1020
www.duanemorris.com
William B Dietrich, President

3249 **William Talbott Hillman Foundation**
310 Grant Street
Suite 2000
Pittsburgh, PA 15219
412-338-3466
Fax: 212-792-2677
foundation@hillmanfo.com
hillmanfamilyfoundations.org
David K. Roger, President
Lisa R. Johns, Treasurer and Senior Program Off
Lauri K. Fink, Senior Program Officer
D.Tyler Gourley, Program Officer

3250 **William V and Catherine A McKinney Charitable Foundation**
20 Stanwix St
Pittsburgh, PA 15222-4802
412-644-8332
Fax: 412-644-6058
verizon.com
William M Schmidt, Senior Vice President

Rhode Island

3251 **Arc South County Chapter**
2 Barber Avenue
Warwick, RI 02886-3549
401-480-9355
paul@pence.com
www.riroads.com

3252 **Arc of Blackstone Valley**
500 Prospect St.
Wing B, Suite 203
Pawtucket, RI 02860- 4332
401-727-0150
800-257-6092
Fax: 401-727-1545
contact@bvcriarc.org
www.bvcriarc.org
Kathleen O'Neill, President
Thomas E. Hodge, Vice President
John J. Padien III, Chief Executive Officer
Katherine S. Hunt, Chief Operating Officer
A private nonprofit organization providing residential, developmental, employment and recreational programs and services to more then 400 individuals with intellectual and related disabilities

3253 **Arc of Northern Rhode Island**
The Homestead Group Administrative Offices
68 Cumberland St
Suite 200
Woonsocket, RI 02895-3323
401-765-3700
Fax: 401-765-1124
arcofnri.org

3254 **Champlin Foundations**
2000 Chapel View Boulevard
Suite 350
Cranston, RI 02920
401-944-9200
Fax: 401-944-9299
Jonathan K. Farnum, Distribution Committee
John Gorham, Distribution Committee
Dione D. Kenyon, Distribution Committee
Lisa P. Koelle, Distribution Committee
Giving in the Rhode Island area. Champlin does not give grants to individuals, only to RI tax-exempt organizations.

3255 **CranstonArc**
The Keystone Group
PO Box 20130
Cranston, RI 02920-942
401-941-1112
Fax: 401-383-8751
info@accesspointri.org
www.accesspointri.org
Thomas Kane, President & CEO
Kevin McHale, Chief Operating Officer
Maureen Russo, Director of Human Resources
Gary Paulhus, Director of Clinical Services
Mission is to empower persons with differing ablilites to claim and enjoy their right to dignity and respect through their lives.

3256 **Down Syndrome Society of Rhode Island**
4635 Post Road
Warwick, RI 02818
401-463-5751
Fax: 401-463-5337
TTY: 800-745-5555
coordinatordssri@verizon.net
www.dssri.org
Claudia M. Lowe, Coordinator
Marilyn Blanche
Jeff DiMillio
Gail Doyle
The Down Syndrome Society of Rhode Island (DSSRI) is dedicated to promoting the rights, dignity and potential of all individuals with Down syndrome through advocacy, education, public awareness, and support.

3257 **Frank Olean Center**
93 Airport Rd
Westerly, RI 02891-3420
401-596-2091
Fax: 401-596-3945
info@oleancenter.org
oleancenter.org
Joan Gradilone, President
Tony Vellucci, Executive Director
Rick Harley, Vice President
Christine Martone, Secretary
A non-profit organization representing and providing services and supports to persons with developmental disabilities and their families throughout Southern Rhode Island and Southeastern Connecticut.

3258 **Horace A Kimball and S Ella Kimball Foundation**
23 Broad Street
Westerly, RI 02891-1879
401-348-1238
Fax: 401-364-3565
www.hkimballfoundation.org
Thomas F Black III, President
Norman D. Baker, Jr., Secretary and Treasurer
Edward C. Marth, Foundation Trustees
Makes grants almost exclusively to Rhode Island operatives (charities) or those benefitting Rhode Island residents and causes.

3259 **James L. Maher Center**
120 Hillside Avenue
Newport, RI 02840
401-846-0340
Fax: 401-849-4267
www.mahercenter.org

Jack Casey, President
William Maraziti, Executive Director
Barbara Burns, President
John S Dugan, Secretary

The mission is to advance independence and opportunity for children and adults with developmental disabilities and their families.

3260 **Rhode Island Arc**
99 Bald Hill Rd
Cranston, RI 02920-2647
401-463-9191
Fax: 401-463-9244
riarc@compuserve.com

Mary Lou Mc Caffray, Executive Director

3261 **Rhode Island Foundation**
One Union Station
Providence, RI 02903-1758
401-274-4564
Fax: 401-331-8085
info@rifoundation.org
rifoundation.org

Neil Steinberg, President & CEO
Wendi DeClercq, Executive Assistant
James S. Sanzi, Esq., Vice President of Development
Pamela Tesler Howitt, Senior Development Officer

The Rhode Island Foundation works to build a better Rhode Island as a philanthropic resource, for people, communities, organizations, and programs.

South Carolina

3262 **Arc of South Carolina**
1202 12th Street
Cayce, SC 29033
803-748-5020
Fax: 803-445-1026
TheArc@ArcSC.org
www.arcsc.org

Margie Williamson, Executive Director
Caroline Kistler, Project Director
Carly Prince, Case Manager
Hilary Bell, Case Manager

The Arc of South Carolina advocates for and alongside people with cognitive, intellectual and developmental disabilities and their families.

3263 **Center for Disability Resources**
University of South Carolina School of Medicine
Department of Pediatrics
8301 Farrow Rd.
Columbia, SC 29208
803-935-5231
Fax: 803-935-5059
david.rotholz@uscmed.sc.edu
uscm.med.sc.edu/cdrhome

3264 **Colonial Life and Accident Insurance Company Contributions Program**
1200 Colonial Life Blvd W
Columbia, SC 29210-7670
803-798-7000
Fax: 803-731-2618

Randy Horn, President and Chief Executive Of
Bill Deeham, Senior Vice President of Sales
Tim Arnold, Senior Vice President of Sales a
John Garrison, Vice President, General Counsel

Tennessee

3265 **Arc of Anderson County**
728 Emory Valley Road, Suite 42
P.O. Box 4823
Oak Ridge, TN 37831-4823
865-481-0550
arc@arcaid.org
www.thearcandersoncounty.com

Sally Browning, President
Dargie Arwood, Executive Director
Ginny Miceli, President
Elizabeth Bonner, Vice President

The Arc of Anderson County provides support and advocacy to people with cognitive, intellectual and developmental disabilities. The Arc provides support, information and training for families and caregivers of adults and children with these disabilities.

3266 **Arc of Davidson County**
111 N Wilson Blvd
Nashville, TN 37205-2411
615-248-4112
Fax: 615-322-9184
arcdc.org

Kate Deitzer, President
Cynthia Gardner, Vice President
Thom Druffel, Treasurer
Elizabeth Ralph, Secretary

Provides services to adults and children with intellectual and developmental disabilities.

3267 **Arc of Hamilton County**
4613 Brainerd Rd
Chattanooga, TN 37411-3826
423-624-6887
800-624-6887
Fax: 423-624-3974
arcofhamilton@aol.com
thearchc.org

Shawn Ellis, Executive Director

Provides assistance to individuals and families with developmental disabilities, in the form of advocacy, information, and support coordination

3268 **Arc of Tennessee**
151 Athens Way
Suite 100
Nashville, TN 37228-1367
615-248-5878
800-835-7077
Fax: 615-248-5879
info@thearctn.org
thearctn.org

John Lewis, President
John Shouse, Vice President
Donna Lankford, Secretary
Ann Curl, Treasurer

Advocacy, information, referral and support for people with intellectual and developmental disabilities and their families.

3269 **Arc of Washington County**
110 East Mountcastle Drive
Johnson City, TN 37601-7557
423-928-9362
Fax: 423-928-7431
kim@arcwc.org
www.arcwc.org

Malessa Fleenor, Executive Director
Kim Reid, Human Resources, Quality Assuran
Kim Wheeler, Respite Coordinator
Linda Tilson, Family Support Program Manager

Is a non-profit organization that serves individuals with disabilities and their families. They have an independent support coordination service, as well as, early intervention, family support and respite services.

3270 **Arc of Williamson County**
129 W Fowlkes St
Suite 151
Franklin, TN 37064-3562
615-790-5815
Fax: 615-790-5891
sbbarc@thearcwc.org
thearcwc.org

Donna Isbell, President
Steve Cassidy, Vice President
Ashley Coulter, Secretary
Jan Lincoln, Treasurer

The Arc is a family-based organization committed to securing for all people with intellectual, developmental, or other disabilities the opportunity to choose and realize their goals of where and how they live, learn, work, and play.

3271 **Arc-Diversified**
453 Gould Dr
Cookeville, TN 38506
931-432-5981
800-239-9029
Fax: 931-432-5987

3272 **Benwood Foundation**
736 Market St
Suite 1600
Chattanooga, TN 37402-4812
423-267-4311
Fax: 423-267-9049
info@benwood.org
benwood.org

Sarah Morgan, President
Kristy Huntley, Program & Financial Officer
Connie Perrin, Accounting & Grants Manager
Jeff Pfitzer, Program Officer

Benwood Foundation seeks to stimulate creative and innovative efforts to build and strengthen the Chattanooga community.

3273 **Community Foundation of Greater Chattanooga**
1270 Market St
Chattanooga, TN 37402-2713
423-265-0586
Fax: 423-265-0587
info2@cfgc.org
cfgc.org

Peter T. Cooper, President
Rebecca Underwood, Vice President, Finance & Admini
Marty Robinson, Vice President, Donor Relations
Rebecca Smith, Director of Scholarships

A non-profit organization which receives, holds, invests and distributes assets contributed by individuals and organizations for the benefit of Chattanooga, its citizens and its institutions.

3274 **Education and Auditory Research Foundation**
PO Box 330867
Nashville, TN 37203-7506
615-627-2724
800-545-4327
Fax: 615-627-2728
www.earfoundation.org

Michael Glasscock, President

Provides the general public support services promoting the integration of the hearing and balance impaired into mainstream society; to provide practicing ear specialists continuing medical education courses and related programs specifically regarding rehabilitation and hearing preservation; to educate young people and adults about hearing preservation and early detection of hearing loss, enabling them to prevent at an early age hearing and balance disorders.

3275 **International Paper Company Foundation**
6400 Poplar Ave
Memphis, TN 38197
901-419-9000
800-207-4003
Fax: 901-419-4439
internationalpaper.comm@ipaper.com
internationalpaper.com

Mark S Sutton, Chairman & CEO
David J Bronczek, President & CEO
C. Cato Ealy, Senior Vice President, Corporate
William P. Hoel, Senior Vice President

The Foundation's primary focus is education-specifically environmental education, iliteracy programs for young children and minority career development opportunities for college bound youth.

3276 **Montgomery County Arc**
1825 K Street
NW, Suite 1200
Washington, DC 20006-2145
202-534-3700
800-433-5255
Fax: 202-534-3731
info@thearc.org
www.thearc.org

Ronald Brown, President
Elise McMillan, Vice President
Peter V Berns, Chief Executive Officer
M.J. Bartelmay, Secretary

Organization works to ensure that the estimated 7.2 million Americans with intellectual and developmental disabilities have the services and supports they need to grow, develop and live in communities across the nation.

Texas

3277 **Abell-Hangar Foundation**
P.O. Box 430
Midland, TX 79702-0430
432-684-6655
Fax: 432-684-4474
abell-hanger.org

David L Smith, Executive Director

The Foundation makes grants to nonprofit organizations, which are involved in such undertakings for public welfare, including but not limited to, education, health services, human services, arts and cultural activities and community or social benefit.

3278 **Albert & Bessie Mae Kronkosky Charitable Foundation**
112 East Pecan
Suite 830
San Antonio, TX 78205-1574
210-475-9000
888-309-9001
Fax: 210-354-2204
kronkosky.org

Palmer Moe, Managing Director

Mission is to produce profound good that is tangible and measurable in Bandera, Bexar, Comal, and Kendall counties in Texas by implimenting the Kronkosky's charitable purposes.

3279 **American Express Foundation**
P.O. Box 981540
El Paso, TX 79998-1540
800-528-4800
TTY: 800-221-9950
americanexpress.com

Kenneth I Chenault, Chairman and Chief Executive Off
L. Kevin Cox, Chief Human Resources Officer
Marc D. Gordon, Executive Vice President and Chi
John D. Hayes, Executive Vice President and Chi

Grants are awarded in the three program areas: Community Service, Cultural Heritage, and Economic Independence. Most grants are made for projects operating where the company has a major employee or market presence.

3280 **Arc of Texas, The**
8001 Centre Park Dr
Suite 100
Austin, TX 78754-5118
512-454-6694
800-252-9729
Fax: 512-454-4956
www.thearcoftexas.org

Charlie Huber, President
John Schneider, Vice President
Amy Mizcles, Executive Director
Terri Schonfeld, Secretary

The Arc of Texas creates opportunities for all people with intellectual and developmental disabilities to actively participate in their communities and make the choices that affect their lives in a positive manner.

3281 **BA and Elinor Steinhagen Benevolent Trust**
Chase Bank of Texas
700 North St.
Suite D
Beaumont, TX 77701-3928 409-832-6565
Fax: 409-832-7532
www.setxnonprofit.org

Jean Moncla, CTFA, President
Ivy Pate, Treasurer
Chester Jourdan, Executive Director
Kristi Stott, Administrative Assistant

3282 **Brown Foundation**
P.O. Box 130646
Houston, TX 77219-0646 713-523-6867
Fax: 713-523-2917
bfi@brownfoundation.org
brownfoundation.org

Nancy Pittman, Executive Director
The purpose of the Brown Foundation is to distribute funds for public charitable purposes, principally for support, encouragement and assistance to education, the arts and community service.

3283 **CH Foundation**
P.O. Box 94038
Lubbock, TX 79493-4038 806-792-0448
Fax: 806-792-7824
ksanford@chfoundation.com
www.chfoundationlubbock.com

Kay Sanford, Executive Director
Heather Hocker, Grants Administrator
Cheryl Sanford, Administrative Assistant
Mission of the CH foundation is to significantly improve human services and cultural and educational opportunities for the residents of the South Plain of Texas.

3284 **Cockrell Foundation**
1000 Main St
Suite 3250
Houston, TX 77002-6338 713-209-7500
Ernest H. Cockrell, President
Nancy Williams, Executive Vice President
Purpose is for giving for higher education at the University of Texas at Austin; support also for cultural programs, social services, youth services and health care. Limitations are giving in Houston, Texas and no grants are awarded to individuals.

3285 **Communities Foundation of Texas**
5500 Caruth Haven Ln
Dallas, TX 75225-8146 214-750-4222
Fax: 214-750-4210
jsmith@cftexas.org
cftexas.org

Brent E. Chrisopher, President and Chief Executive Of
Elizabeth W. Bull, Senior Vice President and Chief
Jeverley R. Cook, Ph.D., Executive Director, W.W. Caruth,
John Fitzpatrick, Executive Director
Mission is to improve lives, we serve the community by investing wisely and making effective charitable grants.

3286 **Community Foundation of North Texas**
306 West 7th
Suite 1045
Fort Worth, TX 76102-4906 817-877-0702
Fax: 817-632-8711
cfntx.org

Nancy E. Jones, President
Rob Miller, Director of Finance
Vicki Andrews, Director of Operations/Donor Ser
Rose Bradshaw, Executive Vice President
Community Foundation is a tax exempt organization that provides stewardship for many individual charitable funds. With its specialized services, Community Foundation of North Texas gives donors efficient charitable fund administration.

3287 **Cullen Foundation**
601 Jefferson St
40th Floor
Houston, TX 77002-7900 713-651-8837
Fax: 713-651-2374
cullenfdn.org

Isaac Arnold, Jr, President
Wilhelmina E Robertson, Vice President and Secretary
Meredith T Cullen, Assistant Secretary
Bert L. Campbell, Director
Grants are restricted to Texas-based organizations for programs in Texas, primarily in the Houston area.

3288 **Curtis & Doris K Hankamer Foundation**
Ste 530
9039 Katy Fwy
Houston, TX 77024-1656 713-461-8140
Gregory A Herbst, Manager

3289 **Dallas Foundation**
3963 Maple Avenue
Ste. 390
Dallas, TX 75219-4447 214-741-9898
Fax: 214-741-9848
info@dallasfoundation.org
dallasfoundation.org

Mary M Jalonick, President & CEO
Gary W. Garcia, Senior Director of Development
Dawn Townsend, Director of Marketing & Communic
William T. Solomon, Jr., Chief Financial Officer
Serves as a leader, catalyst and resource for philanthropy by providing donors with a flexible means of making gifts to charitable causes that enhance our community.

3290 **David D & Nona S Payne Foundation**
P.O. Box 174
Pampa, TX 79066-174 806-665-0063
Vanessa G Buzzard, Director
The David & Nona S Payne Foundation was established in August 1980. Mrs Payne established the foundation and did much of her charitable giving in honor of her late husband.

3291 **El Paso Natural Gas Foundation**
P.O. Box 2511
Houston, TX 77252-2511 713-420-2600
Fax: 713-420-5312
foundation@elpaso.com
www.kindermorgan.com

Douglas Foshee, CEO
Focuses on the areas in locations where we have significant facilities or concentrated employees. Primary area of focus is Civic and Community, Education and Health and Human Services. Secondary area of focus is Arts and Culture and Environment.

3292 **Epilepsy Foundation of Southeast Texas**
2401 Fountain View Dr
Suite 900
Houston, TX 77057-4821 713-789-6295
888-548-9716
info@eftx.org
www.epilepsy.com/texas

Donna Stahlhut, CEO
Rebecca Moreau, Program Director
Amanda Walker Rockwell, Senior Development Coordinator
Shannon Robbins, Assistant Director
The Epilepsy Foundation of Southeast Texas is a non-profit organization devoted to improving the lives of people with epilepsy in Texas. Services offered by the foundation include public education programs, medical care, therapy and recreation programs.

3293 **Epilepsy Foundation: Central and South Texas**
10615 Perrin Beitel Rd
Suite 602
San Antonio, TX 78217 210-653-5353
888-606-5353
Fax: 210-653-5355
staff@efcst.org
www.efcst.org

Ariel Robbins, Program Manager
The Epilepsy Foundation of Central & South Texas is a voluntary health organization serving people with epilepsy. Services of-

fered include youth programs, seizure clinics, support groups, referrals and more.

3294 **Harris and Eliza Kempner Fund**
2201 Market St
12th Floor
Galveston, TX 77553-1529 409-765-6671
Fax: 409-765-9098
kempnercapital.com

Diana L. Bartula, Vice President, Chief Compliance
V. Delynn Greene, Vice President, Head Trader, Ope

Mission is to further the vision and heritage of the Kemper Family's commitment to philanthropy and sense of responsibility to society.

3295 **Hillcrest Foundation**
Bank of America
P.O. Box 830241
Dallas, TX 75283 214-209-1965
Daniel Kelly, VP

3296 **Hoblitzelle Foundation**
5556 Caruth Haven Lane
Suite 200
Dallas, TX 75225-8020 214-373-0462
kstone@hoblitzelle.org
www.hoblitzelle.org

William T Solomon, Chairman
Caren H. Prothro, Vice Chairman
J. McDonald Williams, Treasurer
Karl Hoblitzelle, Founder

Grants made by the directors are usually focused on specific, non-recurring needs of the educational, social service, medical, cultural, and civic organizations in Texas, particularly in the Dallas area.

3297 **Hogg Foundation for Mental Health**
3001 Lake Austin Blvd.
Austin, TX 78703 512-471-5041
hogg-operations@austin.utexas.edu
hogg.utexas.edu

Octavio N. Martinez Jr., Executive Director
Vicky Coffee, Director, Programs
Colleen Horton, Director, Policy
Crystal Viagran, Director, Finance & Operations

The Hogg Foundation for Mental Health is a nonprofit organization that is dedicated to the advancement of mental wellness for the people of Texas through outreach programs, conferences, seminars, research grants, and more.

3298 **Houston Endowment**
600 Travis St
Suite 6400
Houston, TX 77002-3003 713-238-8100
Fax: 713-238-8101
houstonendowment.org

Ann B Stern, President
Sheryl L Johns, Vice President for Admin
F. Xavier Pena, Vice President for Finance and G
Lisa A. Hall, Vice President for-Programs

A private philanthropic foundation that improves life for people of the greater Houston area through its contributions to charitable organizations and educational institutions.

3299 **John G & Marie Stella Kennedy Memorial Foundation**
555 N Carancahua
Suite 1700, Tower II
Corpus Christi, TX 78401-0851 361-887-6565
Fax: 361-887-6582

Judge J. A. Garcia, President and Director
Marc A. Cisneros, Chief Executive Officer
Sylvia Whitmore, Chief Operating Officer
Gloria Hicks, Secretary and Director

To advance and nurture activities that contribute to the foundation's core, Catholic values.

3300 **John S Dunn Research Foundation**
3355 West Alabama
Suite 990
Houston, TX 77098-1722 713-626-0368
Fax: 713-626-3866
jsdrf@swbell.net
johnsdunnfoundation.org

J. Dickson Rogers, President
Dan S. Wilford, Vice President
John R. Wallace, Secretary and Treasurer
John S. Dunn, Trustee

3301 **Lola Wright Foundation**
515 Congress Avenue
10th Floor
Austin, TX 78701 512-397-2001
amber.carden@ustrust.com
fdnweb.org/lolawright

Wilford Flowers, President and Director
Paul Hilgers, Vice-President and Director
Ron Oliveira, Secretary and Director
Jay Stewart, Director

3302 **Meadows Foundation**
3003 Swiss Ave
Dallas, TX 75204-6049 214-826-9431
800-826-9431
Fax: 214-827-7042
www.mfi.org

Linda P Evans, President and CEO
Tom Gale, Vice President and Chief Investm
Paula Herring, Vice President and Treasurer
Laura Bowers, Corporate Secretary

The Meadows Foundation exists to assist people and institutions of Texas improve the quality and circumstances of life for themselves and future generations.

3303 **Moody Foundation**
2302 Post Office St
Suite 704
Galveston, TX 77550-1994 409-797-1500
colleent@moodyf.org
moodyf.org

Frances Moody-Dahlderg, Executive Director
Jamie G. Williams, Human Resources Director
Garrik Addison, Chief Financial Officer
Samantha Seale, Scholarship Administrator

Created for the perpetual benefit of present and future generations.

3304 **Pearle Vision Foundation**
2534 Royal Ln
Dallas, TX 75229-3884 214-821-7770
www.pearlevision.com

Leo Priolo Jr, Owner

Organization dedicated to sight preservation through vision research and education.

3305 **San Antonio Area Foundation**
303 Pearl Parkway
Suite 114
San Antonio, TX 78215 210-225-2243
Fax: 210-225-1980
info@saafdn.org
saafdn.org

Marie Smith, Chair
G.P. Singh, Vice Chair
Michelle R. Scarver, Secretary
Luis de la Garza, Treasurer

The San Antonio Area Foundation aspires to significantly enhance the quality of life in our community by providing outstanding service to donors, producting significant asset growth, strengthning community collaboration and managing an exemplary grants program.

3306 **Shell Oil Company Foundation**
40 Bank Street
London, TX 77252-2463 281-544-7171
Fax: 713-241-3329
info@shellfoundation.org
www.shellfoundation.org
Malcolm Brinded, Chairman
Ben van Beurden, Trustee
William Kalema, Trustee
Hugh Mitchell, Trustee
A not-for-profit foundation funded by donations from Shell Oil Company and other participating Shell companies and subsidiaries.

3307 **South Texas Charitable Foundation**
P.O. Box 2459
Victoria, TX 77902 512-573-4383
Rayford L Keller, Secretary

3308 **Sterling-Turner Foundation**
5850 San Felipe Street
Suite 125
Houston, TX 77057-3292 713-237-1117
Fax: 713-223-4638
jeannie.arnold@stfdn.org
www.sterlingturnerfoundation.org
T. R. Reckling, President
Isla C. Reckling, Treasurer
Patricia Stilley, Executive Director
Christiana R McConn, Secretary
Sterling Turner Foundation is a private trust which can assist any Section 501 (c) (3) organization in the state of Texas. The Foundation is not permitted to assist any individuals

3309 **TLL Temple Foundation**
109 Temple Blvd
Lufkin, TX 75901-7321 936-639-5197
Wayne Corley, Executive Director

3310 **William Stamps Farish Fund**
Ste 1250
1100 Louisiana St
Houston, TX 77002-5232 713-757-7313
Terry Ward, Manager

Utah

3311 **Arc of Utah**
18585 Coastal Hwy # 19
Rehoboth Beach, DE 19971 801-364-5060
800-371-3060
Fax: 801-364-6030
gacosta@dunndunn.com
www.bewitchedtattoos.com
Kathy Scott, Executive Director
The Arc of Utah advocates for and with cognitive, intellectual and developmental disabilities and their families through awareness, outreach, education, support and public policy.

3312 **Marriner S Eccles Foundation**
79 S Main St
Salt Lake City, UT 84111-1929 801-532-0934
Shannon K Toronto

3313 **Questar Corporation Contributions Program**
333 South State Street
P.O. Box 45433
Salt Lake City, UT 84145-0433 801-324-5000
Ronald W Jibson, President & CEO
Craig C Wagstaff, Executive vice president
Micheal Dunn, Executive vice president
Brady Rasmussen, Executive Vice President
Focuses on promoting a healthy environment by investing in and fulfilling its corporate responsibility to support the well-being of communitites where Questar and its subsidiaries conduct business.

Vermont

3314 **Vermont Community Foundation**
3 Court Street
Middlebury, VT 05753 802-388-3355
Fax: 802-388-3398
info@vermontcf.org
www.vermontcf.org
Stuart Comstock-Gay, President
Nina McDonnell, Grants Administrator
Janet McLaughlin, Special Projects Director
Jen Peterson, Vice President for Program and G
Helps build and manage charitable funds created by individuals, families, groups, organizations, and institutions to improve the quality of life in Vermont.

Virginia

3315 **Arc of Virginia**
2147 Staples Mill Road
Richmond, VA 23230 804-649-8481
Fax: 804-649-3585
info@thearcofva.org
www.thearcofva.org
Howard Cullum, President
Shareen Young-Chavez, President-Elect
Marisa Laios, Vice President
Donalda Lovelace, Secretary
The Arc of Virginia advocactes for individuals with developmental disabilities and their families, so they may all lead productive and fulfilling lives.

3316 **Beacon Tree Foundation**
9201 Arboretum Pkwy.
Suite 140
N. Chesterfield, VA 23236 800-414-6427
info@beacontree.org
beacontree.org
Michelle Etheridge, President
Beacon Tree Foundation is dedicated to being an advocate for the family, providing education about treatment and financial resources to help heal children and teens struggling with mental health issues and to provide hope for the future.

3317 **Camp Foundation**
P.O. Box 813
Franklin, VA 23851 757-562-3439
Bobby B Worrell, CEO

3318 **Community Foundation of Richmond & Central Virginia**
7501 Boulder View Drive
Suite 110
Richmond, VA 23225- 4047 804-330-7400
Fax: 804-330-5992
info@tcfrichmond.org
tcfrichmond.org
Darcy Oman, President
Bobby Thalhimer, Senior Advisor
Molly Dean Bittner, Vice President
Lisa Pratt O'Mara, Vice President
The Community Foundation provides effective stewardship of philanthropic assets entrusted to its care by donors who wish to enhance the quality of community life.

3319 **John Randolph Foundation**
112 North Main Street
P.O. Box 1606
Hopewell, VA 23860- 1161 804-458-2239
Fax: 804-458-3754
lsharpe@johnrandolphfoundation.org
www.johnrandolphfoundation.org
Lisa H. Sharpe, Executive Director
M. Stephen Cates, Director of Finance and Accounti
Kiffy Werkheiser, Development Program Officer
Tammy E. McCollum, Administrative Associate

The John Randolph Foundation is a community-based Foundation working to improve the health and quality of life for residents of Hopewell and surrounding areas through Grants and Scholarships.

3320 National Right to Work Legal Defense Foundation
8001 Braddock Rd.
Springfield, VA 22160
703-321-8510
800-336-3600
Fax: 703-321-9319
nrtw.org

Raymond LaJeunesse, Vice President & Legal Director
Byron S. Andrus, Staff Attorney
Matthew B. Gilliam, Staff Attorney
Amanda K. Freeman, Staff Attorney

The National Right to Work Legal Defense Foundation is a non-profit, charitable organization. Its mission is to eliminate coercive union power and compulsory unionism abuses through strategic litigation, public information, and education programs.
1968

3321 Norfolk Foundation
101 W. Main Street,
Suite 4500
Norfolk, VA 23510-2103
757-622-7951
Fax: 757-622-1751
mbrunson@hamptonroadscf.org
www.hamptonroadscf.org

Deborah M DiCroce, Ed.D., President and CEO
Tim McCarthy, Chief Financial Officer
Kay A. Stine, CFRE, Vice President for Development
Lynn Watson Neumann, Director of Gift Planning

The mission of the Norfolk Foundation is to inspire philanthropy and transform the quality of life in southeastern Virginia.

3322 Robey W Estes Family Foundation
Robey W Estes Jr
3901 West Broad Street
P.O. Box 25612
Richmond, VA 23230-5612
866-378-3748
estes-express.com

Robey W Estes Jr, President and CEO

3323 Virginia Beach Foundation
Suite 4500
101 W. Main Street,
Virginia Beach, VA 23454
757-422-5249
Fax: 757-422-1849
mbrunson@hamptonroadscf.org
www.hamptonroadscf.org

Deborah M DiCroce, President
Tim McCarthy, Chief Financial Officer

Mission is to stimulate the establishment of endowments to serve the people of Virgina Beach now and in the future. Respond to changing, emerging, community needs. Provide a vehicle and a service for donors with varied interests. Serve as a resource, broker, catalyst and leader in the community.

Washington

3324 Arc of Washington State
2638 State Avenue NE
Olympia, WA 98506-4880
360-357-5596
888-754-8798
Fax: 360-357-3279
info@arcwa.org
arcwa.org

Cindy O'Neill, Board President
Sue Elliott, Executive Director
Angie Ziska, Secretary
Martha Schulte, Treasurer

Mission is to advocacte for the rights and full participation of all people with intellectual and developmental disabilities.

3325 Ben B Cheney Foundation
3110 Ruston Way
Suite A
Tacoma, WA 98402-5308
253-572-2442
Info@benbcheneyfoundation.org
benbcheneyfoundation.org

Bradbury F. Cheney, President
Piper Cheney, Vice President
Carolyn J. Cheney, Secretary Treasurer
Allan L. Undem, Board Member

The Foundation makes grants in communities where the Cheney Lumber Company was active. The Foundation's goal is to improve the quality of life in those communities by making grants to a wide range of activities.

3326 Community Foundation of North Central Washington
9 South Wenatchee Ave
Wenatchee, WA 98801-3332
509-663-7716
Fax: 888-317-8314
info@cfncw.org
www.cfncw.org

Beth Stipe, Executive Director
Kristy Harris, Chief Financial Officer
Lila R. Edlund, Director of Administration
Jennifer Dolge, Director of Donor Services and C

Assists donors by helping identify their specific charitable and goals and provide grants and scholarships that help groups and people address critical issues in North Central Washington

3327 Glaser Progress Foundation
1601 Second Avenue
Suite 1080
Seattle, WA 98101-9223
206-728-1050
Fax: 206-728-1123

Martin Collier, Executive Director
Mitchell Fox, Program Officer
Melessa Rogers, Operations Manager

The Glaser Prograss Foundation focuses on four program areas: measuring progress, animal advocacy, independent media and global HIV/AIDS.

3328 Greater Tacoma Community Foundation
950 Pacific Avenue
Suite 1100
Tacoma, WA 98402-4423
253-383-5622
Fax: 253-272-8099
info@gtcf.org
www.gtcf.org

Rose Lincoln Hamilton, President and CEO
Shirley Brockmann, CPA, Vice President Finance & Adminis
Elyse Rowe, Chief of Strategy and Community
Gina Anstey, Vice President, Grants

Mission is fostering generosity by connecting people who care with causes that matter, forever enriching our community.

3329 Inland Northwest Community Foundation
421 West Riverside Avenue
Suite 606
Spokane, WA 99201- 0405
509-624-2606
888-267-5606
Fax: 509-624-2608
admin@inwcf.org
www.inwcf.org

Mark Hurtubise, Ph.D., J.D., President and CEO
Troy Braga, CPA, Controller
P J Watters, Director of Gift Planning
Molly Sanchez, Director of Community Engagement

Serving 20 counties throughout Eastern Washington and Northern Idaho, mission is to foster vibrant and sustainable communities in the Inland Northwest.

3330 **Medina Foundation**
801 2nd Ave
Suite 1300
Seattle, WA 98104-1517
206-652-8783
Fax: 206-652-8791
info@medinafoundation.org
www.medinafoundation.org
Jennifer Teunon, Executive Director
Jessica Case, Program Officer
Aana Lauckhart, Program Officer
Alexia Cameron, Grants Administrator
A family foundation that works to foster positive change in the Greater Puget Sound area. The Foundation strives to improve the human condition by supporting organizations that provide critical services to those in need.

3331 **Norcliffe Foundation**
999 3rd Ave
Suite 1006
Seattle, WA 98104-4001
206-682-4820
Fax: 206-682-4821
arline@thenorcliffefoundation.com
www.thenorcliffefoundation.com
Arline Hefferline, Foundation Manager
Nora P. Kenway, President
Geographic area of funding limited to the Puget Sound Region in and around Seattle, Washington.

3332 **Stewardship Foundation**
1145 Broadway
Suite 1500
Tacoma, WA 98402-1278
253-620-1340
Fax: 253-572-2721
info@stewardshipfdn.org
www.stewardshipfdn.org
William T. Weyerhaeuser, Chair
Gail T. Weyerhaeuser, Vice Chair and Treasurer
Chi- Dooh, Director
J. Derek McNeil, Director
Christian, evangelical organizations - national or international impact.

3333 **Weyerhaeuser Company Foundation**
33663 Weyerhaeuser Way South
Federal Way, WA 98003
253-924-2345
800-525-5440
www.weyerhaeuser.com
Daniel S Fulton, President & CEO
Patricia M Bedient, EVP & CFO
Sandy D McDade, SVP & General Counsel
John A Hooper, SVP, Human Resources
Although the foundation does fund programs for disabled persons from time to time, it is not a specific priority for the foundation. Since it was formed in 1948, the foundation has given more than $81.1 million to nonprofit organizations and is one of the oldest funds for corporate philanthropy in the country. Nearly all of its contributions have been made within the communities where Weyerhaeuser employees live and work and awards approximately 600 grants annually.

West Virginia

3334 **Arc Of West Virginia, The**
912 Market Street
Parkersburg, WV 26101-4737
304-422-3151

3335 **Bernard McDonough Foundation**
311 Fourth Street
Parkersburg, WV 26101-5315
304-424-6280
Fax: 304-424-6281
www.mcdonoughfoundation.org
Robert W Stephens, Ed.D., President
Mary Riccobene, Vice President
Francis C. McCusker, Treasurer
Katrina Valentine, Corporate Secretary
Directors and officers continue the legacy of the McDonoughs by providing grants that create a healthier, more educated and culturally appreciative citizenry.

3336 **High Technology Foundation**
1000 Galliher Dr.
Suite 1000
Fairmont, WV 26554
304-363-5482
877-363-5482
info@wvhtf.org
www.wvhtf.org
Frank W. Blake, Chair
James L. Estep, President & CEO
High Technology Foundation is dedicated to maximizing economic development in West Virginia through the high-technology business sector.

Wisconsin

3337 **Arc of Dunn County**
2602 Hils Court
Menomonie, WI 54751-4160
715-235-7373
Fax: 715-233-3565
www.arcofdunncounty.org
Rebecca Cooper, Executive Director
Kathy Lausted, Guardianship Director
Advocating for the rights of citizens with disabilities.

3338 **Arc of Eau Claire**
4800 Golf Road
Suite 450
Eau Claire, WI 54701-6130
715-833-1735
Fax: 715-833-1215
frcec@frcec.org
www.frcec.org
Brook Steele, President
Melanie Koehler, Vice President
Dr. Jennifer Eddy, Secretary
Dr. Emily Smith-Nguyen, Treasurer
Mission is to provide programs and services that build on family strengths through prevention, education, support and networking in collaboration with other resources in the community.

3339 **Arc of Fox Cities**
211 E. Franklin St.
Suite A
Appleton, WI 54911
920-735-0943
Fax: 920-725-1531
info@arcfoxcities.com
arcfoxcities.com
Laura McCormick, President
Todd Klauer, Vice President
Bryan Mueller, Secretary
Rico Tomasi, Treasurer
Mission statement is to utilize advocacy, respect and concern to empower all people with disabilities to have the opportunity to choose and realize their goal of a full life and a secure future.

3340 **Arc of Racine County**
6214 Washington Ave
Suite C-6
Racine, WI 53404-3350
262-634-6303
info@thearcofracine.org
www.thearcofracine.org
Peggy Foreman, Executive Director
Alison Henry, Program Manager
Ross Gietzel, Program Assistant
The Arc of Racine's mission is to advocate for and provide information and services to improve lives.

3341 **Arc of Wisconsin Disability Association**
2800 Royal Ave
Suite 202
Monona, WI 53713-1518
608-222-8907
877-272-8400
Fax: 608-222-8908
arcw@att.net
John Beisbier, President
Donna Auchue, Vice President
Tina Beauprey, Secretary
The Arc-Wisconsin strives to be a major force in advocating and promoting self-determined quality of life opportunities for

poeple with developmental and related disabilities and their families.

3342 **Arc-Dane County**
6602 Grand Teton Plz
Madison, WI 53719-1091
608-833-1199
Fax: 608-833-1307
arcdanecounty@gmail.com
arcdanecounty.org

Ken Hobbs, President
John Leemkuil, Vice President
Mark Lederer, Secretary
Todd Grundahl, Treasurer

The Arc-Dane County is a non-profit organization whose primary objective is to support children and adults with developmental disabilities and their families through advocacy to assure these individuals are offered the same opportunities and have the rights due all people. The Arc-Dane County provides numerous services through education, overall support, and legislation that assists those individuals with developmental disabilities be it within their homes, communities, or at work.

3343 **Faye McBeath Foundation**
101 W. Pleasant Street
Suite 210
Milwaukee, WI 53212- 3157
414-272-2626
Fax: 414-272-6235

P. Michael Mahoney, Chair
Mary T. Kellner, Vice Chair
Gregory M. Wesley, Secretary
Scott E. Gelzer, Executive Director

A private independent foundation providing grants to tax exempt nonprofit organizations principally the metropolitan Milwaukee area.

3344 **Helen Bader Foundation**
233 North Water Street
4th Floor
Milwaukee, WI 53202- 5761
414-224-6464
Fax: 414-224-1441
info@hbf.org
www.hbf.org

Daniel J. Bader, President/CEO
Lisa G. Hiller, VP, Administration
Maria Lopez Vento, VP, Programs and Partnerships
Robert Tobon, Director, Foundation Relations

Strives to be a philanthropic leader in improving the quality of life of the diverse communities in which it works. The Foundation makes grants, convenes partners, and shares knowledge to affect emerging issues in key areas.

3345 **Johnson Controls Foundation**
5757 N Green Bay Ave
P.O. Box 591
Milwaukee, WI 53201- 4408
414-524-1200
800-333-2222
Fax: 414-524-2077
johnsoncontrols.com

Stephen A Molinaroli, Chairman, President and CEO
Dr. Breda Bolzenius, Vice President, Vice Chairman
Kim Metcalf-Kupres, Vice President and Chief Marketi
R. Bruce McDonald, Executive Vice President and CF

Organized and directed to be operated for charitable purposes which include the distribution and application of financial support to soundly managed and operated organizations or causes which are fundamentally philanthropic.

3346 **Lynde and Harry Bradley Foundation**
1241 N Franklin Pl
Milwaukee, WI 53202-2901
414-291-9915
Fax: 414-291-9991
www.bradleyfdn.org

Dennis J. Kuester, Chairman
David V. Uihlein, Vice Chairman
Michael W. Grebbe, President and CEO
Patrick J. English, Chief Investment Officer

The Foundation's programs support limited, competent government; a dynamic marketplace for economic, intellectual and cultural activity; a vigorus defense at home and abroad, of American ideas and institutions; and scholarly studies and academic achievement.

3347 **Milwaukee Foundation**
101 W Pleasant St
Suite 210
Milwaukee, WI 53212-3963
414-272-5805
Fax: 414-272-6235
info@greatermilwaukeefoundation.org
www.greatermilwaukeefoundation.org

Ellen M Gilligan, President and CEO
Marcus White, Vice President
Kathryn J. Dunn, Vice President
Danae Davis, Executive Director

Guided by three tenets- helping donors create personal legacies of giving that last beyond their lifetimes, investing donor funds for maximum return with minimal risk, and playing a leadership role tackling the communities most challenging needs.

3348 **Northwestern Mutual Life Foundation**
720 E Wisconsin Ave
Milwaukee, WI 53202-4703
414-271-1444
www.northwesternmutual.com

John E Schlifske, Chairman and CEO
Gregory C. Oberland, President
Michael G. Carter, Executive Vice President and CFO
Joann M. Eisenhart, Senior Vice President - Human Re

3349 **Patrick and Anna M Cudahy Fund**
70 E. Lake St.,
Suite 1120
Chicago, Il 60601
312-422-1442
Fax: 312-641-5736
laurenkrieg@cudahyfund.org
cudahyfund.org

Janet S Cudahy MD, President
Lauren Krieg, Executive Director

A general purpose foundation which primarily supports organizations in Wisconsin and the metropolitan Chicago area. Interests are social service, youth, and education with some giving for the arts, and other areas.

3350 **SB Waterman & E Blade Charitable Foundation**
Marshall & Ilsley Trust Company
111 E. Kilbourn Ave.,
Milwaukee, WI 53202-2980
414-287-8700
Fax: 414-765-8200

Thomas C Boettcher, Director

Giving primarily to health associations. Geographical focus is Wisconsin.

Wyoming

3351 **Arc of Natrona County**
314 W. Midwest Ave
P.O. Box 393
Casper, WY 82601
307-577-4913
800-433-5255
Fax: 307-577-4014
info@thearc.org
arcofnatronacounty.org

Beau Covert, President
Dr. Nathan Edwards, Vice President
Kelley Reimer, Treasurer
Colbi Maddox, Secretary

Organization works to ensure that the estimated 7.2 million Americans with intellectual and developmental disabilities have the services and supports they need to grow, develop and live in communities across the nation.

Funding Directories

3352 **Chronicle Guide to Grants**
318 S. Lee Street
Alexandria, DC 20037-1146
202-466-1200
800-287-6072
Fax: 202-452-1033
help@philanthropy.com
heideninc.com

Phil Semas, Manager
Edward J. Heiden, President
A computerized research tool, on floppy disks or a CD-ROM, for immediate use on any IBM compatible personal computer. Offers electronic listings of 10,000 grants from hundreds of foundations, with a subscription that offers 1,000 plus new listings every two months. Each listing offers grant information as well as names, addresses and phone numbers of the grant-making organizations. *$295.00*

3353 **College Student's Guide to Merit and Other No-Need Funding**
Reference Service Press
5000 Windplay Dr
Suite 4
El Dorado Hills, CA 95762-9319
916-939-9620
Fax: 916-939-9626
info@rspfunding.com
www.rspfunding.com

Gail Schlachter, Founder
R. David Weber, Editor
Sandy Hirsh, Editor
Sandy Perez, Funding Finder
More than 1,200 funding opportunities for currently-enrolled or returning college students are described in this directory. *$32.50*
450 pages
ISBN 1-588410-41-2

3354 **Community Health Funding Report**
CD Publications
8204 Fenton St
Silver Spring, MD 20910-4502
301-588-6380
800-666-6380
Fax: 301-588-6385
www.cdpublications.com

Michael Gerecht, President
The once twice-monthly report is now web-based to allow for breaking news updates and up the the minute information about funding, including: public and private grant announcements; reports on successful health programs nationwide; interviews with grant officials; plus national news on health policy topics affecting various organizations. *$439.00*
Web-based

3355 **Directory of Financial Aids for Women**
Reference Service Press
2310 Homestead Rd
Suite C1 #219
Los Altos, CA 94024
650-861-3170
Fax: 650-861-3171
info@rspfunding.com
www.rspfunding.com

Gail Schlachter, Founder
R. David Weber, Editor
Sandy Hirsh, Editor
Sandy Perez, Funding Finder
Funding programs listed support study, research, travel, training, career development, or innovative effort at any level; descriptions of more than 1,700 funding programs - representing billions of dollars in financial aid set aside for women; also an annotated bibliography of 60 key directories that identify even more financial aid opportunities and a set of indexes that let you search the directory by title, sponser, researching, tenability, subject, and deadline. *$45.00*
578 pages Biennial
ISBN 1-588410-00-5

3356 **Disability Funding News**
8204 Fenton St
Silver Spring, MD 20910-4502
301-588-6380
800-666-6380
Fax: 301-588-6385
www.cdpublications.com

Michael Gerecht, President

3357 **FC Search**
Foundation Center
79 fifth Avenue
New York, NY 10003-3034
212-620-4230
800-424-9836
Fax: 212-807-3677
order@foundationcenter.org
foundationcenter.org

Bradford K Smith, President
Lisa Philip, Vice President for Strategic Phi
Jen Bokoff, Director of GrantCraft
Lawrence T. McGill, Vice President for Research
Provides access to the Foundation Center's comprehensive database of funders in a convenient CD-ROM format. *$1845.00*

3358 **Federal Grants & Contracts Weekly**
LRP Publications
360 Hiatt Drive
Palm Beach Gardens, FL 33418-1718
800-341-7874
Fax: 561-622-2423
custserve@lrp.com
www.lrp.com

Kelly Sullivan, Editor
Kenneth F. Kahn, President
The latest funding announcements of federal grants for project opportunities in research, training and services. Provides profiles of key programs, tips on seeking grants, updates on legislation and regulations, budget developments and early alerts to upcoming funding opportunities. *$340.00*
Weekly

3359 **Financial Aid for Asian Americans**
Reference Service Press
2310 Homestead Rd
Suite C1 #219
Los Altos, CA 94024
650-861-3170
Fax: 650-861-3171
info@rspfunding.com
www.rspfunding.com

Gail Schlachter, Founder
R. David Weber, Editor
Sandy Hirsh, Editor
Sandy Perez, Funding Finder
This is the source to use if you are looking for financial aid for Asian Americans; nearly 1,000 funding opportunities are described. *$35.00*
336 pages
ISBN 1-588410-02-1

3360 **Financial Aid for Hispanic Americans**
Reference Service Press
2310 Homestead Rd
Suite C1 #219
Los Altos, CA 94024
650-861-3170
Fax: 650-861-3171
info@rspfunding.com
www.rspfunding.com

Gail Schlachter, Founder
R. David Weber, Editor
Sandy Hirsh, Editor
Sandy Perez, Funding Finder
Nearly 1,300 funding programs open to Americans of Mexican, Puerto Rican, Central American, or other Latin American heritage are described here. *$37.50*
472 pages
ISBN 1-588410-03-X

3361 **Financial Aid for Native Americans**
Reference Service Press
2310 Homestead Rd
Suite C1 #219
Los Altos, CA 94024
650-861-3170
Fax: 650-861-3171
info@rspfunding.com
www.rspfunding.com

Gail Schlachter, Founder
R. David Weber, Editor
Sandy Hirsh, Editor
Sandy Perez, Funding Finder

Detailed information is provided on 1,500 funding opportunities open to American Indians, Native Alaskans, and Native Pacific Islanders. *$37.50*
562 pages
ISBN 1-588410-04-8

3362 **Financial Aid for Research and Creative Activities Abroad**
Reference Service Press
2310 Homestead Rd
Suite C1 #219
Los Altos, CA 94024
650-861-3170
Fax: 650-861-3171
info@rspfunding.com
www.rspfunding.com

Gail Schlachter, Founder
R. David Weber, Editor
Sandy Hirsh, Editor
Sandy Perez, Funding Finder

Described here are 1,200 funding programs (scholarships, fellowships, grants, etc.) available to support research, professional, or creative activities abroad. *$45.00*
378 pages
ISBN 1-588410-82-5

3363 **Financial Aid for Veterans, Military Personnel and their Dependents**
Reference Service Press
2310 Homestead Rd
Suite C1 #219
Los Altos, CA 94024
650-861-3170
Fax: 650-861-3171
info@rspfunding.com
www.rspfunding.com

Gail Schlachter, Founder
R. David Weber, Editor
Sandy Hirsh, Editor
Sandy Perez, Funding Finder

According to Reference Book Review, this directory (with its 1,100 entries) is the most comprehensive guide available on the subject. *$40.00*
392 pages
ISBN 1-588410-43-9

3364 **Financial Aid for the Disabled and Their Families**
Reference Service Press
2310 Homestead Rd
Suite C1 #219
Los Altos, CA 94024
650-861-3170
Fax: 650-861-3171
info@rspfunding.com
www.rspfunding.com

Gail Schlachter, Founder
R. David Weber, Editor

This directory, which Children's Bookwatch calls invaluable describes more than 1,100 financial aid opportunities available to support persons with disabilities and members of their families. Updated every 2 years. *$37.50*
508 pages Every other yr.
ISBN 1-588410-01-3

3365 **Foundation & Corporate Grants Alert**
LRP Publications
360 Hiatt Drive
Palm Beach Gardens, FL 33418-1718
800-341-7874
Fax: 561-622-2423
custserve@lrp.com
www.lrp.com

Kelly Sullivan, Editor
Kenneth F. Kahn, President

A complete guide to foundation and corporate grant opportunities for nonprofit organizations. Tracks developments and trends in funding and provides notification of changes in foundations' funding priorities. *$245.00*
Monthly
ISSN 1062-46 6

3366 **Foundation 1000**
Foundation Center
79 fifth Avenue
New York, NY 10003-3076
212-620-4230
800-424-9836
Fax: 212-807-3691
order@foundationcenter.org
www.foundationcenter.org

Bradford K Smith, President
Lisa Philip, Vice President for Strategic Phi
Jen Bokoff, Director of GrantCraft
Lawrence T. McGill, Vice President for Research

Offers comprehensive information on the 1000 largest foundations in the US. *$195.00*

3367 **Foundation Directories**
Foundation Center
79 fifth Avenue
New York, NY 10003-3034
212-620-4230
800-424-9836
Fax: 212-807-3677
order@foundationcenter.org
foundationcenter.org

Bradford K Smith, President
Lisa Philip, Vice President for Strategic Phi
Jen Bokoff, Director of GrantCraft
Lawrence T. McGill, Vice President for Research

Lists key facts on the top 20,000 US foundations. *$125.00*
ISBN 0-87954 -36-1

3368 **Foundation Grants to Individuals**
Foundation Center
79 fifth Avenue
New York, NY 10003-3034
212-620-4230
800-424-9836
Fax: 212-807-3677
order@foundationcenter.org
foundationcenter.org

Bradford K Smith, President
Lisa Philip, Vice President for Strategic Phi
Jen Bokoff, Director of GrantCraft
Lawrence T. McGill, Vice President for Research

The only publication that provides extensive coverage of foundation funding prospects for individual grantseekers. *$40.00*
Biennially

3369 **From the State Capitals: Public Health**
Wakeman/Walworth
P.O. Box 7376
Alexandria, VA 22307-376
703-768-9600
Fax: 703-768-9690

Mark Willen, Editor

Digest of state and municipal health care financing and cost containment measures, includes medical legislation, disease control, etc. *$245.00*
6 pages

3370 **Grant Guides**
Foundation Center
79 fifth Avenue
New York, NY 10003-3034
212-620-4230
800-424-9836
Fax: 212-807-3677
order@foundationcenter.org
foundationcenter.org

Bradford K Smith, President
Lisa Philip, Vice President for Strategic Phi
Jen Bokoff, Director of GrantCraft
Lawrence T. McGill, Vice President for Research

Provides descriptions of actual foundation grants awarded in various subject fields. *$35.00*
ISBN 0-87954 -90-6

3371 **Guide to Funding for International and Foreign Programs**
79 fifth Avenue
New York, NY 10003-3034
212-620-4230
800-424-9836
Fax: 212-807-3677
order@foundationcenter.org
foundationcenter.org

Bradford K Smith, President
Lisa Philip, Vice President for Strategic Phi
Jen Bokoff, Director of GrantCraft
Lawrence T. McGill, Vice President for Research

Grantmakers featured in this guide provide funding for international relief, disaster assistance, human rights, civil liberties, community development, conferences, and education. *$190.00*

3372 **Guide to US Foundations their Trustees, Officers and Donors**
Foundation Center
79 fifth Avenue
New York, NY 10003-3034
212-620-4230
800-424-9836
Fax: 212-807-3677
order@foundationcenter.org
foundationcenter.org

Bradford K Smith, President
Lisa Philip, Vice President for Strategic Phi
Jen Bokoff, Director of GrantCraft
Lawrence T. McGill, Vice President for Research

Provides crucial facts on grantmaking. Each entry includes contact information, current assets, annual contributions, officers, donors and more. *$135.00*

3373 **High School Senior's Guide to Merit and Other No-Need Funding**
Reference Service Press
2310 Homestead Rd
Suite C1 #219
Los Altos, CA 94024
650-861-3170
Fax: 650-861-3171
info@rspfunding.com
www.rspfunding.com

Gail Schlachter, Founder
R. David Weber, Editor
Sandy Hirsh, Editor
Sandy Perez, Funding Finder

Here's your guide to 1,100 funding programs that never look at income level when making awards to college bound high school seniors. *$29.95*
400 pages
ISBN 1-588410-44-X

3374 **How to Pay for Your Degree in Business & Related Fields**
Reference Service Press
2310 Homestead Rd
Suite C1 #219
Los Altos, CA 94024
650-861-3170
Fax: 650-861-3171
info@rspfunding.com
www.rspfunding.com

Gail Schlachter, Founder
R. David Weber, Editor
Sandy Hirsh, Editor
Sandy Perez, Funding Finder

If you need funding for an undergraduate or graduate degree in business or related fields, this is the directory to use (500+ funding programs described). *$30.00*
290 pages
ISBN 1-588411-45-1

3375 **How to Pay for Your Degree in Education& Related Fields**
Reference Service Press
2310 Homestead Rd
Suite C1 #219
Los Altos, CA 94024
650-861-3170
Fax: 650-861-3171
www.rspfunding.com

Gail Schlachter, Founder
R. David Weber, Editor
Sandy Hirsh, Editor
Sandy Perez, Funding Finder

Here's hundreds of funding opportunities available to support undergraduate and graduate students preparing for a career in education, guidance etc. *$30.00*
250 pages
ISBN 1-588411-46-x

3376 **National Directory of Corporate Giving**
Foundation Center
79 fifth Avenue
New York, NY 10003-3034
212-620-4230
800-424-9836
Fax: 212-807-3677
order@foundationcenter.org
foundationcenter.org

Bradford K Smith, President
Lisa Philip, Vice President for Strategic Phi
Jen Bokoff, Director of GrantCraft
Lawrence T. McGill, Vice President for Research

Offers over 2,000 corporate funders, current giving reviews and profiles of sponsoring companies. *$195.00*

3377 **Older Americans Report**
Business Publishers
2222 Sedwick Drive
Durham, NC 27713-1995
240-514-0600
800-223-8720
Fax: 800-508-2592
custserv@bpinews.com
www.bpinews.com

Leonard Eiser, Publisher

Follows all programs and funding sources in education, housing, job training, therapy, Social Security Supplemental Security Income, Medicare, Medicaid and more of importance to persons with disabilities. Also covers the latest on the Americans with Disabilities Act. Publishes a newsletter. *$327.00*

3378 **Student Guide**
US Department of Education
400 Maryland Avenue SW
Washington, DC 20202
202-401-2000
800-872-5327
Fax: 202-401-0689
TTY: 800-437-0833
customerservice@inet.ed.gov
ed.gov

Arne Duncan, Secretary of Education
Jim Shelton, Deputy Secretary
Ted Mitchell, Under Secretary

Government Agencies

Federal

3379 **Administration on Aging**
Administration for Community Living
330 C St. SW
Washington, DC 20201 202-401-4634
aclinfo@acl.hhs.gov
acl.gov/about-acl/administration-aging
Edwin Walker, Deputy Assistant Secretary for Aging
Administers the Older Americans Act of 1965 to assist states and local communities in developing programs and services for older persons.

3380 **Administration on Children, Youth and Families**
330 C St. SW
Washington, DC 20201 202-401-4634
www.acf.hhs.gov/acyf
Amanda Barlow, Acting Commissioner
Responsible for federal programs that support social services for children, youth, and families; protective services for at-risk youth; and adoption services for children with special needs.

3381 **Administration on Disabilities**
Administration for Community Living
330 C St. SW
Washington, DC 20201 202-401-4634
aclinfo@acl.hhs.gov
acl.gov
Alison Barkoff, Acting Administrator, ACL
Ensures that individuals with disabilities and their families participate in the design of and have access to culturally competent services, supports, and other assistance and opportunities that promote independence, productivity, and integration and inclusion into the community.

3382 **Americans with Disabilities Act Information and Technical Assistance**
US Department of Justice
950 Pennsylvania Ave. NW
9th Floor
Washington, DC 20530 202-307-0663
800-514-0301
Fax: 202-307-1197
TTY: 800-514-0383
www.ada.gov
Rebecca B. Bond, Chief
Anne Raish, Principal Deputy Chief
The ADA assures that Americans with disabilities have the same opportunities as all Americans. To this end, the Justice Department produces publications and conducts programs to increase compliance of the ADA nationwide.

3383 **Centers for Medicare and Medicaid Services**
7500 Security Blvd.
Baltimore, MD 21244 410-786-3000
877-267-2323
TTY: 866-226-1819
www.cms.gov
Chiquita Brooks-LaSure, Administrator
Jonathan Blum, Principal Deputy Administrator
Karen Jackson, Chief Operating Officer
Responsible for administering Medicare, Medicaid, and the Children's Health Insurance Program. Formerly the Health Care Financing Administration.

3384 **Civil Rights Division/Disability Rights Section**
US Department of Justice
950 Pennsylvania Ave. NW
9th Floor
Washington, DC 20530 202-307-0663
800-514-0301
Fax: 202-307-1197
TTY: 800-514-0383
www.ada.gov
Rebecca B. Bond, Chief
Anne Raish, Principal Deputy Chief
The US Department of Justice answers questions about the Americans with Disabilities Act (ADA) and provides free materials by mail and fax through the ADA Information Line.

3385 **Committee for Purchase from People Who Are Blind or Severely Disabled**
1401 S Clark St.
Suite 715
Arlington, VA 22202-3259 703-603-7740
800-999-5963
Fax: 703-603-0655
info@abilityone.gov
www.abilityone.gov
Tina Ballard, Executive Director & CEO
Kimberly Zeich, Deputy Executive Director & COO
Kelvin Wood, Chief of Staff
George Govan, Chief Financial Officer
A federal agency that administers the Javits-Wagner-O'Day Program, directing federal agencies to purchase products and services from nonprofit agencies that employ people who are blind or have other severe disabilities. Provides a wide range of vocational options to individuals with severe disabilities.

3386 **Equal Opportunity Employment Commission**
131 M St. NE
Washington, DC 20507 202-663-4900
800-669-4000
TTY: 800-669-6820
info@eeoc.gov
www.eeoc.gov
Charlotte A. Burrows, Chair
Janet Dhillon, Commissioner
Keith E. Sonderling, Commissioner
Andrea R. Lucas, Commissioner
This agency is responsible for enforcing workplace anti-discrimination laws, including the Americans with Disabilities Act (ADA) and the Rehabilitation Act.

3387 **Federal Communications Commission**
45 L St. NE
Washington, DC 20554 202-418-0500
888-225-5322
Fax: 866-418-0232
fccinfo@fcc.gov
fcc.gov
Jessica Rosenworcel, Acting Chair
Brendan Carr, Commissioner
Geoffrey Starks, Commissioner
Nathan Simington, Commissioner
Enforces ADA telecommunications provisions which require that companies offering telephone service to the general public must offer telephone relay services to individuals who use text telephones or similar devices. Also enforces closed captioning rules, hearing compatibility and access to equipment and services for people with disabilities.

3388 **Health Resources and Services Administration (HRSA)**
US Department of Health and Human Services
5600 Fishers Lane
Rockville, MD 20857 301-443-2216
877-464-4772
TTY: 877-897-9910
www.hrsa.gov
Diana Espinosa, Deputy Administrator
Jordan Grossman, Chief of Staff
The Health Resources and Services Administration provides programs for people with HIV/AIDS, pregnant women, mothers, and other individuals in need of high quality primary health care.

3389 **National Cancer Institute**
9609 Medical Center Dr.
Rockville, MD 20850 800-422-6237
TTY: 800-332-8615
nciinfo@nih.gov
www.cancer.gov
Norman E. Sharpless, Director
Douglas R. Lowy, Principal Deputy Director
James Doroshow, Deputy Director, Clinical & Translational Research
Dinah S. Singer, Deputy Director, Scientific Strategy & Development

The National Cancer Institute conducts and supports research, training, health information dissemination, and programs related to cancer, cancer rehabilitation, and the care of cancer patients.

3390 National Coalition of Federal Aviation Employees with Disabilities
Federal Aviation Administration
6500 South MacArthur, AML-4023
RRF Building-185
Oklahoma City, OK 73169
405-954-6877
www.ncfaed.org

Gregory A. Brooks, National President

NCFAED works on improving work conditions for employees; expanding National Coalition to serve all FAA employees; promoting equal opportunity for people with disabilities in the FAA workplace; assisting the FAA in its commitment to remove physical and attudinal barriers which inhibit opportunities for people with disabilities; and aligning with internal and external organizations to attract future generations of people with disabilities to the FAA as employees.

3391 National Council on Disability
1331 F St. NW
Suite 850
Washington, DC 20004
202-272-2004
Fax: 202-272-2022
TTY: 202-272-2074
www.ncd.gov

Andres Callegos, Chair
James T. Brett, Vice Chair
Anne Sommers McIntosh, Executive Director
Joan M. Durocher, General Counsel

Federal agency led by members appointed by the President of the United States and confirmed by the United States Senate. The overall purpose of the National Council is to promote policies, programs, practices and procedures that guarantee equal opportunities to persons with disabilities.

3392 National Eye Institute
National Institutes of Health
31 Center Dr.
MSC 2510
Bethesda, MD 20892-2510
301-496-5248
800-411-1222
2020@nei.nih.gov
www.nei.nih.gov

Michael F. Chiang, Director
Santa Tumminia, Deputy Director
Brian Trent, Associate Director, Management & Executive Officer
Brian Brooks, Clinical Director

As part of the federal government's National Institutes of Health (NIH), the National Eye Institute finances intramural and extramural research on eye diseases and visual disorders.

3393 National Institute of Arthritis and Musculoskeletal and Skin Diseases
National Institutes of Health
31 Center Dr., MSC 2350
Building 31, Room 4C02
Bethesda, MD 20892-2350
301-496-8190
877-226-4267
Fax: 301-480-2814
TTY: 301-565-2966
www.naims.nih.gov

Lindsey A. Criswell, Director
Robert H. Carter, Deputy Director
Rick Phillips, Executive Officer
John O'Shea, Scientific Director, Intramural Research

The mission of the National Institute of Arthritis and Musculoskeletal and Skin Diseases is to advance understanding and treatment of diseases of the bones, joints, muscles, and skin by supporting research, training scientists, and disseminating information on such diseases.

3394 National Institute of Diabetes and Digestive and Kidney Diseases
National Institutes of Health
31 Center Dr.
Bethesda, MD 20892
800-860-8747
TTY: 866-569-1162
healthinfo@niddk.nih.gov
www.niddk.nih.gov

Griffin P. Rodgers, Director
Gregory G. Germino, Deputy Director
Camille Hoover, Executive Officer
Elise Goodwin, Deputy Executive Officer

The National Institute of Diabetes and Digestive and Kidney Diseases conducts and supports research, training, and science-based information dissemination on diabetes, digestive diseases, and kidney, urologic, and hematologic diseases.

3395 National Institute of Mental Health
National Institutes of Health
6001 Executive Blvd.
Room 6200, MSC 9663
Bethesda, MD 20892-9663
866-615-6464
TTY: 866-415-8051
nimhinfo@nih.gov
www.nimh.nih.gov

Joshua A. Gordon, Director
Shelli Avenevoli, Deputy Director

The mission of the National Institute of Mental Health is to advance the prevention, recovery, and cure of mental illnesses through basic and clinical research.

3396 National Institute of Neurological Disorders and Stroke
National Institutes of Health
PO Box 5801
Bethesda, MD 20824
800-352-9424
TTY: 711
www.ninds.nih.gov

Walter J. Koroshetz, Director
Nina Schor, Deputy Director

The mission of the National Institute of Neurological Disorders and Stroke is to reduce the burden of neurological disease by supporting neuroscience research, funding and conducting training and career development programs, and disseminating scientific information on neurological health.

3397 National Institute on Aging
31 Center Dr., MSC 2292
Building 31, Room 5C27
Bethesda, MD 20892
800-222-2225
TTY: 800-222-4225
niaic@nia.nih.gov
www.nia.nih.gov

Richard J. Hodes, Director
Patrick Shirdon, Director, Management
Lisa Mascone, Deputy Director, Management
Luigi Ferrucci, Scientific Director

The National Institute on Aging (NIA) is the primary federal agency engaged in researching Alzheimer's disease, providing resources to scientists and educating the public on the results of studies.

3398 National Institute on Deafness and Other Communication Disorders
National Institutes of Health
31 Center Dr.
MSC 2320
Bethesda, MD 20892-2320
301-827-8183
800-241-1044
Fax: 301-770-8977
TTY: 800-241-1055
nidcdinfo@nidcd.nih.gov
www.nidcd.nih.gov

Debara L. Tucci, Director
Judith A. Cooper, Deputy Director
Timothy J. Wheeles, Executive Officer
Lisa Portnoy, Deputy Executive Officer

The National Institute on Deafness and Other Communication Disorders supports and conducts research to help prevent, detect and diagnose disabilities that affect hearing, balance, taste, smell, voice, speech, and communication.

3399 National Institute on Disability, Independent Living, and Rehabilitation Research (NIDILRR)
Administration for Community Living
330 C St. SW
Washington, DC 20201 202-401-4634
nidilrr-mailbox@acl.hhs.gov
acl.gov

Anjali Forber-Pratt, Director
Kristi Hill, Deputy Director
Phillip Beatty, Director, Office of Research Sciences
Sarah Ruiz, Associate Director, Office of Research Sciences

Serving as the federal government's disability research agency, NIDILRR provides research, training, and technical assistance to maximize the full inclusion of individuals with disabilities into society; promotes the use of rehabilitation technology for individuals with disabilities; and ensures the distribution of practical scientific and technological information in usable formats.

3400 Office of Disability Employment Policy
US Department of Labor
200 Constitution Ave. NW
Washington, DC 20210 202-693-7880
866-633-7365
odep@dol.gov
www.dol.gov/agencies/odep

Bryan Ballmann, Executive Officer
John Tambornino, Senior Advisor
Melissa Turner, Special Assistant

Non-regulatory federal agency that promotes and develops policies that increase employment opportunities for people with disabilities.

3401 Office of Fair Housing and Equal Opportunity
US Department of Housing & Urban Development
451 7th St. SW
Washington, DC 20410 202-708-1112
TTY: 202-708-1455
www.hud.gov/program_offices

Jeanine Worden, Acting Assistant Secretary

The Office of Fair Housing and Equal Opportunity (FHEO) enforces and develops laws and policies that eliminate housing discrimination and ensure that all Americans have equal access to housing. The laws enforced by FHEO include Titles II and III of the Americans with Disabilities Act and Section 504 of the Rehabilitation Act.

3402 Office of Retirement and Disability Policy (ORDP)
Social Security Administration
1100 West High Rise
6401 Security Blvd.
Baltimore, MD 21235 800-772-1213
TTY: 800-325-0778
www.ssa.gov/policy

Kilolo Kijakazi, Deputy Commissioner
Stephen G. Evangelista, Assistant Deputy Commissioner
Gina P. Clemons, Associate Commissioner, Office of Disability Policy

Serves as the principal advisor to the Commissioner of Social Security on major policy issues, including those relating to disability policy.

3403 Office of Special Education Programs
US Department of Education
400 Maryland Ave. SW
Washington, DC 20202-7100 202-245-7459
800-872-5327
Fax: 202-401-0689
TTY: 800-437-0833
www2.ed.gov/about/offices/list/osers/osep

David Cantrell, Assistant Secretary
Melanie Winston, Executive Officer

Assists infants, toddlers, children and youth with disabilities by providing leadership and financial support to states and local districts.

3404 President's Committee on People with Intellectual Disabilities
Administration for Community Living
330 C St. SW
Washington, DC 20201 202-401-4634
acl.gov

3405 Rehabilitation Services Administration
US Department of Education
400 Maryland Ave. SW
Washington, DC 20202 202-245-7468
800-872-5327
Fax: 202-401-0689
TTY: 800-437-0833
www2.ed.gov

David Cantrell, Assistant Secretary
Melanie Winston, Executive Officer

The Rehabilitation Services Administration (RSA) oversees formula and discretionary grant programs that help individuals with physical or mental disabilities obtain employment and live more independently through the provision of such supports as counseling, medical and psychological services, job training and other individualized services.

3406 Social Security Administration
1100 West High Rise
6401 Security Blvd.
Baltimore, MD 21235 800-772-1213
TTY: 800-325-0778
www.ssa.gov

Andrew M. Saul, Commissioner
David F. Black, Deputy Commissioner

Administers old age, survivors, and disability insurance programs under Title II of the Social Security Act. Also administers the federal income maintenance program under Title XVI of the Social Security Act. Maintains network of local/regional offices nationwide.

3407 Substance Abuse and Mental Health Services Administration (SAMHSA)
US Department of Health and Human Services
5600 Fishers Lane
Rockville, MD 20857 877-726-4727
TTY: 800-487-4889
samhsainfo@samhsa.hhs.gov
www.samhsa.gov

Tom Coderre, Acting Assistant Secretary
Sonia Chessen, Chief of Staff

SAMHSA aims to advance substance use and mental health services and improve the lives of people living with mental and substance use disorders.

3408 US Department of Education: Office for Civil Rights
400 Maryland Ave. SW
Washington, DC 20202-1100 800-421-3481
800-872-5327
Fax: 202-453-6012
TTY: 800-877-8339
ocr@ed.gov
www2.ed.gov/about/offices/list/ocr

Suzanne Goldberg, Acting Assistant Secretary
Randolph Wills, Deputy Assistant Secretary, Enforcement
Monique Dixon, Deputy Assistant Secretary, Policy
Laurie Monk, Deputy Assistant Secretary, Management & Planning

Prohibits discrimination in programs and activities funded by the Department of Education. Investigates complaints and provides technical assistance to individuals and entities with rights and responsibilities under Section 504.

3409 US Department of Labor: Office of Federal Contract Compliance Programs
200 Constitution Ave. NW
Washington, DC 20210 866-487-2365
TTY: 877-889-5627
webmaster@dol.gov
www.dol.gov/agencies/ofccp

Jenny R. Yang, Director
Dariely Rodriguez, Chief of Staff

Prohibits contractors and subcontractors from discriminating against applicants or employees.

3410 **US Department of Transportation**
1200 New Jersey Ave. SE
Washington, DC 20590
202-366-4000
855-368-4200
TTY: 800-877-8339
www.dot.gov

Pete Buttigieg, Secretary
Polly Trottenberg, Deputy Secretary
Laura Schiller, Chief of Staff
Carlos Monje, Senior Advisor

Enforces ADA provisions that require nondiscrimination in public and private mass transportation systems and services.

3411 **US Department of Veterans Affairs**
810 Vermont Ave. NW
Washington, DC 20420
800-698-2411
TTY: 711
www.va.gov

Denis McDonough, Secretary
Tanya J. Bradsher, Chief of Staff

The Department of Veterans Affairs provides programs for veterans and their families. Programs include health care, rehabilitation services, compensation for disabilities, veterans benefits, and more.

3412 **US Office of Personnel Management**
1900 E St. NW
Washington, DC 20415-1000
202-606-1800
TTY: 800-877-8339
opm.gov

Kathleen McGettigan, Acting Director

Provides human resources leadership and support to federal agencies. Administers a merit system for federal employment that includes recruiting, examining, training, and promoting people on the basis of knowledge and skills, regardless of sex, race, religion or other factors.

Alabama

3413 **Alabama Council For Developmental Disabilities**
RSA Union Building
RSA Union Building
PO Box 301410
Montgomery, AL 36130- 1410
334-242-3973
800-232-2158
Fax: 334-242-0797
Myra.Jones@mh.alabama.gov
www.acdd.org

Stefan Eisen, Jr., Chair, Parent Advocate
Sophia Whitted, Fiscal Manager
Elmyra Jones-Banks, Executive Director
Shungulla Moorey, Office Manager

Serves as an advocate for Alabama's citizens with developmental disabilities and their families; to empower them with the knowledge and opportunity to make informed choices and exercise control over their own lives; and to create a climate for positive socialchange to enable them to be respected, independent and productive integrated members of society.

3414 **Alabama Department of Public Health**
The RSA Tower, 201 Monroe Street
PO Box 303017
Montgomery, AL 36130-3017
334-206-5300
800-ALA-1818
www.adph.org

Kathy Vincent, Staff Assistant
Donald E Williamson, Administrator

Provides professional services for the improvement and protection of the public's health through disease prevention and the assurance of public health services to resident and transient populations of the state regardless of social circumstances or the ability to pay.

3415 **Alabama Department of Rehabilitation Services**
602 S Lawrence St.
Montgomery, AL 36104
334-293-7500
800-441-7607
Fax: 334-293-7383
www.rehab.alabama.gov

Jane E. Burdeshaw, Commissioner

To enable Alabama's children and adults with disabilities to achieve their maximum potential.

3416 **Alabama Department of Senior Services**
201 Monroe Street
RSA Tower Suite 350
Montgomery, AL 36140
334-242-5743
877-425-2243
Fax: 334-242-5594
Ageline@adss.alabama.gov

Irene Collins, Executive Director
Thomas Ray Edwards, Board Chairman
Dr. Horace Patterson, Vice-Chair

The mission of the Alabama Department of Senior Services is to promote the independence and dignity of those we serve through a comprehensive and coordinated system of quality services

3417 **Alabama Disabilities Advocacy Program**
University of Alabama
P.O. Box 870395
Tuscaloosa, AL 35487-0395
205-348-4928
800-826-1675
Fax: 205-348-3909
adap@adap.ua.edu

Anita Davidson, Legal Assistant
Janet Owens, Accounting Specialist
James Tucker, Director
Rosemary Beck, Information Systems Administrato

The federally mandate statewide protection and advocacy system serving eligible individuals with disabilities in Alabama. ADAP has five program components: Protection and Advocacy for persons with developmental disabilities (PADD), Protection and Advocacy for Individuals with Mental Illness (PAIMT), Protection and Advocacy of Individual Rights (PAIR), Protection and Advocacy for Assistive Technology (PAAT) and Protection & Advocacy For Beneficiaries of Social Security (PABSS).

3418 **Alabama Division of Rehabilitation and Crippled Children**
602 S Lawrence Street
Montgomery, AL 36104
334-293-7500
800-441-7607
Fax: 334-293-7383
www.rehab.state.al.us

Cary F Boswell, Commissioner
Steven Kayes, Board Member
Jimmie Varnado, Board Member

3419 **Alabama Governor's Committee on Employment of Persons with Disabilities**
602 S Lawrence St.
Montgomery, AL 36104
334-293-7500
800-441-7607
Fax: 334-293-7383
www.rehab.alabama.gov

Jane E. Burdeshaw, Commissioner

The Alabama Governor's Committee on Employment of People with Disabilities (AGCEPD) is a program of the Alabama Department of Rehabilitation Services (ADRS).

3420 **Alabama State Department of Human Resources**
Childcare Services Division
50 North Ripley Street
Montgomery, AL 36130
334-242-1310
Fax: 334-353-1115
barry.spear@dhr.alabama.gov
www.dhr.state.al.us

Nancy T. Buckner, Commissioner
Nancy Jinright, Chief of Staff/Ethics Officer
John Hardy, Communications
Conitha King, Finance

Partners with communities to promtoe family stability and provide for the safety and self-sufficiency of vulnerable Alabamians.

3421 Client Assistance Program: Alabama
400 South Union Street
Suite 465
Montgomery, AL 36104 334-263-2749
800-288-3231
Fax: 334-230-9765
rachel.hughes@rehab.alabama.gov
www.sacap.alabama.gov
Rachel Hughes, Director/Advocate

3422 Disability Determination Service: Birmingham
P.O. Box 830300
Birmingham, AL 35283-0300 205-989-2100
800-292-8106
Fax: 205-989-2295
ssa.gov
Tommy Warren, Executive Director
Janet Cox, Owner

3423 Social Security: Mobile Disability Determination Services
PO Box 2371
Mobile, AL 36652-2371 251-433-2820
800-292-6743
Fax: 251-436-0599
www.ssa.gov
Tommy Warren, Executive Director
Jack Miller, Office Manager

3424 South Central Alabama Mental Health (SCAMHC)
19815 Bay Branch Rd.
Andalusia, AL 36420 334-222-2523
877-530-0002
www.scamhc.org

3425 Workers Compensation Board Alabama
649 Monroe Street
Montgomery, AL 36131 334-242-2868
800-528-5166
Fax: 334-353-8262
webmaster@labor.alabama.gov
labor.alabama.gov/wc
Charles DeLamar, Director
Al Pelham, Supervisor
Sandy Hallmark, Supervisor
Peggy Barton, Supervisor
The Workers' Compensation Division is responsible for the administration of the Alabama Workers' Compensation Law to ensure proper payment of benefits to employees injured on the job and encourage safety in the work place

Alaska

3426 ATLA
2217 E Tudor Rd
Ste 4
Anchorage, AK 99507-1068 907-563-2599
800-723-2852
Fax: 907-563-0699
www.atla.biz
Kathy Privratsky, Executive Director
Mystie Rail, Commissioner
Margaret Cisco, AT Specialist
Assistive Technology sales and services. ATLA is Alaska's only assistive technology resource center.

3427 Alaska Commission on Aging
150 Third Street #103
PO Box 110693
Juneau, AK 99811- 0693 907-465-3250
Fax: 907-465-1398
dhss.alaska.gov/acoa
Mary Shields, Chair
Rolf Numme, Vice Chair
Denise Daniello, Executive Director
Sherice Cole, Admin Assistant II
Works to promote and protect the health and well-being of Alaskans.

3428 Alaska Department of Handicapped Children
Ste 314
1231 Gambell St
Anchorage, AK 99501-4664 907-346-1995
Gregory Lee, CEO

3429 Alaska Division of Vocational Rehabilitation:
801 W. 10th Street,
Suite A
Juneau, AK 99801-1878 907-465-2814
800-478-2815
Fax: 907-465-2856
dawn.duval@alaska.gov
labor.alaska.gov
Dianne Blummer, Commissioner
David G Stone, Deputy commissioner
John Cannon, Director
Provides comprehensive services to people with disabilities to assist in achieving an employment outcome.

3430 Client Assistance Program: Alaska
2900 Boniface Pkwy
Ste 100
Anchorage, AK 99504-3195 907-333-2211
800-478-0047
Fax: 907-333-1186
www.icdri.org/legal/AlaskaCAP.htm
Pam Stratton, Executive Director
We provide informatory referral to other programs in Alaska that are funded under the Rehabilitation Act of 1973 as amended; Individual assistance or advocacy, if an individual with disability has applied for or received services from an agency funded under the Rehabilitation Act and has concerns or questions we will work with them to help resolve their concerns with the agency.

3431 Department Of Health & Social Services - Division Of Behaviorial Health
350 Main Street
Suite 214
Juneau, AK 99801-1149 907-465-3370
800-465-4828
Fax: 907-465-2668
www.alaska.gov
Albert E. Wall, Director
Stacy Toner, Division Operations Manager
Liz Clement, Program Coordinator
The division plans for and provides appropriate prevention, treatment and support for families impacted by mental disorders or developmental disabilities while maximizing self-determination. Community based services are provided by grantees. Inpatient services are provided in two division operated facilities.

3432 Governor's Committee on Employment and Rehabilitation of People with Disabilities
Division of Vocational Rehabilitation (DVR)
801 W 10th Street
Suite A
Juneau, AK 99801-1878 907-465-2814
800-478-2815
Fax: 907-465-2815
dawn.duval@alaska.gov
www.labor.state.ak.us/dvr
Cheryl Walsh, Executive Director
Carries on a continuing program to promote the employment and rehabilitation of citizens with disabilities in the State of Alaska. Advocates for a comprehensive statewide system for access to assistive technology. Obtains and maintains cooperation with public and private groups and individuals in this field.

3433 **Governor's Council on Disabilities and Special Education**
3601 C Street
Suite 740
Anchorage, AK 99524-0249
907-269-8990
888-269-8990
Fax: 907-269-8995
GCDSE@alaska.gov
www.hss.state.ak.us/gcdse/

Patrick Reinhart, Executive Director
Rich Sanders, Planner III
Britteny M Howell, M.A., ABD, Research Analyst III
Lanny Mommsen, Health Program Manager

The Governor's Council on Disabilities & Special Education was created to meet Alaska's diverse needs.

3434 **Protection & Advocacy System: Alaska**
Disability Law Center of Alaska
3330 Arctic Blvd
Ste 103
Anchorage, AK 99503-4580
907-565-1002
800-478-1234
Fax: 907-565-1000
akpa@dlcak.org

Deborah Smith, President
James M Shine Sr

Deals with rights of the disabled. Works in conjunction with agencies, law offices and family members.

3435 **Protection & Advocacy for Persons with Developmental Disabilities: Alaska**
Advocacy Services of Alaska
Ste 101
615 E 82nd Ave
Anchorage, AK 99518-3100
907-222-2652
866-275-7273
Fax: 907-677-8777
TTY: 866-232-4525

Greg Schomaker, Manager

3436 **Workers Compensation Division**
Department of Labor & Workforce Development
PO Box 115512
Juneau, AK 99811-5512
907-465-2790
Fax: 907-465-2797
workerscomp@alaska.gov
www.labor.state.ak.us/wc

Clark Bishop, Commissioner
Trena Heikes, Division Director
Michael Monagle, Director

The Division of Workers' Compensation is the agency charged with the administration of the Alaska Workers' Compensation Act (Act). The Act provides for the payment by employers or their insurance carriers of medical, disability and reemployment benefits to injured workers

Arizona

3437 **Arizona Department of Economic Security**
1717 W Jefferson
Phoenix, AZ 85007
602-542-4791
www.azdes.gov

Michael Trailor, Director

The Department of Economic Security is a human service agency providing services in six areas: Aging and Community Services, Benefits and Medical Eligibility, Child Support Enforcement, Children and Family Services, Developmental Disabilities and Employment and Rehabilitation Services.

3438 **Arizona Department of Health Services**
150 North 18th Avenue
Ste 330
Phoenix, AZ 85007-3243
602-542-1025
Fax: 602-542-0883
www.azdhs.gov

Will Humble, Director
Neal Young, Director
Lynne Smith, Chief Exeuctive Officer
Rex Critchfield, Manager

The mission of Children's Rehabilitative Services is to improve the quality of life for children by providing family-centered medical treatment, rehabilitation, and related support services to enrolled individuals who have certain medical, handicapping, or potentially handicapping conditions.

3439 **Arizona Division of Aging and Adult Services**
1789 West Jefferson Street
Site Code 950A
Phoenix, AZ 85007-3202
602-542-4446
Fax: 602-542-6655
www.azdes.gov

Rex Critchfield, Manager
Neal Young, Director
Lynne Smith, Chief Executive Officer
Will Humble, Director

The Division supports at-risk Arizonans to meet their basic needs and to live safely, with dignity and independence.

3440 **Arizona Rehabilitation State Services for the Blind and Visually Impaired**
4620 N 16th St, B-106
Ste 100
Phoenix, AZ 85016-5121
602-266-9579
Fax: 602-264-7819
www.azdes.gov

Paul Howell, Vocational Rehab Supervisor
Suzanne Sayre f, Rehab Counselor for Blind

Offers clients a conservation program, eye examinations, treatments, counseling, social work, psychological testing and evaluation, professional training, computer training and more for the visually impaired. The staff includes 56 full time employees.

3441 **Developmental Disability Council: Arizona**
2828 N Country Club Rd
Ste 100
Tucson, AZ 85716-3202
602-542-4049
800-889-5893
Fax: 602-542-5320
www.cpes.com

David A Berns, Manager
Nebal Chavez, Executive Director
Susan Madison, Manager

The mission of the GovernorOs Council on Developmental Disabilities is to bring together persons with disabilities representing Arizona cultural diversity and their families and other community members, to protect rights, eliminate barriers, and jointly promote equal opportunities

3442 **Governor's Council on Developmental Disabilities**
1700 West Wasington Street
Suite 420
Phoenix, AZ 85007
520-325-9688
877-665-3176
Fax: 520-325-3561
lclausen@azdes.gov
azgovernor.gov/DDPC/

Larry Clausen, Executive Director
Shelly Adams, Executive Secretary

The purpose of the council is to advocate for and assure that individuals with developmental disabilities and their families participate in the design of and have access to culturally competent services, supports and provides opportunities to become integrated and included in the community.

3443 **International Dyslexia Association: Arizona Branch**
Meredith Puls AZ-IDA
985 W. Silver Spring Place
Oro Valley, AZ 85755-6548
480-941-0308
arizona.ida@gmail.com

Meredith Puls, President
Rebekah Dyer, Vice President
Melissa A. L. Pallister, Treasurer
Sue Noel, Secretary

Provides free information and referral services for diagnosis and tutoring for parents, educators, physicians, and individuals with dyslexia. Membership includes yearly journal and quarterly newsletter, and Pennsylvania newsletter; discounts to conferences and events.

3444 Protection & Advocacy for Persons with Disabilities: Arizona
Arizona Center for Disability Law
5025 E Washington St
Suite 202
Phoenix, AZ 85034
602-274-6287
800-927-2260
Fax: 602-274-6779
TTY: 602-274-6287
center@azdisabilitylaw.org
www.azdisabilitylaw.org

Anthony DiRienzi, President
Art Gode, Vice President
J. J. Rico, Executive Director
John Chalmers, Treasurer

The Center provides disability-related legal information and advice to individuals who need their services and assistance. In addition to limited legal representation, their goal is to provide efficient, streamlined services to educate people with disabilities and their support on how to enforce their legal rights through self-advocacy. Guides and documents are available online by selecting Self-Advocacy Materials button on the homepage.

3445 Social Security: Phoenix Disability Determination Services
Social Security Admission
4000 North Central Avenue
Suite 1800
Phoenix, AZ 85714
520-638-2000
800-772-1213
TTY: 800-325-0778
www.ssa.gov

3446 Social Security: Tucson Disability Determination Services
4710 South Palo Verde Road
Tucson, AZ 85714-2030
520-638-2000
800-772-1213
TTY: 800-325-0778
www.ssa.gov

Arkansas

3447 Arkansas Assistive Technology Projects
Increasing Capabilities Access
900 W.7th Street
Little Rock, AR 72201-4538
501-666-8868
800-828-2799
Fax: 501-666-5319
info@ar-ican.org

Eddie Schmeckenbecher, Supervisor
Essie Hardin, Secretary
Bryan Ayres, Advisory Counsel
Billy Altom, Advisory Counsil

A consumer responsive, statewide program promoting assistive technology devices and sources for persons of all ages with all disabilities. Referral and information services provide information about devices, where to obtain them and their cost.

3448 Arkansas Division of Aging & Adult Services
Department of Human Services
PO Box 1437
Slot-S-530
Little Rock, AR 72203-1437
501-682-2441
Fax: 501-682-8155
aging.services@arkansas.gov
www.state.ar.us/dhs/aging

Craig Cloud, Director
Stephenie Blocker, Assistant Director
Brad Nye, Assistant Director
Brian Bowen, Assistant Director

The division provides services geared for adults and the elderly including supervised living, home delivered meals, adult day care, senior centers, personal care, household chores, and adult protective services.

3449 Arkansas Division of Developmental Disabilities Services
Donaghey Plaza
PO Box 1437
Little Rock, AR 72203-1437
501-682-1001
Fax: 501-682-8820

Charlie Green, Manager

State agency to assist persons with developmental disabilities and their family in obtaining appropriate assistance and services.

3450 Arkansas Division of Services for the Blind
Department Of Health and Human Services
700 Main St
Little Rock, AR 72203-4608
501-682-5463
800-960-9270
Fax: 501-682-0366
TTY: 800-285-1131
humanservices.arkansas.gov/dsb

Terry Sheeler, Chairman
Dickie Walker, Vice Chairman
Sandy Edwards, Secretary
Harold Brewer, Ex-Officio Member

State program which offers services in the areas of health, counseling, social work, self help and education for the visually and multihandicapped. The staff includes 4 full time and 13 part time members including mobility specialists and rehabilitation teachers.

3451 Arkansas Governor's Developmental Disabilities Council
5800 West 10th Street
Suite 805
Little Rock, AR 72204- 1763
501-661-2589
855-627-7580
Fax: 501-661-2399
ddcouncil.org

Regina Wilson, Executive Director
Teresa Sandar, Family Services Coordinator
Lee Russell, Information Oficer
Michelle Boyd, Administrative Assistant

A federally-funded state agency established to bring the perspective of individuals with developmental disabilities and his or her family or natural support system to policy makers and make improvements to the service system.

3452 Baptist Health Rehabilitation Institute
Baptist Heath
9601 Baptist Health Dr.
Little Rock, AR 72205-7299
501-202-1839
888-BAP-TIST
Fax: 501-202-7352
www.baptist-health.com

Ellen Callaway, Director, Rehabilition Therapy

Acute rehab facility serving patients with ortho, spinal cord injury, brain injury, CVA, arthritis, cardiac and generalized weakness; JCAHO and CARF accredited; 17 outpatient therapy centers throughout central Arkansas.

3453 Children's Medical Services
P.O. Box 1437
Little Rock, AR 72203-1437
501-682-8207
800-482-5850
Fax: 501-682-8247
www.cms-kids.com

Nancy Holder, Program Director
Iris Fehr, Nursing Director
Rodney Farley, Parent Activities Coordinator

A collection of programs for eligible children with special needs. Each one of our programs and services are family-centered and designed to help children with a variety of conditions and needs.

3454 President's Committee on People with Disabilities: Arkansas
7th & Main St
Little Rock, AR 72203

3455 **Social Security: Arkansas Disability Determination Services**
701 Pulaski Street
Little Rock, AR 72201-3990
501-682-3030
800-772-1213
Fax: 501-682-7553
www.socialsecurity.gov

Arthur Boutiette, COO

California

3456 **California Department of Aging**
1300 National Drive
Suite 200
Sacramento, CA 95834-1992
916-419-7500
Fax: 916-928-2267
TTY: 800-735-2929
webmaster@aging.ca.gov
aging.ca.gov

Lora Connoly, Director
Diane Paulsen, Chief Deputy Director
Anna Esparza, Executive Assistant
Chisorom Okwuosa, Chief Counsel

The Department contracts with the network of Area Agencies on Aging, who directly manage a wide array of federal and state-funded services that help older adults find employment; support older and disabled individuals to live as independently as possible in the community; promote healthy aging and community involvement; and assist family members in their vital care giving role

3457 **California Department of Handicapped Children**
714 P Street
Rm 323
Sacramento, CA 95814-6401
916-445-4171
Maridee Gregory
Diana Bonta, Chief Executive Officer

3458 **California Department of Rehabilitation**
721 Capitol Mall
Sacramento, CA 95814-3510
916-324-1313
800-952-5544
TTY: 916-558-5807
externalaffairs@dor.ca.gov

Joe Xavier, Director
David Supkofl, Manager

Assists people with disabilities, particularly those with severe disabilities, in obtaining and retaining meaningful employment and living independently in their communities. The department develops, purchases, provides and advocates for programs and services in vocational rehabilitation, habilitation and independent living with a priority on serving persons with all disabilities, especially those with the most severe disabilities.

3459 **California Governor's Committee on Employment of People with Disabilities**
Employment Development Department
800 Capitol Mall
PO Box 826880
Sacramento, CA 94280-0001
916-654-8055
800-695-0350
Fax: 916-654-9821
TTY: 916-654-9820
www.edd.ca.gov

Charlie Kaplan, Staff Director

GCEPD works to eliminate the barriers that preclude equal consideration for employment opportunities for people with disabilities. The Governor's Committee is responsible for providing leadership to increase the numbers of people with disabilities in the California workforce.

3460 **California Protection & Advocacy: (PAI) A Nonprofit Organization**
Protection and Advocacy (PA I)
1831 K Street
Sacramento, CA 95811-4114
916-504-5800
800-776-5746
Fax: 916-504-5802
SERVICES@DISABILITYRIGHTSCA.ORG
www.disabilityrightsca.org

Catherine Blakemore, Executive Director
Andrew Mudryk, Deputy Director
Alan Gildestein, Managing Attorney
Sujatha Branch, Associate Managing Attorney

Advancing the human and legal rights of people with disabilities.

3461 **California State Council on Developmental Disabilities**
1507 21st Street
Suite 210
Sacramento, CA 95811-5297
916-322-8481
866-802-0514
Fax: 916-443-4957
council@scdd.ca.gov
www.scdd.ca.gov

April Lopez, Chairperson
Jenny Ning Yang, Interim Vice-Chairperson
Tammy Eudy, Office Assistant
Robin Maitino, Executive Assistant

The State Council on Developmental Disabilities (SCDD) is established by state and federal law as an independent state agency to ensure that people with developmental disabilities and their families receive the services and supports they need.

3462 **Client Assistance Program: California**
CA Health and Human Services Agency Dept of Rehab
721 Capitol Mall
PO Box 944222
Sacramento, CA 95814
916-324-1313
800-952-5544
Fax: 916-558-5391
TTY: 916- 558-580
capinfo@dor.ca.gov
www.dor.ca.gov

Tony P Sauer, Director

We have a three-pronged mission to provide services and advocacy that assist people with disabilities to live independently, become employed and have equality in the communities in which they live and work.

3463 **International Dyslexia Association: Central California Branch**
4594 E Michigan Ave
Fresno, CA 93703-1556
559-251-9385
800-222-3123
Fax: 599-252-1216
info@dyslexiaida.org
dyslexiaida.org

Joy Moody, President

Provides free information and referral services for diagnosis and tutoring for parents, educators, physicians, and individuals with dyslexia. Membership includes yearly journal and quarterly newsletter, and Pennsylvania newsletter; discounts to conferences and events.

3464 **Long Beach Department of Health and Human Services**
2525 Grand Avenue
Long Beach, CA 90815-1765
562-570-4000
Fax: 562-570-4049
www.longbeach.gov/health/

Ron Arias, Executive Director
Michael Johnson, Manager

The Long Beach Department of Health and Human Services (Health Department) has been improving the health of the Long Beach community for over a century.

3465 **Los Angeles County Department of Health Services**
313 N Figueroa Street
Los Angeles, CA 90012-2602
213-240-8101
800-427-8700
Fax: 213-250-4013

Mitchell H Katz, MD, Director
Hal F. Yee, Jr., M.D., Ph.D., Chief Medical Officer
Allan Wecker, Chief Financial Officer
Alexander Li, M.D., Deputy Director

Los Angeles County Department of Health Services is one of the US's largest publicly supported health systems.The system is the main provider of health care for the area's poor and uninsured. It provides general medical and surgical care and is affiliated with the medical school at USC. The system also manages the Emergency Medical Services (EMS) Agency and the Community Health Plan HMO, a low-cost managed care plan for members of Medicaid and other state-funded programs.

3466 **Social Security: California Disability Determination Services**
3164 Garrity Way
Richmond, CA 94806-1983
800-772-1213
TTY: 800-325-0778
www.ssa.gov

Sally Keen, San Francisco Regional PDF Coord

3467 **Social Security: Fresno Disability Determination Services**
Social Security
1052 C St
Fresno, CA 93706-3245
559-487-5391
800-772-1213
Fax: 510-970-2947
TTY: 800-325-0778
www.ssa.gov

Sally Keen, Regional PDF Coordinator

3468 **Social Security: Oakland Disability Determination Services**
P.O. Box 24225
Oakland, CA 94623-1225
510-622-3506
800-772-1213
TTY: 800-325-0778
www.ssa.gov

3469 **Social Security: Sacramento Disability Determination Services**
P.O. Box 997121
Suite A
Sacramento, CA 95899-7121
916-515-4400
800-772-1213
Fax: 916-263-5310
TTY: 916-381-9445
ssa.gov

3470 **Social Security: San Diego Disability Determination Services**
P.O. Box 85326
San Diego, CA 92186-5326
619-278-4300
800-772-1213
Fax: 619-278-4303
TTY: 800-325-0778
www.ssa.gov

Colorado

3471 **Colorado Department of Aging & Adult Services**
1575 Sherman St
10th Floor
Denver, CO 80203-1702
303-866-5700
Fax: 303-620-2696
cdhs.communications@state.co.us

Reggie Bicha, Executive Director

A department providing services to the elderly.

3472 **Colorado Developmental Disabilities Council**
1120 Lincoln
Suite 706
Denver, CO 80203
720-941-0176
Fax: 720-941-8490
cddpc.email@state.co.us
coddc.org

Katherine Carol, Chairperson
Irene Aguilar, Colorado Senate
Marcia Tewell, Executive Director
Lionel Llewellyn, Administrative Assistant

The mission is to advocate in collaboration with and on behalf of people with developmental disabilities for the establishment and implementation of public policy which will further their independence, productivity and integration.

3473 **Colorado Division of Mental Health**
3824 W. Princeton Circle
Denver, CO 80236-3111
303-866-7400
Fax: 303-866-7428
colorado.gov

Patrick K. Fox, Director

Administration of public health program

3474 **Colorado Health Care Program for Children with Special Needs**
4300 Cherry Creek Drive south
Denver, CO 80246-1530
303-692-2370
800-886-7689
Fax: 303-753-9249
cdphe.psdrequests@state.co.us
www.colorado.gov/cdphe/hcp

Christopher Stanley, Board member
Angie Goodger, HCP Consultant
Kelsey Minor, HCP Consultant
Jennie Munthali, HCP Section Manager

Provides information and state aid to children with disabilities.

3475 **Division of Workers' Compensation Department of Labor & Employment**
633 17th Street
Suite 201
Denver, CO 80202-3660
303-318-8700
800-388-5515
888-390-7936
Fax: 303-575-8882
cdle_workers_compensation@state.co.us
www.colorado.gov/cdle

Ellen Golombek, Executive Director

Infomation regarding Division Rules and procedures for Claimants, Employers, Adjusters, and parties to claim.

3476 **Eastern Colorado Services for the Disabled**
P. O. Box 1682
617 South 10th Avenue
Sterling, CO 80751-3168
970-522-7121
Fax: 970-522-1173
rhonda@ecsdd.org
www.easterncoloradoservices.org

Rhonda Roth, Executive Director
Traci Schrade, Finance Director
Melissa Dassaro, Case Management Director
Dave Fast, PHR, Human Resources

Case coordination, infant stimulation, family support, residential and vocational programs.

3477 **International Dyslexia Association: Rocky Mountain Branch**
740 Yale Rd.
Boulder, CO 80305-5010
303-721-9425
855-5ID- RMB
Fax: 303-721-9425
ida_rmb@yahoo.com
www.dyslexia-rmbida.org

Karen Leopold, President
Lynn Kuhn, Secretary
Yona Sammartino, Administrative Director
Julie Bottom, Board of Director

Provides free information and referral services for diagnosis and tutoring for parents, educators, physicians, and individuals with dyslexia. Membership includes yearly journal and quarterly newsletter, and Pennsylvania newsletter; discounts to conferences and events.

3478 **Legal Center for People with Disabilities& Older People**
455 Sherman St
Ste 130
Denver, CO 80203-4403
303-722-0300
800-288-1376
Fax: 303-722-0720
TTY: 303-722-3619

John R. Posthumus, President
Stephen P. Rickles, Vice President
Nancy Tucker, Secretary
John Paul Anderson, Treasurer

Uses the legal system to protect and promote the rights of people with disabilities and older people in Colorado through direct legal representation, advocacy, education and legislative analysis. The Legal Center is Colorado's Protection and Advocacy System. We are also the State Ombudsman for nursing homes and assisted living facilities. Call for a free publications and products list.

Connecticut

3479 **Connecticut Board of Education and Servicefor the Blind**
184 Windsor Avenue
Windsor, CT 06095-4536
860-602-4000
800-842-4510
Fax: 860-602-4020
TTY: 860-602-4221
brian.sigman@CT.GOV
www.ct.gov/besb/site/default.asp

Amy Porter, Commissioner

Offers rehabilitative services and information for persons with legal blindness and childrenwhonare visually impaired that are residents of Connecticut.

3480 **Connecticut Commission on Aging**
210 Capitol Avenue
Hartford, CT 06106
860-240-5200
Fax: 860-240-5204

Julia Evans Starr, Executive Director
Deborah Migneault, Senior Policy Analyst
Alyssa Norwood, Project Manager
Christianne Kovel, Communications Specialist

Advocates on beha;f of elderly persons in Connecticut by regularly monitoring their status, assessing the impact of current and propsed initiatives, and conducting activities which promote the interests of these individuals and report to the Governor and the Legislature.

3481 **Connecticut Department of Children and Youth Services**
505 Hudson Street
Hartford, CT 06106
860-550-6300
Fax: 860-724-2001
Commissioner.dcf@ct.gov
www.ct.gov

Gary Scappini, Manager
Bruce Douglas, Executive Director

3482 **Connecticut Developmental Disabilities Council**
263 Farmington Avenue
Farmington, CT 6030
860-679-1561
800-653-1134
Fax: 860-679-1571
TTY: 860-679-1502
ctkasa.org

Ed Preneta, Executive Director

Kids As Self Advocates (KASA) is a national grassroots network that helps youth with special needs and their friends become self-advocates, helps other people in the community understand what it's like to live with special health care needs.

3483 **Connecticut Office of Protection and Advocacy for Persons with Disabilities**
60B Weston Street
Suite B
Hartford, CT 06120-1551
860-297-4300
800-842-7303
Fax: 860-566-8714
TTY: 860-297-4320
www.ct.gov/opapd

Craig B Henrici, Executive Director
Alexandria Bode, Board Member
Thomas Behrendt, Board Member
John Clausen, Board Member

Provides information, referrals, advocacy assistance & limited legal services to people with disabilities in the state of Connecticut whose civil rights have been violated or who are experiencing the difficulty securing relevant support services. P & A supports the development of community advocacy groups by providing training & technical assistance. P & A is responsible for investigating abuse & neglect of all individuals with intellectual disability ages 18-59.

3484 **Social Security: Hartford Area Office**
960 Main Street
2nd Floor
Hartford, CT 06103-1228
877-619-2851
800-772-1213
Fax: 860-566-1795
TTY: 860-525-4967
www.ssa.gov

Jan Gilbert, Professional Relations Coord.

Delaware

3485 **Delaware Assistive Technology Initiative (DATI)**
461 Wyoming Road
Newark, DE 19716-0269
302-831-0354
Fax: 302-831-4690
TTY: 800-870-3284
dati@asel.udel.edu
www.dati.org

Beth Mineo, Project Director
Joann McCafferty, Staff Assistant

The Delaware Assistive Technology Initiative (DATI) connects Delawareans who have disabilities with the tools they need in order to learn, work, play and participate in community life safely and independently. DATI services include: Equipment demonstration centers in each county; no-cost, short-term equipment loans that let you try before you buy; Equipment Exchange Program; AT workshops and other training sessions; advocacy for improved AT access policies and funing and several more.

3486 **Delaware Client Assistance Program**
United Cerebral Palsy Association
254 E Camden Wyoming Ave
Camden, DE 19934-1303
302-698-9336
800-640-9336
Fax: 302-698-9338
icdri.org/legal/DelawareCAP.htm

Melissa Shahan, Executive Director

Provides advocacy services for persons involved with programs covered under the Rehabilitation Act of 1973 as amended, information and referrals on ADA, Title I.

3487 **Delaware Department of Health and Social Services**
Administration Building D HS S Campus
1901 N Du pont Highway
Main Building
New Castle, DE 19720-1160
302-255-9040
800-464-4357
Fax: 302-255-4429
TTY: 302-744-4556
dhssinfo@state.de.us
www.dhss.delaware.gov

Rita Landgraf, Cabinet Secretary
Henry Smith III, Deputy secretary

Provides most of the human services available through Delaware State Government, including Medicaid, the Children's Health Insurance Program, food stamps, welfare-to-work, vaccines for children, child support enforcement, public health programs, and general services for the aging. Also for individuals with developmental and physical disabilities, visual impairements, mental illness and other vulnerable populations.

3488 **Delaware Department of Public Instructing**
Townsend Building
401 Federal Street
Dover, DE 19901- 1402
302-735-4000
800-433-5292
Fax: 302-739-4654
deeds@doe.k12.de.us
http://www.doe.k12.de.us
Mark T. Murphy, Secretary of Education
David J. Blowman, Deputy Secretary
Mary Kate McLaughlin, Chief of Staff
Penny Schwinn, Chief Accountability Officer
A publicly funded, state agency that gives information about local facilities and administers supplemental funds for visually handicapped students in local schools. It also maintains special teachers of sight conservation and Braille programs for both children and adults.

3489 **Delaware Developmental Disability Council**
410 Federal Street 2nd Floor
Suite 2
Dover, DE 19901- 3640
302-739-3333
800-464-4357
Fax: 302-739-2015
pat.maichle@state.de.us
Barbara Monaghan, Council Chair
Patricia L. Maichle, Senior Administrator
Kristin Cosden, Social Service Administrator
Stefanie Lancaster, Administrative Officer
Working to ensure that people with developmental disabilities enjoy the same quality of life as the rest of society.

3490 **Delaware Division for the Visually Impaired**
1901 North Dupont Highway
New Castle, DE 19720-1160
302-255-9800
Fax: 302-255-4441
dhssinfo@state.de.us
www.dhss.delaware.gov/dvi/
Rita Landgraf, Secretary
Henry Smith, Deputy Secretary
Betsy Deldeo, Office Manager
State agency serving the visually impaired persons from birth, with or without other handicaps. Services offered include vocational rehabilitation, independent living, orientation and mobility, technology assessment, transition from school to work.

3491 **Delaware Protection & Advocacy for Persons with Disabilities**
Arc of Delaware
144 E Market St
Georgetown, DE 19947-1411
302-856-6019
Fax: 302-856-6133
Becky Allen, Executive Director

3492 **Delaware Workers Compensation Board**
Industrial Accident Board de dept
4425 North Market Street
Wilmington, DE 19802-1307
302-761-8085
Fax: 302-761-6601
www.delawareworks.com
James Cagle, Manager
The Office of Workers' Compensation administers and enforces state laws, rules and regulations regarding industrial accidents and illnesses.

3493 **Social Security: Wilmington Disability Determination**
U S Department of Health and Human Services
1528 S 16th Street
Wilmington, NC 28401-3908
866-964-6227
800-772-1213
Fax: 910-254-3444
TTY: 910-815-4695
www.socialsecurity.gov
J Allen Murphy, Founder
Vickie O'Brien, Manager

3494 **The Division for the Visually Impaired**
Herman M. Holloway, Sr. Campus
1901 N Dupont Hwy
New Castle, DE 19720
302-255-9800
Fax: 302-255-4441
dhssinfo@state.de.us
dhss.delaware.gov
Alan Wingrove, General Manager
Romy Mikhail, Customer Service, Quality & ISO Manager
The Division for the Visually Impaired provides educational, vocational and technical support to people with visual impairments. Some programs offered include education, employment support, guidance for living independently and using assistive devices, business enterprise programs, volunteer opporunities and more.

District of Columbia

3495 **District of Columbia Department of Handicapped Children**
D C General Hospital
Bldg 10
1900 Massachusetts Ave SE
Washington, DC 20003- 2542
202-541-6337
Fax: 202-675-7694
Jacqueline Mcmorris, Acting Chief
Nayab Ali, MD

3496 **District of Columbia Office on Aging**
500 K Street NE
Washington, DC 20002-2714
202-724-5622
Fax: 202-724-4979
TTY: 202-724-8925
dcoa@dc.gov
dcoa.dc.gov
John M Thompson, Executive Director
Deborah Royster, General Counsel
Tanya Reid, Executive Assistant
Camile Williams, Chief of Staff
Serves the District of Columbia residents 60 years of age and older. Contact the Information and Assistance Unit for more information about innovative programs and services offered by the Office.

3497 **Information, Protection & Advocacy for Persons with Disabilities**
IPACHI
220 I Street, N.E.
Suite 130
Washington, DC 20002
202-547-0198
Fax: 202-547-2083
jbrown@uls-dc.org
www.acf.hhs.gov/programs/add/states/pas.html
Jane Brown, Executive Director
Ronald Tyson, Information/Referral
Offers services and support for persons with disabilities in the Washington, DC area.

3498 **Information, Protection and Advocacy Center for Handicapped Individuals**
220 I Street, N.E.
Suite 130
Washington, DC 20002-2340
202-547-0198
Fax: 202-547-2083
jbrown@uls-dc.org
www.acf.hhs.gov/programs/add/states/pas.html
Jane Brown, Executive Director
Serves all persons with disabilities in the DC, Maryland and Virginia areas offering them legal representation and advocacy, information and referrals and several publications.

3499 **International Dyslexia Association of DC**
40 York Rd., 4th Floor
Baltimore, MD 21204-1016
410-296-0232
800-222-3123
Fax: 410-321-5069
info@dyslexiaida.org
dyslexiaida.org
Ruth R Tifford LCSW, President

Provides free information and referral services for diagnosis and tutoring for parents, educators, physicians, and individuals with dyslexia. Membership includes yearly journal and quarterly newsletter, and Pennsylvania newsletter; discounts to conferences and events.

3500 **Public Technology Institute**
660 North Capitol St. NW
Suite 400
Washington, DC 20001
202-626-2400
info@pti.org
www.pti.org

Alan R. Shark, Executive Director
Leonard Scott, Director, Public Safety Technology Programs
Susan Cable, Program Manager, Citizen-Engaged Communities

Supports local government executives and elected officials through research, education, consulting services, and recognition programs. Research includes how technology can better benefit people with disabilities.
28 pages

3501 **Wage and Hour Division of the Employment Standards Administration**
US Department of Labor
200 Constitution Ave NW
Washington, DC 20210-1
202-693-5000
866-487-2365
Fax: 202-219-8822
TTY: 877-889-5627
webmaster@dol.gov
www.dol.gov

Hilda Solis, Secretary of Labor
Seth Harris, Deputy Secretary
Elizabeth Kim, Executive Secretariat Director
Betsey Stevenson, Chief Economist

Administers regulations governing the employment of individuals with disabilities in sheltered workshops and the disabled workers industries.

3502 **Washington Hearing and Speech Society**
2150 N 107th St, Suite 205
Seattle, WA 98133-2633
206-209-5271
Fax: 206-367-8777
office@wslha.org
www.wslha.org

Paul Diez, President
Judith Bernier, Secretary
Julie Leonardo, Treasurer
Lesley Stephens, Clinical SLP

Offers individuals with hearing or speech impairments, in the DC area, speech, reading classes, audiological services and new aids.

3503 **Well Mind Association of Greater Washington**
18606 New Hampshire Ave
Ashton, MD 20861-9789
301-774-6617
Fax: 301-946-1402

3504 **Workers Compensation Board: District of Columbia**
4058 Minnesota Avenue, NE,
Washington, DC 20019-5626
202-724-7000
202-698-4817
Fax: 202-673-6993
does@dc.gov

Deborah A Carroll, Director

The Workers' Compensation Program processes claims and monitors the payment of benefits to injured private-sector employees in the District of Columbia

Florida

3505 **ARC Gateway**
3932 North 10th Avenue
Pensacola, FL 32503-2807
850-434-2638
Fax: 850-438-2180
info@arc-gateway.org
www.arc-gateway.org

Peter Mougey, President
Patricia Young, Vice President
Lynn Erickson, Secretary
Donna Fassett, Executive Director

ARC Gateway is a non-profit organization that serves children who have or are at risk of developmental disabilities as well as adults with developmental disabilitie

3506 **Assistive Technology Educational Network of Florida**
1207 S Mellonville Avenue
Sanford, FL 32771-2240
800-558-6580
Fax: 407-320-2379
Diane_Penn@scps.k12.fl.us
www.icdri.org/Assistive%20Technology/aten.htm

Dee Wright, Executive Secretary
Diane Penn, MA, Technology Specialist

Provides state-wide information, awareness and training for students, family members, teachers and other professionals in the area of assisted technology; a quarterly newsletter and a network of specialists (Local Assistive Technology Specialists) trained by ATEN to provide support at the district level.

3507 **Bureau Of Exceptional Education And Student Services**
325 West Gaines Street Suite 614
Tallahassee, FL 32399
850-245-0475
Fax: 850-245-0953
Monica.Verra-Tirado@fldoe.org
www.fldoe.org

Pam Stewart, Education Commissioner
Monica Verra Tirado, Bureau Chief
Chatherine Aponte Gray, Administrative Assistant
Tonya Milton, Program Planner

Provides consultative services for the establishment and operation of school programs for visually impaired students. Provides assistance for in-service teacher training through state or regional workshops or technical assistance to individual programs.

3508 **Department of Health & Rehabilitative Services**
1317 Winewood Blvd
Building 1
Tallahassee, FL 32399-700
850-487-1111
Fax: 850-922-2993
www.dcf.state.fl.us

David Wilkins, Secretary
Ramin Kouzehkanani, Deputy Secretary
John Bryant, Manager

The Florida Department of Children and Families has adopted an integrated approach to programs and services as we work to help improve the lives of individuals and families.

3509 **Disability Rights Florida**
2473 Care Dr.
Suite 200
Tallahassee, FL 32308
850-488-9071
800-342-0823
Fax: 850-488-8640
TTY: 800-346-4127
www.disabilityrightsflorida.org

Peter Sleasman, Executive Director
Ann Siegel, Legal Director
Cherie E. Hall, Director, Operations
Tony DePalma, Director, Public Policy

A federally mandated Protection & Advocacy (P&A) organization working to ensure the safety, well-being and success of people with disabilities.

3510 **Division of Workers Compensation**
200 East Gaines Street
Tallahassee, FL 32399-0318
850-413-3089
877-693-5236
Fax: 850-413-2950
Tanner.Holloman@myfloridacfo.com
Tanner Holloman, Division Director
Andrew Sabolic, Assistant Director
Terry Kester, Chief Information Officer
Robin Delaney, Bureau Chief of Compliance
To actively ensure the self-execution of the workers' compensation system through education and informing all stakeholders of their rights and responsibilities, leveraging data to deliver exceptional value to our customers and stakeholders, and holding parties accountable for meeting their obligations.

3511 **Florida Adult Services**
1317 Winewood Boulevard
Building 1, Room 202
Tallahassee, FL 32399-700
850-488-2881
800-962-2873
800-273-8255
Fax: 850-922-4193
www.myflfamilies.com
Robert Anderson, State Director
Jan Chaney, Administrative Assistant
Roy Car, Data/Systems
Lindsay Conrad, HCDA and CCDA
The Florida Department of Children and Families has adopted an integrated approach to programs and services as we work to help improve the lives of individuals and families.

3512 **Florida Department of Handicapped Children**
4030 Esplanade Way
Suite 380
Tallahassee, FL 32399-7016
850-488-4257
866-273-2273
Fax: 850-245-1075
www.apd.myflorida.com
Mike Gresham, Executive Director
John Bryant, Manager
The APD works in partnership with local communities and private providers to assist people who have developmental disabilities and their families.

3513 **Florida Department of Mental Health and Rehabilitative Services**
1317 Winewood Blvd
Building 1
Tallahassee, FL 32399-700
850-487-1111
Fax: 850-922-2993
www.dcf.state.fl.us
David Wilkins, Secretary
Ramin Kouzehkanani, Deputy Secretary

3514 **Florida Developmental Disabilities Council**
124 Marriott Drive
Suite 203
Tallahassee, FL 32301-2981
850-488-4180
800-580-7801
Fax: 850-922-6702
TTY: 888-488-863
fddc@fddc.org
fddc.org
Sylvia James Miller, Council Chair & Parent Advocate
Tricia Riccardi, Council Vice-Chair
Debra Dowds, Executive Director
Vanda Bowman, Staff Assistant
To advocate and promote meaningful participation in all aspects of life for Floridians with developmental disabilities.

3515 **Florida Division of Vocational Rehabilitation**
4070 Esplanade Way
Building 1
Tallahassee, FL 32399- 7016
850-245-3399
800-451-4327
Fax: 850-245-3316
TTY: 850-488-2867
rehabworks.org
Bill Palmer, Manager
Linda Parnell, Manager
Aleisa Mckinlay, Director
Don Chester, Counsil Member
State agency serving individuals with physical or mental disabilities that interfere with them keeping or maintaining employment.

3516 **International Dyslexia Association: Florida Branch**
40 York Rd., 4th Floor
Baltimore, MD 21204-3896
410-296-0232
800-222-3123
Fax: 410-321-5069
ear228@aol.com
dyslexiaida.org
Kristen Penczek, Executive Director
David Holste, Director Of Operations
Stacy Friedman, Manager of Operation
Cyndi Powers, Office Manager
Provides free information and referral services for diagnosis and tutoring for parents, educators, physicians, and individuals with dyslexia. Membership includes yearly journal and quarterly newsletter, and Pennsylvania newsletter; discounts to conferences and events.

3517 **Social Security Administration**
2002 Old Saint Augustine Rd
Suite B12
Tallahassee, FL 32301-4861
850-942-8978
800-772-1213
Fax: 850-942-8980
ssa.gov
Carrie Tucker, Operations Supervisor
Sheila Lee, Management Support Specialist
Administers the Title II and Title XVII disability programs. To be insured for Title II benefits, applicants must have worked in covered employment for at least five of the last ten years prior to becoming disabled. To be eligible for Title XVII disability benefits, applicants must meet an income and resource test.

3518 **Social Security: Miami Disability Determination**
Social Security
11401 W Flagler St
Miami, FL 33174-1023
305-226-0449
800-772-1213
TTY: 800-325-0778
www.ssa.gov
Robert L Meekins, Deputy General for Executive Ope

3519 **Social Security: Orlando Disability Determination**
Social Security
P.O. Box 144040
Orlando, FL 32814-2231
407-648-6673
800-342-2065
TTY: 407-245-7057
www.ssa.gov
John C Massolio Jr, Founder
Neil Bush, President

3520 **Social Security: Tampa Disability Determination**
Social Security Administration
PO Box 340572
Tampa, FL 33694-572
813-878-2906
800-772-1213
www.dbsatampabay.org
John Balcomb, President
Carol Yaros, 1st Vice President
Cheryl McGhan, 2nd Vice President
Neil Bush, Treasurer
The Depression and Bipolar Support Alliance Tampa Bay, is a nonprofit and all volunteer organization for individuals, family and friends of those who have been diagnosed with bipolar disorder, depression and other affective disorders.

Georgia

3521 **ADA Technical Assistance Program**
Southeast Disability & Business Technical Assist.
1419 Mayson Street NE
Atlanta, GA 30324
404-541-9001
800-949-4232
Fax: 404-541-9002
ADAsoutheast@law.syr.edu
www.sedbtac.org

Pamela Williamson, Project Director
Cheri Hofmann, Information Specialist
Cyndi Smith, Office Assistant
Marsha Schwanke, Web Manager
One of ten regional centers funded by NIDRR, to provide information and technical assistance to assist in voluntary compliance with the Americans with Disabilities Act, and accessible education-based information technology.

3522 **Division of Birth Defects and Developmental Disabilities**
1600 Clifton Road
Atlanta, GA 30333-4027
404-498-3800
800-232-4636
TTY: 888-232-6348
cdcinfo@cdc.gov
www.cdc.gov

Coleen A Boyle, Director
The mission of CDC's National Center on Birth Defects and Developmental Disabilities (NCBDDD) is to promote the health of babies, children and adults and to enhance the potential for full, productive living.

3523 **Georgia Advocacy Office**
One West Court Square
Suite 625
Decatur, GA 30030
404-885-1234
800-537-2329
Fax: 404-378-0031
info@thegao.org
thegao.org

Ruby Moore, Executive Director
Crystal Rasa, Program Manager
Mona Givens, Director of Investigation
Olwyn Mayer, Chief Operating Officer
Protection and advocacy services for Georgians with disabilities.

3524 **Georgia Client Assistance Program**
Division of Rehabilitation Services
2 Peachtree Street NW
Suite 29-250
Atlanta, GA 30303- 3141
404-656-4507
800-822-9727
Fax: 404-651-6880
dhs.georgia.gov/

Mark Trail, Manager
Robertiena Fletcher, Chair
Franklin G Auman, Vice Chair
Monica Walters, Secretary
Helps eligible persons with complaints, appeals and understanding available benefits under the 1992 Rehabilitation Act Amendments and Title I of the Americans with Disabilities Act. CAP investigates complaints, mediates conflict, represents complainants in appeals, provides legal services if warranted, advocates for due process, identifies and recommends solutions to system problems, advises of benefits available under the 1992 Rehab Act Amendments and Americans with Disabilities Act.

3525 **Georgia Council On Developmental Disabilities**
2 Peachtree St N.W.
26th Floor, Suite 246
Atlanta, GA 30303-3141
404-657-2126
888-275-4233
Fax: 404-657-2132
TTY: 404-657-2133
eric.jacobson@gcdd.ga.gov
www.gcdd.org

Eric E. Jacobson, Executive Director
Caitlin Childs, Organizing Director
Dottie Adams, Family/Individual Support Dir.
Valerie Meadows Suber, Public Information Director
The Georgia Council on Developmental Disabilities collaborates with Georgia's citizens, public and private advocacy organizations and policymakers to positively influence public policies that enhance the quality of life for people with disabilities and their families. GCDD provides this through education and advocacy activities, program implementation, funding and public policy analysis and research.
Quartlery

3526 **Georgia Department of Aging**
2 Peachtree Street NW
33rd Floor
Atlanta, GA 30303-3142
404-657-5258
866-552-4464
Fax: 404-657-5285
dhs.georgia.gov/

Stephen Dolinger, President
Andrea Fuller-Ruffin, Administrator
The Division of Aging Services (DAS) works to continuously improve the effectiveness and efficiency of services.

3527 **Georgia Department of Handicapped Children**
2600 Skyland Dr NE
Atlanta, GA 30319-3640
404-679-1625
Fax: 404-679-1630

Ron Jackson, Manager
Frank Koues, Auditor

3528 **Georgia Division of Mental Health, Developmental Disabilities & Addictive Diseases**
Two Peachtree Drive NW
24th Floor
Atlanta, GA 30303-3142
404-657-2252
800-715-4225
Fax: 404-657-2310
mhddad.dhr.georgia.gov

Kimberly Ryan, Board Member
David Glass, Board member
Ellice P. Martin, Board Member
Kimberly Carroll-Hawkins, Board Member
MHDDAD provides treatment and support services to people with mental illnesses and addictive diseases, and support to people with developmental disabilities. MHDDAD serves people of all ages with the most severe and likely to be long-term conditions.

3529 **Georgia State Board of Workers' Compensation**
270 Peachtree St NW
Atlanta, GA 30303-1299
404-656-3875
800-533-0682
Fax: 404-657-1767
sbwc.georgia.gov

Frank McKay, Chairman
Elizabeth Gobeil, Director
Delece A. Brooks, Executive Director
Martine Schweitzer, Administrative Assistant
To provide superior access to the Georgia Workers' Compensation program for injured workers and employers in a manner that is sensitive, responsive, and effective and to insure efficient processing and swift, fair resolution of claims, while encouraging workplace safety and return to work.

3530 **International Dyslexia Association: Georgia Branch**
1951 Greystone Rd.
Atlanta, GA 30318
404-256-1232
info@idaga.org
www.idaga.org

Jennifer Kopp, President
jennings Miller, Vice-President
Robert Moore, Treasurer
Susie McDaniel, Corresponding Secretary
Provides free information and referral services for diagnosis and tutoring for parents, educators, physicians, and individuals with dyslexia. Membership includes yearly journal and quarterly newsletter, and Pennsylvania newsletter; discounts to conferences and events.

3531 Social Security: Atlanta Disability Determination
401 W Peachtree St NW
Suite 2860 Flr 28
Atlanta, GA 30308-3538
800-772-1213
TTY: 800-325-0778
www.socialsecurity.gov

3532 Social Security: Decatur Disability Determination
2853 Candler Rd
Suite 8
Decatur, GA 30034-1421
800-772-1213
TTY: 800-325-0778
ssa.gov

Hawaii

3533 Assistive Technology Resource Centers of Hawaii
200 North Vineyard Boulevard
Suite 430
Honolulu, HI 96817-5362
808-532-7110
800-645-3007
Fax: 808-532-7120
TTY: 808-532-7113
atrc-info@atrc.org
www.atrc.org

Barbara Fischlowitz-Leong, Executive Director
Jodi Asato, Deputy Director
Edna Kaahaaina, Office Manager
Joseph Go, Assistive Technology Trainer
Provides information and referral to anyone interested in assistive technology devices and services. Operates equipment loan. Bank Provides training to consumer and professional groups including self-advocacy skills for consumers and family members. Works to ensure that schools, vocational rehabilitation agencies and health insurers provide assessments, funding and training in the use of assistive technology devices and services for their clients. Low-interest loan programs available.

3534 Diabetes Network of East Hawaii
1221 Kilauea Ave
Suite 70
Hilo, HI 96720-4264
808-935-1673
Fax: 808-935-6760

Steve Fukunada, Manager

3535 Disability and Communication Access Board
1010 Richards St
Suite 118
Honolulu, HI 96813
808-586-8121
Fax: 808-586-8129
dcab@doh.hawaii.gov
hawaii.gov/health/dcab

Francine Wai, Executive Director
Bill-Wayne Nakamatsu, Parking Program Specialist
Provides ADA coordination for state & county government; reviews state & county construction documents to appropriate federal & state accessibility guidelines; credentials American sign language interpreters; coordinates parking for persons with disabilites; coordinates information & referral for consumers, parents and others seeking disability related information.

3536 Hawaii Assistive Technology Training and
200 North Vineyard Boulevard
Suite 430
Honolulu, HI 96817-5362
808-532-7110
800-645-3007
Fax: 808-532-7120
atrc-info@atrc.org
www.atrc.org

Barbara Fischlowitz-Leong, Executive Director

3537 Hawaii Department for Children With Special Needs
Department of Health
741 Sunset Avenue
Honolulu, HI 96816-2343
808-733-9070
Fax: 808-733-9068
patricia.heu@doh.hawaii.gov
health.hawaii.gov

Patricia Heu, Manager
Karen Mak, Manager
Children with Special Health Needs Branch (CSHNB) is working to assure that all children and youth with special health care needs (CSHCN) will reach optimal health, growth, and development, by improving access to a coordinated system of family-centered health care services and improving outcomes, through systems development, assessment, assurance, education, collaborative partnerships, and family support.

3538 Hawaii Department of Health, Adult Mental Health Division
P.O. Box 3378
Honolulu, HI 96801-3378
808-586-4686
Fax: 808-586-4745

3539 Hawaii Department of Human Services
Hawaii Department of Human Serv
P.O. Box 339
Honolulu, HI 96813
808-586-4892
Fax: 808-586-4890
dhs@dhs.hawaii.gov
humanservices.hawaii.gov

Rachael Wong, Director
Pankaj Bhanot, Deputy Director
Lisa Nakao, Admin Assis. & Legislative Coor.
Scott Nakasone, Acting Administrator
To provide timely, efficient and effective programs, services and benefits for the purpose of achieving the outcome of empowering Hawaii's most vulnerable people; and to expand their capacity for self-sufficiency, self-determination, independence, healthy choices, quality of life, and personal dignity.

3540 Hawaii Disability Compensation Division Department of Labor and Industrial Relations
830 Punchbowl Street
Room 209
Honolulu, HI 96813-5095
808-586-9200
Fax: 808-586-9219
dlir.director@hawaii.gov
hawaii.gov/labor

Walter Kawamura, Administrator
Clyde Imada, Workers Comp Chief
The Disability Compensation Division (DCD) administers the Workers' Compensation (WC) law, the Temporary Disability Insurance (TDI) law, and the Prepaid Health Care (PHC) law. All employers with one or more employees, whether working full-time or part-time, are directly affected.

3541 Hawaii Disability Rights Center
1132 Bishop Street
Suite 2102
Honolulu, HI 96813-3701
808-949-2922
800-882-1057
Fax: 808-949-2928
info@hawaiidisabilityrights.org
hawaiidisabilityrights.org

John Dellera, Executive Director
Ann Collins, Director Of Operations
IT IS THE POLICY OF HDRCto advocate for as many people with disabilities in the State of Hawaii, on as wide a range of disability rights issues, as our resources allow; and to resolve rights violations with the lowest feasible level of intervention; but, if necessary, to also provide full legal representation to protect the rights of people with disabilities, consistent with authorizing statutes and Center priorities.

3542 **Hawaii Executive Office on Aging**
250 South Hotel Street
Suite 406
Honolulu, HI 96813-2831
808-586-0100
800-468-4644
Fax: 808-586-0185
hawaii.gov/health/eoa

Noemi Pendleton, Manager
Virginia Pressler, Director
Keith Y. Yamamoto, Deputy Director
Danette Wong Tomiyasu, Deputy Director

State unit on aging responsible for policy formulation, program development, planning, information dissemination, advocacy and other activities, for persons age 60 and over.

3543 **Hawaii State Council on Developmental Disabilities**
919 Ala Moana Blvd
Suite113
Honolulu, HI 96814-4920
808-586-8100
Fax: 808-586-7543

Waynette K Y Cabral, Executive Administrator
Joe Shacter, Planner
Debbie Miyasaka Gushiken, Community & Legislative Liaison
Susan Kawano, Secretary

The mission of the council is to support people with developmental disabilities to control their own destiny and determine the quality of life they desire. The Council: engages in analysis and policy development; provides training in legislative advocacy and leadership development for individuals with disabilities and their families; demonstrates new approaches to services and supports; informs policymakers about developmental disability issues; and fosters interagency collaboration.

3544 **International Dyslexia Association: Hawaii Branch**
913 Alewa Dr.
Honolulu, HI 96817-1610
808-538-7007
hida@dyslexia-hawaii.org

Charles Bering, President
Deborah Knight, Vice President
Laurie Moore, Treasurer
Margaret Higa, Executive Director

Provides free information and referral services for diagnosis and tutoring for parents, educators, physicians, and individuals with dyslexia. Membership includes yearly journal and quarterly newsletter. Call for conference dates.

3545 **Social Security: Honolulu Disability Determination**
Social Security
300 Ala Moana Blvd
Honolulu, HI 96850-1
808-541-3600
800-772-1213
TTY: 800-825-0778
hivrsbd@kestrok.com
www.ssa.gov

Neil Shim, Administrator

3546 **State Planning Council on Developmental Disabilities**
919 Ala Moana Blvd
Room 101
Honolulu, HI 96814-4920
808-586-8121
Fax: 808-586-8129
TTY: 808-586-8121
dcab@doh.hawaii.gov
hawaii.gov/health/dcab

Michael Okamoto, Chairperson
Peter Fritz, Vice Chairperson
Francine Wai, Executive Director
Debbra Jackson, Planning and ADA Cooordinator

Consists of 25 Hawaii residents appointed by the governor. The council addresses the needs of the people with developmental disabilities: specifically, develops a state plan that sets the priorities for persons with developmental disabilities.

Idaho

3547 **Idaho Commission on Aging**
341 W Washington
Boise, ID 83702-1
208-334-3833
800-926-2588
Fax: 208-334-3033
ICOA@aging.idaho.gov
www.idahoaging.com

Sam Haws, Administrator
Cathy Hart, State Ombudsman
Jeff Weller, Deputy Administrator
Raul Enriquez, Program Specialist

There number one priority is to provide the best possible service through this single point of entry website where people of all incomes and ages can obtain information on a full range of long-term care support programs and services.

3548 **Idaho Council on Developmental Disabilities**
Health and Wellfare
700 W. State Street
Suite 119
Boise, ID 83702-5868
208-334-2178
800-544-2433
Fax: 208-334-3417
info@icdd.idaho.gov
icdd.idaho.gov

Jim Baugh, Council Member
Christine Pisani, Executive Director
Tracy Warren, Program Specialist/Planner
Deborah Daniels, Management Assistant

The mission of the Idaho Council on Developmental Disabilities is to promote the capacity of people with developmental disabilities and their families to determine, access, and direct the services and/or support they need to live the lives they choose, and to build the communities ability to support their choices.

3549 **Idaho Department of Handicapped Children**
Statehouse
Boise, ID 83720-1
208-334-8000
Thomas Bruck, Chief
Sandy Frazier, Manager

3550 **Idaho Disability Determinations Service**
PO Box 21
Boise, ID 83707-0021
208-327-7333
800-626-2681
Fax: 208-327-7331
TTY: 800-377-3529
labor.idaho.gov

Roger B Madsen, Director
Rogelio Valdez, Executive Director

Under contract with the Social Security Administration, makes determinations of medical eligibility for disability benefits.

3551 **Idaho Industrial Commission**
P.O. Box 83720
Boise, ID 83720-0041
208-334-6000
800-950-2110
Fax: 208-334-2321
mholbrook@iic.idaho.gov
www.iic.idaho.gov

Mindy Montgomery, Manager
Beth Kilian, Commission Secretary

Free rehabilitation services to workers' who have suffered on the job injuries in Idaho. Field offices throughout the state.

3552 **Idaho Mental Health Center**
1720 Westgate Dr
Boise, ID 83704-7164
208-334-0808
800-926-2588
Fax: 208-334-0828

Richard Armstrong, Director
Darrell Kerby, Chairperson
Tom Stroschein, Vice Chair
Stephen Weeg, Board Member

The State of Idaho provides state funded and operated community based mental health care services through Regional Behavioral Health Centers (RBHC) located in each of the seven geographical regions of the state. Each RBHC provides mental health services through a system of care that is both community-based and consumer-guided.

Illinois

3553 Attorney General's Office: Disability Rights Bureau & Health Care Bureau
100 W Randolph Street
Chicago, IL 60601-3218
312-814-3000
877-305-5145
Fax: 312-793-0802
TTY: 800-964-3013
illinoisattorneygeneral.gov

Lisa Madigan, Manager
Raymond Throlkeld, Chief Health Care Bureau

Information on Illinois' Comprehensive Health Insurance Plan and architectural accessibility. Enforcement of Illinois' access law and standards and other disability rights laws. Information on initiatives such as: Opening the Courthouse Doors to People with Disabilities; the abuse, neglect or financial exploitation of people with disabilities and voter accessibility. Other information and referrals.

3554 Client Assistance Program (CAP)
Illinois State Board of Education
100 South Grand Ave. E.
Springfield, IL 62794
217-524-0695
800-641-3929
888-460-5111
Fax: 217-524-1184
dhs.cap@illinois.gov
www.dhs.state.il.us

James T. Dimas, Secretary
Francisco Alvarado, Manager
Quinetta L. Wade, Rehabilitation Services

The Client Assistance Program (CAP) helps people with disabilities receive quality Vocational Rehabilitation services by advocating for their interests and helping them identify resources, understand procedures, resolve problems, and protect their rights in the rehabilitation process, and employment.

3555 Equip for Equality
20 North Michigan Avenue
Suite 300
Chicago, IL 60602- 4861
312-341-0022
800-537-2632
Fax: 312-541-7544
TTY: 800-610-2779
contactus@equipforequality.org
equipforequality.org

Zena Naiditch, President/CEO
Barry C Taylor, Vice President
Lia Burkey, Administrative Assistant
Thomas Fischer, Special Assistant to President

Equip for equality is an independent, private, not-for-profit organization designated by the Governor in 1985 to implement the federally mandated Protection and Advocacy (P&A) System in Illinois. The mission of Equip for Equality is to advance the human and civil rights of children and adults with disabilities in Illinois.

3556 Equip for Equality - Carbondale Office
300 East Main St
Suite 18
Carbondale, IL 62901
618-457-7930
800-758-0559
Fax: 618-457-7985
TTY: 800-610-2779
contactus@equipforequality.org
equipforequality.org

Zena Naiditch, President/CEO
Barry C Taylor, Vice President
Lia Burkey, Administrative Assistant
Thomas Fischer, Special Assistant to President

Equip for equality is an independent, private, not-for-profit organization designated by the Governor in 1985 to implement the federally mandated Protection and Advocacy (P&A) System in Illinois. The mission of Equip for Equality is to advance the human and civil rights of children and adults with disabilities in Illinois.

3557 Equip for Equality - Moline Office
1515 Fifth Ave
Suite 420
Moline, IL 61265
309-786-6868
800-758-6869
Fax: 309-797-8710
TTY: 800-610-2779
contactus@equipforequality.org
equipforequality.org

Zena Naiditch, President/CEO
Barry C Taylor, Vice President
Lia Burkey, Administrative Assistant
Thomas Fischer, Special Assistant to President

Equip for equality is an independent, private, not-for-profit organization designated by the Governor in 1985 to implement the federally mandated Protection and Advocacy (P&A) System in Illinois. The mission of Equip for Equality is to advance the human and civil rights of children and adults with disabilities in Illinois.

3558 Equip for Equality - Springfield Office
1 West Old State Capitol Plaza
Suite 816
Springfield, IL 62701
217-544-0464
800-758-0464
Fax: 217-523-0720
TTY: 800-610-2779
contactus@equipforequality.org
equipforequality.org

Zena Naiditch, President/CEO
Barry C Taylor, Vice President
Lia Burkey, Administrative Assistant
Thomas Fischer, Special Assistant to President

Equip for equality is an independent, private, not-for-profit organization designated by the Governor in 1985 to implement the federally mandated Protection and Advocacy (P&A) System in Illinois. The mission of Equip for Equality is to advance the human and civil rights of children and adults with disabilities in Illinois.

3559 Illinois Assistive Technology Project
1 West Old State Capitol Plaza
Suite 100
Springfield, IL 62701-1200
217-522-7985
800-852-5110
Fax: 217-522-8067
TTY: 217-522-9966
iatp@iltech.org
iltech.org

Wilhelmina Gunther, Executive Director
Shelly Lowe, Finance/Personnel Manager
Yvonne Miller, Administrative Assistant
Barbara Howell, Administration

Directed by and for people with disabilities and their family members. As a federally mandated program, IATP strives to break down barriers and change policies that make getting and using technology difficult. IATP offers solutions to help people find what is available in products and services that will best meet their needs, where to find it, and how to get it.

3560 Illinois Council on Developmental Disability
State of Illinois Center
100 W Randolph St
16-100
Chicago, IL 60601-3218
312-814-2121
800-843-6154
Fax: 312-814-7441
www2.illinois.gov

Sheila T. Romano, Executive Director
Dennis Sienko, Manager

The Illinois Council on Developmental Disabilities (ICDD) is dedicated to leading change in Illinois so that all people with developmental disabilities are able to exercise their rights to freedom and equal opportunity.

3561 **Illinois Department of Mental Health and Developmental Disabilities**
Suite 3b
314 E Madison
Springfield, IL 62701 217-782-6680
Fax: 217-524-3834

Karen Perrin, Manager
Lori Stone, Director

3562 **Illinois Department of Rehabilitation**
100 South Grand Avenue East
Springfield, IL 62762-1304 217-782-6680
800-843-6154
Fax: 217-524-3834
TTY: 800-447-6404
DHS.WEBBITS@ILLINOIS.GOV
www.dhs.state.il.us/page.aspx?item=29736

Robert Kilbury, Director
Timothy Martin, Manager
DHS's Division of Rehabilitation Services is the state's lead agency serving individuals with disabilities. DRS works in partnership with people with disabilities and their families to assist them in making informed choices to achieve full community participation through employment, education, and independent living opportunities.

3563 **Illinois Department on Aging**
One Natural Resources Way
Suite 100
Springfield, IL 62702-1271 217-785-2870
800-252-8966
Fax: 217-785-4477
TTY: 888-206-1327
www2.illinois.gov

John K. Holton, Director
Jennifer Reif, Deputy Director
Matthew Ryan, Chief of Staff
Bradley A. Rightnowar, General Counsil
The MISSION of the Illinois Department on Aging is to serve and advocate for older Illinoisans and their caregivers by administering quality and culturally appropriate programs that promote partnerships and encourage independence, dignity, and quality of life.

3564 **International Dyslexia Association: Illinois Branch**
751 Roosevelt Rd.
Suite 116
Glen Ellyn, IL 60137 630-469-6900
Fax: 630-469-6810
www.readibida.org

Jo Ann Paldo, President
Foley Burckardt, Vice President
Joan Budovec, Treasurer
Sherry Grobe, Secretary
Provides free information and referral services for diagnosis and tutoring for parents, educators, physicians, and individuals with dyslexia in Illinois. Membership includes yearly journal and quarterly newsletter.

3565 **Social Security: Springfield Disability Determination**
3112 CONSTITUTION DR
Springfield, IL 62704-1323 877-279-9504
800-772-1213
TTY: 800-325-0778
ssa.gov

3566 **Workers Compensation Board Illinois**
100 W Randolph St
Ste 8-200
Chicago, IL 60601-3227 312-814-6611
866-352-3033
Fax: 312-814-6523
infoquestions.wcc@illinois.gov
www2.illinois.gov

Joann Fratianni, Chairman
The Illinois Workers' Compensation Commission resolves disputes between employees and employers regarding work-related injuries and illnesses.

Indiana

3567 **Indiana Client Assistance Program**
4701 N. Keystone Avenue
Suite 222
Indianapolis, IN 46204-1191 317-722-5555
800-622-4845
Fax: 317-722-5564
TTY: 317-722-5555
www.icdri.org/legal/IndianaCAP.htm

Michael Burks, Chairman
Wen Lu, Secretary and Treasurer

3568 **Indiana Developmental Disability Council**
402 West Washington Street
Room E145
Indianapolis, IN 46204-2801 317-232-7770
Fax: 317-233-3712
www.in.gov

Katrina Gossett, Chair
Dawn Adams JD, Agency representative
Suellen Jackson-Boner, Executive Director
Christine Dahlberg, Deputy Director
The Indiana Governor's Council is an independent state agency that facilitates change. Our mission is to promote public policy which leads to the independence, productivity and inclusion of people with disabilities in all aspects of society

3569 **Indiana Protection & Advocacy Services Commission**
4701 N. Keystone Avenue
Suite 222
Indianapolis, IN 46205-1561 317-722-5555
800-622-4845
Fax: 317-722-5564
ExecutiveDirector@ipas.in.gov
www.in.gov/ipas

Dawn Adams, Executive Director
Milo Gray, Client & Legal Services Director
Gary Richter, Support Services Director
Karen Pedevilla, Education/Training Director
An independent state agency established to protect and promote the rights of individuals with disabilities through empowerment and advocacy.

3570 **Indiana State Commission for the Handicapped**
P.O. Box 1964
Indianapolis, IN 46206 317-233-1292

3571 **International Dyslexia Association: Indiana Branch**
Fisher, IN 46038 317-926-1450
www.ida-indiana.org

Kim Haughee, President
Sara Silvey, Vice President
Ginger Lentz, Secretary
Woody Sears, Treasurer
The Indiana Branch was formed to help the members of the learning disabilities community in Indiana. Promotes understanding and facilitate treatment of the Specific Language Disability (Dyslexia) in children and adults, promotes teacher training and educational intervention strategies for dyslexic students and to foster effective teaching, supports research in the field and early identification of dyslexia, serves as a clearinghouse for information and to actively disseminate knowledge.

Iowa

3572 **Governor's Developmental Disability Council**
617 East Second Street
Des Moines, IA 50309-1831 515-281-9082
800-452-1936
Fax: 515-281-9087
http://idaction.com/

Becky Harker, Executive Director
Rik Shannon, Public Policy Manager
Janet Shoeman, Program Planner/Contract Manager
Fran Morris, Council Secretary
The Council identifies, develops and promotes public policy and support practices through capacity building, advocacy, and sys-

tems change activities. The purpose is to ensure that people with developmental disabilities and their families are included in planning, decision making, and development of policy related to services and supports that affect their quality of life and full participation in communities of their choice.

3573 **International Dyslexia Association: Iowa Branch**
P.O. Box 11188
Cedar Rapids, IA 52410-1188
765-507-9432
info@iowaida.org
ia.dyslexiaida.org

Denise Little, President
Tricia Krsek, Vice President
Genevieve Monthie, Secretary
Wayne Wunschel, Treasurer
The purpose of the Iowa Branch of IDA is to increase awareness of dyslexia and promote services that address the importance of diagnosis and remediation for those not meeting their reading potential. Providese services and assistance in a way that promotes unity, support, and cooperation among those who work with these individuals so that all communities in Iowa benefit from the skills and talents of its citizens.

3574 **Iowa Child Health Specialty Clinics**
100 Hawkins Drive
Room 247 CDD
Iowa City, IA 52242-1016
319-356-1117
866-219-9119
Fax: 319-356-3715
kathy-colbert@uiowa.edu
www.chsciowa.org

Jeffrey Lobas, Director
Brian Wilkes, Director Of Operations
Child Health Specialty Clinics has a mission to improve the health, development, and well-being of Iowa's children and youth with special health care needs in partnership with families, service providers, and communities.

3575 **Iowa Commission of Persons with Disabilities**
Department of Human Rights
Lucas State Office Bldg, 2nd Floor
Des Moines, IA 50319- 2006
515-242-6171
888-219-0471
Fax: 515-242-6119
TTY: 888-219-0471
www.state.ia.us/dhr/pd

Jill Fulitano-Avery, Administrator
To equalize opportunities for full participation in employment and other areas of the state's economic, educational, social and political life for Iowans with disabilities.

3576 **Iowa Compass**
Center for Disabilities & Development
100 Hawkins Dr
Suite S295
Iowa City, IA 52242-1011
800-779-2001
TTY: 877-686-0032
iowa-compass@uiowa.edu
www.iowacompass.org

Michael Lightbody, Project Director
Carolyn Petitgout, CRS, Admin Services Coordinator & Database Editor
Iowa Compass offers free information and program referrals to thousands of unique local, state and national organizations serving people with complex health related conditions and disabilities.
BiMonthly

3577 **Iowa Department for the Blind**
State Of Iowa
524 4th Street
Des Moines, IA 50309-2364
515-281-1333
800-362-2587
Fax: 515-281-1263
TTY: 515-281-1355
information@blind.state.ia.us
www.IDBonline.org

Richard Sorey, Director
Jodi Aldini, Library Support Staff
Julie Aufdenkamp, Transition Specialist, Transitio
Jessica Badding, Vocational Rehabilitation Counse
Mission is to be the means for persons who are blind to obtain univeral access and full participation as citizens in whatever roles they may choose.

3578 **Iowa Department of Human Services**
1305 E Walnut St
Des Moines, IA 50319-114
515-242-6510
800-972-2017
Fax: 515-281-4597

Terry E Branstad, Governor
Charles M Palmer, Director
Sally Titus, Deputy Director
Richard Shults, Division Administrator
Help individuals and families to achieve stable and healthy lives.

3579 **Iowa Department on Aging**
510 E 12th Street
Suite 2
Des Moines, IA 50319-9025
515-725-3333
800-532-3213
Fax: 866-236-1430
www.aging.iowa.gov

Donna K. Harvey, Director
Danika Welch, Executive Secretary
Joel Wulf, Administrator
Jeanne Yordi, State Long Term Care Ombudsman

3580 **Iowa Protection & Advocacy for the Disabled**
400 East Court Avenue
Suite 300
Des Moines, IA 50309
515-278-2502
800-779-2502
Fax: 515-278-0539
info@DRIowa.org
disabilityrightsiowa.org

Christine Glosser, President
Todd Lantz, Vice President
Jane Hudson, Executive Director
Cyndy Miller, Senior Staff Attorney
Disability Rights IOWA aims to defend and promote the human and legal rights of Iowans who have disabilities and mental illness.

3581 **Social Security: Des Moines Disability Determination**
Social Security Administration
Riverpoint Office Complex
455 SW 5TH ST STE F
Des Moines, IA 50309-2115
515-284-4260
800-772-1213
Fax: 515-284-4394
TTY: 800-325-0778
ssa.gov

Leroy Brown, Manager

3582 **Workers Compensation Board Iowa**
1000 East Grand Avenue
Des Moines, IA 50319-0209
515-281-5387
Fax: 515-281-6501
www.iowaworkforce.org

Joseph S Cortese II, Commissioner
Janna E. Martin, Commissioner
Sandy Breckenridge, Administrative Secretary
Jolene Doll, Support Staff
The Workers' Compensation Act is a part of the Iowa Code designed to provide certain benefits to employees who receive injury (85), occupational disease (85A) or occupational hearing loss (85B) arising out of and during the course of their employment.

Kansas

3583 **Beach Center on Families and Disability**
University of Kansas
1200 Sunnyside Ave.
Room 3134
Lawrence, KS 66045-7534
785-864-7600
866-783-3378
beachcenter@ku.edu
www.beachcenter.org

Michael Wehmeyer, Director

A federally funded center that conducts research and training in the factors that contribute to the successful functioning of families with members who have disabilities.

3584 **International Dyslexia Association: Kansas/Missouri Branch**
16628 Bond St.
Overland Park, KS 66221
816-945-2665
ksmoida@gmail.com
ksmo.dyslexiaida.org

Cathy Denesia, President
Holly Aranda, Vice President
Nora Wolf, Treasurer
Richard Bradford, Regional Representative

Provides free information and referral services for diagnosis and tutoring for parents, educators, physicians, and individuals with dyslexia in Illinois. Membership includes yearly journal and quarterly newsletter.

3585 **Kansas Advocacy and Protective Services**
214 SW 6th Ave.,
Ste 100
Topeka, KS 66603-3726
785-273-9661
877-776-1541
Fax: 785-273-9414
TTY: 877-335-3725
www.drckansas.org/

Rocky Nichols, Executive Director
Debbie White, Deputy Director
Lane Williams, Deputy Director
Catherine Johnson, Disability Rights Attorney

Protection and advocacy for persons with disabilities.

3586 **Kansas Client Assistance Program**
635 SW Harrison
Suite 100
Topeka, KS 66603
785-273-9661
877-776-1541
Fax: 785-273-9414
TTY: 877-335-3725
rocky@drckansas.org
www.icdri.org/legal/KansasCAP.htm

3587 **Kansas Commission on Disability Concerns**
900 SW Jackson
Suite 100
Topeka, KS 66612-1246
785-296-1722
800-295-5232
Fax: 785-296-1795
KCDCoffice@ks.gov
kcdcinfo.ks.gov

Martha Gabehart, Executive Director
Kerrie Bacon, Employment Liaison

The Kansas Commission on Disability Concerns provides disability-related supports and information to the people of Kansas. The commission offers legislative advocacy, education and resource networking to ensure full and equal citizenship for all Kansans with disabilities.

3588 **Kansas Department on Aging**
503 S Kansas Ave
New England Building
Topeka, KS 66603- 3404
785-296-4986
800-432-3535
Fax: 785-296-0256
TTY: 785-291-3167
wwwmail@kdads.ks.gov
www.kdads.ks.gov

Kathy Greenlee, Manager
Barbara Conant, Public Information Officer
Kari Bruffett, Secretary

Services and information for Kansas seniors, over age 60.

3589 **Kansas Developmental Disability Council**
Disability Rights Center of Kansas
915 SW Harrison
DSOB Rm 141
Topeka, KS 66612-3726
785-296-2608
877-431-4604
Fax: 785-296-2861
TTY: 877-335-3725
sgieber@kcdd.org
www.kcdd.org/

Steve Gieber, Executive Director
Craig Knutson, Public Policy Coordinator
Charline Cobbs, Senior Administrative Assistant

The purpose of the Kansas Council on Developmental Disabilities (KCDD) is to support people of all ages with developmental disabilities so they have the opportunity to make choices regarding both their participation in society, and their quality of life.

Kentucky

3590 **Kentucky Cabinet for Health and Family Services**
275 E Main St.
Frankfort, KY 40621
502-564-5497
800-372-2973
Fax: 502-564-9523
chfs.ky.gov

Jeffrey D. Howard, Commissioner

Oversees program areas relating to aging, behavioral/developmental health, children with special needs, family resources, medicaid, public health, and more.

3591 **Kentucky Council on Developmental Disability**
1151 So. Fourth Street
Louisville, KY 40203
502-584-1239
800-372-2973
Fax: 502-584-1261
info@councilondd.org
councilondd.org

Richard Bush, President
Dave Fowler, Treasurer
Missy Kinnaird, Secretary
Donovan Fornwalt, Chief Executive Officer

Implementation of Developmental Disabilities Planning Council responsible under P.L. 101-496.

3592 **Kentucky Office for the Blind**
275 E Main St
Frankfort, KY 40621
502-564-4754
800-321-6668
Fax: 502-564-2951
TTY: 502-564-2929
blind.ky.gov

Cora McNabb, Executive Director
Deanna Doll, Vocational Rehabilitation Counselor
Tonisha Everhart, Vocational Rehabilitation Counselor

Provides career services and assistance to adults with severe visual handicaps who want to become productive in the home or work force. The office also runs a Client Assistance Program established to provide advice, assistance and information available from rehabilitation programs to persons with handicaps.

3593 **Kentucky Office of Aging Services**
Cabinet for Health Services
275 East Main Street
Suite 1E-B
Frankfort, KY 40621
502-564-6930
Fax: 502-564-4595
TTY: 888-642-1137
David.Boswell@ky.gov
Deborah Anderson, Commissioner
Chris Harbeck, Executive Secretary
Marnie Mountjoy, Staff Assistant
Kristi Gentry, Executive Staff Advisor
The Kentucky Office of Aging Services is the state agency directly responsible for programs and services for people with disabilities. Efforts are made to fully integrate the service response information that considers broad farmiliar implications.

3594 **Kentucky Protection & Advocacy**
100 Fair Oaks Ln 3rd Fl
Frankfort, KY 40601-1108
502-564-2967
800-372-2988
Fax: 502-564-0848
kypa.net
Marsha Hockensmith, Executive Director
Protection and advocacy, Kentucky's federally-mandated protection and advocacy system, protects & promotes the disability rights of individuals through free legally-based advocacy, technical assistance, and education.

3595 **Social Security: Frankfort Disability Determination**
Social Security
140 Flynn Avenue
Frankfort, KY 40601
866-964-1724
800-772-1213
Fax: 502-226-4519
TTY: 502-226-4519
www.ssa.gov
Stephen Jones, Director
Burton Sisk, Manager

3596 **Social Security: Louisville Disability Determination**
Social Security
601 W Broadway
Room 101
Louisville, KY 40202-2227
866-716-9671
800-772-1213
TTY: 502-582-5238
ssa.gov

Louisiana

3597 **Louisiana Assistive Technology Access Network**
3042 Old Forge Dr.
P O Box 14115
Baton Rouge, LA 70898
225-925-9500
800-270-6185
Fax: 225-925-9560
www.latan.org/
Jim Parks, President & CEO
Sandee Winchell, Executive Director
An information and training resource on Assistive Technology for the State of Louisiana. LATAN operates three regional centers to provide better access for consumers.

3598 **Louisiana Center for Dyslexia and Related Learning Disorders**
PO Box 2050
Thibodaux, LA 70310-1
985-448-4214
Fax: 985-448-4423
karen.chauvin@nicholls.edu
www.nicholls.edu
Karen Chauvin, Director
Jason Talbot, Assessment & Research Coor
Ashley D Munson, Senior Program Coordinator
Sue Benoit, Administrative Coordinator 3
Provides free information and referral services for diagnosis and tutoring for parents, educators, physicians and individuals with dyslexia. The voice of our membership is heard in 48 countries.
Membership includes yearly journal and quarterly newsletter. Call for conference dates.

3599 **Louisiana Department of Aging**
Office of Elderly Affairs
PO Box 629
Baton Rouge, LA 70821-0629
225-342-9500
Fax: 225-342-5568
robin.wagner@la.gov
new.dhh.louisiana.gov/
Tara LeBlanc, Assistant Secretary
Robin Wagner, Deputy Assistant Secretary
Kirsten Clebart, Director
Annie Olivier, Director-Program Operation
Serves as a focal point for Louisiana's senior citizens and administers a broad range of home and community based services through a network of 37 Area Agencies on Aging. Serve as the focal point for the development, implementation, and administration of the public policy for the state of Louisiana, and address the needs of the state's elderly citizens.

3600 **Louisiana Department of Health - Mental Health Services**
PO Box 629
Baton Rouge, LA 70821-0629
225-342-9500
888-342-6207
Fax: 225-342-5568
ldhinfo@la.gov
new.dhh.louisiana.gov
Rebekah Gee, Ph.D, Secretary
Michelle Alletto, Deputy Secretary
Jimmy Guidry, Ph.D, State Health Officer
Andrew Tuozzolo, Chief of Staff
The Office of Behavioral Health's mental health services provide a variety of treatments for people who have different types of mental illnesses.Also offered are treatment clinics and family support services.

3601 **Louisiana Developmental Disability Council**
PO Box 3455
626 Main Street, Suite A
Baton Rouge, LA 70821-3455
225-342-6804
800-450-8108
Fax: 225-342-1970
shawn.fleming@la.gov
www.laddc.org
Sandra Sam Beech, Chairperson
Brenda Cosse, Vice Chairperson
Sandee Winchell, Executive Director
Shawn Fleming, Deputy Director
The Council's mission is to lead and promote advocacy, capacity building, and systemic change toimprove the quality of life for individualswith developmental disabilities and their families.

3602 **Louisiana Learning Resources System**
2525 Wyandotte St
Baton Rouge, LA 70805-6464
225-355-6197
Fax: 225-357-3508
Bobbie Robertson, Administrator
Provides consultation on educational seOrvices for local schools, offers psychological testing and evaluation, maintains resource rooms in district schools and more for the blind and handicapped throughout the state.

3603 **Social Security: Baton Rouge Disability Determination**
Department of Social Services
5455 Bankers Ave
Baton Rouge, LA 70808
866-613-3070
800-772-1213
Fax: 225-219-9399
TTY: 225-382-2090
adren.wilson@dss.state.la.us
www.ssa.gov
Shirley Williams, Director
Ann Williamson, Manager

3604 **Workers Compensation Board Louisiana**
1001 North 23rd Street
Post Office Box 94094
Baton Rouge, LA 70804-9094
225-342-3111
800-259-5154
Fax: 225-342-7960
owd@lwc.la.gov
www.laworks.net

Curt Eysink, Executive Director
Carey Foy, Deputy Executive Director
Renee Ellender Roberie, Chief Financial Officer
Bryan Moore, Director

The Louisiana Workforce Commission's vision is to make Louisiana the best place in the country to get a job or grow a business, and our goal is to be the country's best workforce agency.

Maine

3605 **Maine Assistive Technology Projects**
University of Maine at Augusta
Georgia Institute of Technology
490 Tenth Street
Atlanta, GA 30332-0156
404-894-4960
Fax: 404-894-9320
catea@coa.gatech.edu
assistivetech.net

3606 **Maine Bureau of Elder and Adult Services**
11 State House Station
41 Anthony Avenue
Augusta, ME 04333
207-287-9200
800-262-2232
Fax: 207-287-9229
www.maine.gov

Ricker Hamilton, Director
AnnMarie Stevens, Administrative Assistant
Lois Emerson, Office Specialist I
Maureen Hill, Office Associate II

Adult Protective Services (APS), is responsible for providing or arranging for services to protect incapacitated and/or dependent adults in danger.

3607 **Maine Department of Health and Human Services**
221 State Street
Augusta, ME 04333-0040
207-287-3707
Fax: 207-287-3005
www.maine.gov/dhhs

Mary C. Mayhew, Commissioner
Sam Adolphsen, Chief Operating Officer
Ricker Hamilton, Deputy Commissioner of Programs
Alec Porteous, Deputy Commissioner of Finance

Provision of an array of services to people with nental illness, substance abuse issues, children with special needs and people with developmental disabilities.

3608 **Maine Developmental Disabilities Council**
225 Western Avenue
Suite 4
Augusta, ME 04330
207-287-4213
800-244-3990
Fax: 207-287-8001
nancy.e.cronin@maine.gov
www.maineddc.org

Nancy Cronin, Executive Director
Rachel Dyer, Associate Director
Erin Howes, Office Manager

The MDDC is a partnership of people with disabilities, their families, and agencies which identifies barriers to community inclusion, self-determination, and independence, and acts to effect positive change.

3609 **Maine Division for the Blind and Visually Impaired**
21 Enterprise Dr
Suite 2
Augusta, ME 04333-0073
207-624-5120
800-760-1573
Fax: 207-624-5133
TTY: 800-633-0770
mdol@maine.gov
www.maine.gov/rehab/dbvi

Harold Lewis, Director
Sandra Cavanaugh, Executive Director

Works to bring about full access to employment, independence and community integration for people with disabilities in Maine.

3610 **Maine Office of Elder Services**
State of Maine
11 State House Station
41 Anthony Avenue
Augusta, ME 04333
207-287-9200
800-262-2232
Fax: 207-287-9229
TTY: 800-606-0215
mdol@maine.gov

James Martin, Director
Gary Wolcott, Associate Director
Romaine Turyn, Aging Service Manager
Elizabeth Gattine, Long Term Care Service Manager

The Office of Elder Services (OES), an Office within the Maine Department of Health and Human Services, promotes programs and services for older adults, their families and for people with disabilities.

3611 **Maine Workers' Compensation Board**
27 State House Station
Augusta, ME 04333
207-287-3751
888-801-9087
Fax: 207-287-7198
TTY: 877-832-5525
www.maine.gov/wcb

Paul H Sighinolfi, Executive Director
Lindsay Lizzotte, Secretary Specialist
Gary Koocher, Management Representative
Ron Green, Labor Representative

The general mission of the Maine Workers' Compensation Board is to serve the employees and employers of the State fairly and expeditiously by ensuring compliance with the workers' compensation laws, ensuring the prompt delivery of benefits legally due, promoting the prevention of disputes, utilizing dispute resolution to reduce litigation and facilitating labor-management cooperation.

3612 **Social Security: Maine Disability Determination**
330 Civic Center Dr
Suite 4
Augusta, ME 04330-6325
866-882-5422
800-772-1213
TTY: 207-623-4190
ssa.gov

Louis Tepin, Manager

This office makes the medical determination about whether a consumer is disabled and, therefore, medically eligible for Social Security benefits. Legally, an individual is considered disabled if he or she is unable to do any substantial gainful work activity because of a medical condition (or conditions), that has lasted, or can be expected to last for at least 12 months, or that is expected to result in death.

Maryland

3613 **Health Resources & Services Administration: State Bureau of Health**
5600 Fishers Lane
Rockville, MD 20857
301-443-2216
877-464-4772
TTY: 877-897-9910
www.hrsa.gov

Diana Espinosa, Deputy Administrator
Jordan Grossman, Chief of Staff

Through appropriated funds, supports education programs, credentialing analysis, and development of human resources needed to staff the U.S. health care system.

3614 International Dyslexia Association: Maryland Branch
International Dyslexia Association
P.O. Box 233
Brookland, MD 21022-0233
800-509-4980
md.dyslexiaida.org

Annette Fallon, President
Karen Fallon, Vice President
Timothy Yearick, Secretary
Jonathan Grimmel, Treasurer
Nonprofit organization providing free information and referral services for diagnosis and tutoring for parents, educators, physicians, and individuals with dyslexia. Membership includes yearly journal and quarterly newsletter. Call for conference dates.

3615 Maryland Client Assistance Program Division of Rehabilitation Services
2301 Argonne Drive
Baltimore, MD 21218-1628
410-554-9442
888-554-0334
Fax: 410-554-9362
TTY: 443-798-2840
dors@maryland.gov
dors.maryland.gov

Suzanne R. Page, DORS Director
Helps individuals with disabilities understand the rehabilitation process and receives appropriate and quality services from the Division of Rehabilitation Services and other programs and facilities providing services under the Rehabilitation Act of 1973.

3616 Maryland Department of Aging
State Office Building
301 West Preston Street
Suite 1007
Baltimore, MD 21201- 2393
410-767-1100
800-243-3425
Fax: 410-333-7943
www.mdoa.state.md.us/

Stuart Rosenthal, Chair
Sharonlee J. Vogel, Vice-Chair
Rona E. Kramer, Secretary
Sandie Callis, Commissiom Member
The Department of Aging protects the rights and quality of life of older persons in Maryland. To meet the needs of senior citizens, the Department administers programs throughout the State, primarily through local area agencies on aging.

3617 Maryland Department of Handicapped Children
201 W Preston St
Unit 50
Baltimore, MD 21201-2301
410-335-6470
www.msa.md.gov

Judson Force, Director
Children's Medical Services is a joint federal/state/local program which assists in obtaining specialized medical, surgical and related habilitative/rehabilitative evaluation and treatment services for children with special health care needs and their families. To be eligible for the program's services, an individual must be a resident of Maryland, younger than 22 years, have or be suspected of having an eligible medical condition and meet both medical and financial criteria.

3618 Maryland Developmental Disabilities Council
217 E Redwood Street
Suite 1300
Baltimore, MD 21202-3313
410-767-3670
800-305-6441
Fax: 410-333-3686
www.md-council.org

Brian Cox, Executive Director
Catherine Lyle, Deputy Director
Rachel London, Director, Children & Family Poli
Kelley Malone, Director of Communications
A public policy organization comprised of people with disabilities and family members who are joined by state officials, service providers and other designated partners. The Council is an independent, self-governing organization that represents the interests of people with developmental disabilities and their families.

3619 Maryland Division of Mental Health
201 W. Preston Street
Baltimore, MD 21201
410-767-6500
877-463-3464
dhmh.healthmd@maryland.gov

Norma Pinette, Executive Director
Van T. Mitchell, Secretary
Our Public Health Services Division oversees vital public services to Maryland residents including infectious disease and environmental health concerns, family health services and emergency preparedness and response activities.

3620 Maternal and Child Health Bureau - Health Resources and Services Administration
5600 Fishers Lane
Rockville, MD 20857
301-443-2170
www.hrsa.gov

Michael Warren, Associate Administrator
Laura Kavanagh, Deputy Associate Administrator
James Resnick, Executive Officer
Offers information, books and pamphlets to professionals, parents and children facing health issues or disabilities.

3621 Social Security: Baltimore Disability Determination
711 West 40th Street
Ste 415 Rotunda Mall
Baltimore, MD 21211-2120
800-772-1213
TTY: 800-325-0778
ssa.gov

3622 Workers Compensation Board Maryland
10 East Baltimore Street
Baltimore, MD 21202-1641
410-864-5100
800-492-0479
Fax: 410-333-8122
info@wcc.state.md.us
www.wcc.state.md.us

R. Karl Aumann, Chairperson
Mary K. Ahearn, Chief Executive Officer
David E. Jones, Chief Financial Officer
Joyce McNemar, Chief Information Officer

Massachusetts

3623 Center for Public Representation
22 Green Street
Northampton, MA 01060-3708
413-586-6024
Fax: 413-586-5711
info@cpr-ma.org
centerforpublicrep.org

Bob Agoglia, President
Nickie Chandler, Clerk/Treasurer
Bob Riedel, Director
Neal Rosen, Esq., Director
The Center seeks to improve the quality of lives of people with mental illness and other disabilities through the systemic enforcement of their legal rights while promoting improvements in services for citizens with disabilities

3624 Massachusetts Assistive Technology Partnership
Children s Hospital Boston
1295 Boylston St
Suite 310
Boston, MA 02215-3407
617-355-7820
800-848-8867
Fax: 617-355-6345

Marylyn Howe, Project Director
Pat Hill, Training Coordinator
A statewide program promoting assistive technology devices and services for persons with all disabilities.

3625 **Massachusetts Client Assistance Program**
Massachusetts Office on Disability
1 Ashburton Pl
Suite 1305
Boston, MA 02108-1518
617-727-7440
800-322-2020
www.mass.gov/anf/employment-equal-access-disa
Barbara Lybarger, Assistant Director
Myra Berloff, Director
Michael Dumont, Assistant Director
Jeffrey Dougan, Assistant Director
Provides advocacy and information services.

3626 **Massachusetts Department of Mental Health**
25 Staniford St.
Boston, MA 02114-2503
617-626-8000
TTY: 617-727-9842
dmhinfo@massmail.state.ma.us
www.mass.gov/dmh
Joan Mikula, Commissioner
The Massachusetts Department of Mental Health, as the State Mental Health Authority, assures and provides access to services and supports to meet the mental health needs of individuals of all ages, enabling them to live, work and participate in their communities. The Department establishes standards to ensure effective and culturally competent care to promote recovery. The Department sets policy, promotes self-determination, protects human rights and supports mental health training and research.

3627 **Massachusetts Developmental Disabilities Council**
100 Hancock Street
Second Floor, Suite 201
Quincy, MA 02169-4398
617-770-7676
Fax: 617-770-1987
TTY: 617-770-9499
www.state.ma.us/mddc/
Daniel Shannon, Executive Director
Faith Behum, Disability Policy Specialist
Kristin Britton, Director of Public Policy
Adelia DelTrecco, Member Services Coordinator
Group of citizens which analyzes needs of people with severe, lifelong disabilities and works to improve public policy. MDDC produces several publications and has committees and a grants program to study and advocate for changes in the service system.

3628 **Social Security: Boston Disability Determination**
110 Chauncy Street
Boston, MA 02111
617-727-7600
800-772-1213
TTY: 800-882-2040
www.socialsecurity.gov
Michael F. Bertrand, Commissioner

3629 **Workers Compensation Board Massachusetts**
Rm 211
1 Ashburton Pl
Boston, MA 02108-1518
617-626-7122
Fax: 617-727-1090
www.state.ma.us/dia
Russell Gilfus, Manager
The Massachusetts Workers' Compensation system is in place to make sure that workers are protected by insurance if they are injured on the job or contract a work-related illness. Under this system, employers are required by Massachusetts General Laws c. 152, 25A to provide workers' compensation (WC) insurance coverage to all their employees.

Michigan

3630 **Department of Blind Rehabilitation**
Western Michigan University
1903 W Michigan Ave
Kalamazoo, MI 49008-5218
269-387-3455
Fax: 269-387-3567
g.dennis@wmich.edu
www.wmich.edu/visionstudies
James Leja, Chair
Charles Adams, Faculty Specialist I
Gayla Dennis, Office Coordinator
Jeannyne Depoian, Office Associate
The Department of Blindness and Low Vision Studies at Western Michigan University is recognized internationally as the oldest, largest and best program of its kind. It originated in 1961 with a graduate degree in Orientation and Mobility, responding to the need for professionals to rehabilitate the many military personnel blinded during World War Two and the Korean War.

3631 **Michigan Association for Deaf and Hard of Hearing**
5236 Dumond Court
Suite C
Lansing, MI 48917-6001
517-487-0066
800-968-7327
Fax: 517-487-0202
TTY: 517-487-2586
info@madhh.org
www.madhh.org
Nancy Asher, Executive Director
Pat Walton, Office Manager
MADHH is a statewide collaboration agency dedicated to improving the lives of people who are deaf and hard of hearing through leadership in education, advocacy & services. Interpreter IC print-out, assistive devices available.

3632 **Michigan Association for Deaf, and Hard of Hearing**
5236 Dumond Court
Suite C
Lansing, MI 48917-6001
517-487-0066
800-968-7327
Fax: 517-487-2586
www.madhh.org
Nancy Asher, Executive Director
Pat Walton, Office Manager
MADHH is a statewide collaboration agency dedicated to improving the lives of people who are deaf and hard of hearing through leadership in education, advocacy and services.

3633 **Michigan Client Assistance Program**
4095 Legacy Pkwy
Ste 500
Lansing, MI 48911-4264
517-487-1755
800-288-5923
Fax: 517-487-0827
TTY: 800-288-5923
molson@mpas.org
www.mpas.org
Kate Pew Wolters, President
Thomas Landry, Ist Vice President
John McCulloch, 2nd Vice President
Elmer L. Cerano, Executive Director
The Client Assistance Program (CAP) assists people who are seeking or receiving services from Michigan Rehabilitation Services, Consumer Choice Programs, Michigan Commission for the Blind, Centers for Independent Living, and Supported Employment and Transition Programs. The CAP program is part of Michigan Protection and Advocacy Service, Inc.

3634 **Michigan Coalition for Staff Development and School Improvement**
12236 6 1/2 Mile Road
MCES
Battle Creek, MI 49014-1062
269-967-2086
800-444-2014
Fax: 517-371-1170

3635 **Michigan Commission for the Blind - Gaylord**
Ste 102
209 W 1st St
Gaylord, MI 49735-1386
989-732-2448
800-292-4200
Fax: 989-731-3587
www.michigan.gov

Judy Terwilliger, Manager

The mission of the Michigan Commission for the Blind (MCB) is to provide opportunity to individuals who are blind or visually impaired to achieve employability and/or function independently in society. The MCB vision is that someday it will be said that Michigan is a great place for blind people to live, learn, work, raise a family, and enjoy life

3636 **Michigan Commission for the Blind**
Michigan Dept Of Energy, Labor & Economic Growth
PO Box 30652
Lansing, MI 48909-8152
517-373-2062
800-292-4200
Fax: 517-335-5140
TTY: 517-373-4025
turneys@michigan.gov
www.michigan.gov/mcb

Patrick Cannon, State Director

The Michigan Commision for the blind is a state government agency that provides state and federally funded training and other services to individuals who are legally blind (blind and visually impaired). Services are provided to people of all ages throughout the state of Michigan toward the goal of employment and/or independence.

3637 **Michigan Commission for the Blind Training Center**
PO Box 30652
Lansing, MI 48909
517-373-2062
800-292-4200
Fax: 517-335-5140
TTY: 517-373-4025
mossc@michigan.gov
www.michigan.gov/mcb

Cheryl L Heibeck, Director
Bruce Schultz, Assistant Director

Residential facility that provides instruction to legally blind adults in Braille, computer operation and assistive technology, handwriting, cane travel, cooking, personal management, industrial arts and also crafts. During training students will develop career plans which may include work experience, internships, volunteer opprtunities and even part-time paid employment.

3638 **Michigan Commission for the Blind: Escanaba**
305 Ludington St
State Office Bldg., 1st Floor
Escanaba, MI 49829-4029
906-786-8602
800-323-2535
Fax: 906-786-4638
michigan.gov/mcb

Bernie Kramer, Manager

The mission of the Michigan Commission for the Blind (MCB) is to provide opportunity to individuals who are blind or visually impaired to achieve employability and/or function independently in society. The MCB vision is that someday it will be said that Michigan is a great place for blind people to live, learn, work, raise a family, and enjoy life

3639 **Michigan Commission for the Blind: Flint**
125 E Union St
Seventh Floor
Flint, MI 48502-2041
810-760-2030
800-292-4200
Fax: 810-760-2032

Debbie Wilson, Manager

Vocational and Independent living skills training for individuals who are legally blind.

3640 **Michigan Commission for the Blind: Grand Rapids**
250 Ottawa Avenue
Grand Rapids, MI 49503-4029
906-786-8602
800-323-2535
Fax: 906-786-4638
michigan.gov/mcb

Bernie Kramer, Manager

The mission of the Michigan Commission for the Blind (MCB) is to provide opportunity to individuals who are blind or visually impaired to achieve employability and/or function independently in society. The MCB vision is that someday it will be said that Michigan is a great place for blind people to live, learn, work, raise a family, and enjoy life

3641 **Michigan Council of the Blind and Visually Impaired (MCBVI)**
Neal Freeling
350 Ottawa Ave NW
Grand Rapids, MI 49503-2316
616-356-0180
800-292-4200
Fax: 616-356-0199
michigan.gov/mcb

Bernie Kramer, Manager

MCBVI is a diverse group of very friendly people from around the state working together to improve the lives of all citizens who are blind or visually impaired.

3642 **Michigan Department of Handicapped Children**
3423 N Martin Luther King Jr Blvd
Lansing, MI 48906-2934
517-484-9312
Fax: 517-484-9836

Alan Curtiss, President
Bobbie Butler, Manager

3643 **Michigan Developmental Disabilies Council**
201 Townsend Street
Suite 120
Lansing, MI 48910-1646
517-335-3158
Fax: 517-335-2751
TTY: 517-335-3171
mdch-dd-council@michigan.gov
www.michigan.gov/ddcouncil

Nick Lyon, Director
Nancy Grijalva, Assistant
Tim Becker, Chief Deputy Director
Trish Ray, Assistant

The Michigan DD Council is a group of citizens from across the state. Its membership is made up of: people with developmental disabilities; people from families who have, among their members, people with developmental disabilities; and professionals from state and local agencies charged with assisting people with developmental disabilities.

3644 **Michigan Office of Services to the Aging**
P.O. Box 30676
Lansing, MI 48909-8176
517-373-8230
Fax: 517-373-4092
OSAInfo@michigan.gov
www.michigan.gov/osa

Wendi Middleton, Division Director
Kari Sederburg, Director
Carol Dye, Senior Executive Assistant
Annette Gamez, Executive Assistant

State unit on aging; allocates and monitors state and federal funds for the Older American Act services: nutrition, community services, administers home and community based waiver, develops programs through Area Agencies on Aging, advocates on behalf of seniors with legislature, governor, state departments, federal government, responsible for state planning of aging services, develops formula for distribution of state and federal funds.

3645 **Michigan Protection & Advocacy Service**
4095 Legacy Pkwy
Ste 500
Lansing, MI 48911-4264
517-487-1755
800-288-5923
Fax: 517-487-0827
molson@mpas.org
www.mpas.org

Kate Pew Wolters, President
Thomas Landry, Ist Vice President
John McCulloch, 2nd Vice President
Elmer L. Cerano, Executive Director

People with disabilities have to deal with a wide variety of issues. TThey try to answer any questions you may have relating to disability. They have experience in the following areas: discrimination in education, employment, housing, and public places; abuse and neglect; Social Security benefits; Medicaid, Medicare and other insurance; housing; Vocational Rehabilitation; HIV/AIDS issues; and many other disability-related topics

3646 **Michigan Rehabilitation Services**
300 N. Washington Sq.
Lansing, MI 48913
517-335-4590
888-784-7328
Fax: 517-373-0059
TTY: 517-373-4035
zimmermanng@michigan.org
www.michigan.org

George Zimmermann, Vice President
Michelle Begnoche, Communications Specialist
Bonnie Fink, Travel Consultant Coordinator
David Lorenz, Public and Industry Relations Ma

A state and federally funded program that helps persons with disabilities prepare for and fund a job that matches their interests and abilities. Assistance is also available to workers with disabilities who are having difficulty keeping a job. A person is eligible for MRS services if he or she has a disability, is unemployed and needs vocational rehabilitation services to prepare for and find a job or independent living services.

3647 **Social Security Administration**
1100 West High Rise
6401 Security Blvd.
Baltimore, MD 21235-3878
517-393-3876
800-772-1213
Fax: 517-393-4686
TTY: 800-325-0778
jennifer.bower@ssa.gov
ssa.gov

Tiffany L. Flick, Executive Secretary
Michael J. Astrue, Commissioner
Carolyn W. Colvin, Deputy Commissioner

We deliver services through a nationwide network of over 1,400 offices that include regional offices, field offices, card centers, teleservice centers, processing centers, hearing offices, the Appeals Council, and our State and territorial partners, the Disability Determination Services. We also have a presence in U.S. embassies around the globe. For the public, we are the face of the government. The rich diversity of our employees mirrors the public we serve.

3648 **State of Michigan Workers' Compensation Agency**
PO Box 30016
Lansing, MI 48909-7516
888-396-5041
Fax: 517-322-1808
wcinfo@michigan.gov
www.michigan.gov/wca/

Mark C. Long, Director
Jack A. Nolish, Deputy Director
Julie Lenneman, Administrative Assistant
Ted Day, Division Manager

Michigan's injured workers and their employers are governed by the Workers' Disability Compensation Act. This Act was first adopted in 1912 and provides compensation to workers who suffer an injury on the job and protects employers' liability. The mission of the Workers' Compensation Agency is to efficiently administer the Act and provide prompt, courteous and impartial service to all customers.

Minnesota

3649 **International Dyslexia Association: Upper Midwest Branch**
International Dyslexia Association
5021 Vernon Ave. S
Suite 159
Minneapolis, MN 55436-2102
612-486-4242
info.umw@dyslexiaida.org
umw.dyslexiaida.org

Tom Strewler, President
Donna Burns, Member at Large
Jennifer Bennett, Secretary
Brian Pittenger, Treasurer

The Upper Midwest Branch of the International Dyslexia Association serves the residents of Minnesota, North Dakota, South Dakota, and Winnipeg, Canada. They offer local educational conferences about dyslexia and related subjects, Orton-Gillingham training for teachers, tutors, and parents, quarterly speaker series, member discounts on conferences, information line, and tutor referral.

3650 **Minnesota Assistive Technology Project**
STAR
358 Centennial Office Building
658 Cedar Street
Saint Paul, MN 55155-1402
651-201-2640
888-234-1267
800-627-3529
Fax: 651-282-6671
star.program@state.mn.us

Chuck Rassbach, Program Director
Kim Moccia, Program Coordinator
Jennie Delisi, Resource Specialist
Joan Gillum, Contracts Coordinator

A statewide program promoting assistive technology devices and services for persons of all ages with all disabilities.

3651 **Minnesota Board on Aging**
P.O. Box 64976
Saint Paul, MN 55164-0976
651-431-2500
800-882-6262
800-333-2433
Fax: 651-431-7453
TTY: 800-627-3529
www.mnaging.org

Don Samuelson, Chair
Jean Wood, Executive Director
Leonard Axelrod, Board Member
Tracy Keibler, Board Member

A state unit on aging for the state of Minnesota. Funds 14 area agencies on aging throughout the state that provide services at the local level. The mission is to keep older people in the homes or places of residence for as long as possible.

3652 **Minnesota Children with Special Needs, Minnesota Department of Health**
P.O. Box 64882
Saint Paul, MN 55164-0882
651-201-3650
800-728-5420
Fax: 651-201-3655
TTY: 651-201-5797
health.cyshn@state.mn.us

Dr. Edward Ehlinger, Commissioner
Daniel L. Pollock, Deputy Commissioner
Jeanne F. Ayers, Assistant Commissioner
Barb Dalbec, Director

Minnesota Children with Special Health Needs (MCSHN) provides leadership through partnerships with families and other key stakeholders to improve the access and quality of all systems impacting children and youth with special health care needs and their families.

3653 **Minnesota Department of Human Services: Behavioral Health Division**
P.O. Box 64981
Saint Paul, MN 55164
651-431-2225
800-366-5411
Fax: 651-431-7418
dhs.info@state.mn.us
mn.gov/dhs/adult-mental-health

Emily Piper, Commissioner
Charles E. Johnson, Deputy Commissioner
Amy Dellwo, Acting Chief of Staff
Nathan Moracco, Assistant Commissioner for Health Care

Oversees the provision of services to people with mental illness in the state of Minnesota. Services are provided on the local level through a network of 87 county social service departments.

3654 **Minnesota Department of Labor & Industry Workers Compensation Division**
443 Lafayette Rd N
Saint Paul, MN 55155-4301
651-284-5005
800-342-5354
TTY: 651-297-4198
dli.communications@state.mn.us
doli.state.mn.us
Ken Petersom, Commissioner
Jessica Looman, Deputy Commissioner
James Honerman, Communications
Wendy Legge, General Counsil
To reduce the impact of work related injuries for employees and employers. Advice is given and questions answered on the toll-free number.

3655 **Minnesota Disability Law Center**
430 1st Avenue North
Suite 300
Minneapolis, MN 55401- 1780
612-334-5970
800-292-4150
Fax: 612-334-5755
TTY: 612-332-4668
website@mylegalaid.org
mylegalaid.org/about/our-work/disability-law
Mary L. Knoblauch, Chair
Cathy Haukedahl, Executive Director
Andrea Kaufman, Director of Development
Lisa Cohen, Deputy Director of Operations
Provides free, civil, legal assistance to Minnesotans with disabilities on issues related to their disability.

3656 **Minnesota Governor's Council on Developmental Disabilities**
370 Centennial Office Building
658 Cedar St.
Saint Paul, MN 55155
651-296-4018
877-348-0505
Fax: 651-297-7200
TTY: 800-627-3529
admin.dd@state.mn.us
mn.gov/mnddc
John Hoffman, Chair
Colleen Wieck, PhD, Executive Director
Andrei Hahn, Planner
The mission of the Minnesota Governor's Council on Developmental Disabilities is to provide information, education, and training that will lead to increased independence, productivity, integration and inclusion for people with developmental disabilities and their families.

3657 **Minnesota Protection & Advocacy for Persons with Disabilities**
Minnesota Disability Law Center
2324 University Avenue West
Suite 101B
Saint Paul, MN 55114-1742
651-228-9105
800-292-4150
Fax: 651-222-0745
statesupport@mnlegalservices.org
Mary Kaczorek, Supervising Attorney
Ann Conroy, Office Manager
Elsa Marshall, Education for Justice Coordinato
Emily Good, Legal Project Manager
Provide public legal information on legal issues impacting the rights of low-income Minnesotans

3658 **Minnesota State Council on Disability (MSCOD)**
121 E 7th Place
Suite 107
Saint Paul, MN 55101-2114
651-361-7800
800-945-8913
Fax: 651-296-5935
council.disability@state.mn.us
www.disability.state.mn.us
Joan Willshire, Executive Director
Linda Gremillion, Business Operations Manager
Margot Imdieke Cross, Accessibility Specialist
David Fenley, Legislative Coordinator
The MSCOD collaborates, advocates, advises and provide technical information to expand opportunities, increase the quality of life and empower all persons with disabilities. This mission is accomplished by: providing information, referral and technical assistance to thousands of individuals every year via email, letter or telephone; through trainings on a variety of disability related topics; through publications and its web site; and through its advocacy and advisory work.

3659 **Minnesota State Services for the Blind**
2200 University Avenue West
Suite 240
Saint Paul, MN 55114-1840
651-539-2300
800-652-9000
Fax: 651-649-5927
TTY: 651-642-0506
star.program@state.mn.us
http://mn.gov/deed/job-seekers/blind-visual-i
Richard Strong, Executive Director
Kenneth Trebelhorn, Council Member
Jan Bailey, Chair
Steve Jacobson, Council Member
State agency serving blind and visually impaired persons with rehabilitation, information access, assistive technology, training and job placement services. Extensive older blind program.

3660 **Social Security: St. Paul Disability Determination**
5210 Perry Robinson
Lansing, MI 48911-3878
877-512-5944
800-772-1213
Fax: 517-393-4686
TTY: 800-325-0778
jennifer.bower@ssa.gov
www.ssa.gov
Karena L. Kilgore, Executive Secretary
Carolyn W. Colvin, Commissioner
Carolyn W. Colvin, Deputy Commissioner
James A. Kissko, Chief of Staff
We deliver services through a nationwide network of over 1,400 offices that include regional offices, field offices, card centers, teleservice centers, processing centers, hearing offices, the Appeals Council, and our State and territorial partners, the Disability Determination Services. We also have a presence in U.S. embassies around the globe. For the public, we are the face of the government. The rich diversity of our employees mirrors the public we serve.

Mississippi

3661 **International Dyslexia Association: Louisiana Branch**
1217 N. 32nd Ave.
Hattiesburg, MS 39401
601-467-1662
carla.carlos4dys@gmail.com
la.dyslexiaida.org
Carla Carlos, President
Lisa Best, Treasurer
Gale Pick, Secretary
Georgann Mire, Vice President of Education
Provides free information and referral services for diagnosis and tutoring for parents, educators, physicians, and individuals with dyslexia in Illinois. Membership includes yearly journal and quarterly newsletter.

3662 **Mississippi Assistive Technology Division**
1281 Highway 51
PO Box 1698
Jackson, MS 39215-1698
601-853-5160
800-443-1000
Fax: 601-853-5158
www.mdrs.ms.gov
Jean Massey, Superintendent of Education
Carey Wright, Superintendent of Education
Jack Virden, Chairman
Diana Mikula, Executive Director
A statewide program promoting assistive technology devices and services for persons of all ages with all disabilities.

3663 **Mississippi Client Assistance Program**
Mississippi Department of Rehabilitation Services
500-G East Woodrow Wilson Drive
P.O. Box 4958
Jackson, MS 39296
601-982-7051
Fax: 601-982-1951
www.msdisabilities.com

Dr. Ken Cleveland, President
Presley Posey, Executive Director
Dr. Michael Ogburn, Executive Director
David Cleland, Executive Director

Advocacy program for clients/client applicants for state of MS vocational services.

3664 **Mississippi Department of Mental Health**
1101 Robert E Lee Bldg
239 North Lamar Street
Jackson, MS 39201
601-359-1288
877-240-8513
Fax: 601-359-6295
TTY: 601-359-6230
www.dmh.ms.gov

Sampat Shivengi, M.D., Chair
George N. Harrison, Vice Chair
Edwin C. Legrand, Executive Director
Kris Jones, Bureau Director of Quality Manag

Administers Mississippi's public programs of serving persons with mental illness, developmental disabilities, alcohol and substance abuse problems, and alzheimer's disease and related dementia.

3665 **Mississippi Division of Aging and Adult Services**
Mississippi Department Of Human Services
750 North State Street
Jackson, MS 39202-3033
601-355-5536
800-345-6347
877-882-4916
Fax: 601-359-3664
www.mdhs.state.ms.us/

Donald R. Taylor, Executive Director
Julia M. Todd, Director
Judy Collins, Director
Mary Scott, Director

Protects the rights of older citizens while expanding their opportunities and access to quality services.

3666 **Mississippi State Department of Health**
Children s Medical Program
570 East Woodrow Wilson Drive
Post Office Box 1700
Jackson, MS 39216-1700
601-576-7400
866-458-4948
Fax: 601-364-7447
web@HealthyMS.com
www.msdh.state.ms.us

Larry Clark, Director
Vickey Berryman, Director, Bureau of Licensure
Jim Craig, Director, Office of Health Pro
Tim Darnell, Director, MSDH Field Services

Financial assistance to families of children with physical handicaps. Rehabilitative in nature and has as its goal the correction or reduction of physical handicaps. Eligibility determined by diagnosis and provided to children from birth to age twenty-one. Financial eligibility is determined by factors of family income, family size, estimated cost of treatment and family liabilities. Categories include, but are not limited to: orthopedic, congenital heart defects, cerebral palsy, etc.

3667 **Mississippi: Workers Compensation Commission**
1428 Lakeland Dr
P.O. Box 5300, 39296-5300
Jackson, MS 39216-4718
601-987-4200
866-473-6922
Fax: 601-987-4220
www.mwcc.state.ms.us

Liles Williams, Chairman
John Junkin, Commissioner
Debra Gibbs, Commissioner
Cindy Polk Wilson, Administrative Judge

Our goal is to provide the public with useful information regarding Workers' Compensation in the state of Mississippi.

Missouri

3668 **Institute for Human Development**
University of Missouri-Kansas City
215 W. Pershing Road
6th floor
Kansas City, MO 64108- 2639
816-235-1770
800-444-0821
Fax: 888-503-3107
TTY: 800-452-1185
beckmanncc@umkc.edu
www.ihd.umkc.edu

Carl F. Calkins, Ph.D., Director
Kay Conklin, Training Director
Cindy Beckmann, Assistant to the Director
Kathy Fuger, Director, Early Childhood and Yo

A statewide program promoting person-centered planning and services for persons of all ages with all disabilities.

3669 **Missouri Division Of Developmental Disabilities**
Missouri Department Of Mental Health
1706 E. Elm St.
P.O. Box 687
Jefferson City, MO 65102
573-751-4122
800-364-9687
Fax: 573-751-8224
ddmail@dmh.mo.gov
www.dmh.mo.gov

Jay Nixon, Governor
Keith Schafer, Ed.D., Director
Bob Bax, Deputy Director
Rikki J. Wright, J.D., General Counsel

The Missouri Department of Mental Health was first established as a cabinet-level state agency by the Omnibus State Government Reorganization Act, effective July 1, 1974. State law provides three principal missions for the department: (1) the prevention of mental disorders, developmental disabilities, substance abuse, and compulsive gambling; (2) the treatment, habilitation, and rehabilitation of Missourians who have those conditions; and (3) the improvement of public understanding and attitudes

3670 **Missouri Protection & Advocacy Services**
925 S Country Club Dr
Jefferson City, MO 65109-4510
573-893-3333
866-777-7199
Fax: 573-893-4231
TTY: 800-735-2966
moadvocacy.org

Joe Wrinkle, Chair
Barbara H. French, Vice Chair
Shawn De Loyola, Executive Director
Susan Pritchard-Green, Secretary/Treasurer

MO P&A potects the rights of individuals with disabilities by providing advocacy and legal services for disability related issues. As Missouri's Protection and Advocacy system, Mo P&A investigates allegations of abuse, neglect, death, and violations of rights against individuals with disabilities. Those who contact Mo P&A can receive information, referrals, advocacy services or legal counsel provided through one of nine federally-funded programs.

3671 **Missouri Rehabilitation Services for the Blind**
615 Howerton Court
PO Box 2320
Jefferson City, MO 65102-2320
573-751-3221
800-592-6004
Fax: 573-751-3091
askrsb@dss.mo.gov
www.dss.mo.gov/fsd/rsb/

Mark Laird, Executive Director
Ronald J. Levy, Director
Brian Kinkade, Deputy Director
Jennifer Tidball, Division Director

Offers services for the totally blind, legally blind, visually impaired, including counseling, educational, recreational, rehabilitation, computer training and professional training services.

3672 **Social Security: Jefferson City Disability Determination**
129 SCOTT STATION ROAD
Jefferson City, MO 65101-4421
877-405-9803
800-772-1213
Fax: 517-393-4686
TTY: 800-325-0778
jennifer.bower@ssa.gov
www.ssa.gov

Karena L. Kilgore, Executive Secretary
Carolyn W. Colvin, Commissioner
Carolyn W. Colvin, Deputy Commissioner
James A. Kissko, Chief of Staff

We deliver services through a nationwide network of over 1,400 offices that include regional offices, field offices, card centers, teleservice centers, processing centers, hearing offices, the Appeals Council, and our State and territorial partners, the Disability Determination Services. We also have a presence in U.S. embassies around the globe. For the public, we are the face of the government. The rich diversity of our employees mirrors the public we serve.

3673 **Workers Compensation Board Missouri**
Department of Labor and Industrial Realtions
421 East Dunkin Street
P.O. Box 58
Jefferson City, MO 65102-0058
573-751-4231
800-775-2667
800-320-2519
Fax: 573-751-4945
workerscomp@labor.mo.gov
labor.mo.gov/DWC/

Butch Albert, Chairman
James Avery, Commissioner
Curtis E. Chick, Commissioner
Ryan McKenna, Department Director

The Missouri Division of Workers' Compensation administers the programs providing services to all stake holders including workers who have been injured on the job or been exposed to occupational disease arising out of and in the course of employment. The Division makes sure that an injured worker receives benefits that he/she is entitled to under the Missouri Workers' Compensation law. The Division's Administrative Law Judges have the authority to approve settlements or issue awards after a hear

Montana

3674 **Addictive & Mental Disorders Division**
555 Fuller Ave
PO Box 202905
Helena, MT 59620-2905
406-444-3964
Fax: 406-444-4435
http://www.dphhs.mt.gov/amdd/

Lou Thompson, Administrator
Joan Cassidy, Chemical Dependency Bureau Chief
E. Lee Simes, Medical Director
Deb Matteucci, Behavioral Health Program Facili

The mission of the Addictive and Mental Disorders Division (AMDD) of the Montana Department of Public Health and Human Services is to implement and improve an appropriate statewide system of prevention, treatment, care, and rehabilitation for Montanans with mental disorders or addictions to drugs or alcohol.

3675 **Disability Rights Montana**
1022 Chestnut Street
Helena, MT 59601-890
406-449-2344
800-245-4743
Fax: 406-449-2418
TTY: 406-449-2344
advocate@disabilityrightsmt.org
www.disabilityrightsmt.org/janda3/

Bernadette Franks-Ongoy, Executive Director
Kelli Kaufman, Director of Finance & Administra
Steve Heaverlo, Director of Programs/Advocacy Sp
Laurie t Danforth, Paralegal/Executive Suppor

Protects and advocates the human and legal rights of Montanans with mental and physical disabilities while advancing dignity, equality, and self-determination. Designated federal P&A, with AT, CAP, PADD, PAIMI and PAIR programs. Advocacy and legal services for abuse, neglect, rights violations, access, discrimination in employment, accommodations and housing, and assistance with vocational rehabilitation/visual services.

3676 **MonTECH**
029 McGill Hall
University of Montana
Missoula, MT 59803
406-243-5751
877-243-5511
Fax: 406-243-4730
montech@ruralinstitute.umt.edu
montech.ruralinstitute.umt.edu

Anna Goldman, Program Director
Chris Clasby, Program Coordinator
Leslie Mullette

Specializing in Assistive Technology and oversee a variety of AT related grants and contracts. The overall goal is to develop a comprehensive, statewide system of assistive technology related assistance. Striving to ensure that all people in Montana with disabilities have equitable access to assistive technology devices and services in order to enhance their independence, productivity and quality of life.

3677 **Montana Blind & Low Vision Services**
111 N Last Chance Gulch, Suite 4C
PO Box 4210
Helena, MT 59604-4210
406-444-2590
877-296-1197
Fax: 406-444-3632
dphhs.mt.gov

Lou Thompson, Administrator
Joan Cassidy, Chemical Dependency Bureau Chief
E. Lee Simes, Medical Director
Deb Matteucci, Behavioral Health Program Facili

Mission: promoting work and independence for Montanans with disabilities.

3678 **Montana Council on Developmental Disabilities**
2714 Billings Ave
Helena, MT 59601-9767
406-443-4332
866-443-4332
Fax: 406-443-4192
www.mtcdd.org

Deborah Swingley, CEO/Executive Director
Dee Burrell, Contract Manager

The Council is made up of Montanans both with and without developmental disabilities, who believe in improving the lives of Montana's citizens who have a disability. We concentrate on issues related to self-determination, education, employment, transportation, housing, recreation, health care, community inclusion and the overall quality of life of people with developmental disabilities. As a Council we are committed to both question, and action as we work to discover and promote creative ways t

3679 **Montana Department of Aging**
Room 210
111 Sanders
Helena, MT 59604
406-444-7734
Fax: 406-444-3465
www.agingcare.com

Keith Messmer, Manager
Jeff Sturm, President

3680 **Montana Department of Handicapped Children**
111 North Sanders Street
Helena, MT 59620
406-444-7734
Fax: 406-444-3465
dphhs.mt.gov

Keith Messmer, Manager

3681 Montana Protection & Advocacy for Persons with Disabilities
1022 Chestnut Street
Helena, MT 59601-820
406-449-2344
800-245-4743
Fax: 406-449-2418
TTY: 406-449-2344
advocate@disabilityrightsmt.org
www.disabilityrightsmt.org/janda3/

Susie McIntyre, President
Will Warberg, Sales and Marketing Manager
Bernadette Franks-Ongoy, Executive Director
Kelli Kaufman, Director of Finance & Administra

Disability Rights Montana is the federally-mandated civil rights protection and advocacy system for Montana. We have the legal authority to represent almost any person with a disability.

3682 Montana State Fund
P.O. Box 4759
Helena, MT 59604-4759
406-495-5000
800-332-6102
Fax: 406-495-5020
TTY: 406-495-5030
www.montanastatefund.com

Elizabeth Best, Chairman

Montana State Fund is committed to the health and economic prosperity of Montana through superior service, leadership and caring individuals, working in an environment of teamwork, creativity and trust.

3683 Social Security: Helena Disability Determination
10 W 15th St
Ste 1600
Helena, MT 59626-9704
406-441-1270
800-772-1213
TTY: 406-441-1278
www.socialsecurity.gov

Karena L. Kilgore, Executive Secretary
Carolyn W. Colvin, Commissioner
Carolyn W. Colvin, Deputy Commissioner
James A. Kissko, Chief of Staff

Social Security offers online information and services to third parties who do business with them.

Nebraska

3684 Nebraska Advocacy Services
134 S 13th St
Suite 600
Lincoln, NE 68508-1930
402-474-3183
800-422-6691
Fax: 402-474-3274
info@disabilityrightsnebraska.org
www.disabilityrightsnebraska.org

Jill Flagel, Chairperson
Mary Angus, Vice-Chairperson
Timothy F. Shaw, Chief Executive Officer
Eric Evans, Chief Operating Officer

Offers protection and advocacy services to people with developmental disabilities or mental illness. Direct assistance provided if issue within broad case priorities. Sliding scale fee. Information and referral at no cost.

3685 Nebraska Client Assistance Program
301 Centennial Mall South
P. O. Box 94987
Lincoln, NE 68509-4987
402-471-3656
800-742-7594
Fax: 402-471-3656
victoria.rasmussen@nebraska.gov
www.cap.state.ne.us/

3686 Nebraska Commission for the Blind & Visually Impaired
4600 Valley Rd
Suite 100
Lincoln, NE 68510-4844
402-471-2891
877-809-2419
Fax: 402-471-3009
kathy.stephens@nebraska.gov
ncbvi.state.ne.us

Pearl Van zandt, Executive Director
Carlos Servan, Deputy Director
Bob Deaton, Deputy Director
Barbara Loos, Chairman

Offers services for the totally blind, legally blind, visually impaired, and more with health, counseling, educational, recreational, rehabilitation, computer training and professional training services.

3687 Nebraska Department of Health & Human Services of Medically Handicapped Children's Prgm
301 Centennial Mall S
5TH Floor
Lincoln, NE 68508-2529
402-471-3121
800-383-4278
Fax: 402-471-3577
dhhs.ne.gov

Kerry Winterer, Chief Executive Officer
Amy Borer, Admininstrative Assistant,Divisi
Dan Howell, CEO,Beatrice State Developmental

Maternal and child health, Title V, children with special health care needs; community based, statewide programs to facilitate diagnoses and care of children with disabilities and chronic medical conditions.

3688 Nebraska Department of Health and Human Services, Division of Aging Services
P.O. Box 95026
301 Centennial Mall South
Lincoln, NE 68509-5026
402-471-2115
800-942-7830
Fax: 402-471-3577
dhhs.ne.gov

Kerry Winterer, Chief Executive Officer
Amy Borer, Admininstrative Assistant,Divisi
Dan Howell, CEO,Beatrice State Developmental

The Council focuses on persons who experience a severe disability that occurs before the individual attains the age of 22, which includes persons with physical disabilities, mental/behavioral health conditions and persons that are served by the current state developmental disabilities system.

3689 Nebraska Department of Mental Health
4545 South 86th Street
Lincoln, NE 68526-2529
402-483-6990
888-210-8064
Fax: 402-483-7045
www.nmhc-clinics.com

Jill Zlomke McPherson, Executive Director
Thomas I. McPherson, Technical Coordinator
Lee Zlomke, Clinical Director
Lisa Logsden, Staff Psychologist

Nebraska Mental Health Centers is a family mental health clinic for people from all walks of life. Among the many services we provide are psychological evaluations, individual and group counseling, substance abuse care, neuropsychological services, domestic violence group intervention and help for victims of domestic violence, treatment for eating disorders, an ADHD clinic, Women's Counseling and much more.

3690 Nebraska Planning Council on Developmental Disabilities
Department of Health and Human Services
P.O. Box 95026
Lincoln, NE 68509-5026
402-471-2115
Fax: 402-471-3577
TTY: 402-471-9570
dhhs.ne.gov/developmental_disabilities/Pages/

Mary Gordon, Executive Director
Kerry Winterer, Chief Executive Officer
Amy Borer, Admininstrative Assistant,Divisi
Dan Howell, CEO,Beatrice State Developmental

The Council focuses on persons who experience a severe disability that occurs before the individual attains the age of 22, which includes persons with physical disabilities, mental/behavioral health conditions and persons that are served by the current state developmental disabilities system.

3691 Nebraska Workers' Compensation Court
State of Nebraska
P.O. Box 98908
Lincoln, NE 68509-8908
402-471-6468
800-599-5155
Fax: 402-471-8231
www.wcc.ne.gov/
Glenn W. Morton, Administrator
Susan K. Davis, Public Information Manager
Jacqueline J Boesen, General Counsel
Randall Cecrle, Information Technology Manager
It is the web site of the Nebraska Workers' Compensation Court. The court maintains this web site to enhance public access and provide general information regarding workers' compensation in Nebraska.

3692 Social Security: Lincoln Disability Determination
Department of Education
P.O. Box 94987
Lincoln, NE 68509-4987
402-471-2295
800-772-1213
TTY: 402-471-3659
www.socialsecurity.gov
Karena L. Kilgore, Executive Secretary
Carolyn W. Colvin, Commissioner
Carolyn W. Colvin, Deputy Commissioner
James A. Kissko, Chief of Staff
Social Security offers online information and services to third parties who do business with them.

Nevada

3693 Aging and Disability Services Division
3416 Goni Rd
Suite D 132
Carson City, NV 89706-8008
775-687-4210
800-992-0900
Fax: 775-687-0574
adsd@adsd.nv.gov
adsd.nv.gov
Jane Gruner, Administrator
Tina Gerber-Winn, Deputy Administrator
Michele Ferral, Deputy Administrator
Jill Berntson, Deputy Administrator
Provides services for seniors in Nevada including community based care. advocacy and volunteer programs. Call write or e-mail for more information.

3694 Nevada Assistive Technology Project
Ste 32
3656 Research Way
Carson City, NV 89706-7932
775-687-4452
888-337-3839
Fax: 775-687-3292
Todd Butterworth, Manager
Serves all ages and all disabilities through partnerships with community organizations. The NATP provides training, advocacy, funding, information and referral services, a newsletter and weekly television show.

3695 Nevada Bureau of Vocational Rehabilitation
500 East Third Street
Carson City, NV 89713
775-684-0400
Fax: 775-684-4184
TTY: 775-684-0360
detr.state.nv.us
Maureen Cole, Administrator
Melaine Mason, Deputy Administrator, Operations
Janice John, Deputy Administrator, Programs
Mechelle Merrill, Rehabilitation Chief II
Bureau of Vocational Rehabilitation is a state and federally funded program designed to help people with disabilities become employed and to help those already employed perform more successfully through training, counseling and other support methods.

3696 Nevada Community Enrichment Program (NCEP)
2550 University Avenue
Suite 330N
Saint Paul, MN 55114
651-645-7271
800-466-7722
Fax: 651-645-0541
TTY: 800-627-352
info@accessiblespace.org
Mark E. Hamel, Esq., Chair
Kay Knutson, Vice Chair
John W. Adams, MBA, Secretary
Mary Lindgren, Board Member
Comprehensive neurological rehabilitation and life skills training.

3697 Nevada Developmental Disability Council
896 W. Nye Ln.
Suite 202
Carson City, NV 89703
775-687-8619
Fax: 775-684-8626
www.nevadaddcouncil.org
Jodi Thornley, Chairman
Santa Perez, Vice Chairman
Sherry Manning, Executive Director
Kari Horn, Project Manager
The mission of the Nevada Developmental Disabilities Council is to provide resources at the community level which promote equal opportunity and life choices for people with disabilities through which they may positively contribute to Nevada society.

3698 Nevada Disability Advocacy and Law Center -Sparks/Reno Office
2820 West Charleston
Boulevard #11
Las Vegas, NV 89102
702-257-8150
888-349-3843
Fax: 702-257-8170
lasvegas@ndalc.org
www.ndalc.org
Reggie Bennettr, Secretary/Treasurer
Jana Spoor, President
John Miller, Vice President
Bob Bennett, Chairman
Nevada's protection and advocacy system for the human legal and service rights of individuals with disabilities. NDALC has offices in Reno/Sparks and Las Vegas, with services provided statewide.

3699 Nevada Division for Aging: Las Vegas
175 Berkeley Street
Boston, MA 02116
888-398-8924
libertymutual.com
Michael J. Babcockrs, Director
Marian L. Heard, Director
Martn P. Slark, Director
Develops, coordinates and delivers a comprehensive support service system in order for Nevada' senior citizens to lead independent, meaningful and dignified lives.

3700 Nevada Division of Mental Health and Developmental Services
5865 Lakeshore Road
Buford, GA 30518
770-945-4441
Fax: 678-482-1965
Keith Mixon, CEO/President
Offers treatment, prevention, education, habitation and rehabilitation for mental disorders. Works with advocacy groups, families, agencies and the community.

3701 **Social Security: Carson City Disability Determination**
1170 Harvard Way
Reno, NV 89502-2107
775-784-5221
800-772-1213
Fax: 775-784-5501
TTY: 800-325-0778
www.socialsecurity.gov

Karena L. Kilgore, Executive Secretary
Carolyn W. Colvin, Commissioner
Carolyn W. Colvin, Deputy Commissioner
James A. Kissko, Chief of Staff

Social Security offers online information and services to third parties who do business with them.

3702 **State of Nevada Client Assistance Program**
1631 W. Craig Rd.
Suite # 9-162
North Las Vegas, NV 89032-3767
702-635-4020
800-633-9879
800-633-9879
Fax: 702-642-7020
TTY: 800-633-9879

3703 **Workers Compensation Board Nevada**
1301 North Green Valley Parkway
Suite 200
Henderson, NV 89074
702-486-9000
Fax: 775-687-6305
dirweb.state.nv.us

New Hampshire

3704 **New Hampshire Workers Compensation Board**
46 Donovan St
Concord, NH 03301-2624
603-225-2841
800-698-2364
Fax: 603-226-6903
www.nhprimex.org

Ty Gagne, CEO
Jonathan Kipp, Operations Manager
Julie Converse, Director of Finance
Carl Weber, Director of Member Services

Primex3 stands ready to provide our school, municipal, and county government members with the most comprehensive coverages and services available to New Hampshire local government.

3705 **New Hampshire Assistive Technology Partnership Project**
Department of Education
10 West Edge Drive
Suite 101
Durham, NH 03824
603-862-4320
Fax: 603-862-0555
atinnh.org

Jan Nisbet, Director
Mary Schuh, Associate Director
Eve Fralick, Associate Director

The goal of the New Hampshire Assistive Technology Partnership Project is to increase access to assistive technology through the creation and support of consumer driven systems for the provision of state-of-the-art assistive technology products and services for citizens with disabilities in the state of New Hampshire.

3706 **New Hampshire Bureau of Developmental Services**
Department of Health and Human Services
129 Pleasant St
Concord, NH 03301-3852
603-271-5034
Fax: 603-271-5166
www.dhhs.nh.gov

Matthew Ertas, Director
Peggy Sue Greenwood, Administrative Assistant

Developmental Services promotes opportunities for normal life experiences for persons with developmental disabilities and aquired brain disorders in all areas of community life: employment, housing, recreation, social relationships and community association. Services and supports are organized throught a central state office and ten private nonprofit community area agencies. Family support is provided to families of children with chronic health conditions or are developmentally disabled.

3707 **New Hampshire Client Assistance Program**
121 South Fruit Street
Suite 101
Concord, NH 03301-8518
603-271-2773
800-852-3405
Fax: 603-271-2837
Disability@nh.gov
www.state.nh.us/disability/caphomepage.html

Bill Hagy, Ombudsman
John Richards, Executive Director
Jillian Shedd, Accessibility Coordinator
Gayle Baird, Accountant

The Commission's goal is to remove the barriers, architectural, attitudinal or programmatic, that bar persons with disabilities from participating in the mainstream of society.

3708 **New Hampshire Commission for Human Rights**
64 South Street
Concord, NH 03301-8501
603-225-3431
800-735-2964
Fax: 603-224-3766
webmaster@nh.gov
www.nh.gov

Peggy Mc Allister, Executive Director

Enforces New Hampshire law against discrimination in housing, employment or public accomodations. Disability discrimination is prohibited under New Hampshire law. Takes formal charges and investigates them.

3709 **New Hampshire Department of Mental Health**
129 Pleasant Street
Concord, NH 03301-3852
603-226-0111
Fax: 603-271-5058
www.dhhs.nh.gov

Donald Shumway, Director
Paul Garmon
Tim Rourke, Religious Leader

3710 **New Hampshire Developmental Disabilities Council**
2 1/2 Beacon Street
21 Fruit Street
Concord, NH 03301- 4447
603-271-3236
800-852-3345
800-852-3236
Fax: 603-271-1156
TTY: 800-735-2964
nhddc.org

Kristen McGraw, Chairman
Katherine Epstein, Vice-Chair
Carol Stamatakis, Executive Director
David Ouellette, Project Director

Offers information, referral and support services to disabled persons. A federally funded state agency.

3711 **New Hampshire Division of Elderly and Adult Services**
Bureau of Elderly & Adult Services
129 Pleasant St
Concord, NH 03301-3852
603-271-4680
800-351-1888
Fax: 603-271-4643
pio@dhhs.state.nh.us
www.dhhs.state.nh.us

Nicholas A. Toumpas, Comissioner
Mary Maggioncaida, Administrator
Marilee Nihan, Deputy Commissioner
Sheri Rockburn, Chief Financial Officer

The Bureau of Elderly and Adult Services provides a variety of social and long-term supports to adults age 60 and older and to adults between the ages of 18 and 60 who have a chronic illness or disability. These services range from home care, meals on wheels, care management, transportation assistance and assisted living to nursing home care.

3712 **New Hampshire Governor's Commission on Disability**
121 South Fruit Street
Suite 101
Concord, NH 03301-8518
603-271-2773
800-852-3405
Fax: 603-271-2837
Disability@nh.gov
www.nh.gov/disability
Paul Van Blarigan, Chairman
Charles J. Saia, Executive Director
Michael Coe, Accessibility Coordinator
Carol Conforti-Adams, Information and Referral Special
The Commission's goal is to remove the barriers, architectural, attitudinal or programmatic, that bar persons with disabilities from participating in the mainstream of socie

3713 **New Hampshire Protection & Advocacy for Persons with Disabilities**
Disabilities Rights Center, Inc
64 North Main Street
Suite 2, 3rd Floor
Concord, NH 03301-4913
603-228-0432
800-834-1721
Fax: 603-225-2077
TTY: 800-834-1721
advocacy@drcnh.org
drcnh.org
Paul Levy, President
Joanne Malloy, Vice President
Richard Cohen, Executive Director
Aaron Ginsberg, Staff Attorney
Legal services for individuals with disabilities; I & R.

3714 **Social Security: Concord Disability Determination**
Ste 100
70 Commercial St
Concord, NH 03301-5005
603-224-1939
800-772-1213
TTY: 800-325-0778
www.ssa.gov
Karena L. Kilgore, Executive Secretary
Carolyn W. Colvin, Commissioner
Carolyn W. Colvin, Deputy Commissioner
James A. Kissko, Chief of Staff
Social Security offers online information and services to third parties who do business with them.

3715 **Workers Compensation Board New Hampshire**
PO Box 2076
95 Pleasant Street
Concord, NH 03301
603-271-3176
800-272-4353
Fax: 603-271-2668
workerscomp@labor.state.nh.us
www.nh.gov/labor
Kathryn J. Barger, Director, Workers' Compensation
George N. Copadis, Commissioner of Labor
David M. Wihby, Deputy Commissioner
The Department of Labor monitors Employers, Workers Compensation, and Insurance Carriers to insure that they are in compliance with NH Labor laws. These laws range from minimum wage, overtime, safety issues and workers compensation.

New Jersey

3716 **Division of Developmental Disabilities**
210 South Broad Street
3rd Floor
Trenton, NJ 08608
609-292-9742
800-922-7233
Fax: 609-777-0187
TTY: 609-633-7106
advocate@drnj.org
www.njpanda.org
James W Smith Jr, Executive Director
New Jersey's designated protection and advocacy system for poeple with disabilities and provides legal, nonlegal individual and systems advocacy.

3717 **International Dyslexia Association: New Jersey Branch**
P.O. Box 32
Long Valley, NJ 07853
908-876-1179
Fax: 908-876-3621
njida@msn.com
nj.dyslexiaida.org
Patricia Barden, President
Provides free information and referral services for diagnosis and tutoring for parents, educators, physicians, and individuals with dyslexia in Illinois. Membership includes yearly journal and quarterly newsletter.

3718 **New Jersey Commission for the Blind and Visually Impaired**
153 Halsey St, Fl 6
PO Box 47017
Newark, NJ 7101-4701
973-648-3333
877-685-8878
Fax: 973-693-5046
www.state.nj.us/humanservices/cbvi
Daniel B. Frye, J.D., Executive Director
Bernice Davis, Executive Assistant
Edward Szajdecki, Manager
John Walsh, Chief of Program Administration
The mission of the New Jersey Commission for the Blind and Visually Impaired is to promote and provide services in the areas of education, employment, independence and eye health through informed choice and partnership with persons who are blind or visually impaired, their families and the community. Serves Bergen, Essex, Hudson, Morris, Passaic, Sussex and Warren Counties.

3719 **New Jersey Department of Aging**
210 South Broad Street
3rd Floor
Trenton, NJ 08608
609-292-9742
800-922-7233
Fax: 609-777-0187
TTY: 609-633-7106
advocate@drnj.org
www.drnj.org
Walter Anthony Woodberry, Chairman
Andrew McGeady, Vice Chairman
Linda K. Soley, Treasurer
Leah Ziskin, Secretary

3720 **New Jersey Department of Health/Special Child Health Services**
New Jersey Department of Health and Senior Service
P.O. Box 360
Trenton, NJ 08625-0360
609-777-7778
Fax: 609-292-3580
www.nj.gov/health/fhs/sch/
Jennifer Velez, ESQ, Commissioner
Provides services for New Jersey children that will prevent or reduce the effects of a developmental delay, chronic illness or behavioral disorder.

3721 **New Jersey Division of Mental Health Services**
Department Human Services
222 South Warren Street
P.O. Box 700
Trenton, NJ 8625- 700
609-292-3717
800-382-6717
Fax: 609-341-3333
www.state.nj.us/humanservices
Jennifer Velez, ESQ, Commissioner
Lynn A. Kovich, Assistant Commissioner
Oversees the public mental health system for the state of New Jersey. Operates six regional and specialty psychiatric hospitals, and contracts with over 125 not-for-profit agencies to provide a comprehensive system of community mental health services throughout all counties in the state.

3722 **New Jersey Governor's Liaison to the Office of Disability Employment Policy**
1 John Fitch Plaza
P. O.Box 110
Trenton, NJ 08625-110
609-659-9045
Fax: 609-633-9271
Constituent.Relations@dol.state.nj.us
lwd.state.nj.us/labor

Harold J. Wriths, Commissioner
Frederick J. Zavaglia, Chief of Staff
Aaron R. Fichtner, Ph.D., Deputy Commissioner
Brian T. Murray, Director of Communications & Mar

The Division of Vocational Rehabilitation Services provides vocational rehabilitation services to prepare and place in employment eligilbe individuals with disabilities who, because of their disabling conditions, would otherwise be unable to secure and/or mantain employment

3723 **New Jersey Protection & Advocacy for Persons with Disabilities**
210 South Broad Street
3rd Floor
Trenton, NJ 08608
609-292-9742
800-922-7233
Fax: 609-777-0187
TTY: 609-633-7106
advocate@drnj.org
www.drnj.org

Walter Anthony Woodberry, Chairman
Andrew McGeady, Vice Chairman
Linda K. Soley, Treasurer
Leah Ziskin, Secretary

3724 **Regional ADA Technical Assistance Center**
United Cerebral Palsy Associations of New Jersey
201 Dolgen Hall
Ithaca, NY 14853
607-255-6686
800-949-4232
Fax: 607-255-2763
northeastada@cornell.edu
www.northeastada.org

LaWanda H. Cook, Ph.D., Extension Associate/Training Spe
Hannah Rudstam, Ph.D., Director of Training
Erin Sember-Chase, Project Coordinator and Technic
Luz Semeah, Technical Assistance

3725 **Social Security Administration**
1100 West High Rise
6401 Security Blvd.
Baltimore, MD 21235
800-772-1213
TTY: 800-325-0778
www.ssa.gov

Karena L. Kilgore, Executive Secretary
Carolyn W. Colvin, Commissioner
Carolyn W. Colvin, Deputy Commissioner
James A. Kissko, Chief of Staff

Social Security disability is a social insurance program that workers and employers pay for with their Social Security taxes. Eligibility is based on your work history, and the amount of your benefit is based on your earnings. Social Security also has a disability program for people with limited income and resources- the Supplemental Security Income (SSI) program. For more information on these federal programs, please call our nationwide toll-free number.

New Mexico

3726 **New Mexico Aging and Long-Term Services Department**
2550 Cerrillos Rd
P.O. Box 27118
Santa Fe, NM 87505-3260
505-476-4799
866-451-2901
Fax: 505-476-4836
www.nmaging.state.nm.us

Miles Copeland, Deputy Secretary
Retta Ward, Secretary
Jason Sanchez, Administrative Services Division
Greg Rockstroh, IT Manager

Information and services for seniors, people with disabilities and their families.

3727 **New Mexico Client Assistance Program**
1720 Louisiana Blvd NE
Site 204
Albuquerque, NM 87110- 7070
505-256-3100
800-432-4682
Fax: 505-256-3184
info@drnm.org
www.drnm.org

Katie Toledo, Chairperson
Cyndy Costanza, Vice Chairperson
Jeanne A. Hamrick, President
Larry Rodriguez, Vice President

The mission of Disability Rights New Mexico (DRNM) is to protect, promote and expand the legal and civil rights of persons with disabilities. DRNM is an independent, private nonprofit agency operating federally mandated and other advocacy programs in pursuit of this mission.

3728 **New Mexico Commission for the Blind (NMCFTB)**
2905 Rodeo Park Dr E
Bldg 4, Suite 100
Santa Fe, NM 87505
505-476-4479
888-513-7968
www.cfb.state.nm.us

Greg Trapp, Executive Director

Offers services for the totally blind, legally blind, visually impaired, and more with health, counseling, educational, recreational, rehabilitation, computer training and professional training services.

3729 **New Mexico Department of Health: Children's Medical Services**
1190 S Saint Francis Dr
Santa Fe, NM 87505-4173
505-841-6100
800-797-3260
Fax: 505-827-2530

Gloria Bonner, Program Manager
Susan Baum, Medical Director
Freida Adams, Nurse Coordinator
Kim Love, Operations Manager

Title V MCH Program for children with special health care needs from birth to age 21 years. Services provided include: diagnosis, medical intervention, clinics and service coordination.

3730 **New Mexico Governor's Committee on Concerns of the Handicapped**
491 Old Santa Fe Trl
Santa Fe, NM 87501-2753
505-476-0412
877-696-1470
Fax: 505-827-6328
gcd@state.nm.us
www.gcd.state.nm.us/

Susan Gray, Chair
Curtiss Wilson, Vice Chair
Jim Parker, Director
Karen Courtney-Peterson, Chief Financial Officer

3731 **New Mexico Protection & Advocacy for Persons with Disabilities**
1720 Louisiana Blvd NE
Site 204
Albuquerque, NM 87110- 7070
505-256-3100
800-432-4682
Fax: 505-256-3184
info@drnm.org
www.drnm.org

Katie Toledo, Chairperson
Cyndy Costanza, Vice Chairperson
Jeanne A. Hamrick, President
Larry Rodriguez, Vice President

The mission of Disability Rights New Mexico (DRNM) is to protect, promote and expand the legal and civil rights of persons with disabilities. DRNM is an independent, private nonprofit agency operating federally mandated and other advocacy programs in pursuit of this mission.

3732 **New Mexico Technology Assistance Program**
625 Silver Ave SW
Suite 100 B
Albuquerque, NM 87102
505-841-4464
877-696-1470
Fax: 505-841-4467
www.tap.gcd.state.nm.us
Tracy Agiovlasitis, Program Manager
Examines and works to eliminate barriers to obtaining assistive technology in New Mexico. Has established a statewide program for coordinating assistive technology services; is designed to assist people with disabilities to locate, secure, and maintain assistive technology.

3733 **New Mexico Workers Compensation Administration**
2410 Centre Avenue SE
P.O. Box 27198
Albuquerque, NM 87125-7198
505-841-6000
800-255-7965
Fax: 505-841-6009
www.workerscomp.state.nm.us/
Ned S. Fuller, Director
Robert E. Doucette, Executive Deputy Director
Darin A. Childers, General Counsel
Thomas E. Dow, Executive Deputy Director
Regulates workers' compensation in New Mexico.

3734 **Social Security: Santa Fe Disability Determination**
6401 Security Blvd.
Baltimore, MD 21235
800-772-1213
TTY: 800-325-0778
www.socialsecurity.gov
Karena L. Kilgore, Executive Secretary
Carolyn W. Colvin, Commissioner
Carolyn W. Colvin, Deputy Commissioner
James A. Kissko, Chief of Staff

3735 **Southwest Branch of the International Dyslexia Association**
International Dyslexia Association
3915 Carlisle Blvd. NE
Albuquerque, NM 87107
505-255-8234
800-222-3123
Fax: 505-262-8547
swida@southwestida.org
Carolee Dean, President
Claudia Gutierrez, Vice President
Michelle Wick, Recording Secretary
Erin Brown, Corresponding Secretary
Provides free information and referral services for diagnosis and tutoring for parents, educators, physicians, and individuals with dyslexia. The voice of our membership is heard in 48 countries. Membership includes yearly journal and quarterly newsletter. Call for conference dates.

3736 **Workers Compensation Board New Mexico**
2410 Centre Avenue SE
P.O. Box 27198
Albuquerque, NM 87125-7198
505-841-6000
800-255-7965
Fax: 505-841-6009
www.workerscomp.state.nm.us/
Ned S. Fuller, Director
Robert E. Doucette, Executive Deputy Director
Darin A. Childers, General Counsel
Thomas E. Dow, Executive Deputy Director
Regulates workers' compensation in New Mexico.

New York

3737 **Albany County Department for Aging and Albany Social Services**
112 State Street
Room 900
Albany, NY 12207-2304
518-447-7000
Fax: 518-447-7188
aging@albanycounty.com
albanycounty.com
George Brown, Commissioner
Judy L. Coyne, Commissioner
Kathleen M. Dalton, Ph.D., Commissioner
The Point of Entry access line provides information and assistance and comprehensive referrals, and or assessments for the elderly, adults and children with disabilities, their family, or service providers.

3738 **Jawonio**
260 N Little Tor Road
New City, NY 10956-2627
845-708-2000
Fax: 845-634-7731
TTY: 845-639-3521
www.jawonio.org
Jill A. Warner, Executive Director & CEO
Matthew Shelly, Chief Program Officer
Diana Hess, Chief Communications Officer
Joseph Bloss, Chief Financial Officer
A dedicated community resource providing services to more than 500 children and adults annually. Provide early intervention, day care and pre-school special ed to our children. Job training, day habilitation, recreation, medical and service coordination for adults.

3739 **Jawonio Vocational Center**
260 N Little Tor Rd
New City, NY 10956-2627
845-708-2000
Fax: 845-634-7731
TTY: 845-639-3521
jawonio.org
Jill A. Warner, Executive Director & CEO
Matthew Shelly, Chief Program Officer
Diana Hess, Chief Communications Officer
Joseph Bloss, Chief Financial Officer
A dedicated community resource providing services to more than 500 children and adults annually. Provide early intervention, day care and pre-school special ed to our children. Job training, day habilitation, recreation, medical and service coordination for adults.

3740 **NYS Commission on Quality of Care & Advocacy for Persons with Disabilities**
401 State St
Schenectady, NY 12305-2300
518-388-2892
Fax: 518-388-2890
Andrew M. Cuomo, Governor
Roger Bearden, Chair
Bruce Blower, Member
Patricia Okoniewski, Member

3741 **NYSARC**
393 Delaware Ave
Delmar, NY 12054-3094
518-439-8311
800-724-2094
Fax: 518-439-1893
info@nysarc.org
nysarc.org
Laura J. Kennedy, President
Patricia Campanella, Senior Vice President
Joseph M. Bognanno, Vice President
Lori Martindale, Treasurer

3742 **National Alliance on Mental Illness of New York State**
99 Pine Street
Suite 302
Albany, NY 12207-1336
518-462-2000
800-950-3228
Fax: 518-462-3811
info@naminys.org
www.naminys.org

Sherry Grenz, President
Wend Burch, Executive Director
Sharon Clairmont, Finance & Business Office Dir.
Matthew Shapiro, Development/Events Coordinator

3743 **New State Office of Mental Health Agency**
Office of Mental Health
44 Holland Ave
Albany, NY 12229
518-474-4403
800-597-8481
Fax: 518-474-2149
www.omh.ny.gov

Mike Hogan, Commissioner
Promoting the mental health of all New Yorkers with a particular focus on providing hope and recovery for adults with serious mental illness and children with serious emotional disturbances.

3744 **New York Client Assistance Program**
855 Central Avenue
Suite 110
Albany, NY 12206
518-459-6422
Fax: 518-459-7847
TTY: 518-459-6422
www.nls.org

3745 **New York Department of Handicapped Children**
Department of Heath Education
Corning Tower
Empire State Plaza
Albany, NY 12237
518-456-0665
866-881-2809
Fax: 518-456-1126
www.health.ny.gov

Andrew M. Cuomo, Governor
Dr James B. Crucetti, MD, MPH, Commissioner
Howard Zucker, Acting Commissioner

3746 **New York State Commission for the Blind**
52 Washington St
Rensselaer, NY 12144-2796
518-473-7793
866-871-3000
Fax: 518-486-7550
www.ocfs.state.ny.us

Madeline Raciti, Manager
Offers services for the totally blind, legally blind, visually impaired, and more with health, counseling, educational, recreational, rehabilitation, computer training and professional training services.

3747 **New York State Commission on Quality of Care**
401 State St
Schenectady, NY 12305-2300
518-388-2892
Fax: 518-388-2890

Andrew M. Cuomo, Governor
Roger Bearden, Chair
Bruce Blower, Member
Patricia Okoniewski, Member

3748 **New York State Congress of Parents and Teachers**
1 Wembley Ct
Albany, NY 12205-6258
518-452-8808
877-569-7782
Fax: 518-452-8105
pta.office@nyspta.org
nyspta.org

Bonnie Russell, President
Gracemarie Rozea, First Vice President
Judy Van Harren, Secretary
Penny Hollister, Vice President
Parent Teacher Association and PTA are registered service marks of the National Congress of Parents and Teachers (National PTA). Only those groups chartered by the New York State PTA are entitled to use the name PTA. Any other use constitutes trademark infringement.

3749 **New York State Office of Advocates for Persons with Disabilities**
Ste 1001
1 Empire State Plz
Albany, NY 12223-1100
518-449-7860
800-522-4369
Fax: 518-473-6005

Gary O'Brien, Chair Commissioner
Provides information and referral services; administers NYS Tech Art Project; promotes implementation of disability-related laws.

3750 **New York State Office of Mental Health**
44 Holland Ave
Albany, NY 12229-1
518-474-4403
800-597-8481
Fax: 518-474-2149
www.omh.state.ny.gov in

Michael Hogan, Ph.D.
Promoting the mental health of all New Yorkers with a particular focus on providing hope and recovery for adults with serious mental illness and children with serious emotional disturbances.

3751 **New York State TRAID Project**
New York State Commisionon Qualityof Careand Advoc
Ste 1001
1 Empire State Plz
Albany, NY 12223-1100
518-449-7860
800-522-4369
Fax: 518-473-6005

Cliff Sigfride, Manager

3752 **Parent to Parent of New York State**
500 Balltown Rd
Schenectady, NY 12304-2247
518-381-4350
800-305-8817
Fax: 518-393-9607
mjuda@ptopnys.org
parenttoparentnys.org

Louise Nitto, President
Jim Costello, Vice President
Elizabeth Smithmeyer, Secretary
Michele Juda, Executive Director
Parent to Parent of NYS, which began in 1994, is a statewide not for profit organization established to support and connect families of individuals with special needs. The 13 offices, located throughout NYS, are staffed by Regional Coordinators, who are parents or close relatives of individuals with special needs.

3753 **Protection and Advocacy Agency of NY**
401 State St
Schenectady, NY 12305-2303
518-388-2892
Fax: 518-388-2890

Andrew M. Cuomo, Governor
Roger Bearden, Chair
Bruce Blower, Member
Patricia Okoniewski, Member

3754 **Regional Early Childhood Director Center**
89 Washington Ave.
Room 580 EBA
Albany, NY 12234
518-474-2925
800-222-5627
accesadm@mail.nysed.gov
www.acces.nysed.gov

3755 **Schools And Services For Children With Autism Spectrum Disorders.**
116 E 16th St
5th Floor
New York, NY 10003-2164
212-677-4650
Fax: 212-254-4070

Ellen Miller-Wachtel, Chairman
Shon E. Glusky, President
Owen P. J. King, Treasurer
Rachel Howard, Executive Director
This publication fun resource for children provides extreme coverage of services for children with autism, asbergez syndrome, and/or PDD.

3756 **Singeria/Metropolitan Parent Center**
2082 Lexington Ave.
4th Floor
New York, NY 10035
212-643-2840
866-867-9665
Fax: 212-496-5608
intake@sinergiany.org
sinergiany.org
Len Torres, President
Johnny C. Rivera, Vice President
Paola Jordan, Treasurer
Donald Lash, Executive Director

3757 **Social Security: Albany Disability Determination**
1 Clinton Ave
Albany, NY 12207
518-431-4051
800-772-1213
TTY: 518-431-4050
www.ssa.gov
Karena L. Kilgore, Executive Secretary
Carolyn W. Colvin, Commissioner
Carolyn W. Colvin, Deputy Commissioner
James A. Kissko, Chief of Staff

3758 **State Agency for the Blind and Visually Impaired**
52 Washington St
Rensselaer, NY 12144-2834
518-473-7793
866-871-3000
Fax: 518-486-7550
info@ocfs.state.ny.us
www.ocfs.state.ny.us

3759 **State Education Agency Rural Representative**
89 Washington Avenue
Albany, NY 12234
518-474-3852
Fax: 518-473-2860
RegentsOffice@mail.nysed.gov
www.nysed.gov
Merryl H. Tisch, Chancellor
Anthony S. Bottar, Vice Chancellor

3760 **State Mental Health Representative for Children and Youth**
44 Holland Ave
Albany, NY 12229
518-473-6328
www.rcybc.ca
David Woodlock, Deputy Commissioner

3761 **United We Stand of New York**
98 Moore St
Brooklyn, NY 11206-3326
718-302-4313
Fax: 718-302-4315
uwsofny@aol.com
Lourdes Rivera-Putz, Executive Director
Lourdes Figueroa, Intake/Receptionist
Carmen Soltero, Outreach/Trainer
Martha Vizcarrondo, Family Support Associate
Assists families with improving the quality of life for all individuals with disabilities.

3762 **University Afiliated Program/Rose F Kennedy Center**
1971
1300 Morris Park Avenue
Bronx, NY 10461
718-430-2000
www.einstein.yu.edu
Maris D. Rosenberg, Interim Director
Christine M. Baric, Assistant Director
John J. Foxe, Director
Robert W. Marion, Director

3763 **University of Rochester Medical Center**
601 Elmwood Ave
Rochester, NY 14642
585-275-8762
Fax: 585-275-3366
phil_davidson@urmc.rochester.edu
www.rochester.edu
Brad Berk, MD, PhD, CEO

3764 **VESID**
New York State Education Department
89 Washington Ave.
Room 580 EBA
Albany, NY 12234
800-222-5627
Fax: 518-474-8802
accesadm@mail.nysed.gov
www.acces.nysed.gov/vr/
Dr Rebecca Cort, Deputy Commissioner
Vocational and educational services for individuals with disabilities.

3765 **VSA Arts of New York City**
2700 F Street, NW
Washington, DC 20566
202-467-4600
800-444-1324
Fax: 717-225-6305
bbvsanyc@msn.com
David M. Rubenstein, Chairman
Deborah F. Rutter, President
Christoph Eschenbach, Music Director
Roger L. Stevens, Founding Chairman
Provides art, educational and creative expression experiences to thousands of children, youth, and adults with disabilities who reside in the five boroughs of New York City. It provides opportunities for people with disabilities to demonstrate their accomplishments in the arts and foster increased understanding and acceptance.

3766 **Westchester Institute for Human Development**
Cedarwood Hall
Valhalla, NY 10595
914-493-8150
info@WIHD.org
www.wihd.org
William H. Bave, Chairman
Pamela Thornton, Vice Chairman
Ansley Bacon PhD, President/CEO
David M.C. Stern, Treasurer
WIHD advances policies and practices that foster the healthy development and ensure the safety of all children, strengthen families and communities, and promote health and well-being among people of all ages with disabilities and special health care needs.

3767 **Workers Compensation Board New York**
PO Box 5205
328 State Street
Schenectady, NY 12305-2318
518-462-8880
877-632-4996
Fax: 518-473-1415
www.wcb.ny.gov
Andrew M. Cuomo, Governor
Robert E. Beloten, Chairman
Richard A. Bell, Commissioner

North Carolina

3768 **Developmental Disability Services Section**
Building 325n
Albemarle
Raleigh, NC 27699
919-420-7901
Fax: 919-420-7917
www.dhhs.state.nc.us/mhddsas/
Diana Simmons, Human Resources Manager
Ureh N. Lekwauwa, Chief, Clinical Policy
Courtney Cantrell, Acting Director
Jim Jarrard, Deputy Director
Makes policies and monitors public services and supports to people with mental illness, developmental disabilities and substance abuse throughout North Carolina.

3769 **International Dyslexia Association: North Carolina Branch**
NC
nc.dyslexiaida.org
Kris Cox, President
Provides free information and referral services for diagnosis and tutoring for parents, educators, physicians, and individuals with dyslexia in Illinois. Membership includes yearly journal and quarterly newsletter.

3770 **North Carolina Workers Compensation Board**
4340 Mail Service Center
Raleigh, NC 27699-4340
919-807-2501
800-688-8349
Fax: 919-508-8210
infospec@ic.nc.gov
www.ic.nc.gov

Julian Bunn, Owner

3771 **North Carolina Assistive Technology Project**
1110 Navaho Dr
Suite 101
Raleigh, NC 27609-7322
919-872-2298
Fax: 919-850-2792

Ricki Cook, Project Director
Annette Lauber, Funding Specialist
Jacquelyne Gordon, Consumer Resource Specialist
Tony Hiatt, Executive Director

The North Carolina Assistive Technology Project exists to create a statewide, consumer-responsive system of assistive technology services for all North Carolinians with disabilities. The project's activities impact children and adults with disabilities across all aspects of their lives.

3772 **North Carolina Children & Youth Branch**
North Carolina Public of Health
1928 Mail Service Ctr
Raleigh, NC 27699-1900
919-839-6262
Fax: 919-733-8034

Lawrence J Wheeler, Manager
Cathy Kluttz, Unit Manager Special Service
Dianne Tyson, Help Line Manager
Ran Coble, Executive Director

3773 **North Carolina Client Assistance Program**
2806 Mail Service Ctr
Raleigh, NC 27699-2806
919-855-3600
800-215-7227
Fax: 919-715-2456
nccap@dhhs.nc.gov
cap.state.nc.us

John Marens, Director
Diane Rawdarowicz, Client Advocate
Sharon Wisner, Client Advocate
Tami Andrews, Processing Assistant

A federally funded program designed to assist individuals with disabilities in understanding and using rehabilitation services. CAP serves as an integral part of the rehabilitation system by advising and informing individuals of all services and benefits available to them through programs authorized under both the Rehabilitation Act and Title 1 of the Americans with Disabilities Act.

3774 **North Carolina Developmental Disabilities**
3125 Poplarwood Court
Suite 200
Raleigh, NC 27604-7368
919-850-2901
800-357-6916
Fax: 919-850-2915
Info@nccdd.org
www.nc-ddc.org

Caroline Valand, Executive Director

A planning council established to assure that individuals with developmental disabilities and their families participate in the planning of and have access to culturally competent services, supports, and other assistance and opportunities that promote independence, productivity, and integration and inclusion into the community; and to promote, through systemic change, capacity building and advocacy activities, a consumer and family-centered comprehensive system.

3775 **North Carolina Division of Aging**
2101 Mail Service Ctr
Raleigh, NC 27699-2001
919-855-4800
Fax: 919-733-0443
ncdhhs.gov

Dennis Streets, Manager
Jim Slate, Director
Laketha Miller, Controller
Emery Edwards Milliken, General Counsel

3776 **North Carolina Industrial Commission**
4340 Mail Service Center
Raleigh, NC 27699-4340
919-807-2501
800-688-8349
Fax: 919-508-8210
infospec@ic.nc.gov
www.ic.nc.gov

J Howard Bunn Jr, Chairman
Peg Dorer, Executive Director

3777 **Social Security Administration**
4701 Old Wake Forest Rd
Raleigh, NC 27609-4919
877-803-6311
800-772-1213
800-325-0778
Fax: 919-790-2860
TTY: 919-790-2773
www.socialsecurity.gov

Karena L. Kilgore, Executive Secretary
Carolyn W. Colvin, Commissioner
Carolyn W. Colvin, Deputy Commissioner
James A. Kissko, Chief of Staff

Provides information on how to obtain social security through a disability.

North Dakota

3778 **Division of Mental Health and Substance Abuse**
600 East Boulevard Avenue
Dept 325
Bismarck, ND 58505- 0250
701-328-2310
800-472-2622
Fax: 701-328-2359
dhseo@nd.gov
www.nd.gov/humanservices

Dennis Goetz, Executive Director
Kerry Wicks, Executive Director
Andrew J. McLean, Medical Director
Alex Schweitzer, Superitendent

The Department of Human Services' Mental Health and Substance Abuse Services Division provides leadership for the planning, development, and oversight of a system of care for children, adults, and families with severe emotional disorders, mental illness, and/or substance abuse issues.

3779 **North Dakota Workers Compensation Board**
50 E Front Ave
Bismarck, ND 58504
701-328-3800
800-777-5033
Fax: 701-329-9911
TTY: 701-328-3786

Brent Edison, Director

3780 **North Dakota Client Assistance Program**
400 East Broadway
Suite 409
Bismarck, ND 58501-4071
701-328-2950
800-472-2670
Fax: 701-328-3934
panda@nd.gov
www.ndpanda.org/cap

Dennis Lyon, CEO
Janelle Olson, Advocate
Paula Rustad, Office Assistant
Angie Dubovoy, Advocate

CAP assists clients and client applicants of North Dakota Vocational Rehabilitation services, Tribal Vocational Rehabilitation, or Independent Living services.

3781 **North Dakota Department of Human Resources**
1237 W Divide Ave
Suite 6
Bismarck, ND 58501-1208
701-328-5300
800-451-8693
Fax: 701-328-5320
dhsaging@nd.gov
www.nd.gov

Shane Goettle, Manager

3782 **North Dakota Department of Human Services**
600 E Boulevard Ave
Dept 325
Bismarck, ND 58505-0250
701-328-2310
800-472-2622
Fax: 701-328-2359
dhseo@nd.gov
www.nd.gov/dhs

Carol K Olson, Executive Director
Dennis Goetz, Executive Director
Kerry Wicks, Executive Director
Andrew J. McLean, Medical Director

Provides services that help vulnerable North Dakotans of all ages to maintain or enhance their quality of life, which may be threatened by lack of financial resources, emotional crises, disabling conditions, or an inability to protect themselves.

3783 **Protection & Advocacy Project**
1984
400 East Broadway
Suite 409
Bismarck, ND 58501-4071
701-328-2950
800-472-2670
Fax: 701-328-3934
panda@nd.gov
ndpanda.org

Teresa Larsen, Executive Director
Janelle Olson, Advocate
Paula Rustad, Office Assistant
Angie Dubovoy, Advocate

The Protection and Advocacy is a state agency whose purpose is to advocate for and protect the rights of people with disabilities. The Protection and Advocacy Project has programs to serve people with developmental disabilities, mental illnesses and other types of disabilities. The projects programs and services are free to eligible individuals.

3784 **Social Security: Bismarck Disability Determination**
1680 E Capitol Ave
Bismarck, ND 58501-5603
701-250-4200
800-772-1213
TTY: 701-250-4620
ssa.gov

Karena L. Kilgore, Executive Secretary
Carolyn W. Colvin, Commissioner
Carolyn W. Colvin, Deputy Commissioner
James A. Kissko, Chief of Staff

3785 **Workers Compensation Board North Dakota**
1600EastCenturyAvenue
Suite1
Bismarck, ND 58503-649
701-328-3800
800-777-5033
Fax: 701-328-3820
www.workforcesafety.com

Sandy Blunt, CEO

Ohio

3786 **Epilepsy Council of Greater Cincinnati**
Ste 550
895 Central Ave
Cincinnati, OH 45202-5700
513-721-2905
877-804-2241
Fax: 513-721-0799
ecgc@fuse.net

Kathy Stewart, Executive Director

3787 **International Dyslexia Association: Central Ohio Branch**
P.O. Box 1601
Westerville, OH 43086
614-899-5711
coh.dyslexiaida.org

Mike McGovern, President
Blythe Wood, Vice President
Chris Lowe, Secretary
Diana McGovern, Treasurer

Provides free information and referral services for diagnosis and tutoring for parents, educators, physicians, and individuals with dyslexia. Membership includes yearly journal and quarterly newsletter.

3788 **Ohio Bureau for Children with Medical Handicaps**
Ohio Department of Health
246 N. High St
P.O. Box 1603
Columbus, OH 43215-1603
614-466-3543
800-755-4769
Fax: 614-728-3616
bcmh@odh.ohio.gov
www.odh.ohio.gov

John R. Kasich, Governor
James Bryant Md, Bureau Chief
Alvin Jackson, MD, Director
Lance D. Himes, Interim Director

Provides funding for the diagnosis, treatment and coordination of services for eligible Ohio children, under age 21, with medical handicaps; conducts quality assurance activities to establish standards of care and determine unmet needs of children with handicaps and their families; collaborates with public health nurses to increase access to care; and assists families to access and use third party resources. Conducts a separate program for adults with cystic fibrosis.

3789 **Ohio Bureau of Worker's Compensation**
30 W Spring St
Columbus, OH 43215-2256
800-335-0996
Fax: 877-321-9481
TTY: 800-292-4833
ombudsperson@bwc.state.oh.us
www.bwc.ohio.gov

Stephen Buehrer, Administrator/CEO
Dale Hamilton, Chief Operating Officer (COO)
Kevin Abrams, Chief of Employers Services
Toni Brokaw, Chief of Human Resources

To provide a quality, customer-focused workers' compensation insurance system for Ohio's employers and employees.

3790 **Ohio Client Assistance Program**
50 W. Broad St.
Suite 1400
Columbus, OH 43215-5923
614-466-7264
800-282-9181
Fax: 614-752-4197
TTY: 614-728-2553
www.olrs.ohio.gov

Donald Bishop, Executive Director

3791 **Ohio Department of Aging**
1982
50 W Broad St
Fl 9
Columbus, OH 43215-3363
614-466-5500
866-243-5678
888-243-5678
Fax: 614-466-5741
TTY: 614-466-6191
www.aging.ohio.gov

Bonnie Kantor-Burman, Director
John Ratliff, Public Information Officer

The department serves and represents about 2 million Ohioans age 60 & older. They advocate for the needs of all older citizens with emphasis on improving the quality of life, helping senior citizens live active, healthy, & independent lives, & promoting positive attitudes toward aging & older people. Committed to helping the frail elderly who choose to remain at home by providing home & community based services, their goal is to promote the level of choice, independence & self-care.

3792 **Ohio Department of Mental Health**
30 E Broad St
8th Floor
Columbus, OH 43215-3414
614-466-4775
877-275-6364
Fax: 614-752-8410

Michael Hogan, Director
Christine Vincenty, Manager

3793 **Ohio Developmental Disabilities Council**
899 E Broad St, Ste 203
Columbus, OH 43205
614-466-5205
800-766-7426
Fax: 614-466-0298
www.ddc.ohio.gov

Carolyn Knight, Executive Director
Mark Seifarth, Chair
Robert Shuemak, Vice Chair
Kimberly Stults, Secretary

The Ohio Developmental Disabilities Council is one of 55 councils found in all states and territories which provides funding for systems change grant projects. The DD Council is a planning and advocacy agency that seeks to improve the lives of Ohioans with disabilities.

3794 **Ohio Developmental Disability Council (ODDC)**
899 E Broad St, Ste 203
Columbus, OH 43205
614-466-5205
800-766-7426
Fax: 614-466-0298
www.ddc.ohio.gov

Carolyn Knight, Executive Director
Mark Seifarth, Chair
Robert Shuemak, Vice Chair
Kimberly Stults, Secretary

3795 **Ohio Governor's Council on People with Disabilities**
400 E Campus View Blvd
Columbus, OH 43235-4685
614-438-1200
800-282-4536
gcpd.ohio.gov

Jacqueline Romer-Sensky, Chairman
Jack Licate, Vice Chairman
Kevin Miller, Executive Director
Bill Bishilany, Assistant Executive Director

The Governor's Council on People with Disabilities exists to: Advise the Governor and General Assembly on statewide disability issues, promote the value of diversity, dignity and the quality of life for people with disabilities, be a catalyst to create systemic change promoting awareness of disability-related issues that will ultimately benefit all citizens of Ohio, Educate and advocate for: partnerships at the local, state and national level, promotion of equality, access and independence.

3796 **Ohio Rehabilitation Services Commission**
400 E Campus View Blvd
Columbus, OH 43235-4604
614-438-1200
800-282-4536
ohio.gov

Kevin Miller, Executive Director

RSC is Ohio's state agency that provides vocational rehabilitation (VR) services to help people with disabilities become employed and independent. We also offer a variety of services to Ohio businesses, resulting in quality jobs for individuals who have disabilities.

3797 **Ohio Women, Infants, & Children Program - Ohio Department of Health**
246 N High St
Columbus, OH 43215-2406
614-644-8006
Fax: 614-564-2470

Michele Frizzell, Chief, Bureau of Nutrition Svcs.

3798 **Social Security: Columbus Disability Determination**
90 E Washington Bridge Rd
Suite 140
Worthington, OH 43085
614-888-5339
800-772-1213
TTY: 614-288-0226
www.socialsecurity.gov

Karena L. Kilgore, Executive Secretary
Carolyn W. Colvin, Commissioner
Carolyn W. Colvin, Deputy Commissioner
James A. Kissko, Chief of Staff

Oklahoma

3799 **Oklahoma Workers Compensation Board**
Department of Labor
3017 N. Stiles, Suite 100
Oklahoma City, OK 73105
405-521-6100
888-269-5353
Fax: 405-521-6018
labor.info@labor.ok.gov
www.ok.gov/odol

Jim Marshall, Chief of Staff
Mark Costello, Commissioner of Labor
Lizzette McNeill, Communications Director
Stacy Bonner, Deputy Commissioner

3800 **Oklahoma Client Assistance Program/Office of Disability Concerns**
2401 NW 23rd Street
Suite 90
Oklahoma City, OK 73107- 2431
405-521-3756
800-522-8224
Fax: 405-522-6695
www.ok.gov

Todd Lamb, Governor
Gary Jones, Auditor and Inspector
E. Scott Pruitt, Attorney General
Ken Miller, Treasurer

CAP informs and advises applicants and consumers about the vocational rehabilitation process and services available under the Federal Rehabilitation Act, including services provided by DVR and DVS. CAP staff can help you communicate concerns to the DVR/DVS and assist you with administrative, mediation, fair hearing, legal and other solutions

3801 **Oklahoma Department of Human Services Aging Services Division**
25 Sigourney Street, 10th Floor
Hartford, CT 06106
405-521-3646
866-218-6621
800-522-7233
Fax: 860-424-5301

Margaret Ger Murkette, MSW, Director
Ed Lake, Director

3802 **Oklahoma Department of Labor**
3017 N. Stiles
Suite 100
Oklahoma City, OK 73105-5206
405-521-6100
888-269-5353
Fax: 405-521-6018
www.labor.ok.gov

Mark Castello, Commissioner
Jim Marshall, Chief of Staff
Stacy Bonner, Deputy Commissioner
Don Schooler, General Counsel

3803 **Oklahoma Department of Mental Health & Substance Abuse Services**
1200 NE 13th Street
P.O. Box 53277
Oklahoma City, OK 73152-3277
405-522-3908
800-522-9054
Fax: 405-522-3650
TTY: 405-522-3851
www.odmhsas.org

J. Andy Sullivan, Chairperson
Gail Henderson, Vice-Chair
Terri White, Commissioner
Durand Crosby, Chief Operating Officer

State agency providing mental helath, substance abuse and domestic violence services.

3804 **Oklahoma Department of Rehabilitation Services**
3535 NW 58th St.
Suite 500
Oklahoma City, OK 73112-4824
405-951-3400
800-845-8476
Fax: 405-951-3529
info@okdrs.gov
www.okrehab.org
Melinda Fruendt, Executive Director
The Oklahoma Department of Rehabilitation Services (DRS) provides assistance to Oklahomans with disabilities through vocational rehabilitation, employment, independent living, residential and outreach programs, and the determination of medical eligibility for disability benefits.

3805 **Workers Compensation Board Oklahoma**
1915 N Stiles Ave
Oklahoma City, OK 73105-4918
405-522-8600
800-522-8210
Leroy E Young, D.O., Chairman
Joyce Sanders, Supervisor
Michael J. Harkey, Vice Presiding Judge
Katrina Stephenson, Assistant Court Clerk

Oregon

3806 **International Dyslexia Association: Oregon Branch**
International Dyslexia Association
P.P. Box 2609
Portland, OR 97208-2609
503-228-4455
info@orbida.org
or.dyslexiaida.org
Jane Cooper, President
Danielle Thompson, Vice President
Anne Mauboussin, Treasurer
Christy Coss, Secretary
Provides free information and referral services for diagnosis and tutoring for parents, educators, physicians, and individuals with dyslexia. Membership includes yearly journal and quarterly newsletter.

3807 **Office of Vocational Rehabilitation Services (OVRS)**
500 Summer St NE
Salem, OR 97301-1063
503-945-5944
Fax: 503-378-2897
TTY: 503-945-6214
www.oregon.gov/dhs
Erinn Kelley-Siel, Director
Gene Evans, Communication Director
Eric Moore, Chief Financial Officer
Jim Scherzinger, Chief Operating Officer
The mission of OVRS to assist Oregonians with disabilities to achieve and maintain employment and independence.

3808 **Oregon Advocacy Center**
620 SW 5th Ave
5th Floor
Portland, OR 97204-1428
503-243-2081
800-452-6094
Fax: 503-243-1738
TTY: 800-556-5351
Robert Joondeph, Executive Director
Barbara Herget, Operations Director
The protection and advocacy system for Oregon.

3809 **Oregon Client Assistance Program**
620 SW 5th Ave
5th Floor
Portland, OR 97204-1420
503-243-2081
Fax: 503-243-1738
TTY: 800-556-5351
Robert Joondeph, Executive Director

3810 **Oregon Department of Mental Health**
500 Summer St NE
Salem, OR 97301-1063
503-945-5944
Fax: 503-378-2897
TTY: 503-945-6214
www.oregon.gov/DHS
Erinn Kelley-Siel, Director
Gene Evans, Communication Director
Eric Moore, Chief Financial Officer
Jim Scherzinger, Chief Operating Officer
Sets out the purpose and guides the activities of our large, complex organization. Vision is for better outcomes for clients and communities through collaboration, integration and shared responsibility.

3811 **Oregon Technology Access for Life**
2225 Lancaster Drive NE
Salem, OR 97305-1396
503-361-1201
800-677-7512
Fax: 503-370-4530
TTY: 503-361-1201
www.accesstechnologiesinc.org
Laurie Brooks, President
A statewide program promoting assistive technology devices and services for persons of all ages with all disabilities.

3812 **Social Security: Salem Disability Determination**
90 E Washington Bridge Rd
Suite 140
Worthington, OH 43085-3772
614-888-5339
800-722-1213
TTY: 614-288-0226
www.socialsecurity.gov
Karena L. Kilgore, Executive Secretary
Carolyn W. Colvin, Commissioner
Carolyn W. Colvin, Deputy Commissioner
James A. Kissko, Chief of Staff

3813 **Vocational Rehabilitation Agency: Oregon Commission for the Blind**
535 SE 12th Ave.
Portland, OR 97214-2408
971-673-1588
888-202-5463
Fax: 503-234-7468
ocb.mail@state.or.us
www.oregon.gov/blind
Dacia Johnson, Executive Director
A resource for visually impaired Oregonians, as well as their families, friends, and employers. Nationally recognized programs and staff that make a difference in people's lives every day.

3814 **Washington County Disability, Aging and Veteran Services**
Ste 208
180 E Main St
Hillsboro, OR 97123-4054
503-640-3489
Fax: 503-693-6124
Jeff Hill, Director
Janet Long, Support Staff
Provides services to individuals through the Older Americans Act, state in home care services and represent, veterans in benefit claims process with Federal VA.

Pennsylvania

3815 **Disability Rights of Pennsylvania (DRP)**
Harrisburg Office
301 Chestnut St
Suite 300
Harrisburg, PA 17101
717-839-5235
800-692-7443
Fax: 717-236-0192
TTY: 877-375-7139
ldo@disabilityrightspa.org
www.disabilityrightspa.org
Jeneice Davis, Chairman
Peri Jude Radecic, CEO
Kelly Darr, Legal Director
Judy Banks, Programs Director

The Disability Rights of Pennsylvania is a statewide, non-profit corporation dedicated to advancing and protecting the civil rights of adults and children with disabilities by ensuring access to community services, a full and inclusive education and the freedom to live free of discrimination, abuse and neglect.

3816 **International Dyslexia Association: Pennsylvania Branch**
1062 E. Lancaster Ave.
Suite 15A
Rosemont, PA 19010
610-527-1548
855-220-8885
www.pbida.org

Lisa Goldstein, President
Tracy Bowes, Office Manager

Provides free information and referral services for diagnosis and tutoring for parents, educators, physicians, and individuals with dyslexia. Membership includes yearly journal and quarterly newsletter, and Pennsylvania newsletter.

3817 **Mental Health Association in Pennysylvania**
1414 N Cameron St
1st Floor
Harrisburg, PA 17103-1049
717-346-0549
855-220-8885
Fax: 717-236-0192
www.mhapa.org

Julia Walker, Esq., President
Michael Brody, President & CEO
Marge Dailey, Director of Human Resources
Anthony Schweitzer, Treasurer

The Mental Health Association in Pennysylvania is a non-profit providing services to those struggling with mental health issues. Services include advocacy, education and public policy.

3818 **Pennsylvania Workers Compensation Board**
651 Boas Street
Room 1700
Harrisburg, PA 17121-2510
717-787-5279
Fax: 717-772-0342
dli.state.pa.us

Joseph Brimmeier, CEO

3819 **Pennsylvania Bureau of Blindness & Visual Services**
Department of Pennsylvania
1521 N 6th St
Harrisburg, PA 17102
717-787-3201
800-622-2842
Fax: 717-787-3210
www.dli.state.pa.us

David Denotaris, Director
Jennifer Cave, Clerk Typist 3

Offers services for the totally blind, legally blind, visually impaired, and more with health, counseling, educational, recreational, rehabilitation, computer training and professional training services.

3820 **Pennsylvania Client Assistance Program**
1515 Market Street
Suite 1300
Philadelphia, PA 19102- 1819
215-557-7112
888-745-2357
Fax: 215-557-7602
www.equalemployment.org

Stephen S. Pennington, Executive Director
Jamie C Ray, Assistant Director
Margaret Passio-McKenna, Senior Advocate
Lee Lippi, Advocate

The Pennsylvania Client Assistance Program is dedicated to ensuring that the rehabilitation system in Pennsylvania is open and responsive to your needs. CAP help is provided to you at no charge, regardless of income. CAP helps people who are seeking services from the Office of Vocational Rehabilitation, Blindness and Visual Services, Centers for Independent Living and other programs funded under federal law.

3821 **Pennsylvania Department of Aging**
555 Walnut St
5th Floor
Harrisburg, PA 17101-1919
717-783-1550
Fax: 717-783-6842
aging@pa.gov
www.aging.state.pa.us

Nora Eisenhower, Manager

3822 **Pennsylvania Department of Children with Disabilities**
P.O. Box 2675
Harrisburg, PA 17105-2675
717-787-2600
Fax: 717-772-0323
www.pachildren.state.pa.US

Tom Corbett, Governor
Shelly Yanoff, Commission Chair

3823 **Pennsylvania Developmental Disabilities Council**
605 South Drive
Room 561
Harrisburg, PA 17120
717-789-6057
877-685-4452
TTY: 717-705-0819
www.paddc.org

Amy High, Vice Chairperson
Graham Mulholland, Executive Director
Sandra Amador Dusek, Deputy Director

3824 **Public Interest Law Center of Philadelphia**
United Way Building, 2nd Floor
1709 Benjamin Franklin Parkway
Philadelphia, PA 19103-5153
215-627-7100
Fax: 215-627-3183
pilcop.org

Eric J. Rothschild, Chair
Brian T. Feeney, Vice Chair
Jennifer R. Clarke, Executive Director
Latrice Brooks, Director of Administration

A non-profit, public interest law firm with a Disabilities Project specializing in class action suits brought by individuals and organizations.

3825 **Social Security: Harrisburg Disability Determination**
Suite 160
90 E Washington Bridge Rd
Worthington, OH 17101-1925
614-888-5339
800-722-1213
TTY: 614-288-0226
ssa.gov

Karena L. Kilgore, Executive Secretary
Carolyn W. Colvin, Commissioner
Carolyn W. Colvin, Deputy Commissioner
James A. Kissko, Chief of Staff

3826 **Workers Compensation Board Pennsylvania**
651 Boas Street
Room 1700
Harrisburg, PA 17121-2510
717-787-5279
Fax: 717-772-0342
www.dli.state.pa.us

Tom Corbett, Governor
Julia K. Hearthway, Secretary
Joseph Brimmeier, CEO

Rhode Island

3827 **Department of Behavioral Healthcare, Developmental Disabilities and Hospitals**
The Hazard Building
41 West Rd.
Cranston, RI 02920
401-462-3201
www.bhddh.ri.gov

Rebecca Boss, Director
Michelle Place, Assistant to the Director

State department responsible for creating and administering systems of care for individuals with disabilities, specifically focused on mental health and mental illness, developmental disabilities, substance abuse and long term hospital care.

3828 **Rhode Island Department Health**
3 Capitol Hl
Providence, RI 02908-5097 401-222-3855
Fax: 401-222-6548
Mary Salerno, Manager
Patricia Nolan, Executive Director
Pamela Corcoran, Disability Health Program

3829 **Rhode Island Department of Elderly Affairs**
74 West Road
Hazard Bldg, 2nd Floor
Cranston, RI 02920- 3001 401-462-3000
Fax: 401-462-0740
Corrine Russo, Manager

3830 **Rhode Island Department of Mental Health**
Cottage 405 Court B
Cranston, RI 02920 401-462-2003
Fax: 401-462-2008
www.butler.org
George W. Shuster, Chairman
Dennis D. Keefe, President & CEO
Reed Cosper, Manager

3831 **Rhode Island Developmental Disabilities Council**
400 Bald Hill Rd
Suite 515
Warwick, RI 02886-1692 401-737-1238
Fax: 401-737-3395
TTY: 401-737-1238
riddc@riddc.org
www.riddc.org
Charles Zawacki, Chairperson, Individual & Family
John Susa, Chairperson, Executive Committee
Anne Frank, Chairperson, Individual & Family
Mary Okero, Executive Director
The Rhode Island Developmental Disabilities Council works to make Rhode Island a better place for people with developmental disabilities to live, work, go to school, and be part of their community.

3832 **Rhode Island Disability Law Center**
275 Westminster St
Suite 401
Providence, RI 02903-3434 401-831-3150
800-733-5332
Fax: 401-274-5568
TTY: 401-831-5335
info@ridlc.org
www.ridlc.org
Raymond A Marcaccio, Esq., Chair
Raymond L Bandusky, Executive Director
Darby Castigliego, Director of Finance & Administration
Minerva Doti, Intake Advocate
The Rhode Island Disability Law Center (RIDLC) provides free legal assistance to persons with disabilities. Services include individual representation to protect rights or to secure benefits and services, self-help information, educational programs and administrative and legislative advocacy.

3833 **Rhode Island Governor's Commission on Disabilities**
John O Pastore Center
Warwick City Hall
3275 Post Road
Warwick, RI 02920-3049 401-738-2000
Fax: 401-462-0106
www.warwickri.gov
Bob Cooper, Executive Secretary
The Commision is responsible for: coordinating compliance by state agencies with federal and state disablity right laws; approving or modifying state and local goverment agency's open meeting accessibility for persons with disabilities transition plans; assisting local boards of canvassers to ensure accessible polling places locations; aproving or rejecting requests to waive the state building code's standards for accessibility at facilities to be leased by state agencies...

3834 **Rhode Island Parent Information Network**
1210 Pontiac Avenue
Cranston, RI 02920 401-270-0101
800-464-3399
Fax: 401-270-7049
info@ripin.org
ripin.org
Kathleen DiChiara, Chairman
Ammala Douangsavanh, Vice Chairman
Stephen Brunero, Executive Director
Matthew Cox, Associate Exeutive Director
A nonprofit organization established by parents and concerned professionals providing culturally appropriate information, training and support for families and professionals designed to improve educational and life outcomes for all children. Serving the State of Rhode Island.

3835 **Rhode Island Services for the Blind and Visually Impaired**
40 Fountain St
Providence, RI 02903-1830 401-421-7005
800-752-8088
Fax: 401-421-9259
TTY: 401-421-7016
www.ors.ri.gov
Kathleen Grygiel, Administrator
Ronald Racine, Associate Director
Laurie DiOrio, Acting Associate Director
JoAnn Nannig, Assistant Administrator of VR
Offers services for the totally blind, legally blind, visually impaired, and more with health, counseling, educational, recreational, rehabilitation, computer training and professional training services.

3836 **Services for the Blind and Visually Impaired**
40 Fountain St
Providence, RI 02903-1830 401-421-7005
Fax: 401-222-1328
TTY: 401-421-7016
www.ors.ri.gov
Kathleen Grygiel, Administrator
Ronald Racine, Associate Director
Laurie DiOrio, Acting Associate Director
JoAnn Nannig, Assistant Administrator of VR
Offers services for the blind and visually impaired.

3837 **Social Security: Providence Disability Determination**
Social Security
40 Fountain Street
6th Floor
Providence, RI 02903-3246 401-222-3182
800-772-1213
Fax: 401-222-3868
TTY: 401-273-6648
Deborah.A.Cannon@ssa.gov
www.ssa.gov
Karena L. Kilgore, Executive Secretary
Carolyn W. Colvin, Commissioner
Carolyn W. Colvin, Deputy Commissioner
James A. Kissko, Chief of Staff
We deliver services through a nationwide network of over 1,400 offices that include regional offices, field offices, card centers, teleservice centers, processing centers, hearing offices, the Appeals Council, and our State and territorial partners, the Disability Determination Services. We also have a presence in U.S. embassies around the globe. For the public, we are the face of the government. The rich diversity of our employees mirrors the public we serve.

3838 **Workers Compensation Board Rhode Island**
1 Dorrance Plz
Providence, RI 02903-3973 401-458-5000
Fax: 401-222-3121
George E Healy Jr, Manager
George Healy Jr, Manager

South Carolina

3839 Protection & Advocacy for People with Disabilities
Ste 208
3710 Landmark Dr
Columbia, SC 29204-4034
803-782-0639
866-275-7273
Fax: 803-790-1946
TTY: 866-232-4525
info@pandasc.org
protectionandadvocacy-sc.org

Gloria Prevost, Executive Director
Anne Trice, Director of Administration
J. Ashley Twombley, Chair
Sherry Williams, Vice-Chair

An independent, nonprofit organization responsible for safe guarding rights of South Carolinians with disabilities and other handicapped individuals without regard to age, income, severity of disability, sex, race, or religion.

3840 Social Security: West Columbia Disability Determination
P.O. Box 60
Columbia, SC 29171-0060
803-896-6400
800-772-1213
Fax: 803-822-4318
TTY: 800-325-0078
www.socialsecurity.gov

Karena L. Kilgore, Executive Secretary
Carolyn W. Colvin, Commissioner
Carolyn W. Colvin, Deputy Commissioner
James A. Kissko, Chief of Staff

We deliver services through a nationwide network of over 1,400 offices that include regional offices, field offices, card centers, teleservice centers, processing centers, hearing offices, the Appeals Council, and our State and territorial partners, the Disability Determination Services. We also have a presence in U.S. embassies around the globe. For the public, we are the face of the government. The rich diversity of our employees mirrors the public we serve.

3841 South Carolina Assistive Technology Project
Midlands Center
8301 Farrow Road
Columbia, SC 29203
803-935-5263
800-915-4522
Fax: 803-935-5342
TTY: 803-935-5263
jjendron@usit.net
www.sc.edu/scatp/

Carol Page, Ph.D, CCC-SLP, A, Program Director
Janet Jendron, Program Coordinator
Mary Alice Bechtler, Program Coordinator
Lydia Durham, Administrative Assistant

A statewide program promoting assistive technology devices and services for persons of all ages with all disabilities. Recently a statewide AT resource, demonstrations and equipment loan center and lab annual expo and training and workshops on a variety of disabilities and technology topics.

3842 South Carolina Client Assistance Program
Governor's Office oe Executive Policy & Programs
1205 Pendleton St
Columbia, SC 29201-3756
803-734-0285
800-868-0040
Fax: 803-734-0546
TTY: 803-734-1147
cap@oepp.sc.gov

Denise Riley Pensmith, MSW, Executive Director
Cindy Popenhagen, Administrative Assistant

The Client Assistance Program (CAP) helps citizens of the State by acting as advocates regarding services provided by the Vocational Rehabilitation Department (VR), Commission for the Blind, and all Independent Living programs and projects funded under the Rehabilitation Act of 1973. As advocates, CAP staff can investigate, negotiate, mediate, and pursue administrative, and other remedies to ensure that clients' rights are protected.

3843 South Carolina Commission for the Blind (SCCB)
1430 Confederate Ave.
Columbia, SC 29201-79
803-898-8734
publicinfo@sccb.sc.gov
www.sccb.state.sc.us

3844 South Carolina Department of Children with Disabilities
2600 Bull St
Columbia, SC 29201-1708
803-434-4260

Miroslav Cuturic, Director
Peter Getz, Administrator

3845 South Carolina Department of Mental Health
Office of Administration
PO Box 485
Columbia, SC 29202
803-898-8581
800-273-8255
TTY: 800-647-2066
webmaster@scdmh.org
scdmh.net

Mark W. Binkley, Interim State Director

The S.C. Department of Mental Health gives priority to adults, children, and their families affected by serious mental illnesses and significant emotional disorders. We are committed to eliminating stigma and promoting the philosophy of recovery, to achieving our goals in collaboration with all stakeholders, and to assuring the highest quality of culturally competent services possible.

3846 South Carolina Developmental Disabilities Council
Office of the Governor
1205 Pendleton St
Suite 461
Columbia, SC 29201-3756
803-734-0465
Fax: 803-734-1409
TTY: 803-734-1147
jvancleave@oepp.sc.gov
www.scddc.state.sc.us

Valarie Bishop, Executive Director
Cheryl English, Program Information Coordinator
Kimberly Johnson Fontanez, Grants Administrator
Esther Williams, Administrative Support Specialis

The mission of the South Carolina Developmental Disabilities Council is to provide leadership in advocating, funding and implementing initiatives which recognize the inherent dignity of each individual, and promote independence, productivity, respect and inclusion for all persons with disabilities and their families.

3847 Workers Compensation Board: South Carolina
PO Box 1715
Columbia, SC 29202-1715
803-737-5700
Fax: 803-737-5768
www.state.sc.us/wcc

Gary Cannon, Executive Director
Kim Balleutine, Admin. Assistant

South Dakota

3848 Children's Special Health Services Program
600 E Capitol Ave
Pierre, SD 57501-2536
605-773-3361
800-738-2301
Fax: 605-773-5683
DOH.info@state.sd.us
www.doh.sd.gov

Dianne Weyer, Manager
Barb Hemmelman, Program Manager

Health KiCC is a program, funded through federal and state monies, that provides financial assistance for medical appointments, procedures, treatments, medications and travel reimbursement for children with certain chronic health conditions.

3849 Division of Labor and Management
South Dakota Department of Labor
700 Governors Dr
Pierre, SD 57501-2291
605-773-3101
Fax: 605-773-6184
dlr.sd.gov

Sara Minton, Executive Director
Pamela S Roberts, Secretary
Marcia Hultman, Deputy Secretary of Labor and D
Lyle Harter, Director of Administrative Servi
Our mission is to promote economic opportunity and financial security for individuals and businesses through quality, responsive and expert services; fair and equitable employment solutions; and safe and sound business practices.

3850 Health KiCC
South Dakota Department of Health
600 E Capitol Ave
Pierre, SD 57501-2536
605-773-3361
800-738-2301
Fax: 605-773-5683
DOH.info@state.sd.us
www.doh.sd.gov

Dianne Weyer, Manager
Health KiCC is a program, funded through federal and state monies, that provides financial assistance for medical appointments, procedures, treatments, medications and travel reimbursement for children with certain chronic health conditions.

3851 South Dakota Advocacy Services
221 S Central Ave
Ste. 38
Pierre, SD 57501-2479
605-224-8294
800-658-4782
Fax: 605-224-5125
sdas@sdadvocacy.com
sdadvocacy.com

Sandy Stocklin Hook, Partners Coordinator
Designated protection and advocacy progam for South Dakota providing legal, administrative, mediation and other services to elgible persons with disabilities in the state.

3852 South Dakota Department of Aging
700 Governors Dr
Pierre, SD 57501-2291
605-773-3656
866-854-5465
Fax: 605-773-4085

Marilyn Kinsman, Division Director
Lynne Valenti, Deputy Secretary
Amy Iversen-Pollreisz, Deputy Secretary
Kristin Kellar, Communications Director
The Division of Adult Services and Aging (ASA) provides home and community service options to individuals 60 years of age and older and 18 years of age and older with physical disabilities, regardless of income.

3853 South Dakota Department of Human Services
Hillsview Plaza
3800 E Hwy 34
Pierre, SD 57501
605-773-5990
Fax: 605-773-5483
infodhs@state.sd.us
dlr.sd.gov

Shawnie Rechtenbaugh, Secretary
Provides resources for individuals with developmental disabilities, including rehabilitation services, services for the blind and visually impaired, and long-term services and supports.

3854 South Dakota Department of Social Services Division of Behavioral Health
700 Governors Dr.
Pierre, SD 57501
605-367-5236
855-878-6057
Fax: 605-773-7076
DSSbh@state.sd.us
dss.sd.gov/behavioralhealth

Laurie Gill, Secretary
Brenda Tidbull-Zeltinger, Deputy Secretary
Tiffany Wolfgang, Division Director
South Dakota's state mental health authority.

3855 South Dakota Division of Rehabilitation
700 Governors Dr
Pierre, SD 57501-2291
605-773-3101
Fax: 605-773-6184
www.sdjobs.org

Sara Minton, Executive Director
Pamela S Roberts, Secretary
Marcia Hultman, Deputy Secretary of Labor and D
Lyle Harter, Director of Administrative Servi
Offers diagnosis, evaluation and physical restoration services, counseling, social work, educational and professional training, employment and rehabilitation services for the disabled.

3856 Workers Compensation Board: South Dakota
700 Governors Dr
Pierre, SD 57501-2291
605-773-3101
Fax: 605-773-6184
www.sdjobs.org

Sara Minton, Executive Director
Marcia Hultman, Secretary
Lyle Harter, Director of Administrative Servi
Bret Afdahi, Director of the Division of Bank
Our mission is to promote economic opportunity and financial security for individuals and businesses through quality, responsive and expert services; fair and equitable employment solutions; and safe and sound business practices.

Tennessee

3857 Disability Determination Services
400 Deaderick St
Nashville, TN 37243-1403
800-342-1117
DHS.CustomerService@tn.gov
www.tennessee.gov

Thea Smith, Human Resources Program Specialist
Wendy Davis, Finance & Administration
Cherrell Campbell-Street, Assistant Commissioner
The Disability Determination Services is a branch of the Division of Rehabilitation Services in the Department of Human Services. Its main responsibility is to process Social Security and Supplemental Security Income disability claims.

3858 International Dyslexia Association: Tennessee Branch
Knoxville, TN
865-207-4918
msamwood@bellsouth.net
www.tnida.org

Emily Dempster, President
Erin Alexander, Senior Vice President
Nikki Davis, Secretary
Sharon Dytrt, Treasurer
The Tennessee Branch of the International Dyslexia Association (TN-IDA) was formed to increase awareness about Dyslexia in the state of Tennessee. TN-IDA supports efforts to provide information regarding appropriate language arts instruction to those involved with language-based learning differences and to encourage the identity of these individuals at-risk for such disorders as soon as possible.

3859 Tennessee Assistive Technology Projects
Citizens Plaza State Office Buildin
511 Union St.
Nashville, TN 37219-1403
615-313-5183
800-732-5059
TTY: 615-313-5695
TN.TTAP@tn.gov
www.tn.gov

Bill Haslam, Governor
Raquel Hatter, Commissioner
Beth White, Manager
Julie Oden, Manager
A statewide program promoting assistive technology devices and services for persons of all ages with all disabilities.

3860 **Tennessee Client Assistance Program**
Tennessee Protection and Advocacy
P.O. Box 121257
Nashville, TN 37212-1257
615-298-1080
800-342-1660
Fax: 615-298-2046

Shirley Shea, Executive Director
Doris Lopez, Assistant Executive Director

3861 **Tennessee Commission on Aging and Disability**
502 Deaderick Street
9th Floor
Nashville, TN 37243-860
615-741-2056
Fax: 615-741-3309
www.tn.gov/aging.html

Richard M. Honn, Executive Director
Ryan Ellis, Aging Info. & Data Director
Kathy Zamata, Aging Program Director
Richard Presler, Fiscal Director

3862 **Tennessee Council on Developmental Disabilities**
500 James Robertson Pkwy
1st Floor
Nashville, TN 37243
615-532-6615
Fax: 615-532-6964
tnddc@tn.gov
tn.gov/cdd

Wanda Willis, Executive Director
Lynette Porter, Deputy Director
Alicia Cone, Director of Grant Program
Lauren Pearcy, Director of Public Policy

The council is a state agency that leads initiatives to improve disability policies by educating policymakers and the public about best practices in disability services, facilitating collaboration across organizations, and producing educational publications on the subject.

3863 **Tennessee Department of Children with Disabilities**
511 Union St.
Nashville, TN 37219-9004
615-741-9701
800-861-1935
Fax: 615-253-5216
www.tn.gov

Ruth S Letson, Manager
Haticile Buchanan, Manager
Mary Beth Franklyn, CS Program Director
Kristi Faulkner, Special Counsel to the Commissio

Tennessee's children thrive in safe, healthy and stable families. Families thrive in healthy, safe and strong communities. Tennessee's citizens benefit from the best child welfare and juvenile justice agency in the country.

3864 **Tennessee Department of Mental Health**
500 Deaderick Street
Nashville, TN 37243-3400
615-532-6597
800-560-5767
Fax: 615-532-6514

Doug Varney, Commissioner
Grant Lawrence, Director Office of Communication
Bob Grunow, Deputy Commissioner
Howard Burley, Asst Commissioner Clinical Ldrsp

TDMH is the state's mental health and substance abuse authority. Its mission is to plan for and promote the availability of a comprehensive array of quality prevention, early intervention, treatment, habilitation, and rehabilitation services and supports based on the needs and choices of individuals and families served. Responsible for policy, and oversight, and for advocacy of the consumer within the state.

3865 **Tennessee Division of Rehabilitation**
400 Deaderick St
Nashville, TN 37243-1403
615-313-4700
800-270-1349
TTY: 615-313-5695
http://www.tn.gov

Patsy Matthews, Commissioner
Randall Beasley, Manager
Raquel Hatter, Commissioner
Bill Haslam, Givernor

Offers rehabilitation, medical and therapeutic information and referrals to the disabled.

3866 **Workers Compensation Division Tennessee**
Dept of Labor & Workforce Development
220 French Landing Drive
1st Floor
Nashville, TN 37243- 1002
615-741-6642
800-332-2667
Fax: 615-532-1468
wc.info@tn.gov
www.tn.gov/labor-wfd/wcomp.html

Karla Davis, Commissioner
Alisa Malone, Deputy Commissioner
Stephanie Mitchell, General Counsel
Ron Jones, Administrator of Fiscal Services

We administer the workers' compensation system and promote a better understanding of the program's benefits by informing employees and employers of their rights and responsibilities. Workers' Compenstation administers a mediation program for disputed claims, encourage workplace safety, participate in a public awareness campaign concerning fraud, and oversee an information awareness program for educating the public on laws and regulations which define workers' compensation requirements. We ensure

Texas

3867 **Disability Policy Consortium**
2222 West Braker Lane
Austin, TX 78758-1024
512-454-4816
800-252-9108
Fax: 512-323-0902
disabilitytx.org

Mary Faithful, Executive Director
Roberta Rosenberg-Roque, Manager

An independent group of statewide advocacy organizations that strives to achieve the development and full implementation of public policy that promotes and supports the rights, inclusion, integration and independence of Texans with disabilities.

3868 **Disability Rights Texas**
2222 West Braker Lane
Austin, TX 78758-1024
512-454-4816
866-362-2851
www.disabilityrightstx.org

Mary Faithfull, Executive Director
Patty Anderson, Deputy Director

A federally designated legal protection and advocacy agency (P&A) for people with disabilities in Texas. Helps people with disabilities understand and exercise their rights under the law, ensuring their full and equal participation in society.

3869 **Division of Special Education**
1701 Congress Ave.
Austin, TX 78701-1402
512-463-9414
Fax: 512-463-9838
teainfo@tea.state.tx.us
www.tea.state.tx.us

Cory Green, Federal & State Education Policy
Donna Bahorich, Chair
Ruban Cortez Jr., Secretary

The Texas Education Agency is the state agency that oversees primary and secondary public education. It is headed by the commissioner of education. The mission of TEA is to provide leadership, guidance and resources to help schools meet the educational needs of all students

3870 **Easterseals Central Texas**
2324 Ridepoint Dr.
Suite F1
Austin, TX 78754
512-615-6800
Fax: 512-615-7121
www.easterseals.com/centraltx

Tod Marvin, President

Easterseals provides a wealth of programs and services to help promote independence and create opportunities for people with disabilities.

3871 **Easterseals North Texas**
1424 Hemphill St.
Fort Worth, TX 76104
888-617-7171
www.easterseals.com/northtexas
Tod Marvin, President
Jennifer Friesen, Vice President, Programs & Services
Easterseals provides a wealth of programs and services to help promote independence and create opportunities for people with disabilities.

3872 **El Valle Community Parent Resource Center**
Ste J
530 S Texas Blvd
Weslaco, TX 78596-6262
956-969-0215
800-680-0255
Fax: 956-968-7102
Robert Garza, Owner

3873 **Grassroots Consortium**
Greenroots Consortium
6202 Belmark St
Houston, TX 77087-6324
713-643-9576
Fax: 713-643-6291
Speckids@aol.com
Agnes A Johnson, Director

3874 **International Dyslexia Association: Austin Branch**
Austin, TX
512-452-7658
aus.dyslexiaida.org
Mary Bach, President
Karen Monteith, Vice President
Herman H. Klare, Treasurer
Kristie Beavers, Executive Director
Provides free information and referral services for diagnosis and tutoring for parents, educators, physicians, and individuals with dyslexia in Illinois. Membership includes yearly journal and quarterly newsletter.

3875 **National Alliance on Mental Illness (Texas)**
P.O. Box 300817
Austin, TX 78703
512-693-2000
Fax: 512-693-8000
officemanager@namitexas.org
namitexas.org
John Dornheim, President
Holly Doggett, Executive Director
Greg Hansch, Public Policy Director
NAMI Texas is the state headquarters of the National Alliance on Mental Illness, a national nonprofit that aims to improve the lives of all persons affected by mental illness. NAMI Texas oversees over 25 local affiliates throughout the state. NAMI Texas raises awareness about mental illness through the dissemination of information, and seeks to address the mental health needs of Texans through education and support programs for persons with mental illness, families, friends, and professionals.

3876 **Parent Connection**
1020 Riverwood Ct
Conroe, TX 77304-2811
936-756-8321
800-839-8876
parentCNCT@aol.com
http://www.parentingaspergerscommunity.com/pu
Dave Angel, Founder
Includes parenting help and Aspergers advice, including parenting tips, tricks and techniques to help your child with Aspergers. Our worldwide membership base is helping parents to understand their child with Aspergers better and make their home & family life a better place to be.

3877 **Parents Supporting Parents Network**
8001 Centre Park Drive
Suite 100
Austin, TX 78754
512-454-6694
800-252-9729
Fax: 512-454-4956
secretary@thearcoftexas.org
www.thearcoftexas.org
Charlie Huber, President
John Schneider, Vice-President
Nancy Lepley, Treasurer
Terri Schonfeld, Secretary
Since our founding in 1950 by a group of parents of children with intellectual and developmental disabilities, The Arc at the local, state and national level has been instrumental in the creation of virtually every program, service, right, and benefit that is now available to more than half a million Texans with intellectual and developmental disabilities. Today, The Arc continues to advocate for including people with intellectual and developmental disabilities in all aspects of society.

3878 **Partners Resource Network**
Ste B
1090 Longfellow Dr
Beaumont, TX 77706-4819
409-898-4684
800-866-4726
Fax: 409-898-4869
partnersresource@sbcglobal.net
partnerstx.org
Janice Meyer, Executive Director
Statewide network of three parent training and information centers.

3879 **Social Security: Austin Disability Determination**
P.O. Box 149198
Austin, TX 78714-9198
512-437-8311
800-772-1213
800-252-9627
Fax: 512-437-8595
TTY: 512-916-5958
dan.tippit@ssa.gov
www.ssa.gov
Karena L. Kilgore, Executive Secretary
Carolyn W. Colvin, Commissioner
Carolyn W. Colvin, Deputy Commissioner
James A. Kissko, Chief of Staff
We deliver services through a nationwide network of over 1,400 offices that include regional offices, field offices, card centers, teleservice centers, processing centers, hearing offices, the Appeals Council, and our State and territorial partners, the Disability Determination Services. We also have a presence in U.S. embassies around the globe. The rich diversity of our employees mirrors the public we serve.

3880 **Statewide Information at Texas School for the Deaf**
1102 S Congress Ave
Austin, TX 78704-1728
512-462-5353
Fax: 512-462-5353
webmaster@tsd.state.tx.us
www.tsd.state.tx.us
Sonia Karimi Bridges, Video Communication Specialist
Avonne Brooker-Rutowski, Program Specialist
David Coco, Program Specialist
Lisa Crawford, Parent Liason
Welcome to Texas School for the Deaf, a place where students who are deaf or hard of hearing including those with additional disabilities, have the opportunity to learn, grow and belong in a culture that optimizes individual potential and provides accessible language and communication across the curriculum. Our educational philosophy is grounded in the belief that all children who are deaf and hard of hearing deserve a quality language and communication-driven program that provides education tog

3881 **Texas Advocates Supporting Kids with Disabilities**
P.O. Box 162685
Austin, TX 78716-2685
512-310-2102
Fax: 512-310-2102
ASKTASK@aol.com

3882 **Texas Commission for the Blind**
P.O. Box 149198
Austin, TX 78714-9198
512-459-8575
800-252-5204
Fax: 512-424-4730
www.dars.state.tx.us
Canzata Crowder, Manager
Offers services for the totally blind, legally blind, and visually impaired, with counseling, educational, recreational, rehabilitation, computer training and professional training services.

3883 Texas Commission for the Deaf and Hard of Hearing
D AR S
P.O. Box 149198
Austin, TX 78714-9198
512-407-3250
800-628-5115
Fax: 512-424-4730
TTY: 512-407-3251
www.dars.state.tx.us

Veronda L. Durden, Commissioner
Glenn Neal, Deputy Commissioner
David Myers, Executive Director
Daniel Bravo, Chief Operating Officer

3884 Texas Council for Developmental Disabilities
6201 E Oltorf St
Suite 600
Austin, TX 78741-7509
512-437-5432
800-262-0334
Fax: 512-437-5434
TTY: 512-437-5431
tcdd@tcdd.texas.gov
txddc.state.tx.us

Mary Durheim, Chairman
Andrew D. Crim, Vice Chairman
Roger Webb, Executive Director
Koren Vogel, Executive Assistant

The Texas Council for Developmental Disabilities is a 27-member board dedicated to ensuring that all Texans with developmental disabilities, about 411,479 individuals, have the opportunity to be independent, productive and valued members of their communities. The mission of the Texas Council for Developmental Disabilities is to create change so that all people with disabilities are fully included in their communities and exercise control over their own lives.

3885 Texas Department of Human Services
701 W 51st St
P.O. Box 149030
Austin, TX 78751-2312
512-438-3011
888-834-7406
Fax: 512-472-0603
TTY: 888-425-6889
mail@dads.state.tx.us
www.dads.state.tx.us

Jon Weizenbaum, Commissioner
Kristi Jordan, Associate Commissioner
Chris Adams, Deputy Commissioner
Elisa J. Garza, Assistant Commissioner for Acces

3886 Texas Department on Aging
701 W 51st St
P.O. Box 149030
Austin, TX 78751-2312
512-438-3011
800-252-9240
www.dads.state.tx.us

Jon Weizenbaum, Commissioner
Kristi Jordan, Associate Commissioner
Chris Adams, Deputy Commissioner
Elisa J. Garza, Assistant Commissioner for Acces

3887 Texas Federation of Families for Children's Mental Health
Ste 505
7701 N Lamar Blvd
Austin, TX 78752-1000
512-407-8844
866-893-3264
Fax: 512-407-8266
www.txffcmh.org

Patti Derr, Executive Director
Pat Calley, Chairperson
S Barron, Operations Director

3888 Texas Governor's Committee on People with Disabilities
1100 San Jacinto Blvd
P.O. Box 12428
Austin, TX 78701- 1935
512-463-2000
Fax: 513-463-5745
www.governor.state.tx.us/disabilities

Angela English, LPC, LMFT, Executive Director
Erin Lawler, JD, MS, Accessibility and Disability Rig
Nancy Van Loan, Executive Assistant
Jo Virgil, MS, Community Outreach and Informati

The Governor's Committee on People with Disabilities is within the office of the Governor. The committee's mission is to further opportunities for persons with disabilities to enjoy full and equal access to lives of independence, productivity, and self-determination. The committee is composed of 12 members appointed by the governor and of nonvoting ex officio members.

3889 Texas Health and Human Services (HHS)
Brown-Heatly Building
4900 N Lamar Blvd.
Austin, TX 78751-3247
512-424-6500
TTY: 512-424-6597
hhs.texas.gov

Courtney N. Phillips, Executive Commissioner
Cecile Young, Chief Deputy Executive Commissioner
John Hellerstedt, Commissioner, Department of State Health Services
Sonja Gaines, Dep. Exec. Commissioner, Intellectual & Developmental

Responsible for health services in the state of texas, including mental health and substance abuse treatment.

3890 Texas Respite Resource Network
P.O. Box 149030
710 West 51st Street
Austin, TX 78714- 9030
512-438-5555
Fax: 512-438-4374
archrespite.org

Jill Kagan, Program Director
Liz Newhouse, Assistant Director
Mike Mathers, Executive Director
Maggie Edgar, Senior Consultant

A state clearinghouse and technical assistance network for respite in Texas. TRRN identifies, initiates and improves respite options for families caring for individuals with disabilities on the local, state and national levels. TRRN provides training/technical assistance to programs/groups wanting to establish respite services.

3891 Texas Technology Access Project
Center for Disabilities Studies
10100 Burnet Rd
Austin, TX 78758-4445
512-232-0740
800-828-7839
Fax: 512-232-0761
TTY: 512-232-0762
rogerlevy@austin.utexas.edu
techaccess.edb.utexas.edu

Roger Levy, Program Director
Darlene West, Assistive Technology Coordinator
Steve Thomas, Operations and External Relation
Darlene West, Assistive Technology Specialist

Their mission is to increase access for people with disabilities to assistive technology that provides them more control over their immediate environments and an enhanced ability to function independently.

3892 Texas UAP for Developmental Disabilities
University of Texas
1 University Station
Austin, TX 78712
512-471-3434
800-828-7839
www.utexas.edu

Gregory L. Fences, President
Judith H. Langlois, Executive Vice President and Pr
Gregory J. Vincent, Vice President
Patricia C. Ohlendorf, Vice President

Welcome to The University of Texas at Austin. Founded in 1883, UT is one of the largest and most respected universities in the nation. Ours is a diverse learning community, with students from every state and more than 100 countries. We're a university with world talent and Texas traditions. Discover more about us online and come visit our beautiful campus in person.

3893 **Texas Workers Compensation Commission**
333 Guadalupe
P.O. Box 149104
Austin, TX 78701-1645
512-676-6000
800-578-4677
800-252-3439
Fax: 512-804-4401
TTY: 512-322-4238
WebStaff@tdi.state.tx.us
www.tdi.texas.gov

Robert Shipe, Executive Director
Rod Bordelon, Commissioner
Workers' compensation is a state-regulated insurance program that pays medical bills and replaces some lost wages for employees who are injured at work or who have work-related diseases or illnesses.

3894 **United Cerebral Palsy of Texas**
National Cerebral Palsy of American
Ste 145
1016 La Posada Dr
Austin, TX 78752-3828
512-472-8696
800-798-1492
Fax: 512-472-8026

Jean Langendorf, Executive Director
Offers a unique array of programs and services designed for one specific purpose: to ensure that people with cerebral palsy and similar disabilities have the opportunity to participate fully and equally in every aspect of our society.

Utah

3895 **Access Utah Network**
Ste 100
155 S 300 W
Salt Lake City, UT 84101-1288
801-533-4636
800-333-8824
Fax: 801-533-3968

Mark L. Smith, Information Specialist
Access Utah Network is Utah's prime source for information and referral for individuals with disabilities and their caregivers since 1990. Our operators can provide you with the information you need to find accessible housing, assistive technology and financial and social supports needed to live independently with a disability. Call us or explore our web site today to see how Access Utah Network can help you become more independent.

3896 **Social Security: Salt Lake City Disability Determination**
Social Security
P.O. Box 144032
Salt Lake City, UT 84111-4032
801-321-6500
800-772-1213
800-221-3493
Fax: 801-321-6599
TTY: 801-524-5047
Dave.Carlson@ssa.gov
www.ssa.gov

Karena L. Kilgore, Executive Secretary
Carolyn W. Colvin, Commissioner
Carolyn W. Colvin, Deputy Commissioner
James A. Kissko, Chief of Staff
We deliver services through a nationwide network of over 1,400 offices that include regional offices, field offices, card centers, teleservice centers, processing centers, hearing offices, the Appeals Council, and our State and territorial partners, the Disability Determination Services. We also have a presence in U.S. embassies around the globe. The rich diversity of our employees mirrors the public we serve.

3897 **Utah Assistive Technology Projects**
Utah State University
6855 Old Main Hl
Logan, UT 84322-6855
435-797-3824
800-524-5152
TTY: 435-797-2355
www.uatpat.org

Sachin Pavithran, Program Director
Alma Burgess, UATP Data Collection Coordinator
Clay Christensen, Lab Coordinator
Marilyn ' Hammond, Executive Director
A statewide program promoting assistive technology devices and services for persons of all ages with all disabilities.

3898 **Utah Client Assistance Program**
205 N 400 W
Salt Lake City, UT 84103-1125
801-363-1347
800-662-9080
Fax: 801-363-1437
www.disabilitylawcenter.org

Bryce Fifield Ph.D, President
Jared Fields, Vice President
Barbara M. Campbell, Treasurer
Kevin Murphy, Board Member
Since 1979, the Disability Law Center (DLC) has helped thousands of Utahns with disabilities and their families. The DLC has broad statutory powers to safeguard the human and civil rights of persons with disabilities. We provide self-advocacy assistance, legal services, disability rights education, and public policy advocacy on behalf of the more than 400,000 Utah residents with disabilities. Our services are available statewide and without regard for ability to pay.

3899 **Utah Department of Aging and Adult Services**
195 North 1950 West
Salt Lake City, UT 84116
801-538-3910
877-424-4640
Fax: 801-538-4395
debooth@utah.gov

Nels Holmgren, Director
Michael S. Styles, Assistant Director
Michelle Benson, Director
Sarah Brenna, Director
The department administers a wide variety of home and community-based services for Utah residents who are 60 or older. Programs and services are primarily delivered by a network of 12 Area Agencies on Aging which reach all geographic areas of the state. Their goal is to provide services that allow people to remain independent.

3900 **Utah Department of Human Services: Division of Services for People with Disabilities**
195 North 1950 West
Salt Lake City, UT 84116
801-538-4200
844-275-3773
Fax: 801-538-4279
dhsinfo@utah.gov
dspd.utah.gov

3901 **Utah Division Of Substance Abuse & Mental Health**
Utah Department of Human Services
195 No. 1950 West
Salt Lake City, UT 84116-1550
801-538-4171
Fax: 801-538-4016
WWW.DHS.UTAH.GOV

Lana Stohl, Executive Director

3902 **Utah Division of Services for the Disabled**
195 North 1950 West
Salt Lake City, UT 84116
801-538-3910
877-424-4640
Fax: 801-538-4395

Paul T. Smith, Division Director
Clay Hiatt, Fiscal Management
Offers services for the totally blind, legally blind, visually impaired, and more with health, counseling, educational, recreational, rehabilitation, computer training and professional training services.

3903 **Utah Governor's Council for People with Disabilities**
155 S 300 W
Suite 100
Salt Lake City, UT 84101-1288
801-533-4636
Fax: 801-533-3968
www.gcpd.org/

Mark Smith, Manager
Angela Allen, Administrative Secretary

3904 **Utah Labor Commission**
160 E 300 S
3rd Floor
Salt Lake City, UT 84114-6600
801-530-6800
800-222-1238
Fax: 801-530-6390
laborcom@utah.gov
laborcommission.utah.gov

Jaceson R Maughan, Commissioner
Alison Adams-Perlac, Director
Britton Beims, Employment Discrimination Investigation
Michael Barrett, MSHR, Outreach & Education Coordinator

The Utah Labor Commission is a regulatory agency that works to ensure safety in the workplace. The commission also offers services related to workplace injuries, wage issues, descrimination and industrial accidents.

3905 **Utah Protection & Advocacy Services for Persons with Disabilities**
Disability Law Center
205 N 400 W
Salt Lake City, UT 84103-1125
801-363-1347
800-662-9080
Fax: 801-363-1437
www.disabilitylawcenter.org

Bryce Fifield Ph.D, President
Jared Fields, Vice President
Barbara M. Campbell, Treasurer
Kevin Murphy, Board Member

Since 1979, the Disability Law Center (DLC) has helped thousands of Utahns with disabilities and their families. The DLC has broad statutory powers to safeguard the human and civil rights of persons with disabilities. We provide self-advocacy assistance, legal services, disability rights education, and public policy advocacy on behalf of the more than 400,000 Utah residents with disabilities. Our services are available statewide and without regard for ability to pay.

Vermont

3906 **Disability Law Project**
57 N Main St
Rutland, VT 05701-3246
800-889-2047
Fax: 802-775-0022
nbreiden@vtlegalaid.org
vtlegalaid.org

Nanci Smith, President
Jessica Porter, Vice President/Secretary
John Holme, Treasurer
Eric Avildsen, Executive Director

Legal services (protection and advocacy) for people with disabilities on legal issues arising from disability. Statewide. Adults and children. Employment, education, discrimination, housing, public benefits, health care.

3907 **Disability Rights Vermont**
141 Main Street
Suite 7
Montpelier, VT 05602-2916
802-229-1355
800-834-7890
Fax: 802-229-1359
TTY: 800-889-2047
info@disabilityrightsvt.org
www.disabilityrightsvt.org

Sarah Wendell-Launderville, President
David Gallagher, Vice president
Crocker Paquin, Treasurer
Michael Sabourin, Secretary

Advocacy and legal services for people with mental illness on legal issues arising, out of disabilities. Children and adults.

3908 **Social Security: Vermont Disability Determination Services**
Ste 6
93 Pilgrim Park Rd
Waterbury, VT 05676-1729
802-241-2463
800-734-2463
800-772-1213
Fax: 802-241-2492
www.ssa.gov

Karena L. Kilgore, Executive Secretary
Carolyn W. Colvin, Commissioner
Carolyn W. Colvin, Deputy Commissioner
James A. Kissko, Chief of Staff

We deliver services through a nationwide network of over 1,400 offices that include regional offices, field offices, card centers, teleservice centers, processing centers, hearing offices, the Appeals Council, and our State and territorial partners, the Disability Determination Services. We also have a presence in U.S. embassies around the globe. The rich diversity of our employees mirrors the public we serve.

3909 **Vermont Assistive Technology Projects**
103 S Main St
Weeks Building
Waterbury, VT 05671-2305
800-750-6355
800-750-6355
Fax: 802-871-3048
TTY: 802-241-1464
atp.vermont.gov

Amber Fulcher, Program Director
Sharon Alderman, Assistive Technology Reuse Coord
Emma Cobb, Assistive Technology Services Co
Dan Gilman, ATP, Assistive Technology Access Spec

Increase awareness and change policies to insure assistive technology (AT) is available to all Vermonters with disabilities. Our Commitment is to enable Vermonters with disabilities to have greater independence, productivity, and confidence. To provide them with a clear and direct avenue toward integration and inclusion within the work force and community.

3910 **Vermont Client Assistance Program**
57 N Main St
Rutland, VT 05701-3246
802-775-0021
800-769-7459
www.vocrehabvermont.org/html/clientassistance

Patrick Flood, Commissioner

The Client Assistance Program (CAP) is an independent advocacy program to help if you are applying for or receiving services from one of the following sources: Division of Vocational Rehabilitation (VR); Vermont Center for Independent Living (VCIL); Division for the Blind and Visually Impaired (DBVI); Vermont Association of Business, Industry & Rehabilitation (VABIR); Vermont Association for the Blind and Visually Impaired (VABVI); Supported Employment Programs; Transition Programs.

3911 **Vermont Department of Aging**
103 S Main St
Weeks Building
Waterbury, VT 05671-1601
802-241-2401
Fax: 802-871-3281
TTY: 802-241-3557
dail.vermont.gov

Susan Wehry, Commissioner
Marybeth McCaffrey, Director
Linda Henzel, Executive Staff Assistant
Adele Edelman, Assistant Division Director

3912 **Vermont Department of Developmental and**
103 S Main St
Weeks Building
Waterbury, VT 05671-1601
802-241-2401
Fax: 802-871-3281
TTY: 802-241-3557
dail.vermont.gov

Jonathan Wood, Manager

3913 **Vermont Department of Disabilities, Aging and Independent Living**
Aging and Disabilities
103 S Main St
Waterbury, VT 05671-1601 802-241-2401
Fax: 802-241-2325
dail.vermont.gov
Susan Wehry, Commissioner
Camille George, Deputy Commissioner

3914 **Vermont Department of Health: Children with Special Health Needs**
Vermont Department Of Health
108 Cherry Street
Burlington, VT 05402-70 802-863-7200
800-464-4343
Fax: 802-865-7754
healthvermont.gov
Harry Chen, M.D., Commissioner
Barbara Cimaglio, Deputy Commissioner for Alcohol
Tracy Dolan, Deputy Commissioner for Public H
Dixie Henry, Esq., Senior Policy and Legal Advisor
Multidisciplinary clinics and family support for children with chronic conditions, birth to age 21 years.

3915 **Vermont Developmental Disabilities Council**
103 S Main St
Waterbury, VT 05671-9800 082-241-2220
Cynthia D LaWare, Secretary
The mission of VTDDC is to facilitate connections and to promote supports that bring people with developmental disabilities into the heart of Vermont Communities.

3916 **Vermont Division for the Blind & Visually Impaired**
Agency of Human Svcs Dept Disabilities, Aging & IL
103 S Main St
Weeks Building
Waterbury, VT 5671-2304 802-871-3038
800-405-5005
888-405-5005
Fax: 802-871-3048
www.dbvi.vermont.gov
Fred Jones, Director
Scott Langley, Counselor
Heather Allen, Administrative Assistant
Paul Putnam, Rehabilitation Associate
Offers services for the totally blind, legally blind, visually impaired, and more with health, counseling, educational, recreational, rehabilitation, computer training and professional training services.

3917 **Vermont Division of Disability & Aging Services**
103 S Main St
Weeks Building
Waterbury, VT 05671-1601 802-241-2401
Fax: 802-871-3281
TTY: 802-241-3557
www.dail.vermont.gov
Susan Wehry, Commissioner
Marybeth McCaffrey, Director
Linda Henzel, Executive Staff Assistant
Adele Edelman, Assistant Division Director
Provides services to adults and children with developmental disabilities all to the aging.

3918 **Workers Compensation Board Vermont**
Department of Labor
5 Green Mountain Drive
PO Box 488
Montpelier, VT 05601- 0488 802-828-4000
Fax: 802-828-4022
labor.vermont.gov
Deborah Bruce, Human Resource Administrator
Allen Evans, Executive Director Workforce Dev
Annie Noonan, Commissioner
Erika Wolf?ng, Principal Assistant
Welcome to the Vermont Department of Labor's website. VDOL's primary focus is to provide services that assist businesses, workers, and job seekers.

Virginia

3919 **Aging and Disability Services**
2100 Washington Blvd
4th Floor
Arlington, VA 22204 703-228-1700
TTY: 703-228-1788
arlaaa@arlingtonva.us
aging-disability.arlingtonva.us
Anita Friedman, Director, Department of Human Services
The Aging and Disability Services Division offers care coordination, home care, and supportive services to the aging residents of Arlington. Services are provided to adults over 60, adults with developmental disabilities and their caregivers.

3920 **International Dyslexia Association: Virginia Branch**
3126 West Cary St.
Suite 102
Richmond, VA 23221 866-893-0583
va.dyslexiaida.org
Lisa Snidery, President
Lisa Harrah, Vice President
Robin Hegner, Secretary
Mark Whitehurst, Treasurer
Provides free information and referral services for diagnosis and tutoring for parents, educators, physicians, and individuals with dyslexia in Illinois. Membership includes yearly journal and quarterly newsletter.

3921 **Virginia Department for the Blind and Vision Impaired (DBVI)**
401 Azalea Ave.
Richmond, VA 23227 804-371-3151
800-622-2155
www.vdbvi.org
Raymond E. Hopkins, Commissioner
Rick L. Mitchell, Deputy Commissioner, Services
Matt Koch, Deputy Commissioner, Enterprises
Wallica Gaines, Deputy Commissioner, Administration
Offers services for the totally blind, legally blind, visually impaired, and more with health, counseling, educational, recreational, rehabilitation, computer training and professional training services.

3922 **Virginia Department of Mental Health**
P.O. Box 1797
Richmond, VA 23218-1797 804-786-3921
Fax: 804-371-6638
TTY: 804-371-8977
www.dbhds.virginia.gov
Debra Ferquson, Commissioner
John Pezzoli, Deputy Commissioner
Daniel Herr, Assistant Commissioner of Behavi
Connie Cochran, Assistant Commissioner of Develo
Available to citizens statewide, Virginia's public mental health, intellectual disability and substance abuse services system is comprised of 16 state facilities and 40 locally-run community services boards (CSBs) The CSBs and facilities serve children and adults who have or who are at risk of mental illness, serious emotional disturbance, intellectual disabilities, or substance abuse disorders.

3923 **Virginia Developmental Disability Council**
103 S Main St
Waterbury, VT 05671-9800 082-241-2220
Cynthia D LaWare, Secretary
The mission of VTDDC is to facilitate connections and to promote supports that bring people with developmental disabilities into the heart of Vermont Communities.

3924 **Virginia Office Protection and Advocacy for People with Disabilities**
1512 Willow Lawn
Suite 100
Richmond, VA 23230-3034
804-225-2042
800-552-3962
Fax: 804-662-7057
info@dLCV.org
disabilitylawva.org

Coleen Miller, Executive Director
LaToya Blizzard, Deputy Director
Mickie Chapman, IT Specialist
Melissa Charnes-Gibson, Staff Attorney

Through zealous and effective advocacy and legal representation to: protect and advance legal, human, and civil rights of persons with disabilities; combat and prevent abuse, neglect, and discrimination; and promote independence, choice, and self-determination by persons with disabilities.

3925 **Virginia Office for Protection & Advocacy**
5005 Mitchelldale
Suite #100
Houston, TX 77092-3034
713-574-5287
866-964-2867
Fax: 281-476-7800
info@dLCV.org

V Coleen Miller, Executive Director
Rusty Hill, Administrative Assistant
LaToya Blizzard, Deputy Director for Fiscal and O
Mickie Chapman, Information Technology Specialis

An independent state agency that helps ensure that the rights of persons with disabiltiies in the Commonwealth are protected. The mission of DRVD is to provide zealous and effective advocacy and legal representation to protect and advance legal, human and civil rights of persons with disabilities, combat and prevent abuse, neglect and discrimination, and promote independence, choice and self-determination by persons with disabilities.

3926 **Virginia Office for Protection and Advocacy**
5005 Mitchelldale
Suite #100
Houston, TX 77092-3034
713-574-5287
866-964-2867
Fax: 281-476-7800
info@dLCV.org

V Coleen Miller, Executive Director
Rusty Hill, Administrative Assistant
LaToya Blizzard, Deputy Director for Fiscal and O
Mickie Chapman, Information Technology Specialis

An independent state agency that helps ensure that the rights of persons with disabiltiies in the Commonwealth are protected. The mission of DRVD is to provide zealous and effective advocacy and legal representation to protect and advance legal, human and civil rights of persons with disabilities, combat and prevent abuse, neglect and discrimination, and promote independence, choice and self-determination by persons with disabilities.

3927 **Virginia's Developmental Disabilities Planning Council**
Stae Agency
1100 Bank Street
7th Floor
Richmond, VA 23219-3426
804-786-0016
800-846-4464
Fax: 804-662-7662
TTY: 800-811-7893
info@vbpd.virginia.gov
www.vaboard.org

Korinda Rusinyak, Chairman
Charles Meacham, Vice Chairman
Dennis Manning, Secretary
Heidi L. Lawyer, Executive Director

To create a Commonwealth that advances opportunities for independence, personal decision-making and full participation in community life for individuals with developmental disabilities.

Washington

3928 **DSHS/Aging & Adult Disability Services Administration**
P.O. Box 45130
Olympia, WA 98504-5130
360-902-7797
800-737-0617
Fax: 360-902-7848
TTY: 800-737-7931

Dan Murphy, Director
Bea Rector, Project Director
Tamarra Paradee, Executive Secretary
Bill Moss, Director

The Aging and Disability Services Administration assists children and adults with developmental delays or disabilities, cognitive impairment, chronic illness and related functional disabilities to gain access to needed services and supports by managing a system of long-term care and supportive services that are high quality, cost effective, and responsive to individual needs and preferences.

3929 **Disability Rights: Washington**
315 5th Avenue South
Suite 850
Seattle, WA 98104-2691
206-324-1521
800-562-2702
Fax: 206-957-0729
TTY: 206-957-0728
info@dr-wa.org
www.disabilityrightswa.org

Mark Stroh, Executive Director
David Carison, Director of Legal Advocacy
Emily Cooper, Staff Attorney
Charlotte Cunningham, Staff Attorney

WPAS is a private, non-profit right protection agency for persons with disabilities residin in Washington state. Our advocacy services include information referral, technical assistance, training, publications and systemic advocacy.

3930 **International Dyslexia Association: Washington State Branch**
P.O. Box 27435
Seattle, WA 98165
info@wabida.org
wabida.org

Kristie English, President
Jessica Ruger, Vice President
Beverly Wolf, Treasurer
Bonnie Meyer, Secretary

Provides free information and referral services for diagnosis and tutoring for parents, educators, physicians, and individuals with dyslexia in Arkansas, Idaho, Montana and Washington state. Membership includes yearly journal and quarterly newsletter.

3931 **Social Security: Olympia Disability Determination**
Social Security
P.O. Box 9303-MS-45550
Olympia, WA 98507
360-664-7356
800-772-1213
800-562-6074
Fax: 360-586-0851
TTY: 800-325-0778
Jennifer.Elsen@ssa.gov
www.ssa.gov

Karena L. Kilgore, Executive Secretary
Carolyn W. Colvin, Commissioner
Carolyn W. Colvin, Deputy Commissioner
James A. Kissko, Chief of Staff

We deliver services through a nationwide network of over 1,400 offices that include regional offices, field offices, card centers, teleservice centers, processing centers, hearing offices, the Appeals Council, and our State and territorial partners, the Disability Determination Services. We also have a presence in U.S. embassies around the globe. The rich diversity of our employees mirrors the public we serve.

3932 WA Department of Services for the Blind
4565 7th Avenue SE
PO Box 40933
Lacey, WA 98503
360-725-3830
800-552-7103
Fax: 360-407-0679
info@dsb.wa.gov
www.dsb.wa.gov

Sue Ammeter, council chair
Nancy Kim
Veronica Baca, Council Member
Michael Cunningham, Council Member
Vocational rehabilitation for the blind.

3933 Washington Client Assistance Program
2531 Rainier Ave S
Seattle, WA 98144-5328
206-721-5999
800-544-2121
888-721-6072
Fax: 206-721-4537
TTY: 206-721-6072
www.washingtoncap.org

Jerry Johnson, Executive Director
Bob Huven, rehabilitation coordinator
Advocacy and information assistance for persons of disability seeking services through vocational rehabilitation or other program under the 1973 Rehabilitation Act as commented. We provide counseling.

3934 Washington Developmental Disability
2600 Martin Way E
Suite F
Olympia, WA 98506-4974
360-586-3560
800-634-4473
Fax: 360-586-2424
Ed.Holen@ddc.wa.gov
www.ddc.wa.gov

Diana Zottman, Chairman
Ed Holen, Executive Director
Brain Dahl, Support Coordinator
Aziz Aladin, Budget & Fiscal Director
Developmental Disabilities Council members are appointed by the Governor to plan comprehensive services for the State of Washington's citizens with developmental disabilities.

3935 Washington Governor's Committee on Disability Issues & Employment
605 Woodland Square Loop SE
Lacey, WA 98503
360-438-3168
Fax: 928-447-6579
gcdetz@gmail.com
www.gcde.org

Martin Haule, Director
Toby Olson, Manager

3936 Washington Office of Superintendent of Public Instruction
600 Washington St. S.E.
P. O. Box 47200
Olympia, WA 98504-7200
360-725-6000
TTY: 360-644-3631
www.k12.wa.us

Randy Dorn, State Superintendent
Gil Mendoza, Deputy Superintendent
JoLynn Berge, Assistant Superintendent
Ken Kanikeberg, Chief of Staff
The Office of Superintendent of Public Instruction (OSPI) is the primary agency charged with overseeing K-12 education in Washington state. OSPI works with the state's 296 school districts to administer basic education programs and implement education reform on behalf of more than one million public school students.

3937 Washington State Developmental Disabilities Council
2600 Martin Way E
Suite F
Olympia, WA 98506-4974
360-586-3560
800-634-4473
Fax: 360-586-2424
Ed.Holen@ddc.wa.gov
www.ddc.wa.gov

Diana Zottman, Chairman
Ed Holen, Executive Director
Brain Dahl, Support Coordinator
Aziz Aladin, Budget & Fiscal Director
Developmental Disabilities Council members are appointed by the Governor to plan comprehensive services for the State of Washington's citizens with developmental disabilities.

3938 Workers Compensation Board Washington
State of Washington
7273 Linderson Way SW
Tumwater, WA 98501-5414
360-902-5800
800-547-8367
Fax: 360-902-5798
TTY: 360-902-5797
www.lni.wa.gov

Judy Schurke, Director
Lisa Rodriguez, Executive Assistant
Vickie Kennedy, Special Assistant
Tamara Jones, Dir of Government Relations
&I is a diverse state agency dedicated to the safety, health and security of Washington's 3.2 million workers. We help employers meet safety and health standards and we inspect workplaces when alerted to hazards. As administrators of the state's workers' compensation system, we are similar to a large insurance company, providing medical and limited wage-replacement coverage to workers who suffer job-related injuries and illness. Our rules and enforcement programs also help ensure workers are pai

West Virginia

3939 Bureau of Employment Programs Division of Workers' Compensation
State of West Virginia
407 Virginia Street East
Charleston, WV 25301-2531
304-357-0101
800-628-4265
Fax: 304-357-0788
helpdesk@kanawha.us
kanawha.us

Patricia Starkey, Manager
Vern Cormick, Manager
Michael ' Campbell, Director of IT
Larry McDonnell, Chief Webmaster
Kanawha County today is an exciting technology center that is earning recognition in information technology, medical research, chemical synthesis research, and telecommunications.

3940 Disability Determination Section
Ste 500
500 Quarrier St
Charleston, WV 25301-2913
304-343-5055
800-772-1213
800-344-5033
Fax: 304-353-4212
www.ssa.gov

Karena L. Kilgore, Executive Secretary
Carolyn W. Colvin, Commissioner
Carolyn W. Colvin, Deputy Commissioner
James A. Kissko, Chief of Staff
We deliver services through a nationwide network of over 1,400 offices that include regional offices, field offices, card centers, teleservice centers, processing centers, hearing offices, the Appeals Council, and our State and territorial partners, the Disability Determination Services. We also have a presence in U.S. embassies around the globe. The rich diversity of our employees mirrors the public we serve.

3941 **Social Security: Charleston Disability Determination**
Social Security
500 Quarrier Street
Suite 500
Charleston, WV 25301-2913
304-343-5055
800-772-1213
800-344-5033
Fax: 304-353-4212
www.ssa.gov

Karena L. Kilgore, Executive Secretary
Carolyn W. Colvin, Commissioner
Carolyn W. Colvin, Deputy Commissioner
James A. Kissko, Chief of Staff

We deliver services through a nationwide network of over 1,400 offices that include regional offices, field offices, card centers, teleservice centers, processing centers, hearing offices, the Appeals Council, and our State and territorial partners, the Disability Determination Services. We also have a presence in U.S. embassies around the globe. The rich diversity of our employees mirrors the public we serve.

3942 **West Virginia Advocates**
1207 Quarrier St
Suite 400
Charleston, WV 25301-1826
304-346-0847
800-950-5250
Fax: 304-346-0867
kellie.l.aikman@wv.gov
wvadvocates.org

Terry Dilcher, President
John Galloway, Treasurer
Don Neurman, Secretary
Clarice Hausch, Executive Director

West Virginia Advocates, Inc. (WVA) is the federally mandated protection and advocacy system for people with disabilities in West Virginia. WVA is a private, nonprofit agency. Our services are confidential and free of charge.

3943 **West Virginia Client Assistance Program**
West Virginia Advocates
1900 Kanawha Blvd E
Room 9
Charleston, WV 25305-1
304-558-3780
Fax: 304-558-4092

Clarice Hausch, Executive Director

3944 **West Virginia Department of Aging**
1900 Kanawha Blvd. East
Charleston, WV 25305
304-558-3317
877-987-3646
Fax: 304-558-5609
www.wvseniorservices.gov

Robert E. Roswall, Commissioner
Nel Kimble

The information we offer is tailored to those who are seeking to locate programs and services for themselves or their loved ones and also for professionals who may be looking for up-to-date information relating to the field of aging.

3945 **West Virginia Department of Children with Disabilities**
Children with Special Health Care Needs
One Davis Square
Suite 100 East
Charleston, WV 25301- 1757
304-558-0684
Fax: 304-558-1130
DHHRSecretary@wv.gov
www.dhhr.wv.gov

Douglas M. Robinson, Deputy Commissioner
Virginia Mahan, Executive Secretary
Karen Villanueva-Matkovich, General Counsel
Melissa Rosen, CFO

The Bureau for Public Health directs public health activities at all levels within the state to fulfill the core functions of public health: the assessment of community health status and available resources; policy development resulting in proposals to support and encourage better health; and assurance that needed services are available, accessible, and of acceptable quality.

3946 **West Virginia Department of Health**
One Davis Square
Suite 100 East
Charleston, WV 25301
304-558-0684
Fax: 304-558-1130
DHHRSecretary@wv.gov
www.dhhr.wv.gov

Douglas M. Robinson, Deputy Commissioner
Virginia Mahan, Executive Secretary
Karen Villanueva-Matkovich, General Counsel
Melissa Rosen, CFO

The Bureau for Public Health directs public health activities at all levels within the state to fulfill the core functions of public health: the assessment of community health status and available resources; policy development resulting in proposals to support and encourage better health; and assurance that needed services are available, accessible, and of acceptable quality.

3947 **West Virginia Developmental Disabilities Council**
110 Stockton St
Charleston, WV 25387
304-558-0416
Fax: 304-558-0941
TTY: 304-558-2376
dhhrwvddc@wv.gov
www.ddc.wv.gov

Diana Zottman, Chairman
Ed Holen, Executive Director
Brain Dahl, Support Coordinator
Laurie Bahr, Budget & Fiscal Director

Working to assure that West Virginians with developmental disabilities receive the services, supports, and other forms of assistance they need to exercise self-determination and achieve independence, productivity, integration, and inclusion in the community.

6-8 pages Quarterly Newsl

3948 **West Virginia Division of Rehabilitation Services**
107 Capitol Street
Charleston, WV 25301-2609
304-356-2060
800-642-8207
www.wvdrs.org

Donna L. Ashworth, Acting Director
Kay Goodwin, Cabinet Secretary

DRS' mission is to enable and empower individuals with disabilities to work and to live independently.

Wisconsin

3949 **Disability Rights Wisconsin: Milwaukee Office**
Ste 3230
6737 W Washington St
Milwaukee, WI 53214-5651
414-773-4646
800-708-3034
Fax: 414-773-4647
TTY: 888-758-6049
info@drwi.org
disabilityrightswi.org

Ted Skemp, President
Beth Moss, Vice President
Susan Gramling, Secretary
Dan Idzikowski, Executive Director

The protection and advocacy agency for people with disabilities in Wisconsin. DRW provides guidance, advice, investigation, negotiation and in some cases legal representation to people with disabilities and their families. Local and state level systems advocacy and training are also provided.

3950 **International Dyslexia Association: Wisconsin Branch**
1616 Graham Ave.
Eau Claire, WI 54701
608-355-0911
wi.dyslexiaida.org

Tammy Tillotson, President
Kimberly Chan, Treasurer
Pattie Huse, Secretary
Ann Malone, Director

Provides free information and referral services for diagnosis and tutoring for parents, educators, physicians, and individuals with dyslexia in Illinois. Membership includes yearly journal and quarterly newsletter.

3951 **Social Security: Madison Field Office**
6011 Odana Rd
Madison, WI 53719-1101
866-770-2262
800-772-1213
Fax: 608-270-1021
TTY: 800-325-0778
wi.fo.madison@ssa.gov
www.ssa.gov

3952 **West Virginia Department of Health**
One Davis Square
Suite 100 East
Charleston, WV 25301
304-558-0684
800-441-4576
Fax: 304-558-1130
DHHRSecretary@wv.gov
www.dhhr.wv.gov

Rocco S. Fucillo, Cabinet Secretary
Susan Shelton Perry, Deputy Secretary for Legal Servi
Ellen Cannon, Privacy Officer
Virginia Mahan, Executive Secretary

The Department of Health and Family Services operates the federal Title V Maternal and Child Health Block Grant Program for Children with Special Health Care Needs. The program provides program monitoring, consultation and technical assistance to five regional CSHCN centers throughout Wisconsin; a Birth Defects Monitoring and Surveillance Program and a Universal Newborn Hearing Screening Program.

3953 **Wisconsin Board for People with Developmental Disabilities (WBPDD)**
201 W Washington Ave
Suite 111
Madison, WI 53703-2796
608-266-7826
888-332-1677
Fax: 608-267-3906
TTY: 608-266-6660
wcdd.org

Jennifer Ondrejka, Manager
Joshua Ryf, Office Manager

Statewide systems advocacy group for people with developmental disabilities in Wisconsin.

3954 **Wisconsin Bureau of Aging**
State Office of Wisconsin
1 West Wilson Street
Madison, WI 53703
608-266-1865
Fax: 608-267-3203
TTY: 888-701-1251
DHSwebmaster@wisconsin.gov

Donna Mc Dowell, Executive Director
Gail Schwersenska, Section Chief
Dennis G. Smith, Secretary

Keeps and updates information and printed materials on senior housing directories, nursing home listings, and home care agencies.

3955 **Wisconsin Coalition for Advocacy: Madison Office**
16 N Carroll St
Suite 400
Madison, WI 53703-2762
608-267-0214
800-928-8778
Fax: 608-267-0368

Kim Hogan, Intake Specialist
Mr Lynn Breedlove, Executive Director

The protection and advocacy agency for people with disabilities in Wisconsin. WCA provides guidance, advice, investigation, negotiation and in some cases legal representation to people with disabilities and their families. Local and state level systems advocacy and training are also provided.

3956 **Wisconsin Governor's Committee for People with Disabilities**
1 West Wilson Street
Madison, WI 53703
608-266-1865
877-865-3432
Fax: 608-266-3386
TTY: 888-701-1251
DHSwebmaster@wisconsin.gov

Donna Mc Dowell, Executive Director
Gail Schwersenska, Section Chief
Dennis G. Smith, Secretary

To advise the Governor and state agencies on problems faced by people with disabilities; to review legislation affecting people with disabilities; to promote effective operation of publicly-administered or supported programs serving people with disabilities; to promote the collection, dissemination and incorporation of adequate information about persons with disabilities for purposes of public planning at all levels of government.

3957 **Workers Compensation Board Wisconsin**
Room C100, 201 E. Washington Avenue
P. O. Box 7901
Madison, WI 53707-7901
608-266-1340
Fax: 608-267-0394
dwd.wisconsin.gov/wc

Reggie Newson, Secretary
Jonathan Barry, Deputy Secretary
John Metcalf, Division Administrator
Brain Krueger, Deputy Administrator

The Worker's Compensation Division administers programs designed to ensure that injured workers receive required benefits from insurers or self-insured employers; encourage rehabilitation and reemployment for injured workers; and promote the reduction of work-related injuries, illnesses, and deaths.

Wyoming

3958 **Social Security: Cheyenne Disability Determination**
Social Security
821 W Pershing Blvd
Cheyenne, WY 82002-1
307-777-7341
800-438-5788
Fax: 307-637-0247
Jeff.Graham@ssa.gov
ssa.gov

Karena L. Kilgore, Executive Secretary
Carolyn W. Colvin, Commissioner
Carolyn W. Colvin, Deputy Commissioner
James A. Kissko, Chief of Staff

We deliver services through a nationwide network of over 1,400 offices that include regional offices, field offices, card centers, teleservice centers, processing centers, hearing offices, the Appeals Council, and our State and territorial partners, the Disability Determination Services. We also have a presence in U.S. embassies around the globe. The rich diversity of our employees mirrors the public we serve.

3959 **WY Department of Health: Mental Health and Substance Abuse Service Division**
401 Hathaway Building
Cheyenne, WY 82002-1
307-777-7656
800-535-4006
Fax: 307-777-7439
TTY: 307-777-5581
www.health.wyo.gov

Thomas O. Forslund, Director
Lee Clabots, Deputy Director
Bob Peck, Chief Financial Officer
Heather Babbitt, Senior Administartor

State office responsible for purchase of service and program development policy.

3960 **Workers Compensation Board Wyoming**
350 South Washington Street
PO Box 1068
Afton, WY 83110-3004
307-886-9260
Fax: 307-886-9269

3961 **Wyoming Client Assistance Program**
Protection and Advocacy System
2nd Fl
320 W 25th St
Cheyenne, WY 82001-3069
307-632-2682
877-854-5041
Fax: 307-638-0815
wypanda@vcn.com
ap.org

Jeanne Thobro, Manager
Jeanne A Thobro, Executive Director

3962 **Wyoming Department of Aging**
State Department of Wyoming
401 Hathaway Building
Cheyenne, WY 82002-1
307-777-7656
800-442-2766
Fax: 307-777-7439
wyaging@wyo.gov
health.wyo.gov

Thomas O. Forslund, Director
Lee Clabots, Deputy Director
Bob Peck, Chief Financial Officer
Heather Babbitt, Senior Administartor

The Wyoming Department of Health's Aging Division is committed to providing care, ensuring safety and and promoting independent choices for Wyoming's older adults

3963 **Wyoming Developmental Disability Council**
122 W 25th St
1st. Fl. West, Herschler Building,
Cheyenne, WY 82002
307-777-7230
800-438-5791
Fax: 307-777-5690
wgcdd@wyo.gov

Shannon Buller, Executive Director
Von Maul, Administrative Assistant
Sam Janney, Public Information Officer
Calob Taylor, Grants & Policy Analyst

Our purpose is to assure that individuals with developmental disabilities and their families participate in and have access to needed community services, individualized supports and other forms of assistance that promote independence, productivity, integration and inclusion in all facets of community life.

3964 **Wyoming Protection & Advocacy for Persons with Disabilities**
7344 Stockman Street
Cheyenne, WY 82009
307-632-3496
Fax: 307-638-0815
wypanda@wypanda.com
wypanda.com

Tori Rosenthal, President
Jeanne A Thobro, Executive Director

Wyoming Protection & Advocacy System, Inc. (P&A), established in 1977, is the official non-profit corporation authorized to implement certain mandates of several federal laws. Enacted by Congress, these laws provide various protection and advocacy services.

Independent Living Centers

Alabama

3965 **Birdie Thornton Center**
2350 Hine Street
Athens, AL 35611
256-232-0366
Fax: 256-230-9398

Kristy Allen King, Program Director
Heather Mereidth, Program Professional, QMRP
Rabieb Clem, Senior Aid
Kay Green, Training Specialist

The Birdie Thornton Center is devoted to providing care, education, and training to adults with developmental delays and disabilities.

3966 **Independent Living Center of Mobile**
5301 Moffett Rd
Suite 110
Mobile, AL 36618-2926
251-460-0301
Fax: 251-341-1267
TTY: 251-460-2872
Michaeld@ilcmobile.org
ilcmobile.org

Michael Davis, Executive Director
Darmita Flood, Administrative Assistant
Barbara Hattier, ILS/Transportation Coordinator
James Flora, ILS/Outreach Specialist

Helping people with disabilities become independent.

3967 **Independent Living Resources Of Greater Birmingham: Alabaster**
120 Plaza Cir, Suite C
P. O. Box 2048
Alabaster, AL 35007-7034
205-685-0570
Fax: 205-251-0605
TTY: 205-685-0570
www.ilrgb.org

Kathy Lovell, President
Phil Klebine, Vice President
Susan Parker, Secretary
Milton Moats, Treasurer

The mission of this Independent Living Center is to empower people with disabilities to fully participate in the community.

3968 **Independent Living Resources of Greater Birmingham: Jasper**
300 Birmingham Ave
PO Box 434
Jasper, AL 35502-3811
205-387-0159
Fax: 205-387-0162
TTY: 205-387-0159
www.ilrgb.org

Kathy Lovell, President
Phil Klebine, Vice President
Susan Parker, Secretary
Milton Moats, Treasurer

The purpose of this Independent Living Center is to empower people with disabilities to fully participate in the community.

3969 **Independent Living Resources of Greater Birmingham**
1418 6th Avenue North
Birmingham, AL 35203-1317
205-251-2223
Fax: 205-251-0605
TTY: 205-251-2223

Kathy Lovell, President
Phil Klebine, Vice President
Susan Parker, Secretary
Milton Moats, Treasurer

The mission of this Independent Living Center is to empower people with disabilities to fully participate in the community.

3970 **Montgomery Center for Independent Living**
600 S Court St
Montgomery, AL 36104-4106
334-240-2520
Fax: 334-240-6869
TTY: 334-240-2520
mcil@bellsouth.net
www.cilmontgomery.org

Scott Renner, Executive Director
Barbara F. Crozier, President
Kenneth Marshall, Vice President
Vickie P. FitzGerald, Secretary

Encourgaes people with disabilities to support one another in reaching their own independent living goals.

3971 **State of Alabama Independent Living/Homebound Service (SAIL)**
Alabama Department of Rehabilitation Services
602 S Lawrence St.
Montgomery, AL 36104
www.rehab.alabama.gov
Lisa Alford, Director

The following services are provided to Alabamians with significant disabilities: specialized in-home education and counseling; attendant care; training; and medical services.

Alaska

3972 **Access Alaska: ADA Partners Project**
1217 East 10th Ave
Suite 105
Anchorage, AK 99501-2044
907-248-4777
800-770-4488
888-462-1444
Fax: 907-263-1942
TTY: 907-248-8799
info@accessalaska.org
accessalaska.org

Lorali Simon, President
Mike O'Neill, Vice President
Jim Duffield, Treasurer
Eric Spangler, Member

Assisting Alaskans with disabilities to live independently in the community of their choice.

3973 **Access Alaska: Fairbanks**
526 Gaffney Rd
Suite 100
Fairbanks, AK 99701-4914
907-479-7940
800-770-7940
Fax: 907-474-4052
TTY: 907-474-8619
info@accessalaska.org
accessalaska.org

Lorali Simon, President
Mike O'Neill, Vice President
Jim Duffield, Treasurer
Eric Spangler, Member

A local non profit agency using its resources to actively promote a society where persons with disabilities can live and work independently in the community of their choice.

3974 **Access Alaska: Mat-Su**
1075 Check St,
Suite 109
Wasilla, AK 99654-6937
907-357-2588
800-770-0228
Fax: 907-357-5585
info@accessalaska.org
accessalaska.org

Lorali Simon, President
Mike O'Neill, Vice President
Jim Duffield, Treasurer
Eric Spangler, Member

Provides independent living services to persons with significant disabilities. Mission is to encourage and promote the total integration of persons with disabilities into the community of their choice. Services include independent living skills training, information and referral, advocacy, peer support, and at home modifications.

3975 **Alaska SILC**
Ste 206
1217 East 10th Ave
Anchorage, AK 99501-1760
907-248-4777
800-770-4488
888-294-7452
Fax: 907-263-1942
info@accessalaska.org
www.alaskasilc.org

Jim Beck, Executive Director
Lorali Simon, President
Mike O'Neill, Vice President
Jim Duffield, Treasurer

The Alaska Statewide Independent Living is committed to promoting a philosophy of consumer control, peer support, self help, self determination, equal access, and individual and systems advocacy, in order to maximize leadership, empowerment, independence, productivity, and to support full inclusion and integration of individuals with disabilities into the mainstream of American society.

3976 **Arctic Access**
P.O. Box 930
Kotzebue, AK 99752-930
907-412-0695
877-442-2393
TTY: 907-442-2393

Roger Wright Jr, Executive Director
Russell Williams, Jr, Elder & Disability Resource Coor
Audrey Aanes

The Arctic Access Independent Living Center provides services and opportunities for elders and others with disabilities so they may remain in their village and be as active as possible with their families and commuities in the North West Arctic and Bering Straits Regions of Alaska.

3977 **Hope Community Resources**
540 W Intl Airport Rd
Anchorage, AK 99518-1105
907-561-5335
800-478-0078
Fax: 907-564-7429
info@hopealaska.org
hopealaska.org

Robert Owens, President
John Dittrich, Vice President
Eugene 'Gene' Bates, Treasurer
Stephen P. Lesko, Executive Director

Provider of services to individuals who experience a disability.

3978 **Kenai Peninsula Independent Living Center**
265 E. Pioneer Suite 201
P.O. Box 2474
Homer, AK 99603- 2474
907-235-7911
800-770-7911
Fax: 907-235-6236
peninsulailc.org

Candy Norman, President
Mike Harmer, Vice President

Offers peer counseling, disability education and awareness, attendant care registry and information on accessible housing.

3979 **Kenai Peninsula Independent Living Center: Seward**
201 Third Avenue, Suite 101Bs
P. O. Box 3523
Seward, AK 99664-3523
907-224-8711
Fax: 907-224-7793
www.peninsulailc.org

Candy Norman, President
Mike Harmer, Vice President

Offers peer counseling, disability, education and awareness, attendant care registry and information on accessible housing.

3980 **Keni Peninsula Independent Living Center: Central Peninsula**
47255 Princeton Avenue
Suite 8
Soldotna, AK 99669
907-262-6333
Fax: 907-260-4495
www.peninsulailc.org

Candy Norman, President
Mike Harmer, Vice President

Offers peer counseling, disability education and awareness, attendant care registry and information on accessible housing.

3981 **Southeast Alaska Independent Living**
3225 Hospital Drive
Suite 300
Juneau, AK 99801-7863
907-586-4920
800-478-7245
Fax: 907-586-4980
TTY: 907-523-5285
info@sailinc.org
sailinc.org

Robert Purvis, President
Jeff Irwin, Vice President
Suzanne Williams, Secretary
Mary Gregg, Treasurer

To empower consumers with disabilities by providing services and information to support them in making choices that will positively affect their independence and productivity in society.

3982 **Southeast Alaska Independent Living: Ketchikan**
602 Dock St
Suite 107
Ketchikan, AK 99901-6574
907-225-4735
888-452-7245
Fax: 907-247-4735
ketchikan@sailinc.org
www.sailinc.org

Robert Purvis, President
Jeff Irwin, Vice President
Suzanne Williams, Secretary
Mary Gregg, Treasurer

To empower consumers with disabilities by providing services and information to support them in making choices that will positively affect their independence and productivity in society.

3983 **Southeast Alaska Independent Living: Sitka**
514 Lake St
Suite C
Sitka, AK 99835-7405
907-747-6859
888-500-7245
Fax: 907-747-6783
sitka@sailinc.org
www.sailinc.org

Robert Purvis, President
Jeff Irwin, Vice President
Suzanne Williams, Secretary
Mary Gregg, Treasurer

To empower consumers with disabilities by providing services and information to support them in making choices that will positively affect their independence and productivity in society.

Arizona

3984 **ASSIST! to Independence**
P.O. Box 4133
Tuba City, AZ 86045-4133
928-283-6261
888-848-1449
Fax: 928-283-6284
TTY: 928-283-6672
assist01@frontiernet.net
www.assisttoindependence.org

Michael Blatchford, Executive Director
Priscilla Lane, IL Services Coordinator/Dep Dir

A community based, American Indian owned and operated non-profit agency that was established by and for people with disabilities and chronic health conditions to help fill some of the gaps in service delivery.

3985 **Arizona Bridge to Independent Living**
5025 E Washington St
Suite 200
Phoenix, AZ 85034-7439
602-256-2245
800-280-2245
Fax: 602-254-6407
www.abil.org

Mary Slaughter, Chairman
Brad Wemhaner, Vice Chairman
Michael Somsan, Secretary
Jim Winterton, Treasurer

ABIL offers and promotes programs designed to empower people with disabilities to take personal responsibility so they may achieve or continue independent lifestyles within the community.

3986 **Arizona Bridge to Independent Living: Phoenix**
1229 E.Washington St.
Suite D405
Phoenix, AZ 85034
602-296-0551
800-280-2245
Fax: 602-256-0184
TTY: 602-296-0591
www.abil.org

Mary Slaughter, Chairman
Brad Wemhaner, Vice Chairman
Michael Somsan, Secretary
Jim Winterton, Treasurer

ABIL offers and promotes programs designed to empower people with disabilities to take personal responsibility so they may achieve or continue independent lifestyles within the community.

3987 **Arizona Bridge to Independent Living: Mesa**
2150 S Country Club Dr
Suite 10
Mesa, AZ 85210-6879
480-655-9750
800-280-2245
Fax: 480-655-9751
TTY: 480-655-9750
www.abil.org

Mary Slaughter, Chairman
Brad Wemhaner, Vice Chairman
Michael Somsan, Secretary
Jim Winterton, Treasurer

ABIL offers and promotes programs designed to empower people with disabilities to take personal responsibility so they may achieve or continue independent lifestyles within the community.

3988 **Community Outreach Program for the Deaf**
268 W Adams St
Tucson, AZ 85705-6534
520-792-1906
Fax: 520-770-8554
TTY: 520-792-1906
request@copdaz.org
copdaz.org

Anne Levy, Executive Director

A non-profit organization, which has been serving the needs of people in Southern Arizona who are deaf or hard of hearing.

3989 **DIRECT Center for Independence**
1001 N Alvernon Way
Tucson, AZ 85711
520-624-6452
800-342-1853
Fax: 520-792-1438
direct@directilc.org
www.directilc.org

Vicki Cuscino, President

A non-consumer directed, community-based advocacy organization, that promotes independent living and offers a variety of programs for all people with disabilities which encourage them to achieve their full potential and to participate in the community.

3990 **New Horizons Independent Living Center: Prescott Valley**
8085 E Manley Dr
Prescott Valley, AZ 86314-6154
928-772-1266
800-406-2377
Fax: 928-772-3808
TTY: 928-772-1266

Deborah Henderson, Office Manager
Liz Toone, Executive Director
Nick Perry, President
Jim Stobbs, Vice President

To provide services and advocacy which empower and enable people with disabilities to self-determine the goals and activities of their lives.

3991 **Services Maximizing Independent Living and Empowerment (SMILE)**
1931 South Arizona Ave
Suite 4
Yuma, AZ 85364-5721
928-329-6681
855-209-8363
Fax: 928-329-6715
TTY: 928-782-7458
info@smile-az.org
www.smile-az.org

Laura Duval, Executive Director
Brenda Howard, Finance Manager/ Admin Assistant
Shawnnita Miranda, Advocate/ Home modification Mana
Brandon Howard, Outreach Coordinator, Technology

SMILE continually advocates for the Independent Living Philosophy, both individually and system wide. The Board and staff constantly strives to improve the system by writing letters, training staff, providing services, and creating public awareness as to the services and opportunities open to people who have disabilities.

3992 **Sterling Ranch: Residence for Special Women**
Sterling Ranch
P.O. Box 36
Skull Valley, AZ 86338-36
928-442-3289
Fax: 928-442-9272
www.sterlingranch.info

Russell Dryer, Executive Director
Trent Nichel, Manager

A nonprofit residence for women with developmental disabilities which has been in operation since 1947. As a small facility (19 residents) the orientation is personal and family-like. Offers activities that range from gardening, quilting, academics, sign-language, crafts and a myriad of field trips and excursions. Private rooms and spacious living on 4 1/2 acres.

Arkansas

3993 **Arkansas Independent Living Council**
11324 Arcade Drive
Suite 7
Little Rock, AR 72212
501-372-0607
800-772-0607
Fax: 501-372-0598
arkansasilc@att.net
www.ar-silc.org

Sha Stephens, Executive Director
Cheryl, Director
Brenda Stinebuck, Chair
Liz Adams, Vice Chair

A non-profit organization promoting independent living for people with disabilities.

3994 **Delta Resource Center for Independent Living**
11324 Arcade Drive
Little Rock, AR 72212-6249
501-372-0607
800-772-0607
Fax: 501-372-0598
drcilar@yahoo.com
www.ar-silc.org

Sha Stephens, Executive Director
Katy Morris, Director
Cheryl, Director
Brenda Stinebuck, Chair

Provides services, support, and advocacy which enables people with severe disabilities to live as independently as possible within their family and community.

3995 **Mainstream**
300 S Rodney Parham Rd.
Suite 5
Little Rock, AR 72205
501-280-0012
800-371-9026
Fax: 501-280-9267
TTY: 501-280-9262
www.mainstreamilrc.com

Rita Byers, Executive Director

A non-residential, consumer-driven independent living resource center for persons with disabilities. Mainstream operates with the conviction that people with disabilities have the right and responsibility to make choices, to control their lives and to participate fully and equally in the community. Mainstream offers the following services free of charge: Advocacy, Peer Support, Training and Education, Information and Referral, Ramp program, and more.
1988

3996 **Our Way: The Cottage Apt Homes**
9175 Greenback Lane
Orangevale, CA 95662-6616
501-225-5030
888-879-9584
Fax: 501-225-5190
rentthecottages.com

Katrina Williams, Manager
Crystal Brown, Assistant Manager

Advocacy and information services. One bedroom apartments for mobility impaired and elderly 62 years or older persons.
Based on income

3997 **Sources for Community IL Services**
1918 N Birch Ave
Fayetteville, AR 72703-2408
479-442-5600
888-284-7521
Fax: 479-442-5192
TTY: 479-251-1378
jmather@arsources.org
www.arsources.org

Brent Williams, PhD, President
Elise Burt, Treasurer
Burke Fanari, Secretary
Jim Mather, Executive Director

Provides services, support, and advocacy for individuals with disabilities, their families and the community.

3998 **Spa Area Independent Living Services**
621 Albert Pike
Hot Springs, AR 71913
501-624-7710
800-255-7549
Fax: 501-624-7003

Dejan S. Vojnovic, President
Joseph E. Anderson, Vice President - Real Estate
Bryan S. Cox, Vice President - Technology
Brenda Stinebuck, Executive Director

Provides services and advocacy by and for persons with all types of disabilities. The goal is to assist individuals with disabilities to achieve thier maximum potential within their families and communities.

California

3999 **Access Center of San Diego**
8885 Rio San Diego Dr
Suite 131
San Diego, CA 92108-1625
619-293-3500
800-300-4326
Fax: 619-293-3508
TTY: 619-293-7757
info@a2isd.org
www.a2isd.org

Louis Frick, Executive Director
Derek Parker, Chair
Jacquelyn E. Nash, Vice Chair
Nick Bradley, Treasurer

Access to Independence is an independent living center (ILC), a nonresidential, cross-disability, non-profit corporations that provide services to people with disabilities to help maximize their independence and fully integrate into their communities. Access to Independence is one of 391 ILCs across the country and one of 29 serving Californians. Like all ILCs, Access to Independence offers required federal and state programs and services to people of all disability types and ages at no charge.

4000 **Access to Independence**
8885 Rio San Diego Drive
Suite 131
San Diego, CA 92108- 1625
619-293-3500
800-300-4326
Fax: 619-293-3508
TTY: 619-293-7757
info@a2isd.org
www.a2isd.org

Louis Frick, Executive Director
Derek Parker, Chair
Jacquelyn E. Nash, Vice Chair
Nick Bradley, Treasurer

A community resource for people with disabilities to lead independent lives.

4001 **Access to Independence of Imperial Valley**
101 Hacienda Drive
Suite 13
Calexico, CA 92231-2875
760-768-2044
866-976-3515
Fax: 760-768-4977
TTY: 619-293-7757
info@a2isd.org

Louis Frick, Executive Director
Derek Parker, Chair
Jacquelyn E. Nash, Vice Chair
Nick Bradley, Treasurer

A community resource for people with disabilities to lead independent lives.

4002 **Access to Independence of North County**
209 E Broadway
Vista, CA 92084-6005
760-643-0447
Fax: 760-435-9206
info@a2isd.org

Louis Frick, Executive Director
Derek Parker, Chair
Jacquelyn E. Nash, Vice Chair
Nick Bradley, Treasurer

A community resource for people with disabilities to lead independent lives.

4003 **Beaumont Senior Center: Community Access Center**
1310 Oak Valley Parkway
Beaumont, CA 92223-2218
951-769-8524
Fax: 951-769-8519
TTY: 909-769-2794

Laurie Hoirup, Director

A non profit organization; one of 29 similar programs throughout the state of California CAC is a community resource, advocate, and educator for Riverside County residents with disabilities.

4004 **California Foundation For Independent Living Centers**
1234 H Street
Suite 100
Sacramento, CA 95814-1912
916-325-1690
Fax: 916-325-1699
TTY: 916-325-1695
cfilc@cfilc.org
www.cfilc.org

Robert Hand, Chairperson
Ana Acton, Vice Chairperson
Tink Miller, Executive Director
Kim Cantrell, Program Director

Community Rehabilitation Services, Inc. (CRS) is a private, non-profit agency established in 1974 to assist persons with disabilities within the East/North East areas of Los Angeles County to enhance their options for living independently. Any person who is 18 yrs of age or more with physical, sensory, mental/emotional or developmental disabilities can work with us to become more self-sufficient. Our intake procedures provide an orientation to the staff, facilities and services at CRS.

4005 **California Foundation for Independent Living Centers**
1235 H Street
Suite 100
Sacramento, CA 95814-1913
916-325-1690
Fax: 916-325-1699
TTY: 916-325-1695
cfilc@cfilc.org
www.cfilc.org

Robert Hand, Chairperson
Ana Acton, Vice Chairperson
Tink Miller, Executive Director
Kim Cantrell, Program Director

CFILC's mission is to support independent living centers in their local communities through advocating for systems change and promoting access and integration for people with disabilities.

4006 **California State Independent Living Council (SILC)**
1235 H Street
Suite 100
Sacramento, CA 95814-4010
916-325-1690
866-866-7452
Fax: 916-325-1699
TTY: 866-745-2889
www.calsilc.org

Susan M. Madison, Chairman
Eli Gelardin, Vice Chairman
Liz Pazdral, Executive Director
Caroline Kuhn, Staff Services Analyst

To maximize options for independence for persons with disabilities

4007 **Center for Independence of the Disabled**
Suite 103
2001 Winward Way
San Mateo, CA 94404-3062
650-645-1780
Fax: 650-645-1785
TTY: 650-522-9313
http://www.cidsanmateo.org

Brad Friedman, Co-President
Laura Whitsitt Hillyard, Co-President
Thomas J. Devine, Vice President
John Horgan, Secretary

Increase the social, educational, and economic participation of persons with disabilities in San Mateo County, and to encourage, support, and provide options for self determination, equal access and freedom of choice.

4008 **Center for Independence of the Disabled- Daly City**
Ste 256
355 Gellert Blvd
Daly City, CA 94015-2675
650-991-5124
Fax: 650-757-2075
TTY: 650-991-5182
dalycity5@aol.com
www.cidbelmont.org

Kent Mickelson, Director

The Daly City Branch office fulfills its mission by serving disabled consumers in Brisbane, Colma, Daly City, El Granada, Half Moon Bay, Montara, Moss Beach, Pacifica, Pescadero, Princeton and South San Francisco. Our mission is to increase the social, educational, economic, social and political participants of persons with disabilities in San Mateo county, California.

4009 **Center for Independent Living**
Suite 103
2001 Winward Way
San Mateo, CA 94404
650-645-1780
Fax: 650-645-1785
TTY: 510-522-9313
bburgess@cilberkeley.org
www.cidsanmateo.org

Beatrice Burgess, Interim Executive Director
Jody Yarborough, President
Michael Levinson, Vice President

The Center for Independent Living, Inc (CIL) is a national leader in helping people with disabilities live independently and become productive members of society. Advocates for greater accessibility in communities, designing techniques in independent living and providing direct services to people with disabilities.
1972

4010 **Center for Independent Living: East Oakland**
Suite 100
3075 Adeline Street
Berkeley, CA 94703-2403
510-841-4776
Fax: 510-841-6168
info@cilberkeley.org
www.cilberkeley.org

Melissa Male, Chair
Bea Worthen, Vice-Chair
Paul Hippolitus, Secretary

A national leader in helping people with disabilities live independently and become productive, fully participating members of society.

4011 **Center for Independent Living: Oakland**
Suite 100
3075 Adeline Street
Berkeley, CA 94703-1285
510-841-4776
Fax: 510-841-6168
TTY: 510-444-1837
info@cilberkeley.org
cilberkeley.org

Melissa Male, Chair
Bea Worthen, Vice-Chair
Paul Hippolitus, Secretary
Ted Dienstfrey, Finance Committee

A national leader in supporting disabled people in their efforts to lead independent lives.

4012 **Center for Independent Living: Tri-County**
2822 Harris Street
Eureka, CA 95503
707-445-8404
877-576-5000
Fax: 707-445-9751
TTY: 707-445-8405
aa@tilinet.org
www.tilinet.org

Gail Pascoe, President
Linda Arnold, Vice President
Kevin O'Brien, Treasurer
Chris Jones, Executive Director

4013 **Center for Independent Living:Fresno**
3475 Wesy Shaw Ave
Suite 101
Fresno, CA 93711
559-276-6777
Fax: 559-276-6778
TTY: 559-276-6779

Bob Hand, Manager

4014 **Center for Independent Living; Oakland**
1904 Franklin Street
Suite 320
Oakland, CA 94612-2324
510-763-9990
Fax: 510-763-4910
TTY: 510-536-2271
info@cilberkeley.org
cilberkeley.org

Melissa Male, Chair
Bea Worthen, Vice-Chair
Hank Stratford, Treasurer
Paul Hippolitus, Secretary

Independent living center to maximise the options for independence for persons with disabilities.

4015 **Center of Independent Living: Visalia**
121 E Main
Suite 101
Visalia, CA 93291-6262
559-622-9276
Fax: 559-622-9638

Fran Phillips, Executive Directorram Manager
Renee Ezelle, Manager

4016 **Central Coast Center for IL: San Benito**
1234 H Street
Suite 100
Sacramento, CA 95814-1914
916-325-1690
Fax: 916-325-1699
TTY: 916-325-1695
www.cfilc.org

Ana Acton, Chairperson
Larry Grable, Vice Chairperson
Nayana Shah, Treasurer
Jessie Lorenz, Secretary

To advocate for barrier-free access and equal opportunity for people with disabilities to participate in the community life by increasing the capacity of Independent Living Centers to achieve their missions.

4017 **Central Coast Center for Independent Living**
318 Cayuga St.
Suite 208
Salinas, CA 93901-2600
831-757-2968
Fax: 831-757-5549
TTY: 831-757-3949
cccil.org

Jennifer L. Williams, President
Elsa Quezada, Executive Director
Brenda Cardoza, Information and Referral Special
Gabriel Garcia, Independent Living Specialist

CCCIL promotes the independence of people with disabilities by supporting their equal and full participation in community life. CCCIL provides advocacy, education and support to all people with disabilities, their families and the community.

4018 **Central Coast Center: Independent Living - Santa Cruz Office**
1350 - 41st Avenue
Suite 101
Capitola, CA 95010-3930
831-462-8720
Fax: 831-462-8727
TTY: 831-462-8729
www.cccil.org

Jennifer L. Williams, President
Elsa Quezada, Executive Director
Brenda Cardoza, Information and Referral Special
Gabriel Garcia, Independent Living Specialist

CCCIL promotes the independence of people with disabilities by supporting their equal and full participation in community life. CCCIL provides advocacy, education and support to all people with disabilities, their families and the community.

4019 **Central Coast for Independent Living**
1111 San Felipe Rd
Suite 107
Hollister, CA 95023-2814
831-636-5196
Fax: 831-637-0478
TTY: 831-637-6235
www.cccil.org

Jennifer L. Williams, President
Elsa Quezada, Executive Director
Brenda Cardoza, Information and Referral Special
Gabriel Garcia, Independent Living Specialist

CCCIL promotes the independence of people with disabilities by supporting their equal and full particpation in community life. CCCIL provides advocacy, education and support to all people with disabilities, their families and the community.

4020 **Central Coast for Independent Living: Watsonville**
18 W. Beach St.
Suite Y
Watsonville, CA 95076-4371
831-724-2997
Fax: 831-724-2915
TTY: 831-786-0915
www.cccil.org

Jennifer L. Williams, President
Elsa Quezada, Executive Director
Brenda Cardoza, Information and Referral Special
Gabriel Garcia, Independent Living Specialist

An advocacy and information center organized by and for people with disabilities that strives to make our communities more accessible and to empower people with disabilities with information and skills to live fulfilling lives in our communities.

4021 **Communities Actively Living Independent and Free**
634 S Spring St
2nd Floor
Los Angeles, CA 90014-3921
213-627-0477
Fax: 213-627-0535
TTY: 213-623-9502
info@calif-ilc.org

Lillibeth Navarro, Founder & Executive Director
Alex San Martin, Temporary Chair
Fernando Roldan, Board Secretary
Ben Rockwell, Temporary Board Treasurer

Envisions a culturally diverse independent living center designed to empower the Disability Community.

4022 **Community Access Center**
6848 Magnolia Ave
Suite 150
Riverside, CA 92506-2858
951-274-0358
Fax: 951-274-0833
TTY: 951-274-0834
execdir@ilcac.org
www.ilcac.org

Mark Dyer, President
Janet Newcomer, Vice President
Perry Halteman, Secretary
Chuck Reutter, Treasurer

A non-profit organization; one of 29 similar programs throughout the state of California. CAC is a community resource, advocate, and educator for Riverside County residents with disabilities.

4023 **Community Access Center: Indio Branch**
83233 Indio Blvd
Indio, CA 92201-4748
760-347-4888
Fax: 760-347-0722
TTY: 760-347-6802
pmgr3@ilcac.org
www.ilcac.org

Mark Dyer, President
Janet Newcomer, Vice President
Perry Halteman, Secretary
Chuck Reutter, Treasurer

To empower persons with disabilities to control their own lives, create an accessible community and advocate to achieve complete social, economic, and political integration. We implement this vision by providing information, supportive services and independent living skills training.

4024 **Community Access Center: Perris**
371 Wilkerson Ave
Perris, CA 92570-2241 951-443-1158
Fax: 951-443-2608
TTY: 951-443-1158
www.ilcac.org

Mark Dyer, President
Janet Newcomer, Vice President
Perry Halteman, Secretary
Chuck Reutter, Treasurer
Community Access Center empowers persons with disabilities to control their own lives, create an accessible community and advocate to achieve complete social, economic, and political integration. CAC also implements this vision by providing information, suportive services and independent living skills training.

4025 **Community Rehabilitation Services**
844 E. Mission Road
Suite A & B
San Gabriel, CA 91776- 2759 323-266-0453
Fax: 626-614-1590
TTY: 323-266-3016

Frances Garcia, Executive Director
CRS is an independent living center that provides free services to persons with disabilities in the areas of advocacy, housing and independent living skills; assistive technology, employment, personal assistant services, peer counseling and information and referral.

4026 **Community Resources for Independence: Mendocino/Lake Branch**
Ste B
415 Talmage Rd
Ukiah, CA 95482-7486 707-463-8875
Fax: 707-463-8878
TTY: 707-463-4498

Tanner Silva, Manager
A non-profit corporation established by a group of disabled and non-disabled individuals to advance the rights of persons with disabilities to equal justice, access, opportunity and participation in the communities.

4027 **Community Resources for Independence: Napa**
Ste 208
1040 Main St
Napa, CA 94559-2605 707-258-0270
Fax: 707-258-0275
TTY: 707-257-0274

Tyler Stanley, Manager
Matthew Shultz, Independent Living Advocate
A non-profit corporation established by a group of disabled and non-disabled individuals to advance the rights of persons with disabilities to equal justice, access, opportunity and participation in the communities.

4028 **Community Resources for Independent Living: Hayward**
3311 Pacific Ave
Livermore, CA 94550-5013 925-371-1531
Fax: 925-373-5034
TTY: 925-371-1533
info@cril-online.org
crilhayward.org

Sheri Burns, Executive Director
Michael Galvan, PhD., Program Director
April Monroe, Finance Director
Esperanza Diaz-Alvarez, IL Coor - Travel Trainer & PAS
CRIL offers independent living services at no charge to persons with disabilities living in southern and eastern Alameda county. CRIL is also a resource for disability awareness education and training, advocacy and technical advice.

4029 **Community Resources for Independent Living**
39155 Liberty St
Suite A100
Fremont, CA 94538-1503 510-794-5735
crilhayward.org

Sheri Burns, Executive Director
Michael Galvan, PhD., Program Director
April Monroe, Finance Director
Esperanza Diaz-Alvarez, PAS Coordinator/Benefits Advocat
Community Resources for Independent Living is a peer-based disability organization that advocates and provides resources for people with disabilities to improve lives and make communities fully accessible.

4030 **DRAIL (Disability Resource Agency for Independent Living)**
501 W Weber Ave
Ste 200-A
Stockton, CA 95203-6239 209-477-8143
Fax: 209-477-7730
TTY: 209-465-5643
barry@drail.org
www.drail.org

Terry Gray, President
Michael Kim Cornelius, Treasurer
Adeline Bagwell, Secretary
Barry Smith, Executive Director
A non-profit corporation that is community based, consumer controlled, consumer choice, cross disability center for independent living.

4031 **Dayle McIntosh Center: Laguna Niguel**
24031 El Toro Road
Suite 300
Laguna Hills, CA 92653-3632 949-460-7784
800-422-7444
Fax: 949-334-2302
TTY: 800-735-2929
www.daylemc.org

Libby Partain, President
Cindy McLeroy, Vice President
Eva Casas-Sarmiento, Secretary
Michael Ryan, Treasurer
DMC advances empowerment and inclusion of all persons with disabilities. DMC is the largest Independent Living Center in California, and was named in memory of a young woman with a severe physical disability who worked to found the center.

4032 **Disability Resource Agency for Independent Living: Modesto**
920-12th Street
Modesto, CA 95354-543 209-521-7260
Fax: 209-521-4763
TTY: 209-576-2409
larry@drail.org
www.drail.org

Terry Gray, President
Michael Kim Cornelius, Treasurer
Adeline Bagwell, Secretary
Barry Smith, Executive Director
A non-profit corporation that is community based, consumer controlled, consumer choice, cross disability center for independent living.

4033 **Disability Services & Legal Center**
521 Mendocino Ave.
Santa Rosa, CA 95401-1649 707-528-2745
Fax: 707-528-9477
TTY: 707-528-2151
www.disabilityserviceandlegal.org

Adam Brown, Chairman
Shirley Johnson-Foell, Board President
Jack Geary, Board Member
Ben Karpilow, Board Secretary
A non-profit corporation established by a group of disabled and non-disabled individuals to advance the rights of persons with disabilities to equal justice, access, opportunity and participation in the communities.

4034 **Disabled Resources Center**
2750 E Spring St
Suite 100
Long Beach, CA 90806-2263
562-427-1000
Fax: 562-427-2027
TTY: 562-427-1366
info@drcinc.org
drcinc.org

C. Timothy Lashlee, President
Dora Hogan, Vice President
Finola Campbell, Treasurer
Dolores Nason, Executive Director

To empower people with disabilities to live independently in the community, to make their own decisions about their lives and to advocate on their own behalf.

4035 **FREED Center for Independent Living**
2059 Nevada City Hwy
Suite 102
Grass Valley, CA 95945- 3227
530-477-3333
800-655-7732
Fax: 530-477-8184
TTY: 530-477-8194
freed.org

Ana Acton, Executive Director

To eliminate barriers to full equality for people with disabilities through programs which promote independent living.

4036 **FREED Center for Independent Living: Marysville**
508 J St
Marysville, CA 95901-5636
530-742-4476
TTY: 530-742-4474
freed.org

Claudia Hallis, Manager

To eliminate barriers to full equality for people with disabilities through programs which promote independent living.

4037 **First Step Independent Living**
1174 Nevada St
Redlands, CA 92374-2893
800-362-0312

4038 **Independent Living Center of Kern County**
5251 Office Park Dr
Suite 200
Bakersfield, CA 93309
661-325-1063
877-688-2079
800-529-9541
Fax: 661-325-6702
TTY: 661-325-6702
info@ilcofkerncounty.org
www.ilcofkerncounty.org

Jimmie Soto, Executive Director
Tammy Hartsch, Finance Manager
Harvey Clowers, Special Projects and AT Coordina
Olivia Kent, Systems Change Advocate

A consumer-based consumer-directed non-profit agency assisting persons with disabilities to live independently in their community. The ILCKC presently offers a wide range of services to a growing population of persons with disabilities.

4039 **Independent Living Center of Lancaster**
606 East Avenue K4
Lancaster, CA 93535-2844
661-942-9726
Fax: 661-945-5690
TTY: 661-723-2509
www.ilcsc.org

Taura Jacob, Manager
Marcy Hernandez
Niyanta Dave

ILCSC is a non-profit, consumer based, non-residential agency providing a wide range of services to a growing population of people with disabilities. ILCSC is dedicated to empowering persons with disabilities to exercise indpendence-pofessionally, personally and creatively-while striving to educate the community on their needs.

4040 **Independent Living Resource Center**
7425 El Camino Real
Suite R
Atascadero, CA 93422-4656
805-464-3203
Fax: 805-462-1166
TTY: 805-462-1162
info@ilrc-trico.org
www.ilrc-trico.org

Kit McMillion, President
Larry Laborde, Vice President
Dani Anderson, Executive Director
Jennifer Griffin, Business Manager

To assist and encourage individuals to achieve their optimal level of self-sufficiency while eliminating the architectural, communication and attitudinal barriers which prevent them from full participation in the community.

4041 **Independent Living Resource Center: Santa Barbara**
423 W Victoria St
Santa Barbara, CA 93101-3619
805-284-9051
Fax: 805-963-1350
TTY: 805-963-0595
info@ilrc-trico.org
www.ilrc-trico.org

Kit McMillion, President
Larry Laborde, Vice President
Dani Anderson, Executive Director
Jennifer Griffin, Business Manager

To assist and encourage individuals to achieve their optimal level of self-sufficiency while eliminating the architectural, communication and attitudinal barriers which prevent them from full participation in the community.

4042 **Independent Living Resource Center: San Francisco**
825 Howard Street
San Francisco, CA 94103-4128
415-543-6222
Fax: 415-543-6318
TTY: 415-543-6698
info@ilrcsf.org
ilrcsf.org

Juma Byrd, President
Kolya Kirienko, Vice President
Ben MacMullan, Treasurer
Will Simpson, Secretary

To ensure that people with disabilities are full social and economic partners, both within their families and in a fully accessible community.

4043 **Independent Living Resource Center: Santa Maria Office**
327 East Plaza Dr
Suite 3A
Santa Maria, CA 93454-6930
805-354-5948
Fax: 805-349-2416
TTY: 805-925-0015
info@ilrc-trico.org
www.ilrc-trico.org

Kit McMillion, President
Larry Laborde, Vice President
Dani Anderson, Executive Director
Jennifer Griffin, Business Manager

To assist and encourage individuals to achieve their optimal level of self-sufficiency while eliminating the architectural, communication and attitudinal barriers which prevent them from full participation in the community.

4044 **Independent Living Resource Center: Ventura**
1802 Eastman Ave
Suite 112
Ventura, CA 93003-5759
805-256-1036
Fax: 805-650-9278
TTY: 805-650-5993
info@ilrc-trico.org
www.ilrc-trico.org

Kit McMillion, President
Larry Laborde, Vice President
Dani Anderson, Executive Director
Jennifer Griffin, Business Manager

An organization of, by and for persons with disabilities who reside or work in the service area. Purpose is to assist and encourage individuals to achieve their optimal level of self-sufficiency while eliminating the architectural, communication and attitudinal barriers which prevent them from full participation in the community.

4045 **Independent Living Resource of Contra Coast**
1850 Gateway Blvd
Suite 120
Concord, CA 94520-3293
925-363-7293
Fax: 925-363-7296
www.ilrscc.org

Sarah BirdwelL, Board President
Kathy Mitsopoulos, Board Vice President
Teri Ruggiero, Board Secretary
Susan Rotchy, Executive Director
Offers workshops, services are accessible to individuals with cognitive disabilities, physical disabilities, deaf and hard of hearing, emotional disabilities, visual impairments, learing disabilities and seniors.

4046 **Independent Living Resource of Fairfield**
470 Chadbourn Rd
Ste. B
Fairfield, CA 94534
707-435-8174
Fax: 707-435-8177
www.ilrscc.org

Sarah BirdwelL, Board President
Kathy Mitsopoulos, Board Vice President
Teri Ruggiero, Board Secretary
Susan Rotchy, Executive Director
To empower people with disabilities to: control their own lives, provide advocacy and support for individuals with disabilities to live independently, create an accessible community free of physical and attitudinal barriers.

4047 **Independent Living Resource: Antioch**
3727 Sunset Lane
#103
Antioch, CA 94509-1761
925-754-0539
TTY: 925-755-0934
www.ilrscc.org

Sarah BirdwelL, Board President
Kathy Mitsopoulos, Board Vice President
Teri Ruggiero, Board Secretary
Susan Rotchy, Executive Director
Non-profit organizations run and controlled by persons with disabilities. They are non-residential, community-based centers where people with disabilities can receive assistance with a variety of daily living issues and learn the skills they need to take controll of their lives from people who have had similar experiences living with a disability.

4048 **Independent Living Resource: Concord**
1850 Gateway Blvd
Suite 120
Concord, CA 94520-3293
925-363-7293
Fax: 925-363-7296
gilc@ilrccc.org
www.ilrscc.org

Sarah BirdwelL, Board President
Kathy Mitsopoulos, Board Vice President
Teri Ruggiero, Board Secretary
Susan Rotchy, Executive Director
To empower people with disabilities to: control their own lives, provide advocacy and support for individuals with disabilities to live independently, create an accessible community free of physical and attitudinized barriers.

4049 **Independent Living Resources (ILR)**
Bldg 2a
101 Broadway
Richmond, CA 94804-1945
510-233-7400
info@ilrccc.org

Marvin Dyson, Manager
Provides services to meet the diverse needs of people who have a variety of disabilities in all age groups.

4050 **Independent Living Service Northern California: Redding Office**
169 Hartnell Ave
Suite 128
Redding, CA 96002-1849
530-242-8550
800-464-8527
Fax: 530-241-1454
TTY: 530-242-8550
actionctr.org

Lauri Evans, President
Frank Smith, Vice President
Evan Levang, Executive Director
Tracy Barker, Program Manager
Independent Living Services of Northern California is a private non profit organization that provides support services to help empower community members with disabilities.

4051 **Independent Living Services of Northern California**
Jennifer Roberts Building
1161 East Ave
Chico, CA 95926-1018
530-893-8527
800-464-8527
Fax: 530-893-8574
TTY: 530-893-8527
actionctr.org

Lauri Evans, President
Frank Smith, Vice President
Evan Levang, Executive Director
Tracy Barker, Program Manager
Independent Living Services of Northern California is a private, non profit organization that provides support services to help empower community members with disabilities.

4052 **Marin Center for Independent Living**
710 4th St
San Rafael, CA 94901-3213
415-459-6245
Fax: 415-459-7047
TTY: 415-459-7027
marincil.org

Chris Schultz, President
Joe Brnnett, Vice President
Eli Gelardin, Executive Director
Susan Malardino, Deputy Director
A non-profit organization that provides advocacy and services for seniors and persons with disabilities.

4053 **Mother Lode Independent Living Center (DRAIL: Disability Resource Agency for Independent**
Living)
67 Linoberg St
Suite A.
Sonora, CA 95370-4646
209-532-0963
Fax: 209-532-1591
TTY: 209-288-3309
barry@drail.org
www.drail.org

Terry Gray, President
Michael Kim Cornelius, Treasurer
Adeline Bagwell, Secretary
Barry Smith, Executive Director
DRAIL is a non-profit, community based, consumer controlled, cross disability center for independent living.

4054 **Placer Independent Resource Services**
11768 Atwood Rd
Suite 29
Auburn, CA 95603
530-885-6100
800-833-3453
Fax: 530-885-3032
TTY: 530-885-0326
lbrewer@pirs.org
pirs.org

Eldon Luce, President
Michael Cummings, Vice President
Dan Roye, Director
Peter Beckh, Treasurer
A non profit independent living center whose mission is to advocate, empower, educate and provide services for people with disabilities that would enable them to live more independently.

4055 **Resources for Independent Living**
420 i St, Level B.
Suite 3
Sacramento, CA 95814-2319
916-446-3074
Fax: 916-446-2443
leonc@ril-sacramento.org
www.ril-sacramento.org

Ramona Garcia, Board Chairperson
Francisco Godoy, Vice Chairperson
Joanne Bodine, Treasurer
Frances Gracechild, Executive Director

Promoting the socio-economic independence of persons with disabilities by providing peer-supported, consumer-directed independent living services and advocacy.

4056 **Rolling Start**
570 W 4th St
Suite 107
San Bernardino, CA 92401-1438
909-884-2129
Fax: 909-386-7446
TTY: 909-884-7396

John Anaya, Chairperson
Kathi Pryor, Treasurer
Francis Bates, Executive Director
Tony Chavez, Deputy Director

Empowers and educates people with disabilities to achieve the independent life of their choice.

4057 **Rolling Start: Victorville**
17330 Bear Valley Road
Suite A102
Victorville, CA 92395
760-843-7959
Fax: 760-843-7977
TTY: 760-951-8175

John Anaya, Chairperson
Kathi Pryor, Treasurer
Francis Bates, Executive Director
Tony Chavez, Deputy Director

Empowers and educates people with disabilities to achieve the independent life of their choice.

4058 **Services Center For Independent Living**
107 S Spring Street
Claremont, CA 91711-549
909-621-6722
800-491-6722
Fax: 909-445-0727
TTY: 949-445-0726
www.scil-ilc.org

Larry Grable, Executive Director
Janice Ornelas, Independent Living Specialist
Angela Nwokike, System Change Advocate
Albert Gonzales, Benefits Specialist

Dedicated to expanding access, information and resources to help increase independence and enhance the quality of life for the East San Gabriel Valley residents with disabilities.

4059 **Silicon Valley Independent Living Center**
25 N. 14th St.
Suite 1000, 10th floor
San Jose, CA 95112
408-894-9041
Fax: 669-231-4795
info@svilc.org
svilc.org

Patricia Kokes, President
Richard A. Wentz, Vice President
Gabe Lopez, Treasurer
Nayana Shah, Executive Director

A private, consumer-driven, nonprofit corporation that offers quality services to individuals with disabilities in Silicon Valley.

4060 **Silicon Valley Independent Living Center: South County Branch**
7881 Church Street
Suite C
Gilroy, CA 95020-7346
408-843-9100
Fax: 408-842-4791
TTY: 408-842-2591
info@svilc.org
svilc.org

Patricia Kokes, President
Richard A. Wentz, Vice President
Gabe Lopez, Treasurer
Nayana Shah, Executive Director

A private, consumer-driven, non-profit corporation that offers quality services to individuals with disabilities in Silicon Valley.

4061 **Southern California Rehabilitation Services**
7830 Quill Dr
Suite D
Downey, CA 90242-3440
562-862-6531
Fax: 562-923-5274
TTY: 562-869-0931
scrs-ilc.org

Lisa Hayes, President
Michael Strong, Vice President
Carol Trees, Secretary/Treasurer
Chad Williams, Board Member

Empowers persons with disabilities to achieve their personalized goals through community education and individualized services that provide the knowledge, skills, and confidence building to maximize their quality of life.

4062 **Through the Looking Glass**
3075 Adeline St.
Ste. 120
Berkeley, CA 94703
510-848-1112
800-644-2666
Fax: 510-848-4445
TTY: 510-848-1005
tlg@lookingglass.org
www.lookingglass.org

Maureen Block, J.D., Board President
Thomas Spalding, Board Treasurer
Alice Nemon, D.S.W., Board Secretary
Karen Fessel, Ph.D., Executive Director

To create, demonstrate and encourage non-pathological and empowering reesources and model early intervention services for families with disability issues in parent or child which integrate expertise derived from personal disability experience and disability culture.

4063 **Tri-County Independent Living Center**
2822 Harris Street
Eureka, CA 95503
707-445-8404
877-576-5000
Fax: 707-445-9751
TTY: 707-445-8405
aa@tilinet.org
www.tilinet.org

Gail Pascoe, President
Linda Arnold, Vice President
Kevin O'Brien, Treasurer
Chris Jones, Executive Director

Promotes the philosophy of independent living, to connect individuals to services, and to create and accessible community, so that people with disabilities can have control over their lives and full access to the communities in which they live.

4064 **Westside Center for Independent Living**
12901 Venice Blvd
Los Angeles, CA 90066-3509
310-390-3611
888-851-9245
Fax: 310-390-4906
TTY: 310-398-9204
www.wcil.org

David Geffen, President
Chris Knauf, 1st Vice President
Brenda Green, Secretary
Aliza Barzilay, Executive Director

The Westside Center for Independent Living (WCIL) helps people living with disabilities maintain self-sufficient and productive lives through non-residential peer support services and training programs. Independent Living promotes self-determination, community living, full participation in community life and access to the same opportunities and resources available to people without disabilities.

Colorado

4065 Atlantis Community
201 S Cherokee St
Denver, CO 80223-1836
303-733-9324
Fax: 303-733-6211
TTY: 303-733-0047
info@atlantiscommunity.org
David Hays, Manager
Provide direct services, and to empower people with disabilities integrating, with full and equal rights, into all parts of society including employment, affordable, accessible, housing, transportation, recreation, communication, education, and public places while exercising and exerting choice and self determination.

4066 Center for Independence
740 Gunnison Ave
Grand Junction, CO 81501-3222
708-588-0833
Fax: 708-588-0406
center-for-independence.org
Linda Taylor, Executive Director
The Center for Independence works to promote community solutions and to empower individuals with disabilities to live independently.

4067 Center for People with Disabilities
615 Main St
Longmont, CO 80501-4983
303-772-3250
Fax: 303-772-5125
TTY: 303-772-3250
info@cpwd.org
www.cpwd-ilc.org
Dale Gaar, Board President
Deborah.A Conley, Board Vice President
Nancy Phares-Zook, Board Secretary
Tony Adams, Board Treasurer
Provides resources, information, and advocacy to assist people with disabilities in overcoming barriers to independent living.

4068 Center for People with Disabilities: Pueblo
1304 Berkley Ave
Pueblo, CO 81004-3002
719-546-1271
800-659-3656
Fax: 719-546-1374
ivaleneamidei@yahoo.com
www.ilcpueblo.org
Larry Williams, Executive Director
One of the 10 centers for independent living in Colorado founded under Title VII of the Rehabilitation Act of 1973 as amended in 1978. All new centers under this Independent Living (CIL) Title of the Act received initial and ongoing grants through this new Federal Program created by the Act.

4069 Center for People with Disabilities: Boulder
1675 Range St
Boulder, CO 80301-2722
303-442-8662
888-929-5519
Fax: 303-442-0502
info@cpwd.org
www.cpwd-ilc.org
Dale Gaar, Board President
Deborah.A Conley, Board Vice President
Nancy Phares-Zook, Board Secretary
Tony Adams, Board Treasurer
Providing resources, information and advocacy to people with disabilities. Assist people with disabilities in transitioning from nursing homes to independent living in the community. Also provide personal assistance services.

4070 Colorado Springs Independence Center
729 South Tejon Street
Colorado Springs, CO 80903
719-471-8181
Fax: 719-471-7829
TTY: 719-471-2076
www.theindependencecenter.org
Billy A., Chair Elect
Billy B., Secretary
Dean C., Treasurer
To empower persons with disabilities to maximize their independence within the community and to remove barriers which impact their quality of life, while encouraging them to live independently in their community.

4071 Connections for Independent Living
1331 8th Avenue
Greeley, CO 80631-4027
970-352-8682
800-887-5828
Fax: 970-353-8058
TTY: 970-352-8682
pattid4z@yahoo.com
www.connectionsforindependentliving.org
Beth Danielson, Executive Director
Michael Stevens, Director of Services
Alicia Garza, Director
Dianna Shmidl, Community Transition Specialist
Certified IL Center, I and R advocacy, peer support, skills training, sign language interpretations, reader services, housing. Cross-disability, all ages.

4072 Denver CIL
Ste 100
777 Grant St
Denver, CO 80203-3501
303-837-1020
Fax: 303-837-0859
www.denverhousing.org
Greg Beran, Owner
Ismael Guerrero, Executive Director
Joshua Crawley, Agency Counsel
Nichole Ford, Chief Financial Officer
Provides resources, information, and advocacy to assist people with disabilities in overcoming barriers to independent living.

4073 Disability Center for Independent Living
4821 East 38th Avenue
Denver, CO 80207-1232
303-320-1345
Fax: 303-320-1345
TTY: 303-322-2330
avillasenor.dcil@gmil.com
www.accil.net
Larry Williams, Executive Director
John Wooster, Consultant
Anthony Gonzales, Housing Coordinator
Jenna Emery, OBI Specialist
Independent living center providing quality services for people with disabilities.

4074 Disabled Resource Services
1017 Robertson Street
Unit B
Fort Collins, CO 80524-3915
970-482-2700
Fax: 970-449-6972
TTY: 970-407-7060
disabledresourceservices.org
George Tremblay, Chairman
John Weins, Vice Chairman
Nancy Jackson, Executive Director
Marj Grell, Office Manager
To empower individuals with disabilities to achieve their maximum level of independence and to gain personal dignity within society. Disabled Resource Services, as a private non-profit state certified center for independent living, is dedicated to working with individuals with all types of disabilities in Larimer County to promote their independence and equality through services which support advocacy, awareness and access to their community.

4075 **Disbled Resource Services**
640 E Eisenhower Blvd
Loveland, CO 80537-3954
970-667-0816
Fax: 970-593-6582
disabledresourceservices.org

George Tremblay, Chairman
John Weins, Vice Chairman
Nancy Jackson, Executive Director
Marj Grell, Office Manager

To empower individuals with disabilities to achieve their maximum level of independence and to gain personal dignity within society.

4076 **Greeley Center for Independence**
2780 28th Ave
Greeley, CO 80634-7803
970-339-2444
800-748-1012
Fax: 970-339-0033
gciinc@gciinc.org
www.gciinc.org

Chari Armagost, Chief Financial Officer
Sarita Reddy, PH. D, Executive Director
Rob Rabe, Director of Outpatient Service
Dee Seekamp, Director of Nursing

Provides places of growth, transition and encouragement, where people with temporary and permanent disabilities can reach toward their maximum potential of personal independence and wellness.

4077 **Independent Life Center**
P.O. Box 612
Craig, CO 81626-612
970-826-0833
888-526-0833
Fax: 970-826-0832
TTY: 970-826-0833

Larry Williams, Executive Director
John Wooster, Consultant
Anthony Gonzales, Housing Coordinator
Jenna Emery, OBI Specialist

Provides resources, information, and advocacy to assist people with disabilities in overcoming barriers to independent living.

4078 **Southwest Center for Independence**
3473 Main Avenue
#23
Durango, CO 81301-5474
970-259-1672
866-962-2158
Fax: 970-259-0947
TTY: 970-259-1672
swindependence.org/

Martha Mason, Executive Director
Mariellen Walz, Chair
Patricia Ziegler, Assistant Director
Jason Armstrong, Treasurer

Empowering individuals with disabilities and their families to achieve their maximum level of independence in work, play and other areas of life.

4079 **Southwest Center for Independence: Cortez**
2409 East Empire Street
PO Box 640
Cortez, CO 81321-9164
970-570-8001
866-962-2158
Fax: 970-565-7169
director@swilc.org
swindependence.org/

Mariellen Walz, Chair
Johnny Bulson, Vice Chair
Jason Armstrong, Treasurer
Martha Mason, Executive Director

Empowers individiuals with disabilities and their families to achieve their maximum level of independence in work, play and other areas of life.

Connecticut

4080 **Center for Disability Rights**
764-B Campbell Ave
764 Campbell Ave
W Haven, CT 06516- 3786
203-934-7077
Fax: 203-934-7078
TTY: 203-934-7079
info@cdr-ct.org
cdr-ct.org

Marc Gallucci, Executive Director
Chris Zurcher, Consumer Relations
Dana Canevari, I&R Specialist
Susan St. John, Administrative Assistant

Resources, information, and advocacy to assist people with disabilities in overcoming barriers to independent living.

4081 **Center for Independent Living SC**
26 Palmers Hill Rd
Stamford, CT 06902-2113
203-353-8550
Fax: 203-353-1423
TTY: 203-353-8550

Dana Canevari, Director

Provides resources, information, and advocacy to assist people with disabilities in overcoming barriers to independent living.

4082 **Chapel Haven**
1040 Whalley Ave
New Haven, CT 06515-1740
203-397-1714
Fax: 203-937-2466
admissions@chapelhaven.org
chapelhaven.org

Michael Storz, President

The only combined state-accredited special education facility and independent living facility for adults with cognitive disabilities.

4083 **Connecticut State Independent Living Council**
151 New Park Ave
Hartford, CT 06106
860-523-0126
Fax: 860-523-5603
info@ctsilc.org
ctsilc.org

Katherine Pellerin, President
Keith Mullinar, Vice President
Alexia Bouckoms, Treasurer
Daria Smith, Executive Director

The mission of the council is to promote equal access, opportunities, and social inclusion for people with disabilities in all spheres of society.

4084 **Disabilities Network of Eastern Connecticut**
19 Ohio Avenue
Suite 2
Norwich, CT 06360-2111
860-823-1898
Fax: 860-886-2316
CFerry@dnec.org
dnec.org

Katherine Pellerin, President
Robert Davidson, Vice President
Jane O'Friel, Secretary/Treasurer
Cathy Ferry, Executive Director

Dedicated to supporting and advancing the rights of individuals with disabilities. The goal is to creat a completely inclusive society where people live together in communities regardless of their abilities.

4085 **Disability Resource Center of Fairfield County**
80 Ferry Blvd
Suite 205
Stratford, CT 06615-6079
203-378-6977
Fax: 203-375-2748
TTY: 203-378-3248
www.accessinct.org

Ethel M R, President
Thomas D, Vice-President
Anthony Lacava, Executive Director
Glenn Calaffin, Program Director

A crosss-disability resource and advocacy organization for people with disabilities that has provided unique, consumer-directed services both for individuals and for the communities of Fairfield County.

4086 Independence Northwest Center for Independent Living
1183 New Haven Rd
Suite 200
Naugatuck, CT 06770-5033
203-729-3299
Fax: 203-729-2839
TTY: 203-729-1281
info@independencenorthwest.org
www.independencenorthwest.org

Maureen Mayo, President
Tom Ford, Vice President
Charles Marino, Treasurer
Jaff Laliberte, Secretary
Provides services in such areas as peer counseling, advocacy, independent living skills training and information and referral.

4087 New Horizons Village
37 Bliss Rd
Unionville, CT 06085
860-673-8893
Fax: 860-675-4369
Michael.Shaw@NewHorizonsVillage.com
newhorizonsvillage.com

Carolyn Fields, Administrator
A 68 unit apartment complex designed for people who have severe physical disabilities.

Delaware

4088 Freedom Center for Independent Living
400 N Broad St
Middletown, DE 19709-1089
302-376-4399
866-687-3245
Fax: 302-376-4395
TTY: 302-376-4397
info@fcilde.org
fcilde.org

Hersernest Cole, Executive Director
Lillian Evans, Independent Living Specialist
Protects the Civil Rights and promote the empowerment of persons with disabilities and their families through our independent living philosophy.

4089 Independent Living
Apt 210
1800 N Broom St
Wilmington, DE 19802-3854
302-429-6693
Fax: 302-429-8031
TTY: 302-429-8034

Susan Cycyk, Executive Director
Providing skilled support and caring guidance to adults with disabilities. Our case management services include: daily living skills training, medical coordination, transportation assistance, financial management, housing assistance, and vocational/educational planning.

4090 Independent Resource Georgetown
Ste 37
410 S Bedford St
Georgetown, DE 19947-1850
302-854-9330
Fax: 302-854-9408
TTY: 302-854-9340

Larry Henderson, Director
Pat Boyd, Manager
Provides independent living services to persons who experience a significant disability. Offers skills training, individually and in small groups, peer support/peer counseling and information and referral services. Strives to remove the architectural and attitudnal barriers through individual and systems advocacy.

4091 Independent Resources: Dover
154 South Governor's Avenue
Dover, DE 19904-7311
302-735-4599
Fax: 302-735-5623
TTY: 302-735-5629
lhenderson@independentresources.org
www.iri-de.org

Tes DelTufo, Office Director
Carolyn Miller, IL Specialist
Debbie Justice, IL Specialist
Barty Rochester, Peer Support Coordinator
Private, non-profit, consumer-controlled, community based organization providing services and advocacy by and for persons with all types of disabilities. Their goal is to assist individuals with disabilities to achieve their maximum potential within their families and communities.

4092 Independent Resources: Wilmington
6 Denny Rd
Suite 101
Wilmington, DE 19809-3444
302-765-0191
Fax: 302-765-0195
TTY: 302-765-0194
www.iri-de.org

Larry D Henderson, Executive Director
Phyllis Farrare, Director of Operations
Private, non-profit, consumer-controlled, community based organization providing services and advocacy by and for persons with all types of disabilities. Their goal is to assist individuals with disabilities to achieve their maximum potential within their families and communities.

4093 Mosaic Of De
4980 S. 118TH ST
Omaha, NE 68137
302-456-5995
877-366-7242
Fax: 402-896-1511
info@mosaicinfo.org
mosaicinfo.org

Terry Olson, Executive Director
Linda Timmons, President and CEO
Raul Saldivar, Chief Operating Officer
Cindy Schroeder, Chief Financial Officer
Provides services to adults with developmental disabilities who reside in homes and apartments. Services are designed to provide them with opportunities for choices and participation in the life of their communities. Supports are geared to assist each individual in becoming more independent in activities of daily living, vocational skills, community mobility and transportation, and recreation and leisure activities.

District of Columbia

4094 District of Columbia Center for Independent Living
1400 Florida Ave NE
Washington, DC 20002-5032
202-388-0033
Fax: 202-398-3018
info@dccil.org
dccil.org

Rev. Patric Hailes Fears, President
Dr. John Thompson, Vice President
Carl Bartels, Treasurer
Angela Washington, Secretary
Mission is to maximize the leadership, empowerment, independence, and productivity of individuals with disabilities, and to integrate these individuals into the mainstream of American society.

4095 **National Council on Independent Living**
2013 H St. NW
6th Floor
Washington, DC 20006
202-207-0334
844-778-7961
Fax: 202-207-0341
TTY: 202-207-0340
ncil@ncil.org
www.ncil.org

Kelly Buckland, Executive Director
Tim Fuchs, Director, Operations
Cara Liebowitz, Coordinator, Development
Eleanor Canter, Coordinator, Communications

A national cross-disability grassroots organization, NCIL advances independent living and the rights of people with disabilities through consumer-driven advocacy.

Florida

4096 **Ability 1st**
1300 E. Green Street
Pasadena, CA 91106
626-396-1010
877-768-4600
Fax: 626-396-1021
info@abilityfirst.org
abilityfirst.org

Steve Brockmeyer, Chairman
John Kelly, Vice Chairman
Lori.E Gangemi, President
Kevin Schaffels, CFO

To empower persons with disabilities to live independently and participate actively in their community.

4097 **Adult Day Training**
Goodwill Industries - Suncoast
10596 Gandy Blvd N
St Petersburg, FL 33702-1422
727-523-1512
888-279-1988
Fax: 727-563-9300
TTY: 727-579-1068
gw.marketing@goodwill-suncoast.com
www.goodwill-suncoast.org

Oscar J. Horton, Chairman
Martin W. Gladysz, Vice Chairman
Heather Ceresoli, Vice Chairman
Deborah.A Passerini, President

An innovative program which uses job skills to teach self-help, daily living, communication, mobility, travel, decision-making, behavioral and social skills. This focus provides concrete, transferable experiences to help prepare individuals for greater community inclusion by achieving the highest possible degree of independence in their daily life, increasing their confidence and supporting their successful transitions to less structured, self-sufficient environments.

4098 **CIL of Central Florida**
720 N Denning Dr
Winter Park, FL 32789-3020
407-623-1070
Fax: 407-623-1390
info@cilorlando.org
cilorlando.org

Jason Vennings, Development Director
Kim Byerly, Chair
Cheryl Stone, Secretary
Don Pirozzoli, M.S., Programs Director

A private, non-profit organization dedicated to helping people with disabilities achieve their self-determined goals for independent living.

4099 **Caring and Sharing Center for Independent Living**
12552 Belcher Rd S
Largo, FL 33773-3014
727-539-7550
866-539-7550
Fax: 727-539-7588
www.disabilityachievementcenter.org

Barbara Dandro, Treasurer
Mary Bucca, Secretary
Patricia Bell, Director
Dennis Shelt, Director

Empowering people with disabilities.

4100 **Caring and Sharing Center: Pasco County**
12552 Belcher Rd S
Largo, FL 33773-3014
727-539-7550
866-539-7550
Fax: 727-539-7588
www.disabilityachievementcenter.org

Barbara Dandro, Treasurer
Mary Bucca, Secretary
Patricia Bell, Director
Dennis Shelt, Director

Empowering people with disabilities.

4101 **Center for Independent Living in Central Florida**
720 N Denning Dr
Winter Park, FL 32789-3095
407-623-1070
Fax: 407-623-1390
info@cilorlando.org
cilorlando.org

Jason Vennings, Development Director
Kim Byerly, Chair
Cheryl Stone, Secretary
Don Pirozzoli, M.S., Programs Director

In partnership with the community, promotes personal right snad responsiblities among people with all disabilities.

4102 **Center for Independent Living of Broward**
4800 N State Road 7
Suite 102
Lauderdale Lakes, FL 33319-5811
954-722-6400
888-722-6400
Fax: 954-735-1958
cilb@cilbroward.org
www.cilbroward.org

Craig Lilienthal, President
Christopher Sharp, VP
Shea Smith, Treasurer
Laurie Menekou, Secretary

Offers assistance to people with disabilities in fulfilling the goals of independence and self-sufficiency.

4103 **Center for Independent Living of Florida Keys**
103400 Overseas Hwy
Suite 243
Key Largo, FL 33037-2849
305-453-3491
877-335-0187
Fax: 305-453-3488
TTY: 305-453-3491
cilkeys@cilkeys.org
www.cilofthekeys.org

Brenda K Pierce, Executive Director

Offers assistance to persons with disabilities in acquiring independent living and self-advocacy skills in order to obtain and maintain independence and self-sufficiency.

4104 **Center for Independent Living of N Florida**
1823 Buford Ct
Tallahassee, FL 32308-4465
850-575-9621
Fax: 850-575-5740
TTY: 850-575-5245
cilnf@nettally.com
www.ability1st.info

Judith Barrett, Executive Director

Offers assistance to persons with disabilities in acquiring independent living and self-advocacy skills in order to obtain and maintain independence and self-sufficiency

4105 **Center for Independent Living of NW Florida**
3600 N Pace Blvd
Pensacola, FL 32505-4240
850-595-5566
877-245-2457
Fax: 850-595-5560
cil-drc@cil-drc.org
cil-drc.org

James Hicks, President
Kathleen Wilks, Secretary
John Bouchard, Treasurer
Frank Cherry, Executive Director

Provides services such as information and referral, peer counseling, housing, advocacy, training, independent living skills training, free wheelchairs, loan locker, assistive technology.

4106 **Center for Independent Living of North Central Florida**
3445 NE 24th Street
Ocala, FL 34470-9214
352-368-3788
877-232-8261
Fax: 352-629-0098
www.cilncf.org

Joe Dyke, President
Robert Miller, Vice President
David Christie, Treasurer
Jim Gorske, Secretary

Empowers people with disabilities to exert their individual rights to live as independently as possible, make personal life choices and achieve full community inclusion.

4107 **Center for Independent Living of North Central Florida**
222 SW 36th Ter
Gainesville, FL 32607-2863
352-378-7474
800-265-5724
Fax: 352-378-5582
TTY: 352-372-3443
www.cilncf.org

Joe Dyke, President
Robert Miller, Vice President
David Christie, Treasurer
Jim Gorske, Secretary

Empowering people with disabilities to exert their individual rights to live as independently as possible, make personal life choices and achieve full community inclusion.

4108 **Center for Independent Living of S Florida**
6660 Biscayne Blvd
Miami, FL 33138-6285
305-751-8025
Fax: 305-751-8944
TTY: 305-751-8891
soflacil.org

Alvin W. Roberts, President
Gregg Goldfarb, Vice President
Timothy Werner, Ph.D, Secretary
Jay Weiss, M.B.A., Treasurer

A community based non for profit, independent living center serving people of all ages with any type of disability. Services: Basic education, GED preperation, American sign language advocacy, peer support, information and referral, independent living skills training, housing assistance, transportation assistance, home modiifications, transition from nursing facility to the community assisatnace filing ADA complaints, accessibility surveys, diability awareness traing.

4109 **Center for Independent Living of SW Florida**
2321 Bruner Ln
Fort Myers, FL 33912-1904
239-277-1447
800-435-7352
Fax: 239-277-1647

Ronald J Muschong, Interim Executive Director

Helping people with disabilities achieve independence and self-determination in their lives.

4110 **Coalition for Independent Living Options: Okeechobee**
1680 SW Bayshore Boulevard
Suite 231
Port St. Lucie, FL 34984
772-878-3500
Fax: 772-878-3344
www.cilo.org

Scott Shoemaker, President
Sharon D'Eusanio, Vice President
Joseph Fields Jr., Esquire, Secretary
Genevieve Cousminer,Esq, Executive Director

Private non-profit promoting independences for people with disabilities in Palm Beach, Martin, St. Lucie & Okeechobee Counties. Services include advocacy, independent living skills & training, peer support, after school & summer programs for teens, crime victim support services, and veterans transition services.

4111 **Coalition for Independent Living Options: Fort Pierce**
6800 Forest HIll Boulevard
West Palm Beach, FL 33413
561-966-4288
Fax: 561-966-0441
www.cilo.org

Scott Shoemaker, President
Sharon D'Eusanio, Vice President
Joseph Fields Jr., Esquire, Secretary
Genevieve Cousminer,Esq, Executive Director

Private non-profit promoting independences for people with disabilities in Palm Beach, Martin, St. Lucie & Okeechobee Counties. Services include advocacy, independent living skills & training, peer support, after school & summer programs for teens, crime victim support services, and verterans transition services.

4112 **Coalition for Independent Living Options**
6800 Forest HIll Boulevard
West Palm Beach, FL 33413-3310
561-966-4288
Fax: 561-966-0441
www.cilo.org

Scott Shoemaker, President
Sharon D'Eusanio, Vice President
Joseph Fields Jr., Esquire, Secretary
Genevieve Cousminer,Esq, Executive Director

Private non-profit promoting independences for people with disabilities in Palm Beach, Martin, St. Lucie & Okeechobee Counties. Services include advocacy, independent living skills & training, peer support, after school & summer programs for teens, crime victim support services, and verterans transition services.

4113 **Coalition for Independent Living Options: Stuart**
1680 SW Bayshore Boulevard
Suite 231
Port St. Lucie, FL 34984
772-878-3500
Fax: 772-878-3344
www.cilo.org

Scott Shoemaker, President
Sharon D'Eusanio, Vice President
Joseph Fields Jr., Esquire, Secretary
Genevieve Cousminer,Esq, Executive Director

Private non-profit promoting independences for people with disabilities in Palm Beach, Martin, St. Lucie & Okeechobee Counties. Services include advocacy, independent living skills & training, peer support, after school & summer programs for teens, crime victim support services, and verterans transition services.

4114 **Disability Resource Center**
300 W. 5th St.
Panama City, FL 32401-4704
850-769-6890
Fax: 850-769-6891
outreach@drcpc.org
www.drcpc.org

Robert Cox, Executive Director
Becky Cadwell, Independent Living Specialist

They are commiteed to collaborating with other disability/consumer-focused organizations in their community

4115 **Lakeland Adult Day Training**
3033 Drane Field Rd
Suite 5
Lakeland, FL 33811-3305
863-701-1351
TTY: 863-701-1356
gw.marketing@goodwill-suncoast.com
www.goodwill-suncoast.org

Oscar J. Horton, Chairman
Martin W. Gladysz, Vice Chairman
Heather Ceresoli, Vice Chairman
Deborah.A Passerini, President

An innovative program which uses job skills to teach self-help, daily living, communication, mobility, travel, decision-making, behavioral and social skills. This focus provides concrete, transferable experiences to help prepare individuals for greater community inclusion by achieving the highest possible degree of independence in their daily life, increasing their confidence and supporting their successful transitions to less structured, self-sufficient environments.

4116 **Lighthouse Central Florida**
215 E New Hampshire St
Orlando, FL 32804-6403
407-898-2483
Fax: 407-895-5255
lvaneepoel@lcf-fl.org
www.lighthousecentralflorida.com

Alex B. Hull, Chair
David Stahl, Vice Chair
Paul Prewitt, Secretary
Nancy L. Urbach, Treasurer

Promote the independence and success of people living with vision impairment.

4117 **Miami-Dade County Disability Services and Independent Living (DSAIL)**
701 NW 1st Court
Miami, FL 33136-1647
786-469-4600
Fax: 305-547-7355
www.miamidade.gov

Michael Moxam, Manager
Lucia Davis-Raiford, Director

Offers information and referral services serving all types of disabilities with the goal of assisting the disabled acquiring independence and control over their lives. Teaches independent living skills, job readiness and placement, home health care, sensitivity training, training in ASL and Braille, counsel people with disabilities or wide range of problems.

4118 **Ocala Adult Day Training**
2920 W Silver Springs Blvd
Ocala, FL 34475-5654
352-629-0456
TTY: 352-629-0874
gw.marketing@goodwill-suncoast.com
www.goodwill-suncoast.org

Oscar J. Horton, Chairman
Martin W. Gladysz, Vice Chairman
Heather Ceresoli, Vice Chairman
Deborah.A Passerini, President

An innovative program which uses job skills to teach self-help, daily living, communication, mobility, travel, decision-making, behavioral and social skills. This focus provides concrete, transferable experiences to help prepare individuals for greater community inclusion by achieving the highest possible degree of independence in their daily life, increasing their confidence and supporting their successful transitions to less structured, self-sufficient environments.

4119 **Pinellas Park Adult Day Training**
7601 Park Blvd
Pinellas Park, FL 33781-3704
727-541-6205
TTY: 727-544-5835
gw.marketing@goodwill-suncoast.com
www.goodwill-suncoast.org

Oscar J. Horton, Chairman
Martin W. Gladysz, Vice Chairman
Heather Ceresoli, Vice Chairman
Deborah.A Passerini, President

An innovative program which uses job skills to teach self-help, daily living, communication, mobility, travel, decision-making, behavioral and social skills. This focus provides concrete, transferable experiences to help prepare individuals for greater community inclusion by achieving the highest possible degree of independence in their daily life, increasing their confidence and supporting their successful transitions to less structured, self-sufficient environments.

4120 **SCCIL at Titusville**
571-W Haverty Court
Rockledge, FL 32955
321-633-6011
Fax: 321-633-6472
TTY: 706-724-6324
jilldunham9@gmail.com
www.virtualcil.net

Jill Dunham-Schuller, Executive Director

Directory of Independent Living Centers throughout the United States.

4121 **Self Reliance**
8901 N Armenia Ave
Tampa, FL 33604-1041
813-375-3965
Fax: 813-375-3970
TTY: 813-375-3972
bruehl@self-reliance.org
www.self-reliance.org

Finn Kavanagh, Executive Director
Michele Pineda, Director of Finance & Operations
Gary Martoccio, Programs Director
Kim Albritton, Chairperson

A cross disability agency providing services to both children and adults with disabilities to identify and overcome barriers to independence in their lives. Self Reliance also promotes independence through empowering persons with disabilities and improving the communities in which they live.

4122 **Space Coast Center for Independent Living**
571 Haverty Court, Suite W.
Rockledge, FL 32955
321-633-6011
Fax: 321-633-6472
spacecoastcil.org

Michael Lavoie, President
Howard Fetes, VP
Jason Miller, Treasurer/Secretary

Provides overall services for individuals with al types of disabilities. Offers peer support, advocacy, skills training, accessibility surveys, support groups, transportation, specialized equipment and sign language interpreter referral services and home modifications.

4123 **Suncoast Center for Independent Living, Inc.**
3281 17th Street
Sarasota, FL 34235
941-351-9545
Fax: 941-316-9320
Info@scil4u.org
www.scil4u.org

Kevin Sanderson, Chair
Michael Fluker, Executive Director
Vicke Mack, Treasurer
Scott Biehler, Secretary

Helping people with disabilities live independently.

4124 **disAbility Solutions for Independent Living**
119 S Palmetto Ave
Suite 180
Daytona Beach, FL 32114- 4369
386-255-1812
866-310-1039
Fax: 386-255-1814
TTY: 386-252-6222
info@dsil.org
www.dsil.org

Julie M Shaw, Executive Director

To maximize the leadership, empowerment, independence and productivity of individuals with disabilities, to promote and attain integration and full inclusion of individuals with disabilities in all aspects of our society; accomplished through consumer control, peer support, education, self-determination, equal access and individual and systems advocacy

Georgia

4125 Arms Wide Open
5036 Snapfinger Woods Dr.
Suite 205
Decatur, GA 30035- 1677
678-404-7696
Fax: 770-498-2778
kenmorris@armswideopen.org
www.armswideopen.org

Ken Morris, Director
Arms Wide Open operates a durable medical equipment loan program and a life care program. The mission of Arms Wide Open is to provide support services to the aged, disabled and chronically ill for the purpose of helping them to avoid institutional placement.

4126 Bain, Inc. Center For Independent Living
316 W Shotwell St.
Bainbridge, GA 39819-3906
229-246-0150
888-830-1530
Fax: 229-246-1715
TTY: 888-830-1530
www.baincil.org

Virginia Harris, Executive Director
Malissa Thompson, Program Manager
Tomonia Becon, Nursing Home Transition Coordina
Dameca Fillingame, President
A non-residential Center for Independent Living serving eleven counties throughout Southwest. BAIN is a non-profit, community based resource and advocacy center run by and for individuals with disabilities.

4127 DisAbility LINK
1901 Montreal Rd.
Suite 102
Tucker, GA 30084
404-687-8890
Fax: 404-687-8298
TTY: 711
www.disabilitylink.org

Kim Gibson, Executive Director
Ken Mitchell, Assistant Director
Joseph Bryant, Director, Finance
Committed to promoting the rights of all people with disabilities.

4128 Disability Connections
170 College St
Macon, GA 31201-1656
478-741-1425
800-743-2117
Fax: 478-755-1571
disabilityconnections.com

Jerilyn Leverett, Executive Director
A private non-profit organization that looks to enable all people with disabilities to attain and have access to all opportunities in life.

4129 Division of Rehabilitation Services
Georgia Department of Labor
410 Mall Blvd
Suite B
Savannah, GA 31406-4869
912-356-2226
Fax: 912-356-2875
TTY: 912-356-2940
dol.state.ga.us

Mark Bultler, Commissioner
Jody Lane, Manager
George Foley, Manager
Vocational rehabilitation services.

4130 Living Independence for Everyone (LIFE)
5105 Paulsen Street
Suite 143-B
Savannah, GA 31405
912-920-2414
800-948-4824
Fax: 912-920-0007
www.lifecil.com

Mark Schreiber, President
Stuart Klugler, Vice President
John Paul Berlon, Secretary
Cheryl Brackin, Board Member
The Southeast's Regional disability resource center that offers a wide range of resources, education, and advocacy to the community to help level the playing field for people with disabilities to create a world in which everyone can fully participate.

4131 Multiple Choices Center for Independent Living
145 Barrington Dr.
Athens, GA 30605-3133
706-850-4025
www.multiplechoices.us

Doug Hatch, President
Donald Veater, VP
Elllen Des Jardines, Secretary
William Holley, Executive Director
To break down all barriers to inclusion by enhancing the equality of life and empowering people with disabilities through advocacy, education and training.

4132 North District Independent Living Program
Ste 209
311 Green St NW
Gainesville, GA 30501-3364
770-535-5930
Sharon McCurry, Coordinator
Cindy Hanna, Executive Director
Information and referral, advocacy, peer counseling, service coordination and ADA consultation.

4133 Southwest District Independent Living Program
P.O. Box 1606
Albany, GA 31702-1606
229-430-4170
Fax: 229-430-4466

Bill Layton, Director
Diane Davis, Executive Director
Offers peer counseling, disability education and awareness, attendant care registry, and information on accessible home for the disabled.

4134 Statewide Independent Living Council of Georgia
315 West Ponce de Leon Avenue
Suite 600
Decatur, GA 30030-2617
770-270-6860
888-288-9780
Fax: 770-270-5957
shellys5@hotmail.com
silcga.org

Steve Oldaker, President
Angela Denise Davis, Vice President
Mark Schreiber, Treasurer
Scott Osborne, Secretary
Founded to ensure that people with disabilities have opportunities to live as independently as possible.

4135 Walton Options for Independent Living
948 Walton Way
Augusta, GA 30901-519
706-724-6262
877-821-8400
Fax: 706-724-6729
TTY: 706-724-6262
tjohnston@waltonoptions.org
www.waltonoptions.org

Tiffany Cilford, Executive Director
Ann Campbell-Kelly, Special Projects Coordinator
Alyson Schwartz, Special Projects Coordinator
Sam Creech, Director-Information Technology
Services include individual and systems advocacy, peer support, skills training (including basic computer and return to work skills), information and referral services and transition from institutions back to the community.

Hawaii

4136 Center For Independent Living- Kauai
State Office Building 3060 Eiwa Str
Lihue, HI 96766-6529
808-274-3484
Fax: 808-245-3485
kauaiddc@pixi.com

Humberto Blanco, Administrator
Teri Yamashiro, IL Specialist
Offers peer counseling, disability education, attendant care registry, outreach services and advocacy.

4137 **Hawaii Center For Independent Living**
1055 Kinoole Street
Suite 105 le St
Hilo, HI 96720-3872
808-935-3777
800-420-6928
TTY: 808-935-7888
www.cil-hawaii.org
Gordon Fuller, Executive Director
Provides an array of support services for people with all types of disabilities of any age.

4138 **Hawaii Center for Independent Living-Maui**
220 Imi Kala Street
Suite 103
Wailuku, HI 96793-1209
808-242-4966
866-303-4245
800-420-6928
Fax: 808-244-6978
TTY: 808-242-4968
www.cil-hawaii.org
Clytie Nishihara, Manager
T Lay, Administrative Assistant
Offers disability education and awareness, advocacy and counseling.

4139 **Hawaii Centers for Independent Living**
200 N. Vineyard Blvd Bldg. A501
Honolulu, HI 96817-3950
808-522-5400
800-420-6928
Fax: 808-522-5427
www.cil-hawaii.org
Cheryl Mizusaawa, Executive Director
M.J. (Kimo) Keawe, COO & Executive Director
Our staff and Board of directors are excellent advocates with the disabled community. We will connect you with resources to make your own choices for housing, employment, and personal care and to find assistive devices and technology to improve quality of life. On both the islands of Oahu and Hawaii, we have an independent living specialist who is fluent in American sign language and is well known in the deaf community.

4140 **Kauai Center for Independent Living**
4340 Nawiliwili Rd.
Lihue, HI 96766-6529
808-246-4800
800-420-6928
Fax: 808-245-7218
www.cil-hawaii.org
Laurao Tobosa, Program Coordinator
Provides a variety of support services for people with all types of disabilities.

Idaho

4141 **American Falls Office: Living Independently for Everyone (LIFE)**
250 S. Skyline
Idaho Falls, ID 83402-4508
208-529-8610
Fax: 208-529-6804
diane@idlife.org
www.idlife.org
Dean Nilson, Executive Director
Tina Noreen, Programs Coordinator
Mickey Palmer, Fiscal Intermediary Manager
Enables people with disabilities to manage their own lives, make their own choices, and give information and knowledge to assist in living with dignity and bravado.

4142 **Dawn Enterprises**
280 Cedar Street P.O. Box 388
Blackfoot, ID 83221-388
208-785-5890
Fax: 208-785-3095
dawnent.org
Donna Butler, Executive Director
Teresa Oakes, Assistant Director/Fiscal Coordi
To assist individuals of Southeastern Idaho with mental, physical or social disabilities in achieving independence through employment training, skill training, social development, or living enhancements up to each individual's maximum capability.

4143 **Disability Action Center NW**
505 N Main St
Moscow, ID 83843-2615
208-883-0523
800-475-0070
Fax: 208-883-0524
www.dacnw.org
Larry Topp, President
Jean Coil, Vice President
Mark Leeper, CEO
Karl Johanson, Treasurer
A non-profit community partnership working to promote the independence and equality of all individuals with disabilities in all aspects of society. *$45.00*

4144 **Disability Action Center NW: Coeur D'Alene**
7560 N Government Way
Suite 1
Coeur D Alene, ID 83815- 4069
208-664-9896
800-854-9500
Fax: 208-666-1362
www.dacnw.org
Larry Topp, President
Jean Coil, Vice President
Mark Leeper, CEO
Karl Johanson, Treasurer
A non-profit community partnership working to promote the independence and equality of all individuals with disabilities in all aspects of society.

4145 **Disability Action Center NW: Lewiston**
330 5th Street
Suite A1
Lewiston, ID 83501-2086
208-746-9033
800-746-9033
Fax: 208-746-1004
www.dacnw.org
Larry Topp, President
Jean Coil, Vice President
Mark Leeper, CEO
Karl Johanson, Treasurer
A non-profit community partnership working to promote the independence and equality of all individuals with disabilities in all aspects of society.

4146 **Idaho Falls Office: Living Independently for Everyone (LIFE)**
250 S. Skyline
Idaho Falls, ID 83402-3702
208-529-8610
800-631-2747
Fax: 208-232-2753
www.idlife.org
Dean Nielson, Executive Director
Tina Noreen, Programs Coordinator
Mickey Palmer, Fiscal Intermediary Manager
Enables people with disabilities to manage their own lives, make their own choices, and give information and knowledge to assist in living with dignity and bravado.

4147 **LIFE: Fort Hall**
1333 Moursund
Houston, TX 77019
713-520-0232
Fax: 713-520-5785
TTY: 713-520-0232
www.ilru.org
Lex Frieden, Director
Enables people with disabilities to manage their own lives, make thier own choices, and give information and knowledge to assist in living with dignity and bravado.

4148 **Living Independence Network Corporation**
1878 W Overland Rd
Boise, ID 83705-3142
208-336-3335
Fax: 208-384-5037
info@lincidaho.org
lincidaho.org
Roger Howard, Executive Director
A non-profit organization empowering people with disabilities to achieve their desired level of independence.

4149 **Living Independence Network Corporation: Twin Falls**
1182 Eastland Dr North
Suite C
Twin Falls, ID 83301-8972
208-733-1712
Fax: 208-733-7711
info@lincidaho.org
www.lincidaho.org

Melva Heinrich, Executive Director

A non-profit organization empowering people with disabilities to achieve their desired level of independence.

4150 **Living Independence Network Corporation: Caldwell**
1609 Kimball Ave
Ste. 201
Caldwell, ID 83605-6965
208-454-5511
Fax: 208-454-5515
TTY: 208-454-5511
info@lincidaho.org
www.lincidaho.org

Heidi Caldwell, Executive Director

A non-profit organization empowering people with disabilities to achieve their desired level of independence.

4151 **Living Independent for Everyone (LIFE): Pocatello Office**
640 Pershing Ave
PO Box 4185
Pocatello, ID 83201-3702
208-232-2747
800-631-2747
Fax: 208-232-2753
TTY: 208-232-2747
tracy@idlife.org
www.idlife.org

Dean Nielson, Executive Director
Mickey Palmer, Fiscal Intermediary Manager
Tina Noreen, Programs Coordinator

Enables people with disabilities to manage thier own lives, make their own choices, and give information and knowledge to assist in living with dignity and bravado.

4152 **Living Independently for Everyone (LIFE): Blackfoot Office**
Living Independently for Everyone (LIFE): Pocate
570 W. Pacific
P.O. Box 86
Blackfoot, ID 83221-86
208-785-9648
Fax: 208-785-2398
lori@idlife.org
www.idlife.org

Dean Nielson, Executive Director
Tina Noreen, Programs Coordinator
Mickey Palmer, Fiscal Intermediary Manager

Enable people with disabilities to manage their own lives, make their own choices, and give information and knowledge to assist in living with dignity and bravado.

4153 **Living Independently for Everyone: Burley**
2311 Park Ave
Suite 7
Burley, ID 83318-2170
208-678-7705
Fax: 208-678-7771
www.idlife.org

Dean Nielson, Executive Director
Mickey Palmer, Fiscal Intermediary Manager
Tina Noreen, Programs Coordinator

Enables people with disabilities to manage their own lives, make their own choices, and give information and knowledge to assist in living with dignity and bravado.

4154 **Southwestern Idaho Housing Authority**
1108 W Finch Dr
Nampa, ID 83651-1732
208-467-7461
Fax: 208-463-1772

David W Patten, Manager

Offers housing for rent and section/8

Illinois

4155 **Access Living of Metropolitan Chicago**
115 W Chicago Ave
Chicago, IL 60654-3209
312-640-2100
800-613-8549
Fax: 312-640-2101
TTY: 312-640-2102
accessliving.org

Marca Bristo, CEO
Bhuttu Mathews, Disability Resources Coordinator
Gary Arnold, Public Relations Coordinator
Daisy Feidt, Executive Vice President

Established in 1980,access living is a change agent commited to fostering an incusive society that enables Chicagoans with disabilities to live fully engaged and self-directed lives. Nationally recognized as a leading force in the disability community. Access Living challenges stereotypes, protects civil rights, and champions social reform.

4156 **Center on Deafness**
3444 Dundee Rd
Northbrook, IL 60062-2258
847-559-0110
Fax: 847-559-8199
TTY: 847-559-9493
www.centerondeafness.org

Bonnie Simon, Executive Director
Donna Gomez, Residential Services/ Adult Plac
Brandi Buie, School Intake
David Wood, Coordinator

COD is dedicated to providing quality services for persons who are deaf or hard of hearing and their families, through educational, vocational, and residential services in a therapuetic, community-based environment

4157 **Community Residential Alternative**
Coleman Tri- County Services
22 Veterans Drive, ST. A
P.O. Box 869
Harrisburg, IL 62946-2017
618-252-0275
Fax: 618-252-2389
TTY: 618-269-4211
cts.62946@frontier.com
colemantricounty.tripod.com

Samantha Austin, Executive Director

Six bed group home that provides a residential alternative for the developmentally disabled adult. This program is designed to promote independence in daily living skills, economic self-sufficiency, and integration into the community.

4158 **Division of Rehabilitation Services**
Department of Human Services
100 South Grand Avenue East
Springfield, IL 62762-2625
217-782-2093
800-843-6154
Fax: 217-524-2471
DHS.WebBits@illinois.gov
www.dhs.state.il.us

Carol Adams, President

Provides medical, therapeutic and counseling services for the disabled, as well as employment services.

4159 **DuPage Center for Independent Living**
3130 Finley Rd.
Ste. 500
Downers Grove, IL 60515-5877
630-469-2300
Fax: 630-469-2606
TTY: 630-469-2300
www.dupagecil.org

Charles Stack, Board President
Bette Lawrence Water, Vice President
John Lausas, Treasurer
Jeff Gullang, Secretary

A non residential, community based, not for profit agency wich provides advocacy and services to persons with disabilities in DuPage County.

4160 **Fite Center for Independent Living**
1230 Larkin Ave
Elgin, IL 60123-6200
847-695-5818
Fax: 847-695-5892

Linda Bradford-Foster, Chairman, Board Treasurer
Gracia Bittner, Board Secretary

Provides services to people with disabilities in Kane, Kendall and McHenry counties. Our non-residential agency provides independent living skills training, advocacy, systemic + individual peer counseling, information and referral and housing services. Also provides technical assistance to businesses and agencies to work with people with disabilities. Locations in Elgin and Aurora. Please call for further details.

4161 **Illinois Department of Rehab Services**
Department of Human Services
100 South Grand Avenue East
Springfield, IL 62762-1
217-782-2093
800-843-6154
Fax: 217-524-2471
DHS.WebBits@illinois.gov
www.dhs.state.il.us

Carol Adams, President
Karen Perrin, Manager

The state's lead agency serving individuals with disabilities. DRS works in partnership with people with disabilities and their families to assist them in making informed choices to achieve full community participation through employment, education, and independent living opportunities.

4162 **Illinois Valley Center for Independent Living**
18 Gunia Dr
La Salle, IL 61301-9780
815-224-3126
800-822-3246
Fax: 815-224-3576
ivcil@ivcil.com
ivcil.com

John Hurst, President
Gary Rydleski, Vice President
Sue Faber, Secretary
Danielle Furar, Treasurer

A nonprofit service and advocacy organization that assists persons with disabilities in opening doors to their independence.

4163 **Illinois and Iowa Center for Independent Living**
501 11th St.
PO Box 6156
Rock Island, IL 61231-6156
309-793-0090
877-541-2505
855-744-8918
Fax: 309-793-5198
www.iicil.com

Liz Sherwin, Executive Director
Alfonso Ayew-Ew, Blind Independent Living Skill S
Eddie Williams, CommunityReintegration Advocate
Hershel Jackson, Deaf & Hard of Hearing Advocate

To create and maintain independence options for people with disabilities by advocating for civil rights, providing services, and promoting full participation of disabled individuals in all aspects of the community.

4164 **Impact Center for Independent Living**
2735 E Broadway
Alton, IL 62002-1859
618-462-1411
888-616-4261
Fax: 618-474-5309
staff@impactcil.org
impactcil.org

Susy Woods, President
Judy O'Malley, Vice President
Bishop Samuel White, Treasurer
Cathy Contarino, Executive Director

Promotes pride and respect for people with disabilities by sharing the tools that are necessary to take control of one's own life.

4165 **Jacksonville Area CIL: Havana**
220 W Main St
Havana, IL 62644-1138
309-543-6680
877-759-2187
Fax: 309-543-6711
info@jacil.org
www.jacil.org

Phil Foxworth, President
Mark Arnold, Vice President
Ruth Lanier, Secretary
Joe Vieira, Treasurer

Committed to enabling persons with disabilities to gain effective control and director of their own lives in the home, in the workplace and in the community.

4166 **Jacksonville Area Center for Independent Living**
15 Permac Road
Jacksonville, IL 62650-2071
217-245-8371
Fax: 217-245-1872
TTY: 217-245-8371
info@jacil.org
www.jacil.org

Phil Foxworth, President
Mark Arnold, Vice President
Ruth Lanier, Secretary
Joe Vieira, Treasurer

Committed to enabling persons with disabilities to gain effective control and direction of their own lives in the home, in the workplace and in the community.

4167 **LIFE Center for Independent Living**
2201 Eastland Dr
Suite 1
Bloomington, IL 61704
309-663-5433
888-543-3245
Fax: 309-663-7024
TTY: 309-663-5433
rickielee@lifecil.org
www.lifecil.org

Rickielee Benecke, Executive Director
Jill Doran, Associate Director
Brianne Anderson, Office Manager

A community-based, not-for-profit, non-residential organization that promotes disability rights, equal access, and full community participation for persons with disabilities.

4168 **LINC-Monroe Randolph Center**
Ste 4
1514 S Main St
Red Bud, IL 62278-1382
618-282-3700
Fax: 618-282-2740
TTY: 618-282-3700

Violete Nast, Manager

4169 **Lake County Center for Independent Living**
377 N Seymour Ave
Mundelein, IL 60060-2322
847-949-4440
Fax: 847-949-4445
TTY: 847-949-0641
lindsey@lccil.org
www.lccil.org

Kelli Brooks, Executive Director
Andy Balint, Director of Finance
Lety Cruz, Bilingual Program Assistant
Jenny Farley, Youth Leadership Advocate

Lake County Center for Indepdendent Living is a disability rights organization governed and staffed by a majority of people with disabilities. LCCIL offers services and advocacy that promote a fully accessible society, which expects participation by persons with disabilities.

4170 **Life Center for Independent Living: Pontiac**
318 West Madison Street
Pontiac, IL 61764-1785
815-844-1132
Fax: 815-844-1148
lifecil@lifecil.org
lifecil.org

Gail Kear, Executive Director
Jill Doran, Associate Director
Brianne Anderson, Office Manager
Rickielee Benecke, Disability Rights Advocate

A community-based, not-for-profit, non-residential organization that promotes disability rights, equal access, and full community participation for persons with disabilities.

4171 **Living Independently Now Center (LINC)**
120 E a St
Belleville, IL 62220-1401
618-235-9988
Fax: 618-233-3729
TTY: 618-235-9988
info@lincinc.org
www.lincinc.org

Linda Conley, President
Ron Tialdo, Vice-President
Lynn Jarman, Executive Director
Robert Rahlfs, Treasurer
Empowers persons with disabilities to live independently and to promote accessibility and inclusion in all areas.

4172 **Living Independently Now Center: Sparta**
Western Egyptian Building
207 West 4th Street
Waterloo, IL 62298
618-317-4028
info@lincinc.org
www.lincinc.org

Linda Conley, President
Ron Tialdo, Vice-President
Lynn Jarman, Executive Director
Robert Rahlfs, Treasurer
Empowers persons with disabilities to live independently and to promote accessibility and inclusion in all areas.

4173 **Living Independently Now Center: Waterloo**
Western Egyptian Building
207 West 4th Street
Waterloo, IL 62298-1336
618-317-4028
info@lincinc.org
www.lincinc.org

Linda Conley, President
Ron Tialdo, Vice-President
Lynn Jarman, Executive Director
Robert Rahlfs, Treasurer
Empowers persons with disabilities to live independently and to promote accessibility and inclusion in all areas.

4174 **Mosaic: Pontiac**
4980 S. 118th St.
Omaha, NE 68137
877-366-7242
Fax: 402-896-1511
www.mosaicinfo.org

Max Miller, Chairperson
James Zils, Vice Chairperson
Lisa Negstad, 2nd Vice Chairperson
Kathy Patrick, Secretary
A faith-based organization serving people with developmental disabilities.

4175 **Opportunities for Access: A Center for Independent Living**
4206 Williamson Pl
Suite 3
Mount Vernon, IL 62864-6705
618-244-9212
Fax: 618-244-9310
TTY: 618-244-9575
ofacil.org

Michael Egbert, Executive Director
Serves, trains and provides information to persons with disabilities, family members and significant others and service providers. Services include: advocacy, information and referral, peer support, skills training, volunteer programs and other related services. Services are free. A cross disability community based, non-residential, nonprofit organization serving Clay, Clinton, Edwards, Effingham, Fayette, Hamilton, Jasper, Jefferson, Marion, Wabash, Washington, Wayne and White Counties.

4176 **Options Center for Independent Living: Bourbonnais**
22 Heritage Dr
Suite 107
Bourbonnais, IL 60914-2510
815-936-0100
Fax: 815-936-0117
TTY: 815-936-0132
www.optionscil.org

Mark Mantarian, President
Ronald D. Smith, Vice President
Dina Raymond, Co-Secretary
Daniel Brough, Treasurer
A non-residential, not-for-profit, community-based organization that promotes independent living for people with disabilities.

4177 **Options Center for Independent Living: Watseka**
103 Laird Ln
Suite 103
Watseka, IL 60970
815-432-1332
Fax: 815-432-1360
TTY: 815-432-1361

Mark Mountain, President
Ronald D. Smith, Vice President
Dina Raymond, Co-Secretary
Daniel Brough, Treasurer
A non-residential, not-for-profit, community-based organization that promotes independent living for people with disabilities.

4178 **PACE Center for Independent Living**
1317 E Florida Ave
Urbana, IL 61801-6007
217-344-5433
Fax: 217-344-2414
TTY: 217-344-5024
info@pacecil.org
pacecil.org

Evelyn Brown, President
Fred Neubert, Vice President
Nancy McClellan-Hickey, Executive Director
Arland Stratton, Treasurer
Promotes the full participation of people with disabilities in the rights and responsibilities of society. Provides services, which assist people with disabilities in achieving or maintaining independence.

4179 **Progress Center for Independent Living**
7521 Madison St
Forest Park, IL 60130-1407
708-209-1500
Fax: 708-209-1735
TTY: 708-209-1826
info@progresscil.org
www.progresscil.org

Anne Gunter, Independent Living Advocate
Kim Liddell, Independent Living Advocate
Horacio Esparza, Executive Director
Art Johnson, Home Services Team Coordinator
A community-based, non-profit, non-residential, service and advocacy organization operated for people with disabilities, by people with disabilities.

4180 **Progress Center for Independent Living: Blue Island**
12940 Western Ave
Blue Island, IL 60406-3766
708-388-5011
Fax: 708-388-5016
TTY: 708-389-8250
info@progresscil.org
www.progresscil.org

Horacio Esparza, Executive Director
Anne Gunter, Independent Living Advocate
Kim Liddell, Independent Living Advocate
Art Johnson, Home Services Team Coordinator
A community-based, non-profit, non residential, service and advocacy organization operated for people with disabilities, by people with disabilities.

4181 **Regional Access & Mobilization Project**
202 Market St
Rockford, IL 61107-3954
815-968-7467
Fax: 815-968-7612
TTY: 815-968-2401
rampcil.org

Shari Snyder, President
Tina Kaatz, Vice President
Craig Fetty, Secretary
Sharon Wyland, Treasurer

To promote an accessible society that allows and expects full participation by people with disabilities.

4182 **Regional Access & Mobilization Project: Belvidere**
530 S State St
Suite 103
Belvidere, IL 61008-3711
815-544-8404
Fax: 815-544-1896
TTY: 815-544-8404
rampcil.org

Shari Snyder, President
Tina Kaatz, Vice President
Craig Fetty, Secretary
Sharon Wyland, Treasurer

Promote an accessible society that allows and expects full participation by people with disabilities.

4183 **Regional Access & Mobilization Project: De Kalb**
115 N First Street
Dekalb, IL 60115-3055
815-756-3202
Fax: 815-756-3556
TTY: 815-756-4263
rampcil.org

Shari Snyder, President
Tina Kaatz, Vice President
Craig Fetty, Secretary
Sharon Wyland, Treasurer

Promotes an accessible society that allows and expects full partiipation by persons with disabilities.

4184 **Regional Access & Mobilization Project: Freeport**
2155 W Galena Ave
Freeport, IL 61032-3013
815-233-1128
Fax: 815-233-0743
TTY: 815-233-1128
rampcil.org

Shari Snyder, President
Tina Kaatz, Vice President
Craig Fetty, Secretary
Sharon Wyland, Treasurer

Promotes an accessible society that allows and expects full partiipation by persons with disabilities.

4185 **Soyland Access to Independent Living (SAIL)**
2449 E Federal Dr
Decatur, IL 62526-2160
217-876-8888
800-358-8080
Fax: 217-876-7245
TTY: 217-876-8888
jwooters@decatursail.com
www.decatursail.com

Jeri J Wooters, Executive Director
Betty Watkins, Rural Outreach Coordinator

A community-based, non-residential Center for Independent Living whose purpose is to promote and practice independent living for all people with disabilities.

4186 **Soyland Access to Independent Living: Charleston**
757 Windsor Rd
Charleston, IL 61920-7474
217-345-7245
Fax: 217-345-7226
TTY: 217-345-7245
triplec@consolidated.net
www.decatursail.com

Betty Watkins, Rural Outreach Coordinator
Jeri J Wooters, Executive Director

A community-based, non-residential Center for Independent Living whose purpose is to promote and practice independent living for all people iwth disabilities.

4187 **Soyland Access to Independent Living: Shelbyville**
1810 W.S. 3rd ST P.O. Box 650
Shelbyville, IL 62565-650
217-774-4322
Fax: 217-774-4368
TTY: 217-774-4322
sailsel@consolidated.net
www.decatursail.com

Jeri J Wooters, Executive Director
Betty Watkins, Rural Outreach Coordinator

A community-based, non-residential Center for Independent Living whose purpose is to promote and practice independent living for all people with disabilities.

4188 **Soyland Access to Independent Living: Sullivan**
1102 W Jackson St
Sullivan, IL 61951-1067
217-728-3186
Fax: 217-728-2299
TTY: 217-728-3186
sulsail@wireless111.com
www.decatursail.com

Betty Watkins, Rural Outreach Coordinator
Jeri J Wooters, Executive Director

A community-based, non-residential Center for Independent Living whose purpose is to promote and practice independent living for all people with disabilities.

4189 **Springfield Center for Independent Living**
330 South Grand Ave W
Springfield, IL 62704-3716
217-523-4032
800-447-4221
Fax: 217-523-0427
TTY: 217-523-4032
scil@scil.org
scil.org

Pete Roberts, Executive Director
Susan Coopers, Program Director
Denise Groesch, Reintegration Coordinator
Kathryn Cline, Business Manager

To increase opportunities for equality, integration and independence for all persons with disabilities through advocacy, services, and public education.

4190 **Stone-Hayes Center for Independent Living**
39 N Prairie St
Galesburg, IL 61401-4613
309-344-1306
888-347-4245
Fax: 309-344-1305
TTY: 309-344-1306

Vanya Peterson, Executive Director
Michael Bohnenkamp, Associate Director
John Hunigan, Office Manager
Lynn Voeller, Independent Living Associate

The purpose of INCIL is to facilitate the collaboration of all Centers for Independent Living in Illinois for promoting, through the Independent Living Movement, equal opportunities and civil rights for all persons with disaibilities.

4191 **West Central Illinois Center for Independent Living**
639 York St.
Suite 204
Quincy, IL 62301-1065
217-223-0400
Fax: 217-223-0479
TTY: 217-223-0475
info@wcicil.org
www.wcicil.org

Glenda Hackemack, Executive Director
Dale Winner, Information & Referral Coordinat
Dustin Gorde Director of Community, Jenny
Kelly Transition Co-Ordinato

A not-for-profit advocacy center funded by state and federal grants to provide services to people with disabilities.

4192 **West Central Illinois Center for Independent Living: Macomb**
440 N Lafayette St
Macomb, IL 61455-1512
309-833-5766
Fax: 309-833-4690
TTY: 217-223-0475
info@wcicil.org
www.wcicil.org

Glenda Hackemack, Executive Director
Dale Winner, Information & Referral Coordinat
Dustin Gorde Director of Community, Jenny
Kelly Transition Co-Ordinato

A not-for-profit advocacy center funded by state and federal grants to provide services to people with disabilities.

4193 **Will Grundy Center for Independent Living**
2415 W Jefferson St
Suite A
Joliet, IL 60435-6464
815-729-0162
Fax: 815-729-3697
TTY: 815-729-2085
will-grundycil.org

Elaine Sommer, President
Chris Boyk, Vice President
Dianne Mundle, Treasurer
Rhonda Price, Secretary

A cross-disability, community based organization that strives for equalityand empowerment of persons with disabilities in the Will and Grundy County areas.

Indiana

4194 **Assistive Technology Training and Information Center (ATTIC)**
1721 Washington Ave
Vincennes, IN 47591-4823
812-886-0575
877-96A-8842
Fax: 812-886-1128
inbox@atticindiana.org
www.atticindiana.org

Patricia Stewart, Executive Director
Rebecca Anderson, Assistant Director
Mark Schmitt, Fiscal Controller
Jackie Evans, Independent Living Coordinator

ATTIC provides support, information and education for individuals with disabilities and for families of children with special needs, and the professionals who assist these families. All disabilities, all ages.

4195 **DAMAR Services**
6067 Decatur Blvd.
Indianapolis, IN 46241
317-856-5201
Fax: 317-856-2333
info@damar.org
damar.org

Gail Shiel, Chairman
Rick Torbeck, Vice Chairman
Jim Dalton, Psy.D., HSPP, President and CEO
Richard L. Harcourt, Vice President & CFO

Builds better futures for children and adults facing life's greatest developmental and behavioral challenges.

4196 **Everybody Counts Center for Independent Living**
3616 Elm St
Room 3
East Chicago, IN 46410-7097
219-229-5055
888-769-3636
Fax: 219-769-5326
TTY: 219-756-3323
info@everybodycounts.org
everybodycounts.org

Teresa Torres, Executive Director
Emma Lewis Sullivan, On Loan Consultant
Mark Torres, Systems Manager
Jodi Hawn, Administrative Assistant

A nonprofit corporation dedicated to the achievement of maximum independence and enhanced quality of life for persons with disabilities.

4197 **Four Rivers Resource Services**
Hwy. 59 South
P.O. Box 249
Linton, IN 47441-249
812-847-2231
Fax: 812-847-8836
fourrivers@frrs.org
frrs.org

Stephen Sacksteder, Executive Director
Robin Duncan, Chief Financial Officer
Dean Dorrell, Information Systems Director
Jessica Davis, Development Coordinator

FRRS is established to enable individuals with disabilities and other challenges to attain self independence and natural interdependence, inclusion in normal life experiences and opportunities, and general life enrichment, by working in partnership with them, their families and the communities in and around Greene, Sullivan, Daviess, and Martin Counties.

4198 **Future Choices Independent Living Center**
309 N High St
Muncie, IN 47305-1618
765-741-8332
866-741-3444
Fax: 765-741-8333
futurechoices.org

Beth Y. Quarles, President

Provides unlimited options for minorities, youth, and Hoosiers with disabilities.

4199 **Independent Living Center of Eastern Indiana (ILCEIN)**
1818 W Main St
Richmond, IN 47374-3822
765-939-9226
877-939-9226
Fax: 765-935-2215
www.ilcein.org

Jim McCormick, Executive Director
Dean Turner, Administrative Director
Ann Barnhart, Compliance Manager
Michelle Satterfield, Service Coordinator

Serving Fayette, Franklin, Henry, Decatur, Rush, Union and Wayne Counties.

4200 **Indianapolis Resource Center for Independent Living**
5302 East Washington Street
Indianapolis, IN 46219
317-926-1660
866-794-7245
Fax: 317-926-1687
info@abilityindiana.org
www.abilityindiana.org

Judy Townsend, President
Dave Trulock, Vice President
Jacqueline Troy, Treasurer
Don Lane, Secretary

Provides services, support and information to people with disabilities to help insure equal access to all aspects of community life.

4201 **League for the Blind and Disabled**
5821 S Anthony Blvd
Fort Wayne, IN 46816-3701
260-441-0551
800-889-3443
Fax: 260-441-7760
TTY: 800-889-3443
the-league@the-league.org
the-league.org

David A. Nelson, CEO/President
Catherine Collins, Chair
Anne Palmer, Administrative Assistant
Kevin Showalter, Youth Services Coordinator

To provide and promote opportunities that empower people with disabilities to achieve their potential.

4202 **Martin Luther Homes of Indiana**
Mosaic
26 N Brown Ave
Terre Haute, IN 47803-1523
812-235-3399
Fax: 812-235-1590

4203 **Ruben Center for Independent Living**
5302 East Washington Street
Indianapolis, IN 46219-3227
317-926-1660
Fax: 317-926-1687
TTY: 219-397-6496
info@abilityindiana.org
www.abilityindiana.org

Judy Townsend, President
Dave Trulock, Vice President
Jacqueline Troy, Treasurer
Don Lane, Secretary

An independent living center providing support, information and education.

4204 **SILC, Indiana Council on Independent Living (ICOIL)**
P.O. Box 7083
Indianapolis, IN 46207-7083
317-232-1303
800-545-7763
Fax: 317-232-6478

Nancy Young, Program Director
Richard Simers, SILC Chairperson

4205 **Southern Indiana Center for Independent Living**
1494 W. Main Street
PO Box 308
Mitchell, IN 47446-1943
812-277-9626
800-845-6914
Fax: 812-277-9628
sicilindiana.org

Al Tolbert, Executive Director
Darlene Webster, Independent Living Center Direct

SICIL is a consumer controlled, community based, cross-disability, non-residential and not for profit organization that promotes and practices the philosophy of independent living: consumer control, peer support, self-help, self-determination, equal access, and individual and community advocacy. SICIL also promotes accesible and affordable housing, recreation and transportation.

4206 **Wabash Independent Living Center & Learning Center (WILL)**
1 Dreiser Square
Terre Haute, IN 47807
812-298-9455
877-915-9455
Fax: 812-299-9061
TTY: 877-915-9455
info@thewillcenter.org
www.thewillcenter.org

Don Rogers, Chairman
Jody Pomfret, Vice Chairman
Kevin Burke, Treasurer
Peter Ciancone, Secretary-Executive Director

To empower people with disabilities to ensure that they have full and complete access to community resources to promote their independence

Iowa

4207 **Black Hawk Center for Independent Living**
2800 Falls Ave.
P.O. Box 2275
Waterloo, IA 50701-2275
319-291-7755
888-291-7754
Fax: 319-291-7781
TTY: 800-735-2942

4208 **Central Iowa Center for Independent Living**
655 Walnut St
Suite 131
Des Moines, IA 50309-3930
515-243-1742
888-503-2287
Fax: 515-243-5385

Bob Jeppesen, Executive Director
Frank Strong, Associate Director
Crystal Toman, Office Coordinator
Dee Howard, Independent Living Specialist

CICIL is a community based, non-profit, non-residential program serving persons with disabilities. CICIL assists all persons, regardless of disability in making choices about their own lives and in experiencing success in achieving independence.

4209 **Evert Conner Rights & Resources CIL**
730 S Dubuque St
Iowa City, IA 52240-4202
319-338-3870
800-982-0272
Fax: 319-354-1799

Scott Gill, Executive Director

Provides community services like disability awareness training and classroom presentations. Individual services include independent living skills training and peer counseling. All services are custom designed to support the independence of people with disabilities in their own community.

4210 **Hope Haven**
1800 19th St
PO Box 70
Rock Valley, IA 51247-1098
712-476-2737
Fax: 712-476-3110
hopehaven.org

Dr. Kent Eric Eknes, President
Ron Boote, Vice President
David Vanningen, Executive Director
Calvin Helmus, Chief Operating Officer

Unleashes the potential in people through work and life skills so that they may enjoy a productive life in their community.

4211 **League of Human Dignity, Center for Independent Living**
1520 Avenue M
Council Bluffs, IA 51501-1185
712-323-6863
Fax: 712-323-6811
Cinfo@leagueofhumandignity.com
www.leagueofhumandignity.com

Carrie England, Director

League of Human Dignity actively promotes the full integration of individuals with disabilities into society. To this end, the League will advocate their needs and rights, and provide quality services to involve these persons in becoming and remaining independent citizens.

4212 **Martin Luther Homes of Iowa**
P.O. Box 2316
Princeton, NJ 08543-2316
877-843-7953
Fax: 563-568-3992
www.rwjf.org

Mary Lynn ReVoir, Project Director
Fred Naumann III, Communications
Richard Wicks, Executive Director

4213 **South Central Iowa Center for Independent Living**
117 1st Ave W
Oskaloosa, IA 52577-3243
641-672-1867
800-651-7911
Fax: 641-672-1867
brookie43@gmail.com
www.iowasilc.org/cilinfo.html

Deb Philpot, Executive Director

Provides services, support, information and referral to people with disabilities to help insure equal access to all aspects of community life.

4214 **Three Rivers Center for Independent Living**
900 Rebecca Avenue
Pittsburgh, PA 15221-2938
412-371-7700
800-633-4588
Fax: 412-371-9430
TTY: 412-371-6230
lgray@trcil.org

Stanley A. Holbrook, President & Executive Director
Lisa Wilson, HR Program Manager
Rachel Rogan, Director of Waiver Services
Charles Keenan, TRCIL Real Properties Board

Providing a wide array of services to assist individuals and families in achieving positive life goals.

Kansas

4215 Advocates for Better Living For Everyone (A.B.L.E.)
Ste C
521 Commercial St
Atchison, KS 66002
913-367-1830
888-845-2879
Fax: 913-367-1830

Ken Gifford, President & CEO
A not for profit agency providing services within the State of Kansas. ABLE looks to assist people with disabilities as well as any other member of the community to live an integrated, quality life with dignity, respect, and independence.

4216 Center for Independent Living SW Kansas: Liberal
1023 N Kansas Ave
Suite 2
Liberal, KS 67901-2655
620-624-5500
800-327-4048
Fax: 620-624-6576
TTY: 620-624-5500
www.cilswks.org

Victor Otero, Manager
Crystal Tharp, Independent Living Advocate
Dedicated to helping people achieve full participation in society.

4217 Center for Independent Living Southwest Kansas
P.O. Box 2090
Garden City, KS 67846-2090
620-276-1900
800-736-9443
Fax: 620-271-0200

Troy Horton, Executive Director
Dedicated to helping people achieve full participation in society.

4218 Center for Independent Living Southwest Kansas: Dodge City
2601 Central Ave
Dodge City, KS 67801-6200
620-227-6660
800-326-1366
Fax: 620-227-8185
TTY: 620-227-6660

Mary Jane Sandoval, Independent Living Advocate
Dedicated to helping people achieve full participation in society

4219 Coalition for Independence
4911 State Ave
Kansas City, KS 66102-1749
913-321-5140
866-201-3829
Fax: 913-321-5182
TTY: 913-321-5216
cfi-kc.org

Clarence Smith, Executive Director
Laarni Sison, Executive Assistant
Claire Marr, Lead Independent Living Speciali
Shauna Garrett, Lead Accountant
Facilitates positive and responsible independence for all people with disabilities by acting as an advocate for individuals with disabilities, providing services, and promoting accessibility and acceptance.

4220 Cowley County Developmental Services
P.O. Box 618
Arkansas City, KS 67005-618
620-442-5270
866-442-5270
Fax: 620-442-5623

Bill Brooks, Executive Director
Provides services for persons with developmental disabilities in Cowley County..

4221 Independence
2001 Haskell Ave
Lawrence, KS 66046-3249
785-841-0333
888-824-7277
Fax: 785-841-1094
comment@independenceinc.org
independenceinc.org

Karen McGrath, President
Bruce Passman, Vice President
Sandra London, Lieb
Athena Johnson, Secretary

Provides advocacy, services, and education for people with disabilities and our communities.

4222 Independent Connection
1710 W. Schilling Road
P.O. Box 1160
Salina, KS 67402- 1160
785-827-9383
800-526-9731
Fax: 785-823-2015
TTY: 785-827-9383
www.occk.com

Shelia Nelson-Stout, President/CEO
Deanna L. Lamer, Senior Director,Human Resources
Tasha Suppes, Human Resources Coordinator
Dedicated to helping people with physical or mental disabilities remove barriers to employment, independent living, and full participation in their communities.

4223 Independent Connection: Abilene
Suite 221
300 N. Cedar St.
Abilene, KS 67410
785-263-2208
Fax: 785-263-3795
TTY: 785-263-2208
www.occk.com

Shelia Nelson-Stout, President/CEO
Deanna L. Lamer, Senior Director,Human Resources
Tasha Suppes, Human Resources Coordinator
Dedicated to helping people with physical or mental disabilities remove barriers to employment, independent living, and full participation in their communities.

4224 Independent Connection: Beloit
501 W 7th St
Beloit, KS 67420-2107
785-738-5423
Fax: 785-738-3320
TTY: 785-738-5423
www.occk.com

Shelia Nelson-Stout, President/CEO
Deanna L. Lamer, Senior Director,Human Resources
Tasha Suppes, Human Resources Coordinator
Dedicated to helping people with physical or mental disabilities remove barriers to employment, independent living, and full participation in their communities.

4225 Independent Connection: Concordia
1502 Lincoln St
Concordia, KS 66901-4830
785-243-1977
Fax: 785-243-4524
TTY: 785-243-1977
www.occk.com

Shelia Nelson-Stout, President/CEO
Dedicated to helping people with physical or mental disabilities remove barriers to employment, independent living, and full participation in their communities.

4226 Independent Living Resource Center
3033 W 2nd St N
Wichita, KS 67203-5357
316-942-6300
800-479-6861
Fax: 316-942-2078
ilrcks.org

Jean Shuler, President
Angie Schmidt, Vice Chairman
Derrick Prichard, Secretary/Treasurer
James Thayer, Board Member
Empower people with disabilities to lead independent lives by providing advocacy, education and direct services. Serve people with all types of disabilities; permanent or temporary, physical disabilities, mental disabilities, and developmental disabilities.

4227 Kansas Services for the Blind & Visually Impaired
2601 SW East Circle Dr N
Topeka, KS 66606-2445
785-296-3738
800-547-5789
Fax: 785-291-3138
srskansas.org

Dennis Ford, Manager
Michael Donnelly, Director
Helps persons who are blind or visually to improve their quality of life. KSBVI provides people with an array of services and ex-

periences aimed at overcoming not only the physical difficulties brought on by the loss of vision, but also the fear of change associated with vision loss. KSBVI can also help with job search and retention activities; life skills training; access to medical services; and technical assistance..

4228 **LINK: Colby**
505 N Franklin Ave
Suite G
Colby, KS 67701-2342
785-462-7600
800-736-9418
TTY: 785-462-7600
brianatwell@linkinc.org
www.linkinc.org

Brian Atwell, Executive Director

Promotes and supports the civil rights of people with disabilities and empowers them to achieve a life of independence and equality..

4229 **Living Independently in Northwest Kansas: Hays**
2401 E 13th St
Hays, KS 67601-2663
785-625-6942
800-596-5926
Fax: 785-625-2334
TTY: 785-625-6942
brianatwell@linkinc.org
www.linkinc.org

Brian Atwell, Executive Director

Promotes and supports the civil rights of people with disabilities and empowers them to achieve a life of independence and equality.

4230 **Prairie IL Resource Center**
103 W 2nd St
Pratt, KS 67124-2644
620-672-9600
Fax: 620-672-9601
info@pilr.org
www.pilr.org

Dave Mullins, President
Stephanie Guthrie, Vice President
Chris Owens, Executive Director
Roger Frischenmeyer, Independent Living Specialist

To achieve the full inclusion and acceptance of people with disabilities through education and advocacy

4231 **Prairie Independent Living Resource Center**
17th S Main St
Hutchinson, KS 67501
620-663-3989
888-715-6818
Fax: 620-663-4711
TTY: 620-663-9920
info@pilr.org
www.pilr.org

Dave Mullins, President
Stephanie Guthrie, Vice President
Chris Owens, Executive Director
Roger Frischenmeyer, Independent Living Specialist

To achieve the full conclusion and acceptance of people with disabilities through education and advocacy

4232 **Resource Center for Independent Living**
104 S. Washington Ave.
Iola, KS 66749-8805
620-365-8144
877-944-8144
Fax: 620-365-7726
rcilinc.org

Chad Wilkins, Executive Director

Committed to working with individuals, families, and communities to promote independent living and individual choice to persons with disabilities.

4233 **Resource Center for Independent Living, Inc. (RCIL)**
409 Columbia St.
Utica, NY 13503-210
315-797-4642
800-580-7245
Fax: 315-797-4747
TTY: 315-797-5837
rcilinc.org

Chad Wilkins, Executive Director

Committed to working with individuals, families, and communities to promote independent living and individual choice to persons with disabilities. As a center for independent living in Kansas, we provide advocacy, peer counseling, information and referral, independent living skills training and deinstitutionalization. In addition to these services, we also provide HOBS payroll services and a variety of programs benefiting individuals with disabilities.

4234 **Resource Center for Independent Living: Emporia**
215 West Sixth Avenue
Suite 202
Emporia, KS 66801-2886
620-342-1648
888-261-4024
Fax: 620-342-1821
info@rcilinc.org
rcilinc.org

Deone Wilson, Executive Director
Beth Combes, Information & Outreach Coordinat
Amy Richardson, Targeted Case Manager
Trevor Larson, Office Assistant

Committed to working with individuals, families, and communities to promote independent living and individual choice to persons with disabilities.

4235 **Resource Center for Independent Living: Arkansas City**
P.O. Box 257
1137 Laing
Osage City, KS 66523
785-528-3105
800-580-7245
Fax: 785-528-3665
TTY: 785-528-3106
info@rcilinc.org
rcilinc.org

Deone Wilson, Executive Director
Tania Harrington, Director of Quality Assurance
Adam Burnett, Director of Core Services
Mike Pitts, Finance Committee Chairperson

Committed to working with individuals, families, and communities to promote independent living and individual choice to persons with disabilities.

4236 **Resource Center for Independent Living: Burlington**
P.O. Box 257
1137 Laing
Osage City, KS 66523
785-528-3105
800-580-7245
Fax: 785-528-3665
TTY: 785-528-3106
info@rcilinc.org
rcilinc.org

Deone Wilson, Executive Director
Tania Harrington, Director of Quality Assurance
Adam Burnett, Director of Core Services
Mike Pitts, Finance Committee Chairperson

Committed to working with individuals, families, and communities to promote independent living and individual choice to persons with disabilities.

4237 **Resource Center for Independent Living: Coffeyville**
P.O. Box 257
1137 Laing
Osage City, KS 66523
785-528-3105
800-580-7245
Fax: 785-528-3665
TTY: 785-528-3106
info@rcilinc.org
rcilinc.org

Deone Wilson, Executive Director
Tania Harrington, Director of Quality Assurance
Adam Burnett, Director of Core Services
Mike Pitts, Finance Committee Chairperson

Committed to working with individuals, families, and communities to promote independent living and individual choice to persons with disabilities.

4238 **Resource Center for Independent Living: El Dorado**
615 1/2 N Main St
El Dorado, KS 67042-2027
316-322-7853
800-960-7853
Fax: 316-322-7888
info@rcilinc.org
rcilinc.org

Macy Gaines, Independent Living Specialist
Doris Hammons, Targeted Case Manager
Shirley Mullin, Targeted Case Manager
Barbara Ehret, Office Assistant

Committed to working with individuals, families, and communities to promote independent living and individual choice to persons with disabilities.

4239 **Resource Center for Independent Living: Ft Scott**
P.O. Box 257
1137 Laing
Osage City, KS 66523
785-528-3105
800-580-7245
Fax: 785-528-3665
TTY: 785-528-3106
info@rcilinc.org
rcilinc.org

Deone Wilson, Executive Director
Tania Harrington, Director of Quality Assurance
Adam Burnett, Director of Core Services
Mike Pitts, Finance Committee Chairperson

Committed to working with individuals, families, and communities to promote independent living and individual choice to persons with disabilities.

4240 **Resource Center for Independent Living: Ottawa**
233 W 23rd Street
Ottawa, KS 66067-3533
785-242-1805
800-995-1805
Fax: 785-242-1448
rcilinc.org

Chad Wilkins, Executive Director

Committed to working with individuals, families, and communities to promote independent living and individual choice to persons with disabilities.

4241 **Resource Center for Independent Living: Overland Park**
Ste 100
10200 W 75th St
Shawnee Mission, KS 66204-2242
913-362-6618
877-439-2847
Fax: 913-677-2742
rcilinc.org

Chad Wilkins, Executive Director

RCIL is committed to working with individuals, families, and communities to promote independent living and individual choice to persons with disabilities.

4242 **Resource Center for Independent Living: Topeka**
1507 S.W. 21stStreet
Suite 203
Topeka, KS 66604-2356
785-267-1717
877-719-1717
Fax: 785-267-1711
info@rcilinc.org
rcilinc.org

Rosie Cooper, Director of Independent Living S
Stuart Jones, Assistive Technology Specialist
Mikel McCary, Assistive Technology Specialist
Mandy Smith, Finance Committee Chairperson

Committed to working with individuals, families, and communities to promote independent living and individual choice to persons with disabilities.

4243 **Southeast Kansas Independent Living (SKIL)**
1801 Main
P.O. Box 957
Parsons, KS 67357-957
620-421-5502
800-688-5616
Fax: 620-421-3705
TTY: 620-421-0983
skil@skilonline.com
www.skilonline.com

Nancy Varner, Chairman
Janet Spillman, Vice Chairman
Shari Coatney, CEO/President
Olivia Lyons, Secretary/Treasurer

To empower, integrate and maximize independence for all persons with disabilities.

4244 **Southeast Kansas Independent Living: Independence**
107 East Main
P.O. Box 944
Independence, KS 67301-944
620-331-1006
866-927-1006
Fax: 620-331-1257
TTY: 620-331-1006
skilindy@skilonline.com
www.skilonline.com

Nancy Varner, Chairman
Janet Spillman, Vice Chairman
Shari Coatney, CEO/President
Olivia Lyons, Secretary/Treasurer

To empower, integrate and maximize independence for all persons with disabilities.

4245 **Southeast Kansas Independent Living: Chanute**
2 W. Main
P.O. Box 645
Chanute, KS 66720-645
620-431-0757
866-927-0757
Fax: 620-431-7274
TTY: 620-431-0757
skilchanute@skilonline.com
www.skilonline.com

Nancy Varner, Chairman
Janet Spillman, Vice Chairman
Shari Coatney, CEO/President
Olivia Lyons, Secretary/Treasurer

To empower, integrate and maximize independence for all persons with disabilities.

4246 **Southeast Kansas Independent Living: Columbus**
123 N. Kansas
P.O. Box 478
Columbus, KS 66725-1801
620-429-3600
866-927-3600
Fax: 620-429-1027
skilcolumbus@skilonline.com
www.skilonline.com

Nancy Varner, Chairman
Janet Spillman, Vice Chairman
Shari Coatney, CEO/President
Olivia Lyons, Secretary/Treasurer

To empower, integrate and maximize independence for all persons with disabilities.

4247 **Southeast Kansas Independent Living: Fredonia**
623 Monroe
P.O. Box 448
Fredonia, KS 66736-448
620-378-4881
866-927-4881
Fax: 620-378-4851
TTY: 620-378-4881
skilfredonia@skilonline.com
www.skilonline.com

Nancy Varner, Chairman
Janet Spillman, Vice Chairman
Shari Coatney, CEO/President
Olivia Lyons, Secretary/Treasurer

To empower, integrate and maximize independence for all persons with disabilities.

4248 **Southeast Kansas Independent Living: Hays**
510 W. 29thStreet, Suite A
PO Box 366
Hays, KS 67601-366
785-628-8019
800-316-8019
Fax: 785-628-3116
TTY: 785-628-3128
skilhays@skilonline.com
www.skilonline.com

Nancy Varner, Chairman
Janet Spillman, Vice Chairman
Shari Coatney, CEO/President
Olivia Lyons, Secretary/Treasurer

To empower, integrate and maximize independence for all persons with disabilities.

4249 **Southeast Kansas Independent Living: Pittsburg**
1403 N. Broadway
P.O. Box 1706
Pittsburg, KS 66762-1706
620-231-6780
866-927-6780
Fax: 620-232-9915
TTY: 620-231-6780
skilpittsburg@skilonline.com
www.skilonline.com

Nancy Varner, Chairman
Janet Spillman, Vice Chairman
Shari Coatney, CEO/President
Olivia Lyons, Secretary/Treasurer

To empower, integrate and maximize independence for all persons with disabilities.

4250 **Southeast Kansas Independent Living: Sedan**
113 West Main
P.O. Box 340
Sedan, KS 67361-340
620-725-3990
866-906-3990
Fax: 620-725-3942
TTY: 620-725-3990
skilsedan@skilonline.com
www.skilonline.com

Nancy Varner, Chairman
Janet Spillman, Vice Chairman
Shari Coatney, CEO/President
Olivia Lyons, Secretary/Treasurer

To empower, integrate and maximize independence for all persons with disabilities.

4251 **Southeast Kansas Independent Living: Yates Center**
119 W. Butler
P.O. Box 129
Yates Center, KS 66783-129
620-625-2818
866-927-2818
Fax: 620-625-2585
www.skilonline.com

Nancy Varner, Chairman
Janet Spillman, Vice Chairman
Shari Coatney, CEO/President
Olivia Lyons, Secretary/Treasurer

To empower, integrate and maximize independence for all persons with disabilities.

4252 **Three Rivers Independent Living Center**
504 Miller Drive
P.O. Box 408
Wamego, KS 66547-0408
785-456-9915
800-555-3994
Fax: 785-456-9923
TTY: 785-456-9915
reception@threeriversinc.org
www.threeriversinc.org

Audrey Schremmer-Philips, Executive Director
Keyna Steinbrock, IL Specialist
Erica Christie, Director of Supports & Services
Rebel Eichelberger, Senior Accountant

A nonprofit organization promoting the self reliance of individuals with disabilities through education, advocacy, training and support.

4253 **Three Rivers Independent Living Center: Clay**
719 5th Street
P.O. Box 33
Clay Center, KS 67432-0033
785-632-6117
Fax: 785-632-6117
TTY: 785-632-6117
reception@threeriversinc.org
www.threeriversinc.org

Audrey Schremmer-Philips, Executive Director
Keyna Steinbrock, IL Specialist
Erica Christie, Director of Supports & Services
Rebel Eichelberger, Senior Accountant

A non-profit organization promoting the self reliance of individuals with disabilities through, education, advocacy, training and support.

4254 **Three Rivers Independent Living Center: Manhattan**
401 Houston St.
Manhattan, KS 66502
785-776-9294
800-432-2703
Fax: 785-776-9479
reception@threeriversinc.org
www.threeriversinc.org

Audrey Schremmer-Philips, Executive Director
Keyna Steinbrock, IL Specialist
Erica Christie, Director of Supports & Services
Rebel Eichelberger, Senior Accountant

A non profit organization promoting the self reliance of individuals with disabilities through education, advocacy, training and support.

4255 **Three Rivers Independent Living Center: Seneca**
416 Main St
Seneca, KS 66538-1926
785-336-0222
Fax: 785-336-0288
reception@threeriversinc.org
www.threeriversinc.org

Audrey Schremmer-Philips, Executive Director
Keyna Steinbrock, IL Specialist
Erica Christie, Director of Supports & Services
Rebel Eichelberger, Senior Accountant

A non profit organization promoting the self reliance of individuals with disabilities through education, advocacy, training and support.

4256 **Three Rivers Independent Living Center: Topeka**
P.O. Box 4152
Topeka, KS 66604-4152
785-273-0249
Fax: 785-273-0249
reception@threeriversinc.org
www.threeriversinc.org

Audrey Schremmer-Philips, Executive Director
Keyna Steinbrock, IL Specialist
Erica Christie, Director of Supports & Services
Rebel Eichelberger, Senior Accountant

A non profit organization promoting the self reliance of individuals with disabilities through education, advocacy, training and support.

4257 **Topeka Independent Living Resource Center**
501 SW Jackson St
Suite 100
Topeka, KS 66603-3300
785-233-4572
Fax: 785-233-1561
TTY: 785-233-4572
tilrcweb@tilrc.org
tilrc.org

Mike Oxford, Executive Director
Evan Korynta, Operations Manager
Angie Harter, Independent Living Advocacy Staf
Carol Doss, Independent Living Advocacy Staf

A civil and human rights organization that advocates for justice, equality and essential services for a fully integrated and accessible society for all people with disabilities.

4258 **Whole Person: Nortonville**
7301 Mission Road
Suite 135
Prairie Village, KS 66208- 3006
913-262-1294
877-767-8896
Fax: 913-262-2392
info@thewholeperson.org
www.thewholeperson.org
Rick O'Neal, President
Jim Atwater, Vice President
MIchelle Ford, Secretary
Timothy L. Urban, Treasurer
Assists people with disabilities to live independently and encourages change within the community to expand opportunities for independent living.

4259 **Whole Person: Nortonville, The**
7301 Mission Road
Suite 135
Prairie Village, KS 66208- 3006
913-262-1294
877-767-8896
Fax: 913-262-2392
info@thewholeperson.org
www.thewholeperson.org
Rick O'Neal, President
Jim Atwater, Vice President
MIchelle Ford, Secretary
Timothy L. Urban, Treasurer
Assists people with disabilities to live independently and encourages change within the community to expand opportunities for independent living.

4260 **Whole Person: Prairie Village**
7301 Mission Rd
Prairie Village, KS 66208-3006
913-262-1294
Fax: 913-262-2392
info@thewholeperson.org
www.thewholeperson.org
Rick O'Neal, President
Jim Atwater, Vice President
MIchelle Ford, Secretary
Timothy L. Urban, Treasurer
Assists people with disabilities to live independently and encourages change within the community to expand opportunities for independent living.

4261 **Whole Person: Prairie Village, The**
7301 Mission Road
Suite 135
Prairie Village, KS 66208- 3006
913-262-1294
877-767-8896
Fax: 913-262-2392
info@thewholeperson.org
www.thewholeperson.org
Rick O'Neal, President
Jim Atwater, Vice President
MIchelle Ford, Secretary
Timothy L. Urban, Treasurer
Assists people with disabilities to live independently and encourages change within the community to expand opportunities for independent living.

4262 **Whole Person: Tonganoxie**
7301 Mission Road
Suite 135
Prairie Village, KS 66208- 3006
913-262-1294
877-767-8896
Fax: 913-262-2392
info@thewholeperson.org
www.thewholeperson.org
Rick O'Neal, President
Jim Atwater, Vice President
MIchelle Ford, Secretary
Timothy L. Urban, Treasurer
Assists people with disabilities to live independently and encourages change within the community to expand opportunities for independent living.

Kentucky

4263 **Center for Accessible Living**
501 S. 2nd Street
Ste 200
Louisville, KY 40202-2121
502-589-6620
888-813-8497
Fax: 502-589-3980
TTY: 502-589-6690
www.calky.org
Jan Day, CEO
Michael Markiewicz, Chief Financial Officer
Jeanne M. Gallimore, Branch Director
Susan Tharpe, Coordinator of Services
To assist the individuals with disabilities who seek to live independently.

4264 **Center for Accessible Living: Murray**
1051 N 16th St
Suite C
Murray, KY 42071-8511
270-753-7676
888-261-6194
Fax: 270-753-7729
TTY: 270-767-0549
www.calky.org
Jeanne M. Gallimore, Branch Director
Susan Tharpe, Coordinator of Services
Jan Day, CEO
Michael Markiewicz, Chief Financial Officer
To assist the individuals with disabilities who seek to live independently.

4265 **Center for Independent Living: Kentucky Department for the Blind**
Independent Living Office
Rear
409 N Miles St
Elizabethtown, KY 42701-1834
270-766-5126
Buel E Stalls Jr, Office Manager and IL Specialist
Nancy Bachuss, Manager
Offers peer counseling, attendant care registry and other services to the community as they relate to the blind community. The Murray office is an independent living regional office which covers 20 far western counties of Kentucky..

4266 **Disability Coalition of Northern Kentucky**
Ste 219
525 W 5th St
Covington, KY 41011-1293
859-431-7668
Fax: 859-431-7688
TTY: 800-648-6057
Kitt Heeg, Executive Director
Empowering people with disabilities through education, networking, and positive attitudes..

4267 **Disability Resource Initiative**
624 Eastwood St
Bowling Green, KY 42103-1602
270-796-5992
877-437-5045
Fax: 270-796-6630
Marilyn Mitchell, Executive Director
Tracy Cole, Independent Living Specialist
Steve Burchett, IT Specialist
Jenny McCallister, Administrative Assistant
One of the most important premises in Independent Living is that people with disabilities are the most knowledgable about their own needs. Because of this all of their services are designed to be consumer-driven. Within each service, Center Staff work with both participant and provider to achieve and maintain an Independent Lifestyle.

4268 **Independence Place**
1093 S. Broadway
Suite 1218
Lexington, KY 40504-1787
859-266-2807
877-266-2807
Fax: 859-335-0627
TTY: 800-648-6056
info@independenceplaceky.org
www.independenceplaceky.org

Michael Fein, Chairman
Carla Webster, Vice Chairwoman
Pamela Roark-Glisson, Executive Director
Orissa Mason, Consumer Services Coordinator

To assist people with disabilities to achieve their full potential for community inclusion through improving access, choice and equal opportunity.

4269 **Pathfinders for Independent Living**
105 E Mound St
Harlan, KY 40831-2355
606-573-5777
877-340-PATH
Fax: 606-573-5739
TTY: 606-573-5777

Sandra Goodwyn, Executive Director
Andrew Saylor, Director of IT (Internal) and Fi
Stacy Marple, Director of IT (External)
Ron Walker, Public Affairs Specialist

They publish a newsletter called LifeLine 4-5 times a year. Most articles are written by Sandra Goodwyn. Editor is Andrew Saylor. Serves people with disabilities to maintain as much independence as they desire

4270 **SILC Department of Vocational Rehabilitation**
209 Saint Clair St
Frankfort, KY 40601-1817
502-564-4440
800-372-7172
Fax: 502-564-6745
sarahf.richardson@ky.gov

Sarah Richardson, SILC Liaison

We recognize and respect the contributions of all individuals as a necessary and vital part of a productive society..

Louisiana

4271 **New Horizons: Central Louisiana**
Ste 18
2406 Ferrand St
Monroe, LA 71201-3236
318-323-4374
800-428-5505
Fax: 318-323-5445
nhilc@nhilc.org
www.nhilc.org

Alan Loosley, President
Sharon Geddes, Vice-President
Clint Snell, Vice-President for Finance
Mary Russell, Secretary

A private, non-profit, non-residential, consumer-controlled, community-based organization that enables people with disabilities to live independently.

4272 **New Horizons: Northeast Louisiana**
3717 Government Street
Suite 7
Alexandria, LA 71301-4037
318-484-3596
888-361-3596
Fax: 318-484-3640
nhilc@nhilc.org
www.nhilc.org

Alan Loosley, President
Sharon Geddes, Vice-President
Clint Snell, Vice-President for Finance
Mary Russell, Secretary

A private, non-profit, non-residential, consumer controlled, community based organization that enables people with disabilities to live independently.

4273 **New Horizons: Northwest Louisiana**
1111A Hawn Avenue
Shreveport, LA 71106-6144
318-671-8131
877-219-7327
Fax: 318-688-7823
www.nhilc.org

Alan Loosley, President
Sharon Geddes, Vice-President
Clint Snell, Vice-President for Finance
Mary Russell, Secretary

A private, non-profit, non-residential, consumer-controlled, community based organization that enables people with disabilities to live independently.

4274 **Resources for Independent Living: Baton Rouge**
New Orleans Resources for Independent Living
3233 South Sherwood Forest Blvd.
Suite 101A
Baton Rouge, LA 70816
225-753-4772
877-505-2260
Fax: 225-753-4831
www.noril.org

Yavonka G. Archaga, Executive Director
Alisha S. Hammond, Assistant Director
Rosie Calvin, Program Manager
Deonne T. Bailey, Core Service Manager

RIL provides quality services to individuals with disabilities to assist with living independent. RIL also offers services to inculde information and referral, advocacy, peer support and independent living skills training.

4275 **Resources for Independent Living: Metairie**
2001 21st Street Kenner
Kenner, LA 70062
504-522-1955
877-505-2260
Fax: 504-522-1954

Yavonka G. Archaga, Executive Director
Alisha S. Hammond, Assistant Director
Rosie Calvin, Program Manager
Deonne T. Bailey, Core Service Manager

RIL provides quality services to individuals with disabilities to assist with living independently. RIL also offers an array of services to include information and referral, advocacy, peer support and independent living skills training.

4276 **Southwest Louisiana Independence Center: Lake Charles**
2016 Oak Park Boulevard
Lake Charles, LA 70601-5391
337-477-7198
888-403-1062
Fax: 337-477-7198
TTY: 337-477-7198
www.slic-la.org

4277 **Southwest Louisians Independence Center: Lafayette**
850 Kaliste Saloom Rd
Suite 118
Lafayette, LA 70508-4230
337-269-0027
888-516-5009
Fax: 337-233-7660
www.slic-la.org

4278 **Volunteers of America of Greater New Orleans**
4152 Canal St.
New Orleans, LA 70119
504-482-2130
Fax: 504-482-1922
voagno.org

Robert C. Rhoden, Chair
Wayne M. Baquet, Chair Elect
James M. Le Blanc, President/CEO
Geoffrey C. Artigues, Treasurer

Volunteers of America Greater New Orleans offers many services that aim to improve the lives of children, youth, and families.

4279 **W Troy Cole Independent Living Specialist**
Ste H
1900 Lamy Ln
Monroe, LA 71201-9200
318-323-4374
Katherine Carnell, Manager

Maine

4280 **Alpha One: Bangar**
3300 Ponce de Leon Blvd.
Coral Gables, FL 33134
305-567-9888
877-228-7321
Fax: 305-567-1317
info@alpha-1foundation.org
www.alpha1.org

John W. Walsh, President & CEO, Co-founder
Marcia F. Ritchie, Vice President/ COO
Marsha A. Carnes, Director of Program Evaluation
Robert Campbell, Communications Manager

Committed to being a leading enterprise providing the community with information, services and products that create opportunities for people with disabilities to live independently. Provides many services including adaptive and mobility equipment selection, peer support, advocacy, information and referral services, adapted drive evaluation and training, and consumer directed personal assistance.

4281 **Alpha One: South Portland**
127 Main St
South Portland, ME 04106-2647
207-767-2189
800-640-7200
Fax: 207-799-8346
TTY: 207-767-5387
www.alphaonenow.com

Dennis Stubbs, Chairman
Bob McPhee, Vice-Chairman
Darlene Stewart, Independent Living Specialist
Ketra S Crosson, Aroostook County Coordinator

Committed to being a leading enterprise providing the community with information, services and products that create opportunities for people with disabilities to live independently. Offers adaptive equipment loan program, independent living skills instruction, adapted driver evaluation and training, information and referral services, peer support, advocacy, access design consultation, and more.

4282 **Motivational Services**
71 Hospital Street
P.O. Box 229
Augusta, ME 04332-0229
207-626-3465
Fax: 207-626-3469
TTY: 207-621-2542
www.mocomaine.com

Connie Dunn, President
Grace Leonard, Vice President/Secretary
Faith Madore, Treasurer
Richard Weiss, Executive Director

Improving the lives of people with disabilities through housing, employment and community support.

4283 **Shalom House**
106 Gilman St
Portland, ME 04102-3034
207-874-1080
Fax: 207-874-1077
TTY: 207-842-6888
generalmail@shalomhouseinc.org
shalomhouseinc.org

Megan Lewis, Human Resources Manager
Mary Haynes-Rodgers, Executive Director
Kristine Lausier, Quality Assurance Administrator
Jane Collette, Accounting Manager

Offers hope for adults living with severe mental illness by providing a choice of quality housing and support services that help people lead stable and fulfilling lives in the community.

Maryland

4284 **Broadmead**
13801 York Rd
Cockeysville, MD 21030-1899
410-527-1900
877-STA-HOME
www.broadmead.org

Ann H. Heaton, Chair
John E. Howl, Chief Executive Officer
Patricia Gordon, Chief Financial Officer/Treasure
Douglas Bareis, Director of Support Services

To provide continuing care services to a diverse group of seniors in a warm, congenial community founded and operated in the spirit of the Religious Society of Friends.

4285 **Eastern Shore Center for Independent Living**
309 Sunburst Highway
Suite 13
Cambridge, MD 21613-2050
410-221-7701
800-705-7944
Fax: 410-221-7714
TTY: 410-221-4150
www.autismspeaks.org

Liz Feld, President
Alec M. Elbert, Chief Strategy & Dev Officer
Jamitha Fields, VP, Community Affairs
Lisa Goring, EVP, Programs and Services

ESCIL provides services to people with all disabilities regardless of age, religion, gender, ethnicity, race or national origin. In addition to the core services of information and referral, skills training, peer support and advocacy, ESCIL also offers assistance with accessibility modifications, Americans with Disabilities Act education and training, housing referrals and counseling, transportation referral and information, Brailling capabilities, Personal Attendent Services referral, and more.

4286 **Freedom Center**
14 W. Patrick Street
Suite 10
Frederick, MD 21701
301-846-7811
Fax: 301-846-9070
advocate@thefreedomcenter-md.org
thefreedomcenter-md.org

Jamey George, Executive Director
Russell Holt, President
Patrick Mcmurtray, Vice-President
Craig Shafer, Treasurer

A walk in center for independent living, provides services and supports to empower individuals with disabilities to lead self-directed, independent, and productive lives in a barrier-free community.

4287 **Housing Unlimited**
Ste G1
1398 Lamberton Dr
Silver Spring, MD 20902-3435
301-592-9314
Fax: 301-592-9318
information@housingunlimited.org
www.housingunlimited.org

Nancy Cohen, President Emerita
Russell Phillips, President
Robyn S. Raysor, Vice President
Johnnie Mae Armstrong, Treasurer

To address the housing crisis for adults with psychiatric disabilities who reside in Montgomery County, Maryland.

4288 **Independence Now**
12301 Old Columbia Pike
Suite 101
Silver Spring, MD 20904-1656
301-277-2839
Fax: 301-625-9777
info@innow.org
innow.org

Robert Watson, President
Sarah Sorensen, Executive Director
Todd Thorpe, Director of Operations
Trish Foley, Director of Community Services

A nonprofit organization created by people with disabilities and provides services that promote independence and the inclusion of people with disabilities in their communities.

4289 **Independence Now: The Center for Independent Living**
12301 Old Columbia Pike
Suite 101
Silver Spring, MD 20904
301-277-2839
Fax: 301-625-9777
info@innow.org
innow.org

Robert Watson, President
Sarah Sorensen, Executive Director
Todd Thorpe, Director of Operations
Trish Foley, Director of Community Services

A nonprofit organization created by people with disabilities to provide services that promote independence and the inclusion of people with disabilities within their communities.

4290 **Making Choices for Independent Living**
Ste 202
1118 Light St
Baltimore, MD 21230-4152
410-234-8195
888-560-2221

Jimmie Joku Cooper, Owner

Provides services to help empower people with disabilities to lead self-directed, independent and productive lives in the community and protect their civil rights.OUTOF ORDER.

4291 **Resources for Independence**
30 N. Mechanic Street
Unit B
Cumberland, MD 21502-2705
301-784-1774
800-371-1986
Fax: 301-784-1776
www.rficil.org

Lori Magruder, Executive Director
John Michaels, Assistant Director
Robert Cannon, Benefits Counselor
Sherry Williams, Finance Director

Private, non-profit, consumer-controlled, community-based organization providing services and advocacy by and for persons with all type of disabilities. Their goal is to create opportunities for independence, and to assist individuals with disabilities to achieve their maximum level of independent functioning within their families and communities.

4292 **Southern Maryland Center for LIFE**
P.O. Box 657
Charlotte Hall, MD 20622-657
301-884-4498
Fax: 301-884-6099
www.somd.com

Marie Robinson, Executive Director
Carrie Lanthier, Administrative Assistant

A non-profit community based organization which provides services to disabled people who live or work in the tri-county area. Our mission is to empower people with disabilities to lead self-directed, independent, and productive lives in their community.

Massachusetts

4293 **Adlib**
215 North St
Pittsfield, MA 01201-4644
413-442-7047
800-232-7047
Fax: 413-443-4338
adlib@adlibcil.org
adlibcil.org

Linda Febles, President
Michael Hinkley, Vice President
Allison Bedard, Treasurer
Shannon Miller, Secretary/Clerk

Offers information and referral services, independent living skills training, peer counseling, individual and group advocacy services available to all people with disabilities. Access consultation provided to businesses, agencies and institutions in accordance to the Americans with Disabilities Act.

4294 **Arc of Cape Cod**
P.O. Box 428
171 Main Street
Hyannis, MA 02601-428
508-790-3667
Fax: 508-775-5233
info@arcofcapecod.org
www.arcofcapecod.org

4295 **Boston Center for Independent Living**
5th Floor
60 Temple Place
Boston, MA 02111-1324
617-338-6665
Fax: 617-338-6661
TTY: 617-338-6662
www.bostoncil.org

Sergio Goncalves, Chairman
Linda Landry, Vice Chairman
Stacey Zelbow, Treasurer
Bill Henning, Executive Director

A frontline civil rights organization led by people with disabilities that advocates to eliminate discrimination, isolation and segregation by providing advocacy, information and referral, peer support, skills training, and PCA services in order to enhance the independence of people with disabilities.

4296 **Cape Organization for Rights of the Disabled (CORD)**
106 Bassett Ln.
Hyannis, MA 02601
508-775-8300
800-541-0282
Fax: 508-775-7022
TTY: 508-775-8300
cordinfo@cilcapecod.org
www.cilcapecod.org

Coreen Brinckerhoff, CEO & Chair
Mike Magnant, President & COO
Gretchen Arvanitopoulos, Vice President
Cathy Taylor, Director, Services

The Cape Organization for the Rights of the Disabled is dedicated to advancing independence, productivity, and integration of people with disabilities into mainstream society. CORD is the Center for Independent Living (CIL) and is a member of the Aging and Disability Resources Consortium (ADRC) serving Cape Cod and the Islands.

4297 **Center for Living & Working: Fitchburg**
76 Summer Street
Suite 110
Fitchburg, MA 01420-5785
978-345-1568
TTY: 978-345-1568
centerlwA@centerlw.org
www.centerlw.org

Cindy Purcell, Board President
Mary Ann Donovan, Treasurer
Ed Roth, Secretary
Jim O'Day, Advisor to CLW Board of Director

The Center for Living and Working is a non-profit Independent Living Center which takes its direction from persons with disabilities. The Center advocates to empower persons with disabilities to take active roles in their lives and in their community in which they live. Also provides comprehensive and innovative programs and services in order to maximize individual independence and opportunities.

4298 **Center for Living & Working: Framingham**
484 Main St
Suite 345
Worcester, MA 01608-1824
508-798-0350
Fax: 508-797-4015
TTY: 508-755-1003
opsearch@centerlw.org
www.centerlw.org

Cindy Purcell, Board President
Mary Ann Donovan, Treasurer
Ed Roth, Secretary
Jim O'Day, Advisor to CLW Board of Director

The Center for Living and Working is a non-profit Independent Living Center which takes its direction from persons with disabilities. The Center advocates to empower persons with disabilities to take active roles in their lives and in their community in which they live. Also provides comprehensive and innovative programs and services in order to maximize individual independence and opportunities.

4299 Center for Living & Working: Worcester
484 Main St
Suite 345
Worcester, MA 01608-1824
508-798-0350
Fax: 508-797-4015
TTY: 508-755-1003
opsearch@centerlw.org
www.centerlw.org

Cindy Purcell, Board President
Mary Ann Donovan, Treasurer
Ed Roth, Clerk/Secretary
Jim O'Day, Advisor to CLW Board of Director

The Center for Living and Working is a non-profit Independent Living Center which takes its direction from persons with disabilities. The Center advocates to empower persons with disabilities to take active roles in their lives and in their community in which they live. Also provides comprehensive and innovative programs and services in order to maximize individual independence and opportunities.

4300 Developmental Evaluation and Adjustment Facilities
215 Brighton Ave
Allston, MA 02134-2013
617-254-4041
800-886-5195
Fax: 617-254-7091
info@deafinconline.org
deafinconline.org

Sharon L. Applegate, Executive Director
Kelly Kim, President
John Sullivan, Treasurer
Kendra Timko-Hochkeppel, Vice President

Encourages and empowers deaf, hard of hearing, deafblind and late-deafened individuals to lead independent and productive lives.

4301 Independence Associates
100 Laurel Street
1st Suite 122
East Bridgewater, MA 02301-4012
508-583-2166
800-649-5568
Fax: 508-583-2165
info@iacil.org
iacil.org

Mark Lewis, President
James Clark, Treasurer
Anita Ashdon, Secretary
Steven Higgins, Executive Director

Provides comprehensive services which will enhance the range of acceptable options available to the consumer and improve the quality of life of persons with disabilities; to work on behalf of the objective of the disablility rights and independent living movement.

4302 Independent Living Center of Stavros: Greenfield
55 Federal St
Greenfield, MA 01301-2546
413-774-3001
www.stavros.org

Glenn Hartmann, President
Nancy Bazanchuk, Vice President
Donna M. Bliznak, Treasurer
Greta Biagi, Clerk

Promoting independence and access in the communities for persons with disabilities and deaf people.

4303 Independent Living Center of Stavros: Springfield
210 Old Farm Road
Amherst, MA 01002-2704
413-256-0473
800-804-1899
Fax: 413-256-0190
www.stavros.org

Glenn Hartmann, President
Nancy Bazanchuk, Vice President
Donna M. Bliznak, Treasurer
James Kruidenier, Executive Director

Promoting independence and access in the communities for persons with disabilities and deaf people.

4304 Independent Living Center of the North Shore & Cape Ann
27 Congress St
Suite 107
Salem, MA 01970-5577
978-741-0077
888-751-0077
Fax: 978-741-1133
ilcnsca.org

Mary Margaret Moore, Executive Director
Marion A Dawicki, President
Patricia Cox, Vice President
Joe Karaman, Treasurer

A service and advocacy center run by and for people with disabilities that supports the struggle of people who have all types of disabilities to live independently and participate fully in community life.

4305 MetroWest Center for Independent Living
280 Irving Street
Framingham, MA 01702-7306
508-875-7853
Fax: 508-875-8359
TTY: 508-875-7853
info@mwcil.org
mwcil.org

Youcef J. Bellil, President
Michael Kennedy, Vice President
Edward J. Carr, Treasurer
Penny Kelley, Secretary

To help individuals with disabilities become productive and contributing members of the community and to eliminate barriers within the community that impede this process.

4306 Multi-Cultural Independent Living Center of Boston
329 Centre Street
Jamaica Plain, MA 02130-1232
617-942-8060
Fax: 617-942-8630
TTY: 617-288-2707
info@milcb.org
milcb.org

Derrick Dominique, Executive Director
Ana Ortiz, Director of Services
Eleanor Slaughter, Senior IL Advocate
Louise Beach, Community Outreach Coordinator

Seeks to create opportunities for people with disabilities and their families in unserved/under-served populations and cultures who reside in Boston's inner city.

4307 Northeast Independent Living Program
20 Ballard Rd
Lawrence, MA 01843-1018
978-687-4288
Fax: 978-689-4488
TTY: 978-687-4288
help@nilp.org
nilp.org

June Cowen, Executive Director
Nanette Goodwin, Assistant Director
Lisa DiGiuseppe, Director of Finance
Jim Lyons, Director, Community Development

A consumer controlled Independent Living Center providing Advocacy and Services to people with all disabilities in the greater Merrimack Valley who wish to live as independently as possible in the commuity.

4308 Renaissance Clubhouse
176 Walker St
2nd Floor
Lowell, MA 01854-3126
978-454-7944
Fax: 978-937-7867
renclub1@gmail.com

Elaine Walker, Executive Director
Pammy Sadoie, Assistant Director

Offers daily structure, assistance wtih jobs, retirement, and housing.

4309 **Southeast Center for Independent Living**
66 Troy Street
Suite 3
Fall River, MA 02720-3023
508-679-9210
Fax: 508-677-2377
TTY: 508-679-9210
scil@secil.org
secil.org

Lisa M Pitta, Executive Director
Damase Cote, President
Paul Remy, Vice President
Debbie Pacheco, Treasurer / Secretary

The Philosophy of Independent Living, maintains that individuals with disabilities have the right to choose services and make decisions for themselves. This belief is the foundation and guiding principle of all of SCIL's policies and operations. SCIL provides training, information and support to help consumers achieve individual goals, experience personal growth and participate fully in community life.

4310 **Student Independent Living Experience Massachusetts Hospital School**
560 Harrison Avenue
Suite 600
Boston, MA 02118-2447
617-338-6409
800-843-5879
TTY: 800-328-3202
www.mass.gov

Michigan

4311 **Ann Arbor Center for Independent Living**
3941 Research Park Drive
Ann Arbor, MI 48108-6852
734-971-0277
Fax: 734-971-0826
www.annarborcil.org

Carolyn Grawi, Executive Director
Chris Baty, Theater Coordinator
Bryan Wilkinson, Director of Operations and Sales
Shirley Coombs, Chief Financial Officer

AACIL assists people with disabilities and their families in living full and productive lives. AACIL assures the equality of opportunity, full participation, independent living and economic self-sufficiency of people with disabilities in the community.

4312 **Arc Michigan**
1325 S Washington Ave
Lansing, MI 48910-1652
517-487-5426
800-292-7851
Fax: 517-487-0303
dhoyle@arcmi.org
arcmi.org

Donald Teegarden, President
Laurel Robb, Vice President
Dohn Hoyle, Executive Director
Sherri Boyd, Associate Director

Exists to empower local chapters of The ARC to assure that citizens with developmental disabilities are valued and that they and their families can participate fully in and contribute to the life of their community.

4313 **Arc/Muskegon**
601 Terrace Street
Suite 101
Muskegon, MI 49440-2197
231-777-2006
Fax: 231-777-3507
info@arcmuskegon.org
www.arcmuskegon.org

Tim Michalski, President
Brenda McCarthy Wiener, Vice President
Margaret O'Toole, Executive Director
Janis Milliron, Administrative Assistant

Offers information and referral, advocacy services and peer counseling.

4314 **Bad Axe: Blue Water Center for Independent Living**
614 N Port Crescent Street
P.O. Box 29
Bad Axe, MI 48413-1207
989-269-5421
810-987-9337
Fax: 989-269-5422
info@bwcil.org
www.bwcil.org

Karen Massaro-Mundt, President
Chuck Wanninger, Treasurer
Jim Whalen, Executive Director
Bill Farris, Administrative Assistant

A non-profit, consumer-based organization that advocates, informs and supports persons with disabilities in the community.

4315 **Bay Area Coalition for Independent Living**
Ste 17
701 S Elmwood Ave
Traverse City, MI 49684-3185
231-929-4865
Fax: 231-929-4896
steve@bacil.org

Steve Wade, Director

4316 **Capital Area Center for Independent Living**
2812 N. Martin Luther King Jr. Blvd
Lansing, MI 48906
517-999-2760
877-652-3777
Fax: 517-999-2767
TTY: 800-649-3777
www.cacil.org

Mark Pierce, Executive Director
Jeffrey Gass, Financial Manager
Justine Bond, Independent Living Specialist
Jean Harris, Program Coordinator

CACIL provide training, mentoring, and referrals to help people with disabilities and their families live productive lives.

4317 **Caro: Blue Water Center for Independent Living**
1184 Cleaver Rd
Caro, MI 48723-1143
989-673-3678
810-987-9337
Fax: 989-673-3656
info@bwcil.org
www.bwcil.org

Karen Massaro-Mundt, President
Chuck Wanninger, Treasurer
Jim Whalen, Executive Director
Bill Farris, Administrative Assistant

A non-profit, consumer-based organization that advocates, informs and supports persons with disabilities in the community.

4318 **Center for Independent Living of Mid-Michigan**
3941 Research Park Drive
Ann Arbor, MI 48108-6832
734-971-0277
Fax: 734-971-0826
www.annarborcil.org

Carolyn Grawi, Executive Director
Chris Baty, Theater Coordinator
Bryan Wilkinson, Director of Operations and Sales
Shirley Coombs, Chief Financial Officer

Comprised of over 51 percent of people with disabilities, and advocates for the rights of people with disabilities in the Mid-Michigan area. Call for information on disability issues or for assistance in obtaining services, within your community..

4319 **Community Connections of Southwest Michigan**
5671 N. Skeel Ave.
Suite 8
Oscoda, MI 48750
989-569-6001
800-578-4245
Fax: 269-925-7141

Kathy Ellis, Director

An advocacy organization that teaches and empowers people with disabilities to make choices about living life to the fullest, controlling and directing their own lives and asserting their rights and responsibilites within their Berrien County communities..

4320 Cristo Rey Handicappers Program
1717 N High St
Lansing, MI 48906-4529
517-372-4700
Fax: 517-372-8499
www.cristo-rey.org

Marlene M Berens, Manager

To care for the spiritual and social needs of individuals and families by offering services that encourage self-sufficiency and recognize the dignity of the human person..

4321 Detroit Center for Independent Living
1042 Griswold
Suite 2
Port Huron, MI 48060
810-987-9337
810-987-9337
Fax: 810-987-9548
info@bwcil.org
www.bwcil.org

Karen Massaro-Mundt, President
Chuck Wanninger, Treasurer
Jim Whalen, Executive Director
Bill Farris, Administrative Assistant

BWCIL is a consumer-based organization designed to serve persons with disabilities who have physical, psychiatric, sendory, cognitive, and multiple disabilities through the provision of advocacy, information and referral, service provision, and the promotion of needed services so to maximize the individual's optimal level of independence.

4322 Disability Advocates of Kent County
3600 Camelot Drive SE
Grand Rapids, MI 49546-8103
616-949-1100
Fax: 616-949-7865
contact@dakc.us
disabilityadvocates.us

David Bulkowski, JD, Executive Director
Denise Borges, Employment Specialist
Jackson Botsford, Accessibility Specialist
Katie Foreman, Independent Living Specialist

Exists to advocate, assist, educate and inform on independent living options for persons with disabilities and to create a barrier-free society for all.

4323 Disability Connection
27 E. Clay Avenue
Muskegon, MI 49442
231-722-0088
866-322-4501
Fax: 231-722-0066
dcilmi.org

John Wahlberg, President
Michael Hamm, Vice President
Tamera Collier, Executive Director
Tom Munn, Associate Director

To advocate, educate, empower, and provide resources for persons with disabilities and promote accessible communities.

4324 Disability Network Southwest Michigan
517 E Crosstown Pkwy
Kalamazoo, MI 49001-2867
269-345-1516
Fax: 269-345-0229
info@dnswm.org
www.dnswm.org

Cameron J. Lambe, Chair
Cheri Stoltzner, Vice Chair
Joel W Cooper, President
Kevin Klute, Treasurer

To educate and empower people with disabilities to create change intheir own lives, and to advocate for social change to create inclusive communities. As a center for independent living, they are part of the disability rights movement.

4325 Disability Network of Mid-Michigan
1705 S. Saginaw Road
Midland, MI 48640-6825
989-835-4041
800-782-4160
Fax: 989-835-8121
dnmm.org

Tom Provoast, President
Dr. Barbara Gibson, Vice President
David Emmel, Executive Director
Steven Locke, Associate Director

To promote and encourage independence for all people with disabilities.

4326 Disability Network of Oakland & Macomb
16645 15 Mile Rd
Clinton Township, MI 48035-2206
586-268-4160
800-284-2457
Fax: 586-285-9942
info@dnom.org
dnom.org

Andrew Maurer, Chairperson
Randy Charon, Vice Chairperson
Kellie Boyd, Executive Director
Kelly Winn, Director of Operations

Commited to advancing personal choice, independence, and positive social change for persons with disabilities through advocacy, education and outreach.

4327 Disability Network/Lakeshore
426 Century Lane
Holland, MI 49423-2200
616-396-5326
800-656-5245
Fax: 616-396-3220
TTY: 616-396-5326
info@dnlakeshore.org
dnlakeshore.org

Michelle Chaney, President
Amber Marcy, Vice President
Brian Dykhuis, Treasurer
Todd Whiteman, Executive Director

A cross-disability, community-based organization providing advocacy, education, and information and referral to persons with disabilities in Ottawa and Allegan counties.

4328 Grand Traverse Area Community Living Management Corporation
935 Barlow St
Traverse City, MI 49686-4250
231-932-9030
www.gtaclmc.org

Mary Jean Brick, Administrative Director

We are a training home for individuals with developmental disabilities over the age of 18

4329 Great Lakes/Macomb Rehabilitation Group
Apt 104
4 E Alexandrine St
Detroit, MI 48201-2032
313-832-3371
Fax: 313-832-3850

Jeannie Meece-Brooks, Contact

Independent living center. .

4330 JARC
30301 Northwestern Hwy
Suite 100
Farmington Hills, MI 48334-3277
248-538-6611
877-767-7781
Fax: 248-538-6615
jarc@jarc.org
jarc.org

Ronald Applebaum, President
Richard A. Loewenstein, Chief Executive Officer
Randy P. Baxter, Chief Financial Officer
Rena Friedberg, CFRE, Chief Development Officer

A nonprofit, nonsecretarian agency dedicated to enabling people with disabilities to live full, dignified lives in the community, and to providing support and advocacy for their families.

4331 Lapeer: Blue Water Center for Independent Living
392 West Nepessing Street
Lapeer, MI 48446-2192
810-664-9098
810-987-9337
Fax: 810-664-0937
info@bwcil.org
www.bwcil.org

Karen Massaro-Mundt, President
Chuck Wanninger, Treasurer
Jim Whalen, Executive Director
Bill Farris, Administrative Assistant

A non-profit, consumer-based organization that advocates, informs and supports persons with disabilities in the community.

4332 **Livingston Center for Independent Living**
3075 E Grand River Ave
Suite 108
Howell, MI 48843-6585
517-545-1741
Fax: 517-548-1751
www.virtualcil.net

Dan Durci, Director
Independent living skills training and empowerment training for persons with disabilities..

4333 **Michigan Commission for the Blind: Independent Living Rehabilitation Program**
235 S. Grand Ave.
P.O. Box 30037
Lansing, MI 48909-1254
989-758-1765
800-292-4200
Fax: 989-758-1405
www.michigan.gov

Debbie Wilson, Manager
Patrick Cannon, Agency Director
Rehabilitation teaching, independent living skills for persons over 55 with severe vision loss.

4334 **Michigan Commission for the Blind: Detroit**
Ste 4-450
3038 W Grand Blvd
Detroit, MI 48202-6012
313-456-1646
Fax: 313-456-1645
mcnealg@michigan.gov

Gwen McNeal, Supervisor
Shawnese Laury-Johnson, Assistant East Region Manager
Promotes the inclusion of people with legal blindness into our communities on a full and equal basis through empowerment, education, participation, and choice..

4335 **Monroe Center for Independent Living**
1285 N Telegraph Rd
Monroe, MI 48162-3368
734-242-5919
mrawlings@aacil.org
monroecil.tripod.com

Linda Maier, Manager
To act as a catalyst for personal and social change through the empowerment of people with disabilities; and, to replace the perception of disability as tragic with a disability culture promoting pride, power and personal style.

4336 **Port Huron: Blue Water Center for Independent Living**
1042 Griswold St
Suite 2
Port Huron, MI 48060-5431
810-987-9337
810-987-9337
Fax: 810-987-9548
info@bwcil.org

Karen Massaro-Mundt, President
Chuck Wanninger, Treasurer
Jim Whalen, Executive Director
Bill Farris, Administrative Assistant
A non-profit, consumer-based organization that advocates, informs and supports persons with disabilities in the community.

4337 **Sandusky: Blue Water Center for Independent Living**
103 East Sanilac Road
Suite 3
Sandusky, MI 48471-1615
810-648-2555
810-987-9337
Fax: 810-648-2583
info@bwcil.org

Karen Massaro-Mundt, President
Chuck Wanninger, Treasurer
Jim Whalen, Executive Director
Bill Farris, Administrative Assistant
A non-profit, consumer-based organization that advocates, informs and supports persons with disabilities in the community.

4338 **Southeastern Michigan Commission for the Blind**
4450 Grandy St
Detroit, MI 48207
313-456-0334
877-932-6424
Fax: 313-456-1645
www.michigan.gov

Patrick Cannon, Executive Director
Pat Bragg, Manager
Vocational rehabilitation agency. Personal adjustment vocational assessment and training, job placement and follow-up services. .

4339 **Superior Alliance for Independent Living (SAIL)**
1200 Wright Street
Suite A
Marquette, MI 49855
906-228-5744
800-379-7245
Fax: 906-228-5573
TTY: 906-228-5744
www.upsail.com

Elgie Dow, President
Aaron Andres, Vice President
Amy Maes, Executive Director
Judy Vivian, Finance Director
Promotes the inclusion of people with disabilities into our communities on a full and equal basis through empowerment, education, participation and choice.

4340 **disAbility Connections**
409 Linden Ave
Jackson, MI 49203-4065
517-782-6054
Fax: 517-782-3118
www.disabilityconnect.org

Michael Jackson, President
James Gorse, Vice President
Lesia Pikaart, Executive Director
Joann Lucas, Associate Director
Supporting Jackson County residents in their efforts to lead independent, fulfilling, productive lives.

Minnesota

4341 **Access North Center for Independent Living of Northeastern MN**
1309 East 40th Street
Hibbing, MN 55746
218-262-6675
800-390-3681
Fax: 218-262-6677
info@accessnorth.net
www.accessnorth.net

Donald Brunette, Executive Director
Patty Baratto, Administrative Assistant
Assists individuals to live independently, pursue meaningful goals, and have equal opportunities and choices. Other offices are located in Duluth, Brainerd, Walker & Aitkin.

4342 **Accessible Space, Inc.**
2550 University Avenue West
Suite 330N
Saint Paul, MN 55114-1085
651-645-7271
800-466-7722
Fax: 651-645-0541
TTY: 800-627-3529
info@accessiblespace.org
www.accessiblespace.org

Mark E. Hamel, Esq., Chairman
Kay Knutson, Vice Chairman
Steve Schugel, Treasurer
John W. Adams, Secretary
Accessible, rent-subsidized apartments for very low-income adults with qualifying physical disabilities as well as seniors. Accessible Space, Inc., sponsors, develops and manages housing & ASI apartments are rent based on income and are located across the country.

4343 **Courage Center**
800 E. 28th St.
Minneapolis, MN 55407-4298
612-863-4200
866-880-3550
Fax: 763-520-0577
TTY: 763-520-0245
couragekenny@allina.com
www.allinahealth.org
Jan Malcolm, CEO
Alice Johnson, Chief Financial Officer
Stephen Bariteau, Chief Development Officer
Pamela J. Lindemoen, Executive Vice President of Oper
A nonprofit rehabilitation and resource center that advances the lives of children and adults experiencing barriers to health and independence. Specialize in treating brain injury, spinal cord injury, stroke, chronic pain, autism and disabilities experienced since birth.

4344 **Freedom Resource Center for Independent Living: Fergus Falls**
125 W Lincoln Avenue
Suite 7
Fergus Falls, MN 56537-2152
218-998-1799
800-450-0459
Fax: 218-998-1798
freedom@freedomrc.org
www.freedomrc.org
Nate Aalgaard, Executive Director
Angie Bosch, Office Coordinator
Mark Mark Bourdon Bourdon, Program Director
Andrea Nelson, Independent Living Advocate
Freedom Resource Center assists people in working towards goals they establish for themselves.

4345 **Metropolitan Center for Independent Living**
Ste 16
1600 University Ave W
Saint Paul, MN 55104-3825
651-646-8342
Fax: 651-603-2006
TTY: 651-603-2001
homeramps@gmail.com

4346 **Minnesota Association of Centers for Independent Living**
215 North Benton Drive
Sauk Rapids, MN 56379
320-529-9000
888-529-0743
Fax: 320-529-0747
ilicil@independentlifestyles.org
independentlifestyles.org
Cara Ruff, Executive Director
Jay Keller, Board Chairman
Pamela Kotzenmacher, Treasurer
Autumn Gould, Attorney
A non-profit organization whose purpose is to advocate for the independent living needs of people with disabilities who are citizens of the State of Minnesota

4347 **OPTIONS**
Ste B
123 S Main St
Crookston, MN 56716-1970
218-281-5722
Fax: 218-281-5722
TTY: 218-281-5722
Gordie Haug, Manager
Provides people with disabilities advocacy, information, skills training and peer mentoring relationships to help them achieve their personal goals of how and where they live their lives.

4348 **Options Interstate Resource Center for Independent Living**
2200 2nd Street SW
Rochester, MN 55902-1887
507-285-1815
800-726-3692
Fax: 218-773-7119
TTY: 218-773-6100
options@myoptions.info
www.macil.org
Vicki Dalle Molle, President
Randy Sorensen, Executive Director
Located in Minnesota, but also serves North Dakota..

4349 **Perry River Home Care**
330 High Way Pen S
Saint Cloud, MN 56304
320-255-1882
Fax: 320-255-5137
Berna Florentine, CEO
Ken Figge, President
Courtney Salzi, Administrator
Offers skilled nursing services RN, LPN, TV Therapy, Pediatrics, Rehabilitation Services, PT, OT, ST, Paraprofessional staff, Home Health Aides, Homemakers, Personal Care Attendents, Companions, Live-ins, Sleep overs, Respite care, Extended hours.

4350 **SMILES**
820 Winnebago Ave
Suite 1
Fairmont, MN 56031-3619
507-345-7139
888-676-6498
Fax: 507-235-3488
www.smilescil.org
Brain Koch, President
Doug Robinson, Vice President
Alan Augustin, Executive Director
Helen Mitchell, Administrative Assistant
A nonprofit organization committed to providing a wide array of services that assist individuals with disabilities that live independently, pursue meaningful goals, and enjoy the same opportunities and choices as all persons.

4351 **SMILES: Mankato**
709 S. Front Street
Suite 7
Mankato, MN 56001-3887
507-345-7139
888-676-6498
Fax: 507-345-8429
smiles@smilescil.org
smilescil.org
Brain Koch, President
Doug Robinson, Vice President
Alan Augustin, Executive Director
Helen Mitchell, Administrative Assistant
A nonprofit organization committed to providing a wide array of services that assist individuals with disabilities that live independently, pursue meaningful goals, and enjoy the same oportunities and choices as all persons.

4352 **Southeastern Minnesota Center for Independent Living: Red Wing**
2200 2nd Street SW
Rochester, MN 55902
507-285-1815
888-460-1815
Fax: 507-288-8070
semcil@semcil.org
www.semcil.org
Brian Koch, President
Doug Robinson, Vice President
Alan Augustin, Executive Director
Helen Mitchell, Administrative Assistant
Non profit organization that assists people with disabilities to become independent and productive community members.

4353 **Southeastern Minnesota Center for Independent Living: Rochester**
2200 Second Street SW
Rochester, MN 55902-3980
507-285-1815
888-460-1815
Fax: 507-288-8070
semcil@semcil.org
www.semcil.org
Brain Koch, President
Doug Robinson, Vice President
Alan Augustin, Executive Director
Helen Mitchell, Administrative Assistant
A non profit organization that assists people with disabilities to become independent and productive community members.

4354 **Southwestern Center for Independent Living**
2864 S Nettleton Ave
Suite 700
Springfield, MO 65807
417-886-1188
800-676-7245
Fax: 417-886-3619
TTY: 417-886-1188
scil@swcil.org
www.swcil.org

Randy Custer, Board President
Emilio Vela, CEO
Shannon Porter, Deputy Director
Lacee Thompson, Director of Operations
SWCIL is a private, non-profit community-based organization providing independent living services to assist people with disabilities in obtaining and maintaining the greatest control over their lives. Services are available in southwestern Minnesota to persons of all ages, with any disability. Services include community access, education & outreach, mental health counseling, youth services, transition services and more.

4355 **Vinland Center Lake Independence**
3675 Ihduhapi Road
Loretto, MN 55357-308
763-479-3555
866-956-7612
Fax: 763-479-2605
vinland@vinlandcenter.org
www.vinlandcenter.org

Gerald Seck, President
Mary Roehl, Executive Director
Colleen Larson, Operations Manager
Debbie Larson, Accounting Manager
A Minnesota based rehabilitation center which offers services in three distinct service areas: vocational rehabilitation; inclusive community programs; and for people with cognitive disabilities, specially adapted chemical dependency treatment.

Mississippi

4356 **Alpha Home Royal Maid Association for the Blind**
PO Drawer 30
Hazlehurst, MS 39083-30
601-894-1771
Fax: 601-894-2993

Howard Becker, Director
Offers attendant care registry, information on accessible housing and referrals.

4357 **Gulf Coast Independent Living Center**
18 JM Tatum Industrial Drive
Hattiesburg, MS 39401-8341
601-544-4860
Fax: 601-582-2544

Albert Holifield, Executive Director
Independent living center.

4358 **Jackson Independent Living Center**
1981 Hollywood Dr
Jackson, TN 38305-2131
731-668-2211
800-848-0298
Fax: 731-668-0406
TTY: 601-351-1585
information@jcil.tn.org
www.j-cil.com/contact-us.html

Denea Smith, Director
Timothy Jackson
Provides services to consumers with severe disabilities.

4359 **LIFE of Mississippi**
1304 Vine St
Jackson, MS 39202-3429
601-969-4009
800-748-9398
Fax: 601-969-1662
TTY: 800-748-9398
www.lifeofms.com

Augusta Smith, Executive Director
Margie Moore, Project Coordinator
Densie Smith, Assistant
Christine Woodell, ADA Consultant
To empower people wit significant disabilities to be as independent and as fully involved in their communities as they can and want to be.

4360 **LIFE of Mississippi: Biloxi**
2030 Pass Road
Suite C
Biloxi, MS 39531
228-388-2401
Fax: 228-338-2413
www.lifeofms.com

Augusta Smith, Executive Director
Ruby Jackson, I.L. Specialist
Kim Allison, IL Specialist/ B2I
Christine Woodell, ADA Coordinator
To empower people with significant disabilities to be as independent and as fully involved in their communities as they can and want to be.

4361 **LIFE of Mississippi: Greenwood**
502a W Park Ave
Greenwood, MS 38930-2906
662-453-9940
Fax: 662-453-9934
www.lifeofms.com

Augusta Smith, Executive Director
Pam Wraggs, I.L. Specialist
Ruth Elliott, IL Specialist Assistant
Christine Woodell, ADA Consultant
To empower people with significant disabilities to be as independent and as fully involved in their communities as they can and want to be.

4362 **LIFE of Mississippi: Hattiesburg**
710 Katie Ave
Hattiesburg, MS 39401-4377
601-583-2108
www.lifeofms.com

Augusta Smith, Executive Director
Margie Moore, Project Coordinator
Densie Smith, Assistant
Christine Woodell, ADA Consultant
To empower people with significant disabilities to be as independent and as fully involved in their communities as they can and want to be.

4363 **LIFE of Mississippi: McComb**
915-A S. Locust Street
McComb, MS 39648-4817
601-684-3079
www.lifeofms.com

Augusta Smith, Executive Director
Margie Moore, Project Coordinator
Densie Smith, Assistant
Christine Woodell, ADA Consultant
To empower people with significant disabilities to be as independent and as fully involved in their communities as they can and want to be.

4364 **LIFE of Mississippi: Meridian**
Ste 103a
2440 N Hills St
Meridian, MS 39305-2653
601-485-7999
www.lifeofms.com

Augusta Smith, Executive Director
Margie Moore, Project Coordinator
Densie Smith, Assistant
Christine Woodell, ADA Consultant
To empower people with significant disabilities to be as independent and as fully involved in their communities as they can and want to be.

4365 **LIFE of Mississippi: Oxford**
Ste 5
404 Galleria Dr
Oxford, MS 38655-4383
662-234-7010
www.lifeofms.com

Augusta Smith, Executive Director
Margie Moore, Project Coordinator
Densie Smith, Assistant
Christine Woodell, ADA Consultant
To empower people with significant disabilities to be as independent and as fully involved in their communities as they can and want to be.

4366 **LIFE of Mississippi: Tupelo**
1051 Cliff Gookin Blvd
Tupelo, MS 38801-6739
662-844-6633
Fax: 662-844-6803
www.lifeofms.com

Emily Word, Regional Coordinator
Ronnie Jernigan, I.L. Specialist/HOT
Wayne Lauderdale, I.L. Specialist
Tara Christian, I.L. Specialist Assistant
To empower people with significant disabilities to be as independent and as fully involved in their communities as they can and want to be.

Missouri

4367 **Access II Independent Living Center**
101 Industrial Parkway
Gallatin, MO 64640-1280
660-663-2423
888-663-2423
Fax: 660-663-2517
access@accessii.org
www.accessii.org

Heather Swymeler, Executive Director
Brandy Gannan, Program Manager
Amber Wells, Financial Director
Dawn Ernat, In-Home Director
The mission of Access II is to remove architectural and attitudinal barriers that limit the independence of persons with disabilities, promote a positive change in attitudes about disability and persons with disabilities, and encourage greater independence for persons with disabilities within our communities. As a Center for Independent Living, Access II is comitted to the provision of a full range of independent living services.

4368 **Bootheel Area Independent Living Services**
PO Box 326
Kennett, MO 63857-326
573-888-0002
888-449-0949
Fax: 573-888-0708
TTY: 573-888-0002
tshaw@bails.org
www.bails.org

Tim Shaw, Executive Director
BAILS goal is to foster an open, barrier free society flor all people regardless of their disability. BAILS service area is predominantly rural and includes the Southeast Missouri counties of: Dunklin, New Madrid, Pemiscot and Stoddard.

4369 **Coalition for Independence: Missouri Branch Office**
6724 Troost Ave
Ste. 408
Kansas City, MO 66131
816-822-7432
Fax: 816-363-3469
TTY: 913-321-5126

Clarenece Smith, Executive Director
Coalition For Independence (CFI) is to facilitate positive and responsible independence for all people with disabilities by acting as an advocate for individuals with disabilities, providing services, and promoting accessibility and acceptance.

4370 **Delta Center for Independent Living**
PO Box 550
Suite #107
St. Peters, MO 63376-5608
636-926-8761
866-727-3245
Fax: 636-447-0341
info@dcil.org
www.dcil.org

Jennifer Mueller-Sparrow, President
Don Whalen, Vice President
Otis Pitts, Secretary
Bob Zeffert, Treasurer
A non profit corporation which assists people with significant disabilities who want to live more independently.

4371 **Disability Resource Association**
130 Brandon Wallace Way
Festus, MO 63028-1726
636-931-7696
Fax: 636-931-4863
TTY: 636-937-9016
dra@disabilityresourceassociation.org
www.disabilityresourceassociation. org

Craig Henning, Executive Director
Nancy Pope, Assistant Director
Suzan Weller, Director/Resource Developer
Independent Living Cener.

4372 **Easterseals Midwest**
11933 Westline Industrial Dr.
St. Louis, MO 63146
800-200-2119
Fax: 314-394-4007
info@esmw.org
www.easterseals.com/midwest

Wendy Sullivan, Chief Executive Officer
Jeff Arledge, Chief Financial Officer
Tom Barry, Chief Development Officer
Laurel Taylor, Chief Human Resources Officer
Easterseals Midwest helps people with disabilities live and work with dignity in their communities. Programs include community living and independent supported living arrangement services, with support in the following areas: housing, health and safety, money management, nutrition, transportation, and more.

4373 **Independent Living Center of Southeast Missouri**
511 Cedar St
Poplar Bluff, MO 63901-7301
573-686-2333
888-890-2333
Fax: 573-686-0733
TTY: 573-776-1178
info@ilcsemo.org
www.ilcsemo.org

Bruce Lynch, Executive Director
Debbie Hardin, Independent Living Director
To make Southeast Missouri barrier free for all persons with disabilities, enabling them to live more independently, extending their rights to control and direct their own lives and empowering them to live more producitve lives.

4374 **Midland Empire Resources for Independent Living (MERIL)**
4420 South 40th St
Saint Joseph, MO 64503-2157
816-279-8558
800-637-4548
Fax: 816-279-1550
TTY: 816-279-4943
www.meril.org

Dr. Robert Bush, Chair
Jaren Pippitt, Vice Chair
Wayne Crawford, Secretary
J. Robert Brown, Treasurer
Designed to promote independent living and to enhance the quality of life for persons with disabilities by empowering them to control and direct their lives.

4375 **Northeast Independent Living Services**
909 Broadway
Suite 350
Hannibal, MO 63401
573-221-8282
877-713-7900
Fax: 573-221-9445
www.neilscenter.org

Rose McNally, President
Dawn Davis, Vice President
Brooke Kendrick, Executive Director
Tara Fortner, Finance Director
To empower persons with disabilities to live as full and productive members of society.

4376 **On My Own**
428 E Highland Ave
Nevada, MO 64772-2609
417-667-7007
800-362-8852
Fax: 417-667-6262
www.omoinc.org

Jennifer Gundy, Executive Director
A non profit independent living center.

4377 **Ozark Independent Living**
109 Aid Ave
West Plains, MO 65775-3529
417-257-0038
888-440-7500
Fax: 417-257-2380
TTY: 888-440-7500
info@ozarkcil.com
ozarkcil.com

Michael Conner, Vice Chair
Scott Schneider, Secretary/Treasurer
Cindy Moore, Executive Director
Jane Kramer, Special Education Teacher

OIL?was created to provide independent living services to persons with disabilities who reside in the following counties in Missouri: Oregon Ozark, Shannon, Wright, Howell, Texas, and Douglas. OIL is non-profit, on-residential supported by grants, donations, and volunteers

4378 **Paraquad**
5240 Oakland Ave
Saint Louis, MO 63110-1436
314-289-4200
Fax: 314-289-4201
TTY: 314-289-4252
contactus@paraquad.org
www.paraquad.org

Robert Funk, Executive Director

Paraquad works to empower people with disabilities to increase their independence through choice and opportunity.

4379 **Places for People**
4130 Lindell Blvd
Saint Louis, MO 63108-2914
314-535-5600
Fax: 314-535-6037
www.placesforpeople.org

Kevin Kissling, President
Robin Kolker Adkins, Vice President
Joe Yancey, Executive Director
Dennis Wells, Secretary

Places for People provides individualized, high quality and effective services to adults with serious and persistent mental disorders to assist them in living, working and socializing responsibility to serve those individuals who rely on public funding.

4380 **RAIL**
3024 Dupont Circle
Jefferson City, MO 65109
573-526-7039
877-222-8963
888-667-2117
Fax: 573-751-1441
mo.silc@vr.dese.mo.gov
www.mosilc.org

Chris Camene, Chairperson
Jessica Hatfield, Vice-Chairperson
Barrnie Cooper, Secretary/Treasurer
Teresa Myers, Executive Director

RAIL is an Independent Living Center, one of twenty-two in the State of Missouri, RAIL's Mission is to assist persons with disabilities to live as independently as they choose within the communities of their choice. RAIL offers four core services which are: Advocacy, Peer Support, Information & Referral, and Independent Living Skills Training. RAIL is a Consumer Services Directed Program vendor

4381 **SEMO Alliance for Disability Independence**
1913 Rusmar St
Cape Girardeau, MO 63701-7623
573-651-6464
800-898-7234
Fax: 573-651-6565
TTY: 573-651-6464
www.sadi.org

Timothy D. Woodard, President
Michelle Spooler, Vice-President
Leemon Priest, Secretary
Janet Wilson, Treasurer

A community based, non-profit, nonresidential center for independent living that is committed to providing services to persons with disabilities to enable them to remain in their own home and community, not an institution.

4382 **Services for Independent Living**
1401 Hathman Place
Columbia, MO 65201-5552
573-874-1646
800-766-1968
Fax: 573-874-3564
TTY: 573-874-4121
www.silcolumbia.org

Dan Dunham, President
Bonnie Gregg, Vice President
Amy Henderson, Treasurer
Barbara Hammer, Secretary

A non-residential, community-based center for independent living. Provides individualized and group services to persons with severe disabilities in the Mid-Missouri area; works to help people with disabilities achieve their highest potential in independent living and community life.

4383 **Southwest Center for Independent Living (S CIL)**
2864 S Nettleton Ave
Springfield, MO 65807-5970
417-886-3619
800-676-7245
Fax: 417-886-3619
TTY: 417-886-1188
scil@swcil.org
www.swcil.org

Amy C. Lewis, President
Mark Grantham, Vice President
Gary Maddox, Chief Executive Officer
Lacee Thompson, Administrative Assistant

Provides services, advocacy, and resources for people with any disability in Christian, Dallas, Greene, Lawrence, Polk, Stone, Taney and Webster Counties of Southwest Missouri.

4384 **Sunnyhill, Inc.**
11140 So. Towne Square
Ste. 100
Saint Louis, MO 63123
314-845-3900
www.sunnyhillinc.org

Donny Mitchell, Chief Operating Officer
Amy Wheeler, Vice President, Program Services
Luke Mraz, Director, Development & Community Partnerships
Tamico Jones, Director, Advocacy

Services are provided to adults and children with developmental disabilities. Supported living arrangements are located in St. Louis city, St. Louis county and St. Charles County. Group home and camp services are located in Dittmer, MO. Travel program also available.

4385 **Tri-County Center for Independent Living**
1420 HWY 72 East
Rolla, MO 65401
573-368-5933
Fax: 573-368-5991
TTY: 573-368-5933
www.tricountycenter.com

Victoria Evans, Executive Director

Mission is to eliminate physical and attitudinal barriers through the power of advocacy, enlightenment, and reformation.

4386 **West Central Independent Living Solutions**
610 N Ridgeview Dr
Suite B
Warrensburg, MO 64093-9323
660-422-7883
800-236-5175
Fax: 660-422-7895
TTY: 660-422-7894
info@w-ils.org
www.w-ils.org

David De Frain, President
James Piatt, Vice President
Kathy Kay, Executive Director
Julie Steele, Director of Operations

Works to empower people with disabilities to become more independent by providing independent living skills training, peer support, information and referral and advocacy. West Central Independent Living Solutions now has satellite offices in Sedalia, MO and Lexington.

4387 **Whole Person, The**
3710 Main Street
Kansas City, MO 64111-7501
816-225-0301
800-878-3037
Fax: 816-931-0529
TTY: 816-561-0304
info@thewholeperson.org
www.thewholeperson.org

Rick O'Neal, President
Jim Atwater, Vice President
Julie Dejean, CEO
Mike Wiley, COO

The Whole Person, assists people with disabilities to live independently and encourages change within the community to expand opportunities for independent living.

4388 **Whole Person: Kansas City**
3710 Main Street
Kansas City, MO 64111-7501
816-561-0304
800-878-3037
Fax: 816-931-0529
TTY: 816-627-2202
info@thewholeperson.org
www.thewholeperson.org

Rick O'Neal, President
Jim Atwater, Vice President
Julie Dejean, CEO
Mike Wiley, COO

Assists people with disabilities to live independently and encourages change within the community to expand opportunities for independent living.

Montana

4389 **Living Independently for Today and Tomorrow**
1201 Grand Avenue
Suite 1
Billings, MT 59102-2033
406-259-5181
800-669-6319
Fax: 406-259-5259
TTY: 406-245-1225
www.liftt.org

Bobbie Becker, Executive Director
Martha Carstensen, Program Director

LIFTT's Independent living program works with people with disabilities so they can live independently and have access to the community. LIFTT staff, most of whom have disabilities, serve as mentors to people as they work to achieve the goals they have set for themselves.

4390 **Montana Independent Living Project, Inc.**
825 Great Northern Blvd
Suite 105
Helena, MT 59601-4715
406-442-5755
800-735-6457
Fax: 406-442-1612
TTY: 406-442-5755
bmaffit@milp.us
www.milp.us

Bob Maffit, Executive Director
Les Clark, Independent Living Specialist
Charlene White, Financial Manager
Marie Largent, Office Manager

A not-for-profit agency that provides services that promote independence for people with disabilities.

4391 **North Central Independent Living Services**
1120 25th Ave
Black Eagle, MT 59414-1037
406-452-9834
800-823-6245
Fax: 406-453-3940

Tom Osborn, Executive Director

North Central Independent Living Services is located in Great Falls and provides services from Glacier County across the Hi-Line to the North Dakota border. A satellite office is set up in Glasgow.

4392 **Summit Independent Living Center: Kalipsell**
1203 Highway 2 W.
Suite #35
Kalispell, MT 59901-6020
406-257-0048
800-995-0029
Fax: 406-257-0634
TTY: 406-257-0048
webmaster@bils.org
www.summitilc.org

Steve Hackler, President
Larry Riley, Vice President
Jenny Montgomery, Secretary
Flo Kiewel, Manager

To promote community awareness, equal access, and the independence of people with disabilities through advocacy, education, and the advancement of civil rights.

4393 **Summit Independent Living Center: Hamilton**
316 North 3rd St
Suite #113
Hamilton, MT 59840-2479
406-363-5242
800-398-9013
Fax: 406-375-9035
webmaster@bils.org
www.summitilc.org

Steve Hackler, President
Larry Riley, Vice President
Jenny Montgomery, Secretary
Joanne Berwolf, Manager

To promote community awareness, equal access, and the independence of people with disabilities through advocacy, education, and the advancement of civil rights.

4394 **Summit Independent Living Center: Missoula**
700 SW Higgins Ave
Suite #101
Missoula, MT 59803-1489
406-728-1630
800-398-9002
Fax: 406-829-3309
missoula@summitilc.org
www.summitilc.org

Steve Hackler, President
Larry Riley, Vice President
Jenny Montgomery, Secretary
Mike Mayer, Executive Director

To promote community awareness, equal access, and the independence of people with disabilities through advocacy, education, and the advancement of civil rights.

4395 **Summit Independent Living Center: Ronan**
124 Main St.
Ronan, MT 59864-2718
406-215-1604
866-230-6936
Fax: 406-552-1028
ronan@summitilc.org
www.summitilc.org

Steve Hackler, President
Larry Riley, Vice President
Jenny Montgomery, Secretary
Gary Stevens, Manager

To promote community awareness, equal access, and the independence of people with disabilities through advocacy, education, and the advancement of civil rights.

Nebraska

4396 **Center for Independent Living of Central Nebraska**
3335 West Capital Street
Grand Island, NE 68803-1730
308-382-9255
877-400-1004
Fax: 308-384-7832
TTY: 308-382-9255
jthomas@cilne.org
www.cilne.org

Joni Thomas, Executive Director
Irene Britt, Western Program Manager
Lesia Gracia, Independent Living Specialist
Mike Niece, Driving Program Coordinator

Offers independent living skills training, peer sharing, information and referral, housing counseling and referral, accessibility and barrier removal consultation including ADA training and technical assistance, driver education and training, assistive technology services including demonstration and equipment loan, and a free lending library of adapted toys and ability switches for children with severe disabilities. Serves all diabilities and all ages.

4397 **League of Human Dignity: Lincoln**
1701 P St
Lincoln, NE 68508-1799
402-441-7871
888-508-4758
Fax: 402-441-7650
TTY: 402-441-7871
info@leagueofhumandignity.com
www.leagueofhumandignity.com

Mike Schafer, CEO
The mission of the League of Human Dignity is to actively promote the full integration of individuals with disabilities into society. To this end, we will advocate their needs and rights, and provide quality services to involve these persons in becoming and remaining independent citizens.

4398 **League of Human Dignity: Norfolk**
400 Elm Ave
Norfolk, NE 68701-4033
402-371-4475
800-843-5785
Fax: 402-371-4625
TTY: 402-371-4475
ninfo@leagueofhumandignity.com
leagueofhumandignity.com

Mike Shafer, CEO
Jean M. Kloppenborg, Norfolk CIL Director
The mission of the League of Human Dignity is to actively promote the full integration of individuals with disabilities into society. To this end, we will advocate their needs and rights, and provide quality services to involve these persons in becoming and remaining independent citizens.

4399 **League of Human Dignity: Omaha**
5513 Center St
Omaha, NE 68106-3001
402-595-1256
800-843-5784
Fax: 402-595-1410
oinfo@leagueofhumandignity.com
www.leagueofhumandignity.com

Mike Schafer, CEO
Bob Gomez, Executive Director
The mission of the League of Human Dignity is to actively promote the full integration of individuals with disabilities into society. To this end, we will advocate their needs and rights, and provide quality services to involve these persons in becoming and remaining independent citizens.

4400 **Mosaic of Axtell Bethpage Village**
1044 23rd Rd.
PO Box 67
Axtell, NE 68924
308-743-2401
Fax: 308-743-2659
www.mosaicinfo.org/axtell

Max Miller, Chairperson
James Zils, Vice Chairperson
Linda Timmons, President/ CEO
Raul Saldivar, COO
Provides services that respect the human diginity and rights of each person. An interdisciplinary team of family, staffmembers and professional consultatns support individuals served in developing personal goals and programs, helping them to fully participate in Axtell's community life. Mosaic at Axtell offers residential and community services.

4401 **Mosaic of Beatrice**
722 S. 12th St.
PO Box 607
Beatrice, NE 68310-607
402-223-4066
Fax: 402-223-4951
www.mosaicinfo.org/beatrice

Max Miller, Chairperson
James Zils, Vice Chairperson
Linda Timmons, President/ CEO
Raul Saldivar, COO
Provides individualized services, living options, work choices, spiritual nurture and advocacy to people with disabilities in more than 250 communities across 14 states and Great Britain through the work of 4,800 employees.

4402 **Mosiac: York**
220 W South 21st St
York, NE 68467-9316
402-362-2180
Fax: 402-362-2961
www.mosaicinfo.org

Max Miller, Chairperson
James Zils, Vice Chairperson
Linda Timmons, President/ CEO
Raul Saldivar, COO
Providing a wide array of services to assist individuals and families in achieving positive life goals. Services to persons with disabilities and other special needs include community living options, training and employment options, spiritual growth and development options, training and counseling support.

Nevada

4403 **Carson City Center for Independent Living**
900 Mallory Way
Carson City, NV 89701
775-841-2580
Sandra Coyle, Owner
Helps consumers continue to live independently in the community through a variety of individual and community services.

4404 **Northern Nevada Center for Independent Living: Fallon**
1919 Grimes St
Suite B
Fallon, NV 89406-3100
775-423-4900
800-885-3712
Fax: 775-423-1399
TTY: 775-423-4900
nncilf@cccomm.net
www.nncil.org

Lisa Bonie, Executive Director
Hilda Velasco, Operations Manager
Joni Inglis, Independent Living Advocate
Deb Maijala, Rural Services Coordinator
Independent Living Center.

4405 **Rural Center for Independent Living**
1895 E Long St
Carson City, NV 89706-3214
775-841-2580
Fax: 775-841-2580
ruralcil@yahoo.com

Dee Dee Foremaster, Executive Director
Advocacy, Benefit Assistance, social security assistance, peer support, housing information and home-less day drop-in center for individuals with disabilities.

4406 **Southern Nevada Center for Independent Living: North Las Vegas**
3100 E Lake Mead Blvd
North Las Vegas, NV 89030-7380
702-649-3822
800-398-0760
Fax: 702-649-5022
TTY: 702-649-3822
sncilnv@aol.com
www.sncil.org

Connie Kratky, President
Elliot Yug, Vice - President
Pamela Rake, Secretary
William Sheehan, Treasurer

SNCIL is committed to removing barriers preventing indpendent living by providing services designed to empower people with disabilities.

4407 **Southern Nevada Center for Independent Living: Las Vegas**
2950 S. Rainbow Blvd.
Suite 220
Las Vegas, NV 89146-5611
702-889-4216
800-870-7003
Fax: 702-889-4574
TTY: 702-889-4216
sncil2@aol.com
www.sncil.org

Connie Kratky, President
Elliot Yug, Vice - President
Pamela Rake, Secretary
William Sheehan, Treasurer

SNCIL is committed to removing barriers preventing Independent Living by providing services designed to empower people with disabilities.

New Hampshire

4408 **Granite State Independent Living Foundation**
21 Chenell Drive
Concord, NH 3301-4079
603-228-9680
800-826-3700
Fax: 603-444-3128
TTY: 603-228-9680
info@gsil.org
www.gsil.org

Ken Traum, Chair
Lorna D. Greer, Vice Chair
Clyde E. Terry, CEO
Deborah Krider, COO

GSIL is a statewide non-profit that recognizes the fact that all of us will need some type of support in the course of the lives. GSIL offers tools and resources so that individuals can participate as fully as the choose in their lives, families and communities. Contact the Independent Living Foundation for referrals to living situations.

New Jersey

4409 **Alliance Center for Independance**
Alliance for Disabled in Action
629 Amboy Ave, First Floor
Edison, NJ 08837-3579
732-738-4388
Fax: 732-738-4416
TTY: 732-738-9644
adacil@adacil.org
www.adacil.org

Colleen Roche, Chair
Bernard Zuckerman, Treasurer
Carole Tonks, Executive Director
Luke Koppisch, Deputy Director

Alliance for Disabled in Action is a private, not-for-profit center for independent living serving people in Middlesex, Somerset and Union Counties of New Jersey. ADA's mission is to support and promote choice, self-direction and independent living in the lives of people with disabilities, with the right of individuals to inclusion in the community as the primary goal.

4410 **Camden City Independent Living Center**
2600 Mount Ephraim Ave
Camden, NJ 8104-3236
856-966-0800
Fax: 856-966-0832
TTY: 856-966-0830
vedasmithccilc@aol.com
www.camdencityilc.org

Bruce Smith, Chairperson
John Quann, Vice Chairperson
Tanya Brown, Treasurer
Veda Smith, Executive Director

Provides services designed to empower people with disabilities. To provide services to individuals with significant disabilities. Services include information referral, advocacy, peer support, and independent living skills training. CCILC services individuals in Camden City

4411 **Center for Independent Living: Long Branch**
279 Broadway
Suite #201
Long Branch, NJ 7740-6940
732-571-4884
Fax: 732-571-4003
TTY: 732-571-4878
www.moceanscil.org

Jennifer Sterner, Vice Chair
Maureen Poling, Secretary
Stan Soden, Director IL Services
Susan Pniewski, IL Transition Specialist

Offers peer support, disability education and personal assistant services. Serving Monmouth and Ocean Counties with information and referrals, advocacy, peer support and independent living instructions.

4412 **Center for Independent Living: South Jersey**
1150 Delsea Drive
Suite #1
Westville, NJ 8093-2251
856-853-6490
800-413-3791
Fax: 856-853-1466
TTY: 856-853-7602

Hazel Lee-Briggs, Executive Director
Danuta Debicki, Program Manager
Terryama Davis, Independent Living Specialist

Dedicated to providing people with disabilities in Gloucester and Camden counties the opportunity to actively participate in society, to provide freedom of choice, to work, to own a home, raise a family and in general, to participate to the fullest extent in day-to-day activities. The center provides information and referrals, advocacy, peer support, and independent living skills training.

4413 **DAWN Center for Independent Living**
66 Ford Road
Suite 121
Denville, NJ 7834-1235
973-625-1940
888-383-3296
Fax: 973-625-1942
TTY: 973-625-1932
info@dawncil.org
www.dawncil.org

Elizabeth Lehmann, President
Gabrielle Waldman, Vice President
Carmela Slivinski, Executive Director
Caroleen Marano, Independent Living Program

DAWN is the Center for Independent Living serving Morris, Sussex and Warren counties. DAWN empowers people with disabilities to strive for equality and to take control of their own lives by providing the tools that encourage independence and self-advocacy, promoting public awareness of the needs, desires and rights to individuals living with disabilities, and offering community activities that create new experiences and opportunities.

4414 **Dial: Disabled Information Awareness & Living**
2 Prospect Village Plaza
Floor 1
Clifton, NJ 7013-1918
973-470-8090
866-277-1733
Fax: 973-470-8171
TTY: 973-470-2521
info@dial-cil.org
www.dial-cil.org

Cynthia DeSouza, President
Anthony Gianduso, Vice President
John Petix, Executive Director
Tim Burns, Secretary

Promotes the full inclusion of all people living with disabilities into society and encourage the consumers and the community at large to seek involvement in this self-governing organization to the fullest extent.

4415 **Disability Rights New Jersey**
New Jersey Protection and Advocacy
210 S. Broad Street
Floor 3
Trenton, NJ 08608-2407
609-292-9742
800-922-7233
Fax: 609-777-0187
TTY: 609-633-7106
advocate@drnj.org
www.drnj.org

Walter Anthony Woodberry, Chair
Andrew McGeady, Vice Chair
Linda K. Soley, Treasurer
Leah Ziskin, Secretary
Assistive Technology Advocacy Center provides assistance to personswith disabilities in helping them to obtain assistive technology devices and/or services.

4416 **Family Resource Associates**
35 Haddon Ave
Shrewsbury, NJ 7702-4007
732-747-5310
Fax: 732-747-1896
info@frainc.org
www.frainc.org

Allan Proske, President
Bill Sheeser, Vice President
John Feeney, Treasurer
Judy Fuller, Secretary
FRA is dedicated to helping children, adolescents and people of all ages with disabilities to reach their fullest potential. FRA also connects individuals to independence through modern therapies and advanced technology. FRA provides direct services to those in the greater Nonmouth/Ocean County area.

4417 **Heightened Independence and Progress: Hackensack**
131 Main St
Suite #120
Hackensack, NJ 7601-7182
201-996-9100
Fax: 201-996-9422
TTY: 201-966-9424
www.hipcil.org

Eileen Goff, President/CEO
Trish Carney, Finance and Development Director
Empowers people with disabilities to achieve independent living through outreach, advocacy and education.

4418 **Heightened Independence and Progress: Jersey City**
35 Journal Square
Suite #703
Jersey City, NJ 7306-4105
201-533-4407
Fax: 201-533-4421
TTY: 201-533-4409
www.hipcil.org

Jean Csaposs, Board Chair
Lottie Esteban, First Vice Chair
Eileen Goff, President/CEO
Trish Carney, Finance and Development Director
Empowering People with Disabilities to Achieve Independent Living through Outreach, Advocacy, and Education.

4419 **Progressive Center for Independent Living**
3525Quakerbridge Rd.
Suite 904
Hamilton, NJ 8619-3710
609-581-4500
877-917-4500
Fax: 609-581-4555
TTY: 609-581-4550
info@pcil.org
www.pcil.org

Norman Smith, President
John Witman, Vice President
Scott Elliott, Executive Director
Jerry Carbone, Training Coordinator
Advocates for the rights of people with disabilities to achieve and maintain independent lifestyles. The Center has programs to assist with employment, transition from school to adult life, and emergency preparedness.

4420 **Progressive Center for Independent Living: Flemington**
4 Walter E Foran Blvd
Suite 410
Flemington, NJ 8822-4669
908-782-1055
877-376-9174
Fax: 908-782-6025
TTY: 908-782-1081
info@pcil.org
pcil.org

Norman Smith, President
John Witman, Vice President
Scott Elliott, Executive Director
Jerry Carbone, Training Coordinator
Advocates for the rights of people with disabilities to achieve and maintain independent lifestyles.

4421 **Project Freedom**
223 Hutchinson Rd
Robbinsville, NJ 8691-3457
609-448-2998
Fax: 609-448-7293
ProjectFreedom1@aol.com
www.projectfreedom.org

Tim Doherty, Executive Director
Norman A. Smith, Assoc Ex Director
Elizabeth Maxwell, Office Manager
Paul Campanella, Property Manager
Dedicated to developing, supporting, and advocating opportunities for independent living persons with disabilities.

4422 **Project Freedom: Hamilton**
715 Kuser Rd
Hamilton, NJ 8619-3924
609-588-9919
Fax: 609-588-8831
cfunk@projectfreedom.org
www.projectfreedom.org

Cecilia Funk, Social Service Coordinator
Judy Wilkinson, Office Manager
Paul Campanella, Property Manager
Dedicated to developing, supporting, and advocating opportunities for independent living persons with disabilities.

4423 **Project Freedom: Lawrence**
1 Freedom Blvd
Lawrence, NJ 8648-4531
609-278-0075
Fax: 609-278-1250
jelsowiny@projectfreedom.org
www.projectfreedom.org

Jacklene Elsowiny, Social Serv Coordinator
Tim Doherty, Executive Director
Stephen Schaefer, CFO
Tracee Battis, Director of Housing Development
Dedicated to developing, supporting, and advocating opportunities for independent living persons with disabilities.

4424 **Total Living Center**
6712 Washington Ave
Egg Harbor Township, NJ 8234-1999
609-645-9547
Fax: 609-813-2318
TTY: 609-645-9593

Jo Hudson, President
Cliff Anderson, Vice President
Cathy Shaner, Secretary
Julia Bonelli, Executive Director
Total Living Center is a non-profit organization whose mission is to empower individuals with significant disabilities to maximize their potential for independence and productivity, to live as fully as possible within the community, taking responsibility for themselves, and sharing this commitment with others.

New Mexico

4425 **Ability Center**
715 E Idaho Ave.
Suite 3E
Las Cruces, NM 88001
575-526-5016
800-376-4372
Fax: 575-526-1202
TTY: 575-210-5272
freedom@theabilitycenter.org
www.theabilitycenter.org

4426 **CASA Inc.**
116 West Baltimore Street
Hagerstown, MD 21740
301-739-4990
Fax: 301-790-0064
casa4@myactv.net
www.casaabq.com

Sherry Donovan, President
Linda Davis, Vice-President
Melinda Marsden, Treasurer
Laura Allis, Secretary

Offers peer counseling and information and referral services.

4427 **CHOICES Center for Independent Living**
200 E 4th St.
Suite #200
Roswell, NM 88201-6237
575-627-6727
800-387-4572
Fax: 575-627-6754
TTY: 505-627-6727

Julia Calvert, Executive Director

Offers many core services including independent living skills training, peer support, information and referral, advocacy and transition.

4428 **New Mexico Technology Assistance Program**
625 Silver Ave SW
Ste. 100 B
Albuquerque, NM 87102
505-841-4464
877-696-1470
Fax: 505-841-4467
Tracy.Agiovlasitis@state.nm.us
www.tap.gcd.state.nm.us

Tracy Agiovlasitis, Program Manager

Examines and works to eliminate barriers to obtaining assistive technology in New Mexico. Has established a statewide program for coordinating assistive technology services; is designed to assist people with disabilities to locate, secure, and maintain assistive technology.

4429 **New Vistas**
1205 Parkway Dr.
Suite A
Santa Fe, NM 87501-2483
505-471-1001
Fax: 505-471-4427
info@newvistas.org
www.newvistas.org

Victor Ortega, President
Libby Gonzales, Vice-President
Gay Romero, Secretary/Treasurer

Partners with and supports people with disabilities and families of children with special needs to enrich their quality of life in New Mexico.

4430 **San Juan Center for Independence**
1204 San Juan Blvd
Farmington, NM 87401
505-566-5827
877-484-4500
Fax: 505-566-5842
TTY: 505-566-5827
sjci@sjci.org
www.sjci.org

Patricia Ziegler, Executive Director
Tim Carver, CFO

SJCI is a New Mexico private non residential, nonprofit corporation that serves people with disabilities. The purpose of SJCI is to provide a variety of community based, consumer driven service to people with disablities to promote independence, self-residence and intergration into the community.

New York

4431 **AIM Independent Living Center: Corning**
271 E 1st St
Corning, NY 14830-2924
607-962-8225
Fax: 607-937-5125
TTY: 607-962-8225
troche@aimcil.com
www.aimcil.com

Rene Snyder, Executive Director
Sabrina Mineo-O'Connell, President
George Spisack, Vice President
Barbara Squires, Treasurer

AIM is a non-profit organization dedicated to people with disabilities, their families, friends, the businesses that serve them and those with an interest in disabilities. The mission of AIM is to support the individuals ability to make independent, self-directing choices through education, advocacy, information and referral.

4432 **AIM Independent Living Center: Elmira**
650 Baldwin St.
Elmira, NY 14901-2216
607-733-3718
Fax: 607-733-0180
TTY: 607-733-7764
troche@aimcil.com
www.aimcil.com

Rene Snyder, Executive Director
Sabrina Mineo-O'Connell, President
George Spisack, Vice President
Barbara Squires, Treasurer

AIM's goal is to enable the consumer to live an independent and comfortable lifestyle in the security of their home environment so they may feel dignity and pride in their achievements while controling their own care.

4433 **ARISE**
635 James St
Syracuse, NY 13203-2661
315-472-3171
Fax: 315-472-9252
TTY: 315-479-6363
info@ariseinc.org
www.ariseinc.org

Tania Anderson, President
Sue Judge, Vice President
Michael Cook, Treasurer
Tom McKeown, Executive Director

Founded in 1979, ARISE's mission is to work with people of all abilities to create a fair and just community in which everyone can fully participate. As a center for independent living, ARISE is a non-profit organization run by and for individuals with disabilities. ARISE serves over 3,000 children and adults with disabilities each year through our programs and services in several broad areas including advocacy, employment, independent living/integrated recreation programs, and much more.

4434 **ARISE: Oneida**
131 Main St
Suite #107
Oneida, NY 13421-1644
315-363-4672
Fax: 315-363-4675
TTY: 315-363-2364
info@ariseinc.org
www.ariseinc.org

Tania Anderson, President
Sue Judge, Vice President
Michael Cook, Treasurer
Tom McKeown, Executive Director

A consumer controlled, non-profit Independent Living Center that promotes the full inclusion of people with disabilities in the community.

4435 ARISE: Oswego
9 Fourth Avenue
Oswego, NY 13126-1803
315-342-4088
Fax: 315-342-4107
TTY: 315-342-8696
info@ariseinc.org
www.ariseinc.org

Tania Anderson, President
Sue Judge, Vice President
Michael Cook, Treasurer
Tom McKeown, Executive Director

A consumer controlled, non-profit Independent Living Center that promotes the full inclusion of people with disabilities in the community.

4436 ARISE: Pulaski
2 Broad St
Pulaski, NY 13142-4446
315-298-5726
Fax: 315-298-5729
info@ariseinc.org
www.ariseinc.org

Tania Anderson, President
Sue Judge, Vice President
Michael Cook, Treasurer
Tom McKeown, Executive Director

A consumer controlled, non-profit Independent Living Center that promotes the full inclusion of people with disabilities in the community.

4437 Access to Independence of Cortland County, Inc.
26 N Main St
Cortland, NY 13045-2198
607-753-7363
Fax: 607-756-4884
info@aticortland.org
www.aticortland.org

Judy Bentley, Chair
Peter Morse-Ackley, Vice Chair
Chad W. Underwood, CEO
Mary E. Ewing, Program Manager

Access to Independence is Cortland County's foremost disability resource. It empowers people to lead independent lives in their community and strives to open doors to full participation and access for all.

4438 Action Toward Independence: Middletown
130 Dolson Avenue
Suite 35
Middletown, NY 10940-6563
845-343-4284
Fax: 845-342-5269

Stephen McLaughlin, Executive Director
Joann Hargabus, Services Director, Orange Cnty.
Gilles Malkine, Services Director, Sullivan Cnty
Cheryl Babcock, Fiscal Manager

Independent living center that serves Orange & Sullivan counties. Provides programs and services to individuals who have disabilities and to their families. These services include peer counseling, individual & systems advocacy, independent living, skills training, information and referral, benefits advisement, recreation and a drop in center. We are designed to enable people with disabilities to achieve independence, inclusion and participation in their communities.

4439 Action Toward Independence: Monticello
309 E Broadway
Suite A
Monticello, NY 12701-8810
845-794-4228
Fax: 845-794-4475
TTY: 845-794-4228
www.atitoday.org

Steve McLaughlin, Executive Director
Joann Hargabus, Director of Services

A not-for-profit, non residential, peer run, referral and advocacy agency for persons with disaiblities in Orange and Sullivan counties. Our services are aimed at promoting accessibility, community integration, and equal opportunity in all aspects of society for persons with all types of disabilities.

4440 BRiDGES
873 Route 45
Suite 108
New City, NY 10956
845-624-1366
Fax: 845-624-1369
info@bridgesrc.org
www.bridgesrc.org

Patricia Ranieri, President
David Jacobsen, Ph.D, Psy.D, Executive Director
Michael Coleman, Director of Finance & Controller
Nanci Goldman, Director of Human Resources

BRiDGES is a community-based non-profit organization that serves people with disabilities. Services provided by them include personal assistance self-employers, independent living services, volunteer opportunities, advocacy and more.

4441 Bronx Independent Living Services
4419 Thrid Avenue
Suite 2C
Bronx, NY 10457
718-515-2800
Fax: 718-515-2844
TTY: 718-515-2803
webmaster@bils.org
www.bils.org

Barbara Linn, President
Anita Richichi, Vice President
Sheldon Mann, Treasurer
Brett L. Eisenberg, Executive Director

BILS is a not-for-profit community agency serving people with all kinds of disabilities. The mission is to empower people with disabilities toward living independent lives. BILS assists individuals by providing advocacy, peer counseling, housing information, and independent living training/counseling.

4442 Brooklyn Center for Independence of the Disabled
27 Smith Street
Suite #200
Brooklyn, NY 11201
718-998-3000
Fax: 718-998-3743
TTY: 718-998-7406
advocate@bcid.org
www.bcid.org

Joan Peters, Executive Director
Sandrina Kingston, Program Director
Princess Davis, Office Manager
Stanley Stephen, Office Assistant

Operated by a majority of people with disabilities, BCID is dedicated to guaranteeing the civil rights of people with disabilities. BCID exists to improve the quality of life of brooklyn residents with disabilities thgouh programs that empower them to gain greater control of their lives and achieve full and equal integration into society.

4443 Capital District Center for Independence
845 Central Ave
South 3
Albany, NY 12206-1342
518-459-6422
Fax: 518-459-7847
TTY: 518-459-6422
info@cdciweb.com
www.cdciweb.com

Laurel Kelley, Executive Director
Dawn Werner, Deputy Director
Judy Zuchero, Program Director
G. W. Barr, Advocate

One of 37 Independent Living Centers in New York State, the Center is a non-residential, community based organization, which primarily serves Albany and Schenectady Counties. The Center's mission is to assist people with disabilities to acquire self-advocacy skills and by teaching through example, consumers achieve greater control over the direction of their lives.

4444 Catskill Center for Independence
6104 State Highway 23
Oneonta, NY 13820
607-432-8000
Fax: 607-432-6907
TTY: 607-432-8000
ccfi@ccfi.us
www.ccfi.us

Chris Zachmeyer, Executive Director
Christine Worden, Assistant Director

One of 37 community-based independent living centers located throughout the state of New York. As an advocacy agency, we provide a vareity of services to people with disabilities, their friends and family members. In addition, we provide advocacy, training, and technical assistance to our community members, organizations, businesses and state and local governments in a variety of disability related areas. Serves Otsego, Delaware and Schoharie counties.

4445 **Center for Community Alternatives**
115 E Jefferson St
Suite #300
Syracuse, NY 13202-2018
315-422-5638
Fax: 315-471-4924
cca@communityalternatives.org
www.communityalternatives.org

Kwame Johnson, President
Susan R. Horn, Esq., Vice-President
Carole A. Eady, Secretary
Marsha Weissman, Executive Director

Promotes reintegrative justice and a reduced reliance on incarceration through advocacy, services and public policy development in pursuit of civil and human rights.

4446 **Center for Independence of the Disabled of New York**
841 Broadway
Suite 301
New York, NY 10003-4708
212-674-2300
Fax: 212-254-5953
TTY: 212-674-5619
info@cidny.org
www.cidny.org

Martin Eichel, President
Anne M. Davis, Vice President
John O'Neill, Vice President
Susan Dooha, Executive Director

To ensure full integration, independence and equal opportunity for all people with disabilities by removing barriers to the social, economic, cultural and civic life of the community.

4447 **Center for Independence of the Disabled of New York**
841 Broadway
Suite 301
New York, NY 10003-4708
212-674-2300
Fax: 212-254-5953
TTY: 212-674-5619
info@cidny.org
www.cidny.org

Martin Eichel, President
Anne M. Davis, Vice President
John O'Neill, Vice President
Susan Dooha, Executive Director

To ensure full integration, independence and equal opportunity for all people with disabilities by removing barriers to the social, economic, cultural and civic life of the community.

4448 **DD Center/St Lukes: Roosevelt Hospital Center**
St Lukes Roosevelt
1000 10th Ave
New York, NY 10019-1192
212-473-2045
Fax: 212-473-0501

Charles Raimondo, VP
Farooq Chaudry, MD

Independent living center that advocates for people with disabilities by assisting with the application process of housing, benefits, etc.

4449 **Finger Lakes Independence Center**
215 5th St
Ithaca, NY 14850-3403
607-272-2433
Fax: 607-272-0902
TTY: 607-272-2433
flic@clarityconnect.com
www.fliconline.org

Lenore Schwager, Executive Director

FLIC assists all people with disabilities, their families and friends to promote independence and make informed decisions in pursuit of their goals. The servides provided are free of charge, and services are primarily served to residents of Tompkins, Schyler counties.

4450 **Harlem Independent Living Center**
289 St. Nicholas Avenue
Suite #21
New York, NY 10027- 4805
212-222-7122
800-673-2371
Fax: 212-222-7199
harlemilc@aol.com
www.hilc.org

Christina Curry, Executive Director
Edward Randolph, Resource Specialist
Dr. Herbert Thornhill, Emeritus
Vanessa J. Young, Chair

A non-profit agency that advocates for people with disabilities by assisting with the application process of housing, benefits, etc. Our services are free of charge.
Monthly

4451 **Independent Living**
5 Washington Terrace
Newburgh, NY 12550
845-565-1162
Fax: 845-565-0567
TTY: 845-565-0337
info@myindependentliving.org
www.myindependentliving.org

Doug J Hovey, President & CEO
Shannon Zawiski, Chief Operating Officer
Emily Robisch, Chief Financial Officer
Julie Stainton, Community Relations & Marketing Manager

A non-profit agency run by people with disabilities for others with disabilities. The agency offers programs and services to enhance quality of life, including benefits advising, personal assistance services, advocacy, employment and mental health services, recovery center, supportive housing and more.

4452 **Long Island Center for Independent Living**
3601 Hempstead Tpke
Suites 208 & 500
Levittown, NY 11756-1331
516-796-0144
Fax: 516-520-1247
TTY: 516-796-0135
licil@aol.com
www.licil.net

Joan Lynch, Executive Director

LICIL is committed to the empowerment of consumers with disabilities. LICIL staff functions as ambassadors to the belief that individuals with disabilities have a responsibility to take an active role in their own lives and self determined view of their futures.

4453 **Massena Independent Living Center**
156 Center St.
Massena, NY 13662-1495
315-764-9442
877-397-9613
Fax: 315-764-9464
mindepli@twcny.rr.com
www.milcinc.org

Jeff Reifensnyder, Executive Director

Provides a variety of non-residential direct services as well as educating the public through community awareness campaigns. Also seeks to address the current appropriate unmet needs of persons experiencing a disability.

4454 **NYS Independent Living Council**
111 Washington Ave
Suite #101
Albany, NY 12210-2280
518-427-1060
877-397-4126
Fax: 518-427-1139
bradw@nysilc.org
www.nysilc.org

Brad Williams, Executive Director
Patty Black, Administrative Assistant

Provides support and technical assistance to 37 independent living centers-community-based organizations directed by and for people with disabilities.

4455 **Nassau County Office for the Physically Challenged**
60 Charles Lindberg Blvd
Uniondale, NY 11553-4812
516-227-7399
www.nassaucountyny.gov

Edward P. Mangano, County Executive

This agency serves as the ADA compliance coordinating office for all Nassau County governmental facilities, programs and services. It also serves in an advisory capacity to local, regional and national policy-making organizations, planning committees and legislative bodies and conducts advocacy as well as direct programs and services to enhance inclusion by people with disabilities to employment, consumerism and transportation.

4456 **North Country Center for Independent Living**
80 Sharron Avenue
Plattsburgh, NY 12901-3827
518-563-9058
Fax: 518-563-0292
TTY: 518-563-9058
andrew@ncci-online.com
www.ncci-online.com

Ted Graser, President
Kathy Latinville, Vice President
Robert Poulin, Executive Director
Deb Piper, Program Director
To empower people with disabilities to live more independent and productive lives, and to promote beneficial policies and community understanding of disability issues.

4457 **Northern Regional Center for Independent Living: Watertown**
210 Court St
Suite #107
Watertown, NY 13601-4546
315-785-8703
800-585-8703
Fax: 315-785-8612
TTY: 315-785-8704
nrcil@nrcil.net
www.nrcil.net

Ronald Griffin, Chair
Michael Simmons, Vice Chair
Melanie Adkins, Secretary
Aileen Martin, Executive Director
A disability rights and resource center that promotes community efforts to end discrimination, segregation, and prejudice against people with disabilities.

4458 **Northern Regional Center for Independent Living: Lowville**
7632 N State St
Lowville, NY 13367-1318
315-376-8696
Fax: 315-376-3404
TTY: 315-376-8696
karenb@nrcil.net
www.nrcil.net

Ronald Griffin, Chair
Michael Simmons, Vice Chair
Melanie Adkins, Secretary
Aileen Martin, Executive Director
A disability rights and resource center that promotes community efforts to end discrimination, segregation, and prejudice against people with disabilities.

4459 **Options for Independence: Auburn**
75 Genesee St
Auburn, NY 13021-3667
315-255-3447
Fax: 315-255-0836
www.ariseinc.org

Tania Anderson, President
Sue Judge, Vice President
Michael Cook, Treasurer
Tom McKeown, Executive Director
Options for Independence is an Independent Living Center which assists people with disabilities to gain opportunities, make their own decisions, pursue activities and become part of comunity life. Options provides a variety of services to all people with disabilities, their families, friends, and service providers in Cayuga and Seneca Counties.

4460 **Putnam Independent Living Services**
1961 Route 6
2nd Floor
Carmel, NY 10512-2324
845-228-7457
Fax: 845-228-7460
TTY: 866-933-5390
info@wilc.org
www.putnamils.org

Joe Bravo, Executive Director
Mildred Caballero-Ho, Deputy Executive Director
Margaret Valenzuela, Program Director, IL Services
Jessica Baumann, Program Director, Educational Ad
A non-profit, community-based advocacy and resource center that serves people with all types of disabilities.

4461 **Regional Center for Independent Living**
497 State St
Rochester, NY 14608-1642
585-442-6470
Fax: 585-271-8558
TTY: 585-442-6470
bdarling@rcil.org
www.rcil.org

Shelly Perrin, Chairperson
Bobbi Wallach, Vice Chairperson
Bruce E Darling, Executive Director
Jennifer Smouse, Director of Finance
To empower people with disabilities to self-advocate, to live independently and to enhance the quality of community life.

4462 **Resource Center for Accessible Living**
727 Ulster Ave
Kingston, NY 12401-1709
845-331-0541
Fax: 845-331-2076
TTY: 845-331-4527
office@rcal.org
www.rcal.org

Paul Scarpati, President
Paula Kindos-Carberry, Co-Vice President
Bernadette Mueller, Co-Vice President
Susan Hoger, RCAL Executive Director
RCAL is a non-profit, community based service and advocacy run by and for people with any type of disability. RCAL is dedicated to assisting and empowering individuals, of all ages, to live independently and participate in all aspects of community life.

4463 **Resource Center for Independent Living**
347 W Main St
Amsterdam, NY 12010-2225
518-842-3561
Fax: 518-842-0905
TTY: 518-842-3593

Shelly Perrin, Chairperson
Bobbi Wallach, Vice Chairperson
Bruce E Darling, Executive Director
Jennifer Smouse, Director of Finance
Peer counseling, advocacy, independent living skills training, information and referral services, self-advocacy training, ADA consultation, home and community based services, community education, benefits advisement and more. All programs and services are available in English and Spanish.

4464 **Southern Adirondack Independent Living**
418 Geyser Rd
Country Club Plaza
Ballston Spa, NY 12020-6002
518-584-8202
Fax: 518-584-1195
www.sail-center.org

Karen Thayer, Executive Director
Anna Livingston, Assistant Director
Barbara Potvin, Executive Assistant
Michele Nicholson, Administrative Assistant
To assist individuals with disabilities to become independent empowered self-advocates.

4465 **Southern Adirondack Independent Living Center**
71 Glenwood Ave
Queensbury, NY 12804-1728
518-792-3537
Fax: 518-792-0979
TTY: 518-792-0505

Karen Thayer, Executive Director
Anna Livingston, Assistant Director
Shirley Dumont, Director of Advocacy
Barbara Potvin, Executive Assistant
To assist individuals with disabilities to become independent empowered self-advocates.

4466 **Southern Tier Independence Center**
135 E Frederick St
Binghamton, NY 13904-1224
607-724-2111
Fax: 607-772-3600
TTY: 607-724-2111
stic@stic-cil.org
www.stic-cil.org

Maria Dibble, Executive Director
Frank Pennisi, Accessibility Services
STIC provides assistance and services to all people with disabilities of all ages to increase their independence in all aspects of integrated community life. STIC also serves their families and friends, and businesses, agencies, and goverments to enable them to better meet the needs of people with disabilities, and finally STIC educates and influences the community in pursuit of full inclusion of people with disabilities.

4467 **Southwestern Independent Living Center**
843 N Main St
Jamestown, NY 14701-3546
716-661-3010
Fax: 716-661-3011
TTY: 716-661-3012
info@ilc-jamestown-ny.org

Marie T Carrubba, Executive Director
Linda Rumbaugh, Independent Living Specialist
Christine Ahlstrom, Independent Living Specialist
Helen Kern, Independent Living Specialist
A non-residential, private, nonprofit agency established to provide services throughout Chautauqua County that will assist individuals with disabilities in reaching maximum independence and an enriched quality of life.

4468 **Staten Island Center for Independent Living, Inc.**
470 Castleton Ave
Staten Island, NY 10301
718-720-9016
Fax: 718-720-9664
TTY: 718-720-9870
ldesantis@siciliving.org
www.siciliving.org

Lorraine DeSantis, Executive Director
Claudia J. Stanton, Office Manager
Michelle Sabatino, Independent Living Specialist
John Mastellone, Community Consultant / Benefits
Mission is to provide all individuals with disabilities the information, life skills training, and facilitative assistance which contributes to independence, individuality, and integration in the community and provides the skills and knowledge necessary to function in the least restrictive, personally fulfilling, most self reliant and productive manner.

4469 **Suffolk Independent Living Organization (SILO)**
2111 Lakeland Ave.
Suite A
Ronkonkoma, NY 11779
631-880-7929
Fax: 631-946-6377
TTY: 631-946-6585
www.siloinc.org/?

Edward Ahern, Manager
Glenn Campbell, Co-Executive Director
A not-for-profit organization that helps the disabled become more independent and more involved in the community by providing them with information on referrals on Housing, Education, Employment and Benefits.

4470 **Taconic Resources for Independence**
82 Washington St
Suite #214
Poughkeepsie, NY 12601-2305
845-452-3913
866-948-1094
Fax: 845-485-3196
tri@taconicresources.org
www.taconicresources.org

Cynthia L. Fiore, Executive Director
Patrick Muller, Program Director
Diane Barkstrom, Program Director/Staff Interpret
Jeanine Byrnes, Coordinator of Deaf & Hard of He
A center for independent living, benefits advisement information, and referral, advocacy, independent living skills, peer counseling, parent advocacy, sign language interpreters.

4471 **Westchester Disabled on the Move**
984 N. Broadway
Suite LL-10
Yonkers, NY 10701-1320
914-968-4717
Fax: 914-968-6137
info@wdom.org
www.wdom.org

Gail Cartenuto Cohn, President
Mattie Trupia, Vice President
Sandra Dolman, Secretary
Chandra Sookdeo, Assistant Recording Secretary
WDOM empowers people with disabilities to control their own lives; advocates for civil rights and a barrier free society; encourages people with disabilities to participate in the political process; educates government, business, other entities, and a society as a whole to understand, accept, and accommodate people with disabilities; creates an environment that inspires self-respect

4472 **Westchester Independent Living Center**
200 Hamilton Avenue
2nd Floor
White Plains, NY 10601- 1809
914-682-3926
Fax: 914-682-8518
TTY: 866-933-5390
Contact@wilc.org
www.wilc.org

Joseph Bravo, Executive Director
A not-for-profit, community-based advocacy and resource center that serves people with all types of disabilities.

North Carolina

4473 **Disability Awareness Network**
609 Country Club Dr.
Suite C
Greenville, NC 27834-6210
252-353-5522
Fax: 252-353-5160
DAWNpittco@aol.com

Jackie Hansley, Owner
Information and referral for diabled persons; peer counseling for diabled persons; advocacy on ADA issues; independent living skills and training.

4474 **Disability Rights & Resources**
5801 Executive Center Dr.
Suite #101
Charlotte, NC 28212-8870
704-537-0550
800-755-5749
Fax: 704-566-0507
TTY: 704-537-0550
mailto@disability-rights.org
www.disability-rights.org

Maura Chavez, President
Marta Fales, Vice President
Holly Howell, Secretary
Rick Griffiths, Treasurer
To guard the civil rights of people wtih disabilities by empowering ourselves and others to live as we choose.

4475 **Joy: A Shabazz Center for Independent Living**
235 N Greene St
Greensboro, NC 27401-2410
336-272-0501
Fax: 336-272-0575
TTY: 336-272-0501

Aaron Shabazz, Executive Director
James Wells, President
Stephen Simpson, Vice-President
B. J. Gerald Covington, Secretary/Treasurer

A non-profit, consumer oriented, Center for Independent Living (CIL) providing advocacy, peer counseling and peer support, independent living skills, training, information and referrals, with other related services for persons with disabilites.

4476 **Live Independently Networking Center**
P.O. Box 1135
Newton, NC 28658-1135
828-464-0331
Fax: 828-464-7375
TTY: 828-464-2838

Donavon Kirby, Deputy Director

Private, nonprofit, federally funded center for independent living located in Western North Carolina.

4477 **Live Independently Networking Center: Hickory**
2830 16th St NE
Apt. 17
Hickory, NC 28601-8606
828-464-0331
Fax: 828-464-7375

4478 **Pathways for the Future Center for Independent Living**
525 Mineral Springs Dr
Sylva, NC 28779-9077
828-631-1167
Fax: 828-631-1169
TTY: 828-631-1167

Barbara Davis, Executive Director

Dedicated to increasing independence, changing attitudes, promoting equal access and building a peer support network in western North Carolina through the use of community education, independent living services and advocacy.

4479 **Western Alliance Center for Independent Living**
30b London Rd
Asheville, NC 28803-2706
828-274-0444
Fax: 828-274-4461
westernalliance.org

Katy Hollingsworth, Manager
Jerry Brewton, Independent Living Specialist

.

4480 **Western Alliance for Independent Living**
108 New Leicester Highway
Asheville, NC 28806
828-298-1977
Fax: 828-298-0875
khollingsworth@disabilitypartners.org
www.disabilitypartners.org

Kathy Hollingsworth, Associate Director
Rosemary Weaver, Independent Living Specialist
Mechelle Holt, Volunteer/Program Coordinator
Eva Reynolds, Emploment Network Coordinator

North Dakota

4481 **Dakota Center for Independent Living: Dickinson**
26-1st street East
Suite 103
Dickinson, ND 58601-5103
701- 48- 436
800-489-5013
Fax: 701- 48- 436
TTY: 800489501363
dcil@ndsupernet.com
www.dakotacil.org

Robin Were, President
Claudia Ziegler, Vice president
Carol Mihulka, Secretary/Treasurer
Royce Schultze, Executive Director

Believes in self-determination for people with disabilities and creates the environment in which it is achieved.

4482 **Dakota Center for Independent Living: Bismarck**
3111 E Broadway Ave
Bismarck, ND 58501-5085
701-222-3636
800-489-5013
Fax: 701-222-0511
TTY: 701-222-3636
maryr@dakotacil.org
www.dakotacil.org

Robin Were, President
Claudia Ziegler, Vice president
Carol Mihulka, Secretary/Treasurer
Royce Schultze, Executive Director

Believes in self-determination for people with disabilities and creates the environment in which it is achieved.

4483 **Fraser**
2902 University Drive South
Fargo, ND 58103-6053
701-232-3301
Fax: 701-237-5775
fraser@fraserltd.org
fraserltd.org

Sandra Leyland, Executive Director
Mark Brodshaug, President
Michael Kirk, Vice President
David A. Laske, Treasurer

Private non-profit, federally funded center for independent living

4484 **Freedom Resource Center for Independent Living: Fargo**
2701 9th Ave S
Suite H
Fargo, ND 58103-8712
701-478-0459
800-450-0459
Fax: 701-478-0510
TTY: 701-478-0459
freedom@freedomrc.org
www.freedomrc.org

Nate Aalgaard, Executive Director
Angie Bosch, Office Coordinator
Mark Mark Bourdon Bourdon, Program Director
Andrea Nelson, Independent Living Advocate

To work toward equality and inclusion for people with disabilities through programs of empowerment, community education, and systems change.

4485 **Resource Center for Independent Living: Minot**
300 3rd Ave SW
Suite F
Minot, ND 58701-4346
701-839-4724
800-377-5114
Fax: 701-838-1677
TTY: 701-839-4724
independencecil@independencecil.org
www.independencecil.org/?

Susan Ogurek, Chair
Scott Burlingame, Executive Director
Dee Tischer, Senior Independent Living Specia
Jamie Hardt, Youth Transition Specialist

A resource center for independent living. Mission is to advocate for the freedom of choice for individuals with disabilities to live independently through the removal of all barriers.

Ohio

4486 **Ability Center of Greater Toledo**
5605 Monroe St.
Sylvania, OH 43560
419-885-5733
Fax: 419-882-4813
www.abilitycenter.org

Tim Harrington, Executive Director
Ash Lemons, Associate Director
Debbie Andriette, Director, Human Resources
Jack Perion, Director, Finance & Operations

To assist people with disabilities to live, work and socialize within a fully accessible community.

4487 **Ability Center of Greater Toledo: Bryan**
1425 East High St.
Suite 108
Bryan, OH 43506
419-633-1400
855-633-1400
Fax: 419-633-1410
www.abilitycenter.org
Tim Harrington, Executive Director
Angie Burton, Manager, Youth Programs
To assist people with disabilities to live, work and socialize within a fully accessible community. The Bryan office serves residents in Defiance, Fulton, Henry, and Williams Counties.

4488 **Access Center for Independent Living**
901 S Ludlow St
Dayton, OH 45402-2614
937-341-5202
Fax: 937-341-5217
TTY: 937-341-5218
info@acils.com
www.acils.com/?
Darrell Price, IL Team Co-Leader
Tonya Banther, IL Team Co-Leader
Melody Burba, Information & Referral Specialis
John Dixon, Information & Referral Specialis
Offers peer counseling, disability education and other services to the community.

4489 **Center for Independent Living Options**
2031 Auburn Avenue
Cincinnati, OH 45219-2436
513-241-2600
Fax: 513-241-1707
TTY: 513-241-7170
cilo.net
Lin Laing, Executive Director
Justin Bifro, President
Brian Frazier, Vice-President
Ed Klene, Treasurer
The oldest center for independent living in Ohio serving individuals with disabilities in the Greater Cincinnati/Northern Kentucky region.

4490 **Fairfield Center for Disabilities and Cerebral Palsy**
681 E 6th Ave
Lancaster, OH 43130-2602
740-653-5501
Fax: 740-653-6046
fcdcp@sbcglobal.net
www.fcdcp.org
David Macioci, President
David Welsh, Vice-President
Mary Snider, Treasurer
Edwin R. Payne, Secretary
Adult Day Program and Transportation. The mission of the Fairfield Center for disabilities and Cerebral Palsy, Inc, is to create a better future for people with a disability by increasing and enhancing their lifestyle opportunities.

4491 **Linking Employment, Abilities and Potential**
2545 Lorain Ave.
Cleveland, OH 44113-3102
216-696-2716
Fax: 216-687-1453
www.leapinfo.org
Charles Heindrichs, President
Brian Roof, Vice President
Vincent Shemo, Treasurer
Betsey Kamm, Secretary
Consumer-directed to ensure a society of equal opportunity for all persons, regardless of disability.

4492 **Mid-Ohio Board for an Independent Living Environment (MOBILE)**
690 S High St
Columbus, OH 43206-1016
614-443-5936
Fax: 614-443-5954
TTY: 614-443-5957
info@mobileonline.org
www.mobileonline.org
Darry Moore, President
Thomas Shapaka, Vice-President
Mark Morton, Treasurer
Warren King, Secretary
A non-profit Center for Independent Living directed by persons with disabilities. MOBILE was founded on principles that affirm the right of persons with disabilities to live their lives with a full measure of liberty and human dignity.

4493 **Ohio Statewide Independent Living Council**
670 Morrison Road
Suite 200
Gahanna, OH 43230-5324
614-892-0390
800-566-7788
Fax: 614-861-0392
www.ohiosilc.org
Kay Grier, Executive Director
Eugene Iacovetta, Special Projects Coordinator
Mary Butler, Systems Change Coordinator
Janae Miller, Office Manager
Committed to promoting a philosophy of consumer control, peer support, self-help, self-determination, equal acess, and individual and systems advocacy, in order to maximize leadership, empowerment, independence, productivity and to support full inclusion and integration of individuals with disabilities into the mainstream of American society.

4494 **Rehabilitation Service of North Central Ohio**
270 Sterkel Blvd
Mansfield, OH 44907-1508
419-756-1133
800-589-1133
Fax: 419-756-6544
info@therehabcenter.org
www.therehabcenter.org
Veronica L. Groff, President/CEO
Susan Baker, Chairman
Dan Wiegand, Vice-Chairman
Scott Donnenwirth, Secretary
Private nonprofit organization providing coordinated, team-oriented comprehensive outpatient rehabilitation services to children and adults of all ages. Serves 8 counties in N/C Ohio. Four umbrella areas of service include medical rehabilitation services, vocational rehabilitation services, behavioral health service and drug and alcohol addiction services. Medical rehabilitation services include physical therapy, occupational therapy, speech therapy and audiology.

4495 **Samuel W Bell Home for Sightless**
3775 Muddy Creek Rd
Cincinnati, OH 45238-2055
513-241-0720
Fax: 513-241-1481
swbellhome@fuse.net
www.samuelbell.org
Timothy Lighthal, President
Kevin Kappa, Vice-President
Miles L.Hoff, Treasurer
James Witte, Secretary
Offers a residential, independent living environment for blind and legally blind adults.

4496 **Services for Independent Living**
25100 Euclid Ave
Suite #105
Cleveland, OH 44117-2663
216-731-1529
Fax: 216-731-3083
TTY: 216-731-1529
www.sil-oh.org
Lynn Hildebrand, Executive Director
Offers support ADA, consultation and education, advocacy, transitional education services, independent living skills training, information and referrals.

4497 **Society for Equal Access: Independent Living Center**
1458 5th St NW
New Philadelphia, OH 44663-1224
330-343-9292
888-213-4452
Fax: 330-602-7425
TTY: 330-602-2557
www.seailc.org
Scott Huston, President
Edna Fillinger, Vice-President
Victoria Eichel, Secretary
Twyla Mccartney, Treasurer
The Society works with individuals to become more independent. Our agency assists with peer support, advocacy, information and

referral, independent living skills and transportation. Our goal is to move those with challenges in the direction ofn independence.

Oklahoma

4498 **Ability Resources**
823 S Detroit Ave
Suite #110
Tulsa, OK 74120-4223
918-592-1235
800-722-0886
Fax: 918-592-5651
www.ability-resources.org
Carla Lawson, Executive Director
To assist people with disabilities in attaining and maintaining their personal independence.

4499 **Green County Independent Living Resource Center**
4100 S.E. Adams Rd
Suite C-106
Bartlesville, OK 74006- 8409
918-335-1314
800-559-0567
Fax: 918-333-1814
TTY: 918-335-1314
Vicki Haws, Executive Director
Independent living skills training, information and referrals, advocacy, a loan library of adaptive equipment and books. Services available to all individuals with disabilities and their family members who reside in Northeastern Oklahoma.

4500 **Oklahomans for Independent Living**
601 East Carl Albert Parkway
McAlester, OK 74501-5410
918-426-6220
800-568-6821
Fax: 918-426-3245
TTY: 918-426-6263
www.oilok.org
Pam Pulchny, Executive Director/ADAspecialist
Terry Yates, Administrative Assistant/Bookke
Leanna Amos, Service Management Specialist
Stephen Strickland, Living Choice Coordinator
OIL encourages individuals of all ages, with all types of disabilities to increase: personal dependence; empowerment and self determiation; and ful integration and participation in their work, community, school and home activities.

4501 **Progressive Independence**
121 N Porter Avenue
Norman, OK 73071-5834
405-321-3203
800-801-3203
Fax: 405-321-7601
TTY: 405-321-2942
www.progind.org
Scott Spray, Chairperson
Teresa Tisdell, Vice Chair
Mark Newman, Treasurer
Mary Dulan, Secretary
Preovides four cores services of Information & Referral, Individaul& Systems Advocacy, Peer Counseling, and Skills Training; in addition, offers accessible computer lab, short term DME loans, ande benefits counseling for SSI/SSDI.

Oregon

4502 **Abilitree**
2680 NE Twin Knolls Dr.
Suite 3
Bend, OR 97701
541-388-8103
Fax: 541-389-2337
TTY: 541-388-8103
www.abilitree.org
Tim Johnson, Executive Director
Greg Sublett, Director of Operations
April O'Meara, Marketing Director
Jen Michelson, Access Manager
CORIL empowers people with disabilities to maximize their independence, productivity and inclusio in community life. CORIL envisions a society where all people have the opportunity to develop their full capabilities with independence, productivity and more meaningful involvment in local community events and activities.

4503 **Eastern Oregon Center for Independent Living**
1021 SW 5th Ave
Ontario, OR 97914-3301
541-889-3119
866-248-8369
Fax: 541-889-4647
eocil@eocil.org
www.eocil.org
Kirt Toombs, Executive Director
EOCIL is a nonprofit community based resource and advocacy center that promotes independent living and equal access for all persons with disabilities. EOCIL serves consumers in the counties of: Baker, Gilliam, Grant, harney, Malheur, Morrow, Umatilla, Union, Wallowa and Wheeler.

4504 **HASL Independent Abilities Center**
305 NE 'E' Street
Grants Pass, OR 97526
541-479-4275
800-758-4275
Fax: 541-479-7261
TTY: 541-479-3588
haslstaff@yahoo.com
www.haslonline.org
Randy Samuelson, Executive Director
To promote public awareness of the special needs and legal rights of individuals with cross-disabilities; to facilitate their integration into society and provide support through advocacy, peer counseling, skills training and information and referral to encourage independence.

4505 **Independent Living Resources**
1839 NE Couch St.
Portland, OR 97232
503-232-7411
Fax: 503-232-7480
TTY: 503-232-8404
info@ilr.org
www.ilr.org/?
Barry Fox-Quamme, Executive Director
May Altman, LCSW, Associate Director
Barbara Norris, Office Manager/Executive Assistant
Amy Camp, Independent Living Specialist
ILR looks to promote the philosophy of Independent Living by creating opportunities, encouraging choices, advancing equal access, and furthering the level of independence for all people with disabilities

4506 **Laurel Hill Center**
2145 Centennial Plaza
Eugene, OR 97401-2474
541-485-6340
Fax: 541-984-3124
TTY: 541-684-6822
info@laurel.org
www.laurel.org
Tom Fauria, President
DAVE Burtner, Vice-President
EDUARDO Sifuentez, Secretary
Lt. Jennifer Bills, Special operations
Provides natoinall-recognized, recovery-focused rehabilitation services in Lane County, Oregon, for people with severe and persistent mental illnesses

4507 **Progressive Options**
611 S.W. Hurbert Street
Suite A
Newport, OR 97365-9678
541-265-4674
Fax: 541-574-4313
TTY: 541-574-1927
progop541@yahoo.com
www.progressive-options.org
Rhonda Walker, Executive Director
Progressive Options seeks to provide free services and support to people with disabilities of all kinds to help them achieve and maintain maximum independence and self-sufficiency in Lincoln County and surrounding areas in Oregon.

4508 **SPOKES Unlimited**
1006 Main St
Klamath Falls, OR 97601-6029
541-883-7547
Fax: 541-885-2469
TTY: 541-883-7547
www.spokesunlimited.org
Wendy Howard, Executive Director
Mission is to enhance the ability of people with disabilities to live more independently.

4509 **Umpqua Valley Disabilities Network**
736 SE Jackson Street
Roseburg, OR 97470-110
541-672-6336
Fax: 541-672-8606
TTY: 541-440-2882
uvdn@uvdn.org
www.uvdn.org
David Fricke, Executive Director
Heather Vialpando, Executive Assistant
UVDN's mission is to promote independent living and community inclusion for people with disabilities.

Pennsylvania

4510 **Abilities in Motion**
210 N 5th St
Reading, PA 19601-3304
610-376-0010
888-376-0120
Fax: 610-376-0021
TTY: 610-228-2301
www.abilitiesinmotion.org
Terry Graul, Board President
David Lerch, Vice-President
Bonnie Milke, Treasurer
Ralph Trainer, Executive Director
Dedicated to advancing the rights of persons with disabilities in orer to promote a full life in the community through the prevention and elimination of physical, psychological, social and attitudinal barriers which serve to deny them the rights and privileges common to the general public.

4511 **Anthracite Region Center for Independent Living**
Pennsylvania Council on Independent Living
8 West Broad St
Suite 228
Hazleton, PA 18201-6418
570-455-9800
800-777-9906
Fax: 570-455-1731
TTY: 570-455-9800
dcorcoran@anthracitecil.org
Irene Mordosky, President
Margo Madden, Vice-President
Rand Martin, Treasurer
Tracy Clark, Secretary
Enables individuals with disabilities to attain their highest possible level of independence.

4512 **Brian's House**
757 Springdale Dr.
Exton, PA 19341-8531
610-399-1175
ekihara@brianshouse.org
brianshouse.org
Diana L. Ramsay, MPP, OTR, FAOT, Resident and Chief Executive Off
Peter M. Shubiak, MA, Executive Vice President and Chi
Lori Plunkett, Executive Director
A non-profit organization that provides residential, vocational and recreational/respite programs for children and adults with intellectual and developmental disabilities.

4513 **Community Resources for Independence**
3410 W 12th St
Erie, PA 16505-3649
814-838-7222
800-530-5541
Fax: 814-838-8491
TTY: 814-838-8115
www.crinet.org
Timothy Finegan, Executive Director
William Essigmann, Administrative Program Manager
Carl Berry, Human Resources Director
Marty Pushchak, Controller
A community based, nonprofit, nonresidential organization that offers services and assistance to enable people with disabilities to expand their options, pursue their goals, and achieve and maintain self-sufficient and producitve lives in the community.

4514 **Community Resources for Independence, Inc., Bradford**
3410 West 12th Street
Erie, PA 16505
814-838-7222
800-530-5541
Fax: 814-838-8491
TTY: 814-838-8115
crinet.org
Timothy J. Finegan, Executive Director
William Essigmann, Administrative Program Manager
Carl Berry, Human Resources Director
Marty Pushchak, Controller
Community Resources for Independence, Inc is committed to preserve, enhance and enrich the quality of life for all people with disabilities.

4515 **Community Resources for Independence: Lewistown**
33 East Hale Street
Suite L
Lewistown, PA 17044-2160
717-248-8011
800-309-0989
Fax: 717-248-8029
www.crinet.org
Timothy Finegan, Executive Director
William Essigmann, Administrative Program Manager
Carl Berry, Human Resources Director
Marty Pushchak, Controller
A community based, nonprofit, nonresidential organization that offers services and assistance to enable people with disabilities to expand their options, pursue their goals, and achieve and maintain self-sufficient and producitve lives in the community.

4516 **Community Resources for Independence: Altoona**
1331 Twelth Ave
Suite #103
Altoona, PA 16601
814-994-2645
866-944-2645
Fax: 814-944-2683
www.crinet.org
Timothy Finegan, Executive Director
William Essigmann, Administrative Program Manager
Carl Berry, Human Resources Director
Marty Pushchak, Controller
A community based, nonprofit, nonresidential organization that offers services and assistance to enable people with disabilities to expand their options, pursue their goals, and achieve and maintain self-sufficient and producitve lives in the community.

4517 **Community Resources for Independence: Clarion**
1200 Eastwood Drive
Suite #1
Clarion, PA 16214-8824
814-297-7141
800-372-0140
Fax: 814-297-7161
www.crinet.org
Timothy J. Finegan, Executive Director
William Essigmann, Administrative Program Manager
Carl Berry, Human Resources Director
Marty Pushchak, Controller
A community based, nonprofit, nonresidential organization that offers services and assistance to enable people with disabilities to expand their options, pursue their goals, and achieve and maintain self-sufficient and producitve lives in the community.

4518 **Community Resources for Independence: Clearfield**
209 E Locust St
Clearfield, PA 16830-2422 814-765-6405
866-619-6405
Fax: 814-765-1269
www.crinet.org

Timothy Finegan, Executive Director
William Essigmann, Administrative Program Manager
Carl Berry, Human Resources Director
Marty Pushchak, Controller
A community based, nonprofit, nonresidential organization that offers services and assistance to enable people with disabilities to expand their options, pursue their goals, and achieve and maintain self-sufficient and producitve lives in the community.

4519 **Community Resources for Independence: Hermitage**
3875 East State St
Suite B
Hermitage, PA 16148-3415 724-347-4121
Fax: 724-347-5966
www.crinet.org

Timothy J. Finegan, Executive Director
William Essigmann, Administrative Program Manager
Carl Berry, Human Resources Director
Marty Pushchak, Controller
A community based, nonprofit, nonresidential organization that offers services and assistance to enable people with disabilities to expand their options, pursue their goals, and achieve and maintain self-sufficient and producitve lives in the community.

4520 **Community Resources for Independence: Lewisburg**
11 Reitz Blvd
Suite #105
Lewisburg, PA 17837-1493 570-524-4314
800-332-4135
Fax: 570-524-9236
www.crinet.org

Timothy J. Finegan, Executive Director
William Essigmann, Administrative Program Manager
Carl Berry, Human Resources Director
Marty Pushchak, Controller
A community based, nonprofit, nonresidential organization that offers services and assistance to enable people with disabilities to expand their options, pursue their goals, and achieve and maintain self-sufficient and producitve lives in the community.

4521 **Community Resources for Independence: Oil City**
250 Elm St
Oil City, PA 16301-1413 814-677-4655
866-209-3882
Fax: 814-677-4915
www.crinet.org

Tim Finegan, Executive Director
William Essigmann, Administrative Program Manager
Carl Berry, Human Resources Director
Marty Pushchak, Controller
A community based, nonprofit, nonresidential organization that offers services and assistance to enable people with disabilities to expand their options, pursue their goals, and achieve and maintain self-sufficient and producitve lives in the community.

4522 **Community Resources for Independence: Warren**
1003 Pennsylvania Ave W
Warren, PA 16365-1837 814-726-3404
866-579-3404
Fax: 814-726-3428
www.crinet.org

Timothy Finegan, Executive Director
William Essigmann, Administrative Program Manager
Carl Berry, Human Resources Director
Marty Pushchak, Controller
A community based, nonprofit, nonresidential organization that offers services and assistance to enable people with disabilities to expand their options, pursue their goals, and achieve and maintain self-sufficient and producitve lives in the community.

4523 **Community Resources for Independence: Wellsboro**
38 Plaza Ln
Wellsboro, PA 16901-1766 570-724-5852
866-401-7911
Fax: 570-724-3945
www.crinet.org

Timothy Finegan, Executive Director
William Essigmann, Administrative Program Manager
Carl Berry, Human Resources Director
Marty Pushchak, Controller
A community based, nonprofit, nonresidential organization that offers services and assistance to enable people with disabilities to expand their options, pursue their goals, and achieve and maintain self-sufficient and producitve lives in the community.

4524 **Freedom Valley Disability Center**
3607 Chapel Road
Suite B
Newtown Square, PA 19073-3602 610-353-6640
800-427-4754
Fax: 610-353-6753
TTY: 610-353-8900

Ann Cope, Executive Director
Assists persons with disabilities in the achievement of independent living goals. Also promotes individual and community options to maximize independence for persons with disabilities. Serves people with disabilities in Chester, Delaware, and Montgomery Counties.

4525 **Institute on Disabilities At Temple Univ.**
Temple University
1755 N. 13th St
Student Center, Rm. 4115
Philadelphia, PA 19122-6099 215-204-1356
Fax: 215-204-6336
iod@temple.edu
www.disabilities.temple.edu

James Earl Davis, Phd, Interim Executive Director
Celia Feinstein, Co-Executive- Director
Amy Goldman, Co-Executive- Director
Ann Marie White, Deputy- Director
Leads by example, creating connections and promoting networks within and among communitites so that people with disabilities are recognized as integral to the fabric of community life.

4526 **Lehigh Valley Center for Independent Living**
713 North 13th Street
Allentown, PA 18102-9121 610-770-9781
800-495-8245
Fax: 610-770-9801
TTY: 610-770-9789
info@lvcil.org
www.lvcil.org

Scott Berman, President
Michelle Mitchell, Vice President
Amy Beck, Executive Director
Cara Steidel, Fiscal Coordinator
Serves persons in Lehigh and Northampton Counties with any type of disability and/or his/her family.

4527 **Liberty Resources**
714 Market St
Suite #100
Philadelphia, PA 19106-2337 215-634-2000
888-634-2155
Fax: 215-634-6628
TTY: 215-634-6630
lrinc@libertyresources.org
www.libertyresources.org

Edwin Bomba, Chairman
Mary Ellen Caffrey, Chairman
Estelle B. Richman, Vice-Chairman
Thomas H. Earle, CEO
A non-profit, consumer driven organization that advocates and promotes Independent Living for persons with disabilities.

4528 **Life and Independence for Today**
503 E Arch St
Saint Marys, PA 15857-1779
814-781-3050
800-341-5438
Fax: 814-781-1917
TTY: 814-781-3050
lift@liftcil.org
www.liftcil.org

Stephen DePrater, President
Linda McKinstry, Vice-President
Larry Caggeso, Treasurer
Hope Weichman, Deputy Director

Offers services to enable people with disabilities to achieve new goals and broaden their horizons. It enables them to achieve and maintain self-sufficient and productive lives.

4529 **Northeastern Pennsylvania Center for Independent Living**
1142 Sanderson Ave
Suite #1
Scranton, PA 18509
570-344-7211
800-344-7211
Fax: 570-344-7218
TTY: 570-344-5275
nepacilinfo@nepacil.org

Robert Treptow, President
Michael Sporer, Secretary
Chris Armone,Esq, Treasurer

Established to assist in removing barriers and expanding independent living options available to people with disabilities.

4530 **South Central Pennsylvania Center for Independence Living**
1019 Logan Blvd
Altoona, PA 16602-2434
814-949-1905
800-237-9009
Fax: 814-949-1909
TTY: 814-949-1912
www.cilscpa.org

Susan Estep, Executive Director

The missio of the Center for Independent Living of South Central PA is to empower people with disabilities to lead independent lives in their commnuitites. The Center covers Bedford, Blair, cambria, Fulton, Huntingdon, Indiana and Somerset counties.

4531 **Three Rivers Center for Independent Living: New Castle**
900 Rebecca Ave
Pittsburgh, PA 15221-9383
412-371-7700
800-633-4588
Fax: 412-371-9430
TTY: 412-371-6230
www.trcil.myfastsite.net/

Kourtney T. Diaz, Chairperson
Shanicka Kennedy, Esq, Vice-Chairperson
Stanley A Holbrook, President
Rachel Rogan, Chief Executive Officer

To empower people with disabilities to enjoy self-directed, personally meaningful lives by providing outstanding consumer controlled services and by advocating for effective community college.

4532 **Three Rivers Center for Independent Livi ng: Washington**
900 Rebecca Ave
Pittsburgh, PA 15221-4425
412-371-7700
800-633-4588
Fax: 412-371-9430
TTY: 412-371-6230
www.trcil.myfastsite.net/

Stanley A Holbrook, President
Kourtney T. Diaz, Chairperson
Shanicka Kennedy, Esq, Vice-Chairperson
Roxanne Huss, Director of Waiver Services

To empower people with disabilities to enjoy self-directed, personally meaningful lives by providing outstanding consumer controlled services and by advocating for effective community college.

4533 **Three Rivers Center for Independent Living**
900 Rebecca Ave
Pittsburgh, PA 15221-2938
412-371-7700
800-633-4588
Fax: 412-371-9430
TTY: 412-371-6230
www.trcil.myfastsite.net/

Stanley A Holbrook, President
Kourtney T. Diaz, Chairperson
Shanicka Kennedy, Esq, Vice-Chairperson
Roxanne Huss, Director of Waiver Services

To empower people with disabilities to enjoy self-directed, personally meaningful lives by providing outstanding consumer controlled services and by advocating for effective community college.

4534 **Tri-County Patriots for Independent Living**
69 East Beau St
Washington, PA 15301-4711
724-223-5115
877-889-0965
Fax: 724-223-5119
TTY: 724-228-4028
www.tripil.com

Kathleen Kleinmann, Chief Executive Officer
Maxine Berton, Administrative Assistant
Jeffry D. Woods, Chief Information Officer
Jan Crockett, Chief Financial Officer

Brings together individuals who share common problems in equal access, education, housing, employment, attendant care, transportation, and access to technology.

4535 **Voices for Independence**
1107 Payne Ave
Erie, PA 16503-1741
814-874-0064
866-407-0064
Fax: 814-874-3497
TTY: 814-874-0064
web@vficil.org
www.vficil.org

Shona Eakin, Executive Director
Edna Anabui, Executive Administrative Assista
Doug McClintock, Director of Finances
Colleen Porath, Accountant

To empower people with disabilities and promote independent living.

Rhode Island

4536 **Arc of Blackstone**
500 Prospect St.
Wing B, Suite 203
Pawtucket, RI 2860- 4396
401-727-0150
800-257-6092
Fax: 401-727-1545
contact@bvcriarc.org
www.bvcriarc.org

Kathleen O'Neill, President
Thomas E. Hodge, Vice-President
Joseph F. McEnness, Treasurer
A. Melanie Cherry, Secretary

Committed to supporting people with developmental disabilities secure the opportunity to choose and realize their goals of where and how they live, learn, work and play

4537 **Franklin Court Assisted Living**
180 Franklin St
Bristol, RI 2809-3352
401-253-3679
Fax: 401-253-5855

Michelle Belmore Cabana, Chief Financial Officer
Brenda Marshall, Administrator
Lynn A. Marshall, Property Manager
Jennifer Morra, Administrative Assistant

Offers local seniors an affordable assisted living option with first-rate services and gracious accommodations.

4538 **IN-SIGHT Independent Living**
43 Jefferson Blvd
Warwick, RI 2888-1078
401-941-3322
Fax: 401-941-3356
cbutler@in-sight.org
www.in-sight.org

Jean Saylor, Chairman
Robert Tyler, Vice-Chairman
James Hahn, Treasurer
Karl Sherry, Secretary
Creating opportunities and choices for people who are blind and visually impaired

4539 **Ocean State Center for Independent Living**
1944 Warwick Avenue
Warwick, RI 2889-2448
401-738-1013
866-857-1161
Fax: 401-738-1083
TTY: 401-738-1015
info@oscil.org
www.oscil.org

Lorna Ricci, Executive Director
OSCIL is a consumer controlled, community based, nonprofit organization established to provide a range of independent living services to enhance, through self direction, the quality of life of Rhode Islander with significant disability and to promote integration into the community.

4540 **Office of Rehabilitation Services**
40 Fountain Street
Providence, RI 02903-1898
401-421-7005
TTY: 401-421-7016
www.ors.ri.gov

Ron Racine, Associate Director
Kathleen Brown, Administrator
Joseph Murphy, Administrator, Vocational Rehabilitation
Laurie DiOrio, Administrator, SBVI
Their goal is to help individuals with physical and mental disabilities prepare for and obtain appropriate employment.

4541 **PARI Independent Living Center**
500 Prospect St
Pawtucket, RI 2860-6259
401-725-1966
Fax: 401-725-2104
TTY: 401-725-1966
www.pari-ilc.org

Leo Canuel, Executive Director
Sue Bilodau, Program Director
Offers information and referral services, personal care attendant services, home modifications, advocacy services and peer counseling, independent living skills training, and recycled equipment.

South Carolina

4542 **Columbia Disability Action Center**
136 Stonemark Lane
Suite #100
Columbia, SC 29210
800-681-6805
Fax: 803-779-5114
TTY: 803-779-0949
www.able-sc.org/

David Dawson, President
Rochelle Gadson, Vice President
Joe Butler, Treasurer
Angela Jacildone, Secretary
A non-profit consumer governed Center for Independent Living. Programs and services support persons with disaibilities in taking full advantage of community resources, enhancing personal opportunities, and determining the direction of their lives.

4543 **Disability Action Center**
330B Pelham Rd
Suite 100 A
Greenville, SC 29615-3116
864-235-1421
800-681-7715
Fax: 864-235-2056
TTY: 864-235-8798
amayne@dacsc.org
www.able-sc.org/

David Dawson, President
Rochelle Gadson, Vice President
Joe Butler, Treasurer
Angela Jacildone, Secretary
Empowering people with disabilities to reach their highest level of independence.

4544 **Graham Street Community Resources**
306 Graham St
Florence, SC 29501-4735
843-665-6674
Fax: 843-665-6674

Faye Thompson, Manager
Promotes independent living and empowers people with disabilities to reach their highest level of independence.

4545 **South Carolina Independent Living Council**
136 Stonemark Lane
Suite #100
Columbia, SC 29210-7318
803-217-3209
800-994-4322
Fax: 803-731-1439
TTY: 803-217-3209
scilc@scilconline.org
www.scsilc.com

Mike Le Fever, President
Committed to equal opportunity, equal access, self determination, independence, and choice for all people with disabilities and pursues these goals by the means available.

4546 **Walton Options for Independent Living: North Augusta**
325 Georgia Ave
North Augusta, SC 29841-3848
803-279-9611
Fax: 803-279-9135
tjohnston@waltonoptions.org
www.waltonoptions.org

Cynthia Anzek, Executive Director
Empowers persons of all ages with all types of disabilities to reach their highest level of independence, community inclusion and employment.

South Dakota

4547 **Adjustment Training Center**
607 N 4th St
Aberdeen, SD 57401-2733
605-229-0263
Fax: 605-225-3455
www.aspiresd.org

Jennifer Gray, Executive Director
Arlette Keller, Director of Service Coordination
Angela Huffman, Director of Nursing
Paul Schumacher, Director of Vocational Services
Offers peer counseling, attendant care registry and referrals.

4548 **Black Hills Workshop & Training Center**
Black Hills Workshop
3650 Range Road
PO Box 2104
Rapid City, SD 57709-2104
605-343-4550
Fax: 605-343-0879
TTY: 800-877-1113
drosby@bhws.com
www.blackhillsworks.org

Brad Saathoff, Chief Executive Officer
Janet Niehaus, VP of Finance
Michelle Aman, VP of Residential Services
Helen Usera, VP of Development
Offers job placement, housing options, case coordination, supported employment and supported living for all disability groups, as well as specialized services for brian injury victims.

4549 **Communication Service for the Deaf: Rapid City**
200 W Cesar Chavez St
Suite 650
Austin, TX 78701-694
844-222-0002
800-642-6410
Fax: 605-394-6609
TTY: 866-273-3323
csd@csd.org
www.c-s-d.org

Dr. Benjamin Soukup, Founder, Chairman & CEO
Christopher Soukup, President
Brad Hermes, Chief Financial Officer
Christina Kokenge, Vice President, Human Resources

A private, nonprofit organization dedicated to providing broad-based services, ensuring public accessibility and increasing public awareness of issues affecting deaf and hard of hearing inividuals.

4550 **Native American Advocacy Program for Persons with Disabilities**
P.O. Box 527
Winner, SD 57580-527
605-842-3977
800-303-3975
Fax: 605-842-3983
TTY: 605-842-3977

Marla Bull Bear, Executive Director
Charles Bull Bear, Specialist
Betty Farr, Il Specialist
Megan L. Garcia, Prevention Specialist

The mission is to encourage a healthy organization that assists Native Americans with disabilities, by providing prevention, education and training, advocacy, support, independent living skills and referrals.

4551 **Prairie Freedom Center for Independent Living: Sioux Falls**
4107 S Carnegie Cr
Suite #9
Sioux Falls, SD 57106-3100
605-362-3550
Fax: 605-367-5639
i-l-c@ilcchoices.org
www.ilcchoices.org

Steve Tripp, President
Cheri Raymond, Vice President
Matt Cain, Executive Director
Laura Staebner, Treasurer

Established to provide basic skills so many of us take for granted: to take care of our own needs and to make our own decisions to be independent.

4552 **Prairie Freedom Center for Independent Li ving: Madison**
4107 S Carnegie Cr
411 SE 10th St
Sioux Falls, SD 57106-3570
605-362-3550
Fax: 605-256-5071
i-l-c@ilcchoices.org
www.ilcchoices.org

Steve Tripp, President
Cheri Raymond, Vice President
Matt Cain, Executive Director
Laura Staebner, Treasurer

Established to provide basic skills so many of us take for granted: to take care of our own needs and to make our own decisions to be independent.

4553 **Prairie Freedom Center for Independent Living: Yankton**
4107 S Carnegie Cr
Suite #107
Sioux Falls, SD 57106-2800
605-362-3550
Fax: 605-668-3060
TTY: 605-668-3060
www.ilcchoices.org

Steve Tripp, President
Cheri Raymond, Vice President
Matt Cain, Executive Director
Laura Staebner, Treasurer

Established to provide basic skills so many of us take for granted: to take care of our own needs and to make our own decisions to be independent.

4554 **South Dakota Assistive Technology Project: DakotaLink**
1161 Deadwood Ave N
Suite #5
Rapid City, SD 57702-382
605-394-6742
800-645-0673
Fax: 605-394-6744
TTY: 605-394-6742
atinfo@dakotalink.net

Pat Czerny, Manager
Patrick Czerny, Technical Services Coordinator
David Scherer, Program Coordinator

DakotaLink, the South Dakota Assistive Technology Program, provides resources and supports to individuals of all ages to ensure greater access to and acquisition of assistive technology devices and services.

4555 **Western Resources for dis-ABLED Independence**
405 East Omaha St
Suite D
Rapid City, SD 57701-2974
605-718-1930
888-434-4943
Fax: 605-718-1933
TTY: 605-718-1930
chad@wril.org
www.wril.org

Jeff Wangen, President
Dennis Coull, Vice-President
Linda Lockner, Secretary
Mike Pendo, Treasurer

WRDI advocates for the rights of equal inclusion of people with disabilities in all aspects of community life. WRDI also strives to identify and promote access to existing resources and to advocate for the development of new resources, which may enable people with disabilities to live more independently.

Tennessee

4556 **Center for Independent Living of Middle Tennessee**
955 Woodland St
Nashville, TN 37206-3753
615-292-5803
866-992-4568
Fax: 615-383-1176
TTY: 615-292-7790

Tom Hopton, Executive Director
Tria Bridgeman, Benefits Analyst-Jackson
Dylan Brown, Benefits Analyst-Nashville
Pattrick Gallaher, Employment Assistant-Nashville

CILMT provides persons with disabilities opportunities to be self advocates and make their own decisions regarding living arrangements, means of transportation, employment, social and recreational activities, as well as other aspects of everyday life. Serves Davidson, Cheatham, Wilson, Robertson, Rutherford, Sumner and Williamson Counties.

4557 **DisAbility Resource Center: Knoxville**
900 E Hill Ave
Suite 205
Knoxville, TN 37915-2567
865-637-3666
Fax: 865-637-5616
TTY: 865-637-6976

Lillian Burch, Executive Director
Nicole Craig, Programme Director
Katherine Moore, Independent Living Specialist
Basil Farris, Employment Coach

DRCTN mission is to empower people with disabilities to fully integrate and participate in the community. DRC is a community-based non-residential program of services designed to assist people with disabilities to gain independence and to assist the community in eliminating barriers of independence.

4558 **Jackson Center for Independent Living**
1981 Hollywood Drive
Jackson, TN 38305-4388
731-668-2211
Fax: 731-668-0406
TTY: 731-664-3970
www.j-cil.com
Glen Barr, Executive Director
JCIL works with people with significant disabilities and the Deaf Community in achieving their Independent Living Goals while assisting the community in eliminating barriers to Independent Living.

4559 **Memphis Center for Independent Living**
1633 Madison Ave
Memphis, TN 38104-2506
901-726-6404
800-848-0298
Fax: 901-726-6521
TTY: 901-726-6404
info@mcil.org
www.mcil.org
Kevin Lofton, Chairman
Marvin Glenn Bailey, Vice-Chairman
Charles M. Weirich, Jr., Board Counsel
MCIL is a community based non-profit organization whose primary mission is to facilitate the full integration of persons with disabilities into all aspects of community life.

4560 **Tennessee Technology Access Program (TTAP)**
400 Deaderick St
14th Fl
Nashville, TN 37243-1403
615-313-5183
800-732-5059
Fax: 615-532-4685
TTY: 615-313-5695
Kevin Wright, Director
TTAP's mission is to maintain a statewide program of technology-rated assistance that is timely, comprehensive and consumer driven to ensure that all Tennesseans with disabilities have the information, services and deices that they need to make choices about where and how they spend their time as independently as possible. .

4561 **Tri-State Resource and Advocacy Corporation**
6925 Shallowford Rd
#300
Chattanooga, TN 37421
423-892-4774
800-868-8724
Fax: 423-892-9866
TTY: 423-892-4774
www.1trac.org
Mark Woofall, Executive Director
Pam Jackson, Independent Living Facilitator
TRAC is dedicated to improving opportunities for individuals wuth disabilities.

Texas

4562 **ABLE Center for Independent Living**
1931 E 37th
St # 1
Odessa, TX 79762-6906
432-580-3439
info@ablecenterpb.org
Marilyn Hancock, Executive Director
Kathleen Story MA, Independent Living Specialist
Britni Veretto, HR Manager
To promote independent living for people with disabilities.

4563 **Austin Resource Center for Independent Living**
825 E. Rundberg Ln
Suite E6
Austin, TX 78753-4813
512-832-6349
800-414-6327
Fax: 512-832-1869
arcil@arcil.com
www.arcil.com
Ross Davis, Chair
Linda Loach, Vice-Chair
Sylvia Davis, Secretary/Treasurer
Vonnye Gardner, Member
Serving people with disabilities, their families and communities throughout Travis and surrounding counties.

4564 **Austin Resource Center: Round Rock**
525 Round Rock West
Suite A120
Round Rock, TX 78681-5020
512-828-4624
Fax: 512-828-4625
sally@arcil.com
www.arcil.com
Ross Davis, Chair
Linda Loach, Vice-Chair
Sylvia Davis, Secretary/Treasurer
Vonnye Gardner, Member
Serving peole with disabilities, their families and communities throughout Travis and surrounding counties.

4565 **Austin Resource Center: San Marcos**
618 South Guadalupe St
Suite #103
San Marcos, TX 78666- 6977
512-396-5790
800-572-2973
Fax: 512-396-5794
sanmarcos@arcil.com
www.arcil.com
Ross Davis, Chair
Linda Loach, Vice-Chair
Sylvia Davis, Secretary/Treasurer
Vonnye Gardner, Member
Serving people with disabilities, their families and communities throughout Travis and suraounding counties.

4566 **Brazoria County Center For Independent Living**
1104D East Mullberry Street
Suite D
Angleton, TX 77515- 3952
979-849-7060
888-872-7957
Fax: 979-849-8465
TTY: 979-849-7060
bccil@neosoft.com
www.hcil.cc
Chamane Barrow, Manager
To promote the full inclusion, equal opportunity and participation of persons with disabilities in every aspect of community life. We believe that people with disabilities have the right to make choices affecting their lives, a right to take risks, a right to fail, and a right to succeed.

4567 **Centre, The**
3550 West Dallas Rd
Houston, TX 77019
713-525-8400
Fax: 713-525-8444
thecenterhouston.org
Bill Coorsh, President
Richard Rosenberg, Vice-President
Lisa F. Schott, Secretary
Glen Shepherd, Treasurer
Provides services for more than 600 children and adults with mental developmental disabilities. The Center also offers a wide array of programs including education, vocational training and job placement services, three different residential options representing both urban and rural living environments, special programs designed to meet the needs of older adults, and a variety of therapeutic support services.

4568 **Crockett Resource Center for Independent Living**
1020 Loop 304 East
Crockett, TX 75835-1806
936-544-2811
Fax: 936-544-7315
TTY: 936-544-2811
crcil@windstream.net
www.crockettresourcecenter.org
Sara Minton, Executive Director
Mary Killough, Chief Financial Officer
Cathy Newsome, Information/Outreach Coordinator
Debbie Oliver, Information and Outreach Coor.
Provides independent living services to cross-disability groups to increase their personal self-determination and minimize dependence on others. Maintain comprehensive information on availability of resources and provides referrals to such resources. Provides instruction to assist people with disabilities to gain

skills that would empower them to live independently. Peer counseling, advocacy - both individual and community by assisting to obtain support services to make changes in society.

4569 **Houston Center for Independent Living (HCIL)**
6201 Bonhomme Rd.
Suite 150-South
Houston, TX 77036
713-974-4621
Fax: 713-974-6927
hcil@neosoft.com

Sandra Bookman, Executive Director
Advocacy organization created by and for people with disabilities (PWD) to empower and protect their rights. Services include but not limited to: peer to peer support, individual and systems advocacy, independent living skills training, information and referral, disability cultural awareness, ASL and Braille classes, ADA technical assistance, Relocation/Transition to Community Services, computer technology training, SSA Work Incentives Technical Assistance, equipment loan program.

4570 **Independent Life Styles**
215 North Benton Drive
Sauk Rapids, MN 56379-1874
320-529-9000
888-529-0743
Fax: 320-529-0747
ilicil@independentlifestyles.org
www.independentlifestyles.org

Karen Ahles, Chair
Jay Keller, Educator
Cara Ruff, Executive Director
Chad Hansen, Community Member
Offers peer counseling, advocacy and other services to the community.

4571 **Independent Living Research Utilization Project**
Institute For Rehabilitation & Research
1333 Moursund
Houston, TX 77030
713-520-0232
Fax: 713-520-5785
TTY: 713-520-0232
ilru@ilru.org
www.ilru.org

Lex Frieden, Director
ILRU is a national center for information, training, research and technical assistance in independent living. Its goal is to expand the body of knowledge in independent living and to improve utilization of results of research programs and demonstration projects in this field. ILRU is a program of The Institute for Rehabilitation and Research, a nationally recognized medical rehabilitation facility for persons with disabilities. TTY phone number: (713) 520-5136.

4572 **LIFE/ Run Centers for Independent Living**
8240 Boston Avenue
Lubbock, TX 79423-2342
806-795-5433
Fax: 806-795-5607
TTY: 806-795-5433
wilmacrain@yahoo.com
www.liferun.org

Michelle Crain, Executive Director
Committed to providing individuals with disabilities the information and skills necessary to become independent and to achieve full inclusion in every aspect of their life.

4573 **Office for Students with Disabilities, University of Texas at Arlington**
701 South Nedderman Drive
Arlington, TX 76019-1
817-272-3364
800-735-2989
Fax: 817-272-1447
TTY: 800-735-2989
helpdesk@uta.edu
www.uta.edu/disability

Penny Acrey, Director
Demarice Ferguson, MS, CRC, Associate Director
Scott Holmes, Assistant Director for Testing
Gilda Williams, BSW, Office Manager
Offers disability counseling and academic accomodation to UT Arlington community.

4574 **Palestine Resource Center for Independent Living**
421 Avenue a St
Palestine, TX 75801-2903
903-729-7505
888-326-5166
Fax: 903-729-7540
TTY: 903-729-7505
prcil@embarqmail.com
www.palestineresourcecenter.org/?

Sara Minton, Executive Director
Mary Killough, Chief Financial Officer
Cathy Newsome, Information/Outreach Coordinator
Debbie Oliver, Information and Outreach Coor.
Provides independent living services to cross-disability groups to increase their personal self-determination and minimize dependence on others. Maintain comprehensive information on availability of resources and provides referrals to such resources. Provides instruction to assist people with disabilities to gain skills that would empower them to live independently. Peer counseling, advocacy - both individual and community by assisting to obtain support services to make changes in society.

4575 **Panhandle Action Center for Independent Living Skills**
417 W. 10th Avenue
Amarillo, TX 79101-4316
806-374-1400
Fax: 806-374-4550
TTY: 806-374-2774
www.panhandleilc.org

Joe Rogers, Executive Director
Alma Benavides, Employment Director
Chris White, Development Director
Cynthia Hammett, Consumer Coordinator & Youth Tra
PILC is a non profit organization dedicated to the advancement of full participation in all aspects of life. PILC services are developed, directed, delivered, and governed primarily by individuals with disabilities.

4576 **REACH of Dallas Resource Center on Independent Living**
8625 King George
Suite 210
Dallas, TX 75235-2286
214-630-4796
Fax: 214-630-6390
TTY: 214-630-5995
reachdallas@reachcils.org
www.reachcils.org

Charlotte A. Stewart, Executive Director
Information and referral, peer support/peer counseling, independent living skills training and advocacy assistance.

4577 **REACH of Denton Resource Center on Independent Living**
405 S. Elm St
Suite 202
Denton, TX 76201-6068
940-383-1062
Fax: 940-383-2742
reachden@reachcils.org
www.reachcils.org

Charlotte A. Stewart, Executive Director
To provide for people with disabilities so that they are enabled to lead self-directed lives and to educate the general public about disability-related topics in order to promote a barrier free community.

4578 **REACH of Fort Worth Resource Center on Independent Living**
1000 Macon Street
Suite 200
Fort Worth, TX 76102-4527
817-870-9082
Fax: 817-877-1622
reachftw@reachcils.org
www.reachcils.org

Charlotte A. Stewart, Executive Director
To provide services for people with disabilities so that they are enabled to lead self-directed lives and to educate the general public about disability-related topics in order to promote a barrier free community.

4579 **RISE-Resource: Information, Support and Empowerment**
755 11th Street
Suite 101
Beaumont, TX 77701-3723
409-832-2599
Fax: 409-838-4499
TTY: 409-832-2599
www.risecil.org

Jim Brocato, Executive Director
Amanda Powe, Relocation Services Specialist
Cheryl Bass, Program Director
Gracie Jackson, Independent Living Specialist
A non-profit center for independent living.

4580 **SAILS**
1028 S Alamo St
San Antonio, TX 78210-1170
210-281-1878
800-474-0295
Fax: 210-281-1759
TTY: 210-281-1878
kbrietzke@sailstx.org
www.sailstx.org

Patricia Byrd, Chair
Dennis Wolf, Vice Chair
Jerry D. King, Treasurer
Donna McBee, Member
SAILS advocates for the rights and empowerment of people with disabilities in San Antonio; as well as surrounding areas. Services are provided to people with disabilities in the following counties: Atacosa, Bandera, Bexar, Calhoun, Comal, DeWitt, Dimmit, Edwards, Frio, Gillespie, Goliad, Gonzalez, Guadalupe, Jackson, Karnes, La Salle, Kendall, Kerr, Kinney, Lavaca, Maverick, Medina, Real, Uvalde, Val Verde, Victoria, Wilson and Zavala.

4581 **Texas Department of Assistive and Rehabilitative Services**
4800 N. Lamar Blvd
Austin, TX 78756
512-472-4138
800-628-5115
Fax: 512-472-0603
TTY: 866-581-9328
dars.inquiries@dars.state.tx.us
www.dars.state.tx.us

Bill West, Manager
Daniel Bravo, Chief Operating Officer
Rebecca Trevino, Chief Financial Officer
Glenn Neal, Deputy Commissioner
Provides technical assistance and other support services to the state's Independent Living Council, Independent Living Centers and Independent Living Counseling programs.

4582 **VOLAR Center for Independent Living**
1220 Golden Key Circle
El Paso, TX 79925-5825
915-591-0800
800-591-0800
Fax: 915-591-3506
TTY: 915-591-0800
volar@volarcil.org
www.volarcil.org

Luis Chew, Executive Director
Danny Monroe, Chief Financial Officer
Nena Garcia, Records Manager/ Bookkeeper
Thelma Hernandez, Office Manager
VOLAR is committed to providing independent living ervices and information and referral, and to developing community options for persons with cross disabilities to empower them to live the kind of lives they choose. VOLAR is an organization of and for people with disabilities, advocating human and civil rights, community options and empowering people to live the lives they choose. Newsletter available.

4583 **Valley Association for Independent Living (VAIL)**
3012 N McColl Road
McAllen, TX 78501
956-668-8245
866-400-8245
Fax: 956-878-1601
info@vailrgv.org
vailrgv.org

Woodie Johnston, Executive Director
Offers information and referral, peer couseling, MS supprt group, independent living skills training, and advocacy, work incentives planning and assistance, transitioning people with disabilities from the nursing home into the community.

4584 **Valley Association for Independent Living: Harlingen**
1824 W. Jefferson Ave
Suite B
Harlingen, TX 78550-5247
956-428-1126
866-400-8245
Fax: 956-428-4339

Soledad Myers, Manager
Provides information and referral, peer counseling, support groups, independent living skills training, community rehab program and advocacy

Utah

4585 **Active Re-Entry**
10 S Fairgrounds Rd
Price, UT 84501
435-637-4950
Fax: 435-637-4952
TTY: 435-637-4950
active@arecil.org
www.arecil.org

Nancy Bentley, Executive Director
Active Re-Entry is a community based program which assists individuals with disabilities to acheive or maintain self-sufficient and productive live in their own communities. Active Re-Entry is committed to promoting the rights, dignity, and quality of life for all persons with disabilities.

4586 **Active Re-Entry: Vernal**
10 S Fairgrounds Rd
Price, UT 84501-9727
435-637-4950
Fax: 435-789-6090
TTY: 435-789-4021
active@arecil.org
www.arecil.org

Heather Moore, President
Active Re-Entry is a community based program which assists individuals with disabilities to achieve or maintain self-sufficient and productive lives in their own communities. We are committed to promoting the rights, dignity, and quality of life for all persons with disabilities.

4587 **Central Utah Independent Living Center**
3445 S Main St
Salt Lake City, UT 84115-2824
801-466-5565
877-421-4500
Fax: 801-466-2363
TTY: 801-373-5044
uilc@uilc.org
www.uilc.org

Debra Mair, Executive Director
Kim Meichle, Assistant Director
Patty Trent, Fiscal Manager
Shauna Brock, Independent Living Specialist
Empowers people with disabilities to reach their full potential in community settings through peer support, advocacy, and education.

4588 **OPTIONS for Independence**
Northern Utah Center for Independent Living
106 East 1120 N
Logan, UT 84341-2215
435-753-5353
Fax: 435-753-5390
TTY: 435-753-5353
www.optionsind.org

Cheryl Atwood, Executive Director
OPTIONS for Independence, the Northern Utah Center for Independent Living serves people of all ages with all types of disabilities. OPTIONS is a nonresidential Center that provides services to individuals with disabilities to facilitate their full participation in the community and raise the understanding of disability issues and access to the community. The Independent Living philosophy is strictly adhered to: consumer control and choice being the focus.

4589 **OPTIONS for Independence: Brigham Satellite**
106 East 1120 N
Logan, UT 84341-3379
435-753-5353
Fax: 435-753-5390
TTY: 435-723-2171
dcrockett@qwestoffice.net
www.optionsind.org

Cheryl Atwood, Executive Director
Deanna Crockett, Manager

OPTIONS is a nonresidential Independent Living Center where people with disabilities can learn skills to gain more control and independence over their lives. OPTIONS raises the vision and capability of the community at large to the point where people of all abilities will have equal access.

4590 **Red Rock Center for Independence**
515 W 300 N
Suite A
Saint George, UT 84770-4578
435-673-7501
800-649-2340
Fax: 435-673-8808
rrci@rrci.org
www.rrci.org

Barbara Lefler, Executive Director
Jerry Salkowe, President
Celeste Sorensen, Secretary
Joseph Gordon, Treasurer

Red Rock Center for Independence assists people with disabilities to live and participate independently.

4591 **Tri-County Independent Living Center**
P.O. Box 428
Ogden, UT 84402-428
801-612-3215
866-734-5678
Fax: 801-612-3732
TTY: 801-612-3215
www.uilc.org

Richard Fox, Chairperson
Kim Price, Vice-Chairperson
Greg Killpack, Secretary/Treasurer
Debra Mair, Executive Director

The mission of the Tri-County ILC is to enhance independence for all people with disabilities. Serves Davis, Weber and Morgan Counties.

4592 **Utah Assistive Technology Program (UTAP) Utah State University**
6855 Old Main Hill
Logan, UT 84322-6855
435-797-3811
800-524-5152
Fax: 435-797-2355
www.uatpat.org

Sachin Pavithran, UATP Program Director
Marilyn Hammond, Utah Assistive Technology Founda
Lois Summers, UATP Staff Assistant/UATF Busine
Alma Burgess, Data Collection Coordinator

Provides expertise, resources, and a structure to enhance and expand AT services provided by private and public agencies in Utah. Occurs through monitoring, coordination, information dissemination, empowering individuals, the identification and removal of barriers, and expanding state resources.

4593 **Utah Independent Living Center**
3445 S Main St
Salt Lake City, UT 84115-4453
801-466-5565
800-355-2195
Fax: 801-466-2363
TTY: 801-466-5565
uilc@uilc.org
www.uilc.org

Debra Mair, Executive Director
Kim Meichle, Assistant Director
Julie Beckstead, Program Coordinator
Patty Trent, Fiscal Manager

Offers information and referral services. To assist persons with disabilities achieve independence by providing services and activities which enhance independent living skillspromote the public's understanding, accomodation, and acceptance of their rights, needs and abilities.

4594 **Utah Independent Living Center: Minersville**
P.O. Box 168
Minersville, UT 84752-168
435-691-7724
rrci@rrci.org
www.rrci.org

Barbara Lefler, Executive Director
Jerry Salkowe, President
Celeste Sorensen, Secretary
Joseph Gordon, Treasurer

To enhance independence for all people with disaibilities.

4595 **Utah Independent Living Center: Tooele**
42 S Main St
Tooele, UT 84074-2132
435-843-7353
Fax: 435-843-7359
TTY: 435-843-7353
www.uilc.org

Debra Mair, Executive Director
Kim Meichle, Assistant Director
Julie Beckstead, Program Coordinator
Patty Trent, Fiscal Manager

Mission is to assist persons with disabilities achieve greater independence by providing services and activities which enhance independent living skills and promote the public's understanding, accomodation, and acceptance of their rights, needs and abilities.

Vermont

4596 **Vermont Assistive Technology Program**
Department of Aging and Independent Living
100 State Street
Montpelier, VT 05602-2305
802-871-3353
800-750-6355
Fax: 802-871-3048
TTY: 802-241-1464
www.atp.vermont.gov/tryout-centers

Julie Tucker, Program Director
David Punia ATP, Information/Education Specialist

Encompasses a state coordinating council for assistive technology issues, regional centers for demonstration, trial and technical support with computer and augmentative communication equipment and regional seating and positioning centers.

4597 **Vermont Center for Independent Living: Bennington**
601 Main St
Bennington, VT 5201-2875
802-447-0574
800-639-1522
info@vcil.org
www.vcil.org

Colleen Arcodia, Peer Advocate Counselor
Michelle Grubb, Finance & Operations Officer
Sarah Launderville, Executive Director
Sue Booth, Business Office Coordinator

Believes that individuals with disabilities have the right to live with dignity and with appropriate support in their own homes, fully participate in their communities, and to control and make decisions about their lives.

4598 **Vermont Center for Independent Living: Chittenden**
11 East State Street
Montpelier, VT 05602
802-229-0501
800-639-1522
Fax: 802-229-0503
TTY: 802-229-0501
info@vcil.org
www.vcil.org

Colleen Arcodia, Peer Advocate Counselor
Nathan Besio, Peer Advocate Counselor
Chanda Beun, Receptionist/Admin Specialist
Sue Booth, Business Office Coordinator

Believes that individuals with disabilities have the right to live with dignity and with appropriate support in their own homes, fully participate in their communities, and to control and make decisions about their lives.

4599 **Vermont Center for Independent Living: Montpelier**
11 E State St
Montpelier, VT 05602-3008
802-229-0501
800-639-1522
Fax: 802-229-0503
info@vcil.org
vcil.org

Colleen Arcodia, Peer Advocate Counselor
Denise Bailey, Direct Services Coordinator
Dhiresha Blose, Development Officer
Sue Booth, Business Office Coordinator

Believes that individuals with disabilities have the right to live with dignity and with appropriate support in their own homes, fully participate in their communities, and to control and make decisions about their lives.

Virginia

4600 **Access Independence**
324 Hope Dr
Winchester, VA 22601-6800
540-662-4452
Fax: 540-662-4474
TTY: 540-662-5556
askai@accessindependence.org
www.accessindependence.org

Donald Price, Executive Director
Brenda Ernst, Independent Living Specialist
Joan Davis, Manager Operations/Rep Payee
Michaela Zaraszczak, Executive Administrative Assis.

Offers support services to persons with disabilities to assist in maintaining or increasing their independence and self-determination. Includes housing assistance, independent living skills training, information, referral services, assistance and representative payee and advocacy.

4601 **Appalachian Independence Center**
230 Charwood Dr
Abingdon, VA 24210-2566
276-628-2979
Fax: 276-628-4931
TTY: 276-676-0920
aicadmin@ntelos.net
aicadvocates.org

Greg Morrell, Executive Director
Donna Buckland, Development Director
Scarlett Cox, Operations Director

Mission is to advocate for and with people with disabilities to promote full participation in society

4602 **Blue Ridge Independent Living Center**
Ste B
1502 Williamson Rd NE
Roanoke, VA 24012-5100
540-342-1231
Fax: 540-342-9505
TTY: 540-342-1231
brilc@brilc.org
brilc.org

Karen Michalski-Karn, Executive Director
Dana Jackson, Program Services Director
Lottie Diomedi, Independent Living Coordinator
Sallee Ebbett, Finance Manager

BRILC assists people with disabilities to live independently. The Center also serves the community at large by helping to create and environment that is accessible to all. BRILC offers a variety of services ranging from referrals to community resources, support services, and direct services. These include peer counseling, support groups, training and seminars, advocacy, education, support services, awareness, aid in obtaining specialized equipment, and much more.

4603 **Blue Ridge Independent Living Center: Christianburg**
210 Pepper Street S
Christiansburg, VA 24073-3571
540-381-8829
Fax: 540-381-8833
TTY: 540-381-9149
brilc@brilc.org
brilc.org

Karen Michalski-Karney, Executive Director
Dana Jackson, Program Services Director
Lottie Diomedi, Independent Living Coordinator
Sallee Ebbett, Finance Manager

Assists people with disabilities to live independently. The center also serves the community at large by helping to create an environment that is accessible to all.

4604 **Blue Ridge Independent Living Center: Low Moor**
P.O. Box 7
Low Moor, VA 24457-7
540-862-0252
Fax: 540-862-0252
TTY: 540-862-0252
brilc.org

Karen Michalski-Karney, Executive Director
Dana Jackson, Program Services Director
Lottie Diomedi, Independent Living Coordinator
Sallee Ebbett, Finance Manager

Assists to help people with disabilities to live independently. The center also serves the community at large by helping to create an environment that is accessible to all.

4605 **Clinch Independent Living Services**
1139C Plaza Drive
Grundy, VA 24614-6780
276-935-6088
800-597-2322
Fax: 276-935-6342
TTY: 276-935-6088

Betty Bevins, Executive Director

Nonprofit organization providing information and referral, peer counseling, advocacy and independent living skills training to persons with disabilities.

4606 **Disability Resource Center**
409 Progress St
Fredericksburg, VA 22401-3337
540-373-2559
800-648-6324
Fax: 540-373-8126
TTY: 540-373-5890
drc@cildrc.org

Debe Fults, Executive Director
Eric Barnes, Equipment Connection Assistant
Grace Marshall, Community Integration Coor.
Janet Lutkewitte, Accounting/IT

Mission is to assist people with disabilities, those who support them, and the community, through information, education and resources, to achieve the highest potential and benefit of independent living.

4607 **ENDependence Center of Northern Virginia**
2300 Claredon Blvd.
Suite 3305
Arlington, VA 22201-3367
703-525-3268
866-849-3852
Fax: 703-525-3585
TTY: 703-525-3553
info@ecnv.org
www.ecnv.org

Cynthia Evans, Director of Community Services
Layo Oyewole, Director of Medicaid Programs
Doris Ray, Director of Advocacy and Outreac
Brewster Thackeray, Executive Director

ECNV is a community-based resource and advocacy enter which is managed by and for people with disabilities. ENCV promotes independent living philosophy and equal access for all persons with disabilities and, like the nearly 400 centers for independent living across the country, ECNV grew from local disability rights and self-help movements.

4608 **Equal Access Center for Independence**
4031 University Drive
Suite #301
Fairfax, VA 22030-3409
703-934-2020
TTY: 703-277-7730
David Sharp, Executive Director
Provides information and referral, peer counseling, advocacy and independent living skills training to persons with disabilities.

4609 **Independence Empowerment Center**
8409 Dorsey Circle
Suite 101
Manassas, VA 20110-4414
703-257-5400
Fax: 703-257-5043
TTY: 703-257-5400
info@ieccil.org
www.ieccil.org
Mary D Lopez, Executive Director
Roberta McEachern, Program Director
Sheree Thomas, Grants Coordinator
Alan Smiley, Service Facilitator
A non-profit Center for Independent Living. One of over 500 centers in the United States with roots in civil rights models of the 1960's.

4610 **Independence Resource Center**
815 Cherry Ave
Charlottesville, VA 22903-3448
434-971-9629
Fax: 434-971-8242
TTY: 434-971-9629
tvandever@ntelos.net
www.charlottesvilleirc.org
Tom Vandever, Executive Director
Brenda Gianniny, Administrator
Carolyn Berry, Participant Services Coordinator
Nate Brown, Senior Peer Advocate
Information and referral services.

4611 **Independent Living Center Network: Department of the Visually Handicapped**
Ste 300
1809 Staples Mill Rd
Richmond, VA 23230-3515
Fax: 804-355-9297
Robert W Partin, Director
Robert Kastenbaum, Partner
Information and referral services.

4612 **Junction Center for Independent Living**
P.O. Box 1210
Norton, VA 24273-913
276-679-5988
Fax: 276-679-6569
TTY: 276-679-5988
jcil1@junctioncenter.org
junctioncenter.org
Dennis Horton, Executive Director
Cindy Mefford, Assistant to the Executive Direc
Joe Brady, Deaf and Hard of Hearing Coordin
Brenda Cowden, Housing Specialist
To assist those who have significant disabilities so that they migh live independently in the least restrictive and most integrated environment possible.

4613 **Junction Center for Independent Living: Duffield**
P.O. Box 408
Duffield, VA 24244-408
276-431-1195
Fax: 276-431-1196
TTY: 276-431-1195
jcil1@junctioncenter.org
Dennis Horton, Executive Director
Cindy Mefford, Assistant to the Executive Direc
Joe Brady, Deaf and Hard of Hearing Coordin
Brenda Cowden, Housing Specialist
To assist those who have significant disabilities so that they might live independently in the least restrictive and most integrated environment possbile.

4614 **Lynchburg Area Center for Independent Living**
500 Alleghany Ave
Suite #520
Lynchburg, VA 24501-2610
434-528-4971
Fax: 434-528-4976
TTY: 434-528-4972
www.lacil.org
Phil Theisen, Executive Director
LACIL is a private non-profit, non-residential consumer driven organization that promotes the efforts of persons with disabilities to live independently in the community and supports the efforts of the community to be open and accessible to all citizens.

4615 **Peidmont Independent Living Center**
Piedmont Living Center
601 S. Belvidere Street
Richmond, VA 23220
804-782-1986
800-828-1140
Fax: 877-VHD- 123
www.vhda.com
Kit Hale, Chairman
Timothy M. Chapman, Vice Chairman
Susan Dewey, Executive Director
Tammy Neale, Chief Learning Officer
Empowering indiviuals with disabilities to become self-sufficient and independent within their communities.

4616 **Peninsula Center for Independent Living**
2021-A Cunningham Drive
Suite #2
Hampton, VA 23666-3320
757-827-0275
Fax: 757-827-0655
TTY: 757-827-8800
iepcil@hvacil.org
www.hvacil.org
Ralph Shelman, Executive Director
IEPCIL is a private non-profit non-residential Agency established to provide services to people with disabilities. The Centers Philosophy is that people with a disability should play a major role in deciding their future.The center provides services to people with disabilities in the cities of Hampton, Newport News, Poquoson, Williamsburg, and counties of James City, York, and Gloucester.

4617 **Piedmont Independent Living Center**
1045 Main Street
Suite #2
Danville, VA 24541-1800
434-797-2530
Fax: 434-797-2568
TTY: 434-797-2530
Clarence Dickerson, Executive Director
Jeanette King, ILS Coordinator/BPAD
Lori Penn, Office Manager
Empowering indiviuals with disabilities to become self-sufficient and independent within their communities.

4618 **Resources for Independent Living**
4009 Fitzhugh Ave
Richmond, VA 23230-3953
804-353-6503
Fax: 804-358-5606
TTY: 804-353-6583
info@ril-va.org
www.ril-va.org
Gerald O'Neill, Executive Director
Marcia Guardino, Program Manager
Kelly Hickok, Community Services Manager
Tom Allen, Chair
Assisting persons who are severly disabled to live independently in the community and to encourage necessary change within the community so independent living is a possibility.

4619 **Valley Associates for Independent Living (VAIL)**
Shenandoah Valley Workforce Investment Board
3210 Peoples Drive
Suite 220
Harrisonburg, VA 22801-869
540-433-6513
888-242-8245
Fax: 540-433-6313
vail@govail.org
www.govail.org

Marcia Du Bois, Executive Director
Bob Satterwhite, Executive Director

VAIL is a not-for-profit, private Center for Independent Living providing advocacy, information and referral, independent living skills training, supported employment, and peer counseling to individuals with disabilities in our planning district.

4620 **Valley Associates for Independent Living: Lexington**
205-B South Liberty St
Harrisonburg, VA 22801-3638
540-433-6513
888-242-8245
Fax: 540-433-6313
TTY: 540-438-9265
vail@govail.org
www.govail.org

Marcia Du Bois, Executive Director

Promoting self-direction among people with disabilities and removing barriers to independence in the community.

4621 **Woodrow Wilson Rehabilitation Center Training Program**
243 Woodrow Wilson Avenue
Fishersville, VA 22939-1500
540-332-7000
800-345-9972
Fax: 540-332-7132
TTY: 800-811-7893
www.wwrc.net

Rick Sizemore, Executive Director

Information & referral services. Six week Virginia residential programs and evaluation services.

Washington

4622 **Alliance for People with Disabilities: Seattle**
1120 E. Terrace St
Suite 100
Seattle, WA 98122
206-545-7055
866-545-7055
Fax: 206-545-7059
TTY: 206-632-3456
info@disabilitypride.org
www.disabilitypride.org

Kimberly Heymann, Executive Director
Elizabeth Kennedy, Executive Assistant
Bhelle Ollero, IL Specialist
Hope Drumond, Program Manager

The Alliance promotes equality and choice for people with disabilities. They provide advocacy, peer support, idependent living skills training, information and referral, transition assistance for youth, civil rights legal aid, assistive technology, training and nursing home transition back into the community.

4623 **Alliance of People with Disabilities: Redmond**
East King County Office
1150 140th Ave NE
Suite 101
Bellevue, WA 98005-3537
425-558-0993
800-216-3335
Fax: 425-558-4773
TTY: 425-861-4773
info@disabilitypride.org
www.disabilitypride.org

Kimberly Heymann, Executive Director
Elizabeth Kennedy, Executive Assistant
Bhelle Ollero, IL Specialist
Hope Drumond, Program Manager

Services include: information and referral, independent living skills training, peer groups, disAbility law project (DLP), access reviews, health insurance advising, and systems advocacy.

4624 **Community Services for the Blind and Partially Sighted Store: Sight Connection**
9709 Third Ave NE
Suite #100
Seattle, WA 98115-2027
206-525-5556
800-458-4888
Fax: 206-525-0422
www.sightconnection.org

Mary Lewis, Secretary
Shannon Grady Martsolf, President/CEO
Miles Otoupal, Chair
Jonathan Avedovech, Vice Chair

Over 300 practical products for living with vision loss selected by certified vision rehabilitation specialists from Community Services for the Blind and Partially Sighted. Easy-to-use online store features large print, large photos, secure transactions, and links to other vision-related resources.

4625 **DisAbility Resource Connection: Everett**
607 SE Everett Mall Way
Suite 6C
Everett, WA 98208-3210
425-347-5768
800-315-3583
Fax: 425-710-0767
TTY: 425-347-5768

Charley Lane, Executive Director

disAbility Resource Connection is all about living your life as you choose. The staff is committed to assisting every individual to connect to resources, connect to skills, connect to life.

4626 **Kitsap Community Resources**
845 8th St
Bremerton, WA 98337-1517
360-478-2301
Fax: 360-415-2706
info@kcr.org
www.kcr.org

Larry Eyer, Executive Director
Irmgard Davis, Fiscal Officer
Rudy Taylor, Board President
Kurt Wiest, Board Vice President

Kitsap Community Resources is a local, non-profit organization dedicated to helping people in need. KCR creates hope and opportunity for low-income Kitsap County Residents by providing resources that promote self-sufficiency.

4627 **Spokane Center for Independent Living**
8817 E. Mission Ave.
Suite 106
Spokane Valley, WA 99212
509-326-6355
Fax: 509-327-2420
info@scilwa.org

William Kane, Executive Director

To improve the self-determination and self-reliance of people with disabilities through systems and individual advocacy, education and independent living services.

4628 **Tacoma Area Coalition of Individuals with Disabilities**
6315 S 19th St
Tacoma, WA 98466-6217
253-565-9000
877-538-2243
Fax: 253-565-5578
TTY: 253-565-3486
www.tacid.org

Ken Gibson, Executive Director
Steve Pierce, CFO
Jo Ann Maxwell, Deputy Executive Director - Phil
Marsha Doman-Masters, Executive Assistant - Administra

Promotes the independence of individuals with disabilities.

West Virginia

4629 Appalachian Center for Independent Living
4710 Chimney Drive
Suite # C
Charleston, WV 25302-4841
304-965-0376
800-642-3003
Fax: 304-965-0377
TTY: 800-642-3003
acil@yahoo.com
www.mtstcil.org

Ann Weeks, President and CEO
Adam Elmer, Chief Financial Officer
Georgetta Stevens, VP, Corporate Operations
Debbie Conley, Board Chair

A resource center for persons with disabilities and their communities. Serves Kanawha, Clay, Boone and Putnam counties.

4630 Appalachian Center for Independent Living: Spencer
811 Madison Avenue
Suite #106
Spencer, WV 25276-1900
304-927-4080
Fax: 304-927-4330
TTY: 800-642-3003
susanacil@yahoo.com
www.mtstcil.org

Ann Weeks, President and CEO
Adam Elmer, Chief Financial Officer
Georgetta Stevens, VP, Corporate Operations
Debbie Conley, Board Chair

A resource center for persons with disabilities and their communities. Serves Jackson, Roane, and Calhoun counties.

4631 Mountain State Center for Independent Living
329 Prince St
Beckley, WV 25801-4515
304-255-0122
Fax: 304-255-0157
TTY: 304-255-0122
aoweeks@mtstcil.org
www.mtstcil.org

Ann Weeks, President and CEO
Adam Elmer, Chief Financial Officer
Georgetta Stevens, VP, Corporate Operations
Debbie Conley, Board Chair

This office provides individual and systems advocacy, independent living skills development, information and referral, peer support, personal assistance services, housing referral and training, transportation. Serves Raleigh counties.

4632 Mountain State Center for Independent Living
821 Fourth Avenue
Huntington, WV 25701-1406
304-525-3324
866-687-8245
Fax: 304-525-3360
TTY: 304-525-3324
aoweeks@mtstcil.org
www.mtstcil.org

Ann Weeks, President and CEO
Adam Elmer, Chief Financial Officer
Georgetta Stevens, VP, Corporate Operations
Debbie Conley, Board Chair

Services provided are: individual and systems advocacy, independent living skills development, information and referral, peer support, personal assistance services, supported employment, community integration program, housing referral and training, transportation. Serves Cabell and Wayne counties.

4633 Northern West Virginia Center for Independent Living
601-603 East Brockway
Suite A & B
Morgantown, WV 26501
304-296-6091
800-834-6408
Fax: 304-292-5217
TTY: 304-296-6091
nwvcil@nwvcil.org
www.mtstcil.org

Ann Weeks, President and CEO
Adam Elmer, Chief Financial Officer
Georgetta Stevens, VP, Corporate Operations
Debbie Conley, Board Chair

NWVCIL is committed to the philosophy that all persons have equal access and unconditional value, that all individuals shall be respected for their uniqueness and shall have the right to live within the community of their choice, having equal access to participate in and contribute to that community.

Wisconsin

4634 Center for Independent Living of Western Wisconsin
2920 Schneider Avenue East
Menomonie, WI 54751-2331
715-233-1070
800-228-3287
Fax: 715-233-1083
TTY: 800-228-3287
www.cilww.com

Tim Sheehan, Executive Director
Kay Sommerfeld, Assistant Director
Tammy Grage, Fiscal & HR Manager
Noelle Johnson, Resource Counselor Camp Quest

Advocates for the full participation in society of all persons with disabilities. Our goal is empwowering individuals to exercise choices to maintain or increase their indpendence. Our strategy is providing consumer-driven services at no cost to persons with disiabilities in Western Wisconsin

4635 Independence First
540 South 1st Street
Milwaukee, WI 53204-1516
414-291-7520
Fax: 414-291-7525
TTY: 414-297-7520
lschulz@independencefirst.org
www.independencefirst.org

Lee Schulz, President and CEO
John Schmid, Chair
Judy Murphy, Vice Chair
Judi Wisla, Secretary

A non-profit agency directed by, and for the benefit of, persons with disabilities, primarily serving the four county metropolitan Milwaukee area.

4636 Independence First: West Bend
735 S Main St
West Bend, WI 53095-3965
262-306-6717
lschulz@independencefirst.org
www.independencefirst.org

Lee Schulz, President and CEO
John Schmid, Chair
Judy Murphy, Vice Chair
Judi Wisla, Secretary

A non-profit agency directed by, and for the benefit of, persons with disabilities, primarily serving the four county Metropolitan Milwaukee area.

4637 Inspiration Ministries
N2270 State Road 67
Walworth, WI 53184-948
262-275-6131
Fax: 262-275-3355
inspirationministries.org

Robin Knoll, President
Richard Hall, Executive Vice President
Craig Pape, VP Ministry Services
Michael Scholl, VP Development

Formerly known as Christian League for the Handicapped, Inspiration Ministries is a vibrant community of adults with disabilities engaged in living, working, leisure and faith activities designed to provide a complete living experience. The campus consists of a modern residential facility offering a range of living accomodations; a work center and resale shop; and Inspiration Center, a retreat/camping center designed to be 100% wheelchair accessible.

4638 **Mid-State Independent Living Consultants: Wausau**
3262 Church Street
Suite #1
Stevens Point, WI 54481-5321
715-344-4210
800-382-8484
Fax: 715-344-4414
TTY: 800-382-8484
milc@milc-inc.org
www.milc-inc.org

Tom Vandehey, President
Becky Paulson, Independent Living Consultant
Working for persons with disabilities towards empowerment to make informed choices.

4639 **Mid-state Independent Living Consultants: Stevens Point**
3262 Church Street
Suite #1
Stevens Point, WI 54481-5321
715-344-4210
800-382-8484
Fax: 715-344-4414
TTY: 800-382-8484
milc@milc-inc.org
www.milc-inc.org

Jenny Fasula, Executive Director
Karalyn Peterson, Resource Director
Committed to enhancing personal and community relationships, providing opportunities for growth, and helping people with varying abilities achieve their personal goals.

4640 **North Country Independent Living**
69 N 28th St.
Suite 28
Superior, WI 54880-5138
715-392-9118
800-924-1220
Fax: 715-392-4636
northcountryil.com

John Nousaine, Executive Director
Gloria Hakkila-Johnson, Assistant Director
Jim Glaeser, Accountant
Russ Stover, Office Assistant
Empowers people with disabilities.

4641 **North Country Independent Living: Ashland**
422 3rd St. W.
Suite #114
Ashland, WI 54806-1553
715-682-5676
800-499-5676
Fax: 715-682-3144
TTY: 715-682-5676
northcountryil.com

John Nousaine, Director
Empowers people with disabilities.

4642 **Options for Independent Living**
555 Country Club Road
Green Bay, WI 54307-1967
920-490-0500
888-465-1515
Fax: 920-490-0700
TTY: 920-490-0600
www.optionsil.com

Thomas Diedrick, Executive Director
Kathryn C. Barry, Assistant Director
Sandra L. Popp, Independent Living Coordinator
Vicky Lasch, Independent Living Coordinator
A non-profit organization committed to empowering people with disabilities to lead independent and productive lives in their community through advocacy, the provision of information, education, technology and related services.

4643 **Options for Independent Living: Fox Valley**
820 West College Ave
Suite #5
Appleton, WI 54914
920-997-9999
888-465-1515
Fax: 920-997-9381
TTY: 920-490-0600
www.optionsil.com

Thomas Diedrick, Executive Director
Kathryn C. Barry, Assistant Director
Sandra L. Popp, Independent Living Coordinator
Vicky Lasch, Independent Living Coordinator
A non-profit organization committed to empowering people with disabilities to lead independent and productive lives in their community through advocacy, the provision of information, education, technology and related services.

4644 **Society's Assets: Elkhorn**
615 E Geneva St
Elkhorn, WI 53121-2301
262-723-8181
800-261-8181
Fax: 262-723-8184
TTY: 866-840-9763
info@societysassets.org
www.societysassets.org

Bruce Nelson, Director
Jill Vigueres, Manager
To ensure the rights of all persons with disabilities to live and function as independently as possible in the community of their choice, through supporting individual's efforts to achieve control over their lives and become integrated into community life.

4645 **Society's Assets: Kenosha**
5455 Sheridan Road
Suite 101
Kenosha, WI 53140-4103
262-657-3999
800-317-3999
Fax: 262-657-1672
TTY: 866-840-9762
info@societysassets.org
www.societysassets.org

Sue Liu, Manager
Bruce Nelsen, Executive Director
To ensure the rights of all persons with disabilities to live and function as independently as possible in the community of their choice, through supporting individuals efforts to achieve controll over their lives and become integrated into community life. Offers home care and independent living services.

4646 **Society's Assets: Racine**
5200 Washinton Ave
Suite #225
Racine, WI 53406-4238
262-637-9128
800-378-9128
Fax: 262-637-8646
TTY: 886-840-9761
info@societysassets.org
www.societysassets.org

Deb Pitsch, Administrator
Karen Olufs, Director Independent Living
Jean Rumachik, Director Home Care Services
Society's Assets assists people with disabilities to live as independently as possible. A non-profit human services agency, Society's Assets provides information and referal, independent living skills training, peer support, advocacy, and supportive home care. Home health care is provided by SAI Home Health Care. The agency serves 5 counties in southeastern Wisconsin and also provides information about interpreters, employment, benefits, home modifications, assistive equipment and accessibility.
Fees vary

Wyoming

4647 **RENEW: Gillette**
35 Fairgrounds Road
Newcastle, WY 82701
307-746-4733
888-253-4653
Fax: 307-746-9701
www.renew-wyo.com

Donna Bombeck, Chairwoman
Carolyn Holso, Vice Chairwoman
Renee Nack, Secretary
Bryan Bergstreser, Treasurer
Empowering persons with disabilities to enrich their lives.

4648 **RENEW: Rehabilitation Enterprises of North Eastern Wyoming**
1969 S Sheridan Ave
Sheridan, WY 82801-6108
307-672-7481
888-309-2020
Fax: 307-674-5117
pr@renew-wyo.com
www.renew-wyo.com

Donna Bombeck, Chairwoman
Carolyn Holso, Vice Chairwoman
Renee Nack, Secretary
Bryan Bergstreser, Treasurer

Multi-disciplinary organization dedicated to the highest possible economic and social independence for persons with disabilities. Extensive referral service, specialized employment placement, occupational therapy, psychological services, evaluation services, and coordination of external services as needed to meet client plans and objectives.

4649 **Rehabilitation Enterprises of North Eastern Wyoming: Newcastle**
35 Fairgrounds Rd
Newcastle, WY 82701-2625
307-746-4733
888-693-9245
Fax: 307-746-9701
www.renew-wyo.com

Donna Bombeck, Chairwoman
Carolyn Holso, Vice Chairwoman
Renee Nack, Secretary
Bryan Bergstreser, Treasurer

Empowering persons with disabilities to enrich their lives.

4650 **Wyoming Services for Independent Living**
1156 South 2nd
Lander, WY 82520-3905
307-332-4889
800-266-3061
Fax: 307-332-2491
TTY: 307-332-7582
www.wysil.org

Susan Hoesel, Business Manager
Donna Langelier, Program Manager
Marcia Henthorn, Program Manager
Valentina Knutson, Independent Living Specialist

Committed to enhancing personal and community relationships, providing opportunities for growth, and helping people with varying abilities achieve thier personal goals.

Law

Associations & Referral Agencies

4651 **Center for Disability and Elder Law, Inc.**
205 W. Randolph
Suite 1610
Chicago, IL 60606
312-376-1880
Fax: 312-376-1885
info@cdelaw.org
www.cdelaw.org

Caroline Manley, Executive Director
Stephanie Ridella Vittands, Staff Attorney
A not-for-profit legal services organization which provids legal services to low income persons residing in Chicago and Cook County, Il., who are either elderly and/or persons with disabilities. CDEL provides legal services by matching qualified candidates with volunteer attorneys who represent them, pro-bono, in a wide range of civil legal matters; and through special initiatives including the Senior Center Initiative (SCI) and the Senior Tax Opportunity program.

4652 **Center for Workplace Compliance**
1501 M Street NW
Suite 400
Washington, DC 20005
202-629-5650
Fax: 202-629-5651
info@cwc.org
cwc.org

Joseph S. Lakis, President
Michael Eastman, Senior Vice President, Policy
Danny Patrella, Vice President, Compliance
Patience Addo, Vice President, Finance
Formerly known as the Equal Employment Advisory Council, it is a nonprofit employer association providing guidance to its member companies on understanding and complying with their affirmative action obligations.
1976

4653 **Chicago Lawyers' Committee for Civil Rights Under Law**
100 N LaSalle Street
Suite 600
Chicago, IL 60602-2400
312-630-9744
Fax: 312-630-1127
info@clccrul.org
www.clccrul.org

Bonnie Allen, Executive Director
Timna Axel, Director, Communications
Aneel Chablani, Chief Counsel
Oi Eng-Crandus, Chief Financial Officer
Promotes and protects civil rights of low-income, minority and disadvantaged people in the social, economic, and political systems of the nation.

4654 **CrescentCare Legal Services**
1631 Elysian Fields Ave.
New Orleans, LA 70117
504-323-2642
www.aidslaw.org

J. Lind, Attorney
J. Johnson, Attorney
J. Holmes, Attorney
C. Terrance, Attorney
The mission of CrescentCare Legal Services (formerly AIDSLAW Louisiana) is to provide excellent, specialized legal services for people living with HIV/AIDS in Louisiana, to improve their quality of life and access to health care, related to their HIV/AIDS status.

4655 **DNA People's Legal Services**
PO Box 306
Window Rock, AZ 86515
928-871-4151
Fax: 928-871-5036
www.dnalegalservices.org

Kathy Gallagher, Development Director
A nonprofit legal aid organization working to protect civil rights, promote tribal sovereignty and alleviate civil legal problems for people who live in poverty in the Southwestern United States.
1967

4656 **Disability Law Colorado**
455 Sherman St.
Suite 130
Denver, CO 80203
303-722-3619
800-288-1376
Fax: 303-722-0720
disabilitylawco.org

Mary Anne Harvey, Executive Director
Alison L. Butler, Esq., Director, Legal Services
Mark Ivandick, Managing Attorney/Program Coordinator
Protects and promotes the rights of people with disabilities and older people in Colorado through direct legal representation, advocacy, education and legislative analysis.

4657 **Disability Rights Advocates**
2001 Center St
4th Floor
Berkeley, CA 94704-1204
510-665-8644
Fax: 510-665-8511
frontdesk@dralegal.org
dralegal.org

Michelle Caiola, Managing Director, Litigation
Kate Hamilton, Managing Director, Development & Operations
Stuart Seaborn, Managing Director, Litigation
Disability Rights Advocates is a non-profit legal center representing people with disabilities, advocating for them when their civil rights have been violated. Their clients include those with mobility, sensory, cognitive, and psychiatric disabilities.

4658 **Disability Rights Education and Defense Fund**
3075 Adeline Street
Suite 210
Berkeley, CA 94703
510-644-2555
Fax: 510-841-8645
info@dredf.org
dredf.org

Susan Henderson, Executive Director
Claudia Center, Legal Director
Silvia Yee, Senior Staff Attorney
Nonprofit organization dedicated to advancing the civil rights of individuals with disabilities through legislation, litigation, informal and formal advocacy and education and training of lawyers, advocates and clients with respect to disability issues. DREDF also provides training, advocacy, technical assistance and referrals for parents of disabled children.

4659 **Disability Rights Texas**
2222 West Braker Lane
Austin, TX 78758-1024
512-454-4816
866-362-2851
www.disabilityrightstx.org

Mary Faithfull, Executive Director
Patty Anderson, Deputy Director
A federally designated legal protection and advocacy agency (P&A) for people with disabilities in Texas. Helps people with disabilities understand and exercise their rights under the law, ensuring their full and equal participation in society.

4660 **Guardianship Services Associates**
41A South Blvd
Oak Park, IL 60302-2777
708-386-5398
Fax: 708-386-5970

Robert R. Wohlgemuth, Executive Director
Information and counseling on guardianship and its alternatives. Can provide direct assistance in obtaining guardianship for disabled adults in Cook County. Also provides information and direct assistance on durable powers of attorney.

4661 **Independence Economic Development**
210 W Truman Road
Independence, MO 64050
816-252-5777
Fax: 816-254-1641
info@inedc.biz
www.iced.org
J.D. Kehrman, President
Jodi Krantz, Vice President
Xander Winkel, Executive Director, Ennovation Center
Sarah Beth Wood, Administrative Assistant
A non-profit, public/private partnership established for the purpose of supporting and enhancing the economic growth of independence.

4662 **Independent Living Research Utilization**
1333 Moursund
Houston, TX 77030-7031
713-520-0232
Fax: 713-520-5785
TTY: 713-520-0232
ilru@ilru.org
ilru.org
Lex Frieden, Director
Richard Petty, Co-Director
Brooke Curtis, Program Coordinator
Vinh Nguyen, Program Director
The ILRU is a national center for information, training, research, and technical assistance in independent living. Its goal is to expand the body of knowledge in independent living and to improve utilization of results of research programs and demonstration projects in this field.

4663 **Judge David L Bazelon Center for Mental Health Law**
1090 Vermont Avenue NW
Suite 220
Washington, DC 20005
202-467-5730
communications@bazelon.org
www.bazelon.org
Holly O'Donnell, CEO
Ira Burnim, Director, Legal
Jennifer Mathis, Director, Policy & Legal Advocacy
Kathy Chamberlain, Deputy Director, External Affairs
A nonprofit organization devoted to improving the lives of people with mental illnesses through changes in policy and law.

4664 **Legal Action Center**
810 1st Street
Suite 200
Washington, DC 20002
202-544-5478
Fax: 202-544-5712
lacinfo@lac.org
www.lac.org
Paul N. Samuels, Director & President
Anita R. Marton, Senior Vice President
Ellen Weber, Vice President, Health Initiatives
Abigail Woodworth, Vice President, External Affairs
The only non-profit law and policy organization in the United States whose sole mission is to fight discrimination against people with histories of addiction, HIV/AIDS, or criminal records, and to advocate for sound public policies in these areas.

4665 **Legal Counsel for Health Jusice**
17 North State Street
Suite 900
Chicago, IL 60602
312-427-8990
Fax: 312-427-8419
legalcouncil.org
Tom Yates, Executive Director
Ellyce Anapolsky, Senior Staff Attorney
Julie Brennan, Program Director
Carrie Chapman, Senior Director, Litigation & Advocacy
Formerly known as the AIDS Legal Council of Chicago, the group provides legal assistance for people with illness and/or disability.

4666 **National Health Law Program (NHeLP)**
3701 Wilshire Blvd
Suite 750
Los Angeles, CA 90010
310-204-6010
www.healthlaw.org
Amy Chen, Senior Attorney
Abigail Coursolle, Senior Attorney
Elizabeth G. Taylor, Executive Director
Jane Perkins, Legal Director
A national public interest law firm that seeks to improve health care for America's working and unemployed poor, minorities, the elderly and people with disabilities. NHeLP serves legal services programs, community-based organizations, the private bar, providers and individuals who work to preserve a health care safety net for the millions of uninsured or underinsured low-income people.
1970

4667 **National Right to Work Legal Defense Foundation**
8001 Braddock Rd.
Springfield, VA 22160
703-321-8510
800-336-3600
Fax: 703-321-9319
nrtw.org
Raymond LaJeunesse, Vice President & Legal Director
Byron S. Andrus, Staff Attorney
Matthew B. Gilliam, Staff Attorney
Amanda K. Freeman, Staff Attorney
The National Right to Work Legal Defense Foundation is a non-profit, charitable organization. Its mission is to eliminate coercive union power and compulsory unionism abuses through strategic litigation, public information, and education programs.
1968

4668 **Ohio Civil Rights Commission (OCRC)**
Rhodes State Office Tower
30 East Broad Street, 5th Floor
Columbus, OH 43215
614-466-2785
888-278-7101
Fax: 614-644-8776
crc.ohio.gov
G. Michael Payton, Executive Director
Darlene Sweeney-Newbern, Director, Regional Operations
Stephanie Bostos-Demers, Chief Legal Counsel
Mary Turocy, Director, Public Affairs and Civic Engagement
Primary function is to enforce state laws against discrimination.

4669 **REACH/Resource Centers on Independent Living**
8625 King George
Suite 210
Dallas, TX 75235-2286
214-630-4796
Fax: 214-630-6390
TTY: 214-630-5995
reachdallas@reachcils.org
www.reachcils.org
Sylvia Hodgins, President
Charlotte A. Stewart, Executive Director
Penny Acrey, Secretary
Gordon Meredith, Treasurer
Providing services for people with disabilities so that they are empowered to lead self-directed lives and educating the general public on disability-related topics in order to promote a barrier-free community.

Resources for the Disabled

4670 **ADA In Details: Interpreting the 2010 Americans with Disabilities Act Stands**
Wiley Publishing
111 River St
Hoboken, NJ 07030-5774
201-748-6000
Fax: 201-748-6088
info@wiley.com
www.wiley.com
Matthe S. Kissner, Chief Executive Officer
Christopher Caridi, Senior Vice President
Helps readers understand the facilities requirements of the Americans with Disabilities Act Accessibility Guidelines. Presents the

technical requirements for accessible elements and spaces in new construction, alterations and additions. *$40.00*
304 pages Paperback 1917
ISBN 9-781119-27-7

4671 **Americans With Disabilities Act Annotated: Legislative History, Regulations & Commentary**
Disability Rights Education and Defense Fund
3075 Adeline Street
Suite 210
Berkeley, CA 94703
510-644-2555
Fax: 510-841-8645
info@dredf.org
dredf.org
Arlene B. Mayerson, Author
Also known as the Blue Book, written in narrative form for both professionals and lay people, this work offers detailed, thorough analysis of all of the law's provisions, encompassing ADA legislative history, the statute and regulations. Available in alternative formats.

4672 **Americans with Disabilities Act Manual**
US Department of Justice
950 Pennsylvania Ave NW
Washington, DC 20530-9
202-307-0663
800-514-0301
Fax: 202-307-1197
TTY: 800-514-0383
www.ada.gov
Rebecca B. Bond, Chief
Zita Johnson Betts, Deputy Chief
Sally Conway, Deputy Chief
James Bostrom, Deputy Chief
An in-depth analysis of the legal and practical implications of the ADA using non-technical language. *$20.00*

4673 **Americans with Disabilities Act: Selected Resources for Deaf**
Gallaudet University Bookstore
800 Florida Avenue NE
Washington, DC 20002-3695
202-651-5000
800-621-2736
Fax: 202-651-5508
clerc.center@gallaudet.edu
www.gallaudet.edu
Priscilla O'Donnell, Bookstore Manager
Iva Williams, Bookstore Secretary
Elaine Vance, Human Resources Director
Marteal Pitts, Circulation Coordinator
This resource identifies programs and publications specific to the ADA and deafness and also lists ADA materials and programs for people with any disability.

4674 **Approaching Equality**
T J Publishers
Ste 108
2544 Tarpley Rd
Carrollton, TX 75006-2288
972-416-0800
800-999-1168
Fax: 301-585-5930
TJPubinc@aol.com
Frank Bowe, Author
Public education laws guarantee special education for all deaf children, but may find the special education system confusing, or are unsure of their rights under current laws. For anyone with an interest in education, advocacy and the deaf community, this book reviews dramatic developments in education of deaf children, youth and adults since COED's 1988 report, Toward Equality.. *$12.95*
112 pages
ISBN 0-93266 -39-6

4675 **Assessment of the Feasibility of Contracting with a Nominee Agency**
Mississippi State University
PO Drawer 6189
Mississippi State, MS 39762
662-325-2001
Fax: 662-325-8989
rrtc@colled.msstate.edu
www.blind.msstate.edu
Michelle Capella McDonnall, Interim Director
Stephanie Hall, Business Manager
Douglas Bedsaul, Research and Training Coordinator
Jacqui Bybee, Research Associate II
Only five State Licensing Agencies currently utilize nominee agreements. This study compared the Pennsylvania BE program with four states that utilize nominee agencies and four states that do not. *$20.00*
152 pages Paperback

4676 **Can America Afford to Grow Old?**
Brookings Institution
1775 Massachusetts Ave NW
Washington, DC 20036-2103
202-797-6000
Fax: 202-797-6004
www.brookings.edu
William Antholis, Managing Director
Steven Bennett, Vice President and Chief Operating Officer
Kimberly Churches, Vice President for Development
Kemal Dervis, Vice President and Director, Global Economy and Development
Social security laws and regulations. *$8.95*
144 pages Paperback
ISBN 0-815700-43-1

4677 **Childcare and the ADA**
Eastern Washington University
Rm 223
705 W 1st Ave
Spokane, WA 99201-3909
509-623-4200
Fax: 509-623-4230
susan.vanmeter@mail.ewu.edu
Nancy Ashworth, Director Child Development
Allen Barrom, Manager
Provides information on how childcare providers must comply with the ADA. Eight videotapes plus an instructional manual with examples of situations and problems.. *$85.00*
Set

4678 **Common ADA Errors and Omissions in New Construction and Alterations**
US Department of Justice
950 Pennsylvania Ave NW
Washington, DC 20530
202-307-0663
800-574-0301
Fax: 202-307-1197
www.ada.gov
Rebecca B. Bond, Chief
Zita Johnson Betts, Deputy Chiefs
James Bostrom, Deputy Chiefs
Sally Conway, Deputy Chiefs
Lists a sampling of common accessibility errors or omissions that have been identified through the Department of Justice's ongoing enforcement efforts.
13 pages

4679 **Commonly Asked Questions About Child Care Centers and the Americans with Disabilities Act**
US Department of Justice
950 Pennsylvania Ave NW
Washington, DC 20530
202-307-0663
800-574-0301
Fax: 202-307-1197
www.ada.gov
Rebecca B. Bond, Chief
Zita Johnson Betts, Deputy Chiefs
James Bostrom, Deputy Chiefs
Sally Conway, Deputy Chiefs
Explains how the requirements of the ADA apply to Child Care Centers. Also describes some of the Department of justice's on-

going enformcement efforts in the child care area and it provides a resource list on sources of information on the ADA.
13 pages

4680 **Commonly Asked Questions About Title III of the ADA**
US Department of Justice
950 Pennsylvania Ave NW
Washington, DC 20530-9
202-307-0663
800-574-0301
Fax: 202-307-1197
TTY: 800-514-0383
www.ada.gov

Rebecca B. Bond, Chief
Zita Johnson Betts, Deputy Chief
Sally Conway, Deputy Chief
James Bostrom, Deputy Chief
A 6-page publication providing information for state and local governments about ADA requirements for ensuring that people with disabilities receive the same services and benefits as provided to others.
on-line

4681 **Commonly Asked Questions About the ADA and Law Enforcement**
US Department of Justice
950 Pennsylvania Ave NW
Washington, DC 20530-9
202-307-0663
800-574-0301
Fax: 202-307-1197
TTY: 800-514-0383
www.ada.gov

Rebecca B. Bond, Chief
Zita Johnson Betts, Deputy Chief
Sally Conway, Deputy Chief
James Bostrom, Deputy Chief
A publication explaining ADA requirements for ensuring that people with disabilities receive the same law enforcement services and protections as provided to others.
13 pages on-line

4682 **Complying with the Americans with Disabilis Act**
Greenwood Publishing Group
130 Cremona Drive
Santa Barbara, CA 93117
805-968-1911
800-368-6868
Fax: 866-270-3856
CustomerService@abc-clio.com
www.greenwood.com

Don Fresh, Author
Peter W Thomas, Co-Author
John Gosden, Library Resource Consultants
Lina Gosden, Library Resource Consultants
A guidebook for management and people with disabilities. This unique guidebook presents a comprehensive analysis of the new Americans with Disabilities Act (ADA), the most significant federal civil rights law in almost 30 years, and its impact on over four million American businesses, state and local governments, non-profit associations, 87 percent of American's private sector jobs, and 22.7 million working-age people with disabilities. *$117.95*
280 pages Hardcover
ISBN 0-899307-14-0

4683 **Court-Related Needs of the Elderly and Persons with Disabilities**
Mental Health Commission
2700 Martin Luther King Jr Ave SE
Washington, DC 20032- 2601
202-282-0027
Fax: 202-373-7982

276 pages

4684 **Criminal Law Handbook on Psychiatric & Psychological Evidence & Testimony**
New York City Bar
42 West 44th Street
New York, NY 10036-6604
212-382-6600
Fax: 212-768-8116
phynes@nycbar.org
www.nycbar.org

Bret Parker, Executive Director
Debra Raskin, President
Alan Rothstein, General Counsel
Maria Cilenti, Director Legislative Affairs
The Criminal Law Handbook provides lawyers, judges and forensic experts with comprehensive, in-depth treatment of admissibility (and limitations on admissibility) of psychiatric and psychological evidence and testimony pertaining to key criminal mental health law standards. *$47.00*

4685 **Department of Justice ADA Mediation Program**
US Department of Justice
950 Pennsylvania Ave NW
Washington, DC 20530
202-307-0663
800-574-0301
Fax: 202-307-1197
TTY: 800-514-0383
www.ada.gov

Rebecca B. Bond, Chief
Zita Johnson Betts, Deputy Chiefs
James Bostrom, Deputy Chiefs
Sally Conway, Deputy Chiefs
Provides an overview of the Department's Mediation Program and examples of successfully mediated cases.
6 pages

4686 **Dimensions of State Mental Health Policy**
Greenwood Publishing Group
130 Cremona Drive
Santa Barbara, CA 93117
805-968-1911
800-368-6868
Fax: 866-270-3856
CustomerService@abc-clio.com
www.greenwood.com

Christopher Hudson, Author
Arthur J Cox, Co-Author
John Gosden, Library Resource Consultants
Lina Gosden, Library Resource Consultants
Introduces students to the emerging field of state mental health policy, its history, current policies, organizational models and required programming knowledge. *$86.95*
320 pages Hardcover
ISBN 0-275932-52-7

4687 **Disability Compliance for Higher Education**
LRP Publications
360 Hiatt Dr
Palm Beach Gardens, FL 33418
561-622-6520
800-341-7874
Fax: 561-622-0757
lrpitvp@lrp.com
www.lrp.com

Kenneth Kahn, CEO
Gives guidance on the most difficult issues faced, such as supporting students with psychological disabilities, ensuring accessibility, understanding OCR rulings, and more. *$57.29*
300 pages

4688 **Disability Discrimination Law, Evidence and Testimony**
ABA Commission on Mental & Physical Disability Law
1050 Connecticut Ave. N.W.
Suite 400
Washington, DC 20036
202-662-1000
800-285-2221
Fax: 202-442-3439
cmpdl@americanbar.org
www.americanbar.org

John W Parry JD, Author
Explains and analyzes key aspects of disability discriminiation law from several different perspectives to guide you through the

myriad federal and state statutes, court cases, and regulations. *$105.00*

694 pages Paperback

ISBN 1-604420-12-8

4689 Disability Law in the United States

William Hein & Company
2350 North Forest Rd.
Getzville, NY 14068-1296
716-882-2600
800-828-7571
Fax: 716-883-8100
mail@wshein.com
www.wshein.com

Dr Bernard D Reams Jr, Author
Peter J McGovern, Co-Author
Jon S Schultz, Co-Author

Offers thousands of pages of information on the laws and legislation affecting the disabled in the United States. Its purpose is to provide a clear and comprehensive mandate to end discrimination against individuals with disabilities and to bring disabled persons into the economic and social midstream of American Life. *$675.00*

5750 pages

ISBN 0-899417-97-3

4690 Disability Under the Fair Employment & Housing Act: What You Should Know About the Law

California Department of Fair Employment & Housing
2218 Kausen Drive
Suite 100
Elk Grove, CA 95758
916-478-7251
800-884-1684
Fax: 916-227-2870
contact.center@dfeh.ca.gov
www.dfeh.ca.gov

Phyllis W Cheng, Director

Intended to highlight and summarize workplace disability laws enforced by the California Department of Fair Employment and Housing. It will familiarize people with the content of these laws, including recent changes and amendments to state statutes and attendent accommodation responsibilities.

4691 Discrimination is Against the Law

California Department of Fair Employment & Housing
2218 Kausen Drive
Suite 100
Elk Grove, CA 95758
916-478-7251
800-884-1684
Fax: 916-227-2870
contact.center@dfeh.ca.gov
www.dfeh.ca.gov

Phyllis Cheng, Director

Enforces California state laws that prohibit harassment and discrimination in employment, housing, and public accomodations and that provide for pregnancy leave and family and personal leave.

4692 Education of the Handicapped: Laws, Legislative Histories and Administrative Document

William S Hein & Co Inc
2350 North Forest Rd.
Getzville, NY 14068-1296
716-882-2600
800-828-7571
Fax: 716-883-8100
mail@wshein.com
www.wshein.com

Bernard D Reams Jr, Editor

Focuses upon Elementary and Secondary Education Act of 1965 and its amendment, Education For All Handicapped Children Act of 1975 and its amendments and acts providing services for the blind, deaf, developmentally disabled, etc. *$2950.00*

55 volumes

ISBN 0-899411-57-6

4693 ElderLawAnswers.com

150 Chestnut Street
4th Floor, Box 15
Providence, RI 02903
617-267-9700
866-267-0947
support@elderlawanswers.com
www.elderlawanswers.com

Harry S Margolis, Founder/President
Mark Miller, Director of Product and Business Development
Ken Coughlin, Managing Editor

Supports seniors, their families and their attorneys in achieving their goals by providing

4694 Employment Discrimination Based on Disability

California Department of Fair Employment & Housing
2218 Kausen Drive
Suite 100
Elk Grove, CA 95758
916-478-7251
800-884-1684
Fax: 916-227-2870
contact.center@dfeh.ca.gov
www.dfeh.ca.gov

Phyllis W Cheng, Director

Prohibits employment discrimination and harassment based on a person's disability or perceived disability. Also requires employers to reasonably accommodate individuals with mental or physical disabilities unless the employer can show that to do so would cause an undue hardship.

4695 Employment Standards Administration Department of Labor (ESA)

200 Constitution Ave NW
Washington, DC 20210-1
800-321-6742
TTY: 877-889-5627
osha.gov

David Michaels, Assistant Secretary
Jordan Barab, Deputy Assistant Secretary
Richard Fairfax, Deputy Assistant Secretary
Deborah Berkowitz, Chief of Staff

Monitors compliance with sub-minimum wage requirements for handicapped workers in sheltered workshops, competitive industry and hospitals and institutions under Section 14 of the Fair Labor Standards Act of 1938.

4696 Enforcing the ADA: A Status Report from the Department of Justice

US Department of Justice
950 Pennsylvania Ave NW
Washington, DC 20530
202-307-0663
800-514-0301
Fax: 203-307-1197
www.ada.gov

Rebecca B. Bond, Chief
Zita Johnson Betts, Deputy Chiefs
James Bostrom, Deputy Chiefs
Sally Conway, Deputy Chiefs

A brief report issued by the Justice Department each quarter providing timely information about ADA cases and settlements, building codes that meet ADA accessibility standards, and ADA technical assistance activities.

4697 Federal Laws of the Mentally Handicapped: Laws, Legislative Histories and Admin. Documents

William Hein & Company
2350 North Forest Rd.
Getzville, NY 14068-1296
716-882-2600
800-828-7571
Fax: 716-883-8100
mail@wshein.com
www.wshein.com

Bernard D Reams Jr, Editor

Chronological compilation of all relevant federal laws dealing with the mentally handicapped along with supporting documentation necessary to create a complete legislative history. *$3500.00*

42 Volume/Set

ISBN 0-899411-06-1

4698 Formed Families: Adoption of Children with Handicaps
Haworth Press
711 Third Avenue
New York, NY 10017
212-216-7800
800-354-1420
Fax: 212-244-1563
subscriptions@tandf.co.uk
www.haworthpress.com

William Cohen, Owner
Provides broad coverage of the issues relating to the adoption of children with handicaps. Concerned professionals can find here all the answers about clinical programs, legal issues, estimates of frequency, and important factors related to positive and negative outcomes of these adoptions. *$74.95*
242 pages Hardcover
ISBN 0-866569-14-6

4699 Free Appropriate Public Education: The Law and Children with Disabilities
Love Publishing Company
9101 E Kenyon Avenue
Suite 2200
Denver, CO 80237
303-221-7333
Fax: 303-221-7444
lpc@lovepublishing.com
www.lovepublishing.com

H Rutherford Turnbull III, Author
Matthew J Stowe, Co-Author
Nancy E Huerta, Co-Author
Includes the 2004 IDEA reauthorization and the proposed regulations. This up-to-the-minute resource brings you the most recent developments in legislation, case law techniques, due process, parent participation and much, much more. *$78.00*
448 pages Hardcover
ISBN 0-891083-25-2

4700 Health Care Quality Improvement Act of 1986
William Hein & Company
2350 North Forest Rd.
Getzville, NY 14068-1296
716-882-2600
800-828-7571
Fax: 716-883-8100
mail@wshein.com
www.wshein.com

Bernard D Reams Jr, Editor
In order to encourage more stringent peer review by doctors and hospitals, and to protect reporting physicians and institutions from retaliatory lawsuits, Congress enacted The Health Care Quality Improvement Act. The Act was also intended to address the increasing incidence of medical malpractice and to prevent the ease with which incompetent practitioners moved from state to state. Hardcover. *$125.00*
721 pages
ISBN 0-899416-93-4

4701 Housing and Transportation of the Handicapped
William Hein & Company
2350 North Forest Rd.
Getzville, NY 14068-1296
716-882-2600
800-828-7571
Fax: 716-883-8100
mail@wshein.com
www.wshein.com

Bernard D Reams Jr, Editor
National laws, recognizing the problems encountered by the handicapped in the areas of Housing and Transportation and providing assistance in an effort to surmount those problems, span more than half a century. *$1552.50*
30000 pages 250 documents
ISBN 0-899412-47-5

4702 Human Resource Management and the Americans with Disabilities Act
Greenwood Publishing Group
130 Cremona Drive
Santa Barbara, CA 93117
805-968-1911
800-368-6868
Fax: 866-270-3856
CustomerService@abc-clio.com
www.greenwood.com

John G Veres, Author
Ronald R Sims, Co-Author
John Gosden, Library Resource Consultants
Lina Gosden, Library Resource Consultants
Concrete advice for human resource professionals on how to cope with the vague, often obscure provisions of the Americans with Disabilities Act. *$107.95*
232 pages Hardcover
ISBN 0-899308-57-9

4703 International Handbook on Mental Health Policy
Greenwood Publishing Group
130 Cremona Drive
Santa Barbara, CA 93117
805-968-1911
800-368-6868
Fax: 866-270-3856
CustomerService@abc-clio.com
www.greenwood.com

John Gosden, Library Resource Consultants
Lina Gosden, Library Resource Consultants
Steve Pearson, Library Resource Consultants
Lou Pingitore, Library Resource Consultants
The first major reference book for academics and practitioners that provides a systematic survey and analysis of mental health policies in twenty representative countries. *$179.95*
512 pages Hardcover
ISBN 0-313275-67-8

4704 Knowing Your Rights
A AR P Fulfillment
601 E St NW
Washington, DC 20049-1
202-434-3525
800-687-2277
Fax: 202-434-3443
TTY: 877-434-7598
member@aarp.org
www.aarp.org

William D. Novelli, CEO
Lynn Smith, Director of Human Resources
Describes how changes in Medicare's reimbursement policies are designed to reduce health care costs and suggests steps that Medicare beneficiaries, their families and friends can take to assure that they continue to receive quality care under the Prospective Payment System.
19 pages

4705 Law Center Newsletter
Public Interest Law Center of Philadelphia
1709 Benjamin Franklin Parkway
United Way Building
Philadelphia, PA 19103
215-627-7100
Fax: 215-627-3183
www.pilcop.org

Eric J Rothschild, Chair
Brian T Feeney, Vice Chair
Jennifer R. Clarke, Executive Director
Ellen S Friedell, Treasurer
Information on mental health, foster care and public education. Provides all updates concerning the law in these areas.

4706 Legal Center for People with Disabilities& Older People
455 Sherman St
Suite 130
Denver, CO 80203
303-722-0300
800-288-1376
Fax: 303-722-0720
TTY: 303-722-3619

Mary Anne Harvey, Executive Director
John R. Posthumus, President
Stephen P. Rickles, Vice President
John Paul Anderson, Treasurer

Uses the legal system to protect and promote the rights of people with disabilities and older people in Colorado through direct legal representation, advocacy, education and legislative analysis. The Legal Center is Colorado's Protection and Advocacy System. We are also the State Ombudsman for nursing homes and assisted living facilities. Call for a free publications and products list.

4707 **Legal Right: The Guide for Deaf and Hard of Hearing People**

National Association of the Deaf
8630 Fenton Street
Suite 820
Silver Spring, MD 20910- 3819
301-587-1789
Fax: 301-587-1791
TTY: 301-587-1789
www.nad.org

Christopher Wagner, Board Chair
Howard A. Rosenblum, Chief Executive Officer
Marc P. Charmatz, Staff Attorney
Lizzie Sorkin, Director of Communications

This revised fifth edition is in easy-to-understand language, offering the latest state and federal statues and administrative procedures that prohibit discrimination against the deaf, hard of hearing and other physically challenged people. *$32.50*
264 pages Paperback
ISBN 1-563680-00-9

4708 **Legal Rights of Persons with Disabilities**

LRP Publications
360 Hiatt Dr
Palm Beach Gardens, FL 33418-7106
561-622-6520
800-341-7874
Fax: 561-622-0757
lrpitvp@lrp.com
www.lrp.com

Kenneth Kahn, CEO

Shows what is required, permitted and guaranteed by federal disability laws-including the ADA, Section 504 of the Rehabilitation Act and the IDEA. Explores the boundaries of accceptable behavior under disability laws and provides guidelines to help clients fulfill their legal obligations. *$365.00*
2722 pages

4709 **Legislative Handbook for Parents**

NAPVI
250 W 64th St
New York, NY 10023
800-284-4422
napvi@lighthouseguild.org
www.napvi.org

Alan R. Morse, President/CEO
Mark G. Ackermann, Executive Vice President
James M. Dubin, Chairman
Joseph A. Ripp, Vice Chairman

A publication for parents who make direct contact with public officials on behalf of their children. Sample letters, do's-and-dont's, and a glossary of legislative terms are some of the topics that are contained in this manual. *$5.50*
24 pages Paperback

4710 **Legislative Network for Nurses**

Business Publishers
2222 Sedwick Drive
Durham, NC 27713
800-223-8720
Fax: 800-508-2592
www.bpinews.com

8 pages Newsl./BiMonthly

4711 **Loving Justice**

Exceptional Parent Library
P.O. Box 1807
Englewood Cliffs, NJ 7632-1207
201-947-6000
800-535-1910
Fax: 201-947-9376
eplibrary@aol.com
www.eplibrary.com

4712 **Making News: How to Get News Coverage of Disability Rights Issues**

Advocado Press
PO Box 406781
Louisville, KY 40204
888-739-1920
Fax: 502-899-9562
www.advocadopress.org

Tari Susan Hartman, Author
Mary Johnson, Co-Author

This book gives examples and tips on how to fight back and get on the front pages, lead the newscasts and influence public debate. *$10.95*
165 pages Paperback
ISBN 0-962706-43-4

4713 **Medicare and Medicaid Patient and Program Protection Act of 1987**

William Hein & Company
2350 North Forest Rd.
Getzville, NY 14068-1296
716-882-2600
800-828-7571
Fax: 716-883-8100
mail@wshein.com
www.wshein.com

Bernard D Reams Jr, Editor

Enables the HHS to protect patients and federal health care programs from censured practitioners. The Act broadens the authority of HHS to exclude practitioners from Medicare and Medicaid programs; strengthens the monetary penalities HHS may impose on violators; provides for criminal penalties in certain cases; and requires states to inform HHS regarding sanctions against health care providers. *$195.00*
3 Volumes
ISBN 0-899416-95-0

4714 **Mental & Physical Disability Law Reporter**

American Bar Association
1050 Connecticut Ave. N.W.
Suite 400
Washington, DC 20036-1019
202-662-1570
800-285-2221
Fax: 202-442-3439
cmpdl@abanet.org
www.abanet.org

Robert M Carlson, Chair
James R Silkenat, President
Jack L Rives, Executive Director
G. Nicholas Casey, Treasurer

Contains over 2,000 summanes per year of federal and state court decisions and legislation that affect persons with mental and physical disabilities. Includes bylined articles by experts in the field regarding disability law developments and trends. *$384.00*
350+ pages BiMonthly

4715 **Mental Disabilities and the Americans with Disabilities Act**

Greenwood Publishing Group
130 Cremona Drive
Santa Barbara, CA 93117
805-968-1911
800-368-6868
Fax: 866-270-3856
CustomerService@abc-clio.com
www.greenwood.com

John Gosden, Library Resource Consultants
Lina Gosden, Library Resource Consultants
Steve Pearson, Library Resource Consultants
Lou Pingitore, Library Resource Consultants

A clear, practical compliance guide, written by a psychologist, to help organizations conform to provisions on mental disabilities in the Americans with Disabilities Act. Hardcover. *$91.95*
216 pages Hardcover
ISBN 0-899308-26-5

4716 **Mental Disability Law, Evidence and Testimony**
ABA Commission on Mental & Physical Disability Law
1050 Connecticut Ave. N.W.
Suite 400
Washington, DC 20036-1019
202-662-1000
800-285-2221
www.abanet.org

Robert M Carlson, Chair
James R Silkenat, President
Jack L Rives, Executive Director
G. Nicholas Casey, Treasurer

Provides a comprehensive analysis of federal and state statues and case law with a disability discrimination focus. *$95.00*
491 pages Paperback
ISBN 1-590318-32-3

4717 **Mental Health Law Reporter**
Business Publishers
2222 Sedwick Drive
Durham, NC 27713
240-514-0600
800-223-8720
Fax: 800-508-2592

Leonard A Eiserer, Publisher
Jeremy Bond, Editor MHLR
Bob Grupe, Editor MHLR
Adam Goldstein, President

MHLR brings you the most timely, focused and thorough information on the legal issues that concern mental health practitioners in mental health litigation. Topics include: malpractice litigation, patient-therapist confidentiality, sexual victimization of patients, the insanity defense, social security administrative case law and much more.. *$286.00*
8 pages Monthly

4718 **Mental and Physical Disability Law Reporter**
American Bar Association
1050 Connecticut Ave. N.W.
Suite 400
Washington, DC 20036-1019
202-662-1000
800-285-2221
service@americanbar.org
www.americanbar.org

Wm T Robinson III, President

The only periodical that comprehensively covers civil and criminal mental disability law and disability discrimination law. *$324.00*
150+ pages Bimonthly

4719 **Mentally Disabled and the Law**
William S Hein & Company
2350 North Forest Rd.
Getzville, NY 14068-1296
716-882-2600
800-828-7571
Fax: 716-883-8100
mail@wshein.com
www.wshein.com

Samuel Brakel, Author
John Parry, Co-Author
Barbara A Weiner, Co-Author

Chapters retained from 1961 and 1971 editions have been substantially rewritten. Two subjects-sterilization and sexual psychopathy-have been integrated into chapters on family law. Three new chapters on treatment rights, provider-patient relationship and rights of mentally disabled persons in the community. Sixteen new tables supplement the existing revised 41. *$92.00*
845 pages
ISBN 0-910059-05-5

4720 **Myths and Facts**
US Department of Justice
950 Pennsylvania Ave NW
Washington, DC 20530-9
202-307-0663
800-514-0301
Fax: 202-307-1197
TTY: 800-514-0383
www.ada.gov

Rebecca B. Bond, Chief
Zita Johnson Betts, Deputy Chief
Sally Conway, Deputy Chief
James Bostrom, Deputy Chief

A 3-page publication dispelling some common misconceptions about the ADA's requirements and implementation.

4721 **NAD Broadcaster**
National Association of the Deaf
8630 Fenton Street
Suite 820
Silver Spring, MD 20910- 3819
301-587-1789
Fax: 301-587-1791
TTY: 301-587-1789
nad.info@nad.org
www.nad.org

Christopher Wagner, Board Chair
Howard A. Rosenblum, Chief Executive Officer
Marc P. Charmatz, Staff Attorney
Lizzie Sorkin, Director of Communications

National newspaper published 11 times a year by the nation's largest organization safeguarding the accessbility and civil rights of 28 million deaf and hard of hearing Americans in education, employment, health care, and telecommunications. Membership: individual $30 per year. *$7.00*

4722 **No Longer Disabled: the Federal Courts & the Politics of Social Security Disability**
Greenwood Publishing Group
130 Cremona Drive
Santa Barbara, CA 93117
805-968-1911
800-368-6868
Fax: 866-270-3856
CustomerService@abc-clio.com
www.greenwood.com

John Gosden, Library Resource Consultants
Lina Gosden, Library Resource Consultants
Steve Pearson, Library Resource Consultants
Lou Pingitore, Library Resource Consultants

This book is a case study of judicial policy making. It focuses on the role of adjudication in the making and refining of federal policy. *$107.95*
208 pages Hardcover
ISBN 0-313254-24-9

4723 **Nolo's Guide to Social Security Disability Getting and Keeping Your Benefits**
NOLO
950 Parker St
Berkeley, CA 94710-2524
800-955-4775
Fax: 800-645-0895
www.nolo.com

David Morton, Author

This guide demystifies the program and tells you everything you need to know about qualifying and applying for benefits, maintaining your benefits, and appealing the denial of a claim. *$25.49*
512 pages paperback
ISBN 1-413311-04-4

4724 **Opening the Courthouse Door: An ADA Access Guide for State Courts**
American Bar Association
1050 Connecticut Ave. N.W.
Suite 400
Washington, DC 20036-1019
202-662-1000
800-285-2221
service@americanbar.org
www.americanbar.org

Wm T Robinson III, President

Practical step-by-step guide walks the reader through the courthouse and court process, presenting a menu of straightforawrd access ideas to enhance communications in court, make the facility more accessbile, and nodify rules and procedures. *$12.00*
78 pages

4725 **PPAL In Print**
Parent Professional Advocacy League
77 Rumford Ave.
Waltham, MA 02453
866-815-8122
Fax: 617-542-7832
info@ppal.net
www.ppal.net
Lisa Lambert, Executive Director
Meri Viano, Associate Director
Joel Khattar, Program Manager
The Parent Professional Advocacy League (PPAL) is a statewide organization focusing on the interests of families with children with mental health needs. PPAL advocates for improved and better access to mental health services for children and their families.

4726 **Power of Attorney for Health Care**
Center for Public Representation
P.O. Box 260049
Madison, WI 53726-49
608-251-4008
800-369-0388
Fax: 606-251-1263
132 pages
ISBN 0-93262 -38-0

4727 **Special EDitions**
Disability Rights Education and Defense Fund
3075 Adeline Street
Suite 210
Berkeley, CA 94703
510-644-2555
Fax: 510-841-8645
info@dredf.org
dredf.org
Susan Henderson, Executive Director
Special news releases by the Disability Rights Education and Defense Fund, available electronically online.
Quarterly

4728 **Summaries of Legal Precedents & Law Review**
Through the Looking Glass
3075 Adeline St
Suite 120
Berkeley, CA 94703
510-848-1112
800-644-2666
Fax: 510-848-4445
TLG@lookingglass.org
www.lookingglass.org
Megan Kirshbaum, Executive Director
Summarizes legal precedents and law review articles relevant to marital custody and child protection situations of parents with diverse disabilities. *$25.00*
24 pages

4729 **TASH Connections**
TASH
1101 15th St. NW
Suite 206
Washington, DC 20005
202-817-3264
Fax: 202-999-4722
info@tash.org
www.tash.org
Julia M. White, Editor
Connections is the online magazine written exclusively for, and by, TASH members, containing articles on new developments in the disability field, while challenging readers to consider issues affecting people with disabilities, their families and advocates.
Quarterly

4730 **Title II & III Regulation Amendment Regarding Detectable Warnings**
U S Department of Justice
950 Pennsylvania Ave NW
Washington, DC 20530-9
202-307-0663
800-514-0301
Fax: 202-307-1197
TTY: 800-514-0383
www.ada.gov
Rebecca B. Bond, Chief
Zita Johnson Betts, Deputy Chief
Sally Conway, Deputy Chief
James Bostrom, Deputy Chief
This document suspends the requirements for detectable warnings at curb ramps, hazardous vehicular areas, and reflecting pools.

4731 **Title II Complaint Form**
US Department of Justice
950 Pennsylvania Ave NW
Washington, DC 20530
202-307-0663
800-514-0301
Fax: 202-307-1197
www.ada.gov
Rebecca B. Bond, Chief
Zita Johnson Betts, Deputy Chiefs
James Bostrom, Deputy Chiefs
Sally Conway, Deputy Chiefs
Standard form for filing a complaint under title II of the ADA or section 504 of the Rehabilitation Act of 1973, which prohibit discrimination on the basis of disability by State and local governments and by recipients of federal financial assistance.

4732 **Title II Highlights**
US Department of Justice
950 Pennsylvania Ave NW
Washington, DC 20530
202-307-0663
800-514-0383
Fax: 202-307-1197
www.ada.gov
Rebecca B. Bond, Chief
Zita Johnson Betts, Deputy Chiefs
James Bostrom, Deputy Chiefs
Sally Conway, Deputy Chiefs
Outline of the key requirements of the ADA for State and local governments. Provides detailed information in bullet format for quick reference.
8 pages

4733 **Title III Technical Assistance Manual and Supplement**
U S Department of Justice
950 Pennsylvania Ave NW
Washington, DC 20530
202-307-0663
800-574-0301
Fax: 202-307-1197
www.ada.gov
Rebecca B. Bond, Chief
Zita Johnson Betts, Deputy Chiefs
James Bostrom, Deputy Chiefs
Sally Conway, Deputy Chiefs
Explains in lay terms what businesses and non-profit agencies must do to ensure access to their goods, services, and facilities.
83 pages

4734 **Toward Independence**
National Council on Disability
81 E. Main Street
Xenia, OH 45385
937-376-3996
Fax: 937-376-2046
info@ti-inc.org
Mary Rose Zink, Chair
Paul Osterfeld, Vice Chair
Mark Schlater, Executive Director
Bob Groskopf, Treasurer
A 1986 report to the U.S. Congress on the federal laws and programs serving people with disabilities, and recommendations for legislation.

4735 **UCP Washington Wire**
United Cerebral Palsy
1825 K Street NW
Suite 600
Washington, DC 20006-1601
202-776-0406
800-872-5827
Fax: 202-776-0414
info@ucp.org
www.ucp.org

Stephen Bennett, President/CEO

Publication that provides a comprehensive source of information on federal legislation, agency regulations, court decisions and other issues of interest to the disability community.

weekly

4736 **US Department of Health and Human Services Office for Civil Rights**
200 Independence Ave SW
Room 509F, HHH Building
Washington, DC 20201
202-619-0403
800-368-1019
TTY: 800-537-7697
ocrmail@hhs.gov
www.hhs.gov

Georgina Verdugo, Director

The Department's civil rights and health privacy law enforcement agency, OCR investigates complaints, enforces rights, and promulgates regulations, develops policy and provides technical assistance and public education to ensure understanding of and compliance with non-discrimination and health information privacy laws.

4737 **US Department of Labor**
200 Constitution Ave NW
Washington, DC 20210
866-487-2365
www.dol.gov

Hilda L Solis, Secretary of Labor
Seth D Harris, Deputy Secretary

To foster, promote, and develop the welfare of the wage earners, job seekers, and retirees of the United States; improve working conditions, advance opportunities for profitable employment; and assure work-related benefits and rights.

4738 **US Department of Labor Office of Federal Contract Compliance Programs**
200 Constitution Ave NW
Washington, DC 20210
312-596-7010
866-487-2365
Fax: 312-596-7044
OFCCP-MW-PreAward@dol.gov
www.dol.gov

Melissa L Speer, Interim Regional Director

To enforce, for the benefit of job seekers and wage earners, the contractual promise of affirmative action and equal employment opportunity required of those who do business with the Federal government.

4739 **University Legal Services AT Program**
Ste 130
220 i St NE
Washington, DC 20002-4364
202-547-4747
877-221-4638
Fax: 202-547-2083
TTY: 202-547-2657
atpdc@uls-dc.org

Jane Brown, Executive Director

Designed to empower individuals with disabilities; to promote consumer involvement and advocacy, and provide information, referral and training as they relate to accessing assistive technology services and devices; and to identify and improve access to funding resources..

4740 **William S Hein & Company**
2350 North Forest Rd.
Getzville, NY 14068-1296
716-882-2600
800-828-7571
Fax: 716-883-8100
mail@wshein.com
www.wshein.com

Kevin Marmion, President

Offers a catalog of periodicals, publications and reprints, microforms and government publications on medical, handicapped and health law.

Libraries & Research Centers

Alabama

4741 **Alabama Institute for Deaf and Blind Library and Resource Center**
205 E South Street
P.O. Box 698
Talladega, AL 35160
256-761-3206
Fax: 256-761-3352
aidb.org
Dr. John Mascia, President
Teresa Lacy, Director, Library & Resource Center
Book collection includes discs, cassettes, Braille and large print. Also closed-circuit TV and magnifiers. Offers Braille production and binding.

4742 **Alabama Radio Reading Service Network (ARRS)**
Public Radio WBHM 90.3 FM
650 11th St S
Birmingham, AL 35233-1
205-934-2606
800-444-9246
Fax: 205-934-5075
wbhm.org
Audrey Atkins, Marketing Manager
Scott E Hanley, General Manager
Theresa Kidd, Office Manager
Michael Krall, Program Director
Services and readings are broadcast over a subcarrier service of public radio WBHM. This is a statewide service devoted to Alabama's blind and handicapped community.

4743 **Alabama Regional Library for the Blind and Physically Handicapped**
Alabama Public Library Service
6030 Monticello Dr
Montgomery, AL 36130-1
334-213-3906
800-392-5671
Fax: 334-213-3993
revans@apls.state.al.us
Mike Coleman, Blind & Physically Handicapped Division
Tim Emmons, Blind & Physically Handicapped Division
Nancy Pack, Director
Kelyn Ralya, Assistant Director
Recreational reading in special format for persons unable to use standard print. Reference materials offered include materials on blindness and other handicaps, films, local subjects and authors.

4744 **Dothan Houston County Library System**
Formerly Houston-Love Memorial Library
445 N Oates St
Dothan, AL 36303
334-793-9767
dhcls@dhcls.org
www.dhcls.org
Jason DeLuc, Library Director
Charlotte Mitchell, Main Library Manager
Offers magnifiers, summer reading programs and more for the blind and physically handicapped. Scanner, software, jaws for Windows.

4745 **Huntsville Subregional Library for the Blind & Physically Handicapped**
Huntsville-Madison County Public Library
915 Monroe St SW
Huntsville, AL 35804-0000
256-532-5980
Fax: 256-532-5994
bphdept@hmcpl.org
www.hmcpl.org
Laurel Best, Executive Director
Talking books for people who are blind or disabled offering reference materials on the blind and other disabilities, large-print photocopier, thermaform duplicator and more.

4746 **Public Library Of Anniston-Calhoun County**
108 E 10th St
Anniston, AL 36201
256-237-8501
library@publiclibrary.cc
publiclibrary.cc

4747 **Technology Assistance for Special Consumers**
UCP Huntsville
1856 Keats Drive
Huntsville, AL 35810
256-859-8300
Fax: 256-859-4332
ucphuntsville.org
Cheryl Smith, Chief Executive Officer
Provide individuals with disabilities, their families and/or advocates, and associated professionals access to assistive technology devices and services to increase independence at home, school, and work.

Alaska

4748 **Alaska State Library Talking Book Center**
State of Alaska
344 W 3rd Ave
Ste 125
Anchorage, AK 99501-2338
907-465-1304
888-820-4525
Fax: 907-269-6580
tbc@alaska.gov
talkingbooks.alaska.gov
Patience Frederiksen, Director, Division of Libraries, Archives & Museums
Freya Anderson, Requisitions Librarian
Ginny Jacobs, Library Assistant
The Alaska State Library Talking Book Center is a cooperative effort between the Library of Congress National Library Service for the Blind and Physically Handicapped and the Alaska State Library to provide print handicapped Alaskans with talking book and Braille service. The Talking Book Center has 55,000 audiobooks that can be checked out to eligible Alaskans whose visual or physical handicap prevents them from reading standard print materials.

Arizona

4749 **Arizona Braille and Talking Book Library**
Arizona State Library
1030 N 32nd St
Phoenix, AZ 85008-5108
602-255-5578
800-255-5578
Fax: 602-286-0444
www.azlibrary.gov
Linda Montgomery, Director
Audio and Braille books and magazines, summer reading program, volunteer-produced audio books, audo described, films and more.

4750 **Books for the Blind of Arizona**
Unit A107
6120 E 5th St
Tucson, AZ 85711-2536
602-792-9153
Fax: 520-886-9839
Betty Evans, Chairperson
Offers large print photocopier, textbooks, recreational, career, vocational, Braille books, talking books, cassettes, large print books and more for the visually impaired K-12, college students and adults..

4751 **Children's Center for Neurodevelopmental Studies**
5430 W Glenn Dr
Glendale, AZ 85301-2628
623-915-0345
Fax: 623-937-5425
admin@ccnsaz.org
www.thechildrenscenteraz.org
Kent Rideout, Executive Director
Dawna Sterner, Preschool & Education Informatio
Catherine Orsak, Therapy Information
Alicia Bolan, Teaching Staff
The Center is a non-profit school and therapy center for children with autism and other developmental delays specializing in the use of sensory integration.

4752 **Flagstaff City-Coconino County Public Library**
300 W Aspen Ave
Flagstaff, AZ 86001-5304 928-779-7670
TTY: 928-214-2417
www.flagstaffpubliclibrary.org

4753 **Fountain Hills Lioness Braille Service**
P.O. Box 18332
Fountain Hills, AZ 85269-8332 480-837-3961
Jean Hauck, Chairperson
Braille and large print books on the subjects of recreation, career and vocations, religion, novels and cookbooks for the visually impaired..

4754 **Prescott Public Library**
215 E Goodwin St
Prescott, AZ 86303-3911 928-777-1500
Fax: 928-771-5829
prescottlibrary.info
Roger Saft, Director
Martha Baden, Public Services Manager
Teresa Vonk, Support Services Manager
Lisa Zierke, Technical Services
Large print, Braille and audio books; magnifiers; text to voice scanner; talking book machine application; toy library for children with special needs; special needs product catalogs; home book delivery; descriptive videos; 43 point PC monitor..

4755 **Special Needs Center/Phoenix Public Library**
1221 N Central Ave
Phoenix, AZ 85004-1867 602-262-4636
TTY: 602-254-8205
www.phoenixpubliclibrary.org

4756 **World Research Foundation**
P.O. Box 20828
Sedona, AZ 86341-8804 928-284-3300
Fax: 928-284-3530
info@wrf.org
wrf.org
Steven A Ross, President
LaVerne Boeckmann, Co-Founder
Large research library of alternative medicine; offers a computer search and printout of specific health issues for a nominal fee.

Arkansas

4757 **Arkansas Regional Library for the Blind and Physically Handicapped**
900 West Capitol Avenue
Suite 100
Little Rock, AR 72201-3108 501-682-2053
www.library.arkansas.gov
J D Hall, Manager of BPH Services
Dwain Gordon, Deputy Director
Danny Koonce, Public Information Specialist
Ruth Hyatt, Manager of Extension Services
Public library books in recorded or Braille format. Popular fiction and nonfiction books for all ages, books and players are on free loan, sent to patrons by mail and may be returned postage free. Anyone who cannot see well enough to read regular print with glasses on or who has a disability that makes it difficult to hold a book or turn the pages is eligible.

4758 **Arkansas School for the Blind**
P.O. Box 668
Little Rock, AR 72203-668 501-296-1810
800-362-4451
Fax: 501-296-1831
www.arkansasschoolfortheblind.org
Khayyam Eddings, Chairperson
Jennifer Benedetti, Elementary Principal
Teresa Doan, Special Education Supervisor
William Harrison, Technology Director
Students at the ASB receive a quality education from specially trained instructors of the Visually Impaired in all academic areas. ASB features a comprehensive Music and Art program, as well as extensive extra-curricular activities. ASB is a proud member of the Arkansas Activities Association and The North Central Association of Schools for the Blind.

4759 **Educational Services for the Visually Impaired**
2402 Wildwood Avenue
Suite 112
Sherwood, AR 72120-5085 501-835-5448
Fax: 501-835-6840
Angyln.Young@arkansas.gov
www.esvi.org
Angyln Young, State Coordinator
Cindy Lester, Data Management Specialist
Cynthia Kelly, ESVI Office Manager
Offers textbooks, Braille books and more to the visually impaired grades K-12 in the Arizona area.

4760 **Library for the Blind and Physically Handicapped SW Region of Arkansas**
P.O. Box 668
2057 North Jackson St
Magnolia, AR 71754-668 870-234-1991
Fax: 870-234-5077
library@cocolib.org
Rhonda Rolen, Director
Dana Thornton, Assistant Director
Becky Verschage, Processing Clerk
Lisa Lewis, Bookkeeping
A free library service that serves adults and children who meet the eligiblity requirements, offers free loan of cassette machine and recorded books, which meet the reading preferences of a highly diverse clientele.

4761 **Northwest Ozarks Regional Library for the Blind and Handicapped**
Fayetteville, AR 72701 479-575-2000
www.uark.edu

California

4762 **Braille Institute Library**
741 N Vermont Ave
Los Angeles, CA 90029-3594 323-663-1111
800-808-2555
Fax: 323-663-0867
la@Brailleinstitute.org
Brailleinstitute.org
Leslie E. Stocker, President
Sally H. Jameson, Vice President of Programs and S
Peter A. Mindnich, Executive Vice President
Reza Rahman, Vice President of Finance/Chief
Braille Institute provides an environment of hope and encouragement for people who are blind and visually impaired through integrated educational, social and recreational programs and services.

4763 **Braille Institute Santa Barbara Center**
2031 De La Vina St
Santa Barbara, CA 93105-3895 805-682-6222
800-272-4553
Fax: 805-687-6141
sb@Brailleinstitute.org
Brailleinstitute.org
Leslie E. Stocker, President
Sally H. Jameson, Vice President of Programs and S
Peter A. Mindnich, Executive Vice President
Reza Rahman, Vice President of Finance/Chief
Offers programs, services and information for persons with visual impairments.

4764 **Braille Institute Sight Center**
741 N Vermont Ave
Los Angeles, CA 90029-3594
323-663-1111
800-808-2555
Fax: 323-663-0867
la@Brailleinstitute.org
Brailleinstitute.org
Sally H. Jameson, Vice President of Programs and S
Leslie E Stocker, President
Peter A. Mindnich, Executive Vice President
Reza Rahman, Vice President of Finance/Chief
Offers help, programs, services and information to the blind and visually impaired children and adults.

4765 **Braille and Talking Book Library: California**
P.O. Box 942837
Sacramento, CA 94237-0001
916-654-0640
800-952-5666
www.library.ca.gov/services/btbl.html
Stacey A. Aldrich, State Librarian
Debbie Newton, Bureau Chief, Administrative Ser
Phyllis Smith, Manager, Human Resources and Bus
Sharleen Finn, Budget Officer, Fiscal Services
Free service for eligible Northern California residents.

4766 **California State Library Braille and Talking Book Library**
PO Box 942837
Sacramento, CA 94237-0001
916-654-0640
800-952-5666
btbl@library.ca.gov
www.btbl.ca.gov

4767 **Clearinghouse for Specialized Media and Translations**
1430 N St
Ste 3207
Sacramento, CA 95814-5901
916-319-0800
Fax: 916-323-9732
www.cde.ca.gov/re/pn/sm
Jonn Paris-Salb, Manager
Provides materials in accessible formats; aural media, Braille, large print, digital talking books and electronic media access technology.

4768 **Dental Amalgam Syndrome (DAMS) Newsletter**
725-9 Tramway Ln NE
Albuquerque, NM 87122-1672
505-291-8239
Fax: 505-294-3339

4769 **Fresno County Free Library Blind and Handicapped Services**
2420 Mariposa Street
Fresno, CA 93721-3640
559-600-7323
800-742-1011
wendy.eisenberg@fresnolibrary.org
www.fresnolibrary.org/tblb
Wendy Eisenberg, Manager
Laurel Prysiazny, County Librarian
Magnifiers, home visits, volunteer-produced cassette books, discs and cassettes.

4770 **Glaucoma Research Foundation**
251 Post St
Ste 600
San Francisco, CA 94108-5017
415-986-3162
800-826-6693
Fax: 415-986-3763
question@glaucoma.org
glaucoma.org
Tom Brunner, President and CEO
Nancy Graydon, Executive Director of Development
Andrew L. Jackson, Director of Communications
Catalina San Agustin, Director of Operations
Clinical and laboratory studies of glaucoma. We work to prevent vision loss from glaucoma by investing in innovative research, education and support with the ultimate goal of finding a cure..

4771 **Herrick Health Sciences Library**
Alta Bates Medical Center
2001 Dwight Way
Berkeley, CA 94704-2608
510-869-6777
Fax: 510-204-4091
www.altabatessummit.org
Laurie Bagley, Librarian
Carol Hirsch-Butler, Administrator
Carolyn Kemp, Regional Manager of Public Relations
Information on rehabilitation, psychiatry and psychoanalysis.

4772 **Kuzell Institute for Arthritis and Infectious Diseases**
Medical Research Institute Of San Francisco
2200 Webster St.
San Francisco, CA 94115-1821
415-561-1734
Edward Byrd, Owner
One of seven units comprising the Medical Research Institute of San Francisco that offers basic and applied research in arthritis and related diseases.

4773 **New Beginnings: The Blind Children's Center**
4120 Marathon St
Los Angeles, CA 90029-3584
323-664-2153
info@blindchildrenscenter.org
blindchildrenscenter.org/document-library
Sarah E. Orth, CEO
Fernanda Armenta-Schmitt, Director, Education & Family Services
The purpose of the Center is to turn initial fears into hope. Helps children and their families become independent by creating a climate of safety and trust. Children learn to develop self confidence and to master a wide range of skills. Services include an infant stimulation program, educational preschool, interdisciplinary assessment services, family services, correspondence program, toll free national hotline and a publication and research service.

4774 **Research & Training Center on Mental Health for Hard of Hearing Persons**
California School of Professional Psychology
Ste 140
6215 Ferris Sq
San Diego, CA 92121-3279
619-282-4443
800-HEA-R619
Fax: 800-642-0266
Raymond J Trybus, Director
Thomas J Goulder, Associate Director
Funded by the National Institute on Disability and Rehabilitation Research, this training center aims to address issues of psychological relevance to persons who are hard of hearing or late deafened (as distinct from prelingually, culturally deaf persons). Also serves as information clearinghouse on this topic.

4775 **Rosalind Russell Medical Research Center for Arthritis**
Suite 600
350 Parnassus Ave
San Francisco, CA 94117
415-476-1141
Fax: 415-476-3526
rrac@medicine.ucsf.edu
Ephraim P Engleman, MD, Center Director
David Wofsy, MD, Associate Director
Paula R. Gambs, Chair
Christine Abele, Volunteer
Arthritis research and its probable causes.

4776 **San Francisco Public Library for the Blindand Print Handicapped**
100 Larkin St
San Francisco, CA 94102-4705
415-557-4400
Fax: 415-557-4252
TTY: 415-557-4433
webmail@sfpl.org
www.sfpl.org
Toni Cordova, Chief of Communications, Program
Toni Bernardi, Special Projects Manager
Laura Lent, Chief of Collections & Technical
Edward Melton, Chief of Branches
Foreign-language books on cassette, children's books on cassettes and more.

4777 **San Jose State University Library**
150 E San Fernando St
San Jose, CA 95112-3580
408-808-2000
Fax: 408-924-1118
www.sjlibrary.org

Don W Kassing, President
Jane Light, Library/Executive Director
Jeff Barber, Security Officer
Luann Budd, Administrative Officer
Information on physical disabilities, accessibility and learning disabilities.

Colorado

4778 **AMC Cancer Research Center**
3401 Quebec Street
Suite 3200
Denver, CO 80207
303-233-6501
800-321-1557
Fax: 303-239-3400
amc.org

Gary Kortz, Chairman
Steven D. Toltz, Treasurer
Cheryl Kisling, Secretary
Karen Padgett, President and CEO
Provides trained counselors who provide understanding and support for cancer patients; information and referral services; and screening programs.

4779 **Boulder Public Library**
1001 Arapahoe Ave
Boulder, CO 80302-6015
303-441-3100
www.boulderlibrary.org

Melinda Mattling, Manager
Priscilla Hudson, Manager
Offers Braille books, cassettes, talking books, large print photocopier, large print books and more for the visually impaired.

4780 **Colorado Talking Book Library**
180 Sheridan Blvd
Denver, CO 80226-8101
303-727-9277
800-685-2136
Fax: 303-727-9281
ctbl.info@cde.state.co.us

Debbie Macleod, Executive Director
Provides free library service to Coloradans of all ages who are unable to read standard print due to visual, physical or learning disabilities whether permanent or temporary. Provides audio, Braille and large-print books and magazines.

4781 **National Jewish Medical & Research Center**
1400 Jackson St
Denver, CO 80206-2762
303-388-4461
877-225-5654
www.nationaljewish.org

Michael Salem, MD, President and CEO
Richard A. Schierburg, Chair
Robin Chotin, Vice Chair
Robin Chotin, Secretary
The only medical center in the country whose research and patient care resources are dedicated to respiratory and immunologic diseases.

Connecticut

4782 **Connecticut Braille Association**
107 Vanderbilt Ave
West Hartford, CT 6110-1514
860-953-4445
Fax: 860-378-0205

Nick Martino, Owner
Offers textbooks, cassettes, large print books, Braille books and more.

4783 **Connecticut Library for the Blind and Physically Handicapped**
231 Capitol Avenue
Hartford, CT 06106-1569
860-757-6500
860-866-4478
Fax: 860-721-2056
ctaylor@cslib.org

Kendall Wiggin, State Librarian
Ursula Hunt, Administrative Assistant
Shelley Delisle, IT Manager
Jane Beaudoin, Administrative Assistant
Network library of the National Library Service for the Blind and Physically Handicapped, Library of Congress. Lends books and magazines in Braille or recorded formats along with the necessary playback equipment, free, for any Connecticut adult or child who is unable to read regular print due to a visual or physical disability. All materials are mailed to and from library patrons by postage-free mail

4784 **Connecticut State Library**
Connecticut State Government
231 Capitol Ave
Hartford, CT 06106-1569
860-757-6500
866-866-4478
Fax: 860-721-2056
isref@cslib.org

Kendall Wiggin, State Librarian
Ursula Hunt, Administrative Assistant
Shelley Delisle, IT Manager
Jane Beaudoin, Administrative Assistant
Discs, cassettes, Braille, reference materials on blindness and other handicaps, closed-circuit TV and large-print photocopier.

4785 **Connecticut Tech Act Project: Connecticut Department of Social Services**
Bureau of Rehabilitations Services
25 Sigourney St
11th Floor
Hartford, CT 06106-5041
860-424-4881
800-537-2549
Fax: 860-424-4850
TTY: 860-424-4839
arlene.lugo@ct.gov
www.cttechact.com

Arlene Lugo, Program Director
Single point of entry, advocacy, information and referral, peer counseling, and access to objective expert advice and consultation for people with disabilities.

4786 **Prevent Blindness Connecticut**
101 Whitney Avenue
New Haven, CT 06510
203-722-4653
800-850-2020
Fax: 203-722-4691

Kathryn Garre-Ayars, President and CEO
Tahesha Bryan, Administrative Assistant
Naomi Hayner, Connecticut Program Manager
Maria Giarratana, Grants Manager
The mission of Prevent Blindness Connecticut is to save sight and prevent blindness through eye screenings, education, safety activities and research.

4787 **Yale University: Vision Research Center**
310 Cedar St, LH 108
PO Box 208023
New Haven, CT 06520- 8023
203-785-2759
800-395-7949
Fax: 203-785-7303
pamela.berkheiser@yale.edu
medicine.yale.edu/pathology

George Shafranov, Chairman
Pam Burkheiser, Manager
Robert J. Alpern, Dean
Vision including studies on growth and development.

Delaware

4788 **Delaware Assistive Technology Initiative (DATI)**
Alfred I. duPont Hospital for Children
461 Wyoming Road
Newark, DE 19716-0269
302-831-0354
800-870-3284
Fax: 302-831-4690
TTY: 302-651-6794
dati@asel.udel.edu
www.dati.org

Beth Mineo Mollica, Director
Sonja Rathel, Project Coordinator

The Delaware Assistive Technology Initiative (DATI) connects Delawareans who have disabilities with the tools they need in order to learn, work, play and participate in community life safely and independently. DATI services include: Equipment demonstration centers in eah county; no-cost, short-term equipment loans that let you try before you buy; Equipment Exchange Program; AT workshops and other training sessions; advocacy for improved AT access policies and funding and several more.

4789 **Delaware Library for the Blind and Physically Handicapped**
Government
121 Duke of York Street
Dover, DE 19901-7430
302-739-4748
800-282-8676
Fax: 302-739-6787
debph@lib.de.us
libraries.delaware.gov

Dr. Annie E. Norman, Director
Sonja Brown, Administrative Specialist
Beth-Ann Ryan, Deputy Director
Diann Colose, Administrative Librarian

Books on cassette and playback equipment are provided to patrons who are unable to read regular printed books.

4790 **Elwyn Delaware**
321 E 11th St.
Wilmington, DE 19801-3417
302-658-8860
info@elwyn.org
elwyn.org

Charles S. McLister, President & CEO, Elwyn

Provides work training, job placement and supported employment, and elder care services.

District of Columbia

4791 **District of Columbia Public Library: Services for the Deaf Community**
District of Columbia Public Library
901 G St NW, Room 215
Washington, DC 20001-4531
202-727-0321
Fax: 202-727-0321
TTY: 202-559-5368
library_deaf_dc@yahoo.com
dclibrary.org

Venetia Demson, Chief Adaptive Services
Janice Roseu, Library for the Deaf Community

Offers reference services through videophone, signers for library programs, sign language classes, information about deafness, print and non-print materials for persons who have hearing disabilities. Book talks on deaf culture and American Sign Language story hours for kids, and Saturday sessions on employment-related skills are offered. Videophones for public use are available at the MLK Library.

4792 **District of Columbia Regional Library for the Blind and Physically Handicapped**
901 G St NW
Washington, DC 20001-4531
202-727-0321
Fax: 202-727-1129
TTY: 202-727-2145
lbphb_2000@yahoo.com
www.dclibrary.org

Richard Reyes-Gavilan, Executive Director
Jonathan Butler, Director of Business Services
Barbara Kirven, Director of Human Resources
Joi Mecks, Director of Communications

Regional library/RPH is network library in the Library of Congress, National Library Services for the Blind and Physically Handicapped.

4793 **Georgetown University Center for Child and Human Development**
P.O. Box 571485
Washington, DC 20057
202-687-5000
Fax: 202-687-8899
TTY: 202-687-5000
gucdc@georgetown.edu
gucchd.georgetown.edu

Phyllis R. Magrab, PhD, Director
John J. DeGioia, President

The Georgetown University Center for Child and Human Development (GUCCHD) was established over 50 years ago to improve the quality of life for all children and youth and their families, especially those with special health care needs, behavioral health challenges, or disabilities. Located in the nation's capital, this center both directly serves vulnerable children and their families, as well as influences local, state, national, and international programs and policy.

4794 **National Institute on Disability, Independent Living, and Rehabilitation Research (NIDILRR)**
Administration for Community Living
330 C St. SW
Washington, DC 20201
202-401-4634
nidilrr-mailbox@acl.hhs.gov
acl.gov

Anjali Forber-Pratt, Director
Kristi Hill, Deputy Director
Phillip Beatty, Director, Office of Research Sciences
Sarah Ruiz, Associate Director, Office of Research Sciences

NIDILRR is the US government's primary disability research agency.

Florida

4795 **Brevard County Talking Books Library**
Brevard County Libraries
2725 Judge Fran Jamieson Way
Viera, FL 32940
321-633-2000
Fax: 321-633-1964
TTY: 321-633-1838
kbriley@brev.org
www.brevardcounty.us/PublicLibraries

Camille Johnson, Manager
Catherine J Schweinsburg, Library Services Director

Subregional library for the blind and physically handicapped, assistive reading devices collection, reference materials on blindness and other handicaps, descriptive videos, CCTV, phonic ear, reading edge and LOUD-R assistive listening devices available.

4796 **Broward County Talking Book Library**
100 S Andrews Ave
Fort Lauderdale, FL 33301-1830
954-357-7444
Fax: 954-357-5548
www.broward.org

Robert E. Cannon, Director
Carolyn Kayne, Manager

Reference materials on blindness and other handicaps, films, closed-circuit TV, discs, cassettes and a book discussion group is offered.

4797 **Dade County Talking Book Library**
Miami Dade Public Library System
101 West Flagler Street
Miami, FL 33130
305-375-2665
800-451-9544
Fax: 305-757-8401
talkingbooks@mdpls.org
www.mdpls.org

Raymond Sanpiago, Executive Director
Lainey Brooks, Development Officer
Sylvia Mora Oria, Assistant Director
Ian D. Rosenior, Operations Administrator

A free Outreach Service of the Miami-Dade Public Library System. A network library, or subregional, of the National Library Service for the Blind and Physically Handicapped, Library of Congress, and of the Florida Bureau of Braille and Talking Books Library Service.

4798 **Florida Division of Blind Services**
Regional Library
325 West Gaines Street
Turlington Building, Suite 1114
Tallahassee, FL 32399-0400
850-245-0300
800-342-1828
Fax: 850-245-0363
dbs.myflorida.com

Mike Gunde, Manager
Susan Roberts, Bureau Chief
Robert Doyle, Director
Edward Hudson, Bureau Chief

Discs, cassettes, closed-circuit TV, large-print photocopier, films, children's books on cassettes and more.

4799 **Florida Instructional Materials Center forthe Visually Impaired (FIMC-VI)**
4210 W Bay Villa Ave
Tampa, FL 33611-1206
813-837-7826
800-282-9193
Fax: 813-837-7979
FloridaBrailleChallenge@gmail.com
www.fimcvi.org

Mary Stoltz, Database Manager
Jeffrey Fitterman, Technology Specialist
Teresa Gutierrez, Administrative Secretary
Kay Ratzlaff, Coordinator

Operates a clearinghouse depository and production center for Braille, large print and digital texts. Provides assistance in assessment of materials and specialized apparatus, organizes and trains volunteers for material production for the visually impaired, and provides professional development for teachers of the visually impaired. Provides electronic texts to NIMAS-eligible students in Florida.

4800 **Hillsborough County Talking Book Library Tampa-Hillsborough County Public Library**
900 N Ashley Dr
Tampa, FL 33602-3704
813-273-3652
Fax: 813-273-3707
TTY: 813-273-3610
www.hcplc.org

Joe Stines, Director of Libraries
Marcee Challener, Assitant Director
David Wullschleger, Chief of Operations
Linda Gillon, Manager of Staff & Administrativ

Serves as the reference hub and resource center for all citzens of Hillsborough County and as the flagship library of the Tampa-Hillsborough County Public Library System.

4801 **Jacksonville Public Library: Talking Books/Special Needs**
303 N Laura St
Jacksonville, FL 32202-3505
904-630-2665
Fax: 904-630-0604
www.jpl.coj.net/lib/talkingbooks.html

Barbara Gubbin, Executive Director

Offers cassettes and digital books, reference materials on blindness and ADA issues, newsline, descriptive videos, and some assistive devices.

4802 **Lee County Library System: Talking Books Library**
2001 N. Tamiami Trail N.E.
North Fort Myers, FL 33903-4855
239-533-4320
800-854-8195
Fax: 239-485-1146
TTY: 239-995-2665
talkingbooks@leegov.com
www.lee-county.com/library

Cynthia N Cobb, Director
Terri Crawford, Deputy Director
Debbie Parrott, Manager
Karen McLeish-Delgado, Librarian

Provides free books and magazines to Lee County residents of all ages who have any disability that prevents them from reading printed material. Books are played on special players provided free by the National Library Service. Circulates low tech assistive aids and devices for temporary loan to Lee County Library card holders. Directs people to assistive technology and disability related resources.

4803 **Louis de la Parte Florida Mental Health Institute Research Library**
University of South Florida
4202 E. Fowler Ave. LIB122
Tampa, FL 33620
813-974-2729
Fax: 813-974-7242
lib.usf.edu/fmhi

William A. Garrison, Dean
Florence Jandreau, CAP, Senior Assistant to the Dean
Claudia Dold, Assistant University Librarian
Tomaro Taylor, Associate University Librarian / Certified Archivist

Information offered on mental illness, autism and pervasive development disabilities mental health research and archives management.

4804 **Orange County Library System: Audio-Visual Department**
101 E Central Blvd
Orlando, FL 32801-2429
407-835-7323
Fax: 407-835-7649
TTY: 407-835-7641
comments@ocls.info
www.ocls.info

Ted Maines, President
Lisa Franchina, Vice President
Bob Tessier, Comptroller
Craig Wilkins, Public Service Administrator

Serves the residents of the Orange County Library District, with headquarters in downtown Orlando.

4805 **Pearlman Biomedical Research Institute**
Mt Sinai Medical Center
1600 NW 10th Ave
Miami Beach, FL 33140
305-674-2121
Fax: 305-674-2198
william-abraham@msmc.com

William Abraham, Director

A 32,000 square feet facility located on the main campus of Mount Sinai. The institute consists of laboratory space, research and administrative offices. The studies conducted within the facility are primarily pre-clinical research.

4806 **Pinellas Talking Book Library for the Blind and Physically Handicapped**
1330 Cleveland St
Clearwater, FL 33755-5103
727-441-8408
Fax: 727-441-8398
TTY: 727-441-3168
contactus@pplc.us
www.pplc.us

William Horne, Chair
Cheryl Morales, Executive Director
David Saari, Facilities Manager
Rosa Rodriguez, Deaf Literacy Coordinator at Saf

The Pinellas Public Library Cooperative serves Pinellas County residents in member cities and the unincorporated county. The Cooperative Office provides cooridination of activities and funding as well as marketing services for the the member counties. The Talking Book Library servces Pinellas, Manatee, and Sarasota counties.

4807 **Talking Book Service: Mantatee County Central Library**
1112 Manatee Avenue West
Bradenton, FL 34206-1000
941-748-4501
Fax: 941-751-7098
www.mymanatee.org

Patricia Schubert, Manager
Offers children's books on disc and cassette and more reference materials for the blind and physically handicapped.

4808 **Talking Books Library for the Blind and Physically Handicapped**
Palm Beach County Library
3650 Summit Blvd
West Palm Beach, FL 33406-4114
561-233-2600
888-780-4962
Fax: 561-233-2627
webmaster@pbclibrary.org
www.pbclibrary.org

John Callahan, Executive Director
Bill Rautenberg, Chair
Harriet Helfman, Vice Chair
John Callahan III, Library Director
Established in 1967, today the County Library system serves Palm Beach County through the Main Library, 2 Regional Libraries, 11 Branch Libraries, a Bookmobile and a library annex. It continues to expand through our involvement with library networks, the Internet, and the World Wide Web.

4809 **Talking Books/Homebound Services**
Brevard County Library System
2725 Judge Fran Jamieson Way
Viera, FL 32940
321-633-2000
Fax: 321-633-1838
kbriley@brev.org
www.brevardcounty.us/PublicLibraries

Kay Briley, Librarian
Camille Johnson, Executive Director
Offers reference materials on blindness and other handicaps. Subregional library for the blind and physically handicapped, assistive reading devices collection, reference materials on blindness and other handicaps; CCTV, phonic ear, reading edge and LOUD-R assistive listening devices available.

4810 **University of Miami: Bascom Palmer Eye Institute**
Department Of Ophthalmalogy
900 NW 17th St
Miami, FL 33136-1119
305-243-2020
888-845-0002
Fax: 305-326-7000
www.bascompalmer.org

Michael Gittelman, CEO
Teresa Spaulding, Manager
Eduardo C. Alfonso, M.D., Professor and Chairman
Jennifer Cohen, Executive Director
Clinical and basic research into blindness and visual impairments.

4811 **University of Miami: Mailman Center for Child Development**
1601 NW 12th Ave
Miami, FL 33136-1005
305-243-6395
Fax: 305-326-7594
pedsinformation@med.miami.edu
pediatrics.med.miami.edu

William Donelan, Vice President for Medical Admin
William W. O'Neill, M.D., Executive Dean, Chief Medical Of
Pascal J. Goldschmidt, M.D., SVP, Dean, CEO
Steven Falcone, M.D., Executive Dean
Focuses on birth defects and children's illnesses.

4812 **West Florida Regional Library**
200 W Gregory St
Pensacola, FL 32502-4822
850-436-5060
Fax: 850-436-5039
TTY: 850-436-5063
hhudson@ci.pensacola.fl.us

Eugene Fischer, Executive Director
Helen Hudson, Outreach Librarian
Offers children's print/Braille books.

Georgia

4813 **Athens Talking Book Center-Athens-Clarke County Regional Library**
2025 Baxter St
Athens, GA 30606-6331
706-613-3655
800-531-2063
Fax: 706-613-3660

Stacey Chandler, Manager
Discs, cassettes, large print books, reference materials on blindness, descriptive videos, films, closed-circuit TV, magnifiers, Braille writer, summer reading programs, cassette books and magazines and more.

4814 **Augusta Talking Book Center**
823 Telfair Street
Augusta, GA 30901-2232
706-821-2600
Fax: 706-724-6762
TTY: 706-722-1639
www.ecgrl.org

Lillie Hamilton, Board Of Trustee
Audrey Bell, Manager
Loran Gray, Board Of Trustee
Brenda Morton, Board Of Trustee
Discs, cassettes, Braille writer, films, large print books, summer reading program, magnifiers and reference materials on blindness and other handicaps.

4815 **Bainbridge Subregional Library for the Blind & Physically Handicapped**
S W Georgia Regional Library
301 S Monroe St
Bainbridge, GA 39819-4029
229-248-2665
800-795-2680
Fax: 229-248-2670
lbph@swgrl.org
www.swgrl.org

Susans Wittle, Manager
Kathy Hutchins, Supervisor
The library houses a large collection of recorded materials as well as reference materials. For recorded and Braille materials that are provided by the National Library Service (NLS) but not currently in stock at the Bainbridge Library, the Regional Library in Atlanta can be contacted to Interlibrary Loan the requested materials.

4816 **Columbus Subregional Library For The Blind And Physically Handicapped**
1120 Bradley Dr
Columbus, GA 31906-2813
706-649-0780
800-652-0782
Fax: 706-649-1914
TTY: 706-649-0974

Dorothy Bowen, Librarian
Braille writer, magnifiers, closed-circuit TV, large-print photocopier, cassette books and magazines, children's books on cassette, home visits and other reference materials on blindness and other handicaps.

4817 **Emory Autism Resource Center**
Emory University
1551 Shoup Ct
Decatur, GA 30033
404-727-8350
Fax: 404-727-3969
tohannon@emory.edu
www.emory.edu/HOUSING/CLAIRMONT/autism.html

James W. Wagner, President
Larry Hagan, IT Manager
Paul B. Pruett, MD, Director of Residency Education
Terri Trotter, Coordinator of Residency Educati
Offers on-line bulletin boards which are relevant to autism.

4818 Emory University Laboratory for Ophthalmic Research
1365b Clifton Rd NE
Atlanta, GA 30322-1013 404-778-4530
Fax: 404-778-4002
pbennet@emory.edu
www.eyecenter.emory.edu
James W. Wagner, President
Larry Hagan, IT Manager
Paul B. Pruett, MD, Director of Residency Education
Terri Trotter, Coordinator of Residency Educati
Various studies into the aspects of blindness.

4819 Georgia Library for the Blind and Physically Handicapped
Georgia Public Library
1800 Century Place
Suite 150
Atlanta, GA 30345-4304 404-235-7200
800-248-6701
Fax: 404-756-4618
georgialibraries.org
Stella Cone, Director
Deborah Scott, Business Manager
Dr. Lamar Veatch, Librarian
Julie Walker, State Librarian
Discs, cassettes, Braille, films, closed-circuit TV, Braille writer, large-print photocopier, cassette books and magazines.

4820 Hall County Library: East Hall Branch and Special Needs Library
127 Main St NW
Gainesville, GA 30501-3614 770-532-3311
Fax: 770-532-4305
TTY: 770-531-2520
info@hallcountylibrary.org
www.hallcountylibrary.org
Adrian Mixson, Manager
Summer reading programs, Braille writer, magnifiers, scanners and readers, audio described videos, closed captioned videos, closed-circuit TV, large-print photocopier, cassette books and magazines, large print books, children's books on cassette, home visits and other reference materials on blindness and other handicaps.

4821 Macon Library for the Blind and Physically Handicapped
Washington Memorial Library
1180 Washington Ave
Macon, GA 31201-1762 478-744-0800
Fax: 478-742-3161
www.co.bibb.ga.us/library
Thomas Jones, Director
Leila Brittain, Finance Officer
Hannah Warren, Office Manager
Viveca Jackson, Librarian, West Bibb Branch
Summer reading programs, Braille writer, magnifiers, closed-circuit TV, large-print photocopier, cassette books and magazines, children's books on cassette, home visits and other reference materials on blindness and other handicaps.

4822 National Center on Birth Defects and Developmental Disabilities
Centers for Disease Control and Prevention
1600 Clifton Rd NE
MS E-87
Atlanta, GA 30333 404-639-3311
800-232-4636
Fax: 404-498-3070
TTY: 888-232-6348
cdcinfo@cdc.gov
www.cdc.gov/ncbddd/
Coleen A. Boyle, PhD, MSHyg, Director
Stephanie Dulin, MBA, Deputy Director
Vicki Kipreos, PMP, Management Officer
Lisa Richardson, MD, Director, Division of Blood Diso
Promotes child development, prevents birth defects and developmental disabilities.

4823 North Georgia Talking Book Center
LaFayette-Walker Public Library
305 S Duke St
La Fayette, GA 30728-2936 706-638-8312
888-506-0509
888-506-0509
Fax: 706-638-4028
www.chrl.org
Tim York, Manager
June DeLong, Library Assistant
Martha McKeehan, Library Assistant
Kaylee Smith, Library Assistant
We offer books on cassette for the visual and physically disabled induvidual, books in Braille, magazines on cassette, zoom text screen magnifier, computer voice program, large-print photocopier, summer reading program, home visits na dother reference materials on blindness and other disabilities.

4824 Oconee Regional Library
801 Bellevue Ave
Dublin, GA 31021-4847 478-272-5710
Fax: 478-275-5381
georgialibraries.org
Stella Cone, Director
Deborah Scott, Business Manager
Dr. Lamar Veatch, Librarian
Leard Daughety, Director
Summer reading programs, Braille writer, magnifiers, closed-circuit TV, large-print photocopier, cassette books and magazines, children's books on cassette, home visits and other reference materials on blindness and other handicaps.

4825 Rome Subregional Library for the Blind and Physically Handicapped
205 Riverside Pkwy
Rome, GA 30161-2922 706-236-4611
888-263-0769
Fax: 706-236-4631
TTY: 706-236-4618
Diana Mills, Librarian
Delana Hickman, Manager
The regional library system serves Floyd and Polk counties. System headquarters are located in Rome, Georgia, within the Rome/Floyd County Library Branch.

4826 South Georgia Regional Library-Valdosta Talking Book Center
300 Woodrow Wilson Dr
Valdosta, GA 31602-2532 229-333-0086
Fax: 229-333-0364
commissioner@lowndescounty.com
sgrl.org
Chuck Gibson, Manager
Summer reading programs, Braille writer, magnifiers, closed-circuit TV, large print photocopier, cassette books and magazines, children's books on cassette, home visits and other reference materials on blindness and other handicaps.

4827 Talking Book Center Brunswick-Glynn County Regional Library
208 Gloucester St
Brunswick, GA 31520-7007 912-267-1212
Fax: 912-267-9597
www.trrl.org
Betty Ransom, Librarian
Joe Shinnick, Executive Director
The Three Rivers Regional Library system is named for 3 rivers that flow through all 7 counties of the library system. The Three Rivers Regional Library system serves patrons in Brantley, Camden, Charlton, Glynn, Long, McIntosh, and Wayne counties in southeast Georgia.

Hawaii

4828 **Assistive Technology Resource Centers of Hawaii (ATRC)**
200 North Vineyard Boulevard
Suite 430
Honolulu, HI 96817-5362
808-532-7110
800-645-3007
Fax: 808-532-7120
TTY: 808-532-7110
atrc-info@atrc.org
www.atrc.org

Barbara Fischlowitz-Leong, Executive Director
Jeff Ah Sam, Technical Assisstant
Jodi Asato, Deputy Director
Edna Kaahaaina, Office Manager

Provides information and training on assistive technology devices, services, and funding resources. Conducts presentations and demonstrations in the community to increase AT awareness and promote self-advocacy among people with disabilities.

4829 **Hawaii State Library for the Blind and Physically Handicapped**
874 Dillingham Blvd
Honolulu, HI 96817-4505
808-845-9221
800-559-4096
Fax: 808-733-8449
honcclib@hawaii.edu
www2.honolulu.hawaii.edu/library

Fusako Miyashiro, Manager

Supported by the Hawaii State Public Library System and the National Library Service for the Blind and Physically Handicapped, Library of Congress. Staff with knowledge of sign language; Special interest periodicals; Books on deafness and sign language; captioned media; Special Services: Radio Reading Service, Talking Books Reader's Club, educational and cultural programs, machine lending agency. Braille, cassette and large type. Regional and National service, quarterly newsletter.

Idaho

4830 **Idaho Assistive Technology Project**
University of Idaho
121 West Sweet Ave
Moscow, ID 83843-2268
208-885-3557
800-432-8324
Fax: 208-885-6145
idahoat@uidaho.edu
www.idahoat.org

Janice Carson, Project Director
Irene Lunsford, Loan Program Manager
Julie Magelky, Loan Program Coordinator
Dan Dyer, Training Coordinator

A federally funded program managed by the Center on Disbailities and Human Development at the University of Idaho. The goal of the IATP is to increase the availability of assistive technology devices and services for Idahoans with disabilities. The IATP offers free trainings and technical assistance, a low-interest loan program, assistive technology assessments for children and agriculture workers, and free informational materials.

4831 **Idaho Commission for Libraries: Talking Book Service**
325 W State St
Boise, ID 83702-6055
208-334-2150
800-458-3271
Fax: 208-334-4016
talkingbooks@libraries.idaho.gov
www.libraries.idaho.gov/tbs

Ann Joslin, Manager
Irene Lunsford, Library Consultant
David Harrell, IT & Telecommunications Resources Manager
Erica Compton, Project Coordinator

Offers audio and Braille books and magazines, equipment, and accessories. All materials are mailed free to users' homes. Service is available free to all Idaho residents with a disability which limits their ability to use print materials.

Illinois

4832 **Chicago Public Library Talking Book Center**
400 S State St
Chicago, IL 60605-1216
312-747-4300
800-757-4654
Fax: 312-747-4962
www.chipublib.org

Linda Johnson Rice, President
Christopher Valenti, Vice President
Cristina Benitez, Secretary
Joselyn Bell, Director, Finance

Summer reading programs, Braille writer, closed-circuit TV, large print photocopier, cassette books and magazines, children's books on cassette, home visits and other reference materials on blindness and other handicaps. Three assistive technology centers designed and equipped for the blind and visually impaired, funded by the National Library Service for the Blind and Handicapped, a division of the Library of Congress. All services FREE!

4833 **Department of Ophthalmology and Visual Science**
1855 W Taylor St
Chicago, IL 60612-7242
312-996-7000
800-625-2013
Fax: 312-996-7770
TTY: 312-413-0123
www.uic.edu

Paula Allen-Meares, Chancellor
Lon S. Kaufman, Vice Chancellor for Academic Aff
Mitra Dutta, Vice Chancellor for Research
Barbara Henley, Vice Chancellor for Student Affa

Offers help, support, information and research for persons with vision problems, including Retinitis Pigmentosa.

4834 **Guild for the Blind**
65 E. Wacker Place
Suite 1010
Chicago, IL 60601-7463
312-236-8569
Fax: 312-236-8128
www.second-sense.org

Brett Christenson, President
Laura Rounce, Vice President
Michael P. Wagner, Treasurer
Toria Emas, Secretary

provides worship on vision rehabilitation, training on computers and other adaptive technology, career counseling, and professional development workshops and offers assistive devices for sale.

4835 **Horizons for the Blind**
125 Erick St.
A103
Crystal Lake, IL 60014
815-444-8800
800-318-2000
Fax: 815-444-8830
mail@horizons-blind.org
www.horizons-blind.org

Camille Caffarelli, Executive Director
Jeff T. Thorsen, First Vice President & Treasurer
Keith Myers, Second Vice President
Maryann Bartkowski, Secretary

Horizons for the Blind is a nonprofit organization working to improve the quality of life for people who are blind or visually impaired by increasing access to consumer products, services, culture, arts, education, and recreation.

4836 **Illinois Early Childhood Intervention Clearinghouse**
51 Gerty Drive
Champaign, IL 61820-7469
217-333-1386
877-275-3227
Fax: 217-244-7732
Illinois-eic@illinois.edu
www.eiclearinghouse.org

Charlton Brandt, Manager
Patricia Traylor, Project Associate

Free lending library of materials related to early childhood and disability. Books, audiovisuals and articles available. Computerized database with more than 31,000 items available to Illinois residents.

4837 **Illinois Machine Sub-Lending Agency**
607 S Greenbriar Rd
Carterville, IL 62918-1602
618-985-8375
800-455-2665
Fax: 618-985-4211
imsastaff@imsa.lib.il.us

Loretta Broomfield, Director

The Illinois Machine Sublending Agency (IMSA) is a division of the Illinois Network of Talking Book and Braille Libraries. The primary responsibility of IMSA is to maintain Talking Book equipment and accessories and to issue Talking Book equipment and accessories to Illinois residents who are registered for the service. IMSA is also the support center for patrons in need of assistance with the Braille and Audio Reading Download (BARD) service.

4838 **Illinois Regional Library for the Blind and Physically Handicapped**
1055 W Roosevelt Rd
Chicago, IL 60608-1559
312-746-9210
800-331-2351
Fax: 312-746-9192

Shawn Thomas, Reference Librarian
Barbara Perkins, Acting Director

Summer reading programs, Braille writer, magnifiers, closed-circuit TV, large-print photocopier, cassette books and magazines, descriptive videos, children's books on cassette, home visits and other reference materials on blindness and other handicaps.

4839 **Mid-Illinois Talking Book Center**
600 High Point Ln
East Peoria, IL 61611-9396
309-694-9200
800-426-0709

Rose Chenoweth, Director
Michelle Moran, Assistant
Rebecca Rollings, Assistant
Jane Furrh, Assistant

Providing a free library service to anyone unable to read regular print because of a visual or physical disability. There are books and magazines on tape and playback equipment; and also in Braille. Books and magazines are mailed free to and from library patrons, wherever they reside.

4840 **National Eye Research Foundation (NERF)**
Ste 207a
910 Skokie Blvd
Northbrook, IL 60062-4033
847-564-4652
800-621-2258
Fax: 847-564-0807
info@nerf.org
www.nerf.org

Joel Tenner, Manager

Dedicated to improving eye care for the public and meeting the professional nees of eye care practitioners; sponsors eye research projects on contact lens applications and eye care problems. Special study sections in such fields as orthokertology, primary eyecare, pediatrics, and through continuing education programs. Provides eye care information for the public and professionals. Educational materials including pamphlets. Program activities include education and referrals.

4841 **National Lekotek Center**
2001 N. Clybourn
Chicago, IL 60614
773-528-5766
800-366-7529
Fax: 773-537-2992
www.lekotek.org

Elaine D. Cottey, Chair
Joanna Horsnail, Chair Elect
Eric Gastevich, Treasurer
Carol Neiger, Secretary

Toy library and play-centered programs for children with special needs and their families with branches in 17 states. Sliding fee scale. Lekotek also has a Toy Resource Helpline that provides individualized assistances in the selection of toys and play materials and general resources for families with children with disabilities.

4842 **Northwestern University Multipurpose Arthritis & Musculoskeletal Center**
420 East Superior Street
Chicago, IL 60611-4296
312-503-8194
Fax: 312-503-1204
www.feinberg.northwestern.edu

Cynthia Barnard, MBA, Director, Quality Strategies
John Vozenilek, MD, Assistant Professor
Eric G. Neilson, MD, Vice President for Medical Affairs
Sherri L. LaVela, PhD, MPH, MBA, Assistant Professor

Conducts biomedical, educational and health services research into musculoskeletal diseases.

4843 **Skokie Accessible Library Services**
Skokie Public Library
5215 Oakton St
Skokie, IL 60077-3680
847-673-7774
Fax: 847-673-7797
TTY: 847-673-8926
www.skokie.lib.il.us

Carolyn A. Anthony, Director
John J. Graham, President
Diana Hunter, Vice President/President Emerita
Karen Parrilli, Secretary

Library services for people with disabilities, including electronic aids, materials in special formats, programs and special services.

4844 **University of Illinois at Chicago: Lions of Illinois Eye Research Institute**
University of Illinois at Chicago
1855 West Taylor Street, m/c 648
Room 3.138
Chicago, IL 60612
312-996-6591
Fax: 312-996-7770
eyeweb@uic.edu
www.uic.edu

Rolanda Geddis, Manager
Paula Allen Meares, Chancellor
Jerry Bauman, Vice President for Health Affairs
James Schmidt, Director of Athletics

Visual impairments and blindness research, including glaucoma studies.

4845 **Voices of Vision Talking Book Center at DuPage Library System**
125 Tower Drive
Burr Ridge, IL 60527-2771
630-734-5055
800-426-0709
Fax: 630-208-0399
info@illinoistalkingbooks.org
www.illinoistalkingbooks.org

Karen L. Odean, Director

Provides library service to persons who are unable to use standard printed material because of visual or physical disabilities. Part of the Illinois network of Talking Book Libraries. The service is free to those who are eligable. Provides books and magazines on audio-cassettes. Special playback equipment needed to use the books is also loaned. Braille books and magazines are also available. The collection includes popular books, classics and children's literature.

Indiana

4846 **Allen County Public Library**
900 Library Plaza
Fort Wayne, IN 46802-3699
260-421-1200
Fax: 260-421-1386
TTY: 260-421-1302
Genealogy@ACPL.Info
www.acpl.lib.in.us

Jeffrey R. Krull, Director
Martin E. Seifert, President
Alan McMahan, Vice President
Paul G. Moss, Secretary

Summer reading programs, Braille writer, magnifiers, closed-circuit TV, large-print photocopier, cassette books and magazines, children's books on cassette, home visits and other reference materials on blindness and other handicaps.

4847 **Bartholomew County Public Library**
536 5th St
Columbus, IN 47201-6225
812-379-1255
Fax: 812-379-1275
library@barth.lib.in.us
barth.lib.in.us

Beth Poor, Executive Director

Summer reading programs, Braille writer, magnifiers, closed-circuit TV, large-print photocopier, cassette books and magazines, children's books on cassette, home visits and other reference materials on blindness and other handicaps.

4848 **Elkhart Public Library for the Blind and Physically Handicapped**
300 S 2nd St
Elkhart, IN 46516-3109
574-522-2223
800-622-4970
Fax: 574-522-2174
www.myepl.org/epl

Connie Jo Ozinga, Executive Director
Barbara G. Anderson, President
Janice E. Dean, Vice-President
Krystal Anderson, Secretary

Summer reading programs, Braille writer, magnifiers, closed-circuit TV, large-print photocopier, cassette books and magazines, children's books on cassette, home visits and other reference materials on blindness and other handicaps.

4849 **Indiana Resource Center for Autism**
2853 E 10th St
Bloomington, IN 47408-2696
812-855-6508
800-825-4733
Fax: 812-855-9630
TTY: 812-855-9396
iidc@indiana.edu
www.iidc.indiana.edu/irca

Dr Cathy Pratt Ph.D., BCBA, Director
Donna Beasley, Administrative Program Secretary
Pamela Anderson, Outreach/Resource Specialist
Marci Wheeler, M.S.W., Social Work Specialist

The Indiana Resource Center for Autism staff conduct outreach training and consultations, engage in research and develop and disseminate information focused on building the capicity of local communities, organizations, agencies and families to support children and adults across the autism spectrum in typical work, school, home and community settings. Please check our website for a complete list of publications.

4850 **Indiana University: Multipurpose Arthritis Center**
School Of Medicine, Rheumatology Division
509 E. 3rd Street
Bloomington, IN 47401-3654
812-855-0516
Fax: 812-855-9943
research.iu.edu

Dr. Kenneth Brandt MD, Director
Carmichael Center, Vice President for Research
Steven A Martin, Associate Vice President for Research
Marisa Pratt, Executve Financial & Operations Officer

The mission of the center is to pursue major biomedical research interests relevant to the rheumatic diseases. Current areas of emphasis include; articular cartilage biology, pathogenesis of articular cartilage breakdown in osteoarthritis, causes of pain and disability in QA, the pathogenesis and treatment of various forms of amyloidosis, the pathogenesis of dermatomyositis, and immunologic and biochemical markers of cartilage breakdown and repair.

4851 **Lake County Public Library Talking Books Service**
1919 W 81st Ave
Merrillville, IN 46410-5488
219-769-3541
Fax: 219-769-0690
www.lcplin.org

Larry Acheff, Manager

Large-print books, descriptive videos, Braille writer, magnifiers, closed-circuit TV, large-print photocopier, cassette books and magazines, children's books on cassette, and other reference materials on blindness and other handicaps.

4852 **Special Services Division: Indiana State Library**
140 N Senate Ave
Indianapolis, IN 46204-2207
317-232-3675
800-622-4970
Fax: 317-253-3209
TTY: 317-232-7763
www.in.gov/isloutage

Roberta Brooker, Manager
Barbara Maxwell, State Librarian
C Ewick, Manager

Circulates a collection of Braille, recorded, and large print books and magazines and the special equipment needed to play the recorded materials to anyone in Indiana who cannot read regular print due to a visual or physical disability.

4853 **St. Joseph Hospital Rehabilitation Center**
700 Broadway
Fort Wayne, IN 46802-1402
260-425-3000
Fax: 260-425-3741
www.stjoehospital.com

Kirk Ray, CEO
Bob Hailes, Vice President

Information offered on rehabilitation.

4854 **Talking Books Service Evansville Vanderburgh County Public Library**
200 SE Martin Luther King Jr Blvd
Evansville, IN 47713- 1802
812-428-8200
866-645-2536
Fax: 812-428-8397
tbs@evpl.org
www.evpl.org

Marcia Learned Au, COO
Connie Davis, Vice President
Marcia Au, Executive Director
Barbara Shanks, Talking Book Manager

The Talking Book Service of the Evansville Vanderburgh Public Library is part of a nationwide network of cooperating libraries headed by the National Library Service & a division of the Library of Congress. This free program provides library services and materials in alternative formats to person who are unable to use standard print material due to a visual or physical handicap.

Iowa

4855 **Iowa Department for the Blind Library**
State Of Iowa
524 4th Street
Des Moines, IA 50309-2364
515-281-1333
800-362-2587
Fax: 515-281-1263
TTY: 515-281-1355
contact@blind.state.ia.us
www.IDBonline.org

Richard Sorey, Director
Mike Hoenig, Chair
Steve Hagemoser, Commision Board Member
Peggy Elliott, Commision Board Member

Summer reading programs, large print, disc, Braille and cassette books and magazines, descriptive videos and reference materials on blindness and other handicaps.

4856 **Iowa Registry for Congenital and Inherited Disorders**
University of Iowa
Department of Epidemiology, Univers
100 BVC, Room W260
Iowa City, IA 52242-5000
319-335-4107
866-274-4237
Fax: 319-335-4030
ircid@uiowa.edu
www.public-health.uiowa.edu/ircid/

Paul Romitti, Ph.D, Director
Kim Keppler-Noreuil, M.D, Clinical Director for Birth Defects
Katherine. Mathews, M.D, Clinical Director for Neuromuscular Disorders
James Torner, Ph.D., Chair

The mission of the Iowa Registry for Congenital and Inherited Disorders is; maintain statewide surveillance for collecting information on selected congenital and inherited disorders in Iowa, monitor annual trends in occurrence and mortality of these disorders, provide data for research studies and educational activities for the prevention and treatment of these disorders.

4857 **Library Commission for the Blind**
State Of Iowa
524 4th Street
Des Moines, IA 50309-2364
515-281-1333
800-362-2587
Fax: 515-281-1263
TTY: 515-281-1355
contact@blind.state.ia.us

Karen A Keninger, Director
Aldini Jodi, Library Support Staff
Barber Kim, Independent Living Supervisor
Bauer Marcia, Rehabilitation Teacher
Summer reading programs, Braille writer, magnifiers, closed-circuit TV, large print photocopier, cassette books and magazines, children's books on cassette and other reference materials on blindness and other handicaps.

Kansas

4858 **Center for the Improvement of Human Functioning**
3100 N Hillside St
Wichita, KS 67219-3904
316-682-3100
Fax: 316-682-5054
information@riordanclinic.org
www.riordanclinic.org

Hugh D Riordan, President
Ron Hunninghake MD, Chief Medical Officer
Brian Riordan, Chief Executive Officer
Medical, research, and educational facility specializing in the treatment of chronic illness.

4859 **Central Kansas Library Systems Headquarters (CSLS)**
1409 Williams St
Great Bend, KS 67530-4020
620-792-4865
800-362-2642
Fax: 620-793-7270
www.ckls.org

Harry Williams, Administrator
Vickie Herl, Adminstrative Manager
Marquita Boehnke, Department Head
Connie Bobbitt, Assistant
Summer reading programs, Braille writer, magnifiers, closed-circuit TV, large-print photocopier, cassette books and magazines, children's books on cassette, home visits and other reference materials on blindness and other handicaps. Assistive technology available. Serving 17 counties in Central Kansas.

4860 **Manhattan Public Library**
629 Poyntz Ave
Manhattan, KS 66502-6131
785-776-4741
800-432-2796
Fax: 785-776-1545
refstaff@mhklibrary.org
manhattan.lib.ks.us

Linda Knupp, Director
John Pecoraro, Assistant Director
Brice Hobrock, President
Thomas Giller, Vice President
Summer reading programs, Braille writer, magnifiers, closed-circuit TV, large-print photocopier, cassette books and magazines, children's books on cassette, home visits and other reference materials on blindness and other disabilities.

4861 **Northwest Kansas Library System Talking Books**
2 Washington Square
Norton, KS 67654-1615
785-877-5148
800-432-2858
Fax: 785-877-5697
www.nwkls.org

George Seamon, Director
Alice Evans, Business Manager & Acquisitions
David Fischer, Technology Consultant
Marry Boller, Children's and Talking Book Consultant

Offers books on disc and cassette. Library of Congress talking book and program for qualified individuals. Also offers descriptive videos to eligible persons.

4862 **South Central Kansas Library System**
321 North Main Street
South Hutchinson, KS 67505-1145
620-663-3211
800-234-0529
Fax: 620-663-9797
sckls.info

Paul Hawkins, Director
Sharon Barnes, Technology Consultant
Larry Papenfuss, Director of Information Technology
Jill Stern, Continuing Education Specialist
Serving public, school, academic and special libraries in 12 counties since 1968, the South Central Kansas Library System (SCKLS) is the "go to" resource for innovative services, quality member awareness and assistance.

4863 **State Library of Kansas**
Esu Memorial Union
300 SW 10th Ave.
Room 312-N
Topeka, KS 66612-1593
620-341-6280
800-362-0699
KTB@ks.gov
kslib.info/talking-books

Cindy Roupe, State Librarian
Michael Lang, Director
Kansas Talking Books provides personalized library support and materials in a specialized format to eligible Kansas residents to ensure that all may read. Features: Audiobooks, magazines and audio equipment mailed directly to your house and returned postage free; special equipment lent to you at no charge; downloadable books from the Braille and Audio Reading Download (BARD) website or by using the new BARD app.

4864 **Topeka & Shawnee County Public Library Talking Books Service**
1515 SW 10th Ave
Topeka, KS 66604-1374
785-580-4400
800-432-2925
Fax: 785-580-4496
TTY: 785-580-4544
www.tscpl.org

Stephanie Hall, Manager
Gina Millsap, Chief Executive Officer
Robert Banks, Chief Operating Officer
Sheryl Weller, Chief Financial Officer
Talking books is a free service that provides cassette and digital books and equipment to people who are unable to read or use standard print materials because of a visual or physical impairment. There are no fees. To apply for Talking Books you must fill out and submit an application, have it certified by the appropriate authority and return it to the library. You can find an application on our website or have one mailed out to you by contacting our office.

4865 **Wichita Public Library/Talking Book Service**
Wichita Public Library
223 S Main St
Wichita, KS 67202-3795
316-261-8500
Fax: 316-262-4540
TTY: 316-262-3972
admin@wichita.lib.ks.us

Cynthia Berner-Harris, Executive Director
Eric J. Larson, Member of the Board
Furnish recorded reading material (books and magazines) for visually and physically challenged citizens.

4866 **Wichita Public Library/Talking Book Service**
223 S Main St
Wichita, KS 67202-3795
316-261-8500
Fax: 316-262-4540
TTY: 316-262-3972
admin@wichita.lib.ks.us

Cynthia Berner-Harris, Executive Director
Eric J. Larson, Member of the Board
Furnish recorded reading material (books and magazines) for visually and physically challenged citizens.

Kentucky

4867 **EnTech: Enabling Technologies of Kentuckiana**
Spaulding University
851 South 3rd Street
Louisville, KY 40203-2115
502-585-9911
800-896-8941
Fax: 502-585-7103
www.spalding.edu

Laura Strickland, Manager
Mary Kaye Steinmietz, Outreach Coordinator
Tori Murden McClure, President

Assistive technology resource and demonstration center, serving persons of all ages and disabilities in Kentucky and Southern Indiana. Services include: assistive technology information, demonstration, evaluation, training, technical support and short-term loan of equipment.

4868 **Kentucky Talking Book Library - Kentucky Dept. for Libraries and Archives**
300 Coffee Tree Road
PO Box 537
Frankfort, KY 40602-0537
502-564-8300
800-372-2968
Fax: 502-564-5773
ktbl.mail@ky.gov
www.kdla.ky.gov

Barbara Penegor, Regional Librarian
Lauren Abner, Field Services
Katherine K. Adelberg, E-Rate Coordinator
Jackie Arnold, Local Records Regional Administrator

Provides library service to those who are physically unable to read print. Audio and Braille books and magazines are available via mail or download.

4869 **Louisville Free Public Library**
301 York Street
Louisville, KY 40203-2257
502-574-1611
Fax: 502-574-1666
lfpl.org

Craig Buthod, Manager

Summer reading programs, Braille writer, magnifiers, closed-circuit TV, large-print photocopier, cassette books and magazines, children's books on cassette, home visits and other reference materials on blindness and other handicaps.

Louisiana

4870 **Central Louisiana State Hospital Medical and Professional Library**
P.O. Box 5031
Pineville, LA 71361-5031
318-484-6200
Fax: 318-484-6501
www.doa.la.gov

Patrick Kelly, CEO
Carol Gee, Manager

Information offered on psychiatry, psychology and mental health.

4871 **Louisiana State Library**
701 North 4th St
Baton Rouge, LA 70802-5345
225-342-4913
800-543-4702
Fax: 225-219-4804
admin@state.lib.la.us
www.state.lib.la.us

Rebecca Hamilton, Assistant Secretary, State Libra
Diane Brown, Deputy State Librarian
Beverly Dugas, Business Manager
Meg Placke, Associate State Librarian

Summer reading programs, Braille writer, magnifiers, closed-circuit TV, large-print photocopier, cassette books and magazines, children's books on cassette. Descriptive videoss and other reference materials on blindness and other handicaps.

4872 **Louisiana State University Genetics Section of Pediatrics**
533 Bolivar St
New Orleans, LA 70112-1349
504-568-6151
Fax: 504-568-8500
postmaster@lsuhsc.edu
www.medschool.lsuhsc.edu

Steve Nelson, MD, Dean
Janis Letourneau, MD, Associate Dean for Faculty & Ins
Cathi Fontenot, MD, Associate Dean for Alumni Affair
Charles Hilton, MD, Associate Dean for Academic Affa

Our goal is to continue building a strong department in which all of the faculty are successful in attracting funding, and committed to establishing productive programs that bring credit to the Department and to the Health Sciences Center as a whole.

4873 **State Library of Louisiana: Services for the Blind and Physically Handicapped**
701 North 4th St
Baton Rouge, LA 70802-5345
225-342-4913
800-543-4702
Fax: 225-219-4804
www.state.lib.la.us

Rebecca Hamilton, Assistant Secretary, State Libra
Diane Brown, Deputy State Librarian
Beverly Dugas, Business Manager
Meg Placke, Associate State Librarian

Summer reading programs, Braille publications, cassette books and magazines, children's books on cassette and other reference materials on blindness and other handicaps. Louisiana Hotlines - quarterly newsletter. Affiliated with National Library Service for the Blind and Physically Handicapped, Washington, DC. Louisiana Voices recording program uses volunteers to record books for the blind.

Maine

4874 **Bangor Public Library**
145 Harlow St
Bangor, ME 04401-4900
207-947-8336
Fax: 207-945-6694
www.bpl.lib.me.us

Barbara Mc Dade, Executive Director
Norman Minsky, President
Franklin E. Bragg II, MD, Vice President
Lee Chick, Treasurer

Summer reading programs, Braille writer, magnifiers, closed-circuit TV, large-print photocopier, cassette books and magazines, children's books on cassette, home visits and other reference materials on blindness and other handicaps.

4875 **Cary Library**
107 Main Street
Houlton, ME 04730-2196
207-532-1302
Fax: 207-532-4350
www.cary.lib.me.us

Iva Sussman, Chair
Forrest Barnes, Treasurer
Gary Hagan, Secretary
Linda Faucher, Library Director

Summer reading programs, Braille writer, magnifiers, closed-circuit TV, large-print photocopier, cassette books and magazines, children's books on cassette, home visits and other reference materials on blindness and other handicaps.

4876 **Lewiston Public Library**
200 Lisbon St
Lewiston, ME 04240-7234
207-513-3004
Fax: 207-784-3011
TTY: 207-200-1511
LPLReference@LewistonMaine.gov
lplonline.org

Rick Speer, Library Director
Marcela Peres, Adult Services Librarian
David Moorhead, Children's Librarian
Beth Martel, Circulation Services Supervisor

Summer reading programs, Braille writer, magnifiers, closed-circuit T.V., large-print photocopier, cassette books and magazines, children's books on cassette, home visits and other reference materials on blindness and other handicaps.

4877 Maine State Library
Maine State
64 State House Sta
Augusta, ME 04333-64
207-287-5650
800-762-7106
Fax: 207-287-5624
TTY: 888-577-6690
benitad@ursus3.ursus.maine.edu
maine.gov

Chris Boynton, Manager
J Gary Nichols, State Librarian
Melora Norman, Manager
Summer reading programs, cassette books and magazines, children's books on cassette, home visits and other reference materials on blindness and other handicaps.
Newsl./BiAnnual

4878 New England Regional Genetics Group
P.O. Box 920288
Needham, MA 02492-4
781-444-0126
Fax: 781-444-0127
mfgnergg@verizon.net
www.nergg.org

Marinell Newtown, President
Jennifer Walsh, Secretary
Merrill Henderson, Treasurer
Mary Frances Garber, MS, CGC, Executive Director
New Englands primary network for collaborative exchange of genetic health information and education.

4879 Portland Public Library
5 Monument Sq
Portland, ME 04101-4072
207-871-1700
Fax: 207-871-1703
reference@portland.lib.me.us
portlandlibrary.com

Stephen J. Podgajny, Executive Director
Clare E. Hannan, Head of Finance and Operations
Linda Albert, Head of Human Resources
Linda Putnam, Head of Reference and Informatio
Summer reading programs, magnifiers, closed-circuit T.V., large-print photocopier, cassette books and magazines, children's books on cassette, home visits and other reference materials on blindness and other handicaps.

4880 Waterville Public Library
73 Elm Street
Waterville, ME 04901-6078
207-872-5433
Fax: 207-873-4779
wplhelpdesk@waterville.lib.me.us
www.watervillelibrary.org

Sarah Sugden, Executive Director
Marnie Terhune, President
William Grant, Treasurer
Cindy Jacobs, Secretary
Summer reading programs, Braille writer, magnifiers, closed-circuit T.V., large-print photocopier, cassette books and magazines, children's books on cassette, home visits and other reference materials on blindness and other handicaps.

Maryland

4881 Johns Hopkins University Dana Center for Preventive Ophthalmology
Wilmer Ophthalmology Institute
600 N Wolfe St
Wilmer Suite 122
Baltimore, MD 21287-9019
410-955-2777
Fax: 410-955-2542
boland@jhu.edu

Harry Quigley, Director
Emily W. . Gower, Ph.D, Director
Joanne . Katz, Sc.D, Director/Professor and Associate Chair
Oliver D. Schein, M.D., MPH, MBA, Director
Established in 1979, the Dana Center for Preventive Ophthalmology is dedicated to improving knowlege of risk factors for ocular disease and public health approaches to the prevention of these diseases and their ensuing visual impairment and blindness worldwide.

4882 Johns Hopkins University: Asthma and Allergy Center
5501 Hopkins Bayview Cir
Baltimore, MD 21224-6821
410-550-0545
Fax: 410-550-1733
jhuallergy@jhmi.edu
hopkins-arthritis.org

Lawrence Lichtenstein, Director
Studies of allergic diseases and individuals with allergic disease, pulmonary diseases and diseases involving inflammation and immunological processes.

4883 Maryland State Library for the Blind and Physically Handicapped
Maryland State Department of Education
415 Park Avenue
Baltimore, MD 21201-3603
410-230-2424
800-964-9209
Fax: 410-333-2095
TTY: 800-934-2541
referenc@lbph.lib.md.us

Jill Lewis, Manager
Diana Jarvis, Administrative Specialist
LaTarsha Wilson, Secretary
Provide comprehensive library services to the eligible blind and physically handicapped residents of the State of Maryland. The vision is to provide innovative and quality services to meet the needs and expectations of the patrons of Maryland.

4884 Montgomery County Department of Public Libraries/Special Needs Library
6400 Democracy Blvd
Bethesda, MD 20817-1638
240-777-0922
TTY: 301-897-2203
montgomerycountymd.gov

Susan F Cohen, Assistant Head Librarian
James Montgomery, Owner
Joseph Eagan, Branch Manager
Serves the library information and reading needs of people with disabilities, family members, students and service providers. Some of its services include books, periodicals, and videos on disability issues, adaptive technology, community information; the National Library for the Blind and Physically Handicapped Talking Book program; large print books; and computer room with adaptive technology.

4885 National Epilepsy Library (NEL)
Epilepsy Foundation
8301 Professional Pl
Landover, MD 20785-7223
866-330-2718
800-332-1000
Fax: 877-687-4878
ContactUs@efa.org
www.epilepsyfoundation.org

Marl A Finucane, Executive Vice President
Patty Dukes, Vice President Operations/Human
Mimi Browne, Director, HRSA programs
Chad Hartman, Director of Major Gifts
Contains information about epilepsy and seizure disorders and serves physicians and other health professionals. Provides in-house bibliographic database (ESDI), searches and documents delivery and interlibrary loans. Maintains the Albert and Ellen Grass Archives.

4886 National Federation of the Blind Jernigan Institute
200 E. Wells St.
at Jernigan Place
Baltimore, MD 21230
410-659-9314
Fax: 410-685-5653
nfb@nfb.org
nfb.org/programs-services

Anil Lewis, Executive Director, Blindness Initiatives
Cutting-edge research and training is conducted through the NFB Jernigan Institute to address the real problems of blindness, such as model education and rehabilitation methods to empower the

blind or improved instruction in Braille. The Jacobus tenBroek Library is also hosted at the NFB headquarters.

4887 **National Institute on Aging**
31 Center Dr, MSC 2292
Building 31, Room 5C27
Bethesda, MD 20892
800-222-2225
TTY: 800-222-4225
niaic@nia.nih.gov
www.nia.nih.gov

Luigi Ferrucci, M.D., Ph.D, Scientific Director
Patrick Shirdon, Director of Management
Michael O'Donnell, Chief Administrative Officer
The National Institute on Aging (NIA) is the primary Federal agency engaged in researching Alzheimer's disease.

4888 **National Rehabilitation Information Center (NARIC)**
8400 Corporate Drive
Suite 500
Landover, MD 20785-2245
301-459-5984
800-346-2742
Fax: 301-459-4263
TTY: 301-459-5984
naricinfo@heitechservices.com
www.naric.com

Mark X. Odum, Project Director
Natalie J. Collier, Library & Acquisitions Manager
Tamara J. Pyle, Library & Information Services Coordinator
NARIC is a federally-funded library and information center that focuses on disability and rehabilitation information.

4889 **Red Notebook**
Friends of Libraries for Deaf Action
2930 Craiglawn Rd
Silver Spring, MD 20904-1816
301-572-5168
Fax: 301-572-5168
TTY: 301-572-5168
folda86@aol.com

Alice L Hagemeyer, MLS, Founder/President
Merrie A. Davidson, Associate
Ricardo Lopez, MS, Associate
Joan Naturale, M.Ed, MLIS, Associate
A binder containing fact sheets, library reprints, announcements and other printed informational materials that are related to both deaf and library issues. It is designed to help build communication among individuals and groups within the deaf community. The focus is on assisting libraries in providing cost-effective and efficient library and information services to these consumers in a unbiased fashion.

4890 **Social Security Library**
U S Social Security Administration
6401 Security Blvd
Baltimore, MD 21235-6401
800-772-1213
TTY: 800-325-0778
www.socialsecurity.gov

Bill Vitek, Manager
Jo B Barnhart, Chief Executive Officer
Information on social security and disability insurance.

4891 **Trace Research and Development Center**
Univ. of Maryland, College of Information Studies
4130 Campus Dr.
College Park, MD 20742
301-405-2043
trace-info@umd.edu
trace.umd.edu

Kate Vanderheiden, Program Manager
Research focused on how standard information and communication technology products may be designed so that more people with disabilities can use them.

4892 **Warren Grant Magnuson Clinical Center**
National Institue Health
9000 Rockville Pike
Bethesda, MD 20892-1
301-496-2563
800-411-1222
Fax: 301-480-2984
TTY: 866-411-1010
prpl@mail.cc.nih.gov
www.cc.nih.gov

John I Gallin, MD, Clinical Center Director
Clare Hastings, PhD, RN, FAA, Chief Nurse Officer
Maureen E. Gormley, MPH, MA, RN, Chief Operating Officer
Maria D. Joyce, MBA, CPA, Chief Financial Officer
Established in 1953 as the research hospital of the National Institutes of Health. Designed so that patient care facilities are close to research laboratories so new findings of basic and clinical scientists can be quickly applied to the treatment of patients. Upon referral by physicians, patients are admitted to NIH clinical studies.

Massachusetts

4893 **Boston University Arthritis Center**
Boston University
715 Albany St
Boston, MA 02118-2526
617-638-4640
Fax: 617-638-5226
www.bumc.bu.edu

Karen Antman, Dean & Provost, Medical School
Meg Aranow, Director
Barbara A. Cole, Associate VP for Research Admin
Christopher Dorney, Director
The Arthritis Center focuses its educational, research and patient care efforts on the diagnosis and treatment of rheumatic diseases. These include the many forms of arthritis; the auto-immune diseases such as Scleroderma, Systemic Lupus, Erythematosus, Rheumatoid Arthritis; localized pain syndromes such as tendonitis, bursitis, and carpal tunnel syndrome; and metabolic bone disorders such as osteoporosis.

4894 **Boston University Center for Human Genetics**
840 Memorial Drive
Suite 101
Cambridge, MA 02139
617-638-7083
Fax: 617-638-7092
amilunsk@bu.edu
www.chginc.org

Aubrey Milunsky, Co-Director
Jeff Milunsky, M.D., F.A.C., Director of Clinical Genetics
Research and molecular diagnosis.

4895 **Boston University Robert Dawson Evans Memorial Dept. of Clinical Research**
75 East Newton St
Boston, MA 02118-2657
617-247-5019
Fax: 617-638-8728

Norman G Levinsky, Director
Jack Ansel, MD
Integral unit of the University Hospital specializing in arthritis and connective tissue studies.

4896 **Braille and Talking Book Library, Perkins School for the Blind**
175 North Beacon Street
Watertown, MA 02472-2751
617-972-3434
800-852-3133
Fax: 617-926-2027
Info@Perkins.org
www.perkins.org

Frederic M. Clifford, Chairman
Philip L. Ladd, Vice Chairman
Dave Power, CEO & President
Michael Schnitman, Secretary
The Braille and Talking Book Library loans Braille and recorded reading materials and the playback equipment necessary to use them. You are eligible for services if you are unable to read print due to a disability.

4897 **Brigham and Women's Hospital: Asthma and Allergic Disease Research Center**
75 Francis St
Boston, MA 02115-6110
617-732-5500
855-278-8010
Fax: 617-730-2858
arc@partners.org
Matthew H Liang, Director
Elizabeth G Nabel, President
Arthur Mombourquette, Vice President of Support Servic
Joel T. Katz, M.D., Director
Integral unit of the hospital focusing research attention on asthma and allergy related disorders.

4898 **Brigham and Women's Hospital: Robert B Brigham Multipurpose Arthritis Center**
Brigham and Women s Hospital
75 Francis St
Boston, MA 02115-6110
617-732-5500
855-278-8010
Fax: 617-432-0979
www.brighamandwomens.org
Matthew H Liang, Director
Elizabeth G Nabel, President
Arthur Mombourquette, Vice President of Support Servic
Joel T. Katz, M.D., Director
Research studies into arthritis and rheumatic diseases.

4899 **Caption Center**
Media Access Group at WGBH
One Guest St.
Boston, MA 02135
617-300-3600
Fax: 617-300-1020
access@wgbh.org
www.wgbh.org/caption
Pat McDonald, Director
The Caption Center was the world's first captioning agency providing access to television for viewers who are visually impaired and/or hard of hearing. The Center develops new solutions and uses closed captioning and descriptive video to promote access to technology .

4900 **Center for Interdisciplinary Research on Immunologic Diseases**
Childrens Hospital Medical Center
300 Longwood Avenue
Boston, MA 02115-5724
617-355-6000
800-355-7944
Fax: 617-355-0443
TTY: 617-730-0152
webteam@tch.harvard.edu
www.childrenshospital.org
Sandra L. Fenwick, President and Chief Executive Officer
Kevin Churchwell, MD, Executive Vice President
Dick Argys, Senior Vice President and Chief Administrative Officer
Jean Mixer, Vice President, Strategy
Organizational research unit of the Children's Hospital that focuses on the causes, prevention and treatments of asthma, infections and allergies.

4901 **Harvard University Howe Laboratory of Ophthalmology**
Massachusetts Eye & Ear Infirmary
243 Charles Street
Boston, MA 02114-3002
617-523-7900
Fax: 617-573-4380
TTY: 617-573-5498
richard.godfrey@schepens.harvard.edu
www.masseyeandear.org/
Wycliffe Grousbeck, Chairman
John Fernandez, President and CEO
Jonathan Uhrig, Treasurer
Lily H. Bentas, Secretary
Development ophthalmology and eye research.

4902 **Laboure College Library**
303 Adams Street
Dorchester Center, MA 02124-5698
617-296-8300
Fax: 617-296-7947
admissions@laboure.edu
laboure.edu
Andrew Callo, Manager
Maureen A. Smith, President
Offers information on physical disabilities, independent living, peer counseling and advocacy.

4903 **Massachusetts Rehabilitation Commission**
600 Washington Street
Boston, MA 02111
617-204-3603
800-245-6543
Fax: 617-727-1354
TTY: 800-245-6543
www.mass.gov/mrc
Elmer C Bartels, Commissioner
Deval L. Patrick, Governor
Timothy P. Murray, Lieutenant Governor
John Polanowicz, Secretary
Vacational Rehabilitation and Independent Living for people with disabilities.

4904 **Schepens Eye Research Institute**
20 Staniford Street
Boston, MA 02114-2508
617-912-0100
Fax: 617-912-0118
geninfo@vision.eri.harvard.edu
John Fernandez, President and CEO
Debra Rogers, Vice President for Ophthalmology
Alan A Ryan, Director Research Finance
Frances Ng, M.B.A., Director of Human Resources
Prominent center for research on eye, vision, and blinding diseases; dedicated to research that improves the understanding, management, and prevention of eye diseases and visual deficiencies; fosters collaboration among its faculty members; trains young scientists and clinicians from around the world; promotes communication with scientists in allied fields; leader in the worldwide dispersion of basic scientific knowledge of vision.

4905 **Talking Book Library at Worcester Public Library**
3 Salem Sq
Worcester, MA 01608-2015
508-799-1730
800-762-0085
Fax: 508-799-1676
www.worcpublib.org
James Izatt, Dept Head
Braille embosser, magnifiers, closed-circuit TV, adapted computers, cassette books and magazines, children's books on cassette, reference materials on blindness and other disabilities.

Michigan

4906 **Artificial Language Laboratory**
Michigan State University
220 Trowbridge Rd
East Lansing, MI 48824-1042
517-353-5940
Fax: 517-353-4766
finaid@msu.edu
www.msu.edu
Dr. John B Eulenberg, Phd, Director
Stephen R. Blosser, BSME, Technical Director
Shawn A. Miller, Laboratory Manager
Rebecca Ann Baird, Editor, Communication Outlook
Multidisciplinary research center in the Audiology & Speech Science department, Michigan State University. Its basic research program includes speech analysis and synthesis. Applied research is carried out on computer-based systems for persons who are blind and for persons with cerebral palsy and head injury. The laboratory develops physical, cognitive and linguistic assessment technology.

4907 **Burger School for the Autistic**
31735 Maplewood St.
Garden City, MI 48135-1993
734-793-1830
Fax: 734-762-8533
garden-city.lib.mi.us

James B Lenze, Library Director
Dan Lodge, Adult Librarian
Lindsay Fricke, Youth Librarian
Marti Boyn Tamaroglio, Library Aide

Burger school for students with autism is the largest public school in the United States that specializes in the education of students with autism.

4908 **Chi Medical Library**
Ingham Regional Medical Center
401 West Greenlawn
Lansing, MI 48910-2819
517-975-6000
irmc.org

Judy Barnes, Manager

Consumer health and patient education collection in books, videotapes, pamphlets. Open to the public.

4909 **Glaucoma Laser Trial**
Sinai Hospital of Detroit: Dept. of Opthalmology
31 Center Drive
Bethesda, MI 20892-2510
301-496-5248
kcl@nei.nih.gov
www.nei.nih.gov

Paul A. Sieving, M.D., Ph.D., Director

The purpose of the trial is to compare the safety and long-term efficacy of argon laser treatment of the trabecular meshwork with standard medical treatment for primary open-angle glaucoma.

4910 **Grand Traverse Area Library for the Blind and Physically Handicapped**
610 Woodmere Ave
Traverse City, MI 49686-3103
231-932-8500
877-931-8558
Fax: 231-932-8578
webmaster@tadl.tcnet.org
www.tadl.org

Metta Lansdale, Library Director
Thomas Kachadurian, President
Jason Gillman, Vice President
Jerry Beasley, Secretary

The LBPH was established as a sub-regional library in 1972 and currently provides services for 783 registered individuals in 16 counties, 171 of these registrants are Grand Traverse County residents. Anyone unable to read regular printed materials because of visual or physical limitations may be eligible.

4911 **Kent District Library for the Blind and Physically Handicapped**
814 West River Center Dr. NE
Comstock Park, MI 49321-3420
616-784-2007
877-243-2466
Fax: 616-336-3256
WyomingYouthStaff@kdl.org
www.kdl.org

Charles R Myers, Chair
Vickie Hoekstra, Vice Chair
Carol Simpson, Secretary
Lance Werner, Director

Summer reading programs, Braille writer, magnifiers, large-print photocopier, cassette books and magazines, children's books on cassette, and other reference materials on blindness and other handicaps.

4912 **Macomb Library for the Blind & Physically Handicapped**
40900 Romeo Plank
Clinton Township, MI 48038-1132
586-226-5020
800-203-5274
Fax: 586-286-0634
mlbph@cmpl.org
www.cmpl.org

Larry Neal, Library Director
Fred L. Gibson, Jr., President
Peter M. Ruggirello, Vice Chairman
Barbara S. Brown, Treasurer

Braille writer, closed-circuit T.V., large-print books, cassette books and magazines, children's books on cassette, other reference materials on blindness and other handicaps, descriptive videos and bifokal kits. Assistive technology including JAWS, Zoomtext, OpenBook, and Duxbury.

4913 **Michigan Braille and Talking Book Library**
P.O. Box 30007
702 W. Kalamazoo St
Lansing, MI 48909-7507
517-373-5614
800-992-9012
Fax: 517-373-5865
btbl@michigan.gov
www.michigan.gov/btbl

Sue Chinault, Manager

Provides library service to people with visual or physical disabilities that are unable to utilize standard print materials. Digital book cartridges (audio books) and/or Braille books are sent directly to the patron's home, completely free of charge. This program is available to all Michigan residents.

4914 **Michigan Library for the Blind and Physically Handicapped**
Genesee District Library
G-4195 Pasadena Rd.
Flint, MI 48504
810-732-1120
866-732-1120
fun@thegdl.org
www.thegdl.org/services/talking-book-center

William Delaney, Chair
David Conklin, Director
Amy Goldyn, Finance Manager
Jerilyn Klich, Human Resources Manager

Offers Genesee County residents with visual or physical impairments a service allowing them to borrow talking books application through the Talking Book Center.

4915 **Michigan's Assistive Technology Resource**
Physically Impaired Association of Michigan
1023 S Us Highway 27
Saint Johns, MI 48879-2423
989-224-0333
800-274-7426
Fax: 989-224-0330
www.cenmi.org

Jeff Diedrich, Manager
Maryann Jones, Coordinator
Barbara Warren, Information Specialist

Provides information services, support materials, technical assistance, and training to local and intermediate school districts in michigan to increase their capacity to address the needs of students with disabilities for assistive technology.

4916 **Mideastern Michigan Library Co-op**
503 S Saginaw St
Suite 711
Flint, MI 48502
810-232-7119
800-641-6639
Fax: 810-232-6639
dhooks@mmlc.info
www.mmlc.info

Denise Hooks, Director
Irene Bancroft, Administrative Specialist

Provides resources and supports for member libraries in the areas of funding, advocacy, educational opportunities for librarians and networking with other libraries. Its members include Library for the Blind and Physically Handicapped, and Braille and Talking Book Library.

4917 **Muskegon Area District Library for the Blind and Physically Handicapped**
4845 Airline Rd
Unit 5
Muskegon, MI 49444-4503
231-737-6248
877-569-4801
Fax: 231-737-6307
TTY: 231-722-4103
madl.org

Stephen Dix, Director
Richard Schneider, Assistant Director
Brenda Hall, Business Manager
Michele Wittkopp, Youth Services Coordinator

Braille typewriter, magnifiers, closed-circuit TV, large-print photocopier, cassette books and magazines, children's books on cassette, home visits and other reference materials on blindness and other handicaps, The Reading Edge, and large print books.

4918 **Northland Library Cooperative**
Library Cooperative/ Library for the blind
220 W. Clinton St.
Charlevoix, MI 49720 231-855-2206
www.nlc.lib.mi.us

Jennifer Dean, Director
Christine Johnston, Executive Director
Roger Mendel, Director
Summer reading programs, Braille writer, magnifiers, closed-circuit TV, large-print photocopier, cassette books and magazines, children's books on cassette and other reference materials on blindness and other handicaps.

4919 **Oakland County Library for the Visually & Physically Impaired**
1200 N Telegraph Rd
Pontiac, MI 48341-1032 248-858-5050
800-774-4542
Fax: 248-858-1153
TTY: 248-452-2247
www.oakgov.com/lvpi

Dave Conklin, Manager
The Oakland County Library for the Visually and Physically Impaired was established in 1974 to provide access to free library service for County residents who are unable to read standard printed material because of a visual impairment or physical limitation.

4920 **St. Clair County Library Special Technologies Alternative Resources (S.T.A.R.)**
210 McMorran Blvd
Port Huron, MI 48060-4014 810-982-3600
800-272-8570
Fax: 810-982-3600
TTY: 810-455-0200
www.sccl.lib.mi.us/LBPH.aspx

Arnold H. Larson, Chairperson
Arlene M. Marcetti, Trustee
Kathleen J. Wheelihan, Trustee
Laurie Crisenbery, Trustee
Offers library services to the blind, deaf and blind, visually disabled, phsyically disabled, and reading disabled.

4921 **University of Michigan: Orthopaedic Research Laboratories**
1500 E. Medical Center Drive
Ann Arbor, MI 48109 734-936-6641
800-211-8181
Fax: 734-647-0003
www.med.umich.edu

Steve Goldstein, Lab Director
Paul Castillo, C.P.A., Chief Financial Officer
Michael ME Johns, M.D., Interim Executive Vice President for Medical Affairs
Quinta Vreede, Chief Administrative Officer,
Develops and studies the causes and treatments for arthritis including new devices and assistive aids.

4922 **Upper Peninsula Library for the Blind**
1615 Presque Isle Ave
Marquette, MI 49855-2811 906-228-7697
800-562-8985
Fax: 906-228-5627
TTY: 906-228-7697
webmaster@uproc.lib.mi.us
www.uplibraries.org

Suzanne Dees, Executive Director
Summer reading programs, Braille writer, magnifiers, closed-circuit T.V., large-print photocopier, cassette books and magazines, children's books on cassette, home visits and other reference materials on blindness and other handicaps.

4923 **Washtenaw County Library for the Blind & Physically Handicapped**
P.O. Box 8645
Ann Arbor, MI 48107-8645 734-222-6860
Fax: 734-222-6803
ewashtenaw.org

Mary Udoji, Manager
Michigan Subregional Library, Library of Congress National Library Service network. General library service for persons unable to use standard print materials for various physical reasons. Lends audio books and listening equipment, large type books, descriptive videos. Provides reference information and programs. Kurzweil scanner with components which convert standard print to Braille, large type or audio and closed circuit TV magnifier on site.

4924 **Wayne County Regional Library for the Blind**
30555 Michigan Ave
Westland, MI 48186-5310 734-727-7300
888-968-2737
Fax: 734-727-7333
TTY: 734-727-7330

Vanessa Morris, Regional Librarian
Sue Steiger, Librarian
Rebecca Farmer, Student Intern
Mariya Webb, Student Intern
Summer reading programs, Braille writer, magnifiers, closed-circuit T.V., large-print photocopier, cassette books and magazines, children's books on cassette, and other reference materials on blindness and other handicaps.

4925 **Wayne State University: CS Mott Center for Human Genetics and Development**
42. W. Warren Avenue
Detroit, MI 48202-1405 313-577-1485
Fax: 313-577-8554
rsokol@med.wayne.edu
www.media.wayne.edu

Robert Sokol, Director
Matthew Lockwood, Director of Communications
Tom Reynolds, Associate Director of Public Relations
Mike Brinich, Associate Director of Communicaitons
Human growth and development disorders.

Minnesota

4926 **Century College**
3300 Century Ave North
White Bear Lake, MN 55110-1252 651-779-3300
800-228-1978
Fax: 651-779-3417
TTY: 651-773-1715
century.edu

Dr. Ron Anderson, President
Steven Ritt, Vice President
Harold M. Johnson, Treasurer
Ralph Olsen, Jr., Secretary
Programs of study - Orthotic Practitioner, Orthotic Technician, Prosethetic Practitioner, Prosthetic Technician. In addition, Century College offers more than 50 other programs in liberal arts, career and occupational programs.

4927 **Communication Center/Minnesota State Services for the Blind**
Services for the Blind
332 Minnesota Street
Suite 200
Saint Paul, MN 55101-1351 651-642-0500
800-652-9000
Fax: 651-649-5927
DEED.CustomerService@state.mn.us
www.mnssb.org

Katie Clark Sieben, Commissioner
Brian Allie, Chief Information Officer
Kim Babine, Director Government Affairs
Richard Strong, Executive Director
Special library service for the blind and physically handicapped providing tape and Braille transcription of textbooks and voca-

tional materials; Minnesota Radio Talking Book providing current newspaper, magazines and best selling books; Dial-in-News, a touch tone phone accessed newspaper service; Library of Congress cassette and phonograph talking book equipment; repair services for special audio reading equipment, with most services free to Minnesota Residents.

4928 **Duluth Public Library**
520 W Superior St
Duluth, MN 55802-1578
218-730-4200
Fax: 218-723-3822
www.duluth.lib.mn.us

Carla Powers, Library Manager
Renee Zurn, Digital & Outreach Manager
Davis Ouse, Public Services Manager
Dave Lull, Technical Services Manager

Main library computer lab contains one Sorenson Relay and accessibility computer with zoom text JAWS software.

4929 **Minnesota Library for the Blind and Physically Handicapped**
Department of Education
1500 Highway 36 West
Roseville, MN 55113
651-582-8200
800-722-0550
Fax: 507-333-4832
charlene.briner@state.mn.us
education.state.mn.us

Catherine A. Durivage, Manager
Rene Perrance, Librarian
Charlene Briner, Chief of Staff
Dr. Brenda Cassellius, Commissioner

Provides books and magazines in Braille, large print, records, and cassettes to qualified residents of Minnesota who have a visual or physical impairment, including reading disabilities due to an organic cause certified by a medical doctor, that prevents residents from reading standard print or physically handling a book. Equipment for in-house use include magnifiers, Braillers, listening equipment, and CCTV. Reference collection for in-house use only on visual impairment topics.

4930 **Special U**
University of Minnesota
P.O. Box 721-Umhc
Minneapolis, MN 55455
612-625-3846
800-276-8642
Fax: 612-624-0997
kdwb-var@umn.edu

Mississippi

4931 **Blind and Physically Handicapped Library Services**
Mississippi Library Commission
3881 Eastwood Dr
Jackson, MS 39211-6473
601-432-4492
877-594-5733
Fax: 601-432-4478
mlcref@mlc.lib.ms.us
www.mlc.lib.ms.us

Shellie Zeigler, BPHLS Director
Christy Williams, Director of Administrative Services Bureau
Gloria Washington, Public Relations Director
Jennifer Walker, Director of Development Services Bureau

BPHLS serves as the MS Regional Library for the Library of Congress, NLS for the Blind and Physically Handicapped. Book collections include audio cassette, CDs, digital books, Braille, large print, children's 18-20 point large print, and standard print reference collection. Descriptive videos, magazines in Braille or on cassette are available, as well as equipment: adaptive workstation, Braille embosser, closed-circuit TV, magnifier, speech input/output, and more. Check for eligibility.

4932 **Mississippi Library Commission**
3881 Eastwood Dr
Jackson, MS 39211-6473
601-432-4111
800-647-7542
Fax: 601-354-4181
TTY: 601-354-6411
mslib@mlc.lib.ms.us
www.mlc.lib.ms.us/index.html

Susan Cassagne, Executive Director
Katherine Buntin, Senior Library Consultant
Tracy Carr, Library Services Bureau Director
David Collins, Grant Program Director

Summer reading programs, Braille writer, magnifiers, closed-circuit T.V., large-print photocopier, cassette books and magazines, children's books on cassette, home visits and other reference materials on blindness and other handicaps.

4933 **Mississippi Library Commission\Talking Book and Braille Services**
3881 Eastwood Dr
Jackson, MS 39211-6473
601-432-4111
800-446-0892
Fax: 601-354-4181
mslib@mlc.lib.ms.us

Susan Cassagne, Executive Director
Katherine Buntin, Senior Library Consultant
Tracy Carr, Library Services Bureau Director
David Collins, Grant Program Director

Library service for the print handicapped Braille, cassette and disc materials (books & periodicals) for children and adults. Large print RG production (copier & printer), Braille embosser and other handicaps.

Missouri

4934 **Assemblies of God Center for the Blind**
1445 N Boonville Ave
Springfield, MO 65802-1894
417-862-2781
855-642-2011
Fax: 417-863-6614
www.blind.ag.org

Paul Weingartner, Director
Caryl Weingartner, Office Administrator
Sarah Sykes, Certified Braille Transcriber
Sharron Stevens, Librarian

Offers Braille and electronic text lending library, Sunday School materials for all ages, Braille and audio periodicals, resource assistance, and resources for blind children and children of blind parents. Children's Braille books with tactile graphics are also avaiable for purchase or loan, as well as books in digital media for adaptive reading services.

4935 **Church of the Nazarene**
Nazarene Publishing House
P.O. Box 843116
Kansas City, MO 64184-3116
816-333-7000
800-877-0700
Fax: 800-849-9827
it@nazarene.org
www.nazarene.org

Dr.Eugenio R Duarte, Board of General Superintendents
Dr.Jerry D. Porter, Board of General Superintendents
Dr. David A Busic, Board of General Superintendents
Dr. David W. Graves, Board of General Superintendents

Offers Braille and large print books. Also offers a lending library and cassettes for the blind.

4936 **Judevine Center for Autism**
1333 W Lockwood Avenue
Saint Louis, MO 63132-3252
314-432-6200
800-780-6545
Fax: 888-507-4453
judevine@judevine.org
www.judevine.org

Becky Blackwell, President

Evaluations and assessments, parent and professional training programs, consultations, workshops, seminars, family support, clinical therapies, adult programs and support, residential services.

4937 **Lutheran Blind Mission**
7550 Watson Rd
Saint Louis, MO 63119-4409 314-918-0415
888-215-2455
Fax: 314-963-0738
blind.mission@blindmission.org
Sherry Lambing, Manager
Dave Andrus, Executive Director
Nancy Crawford, Manager
Offers Christian books in Braille and large print books and cassettes for the blind and visually impaired, on loan, as well as Christian periodicals in Braille, large print and cassette tape.

4938 **University of Missouri: Columbia Arthritis Center**
University of Missouri
1 Hospital Dr
Columbia, MO 65212-1 573-882-4141
Fax: 573-884-3996
www.muhealth.org
James Ross, Chief Executive Officer
Mitch Wasden, Chief Operating Officer
Anita Larsen, Chief Nurse Executive
Jeri Doty, Chief Planning Officer
Research into arthritis and rheumatic diseases. One of the most comprehensive health-care networks in Missouri, our 5 hospitals and numerous clinics, all staffed by University Physicians, offer the finest primary, secondary, and tertiary health-care services. We also provide education for future health-care providers and participate in important research.

4939 **Wolfner Talking Book & Braille Library**
Secretary State Office
600 West Main Street
PO Box 387
Jefferson City, MO 65101-387 573-751-4936
800-392-2614
Fax: 573-526-2985
TTY: 800-347-1379
wolfner@sos.mo.gov
www.sos.mo.gov/wolfner/
Richard J Smith, Division Director
Paul Mathews, Reader Advisor, A-CO
Brandon Kempf, Reader Advisor, CP-G & Wi-Z
Virginia Ryan, Reader Advisor, H-L
Wolfner Library provides reading material for Missouri State residents unable to read standard print due to a visual or physical disability. Book formats are recorded books on digital cartridge and cassette, Braille and some childrens books in large print. Wolfner Library also lends out descriptive videos, playback equipment for the cartridges and cassettes are also on loan.

Montana

4940 **MonTECH**
029 McGill Hall
University of Montana
Missoula, MT 59803 406-243-5751
877-243-5511
montech@ruralinstitute.umt.edu
montech.ruralinstitute.umt.edu
Kathy Laurin PhD, Project Director
Chris Clasby MSW MATP, Project Coordinator
James Poelstra MA, Info Technology Specialist
Specializing in Assistive Technology and oversee a variety of AT related grants and contracts. The overall goal is to develop a comprehensive, statewide system of assistive technology related assistance. Striving to ensure that all people in Montana with disabilities have equitable access to assistive technology devices and services in order to enhance their independence, productivity and quality of life.

4941 **Montana State Library-Talking Book Library**
1515 East 6th Ave
P.O. Box 201800
Helena, MT 59620-1800 406-444-2064
800-332-5087
Fax: 406-444-0266
TTY: 406-444-4799
mtbl@mt.gov
msl.mt.gov/talking_book_library
Christie Briggs, Regional Librarian/Supervisor
Erin Harris, Director Recording and Volunteer Programs
Carolyn Meier, Library Clerk/Circulation
Martin Landry, Readers' Advisor
The Library offers FREE alternative audio and Braille reading materials for Montana citizens who cannot read standard print materials because of a visual, physical or reading handicap. Over 50,000 titles on 4-track cassette, WebBraille, Web0pac, WebBlud, summer reading programs, Braille writer, magnifiers, closed-circuit T.V., large-print photocopier, cassette books and magazines, children's books on cassette, home visits and other reference materials on blindness and other handicaps.

Nebraska

4942 **Nebraska Assistive Technology Partnership Nebraska Department of Education**
Ste C
5143 S 48th St
Lincoln, NE 68516-2261 402-471-0734
888-806-6287
888-806-6287
Fax: 402-471-6052
TTY: 402-471-0734
nlc.nebraska.gov/tbbs/
Steve Miller, Manager
Lilly Blase, Program Coordinator
Provides statewide assistive technology and home modification services for Nebraskans of all ages and disabilities.

4943 **Nebraska Library Commission: Talking Book and Braille Service (TBBS)**
Talking Book and Braille Service
1200 N St
Suite 120
Lincoln, NE 68508-2023 402-471-4038
800-742-7691
Fax: 402-471-6244
nlc.readadv@nebraska.gov
nlc.nebraska.gov/tbbs
David Oertli, Executive Director
Kay Goehring, Reader Services Coordinator
Bill Ainsley, Audio Production Studio Manager
Scott Scholz, Circulation & Audio Prod. Coor.
Provides eligible users with free audio books, audio magazines and Braille via the mail. Also features in-house studios for audiobook production.

Nevada

4944 **Las Vegas-Clark County Library District**
7060 W. Windmill Lane
Las Vegas, NV 89113 702-734-7323
Fax: 702-507-6187
www.lvccld.org
Keiba Crear, Chair
Michael Saunders, Vice Chair
Randy Ence, Secretary
Ydoleena Yturralde, Treasurer
Summer reading programs, Braille writer, magnifiers, closed-circuit T.V., large-print photocopier, cassette books and magazines, children's books on cassette, home visits and other reference materials on blindness and other handicaps.

4945 **Nevada State Library and Archives**
100 North Stewart Street
Carson City, NV 89701-4285 775-684-3313
800-922-2880
Fax: 775-684-3330

Michael Fischer, Director
Ann Brinkmeyer, Head of Government Publications
Kathy Edwards, Government Publications Libraria
Sherry Glick, Library Assistant
Summer reading programs, Braille writer, magnifiers, closed-circuit T.V., large-print photocopier, cassette books and magazines, children's books on cassette, home visits and other reference materials on blindness and other handicaps.

New Hampshire

4946 **New Hampshire State Library: Talking Book Services**
117 Pleasant St
Concord, NH 03301-3852 603-271-3429
800-491-4200
Fax: 603-271-8370
TTY: 800-735-2964
michael.york@dcr.nh.gov
www.nh.gov/nhsl/talking_books

Michael York, State Librarian
Janet Eklund, Administrator of Library Operations
Donna Gilbreth, Supervisor
Marilyn Stevenson, Supervisor
Regional Library for National Library Service for the Blind & Physically Handicapped offers digital and cassette books, magazines on cassette, children's books on digital and on cassette, descriptive videos, playaways, and downloadable digital audio books, and Braille services.

New Jersey

4947 **Autism New Jersey**
500 Horizon Dr.
Suite 530
Robbinsville, NJ 08691 609-588-8200
800-4AU-TISM
Fax: 609-588-8858
information@autismnj.org
www.autismnj.org

Suzanne Buchanan, Executive Director
Ellen Schisler, Associate Executive Director
Elena Graziosi, Manager of Information Services
Autism New Jersey is the largest statewide network of parents and professionals dedicated to improving lives of individuals with autism spectrum disorders. Self-advocates, families, the professionals who work with them, government officials, the media, and concerned state residents all turn to Autism New Jersey for information, compassionate support, and training.

4948 **Children's Specialized Hospital Medical Library - Parent Resource Center**
200 Somerset St.
New Brunswick, NJ 08901 888-244-5373
www.childrens-specialized.org

Warren E. Moore, President & CEO
Charles Chianese, Vice President & Chief Operating Officer
Joseph J. Dobosh Jr., Vice President & Chief Financial Officer
Matthew B. McDonald III, Vice President & Chief Medical Officer
Contains some 3,000 books, and journals specializing in nursing, pediatrics, child neurology, and rehabilitation. Also provides a Parent Resource Center, a special collection of books, videos and pamphlets designed to meet the information needs of parents and families, as well as the local community.

4949 **Christopher & Dana Reeve Foundation**
636 Morris Turnpike
Suite 3A
Short Hills, NJ 07078 973-379-2690
800-225-0292
Fax: 973-912-9433
infospecialist@christopherreeve.org
www.christopherreeve.org

John M Hughes, Chairman
John E McConnell, Vice Chairman
Peter Wilderotter, President & CEO
Maggie Goldberg, Vice President, Policy & Programs
A national clearinghouse for information, referral and educational materials on paralysis. The foundation also offers a free book titled 'Paralysis Resource Guide' in English or Spanish, as well as a free library.

4950 **Eye Institute of New Jersey**
New Jersey Medical School
Suite 6100
PO Box 1709
Newark, NJ 07101-1709 973-972-2065
Fax: 973-972-2068

Jacinta Ogbonna, Administrative director
Department A
Tatiana Forofonova, Program Coordinator
Ophthamology, including research into cornea, retina and neuro-ophthamalogy.

4951 **Mycoclonus Research Foundation**
Apt 17d
200 Old Palisade Rd
Fort Lee, NJ 7024-7060 201-585-0770
Fax: 201-585-0770
http://www.pspinformation.com/index.html

Mark Seiden, VP
Supports clinical and basic research into the cause and treatment of myoclonus; four international workshops facilitated the sharing of information by physicians, scientists, and investigators active in the field, resulted in three publications; supports promising research projects, clinical neurological fellows, with special emphasis on posthypoxic myoclonus and encourages all who are interested in futhering the understanding, treatment, and cure of myoclonus.

4952 **New Jersey Library for the Blind and Handicapped**
2300 Stuyvesant Ave
Trenton, NJ 8618-3226 609-530-4000
800-792-8322
Fax: 609-406-7181
TTY: 609-530-4000
tbbc@njstatelib.org
njlbh.org

Adam Szczepaniak, Director
Maria Baratta, Assistant Director
Information Technology
Summer reading programs, Braille writer, magnifiers, closed-circuit T.V., large-print, cassette, Braille books and magazines, children's books on cassette, and other reference materials on blindness and other handicaps. Provides reading material on audio, cassette, large print and Braille to eligible NJ residents.

New Mexico

4953 **New Mexico State Library for the Blind and Physically Handicapped**
1209 Camino Carlos Rey
Santa Fe, NM 87507-4400 505-476-9700
1 -0 -6 5
Fax: 505-476-9776
TTY: 800-659-4915
lbph@state.nm.us
www.nmstatelibrary.org

David L. Caffey, Chairperson
Norice Lee, Vice Chairperson
Eugene Gant, Public Education Department Appointee
Dean Smith, Professional Member

Summer reading programs, Braille writer, magnifiers, closed-circuit T.V., large-print photocopier, cassette books and magazines, children's books on cassette, home visits and other reference materials on blindness and other handicaps.

New York

4954 Andrew Heiskell Braille and Talking Book Library
New York Public Library
40 W 20th St
New York, NY 10011-4211
212-206-5400
Fax: 212-206-5418
TTY: 212-206-5458
ahlbph@nypl.org
www.nypl.org/locations/heiskell

Tony Marx, President and CEO
Mary Lee Kennedy, Chief Library Officer
Anne L. Coriston, Vice President for Public Service
Jeff Roth, Vice President for Finance and Strategy
The library provides talking books and talking book players to the five boroughs of New York City, and Braille books to New York City and Long Island. These items may be circulated in person or through the mail without charge to the borrower. Deposit collections may be arranged with agencies that provide service to people with visual impairments. The library also circulates large print books and materials in other formats.

4955 Center on Human Policy: School of Education
Syracuse University
302 Huntington Hall
Syracuse, NY 13244
315-443-3851
800-894-0826
Fax: 315-443-4338
thechp@syr.edu
thechp.syr.edu

Alan Foley, Director
The Center on Human Policy is an organization that works to ensure the rights of people with disabilities. This is accomplished through research, teaching, and advocacy in policy.

4956 DREAMMS for Kids
190 Whispering Oaks Dr
Longs, SC 29568-6973
607-539-3027
Fax: 607-539-9930
janet@dreamms.org
www.dreamms.org

Janet Hosmer, Executive Director
DREAMMS is committed to increasing the use of computers, high quality instructional technology, and assistive technologies for students with special needs in schools, homes and the workplace.

4957 Ehrman Medical Library
New York University Medical Center
577 First Avenue
Room 117
New York, NY 10016-6402
212-263-5394
Fax: 212-263-6534
HSL_admin@nyumc.org
hsl.med.nyu.edu

N. Rambo, Chair/Director
D. Peters, Executive Assistant
N. Romanosky, Department

Administrator
J. Williams, Associate Director

Our mission of the Fredrick L. Ehrman Library is to enhance learning, research and patient care and New York University Medical Center by effectively managing knowledge-based resources, providing client-centered information services and education, and extending access through new initiatives in information technology.

4958 Finger Lakes Developmental Disabilities Service Office
44 Holland Avenue
Albany, NY 12229-0001
518-474-3625
866-946-9733
Fax: 585-461-8764
opwdd.ny.gov/

Mike Feeney, Director
Carolyn Bassett, Manager
Andrew M Cuomo, Governor
Information on developmental disabilities.

4959 Helen Keller International
Fl 12
352 Park Ave S
New York, NY 10010-1723
212-532-0544
877-535-5374
Fax: 212-532-6014
info@hki.org
hki.org

Henry C. Barkhorn III, Chairman
Desmond G. FitzGerald, Vice Chairman
Mary Crawford, Secretary
Nonprofit international organization whose mission is to combat the causes and consequences of blindness and malnutrition.

4960 Helen Keller National Center for Deaf - Blind Youths And Adults
141 Middle Neck Rd
Sands Point, NY 11050-1218
516-944-8900
Fax: 516-944-7302
TTY: 516-944-8637
hkncinfo@hknc.org
www.hknc.org

Joseph McNulty, Executive Director
HKNC is the only national vocational and rehabilitation program providing services exclusively to youth and adults who are deaf-blind.

4961 Institute for Basic Research in Developmental Disabilities
1050 Forest Hill Rd
Staten Island, NY 10314-6399
718-494-0600
Fax: 718-698-3803
ibr@opwdd.ny.gov
opwdd.ny.gov

Khalid Iqbal, Department Chairman
Joseph J Maturi, Acting Director
Wojciech Kaczmarski, Research Scientist
Maureen Marlow, Editor, Grants Manager, Communications
The Institute for Basic Research in Developmental Disabilities offers services to New Yorkers with developmental disabilities. Services include research, clinical studies, education, publications, employment supports and more.

4962 Institute for Visual Sciences
221 E 71st St
New York, NY 10021-4139
212-517-0400
Fax: 212-472-0295
www.mmm.edu/

Judson R. Shaver, Ph.D., President
Paul Ciraulo, Executive Vice President for Administration and Finance
Carol L Jackson, Vice President for Student Affairs and Dean of Students
David Podell, Vice President for Academic Affairs & Dean of the Faculty
Ophthalmology with emphasis on the development of care for the eye.

4963 JGB Cassette Library International
15 W 65th St
New York, NY 10023-6601
212-769-6200
800-284-4422
Fax: 212-769-6266
www.guildhealth.org

Jerry Bechhofer, President
Summer reading programs, Braille writer, magnifiers, closed-circuit T.V., large-print photocopier, cassette books and magazines, children's books on cassette, home visits and other reference materials on blindness and other handicaps.

4964 **Nassau Library System**
900 Jerusalem Ave
Uniondale, NY 11553-3097
516-292-8920
Fax: 516-565-0950
outreach@nassaulibrary.org
nassaulibrary.org

Ken Ulric, President
Barbara Behrens, Vice President
Kathy Seyfried, Treasurer
Joe Carroll, Secretary
Information about public library services in Nassau County, including services for people with disabilities and the Senior Connections volunteer project (information and referral for seniors and their families).

4965 **National Braille Association**
95 Allens Creek Road
95 Allens creek road
Suite 202
Rochester, NY 14618
585-427-8260
Fax: 585-427-0263
nbaoffice@nationalBraille.org
www.nationalBraille.org

David Shaffer, Executive Director
Jan Carroll, President
Cindi Laurent, Vice President
Heidi Lehmann, Secretary
Only national organization dedicated to the professional development of individuals who prepare and produce Braille materials.

4966 **New York State Talking Book & Braille Library**
New York State Library and Education
Cultural Education Center
222 Madison Avenue
Albany, NY 12230-1
518-474-5930
800-342-3688
Fax: 518-474-5786
tbbl@mail.nysed.gov

Loretta Ebert, Research library director
Lends audio and Braille books and specialized playback equipment to eligible borrowers with print disabilities. Service is completely free. Serves 55 counties of upstate NY (Westchester and above). Also provides service to schools, nursing homes, and other facilities.

4967 **Postgraduate Center for Mental Health**
124 E 28th St
New York, NY 10016-8402
212-576-4150
Fax: 212-696-1679
www.dvguide.com/newyork/postgrad.html

Marge Slobetz, Assistant Director
Marie Serrano, Manager
Evaluations and psychotherapy by social workers psychologists for children, adolescents, families and couples. Neuropsychological testing and remedation for learning disabilities.

4968 **Rehabilitation Research Library**
Human Resources Center
Albertson, NY 11507
516-741-2010
Fax: 516-746-3298

Amnon Tishler, Research Librarian
Susan Feifer, Manager
Information on rehabilitation and occupational rehabilitation.

4969 **State University of New York Health Sciences Center**
450 Clarkson Avenue
Brooklyn, NY 11203-2098
718-270-1000
Fax: 718-778-5397
www.downstate.edu

Meg O'Sullivan, Assistant Vice President
Jennifer Hayes, Staff Assistant
Child psychiatry research programs.

4970 **Suffolk Cooperative Library System: Long Island Talking Book Library**
Long Island Talking Book Library System
2 Penn Plaza
Suite 1102
New York, NY 10121
212-502-7600
888-545-8331
Fax: 631-286-1647
TTY: 631-286-4546
communications@afb.net
www.afb.org

Carl R Augusto, President & CEO
Kelly Bleach, Chief Administrative Officer
Rick Bozeman, Chief Financial Officer
Robin Vogel, Vice President Resource Development
Offers a variety of support services to its 55 member libraries and other patrons including, an extensive talking book program, assistive technology and other services for people with disabilities.

4971 **United Spinal Association**
75-20 Astoria Blvd
Suite 120
East Elmhurst, NY 11370
718-803-3782
800-444-0120
Fax: 718-803-0414
mkurtz@unitedspinal.org
www.unitedspinal.org

James Weisman, President & CEO
Abby Ross, COO
Information on spinal cord injury and laws and regulations concerning people with disabilities, including veterans.

4972 **Wallace Memorial Library**
Rochester Institute Of Technology
90 Lomb Memorial Dr
Rochester, NY 14623-5603
585-475-2551
Fax: 585-475-7220
TTY: 585-475-2760
twc@rit.edu
wallacecenter.rit.edu

Lynn Wild, Associate Provost for Faculty Development
Shirley Bower, Director RIT Libraries
Julia Lisuzzo, Director of TWC Administration
Steven Wunrow, Director of RIT Production Services
Information on physical disabilities and deafness.

4973 **Xavier Society for the Blind**
Two Penn Plaza,
Suite 1102
New York, NY 10121-4595
212-473-7800
800-637-9193
Fax: 212-473-7801
info@xaviersocietyfortheblind.org
www.xaviersocietyfortheblind.org

Fr. John Sheehan, SJ, Chairman of the Board / CEO
Fr. Claudio Burgaleta, SJ, Vice-President
Mr. Victor Gainor, Secretary
Ms.Margaret O'Brien, Operations Manager
Provides spiritual and inspirational reading material to visually impaired persons in suitable format: Braille, large print and cassette, throughout U.S. and Canada. Services are provided both by way of regular periodical publications sent through the mail and non-returnable; and by means of a lending library where books are returned. All services are provided free.

North Carolina

4974 **Genova Diagnostics**
63 Zillicoa St.
Asheville, NC 28801
828-253-0621
800-522-4762
info@gdx.net
www.gdx.net

Jeffrey Ledford, Chief Executive Officer
Craig Thiel, Chief Financial Officer
Jeff Ellis, Chief Commercial Officer
Ceco Ivanov, Chief Information Officer

Genova Diagnostics specializes in nutritional, metabolic, and toxicant analyses. Genova is committed to helping health care professionals identify nutritional influences on health and disease, and laboratory procedures in nutritional and biochemical testing.

1984

4975 **North Carolina Library for the Blind and Physically Handicapped**

109 East Jones Street
Raleigh, NC 27635-1
919-807-7450
888-388-2460
Fax: 919-733-6910
TTY: 919-733-1462
nclbph@ncdcr.gov

Francine Martin, Manager
Carl Ginger Rush, Secretary
James Benton, President
Dennis Thurman, Vice president

Free loan of large print, Braille, and cassette tape books and magazines and specialized playback equipment to registered eligible North Carolinians. Call for an application form. Collection contains general fiction and nonfiction titles. Registered borrowers may subscribe to receive descriptive videos for a one time fee.

4976 **Pediatric Rheumatology Clinic**

Duke Medical Center
P.O. Box 3212
Durham, NC 27708-3212
919-684-8111
Fax: 919-684-6616
rabin001@mc.duke.edu
www.duke.edu

Rebecca H. Buckley, Medical Director
Michael Duke, Owner

Clinical and laboratory pediatric rheumatoid studies.

4977 **University of North Carolina at Chapel Hill: Neuroscience Research Building**

115 Mason Farm Road
Chapel Hill, NC 27599-7250
919-843-8536
Fax: 919-966-9605
www.med.unc.edu/ophth/

Ricky D. Bass, MBA, MHA, Associate Chair for Administration
Sandy Scarlett, Development Director
Cassandra J. Barnhart, MPH, Manager of Research Administration

An interdepartmental research center on the campus of the UNC-Chapel Hill School of Medicine. Mission is to promote neuroscience research with specific emphasis on developmental, cellular, and disease-related processes.

North Dakota

4978 **North Dakota State Library Talking Book Services**

604 E Boulevard Ave
Bismarck, ND 58505-0800
701-328-4622
800-472-2104
Fax: 701-328-2040
TTY: 800-892-8622
ndsl.lib.state.nd.us

Doris Ott, Manager
Hullen E. Bivins, State Lbirarian
Susan Hammer-Schneider, Head Disability Serves

The Talking Books Program provides patrons with free access to cassette books and magazines. The Talking Books Program is administered by the National Library Service for the Blind and Physically Handicapped.

Ohio

4979 **Case Western Reserve University**

10900 Euclid Ave
Cleveland, OH 44106-4901
216-368-2000
president@case.edu
www.case.edu

Barbara R. Snyder, President
Stanton L. Gerson, MD
W.A. Bud Baeslack, Provost and Executive Vice President
Steven M. Altschuler, M, Chief Executive Officer

Programs which encompass the arts and sciences, engineering, health sciences, law, management, and social work.

4980 **Case Western Reserve University Northeast Ohio Multipurpose Arthritis Center**

11100 Euclid Ave
Cleveland, OH 44106-1716
216-844-3969
888-844-8447

Fred Rothstein, Executive Director

Basic and clinical research into the causes, diagnosis and treatment of arthritis.

4981 **Cincinnati Children's Hospital Medical Center**

University Of Cincinnati Uap
3333 Burnet Ave
Cincinnati, OH 45229-3026
513-636-4200
800-344-2462
Fax: 513-636-2837
TTY: 513-636-4900
www.cincinnatichildrens.org

James Anderson, CEO
James M Anderson, Chief Executive Officer
David Schonfeld, Executive Director
Richard G Azizkhan, Member of the Board

Dedicated to providing the highest level of pediatric care. As Greater Cincinnati's only pediatric hospital, Cincinnati Children's is committed to bringing the very best medical care to children in our community.

4982 **Cleveland FES Center**

11000 Cedar Ave
Suite 230
Cleveland, OH 44106-3056
216-231-3257
Fax: 216-231-3258
TTY: 216-231-3257
fescenter.case.edu

Robert Kirsch, Executive Director
Peckham P Hunter, Director

Research and development center on functional electrical stimulation. Houses the FES Information Center, a resource center with a library. Publications, newsletters and videotapes for persons with disabilities and others interested in electrical stimulation are offered.

4983 **Cleveland Public Library**

325 Superior Ave E
Cleveland, OH 44114-1271
216-623-2800
Fax: 216-623-2800
cpl.org

Felton Thomas, Executive Director
Thomas D. Corrigan, President
Maritza Rodriguez, Vice President
Alan Seifullah, Secretary

Summer reading programs, Braille writer, magnifiers, closed-circuit T.V., large-print photocopier, cassette books and magazines, children's books on cassette, and other reference materials on blindness and other handicaps.

4984 **Ohio Regional Library for the Blind and Physically Handicapped**
National Library Office
800 Vine St
Cincinnati, OH 45202-2009
513-369-6900
800-582-0335
Fax: 513-369-3111
TTY: 516-665-3384
www.cincinnatilibrary.org

Kimber L. Fender, Director
Ross A Wright, President
Paul G Sittenfeld, Vice President
Elizabeth H LaMachhia, Secretary

Summer reading programs, Braille writer, magnifiers, closed-circuit T.V., large-print photocopier, cassette books and magazines, children's books on cassette, and other reference materials on blindness and other handicaps.

4985 **State Library of Ohio: Talking Book Program**
National Library Service in Washington
Ste 100
274 E 1st Ave
Columbus, OH 43201-3692
614-644-7061
800-686-1531
Fax: 614-466-3584
library.ohio.gov

Jo Budler, Manager
Jim Buchman, Dir Patron & Catalog Services
Peter Bates, Deputy Director

A machine-lending agency for the visually impaired. Provides free recorded books, and magazines to approximately 26,000 eligible blind, visually impaired, physically handicapped, and reading disabled Ohio residents.

Oklahoma

4986 **Oklahoma Library for the Blind & Physically Handicapped**
300 NE 18th St
Oklahoma City, OK 73105-3296
405-521-3514
800-523-0288
Fax: 405-521-4582
TTY: 405-521-4672
library@drs.state.ok.us
www.library.state.ok.us

Paul Adams, Library Director
Vicky Golightly, Public Information Officer

Braille writer, magnifiers, closed-circuit T.V., large-print photocopier, cassette books and magazines, children's books on cassette, home visits and other reference materials on blindness and other handicaps.

4987 **Oklahoma Medical Research Foundation**
825 NE 13th St
Oklahoma City, OK 73104-5097
405-271-6673
800-522-0211
Fax: 405-271-7510
contact@omrf.org
www.omrf.org

Dr. Stephen Prescott, President
Mike D. 'Chip' Morgan, Executive VP and COO
Adam Cohen, Senior VP and General Counsel
Lisa Day, VP of Business and Government Affairs

Focuses on arthritis and muscoloskeletal disease research.

4988 **Tulsa City-County Library System: Outreach Services**
Tulsa City: County Library System
400 Civic Centre
Tulsa, OK 74103-3857
918-549-7323
os@tulsalibrary.org
www.tulsalibrary.org

Tracy Warren, Director

Tulsa City-County Library's Outreach Services Department provides library services to individuals that are unable to regularly visit a library, including monthly bookmobile visits and deliveries to residents of senior sites, along with mailing materials to homebound individuals/caretakers residing in their own homes.

Oregon

4989 **Oregon Health Sciences University, Elks' Children's Eye Clinic**
Casey Eye Institute
3181 S.W. Sam Jackson Park Rd.
Portland, OR 97239-3098
503-494-3000
888-222-8311
Fax: 503-494-4286
www.ohsucasey.com

Earl A Palmer, Director
Eleen Reyster, Clinic Manager
James Rosenbaum, Manager

The elks children's eye clinic is the major charitable project of the Oregon State Elks association. The clinic would not be possible without the organization's dedication and commitment to providing eye care for babies and children.

4990 **Oregon Talking Book & Braille Services**
250 Winter St NE
Salem, OR 97301-3950
503-378-5389
800-452-0292
Fax: 503-585-8059
TTY: 503-378-4334
www.oregon.gov/OSL/TBABS/Pages/index.aspx

Mary Kay Dahlgreen, Interim State Librarian
Robin Speer, Fund Development Officer
Susan Westin, Program Manager
Joel Henderson, Admin Program Coordinator

We serve the blind and physically disabled. Cassette books and magazines, Braille books-magazines, for children and adults. Descriptive videos. Audiocassette machines are provided free of charge. Call us for an application.

4991 **Talking Book & Braille Services Oregon State Library**
250 Winter St NE
Salem, OR 97301-3950
503-378-5389
800-452-0292
Fax: 503-585-8059
TTY: 503-378-4334
www.oregon.gov/OSL/TBABS/Pages/index.aspx

Mary Kay Dahlgreen, Interim State Librarian
Robin Speer, Fund Development Officer
Susan Westin, Program Manager
Joel Henderson, Admin Program Coordinator

Braille writer, magnifiers, large-print photocopier, cassette books and magazines, children's books on cassette and Braille books.

Pennsylvania

4992 **Associated Services for the Blind and Visually Impaired**
ASB
919 Walnut Street
Philadelphia, PA 19107-5237
215-627-0600
Fax: 215-922-0692
asbinfo@asb.org
www.asb.org

Karla S. McCaney, President & CEO
Beth Deering, Director, Human Services
Richard Forsythe, Director, Braille Division & Custom Audio
Joyce Robertson, Director, Finance & Information Technology

Associated Services for the Blind and Visually Impaired (ASB), is a private, nonprofit organization working to provide services, education, training, and resources to promote self-esteem, independence, and self determination in people who are blind or visually impaired. In addition, ASB advocates for the rights of blind and visually impaired persons through community actions and public education.

4993 Carnegie Library of Pittsburgh Library for the Blind & Physically Handicapped
4400 Forbes Ave
Pittsburgh, PA 15213-4007
412-622-3114
800-242-0586
Fax: 412-687-2442
info@carnegielibrary.org
carnegielibrary.org

Cathy Chaparro, Manager
Sue Murdock, Manager
Jane Dayton, Assistant Director
Jacqueline Flanagan, Executive Director

Loans recorded books/magazines and playback equipment, large print books and described videos to western PA residents unable to use standard printed materials due to a visual, physical, or physically-based reading disability.

4994 Free Library of Philadelphia: Library for the Blind and Physically Handicapped
1901 Vine Street
Philadelphia, PA 19103
215-686-5322
reardons@freelibrary.org
www.library.phila.gov

Tobey Gordon Dichter, Chair
Richard A. Greenawalt, First Vice Chair
Miriam Spector, Vice Chair
Siobhan A. Reardon, President and Director

Summer reading programs for children and teens. Closed-circuit T.V.for enlarging print for low vision; computers with screen readers and large print; cassette books and magazines; Braille books and magazines; and descriptive videos for the blind and visually impaired. Unique and acclaimed adult education program for all disabilities. State of the art book recording facilities.

4995 Pennsylvania College of Optometry Eye Institute
8360 Old York Rd
Elkins Park, PA 19027-1598
215-780-1400
Fax: 215-780-1336

4996 Reading Rehabilitation Hospital
Box 250
Rr 1
Reading, PA 19607
610-796-6297
Fax: 610-796-6353

Richard Kruczek, CEO
Doug Mehrkam, Owner

Information on physical disabilities, stroke, head injuries, aging and spinal cord injuries.

Rhode Island

4997 Office Of Library & Information Services for the Blind and Physically Handicapped
1 Capitol Hill
4th Floor
Providence, RI 02908-5803
401-574-9300
Fax: 401-574-9320
olis.webmaster@olis.ri.gov
www.olis.ri.gov

Howard Boksenbaum, Chief Library Officer
Chaichin Chen, Library Program Specialist: LORI
Debbie Cullerton, Information Services Technician:
Jeremy Cutler, Information Services Technician

Offers information and services for the visually impaired including reference materials, Braille printers, Braille writers, large-print books and more.

4998 Talking Books Plus
Library for the Blind & Physically Handicapped
1 Capitol Hill
4th Floor
Providence, RI 02908-5803
401-574-9300
Fax: 401-574-9320
olis.webmaster@olis.ri.gov
www.olis.ri.gov

Howard Boksenbaum, Chief Library Officer
Chaichin Chen, Library Program Specialist: LORI
Debbie Cullerton, Information Services Technician:
Jeremy Cutler, Information Services Technician

Offers talking book services for the blind and physically handicapped. Collection includes reference materials, Braille printer, Braille writer, large-print books, adaptive computer workstations and referrals to appropriate agencies/programs for other services.

South Carolina

4999 Medical University of South Carolina Arthritis Clinical/Research Center
171 Ashley Avenue
Charleston, SC 29425-100
843-792-1414
800-424-MUSC
Fax: 843-792-7121
academicdepartments.musc.edu/musc/

Jennie Ariail, Director
Tom Gasque Smith, Associate Director
Dr. David Cole, President
Mark S Sothmann, Ph.D., Vice President for Academic Affairs and Provost

Offers patient care services and basic and clinical research on various types of arthritis and connective tissue diseases.

5000 South Carolina State Library
1500 Senate Street
P.O. Box 11469
Columbia, SC 29211-1469
803-734-8026
Fax: 803-734-4757
reference@statelibrary.sc.gov
statelibrary.sc.gov

Debbie Anderson, Administrative Coordinator
Flora A. DuBose, Administrative Specialist
Leesa Benggio, Acting Director
Paula James, Director of Finance and Administration

Summer reading programs, Braille writer, magnifiers, closed-circuit T.V., large-print photocopier, cassette books and magazines, children's books on cassette, home visits and other reference materials on blindness and other handicaps.

South Dakota

5001 South Dakota State Library
800 Governors Dr
Pierre, SD 57501-2294
605-773-3131
800-423-6665
Fax: 605-773-6962
TTY: 605-773-4950
library@state.sd.us
library.sd.gov

Dr. Lesta V. Turchen, President
Monte Loos, Vice President
Sarah Easter, Secretary
Daria Bossman, State Librarian

Summer reading programs, Braille writer, magnifiers, closed-circuit T.V., large-print photocopier, cassette books and magazines, children's books on cassette, home visits and other reference materials on blindness and other handicaps.

Tennessee

5002 **Tennessee Library for the Blind and Physically Handicapped**
Tennessee State Library Archives
403 7th Ave N
Nashville, TN 37243-1409
615-741-3915
800-342-3308
Fax: 615-532-8856
tlbph.tsla@tn.gov
www.tennessee.gov/tsla/lbph/

Ruth Hemphill, Director
Ed Byrne, Assistant Director
Blake Fontenay, Communications Director

Provides free public library service to residents of Tennessee who are unable to read standard print due to a physical disability. Co-operating library with national network of libraries serving people with print disabilities, operating under the auspices

Texas

5003 **Baylor College of Medicine Birth Defects Center**
One Baylor Plaza
Houston, TX 77030-2348
713-798-4951
Fax: 832-825-3141
www.bcm.edu/obgyn/tcfs

Frank Greenberg, Director
Dr. Paul Klotman, President

One of the few centers in the world that performs fetal surgery. Provides integrated, multidisciplinary care for mothers, carrying babies with genetic or anatomic birth defects requiring therapy before or immediately after birth. This collaboration enable.

5004 **Baylor College of Medicine: Cullen Eye Institute**
Baylor College of Medicine
One Baylor Plaza
Houston, TX 77030-2743
713-798-4951
888-562-3937
Fax: 713-798-1521
http://www.bcm.edu/eye/index.cfm?pmid=0

Dan B. Jones, Professor and Chair
Al Vaughan, Manager
Michael Cassidy, Plant Manager
Dr. Paul Klotman, President

Research activities focus on restoring vision and preventing blindness through a better understanding of the disease.

5005 **Brown-Heatly Library**
4800 N Lamar Blvd
P O Box 149198
Austin, TX 78756-2316
800-252-5204
800-628-5115
www.dars.state.tx.us

Veronda L. Durden, Commissioner
Glenn Neal, Deputy Commissioner
Daniel Bravo, Chief Operating Officer
Rebecca Trevino, Chief Financial Officer

Houses a collection of books, audio and video tapes and periodicals focusing on rehabilitation, disabilities, employment skills and practices and management for the Texas Rehabilitation Commission. Houses materials on developmental and other disabilities.

5006 **Center for Research on Women with Disabilities**
Baylor College of Medicine
One Baylor Plaza
Houston, TX 77030-3411
713-798-5782
800-443-7693
Fax: 713-798-4688
crowd@bcm.tmc.edu
www.bcm.edu/crowd

Kathy Fire, Administrator
Margaret A. Nosek, Executive Director
Martha Mendez, Secretary
Susan Robin Whelen, Investigator

Research organization dedicated to conducting research and promoting, developeing, and disseminating information to expand the life choices of women with disabilities. Conducts research and training activities on issues related to the health, independence

5007 **Christian Education for the Blind**
Suite 702
4200 S Freeway Dr
Fort Worth, TX 76115
817-920-0044
Fax: 817-920-0777
bceb@evl.net

Rodger Dyer, Executive Director

Offers Braille and large print books and cassettes for the visually impaired.

5008 **Houston Public Library: Access Center**
500 McKinney St
Houston, TX 77002-5000
832-393-1313
Fax: 832-393-1474
TTY: 832-393-1539
website@hpl.lib.tx.us
houstonlibrary.org

Rhea Brown Lawson, Director
Roosevelt Weeks, Deputy Director
Greg Simpson, Assistant Director

Offers full library services to the visually and hearing impaired in Houston, TX at no charge. Houses unique and critical services for its users including online access to the Internet in a private and secure area.

5009 **Talking Book Program/Texas State Library**
Talking Book Program
1201 Brazos St.
PO Box 12927
Austin, TX 78711-2927
512-463-5458
800-252-9605
Fax: 512-936-0685
tbp.services@tsl.state.tx.us
www.texastalkingbooks.org

Ava M Smith, Director

Providing free library service to Texans of all ages who are unable to read standard print material due to visual, physical, or reading disabilities-whether permanent or temporary. The program offers more than 80,000 titles in fiction and nonfiction, plus 80 national magazines for adults and children.

5010 **University of Texas Southwestern Medical Center/Allergy & Immunology**
5323 Harry Hines Blvd
Dallas, TX 75390-7208
214-648-3111
www.utsouthwestern.edu

Diane Jeffries, Director
Priscilla Alderman, Executive Assistant
Daniel K Podolsky, President

Mission is to improve the health care in our community, Texas, our nation, and the world through innovation and education. To educate the next generation of leaders in patient care, biomedical science and disease prevention. To conduct high-impact, intern

5011 **University of Texas at Austin Library**
101 E 21st St
Austin, TX 78712-900
512-495-4350
Fax: 512-495-4347
webform@lib.utexas.edu
www.lib.utexas.edu

Douglas Dempster, Manager
Sheldon Ekland-Olson, Chief Executive Officer
Dr. Fred Heath, Vice Provost and Director

Provides access to information for all users, including those with disabilities, in accordance with the overall mission of the General Libraries of the University of Texas at Austin.

Utah

5012 **Utah State Library Division: Program for the Blind and Disabled**
250 North 1950 West
Suite A
Salt Lake City, UT 84116- 7901
801-715-6789
800-662-5540
Fax: 801-715-6767
TTY: 801-715-6721
blind@utah.gov
www.blindlibrary.utah.gov

Donna Morris, Director
Lisa Nelson, Program Manager
Michael Sweeney, Readers Advisor Librarian
Scott Brooks, Multistate Manager

The Program for the Blind and Disabled provides the kinds of materials found in public libraries in formats accessible to the blind and disabled. Books and magazines are available in Braille, in large print, on audio cassettes, and on audio digital books. Services are provided by the Utah State Library Division in cooperation with the Library of Congress, National Library Service for the Blind and Physically Handicapped. Services are provided free of charge to eligible readers.

Vermont

5013 **National Center for PTSD**
VA Medical Center (116D)
215 N Main St
White River Junction, VT 05009
802-296-5132
802-296-6300
Fax: 802-296-5135
ncptsd@va.gov
www.ptsd.va.gov

Paula P Schnurr, PhD, Executive Director
Cybele Merrick, MA, MS, Associate Director for Education
Nancy Bernardy, PhD, Associate Director of Clinical Networking
Lauren Sippel, PhD, Associate Director for Research

The National Center for PTSD works to improve care for America's Veterans and others who suffer from trauma or PTSD. The center engages in researchand provides education and training for diagnosis and treatment of the disorder.

5014 **Vermont Department of Libraries - Special Services Unit**
578 Paine Tpke N
Berlin, VT 05602
802-828-3273
800-479-1711
Fax: 802-828-3109
libraries.vermont.gov/library_for_the_blind

Teresa Faust, Special Services Librarian
Sara Blow, Library Assistant
Jennifer Hart, Librarian
Aidan Sammis, Library Assistant

Regional network library pf the National Library Service for the Blind & Physically Handicapped. The SSU makes available reading material in large print and NLS talking book formats, including these special collections: children's print Braille books, audio described videos and DVDs.

5015 **Vermont Department of Libraries -Special Services Unit**
578 Paine Tpke N
Berlin, VT 05602-9139
802-828-3273
800-479-1711
Fax: 802-828-3109
www.libraries.vermont.gov/ssu

Teresa Faust, Special Services Librarian
Sara Blow, Library Assistant
Jennifer Hart, Librarian
Aidan Sammis, Library Assistant

Virginia

5016 **Access Services**
Fairfax County Public Library
12000 Government Center Pkwy
Suite 123
Fairfax, VA 22035-1
703-324-7329
Fax: 703-222-3193
TTY: 703-324-8365
access@fairfaxcounty.gov
fairfaxcounty.gov

Janice Kuch, Branch Manager
Beena Pandey, Volunteer Coordinator
Ken Plummer, Outreach Manager

Offers talking books, TDD access, assistive devices such as decoders for three-week loans, support groups for people who are visually impaired, adapted computer work station with Braille printer and assistive listening devices.

5017 **Alexandria Library Talking Book Service**
5005 Duke St
Alexandria, VA 22304-2903
703-746-1702
Fax: 703-519-5917
TTY: 703-519-5911
www.alexandria.lib.va.us

Rose T. Dawson, Director
Renee DiPilato, Deputy Director
Linda Wesson, Communications Officer
Kym Robertson, Talking Book Service

Summer reading programs, Braille writer, magnifiers, closed-circuit T.V., large-print photocopier, cassette books and magazines, children's books on cassette, home visits and other reference materials on blindness and other handicaps.

5018 **Arlington County Department of Libraries**
Arlington County Library
1015 N Quincy St
Arlington, VA 22201-4603
703-228-5990
Fax: 703-228-7720
TTY: 703-228-6320
libraries@arlingtonva.us
arlingtonva.us

Diane Kresh, Director
Margaret Brown, Chief
Anne Gable, Administrative Services/Technology Division Chief
Peter Golkin, Public Information Officer

Summer reading programs, Braille writer, magnifiers, closed-circuit T.V., large-print photocopier, cassette books and magazines, children's books on cassette, home visits and other reference materials on blindness and other handicaps.

5019 **Braille Circulating Library for the Blind**
2700 Stuart Ave
Richmond, VA 23220-3305
804-359-3743
Fax: 804-359-4777
bclministries.org

Rev. Brian J Barton, Sr., Executive Director

Offers library materials for the blind and visually impaired on a free-loan basis. Serves the entire USA and 41 foreign countries with cassette tapes, reel to reel tapes, Braille books, large print books along with talking book records.

5020 **Central Rappahannock Regional Library**
1201 Caroline St
Fredericksburg, VA 22401-3701
540-372-1144
Fax: 540-899-9867
TTY: 540-371-9165
webmaster@crrl.org
www.librarypoint.org

Donna Cote, Executive Director
Alison Heartwell, Librarian

Offers reference materials on blindness and other disabilities.

5021 Council for Exceptional Children (CEC)
Council for Exceptional Children
3100 Clarendon Blvd.
Suite 600
Arlington, VA 22201-5332
888-232-7733
TTY: 866-915-5000
service@exceptionalchildren.org
www.exceptionalchildren.org

Chad Rummel, Executive Director
Laurie VanderPloeg, Associate Executive Director, Professional Affairs
Craig Evans, Chief Financial Officer
Sharon Rodriguez, Director, Governance & Executive Services

The Council for Exceptional Children aims to improve the educational success of individuals with disabilities and/or gifts and talents by advocating for appropriate policies, setting professional standards, and providing resources and professional development for special educators.

5022 James Branch Cabell Library
Virginia Commonwealth University
901 Park Avenue
PO Box 842033
Richmond, VA 23284-2033
804-828-1110
866-828-2665
866-828-2665
Fax: 804-828-0151
library@vcu.edu
www.library.vcu.edu

John Birch, Media Specialist II
Wesley Chenault, Head
Yuki Hibben, Assistant Head
Ray Bonis, Coordinator

Provides individualized orientations and assistance with library research and equipment.

5023 Newport News Public Library System
2400 Washington Ave
3rd Floor
Newport News, VA 23607- 4301
757-926-8000
Fax: 757-926-1365
icieszyn@ci.newport-news.va.us
newportnewsva.com

Thomas P. Herbert, P.E., Chair
Wendy C. Drucker, Vice Chair
Sam Workman, Assistant Director of Development
Matt Johnson, Business Retention Coordinator

Summer reading programs, Braille writer, magnifiers, closed-circuit T.V., large-print photocopier, cassette books and magazines, children's books on cassette, home visits and other reference materials on blindness and other handicaps.

5024 Northern Virginia Resource Center for Deafand Hard of Hearing Persons
3951 Pender Dr
Suite 130
Fairfax, VA 22030-6035
703-352-9056
Fax: 703-352-9058
TTY: 703-352-9056
info@nvrc.org
nvrc.org

William Boyd, Chair
Jim Faughnan, Vice Chair
Steve Williams, Treasurer
Donna Grossman, Secretary

Empowering deaf and hard of hearing individuals and their families through education, advocacy and community involvement.

5025 Roanoke City Public Library System
706 S Jefferson St
Roanoke, VA 24016-5191
540-853-2473
Fax: 540-853-1781
main.library@roanokeva.gov
www.roanokegov.com/library

Michael L. Ramsey, President
Barbara Lemon, Vice President

Summer reading programs, Braille writer, magnifiers, closed-circuit T.V., large-print photocopier, cassette books and magazines, children's books on cassette, home visits and other reference materials on blindness and other handicaps.

5026 Staunton Public Library Talking Book Center
1 Churchville Ave
Staunton, VA 24401-3229
540-885-6215
800-995-6215
Fax: 540-332-3906
www.talkingbookcenter.org

Lisa Eye, Reader Advisor
Lynn Harris, President
Daniel Swift, Treasurer
Betsy Little, Secretary

Offers free library service by circulating recorded books, magazines, and playback equipment to individuals unable to use standard print materials because of visual or physical impairment.

5027 University of Virginia Health System General Clinical Research Group
P.O. Box 800787
Charlottesville, VA 22908-0787
434-924-2394
Fax: 434-924-9960
gcrc.med.virginia.edu

Pamela Sprouse, Administrator
Eugene J. Barrett, Program Director
Mary Lee Vance, Associate Director

Provides investigators with the specialized resources necessary to conduct advanced clinical research. The facility includes ten inpatient beds, skilled research nurses, a core assay laboratory, a metabolic kitchen, outpatient facilities, computing and st

5028 Virginia Autism Resource Center
4100 Price Club Blvd
PO Box 842020
Richmond, Virginia, VA 23284-2020
804-674-8888
877-667-7771
877- -
Fax: 804-276-3970
www.varc.org

Carol Schall, Ph.D., Director
Florence McLeod, Administrative Assistant
Dawn Hendricks, Ph.D., Faculty/instructor

VARC promotes and facilitates best practices for those diagnosed within the autism spectrum. Information, resources, and education and training help parents, educators, service providers and medical professionals provide effective support from early childhood through adulthood.

5029 Virginia Beach Public Library Special Services Library
936 Independence Blvd
Virginia Beach, VA 23455-6006
757-385-2680
Fax: 757-464-6741
spaddock@vbgov.com
www.vbgov.com/dept/library

Marcy Sims, Library Director
David Palmer, Public Services Manager
Susan Paddock, Library Manager

A public library for people with visual and physical disabilities, Braille writer, magnifiers, closed-circuit T.V., large-print photocopier, cassette books and magazines, children's books on cassette, and other reference materials on blindness and other d

5030 Virginia Chapter of the Arthtitis Foundation
2201 W. Broad St
Suite 100
Richmond, VA 23220-3937
800-365-3811
800-456-4687
Fax: 804-359-4900
cmogel@arthritis.org
www.arthritis.org/virginia

Gail Norman, Interim President/CEO
Terri Harris, Chief Financial Officer
Nick Turvas, Senior VP of Health/Wellness
Cecil Wallace, Senior VP Policy and Communication

Provides free information, services and counseling to the public. Services include assistance in locating and accessing government and other health care programs for persons with arthritis, referral to doctors specializing in the treatment of arthritis,

5031 **Virginia State Library for the Visually and Physically Handicapped**
395 Azalea Ave
Richmond, VA 23227-3623
804-266-2477
800-552-7015
Fax: 804-266-2478
virginiavoice.org

Paula I. Otto, President
Susan C. Rucker, Secretary/Treasurer
Nicholas B Morgan, Executive Director
Rebecca Emmett, Office Manager
Summer reading programs, Braille writer, magnifiers, closed-circuit T.V., large-print photocopier, cassette books and magazines, children's books on cassette, home visits and other reference materials on blindness and other handicaps.

Washington

5032 **Meridian Valley Clinical Laboratory**
801 SW 16th St
Suite 126
Renton, WA 98057-2632
425-271-8689
855-405-8378
Fax: 425-271-8674
meridian@meridianvalleylab.com
www.meridianvalleylab.com

Dr. Jonathan Wright, Medical Director
A clinical test facility dedicated to providing the most accurate and informative data for patient diagnosis and therapeutic monitoring. With our current research and up-to-date information and various aspects of clinical nutritional medicine, our methodo

5033 **Ophthalmic Research Laboratory Eye Institute/First Hill Campus**
747 Broadway
Seattle, WA 98122-4307
206-386-6000
800-833-8879
TTY: 206-386-2022
www.swedish.org

Bryan Mueller, CEO
Dan Harris, CFO
Heidi Aylsworth, Chief Strategy Officer
Naren Balasubramaniam, Chief Human Resources Officer
Color vision physiology, vision disorders and blindness research.

5034 **Washington Talking Book and Braille Library**
2021 9th Ave
Seattle, WA 98121-2783
206-615-0400
800-542-0866
Fax: 206-615-0437
TTY: 206-615-0418
wtbbl@sos.wa.gov
wtbbl.org

Danielle Miller, Director and Regional Librarian
Amy Ravenholt, Assistant Program Manager
Mandy Gonnsen, Youth Services Librarian
David Gonnsen, Volunteer and Outreach Services
Summer reading programs, Braille writer, magnifiers, closed-circuit T.V., large-print photocopier, cassette books and magazines, children's books, and other reference materials on blindness and other handicaps, online catalog, reference station with assis

West Virginia

5035 **Cabell County Public Library/Talking Book Department/Subregional Library for the Blind**
455 9th St
Huntington, WV 25701-1417
304-528-5700
Fax: 304-528-5739
cabell.lib.wv.us

Judy K. Rule, Director
Angela Straight, Assistant Director
Mary Lou Pratt, Adult Services Coordinator
Breana Brown, Youth Service Manager
Summer reading programs, Braille writer, magnifiers, closed-circuit TV, cassette books and magazines, children's books on cassette reference materials on blindness and other handicaps, enlargers and Arkenstone Reader.

5036 **Division of Rehabilitation Services: Staff Library**
107 Capitol St
Charleston, WV 25301-2609
304-356-2060
800-642-8207
Fax: 304-766-4913
wvdrs.org

Carol Johnson, Manager
Specialized library with information on disabilities and the rehabilitation there of special collections: deaf and hard of hearing, visually impaired/blind, wellness center, literacy and career. The library has assistive devices such as CCTV, scanner and

5037 **Kanawha County Public Library**
123 Capitol St
Charleston, WV 25301-2686
304-343-4646
Fax: 304-348-6530
kanawha.lib.wv.us

Cheryl Morgan, President
Jennifer Pauer, First Vice President
Elizabeth O. Lord, Second Vice President
Michael Albert, Board Member
Summer reading programs, large print PC option, magnifiers, large type books, cassette books, and magazines, children's books on cassette, home visits and other reference materials on blindness and other handicaps

5038 **Ohio County Public Library Services for the Blind and Physically Handicapped**
52 16th St
Wheeling, WV 26003-3671
304-232-0244
Fax: 304-232-6848
wheeling.weirton.lib.wv.us

Jimmie McCamic, Chairman
Michael Baker, Secretary-Treasurer
Greg Marquart, Trustee
Anthony Werner, Trustee
The Ohio Public Library exists to provide books and related materials that will assist the residents of the community in the pursuit of knowledge, information, education, research, and recreation in order to promote an enlightned citizenry and to enrich t

5039 **Talking Book Department, Parkersburg and Wood County Public Library**
3100 Emerson Ave
Parkersburg, WV 26104-2414
304-420-4587
Fax: 304-420-4589

Lindsay Place, Talking Books Dept. Coordinator
Brian Raitz, Director
Free program loaning recorded books and magazines, Braille books and magazines to people who are unable to read or use standard print due to a visual or physical impairment.

5040 **West Virginia Autism Training Center**
Marshall University College Of Educational & Human
Old Main 316
1 John Marshall Drive
Huntington, WV 25755-1
304-696-2332
800-344-5115
Fax: 304-696-2846
www.marshall.edu/atc/

Amanda Plumley, Executive Office Manager
Ginny Painter, Communications Director
Joe Ciccarello, Associate Executive Director
J. T. Schneider, Grants Officer
Provides education, training, and treatment programs for W Virginians who have autism, pervasive devolopmental disorders or Asperger's disease and have formally been registered with the center.

5041 **West Virginia Library Commission**
1900 Kanawha Blvd E
Charleston, WV 25305-9
304-558-2041
800-642-9021
Fax: 304-558-2044
www.librarycommission.wv.gov

Karen Goff, Secretary
Deborah McNeal, Personnel Officer
Steve Tyler, Supervisor
Denise Seabolt, Library Administrative Services Director

Summer reading programs, Braille writer, magnifiers, closed-circuit T.V., large-print photocopier, cassette books and magazines, children's books on cassette, home visits and other reference materials on blindness and other handicaps.

5042 **West Virginia School for the Blind Library**
301 E Main St
Romney, WV 26757-1828
304-822-4840
Fax: 304-822-3370
cjohn@access.mountain.net
wvde.state.wv.us

Patsy Shank, Administrator
Cynthia Johnson, Librarian

Summer reading programs, Braille writer, magnifiers, closed-circuit T.V., large-print photocopier, cassette books and magazines, children's books on cassette, home visits and other reference materials on blindness and other handicaps.

Wisconsin

5043 **Brown County Library**
Central Library Downtown
515 Pine Street
Green Bay, WI 54301-3743
920-448-4400
Fax: 920-448-4376
TTY: 920-448-4400
bc_library@co.brown.wi.us
www.co.brown.wi.us/library

Terry Watermelon, President
Kathy Pletcher, Vice President
Carla Buboltz, Secretary
John Hickey, Financial Secretary

Summer reading programs, Braille writer, magnifiers, closed-circuit TV, large-print photocopier, cassette books and magazines, children's books on cassette, home visits and other reference materials on blindness and other handicaps.

5044 **Eye Institute of the Medical College of Wisconsin and Froedtert Clinic**
925 N 87th St
Milwaukee, WI 53226-4812
414-456-2020
Fax: 414-456-6300
eyecare@mcw.edu
doctor.mcw.edu

Jane D Kivlin, Director
Richard Schultz, MD, Director

A national leader as a full-service academic opthalmology program. Dedicated to the highest quality patient care, education, and vision research, the faculty and staff strive to provide state-of-the-art clinical and surgical patient care in a compassionat

5045 **Wisconsin Regional Library for the Blind& Physically Handicapped**
813 W Wells St
Milwaukee, WI 53233-1436
414-286-3045
800-242-8822
Fax: 414-286-3102
TTY: 414-286-3548
lbph@mpl.org

Marsha J Valance, Manager
Meredith Wittmann, Regional Librarian

Circulates recorded materials, playback equipment and Braille materials to print-handicapped Wisconsin residents.

Wyoming

5046 **Wyoming Services for the Visually Impaired**
Wyoming Department of Education
2300 Capitol Ave
Cheyenne, WY 82002-0050
307-777-7690
Fax: 307-777-6234
jackie.miller@wyo.gov
edu.wyoming.gov/in-the-classroom/special-prog

Ron Micheli, Chairman
Scotty Ratliff, Vice-Chair
Pete Ratliff, Treasurer
Cindy Hill, Superintendent

Services for the Visually Impaired assists people of all ages who have low vision or are blind. The goal is to provide information, education, and support to individuals with low vision in order that they may lead enjoyable and productive lives with maxim

5047 **Wyoming's New Options in Technology (WYNOT) - University of Wyoming**
1000 E University Ave
Laramie, WY 82071-2000
307-766-2761
888-989-9463
Fax: 307-766-2763
TTY: 800-908-7011
wind.uw@uwyo.edu
wind.uwyo.edu/wynot

William MacLean Jr., Ph.D., Executive Director

Designed to develop and implement a consumer oriented statewide system of technology-related assistance for people with disabilities of all ages.

Media, Print

Children & Young Adults

5048 Assistive Technology for Infants and Toddlers with Disabilities Handbook
Idaho Assistive Technology Project
University of Idaho
1187 Alturas Dr.
Moscow, ID 83843- 2268
800-432-8324
Fax: 208-885-6102
idahoat@uidaho.edu
www.idahoat.org

LaRae Rhoads, Author
Ron Seiler, Author
This handbook is designed as a guide for parents and families in Idaho who have infants and toddlers with developmental delays or disabilities.

5049 Assistive Technology for School-Age Children with Disabilities - Handbook
Idaho Assistive Technology Project
University of Idaho
1187 Alturas Dr.
Moscow, ID 83843- 2268
208-885-3557
800-432-8324
Fax: 208-885-6102
idahoat@uidaho.edu
www.idahoat.org

LaRae Rhoads, Author
Ron Seiler, Author
Michelle Doty, Author
A handbook designed to provide guidance and information for parentswho have school-aged children with disabilities, focusing on resources for assistive technologies available for their children.

5050 Children's Understanding of Disability
Routledge (Taylor & Francis Group)
711 Third Ave.
New York, NY 10017
212-216-7800
800-634-7064
Fax: 202-564-7854
enquiries@taylorandfrancis.com
www.routledge.com

Ann Lewis, Author
Children's Understanding of Disability is a valuable addition to the debate surrounding the integration of children with special needs into ordinary schools. Taking the viewpoint of the children themselves, it explores how pupils with severe learning difficulties and their non-disabled classmates interact.Ann Lewis examines what happens when non-disabled children and pupils with severe learning difficulties work together regularly over the course of a year.
Hardcover

5051 Complete IEP Guide: How to Advocate for Your Special Ed Child (8th Edition)
NOLO (Internet Brands)
909 N. Sepulveda Blvd
11th Fl.
El Segundo, CA 90245
310-280-4000
www.nolo.com

Lawrence Siegel, Attorney/Author
This all-in-one guide will help you understand special education law, identify your child's needs, prepare for meetings, develop the IEP and resolve disputes.
384 pages

5052 Don't Call Me Special: A First Look at Disability
Barron's Educational Series
250 Wireless Blvd
Hauppauge, NY 11788
800-645-3476
Fax: 631-494-3723
barrons@barronseduc.com
www.barronseduc.com

Pat Thomas, Author
This picture book explores questions and concerns about physical disabilities in a simple and reassuring way. Youger children can find out about individual disabilities, special equipment that is available to help the disabled, and how people of all ages can deal with disabilities and live happy and full lives.
Paperback

5053 Everything Parent's Guide to Special Education
Adams Media
4868 Innovation Dr
Bldg 2
Fort Collins, CO 80525
855-278-0402
www.adamsmediastore.com

Amanda Morin, Author
This handbook offers parents assistance, advice, and aid on navigating special education for their child, with information on assessment, evaluation, specific needs for specific disabilities, current law, and dealing with parent-school conflict. It includes worksheets, forms, and sample documents to help parents be effective advocates for their child's learning.

5054 It isn't Fair!: Siblings of Children with Disabilities
Praeger - ABC-CLIO
130 Cremona Dr
Santa Barbara, CA 93117
805-968-1911
800-368-6868
Fax: 866-270-3856
CustomerService@abc-clio.com
www.abc-clio.com/praeger

Stanley D. Klein, Editor
Maxwell J. Schleifer, Editor
This book presents a wide range of perspectives on the relationship of siblings to children with disabilities. These perspectives are written in the first person by parents, young adult siblings, younger siblings, and professionals.
200 pages

5055 Life Beyond the Classroom: Transition Strategies for Young People with Disabilities
Brookes Publishing
P.O. Box 10624
Baltimore, MD 21285-0624
410-337-9580
800-638-3775
Fax: 410-337-8539
custserv@brookespublishing.com
www.brookespublishing.com

Paul Wehman, Author
This textbook is an essential guide to planning, designing, and implementing successful transition programs for students with disabilities.
616 pages

5056 Mayor of the West Side
Fanlight Productions
32 Court St
21st Fl.
Brooklyn, NY 11201
718-488-8900
800-876-1710
Fax: 718-488-8642
info@fanlight.com
www.fanlight.com

Judd Ehrlich, Director
What happens when love gets in the way of letting go? As a teenager with multiple disabilities prepares for his Bar Mitzvah, his family and community consider what Mark's life will be like when they are no longer able to protect him.

5057 New Horizons Independent Living Center
8085 E Manley Dr
Prescott Valley, AZ 86314-6154
928-772-1266
800-406-2377
Fax: 928-772-3808
TTY: 928-772-1266
www.nhilc.org

Gale Dean, Executive Director
Alan Loosley, President
Sharon Geddes, Vice President
Mary Russell, Secretary
The mission of New Horizons Independent Living Center is to provide programs and services in Northern Arizona which en-

courage and empower people with disabilities to self-determine the goals and activities of their lives.

5058 **Rolling Along with Goldilocks and the Three Bears**
Woodbine House
6510 Bells Mill Rd
Bethesda, MD 20817
800-843-7323
info@woodbinehouse.com
www.woodbinehouse.com

Cindy Meyers, Author
Carol Morgan, Illustrator
The familiar fairytale with a special needs twist. Ages 3-7.
28 pages

5059 **Shriner's Hospitals for Children Newsletter**
3101 SW Sam Jackson Park Rd
Portland, OR 97201
503-241-5090
Fax: 503-221-3498
www.shrinershospitalforchildren.org

5060 **Sibling Forum: A FRA Newsletter**
Family Resource Associates
35 Haddon Ave
Shrewsbury, NJ 07702-4007
732-747-5310
Fax: 732-747-1896
info@frainc.org
www.frainc.org

Quarterly

5061 **Sibshops: Workshops for Siblings of Children with Special Needs**
Sibling Supporting Project
322-6512 23rd Ave NW
Seattle, WA 98117
206-297-6368
info@siblingsupport.org
www.siblingsupport.org

Don Meyer, Author
Patricia Vadasy, Author
Sibshops is a program that brings together 8-to 13-year-old brothers and sisters of children with special needs. The siblings receive support and information in a recreational setting, so they have fun while they learn.
264 pages

5062 **Special Education Report**
LRP Publications
360 Hiatt Dr
Dept. 150F
Palm Beach Gardens, FL 33418
800-341-7874
Fax: 561-622-2423
custserv@lrp.com
www.lrp.com

Monthly Newsletter

5063 **Special Format Books for Children and Youth Ages 3-19**
New York State Talking Book and Braille Library
Cultural Education Center
222 Madison Ave
Albany, NY 12230-0001
518-474-5935
800-342-3688
Fax: 518-474-7041
tbbl@nysed.gov
www.nysl.nysed.gov/tbbl/index.html

5064 **The Sibling Slam Book: What It's Really Like To Have a Brother or Sister with Special Needs**
Sibling Support Project
6512 23rd Ave NW
Ste 322
Seattle, WA 98117
206-297-6368
info@siblingsupport.org
www.siblingsupport.org

Don Meyer, Author
A brutally honest, non-PC look at the lives, experiences, and opinions of siblings without disabilities who have siblings with disabilities. Formatted like the slam books passed around in many junior high and high schools, this one poses a series of 50 personal questions, with responses drawn from the author's interviews with over 80 teens from across the United States. It reflects experiences that range from positive to negative.

5065 **The Sibling Survival Guide**
Sibling Support Project
6512 23rd Ave. NW
Ste 322
Seattle, WA 98117
206-297-6368
info@siblingsupport.org
www.siblingsupport.org

Don Meyer, Author
Emily Holl, Author
Edited by experts in the field of disabilities and sibling relationships, The Sibling Survival Guide focuses on the topmost concerns identified in a survey of hundreds of siblings.

5066 **Views from Our Shoes**
Sibling Support Project
6512 23rd Ave NW
Ste 322
Seattle, WA 98117
206-297-6368
www.siblingsupport.org

Don Meyer, Author
Siblings share what it is like to have a brother or sister with a disability. Age 9 and up.
106 pages Paperback

5067 **What About Me? Growing Up with a Developmentally Disabled Sibling**
Da Capo Press/ Perseus Books Group
Order Department
210 American Dr
Jackson, TN 38301
800-343-4499
Fax: 800-351-5073
www.perseusbooksgroup.com

Bryna Siegel, Author
Stuart Silverstein, Author
A compassionate and accessible guide on living with and caring for a developmentally disabled sibling.
316 pages Paperback

5068 **What It's Like to be Me**
Friendship Press
P.O. Box 37844
Cincinnati, OH 45222-844
513-948-8733
Fax: 513-761-3722

Community

5069 **'Cultural Life,' Disability, Inclusion, and Citizenship: Moving Beyond Leisure in Isolation**
Routledge (Taylor & Francis Group)
711 Third Ave
New York, NY 10017
212-216-7800
800-634-7064
Fax: 202-564-7854
enquiries@taylorandfrancis.com
www.routledge.com

Simon Darcy, Editor
Jerome Singleton, Editor
This book concentrates on disability citizenship in leisure.
90 pages Hardback

5070 **Active Citizenship and Disability: Implementing the Personalization of Support**
Cambridge University Press
Shaftesbury Rd
Cambridge, UK CB2-8BS
information@cambridge.org
www.cambridge.org

Andrew Power, Author
Janet E. Lord, Author
Allison S. DeFranco, Author
This book provides an international comparative study of the implementation of disability rights law and policy focused on the emerging principles of self-determination and personalisation. The case studies examine how different jurisdictions have reformed disability law and policy and reconfigured how support is administered and funded to ensure maximum choice and independence is accorded to people with disabilities.
518 pages Paperback; Hardcover

5071 **California Community Care News**
Community Residential Care Association of CA
1924 Alhambra Blvd
P.O. Box 163270
Sacramento, CA 95816-9270 916-455-0723
Fax: 916-455-7201
www.crcac.com

Charles W Skoien Jr, Director/Lobbyist
Denise Johnson, Consultant
Forum for the exchange of ideas, information and opinions among clients, families and service providers. Information regarding services and assisted living programs for the elderly, mentally ill and disabled.
Monthly

5072 **Community Disability Services: An Evidence-Based Approach to Practice**
Purdue University Press
Stewart Center 190
504 W State St
West Lafayette, IN 47907-2058 265-494-2038
pupress@purdue.edu
www.thepress.purdue.edu

Ian Dempsey, Editor
Karen Nankervis, Editor
Articles by an array of international experts provide as an excellent resource for professionals and students involved in the area of disability studies. The book is divided into three parts: (1) disability and modern society; (2) working with people who are challenged; and (3) working within a disability-services environment. This approach mirrors the contemporary debate within a practice framework reflecting how individuals, organizations, and communities deal with the problem and solutions.
304 pages Paperback

5073 **Comprehensive Care Coordination for Chronically Ill Adults**
Wiley-Blackwell
111 River St
Hoboken, NJ 07030-5774 201-748-6000
877-762-2974
Fax: 201-748-6088
info@wiley.com
www.wiley.com

Cheryl Schraeder, Editor
Paul S. Shelton, Editor
A combination of theory and case studies, this book presents the growing demographic of chronically ill adults in the U.S., offering models for change and improvement in quality of care; recommendations on relevant and current literature; and descriptions of successful care outcomes.
440 pages Paperback

5074 **Hallmarks and Features of High-Quality Community-Based Services**
Independent Living Research Utilization (ILRU)
1333 Moursund
Houston, TX 77030 713-520-0232
Fax: 713-520-5785
ilru@ilru.org
ilru.org

5075 **Human Exceptionality: School, Community,and Family (12th Edition)**
Cengage Learning
20 Channel Center St
Boston, MA 02210 617-289-7700
Fax: 617-289-7844
www.cengage.com/us

Michael L. Hardman, Author
M. Winston Egan, Author
Clifford J. Drew, Author
An evidence-based testament to the critical role of cross-professional collaboration in enhancing the lives of exceptional individuals and their families. This text's unique lifespan approach combines powerful research, evidence-based practices, and inspiring stories, engendering passion and empathy and enhancing the lives of individuals with exceptionalities.
544 pages Hardcover

5076 **Inclusive Leisure Services (3rd Edition)**
Venture Publishing Inc.
1999 Cato Ave
State College, PA 16801 814-234-4561
Fax: 814-234-1651
www.venturepublish.com

John Dattilo, Author
This text will educate future and current leisure services professionals about attitude development and actions that promote positive attitudes about people who have experienced discrimination and segregation. It provides strategies that will facilitate meaningful leisure participation by all participants, while respecting their rights.
560 pages Hardcover

5077 **Independent Living for Persons with Disabilities and Elderly People**
IOS Press
6751 Tepper Dr
Clifton, VA 20124 703-830-6300
Fax: 703-830-2300
sales@iospress.com
www.iospress.nl

Mounir Mokhtari, Editor
Discusses the need for assistive technology in making homes more accessible for the elderly and people with disabilities. Goes on to suggest the application of these technologies in other areas of the community, such as hospitals and schools, which allow those with disabilities and the elderly to live their lives with some independence and autonomy.
216 pages Softcover

5078 **Independent Living for Physically Disabled People**
People With Disabilities Press (iUniverse)
1663 Liberty Dr
Bloomington, IN 47403 812-330-2909
800-288-4677
Fax: 812-355-4085
media@iuniverse.com
www.iuniverse.com

Nancy M. Crewe, Author
Irving Kenneth Zola, Author
This book describes the philosophy of independent living, from legislative strides to community centres, as well as future trends.
436 pages

5079 **Pathways To Inclusion (2nd Edition)**
Captus Press
1600 Steeles Ave W
Concord, ON, Canada L4K-4M2 416-736-5537
Fax: 416-736-5793
info@captus.com
www.captus.com

John Lord, Author
Peggy Hutchison, Author
Pathways to Inclusion 2nd edition addresses the organizational strategies that have been used in the past and highlights areas for change. Human service organizations are examined, pinpointing common characteristics that have led to improved quality of life for people with disabilities and other vulnerable citizens.
328 pages Paperback

Employment

5080 **A Supported Employment Workbook: Individual Profiling and Job Matching**
Jessica Kingsley Publishers
73 Collier St
London, UK N19BE hello@jkp.com
www.jkp.com

Steve Leach, Author
Created with the goal of helping job developers, this guide offers practical tools and strategies to help job development professionals assist their clients. The workbook includes vocational forms, job analysis forms, and support review charts, and offers aid to

professionals in assisting disabled persons to find and secure stable jobs in their communities.
224 pages Paperback

5081 **Career Success for Disabled High-Flyers**
Jessica Kingsley Publishers
73 Collier St
London, UK N19BE
hello@jkp.com
www.jkp.com
Sonali Shah, Author
Drawing on case studies of 31 disabled adults, this book suggests that individual traits and patterns of behaviour are key factors in career success, and shows that it is often society rather than impairment that hinders professional progression. It will provide role models and valuable insights for young career-minded disabled people.
208 pages Paperback

5082 **Job Success for Persons with Developmental Disabilities**
Jessica Kingsley Publishers
73 Collier St
London, UK N19BE
hello@jkp.com
www.jkp.com
David B. Wiegan, Author
This book provides a comprehensive approach to developing a successful jobs program for persons with developmental disabilities, drawn from the author's extensive experience and real success.
160 pages Paperback

5083 **Making News: How to Get News Coverage of Disability Rights Issues**
The Advocado Press
contact145@advocadopress.org
www.advocadopress.org
165 pages

5084 **Making Self-Employment Work for People with Disabilities**
Brookes Publishing
P.O. Box 10624
Baltimore, MD 21285-0624
410-337-9580
800-638-3775
Fax: 410-337-8539
custserv@brookespublishing.com
www.brookespublishing.com
Cary Griffin, Author
David Hammis, Author
Beth Keeton, Author
Molly Sullivan, Author
Practical support for individuals with significant disabilities in starting and maintaining a small business. Covers building a business plan; pinpointing interests, strengths, and goals; and finding helpful information and support
288 pages

5085 **Road Ahead: Transition to Adult Life for Persons with Disabilities (3rd Edition)**
IOS Press
6751 Tepper Dr
Clifton, VA 20124
703-830-6300
Fax: 703-830-2300
sales@iospress.com
www.iospress.nl
Keith Storey, Editor
Dawn Hunter, Editor
Explores transition planning, assessment, instructional strategies, career development and support, social life, quality of life, supported living, and post-secondary education for people with disabilities.
318 pages

5086 **The Job Developer's Handbook: Practical Tactics for Customized Employment**
Brookes Publishing
P.O. Box 10624
Baltimore, MD 21285-0624
410-337-9580
800-638-3775
Fax: 410-337-8539
custserv@brookespublishing.com
www.brookespublishing.com
Cary Griffin, Author
David Hammis, Author
Tammara Geary, Author
Michael Callahan, Author
One of the most practical employment books available, this forward-thinking guide walks employment specialists step by step through customized job development for people with disabilities, revealing the best ways to build a satisfying, meaningful job around a person's preferences, skills, and goals.
264 pages

General Disabilities

5087 **A Guide to Disability Rights Laws**
U.S. Department of Justice
950 Pennsylvania Ave NW
Washington, DC 20530-0001
202-514-2000
www.ada.gov
Available in Large Print & Braille

5088 **A Practical Guide to Art Therapy Groups**
Routledge (Taylor & Francis Group)
711 Third Ave
New York, NY 10017
212-216-7800
800-634-7064
Fax: 202-564-7854
enquiries@taylorandfrancis.com
www.routledge.com
Diane Fausek, Author
Unique approaches, materials, and device will inspire you to tap into your own well of creativity to design your own treatment plans. It lays out the ingredients and the skills to get the results you want. Includes strategies that have been used for people with Alzheimer's, geri-psychiatric conditions and developmental disabilities.
124 pages Hardcover; Paperback

5089 **A World Awaits You**
Mobility International USA
132 E Broadway
Suite 343
Eugene, OR 97401
541-343-1284
Fax: 541-343-6812
TTY: 541-343-1284
clearinghouse@miusa.org
www.miusa.org
Susan Sygall, Chief Executive Officer
Cindy Lewis, Director, Programs
Publication from Mobility International USA featuring stories from people with disabilities who have participated in international exchange experiences.
Annually

5090 **ADA Guide for Small Businesses**
U.S. Department of Justice, Civil Rights Division
950 Pennsylvania Ave NW
Washington, DC 20530-0001
202-514-4609
Fax: 202-307-1197
TTY: 202-514-0716
www.ada.gov

5091 **ADA Information Services**
U.S. Department of Justice, Civil Rights Division
950 Pennsylvania Ave NW
Washington, DC 20530-0001
202-514-4609
800-514-0301
Fax: 202-307-1197
TTY: 800-514-0383
www.ada.gov

5092 **ADA Pipeline**
DRTAC: Southeast ADA Center
1419 Mayson Street NE
Atlanta, GA 30324
404-385-0636
800-949-4232
Fax: 404-385-0641
www.sedbtac.org

Cyndi Smith, B.S., Office Assistant
Mary Morder, Information Technology Support
Sally Z. Weiss, B.A., Director
Rebecca Williams, B.A., M.S., Information Specialist / Technical Assistance
16 pages Quarterly

5093 **ADA Questions and Answers**
U.S. Department of Justice, Civil Rights Division
950 Pennsylvania Ave NW
Washington, DC 20530-0001
202-514-4609
800-514-0301
Fax: 202-307-1197
TTY: 800-514-0383
www.ada.gov

5094 **ADA Tax Incentive Packet for Business**
US Department of Justice
950 Pennsylvania Ave NW
Washington, DC 20530-9
202-586-5000
800-574-0301
Fax: 202-307-1197
TTY: 800-514-0383
www.ada.gov

James Bostrom, Deputy Chiefs
Zita Johnson Betts, Deputy Chiefs
Sally Conway, Deputy Chiefs
Jana Erickson, Deputy Chiefs
A 13-page packet of information to help businesses understand and take advantage of the tax credit and deduction available for complying with the ADA.

5095 **ADA and City Governments: Common Problems**
US Department of Justice
950 Pennsylvania Ave NW
Washington, DC 20530-9
202-586-5000
800-574-0301
Fax: 202-307-1197
TTY: 800-514-0383
www.ada.gov

James Bostrom, Deputy Chiefs
Zita Johnson Betts, Deputy Chiefs
Sally Conway, Deputy Chiefs
Jana Erickson, Deputy Chiefs
A 9-page document that contains a sampling of common problems shared by city governments of all sizes, provides examples of common deficiencies and explains how these problems affect persons with disabilities.

5096 **ADA-TA: A Technical Assistance Update from the Department of Justice**
US Department of Justice
950 Pennsylvania Ave NW
Washington, DC 20530-9
202-586-5000
800-574-0301
Fax: 202-307-1197
TTY: 800-514-0383
www.ada.gov

James Bostrom, Deputy Chiefs
Zita Johnson Betts, Deputy Chiefs
Sally Conway, Deputy Chiefs
Jana Erickson, Deputy Chiefs
A serial publication that answers Common Questions about ADA requirements and provides Design Details illustrating particular design requirements. The first edition addresses Readily Achievable Barrier Removal and Van Accessible Packing Spaces.

5097 **AEPS Family Report: For Children Ages Birth to Three**
Brookes Publishing
P.O. Box 10624
Baltimore, MD 21285-0624
410-337-9580
800-638-3775
Fax: 410-337-8539
custserv@brookespublishing.com
www.brookespublishing.com

Diane Bricker, Author
Betty Capt, Author
JoAnn Johnson, Author
Kristine Slentz, Author
This is a 64-item questionnaire that asks parents to rank their child's abilities on specific skills. In packages of 10.
28 pages Saddle-stiched

5098 **ARC's Government Report**
Arc of the District of Columbia
817 Varnum St NE
Washington, DC 20017-2144
202-636-2950
Fax: 202-636-2996
www.arcdc.net

Mary Lou Meccariello, Executive Director
Ed Cabatic, Director of Finance
Randy Shingler, Chief Operating Officer
Denize Stanton-Williams, Director of Supports & Services
Reports on government activities related to individuals with disabilities with a focus on persons with developmental disabilities.
$50.00

5099 **ARCA Newsletter**
ARCA - Dakota County Technical College
1300 145th St E
Rosemount, MN 55068-2932
651-423-8301
877-937-3282
Fax: 651-423-7028
dctc.edu

Ron Thomas, President
Offers information on support groups, conventions, books, manuscripts and programs for the rehabilitation professional and the disabled.
Monthly

5100 **Accent on Living Magazine**
Cheever Publishing
P.O. Box 700
Bloomington, IL 61702-700
309-378-2961
800-787-8444
Fax: 309-378-4420

Julie Cheever, Marketing Manager
A magazine published for forty four years, serves physically disabled people, with general interest, travel, and home modification features. *$12.00*
112 pages Quarterly

5101 **Access Design Services: CILs as Experts**
Independent Living Research Utilization ILRU
1333 Moursund
Houston, TX 77030
713-520-0232
Fax: 713-520-5785
ilru@ilru.org
ilru.org

Lex Frieden, Director, ILRU
Richard Petty, Co-Director
Featuring the Access Design Services of Alpha One in Maine, this month's Readings is another of the winners of the recent competition for innovative CIL programs.
10 pages

5102 **Access To Independence Inc.**
Access to Independence
3810 Milwaukee Street
Madison, WI 53714
608-242-8484
800-362-9877
Fax: 608-242-0383
TTY: 608-242-8485
info@accesstoind.org
www.accesstoind.org

Dee Truhn, Executive Director
Jason Belaungy, Assistant Director
Geri, Finances/HR
Janie, Administrative Assistant

Independent Living Center serving people of any age and all types of disabilities in south-central Wisconsin. Empower people with disabilities, through advocacy, education, and support.
24 pages Semi-Annual

5103 **Access for 911 and Telephone Emergency Services**
US Department of Justice
950 Pennsylvania Ave NW
Washington, DC 20530-9
202-586-5000
800-574-0301
Fax: 202-307-1197
TTY: 800-514-0383
www.ada.gov

James Bostrom, Deputy Chiefs
Zita Johnson Betts, Deputy Chiefs
Sally Conway, Deputy Chiefs
Jana Erickson, Deputy Chiefs

A 10-page publication explaining the requirements for direct, equal access to 911 for persons who use teletypewritters (TTYs).

5104 **Achieving Diversity and Independence**
Independent Living Research Utilization ILRU
1333 Moursund
Houston, TX 77030
713-520-0232
Fax: 713-520-5785
ilru@ilru.org
ilru.org

Lex Frieden, Director, ILRU
Richard Petty, Co-Director
10 pages

5105 **Activity-Based Intervention: 2nd Edition**
Brookes Publishing
P.O. Box 10624
Baltimore, MD 21285-0624
410-337-9580
800-638-3775
Fax: 410-337-8539
custserv@brookespublishing.com
readplaylearn.com

Paul H. Brooks, Chairman
Jeffrey D. Brookes, President
Melissa A. Behm, Executive Vice President

This 14 minute video illustrates how activity-based intervention can be used to turn everyday events and natural interactions into opportunities to promote learning in young children who are considered at risk for developmental delays or who have mild to significant disabilities. *$39.00*
ISBN 1-55766 -86-3

5106 **Ad Lib Drop-In Center: Consumer Management, Ownership and Empowerment**
Independent Living Research Utilization ILRU
1333 Moursund
Houston, TX 77030
713-520-0232
Fax: 713-520-5785
ilru@ilru.org
ilru.org

Lex Frieden, Director, ILRU
Richard Petty, Co-Director

Joe describes how Ad Lib ensured consumer control in their Drop-In Center: the DIC came about because of consumer input, and consumers are involved in planning the program; members can choose to become volunteers or paid staff members. All of the staff at the DIC are consumers; and active consumer advisory board helps develop policies and programs and provides input to the Ad Lib board.
10 pages

5107 **Adobe News**
Santa Barbara Foundation
15 E Carrillo St
Santa Barbara, CA 93101-2706
805-963-1873
805-966-2345
Fax: 805-966-2345

Ron Gallo, CEO
8 pages Bi-Annually

5108 **Advocate**
Arc Massachusetts
217 South St
Waltham, MA 02453-2710
781-891-6270
Fax: 781-891-6271
arcmass@arcmass.org
www.arcmass.org

Leo V. Sarkissian, Executive Director
Judy Zacek, Associate Editor
Beth Rutledge, Production Coordinator/Ad
Brenda Asis, Director of Development

Advocate is The Arc of Massachusetts' quarterly newsletter. This is one of the ways in which we inform and educate people about current topics in the field of developmental disabilities. *$20.00*
8-12 pages Quarterly

5109 **American Herb Association Newsletter**
P.O. Box 353
Nevada City, CA 95959-353
530-265-9552
Fax: 530-274-3140
www.ahaherb.com

5110 **Americans with Disabilities Act Checklist for New Lodging Facilities**
US Department of Justice
950 Pennsylvania Ave NW
Washington, DC 20530
202-586-5000
800-574-0301
Fax: 202-307-1197
TTY: 800-514-0383
www.ada.gov

James Bostrom, Deputy Chiefs
Zita Johnson Betts, Deputy Chiefs
Sally Conway, Deputy Chiefs
Jana Erickson, Deputy Chiefs

This 34-page checklist is a self-help survey that owners, franchisors, and managers of lodging facilities can use to identify ADA mistakes at their facilities.

5111 **Americans with Disabilities Act Handbook**
Aspen Publishers
76 9th Ave
7th Floor
New York, NY 10011-4962
212-790-2000
Fax: 212-771-0885
www.aspenpublishers.com

Henry H Perritt Jr Esq, Author
Bob Lemmond, President and CEO
Gustavo Dobles, Vice President & Chief Content Officer
Susan Pikitch, Vice President & CFO

The Americans With Disabilities Act (ADA) Handbook provides comprehensive coverage of the ADA's employment, commercial facilities, and public accommodations provisions as well as coverage of the transportation, communication, and federal, local, and state government requirements. *$599.00*
1671 pages 2X per year
ISBN 0-735531-48-X

5112 **An Interdisciplinary Journal for the Social Study of Health, Illness and Medicine**
Sage Publications
2455 Teller Rd
Thousand Oaks, CA 91320-2218
805-499-0721
800-818-7243
Fax: 805-499-0871
hea.sagepub.com

Alan Radley, Editor
Blaise Simqu, Chief Executive Officer
Quarterly

5113 Annual Report Sarkeys Foundation
530 E Main St
Norman, OK 73071-5823
405-364-3703
Fax: 405-364-8191
susan@sarkeys.org
sarkeys.org

Kim Henry, Executive Director
Lorri Sutton, Executive Assistant
Susan C. Frantz, Senior Program Officer
Linda English Weeks, Senior Program Officer
Yearly

5114 Applied Kinesiology: Muscle Response in Diagnosis, Therapy and Preventive Medicine
Inner Traditions
P.O. Box 388
Rochester, VT 05767-388
802-767-3174
800-246-8648
Fax: 802-767-3726
orders@innertraditions.com
www.InnerTraditions.com

Jessica Arsenault, Sales Associate
Rob Meadows, VP Sales & Marketing
$12.95
144 pages
ISBN 0-892813-28-8

5115 Arc Connection Newsletter
Arc of Tennessee
151 Athens Way
Suite 100
Nashville, TN 37228-1367
615-248-5878
800-835-7077
Fax: 615-248-5879
pcooper@thearctn.org
thearctn.org

Carrie Hobbs Guiden, Executive Director
Peggy Cooper, Membership, Chapter and Communications Manager
Nicole Davidson, Business Manager
Lori Israel, Office Manager

The Arc of Tennessee is a nonprofit organization that offers advocacy, information, referral and support to people with intellectual or developmental disabilities and their families. This is their publication. It is free to members. *$10.00*
12 pages Quarterly

5116 Aromatherapy Book: Applications and Inhalations
2526 Martin Luther King Jr. Way
Berkeley, CA 94704
510-549-4270
Fax: 510-549-4276
info@northatlanticbooks.com
www.northatlanticbooks.com

Minda Armstrong, Print Production Manager
Richard Grossinger, Founding Publisher
Janet Levin, Director of Sales & Distribution
Alla Spector, Director of Finance & Office Operations

A book of practical and researched information about aromatherapy. *$18.95*
400 pages
ISBN 1-556430-73-6

5117 Aromatherapy for Common Ailments
Simon & Schuster
100 Front St
Delran, NJ 8075-1181
856-461-6500
800-323-7445
Fax: 856-824-2402
www.simonsays.com

David Schaeffer, VP

Explains aromatherapy with emphasis on medicinal uses.
96 pages
ISBN 0-671731-34-3

5118 As I Am
Fanlight Productions
32 Court Street
21st Floor
Brooklyn, NY 11201
718-488-8900
800-876-1710
Fax: 718-488-8642
info@fanlight.com
www.fanlight.com

Ben Achtenberg, Owner
Anthony Sweeney, Marketing Director

Three young people with developmental disabilities speak for themselves about their lives, the problems they face and their hopes and expectations for the future. *$99.00*
ISBN 1-572950-58-7

5119 Attitudes Toward Persons with Disabilities
Springer Publishing Company
11 West 42nd Street
15th Floor
New York, NY 10036
212-431-4370
877-687-7476
Fax: 212-941-7842
marketing@springerpub.com
www.springerpub.com

James C. Costello, Vice President, Journal Publishing
Diana Osborne, Production Manager
Megan Larkin, Managing Editor, Journals
Theodore C. Nardin, Chief Executive Officer and Publisher

This volume examines what is known of people's complex and multifaceted attitudes toward persons with disabilities. Divided into five areas of concern: theory, origin of attitudes, attitude measurement, attitudes of specific groups and attitude change.
$38.95
352 pages Hardcover
ISBN 0-82616 -90-1

5120 Authoritative Guide to Self- Help Resourcein Mental Health
Guilford Press
72 Spring St
New York, NY 10012-4019
212-431-9800
800-365-7006
Fax: 212-966-6708
info@guilford.com
www.guilford.com

Linda F Campbell PhD, Author
Thomas P Smith PsyD, Author
Robert Sommer PhD, Author
Bob Matloff, President

Reviews and rates 600+ self-help books, autobiographies, and popular films, and evaluates hundreds of Internet sites. Addresses 28 of the most prevalent clinical disorders and life challenges- from ADHD, Alzheimer's, and anxiety disorders, to marital problems, mood disorders and weight management. Also in cloth at $45.00 (ISBN# 1-57230-506-1) *$25.00*
377 pages Paperback
ISBN 1-572305-80-0

5121 AwareNews
Services for Independent Living
26250 Euclid Ave
Suite 801
Euclid, OH 44132
216-731-1529
Fax: 216-731-3083
sil@stratos.net
www.sil-oh.org

Molly Foos, Executive Director
Katherine Foley, Director of Advocacy
Lisa Marn, Assistant Director
Laura A. Gold, Director
12 pages Quarterly

5122 **Bach Flower Therapy: Theory and Practice**
Inner Traditions
1 Park St
Rochester, VT 05767
802-767-3174
Fax: 802-767-3726
customerservice@InnerTraditions.com
www.innertraditions.com
Ehud Sperling, Owner
Contemporary study of Bach's techniques, intended for practitioners and lay readers alike. Includes lists of symptoms to facilitate diagnosis, ans aims to provide an understanding of psychosomatic elements in relation to physical complaints.
ISBN 0-892812-39-7

5123 **Barrier Free Travel: A Nuts and Bolts Guide for Wheelers and Slow Walkers (3rd Edition)**
Demos Health Publishing
11 W 42nd St
15th Fl
New York, NY 10036
212-683-0072
barrierfreetravel.net
Candy Harrington, Author
Billed as the definitive guide to accessible travel, this indispensable resource contains detailed information about the logistics of planning accessible travel by plane, train, bus and ship. *$19.95*
200 pages Paperback
ISBN 1-932603-83-2

5124 **Beliefs, Values, and Principles of Self Advocacy**
Brookline Books
34 University Rd
Brookline, MA 02445-4533
800-666-2665
Fax: 617-734-3952
brbooks@yahoo.com
www.brooklinebooks.com
48 pages Paperback
ISBN 0-57129 -22-2

5125 **Beliefs: Pathways to Health and Well Being**
Metamorphous Press
P.O. Box 10616
Portland, OR 97296-616
503-228-4972
Fax: 503-223-9117
David Balding, Publisher
Explores behavioral technologies and belief change strategies that can alter beliefs that support unhealthy habbits such as smoking, overeating, and drug use. Also covers the changing of thinking processes that create phobias and unreasonable fears, retraining the immune system to eliminate allergies and to deal optinally with cancer, AIDS, and other diseases. Includes strategies to transform unhealthy beliefs into lifelong constructs of wellness.

5126 **Bench Marks**
Govennor's Council on Developmental Disabilities
1717 W Jefferson St
Phoenix, AZ 85007-3202
602-542-4049
800-889-5893
Fax: 602-542-5320
Micheal Ward, Executive Director
Susan Madison, Manager
Quarterly

5127 **Bodie, Dolina, Smith & Hobbs, P.C.**
21 W Susquehanna Ave
Suite 110
Towson, MD 21204-5218
410-823-1250
877-739-1013
Fax: 443-901-0802
chobbs@bodie-law.com
www.bodie-law.com
Chester Hobbs, Esquire
Thomas G. Bodie, Lawyer
Wallace Dann, Lawyer
Thomas J. Dolina, Lawyer
Law firm; provides estates, trusts and guardianship administration, estate planning, elder law, tax issues, bankruptcy, foreclosures, and real estate issues. *$25.00*
Quarterly

5128 **Body Reflexology: Healing at Your Fingertips**
Parker Publishing Company
Ste 2605
1501 Broadway
New York, NY 10036-5600
212-869-6350
Hy Dubin, President
Features step-by-step instructions of how to send healing flows of energy through the body to relieve back pain, headaches, arthritis, and other afflictions. Illustrated.
343 pages Hardcover
ISBN 0-132997-36-3

5129 **Body Silent: The Different World of the Disabled**
WW Norton & Company
324 State Street
Suite H
Santa Barbara, CA 93101-2364
818-718-9900
800-333-6867
Fax: 818-349-2027
editor@specialneeds.com
www.specialneeds.com
256 pages
ISBN 0-393320-42-1

5130 **Body of Knowledge/Hellerwork**
406 Berry St
Mount Shasta, CA 96067-2548
530-926-2500
theheller@aol.com
www.josephheller.com
Joseph Heller, Owner
Information, referral directory, training and certification.

5131 **Bridge Newsletter**
Arizona Bridge to Independent Living
1229 E Washington St
Phoenix, AZ 85034-1101
602-256-2245
800-280-2245
Fax: 602-254-6407
abil.org
Phil Pangrazio, President & CEO
Regina Mitzel, V. P. & Chief Administrative Officer
Amina Kruck, V.P. of Advocacy
Ann Pasco, V.P. of Operations
12 pages Monthly

5132 **Bridging the Gap: A National Directory of Services for Women & Girls with Disabilities**
Educational Equity Concepts
71 Fifth Avenue
New York, NY 10016-5506
212-725-1803
Fax: 212-725-0947
TTY: 212-725-1803
www.edequity.org
Ellen Rubin, Coordinator Disability Programs
Merle Froschl, Editor
Contains a resource section of publications and videos geared specifically to women and girls with disabilities. Available in print, on cassette, and also in Braille. *$24.95*
ISBN 0-931629-16-0

5133 **Bulletin of the Association on the Handicapped**
Assoc. on Handicapped Student Service Program
P.O. Box 21192
Columbus, OH 43221-0192
614-365-5216
Fax: 614-365-6718

5134 **CDR Reports**
Council for Disability Rights
Ste 1540
20 N Wacker Dr
Chicago, IL 60606-2903
312-201-4800
Fax: 312-444-1977
www.disabilityrights.org
Jo Holzer, Executive Director/Editor
Bruce Moore, Employment Specialist
$15.00
8 pages Monthly

5135 **California Financial Power of Attorney**
NOLO
950 Parker St
Berkeley, CA 94710-2524
510-549-1976
800-955-4775
Fax: 510-548-5902
www.nolo.com
Maira Dizgalvis, Trade Customer Service Manager
Susan McConnell, Director Sales
Natasha Kaluza, Sales Assistant
David Rothenberg, CEO
A plain-English book packed with forms and instructions to give a trusted person the legal authority to handle your financial affairs.
Paperback

5136 **Caring for America's Heroes**
Oklahoma City VA Medical Center
921 NE 13th St
Oklahoma City, OK 73104-5007
405-270-0501
Fax: 405-270-1560
www.oklahoma.va.gov
Steven Gentlin, Director
Kathleen Fogarty, Associate Director
D Robert McCaffree MD, Chief of Staff
Tom Duchene, Plant Manager

5137 **Center for Health Research: Eastern Washington University**
Showalter 209a
Cheney, WA 99004
509-359-2279
800-221-9369
Fax: 509-359-2778
sharon.wilson@mail.ewu.edu

5138 **Center for Libraries and Educational Improvement**
400 Maryland Ave SW
Washington, DC 20202-1
202-260-2226
800-872-5327
Fax: 202-401-0689
TTY: 800-437-0833
www.ed.gov

5139 **Centering Corporation Grief Resources**
7230 Maple Street
Omaha, NE 68134
402-553-1200
866-218-0101
Fax: 402-533-0507
j1200@aol.com
www.centering.org
Joy Johnson, Founder
Dr. Marvin Johnson, Founder
Janet Roberts, Executive Director
Kelsey Novacek, Director of Marketing
A full catalog of all our available bereavement resources. We are a small, non-profit organization providing help to families in crisis situations.
32 pages BiAnnually

5140 **Centers for Disease Control and Prevention**
US Department of Health and Human Services
1600 Clifton Rd NE
Atlanta, GA 30329-4018
404-639-3311
800-232-4636
Fax: 404-498-1177
www.cdc.gov
Robert Delaney, Plant Manager
Publishes an annually updated list of infectious and communicable diseases transmitted through the handling of food in accordance with Section 103 of Title I.

5141 **Child With Special Needs: Encouraging Intellectual and Emotional Growth**
Addison-Wesley Publishing Company
Ste 300
75 Arlington St
Boston, MA 02116-3988
617-848-7500
800-238-9682
Fax: 617-944-7273
www.awprofessional.com
Bill Barke, CEO
Covering all kinds of disabilities — including cerebral palsy, autism, developmental, ADD, and language problems — this guide offers parents specific ways of helping all special needs chidren reach their full intellectual and emotional potential. *$32.00*
496 pages
ISBN 0-201407-26-4

5142 **Chinese Herbal Medicine**
Shambhala Publications
300 Massachusetts Avenue
Boston, MA 02115
617-424-0030
Fax: 617-236-1563
editors@shambhala.com
shambhala.com
Richard Reoch, President
Gives an in-depth look into herbal medicine.
176 pages
ISBN 0-877733-98-8

5143 **Christian Approach to Overcoming Disability: A Doctor's Story**
Haworth Press
10 Alice St
Binghamton, NY 13904-1503
607-722-5857
800-429-6784
Fax: 607-722-6362
orders@haworthpress.com
www.haworthpress.com
William Cohen, Owner
$29.95
128 pages
ISBN 0-789022-57-5

5144 **Closing the Gap**
P.O. Box 68
Henderson, MN 56044
507-248-3294
Fax: 507-248-3810
www.closingthegap.com
Dolores Hagen, Co-Founder
Budd Hagen, Co-Founder
Explores use of microcomputers as personal and educational tools for persons with disabilities.
36+ pages BiMonthly

5145 **Conference of the Association on Higher Education & Disability (AHEAD)**
8015 West Kenton Circle
Suite 230
Huntersville, NC 28078
704-947-7779
Fax: 704-948-7779
www.ahead.org
Stephan Smith, Executive Director
Carol Funckes, Chief Operations Officer
Howard Kramer, Conference Director
Jeremy Jarrell, Director, Innovation and Development
An annual conference focused on aiding and meeting the needs of persons with disabilities attending higher education institutions.

5146 **Constellations**
Minnesota STAR Program
Ste 309
50 Sherburne Ave
Saint Paul, MN 55155-1402
651-296-2771
800-657-3862
Fax: 651-282-6671
star.program@state.mn.us
Chuck Rassbach, Executive Director
Free quarterly publication from the Minnesota STAR Program.
8 pages Quarterly

5147 Coping+Plus: Dimensions of Disability
Greenwood Publishing Group
130 Cremona Drive
Santa Barbara, CA 93117
805-968-1911
800-368-6868
Fax: 866-270-3856
CustomerService@abc-clio.com
www.abc-clio.com

Matt Laddin, Vice President of Marketing
Mike Saltzman, Director-Eastern Territories & National Accounts
James Lingle, International Sales & Marketing
Everyone can learn new or more effective coping skills and strategies to deal with times of loss, crisis and disability. $55-$59.95
280 pages Hardcover
ISBN 0-275945-44-8

5148 Council News
Northern Nevada Center for Independent Living
999 Pyramid Way
Sparks, NV 89431-4471
775-353-3599
Fax: 775-353-3588
www.nncil.org

Lisa Bonie, Executive Director
Hilda Velasco, Operations Manager
Joni Inglis, Independent Living Advocate
Patti Rodriguez, Life Skills Coordinator
NNCIL was founded in 1982 by a small group of people with disabilities, who believe that each person, regardless of the severity of his or her disability, has the potential to grow, develop and share fully the joys and responsibilities of our society.
12 pages Quarterly

5149 Counseling in Terminal Care & Bereavement
Brookes Publishing
P.O. Box 10624
Baltimore, MD 21285-0624
410-337-9580
800-638-3775
Fax: 410-337-8539
custserv@brookespublishing.com
readplaylearn.com

Paul H. Brooks, Chairman
Jeffrey D. Brookes, President
Melissa A. Behm, Executive Vice President
Provides practical suggestions for addressing the needs of patients and family members who are anticipating or currently dealing with grief and bereavement, such as hospice care, hospitals, or at home care. *$34.00*
210 pages Paperback
ISBN 1-85433 -78-7

5150 Creating Wholeness: Self-Healing Workbook Using Dynamic Relaxation, Images and Thoughts
Plenum Publishing Corporation
233 Spring St
7th Floor
New York, NY 10013-1522
212-620-8000
800-644-4831
Fax: 212-460-1575
ainy@aveda.com
www.aveda.edu

232 pages
ISBN 0-306441-72-1

5151 DRS Connection
Disabled Resource Services
Ste 101
424 Pine St
Fort Collins, CO 80524-2421
970-482-2700
Fax: 970-407-7072

Nancy Jackson, Executive Director
4 pages Quaterly

5152 Demand Response Transportation Through a Rural ILC
Independent Living Research Utilization ILRU
1333 Moursund
Houston, TX 77030
713-520-0232
Fax: 713-520-5785
ilru@ilru.org
ilru.org

Lex Frieden, Director, ILRU
Richard Petty, Co-Director
Oklahomans for Independent Living's transportation program was selected as exemplary becuase they marketed it by emphasizing people with disabilities as economic constituency.
10 pages

5153 Developing Organized Coalitions and Strategic Plans
Independent Living Research Utilization ILRU
1333 Moursund
Houston, TX 77030
713-520-0232
Fax: 713-520-5785
ilru@ilru.org
ilru.org

Lex Frieden, Director, ILRU
Richard Petty, Co-Director
10 pages

5154 Dictionary of Congenital Malformations& Disorders
Informa Healthcare
Fl 16
52 Vanderbilt Ave
New York, NY 10017-3846
212-520-2777
Fax: 212-661-5052
orders@crcpress.com
www.tandfonline.com

193 pages
ISBN 0-850705-77-1

5155 Dictionary of Developmental Disabilities Terminology
Brookes Publishing
P.O. Box 10624
Baltimore, MD 21285-0624
410-337-9580
800-638-3775
Fax: 410-337-8539
custserv@brookespublishing.com
www.brookespublishing.com

Paul H. Brooks, Chairman
Jeffrey D. Brookes, President
Melissa A. Behm, Executive Vice President
George S. Stamathis, Vice President & Publisher
With more than 3,000 easy-to-understand entries, this dictionary provides thorough explanations of terms associated with developmental disabilities and disorders. *$55.95*
368 pages Hardcover
ISBN 1-557662-45-2

5156 Directory of Members
American Network of Community Options & Resources
1101 King St
Suite 380
Alexandria, VA 22314-2962
703-535-7850
Fax: 703-535-7860
ancor@ancor.org
ancor.org

Dave Toeniskoetter, President
Chris Sparks, Vice President
Julie Manworren, Secretary/Treasurer
Wendy Swager, Past president
The Directory lists over 600 agencies that provide residential services and supports in 48 states and the District of Columbia. The listings include the name of the Executive Directors, the name, address, and phone number of the agency, describe the types of services that are provided and how many individuals receive services from that agency. *$25.00*
189 pages

5157 **Disability Awareness Guide**
Central Iowa Center for Independent Living
655 Walnut St
Suite 131
Des Moines, IA 50309-3930
515-243-1742
Fax: 515-243-5385
Bob Jeppesen, Executive Director
Frank Strong, Assistant Director Programs
Bob Jepson, Manager
The Disability Awareness Guide contains information about our center; who we are and what we do. It also contains the telephone numbers of local and national agencies and resources available for people with disabilities.

5158 **Disability Rights Movement**
Children's Press
Sherman Tpke
Danbury, CT 6813
800-621-1115
Fax: 800-374-4329
Elena Rockman, Marketing Manager
Author Deborah Kent illuminates both the history of the National Disability Rights Movement and the inspiring personal stories of individuals with various disabilities. *$18.00*
32 pages Hardcover
ISBN 0-53106 -32-3

5159 **Disabled People's International Fifth World Assembly as Reported by Two US Participants**
Independent Living Research Utilization ILRU
1333 Moursund
Houston, TX 77030
713-520-0232
Fax: 713-520-5785
ilru@ilru.org
ilru.org
Lex Frieden, Director, ILRU
Richard Petty, Co-Director
This report describes the international conference on independent living held in Mexico City in December 1998 as experienced by staff members from two U.S. centers. Kaye Beneke interviewed Luis Chew and Marco Antonio Coronado for this edition of Readings in Independent Living.
10 pages

5160 **Disabled We Stand**
Brookline Books
34 University Rd
Brookline, MA 02445-4533
800-666-2665
Fax: 617-734-3952
brbooks@yahoo.com
www.brooklinebooks.com
Paperback
ISBN 0-25331 -80-0

5161 **Disabled, the Media, and the Information Age**
Greenwood Publishing Group
130 Cremona Drive
Santa Barbara, CA 93117
805-968-1911
800-368-6868
Fax: 866-270-3856
CustomerService@abc-clio.com
www.abc-clio.com
Matt Laddin, Vice President of Marketing
Mike Saltzman, Director-Eastern Territories & National Accounts
James Lingle, International Sales & Marketing
A short and easy-to-read overview of how disabled Americans have been portrayed by the media and how images and the role of the handicapped are changing. *$55.00*
264 pages Hardcover
ISBN 0-313284-72-5

5162 **Discovery Newsletter**
North Dakota State Library Talking Book Services
Dept 250
604 E Boulevard Ave
Bismarck, ND 58505-605
701-328-2000
800-843-9948
Fax: 701-328-2040
sbschneider@nd.gov
ndsl.lib.state.nd.us/DisabilityServices.html
Doris Ott, Manager
The North Dakota State Library Disability Services produces the Doscovery Newsletter containing information on services, books, catalogs and of interest to the patron.
6 pages Bi-Annually

5163 **EP Resource Guide**
Exceptional Parent Library
P.O. Box 1807
Englewood Cliffs, NJ 7632-1207
201-947-6000
800-535-1910
Fax: 201-947-9376
eplibrary@aol.com
www.eplibrary.com

5164 **ESCIL Update Newsletter**
Eastern Shore Center for Independent Living
9 Sunburst Ctr
Cambridge, MD 21613-2057
410-221-7701
800-705-7944
Fax: 410-221-7714
Shirley Tarbox, Executive Director
Jean Reed, Administrative Assistant
Lisa Morgan, Director IL Services
6 pages Quarterly

5165 **Easy Things to Make Things Simple: Do It Yourself Modifications for Disabled Persons**
Brookline Books
34 University Rd
Brookline, MA 02445-4533
800-666-2665
Fax: 617-734-3952
brbooks@yahoo.com
www.brooklinebooks.com
160 pages Paperback
ISBN 1-571290-24-9

5166 **Enabling Romance: A Guide to Love, Sex & Relationships for the Disabled**
Ken Kroll, Author
Erica Levy Klein, Author
An uncensored, illustrated guide to intimacy and sexual expression for persons with physical disabilities.

5167 **Encyclopedia of Disability**
Sage Publications
2455 Teller Rd
Thousand Oaks, CA 91320-2218
805-499-0721
info@sagepub.com
www.sagepub.com
Gary L Albrecht, Editor
Blaise Simqu, Chief Executive Officer
A five volume set that covers disabilities A-Z *$850.00*
2500 pages
ISBN 0-761925-65-1

5168 **EveryBody's Different: Understanding and Changing Our Reactions to Disabilities**
Brookes Publishing
P.O. Box 10624
Baltimore, MD 21285-0624
410-337-9580
800-638-3775
Fax: 410-337-8539
custserv@brookespublishing.com
readplaylearn.com
Paul H. Brooks, Chairman
Jeffrey D. Brookes, President
Melissa A. Behm, Executive Vice President
This book discusses the emotions, questions, fears, and stereotypes that people without disabilities sometimes experience when they interact with people who do have disabilities. The author teaches readers to become more at ease with the concept of disability and to communicate more effectively with each other. Features activities and exercises that encourage self-examination, helping people to create more enriching personal relationships and work toward a fully inclusive society.
Paperback
ISBN 1-55766 -59-9

5169 **Everybody's Guide to Homeopathic Medicines**
Jeremy P Tarcher
375 Hudson St
New York, NY 10014-3658 212-366-2000
academic@penguin.com
www.us.penguingroup.com
John Makinson, Chairman and CEO
Coram Williams, CFO
Covers alternative treatments in homeopathic medicines.
375 pages
ISBN 0-874778-43-3

5170 **Everyday Social Interaction: A Program for People with Disabilities**
Brookes Publishing
P.O. Box 10624
Baltimore, MD 21285-0624 410-337-9580
800-638-3775
Fax: 410-337-8539
custserv@brookespublishing.com
readplaylearn.com
Paul H. Brooks, Chairman
Jeffrey D. Brookes, President
Melissa A. Behm, Executive Vice President
This source guides teachers and human services professionals in helping people with disabilities acquire social interaction skills and develop satisfying relationships. Included is a checklist and task analyses that shows how complex skills can be broken down into major components for easy performance monitoring accompanied by tips on social courtesies, rewards, praise, and criticism. *$41.95*
342 pages Paperback
ISBN 1-55766 -58-4

5171 **Family Challenges: Parenting with a Disability**
Aquarius Health Care Videos
P.O. Box 1159
Sherborn, MA 01770-7159 508-650-1616
888-440-2963
Fax: 508-650-4216
aqvideos@tiac.net
www.aquariusproductions.com
Lesile Kussmann, Owner
When a parent has a disability, everyone in the family is affected. For children, these experiences may profoundly influence their lives and views of the world. In this sensitive film, you will hear about different roles that all the family members take on at varying times. *$195.00*

5172 **Force A Miracle**
Writer's Showcase Press

244 pages
ISBN 0-595226-88-4

5173 **Forum**
Coalition for the Education of Disabled Children
165 W Center St
Marion, OH 43302-3742 740-382-7362
800-374-2806
Fax: 740-382-3428
Tracie Wilson, Manager
Leeann Derugen, Manager
Forum is a newsletter reporting on legislative and other developments affecting persons with disabilities.
Quarterly

5174 **Foundation Fundamentals for Nonprofit Organizations**
Foundation Center
Department Ze
79 5th Ave
New York, NY 10003-3034 212-620-4230
800-424-9836
Fax: 212-807-3677
order@foundationcenter.org
www.fdncenter.org
Bradford K. Smith, President
Lisa Philip, Vice President for Strategic Philanthropy
Lawrence T. McGill, Vice President for Research
Lisa Brooks, Director of Knowledge Management Systems
This video is designed to give fundraisers a general overview of the foundation funding process and to introduce them to the many resources available through our libraries and cooperating collections. The video gives clear, step-by-step instructions on how to build a fundraising program. *$24.00*
Video

5175 **Four-Ingredient Cookbook**
Laurel Designs
Apt A
1805 Mar West St
Belvedere Tiburon, CA 94920-1962 Fax: 415-435-1451
Janet Sawyer, Owner
Lynn Montoya, Owner
Simple, easy to follow recipes, each containing four ingredients. Particularly suited to persons with limited physical ability. Includes 400 recipes, appetizers to desserts. *$9.00*

5176 **Frequently Asked Questions About Multiple Chemical Sensitivity**
Independent Living Research Utilization ILRU
1333 Moursund
Houston, TX 77030 713-520-0232
Fax: 713-520-5785
ilru@ilru.org
ilru.org
Lex Frieden, Director, ILRU
Richard Petty, Co-Director
This FAQ covers important information about multiple chemical sensitivity and environmental illness. The FAQ describes the conditions, recommends strategies for improving access, and lists resources for CILs and other organizations. As the fact sheet states, centers must set an example in assuring that all people can enter their offices.
10 pages

5177 **Genetic Disorders Sourcebook**
Omnigraphics
615 Griswold Street
Suite 520
Detroit, MI 48226 610-461-3548
800-234-1340
Fax: 800-875-1340
contact@omnigraphics.com
www.omnigraphics.com
Peter Ruffner, Co-Founder
Fred Ruffner, Co-Founder
Provides information on hereditary diseases and disorders. *$7800.00*
650 pages
ISBN 0-789892-41-1

5178 **Genetic Nutritioneering**
McGraw-Hill Company
2460 Kerper Blvd
Dubuque, IA 52001-2224 563-588-1451
800-338-3987
Fax: 614-755-5654
Kurt Strand, VP
Describes how to modify the expression of genetic traits, potentially preventing heart disease, cancer, arthritis, and hormone-related problems. Features how to slow biological aging and reduce the risk of age-related diseases. *$16.95*
288 pages
ISBN 0-879839-21-X

5179 **Going to School with Facilitated Communication**
Syracuse University, School of Education
230 Huntington Hall
Syracuse, NY 13244-1 315-443-4752
Fax: 315-443-2258
jhrusso@syr.edu
www.soe.syr.edu
Shirley Adamczyk, Administrative Assistant
Rachael Gazdick, Executive Director
Isabelle M. Glod, Administrative Assistant
Angela Flanagan, Development Assistant

A video in which students with autism and/or severe disabilities illustrate the use of facilitated communication focusing on basic principles fostering facilitated communication.
Video

5180 Grief: What it is and What You Can Do
Centering Corporation
7230 Maple Street
Omaha, NE 68134
402-553-1200
866-218-0101
Fax: 402-533-0507
j1200@aol.com
www.centering.org
Joy Johnson, Founder
Dr. Marvin Johnson, Founder
Janet Roberts, Executive Director
Kelsey Novacek, Director of Marketing
General grief information for all grief issues. *$3.50*
32 pages Paperback

5181 Guidelines on Disability
US Department of Housing & Urban Development
451 7th St SW
Washington, DC 20410-1
202-708-1112
TTY: 202-708-1455
portal.hud.gov/hudportal/HUD
Shaun Donovan, Secretary
Helen R. Kanovsky, Acting Deputy Secretary
Jennifer Ho, Senior Advisor to the Secretary
Mike Anderson, Chief Human Capital Officer
Contains information on housing and accessibility for persons with disabilities.

5182 Handbook of Services for the Handicapped
Greenwood Publishing Group
130 Cremona Drive
Santa Barbara, CA 93117
805-968-1911
800-368-6868
Fax: 866-270-3856
CustomerService@abc-clio.com
www.abc-clio.com
Matt Laddin, Vice President of Marketing
Mike Saltzman, Director-Eastern Territories & National Accounts
James Lingle, International Sales & Marketing
A handy reference book offering information and services for disabled individuals. $59.95-$65.00.
291 pages Hardcover
ISBN 0-313213-85-2

5183 Healing Herbs
Rodale Press
33 E Minor St
Emmaus, PA 18098-1
610-967-5171
Fax: 610-967-8963
Maria Rodale, Chairman/Chief Executive Officer
Scott D. Schulman, President
Heather Rodale, Board Member/Vice President/ Leadership Development
Thomas A. Pogash, EVP/Chief Financial Officer
Covers everything from growing the herbs to home remedies.

5184 Helen Keller National Center for Deaf- Blind Youths And Adults
141 Middle Neck Rd
Sands Point, NY 11050-1218
516-944-8900
Fax: 516-944-7302
hkncinfo@hknc.org
www.hknc.org
Joseph McNulty, Executive Director
HKNC is the only national vacational and rehabilitation program providing services exclusively to youth and adults who are deaf-blind.

5185 Hospice Alternative
Harper Collins Publishers/Basic Books
10 E 53rd St
New York, NY 10022-5244
212-207-7000
800-242-7737
Fax: 212-207-7203
Jane Friedman, CEO
An account of the hospice experience. An innovative and humane way of caring for the terminally ill. *$8.95*
256 pages
ISBN 0-46503 -61-0

5186 How to File a Title III Complaint
US Department of Justice
950 Pennsylvania Ave NW
Washington, DC 20530-9
202-307-0663
800-574-0301
Fax: 202-307-1197
TTY: 800-514-0383
www.ada.gov
Rebecca B. Bond, Chief
Zita Johnson Betts, Deputy Chiefs
Sally Conway, Deputy Chiefs
James Bostrom, Deputy Chiefs
This publication details the procedure for filing a complaint under Title III of the ADA.

5187 How to Live Longer with a Disability
Accent Books & Products
PO Box 700
Bloomington, IL 61702-700
309-378-2961
800-787-8444
Fax: 309-378-4420
acmtlvng@aol.com
Raymond C Cheever, Publisher
Betty Garee, Editor
Eleven chapters to help you enjoy every aspect of your life, and live easier and happier. Includes sexuality and disability, getting more from the medical community and benefit programs. Co-authored by Robert Mauro, sociologist and Elle Becker, counselor and psychologist, both disabled. *$11.50*
266 pages Paperback
ISBN 0-19570 -38-8

5188 Ideas for Kids on the Go
Accent Books & Products
PO Box 700
Bloomington, IL 61702-700
309-378-2961
800-787-8444
Fax: 309-378-4420
acmtlvng@aol.com
Raymond C Cheever, Publisher
Betty Garee, Editor
This guide shows kids with physical disabilities how to go for it! Lists products and where to get them, and includes tips from others for having fun and getting ahead. Ages 1-18. *$6.95*
69 pages Paperback
ISBN 0-91570 -17-5

5189 If I Only Knew What to Say or Do
AARP Fulfillment
601 E St NW
Washington, DC 20049-1
202-434-2277
800-424-3410
Fax: 202-434-3443
TTY: 877-434-7598
member@aarp.org
www.aarp.org
Carol Raphael, Chair
Ronald E. Daly, Sr., Board Vice Chair
Jeannine English, President
A. Barry Rand, Chief Executive Officer
Provides a concise discussion of how to help a friend in crisis. Learn what to say and what not to say.

5190 If it Weren't for the Honor: I'd Rather Have Walked
Accent Books & Products
PO Box 700
Bloomington, IL 61702-700
309-378-2961
800-787-8444
Fax: 309-378-4420
acmtlvng@aol.com
Raymond C Cheever, Publisher
Betty Garee, Editor
Revealing, often humorous, highly interesting and important reading. This book offers an account told by the author who was

on the scene and actually saw and participated in many events that paved the way for progress for all those with disabilities. *$14.50*
262 pages Paperback
ISBN 0-91570 -41-8

5191 **Imagery in Healing Shamanism and Modern Medicine**
Shambhala Publications
300 Massachusetts Avenue
Horticultural Hall
Boston, MA 02115 617-424-0030
888-424-2329
Fax: 617-236-1563
editors@shambhala.com
www.shambhala.com
Richard Reoch, President
Patients use self imagery to fight sickness and pain throughout their lives. *$15.95*
272 pages
ISBN 1-570629-34-x

5192 **Independence**
Easterseals
1219 Dunn Ave
Daytona Beach, FL 32114-2405 386-255-4568
877-255-4568
Fax: 386-258-7677
Jeff Blass, Chairman
Austin Brownlee, Chair-Elect
Becky Rutland, Vice Chair
Lynn Sinnott, President/ CEO
4-6 pages Quarterly

5193 **Independent Living Centers and Managed Care: Results of an ILRU Study on Involvement**
Independent Living Research Utilization ILRU
1333 Moursund
TIRR Memorial Hermann Research Cent
Houston, TX 77030-7031 713-520-0232
Fax: 713-520-5785
ilru@ilru.org
www.ilru.org
Lex Frieden, Director, ILRU
Richard Petty, Co-Director
Vinh Nguyen, Program Director
This month's Readings presents findings from an ILRU study of roles centers are taking vis-a-vis managed care. Initiated in spring 1998, we asked Drew Batavia to take the lead in conducting this study for us. We were interested in collecting data on frequency with which centers are contacted by consumers with managed care problems. This is a study that will need to be repeated periodically as our experiences with managed care evolves. Meanwhile, here are the initial findings.
10 pages

5194 **Independent Living Challenges the Blues**
Independent Living Research Utilization ILRU
1333 Moursund
TIRR Memorial Hermann Research Cent
Houston, TX 77030-7031 713-520-0232
Fax: 713-520-5785
ilru@ilru.org
www.ilru.org
Lex Frieden, Director, ILRU
Richard Petty, Co-Director
Vinh Nguyen, Program Director
Patricia's article highlights the Georgia SILC's health care advocacy efforts: the Georgia legislature passed a bill enabling Georgia Bleu to convert to for-profit status without a distribution of assets to similar nonprofit corporations; the Georgia SILC joined other health care advocates in filing a class action law suit to challenge the legality of the conversion; the Georgia SILC continues advocacy efforts to involve people with disabilities in developing and monitoring health care policy.
10 pages

5195 **Independent Living Office**
Department of Housing & Urban Development (HUD)
451 7th St SW
Washington, DC 20410-1 202-863-2800
Ted Tozer, President
Rafael Diaz, Chief Information Officer/Chief Information Officer
Mike Anderson, Chief Human Capital Officer
Shaun Donovan, Secretary
This office within HUD is charged with encouraging the construction of housing that is accessible to handicapped persons. The Office of Independent Living encourages modifications of apartments and other dwellings so that handicapped persons can enter without assistance.

5196 **Information Services for People with Developmental Disabilities**
Greenwood Publishing Group
130 Cremona Drive
Santa Barbara, CA 93117 805-968-1911
800-368-6868
Fax: 866-270-3856
CustomerService@abc-clio.com
www.abc-clio.com
Matt Laddin, Vice President of Marketing
Mike Saltzman, Director - Eastern Territories
James Lingle, International Sales & Marketing
Overviews the information needs of people with developmental disabilities and tells librarians how to meet them. $65.oo-$75.00.
368 pages Hardcover
ISBN 0-313287-80-5

5197 **Innovative Programs: An Example of How CILs Can Put Their Work in Context**
Culture
1333 Moursund
TIRR Memorial Hermann Research Cent
Houston, TX 77030-7031 713-520-0232
Fax: 713-520-5785
ilru@ilru.org
www.ilru.org
Lex Frieden, Director, ILRU
Richard Petty, Co-Director
Vinh Nguyen, Program Director
Another winner in the innovative CIL competition- Steve Brown describes the Talking Books Program of Southeast Alaska Independent Living, discussing their efforts to record the oral history and life experiences of people with disabilities in the larger context of disability culture.
10 pages

5198 **Insurance Solutions: Plan Well, Live Better**
Demos Medical Publishing
11 West 42nd Street
15th Floor
New York, NY 10036 212-683-0072
800-532-8663
Fax: 212-683-0118
support@demosmedical.com
www.demosmedpub.com
Paul Choi, Vice-President of Finance and Operations
Matt Conmy, Sr. Director of Sales
Thomas Hastings, Marketing Manager
Beth Kaufman Barry, Publisher
Learn how to look at various insurance options from a new perspective — including life, disability, health, and long-term care. Concrete information for dealing with potential problems in your coverage, to secure your financial future. *$24.95*
192 pages 2002
ISBN 1-888799-55-2

5199 **International Directory of Libraries for the Disabled**
KG Saur/Division of RR Bowker
121 Chanlon Rd
New Providence, NJ 7974-1541 908-286-1090
800-521-8110
Michael Cairns, CEO
An essential resource for improving the quality and quantity of materials available to the print-handicapped audience. Featuring

talking books, Braille books, large print books as well as production centers for these materials. *$46.00*
257 pages
ISBN 3-59821 -81-1

5200 Issues in Independent Living
Independent Living Research Utilization
1333 Moursund
TIRR Memorial Hermann Research Cent
Houston, TX 77030-7031
713-520-0232
Fax: 713-520-5785
ilru@ilru.org
www.ilru.org
Lex Frieden, Executive Director
Vinh Nguyen, Program Director
This booklet is a report of the National Study Group on the Implications of Health Care Reform for Americans with Disabilities and Chronic Health Conditions.
30 pages

5201 JAMA: The Journal of the American Medical Association
American Medical Association
PO Box 10946
Chicago, IL 60654-4820
312-670-7827
800-262-2350
Fax: 312-464-5909
subscriptions@jamanetwork.com
jama.jamanetwork.com
Howard Bauchner, MD, Editor-in-Chief
Articles cover all aspects of medical research and clinical medicine. *$66.00*

5202 JCIL Advocate Times
Jackson Center for Independent Living
409 Linden Ave
Jackson, MI 49203-4065
517-782-6054
Fax: 517-782-3118
Lesia Pikaart, Executive Director
JoAnn Lucas, Associate Director
Quarterly

5203 Jason & Nordic Publishers, Inc.
PO Box 441
Hollidaysburg, PA 16648-441
814-696-2929
Fax: 814-696-4250
Norma Mc Phee, Owner/CEO
Norma Phee
Turtle Books for children with disabilities present heroes who look like them, have problems like theirs, have similar doubts and feelings in non-threatening, fun stories. They are motivational, bridge the gap and promote understanding among peers and siblings. 22 children's books (grades preK-3) plus Sensitivity and Awareness Guide containing lesson plans, activities, background information keyed to the series. Disabilities include: Down syndrome, cerebral palsy, blindness, deafness and more.

5204 Journal of Social Work in Disabilty & Rehabilitation
Haworth Press
10 Alice St
Binghamton, NY 13904-1503
607-722-5857
800-429-6784
Fax: 607-722-6362
orders@haworthpress.com
www.haworthpress.com
William Cohen, Owner
John T Oardeck PhD, Editor
S Harrington-Miller, Advertising
Presents and explores issues related to disabilities and social policy, practice, research, and theory. Reflecting the broad scope of social work in disabilty practice, this interdisciplinary journal examines vital issues aspects of the field — from innovative practice methods, legal issues, and literature reviews to program descriptions and cuttinf-edge practice research.
Quarterly

5205 Just Like Everyone Else
World Institute on Disability
3075 Adeline St.
Suite 155
Berkeley, CA 94703
510-225-6400
Fax: 510-225-0477
wid@wid.org
www.wid.org
Marcie Roth, Executive Director & CEO
Katherine Zigmont, Senior Director, Operations & Deputy Director
Reggie Johnson, Senior Director, Marketing & Communications
Marsha Saxton, Director, Research
Intended for general audiences, the publication provides perspective, inspiration and information about the Independent Living Movement and the Americans with Disabilities Act.

5206 Keep the Promise: Managed Care and People with Disabilities
American Network of Community Options & Resource
1101 King St
Ste 380
Alexandria, VA 22314-2962
703-535-7850
Fax: 703-535-7860
ancor@ancor.org
www.ancor.org
Dave Toeniskoetter, President
Chris Sparks, Vice President
Julie Manworren, Secretary/Treasurer
Renee L. Pietrangelo, PhD, Chief Executive Officer
This publication presents a detailed review of the process and the lessons learned. Details a way for all stake holders to work together for a state or local system.
119 pages $18 - $22

5207 Keeping Our Families Together
Through the Looking Glass
3075 Adeline St.
Ste. 120
Berkeley, CA 94703-2212
510-848-1112
800-644-2666
Fax: 510-848-4445
TTY: 510-848-1005
tlg@lookingglass.org
www.lookingglass.org
Maureen Block, J.D., Board President
Thomas Spalding, Board Treasurer
Alice Nemon, D.S.W., Board Secretary
Report of the National Task Force on parents with disabilities and their families. Available in Braille, large print or cassette. *$2.00*
12 pages

5208 Learn About the ADA in Your Local Library
US Department of Justice
950 Pennsylvania Ave NW
Washington, DC 20530-9
202-307-0663
800-574-0301
Fax: 202-307-1197
TTY: 800-514-0383
www.ada.gov
Rebecca B. Bond, Chief
Zita Johnson Betts, Deputy Chiefs
Sally Conway, Deputy Chiefs
A 10-page annotated list of 95 ADA publications and one videotape that are available in 15,000 public libraries throughout the country.

5209 LifeLines
Disabled & Alone/Life Services for the Handicapped
1440 Broadway
23rd Floor
New York, NY 10018-2326
212-532-6740
800-995-0066
Fax: 212-532-6740
info@disabledandalone.org
www.disabledandalone.org/lifelines.html
Leslie D. Park, Chair
Rex L. Davidson, Vice President
Lee Alan Ackerman, Executive Director
William G. Shannon, Treasurer

Newsletter providing current and valuable information about lifetime care and planning for persons with disabilities and their families and the organizations serving them. Free upon request.
4-10 pages Biannual

5210 Lifelong Leisure Skills and Lifestyles for Persons with Developmental Disabilities
Brookes Publishing
PO Box 10624
Baltimore, MD 21285-0624
410-337-9580
800-638-3775
Fax: 410-337-8539
custserv@brookespublishing.com
www.readplaylearn.com

Paul H. Brooks, Chairman
Jeffrey D. Brookes, President
Melissa A. Behm, Executive Vice President
This instructional manual offers ideas and detailed examples that describe how to guide individuals of all ages through popular activities using adaptations that foster skill acquisition and inclusion. Some of the concepts explored are home-school-community collaboration, choice making and the dignity of risk, and leisure skill acquisition for the life span. *$35.00*
352 pages Paperback
ISBN 1-55766-47-2

5211 Livin'
Lehigh Valley Center for Independent Living
435 Allentown Dr
Allentown, PA 18109-9121
610-770-9781
Fax: 610-770-9801
info@lvcil.org
www.lvcil.org

Amy Beck, Executive Director
Cara Steidel, Director of Finance
Greg Bott, Director of Development
Jessica DeMaio, Administrative Services Coordinator
4 pages Quarterly

5212 Living in a State of Stuck
Brookline Books
8 Trumbull Rd
Suite B-001
Northampton, MA 01060
413-584-0184
800-666-2665
Fax: 413-584-6184
brbooks@yahoo.com
www.brooklinebooks.com

3rd ed., paper
ISBN 1-571290-27-3

5213 Living in the Community
Independent Living Research Utilization ILRU
1333 Moursund
TIRR Memorial Hermann Research Cent
Houston, TX 77030-7031
713-520-0232
Fax: 713-520-5785
ilru@ilru.org
www.ilru.org

Lex Frieden, Director, ILRU
Richard Petty, Co-Director
Vinh Nguyen, Program Director
James, Lori, and Jamey describe the elements of their successful program to move people out of nursing homes and into the community: providing funding for deposits, first month's rent and other neccessities, including assistive technology; providing training and the other core services before and after consumers leave the nursing home; developing relationships with housing and other service providers.
10 pages

5214 Loud, Proud and Passionate
Mobility International USA
132 E Broadway
Suite 343
Eugene, OR 97401
541-343-1284
Fax: 541-343-6812
TTY: 541-343-1284
clearinghouse@miusa.org
www.miusa.org

Susan Sygall, Chief Executive Officer
Cindy Lewis, Director, Programs
A resource book for international development and women's organization about including women with disabilities in projects in the community. Informs women with disabilities about the efforts and successes of their peers worldwide.

5215 Love: Where to Find It, How to Keep It
Accent Books & Products
PO Box 700
Bloomington, IL 61702-700
309-378-2961
800-787-8444
Fax: 309-378-4420
acmtlvng@aol.com

Raymond C Cheever, Publisher
Betty Garee, Editor
Offers ideas such as how to meet other single people, avoid the wrong type; communications skills and much more for the disabled person wanting to date. *$6.95*
104 pages Paperback
ISBN 0-91570-31-0

5216 MOOSE: A Very Special Person
Brookline Books
8 Trumbull Rd
Suite B-001
Northampton, MA 01060
413-584-0184
800-666-2665
Fax: 413-584-6184
brbooks@yahoo.com
www.brooklinebooks.com

Paperback
ISBN 0-91479-73-5

5217 Mainstream Magazine
2973 Beech St
San Diego, CA 92102-1529
619-232-2727
Fax: 619-234-3155
www.mainstream-mag.com

Cyndi Jones, Executive Director
The authoritative, national voice of people with disabilities, publishes in-depth reports on employment, education, new products and technology, legislation and disability rights advocacy, recreation and travel, disability arts and culture, plus personality profiles and challenging commentary. *$24.00*
Monthly

5218 Making Changes: Family Voices on Living Disabilities
Brookline Books
8 Trumbull Rd
Suite B-001
Northampton, MA 01060
413-584-0184
800-666-2665
Fax: 413-584-6184
brbooks@yahoo.com
www.brooklinebooks.com

216 pages Paperback
ISBN 0-91479-93-

5219 Making Informed Medical Decisions: Where to Look and How to Use What You Find
Patient-Centered Guides
1005 Gravenstein Highway North
Sebastopol, CA 95472-3836
707-827-7019
800-889-8969
Fax: 707-824-8268
orders@oreilly.com

Tim O'Reilly, CEO
Making Informed Medical Decisions acts like a friendly reference librarian, explaining: tips for researching for someone else; medical journal articles; statistics and risk; standard treatment

options; clinical trial; making an ally of your doctor; and determining your own best course. Authors Oster, Thomas, and Joseff-a patient advocate, medical librarian, and medical doctor-also share examples and stories. *$17.95*

280 pages Paperback

ISBN 1-565924-59-2

5220 Making Wise Decisions for Long-Term Care

AARP Fulfillment
601 E St NW
Washington, DC 20049-1
202-434-2277
800-424-3410
Fax: 202-434-3443
TTY: 877-434-7598
member@aarp.org
www.aarp.org

Carol Raphael, Chair
Ronald E. Daly, Sr., Board Vice Chair
Jeannine English, President
A. Barry Rand, Chief Executive Officer

Here's a comprehensive consumer education effort in the area of long-term care.

28 pages

5221 Making a Difference

Georgia Council On Developmental Disabilities
2 Peachtree St N.W.
Suite 26-246
Atlanta, GA 30303-3141
404-657-2126
888-275-4233
Fax: 404-657-2132
TTY: 404-657-2133
eejacobson@dhr.state.ga.us
www.gcdd.org

Eric E Jacobson, Executive Director
Pat Nobbie, Deputy Director
Dottie Adams, Family/Individual Support Dir.
Valerie Meadows Suber, Public Information Director

The Georgia Council on Developmental Disabilities collaborates with Georgia's citizens, public and private advocacy organizations and policymakers to positively influence public policies that enhance the quality of life for people with disabilities and their families. GCDD provides this through education and advocacy activities, program implementation, funding and public policy analysis and research.

5222 Making a Difference: A Wise Approach

Easterseals
141 W Jackson Blvd.
Suite 1400A
Chicago, IL 60604
312-726-6200
800-221-6827
Fax: 312-726-1494
info@easterseals.com
www.easterseals.com

Angela F. Williams, President & CEO
Glenda Oakley, Chief Financial Officer
Marcy Traxler, Senior Vice President, Network Advancement
John Osterlund, Senior Vice President, Development

The town of Wise, Virginia, and its leading citizen, Virgil Craft, personify what Making a Difference is all about when a community supports implementing the provisions of the Americans with Disabilities Act. Craft, a person with a disability, has spent his life giving back to the community. The community, in turn, has supported Craft's efforts to improve the environment, education, healthcare and access for disabled persons. A 16-minute video.

5223 Managing Your Activities

Arthritis Foundation
PO Box 78423
Atlanta, GA 30357-0669
404-237-8771
800-933-7023
Fax: 404-872-0457
help@arthritis.org
www.arthritis.org

John H Klippel, CEO/ President

5224 Managing Your Health Care

Arthritis Foundation
PO Box 78423
Atlanta, GA 30357-0669
404-237-8771
800-933-7023
Fax: 404-872-0457
help@arthritis.org
www.arthritis.org

John H Klippel, CEO/ President

5225 Medical Aspects of Disability: A Handbook For The Rehabilitation Professional

Springer Publishing Company
11 West 42nd Street
15th Floor
New York, NY 10036
212-431-4370
877-687-7476
Fax: 212-941-7842
cs@springerpub.com
www.springerpub.com

Ursula Springer, President
Theodore C. Nardin, CEO/Publisher
Jason Roth, VP/Marketing Director
James C. Costello, Vice President, Journal Publishing

$62.92

744 pages

ISBN 0-826179-71-1

5226 Meeting the Needs of Employees with Disabilities

Resources for Rehabilitation
22 Bonad Road
Ste 19a
Winchester, MA 01890-4330
781-368-9080
Fax: 781-368-9096
orders@rfr.org
www.rfr.org

Susan Greenblatt, Editor

Provides information to help people with disabilities retain or obtain employment. Information on government programs and laws, supported employment, training programs, environmental adaptations and the transition from school to work are included. Chapters on mobility impairment, vision impairment and hearing and speech impairments. *$47.95*

167 pages Biennial

ISBN 0-92971 -13-5

5227 NCD Bulletin

National Council on Disability
1331 F Street Northwest
Suite 850
Washington, DC 20004- 1138
202-272-2004
Fax: 202-272-2022
ncd@ncd.gov
www.ncd.gov

Jeff Rosen, Chairperson
Kamilah Oni Martin-Proctor, Co-Vice Chair
Lynnae Ruttledge, Co-Vice Chair
Rebecca Cokley, Executive Director

Reports on the latest issues and news affecting people with disabilities.

2 pages Monthly

5228 NCDE Survival Strategies for Overseas Living for People with Disabilities

Mobility International USA
132 E Broadway
Suite 343
Eugene, OR 97401
541-343-1284
Fax: 541-343-6812
TTY: 541-343-1284
clearinghouse@miusa.org
www.miusa.org

Susan Sygall, Chief Executive Officer
Cindy Lewis, Director, Programs

This book will provide individuals with disablilities information, resources and guidance on pursuing international exchange opportunities. It addresses disability-related aspects of the international exchange process such as choosing a program, applying, preparing for the trip, adjusting to a new country and returning home.

5229 **National Hookup**
ISC
16 Liberty St
Larkspur, CA 94939-1520 415-924-3549
Fax: 415-927-9556
Russ Bohlke, Manager
Newsletter published by ISC, a national organization of people with physical disabilities. *$6.00*
12-16 pages Quarterly

5230 **New Horizons in Sexuality**
Accent Books & Products
PO Box 700
Bloomington, IL 61702-700 309-378-2961
800-787-8444
Fax: 309-378-4420
acmtlvng@aol.com
Raymond C Cheever, Publisher
Betty Garee, Editor
This manual helps both males and females progress toward a satisfying post-injury relationship. *$7.95*
50 pages Paperback
ISBN 0-91570 -42-6

5231 **New Voices: Self Advocacy By People with Disabilities**
Brookline Books
8 Trumbull Rd
Suite B-001
Northampton, MA 01060 413-584-0184
800-666-2665
Fax: 413-584-6184
brbooks@yahoo.com
www.brooklinebooks.com
274 pages Paperback
ISBN 1-57129 -04-4

5232 **North Star Community Services**
3420 University Ave
Waterloo, IA 50701-2050 319-236-0901
888-879-1365
Fax: 319-236-3701
jmuller@northstarcs.org
www.northstarcs.org
Mark Witmer, Executive Director
Matt Hinders, Director of Operations & Safety
Bridget Hartmann, Director of Human Resources
Terri Davis, Director of Financial Services
North Star Community Services is a rehabilitative services organization with home office in Waterloo, IA and several branch offices in Northeast, Northern and Central Iowa. North Star helps indiviuals with disabilities live and work in their communities. Services include: adult day services, supported community living services, employment services, and case management/service coordination.

5233 **Nothing is Impossible: Reflections on a New Life**
Ballantine Books
1745 Broadway
10th Floor
New York, NY 10019 212-782-9000
rhkidspublicity@randomhouse.com
www.atrandom.com
Edward Warren, Owner
Reeve offers a uniquely powerful message of hope on topics ranging from the controversial stem cell debate to the mind-body connection he credits with his recent physical improvements. *$6.99*
224 pages
ISBN 0-345470-73-7

5234 **Nutritional Desk Reference**
Keats Publishing
P.O. Box 876
New Canaan, CT 06840 203-966-8721
800-323-4900

5235 **Nutritional Influences on Illness:**
Third Line Press
4751 Viviana Dr
Tarzana, CA 91356-5038 818-996-0076
third-line.com
Melvyn R Werbach, Owner
A comprehensive summary of the world's knowledge concerning the relationship between dietary and nutrtional factors and illness. This book does not try to promote any particular school of thought. Instead of the author telling readers his opinion as to what research says, he makes it easy for them to see data for themselves and then form their own opinions.
504 pages
ISBN 0-879835-31-1

5236 **Oregon Perspectives**
Oregon Council on Developmental Disabilities
540 24th Pl NE
Salem, OR 97301-4517 503-945-9941
800-292-4154
Fax: 503-945-9947
www.ocdd.org
Laura Bronson, Office Manager
Beth Kessler, Planning & Communications Coordi
A quarterly publication from the Oregon Council on Developmental Disabilities.

5237 **Organ Transplants: Making the Most of Your Gift of Life**
Patient-Centered Guides
1005 Gravenstein Highway North
Sebastopol, CA 95472-3836 707-827-7000
800-998-9938
Fax: 707-824-8268
orders@oreilly.com
Linda Lamb, Series Editor
Shawnde Paull, Marketing
Tim O'Reilly, CEO
Over 64,000 people in the US are awaiting an organ transplant. Although transplant surgeries are now fairly routine and can give their recipients the gift of new life, the road to getting a transplant can be long and harrowing. Living with immunosuppressive drugs and strong emotional responses can also be more challenging than families imagine. Medical journalist Robert Finn answers the concerns of these families, with the latest facts about transplantation - as well as the stories behind them. *$19.95*
326 pages Paperback
ISBN 1-565926-34-X

5238 **PEAK Parent Center**
917 East Moreno Ave.
Suite 140
Colorado Springs, CO 80903 719-531-9400
Fax: 719-531-9452
info@peakparent.org
www.peakparent.org
Michele Williers, Executive Director
Pam Christy, Director, Parent Training & Information
PEAK Parent Center is Colorado's federally-designated Parent Training and Information Center (PTI). As a PTI, PEAK supports and empowers parents, providing them with information and strategies to use when advocating for their children with disabilities. PEAK works one-on-one with families and educators helping them realize new possibilities for children with disabilities by expanding knowledge of special education and offering new strategies for success.

5239 **Parallels in Time**
MN Governor's Council on Development Disabilities
658 Cedar St
Saint Paul, MN 55155-1603 651-296-4018
877-348-0505
Fax: 651-297-7200
admin.dd@state.mn.us
www.mncdd.org
Colleen Wieck PhD, Executive Director
Parallels in Time traces present attitudes and the treatment of people with disabilities, and supplements the first weekend seesion of Partners in Policymaking. This CD-ROM includes the History of the Parent Movement and the History of the Independent Living Movement, as well as personal stories of self advocates, leaders in the self advocacy movement.

5240 **Part of the Team**
Easterseals
Ste 1800
230 W Monroe St
Chicago, IL 60606-4851 312-726-6800
Fax: 312-726-1494

Janet D Jamieson, Communications Manager
James Williams Jr, Chief Executive Officer

Designed for employers of all sizes, rehabilitation organizations and all others concerned with the employment of people with disabilities. It addresses managers' concerns and questions about supervising persons with disabilities and can be used as a discussion/team-building tool for employees with and without disabilities. The video recognizes people with disabilities as strong contenders for almost any job. *$15.00*

5241 **Partnering with Public Health: Funding& Advocacy Opportunities for CILs and SILCs**
Independent Living Research Utilization ILRU
1333 Moursund
Houston, TX 77030-7031 713-520-0232
Fax: 713-520-5785
ilru@ilru.org
ilru.org

Lex Frieden, Director, ILRU
Richard Petty, Co-Director

Laura Rauscher discusses how CILs and SCILs can use funding from the Centers for Disease Control and partnerships with public health agencies to provide innovative programs promoting the health of people with disabilities.
10 pages

5242 **Peer Counseling: Roles, Functions, Boundaries**
Independent Living Research Utilization ILRU
1333 Moursund
Houston, TX 77030-7031 713-520-0232
Fax: 713-520-5785
ilru@ilru.org
ilru.org

Lex Frieden, Director, ILRU
Richard Petty, Co-Cirector

In this article, the following points were discussed: describing peer support as counseling suggests safeguards and expectations which cannot be provided by nonprofessionals; the purpose of peer counseling is to promote the independent living philosophy and encourage consumers to embrace it; peer counseling cannot and is not intended to help individuals deal with intense emotional stress, whether it is related to their disability or to something else.
10 pages

5243 **Peer Mentor Volunteers: Empowering People for Change**
Independent Living Research Utilization ILRU
1333 Moursund
Houston, TX 77030-7031 713-520-0232
Fax: 713-520-5785
ilru@ilru.org
ilru.org

Lex Frieden, Director, ILRU
Richard Petty, Co-Director

Arizona Bridge to Independent Living (ABIL) in Phoenix, featured in this issue, is another winner in the innovative CIL program competition.
10 pages

5244 **People and Families**
New Jersey Council on Developmental Disabilities
20 West State Street, 6th Floor
P.O. Box 700
Trenton, NJ 08625-0700 609-292-3745
800-792-8858
Fax: 609-292-7114
TTY: 609-777-3238
njcdd@njcdd.org
www.njcdd.org

Elaine Buchsbaum, Chairman
Christopher Miller, Vice Chair
Alison M. Lozano, Ph.D, Executive Director
Shirla Rufo Simpson, M.A., DRCC, Deputy Director

A free magazine for people with disabilities, their families and the public about disability topics such as personal assistance, deinstitutionalization, health care and community living. Published by the New Jersey council on Developmental Disabilities, a federally funded advocacy and policy advisory body. The council has 25 members - 15 consumer/product volunteers and 10 professionals.
48 pages Quarterly

5245 **People with Disabilities & Abuse: Implications for Center for Independent Living**
Independent Living Research Utilization ILRU
1333 Moursund
P.O. Box 700
Houston, TX 77030-7031 713-520-0232
Fax: 713-520-5785
ilru@ilru.org
ilru.org

Lex Frieden, Director, ILRU
Richard Petty, Co-Director
10 pages

5246 **People with Disabilities Who Challenge the System**
Brookes Publishing
P.O. Box 10624
Baltimore, MD 21285-0624 410-337-9580
800-638-3775
Fax: 410-337-8539
custserv@brookespublishing.com
readplaylearn.com

Paul H. Brooks, Chairman
Jeffrey D. Brookes, President
Melissa A. Behm, Executive Vice President
Jeffrey D. Brookes, President

Helpful forms, tables, and case studies plus an emphasis on self-determination point the way to the development of supports so that people who are deaf-blind, have severe to profound physical and cognitive disabilities, or have serious behavior problems can be fully included in the classroom, workplace, and community. *$34.00*
464 pages Paperback
ISBN 1-55766 -29-0

5247 **People's Voice**
Independence CIL
300 3rd Ave SW
Suite F
Minot, ND 58701-4346 701-839-4724
800-377-5114
Fax: 701-838-1677
independencecil@independencecil.org
independencecil.org

Susan Ogurek, Chair
Heather Wittliff, Vice Chair
Scott Burlingame, Executive Director
Emily Rodacker, Secretary/Treasurer
8 pages Quarterly

5248 **Personal Perspectives on Personal Assistance Services**
World Institute on Disability
3075 Adeline St.
Suite 155
Berkeley, CA 94703 510-225-6400
Fax: 510-225-0477
wid@wid.org
www.wid.org

Marcie Roth, Executive Director & CEO
Katherine Zigmont, Senior Director, Operations & Deputy Director
Reggie Johnson, Senior Director, Marketing & Communications
Marsha Saxton, Director, Research

A collection of personal essays that explores a range of perspectives on Personal Assistance Services. Family issues and PAS concerns for people with various different disabilities, of different ages and as members of minority groups are addressed.

5249 **Perspectives**
National Assoc of State Directors of DD Services
113 Oronoco St
Alexandria, VA 22314-2015
703-683-4202
Fax: 703-684-1395
dberland@nasddds.org

Nancy Thaler, Executive Director
Nancy Thaler, Executive Director

Provides a concise summary of national policy developments and initiatives affecting persons with devlopmental disabilities and the programs that serve them. From bills pending before Congress, to the growth in Medicaid-funded services, to changes in federal-state Medicaid policies and the shift of responsibility from Washington to the states, keeps readers in tune with the latest national issues shaping publically funded disability services.
$95.00
Monthly

5250 **Place to Live**
Accent Books & Products
P.O. Box 700
Bloomington, IL 61702-700
309-378-2961
800-787-8444
Fax: 309-378-4420
acmtlvng@aol.com

Raymond C Cheever, Publisher
Betty Garee, Editor
Raymond C Cheever, Publisher

Many disabled people have found that group housing or accessible apartments are the best alternative to living in a nursing home. These articles tell about some of the alternatives people have found so they can live independently. Just one idea might be the answer for better living for you. *$4.95*
64 pages Paperback
ISBN 0-91570 -30-2

5251 **Psychological & Social Impact of Disability**
Springer Publishing Company
11 West 42nd Street
15th Floor
New York, NY 10036
212-431-4370
877-687-7476
Fax: 212-941-7842
cs@springerpub.com
www.springerpub.com

James C. Costello, Vice President, Journal Publishing
Diana Osborne, Production Manager
Megan Larkin, Managing Editor, Journals
$49.95
488 pages
ISBN 0-826122-13-2

5252 **Psychology and Health**
Springer Publishing Company
11 West 42nd Street
15th Floor
New York, NY 10036
212-431-4370
877-687-7476
Fax: 212-941-7842
cs@springerpub.com
www.springerpub.com

James C. Costello, Vice President, Journal Publishing
Diana Osborne, Production Manager
Megan Larkin, Managing Editor, Journals

Content of this book spans a wide range of clinical conditions, including somatization disorders, chronic pain, migraine, anxiety and cancer. *$29.95*
256 pages

5253 **Psychology of Disability**
Springer Publishing Company
11 West 42nd Street,
15th Floor
New York, NY 10036-3915
212-431-4370
877-687-7476
Fax: 212-941-7842
cs@springerpub.com
www.springerpub.com

James C. Costello, Vice President, Journal Publishing
Diana Osborne, Production Manager
Megan Larkin, Managing Editor, Journals
Theodore C Nardin, Chief Executive Officer

Reactions to the disabled. *$27.95*
288 pages
ISBN 0-82613 -40-1

5254 **Quality of Life for Persons with Disabilities**
Brookline Books
8 Trumbull Road
Suite B-001
Northampton, MA 01060
413-584-0184
800-666-2665
Fax: 413-584-6184
brbooks@yahoo.com
www.brooklinebooks.com

James C. Costello, Vice President, Journal Publishing

Quality of life generally refers to a person's subjective experience of his or her life and focuses attention on how the individual with a disabling condition experiences the world. This book presents a comprehensive and international view of this concept as applied to a broad range of settings in which persons with disabilities live, work and play. *$35.00*
Paperback
ISBN 0-91479 -92-1

5255 **REACHing Out Newsletter**
REACH of Dallas Resource on Independent Living
8625 King George
Suite 210
Dallas, TX 75235-2286
214-630-4796
Fax: 214-630-6390
TTY: 214-630-5995
reachdallas@reachcils.org
reachcils.org

Charlotte A. Stewart, Executive Director

Quarterly newsletter from REACH of Dallas Resource Center on Independent Living.
16 pages Quarterly

5256 **RTC Connection**
Research and Training Center
University of Wisconsin Stou
Menomonie, WI 54751
715-232-2236
Fax: 715-232-2251
menz@uwstout.edu

Julie Larson, Program Assistant

Bi-annual reports on disability and rehabilitation research and policy topics.
Newsletter

5257 **Relaxation: A Comprehensive Manual for Adults and Children with Special Needs**
Research Press
2612 N. Mattis Ave.
P.O. Box 7886
Champaign, IL 61822- 9177
217-352-3273
800-519-2707
Fax: 217-352-1221
orders@researchpress.com
www.researchpress.com

Paperback
ISBN 0-878221-86-8

5258 **Resources for People with Disabilities and Chronic Conditions**
Resources for Rehabilitation
Ste 19a
33 Bedford St
Lexington, MA 02420-4330
781-890-6371
Fax: 781-861-7517
Susan Greenblatt
A comprehensive resource directory that helps people with disabilities and chronic conditions achieve their maximum level of independence. Chapters on spinal cord injuries, low back pain, diabetes, hearing and speech impairments, epilepsy, multiple sclerosis. Describes organizations, products and publications. *$49.95*
215 pages Biennial
ISBN 0-92971 -12-7

5259 **Role Portrayal and Stereotyping on Television**
Greenwood Publishing Group
130 Cremona Drive
P O Box 1911
Santa Barbara, CA 93117- 4208
203-226-3571
800-368-6868
805-968-1911
Fax: 866-270-3856
customerservice@abc-clio.com
www.abc-clio.com
214 pages $55 - $59.95
ISBN 0-313248-55-9

5260 **Screening in Chronic Disease**
Oxford University Press
2001 Evans Rd
Cary, NC 27513-2009
800-445-9714
877-773-4325
Fax: 919-677-1303
custserv.us@oup.com
global.oup.com
Thomas Carty, Senior Vice President
Early detection, or screening, is a common strategy for controlling chronic disease, but little information has been available to help determine which screening procedures are worthwhile, until this textbook. *$42.50*
256 pages

5261 **Sexual Adjustment**
Accent Books & Products
P.O. Box 700
Bloomington, IL 61702-700
309-378-2961
800-787-8444
Fax: 309-378-4420
acmtlvng@aol.com
Raymond C Cheever, Publisher
Betty Garee, Editor
Essential information concerning sexual adjustment for the paraplegic male. *$4.95*
73 pages Paperback
ISBN 0-19570 -00-0

5262 **Sexuality and Disabilities: A Guide for Human Service Practitioners**
Haworth Press
2&4 Park Square
Abingdon, FL 33487-1503
561-994-0555
Fax: 561-241-7856
orders@taylorandfrancis.com
159 pages Hardcover
ISBN 1-560243-75-9

5263 **Sickened: The Memoir of a Muchausen by Proxy Childhood**
Bantam Books
1745 Broadway
10th Floor
New York, NY 10019-4039
212-782-9000
Fax: 212-572-6066
crownpublicity@randomhouse.com
www.randomhouse.com
256 pages Hardcover
ISBN 0-553803-07-7

5264 **Socialization Games for Persons with Disabilities**
Charles C. Thomas
2600 S First St
Springfield, IL 62704-4730
217-789-8980
800-258-8980
Fax: 217-789-9130
books@ccthomas.com
www.ccthomas.com
Michael P. Thomas, President
This text will assist those who want to teach severely multiple disabled students by providing information on: general principles of intervention and classroom organization; managing the behavior of students; physically managing students and using adaptive equipment; teaching eating skills; teaching toileting, dressing, and hygiene skills; teaching cognition, communication, and socialization skills; teaching independent living skills; and teaching infants and preschool students. *$38.95*
176 pages Paperback
ISBN 0-398067-46-5

5265 **Sometimes You Just Want to Feel Like a Human Being**
Brookes Publishing
P.O. Box 10624
Baltimore, MD 21285-0624
410-337-9580
800-638-3775
Fax: 410-337-8539
custserv@brookespublishing.com
readplaylearn.com
Paul Brooks, Owner
Case studies of empowering psychotherapy with people with disabilities. This text reveals how counseling can be beneficial to individuals with disabilities of all kinds, including autism, developmental disabilities, sensory impairment, cerebral palsy, or HIV infection. *$26.95*
272 pages Paperback
ISBN 1-55766 -96-0

5266 **South Carolina Assistive Technology Program**
8301 Farrow Road
University Center for Excellence
Columbia, SC 29203-2920
803-935-5263
800-915-4522
Fax: 803-935-5342
carol.page@uscmed.sc.edu
www.sc.edu/scatp/
Carol Page, Ph.D, Program Director
Mary r Alice Bechtle, Program Coordinator
Janet Jendron, Program Coordinator
Lydia Durham, Administrative Assistant
The South Carolina Assistive Technology Program (SCATP) is a federally funded program concerned with getting technology into the hands of people with disabilities so that they might live, work, learn and be a more independent part of the community.We provide an equipment loan and demonstration program, an on-line equipment exchange program, training, technical assistance, publications, an interactive CDROM (SC Curriculum Access through AT), an information listserv and work with various state com
7-8 pages Bi-annually

5267 **Space Coast CIL News**
Space Coast Center for Independent Living
571 Haverty Court,
Suite W
Rockledge, FL 32955-2566
321-633-6011
Fax: 321-633-6472
TTY: 321-784-9008
www.sccil.net
Michael Lavoie, President
Howard Fetes, Vice-President
Non-profit organization that provides services which enable people with disabilities to live as independently as possible.
12 pages Quarterly

5268 **Special Needs Trust Handbook**

Aspen Publishers
7th Fl
76 9th Ave
New York, NY 10011-4962 301-644-3599
800-638-8437
www.aspenpublishers.com

Bob Lemmond, President and CEO
Gustavo Dobles, Vice President and Chief Content Officer
Susan Pikitch, Vice President and Chief Financial Officer
Alan Scott, Vice President & Chief Marketing Office

The Special Needs Trusts Handbook is the single-volume, comprehensive resource that provides information on how to handle the complex requirements of drafting and administering trusts for clients who are mentally or physically disabled, or who wish to provide for others with disabilities. *$245.00*

900 pages
ISBN 0-735572-88-7

5269 **Special Siblings: Growing Up With Someone with A Disability**

Brookes Publishing
P.O. Box 10624
Baltimore, MD 21285-0624 410-337-9580
800-638-3775
Fax: 410-337-8539
custserv@brookespublishing.com
readplaylearn.com

Paul Brooks, Owner

The author reveals what she experienced as the sister of a man with cerebral palsy and developmental disability — and shares what others have learned about being and having a special sibling. Weaving a lifetime of memories and reflections with relevant research and interviews with more than 100 other siblings and experts, McHugh explores a spectrum of feelings — from anger and guilt to love and pride — and helps readers understand the issues siblings may encounter. *$21.95*

256 pages Paperback
ISBN 1-557666-07-5

5270 **TERI**

251 Airport Rd
Oceanside, CA 92058-1321 760-721-1706
teriinc.org

Cheryl Kilmer, CEO & Founder
William E. Mara, Chief Operating Officer
Krysti DeZonia, Ed.D, Director of Education & Research
Joe Michalowski, Chief Financial Officer

A private, nonprofit corporation which has been developing and operating programs for individuals with developmental disabilities since 1980. Offers staff training videos, staff training tools and technique manuals.

5271 **That All May Worship: An Interfaith Welcome to People with Disabilities**

American Association of People with Disabilities
2013 H St. NW
5th Floor
Washington, DC 20006 202-521-4316
800-840-8844
communications@aapd.com
www.aapd.com/publications

Maria Town, President & CEO
Jasmin Bailey, Manager, Business Operations
Christine Liao, Manager, Programs
Rachita Singh, Coordinator, Public Relations & Communications

An interfaith handbook to assist congregations in welcoming people with disabilities to promote acceptance and full participation.

5272 **The Ultimate Guide to Sex and Disability**

Read How You Want Large Print Books
800-797-9277
support@readhowyouwant.com
www.readhowyouwant.com

Miriam Kaufman, Author

For everyone, men and women of all ages and sexual identities, The Ultimate Guide to Sex and Disability covers the span of disabilities - from chronic fatigue and back pain to spinal cord injury, multiple sclerosis, cystic fibrosis, cerebral palsy, and many others.

5273 **To Live with Grace and Dignity**

LRP Publications

Lydia Gans, Author

This book combines photographs and essays to allow the reader to enter some of the real day to day relationships that develop between individuals with disabilities and their personal assistants. The individuals included in this book represent a wide range of ages, disabilities and cultural backgrounds.

72 pages Paperback
ISBN 0-934753-85-7

5274 **Touch/Ability Connects People with Disabilities & Alternative Health Care Pract.**

Independent Living Research Utilization ILRU
1333 Moursund
Houston, TX 77030-7031 713-520-0232
Fax: 713-520-5785
ilru@ilru.org
ilru.org

Lex Frieden, Director, ILRU
Richard Petty, Co-Director

The people at DIRECT center for Independence and Touch/Ability in Tuscon, Arizona, have collaborated to develop a wellness program that makes alternative health care choices available to people with disabilities. The Touch/Ability Wellness program was selected as one of last year's winners in the Innovative CILs competition because of this outcome of increased options open to people with disabilities.

10 pages

5275 **US Role in International Disability Activities: A History**

World Institute on Disability
3075 Adeline St.
Suite 155
Berkeley, CA 94703 510-225-6400
Fax: 510-225-0477
wid@wid.org
www.wid.org

Marcie Roth, Executive Director & CEO
Katherine Zigmont, Senior Director, Operations & Deputy Director
Reggie Johnson, Senior Director, Marketing & Communications
Marsha Saxton, Director, Research

This study serves as an introduction to US involvement in the field of international rehabilitation and disability.

5276 **Understanding and Accommodating Physical Disabilities: Desk Reference**

Greenwood Publishing Group
130 Cremona Drive
P O Box 1911
Santa Barbara, CA 93117- 4208 203-226-3571
800-368-6868
805-968-1911
Fax: 866-270-3856
customerservice@abc-clio.com
www.abc-clio.com

200 pages $52.95 - $55
ISBN 0-899308-14-7

5277 **Vestibular Disorders Association**

Vestibular Disorders Association
5018 NE 15th Ave.
P.O. Box 13305
Portland, OR 97211 503-229-7705
800-837-8428
Fax: 503-229-8064
info@vestibular.org
www.vestibular.org

Cynthia Ryan, MBA, Executive Director
Tony Staser, Development Director
Kerrie Denner, Outreach Coordinator
Karen Ilari, Administrative Support Coordinator

The mission of the Vestibular Disorders Association is to serve people with vestibular disorders by providing access to information, offering a support network, and elevating awareness of the challenges associated with these disorders. They also aim to sup-

port and empower vestibular patients on their journey back to balance. *$15.00*
ISBN 0-963261-15-0

5278 Visions & Values
Idaho Council on Developmental Disabilities
650 W. State St., Room 100
P. O. Box 83720
Boise, ID 83720-5840 208-332-1824
800-544-2433
Fax: 208-334-2307
C. L. Butch Otter, Governor
A quarterly publication from the Idaho Council on Developmental Disabilities.

5279 Weiner's Herbal
Quantum Books
355 Middlesex Avenue
Wilmington, MA 01887-1406 978-988-2470
Fax: 617-577-7282
www.quantumbooks.com
William Szabo, Owner
A-Z index covering all aspects of herbs.
Paperback
ISBN 0-812825-86-1

5280 When the Brain Goes Wrong
Fanlight Productions
32 Court Street,
21st Floor
Brooklyn, NY 11201-1731 718-488-8900
800-876-1710
Fax: 718-488-8642
info@fanlight.com
www.fanlight.com
Ben Achtenberg, Owner
Nicole Johnson, Publicity Coordinator
Anthony Sweeney, Marketing Director
An extraordinary and provocative series of seven short films which profile individuals with a range of brian dysfunctions. The seven brief segments focus on schizophrenia, manic depression, epilepsy, head injury, headaches and addiction. In addition to the personal stories, the segments include interviews with physicians who speak briefly about what is known about the disorders and treatment. #131 *$245.00*
ISBN 1-572951-31-1

5281 Women with Physical Disabilities: Achieving & Maintaining Health & Well-Being
Spina Bifida Association of America
1600 Wilson Blvd.
Suite 800
Arlington, VA 22209-4226 202-944-3285
800-621-3141
Fax: 202-944-3295
sbaa@sbaa.org
www.spinabifidaassociation.org
Ana Ximenes, Chair
Sara Struwe, President & CEO
Cindy Brownstein, CEO
George Sturm, Treasurer
Introduces the critical concept of womens health in the context of physical disabilities. *$42.00*

5282 Work in the Context of Disability Culture
Independent Living Research Utilization ILRU
1333 Moursund
Houston, TX 77030-7031 713-520-0232
Fax: 713-520-5785
ilru@ilru.org
ilru.org
Lex Frieden, Director, ILRU
Richard Petty, Co-Director
Another winner in the innovative CIL competition-Steve Brown describes the Talking Books Program of Southeast Alaska Independent Living, discussing their efforts to record the oral history and life experiences of people with disabilities in the larger context of the disability culture.
10 pages

5283 Your Role in Inclusion Theatre
Houston, TX 713-202-8840
Inclusiontheater@gmail.com
Deborah E. Nowinski, Author/Inclusion Specialist
A guidebook for educators who wish to create a successful theatre environment for individuals of all abilities. The book also includes stories, tips, and games. *$19.95*
192 pages
ISBN 1-517357-49-8

Parenting: General

5284 AEPS Family Report: Birth to Three Years
Brookes Publishing
P.O. Box 10624
Baltimore, MD 21285-0624 410-337-9580
800-638-3775
Fax: 410-337-8539
custserv@brookespublishing.com
www.brookespublishing.com
Diane Bricker, Author
Betty Capt, Author
JoAnn Johnson, Author
Misti Waddell, Author
This Family Report was developed for use in conjunction with the AEPSr for children birth to 3 years to obtain information from parents and other caregivers about their children's skills and abilities across major areas of development. Available in packages of 10.
28 pages Saddle-stitched

5285 AEPS Family Report: For Children Ages Three to Six
Brookes Publishing
P.O. Box 10624
Baltimore, MD 21285-0624 410-337-9580
800-638-3775
Fax: 410-337-8539
custserv@brookespublishing.com
www.brookespublishing.com
Diane Bricker, Author
Betty Capt, Author
JoAnn Johnson, Author
Elizabeth Straka, Author
This is a 64-item questionnaire that asks parents to rank their child's abilities on specific skills. In packages of 10 paperback.
28 pages Saddle-stiched

5286 Adapted Physical Activity
Human Kinetics
1607 N Market St
P.O. Box 5076
Champaign, IL 61820-5076 800-747-4457
Fax: 217-351-1549
info@hkusa.com
www.humankinetics.com

5287 Assistive Technology for Parents with Disabilities Handbook
Idaho Assistive Technology Project
University of Idaho
1187 Alturas Dr.
Moscow, ID 83843- 2268 208-885-3557
800-432-8324
Fax: 208-885-6102
idahoat@uidaho.edu
www.idahoat.org

5288 Babyface: A Story of Heart and Bones
Penguin Books USA
375 Hudson St
New York, NY 10014 212-366-2000
consumerservices@penguinrandomhouse.com
www.penguin.com
Jeanne McDermott, Author
A must read for families that seek insight into coping with a chronic condition. Many useful resources provided.
288 pages Paperback

5289 **Backyards and Butterflies: Ways to Include Children with Disabilities in Outdoor Activities**
Brookline Books
8 Trumbull Rd
Ste B-001
Northampton, MA 01060
413-584-0184
800-666-2665
Fax: 413-584-6184
brbooks@yahoo.com
www.brooklinebks.com

Doreen Greenstein, Author
Suzanne Bloom, Author
An illustrated book with dozens of imaginative ways parents can include children with physical disabilities in outdoor activities. Offers clear concise, how-to directions for constructing homemade toys, utensils, and other items that can be enjoyed outside safely and comfortably.
72 pages Paperback

5290 **Beyond Tears: Living After Losing a Child**
St. Martin's Griffin (Macmillan Publishers)
75 Varick St
New York, NY 10013
212-226-7521
press.inquiries@macmillan.com
us.macmillan.com/smp

Ellen Mitchell, Author
Meant to comfort and give direction to bereaved parents, Beyond Tears is written by nine mothers who have each lost a child. This revised edition includes a new chapter written from the perspective of surviving siblings. The death of a child is that unimaginable loss no parent ever expects to face. In this book, nine mothers share their individual stories of how to survive in the darkest hour.

5291 **Broken Dolls: Gathering the Pieces: Caringfor Chronically Ill Children**
St. Paul Press

Jennifer Travis Cox, Author
Told from the point of view of the author, this book tracks the challenges faced by parents and caregivers of chronically ill-children - both in terms of medical care and emotional impact. It offers advice based on the author's own experiences caring for her child, as well as insights from other families who have gone through the same experience.
164 pages Paperback

5292 **Building the Healing Partnership: Parents, Professionals and Children**
Brookline Books
8 Trumbull Road
Suite B-001
Northampton, MA 01060
413-584-0184
800-666-2665
Fax: 413-584-6184
brbooks@yahoo.com
www.brooklinebooks.com

Paperback
ISBN 0-91479 -63-8

5293 **Children with Disabilities**
Brookes Publishing
P.O. Box 10624
Baltimore, MD 21285-0624
410-337-9580
800-638-3775
Fax: 410-337-8539
custserv@brookespublishing.com
www.brookespublishing.com

Mark L Batshaw MD, Editor
Paul Brooks, Owner
Lauren Rohe, Regional Sales Consultant
Cary Gold, Educational Sales Representative
Extensive coverage of genetics, heredity, pre- and postnatal development, specific disabilities, family roles, and intervention. Features chapters on substance abuse, HIV and AIDS, Down syndrome, fragile X syndrome, behavior management, transitions to adulthood, and health care in the 21st century. Also reveals the causes of many conditions that can lead to developmental disabilities. *$69.95*
912 pages Hardcover
ISBN 1-557665-81-8

5294 **Conditional Love: Parents' Attitudes Toward Handicapped Children**
Greenwood Publishing Group
130 Cremona Drive
P O Box 1911
Santa Barbara, CA 93117- 4208
203-226-3571
800-368-6868
805-968-1911
Fax: 866-270-3856
customerservice@abc-clio.com
www.abc-clio.com

312 pages
ISBN 0-89789 -24-7

5295 **Coordinacion De Servicios Centrado En La Familia**
Brookline Books
8 Trumbull Road
Suite B-001
Northampton, MA 01060
413-584-0184
800-666-2665
Fax: 413-584-6184
brbooks@yahoo.com
www.brooklinebooks.com

34 pages Paperback
ISBN 0-91479 -90-5

5296 **Developing Personal Safety Skills in Children with Disabilities**
Brookes Publishing
P.O. Box 10624
Baltimore, MD 21285-0624
410-337-9580
800-638-3775
Fax: 410-337-8539
custserv@brookespublishing.com
readplaylearn.com

Paul Brooks, Owner
A guide for teachers, parents, and caregivers, this volume explores the issue of personal safety for children with disabilities and offers strategies for empowering and protecting them at home and in school. Recognizing that children with disabilities are vulnerable to abuse, this work explores why children with disabilities need personal safety skills, offers, curriculum ideas and exercises, and advocates the development of self-esteem and assertiveness so that children can protect themselves. *$34.00*
220 pages Paperback
ISBN 1-557661-84-7

5297 **Developmental Disabilities in Infancy and Childhood**
Brookes Publishing
P.O. Box 10624
Baltimore, MD 21285-0624
410-767-6100
800-638-3775
Fax: 410-767-5850
custserv@brookespublishing.com
readplaylearn.com

Paul Brooks, Owner
This two volume set explores advances in assessment and treatment, retains a clinical focus, and incorporates recent developments in research and theory. Can be purchased individually or as a set (Vol. 1: Neurodevelopmental Diagnosis and Treatment Vol. 2: The Spectrum of Developmental Disabilities). *$210.00*
Hardcover
ISBN 1-55766O-CA-P

5298 **Dictionary of Developmental Disabilities Terminology**
Brookes Publishing
P.O. Box 10624
Baltimore, MD 21285-0624
410-337-9580
800-638-3775
Fax: 410-337-8539
custserv@brookespublishing.com
readplaylearn.com

Paul Brooks, Owner
Answers thousands of questions for medical or human services professionals, parents or advocates of children with disabilities,

or students preparing for their careers. Provides thorough explanations of the most common terms associated with disabilities.
$55.95
368 pages Hardcover
ISBN 1-557662-45-2

5299 **Encyclopedia of Genetic Disorders & Birth Defects**
Facts on File
132 W 31st St
17th Floor
New York, NY 10001-3406
800-322-8755
Fax: 800-678-3633
custserv@factsonfile.com
www.infobasepublishing.com/
Mark Donnell, President
Layperson-accessible entries on genetic terminology and genetically-influenced conditions. *$71.50*
474 pages
ISBN 0-816038-09-0

5300 **Exceptional Parent Magazine**
Psy-Ed Corporation
416 Main Street
Johnstown, PA 15901-2032
814-361-3860
877-372-7368
Fax: 814-361-3861
www.eparent.com
Vanessa B Ira, Contributing Writer / Editor
Joseph M. Valenzano, Jr., President, CEO & Publisher
Rick Rader, MD, Editor-in-Chief
Lois Keegan, Human Resources Manager
Magazine that provides information, support, ideas, encouragement, and outreach for parents and families of children with disabilities and the professionals who work with them. *$39.95*
85 pages Monthly

5301 **Face of Inclusion**
Special Needs Project
Ste H
324 State St
Santa Barbara, CA 93101-2364
805-962-8087
800-333-6867
Fax: 805-962-5087
eplibrary@aol.com
www.eplibrary.com
Hod Gray, Owner
A unique and moving parents' perspective of inclusion for administrators, teachers, and parents of children with disabilities. *$99.00*

5302 **Families Magazine**
New Jersey Developmental Disabilities Council
20 West State Street, 6th Floor
P.O. Box 700
Trenton, NJ 08625-0700
609-292-3745
800-792-8858
Fax: 609-292-7114
TTY: 609-777-3238
njcdd@njcdd.org
www.njddc.org
Elaine Buchsbaum, Chairman
Christopher Miller, Vice Chair
Alison M. Lozano, Ph.D, Executive Director
Shirla Rufo Simpson, M.A., DRCC, Deputy Director
Quarterly magazine for people with disabilities, their families and the public, features family profiles, news, columns and the New Jersey Family support councils newsletter.
Quarterly

5303 **Families, Illness & Disability**
Through the Looking Glass
3075 Adeline St
Ste. 120
Berkeley, CA 94703-2212
510-848-1112
800-644-2666
Fax: 510-848-4445
TTY: 510-848-1005
tlg@lookingglass.org
www.lookingglass.org
Maureen Block, J.D., Co-Founder
Karen Fessel, Ph.D., Executive Director

$35.00
320 pages

5304 **Family Interventions Throughout Disability**
Springer Publishing Company
11 West 42nd Street,
15th Floor
New York, NY 10036-3915
212-431-4370
877-687-7476
Fax: 212-941-7842
cs@springerpub.com
www.springerpub.com
Theodore C Nardin, Chief Executive Officer
James C. Costello, Vice President, Journal Publishing
Diana Osborne, Production Manager
Megan Larkin, Managing Editor, Journals
Family attitudes throughout chronic illness and disability. *$31.95*
320 pages
ISBN 0-82615 -80-4

5305 **Family-Centered Service Coordination: A Manual for Parents**
Brookline Books
8 Trumbull Road
Suite B-001
Northampton, MA 01060
413-584-0184
800-666-2665
Fax: 413-584-6184
brbooks@yahoo.com
www.brooklinebooks.com
34 pages Paperback
ISBN 0-91479 -90-5

5306 **Handbook About Care in the Home**
AARP Fulfillment
601 E St NW
Washington, DC 20049-1
202-434-2277
888-687-2277
TTY: 877-434-7598
member@aarp.org
www.aarp.org
24 pages

5307 **LifeLines**
Disabled & Alone/Life Services for the Handicapped
1440 Broadway
23rd Floor
New York, NY 10018-2326
212-532-6740
800-995-0066
Fax: 212-532-6740
info@disabledandalone.org
www.disabledandalone.org/lifelines.html
Leslie D. Park, Chair
Rex L. Davidson, Vice President
Lee Alan Ackerman, Executive Director
William G. Shannon, Treasurer
Newsletter providing current and valuable information about lifetime care and planning for persons with disabilities and their families and the organizations serving them. Free upon request.
4-10 pages Biannual

5308 **Living with a Brother or Sister with Special Needs: A Book for Sibs**
Sibling Support Project
6512 23rd Ave NW
Ste 322
Seattle, WA 98117
206-297-6368
info@siblingsupport.org
www.siblingsupport.org
Don Meyer, Author
Patricia Vadasy, Author
Living with a Brother or Sister with Special Needs focuses on the intensity of emotions that brothers and sisters experience when they have a sibling with special needs, and the hard questions they ask. It talks about the good and not-so-good parts of having a brother or sister who has special needs, and offers suggestions for how to make life easier for everyone in the family.
144 pages Paperback

5309 **Loving & Letting Go**
Centering Corporation
7230 Maple Street
Omaha, NE 68134-5064
402-553-1200
866-218-0101
Fax: 402-533-0507
j1200@aol.com
www.centering.org

Joy Johnson, Founder
Dr. Marvin Johnson, co-Founder
For parents who decide to turn away from aggressive medical intervention for their critically ill newborn. *$5.95*
48 pages Paperback

5310 **Mobility Training for People with Disabilities**
Charles C. Thomas
2600 S First St
Springfield, IL 62704-4730
217-789-8980
800-258-8980
Fax: 217-789-9130
books@ccthomas.com
www.ccthomas.com

Michael P. Thomas, President

5311 **Mother to Be**
Through the Looking Glass
3075 Adeline St
Ste. 120
Berkeley, CA 94703-2212
510-848-1112
800-644-2666
Fax: 510-848-4445
TTY: 510-848-1005
tlg@lookingglass.org
www.lookingglass.org

Maureen Block, J.D., Co-Founder
Karen Fessel, Ph.D., Executive Director
Guide to pregnancy and birth for women with disabilities. *$34.00*
410 pages

5312 **New Language of Toys: Teaching Communication Skills to Children with Special Needs**
Spina Bifida Association of America
1600 Wilson Blvd.
Suite 800
Arlington, VA 22209-4226
202-944-3285
800-621-3141
Fax: 202-944-3295
sbaa@sbaa.org
www.spinabifidaassociation.org

Ana Ximenes, Chair
Sara Struwe, President & CEO
Cindy Brownstein, CEO
George Sturm, Treasurer
A guide for parents and teachers and a reader-friendly resource guide that provides a wealth of information on how play activities affect a child's language development and where to get the toys and materials to use in these activities. *$19.00*

5313 **Newsline**
Federation for Children with Special Needs
529 Main St.
Suite 1M3
Boston, MA 02129
617-236-7210
800-331-0688
Fax: 617-241-0330
fcsninfo@fcsn.org
www.fcsn.org

Pam Nourse, Executive Director
Offers information and resources for families of children with disabilities, as well as event announcements, project updates, news and more.
Quarterly

5314 **On the Road to Autonomy: Promoting Self- Competence in Children & Youth with Disabilities**
Brookes Publishing
P.O. Box 10624
Baltimore, MD 21285-0624
410-337-9580
800-638-3775
Fax: 410-337-8539
custserv@brookespublishing.com
readplaylearn.com

Paul Brooks, Owner
This book provides detailed conceptual, practical, and personal information regarding the promotion of self-esteem, self-determination, and coping skills among children and youth with and without disabilities. *$48.00*
432 pages Paperback
ISBN 1-55766 -35-5

5315 **Pain Erasure**
M Evans and Company
216 E 49th St
New York, NY 10017-1546
212-979-0880
Fax: 212-486-4544

Mary Evans, Owner
This book explains Bonnie Prudden's method for pain relief using myotherapy, a method hailed by doctors and patients.
ISBN 0-345331-02-8

5316 **Parent Centers and Independent Living Centers: Collectively We're Stronger**
Independent Living Research Utilization ILRU
1333 Moursund
Houston, TX 77030-7031
713-520-0232
Fax: 713-520-5785
ilru@ilru.org
ilru.org

Lex Frieden, Director, ILRU
Richard Petty, Co-Director
This article describes several examples of effective working relationships of PTIs and CILs. The examples highlight how parent and consumer organizations have identified complimentary strengths and formed partnerships to better support children with disabilities and their families. These partnerships can also be a very important way of involving youth in the disability movement so they may become leaders of tomorrow.
10 pages

5317 **Parent-Child Interaction and Developmental Disabilities**
Greenwood Publishing Group
130 Cremona Drive
P O Box 1911
Santa Barbara, CA 93117
800-368-6868
805-968-1911
Fax: 866-270-3856
customerservice@abc-clio.com
www.abc-clio.com

395 pages Hardcover
ISBN 0-275928-35-7

5318 **Parenting**
Accent Books & Products
P.O. Box 700
Bloomington, IL 61702-700
309-378-2961
800-787-8444
Fax: 309-378-4420
acmtlvng@aol.com

Raymond C Cheever, Publisher
Betty Garee, Editor
Experienced parents (who are disabled) discuss: raising children from infant to teens, balancing career and motherhood, discipline methods and more when both parents are disabled. *$7.95*
83 pages
ISBN 0-91570 -26-4

5319 **Parenting with a Disability**
Through the Looking Glass
3075 Adeline St
Ste. 120
Berkeley, CA 94703-2212
510-848-1112
800-644-2666
Fax: 510-848-4445
TTY: 510-848-1005
tlg@lookingglass.org
www.lookingglass.org
Maureen Block, J.D., Board President
Rusty Hendlin, M.A., LMFT, Director of Medi-Cal Services
Thomas Spalding, Board Treasurer
Alice Nemon, D.S.W., Board Secretary
International newsletter. Available in Braille, large print or cassette.
3 per year

5320 **Perspectives on a Parent Movement**
Brookline Books
8 Trumbull Rd
Suite B-001
Northampton, MA 1060-4533
413-584-0184
800-666-2665
Fax: 413-584-6184
brbooks@yahoo.com
www.brooklinebooks.com
Paperback
ISBN 0-91479 -74-3

5321 **Sexuality and the Developmentally Handicapped**
Edwin Mellen Press
P.O. Box 450
Lewiston, NY 14092-450
716-754-2266
Fax: 716-754-4056
jrupnow@mellenpress.com
mellenpress.com
Herbert Richardson, Owner
Presents the knowledge, attitudes, and skills pertinent to responding to the sexual problems of developmentally handicapped persons, their families and communities. Details fully documented cases, issues concerning the law, and resource materials available. *$89.95*
245 pages Hardcover
ISBN 0-88946 -32-5

5322 **Shattered Dreams-Lonely Choices: Birth Parents of Babies with Disabilities**
Greenwood Publishing Group
130 Cremona Drive
Santa Barbara, CA 93117-4208
203-226-3571
800-368-6868
805-968-1911
Fax: 866-270-3856
customerservice@abc-clio.com
www.abc-clio.com
208 pages Hardcover
ISBN 0-897892-86-0

5323 **Since Owen, A Parent-to-Parent Guide for Care of the Disabled Child**
Special Needs Project
324 State Street
Suite H
Santa Barbara, CA 93101-2364
818-718-9900
800-333-6867
Fax: 818-349-2027
editor@specialneeds.com
www.specialneeds.com
Hod Gray, Owner
Against the background of his experience as the parent of a severely disabled young man, Callahan writes conscientiously to other parents. *$16.95*
486 pages

5324 **Sleep Better! A Guide to Improving Sleep for Children with Special Needs**
Brookes Publishing
P.O. Box 10624
Baltimore, MD 21285-624
410-337-9580
800-638-3775
Fax: 410-337-8539
custserv@brookespublishing.com
readplaylearn.com
Paul Brooks, Owner
This book offers step-by-step, how to instructions for helping children with disabilities get the rest they need. For problems ranging from bedtime tantrums to night waking, parents and caregivers will find a variety of widely tested and easy-to-implement techniques that have already helped hundreds of children with special needs. *$21.95*
288 pages Paperback
ISBN 1-55766 -15-7

5325 **Something's Wrong with My Child!**
Charles C. Thomas
2600 S First St
Springfield, IL 62704-4730
217-789-8980
800-258-8980
Fax: 217-789-9130
books@ccthomas.com
www.ccthomas.com
Michael P. Thomas, President
This text provides professionals and parents with the opportunity to gain insights into a family that has benefited positively and constructively from the presence of a member with a disability. The author presents a compilation of easy-to-read material that's based on real-life experiences. *$39.95*
234 pages Paperback 1998
ISBN 0-398068-99-8

5326 **Sometimes I Get All Scribbly**
Exceptional Parent Library
P.O. Box 1807
Englewood Cliffs, NJ 7632-1207
201-947-6000
800-535-1910
Fax: 201-947-9376
eplibrary@aol.com
www.eplibrary.com

5327 **Son-Rise: The Miracle Continues**
2080 South Undermountain Road
Sheffield, MA 01257-9643
413-229-2100
877-766-7473
Fax: 413-229-3202
sonrise@option.org
www.son-rise.org
Barry Neil Kaufman, Co-Founder/ Co-Originator/Senior Teacher/Trainer
Samahria Lyte Kaufman, Co-Founder/ Co-Originator/Senior Teacher/Trainer
Bryn Hogan, ATCA Senior Staff
William Hogan, ATCA Senior Staff
Documents Raun Kaufman's astonishing development from a lifeless, autistic child into a highly verbal, lovable youngster with no traces of his former condition. Details Raun's extraordinary progress from the age of four into young adulthood, also shares moving accounts of five families that successfully used the Son-Rise Program to reach their own special children.
372 pages
ISBN 0-915811-53-7

5328 **Special Kids Need Special Parents: A Resource for Parents of Children With Special Needs**
Berkley Publishing Group
375 Hudson Street
New York, NY 10014-3657
212-366-2372
Fax: 212-366-2933
ecommerce@us.penguingroup.com
www.us.penguingroup.com
319 pages Paperback
ISBN 0-425176-62-2

5329 **Special Parent, Special Child**
Exceptional Parent Library
P.O. Box 1807
Englewood Cliffs, NJ 7632-1207
201-947-6000
800-535-1910
Fax: 201-947-9376
eplibrary@aol.com
www.eplibrary.com

Hardcover

5330 **Strategies for Working with Families of Young Children with Disabilities**
Brookes Publishing
P.O. Box 10624
Baltimore, MD 21285-624
410-337-9580
800-638-3775
Fax: 410-337-8539
custserv@brookespublishing.com
readplaylearn.com

Paul Brooks, Owner

This text offers useful techniques for collaborating with and supporting families whose youngest members either have a disability or are at risk for developing a disability. The authors address specific issues such as cultural diversity, transitions to new programs, and disagreements between families and professionals. *$33.00*

272 pages Paperback
ISBN 1-55766 -57-6

5331 **That's My Child**
Exceptional Parent Library
P.O. Box 1807
Englewood Cliffs, NJ 7632-1207
201-947-6000
800-535-1910
Fax: 201-947-9376
eplibrary@aol.com
www.eplibrary.com

5332 **The Complete Guide to Creating a Special Needs Life Plan**
Jessica Kingsley Publishers
73 Collier St
London, UK N19BE
hello@jkp.com
www.jkp.com

Hal Wright, Author

The purpose of special needs planning is to create the best possible life for an adult with a disability. This book provides comprehensive guidance on creating a life plan to transition a special needs child to independence or to ensure they are well cared for in the future.

360 pages

5333 **They Don't Come with Manuals**
Fanlight Productions
32 Court Street, 21st Floor
Brooklyn, NY 11201-1731
718-488-8900
800-876-1710
Fax: 718-488-8642
orders@fanlight.com
www.fanlight.com

Ben Achtenberg, Owner
Anthony Sweeney, Marketing Director
Nicole Johnson, Publicity Coordinator

The parents and adoptive parents in this video speak candidly of their day to day experiences caring for children with physical and mental disabilities. *$145.00*

5334 **They're Just Kids**
Aquarius Health Care Videos
30 Forest Road
P.O. Box 249
Millis, MA 02054-7159
508-376-1244
Fax: 508-376-1245
aqvideos@tiac.net
www.aquariusproductions.com

Lesile Kussmann, President
Joyce Farmer, Assistant Director

The importance and value of inclusion, excellent for anyone working with kids with disabilities. The documentary explores the advantages of the inclusion of disabled children in the classroom, cub scouts and other extracurricular activities. *$99.00*

Video

5335 **To a Different Drumbeat**
Alliance for Parental Involvement in Education
P.O. Box 59
East Chatham, NY 12060-59
518-392-6900
Fax: 518-392-6900

5336 **Uncommon Fathers**
Woodbine House
6510 Bells Mill Rd
Bethesda, MD 20817-1636
301-897-3570
800-843-7323
info@woodbinehouse.com
woodbinehouse.com

Irv Shapell, Owner

Nineteen fathers talk about the life-altering experience of having a child with special needs and offer a welcome, seldom-heard perspective on raising kids with disabilities, including autism, cerebral palsy, and Down syndrome. Uncommon Fathers is the first book for fathers by fathers, but it is also helpful to partners, family, friends, and service providers. *$14.95*

206 pages Paperback
ISBN 0-933149-68-9

5337 **We Can Speak for Ourselves: Self Advocacy by Mentally Handicapped People**
Brookline Books
8 Trumbull Rd
Suite B-001
Northampton, MA 1060-4533
413-584-0184
800-666-2665
Fax: 413-584-6184
brbooks@yahoo.com
www.brooklinebooks.com

246 pages Paperback
ISBN 0-25336 -65-9

5338 **You May Be Able to Adopt**
Through the Looking Glass
3075 Adeline St
Ste. 120
Berkeley, CA 94703-2212
510-848-1112
800-644-2666
Fax: 510-848-4445
TTY: 510-848-1005
tlg@lookingglass.org
www.lookingglass.org

Maureen Block, J.D., Board President
Rusty Hendlin, M.A., LMFT, Director of Medi-Cal Services
Thomas Spalding, Board Treasurer
Alice Nemon, D.S.W., Board Secretary

A guide to the adoption process for prospective mothers with disabilities and their partners. Available in Braille, large print or cassette. *$10.00*

112 pages

5339 **You Will Dream New Dreams**
Kensington Publishing
119 West 40th Street
New York, NY 10018
800-221-2647
www.kensingtonbooks.com

Steven Zacharius, Chairman, President & CEO

A parent's support group in print. The shared narratives come from those with newly diagnosed children, adult disabled children, and everything in between. *$13.00*

278 pages Paperback
ISBN 1-575665-60-3

5340 **Your Child Has a Disability: A Complete Sourcebook of Daily and Medical Care**
Brookes Publishing
P.O. Box 10624
Baltimore, MD 21285-624
410-337-9580
800-638-3775
Fax: 410-337-8539
custserv@brookespublishing.com
readplaylearn.com

Paul Brooks, Owner

Offers expert advice on a wide range of issues-from finding the right doctor and investigating the medical aspects of a child's condition to learning care techniques and fulfilling education requirements. *$24.95*
368 pages Paperback
ISBN 1-557663-74-2

Parenting: Specific Disabilities

5341 **Cancer Clinical Trials: A Commonsense Guide to Experimental Cancer Therapies and Trials**
DiaMedica Inc.
2 Carlson Pkwy N
Ste 165
Minneapolis, MN 55447
763-270-0603
Fax: 763-710-4456
www.diamedica.com

Tomasz M. Beer, Author
Larry W. Axmaker, Author
Cancer Clinical Trials is a comprehensive, no-nonsense, and readable guide for anyone who is considering therapeutic options in addition to standard cancer therapy. The book seeks to share knowledge about cancer clinical trials with people living with cancer, their families and loved ones. It will help readers decide if a clinical trial is a good option for them, to choose an appropriate trial, and to navigate through the clinical trial process.
192 pages

5342 **Different Dream Parenting: A Practical Guide to Raising a Child with Special Needs**
Discovery House Publishers
3000 Kraft Ave SE
P.O. Box 3566
Grand Rapids, MI 49512
800-653-8333
support@dhp.org
dhp.org

Jolene Philo, Author
In Different Dream Parenting, author Jolene Philo offers guidance and encouragement through biblical insights and her own personal experiences. Find spiritual wisdom, practical resources, and tools that can help you become an extraordinary advocate for your child. Discover how you can move beyond the challenges and experience the joy of being your childs biggest and best supporter.
336 pages

5343 **Essential First Steps for Parents of Children with Autism**
Woodbine House
6510 Bells Mill Rd
Bethesda, MD 20817
301-897-3570
800-843-7323
info@woodbinehouse.com
www.woodbinehouse.com

Lara Delmolino, Author
Sandra L. Harris, Author
When autism is diagnosed or suspected in young children, overwhelmed parents wonder where to turn and how to begin helping their child. Drs. Delmolino and Harris, experienced clinicians and ABA therapists, eliminate the confusion and guesswork by outlining the pivotal steps parents can take now to optimize learning and functioning for children ages 5 and younger.
154 pages Paperback

5344 **Final Report: Challenges and Strategies of Disabled Parents: Findings from a Survey (1997)**
Through the Looking Glass
3075 Adeline St
Ste. 120
Berkeley, CA 94703-2212
510-848-1112
800-644-2666
Fax: 510-848-4445
TTY: 510-848-1005
tlg@lookingglass.org
www.lookingglass.org

Linda Toms Barker, Author
Vida Maralani, Author
This milestone TLG-directed report presents findings from the first national survey of parents with disabilities. The report includes a description of parents with disabilities, barriers to parenting among adults with disabilities, transportation issues, personal assistance, adaptive parenting equipment, housing, as well as recommendations for legal and service system changes.

5345 **Pervasive Developmental Disorders: Findinga Diagnosis and Getting Help**
Patient-Centered Guides/O'Reilly Media
1005 Gravenstein Hwy N
Sebastopol, CA 95472
707-827-7019
800-889-8969
Fax: 707-824-8268
orders@oreilly.com
shop.oreilly.com

Mitzi Waltz, Author
This unique book encompassess both the practical aspects as well as ther personal stories and emotional facets of living with PDD-NOS, the most common pervasive developmental disorder. Parents of an undiagnosed child may suspect many things, from autism to servere allergies. Pervasive Developmental Disorders is for parents (or newly diagnosed adults) who struggle with this neurological condition that profoundly impacts the life of child and family.
580 pages Paperback 1999

5346 **Teaching Children with Down Syndrome about Their Bodies, Boundaries, and Sexuality**
Woodbine House
6510 Bell Mills Rd
Bethesda, MD 20817
800-843-7323
info@woodbinehouse.com
www.woodbinehouse.com

Terri Couwenhoven, Author
Drawing on her unique background as both a sexual educator and mother of a child with Down syndrome, the author blends factual information and practical ideas for teaching children with Down syndrome about their bodies, puberty, and sexuality. This book gives parents the confidence to speak comfortably about these sometimes difficult subjects.
332 pages Paperback

5347 **Thinking Differently: An Inspiring Guidefor Parents of Children with Learning Disabilities**
William Morrow Paperbacks (HarperCollins)
195 Broadway
New York, NY 10007
212-207-7000
orders@harpercollins.com
www.harpercollins.com

David Flink, Author
An innovative, comprehensive guide—the first of its kind—to help parents understand and accept learning disabilities in their children, offering tips and strategies for successfully advocating on their behalf and helping them become their own best advocates.

5348 **Your Child in the Hospital: A Practical Guide for Parents (3rd Edition)**
Childhood Cancer Guides/O'Reilly Media
1005 Gravenstein Hwy N
Sebastopol, CA 95472
707-827-7019
800-889-8969
Fax: 707-824-8268
orders@oreilly.com
shop.oreilly.com

Nancy Keene, Author
This book offers advice from dozens of veteran parents on how to cope with a child's hospitalization, relieving anxious parents so they can help dispel their child's fears and concerns. Parents will find easy-to-read tips on preparing their child, handling procedures without trauma, and preventing insurance snafus. The second edition features a journal to help open communication and give the child a measure of control over the experience.
176 pages Paperback

Parenting: School

5349 **Allergy & Asthma Today**
Allergy & Asthma Network
8229 Boone Blvd
Ste 260
Vienna, VA 22182
800-878-4403
Fax: 703-288-5271
canderson@allergyasthmanetwork.org
www.allergyasthmanetwork.org
Tonya Winders, President
Charmayne Anderson, Director, Advocacy
Gary Fitzgerald, Managing Editor
Laurie Ross, Associate Editor
Practical, medical,information for school patients, physicians, caregivers and families.

5350 **Carolina Curriculum for Infants and Toddlers with Special Needs (3rd Edition)**
Brookes Publishing
P.O. Box 10624
Baltimore, MD 21285-0624
410-337-9580
800-638-3775
Fax: 410-337-8539
custserv@brookespublishing.com
www.brookespublishing.com
Nancy M. Johnson-Martin, Author
Susan M. Attermeier, Author
Bonnie J. Hacker, Author
This book includes detailed assessment and intervention sequences, daily routine integration strategies, sensorimotor adaptations, and a sample 24-page Assessment Log that shows readers how to chart a child's individual progress.
504 pages Spiral-bound

5351 **Choosing Outcomes and Accommodations for Children (COACH) (2nd Edition)**
Brookes Publishing
P.O. Box 10624
Baltimore, MD 21285-0624
410-337-9580
800-638-3775
Fax: 410-337-8539
custserv@brookespublishing.com
www.brookespublishing.com
Michael F. Giangreco, Author
Chigee J. Cloninger, Author
Virginia Salce Iverson, Author
A guide to educational planning for students with disabilities, second edition. Focuses on life outcomes such as social relationships and participation in typical home, school, and community activities.
232 pages Spiral bound

5352 **Complete IEP Guide: How to Advocate for Your Special Ed Child (8th Edition)**
NOLO (Internet Brands)
909 N. Sepulveda Blvd
11th Fl.
El Segundo, CA 90245
310-280-4000
www.nolo.com
Lawrence Siegel, Author/Attorney
This all-in-one guide will help you understand special education law, identify your child's needs, prepare for meetings, develop the IEP and resolve disputes.
384 pages

5353 **Exceptional Student in the Regular Classroom (6th Edition)**
Pearson
330 Hudson St
New York, NY 10013
212-641-2400
www.pearsoned.com
Bill R. Gearheart, Author
Mel W. Weishan, Author
Carol J. Gearheart, Author
Offers good, solid information through a practical understandable presentation unencumbered by specialized jargon. Covers topics associated with special learners.
517 pages

5354 **Study Power Workbook: Exercises in Study - Skills to Improve Your Learning and Your Grades**
Brookline Books
8 Trumbull Rd
Ste B-001
Northampton, MA 1060-4533
413-584-0184
800-666-2665
Fax: 413-584-6184
brbooks@yahoo.com
www.brooklinebks.com
Sara Beth Huntley, Author
William Luckie, Author
Wood Smethurst, Author
The techniques in the easy-to-use, self-teaching manual have yielded remarkable success for students from elementary to medical school, at all levels of intelligence and achievement. Key skills covered include: listening, note taking, concentration, summarizing, reading comprehension, memorization, test taking, preparing papers and reports, time management, and more. These abilities are vital to success throughout every stage of learning; the benefits will last a lifetime.

Parenting: Spiritual

5355 **A Good and Perfect Gift: Faith, Expectations, and a Little Girl Named Penny**
Bethany House Publishers (Baker Publishing Group)
6030 E Fulton Rd
Ada, MI 49301
616-676-9185
800-877-2665
Fax: 616-676-9573
bakerpublishinggroup.com
Amy Julia Becker, Author
When her first baby, Penny, is given a frightening diagnosis, Amy Julia's world comes crashing down. Could she continue to trust God's goodness through what felt like personal tragedy? But challenging surprises often lead to unforeseen joy, and disappointments can turn into blessings. This wise and beautiful book is more than a courageous story of raising a child against the odds—it is a journey through the unexpected ups and downs of life and the discoveries that come along the way.
240 pages

5356 **Before and After Zachariah**
Chicago Review Press
814 N Franklin St
Chicago, IL 60610
312-337-0747
800-888-4741
Fax: 312-337-5110
www.chicagoreviewpress.com
Fern Kupfer, Author
This intimate chronicle of one family's life with a severely brain damaged child is recently back in print.
247 pages 1982

5357 **Bethy and the Mouse: A Father Remembers His Children with Disabilities**
Brookline Books
8 Trumbull Rd
Ste B-001
Northampton, MA 1060-4533
413-584-0184
800-666-2665
Fax: 413-584-6184
brbooks@yahoo.com
www.brooklinebks.com
Donald C. Bakely, Author
A moving collection of poetry, photographs, and prose following a father's experiences with two disabled children—one with Down Syndrome and one with an underdeveloped brain.
184 pages Paperback 1999

5358 **Disabled God: Toward a Liberatory Theologyof Disability**
Abingdon Press
2222 Rosa L. Parks Blvd
Nashville, TN 37288
615-749-6615
800-251-3320
orders@abingdonpress.com
www.abingdonpress.com
Nancy L. Eisland, Author
Draws on themes of the disability rights movement to identify people with disabilities as members of a socially disadvantaged minority group rather than as individuals who need to adjust. Highlights the history of people with disabilities in the church and society.
139 pages Paperback 1994

5359 **Farewell, My Forever Child**
CreateSpace, an Amazon Company
4900 Lacross Rd
North Charleston, SC 29406
843-760-8000
www.createspace.com
Kalila Smith, Author
Based on her own experiences following the loss of her 29-year-old daughter, Kalila Smith discusses the complex grief felt by parents who have lost a developmentally disabled child, and offers strategies to help families achieve peace and deal with the loss.
134 pages

5360 **In Time and with Love: Caring for the Special Needs Infant and Toddler**
William Morrow Paperbacks (HarperCollins)
195 Broadway
New York, NY 10007
212-207-7000
orders@harpercollins.com
www.harpercollins.com
Marilyn Segal, Author
Roni Leiderman, Author
Wendy S. Masi, Author
For families and caregivers of preteen and handicapped children in their first three years - more than one hundred tips for adjusting and coping. Part of the Your Child At Play series.
240 pages

5361 **Journal of Disability & Religion**
Routledge (Taylor & Francis Group)
711 Third Ave
New York, NY 10017
212-216-7800
800-354-1420
Fax: 202-564-7854
orders@taylorandfrancis.com
www.tandfonline.com
Quarterly

5362 **Spiritually Able: A Parents Guide to Teaching Faith To Children with Special Needs**
Loyola Press
3441 N Ashland Ave
Chicago, IL 60657
800-621-1008
Fax: 773-281-0555
customerservice@loyolapress.com
www.loyolapress.com
David Rizzo, Author
Both memoir and manual, Spiritually Able: A Parent's Guide to Teaching the Faith to Children with Special Needs is a life-preserver to parents who are seeking ways to grow and nourish a deeper relationship to God and their faith for their child with special needs. Full of tips, advice, and personal accounts, Spiritually Able helps bridge the gap and invites all into the welcoming embrace of the Church.
140 pages

5363 **The Spiritual Art of Raising Children with Disabilities**
Judson Press
P.O. Box 851
Valley Forge, PA 19482
800-458-3766
www.judsonpress.com
Kathleen Deyer Bolduc, Author
In The Spiritual Art of Raising Children with Disabilities, Bolduc uses the metaphor of the mosaic to life as parents of children with disabilities. Readers are walked through the process using the spiritual disciplines to help you recognize God's presence in your life and regain the balance we all need. this book offers readers the unique perspective of a parent raising a child with disabilities and dealing with it through faith and spiritual direction.
192 pages Paperback

5364 **Worst Loss: How Families Heal from the Death of a Child**
Holt Paperbacks (Macmillan Publishers)
75 Varick St
New York, NY 10013
212-226-7521
press.inquiries@macmillan.com
us.macmillan.com/henryholt
Barbara D. Rosof, Author
Combines anecdotal case histories and the latest research to help bereaved parents cope with the loss of a child, offering practical and comforting advice on how to overcome the disabling symptoms of grief.
304 pages 1995

Professional

5365 **American Journal of Physical Medicine & Rehabilitation**
Lippincott, Williams & Wilkins
2001 Market St
Ste 5
Philadelphia, PA 19103-1551
215-521-8300
800-638-3030
Fax: 215-521-8902
orders@lww.com
www.lww.com
Walter R. Frontera, MD, PHD, Editor-in-Chief
Journal of the Association of Academic Psychiatrists. Articles covering research and clinical studies and applications of new equipment, procedures and therapeutic advances.
Monthly

5366 **American Journal of Psychiatry**
American Psychiatric Association
1000 Wilson Blvd
Ste 1825
Arlington, VA 22209-3924
703-907-7322
800-368-5777
Fax: 703-907-1091
ajp@psych.org
ajp.psychiatryonline.org
Robert Freedman, Editor
Peer-reviewed articles focus on developments in biological psychiatry as well as on treatment innovations and forensic, ethical, economic, and social topics.
Monthly

5367 **American Journal of Public Health (AJPH)**
American Public Health Association
800 I St. NW
Washington, DC 20001
202-777-2742
Fax: 202-777-2534
TTY: 202-777-2500
www.apha.org
Georges C. Benjamin, Executive Director
Alfredo Morabia, Editor-in-Chief
Association journal containing editorials, commentary, and analyses on public health.
Monthly

5368 **Art Therapy**
American Art Therapy Association
4875 Eisenhower Ave.
Suite 240
Alexandria, VA 22304
703-548-5860
888-290-0878
Fax: 703-548-5860
info@arttherapy.org
arttherapy.org
Jordan Potash, Editor-in-Chief

Publishes articles on news, developments, ideas and research relating to the field of art therapy.
Quarterly

5369 **CAREERS & the disABLED Magazine**
Equal Opportunity Publications
445 Broad Hollow Rd
Ste 425
Melville, NY 11747-3615
631-421-9421
Fax: 631-421-1352
info@eop.com
www.eop.com
Barbara Capella Loehr, Editor
A career magazine for professional career seekers who have disabilities. Profiles disabled people who have achieved successful careers. Features a career section in Braille, career guide.

5370 **Clinician's Practical Guide to Attention-Deficit/Hyperactivity Disorder**
Brookes Publishing
P.O. Box 10624
Baltimore, MD 21285-0624
410-337-9580
800-638-3775
Fax: 410-337-8539
custserv@brookespublishing.com
www.brookespublishing.com
Marianne Mercugliano, Author
Quick reference volume with comprehensive data on psychoeducational and neuropsychological assessment, related symptoms, drug and counseling therapies and critical issues.
368 pages

5371 **Counseling Parents of Children with Chronic Illness or Disability**
Wiley
111 River St
Hoboken, NJ 07030-5774
201-748-6000
877-762-2974
Fax: 201-748-6088
info@wiley.com
www.wiley.com
Hilton Davis, Author
This book aims to help medical staff and carers relate to parents in ways that facilitate their adaptation to their child's illness. The key to this is in effective communication.
148 pages Paperback

5372 **Creating Options for Family Recovery: A Provider's Guide to Promoting Parental Mental Health**
Employment Options Inc.
82 Brigham St
Marlboro, MA 01752-3137
508-485-5051
Fax: 508-485-8807
options@employmentoptions.org
www.employmentoptions.com
Joanne Nicholson, Author
Toni Wolf, Author
Chip Wilder, Author
Kathleen Biebel, Author
This book seeks to advise professionals and providers on strategies to use when working with families who are dealing with mental illness, assisting them with the promotion of a healthy recovery. The resources in this guide are drawn from over 20 years of research and practice, and the lived experiences of parents, children and family members.
120 pages Paperback

5373 **Cystic Fibrosis: Medical Care**
Lippincott, Williams & Wilkins
16522 Hunters Green Pkwy
Hagerstown, MD 21740
301-223-2300
800-638-3030
Fax: 301-223-2400
orders@lww.com
www.lww.com
David M. Orenstein, Author
Beryl J. Rosenstein, Author
Robert C. Stern, Author
A guide to the medical community to the principles and practices of cystic fibrosis care. After chapters on the molecular and cellular bases of CF and its diagnosis, they cover the major organ systems affected by CF and deal with surgery for CF patients, transplantation (lung and liver), hospitalization, and terminal care. Also included are chapters on special populations, exercise, and laboratory testing.
365 pages

5374 **Disability & Rehabilitation Journal**
Taylor & Francis Online
6000 Broken Sound Pkwy NW
Ste 300
Boca Raton, FL 33487
212-216-7800
800-634-7064
Fax: 212-564-7854
enquiries@taylorandfrancis.com
www.taylorandfrancis.com
Dave Muller, Editor-in-Chief
Peer-reviewed journal offering the latest news, research, and insights on disability and rehabilitation medicine.
Bi-weekly

5375 **Disability Analysis Handbook: Tools for Independent Practice**
American Board of Disability Analysts
4525 Harding Rd.
Second Floor
Nashville, TN 37205
615-327-2984
Fax: 615-327-9235
americanbd@aol.com
www.americandisability.org
Kenneth Anchor, Administrative Officer
Handbook providing information on physical and mental disabilities, including diabetes, substance abuse, aging, nonverbal learning, chronic pain, etc.
396 pages

5376 **Enhancing Everyday Communication for Children with Disabilities**
Brookes Publishing
P.O. Box 10624
Baltimore, MD 21285-0624
410-337-9580
800-638-3775
Fax: 410-337-8539
custserv@brookespublishing.com
www.brookespublishing.com
Jeff Sigafoos, Author & Editor
Michael Arthur-Kelly, Author
Nancy Butterfield, Author
Practical and concise, this introductory guide is filled with real-world tips and strategies for anyone working to improve the communication of children with moderate, severe, and multiple disabilities. Emphasizing the link between behavior and communication, three respected researchers transform up-to-date research and proven best practices into instructional procedures and interventions ready for use at home or in school.
176 pages Paperback

5377 **Ethical Issues In Home Health Care (2nd Edition)**
Charles C. Thomas
2600 S First St
Springfield, IL 62704-4730
217-789-8980
800-258-8980
Fax: 217-789-9130
books@ccthomas.com
www.ccthomas.com
Sheri Smith, Author
Rosalind Ekman Ladd, Author
Lynn Pasquerella, Author
This book will help to answer some of the growing number of ethical questions and more complex issues that home health care nurses face. The cases presented in each chapter of the book are fictionalized situations based on interviews conducted with home health care nurses in both hospital-sponsored and private agencies, in hospices, and in urban and rural settings. Each chapter of the book is devoted to one of the main areas of concern for home health care nurses.
258 pages

5378 **Journal of Public Health**
Oxford Journals, Oxford University Press
2001 Evans Rd
Cary, NC 27513
919-677-0977
800-852-7323
Fax: 919-677-1714
www.oxfordjournals.org
Eugene Milne, Editor
Ted Schrecker, Editor
Scholarly articles on issues that relate to public health and the healthcare system.

5379 **PM&R Journal**
American Academy of Physical Medicine & Rehab
9700 W Bryn Mawr Ave
Ste 200
Rosemont, IL 60018-5701
847-737-6000
877-227-6799
Fax: 847-737-6001
TTY: 800-437-0833
info@aapmr.org
www.pmrjournal.org
Stuart M. Weinstein, Editor-in-Chief
Cathy Mendelsohn, Managing Editor
Covers medical, social and employment aspects of vocational rehabilitation. The content of PM&R includes articles that are contemporary and important to both research and clinical practice. The various sections of the journal include original research such as clinical trials, outcomes studies, and clinically relevant translational science; reviews (narrative and analytical); case presentations; point/counterpoint debates; ethical/legal topics; practice management updates; and statistical themes.
Monthly

5380 **Provider Magazine**
American Health Care Association
1201 L St NW
Washington, DC 20005-4024
202-842-4444
888-656-6669
Fax: 202-842-3860
sales@ahca.org
Joanne Erickson, Editor-in-Chief
Amy Mendoza, Managing Editor
Magazine for long-term healthcare professionals.
Monthly

5381 **Public Health Reports**
Association of Schools & Programs of Public Health
1900 M St NW
Ste 710
Washington, DC 20036
202-296-1099
Fax: 202-296-1252
www.publichealthreports.org
Frederic E. Shaw, Editorn-in-Chief
Sasha M. Ruiz, Acting Managing Editor
PHR is a peer-reviewed journal published on a bi-monthly basis. Each issue offers recurring guest columns such as Local Acts, Global Health Matters, ASPPH From the Schools and Programs of Public Health, Law and the Public's Health, Public Health Chronicles, NCHS Dataline, and the Surgeon General's Perspectives.
Bi-monthly

5382 **Sociopolitical Aspects of Disabilities (2nd Edition)**
Charles C. Thomas
2600 S First St
Springfield, IL 62704-4730
217-789-8980
800-258-8980
Fax: 217-789-9130
books@ccthomas.com
www.ccthomas.com
Willie V. Bryan, Author
Provides understanding of the social and political histories of people with disabilities in the United States. This understanding is pivotal in working with persons with disabilities, to provide background and perspective on current policies and attitudes.
284 pages

5383 **Starting and Sustaining Genetic Support Groups**
Johns Hopkins University Press
2715 N Charles St
Baltimore, MD 21218-4363
410-516-6900
Fax: 410-516-6968
webmaster@jhupress.jhu.edu
www.press.jhu.edu
Joan O. Weiss, Author
Jayne S. Mackta, Author
Guide to the establishment and maintenance of genetic support groups for individuals with genetic disorders and their families. For therapists and group leaders. Discusses practical matters including finding a leader, fund-raising, organizing peer support training programs.
152 pages

5384 **The Essential Brain Injury Guide (5th Edition)**
Brain Injury Association of America
3057 Nutley St.
Suite 805
Fairfax, VA 22031-1931
703-761-0750
Fax: 703-761-0755
info@biausa.org
shop.biausa.org
Susan Connors, President & CEO
Mary S. Reitter, Executive Vice President & COO
Robbie Baker, Vice President & CDO
Marianna Abashian, Director, Professional Services
The expanded and updated Essential Brain Injury Guide 5.0 is a hard cover, 25 chapter, 500-page text that provides information about brain injury, as well as brain injury treatment and rehabilitation. *$135.00*

5385 **What Psychotherapists Should Know about Disabilty**
Guilford Press
370 Seventh Ave
Ste 1200
New York, NY 10001-1020
800-365-7006
Fax: 212-966-6708
info@guilford.com
www.guilford.com
Rhoda Olkin, Author
This comprehensive volume provides the knowledge and skills that mental health professionals need for more effective, informed work with clients with disabilities. Topics addressed include etiquette with clients with disabilities; special concerns in assessment, evaluation, and diagnosis. Filled with clinical examples and observations, the volume also discusses strategies for enhancing teaching, training, and research.
368 pages

5386 **Women with Visible & Invisible Disabilitiees: Multiple Intersections, Issues, Therapies**
Routledge (Taylor & Francis Group)
711 Third Ave
New York, NY 10017
212-216-7800
800-634-7064
Fax: 202-564-7854
enquiries@taylorandfrancis.com
www.routledge.com
Martha E. Banks, Editor
Ellyn Kaschak, Editor
Addresses the issues faced by women with disabilities, examines the social construction of disability, and makes suggestions for the development and modification of culturally relevant therapy to meet the needs of disabled women.
414 pages Hardcover; Paperback

Specific Disabilities

5387 **inMotion Magazine**
Amputee Coalition
601 Pennsylvania Ave. NW
Suite 600, South Bldg.
Washington, DC 20004
888-267-5669
www.amputee-coalition.org
Mary Richards, President & CEO

inMotion Magazine is published bimonthly for amputees, caregivers and health care professionals, offering timely and comprehensive information. Offered both in print and online, free subscription.

Vocations

5388 **Ability Magazine**
P.O. Box 10878
Costa Mesa, CA 92627 www.abilitymagazine.com
Bi-monthly

5389 **Chemists with Disabilities Committee - American Chemical Society**
American Chemical Society
1155 16th St NW
Washington, DC 20036 202-872-4600
800-227-5558
Fax: 202-872-4574
cwd@acs.org
www.acs.org
John Johnston, Ph.D, MBA, Chair
James Schiller, Chair Elect
Paula Christopher, Staff Liaison
Promotes the full involvement of individuals with physical and learning disabilities in educational and career opportunities in the chemical and allied sciences. CWD members help individuals with disabilities to connect with employers and educators of persons with disabilities.

5390 **Demystifying Job Development: Field-Based Approaches to Job Development for the Disabled**
Training Resource Network
266 Roaring Dr.
St. Augustine, FL 32084 Fax: 904-823-3554
www.trn-store.com
David Hoff, Author
Cecilia Gandolfo, Author
Marty Gold, Author
Melanie Jordan, Author
A guide to successful placement of individuals with severe disabilities in quality jobs in the community.
105 pages

5391 **Hiring Idahoans with Disabilities**
Idaho Assistive Technology Project
University of Idaho
1187 Alturas Dr.
Moscow, ID 83843- 8331 208-885-3557
800-432-8324
Fax: 208-885-6102
idahoat@uidaho.edu
Jane Frederickson, Author
Kristen Hagen, Author
The purpose of this handbook is to inform employers in Idaho business and industry about the promise of hiring Idahoans with disabilities.

5392 **Life Beyond the Classroom: Transition Strategies for Young People with Disabilities**
Brookes Publishing
P.O. Box 10624
Baltimore, MD 21285-0624 410-337-9580
800-638-3775
Fax: 410-337-8539
www.brookespublishing.com
Paul Wehman, Author
Specialists in a variety of disciplines use creative and practical techniques to ensure careful transition planning, to build young people's confidence and competence in work skills, and to foster support from businesses and community organizations for training and employment programs.
616 pages

5393 **More Than a Job: Securing Satisfying Careers for People with Disabilities**
Brookes Publishing
P.O. Box 10624
Baltimore, MD 21285-0624 800-638-3775
Fax: 410-337-8539
custserv@brookespublishing.com
www.brookespublishing.com
Paul Wehman, Editor
John Kregel, Editor
This book transforms job placement into career counseling for people with physical and developmental disabilities. It presents step-by-step guidelines for helping people with disabilities to identify their own interests.
384 pages 1998

5394 **OT Practice Magazine**
American Occupational Therapy Association
6116 Executive Blvd.
Suite 200
North Bethesda, MD 20852-4929 301-652-6611
800-729-2682
otpractice@aota.org
www.aota.org/Publications-News/otp.aspx
Sherry Keramidas, Executive Director
Neil Harvison, Chief Officer, Knowledge
Matthew Clark, Chief Officer, Innovation & Engagement
Tricia Hopkins, Chief Officer, Finance & Operations
OT Practice covers professional information on all aspects of occupational therapy practice today. Features include hands-on techniques, continuing education, legislative issues, career advice, job opportunities, and the latest professional news. Also available online.

5395 **Occupational Therapy and Vocational Rehabilitation**
Wiley
111 River St
Hoboken, NJ 07030-5774 201-748-6000
877-762-2974
Fax: 201-748-6088
info@wiley.com
www.wiley.com
Joanne Ross
This book introduces the occupational therapist to the practice of vocational rehabilitation. As rehabilitation specialists, Occupational Therapists work in a range of diverse settings with clients who have a variety of physical, emotional and psychological conditions. This book highlights the contribution, which can be made by occupational therapists in assisting disabled, ill or injured workers to access, remain in and return to work.
280 pages Paperback

5396 **Work and Disability: Contexts, Issues & Strategies for Enhancing Employment Outcomes**
PRO-ED Inc.
8700 Shoal Creek Blvd
Austin, TX 78757-6897 512-451-3246
800-897-3202
Fax: 800-397-7633
general@proedinc.com
www.proedinc.com
Edna Mora Szymanski, Editor
Randall M. Parker, Editor
492 pages

Media, Electronic

Audio/Visual

5397 **A Place for Me**
Educational Productions
9000 SW Gemini Dr
Beaverton, OR 97008-7151
503-644-7000
800-950-4949
Fax: 503-350-7000
custserve@edpro.com
www.teachingstrategies.com
Diane Trister Dodge, Founder/President/Lead Author
Arnitra Duckett, VP, Sales & Strategic Marketing
In this video, parents discuss the issues they face in planning for their child's future. This program is designed to stimulate discussion of these issues and help increase awareness of the options available in your local community.

5398 **Able to Laugh**
Fanlight Productions
32 Court St.
21st Floor
Brooklyn, NY 11201-4421
718-488-8900
800-876-1710
Fax: 718-488-8642
info@fanlight.com
www.fanlight.com
Jonathan Miller, President
Patricio Guzman, Director
Meredith Miller, Sales Manager
Anthony Sweeney, Acquisitions
An exploration of the world of disability as interpreted by six professional comedians who happen to be disabled. It is also about the awkward ways disabled and able-bodied people relate to one another. *$199.00*
ISBN 1-572951-05-2

5399 **Acting Blind**
Fanlight Productions
32 Court St.
21st Floor
Brooklyn, NY 11201-4421
718-488-8900
800-876-1710
Fax: 718-488-8642
info@fanlight.com
www.fanlight.com
Jonathan Miller, President
Patricio Guzman, Director
Meredith Miller, Sales Manager
Anthony Sweeney, Acquisitions
Takes audiences behind the scenes as a company of non-professional actors rehearse a play about life without sight. The performers have no problem imagining themselves in these roles: they are blind themselves. *$229.00*

5400 **Adaptive Baby Care**
Through the Looking Glass
3075 Adeline St
Suite 120
Berkeley, CA 94703-2577
510-848-1112
800-644-2666
Fax: 510-848-4445
TTY: 510-848-1005
tlg@lookingglass.org
www.lookingglass.org
Megan Kirshbaum, Executive Director
Paul Preston, Assoc. Dir
This publication is presented as a catalyst for problem-solving regarding the development of adaptive baby care equipment. This newest publication is designed for parents, family members and professionals. It includes: guidelines for problem-solving baby care barriers; photographs and descriptions of prototypes and resources for adaptive baby care equipment; adaptive baby care techniques; adaptive baby care equipment checklist; commercial product safety commission guidelines; and local and natio
$250.00

5401 **Adaptive Baby Care Equipment Video and Book Through the Looking Glass**
Through the Looking Glass
3075 Adeline St
Suite 120
Berkeley, CA 94703-2577
510-848-1112
800-644-2666
Fax: 510-848-4445
TTY: 510-848-1005
tlg@lookingglass.org
www.lookingglass.org
Stephanie Miyashiro, Board President
Thomas Spalding, Board Treasurer
Alice Nemon, D.S.W., Board Secretary
Christina Jopes, Board Members
Includes Adaptive Baby care Equipment: Guide Lines; Prototypes and Resources, plus a twelve minute video. Available in Braille, large print or cassette. *$79.00*

5402 **All About Attention Deficit Disorders, Revised**
Parent Magic
800 Roosevelt Rd
B-309
Glen Ellyn, IL 60137-5839
630-208-0031
800-442-4453
Fax: 630-208-7366
www.parentmagic.com
Nancy Roe, Administrator/Exec Admin
Thomas Phelan, Owner/President/CEO
A psychologist and expert on ADD outlines the symptoms, diagnosis and treatment of this neurological disorder. Video ($49.95 - 2 parts) and audio cassette ($24.95). Also in DVD format (1 disk-$39.93).

5403 **Autism**
Aquarius Health Care Media
30 Forest Rd
PO Box 249
Millis, MA 2054-1511
508-376-1244
Fax: 508-376-1245
www.nmm.net
Lesile Kussmann, Owner/President/Producer
Kathy Newkirk, Director
Jane Hutchinson, Assoc. Director
This video takes you into the lives of autistic people and their families to understand more about autism. What defines autism and how can we help those living with the disability? Children, teens, and adults are also profiled and we begin to see the varying levels of development and new technology to help these people communicate. Preview Available. *$149.00*
Video

5404 **Basic Course in American Sign Language (B100) Harris Communications, Inc.**
Harris Communications
15155 Technology Dr
Eden Prairie, MN 55344-2273
952-906-1180
800-825-6758
Fax: 952-906-1099
TTY: 800-825-9187
info@harriscomm.com
www.harriscomm.com
Robert Harris, Owner & President
Kevin Horsky, Business Director
Randall Moore, Manager
This series of four one-hour tapes is designed to illustrate the various exercises and dialogues in the text. *$39.95*
Video

5405 **Beginning ASL Video Course**
Harris Communications
15155 Technology Dr
Eden Prairie, MN 55344-2273
952-906-1180
800-825-6758
Fax: 952-906-1099
TTY: 800-825-9187
info@harriscomm.com
www.harriscomm.com

Robert Harris, Owner & President
Kevin Horsky, Business Director
Randall Moore, Manager

You'll watch a family teach you to learn American Sign Language during funny and touching family situations. A total of 15 tapes in the course. *$599.40*
Video

5406 **Blindness**
Landmark Media
3450 Slade Run Dr
Falls Church, VA 22042-3940
703-241-2030
800-342-4336
Fax: 703-536-9540
info@landmarkmedia.com

Michael Hartogs, President/Owner
Joan Hartogs, Owner/Vice President
Peter Hartogs, Vice President
Richard Hartogs, Vice President

Landmark Media is an independent family-owned company currently celebrating our 28th anniversary. We have been fortunate to be able to offer the finest quality educational DVDs available. *$250.00*
Video

5407 **Boy Inside, The**
Fanlight Productions
32 Court St.
21st Floor
Brooklyn, NY 11201-4421
718-488-8900
800-876-1710
Fax: 718-488-8642
info@fanlight.com
www.fanlight.com

Jonathan Miller, President
Patricio Guzman, Director
Meredith Miller, Sales Manager
Anthony Sweeney, Acquisitions

Filmmaker Marianne Kaplan tells the personal and often distressing story of her son Adam, a 12-year-old with Asperger Syndrome, during a tumultuous year in the life of their family.

5408 **Braille Documents**
Metrolina Association for the Blind
704 Louise Ave
Charlotte, NC 28204-2128
704-887-5118
800-926-5466
Fax: 704-372-3872
bschmiel@mabnc.org
www.mabnc.org

Robert Scheffel, President
Richard Hartness, Vice President, Product Design & Development
Barbara Schmiel, Vice President, Accessible Braille Services
Chris Wilkins, Vice President, Information Technology

This production shop creates Braille and large-print documents. We work with our clients to find the most cost effective solutions for their needs. Unlike other modified statement service providers, we accept your existing style of statement or allow you to design your own statement.Documents may be received in electronic data files as encrypted data sent over public networks, data sent to a file transfer protocol drop box, or data sent over a dedicated data line. ABS also accepts paper hardcopi

5409 **Bringing Out the Best**
PO Box 9177
Dept. 11W
Champaign, IL 61826-9177
217-352-3273
800-519-2707
Fax: 217-352-1221
orders@researchpress.com
www.researchpress.com

David Parkinson, Chairman
Russell Pence, President
Gail Salyards, Dir. Of Marketing/President

5410 **Business as Usual**
Fanlight Productions
32 Court St.
21st Floor
Brooklyn, NY 11201-4421
718-488-8900
800-876-1710
Fax: 718-488-8642
info@fanlight.com
www.fanlight.com

Jonathan Miller, President
Patricio Guzman, Director
Meredith Miller, Sales Manager
Anthony Sweeney, Acquisitions

An enlightening documentary, brings a unique international perspective to this struggle. This film examines five innovative programs which create opportunities for people with mental and physical disabilities to own and operate their own businesses. *$145.00*

5411 **Buying Time: The Media Role in Health Care**
Fanlight Productions
32 Court St.
21st Floor
Brooklyn, NY 11201-4421
718-488-8900
800-876-1710
Fax: 718-488-8642
info@fanlight.com
www.fanlight.com

Jonathan Miller, President
Patricio Guzman, Director
Meredith Miller, Sales Manager
Anthony Sweeney, Acquisitions

This video program is a thoughtful and disturbing examination in the role of the media in determining the allocation of health care resources. This program is a powerful tool on ethics, policy, journalism, sociology, medicine and nursing as well as for professional workshops, and continuing education programs. *$99.00*

5412 **Caring for Persons with Developmental Disabilities**
PO Box 9177
Dept. 11W
Champaign, IL 61826-9177
217-352-3273
800-519-2707
Fax: 217-352-1221
www.researchpress.com

David Parkinson, Chairman
Russell Pence, President
Gail Salyards, Dir. Of Marketing/President

5413 **Clockworks**
Learning Corporation of America
6493 Kaiser Dr
Fremont, CA 94555-3610
510-490-7311
Oonchia Chia, Owner

Scotty, who has Down Syndrome, is fascinated by clocks. This film follows him on his adventures of employment in the clock shop.
Film

5414 **Close Encounters of the Disabling Kind**
Mainstream
6930 Carroll Ave
Suite 204
Takoma Park, MD 20912-4468
301-891-8777
Fax: 301-891-8778

Lillie Harrison, Information Programs Clerk
Fritz Rumpel, Editor

A training video that provides a hiring manager with information on how to learn the basics of disability etiquette and, by the end of

the video, seems much better prepared and willing to interview qualified individuals with disabilities. Includes trainer and trainee guides. *$99.95*
Video

5415 Deaf Children Signers
Harris Communications
15155 Technology Dr
Eden Prairie, MN 55344-2273
952-906-1180
800-825-6758
Fax: 952-906-1099
TTY: 800-825-9187
info@harriscomm.com
www.harriscomm.com
Robert Harris, Owner & President
Kevin Horsky, Business Director
Randall Moore, Manager
Graduate to voicing for Deaf children ages 5-11. This unique tape lets eleven young children demonstrate their abilities by signing about what is important to them. *$39.95*
Video

5416 Deaf Culture Series
Harris Communications
15155 Technology Dr
Eden Prairie, MN 55344-2273
952-906-1180
800-825-6758
Fax: 952-906-1099
TTY: 800-825-9187
info@harriscomm.com
www.harriscomm.com
Robert Harris, Owner & President
Kevin Horsky, Business Director
Randall Moore, Manager
Each video in this five-part series features a topic dealing with the unique culture of deaf people. It is an excellent resource for deaf studies programs, Interpreter Preparation programs and Sign Language programs. *$49.95*
Video

5417 Deaf Mosaic
Harris Communications
15155 Technology Dr
Eden Prairie, MN 55344-2273
952-906-1180
800-825-6758
Fax: 952-906-1099
TTY: 800-825-9187
info@harriscomm.com
www.harriscomm.com
Robert Harris, Owner & President
Kevin Horsky, Business Director
Randall Moore, Manager
Deaf Mosaic: Deaf President Now documents the most extraordinary week in deaf history, including interviews with student leaders; exclusive footage of the demonstrations; and an interview with Gallaudet president, Dr. I. King Jordan. *$29.95*
Video

5418 Do You Hear That?
Alexander Graham Bell Association
3417 Volta Pl. NW
Washington, DC 20007
202-337-5220
Fax: 202-337-8314
TTY: 202-337-5221
info@agbell.org
www.agbell.org
Emilio Alonso-Mendoza, Chief Executive Officer
This video shows auditory-verbal therapy sessions of a therapist working individually with 11 children who range in age from 7 months to 7 years old and have hearing aids or cochlear implants.
Video

5419 Doing Things Together
Britannica Film Company
345 4th St
San Francisco, CA 94107-1206
415-928-8466
Fax: 415-928-5027
Dave Bekowich, Owner

Steve went with his parents to an amusement park. He met another boy named Martin who at first was shocked by Steve's prosthetic hand.
Film

5420 Emerging Leaders
Mobility International USA
132 E Broadway
Suite 343
Eugene, OR 97401
541-343-1284
Fax: 541-343-6812
TTY: 541-343-1284
clearinghouse@miusa.org
www.miusa.org
Susan Sygall, Chief Executive Officer
Cindy Lewis, Director, Programs
Pioneering short-term international disability leadership programs in the U.S. and abroad with 2,000 youth, young adults and professionals from over 100 countries.
Video

5421 Face First
Fanlight Productions
32 Court St.
21st Floor
Brooklyn, NY 11201-4421
718-488-8900
800-876-1710
Fax: 718-488-8642
info@fanlight.com
www.fanlight.com
Jonathan Miller, President
Patricio Guzman, Director
Meredith Miller, Sales Manager
Anthony Sweeney, Acquisitions
In this documentary, the stories told reflect the reality faced by all those who are seen as different. Despite their difficult experiences, the survival of the profiled individuals affords comic relief &, by adulthood, they possess unusual strengths that shape their careers in pediatrics, disability care, public speaking, and journalism. *$195.00*

5422 Family-Guided Activity-Based Intervention for Toddlers & Infants
Brookes Publishing
PO Box 10624
Baltimore, MD 21285-0624
410-337-9580
800-638-3775
Fax: 410-337-8539
custserv@brookespublishing.com
Paul Brooks, Owner
This 20-minute video was created to assist early childhood professionals to incorporate therapeutic intervention into daily living. It includes a discussion and demonstration of how intervention professionals actively may involve caregivers in the planning and implementation of activities aimed at encouraging development of a child's target skills *$37.00*
20 Minutes
ISBN 1-55766-19-3

5423 Filmakers Library
124 E 40th St
Suite 901
New York, NY 10016-1798
212-808-4980
Fax: 212-808-4983
www.filmakers.com
Sue Oscar, Co-President
Linda Gottesman, Co-President
Andrea Traubner, Dir., Broadcast Sales
Filmakers Library has been a leading source of outstanding films for the education, library, and non-theatrical markets. Now, as an imprint of award-winning online publisher Alexander Street Press, Filmakers Library is able to offer online streaming access to most of our titles, ensuring that our films receive the greatest possible exposure and accessibility through the most flexible delivery platforms. We market and promote our films throughout the world by direct mail, print advertising, exhib

5424 **Filmakers Library: An Imprint Of Alexander Street Press**
124 E 40th St
Suite 901
New York, NY 10016-1798
212-808-4980
Fax: 212-808-4983
www.filmakers.com

Sue Oscar, Co-President
Linda Gottesman, Co-President
Andrea Traubner, Dir., Broadcast Sales

Filmakers Library has been a leading source of outstanding films for the education, library, and non-theatrical markets. Now, as an imprint of award-winning online publisher Alexander Street Press, Filmakers Library is able to offer online streaming access to most of our titles, ensuring that our films receive the greatest possible exposure and accessibility through the most flexible delivery platforms. We market and promote our films throughout the world by direct mail, print advertising, exhib
$100 - $300

5425 **Films & Videos on Aging and Sensory Change**
Lighthouse International
111 E 59th St
New York, NY 10022-1202
212-821-9200
800-829-0500
Fax: 212-821-9706
info@lighthouse.org

Joanna Mellor, VP Information Services
Tara Cortes, President

An annotated list of over 80 films and videos dealing with age-related sensory change, divided into sections on vision impairment, hearing impairment, and multiple sensory impairments. *$5.00*

5427 **Heart to Heart**
Blind Children's Center
4120 Marathon St
Los Angeles, CA 90029-3584
323-664-2153
info@blindchildrenscenter.org
www.blindchildrenscenter.org

Nancy Chernus-Mansfield, Co-Author
Dori Hayashi, Co-Author

Parents of blind and partially sighted children talk about their feelings. *$35.00*
VHS/DVD

5428 **Helping Hands**
Fanlight Productions
32 Court St.
21st Floor
Brooklyn, NY 11201-4421
718-488-8900
800-876-1710
Fax: 718-488-8642
info@fanlight.com
www.fanlight.com

Jonathan Miller, President
Patricio Guzman, Director
Meredith Miller, Sales Manager
Anthony Sweeney, Acquisitions

The ADA mandates equal access and opportunity for the 43 million people with disabilities in the United States. These individuals may have limited speech, sight or mobility; a developmental disability; or a medical condition which limits some life activities. Many, however, are ready, willing and very able to join the workforce. This video demonstrates that many modifications or adaptations can be made simply by using ingenuity or common sense — such as keeping the aisles clear, etc. *$145.00*
37 Minutes

5429 **Home is in the Heart: Accommodating Peoplewith Disabilities in the Homestay Experience**
Mobility International USA
132 E Broadway
Suite 343
Eugene, OR 97401
541-343-1284
Fax: 541-343-6812
TTY: 541-343-1284
clearinghouse@miusa.org
www.miusa.org

Susan Sygall, Chief Executive Officer
Cindy Lewis, Director, Programs

Provides information and ideas for exchange organizations. Discusses how to recruit homestay families, meet accessibility needs and accommodate international participants with disabilities.
Video

5430 **How Difficult Can This Be ? (Fat City) - Rick Lavoie**
CACLD
PO Box 210
Barnstable, MA 02630-210
508-362-1052
scheduling@ricklavoie.com
www.ricklavoie.com

Rick Lavoie, Film Maker

This unique program allows viewers to experience the same frustration, anxiety and tension that children with learning disabilities face in their daily lives. Teachers, social workers, psychologists, parents and friends who have participated in Richard Lavoie's workshop reflect upon their experience and the way it changed their approach to L.D. children. 1989.

5431 **How We Play**
Fanlight Productions
32 Court St.
21st Floor
Brooklyn, NY 11201-4421
718-488-8900
800-876-1710
Fax: 718-488-8642
info@fanlight.com
www.fanlight.com

Jonathan Miller, President
Patricio Guzman, Director
Meredith Miller, Sales Manager
Anthony Sweeney, Acquisitions

Though most of the people in this new, short documentary are in wheelchairs, and one is blind, they are anything but handicapped. Playing tennis, snorkeling, whitewater canoeing, practicing karate - they are living proof that a disability can be a challenge, not an obstacle. *$99.00*

5432 **I'm Not Disabled**
Landmark Media
3450 Slade Run Dr
Falls Church, VA 22042-3940
703-241-2030
800-342-4336
Fax: 703-536-9540
info@landmarkmedia.com

Michael Hartogs, President
Joan Hartogs, Vice President
Peter Hartogs, Vice President
Richard Hartogs, Vice President

Young people talk about their disabilities and the importance of sports in their lives. The afflictions range from blindness and missing limbs to paralysis. Through physical education and therapy they enjoy freedom of movement and participate in sports such as tennis, basketball, kayaking, skiing, and swimming. *$195.00*
Video

5433 **Imagery Procedures for People with Special Needs**
Research Press
PO Box 9177
Dept. 11W
Champaign, IL 61826-9177
217-352-3273
800-519-2707
Fax: 217-352-1221
rp@researchpress.com
www.researchpress.com

David Parkinson, Chairman
Russell Pence, President
Gail Salyards, Dir. Of Marketing/President

This video was developed at the Groden Center and illustrates imagery based procedures including the use of positive reinforcement, covert modeling, and a self-control triad to assists individuals to self-regulate their behaviors in stressful situations or under conditions that may evoke extreme fear. Recommended for professionals and family members interested in teaching self-control strategies that individuals with autism spectrum disorders can use in community settings. *$195.00*
32 Minutes

5434 In the Middle
Fanlight Productions
c/o Icarus Films
32 Court Street, 21st Floor
Brooklyn, NY 11201
718-488-8900
800-876-1710
Fax: 718-488-8642
info@fanlight.com
www.fanlight.com
Ben Achtenberg, Founder, Owner
Documents the problems and joys shared by Ryanna, who has Spina Bifida, and her parents, teachers and classmates during her first year of being mainstreamed in a Head Start Program. *$99.00*

5435 Include Us
Exceptional Parent Library
PO Box 1807
Englewood Cliffs, NJ 7632-1207
201-947-6000
800-535-1910
Fax: 201-947-9376
eplibrary@aol.com

5436 Intensive Early Intervention and Beyond
PO Box 9177
Dept. 11W
Champaign, IL 61826-9177
217-352-3273
800-519-2707
Fax: 217-352-1221
www.researchpress.com
David Parkinson, Chairman
Russell Pence, President
Gail Salyards, Dir. Of Marketing/President

5437 Invisible Children
Learning Corporation of America
6493 Kaiser Dr
Fremont, CA 94555-3610
510-490-7311
Oonchia Chia, Owner
Renaldo was blind, Mandy was deaf, and Mark had Cerebral Palsy and used a wheelchair. These child-size puppet characters interacted with non-handicapped puppets.
Film

5439 Let's Eat Video
Blind Children's Center
4120 Marathon Street
Los Angeles, CA 90029-3584
323-664-2153
info@blindchildrenscenter.org
blindchildrenscenter.org
Jill Brody, Co-Author
Lynne Webber, Co-Author
Babies and toddlers with visual impairments lack one major avenue of exploration, and this significantly infulences their awareness, perceptions, and anticipation of the food which is presented to them. *$35.00*
VHS/DVD

5440 Look Who's Laughing
Aquarius Health Care Videos
30 Forest Rd
PO Box 249
Millis, MA 2054-1511
508-376-1244
Fax: 508-376-1245
aqvideos@tiac.net
www.aquariusproductions.com
Lesile Kussmann, Owner/President/Producer
Kathy Newkirk, Director
Jane Hutchinson, Assoc. Director
This video is packed with laugh-out-loud comedic moments, but is also full of intelligent and inspiring messages. Look Who's Laughing introduces viewers to some of today's funniest comedians - who just happen to be physically disabled. We hear them talk openly and honestly about their limitations as well as their abilities and talents. Helpful for those who work with the disabled and motivational to both the disabled and able-bodied. Preview option available. *$95.00*
Video

5441 My Body is Not Who I Am
Aquarius Health Care Videos
30 Forest Rd
PO Box 249
Millis, MA 2054-1511
508-376-1244
Fax: 508-376-1245
aqvideos@tiac.net
www.aquariusproductions.com
Lesile Kussmann, Owner/President/Producer
Kathy Newkirk, Director
Jane Hutchinson, Assoc. Director
This thought-provoking video introduces viewers to people who openly discuss the struggles and triumphs they have experienced living in a body that is physically disabled. They talk honestly about the social stigma of their disability and the problems they face in terms of mobility, health care and family relationships, as well as the challenges of emotional and sexual intimacy. Preview option available. *$195.00*
Video

5442 My Country
Aquarius Health Care Videos
30 Forest Rd
PO Box 249
Millis, MA 2054-1511
508-376-1244
Fax: 508-376-1245
aqvideos@tiac.net
www.aquariusproductions.com
Lesile Kussmann, Owner/President/Producer
Kathy Newkirk, Director
Jane Hutchinson, Assoc. Director
By telling the stories of three people with disabilities and their struggle for equal rights under the law, this film draws a powerful parallel between the efforts of disability rights activists and the civil rights struggle of the 1960s. Great for disability awareness programs, and for discussions of disability rights issues. Should be part of every college curriculum on disabilities. Awarded Best of Show Superfest 98. Preview option available. *$195.00*
Video

5443 Narcolepsy
Fanlight Productions
c/o Icarus Films
32 Court Street, 21st Floor
Brooklyn, NY 11201
718-488-8900
800-876-1710
Fax: 718-488-8642
info@fanlight.com
www.fanlight.com
Ben Achtenberg, Founder, Owner
Jason Margolis, Producer
Presents the experiences of three individuals who lives and relationships have been disrupted by narcolepsy. Rental $50/day. *$199.00*
VHS/25 Minutes

5444 No Barriers
Aquarius Health Care Videos
30 Forest Rd
PO Box 249
Millis, MA 2054-1511
508-376-1244
Fax: 508-376-1245
aqvideos@tiac.net
www.aquariusproductions.com
Lesile Kussmann, Owner/President/Producer
Kathy Newkirk, Director
Jane Hutchinson, Assoc. Director
Everyone faces the world with different abilities and disabilities. But everyone has at least one goal in common...to break through their own barriers says Mark Wellman. Mark, a paraplegic, knows this well. No Barriers takes us into Mark's world where he defies the odds for most able bodied individuals by climbing Yosemite's Half Dome and El Capitan. This video is more than inspiring and fun to watch...it helps one make that paradigm shift from can't do to can do! Preview option available *$90.00*
Video

5445 **On The Spectrum**
Fanlight Productions
32 Court St.
21st Floor
Brooklyn, NY 11201-4421
718-488-8900
800-876-1710
Fax: 718-488-8642
info@fanlight.com
www.fanlight.com
Jonathan Miller, President
Patricio Guzman, Director
Meredith Miller, Sales Manager
Anthony Sweeney, Acquisitions
Adults living with Asperger syndrome describe the ways AS has affected their lives, their work and their relationships. They discuss learning to cope with the disorder and the comfort and reinforcement of participating with others 'like them' in an Asperger's support group. 53 min. *$199.00*

5446 **Open for Business**
Disability Rights Education and Defense Fund
3075 Adeline Street
Suite 210
Berkeley, CA 94703-2219
510-644-2555
800-841-8645
Fax: 510-841-8645
info@dredf.org
www.dredf.org
Sue Henderson, Executive Director
Jenny . Kern, Esq, President/Chair
Claudia Center, Esq, Treasurer
Vikki Davis, Secretary
Documentary video captures the drama and emotions of the historic civil rights demonstration of people with disabilities in 1977, resulting in the signing of the 504 Regulations, the first Federal Civil Rights Law protecting people with disabilities. Includes contemporary news footage and news interviews with participants and demonstration leaders. *$179.00*

5447 **Open to the Public**
Aquarius Health Care Videos
30 Forest Rd
PO Box 249
Millis, MA 2054-1511
508-376-1244
Fax: 508-376-1245
aqvideos@tiac.net
www.aquariusproductions.com
Lesile Kussmann, Owner/President/Producer
Kathy Newkirk, Director
Jane Hutchinson, Assoc. Director
Provides an overview of the Americans with Disabilities Act as it applies to state and local governments. The ADA doesn't provide recommendations for solving common problems, but this film could provide enough information for governments to solve some common problems without turning to high-priced consultants. Preview option available. *$125.00*
Video

5448 **Our Own Road**
Aquarius Health Care Videos
30 Forest Rd
PO Box 249
Millis, MA 2054-1511
508-376-1244
Fax: 508-376-1245
aqvideos@tiac.net
www.aquariusproductions.com
Lesile Kussmann, Owner/President/Producer
Kathy Newkirk, Director
Jane Hutchinson, Assoc. Director
This video shows the disabled helping other people who are disabled and portrays the sense of pride they get from helping others. This multicultural program features many different healing techniques, and teaches the importance of helping those who are disabled become independent and productive. *$99.00*

5449 **Outsider: The Life and Art of Judith Scott**
Fanlight Productions
32 Court St.
21st Floor
Brooklyn, NY 11201-4421
718-488-8900
800-876-1710
Fax: 718-488-8642
info@fanlight.com
www.fanlight.com
Jonathan Miller, President
Patricio Guzman, Director
Meredith Miller, Sales Manager
Anthony Sweeney, Acquisitions
Judith Scoot has Down Syndrome, is deaf, and does not speak. Yet after 35 years of institutionalization, with the help of a sister who never gave up on her, she emerged to create a series of sculptures that have fascinated and mystified art experts and collectors around the world. 26 minutes. *$199.00*

5450 **Passion for Justice**
Fanlight Productions
32 Court St.
21st Floor
Brooklyn, NY 11201-4421
718-488-8900
800-876-1710
Fax: 718-488-8642
info@fanlight.com
www.fanlight.com
Jonathan Miller, President
Patricio Guzman, Director
Meredith Miller, Sales Manager
Anthony Sweeney, Acquisitions
An unusually penetrating examination of the question of inclusion, this is an engaging portrait of Bob Perske, the author of Unequal Justice, and a crusader for the legal rights of people with developmental disabilities. A Passion for Justice asks challenging questions about society's responsibility to this population, and about ways to protect everyone's rights to equality and justice. *$99.00*
29 Minutes

5451 **Phoenix Dance**
Fanlight Productions
32 Court St.
21st Floor
Brooklyn, NY 11201-4421
718-488-8900
800-876-1710
Fax: 718-488-8642
info@fanlight.com
www.fanlight.com
Jonathan Miller, President
Patricio Guzman, Director
Meredith Miller, Sales Manager
Anthony Sweeney, Acquisitions
A heroic journey of transformation and healing, Phoenix Dance challenges our expectations of what it means to be disabled. In March, 2001, renowned dancer Homer Avila discovered that the pain in his hip was cancer. A month later, his right leg and most of his hip were amputated. *$199.00*

5452 **Pool Exercise Program - Arthritis Water Exercise / Arthritis Foundation**
Arthritis Foundation Distribution Center
PO Box 932915
Atlanta, GA 31193-2915
440-872-7100
800-283-7800
Fax: 404-872-0457
aforders@arthritis.org
www.arthritis.org
John Klippel, President/CEO
This video features water exercises that will help you increase and maintain joint flexibility, strengthen and tone muscles, and increase endurance. All exercises are performed in water at chest level. No swimming skills are necessary. *$19.50*

5453 **Potty Learning for Children who Experience Delay**
Exceptional Parent Library
PO Box 1807
Englewood Cliffs, NJ 7632-1207
201-947-6000
800-535-1910
Fax: 201-947-9376
eplibrary@aol.com

5454 **Pushin' Forward**
Fanlight Productions
32 Court St.
21st Floor
Brooklyn, NY 11201-4421
718-488-8900
800-876-1710
Fax: 718-488-8642
info@fanlight.com
www.fanlight.com
Jonathan Miller, President
Patricio Guzman, Director
Meredith Miller, Sales Manager
Anthony Sweeney, Acquisitions
Growing up poor and Latino, James Lilly was a gang member and drug dealer until, at fifteen, he was shot in the back and paralyzed. Today, he shares his story with inner city kids, and tells them about one thing that helped him move on; wheelchair racing. In Pushin' Forward he takes on the world's longest wheelchair race, from Fairbanks to Anchorage, Alaska, in six days! 39 minutes. *$229.00*

5455 **Recognizing Children with Special Needs**
Films Media Group
132 W. 31st St
16th Fl.
New York, NY 10001
800-322-8755
Fax: 800-678-3633
custserv@films.com
www.films.com
DVD/Video

5456 **Relaxation Techniques for People with Special Needs**
Research Press
PO Box 9177
Dept. 11W
Champaign, IL 61826-9177
217-352-3273
800-519-2707
Fax: 217-352-1221
rp@researchpress.com
www.researchpress.com
David Parkinson, Chairman
Russell Pence, President
Gail Salyards, Dir. Of Marketing/President
The developers discuss and demonstrate how to use special relaxation procedures with children and adolescents who have developmental disabilities. They emphasize the need for students to learn relaxation as a means of coping with stress and developing self-control. During the scenes of Dr June Groden conducting relaxation training, viewers will see how to correctly use the training procedures, how to use reinforcement during training and how to use guided imagery. 23 minutes. Includes book. *$195.00*
Video

5457 **Right at Home**
Aquarius Health Care Videos
30 Forest Rd
PO Box 249
Millis, MA 2054
508-376-1244
Fax: 508-376-1245
aqvideos@tiac.net
www.aquariusproductions.com
Lesile Kussmann, Owner/President/Producer
Kathy Newkirk, Director
Jane Hutchinson, Assoc. Director
Shows simple solutions for complying with the Fair Hoiusing Act amendments. Emphasizes low-cost, practical solutions, and working with people with disabilities to find the best applicable solution. Ideal for people with disabilities and their families, as well as housing providers, university courses, and disability awareness organizations. Preview option is available. *$99.00*
Video

5458 **Seat-A-Robics**
PO Box 630064
Little Neck, NY 11363-64
718-631-4007
Daria Alinovi, President
Offers a variety of safe, affordable and medically approved video exercise programs that are listed in our video chapter. In addition the company offers two resources. The first Healthy Eating & Facts For Kids is geared specifically to health professionals and educators that work with disabled children ($39.95). The second is a recreational resource guide that stimulates children to be creative and get involved. It keeps them actively engaged while having fun and getting fit ($29.95).

5459 **Shining Bright: Head Start Inclusion**
Brookes Publishing
PO Box 10624
Baltimore, MD 21285-624
410-337-9580
800-638-3775
Fax: 410-337-8539
custserv@brookespublishing.com
Paul Brooks, Owner
This documentary depicts the collaborative efforts of a Head Start and a local education agency to include children with severe disabilities in a Head Start program. This video addresses issues such as support for children with severe health impairments, benefits of participating in Head Start, ability of teachers with a general education background to serve children with severe disabilities, and staff relations. Includes a 28-page saddle-stitched booklet. *$45.00*
23 Minutes
ISBN 1-55766 -95-9

5460 **Small Differences**
Aquarius Health Care Videos
30 Forest Rd
PO Box 249
Millis, MA 2054-1511
508-376-1244
Fax: 508-376-1245
aqvideos@tiac.net
www.aquariusproductions.com
Lesile Kussmann, Owner/President/Producer
Kathy Newkirk, Director
Jane Hutchinson, Assoc. Director
What happens when you give children with and without disabilities a camera and ask them to produce a video about disabilities? The result is an uplifting, award-winning disability video that both children and adults can relate to. The kids interviewed adults and children with physical and sensory disabilities. A top-quality production that increases understanding and awareness. Winner, Columbus International Film & Video Festival. Winner, National Education Media Network. Preview option availabe *$110.00*
Video

5461 **Someday's Child**
Educational Productions
9000 SW Gemini Dr
Beaverton, OR 97008-7151
503-644-7000
800-950-4949
Fax: 503-350-7000
custserv@edpro.com
www.edpro.com
Diane Trister Dodge, Founder/President/Lead Author
Arnitra Duckett, VP, Sales & Strategic Marketing
This video focuses on three families' search for help and information for their children with disabilities.

5462 **Sound & Fury**
Aquarius Health Care Videos
30 Forest Rd
PO Box 249
Millis, MA 2054-1511
508-376-1244
Fax: 508-376-1245
aqvideos@tiac.net
www.aquariusproductions.com
Lesile Kussmann, Owner/President/Producer
Kathy Newkirk, Director
Jane Hutchinson, Assoc. Director
This film takes viewers inside the seldom seen world of the deaf to witness a painful family struggle over a controversial medical technology called the cochlear implant. Some of the family mem-

bers celebrate the implant as a long overdue cure for deafness while others fear it will destroy their language and way of life. This documentary explores this seemingly irreconcilable conflict as it illuminates the ongoing struggle for identity among deaf people today. *$195.00*

Video

5463 **Special Children/Special Solutions**

Option Indigo Press
2080 S Undermountain Rd
Sheffield, MA 1257-9643 413-229-8727
800-714-2779
Fax: 413-229-8727
indigo@option.org

Barry Kaufmans, Owner/Founder/Author
Samahria Kaufmans, Owner/Founder

This four-tape audio series presents concrete, down-to-earth, no-nonsense alternatives which are full of love and acceptance for the special child while being wholly supportive of parents, professionals and helpers who want to reach out. The accepting (nonjudgmental) attitude presented is the basis of all Samahria's work and is the foundation for the nurturing teaching process that has encouraged and helped parents, children and others to accomplish more than most would have believed. *$55.00*

Audio

5464 **Technology for the Disabled**

Landmark Media
3450 Slade Run Dr
Falls Church, VA 22042-3940 703-241-2030
800-342-4336
Fax: 703-536-9540
info@landmarkmedia.com
landmarkmedia.com

Michael Hartogs, President
Joan Hartogs, Vice President
Peter Hartogs, Vice President
Richard Hartogs, Vice President

Physically disabled people cope with the frustrations of a body they cannot control. The computer age has made many disabled more self-reliant; armless feed themselves, the blind read newspapers and the voiceless speak through marvelous technological breakthroughs. *$195.00*

Video

5465 **Three R's for Special Education: Rights, Resources, Results**

Brookes Publishing
PO Box 10624
Baltimore
MD, 21 0624-624 410-337-9580
800-638-3775
Fax: 410-337-8539
custserv@brookespublishing.com

Paul Brooks, Owner

This is a guide for parents, and a tool for educators. Through this video parents learn how to work through the steps of the special education system and work toward securing the best education and services for their children. Reviews the laws to protect children with disabilities in easy to understand language. Also provides a list of national organizations that can offer resources, information and advice to parents. *$49.95*

50 Minutes
ISBN 0-96461 -80-7

5466 **Tools for Students**

Aquarius Health Care Videos
30 Forest Rd
PO Box 249
Millis, MA 2054-1511 508-376-1244
Fax: 508-376-1245
aqvideos@tiac.net
www.aquariusproductions.com

Lesile Kussmann, Owner/President/Producer
Kathy Newkirk, Director
Jane Hutchinson, Assoc. Director

Provides a series of 26 fun occupational therapy sensory processing activities. Designed as an in-home, in-workshop, and in-class exercise leader with students. Activities include: Strenghten the muscles necessary for normal activities, provide the muscles necessary to enhance alertness and concentration, increase the ability to use good posture, help social skills and fitting in and increase coordination; concludes with emphasis on team collaboration between the student, teacher, and parents. *$99.00*

Video

5467 **Twitch and Shout**

Fanlight Productions
c/o Icarus Films
32 Court Street, 21st Floor
Brooklyn, NY 11201 718-488-8900
800-876-1710
Fax: 718-488-8642
info@fanlight.com
www.fanlight.com

Ben Achtenberg, Founder, Owner
Laurel Chitden, Producer

This documentary provides an intimate journey into the startling world of Tourette Syndrome (TS), a genetic disorder that can cause a bizarre range of involuntary movements, vocalizations, and compulsions. Through the eyes of a photojournalist with TS, the film introduces viewers to others who have this puzzling disorder. This is an emotionally absorbing, sometimes, unsettling, and finally uplifting program about people who must contend with a society that often sees them as crazy or bad. *$225.00*

5468 **Video Guide to Disability Awareness**

Aquarius Health Care Videos
30 Forest Rd
PO Box 249
Millis, MA 2054-1511 508-376-1244
Fax: 508-376-1245
aqvideos@tiac.net
www.aquariusproductions.com

Lesile Kussmann, Owner/President/Producer
Kathy Newkirk, Director
Jane Hutchinson, Assoc. Director

President Clinton opens and concludes this informative video about disability awareness. A series of candid interviews with people who have a wide range of disabilities provide personal insights into the issues surrounding visual, hearing, physical and mental disabilities. Video comes with written reference guide and is also available with open or closed captioning. Preview option available. *$195.00*

Video

5469 **Video Intensive Parenting**

Systems Unlimited/LIFE Skills
1556 S 1st Ave
Iowa City, IA 52240-6007 319-356-5412

Geoffrey Lauer, Program Director
Bill Gorman, President
Ginny Kirschling, Public Information Specialist

Parents who have children with special needs share their reactions to their child's diagnosis and how they have learned to cope with their feelings. *$69.95*

5470 **Vital Signs: Crip Culture Talks Back**

Fanlight Productions
32 Court St.
21st Floor
Brooklyn, NY 11201-4421 718-488-8900
800-876-1710
Fax: 718-488-8642
info@fanlight.com
www.fanlight.com

Jonathan Miller, President
Patricio Guzman, Director
Meredith Miller, Sales Manager
Anthony Sweeney, Acquisitions

This edgy, raw video documentary explores the politics of disability through the performances, debates and late-night conversations of artists at a recent national conference of disabilities and the art's. Vital Signs conveys the intensity, variety and vitality of disability culture today. *$225.00*

Video

5471 **What About Me?**
Educational Productions
9000 SW Gemini Dr
Beaverton, OR 97008-7151
503-644-7000
800-950-4949
Fax: 503-350-7000
custserve@edpro.com
www.teachingstrategies.com
Diane Trister Dodge, Founder/President/Lead Author
Arnitra Duckett, VP, Sales & Strategic Marketing
This video focuses on two siblings of children with disabilities. The siblings (Brian and Julie) share their perspectives, their worries, concerns and victories about living with a sibling with a disability.

5472 **When Billy Broke His Head...and Other**
Fanlight Productions
32 Court St.
21st Floor
Brooklyn, NY 11201-4421
718-488-8900
800-876-1710
Fax: 718-488-8642
info@fanlight.com
www.fanlight.com
Jonathan Miller, President
Patricio Guzman, Director
Meredith Miller, Sales Manager
Anthony Sweeney, Acquisitions
When Billy Golfus, an award-winning journalist, became brain damaged as the result of a motor scooter accident, he joined the ranks of the 43 million Americans with disabilities, this country's largest and most invisible minority. He helped create this video, which blends humor with politics and individual experience with a chorus of voices, to explain what it is really like to live with a disability in America. #136 *$195.00*
ISBN 1-57295 -36-2

5473 **When I Grow Up**
Britannica Film Company
345 4th St
San Francisco, CA 94107-1206
415-928-8466
Fax: 415-928-5027
Dave Bekowich, Owner
At a costume party each child was to come as what they wanted to be when they grew up. Some of the children had handicaps, and they talked about why their handicaps would not prevent them from fulfilling their desires.
Film

5474 **When Parents Can't Fix It**
Fanlight Productions
32 Court St.
21st Floor
Brooklyn, NY 11201-4421
718-488-8900
800-876-1710
Fax: 718-488-8642
info@fanlight.com
www.fanlight.com
Jonathan Miller, President
Patricio Guzman, Director
Meredith Miller, Sales Manager
Anthony Sweeney, Acquisitions
This documentary looks at the lives of five families who are raising children with disabilities - the problems they face, how they have learned to cope, and the rewards and stresses of adapting to their child's condition. It explores the medical complexities and financial pressures families encounter, the emotional and physical toll on parents and siblings, and the dangers of child abuse in this population. It offers a very realistic look at different family strengths and coping styles.
58 Min. DVD/VHS
ISBN 1-572958-76-6

5475 **White Cane and Wheels**
Fanlight Productions
32 Court St.
21st Floor
Brooklyn, NY 11201-4421
718-488-8900
800-876-1710
Fax: 718-488-8642
info@fanlight.com
www.fanlight.com
Jonathan Miller, President
Patricio Guzman, Director
Meredith Miller, Sales Manager
Anthony Sweeney, Acquisitions
Carmen and Steve once dreamed of lives on stage and screen, but their plans were cut short by her blindness and his muscular dystrophy. This program is a funny and touching exploration of a relationship filled with frustration, but held together with patience, stubborness, forgiveness, and love. 26 minutes. *$169.00*

Web Sites

5476 **ADA Questions and Answers**
U.S. Department of Justice, Civil Rights Division
950 Pennsylvania Ave NW
Washington, DC 20530-0001
202-514-4609
Fax: 202-307-1197
TTY: 202-514-0716
www.ada.gov

5477 **Ability Jobs**
Ability Magazine
P.O. Box 10878
Costa Mesa, CA 92627
www.abilityjobs.com

5478 **AbleApparel - Affordable Adaptive Clothing and Accessories**
2121 Hillside Ave
New Hyde Park, NY 11040-2712
516-873-6552
Fax: 516-248-7308
www.ableapparel.com
Mary Ann Tenaglia, Partner
Marie Harmon, Partner
Donna Lo Monica, Partner/Designer
AbleApparel is always designing and creating new products that will make Matty's life and others with disabilities a little easier. Most of the people spoken to regardless of age want to be able to wear clothes that are functional, affordable and, above all, fashionable.

5479 **AbleData**
103 W Broad St
Suite 400
Falls Church, VA 22046
301-608-8998
800-227-0216
Fax: 301-608-8958
TTY: 301-608-8912
www.abledata.com
Katherine Belknap, Director
David Johnson, Publications Director
AbleData provides objective information on assistive technology and rehabilitation equipment available from domestic and international sources to consumers, organizations, professionals, and caregivers within the United States. AbleData serves the nation's disability, rehabilitation and senior communities.

5480 **Access Unlimited**
570 Hance Rd
Binghamton, NY 13903-5700
607-669-4822
800-849-2143
Fax: 607-669-4595
www.accessunlimited.com
Thomas Egan, President/Owner
Tom 'TC' Cole, National Sales Manager
Adaptive transportation and mobility equipment for people with disabilities. ccess Unlimited products empower people with disabilities to regain control of their mobility.

5481 **Ai Squared**
130 Taconic Business Park
Manchester Center, VT 05255-9752
802-362-3612
800-859-0270
Fax: 802-362-1670
sales@aisquared.com
www.aisquared.com

David Wu, CEO
Jost Eckhardt, VP of Engineering
Doug Hacker, VP of Business Development
Scott Moore, VP of Marketing

Ai Squared has been a leader in the assistive technology field for over 20 years. Our flagship product, ZoomText, is the world's best magnification and reading software for the vision impaired. We pride ourselves on delivering the highest quality software products and superior technical support.

5482 **Alternatives in Education for the Hearing Impaired (AEHI)**
9300 Capitol Drive
Wheeling, IL 60090-7207
847-850-5490
Fax: 847-850-5493
info@agbms.org
www.agbms.org

Sandra L. Mosetick, Board President Emeritus
Bridget Chevez, Board President
Daniel Konopacki, Treasurer
Debra Trude-Suter, Ph.D., CEO/Executive Director

AEHI is a program of the Alexander Graham Bell Montessori School in Mt. Prospect, IL, that fosters literacy and empowers people with hearing impairments to achieve their full potential through unique educational options. AEHI provides Cued Speech workshops, individualized parental training and support, educational consulting, professional development opportunities, and access to a wide variety of information on Cued Speech and its benefits.

5483 **American Academy of Audiology (AAA)**
11480 Commerce Park Dr.
Suite 220
Reston, VA 20191
703-790-8466
Fax: 703-790-8631
infoaud@audiology.org
www.audiology.org

Patrick E. Gallagher, Executive Director
Kathryn Werner, Vice President, Public Affairs
Amy Miedema, Vice President, Communications & Membership
Dina Santucci, Senior Director, Business Development

The American Academy of Audiology is the world's largest professional organization for audiologists. The Academy is dedicated to providing quality hearing care services through professional development, education, research, and increased public awareness of hearing and balance disorders.

5484 **American Association of People with Disabilities (AAPD)**
2013 H St. NW
5th Floor
Washington, DC 20006
202-521-4316
800-840-8844
communications@aapd.com
www.aapd.com

Maria Town, President & CEO
Jasmin Bailey, Manager, Business Operations
Christine Liao, Manager, Programs
Rachita Singh, Coordinator, Public Relations & Communications

Nonprofit cross-disability member organization dedicated to ensuring economic self-sufficiency and political empowerment for Americans with disabilities. AAPD works in coalition with other disability organizations for the full implementation and enforcement of disability nondiscrimination laws, particularly the Americans With Disabilities Act (ADA) of 1990 and the Rehabilitation Act of 1973.

5485 **American College of Rheumatology, Researchand Education Foundation**
2200 Lake Boulevard NE
Atlanta, GA 30319-5310
404-633-3777
Fax: 404-633-1870
acr@rheumatology.org
www.rheumatology.org

Audrey B. Uknis, MD, President
David I. Daikh, MD, PhD, Foundation President
Jan K. Richardson, PT, PhD, O, ARHP President
E. William St.Clair, MD, Treasurer

The American College of Rheumatology's mission is advancing rheumatology.The organization represents over 8,500 rheumatologists and rheumatology health professionals around the world. The ACR offers its members the support they need to ensure that they are able to continue their innovative work by providing programs of education, research, advocacy, and practice support.

5486 **American Liver Foundation**
39 Broadway
Suite 2700
New York, NY 10006-3054
212-668-1000
Fax: 212-483-8179
www.liverfoundation.org

Ryan Reczek, National Director, Field Development
Rolf Taylor, National Director, Corporate Relations
Pritha Kuchaculla, National Director, Programs
David Ticker, Chief Financial Officer

Is the only national voluntary health organization dedicated to preventing, treating, and curing hepatitis and other liver and gall bladder diseases through research and education.

5487 **American Mobility: Personal Mobility Solutions**
60 Island St
Lawrence, MA 1840-1835
978-794-3030
www.americanmobility.com

David Lacroix, President

Source of Pride Scooters, Jazzy Power Chairs, personal mobility vehicles, and lift and recline chairs.

5488 **American Speech-Language and Hearing Association**
2200 Research Blvd
Rockville, MD 20850-3289
301-296-5700
800-638-8255
Fax: 301-296-8580
TTY: 301-296-5650
actioncenter@asha.org
www.asha.org

Wayne A. Foster, PhD, CCC-SLP/A, Chair, Audiology Advisory Council
Patricia A. Prelock, PhD, CCC-SLP, President
Carolyn W. Higdon, EdD, CCC-SLP, Vice President for Finance
Howard Goldstein, PhD, CCC-SL, Vice President for Science and Research

Exhibits by companies specializing in alternative and augmentative communications products, publishers, software and hardware compinies, and hearing aid testing equipment manufacturers.

5489 **Americans with Disabilities Act: ADA Home Page**
800-514-0301
TTY: 800-514-0383
webmaster@usdoj.gov
www.ada.gov

5490 **Aspies For Freedom (AFF)**
www.aspiesforfreedom.com

Gwen Nelson, Co-Founder
Amy Nelson, Co-Founder

Seeks to change the discourse on autism, including negative treatment in the media. Runs an online chatroom and promotes Autistic Pride Day.

5491 Association for the Cure of Cancer of the Prostate (CaP CURE)-Prostate Cancer Foundation
1250 Fourth St
Suite 360
Santa Monica, CA 90401-1444
310-570-4700
800-757-2873
Fax: 310-570-4701
info@pcf.org
www.pcf.org
Mike Milken, Founder/Chairman
Jonathon Simons, MD, President/CEO
Ralph Finerman, Chief Financial Officer/Treasurer/Secretary
Howard R. Soule, PhD, Executive Vice President /Chief Science Officer
CURE is a nonprofit public charity that is dedicated to supporting prostate cancer research and hastening the conversion of research into cures or controls.

5492 Asthma and Allergy Foundation of America
8201 Corporate Drive
Suite 1000
Landover, MD 20785-2266
800-727-8462
info@aafa.org
www.aafa.org
Lynn Hanessian, Chair
Michele Abu Carrick, LICSW, Co-Chair, Governance
Judi McAuliffe, RN, Co-Chair, Programs & Services
Calvin Anderson, Chair/Finance/Treasurer
AAFA is dedicated to improving the quality of life for people with asthma and allergic diseases through education, advocacy and research.

5493 AudiologyOnline
12333 Sowden Rd.
Ste. B. #79931
Houston, TX 77080-2059
800-753-2160
Fax: 210-579-7010
www.audiologyonline.com
Ted A. Meyer, Chair
Catharine McNally, Chair-Elect
Susan Lenihan, Secretary
Emilion Alonso Mendoza, Chief Exectuive Officer
Online continuing education resources for audiology professionals.

5494 BDRC Newsletter
Birth Defect Research for Children
976 Lake Baldwin Lane
Suite 104
Orlando, FL 32814
407-895-0802
staff@birthdefects.org
www.birthdefects.org
Betty Mekdeci, Executive Director
A monthly electronic newsletter offering the latest news, research, and updates on birth defects.
Monthly

5495 Braille and Audio Reading Download (BARD)
National Library Service
1291 Taylor St NW
Washington, DC 20542
202-707-5100
800-424-8567
888-657-7323
Fax: 202-707-0712
NLSDownload@loc.gov
nlsbard.loc.gov

5496 Cancer Research Institute
29 Broadway
4th Floor
New York, NY 10006
212-688-7515
800-992-2623
Fax: 212-832-9376
info@cancerresearch.org
www.cancerresearch.org
Jill O'Donnell-Tormey, CEO & Director of Scientific Affairs
Lynne Harmer, Director of Grants Administration and Special Events
Alfred R. Massidas, Chief Financial Officer and Director of Human Resources
Alexandra S. Mulvey, Associate Director of Communications
Nonprofit organization dedicated to cancer immunotherapy.

5497 Center on the Social & Emotional Foundations for Early Learning (CSEFEL)
Vanderbilt University 110 Magnolia
Box 328 GPC
Nashville, TN 37203
615-322-8150
Fax: 615-343-1570
ml.hemmeter@vanderbilt.edu
csefel.vanderbilt.edu
Mary-Louise Hemmeter, Principal Investigator
Rob Corso, Project Coordinator
Tweety Yates, Project Coordinator
Glen Dunlap, Key Center Personnel
The center will: focus on promoting the social and emotional developmental of children as a means of preventing challenging behaviors; collaborate with existing T/TA providers for the purpose of ensuring the implementation and sustainability of practices at the local level; provide ongoing identification of training needs and preferred delivery formats of local programs and T/TA providers; disseminate evidence-based practices.

5498 Damon Runyon Cancer Research Foundation
Walter Winchell Foundation
One Exchange Plaza, 55 Broadway
Suite 302
New York, NY 10006-3720
212-455-0500
877-722-6237
info@damonrunyon.org
www.damonrunyon.org
Lorraine Egan, President/Chief Executive Officer
Elizabeth Portland, Director of Development
Marialice C. Pagnotta, Director of the Damon Runyon Broadway Tickets Service
Kimberly Kubert, Director of Special Events
The Damon Runyon Cancer Research Foundation funds early career cancer researchers who have the energy, drive and creativity to become leading innovators in their fields. We identify the best young scientists in the nation and support them through four award programs: our Fellowship, Pediatric Cancer Fellowship, Clinical Investigator and Innovation Awards.

5499 DisAbility Information and Resources
jlubin@eskimo.com
www.makoa.org
Jim Lubin, Creator/Owner
Offers dozens of links to sites with information, services and products for the disabled.

5500 Disability Rights Activist
www.disrights.org

5501 DisabilityAdvisor.com
37 North Orange Ave.
Suite 500
Orlando, FL 32801
321-332-7800
888-393-1010
Fax: 888-985-6060
www.disabilityadvisor.com
Joseph E. Ram, Publisher
Kay Derochie, Editor
Jackie Booth, Ph.D., Editor
DisabilityAdvisor.com provides free information on federal and state disability benefits programs and other resources for readers and their families. This includes disabled children and students, military veterans, injured workers and disabled seniors. Readers are encouraged to submit their questions and comments online. The website also offers information on managing finances, education, parenting, relationships and other issues of interest to the disabled and their friends and families.

5502 DisabilityResources.org
Four Glatter Lane
Dept. IN
Centereach, NY 11720-1032
631-585-0290
Fax: 631-585-0290
Julie Klauber, Co-founder/Managing Editor
Avery Klauber, Co-Founder/Executive Director
Sally Rosenthal, Contributing Editor
Ruth Porfert, Editorial Assistant

Disability Resources, inc. is a nonprofit 501 (c) (3) organization established to promote and improve awareness, availability and accessibility of information that can help people with disabilities live, learn, love, work and play independently.

5503 **Discover Technology**
Houston, TX
713-885-1519
dtinc8888@hotmail.com
www.discovertechnology.com
Amantha Cole, Founder
The primary mission of Discover Technology, Inc.is to create and administer computer labs for persons with disabilities, to encourage communication between persons with and without disabilities and to educate the general population about the disabled population.

5504 **Dynamic Living**
125 Old Iron Ore Road
Bloomfield, CT 06002-1315
860-683-4442
888-940-0605
Fax: 860-243-1910
www.dynamic-living.com
Andrea Tannenbaum, Owner
Kitchen products, bathroom helpers, and unique daily living products that provide a convienient, comfortable, and safe environment for people with disabilities.

5505 **ERIC Clearinghouse on Disabilities and Gifted Education**
www.hoagiesgifted.org/eric

5506 **ElderLawAnswers.com**
150 Chesnut St
4th Floor, Box #15
Providence, RI 02903
866-267-0947
support@elderlawanswers.com
www.elderlawanswers.com
Harry S. Margolis, Founder/President
Ken Coughlin, Editor
Mark Miller, Director of Product and Business Development
Wendy Miki Glaus, Attorney
Provides information about legal issues facing senior citizens and a searchable directory of attorneys.

5507 **Exploring Autism: A Look at the Genetics of Autism**
Box 3445 DUMC
Durham, NC 27710
Fax: 919-684-0952
Chantelle Wolpert, Project Director
Dedicated to helping families who are living with the challenges of autism stay informed about the exciting breakthroughs involving the genetics of autism. Report and explain new genetic research findings. Explain genetic principles as they relate to autism, provide the latest research news, and seek your imput.

5508 **FHI 360**
1825 Connecticut Ave., NW
Suite 800
Washington, DC 20009-5721
202-884-8000
Fax: 202-884-8400
CareerCenterSupport@fhi360.org
www.fhi360.org
Willard Cates Jr, MD, MPH, President Emeritus
Albert J. Siemens, PhD, Chief Executive Officer
Patrick C. Fine, MS, Chief Operating Officer
Robert S. Murphy, MBA, Chief Financial Officer
FHI 360 is a nonprofit human development organization dedicated to improving lives in lasting ways by advancing integrated, locally driven solutions.

5509 **Foundation Fighting Blindness**
7168 Columbia Gateway Dr.
Suite 100
Columbia, MD 21046
410-423-0600
800-683-5555
TTY: 410363713951
info@FightBlindness.org
www.blindness.org
William T. Schmidt, Chief Executive Officer
Valerie Navy-Daniels, Chief Development Officer
Stephen M. Rose, PhD, Chief Research Officer
The Foundation Fighting Blindness (FFB) works to promote research in order to prevent, treat and restore vision. FFB is currently the world's leading private funder of retinal disease research, funding over 100 research grants and 150 researchers.

5510 **Freedom Scientific**
11830 31st Court North
St. Petersburg, FL 33716-1805
727-803-8000
800-444-4443
Fax: 727-803-8001
info@freedomscientific.com
www.freedomscientific.com
Lee Hamilton, President/CEO/Chairman
Mike Self, Sales Representative
Joseph McDaniel, Sales Representative
Bobby Lakey, Sales Representative
Assistive technology for blind and visually impaired computer users.

5511 **Gallaudet University Press**
800 Florida Ave, NE
Washington, DC 20002-3695
202-651-5488
Fax: 202-651-5489
gupress@gallaudet.edu
www.gupress.gallaudet.edu

5512 **Glaucoma Research Foundation**
251 Post Street
Suite 600
San Francisco, CA 94108-5017
415-986-3162
800-826-6693
question@glaucoma.org
www.glaucoma.org
Andrew Iwach, MD, Board Chair/Executive Director
Thomas r M. Brunne, President/CEO
H. Allen Bouch, Vice Chair
Fred H. Brinkmann, Treasurer
Our mission is to prevent vision loss from glaucoma by investing in innovative research, education, and support with the ultimate goal of finding a cure.

5513 **HealthyWomen**
P.O. Box 430
Red Bank, NJ 07701
732-530-3425
877-986-9472
Fax: 732-865-7225
info@healthywomen.org
www.healthywomen.org
Oxana K Pickeral, Ph.D, MBA, Chair
Beth Battaglino, CEO
Phyllis E Greenberger, MSW, Senior Vice President, Science & Health Policy
Amy Takis, Director of Communications & Development
Website providing information for women with disabilities, health professionals, researchers, and caretakers.

5514 **Herb Research Foundation**
5589 Arapahoe Ave
Suite 205
Boulder, CO 80303-8115
303-449-2265
www.herbs.org
Rob McCaleb, President
John Lowe, Director of Research
Research and public education on the health benefits of medicinal plants. Dedicated to world health through the informed use of herbs.

5515 **Hypokalemic Periodic Paralysis Resource Page**
155 West 68th St
Suite 1732
New York, NY 10023-5830
407-339-9499
lfeld@cfl.rr.com
www.periodicparalysis.org
Jacob Levitt, President/Medical Director
Linda Feld, Vice President
Provides understandable information on HKPP, dynamia linkage to several additional sources of helpful information on the Internet, and offers several online networking opportunities.

5516 **INCLUDEnyc**
Formerly Resources for Children with Special Needs
116 E. 16th St.
5th Fl.
New York, NY 10003
212-677-4650
Fax: 202-254-4070
info@includenyc.org
www.includenyc.org
Barbara Glassman, Executive Director
Todd Dorman, Senior Director of Communications and Outreach
Mariko Sakita, Director of Parent & Family Services
Lori Podvesker, Senior Manager of Disability and Education Policy
Provides free services and resources for youth and families with disabilities in all five state boroughs. Organizational services include: Parenting & Advocacy; School and Community Activities; Parent counseling and Training for students with Autism; Medicaid Waiver services; Transition and Adult Services; and Social skills and building relationships.

5517 **Innovation Management Group**
179 Niblick Road
Suite 454
Paso Robles, CA 93446-4845
818-701-1579
800-889-0987
Fax: 818-936-0200
sales@imgpresents.com
www.imgpresents.com

5518 **Interstitial Cystitis Association**
1760 Old Meadow Road
Suite 500
McLean, VA 22102-2651
703-442-2070
800-435-7422
Fax: 703-506-3266
icamail@ichelp.org
www.ichelp.org
Barbara Gordon, Co-Chair/Executive Director
Eric Zarnikow, MBA, Co-Chair
Marilynn Schreibstein, CFO
F. Neal Thompson, Treasurer
The Interstitial Cystitis Association (ICA) advocates for interstitial cystitis (IC) research dedicated to discovery of a cure and better treatments, raises awareness, and serves as a central hub for the healthcare providers, researchers and millions of patients who suffer with constant urinary urgency and frequency and extreme bladder pain called IC. (IC is also referred to as painful bladder syndrome, bladder pain syndrome, and chronic pelvic pain.)

5519 **JoanBorysenko.Com**
PO Box 1300
Tesuque, NM 87574
www.joanborysenko.com
Joan Borysenko, Founder
Publishes resources for credible information about the intersection of mind-body health, positive psychology, and spiritual exploration.

5520 **LD OnLine - WETA Public Television**
2775 S. Quincy Street
Arlington, VA 22206-2269
Fax: 703-998-2060
ldonline@weta.org
www.ldonline.org
Noel Gunther, Executive Director
Christian Lindstrom, Director, Learning Media
Tina Chovanec, Director, Reading Rockets
Lydia Breiseth, Director, Colorin Colorado
LD OnLine seeks to help children and adults reach their full potential by providing accurate and up-to-date information and advice about learning disabilities and ADHD.The site features hundreds of helpful articles, multimedia, monthly columns by noted experts, first person essays, children's writing and artwork, a comprehensive resource guide, very active forums, and a Yellow Pages referral directory of professionals, schools, and products.

5521 **Lighthouse Guild**
250 W 64th St.
New York, NY 10023
212-769-6200
800-284-4422
www.lighthouseguild.org
Calvin W. Roberts, President & CEO
Paul D. Misiti, Chief of Staff
Himanshu R. Shah, Chief Financial Officer
Maura J. Sweeney, Chief Program Officer
Lighthouse Guild is a not-for-profit vision & healthcare organization, addressing the needs of people who are blind or visually impaired, including those with multiple disabilities or chronic medical conditions.

5522 **Lyme Disease Foundation**
PO Box 332
Tolland, CT 6084-332
860-870-0070
Fax: 860-870-0080
www.lyme.org
Karen Forschuer, Chairman
Thomas Forschuer, Executive Director
Provides critical information about tick-borne disease prevention, improves healthcare and funds research for solutions. 500,000 children, adults, and professionals assisted 25 countries.

5523 **Mainstream Living**
333 SW 9th St
Des Moines, IA 50309
515-243-8115
Fax: 515-243-5017
www.mainstreamliving.org

5524 **Mainstream Online Magazine of the Able-Disabled**
www.mainstream-mag.com
Cyndi Jones, Publisher
William G. Stothers, Editor
The leading news, advocacy and lifestyle magazine for people with disabilities.

5525 **Microsoft Accessibility Technology for Everyone**
One Microsoft Way
Redmond, WA 98052-6399
425-882-8080
800-642-7676
Fax: 425-936-7329
TTY: 800-892-5234
www.microsoft.com/enable
William Gates III, Chairman
Steven Ballmer, CEO/Director
Information about accessibility features and options included in Microsoft products.

5526 **MossRehab ResourceNet**
1200 West Tabor Road
Philadelphia, PA 19141-3099
215-456-9900
800-225-5567
www.mossresourcenet.org
John Whyte, Owner
Ruth Lefton, COO
Anthony Allonardo, Director of Technology
MossRehab, a modern, 147-bed facility, offers comprehensive care to people with a broad range of conditions—including stroke, brain injury, orthopaedic and musculoskeletal disabilities, spinal cord dysfunction, pulmonary disorders, amputations, and other forms of disability.

5527 **Multiple Sclerosis National Research Institute**
11350 SW Village Parkway
Port St. Lucie, FL 34987-2352
858-597-3872
866-676-7400
Fax: 858-597-3804
www.ms-research.org
Robin Offord, Chairman
Richard Houghten, President/CEO
Donald B. Cooper, C.F.O
Karen Douthitt, VP & Corporate Secretary
Multiple Sclerosis National Research Institute is a division of Torrey Pines Institute for Molecular Studies, a not-for-profit basic research center dedicated to the discovery and development of innovative research methods that lead to treatments for major medical conditions, including multiple sclerosis, AIDS, Alzheimer's disease, pain, heart disease, many types of cancer, and more.

5528 **National Alliance of the Disabled (NAOTD)**

Walton Dutcher, Executive Director/Operations
Fred Temple, Director
Spike Spikberg, Director
Donna Eustice, Director

The National Alliance OF The DisAbled is an online informational and advocacy organization dedicated to working towards gaining equal rights for the disAbled in all areas of life.

5529 **National Birth Defect Registry**

Birth Defect Research for Children
976 Lake Baldwin Lane
Suite 104
Orlando, FL 32814 407-895-0802
staff@birthdefects.org
www.birthdefects.org

Betty Mekdeci, Executive Director

Data collection project by Birth Defect Research for Children to answer parents' questions about birth defects.

5530 **National Brain Tumor Foundation - National Brain Tumor Society**

55 Chapel Street
Suite 200
Newton, MA 02458-2599 617-924-9997
800-770-8287
Fax: 617-928-9998
info@braintumor.org
www.braintumor.org

Jeffrey Kolodin, Chair
Michael Nathanson, Vice Chair
N. Paul TonThat, Executive Director
Michele Rhee, Director of Program Initiatives

An organization serving people whose lives are affected by brain tumors. The organization is dedicated to promoting a cure for brain tumors, improving the quality of life and giving hope to the brain tumor community by funding meaningful research and providing patient resources, timely information and education.

5531 **National Business & Disability Council**

201 I.U. Willets Road
Albertson, NY 11507-1516 516-465-1516
lfrancis@viscardicenter.org
www.business-disability.com

Michael C. Pascucci, Executive Leadership Team Chairman
Laura Francis, Executive Director
John D. Kemp, President

The NBDC is the leading resource for employers seeking to integrate people with disabilities into the workplace and companies seeking to reach them in the consumer marketplace.

5532 **National Organization on Disability (NOD)**

77 Water St.
13th Floor
New York, NY 10005 646-505-1191
Fax: 646-505-1184
info@nod.org
www.nod.org

Carol Glazer, President
Moeena Das, Chief of Staff
Priyanka Ghosh, Director, External Affairs
Bernard Blake, Manager, Finance & Administration

The National Organization on Disability is a private, nonprofit organization that promotes the full and equal participation of men, women, and children with disabilities in all aspects of American life.

1982

5533 **National Rehabilitation Information Center (NARIC)**

8400 Corporate Drive
Suite 500
Landover, MD 20785-2266 301-459-5984
800-346-2742
Fax: 301-459-4263
TTY: 301-459-5984
www.naric.com

Mark X. Odum, Project Director

Serves both professionals and the general public intersted in disability and rehabilitation.

5534 **National Youth Leadership Network Youth Leader Blog (NYLN)**

nyln.org

5535 **Nebraska Library Commission: Talking Book and Braille Service (TBBS)**

Talking Book and Braille Service
1200 N St
Suite 120
Lincoln, NE 68508-2023 402-471-4038
800-742-7691
Fax: 402-471-6244
nlc.readadv@nebraska.gov
nlc.nebraska.gov/tbbs

David Oertli, Executive Director
Kay Goehring, Reader Services Coordinator
Bill Ainsley, Audio Production Studio Manager
Scott Scholz, Circulation & Audio Prod. Coor.

Provides eligible users with free audio books, audio magazines and Braille via the mail. Also features in-house studios for audiobook production.

5536 **NeuroControl Corporation**

8333 Rockside Rd
Valley View, OH 44125-6134 216-912-0101
800-378-6955
Fax: 216-912-0129

5537 **Newsletter of PA's AT Lending Library**

Temple University Institute on Disabilities
1755 N 13th Street
Student Center, Room 411S
Philadelphia, PA 19122-6024 215-204-1356
800-204-PIAT
Fax: 215-204-6336
TTY: 215-204-1805
iod@temple.edu
www.disabilities.temple.edu/atlend

Celia Feinstein, Co-Executive Director of the Institute on Disabilities
Amy Goldman, Co-Executive Director of the Institute on Disabilities
Ann Marie, Deputy Director
Kristin Ahrens, PA Consumer & Family Training Project Assistant Director

Newsletter from the Assistive Technology Lending Library in Pennsylvania. It is produced quarterly, is free of charge, and is available online only.

4-8 pages Quarterly

5538 **Office of Juvenile Justice and Delinquency Prevention**

810 Seventh St NW
Washington, DC 20531-3718 202-307-5911
800-851-3420
Fax: 301-519-5600
www.ojjdp.gov

Kathi Grasso, Director, Concentration of Federal Efforts Program
Robert Listenbee, Jr., Administrator
Melodee Hanes, Principal Deputy Administrator
Nancy Ayers, Deputy Administrator for Operations

The Office of Juvenile Justice and Delinquency Prevention (OJJDP) provides national leadership, coordination, and resources to prevent and respond to juvenile delinquency and victimization. OJJDP supports states and communities in their efforts to develop and implement effective and coordinated prevention and intervention programs and to improve the juvenile justice system so that it protects public safety, holds offenders accountable, and provides treatment and rehabilitative services tailored

5539 **Osteogenesis Imperfecta Foundation**
804 W. Diamond Ave.
Suite 210
Gaithersburg, MD 20878- 1414
301-947-0083
800-981-2663
Fax: 301-947-0456
bonelink@oif.org
www.oif.org

Mary Beth Huber, Director of Program Services
Tom Costanzo, Director of Finance & Administration
Erika r Ruebensaal Carte, Director of Communications & Development
Tracy Smith Hart, Chief Executive Officer
Strives to improve the quality of life for indivduals with this brittle bone disorder through research, education, awareness, and mutual support.

5540 **Quantum Technologies**
25242 Arctic Ocean Drive
Lake Forest, CA 92630-6217
949-930-3400
Fax: 949-399-4600
www.qtww.com

Dale Rasmussen, Chairman
Alan Niedzwieck, President/Director
W. Brian Olson, Chief Executive Officer
Bradley J. Timon, Chief Financial Officer
Provides access to information and tools for independence to serve the visually impaired and those with a learning disability.

5541 **Regional Resource Centers Program**
1 Quality Street
Suite 721
Lexington, KY 40507
859-257-4921
Fax: 859-257-4353
TTY: 859-257-2903
mike.abell@uky.edu
www.rrcprogram.org

Shauna Crane, RRCP Coordinator
Perry Williams, OSEP, Team Member
Mike Abell, Team Member
Betty Beale, Team Member
The Regional Resource Centers Program provides service to all states as well as the Pacific jurisdictions, the Virgin Islands, and Puerto Rico. The six regional program centers are funded by the federal Office of Special Education Programs (OSEP) to assist state education agencies in the systemic improvement of education programs, practices, and policies that affect children and youth with disabilities.

5542 **Research!America**
1101 King Street
Suite 520
Alexandria, VA 22314-2960
703-739-2577
800-366-2873
Fax: 703-739-2372
info@researchamerica.org
www.researchamerica.org

Hon. John Edward Porter, Chair
Hon. Michael Castle, Vice Chair
Mary Woolley, President/CEO
Barbara Love, Executive Assitant to the President
Builds active public support for more government and private-industry research to find treatments and cures for both physical and mental disorders.

5543 **Social Security Online**
5 Park Centre Court
Suite 100
Owings Mills, MD 21117-1
800-772-1213
TTY: 800-325-0778
www.ssa.gov

Carolyn W. Colvin, Commissioner
James A. Kissko, Chief of Staff
Katherine A. Thornton, Deputy Chief of Staff
Karena L. Kilgore, Executive Secretary,Office of Executive Operations
Official website of the Social Security Administration.

5544 **Special Clothes for Children**
PO Box 333
E. Harwich, MA 02645-333
508-430-2410
Fax: 508-430-2410
TTY: 508-430-2410
lou@lnrmusic.com

A catalog of adaptive clothing for children with disabilities - helping boys and girls with special needs meet the world with pride and confidence since 1987.

5545 **The Arc of the United States**
1825 K St NW
Suite 1200
Washington, DC 20006
202-534-3700
800-433-5255
Fax: 202-534-3731
info@thearc.org
www.thearc.org

Peter Berns, Chief Executive Officer
Ruben Rodriguez, Chief Operating Officer
Julie Ward, Senior Executive Officer, Public Policy
Karen Wolf-Branigin, Senior Executive Officer, Chapter Growth & Affiliates
The Arc promotes and protects the rights of people with intellectual and developmental disabilities and actively supports their inclusion and participation in the community throughout their lifetimes. The Arc's clients include people with autism, Down syndrome, Fragile X syndrome, and various other developmental disabilities. Some services offered by The Arc include public policy advocacy, education and vocational services.

5546 **V Foundation for Cancer Research**
106 Towerview Court
Cary, NC 27513-3595
919-380-9505
800-454-6698
info@jimmyv.org
www.jimmyv.org

Sherrie Mazur, Director of Marketing & Communication
Danielle Smith, Director of Corporate and Market Development
Mark Steudel, Associate Director of Development for Prospect Research
Nick Valvano, President Emeritus
Named after basketball coach and broadcaster, Jim Valvano. The V Foundation funds critical stage research conducted by young researchers at NCI approved cancer research facilities.

5547 **ValueOptions**
240 Corporate Blvd.
Norfolk, VA 23502-4900
757-459-5100
Fax: 501-707-0940
TTY: 877-334-0077
www.valueoptions.com

Heyward R. Donigan, President/CEO
Scott Tabakin, Chief Financial Officer
Kyle A. Raffaniello, Executive Vice President and Chief Strategy Officer
Paul Rosenberg, Executive Vice President and General Counsel
Serves over 22 million people in behavioral healthcare through publicaly funded, federal, and commercial contracts.

5548 **Wardrobe Wagon: The Special Needs Clothing Store**
258B Route 46 E
Fairfield, NJ 7004-2324
973-244-2414
800-992-2737
wardrobew@aol.com
www.wardrobewagon.com

E Oppenberg, President
Bonnie Oppenberg
Jerome Oppenberg, Owner
Wearing apparel for individuals with special clothing needs.

5549 **We Magazine**
130 William St
New York, NY 10038
646-769-2722
Fax: 212-375-6266
TTY: 212-375-6235
sales@wemedia.com

5550 **We Media**
1801 Reston Parkway
Suite 300
Reston, VA 20190-4303 703-880-2659
help@wemedia.com
www.wemedia.com

Andrew Nachison, Founder
Dale Peskin, Founder
Online network for people with disabilities.

5551 **WebABLE**
www.hisoftware.com/press/webable.html

5552 **WheelchairNet**
6425 Penn Ave
Suite 401 BAKSQ, Department of Reha
Philadelphia, PA 15206 412-624-6279
ruffing@pitt.edu
www.wheelchairnet.org

Joseph Ruffing, Communications Specialist
A virtual community of people who care about wheelchairs.

5553 **World Association of Persons with Disabilities**
2441 N Sterling Ave
302W
Oklahoma, OK 73127-2009 405-672-4440
www.wapd.org

Byron R. Kerford, Founder/Leader
Thomas J. Mecke, Executive Director
Sierra Hebron, Director of Human Resources
Ashley Wardle, Director of Internet Marketing
Dedicated to improving the quality of life for those with disabilities.

Toys & Games

General

5554 **Age Appropriate Puzzles**
7756 Winding Way
Fair Oaks, CA 95628-5735
916-961-3507
Fax: 916-961-0765
Cheryl Meyers, President
These unique puzzles teach numerous concepts: picture, name, color and shape recognition. Each of the two themes (holidays, and clothing) comes with self-adhesive stickers that name each picture in English, Hmong, Russian, Spanish and Vietnamese. A notch at each puzzle piece makes grasping and lifting the pieces easy to use., They are designed for children from 18 months and up. Special needs children, preschool through high school would also benefit. *$9.95*

5555 **All-Turn-It Spinner**
AbleNet, Inc.
2625 Patton Road
Roseville, MN 55113-1137
651-294-2200
800-322-0956
Fax: 651-294-2259
customerservice@ablenetinc.com
www.ablenetinc.com
Bill Sproull, Chair of the Board
Jennifer Thalhuber, President & CEO
William Mills, Board of Directors
Paul Sugden, CFO & Trustee
The All-Turn-It Spinner is a random spinner that comes with a dice overlay allowing users to participate in any commercially-available game that require dice. Activate the spinner with its built-in switch or connect an external switch. Overlays are interchangeable with AbleNet designed spinner games or users can create their own overlay. *$89.00*

5556 **Anthony Brothers Manufacturing**
Convert-O-Bike
9 Capper Drive
Dailey Industrial Park,
Pacific, MO 63069-5196
636-257-0533
800-346-6313
Fax: 636-257-5473
www.angelesstore.com
Tim Lynch, Director of Sales
David Curry, General Manager
Michelle Vondera, Customer Service Manager
Sally Perrin, National Account Manager
Manufacture wheeled toys and goods for disabled children.

5557 **Automatic Card Shuffler**
Maxi Aids
42 Executive Blvd.
Farmingdale, NY 11735-4710
631-752-0521
800-522-6294
Fax: 631-752-0689
TTY: 631-752-0738
sales@maxiaids.com
www.maxiaids.com
Elliot Zaretsky, Founder, President & CEO
Allows for hands-free card shuffling. Holds up to two decks at a time. Designed for those with limited hand dexterity. *$13.95*

5558 **Backgammon Set: Deluxe**
Maxi Aids
42 Executive Blvd.
Farmingdale, NY 11735-4710
631-752-0521
800-522-6294
Fax: 631-752-0689
TTY: 631-752-0738
sales@maxiaids.com
www.maxiaids.com
Elliot Zaretsky, Founder, President & CEO
Backgammon game board set featuring raised white dividers and color contrast for players with low vision. *$59.95*

5559 **Board Games: Peg Solitaire**
Maxi Aids
42 Executive Blvd.
Farmingdale, NY 11735-4710
631-752-0521
800-522-6294
Fax: 631-752-0689
TTY: 631-752-0738
sales@maxiaids.com
www.maxiaids.com
Elliot Zaretsky, Founder, President & CEO
This version of the solo board game uses wood marbles and a wood game board with 33 indentations. *$12.95*

5560 **Board Games: Snakes and Ladders**
Maxi Aids
42 Executive Blvd.
Farmingdale, NY 11735-4710
631-752-0521
800-522-6294
Fax: 631-752-0689
TTY: 631-752-0738
sales@maxiaids.com
www.maxiaids.com
Elliot Zaretsky, Founder, President & CEO
A board game for two to four players. Comes with a raised board and wood die Braille spinner. *$65.95*

5561 **Braille Playing Cards**
Maxi Aids
42 Executive Blvd.
Farmingdale, NY 11735-4710
631-752-0521
800-522-6294
Fax: 631-752-0689
TTY: 631-752-0738
sales@maxiaids.com
www.maxiaids.com
Elliot Zaretsky, Founder, President & CEO
Playing cards that offer regular print and Braille on plastic cards for the blind or visually impaired player. *$6.95*

5562 **Braille: Bingo Cards, Boards and Call Numbers**
Maxi Aids
42 Executive Blvd.
Farmingdale, NY 11735-4710
631-752-0521
800-522-6294
Fax: 631-752-0689
TTY: 631-752-0738
sales@maxiaids.com
www.maxiaids.com
Elliot Zaretsky, Founder, President & CEO
Bingo products for the visually impaired. Cards, boards and call numbers in regular print and Braille.

5563 **Braille: Rook Cards**
Maxi Aids
42 Executive Blvd.
Farmingdale, NY 11735-4710
631-752-0521
800-522-6294
Fax: 631-752-0689
TTY: 631-752-0738
sales@maxiaids.com
www.maxiaids.com
Elliot Zaretsky, Founder, President & CEO
This set of cards for Rook, the popular bidding card game with 23 variations, has regular size print and Braille print for the blind/visually impaired player. *$18.95*

5564 **Cards: Musical**
ASB
919 Walnut Street
Philadelphia, PA 19107-5237
215-627-0600
Fax: 215-922-0692
asbinfo@asb.org
www.asb.org
Karla S. McCaney, President & CEO
Beth Deering, Director, Human Services
Richard Forsythe, Director, Braille Division & Custom Audio
Joyce Robertson, Director, Finance & Information Technology
These cards, for all occasions, play music when they are opened, for the visually impaired and blind persons. *$2.50*

5565 **Cards: UNO**
Maxi Aids
42 Executive Blvd.
Farmingdale, NY 11735-4710
631-752-0521
800-522-6294
Fax: 631-752-0689
TTY: 631-752-0738
sales@maxiaids.com
www.maxiaids.com

Elliot Zaretsky, Founder, President & CEO
Traditional card game in Braille for blind or visually impaired players. *$12.97*

5566 **Chess Set: Deluxe**
Maxi Aids
42 Executive Blvd.
Farmingdale, NY 11735-4710
631-752-0521
800-522-6294
Fax: 631-752-0689
TTY: 631-752-0738
sales@maxiaids.com
www.maxiaids.com

Elliot Zaretsky, Founder, President & CEO
Wooden board contains holes for inserting pieces. Black pieces contain a metal tip to distinguish them from white pieces. *$46.95*

5567 **Dice: Jumbo Size**
ASB
919 Walnut Street
Philadelphia, PA 19107-5237
215-627-0600
Fax: 215-922-0692
asbinfo@asb.org
www.asb.org

Karla S. McCaney, President & CEO
Beth Deering, Director, Human Services
Richard Forsythe, Director, Braille Division & Custom Audio
Joyce Robertson, Director, Finance & Information Technology
The large white and black dice are over-sized and have grooved dots to indicate the numbers, for easy reading for the visually handicapped. *$4.95*

5568 **Dominoes with Raised Dots**
Maxi Aids
42 Executive Blvd.
Farmingdale, NY 11735-4710
631-752-0521
800-522-6294
Fax: 631-752-0689
TTY: 631-752-0738
sales@maxiaids.com
www.maxiaids.com

Elliot Zaretsky, Founder, President & CEO
Standard set with tactile pieces for easier identification. *$14.95*

5569 **Early Learning 1**
MarbleSoft
12301 Central Ave NE
Suite 205
Blaine, MN 55434-4902
763-755-1402
888-755-1402
Fax: 763-862-2920
sales@marblesoft.com
www.marblesoft.com

Vicki Larson, Manager
Early learning 2.1 includes four activities that teach prereading skills. Single and dual-switch scanning are built in and special prompts allow blind students to use all levels of difficulty. Includes Matching Colors, Learning Shapes, Counting Numbers and Letter Match. Runs on Windows 98 or later and MAC OS 9 or OSX (classic not required). *$70.00*

5570 **Enabling Devices**
50 Broadway
Hawthorne, NY 10532-2837
914-747-3070
800-832-8697
Fax: 914-747-3480
sales@enablingdevices.com
www.enablingdevices.com

Seth Kanor, President & CEO
Enabling Devices is a company dedicated to developing affordable learning and assistive devices to help people of all ages with disabling conditions. Founded by Steven E. Kanor, Ph.D. and orginally known as Toys for Special Children, the company has been creating innovative communicators, adapted toys and switches for the physically challenged for more than 35 years.

5571 **Four in a Row Game: Tactile**
Maxi Aids
42 Executive Blvd.
Farmingdale, NY 11735-4710
631-752-0521
800-522-6294
Fax: 631-752-0689
TTY: 631-752-0738
sales@maxiaids.com
www.maxiaids.com

Elliot Zaretsky, Founder, President & CEO
Comes with game console, 23 red disks, and 23 yellow disks. Red disks are drilled for tactile identification. *$22.95*

5572 **Hands-Free Controller**
Nintendo
PO Box 957
Redmond, WA 98073-957
800-255-3700
www.nintendo.com

Yoshio Tsuboike, Editor-in-Chief
Nintendo controller for the physically disabled.

5573 **National Lekotek Center**
2001 N. Clybourn Av.
1st Floor
Chicago, IL 60614-3716
773-528-5766
800-366-PLAY
Fax: 773-537-2992
TTY: 773-973-2180
www.lekotek.org

Elaine D. Cottey, Chair
Joanna Horsnail, Chair
Eric Gastevich, Treasurer
Carol Neiger, Secretary
Maximizes the development of children with special needs through play. Supports families through nationwide family play centers, toy lending libraries and computer play programs. Publishes six-page newsletter three times per year.

5574 **New Language of Toys: Teaching Communication Skills to Children with Special Needs**
Spina Bifida Association of America
4590 MacArthur Blvd,NW,
Suite 250
Washington, DC 20007- 4226
202-944-3285
800-621-314
Fax: 202-944-3295
sbaa@sbaa.org
www.spinabifidaassociation.org

Lisa Raman, Director-National Resource Center
Mary Nethercutt, National Walk Director
Christopher Vance, Director of Development
Cindy Brownstein, President /CEO
A guide for parents and teachers and a reader-friendly resource guide that provides a wealth of information on how play activities affect a child's language development and where to get the toys and materials to use in these activities. *$19.00*

5575 **Playing Card Holders**
Maxi Aids
42 Executive Blvd.
Farmingdale, NY 11735-4710
631-752-0521
800-522-6294
Fax: 631-752-0689
TTY: 631-752-0738
sales@maxiaids.com
www.maxiaids.com

Elliot Zaretsky, Founder, President & CEO
A playing card holder for those with arthritis, dexterity issues or visual impairments. Holds up to 15 cards. *$8.95*

5576 Puzzle Games: Cooking, Eating, Community and Grooming
PCI
PO Box 34270
San Antonio, TX 78265-4270
210-670-3866
800-594-4263
Fax: 218-210-3771

Janie Haugen, Program Director
Jeff McLane, President/CEO
Rebecca Phillips, Executive Director

Each game has 63 pieces which are 2 inches in size. The completed full color puzzle is 19 inch x 15 inch. Step 1 - Work the puzzle. Step 2 - Match picture or word cards to the correct space on the puzzle. These puzzles teach basic life skills. *$19.95*

5577 Single Switch Games
MarbleSoft
12301 Central Ave NE
Suite 205
Blaine, MN 55434-4902
763-755-1402
888-755-1402
888-755-1402
Fax: 763-862-2920
sales@marblesoft.com
www.marblesoft.com

Vicki Larson, Manager
Mark Larson

Theres alot of educational software for single switch users, but how about something that's just fun? We've taken some games similar to the ones you enjoyed as a kid and made them work just right for single switch users. Includes Single Switch Maze, A Frog's Life, Switching Lanes, Switch Invaders, Slingshot Gallery and Scurry. Runs on Windows 98 or later and MAC OS9 or OSX (classic not required) *$60.00*

5578 Single Switch Latch and Timer
AbleNet, Inc.
2625 Patton Road
Roseville, MN 55113-1137
651-294-2200
800-322-0956
Fax: 651-294-2259
customerservice@ablenetinc.com
www.ablenetinc.com

Bill Sproull, Chair of the Board
Jennifer Thalhuber, President & CEO
William Mills, Board of Directors
Paul Sugden, CFO & Trustee

A Single Switch Latch and Timer allows a user to activate a battery-operated toy or appliance in the latch, timed seconds and timed minutes modes of control. Choose for one user and one device at a time. *$63.00*

5579 Socialization Games for Persons with Disabilities
Charles C. Thomas
2600 S First St
Springfield, IL 62704-4730
217-789-8980
800-258-8980
Fax: 217-789-9130
books@ccthomas.com
www.ccthomas.com

Michael P. Thomas, President
Nevalyn Nevil, Author
Marna Beatty, Author
David Moxley, Author

This text will assist those who want to teach severely multiple disabled students by providing information on: general principles of intervention and classroom organization; managing the behavior of students; physically managing students and using adaptive equipment; teaching eating skills; teaching toileting, dressing, and hygiene skills; teaching cognition, communication, and socialization skills; teaching independent living skills; and teaching infants and preschool students. *$38.95*

176 pages Paperback
ISBN 0-398067-46-5

5580 Tactile Checkers Set
Maxi Aids
42 Executive Blvd.
Farmingdale, NY 11735-4710
631-752-0521
800-522-6294
Fax: 631-752-0689
TTY: 631-752-0738
sales@maxiaids.com
www.maxiaids.com

Elliot Zaretsky, Founder, President & CEO

A wooden board with peg holes and high-contrast tactile squares. Game pieces are tactile wooden discs with pegs. *$33.92*

5581 Take a Chance
Speech Bin
1965 25th Ave
Vero Beach, FL 32960-3062
772-770-0007
800-477-3324
Fax: 772-770-0006
info@speechbin.com

Jan J Binney, Senior Editor

Card game for practice of commonly misarticulated speech sounds. *$18.75*

16 pages Book & Cards
ISBN 0-93785 -46-7

5582 Tic Tac Toe
Maxi Aids
42 Executive Blvd.
Farmingdale, NY 11735-4710
631-752-0521
800-522-6294
Fax: 631-752-0689
TTY: 631-752-0738
sales@maxiaids.com
www.maxiaids.com

Elliot Zaretsky, Founder, President & CEO

Comes with wooden board with peg holes/grooves and three-dimensional tactile game pieces.

Travel & Transportation

Newsletters & Books

5583 **A World Awaits You**
Mobility International USA
132 E Broadway
Suite 343
Eugene, OR 97401
541-343-1284
Fax: 541-343-6812
TTY: 541-343-1284
clearinghouse@miusa.org
www.miusa.org

Susan Sygall, Chief Executive Officer
Cindy Lewis, Director, Programs
A journal of success stories and tips of people with disabilities participating in international exchange programs.
Annually

5584 **Hostelling North America**
Hostelling International
8455 Colesville Rd.
Suite 1225
Silver Spring, MD 20910
240-650-2100
Fax: 240-650-2094
www.hiusa.org

Russ Hedge, Chief Executive Officer
HI-USA has hostels in major cities, in national and state parks, near beaches, and in the mountains. Hostelling North America is a directory of hostels in U.S. and Canada, including hostels that are accessible.
400 pages

5585 **Sports n' Spokes Magazine**
Paralyzed Veterans of America
801 18th St. NW
Washington, DC 20006-3517
800-424-8200
888-888-2201
TTY: 800-795-4327
info@pva.org
www.sportsnspokes.com

Tom Fjerstad, Editor
Andy Nemann, Assistant Editor
John Groth, Editorial Coordinator
Brittany Martin, Editorial Coordinator
Publication of the PVA, a congressionally chartered veterans service organization. Sports n' Spokes serves as a source for wheelchair sports and recreation.

5586 **United States Department of the Interior National Park Service**
1849 C St. NW
Washington, DC 20240
202-208-6843
www.nps.gov

Shawn Benge, Deputy Director, Operations
Lena McDowall, Deputy Director, Management & Administration
Susan Farinelli, Acting Chief of Staff
Jenny Anzelmo-Sarles, Chief of Public Affairs
Offers an informational packet containing books, guides and tours for the disabled and elderly.

5587 **Wheelin Around e-Guide**
Wheelers Accessible Van Rentals
6614 W Sweetwater Ave.
Glendale, AZ 85304
623-776-8830
800-456-1371
Fax: 623-776-8930
info@wheelersvanrentals.com
www.wheelersvanrentals.com

Associations & Programs

5588 **American Airlines**
1 Skyview Dr.
Fort Worth, TX 76155
682-278-9000
www.aa.com

W. Douglas Parker, Chair & CEO
Robert D. Isom Jr., President
Derek J. Kerr, Executive Vice President & CFO
Maya Leibman, Executive Vice President & CIO
This airline trains employees to make sure that passengers with disabilities enjoy convenient, safe, and comfortable travel.

5589 **American Hotel and Lodging Association**
1250 Eye St. NW
Suite 1100
Washington, DC 20005
202-289-3100
Fax: 202-289-3199
membership@ahla.com
www.ahla.com

Chip Rogers, President & CEO
Kevin Carey, Executive Vice President & COO
Brian Crawford, Executive Vice President, Government Affairs
Rosanna Maietta, Executive Vice President, Communications & Public Relations
Disseminates information, develops and conducts a series of seminars for the hotel and motel industry at state-level association conferences, and develops and distributes an ADA Compliance handbook for use by the lodging industry.

5590 **Amtrak**
1 Massachusetts Ave. NW
Washington, DC 20001
215-856-7924
800-872-7245
TTY: 800-523-6590
www.amtrak.com

William J. Flynn, Chief Executive Officer
Stephen J. Gardner, President
Eleanor D. Acheson, Executive Vice President & General Counsel
Scot Naparstek, Executive Vice President & Chief Operations Officer
Amtrak provides services for passengers with disabilities and works to make facilities more accessible. Contact Amtrak's Special Services Desk at 1-800-USA-RAIL at least 24 hours in advance to arrange for special assistance. The type of equipment and accessibility vary from train to train and station to station.

5591 **Easterseals Project Action Consulting**
1101 Vermont Ave. NW
Suite 510
Washington, DC 20005
202-347-3066
844-227-3772
TTY: 202-347-7385
espaconsulting@easterseals.com
www.projectaction.com

Carol Wright Kenderdine, Assistant Vice President, Mobility & Transportation
Grozda Tisma, Procurement & Special Project Coordinator
Kristi McLaughlin, Consultant
A national technical assistance program designed to improve access to transportation services for people with disabilities and assist transit providers in implementing the Americans with Disabilities Act.

5592 **General Motors Mobility Program for Persons with Disabilities**
GM Mobility Program
PO Box 33170
Detroit, MI 48232
800-323-9935
Fax: 866-234-3036
TTY: 800-833-9935
mobility@gm.com
www.gmmobility.com

5593 **Marriott International**
10400 Fernwood Rd.
Bethesda, MA 20817
301-380-3000
800-228-9290
www.marriott.com

J.W. Marriott Jr., Executive Chairman
Anthony Capuano, Chief Executive Officer
Stephanie Linnartz, President
Leeny Oberg, Executive Vice President & CFO
Marriott International operates 30 brands and 7,000+ properties across 131 countries and territories, with an emphasis on diversity, inclusion, sustainability and social impact.

5594 **MedEscort International**
PO Box 8766
Allentown, PA 18105
800-255-7182
service@medescort.com
www.medescort.com

Craig Poliner, President
MedEscort International serves the health care community throughout the world. They specialize in the long-distance transportation of patients by air ambulance, commercial airline, or other forms of transportation. Other services include pre-trip preparations, bedside to bedside service, ground transportation service, and worldwide travel coordination.

5595 **MossRehab Travel Resources**
Moss Rehabilitation Hospital
60 Township Line Rd.
Elkins Park, PA 19027
215-663-6000
800-225-5667
Fax: 215-663-8891
www.mossrehab.com

Thomas Smith, Chief Operating Officer
Alberto Esquenazi, Chief Medical Officer
Eileen Hartranft, Program Director
Julie Hensler-Cullen, Director, Quality & Education
Offers information and resources for persons with special traveling/accessibility needs.

5596 **Nantahala Outdoor Center**
13077 Hwy. 19 W
Bryson City, NC 28713
828-785-5557
reservations@noc.com
www.noc.com

Colin McBeath, President
Nantahala Outdoor Center offers whitewater rafting adventures on six rivers in the Southeast for all skill levels, as well as kayak and canoe adaptive instruction. NOC can tailor whitewater programs to a variety of skills and ability levels, modify gear, and pace instruction.

5597 **Paralyzed Veterans of America**
801 18th St. NW
Washington, DC 20006-3517
800-424-8200
TTY: 800-795-4327
info@pva.org
www.pva.org

David Zurfluh, National President
Charles Brown, National Senior Vice President
Carl Blake, Executive Director
Shaun Castle, Deputy Executive Director
A national organization serving veterans and individuals with spinal cord injury/disorder (SCI/D), as well as their family members and caregivers.

5598 **Rehabiliation Engineering Research Center on Accessible Public Transportation**
SUNY Buffalo, School of Architecture & Planning
3435 Main St.
Buffalo, NY 14214-3087
716-829-5899
arced@buffalo.edu
www.rercapt.org

Aaron Steinfeld, Co-Director
Jordana Maisel, Co-Director
A partnership between the Robotics Institute at Carnegie Mellon University and the Center for Inclusive Design and Environmental Access at University at Buffalo, the RERC on Accessible Public Transportation conducts research and develops methods to further advance accessible transportation systems and equipment.

5599 **Shilo Inns & Resorts**
11707 NE Airport Way
Portland, OR 97220
503-641-6565
800-222-2244
guestservices@shiloinns.com
www.shiloinns.com

Mark S. Hemstreet, Founder & Owner
Shilo Inns offers special assist rooms at many locations throughout the Western United States. These rooms include larger sized bathrooms equipped with assistance railings and wheelchair access. Special assist dogs are welcome at most Shilo Inns.

5600 **Travelers Aid International**
110 Maryland Ave. NE
Suite 508
Washington, DC 20002
202-546-1127
www.travelersaid.org

Kathleen Baldwin, President & CEO
Edward Powers, Membership Director
Ellen Horton, Communications Director
Lynn Adams, Administrative Coordinator
Provides crisis intervention and casework services, limited financial assistance, protective travel assistance and information and referrals for travelers, transients, and newcomers.

5601 **US Servas**
PO Box 3419
Berkeley, CA 94703-0419
800-509-1450
info@usservas.org
www.usservas.org

Marguerite Hills, Chair
Joanne Ferguson Cavanaugh, Secretary
Steve Kanters, Treasurer
International network that links travelers with hosts in 120+ countries with the hope of building world peace through understanding and friendship.

5602 **Wheelers Accessible Van Rentals**
6614 W Sweetwater Ave.
Glendale, AZ 85304
623-776-8830
800-456-1371
Fax: 623-776-8930
info@wheelersvanrentals.com
www.wheelersvanrentals.com

5603 **Wilderness Inquiry**
1611 County Rd. B West
Suite 315
St. Paul, MN 55113
612-676-9400
Fax: 612-676-9401
info@wildernessinquiry.org
www.wildernessinquiry.org

Kim Keprios, Executive Director
Julie K. Edmiston, Associate Executive Director
Jeff Hanson, Operations Manager
Nell Holden, Business Operations Director
Allows people of all ages and abilities to share the adventure of wilderness travel. This nonprofit organization was formed in 1978 and conducts tours to some of the most beautiful and remote parts of the world.

Tours

5604 **Able Trek Tours**
510 K St.
PO Box 384
Reedsburg, WI 53959
608-524-3021
800-205-6713
Fax: 608-524-8302
staff@abletrektours.com
abletrektours.com

Don Douglas, Owner & President
Able Trek Tours offers vacation programs and charter bus services for individuals with special needs.

5605 **Access Pass**
National Park Service
1849 C St. NW
Washington, DC 20240
202-208-6843
www.nps.gov

Shawn Benge, Deputy Director, Operations
Lena McDowall, Deputy Director, Management & Administration
Susan Farinelli, Acting Chief of Staff
Jenny Anzelmo-Sarles, Chief of Public Affairs

A free passport to federally operated parks, monuments, historic sites, recreation areas, and wildlife refuges for persons who are permanently disabled.

5606 **Accessible Journeys**
35 W Sellers Ave.
Ridley Park, PA 19078
610-521-0339
800-846-4537
Fax: 610-521-6959

Howard McCoy, President & CEO

Accessible Journeys is a vacation planner and tour operator for wheelchair travelers and people with disabilities.

5607 **Anglo California Travel Service**
10620 Creston Dr.
Los Altos, CA 94024
408-257-2257
800-339-4484
Fax: 408-257-2664
anglocalifornia@yahoo.com
www.anglocalifornia.com

Audrey Cooper, Contact
Tony Cooper, Contact

Provides plans for one and two week accessible tours.

5608 **Courier Travel**
532 Duane St.
Glen Ellyn, IL 60137
630-469-0511
info@couriertravelinc.com
www.couriertravelinc.com

Fred Mueller, Owner

Offers specialized assistance for independent travel or tours for persons with disabilities. Vacations include cruises and travel in the USA and abroad.

5609 **Cunard Line**
24303 Town Center Dr.
Suite 200
Valencia, CA 91355
800-728-6273
www.cunard.com

Simon Palethorpe, President

The Cunard Line is a British cruise line providing luxury cruise vacations and ocean travel experiences. The fleet consists of Queen Elizabeth, the Queen Mary 2, and the Queen Victoria. The Cunard Line accommodates guests with disabilities and reduced mobility.

5610 **Dialysis at Sea Cruises**
5230 Land O' Lakes Blvd.
PO Box 1158
Land O' Lakes, FL 34639-9998
813-775-4040
800-544-7604
Fax: 727-372-7490
info@dialysisatsea.com
www.dialysisatsea.com

Steve Debroux, Owner

Has been providing travel opportunities for persons on hemodialysis and CAPD since 1977. Handles all aspects of their travel and medical requirements. Not sold through travel agents. Makes all reservations and coordinates the total set-up and operation of an onboard ship mobile dialysis clinic. Cruises run from seven days to three weeks and have departures from cities around the world on a variety of cruise lines.

5611 **Dvorak Raft Kayak & Fishing Expeditions**
17921 US Hwy. 285
Nathrop, CO 81236
719-539-6851
800-824-3795
info@dvorakexpeditions.com
www.dvorakexpeditions.com

Bill Dvorak, Co-Owner
Jaci Dvorak, Co-Owner

Family owned and operated since 1969, Dvorak offers a wide range of whitewater rafting trips on the Arkansas, Colorado, Dolores, Gunnison, Green, North Platte, Rio Grande, and San Miguel rivers ranging from half-day to multi-day excursions. Provides river trips for people who are deaf, visually impaired, and physically or mentally disabled. Colorado's first Licensed Outfitter.

5612 **Easy Access Travel**
1716 Morning Glory
Carrollton, TX 75007
800-920-8989
debra@easyaccesstravel.com
www.easyaccesstravel.com

Debra Kerper, Owner

Specializes in accessible cruise vacations and land tours for individuals with disabilities.

5613 **Environmental Traveling Companions**
Fort Mason Center
2 Marina Blvd.
Suite C385
San Francisco, CA 94123
415-474-7662
Fax: 415-474-3919
info@etctrips.org
www.etctrips.org

Diane Poslosky, Executive Director
Magen Kuzma, Administrative Director
Benjamin Harwood, Development Director
Jenny Jedeikin, Communications Manager

Provides accessible outdoor experiences for people with disabilities and under-resourced youth.

5614 **Guide Service of Washington**
734 15th St. NW
Suite 701
Washington, DC 20005
202-628-2842
Fax: 202-638-2812
sales@dctourguides.com
www.dctourguides.com

5615 **New Directions For People With Disabilities**
5276 Hollister Ave.
Suite 207
Santa Barbara, CA 93111
805-967-2841
888-967-2841
Fax: 805-964-7344
hello@newdirectionstravel.org
www.newdirectionstravel.org

Dee Duncan, Executive Director

A nonprofit organization providing local, national, and international travel vacations and holiday programs for people with mild to moderate developmental disabilities.

5616 **Norwegian Cruise Line**
7665 Corporate Center Dr.
Miami, FL 33126
305-436-4000
800-327-7030
www.ncl.com

Harry Sommer, President & CEO
David J. Herrera, Senior Vice President, Strategy & Business Development
Chad Berkshire, Senior Vice President, Revenue Management
Isis Ruiz, Senior Vice President & Chief Marketing Officer

Accommodates guests with disabilities and special needs, but advance notice is required. Cruise fares vary.

5617 **ROW Adventures**
PO Box 579
Coeur d'Alene, ID 83816
208-765-0841
800-451-6034
Fax: 208-667-6506
info@rowadventures.com
www.rowadventures.com

Peter Grubb, Co-Founder
Betsy Bowen, Co-Founder
Jonah Grubb, Operations Manager
Michelle Darnell, Assistant Director, Sales & Marketing

Offers one to six day rafting trips to physically disadvantaged people. Designs custom itineraries, or trips with a special focus for small groups. For those with special dietary needs, they prepare special meals. They also offer canoe trips aboard 34' voyager canoes along the trail of Lewis and Clark on Montana's upper Missouri River. Free brochure upon request.

5618 **Sundial Special Vacations**
750 Marine Dr.
Suite 100
Astoria, OR 97103
503-325-4484
800-547-9198
Fax: 503-325-4536
info@sundial-travel.com
www.sundialtour.com
Bruce Conner, Owner
Provides special vacations for developmentally disabled persons. Tour ratio is 1 to 4 depending on capabilities.

5619 **The Guided Tour, Inc.**
7900 Old York Rd.
Suite 111-B
Elkins Park, PA 19027
215-782-1370
Fax: 215-635-2637
director@guidedtour.com
www.guidedtour.com
Ari Segal, Director
Jon Fash, Administrator
Lynsey Trohoske, Administrator
The Guided Tour is a program that offers supervised vacations for adults with developmental disabilities.

5620 **Trips Inc.**
PO Box 10885
Eugene, OR 97440
541-686-1013
800-686-1013
Fax: 541-465-9355
trips@tripsinc.com
www.tripsinc.com
Jim Peterson, Founder & President
Leslie Peterson, Executive Director
Trips Inc. Special Adventures provides travel outings to adults with intellectual and developmental disabilities.

5621 **Ventures Travel**
3600 Holly Lane N
Suite 95
Plymouth, MN 55447
952-852-0107
866-692-7400
Fax: 952-852-0123
www.venturestravel.org
Kayleen Pfitzer, Manager
Seeks to enhance independence and self-esteem and provide necessary supports to facilitate safe and memorable travel experiences for people with developmental disabilities.

5622 **Wilderness Inquiry**
1611 County Rd. B West
Suite 315
St. Paul, MN 55113
612-676-9400
Fax: 612-676-9401
info@wildernessinquiry.org
www.wildernessinquiry.org
Kim Keprios, Executive Director
Julie K. Edmiston, Associate Executive Director
Jeff Hanson, Operations Manager
Nell Holden, Business Operations Director
Allows people of all ages and abilities to share the adventure of wilderness travel. This nonprofit organization was formed in 1978 and conducts tours to some of the most beautiful and remote parts of the world.

Vehicle Rentals

5623 **Accessible Vans Of America**
866-224-1750
www.accessiblevans.com
David Adams, Executive Director
Accessible Vans of America (AVA) is dedicated to providing wheelchair accessible vehicles to people with disabilities.

5624 **Avis Rent A Car System, LLC**
6 Sylvan Way
Parsippany, NJ 07054
973-496-3500
800-352-7900
TTY: 800-331-2323
www.avis.com
Joe Ferraro, President & Chief Executive Officer
Brian Choi, Chief Financial Officer
Izzy Martins, Executive Vice President, Americas
Arthur Orduna, Executive Vice President & Chief Innovation Officer
Avis Access is a program of Avis Rent A Car that provides a full range of complementary products and services to drivers and passengers with physical disabilities. Products or services include transfer boards, hand controls, swivel seats, and more.

5625 **National Car Rental System**
600 Corporate Park Dr.
St. Louis, MO 63105
314-512-5000
www.nationalcar.com
Chrissy Taylor, Chief Executive Officer
Accommodates special requests subject to availability. Offers hand controls, bench seats, extra mirrors and vans with lifts at many major locations.

5626 **Northwest Limousine Service**
Yonkers, NY 10710
914-294-0777
northwestlimony@gmail.com
northwestlimoinc.com

5627 **The Creative Mobility Group, LLC**
32217 Stephenson Hwy.
Madison Heights, MI 48071
248-577-5430
888-940-8337
Fax: 248-577-5450
info@creativemobilitygroup.com
www.creativemobilitygroup.com
Christina Duggan, Contact
Provides wheelchair accessible van rentals, as well as mobility scooter rentals, stairlift rentals, ramp rentals, and wheelchair rentals. Locations in Madison Heights, Michigan; Wayne, Michigan; and Byron Center, Michigan.

5628 **Wheelchair Getaways**
PO Box 1098
Mukilteo, WA 98275
425-353-8213
866-224-1750
Fax: 425-355-6159
www.wheelchairgetaways.com

5629 **Wheelers Accessible Van Rentals**
6614 W Sweetwater Ave.
Glendale, AZ 85304
623-776-8830
800-456-1371
Fax: 623-776-8930
info@wheelersvanrentals.com
www.wheelersvanrentals.com

Veteran Services

National Administrations

5630 **Department of Medicine and Surgery Veterans Administration**
810 Vermont Ave NW
Washington, DC 20420
202-273-8504
800-827-1000
www.va.gov

David J. Shulkin, Secretary
Vivieca Wright, Chief of Staff
Provides hospital and outpatient treatment as well as nursing home care for eligible veterans in Veterans Administration facilities. Services elsewhere provided on a contract basis in the United States and its territories. Provides non-vocational inpatient residential rehabilitation services to eligible legally blinded veterans of the armed forces of the United States.

5631 **Department of Veterans Affairs Regional Office - Vocational Rehab Division**
810 Vermont Ave NW
Washington, DC 20420
202-273-8504
800-827-1000
www.va.gov

David J. Shulkin, Secretary
Vivieca Wright, Chief of Staff
Vocational rehabilitation is a program of services administered by the Department of Veterans Affairs for service members and veterans with service-connected physical or mental disabilities. If persons are compensibly disabled and are found in need of rehabilitation services because they have an employment handicap, this program can prepare them for a suitable job; get and keep that job; assist persons to become fully productive and independent.

5632 **Department of Veterans Benefits**
810 Vermont Ave NW
Washington, DC 20420
202-461-6913
800-827-1000
www.va.gov

David J. Shulkin, Secretary
Vivieca Wright, Chief of Staff
Furnishes compensation and pensions for disability and death to veterans and their dependents. Provides vocational rehabilitation services, including counseling, training, assistance and more towards employment, to blinded veterans disabled as a result of service in the armed forces during World War II, Korea and the Vietnam era; also provides rehabilitation services to certain peace-time veterans.

5633 **Disabled American Veterans Headquarters**
3725 Alexandria Pike
Cold Spring, KY 41076
877-426-2838
feedback@davmail.org
www.dav.org

David W Riley, Chairman
Barry Jesinoski, Executive Director
James Killen, Associate National Communications Director
Randy Reese, Director of Human Resources
Serves America's disabled veterans and their families. Direct services include legislative advocacy; professional counseling about compensation, pension, educational and job training programs and VA health care; and assistance in applying for those entitlements.

5634 **Federal Benefits for Veterans and Dependents**
810 Vermont Ave NW
Washington, DC 20420
202-273-6763
800-827-1000
www.benefits.va.gov

David J. Shulkin, Secretary
Viveca Wright, Chief of Staff
Offers information on benefits for veterans and their families.
93 pages
ISBN 0-16048 -58-

5635 **US Department of Veterans Affairs National Headquarters**
810 Vermont Ave NW
Washington, DC 20420
202-273-5400
800-827-1000
www.va.gov

David J. Shulkin, Secretary
Vivieca Wright, Chief of Staff
A federal agency that provides healthcare services to military veterans at VA medical centers and outpatient clinics located throughout the country; several non-healthcare benefits including disability compensation, vocational rehabilitation, education assistance, home loans, and life insurance; and provides burial and memorial benefits to veterans and family members at 135 national cemeteries.
80 pages

5636 **Veteran's Voices Writing Project**
406 W 34th St
Suite 103
Kansas City, MO 64111-3043
816-701-6844
veteransvoices@sbcglobal.net
www.veteransvoices.com

Deann Mitchell, President
Sheryl Liddle, Vice President
Marianne Watson, Treasurer
Margaret Clark, Editor in Chief
Individuals and organizations united to encourage veterans to write for pleasure and rehabilitation. The organization also maintains speakers' bureau and audio tape versions for the blind. Also offered are numerous monetary awards, articles, book reviews, cartoons and drawings, light verse, poetry and short stories.
$15.00
64 pages Magazine
ISSN 0504-07 9

Alabama

5637 **Alabama VA Benefits Regional Office - Montgomery**
U.S. Department of Veteran Affairs
345 Perry Hill Rd
Montgomery, AL 36109
800-827-1000
Fax: 334-213-3565
montgomery.query@vba.va.gov
www.va.gov

Cory A. Hawthorne, Director
Erica P. Worthington, Assistant Director
Jamie Bozeman, Vocational Rehabilitation & Employment Officer
Lolita McClung-Shepherd, Veterans Service Center Manager
The Veterans Benefits Administration (VBA) provides a variety of benefits and services to Servicemembers, Veterans, and their families.

5638 **Alabama VA Medical Center - Birmingham**
Veterans Health Administration U.S. Dept. of VA
700 S. 19th St
Birmingham, AL 35233
205-933-8101
www.birmingham.va.gov

Thomas Smith, Director
Veterans medical clinic offering disabled veterans medical treatments.

5639 **Central Alabama Veterans Healthcare System**
Veterans Health Administration, U.S. Dept. of VA
215 Perry Hill Rd
Montgomery, AL 36109-3798
334-272-4670
800-214-8387
www.centralalabama.va.gov

Paul Bockelman, Interim Director
Thomas Huettemann, Associate Director for Resources
Linda Townsend-Green, Acting Associate Director, Operations
Vic Malabonga, Chief of Staff
CAVHCS exists to provide excellent services to veterans across the continuum of healthcare. We take pride in providing delivery of timely quality care by staff who demonstrate outstanding customer service, the advancement of health care through research, and the education of tomorrow's health care providers.

5640 **Tuscaloosa VA Medical Center**
Veterans Health Administration, U S Dept. of V A
3701 Loop Rd E
Tuscaloosa, AL 35404-5015
205-554-2000
888-269-3045
Fax: 205-554-2845
www.tuscaloosa.va.gov
John F. Merkle, Medical Center Director
David L. Carden, Associate Director, Nursing & Patient Care Services
Carlos Berry, Chief of Staff
To serve America's Heroes by improving their health and well-being through Veteran and Family Centered Care.

Alaska

5641 **Alaska VA Healthcare System - Anchorage**
1201 North Muldoon Road
Ste 115
Anchorage, AK 99504-5914
907-257-4700
888-353-7574
Fax: 907-561-7183
www.alaska.va.gov
Linda L. Boyle, Interim Director
Shawn Bransky, Associate Director
Veterans medical clinic offering disabled veterans medical treatments.

5642 **DAV Department of Alaska**
2925 Debarr Rd
Room 3101
Anchorage, AK 99508-2983
907-257-4803
Fax: 907-258-9828
www.davmembersportal.org
Pamela F. Beale, Alaska Commander
Robert W. Bingham, Membership Chairman

5643 **Veteran Benefits Administration - Anchorage Regional Office**
U.S. Department of Veteran Affairs
1201 Muldoon Rd
Anchorage, AK 99504
907-257-4803
800-827-1000
anchorage.query@vba.va.gov
www.benefits.va.gov/anchorage
Robert A. McDonald, Secretary of Veterans
Robert D. Snyder, Chief of Staff
The Anchorage Regional Office is remotely managed by the Salt Lake City Regional Office. The VBA operation includes a one-stop Veterans Service Center made up of the merged Adjudication and Veterans Service Divisions. There is also a one person Loan Guaranty Division and a Vocational Rehabilitation and Employment Division.

Arizona

5644 **Carl T Hayden VA Medical Center**
Veterans Health Administration, U S Dept. of V A
650 E Indian School Rd
Phoenix, AZ 85012-1839
602-277-5551
800-554-7174
Fax: 602-222-6472
g.vhacss@forum.va.gov
www.phoenix.va.gov
D Gregg Gordon, President
Marva Greene, Vice President
John Fears, CEO
Linda Herrly MSW, LCSW, Caregiver Support Coordinator

5645 **Northern Arizona VA Health Care System**
Veterans Health Administration, US Dept. of VA
500 Hwy 89N
Prescott, AZ 86313-5001
928-445-4860
800-949-1005
Fax: 928-768-6076
g.vhacss@forum.va.gov
www.prescott.va.gov
Deborah Thompson, Manager

5646 **Southern Arizona VA Healthcare System**
Veterans Health Administration, U S Dept. of V A
3601 S 6th Ave
Tucson, AZ 85723
520-792-1450
800-470-8262
Fax: 520-629-1818
g.vhacss@forum.va.gov
www.tucson.va.gov
Jonathan H. Gardner, MPA, FACHE, Director
Jennifer S Gutowski, MHA, FACHE, Associate Director
Katie A. Landwehr, MBA, Assistant Director
Fabia Kwiecinski, MD, FACP, Chief of Staff
The Southern Arizona VA Health Care System (SAVAHCS) located in Tucson AZ serves over 170,000 Veterans located in eight counties in Southern Arizona and one county in Western New Mexico.

Arkansas

5647 **Eugene J Towbin Healthcare Center**
Veterans Health Administration, U S Dept. of V A
2200 Fort Roots Dr
North Little Rock, AR 72114-1706
501-257-1000
800-827-1000
Fax: 501-257-1779
g.vhacss@forum.va.gov
www.littlerock.va.gov
Michael R. Winn, Director
Toby T. Mathew, MHA/MBA, Deputy Director
Cyril O. Ekeh, MHA, Associate Director
Julie A. Brandt, MSN, RN, CNA-B, Associate Director for Patient Care Service/Nurse Executive
CAVHS is reaching out to veterans through its community-based outpatient clinics in Mountain Home, El Dorado, Hot Springs, Mena, Pine Bluff, Searcy, Conway, Russellville, its Home Health Care Service Center in Hot Springs, and a VA Drop-In Day Treatment Center for homeless veterans in downtown Little Rock.

5648 **Fayetteville VA Medical Center**
Veterans Health Administration, US Dept. of VA
1100 N College Ave
Fayetteville, AR 72703-1944
479-443-4301
800-691-8387
g.vhacss@forum.va.gov
www.fayettevillear.va.gov
W. Todd Grams, Chief Financial Officer
Glenn D. Haggstrom, Principal Executive Director
Stephen W. Warren, Principal Deputy Assistant Secretary
Honor America's Veterans by providing exceptional health care that improves their health and well-being.

5649 **John L McClellan Memorial Hospital**
Veterans Health Administration, US Dept. of VA
4300 W 7th St
Little Rock, AR 72205-5446
501-257-1000
800-827-1000
g.vhacss@forum.va.gov
www.littlerock.va.gov
Michael R. Winn, Director
Toby T. Mathew, MHA/MBA, Deputy Director
Cyril O. Ekeh, MHA, Associate Director
Julie A. Brandt, MSN, RN, CNA-B, Associate Director for Patient Care Service/Nurse Executive
CAVHS is reaching out to veterans through its community-based outpatient clinics in Mountain Home, El Dorado, Hot Springs, Mena, Pine Bluff, Searcy, Conway, Russellville, its Home Health Care Service Center in Hot Springs, and a VA Drop-In Day Treatment Center for homeless veterans in downtown Little Rock.

Throughout its rich 90 year history, CAVHS has been widely recognized for excellence in education, research, and emergency prepardedness, and -first and foremost -for a tradition of quality an

5650 **North Little Rock Regional Office**
Veterans Benefits Administration, U S Dept. of V A
2200 Fort Roots Drive
Building 65
N Little Rock, AR 72114-1756
501-370-3820
800-827-1000
Fax: 501-370-3829
littlerock.query@vba.va.gov
www.va.gov

Eric K. Shinseki, Secretary
Stephen W. Warren, Principal Deputy Assistant Secretary
W. Todd Grams, Chief Financial Officer
Glenn D. Haggstrom, Principal Executive Director

The Little Rock VA Regional Office offers services to veterans in the State of Arkansas and the city of Texarkana in Bowie County, Texas. Based on 2004 information provided by the Office of Policy, Planning, and Preparedness, the veteran population of Arkansas is 268,000 and the city of Texarkana, Texas, has a veteran population of 3,545. With a staff of approximately 124 employees, the Regional Office determines entitlement to disability compensation and pension, survivors' benefits, vocational

California

5651 **Jerry L Pettis Memorial VA Medical Center**
Veterans Health Administration, U S Dept. of V A
11201 Benton St
Loma Linda, CA 92357-1000
909-825-7084
800-741-8387
g.vhacss@forum.va.gov
www.lomalinda.va.gov

Barbara Fallen, RD, MPA, FACHE, Acting Director
Prachi V. Asher, FACHE, Assistant Director
Dwight C. Evans, M.D., Chief of Staff
Shane M. Elliott, MBA, AD for Administration

Since 1977, VA Loma Linda Healthcare System has been improving the health of the men and women who have so proudly served our nation. We consider it our privilege to serve your health care needs in any way we can.

5652 **Long Beach VA Medical Center**
Veterans Health Administration, U S Dept. of V A
5901 E 7th St
Long Beach, CA 90822-5201
562-826-8000
800-827-1000
888-769-8387
g.vhacss@forum.va.gov
www.longbeach.va.gov

Isabel Duff, Medical Center Director
John M. Tryboski, MSN, Associate Director
Anthony DeFrancesco, FACHE, Associate Director
Sherrie Schuldheis, Ph.D., RN, Assistant Director, Systems Redesign

5653 **Los Angeles Regional Office**
Veterans Benefits Administration, U S Dept. of V A
11000 Wilshire Blvd
Los Angeles, CA 90024-3602
800-827-1000
losangeles.query@vba.va.gov
www.va.gov

Eric K. Shinseki, Secretary
Stephen W. Warren, Principal Deputy Assistant Secretary
W. Todd Grams, Chief Financial Officer
Glenn D. Haggstrom, Principal Executive Director

The Los Angeles Regional Office (RO) provides benefits and services to approximately 706,000 veterans residing in the Southern California counties of Los Angeles, San Bernardino, Riverside, Ventura, Santa Barbara, San Luis Obispo, and Kern. VA benefits expenditures for veterans residing within the jurisdiction of the RO exceed $800 million annually. All Loan Guaranty activities for the six counties are under jurisdiction of the Phoenix Regional Office.

5654 **Martinez Outpatient Clinic**
Veterans Health Administration, U S Dept. of V A
150 Muir Rd
Martinez, CA 94553-4668
925-372-2000
800-382-8387
g.vhacss@forum.va.gov
www.va.gov

John H Simms, Director
Brian E. Schuman, Chief of Police

The Martinez Outpatient Clinic offers a full range of medical, surgical, mental health, and diagnostic outpatient services, including nuclear medicine, ultrasound, CT and MRI. The Center for Rehabilitation and Extended Care is located adjacent to the outpatient clinic.

5655 **Oakland VA Regional Office**
Veterans Benefits Administration U S Dept. of V A
1301 Clay Street
12th Floor
Oakland, CA 94612-5217
800-827-1000
oakland.query@vba.va.gov
www.benefits.va.gov/oakland

Geri Spearman, Director

The jurisdiction includes all Northern California, except for Modoc, Lassen, Alpine and Mono counties, which are assigned to the Reno Regional Office. All Loan Guaranty activities are under the jurisdiction of the Phoenix Regional Office. Seven service organizations are collocated on the eleventh floor of the Federal Office building occupied by the regional office.

5656 **Rehabilitation Research and Development Center**
Department of Veteran s Affairs
810 Vermont Avenue, NW
Washington, DC 94304-1207
202-443-0575
Fax: 202-495-6153
tiffany.asqueri@va.gov

Patricia A. Dorn, Ph.D., Acting Director, Rehab R&D Service
Ricardo Gonzalez, Administrative Officer
Gloria Winford, Staff Assistant
Sarah Armstrong, Budget Technician

The VA Center of Excellence on Mobility in Palo Alto, CA is dedicated to developing innovative clinical treatments and assistive devices for veterans with physical disabilities to increase their independence and improve their quality of life. The clinical emphasis of the center is to improve mobility, either ambulation or manipulation, in individuals with neurologic impairments or orthopaedic impairments. We do not publish any printed books, journals or periodicals.

5657 **Sacramento Medical Center**
Veterans Health Administration U S Department of V
10535 Hospital Way
Mather, CA 95655-4200
916-843-7000
800-382-8387
g.vhacss@forum.va.gov
www.northerncalifornia.va.gov

David G. Mastalski, Interim Director
Donna Iatarola, RN, MSN, Associate Director
William T. Cahill, MD, Chief of Staff

It is an integrated health care delivery system, offering a comprehensive array of medical, surgical, rehabilitative, mental health and extended care to veterans in Northern California. The health system is comprised of a medical center in Sacramento; a rehabilitation and extended care facility in Martinez, and seven outpatient clinics.

5658 **San Diego VA Regional Office**
Veterans Benefits Administration, U S Dept. of V A
8810 Rio San Diego Dr
San Diego, CA 92108-1698
858-552-8585
800-827-1000
Fax: 858-552-7436
oakland.query@vba.va.gov
www.benefits.va.gov/sandiego

Janet M Peyton, Administrative Officer

The San Diego VA Regional Office provides benefit services for over 600,000 Veterans and their dependents in the Southern California Counties of Imperial, Orange, Riverside and San Diego. Since the Regional Office shares occupancy of the building with a VA Outpatient Clinic and the Employment Development Department of the State of California, it truly offers a one stop Service Center.

5659 VA Central California Health Care System
Veterans Health Administration, U S Dept. of V A
2615 E Clinton Ave
Fresno, CA 93703-2223
559-225-6100
888-826-2838
Fax: 559-268-6911
g.vhacss@forum.va.gov
www.fresno.va.gov

Joanne Krumberger, Director
Susan Shyshka, Associate Director
Patricia Richardson Ed.D, RN, N, Nursing Executive
Wessel Meyer MB ChB, FCP (SA), Chief of Staff

VA Central California Health Care System (VACCHCS) has been improving the health of the men and women who have so proudly served our nation. We consider it our privilege to serve your health care needs in any way we can.

5660 VA Greater Los Angeles Healthcare System
Veterans Health Administration U S Deptartment of
11301 Wilshire Blvd
Los Angeles, CA 90073-1003
310-478-3711
800-827-1000
Fax: 310-268-4848
g.vhacss@forum.va.gov
www.losangeles.va.gov

Donna M. Beiter, RN, MSN, Director
Christopher Sandles, Assistant Director
Marlene Brewster, RN, MSN, Acting Associate Director, Nursing and Patient Care Services
Carrie J Dekorte, Associate Director for Administration / Operations

The VA Greater Los Angeles Healthcare System is the largest, most complex healthcare system within the Department of Veterans Affairs.GLA consists of three ambulatory care centers, a tertiary care facility and 10 community based outpatient clinics. GLA serves veterans residing throughout five counties: Los Angeles, Ventura, Kern, Santa Barbara, and San Luis Obispo. There are 1.4 million veterans in the GLA service area. GLA is affiliated with both UCLA School of Medicine and USC School of Medici

5661 VA Northern California Healthcare System
Veterans Health Administration, U S Dept. of V A
150 Muir Rd
Martinez, CA 94553-4668
925-372-2000
800-382-8387
g.vhacss@forum.va.gov
www.northerncalifornia.va.gov

David G. Mastalski, Interim Director
Donna Iatarola, RN, MSN, Associate Director
William T. Cahill, MD, Chief of Staff

VA Northern California Health Care System (VANCHCS) is an integrated health care delivery system, offering a comprehensive array of medical, surgical, rehabilitative, mental health and extended care to veterans in Northern California. The health system is comprised of a medical center in Sacramento; a rehabilitation and extended care facility in Martinez, and seven outpatient clinics.

5662 VA San Diego Healthcare System
Veterans Health Administration, U S Dept. of V A
3350 La Jolla Village Dr
San Diego, CA 92161
858-552-8585
800-331-8387
g.vhacss@forum.va.gov
www.sandiego.va.gov

Jeffrey T. Gering, FACHE, Director
Cynthia Abair, MHA, Associate Director
Robert M. Smith, MD, Chief of Staff/Medical Director
Sandra Solem, PhD, RN, Associate Director, Patient Care Services/Nurse Executive

We provide medical, surgical, mental health, geriatric, spinal cord injury, and advanced rehabilitation services. VASDHS has 296 authorized beds, including skilled nursing beds and operates several regional referral programs including cardiovascular surgery and spinal cord injury. The facility also supports three Vet Centers at the following locations: Chula Vista, San Diego, and San Marcos.

Colorado

5663 Boulder Vet Center
4999 Pearl East Circle
Suite 106
Boulder, CO 80301
303-440-7306
877-927-8387
Fax: 303-449-3907
www.va.gov

Gail N Bennett, Office Manager
Michael J Pantaleo, Team Leader
Annette Matlock, Counselor
Collette M Archibald, Counselor

Offers trauma and readjustment from military and civilian life counseling and assistance with disability claims, military benefits and employment are provided.

5664 Colorado/Wyoming VA Medical Center
Veterans Benefits Administration U S Dept. of V A
155 Van Gordon St
Suite 395
Lakewood, CO 80225
303-914-2680
800-827-1000
denver.query@vba.va.gov
www.denver.va.gov

Forest Farley Jr, Medical Center Director
Thomas E Bowen, Chief of Staff

5665 Denver VA Medical Center
Veterans Health Administration, U S Dept. of V A
1055 Clermont St
Suite 6A138
Denver, CO 80220-3808
303-393-2869
888-336-8262
www.denver.va.gov

Lynnette Roth, Executive Director
Peggy Kearns MS, RD, FACHE, Associate Director
Judith Burke RN, MS, NEA-BC, Associate Director, Patient Care Services
Rebecca Keough MPA, VHA-CM, Assistant Director

Construction of our 1.1m sq foot, $800m replacement facility is well under way! Concrete is being poured, steel is being put in, and we're working hard to open in 2015.

5666 Grand Junction VA Medical Center
Veterans Health Administration
2121 North Ave
Grand Junction, CO 81501-6428
970-242-0731
866-206-6415
Fax: 970-244-1300
g.vhacss@forum.va.gov
www.grandjunction.va.gov

Patricia A. Hitt, MS, Acting Director
Michael Murphy, Manager
Randal France, M.D., Chief Psychiatry Service/ Int. Chf. of Staff
Angela T Brothers, AD/ Patient Care Svcs

The VAMC operates 53 beds comprised of 23 acute care and 30 Transitional Care Unit beds. The VAMC provides primary and secondary care including acute medical, surgical, and psychiatric inpatient services, as well as a full range of outpatient services.

Connecticut

5667 Hartford Regional Office
Veterans Benefits Administration
555 Willard Ave
Building 2E
Newington, CT 6111-2631
860-666-6951
800-827-1000
hartford.query@vba.va.gov

Jeanette A Chirico Post, Network Director

The Hartford Regional Office now provides one-stop service to veterans and their families seeking assistance in compensation, pension, and vocational rehabilitation and employment in an accessible campus environment.

5668 **Hartford Vet Center**
25 Elm St
Suite A
Rocky Hill, CT 06067-2305
860-563-8800
877-927-8387
Fax: 860-563-8805
www.va.gov

Donna Hryb LCSW, Team Leader
Pedro Ortiz, Counselor
Amy Otzel, Counselor
Laura Hall, Military Sexual Trauma Counselor

A U.S. Department of Veterans Affairs counseling center offering counseling to Vietnam era and combat veterans. Sexual trauma/harassment counseling, medical screening and benefit referral is available to all veterans.

5669 **VA Connecticut Healthcare System: Newington Division**
Veterans Health Administration U S Department. of
555 Willard Ave
Newington, CT 6111-2631
860-666-6951
800-827-1000
Fax: 860-667-6764
g.vhacss@forum.va.gov
www.connecticut.va.gov

Janice M. Boss, MS, Director
Margaret Veazey, RN, MSN, Associate Director for Patient Care Services
John Callahan, Associate Director
Al Montoya, Assistant Director

The mission of VA Connecticut Healthcare Systems is to fulfill a nation's commitment to its veterans by providing quality healthcare, promoting health through prevention and maintaining excellence in teaching and research. Provides primary, secondary and tertiary care in medicine, geriatrics, neurology, psychiatry and surgery with an operating capacity of 211 hospital beds.

5670 **VA Connecticut Healthcare System: West Haven**
Veterans Health Administration, U S Dept. of V A
950 Campbell Ave
West Haven, CT 06516-2770
203-932-5711
800-827-1000
Fax: 203-937-3868
g.vhacss@forum.va.gov
www.connecticut.va.gov

Janice M. Boss, MS, Director
Margaret Veazey, RN, MSN, Associate Director for Patient Care Services
John Callahan, Associate Director
Al Montoya, Assistant Director

The mission of VA Connecticut Healthcare Systems is to fulfill a nation's commitment to its veterans by providing quality healthcare, promoting health through prevention and maintaining excellence in teaching and research. Provides primary, secondary and tertiary care in medicine, geriatrics, neurology, psychiatry and surgery with an operating capacity of 211 hospital beds.

Delaware

5671 **Delaware VA Regional Office**
Veterans Benefits Administration U S Dept. of V A
1601 Kirkwood Hwy
Wilmington, DE 19805-4917
302-994-2511
800-461-8262
Fax: 302-633-5516
wilmington.query@vba.va.gov
www.wilmington.va.gov

Daniel D. Hendee, FACHE, MHA, Director
Mary Alice Johnson, MS, RN, Associate Director for Patient Care Services
William E. England, Associate Director for Finance and Operations
Enrique Guttin, MD, MMM, CPE, Chief of Staff

We offer comprehensive services ranging from preventive screenings to long-term care. Wilmington VAMC proudly serves Veterans in multiple locations for convenient access to the services we provide.

5672 **Wilmington VA Medical Center**
Veterans Health Administration, US Dept. of VA
1601 Kirkwood Hwy
Wilmington, DE 19805-4917
302-994-2511
800-461-8262
Fax: 302-633-5516
g.vhacss@forum.va.gov
www.wilmington.va.gov

Daniel D. Hendee, FACHE, MHA, Director
Mary Alice Johnson, MS, RN, Associate Director for Patient Care Services
William E. England, Associate Director for Finance and Operations
Enrique Guttin, MD, MMM, CPE, Chief of Staff

We offer comprehensive services ranging from preventive screenings to long-term care. Wilmington VAMC proudly serves Veterans in multiple locations for convenient access to the services we provide.

5673 **Wilmington Vet Center**
2710 Centerville Road
Suite 103
Wilmington, DE 19808- 4917
302-994-1660
877-927-8387
Fax: 302-994-8361
www.va.gov

Joan Spencer, Team Leader
Patricia Elwood, Office Manager
Valerie Feeley, Counselor
Barbara F Blevins, Counselor

Veterans counseling program offering individual counseling services, advocacy services and group counseling. The focus is the counseling of all veterans coping with the aftermath of war, sexual abuse/harassment in the military and all veterans of the Vietnam era. The center also has an active outreach program to seek veterans needing services. Hours of operation are between 8:00 AM - 4:30 PM, Monday - Friday and other times by appointment only. Services are free.

District of Columbia

5674 **Disabled American Veterans**
Legislative HQ
807 Maine Ave SW
Washington, DC 20024
202-554-3501
Fax: 202-554-3581
feedback@davmail.org
www.dav.org

David W Riley, Chairman
Delphine Metcalf-Foster, National Commander
J. Marc Burgess, National Adjutant
Garry J Augustine, Executive Director

Serves America's disabled veterans and their families. Direct services include legislative advocacy; professional counseling about compensation, pension, educational and job training programs and VA health care; and assistance in applying for those entitlements.

5675 **PVA Adaptive Sports**
Paralyzed Veterans of America
801 18th St. NW
Washington, DC 20006-3517
800-424-8200
TTY: 800-795-4327
info@pva.org
www.pva.org/adaptive-sports

David Zurfluh, National President
Charles Brown, National Senior Vice President
Carl Blake, Executive Director
Shaun Castle, Deputy Executive Director

Sports include air guns, bass fishing, billiards, boccia, bowling, golf, handcycling, quad rugby, and trapshooting.

5676 **VA Medical Center, Washington DC**
50 Irving St NW
Washington, DC 20422-1 202-745-8000
800-827-1000
877-328-2621
g.vhacss@forum.va.gov
www.washingtondc.va.gov
Brian A. Hawkins, MHA, Medical Center Director
Bryan C. Matthews, MBA, Associate Medical Center Director
Natalie Merckens, Assistant Medical Center Director
Ross D. Fletcher, MD, Chief of Staff
Acute general and specialized services in medicine, surgery, neurology, and psychiatry.

5677 **Washington DC VA Medical Center**
Veterans Health Administration, U S Dept. of V A
50 Irving St NW
Washington, DC 20422-1 202-745-8000
800-827-1000
877-328-2621
Fax: 202-754-8530
g.vhacss@forum.va.gov
www.washingtondc.va.gov
Brian A. Hawkins, MHA, Medical Center Director
Bryan C. Matthews, MBA, Associate Medical Center Director
Natalie Merckens, Assistant Medical Center Director
Ross D. Fletcher, MD, Chief of Staff
Acute general and specialized services in medicine, surgery, neurology, and psychiatry.

Florida

5678 **Bay Pines VA Medical Center**
Veterans Health Administration, U S Dept. of V A
10000 Bay Pines Blvd
PO Box 5005
Bay Pines, FL 33744 727-398-6661
800-827-1000
888-820-0230
g.vhacss@forum.va.gov
www.baypines.va.gov
Suzanne M. Klinker, Medical Center Director
Kristine Brown, MPH, Associate Director
Teresa Kumar, RN, MSN, CPHQ, Associate Director for Patient / Nursing Services
Keith Neeley, FACHE, Assistant Director
Since 1933, Bay Pines VA Healthcare System has been improving the health of the men and women who have so proudly served our nation. We consider it our privilege to serve your health care needs in any way we can. Our services are available to Veterans living in a ten county catchment area in west central Florida.

5679 **Gainesville Division, North Florida/South Georgia Veterans Healthcare System**
Veterans Health Administration, U S Dept. of V A
1601 SW Archer Rd
Gainesville, FL 32608-1611 352-376-1611
800-324-8387
Fax: 352-379-7445
g.vhacss@forum.va.gov
www.northflorida.va.gov/northflorida
Thomas Wisnieski, MPA, FACHE, Director
Nancy Reissener, Deputy Director
Maureen Wilkes, Associate Director
LeAnne Whitlow, RN, MSHSA, MB, Associate Director, Nursing Service
In addition to our medical centers in Gainesville and Lake City, we offer services in three satellite outpatient clinics and several community-based outpatient clinics across North Florida and South Georgia.

5680 **James A Haley VA Medical Center**
Veterans Health Administration, U S Dept. of V A
13000 Bruce B Downs Blvd
Suite T72
Tampa, FL 33612-4745 813-972-2000
800-827-1000
888-811-0107
g.vhacss@forum.va.gov
www.tampa.va.gov
Kathleen R. Fogarty, Director
Roy L. Hawkins Jr., Deputy Director
David J. VanMeter, Associate Director
Suzanne Tate, Assistant Director
Comprehensive health care is provided through primary care, tertiary care, and long-term care in areas of medicine, surgery, psychiatry, physical medicine and rehabilitation, spinal cord injury, neurology, oncology, dentistry, geriatrics, and extended care.

5681 **Miami VA Medical Center**
Veterans Health Administration, U S Dept. of V A
1201 NW 16th St
Suite B822
Miami, FL 33125-1693 305-575-7000
800-827-1000
888-276-1785
Fax: 305-575-3266
g.vhacss@forum.va.gov
www.miami.va.gov
Paul M. Russo, Director
Mark E. Morgan, Associate Director
Marcia Lysaght, Associate Director, Patient Care Services
P. Gwendolyn Findley, Ph.D., Assistant Director
The Miami VA is an accredited comprehensive medical provider, providing general medical, surgical, inpatient and outpatient mental health services, the Miami VA Healthcare System includes an AIDS/HIV center, a prosthetic treatment center, spinal cord injury rehabilitative center, and Geriatric Research, Education, and Clinical Center (GRECC).

5682 **St. Petersburg Regional Office**
Veterans Benefits Administration, U S Dept. of V A
9500 Bay Pines Blvd
St Petersburg, FL 33708 727-319-7492
800-827-1000
stpete.query@vba.va.gov
www.va.gov
Warren McPherson, Executive Director

5683 **West Palm Beach VA Medical Center**
Veterans Health Administration, U S Dept. of V A
7305 N Military Trl
West Palm Beach, FL 33410-7417 561-422-8262
800-972-8262
Fax: 561-882-6707
g.vhacss@forum.va.gov
www.westpalmbeach.va.gov
Charleen R. Szabo, FACHE, Medical Center Director
Cristy McKillop, FACHE, MHA, Medical Center Associate Director
Gloria A. Bays, MSN, ARNP, NE-BC, Associate Director for Patient Care Services
Deepak Mandi, MD, Chief of Staff
The medical center is a general medical, psychiatric and surgical facility. It is a teaching hospital, providing a full range of patient care services, with state-of-the-art technology as well as education and limited research. Comprehensive healthcare is provided through primary care and long-term care in the areas of dentistry, extended care, medicine, neurology, oncology, pharmacy, physical medicine, psychiatry, rehabilitation and surgery. The West Palm Beach VA Medical Center operates a Blin

Georgia

5684 **Atlanta Regional Office**
Veterans Benefits Administration, U S Dept. of V A
1700 Clairmont Road
Decatur, GA 30033-1210
404-463-3100
800-827-1000
Fax: 404-929-5819
atlanta.query@vba.va.gov
www.va.gov

Chick Krautler, Executive Director

The Atlanta VA Regional Office is responsible for delivering non-medical VA benefits and services to Georgia Veterans and their dependent family members. This is accomplished through the administration of comprehensive and diverse benefit programs established by Congress. Our goal is to deliver these benefits and services in a timely, accurate, and compassionate manner.

5685 **Atlanta VA Medical Center**
Veterans Health Administration, U S Dept. of V A
1670 Clairmont Rd
Decatur, GA 30033-4004
404-321-6111
800-827-1000
Fax: 404-728-7734
g.vhacss@forum.va.gov
www.atlanta.va.gov

Leslie B. Wiggins, Director
Tom Grace, MBA/MHA, Associate Director
Sheila Meuse, PhD, Assistant Director
Sandy Leake, MSN, RN, Associate Director for Nursing/Patient Services

The Atlanta VA Medical Center (VAMC), located on 26 acres in Decatur, is one of eight medical centers in the VA Southeast Network. It is a teaching hospital, providing a full range of patient care services complete with state-of-the-art technology, education, and research.

5686 **Augusta VA Medical Center**
Veterans Health Administration, U S Dept. of V A
950 15th Street Downtown/1 Freedom
Augusta, GA 30904-6258
706-733-0188
800-827-1000
Fax: 706-731-7227
g.vhacss@forum.va.gov

Robert U. Hamilton, MHA, FACHE, Medical Center Director
Richard Rose, Associate Director
Michelle Cox-Henley, MS, RN, Associate Director for Nursing/Patient Services
Luke M. (Mik Stapleton, MD, Chief of Staff

The Charlie Norwood VA Medical Center is a two-division Medical Center that provides tertiary care inmedicine, surgery, neurology, psychiatry, rehabilitation medicine, and spinal cord injury. The Downtown Division is authorized 155 beds (58 medicine, 37 surgery, and 60 spinal cord injury). The Uptown Division, located approximately three miles away, is authorized 315 beds (68 psychiatry, 15 blind rehabilitation and 40 medical rehabilitation. In addition, a 132-bed Restorative/Nursing Home C

5687 **Carl Vinson VA Medical Center**
Veterans Health Administration, U S Dept. of V A
1826 Veterans Blvd
Dublin, GA 31021-3699
478-272-1210
Fax: 478-277-2717
www.dublin.va.gov

John S. Goldman, Director
Gerald M. DeWorth, Associate Director
Sue Preston, RN, Associate Director for Patient and Nursing Services
Nomie Finn, M.D, Chief of Staff

Since 1948, Carl Vinson VA Medical Center has been improving the health of the men and women who have so proudly served our nation. We consider it our privilege to serve your health care needs in any way we can. Services are available to veterans living in the Middle Georgia area.

5688 **Southeastern Paralyzed Veterans of America**
4010 Deans Bridge Rd.
Hephzibah, GA 30815
706-796-6301
800-292-9335
Fax: 706-796-0363
www.southeasternpva.org

Alan Washington, President
Lee Baker, Vice President
Lonnie Burnett, Treasurer
Joseph Gethers, Secretary

Works to maximize the quality of life for its members and all people with SCI/D as a leading adovocate for healthcare, SCI/D research and education, veteran's benefits, and rights, accessibility and the removal of architectural barriers, sports programs, and disability rights.

Hawaii

5689 **Hilo Vet Center**
70 Lanihuli St
Suite 102
Hilo, HI 96720-2067
808-969-3833
877-927-8387
Fax: 808-969-2025
www.va.gov

Felipe Sales, Team Leader
Samuelito Labasan, Office Manager
Peter Ehlich, Counselor
Nancy G Waller, Counselor

Veterans medical clinic offering disabled veterans medical treatments, readjustment and PTSD counseling to combat veterans

5690 **Honolulu VBA Regional Office**
Veterans Benefits Administration, U S Dept. of V A
459 Patterson Road, E-Wing
Honolulu, HI 96819-1522
808-566-1412
800-827-1000
Fax: 808-433-0478
honolulu.query@vba.va.gov
www.vba.va.gov/ro/honolulu

Claude M Kicklighter, Chief of Staff
Alan Furuno, Manager
Alvin Kalawe, Elderly Program Coordinator
Karin Frazier, Women Veteran's Program Coordinator

The Honolulu Regional Office is responsible for administering VA's benefit programs under the leadership and direction of the Under Secretary for Benefits for the Veterans Benefits Administration. Formerly part of the Honolulu VA Medical & Regional Office Center (VAMROC), the Honolulu Regional Office (RO) was renamed as a stand alone RO on June 2, 2003. The office is co-located with the Spark M. Matsunaga Pacific Islands Health Care System medical center, on the grounds of the Tripler Army Medic

5691 **Pacific Islands Health Care System**
Veterans Health Administration, US Dept. of VA
459 Patterson Rd
Honolulu, HI 96819-1522
808-433-0600
800-214-1306
Fax: 808-433-0390
g.vhacss@forum.va.gov
www.hawaii.va.gov

William F. Dubbs, M.D., Acting Director
Brandon K. Yamamoto, Acting Associate Director
Jane Wellman, APRN, Associate Director of Patient Care Services
David M. Bernstein, M.D, Acting Chief of Staff

The VA Pacific Islands Health Care System (VAPIHCS) Honolulu provides a broad range of medical care services, serving an estimated 127,600 veterans throughout Hawaii and the Pacific Islands. The VAPIHCS provides outpatient medical and mental health care through a main Ambulatory Care Clinic on Oahu (Honolulu) and through five Community Based Outpatient Clinics (CBOCs) on the neighboring islands including: Hawaii (Hilo and Kona), Maui, Kauai, and Guam. Traveling clinicians also provide episodi

Idaho

5692 **Boise Regional Office**
Veterans Benefits Administration, U S Dept. of V A
444 W. Fort Street
Boise, ID 83702-4531
800-827-1000
boise.query@vba.va.gov
www.va.gov

Jim Vance, Director
Pat Teague, Service Officer
Tom Ressler, Manager

The Boise Regional Office administers monetary benefits to 17,283 veterans in Idaho, Utah, and Oregon. The Regional Office issued monthly disability and death benefit payments of over $15 million in January 2007. VBA's annual compensation and pension benefits for veterans residing within the RO's jurisdiction now exceed $185 million

5693 **Boise VA Medical Center**
Veterans Health Administration, U S Dept. of V A
500 W Fort St
Boise, ID 83702-4531
208-422-1000
800-827-1000
Fax: 208-422-1326
g.vhacss@forum.va.gov
www.boise.va.gov

Jennifer T Shalz, Chief of Staff

We truly hope to improve your health and well-being and will make your visit or stay as pleasant as possible. We are committed to veterans and the nation and strive to continually enhance the care we provide. We also train future healthcare professionals, conduct research and support our nation in times of emergency. In all of these activities, our employees will respect and support your rights as a patient.

Illinois

5694 **Edward Hines Jr Hospital**
Veterans Health Administration, U S Dept. of V A
5000 South 5th Avenue
Hines, IL 60141
708-202-8387
800-827-1000
Fax: 708-202-2684
g.vhacss@forum.va.gov
www.hines.va.gov

Joan Ricard, FACHE, Hospital Director
Dr. Daniel Zomchek, Associate Director
Carol A. Gouty, RN, MSN, PhD, Associate Director of Patient Care
Karandeep Sraon, Assistant Director

Specialized clinical programs include Blind Rehabilitation, Spinal Cord Injury, Neurosurgery, Radiation Therapy and Cardiovascular Surgery. The hospital also serves as the VISN 12 southern tier hub for pathology, radiology, radiation therapy, human resource management and fiscal services. Hines VAH currently operates 471 beds and six community based outpatient clinics in Elgin, Kankakee, Oak Lawn, Aurora, LaSalle, and Joliet.

5695 **Marion VA Medical Center**
Veterans Health Administration U S Department of V
2401 W Main St
Marion, IL 62959-1188
618-997-5311
800-827-1000
www.marion.va.gov

Paul Bockelman, Medical Center Director
Frank Kehus, Associate Director

The VA Medical Center in Marion, Illinois, is a general medical and surgical facility that operates 55 acute care beds and a 60 bed Community Living Center. Ten Outpatient Clinics that provide primary care and behavioral medicine services are located in Harrisburg; Carbondale; Effingham; and Mt. Vernon, IL; Paducah; Hanson; Owensboro; and Mayfield, Kentucky; Vincennes and Evansville, IN.

5696 **North Chicago VA Medical Center**
Veterans Health Administration, U S Dept. of V A
3001 North Green Bay Rd
North Chicago, IL 60064-3048
847-688-1900
800-393-0865
g.vhacss@forum.va.gov
www.lovell.fhcc.va.gov

Patrick L. Sullivan, Director
Captain Jos, A. Acosta, MC, US, Commanding Officer/Deputy Director
Captain Jami Kersten, Associate Director
Dr. Sarah Fouse, Associate Director of Patient Services/Nurse Executive

The arrangement incorporates facilities, services and resources from the North Chicago VA Medical Center (VAMC) and the Naval Health Clinic Great Lakes (NHCGL). A combined mission of the health care center means active duty military, their family members, military retirees and veterans are all cared for at the facility.

5697 **VA Illiana Health Care System**
Veterans Health Administration, U S Dept. of V A
1900 E Main St
Danville, IL 61832-5198
217-554-3000
800-320-8387
Fax: 217-554-4552
g.vhacss@forum.va.gov
www.danville.va.gov

Emma Metcalf, MSN, RN, Director
Diana Carranza, Associate Director
Alesia Coe, MSN, RN, Associate Director for Patient Care Services
Nirmala Rozario, M.D., Ph.D, Chief of Staff

Since 1898, our buildings, facilities, patients, and missions have changed, but remaining constant is VA Illiana Health Care System's endeavor in improving the health of the men and women who have so proudly served our nation. Being the 8th oldest VA facility, we consider it our privilege to serve your health care needs in any way we can.

Indiana

5698 **Indianapolis Regional Office**
Veterans Benefits Administration
575 N Pennsylvania St
Indianapolis, IN 46204-1563
317-226-7860
800-827-1000
TTY: 800-829-4833
indianapolis.query@vba.va.gov
www.benefits.va.gov/indianapolis

5699 **Richard L Roudebush VA Medical Center**
Veterans Health Administration, U S Dept. of V A
1481 W 10th St
Indianapolis, IN 46202-2803
317-554-0000
800-827-1000
Fax: 317-554-0127
g.vhacss@forum.va.gov
www.indianapolis.va.gov

Thomas Mattice, Director
Jeff Nechanicky, Associate Director
Kimberly Radant, Associate Director for Patient Care Services
Cathy Lee, Assistant Director

Since 1932, Richard L. Roudebush VA Medical Center has been improving the health of the men and women who have so proudly served our nation. We consider it our privilege to serve your health care needs in any way we can. Services are available to more than 196,000 veterans living in a 45-county area of Indiana and Illinois.

5700 **VA North Indiana Health Care System: Fort Wayne Campus**
Veterans Health Administration, U S Dept. of V A
2121 Lake Ave
Fort Wayne, IN 46805-5100
260-426-5431
800-360-8387
g.vhacss@forum.va.gov
www.northernindiana.va.gov

Denise M. Deitzen, Medical Center Director
Audrey L. Frison, MHA, RN, Associate Director
Helen Rhodes MPA, RN, Associate Director for Operations
Ajay Dhawan MD FACHE, Chief of Staff

The Fort Wayne Campus offers primary and secondary medical and surgical services. Primary care clinics are available at both medical center campuses and at Community Based Outpatient Clinics (CBOCs) located in South Bend, Goshen, Peru and Muncie Indiana. Recently completed renovations and construction, and continuous maintenance, ensure an attractive, state-of-the-art healthcare environment.

5701 **VA Northern Indiana Health Care System: Marion Campus**
Veterans Health Administration, U S Dept. of V A
1700 E 38th St
Marion, IN 46953-4568
765-674-3321
800-360-8387
g.vhacss@forum.va.gov
www.northernindiana.va.gov

Denise M. Deitzen, Medical Center Director
Audrey L. Frison, MHA, RN, Associate Director
Helen Rhodes MPA, RN, Associate Director for Operations
Ajay Dhawan MD FACHE, Chief of Staff

The Marion Campus offers a full range of mental health, nursing home care, and extended care services. Primary care clinics are available at both medical center campuses and at Community Based Outpatient Clinics (CBOCs) located in South Bend, Goshen, Peru and Muncie Indiana.

Iowa

5702 **Des Moines VA Medical Center**
Veterans Health Administration, U S Dept. of V A
3600 30th St
Des Moines, IA 50310-5753
515-699-5999
800-294-8387
Fax: 515-699-5862
g.vhacss@forum.va.gov
www.centraliowa.va.gov

Donald Cooper, Director
Susan Martin, Associate Director for Resources and Operations
Tammy Neff, RN, MBA, MSN, M, Acting Associate Director for Patient Services/Nurse Executi
Fredrick Bahls, MD, Chief of Staff

The VA Central Iowa Health Care System (VACIHCS) operates a Veterans Health Administration (VHA) medical facility in Des Moines, with Community Based Outpatient Clinics (CBOCs) in Mason City, Fort Dodge, Knoxville, Marshalltown and Carroll. The medical center provides acute and specialized medical and surgical services, residential outpatient treatment programs in substance abuse and post-traumatic stress and a full range of mental health and long-term care services, as well as sub-acute and r

5703 **Des Moines VA Regional Office**
Veterans Benefits Administration, U S Dept. of V A
210 Walnut Street
Des Moines, IA 50309-2115
515-323-7580
800-827-1000
Fax: 515-323-7580
leander@vba.va.gov
www.va.gov

Rich Anderson, Service Director

The Des Moines VA Regional Office provides Compensation, Pension and Vocational Rehabilitation and Counseling services for all military veterans in the State of Iowa. The Des Moines VA Regional Office currently provides approximately $260 million in benefits to the approximately 270,000 veterans in Iowa.

5704 **Iowa City VA Medical Center**
Veterans Health Administration, U S Dept. of V A
601 Highway 6 West
Iowa City, IA 52240-2202
319-338-0581
800-637-0128
866-687-7382
Fax: 319-339-7171
g.vhacss@forum.va.gov
www.iowacity.va.gov

Barry Sharp, Director
Timothy McMurry, Associate Director for Operations
Dawn Oxley, RN, Associate Director Patient Care Services/Nurse Executive
Stanley Parker, MD, Acting Chief of Staff

Tertiary care facility, affiliated teaching hospital, and research center seving an aging veteran populatiaon in eastern Iowa and western Illinois. Satellite clinics are located in Bettendord, Dubuque, and Waterloo, Iowa and in Quincy and Galesburg, Illinois.

5705 **Knoxville VA Medical Center**
Veterans Health Administration, U S Dept. of V A
1515 W Pleasant St
Knoxville, IA 50138-3399
641-842-3101
800-816-8878
Fax: 641-828-5124
g.vhacss@forum.va.gov
www.centraliowa.va.gov

Claudia M Kicklighter

5706 **VA Central Iowa Health Care System**
3600 30th St
Des Moines, IA 50310-5753
515-699-5999
800-294-8387
Fax: 515-699-5862
www.centraliowa.va.gov

Donald Cooper, Director
Susan Martin, Associate Director for Resources and Operations
Tammy Neff, RN, MBA, MSN, M, Acting Associate Director for Patient Services/Nurse Executi
Fredrick Bahls, MD, Chief of Staff

The VA Central Iowa Health Care System (VACIHCS) operates a Veterans Health Administration (VHA) medical facility in Des Moines, with Community Based Outpatient Clinics (CBOCs) in Mason City, Fort Dodge, Knoxville, Marshalltown and Carroll. The medical center provides acute and specialized medical and surgical services, residential outpatient treatment programs in substance abuse and post-traumatic stress and a full range of mental health and long-term care services, as well as sub-acute and r

Kansas

5707 **Colmery-O'Neil VA Medical Center**
Veterans Health Administration, U S Dept. of V A
2200 SW Gage Blvd
Topeka, KS 66622
785-350-3111
800-574-8387
g.vhacss@forum.va.gov
www.topeka.va.gov

A. Rudy Klopfer, FACHE, Director
John Moon, Associate Director
Nelson L. Dean, RN, BSN, MA, Associate Director for Patient Care Services
Christine M Kleckner, MBA, RD, Assistant Director

Since 1946, the staff of the Colmery-O'Neil VA Medical Center has been serving veterans. Today, we proudly serve our nation's veterans with excellent health care as part of the VA Eastern Kansas Health Care System (VAEKHCS). We consider it our privilege to serve your health care needs in any way we can.

5708 **Dwight D Eisenhower VA Medical Center**
Veterans Health Administration, U S Dept. of V A
4101 4th Street Trafficway
Leavenworth, KS 66048-5014
913-682-2000
800-952-8387
g.vhacss@forum.va.gov
www.leavenworth.va.gov
A. Rudy Klopfer, FACHE, Director
John Moon, Associate Director
Nelson L. Dean, RN, BSN, MA, Associate Director for Patient Care Services
Christine M Kleckner, MBA, RD, Assistant Director
Since 1886, the staff of the Dwight D. Eisenhower VA Medical Center has been serving veterans. Today, we proudly serve our nation's veterans with excellent health care as part of the VA Eastern Kansas Health Care System (VAEKHCS). We consider it our privilege to serve your health care needs in any way we can.

5709 **Kansas VA Regional Office**
Veterans Benefits Administration, U S Dept. of V A
5500 E Kellogg Dr
Wichita, KS 67218-1607
800-827-1000
wichita.query@vba.va.gov
www.benefits.va.gov/wichita
Edgar L Tucker, Medical Center Director

5710 **Robert J Dole VA Medical Center**
Veterans Health Administration, U S Dept. of V A
5500 E Kellogg Dr
Wichita, KS 67218-1607
316-685-2221
800-827-1000
888-827-6881
Fax: 316-651-3666
g.vhacss@forum.va.gov
www.wichita.va.gov
Kevin Inkley, MA, Director
Vicki Bondie, MBA, Associate Director
Carol A. Kaster, MA, RN, Associate Director of Patient Care/Nurse Executive
M. Ganga Hematillake, MD, Chief of Staff
For over 70 years, the Dole VA Medical and Regional office center has been honored to serve Kansas area veterans. The center provides a full range of primary and specialty acute and extended care services to veterans in 59 counties of Kansas. Special emphasis programs include substance abuse, post traumatic stress disorder (PTSD), women's health, spinal cord injury, visual impairment, prosthetic and sensory aids, and homeless services.

Kentucky

5711 **Lexington VA Medical Center**
Veterans Health Administration, U S Dept. of V A
1101 Veterans Dr
Lexington, KY 40502-2235
859-281-4900
800-352-4000
g.vhacss@forum.va.gov
www.lexington.va.gov
Martin J. Traxler, Acting Medical Center Director
Patricia Breeden, MD, Acting Chief of Staff
Laura Faulkner, Acting Associate Medical Center Director
Agnes Therady, RN, NEA-BC, F, Acting Associate Director Patient Care Services
The Lexington Veterans Affairs Medical Center is a fully accredited, two-division, tertiary care medical center with an operating bed complement of 199 hospital beds. Acute medical, neurological, surgical and psychiatric inpatient services are provided at the Cooper Division, located adjacent to the University of Kentucky Medical Center. Other available services include: emergency care, medical-surgical units, acute psychiatry, ICU, progressive care unit, (includes Cardiac Cath Lab) ambulatory s

5712 **Louisville VA Medical Center**
Veterans Health Administration, U S Dept. of V A
800 Zorn Ave
Louisville, KY 40206-1433
502-287-4000
800-376-8387
g.vhacss@forum.va.gov
www.louisville.va.gov
Wayne L. Pfeffer, MHSA, FACHE, Medical Center Director
Douglas V Paxton, Sr, Associate Director / Operations
Pamala Thompson, RN, MSA, MSN, Associate Director for Patient Care Services
Marylee Rothschild, M.D., Chief of Staff
Since 1952, Robley Rex VAMC has been improving the health of the men and women who have so proudly served our nation. We consider it our privilege to serve your health care needs in any way we can. Services are available to more than 166,000 veterans living in a 35-county area of the Kentuckiana area.

5713 **Louisville VA Regional Office**
Veterans Benefits Administration, U S Dept. of V A
800 Zorn Avenue
Louisville, KY 40206-1433
502-287-4000
800-376-8387
louisville.query@vba.va.gov
www.louisville.va.gov
Wayne L. Pfeffer, MHSA, FACHE, Medical Center Director
Douglas V Paxton, Sr, Associate Director / Operations
Pamala Thompson, RN, MSA, MSN, Associate Director for Patient Care Services
Marylee Rothschild, M.D., Chief of Staff
Since 1952, Robley Rex VAMC has been improving the health of the men and women who have so proudly served our nation. We consider it our privilege to serve your health care needs in any way we can. Services are available to more than 166,000 veterans living in a 35-county area of the Kentuckiana area.

Louisiana

5714 **Alexandria VA Medical Center**
Department of Veterans Affairs
2495 Shreveport Highway
Pineville, LA 71360-9004
318-466-4000
800-375-8387
Fax: 318-483-5029
richard.wright2@va.gov
www.alexandria.va.gov
Martin J. Traxler, Medical Center Director
Yolanda Sanders-Jackson, Associate Director
Jose N Rivera, MD, Acting Chief of Staff
Amy Lesniewski, RN MS, Nurse Executive
The VAMC Alexandria is categorized as a primary and secondary care facility. It is a teaching hospital, providing a full range of primary care services with state-of-the-art technology and education. Comprehensive acute and extended health care is provided on a primary and secondary basis in areas of medicine, surgery, psychiatry, physical medicine and rehabilitation, neurology, oncology, dentistry, geriatrics, and extended care. The Medical Center serves a potential veteran population of over 1

5715 **New Orleans VA Medical Center**
Veterans Health Administration, U S Dept. of V A
1601 Perdido St
New Orleans, LA 70112-1262
504-412-3700
800-935-8387
Fax: 504-589-5210
Stacie.Rivera@med.va.gov
www.neworleans.va.gov
John D Church Jr, Medical Director/President
Fernando Rivera, Association Medical Center Direc
Sam Lucero, Special Assistant to Director
Stacie M Rivera, Public Affairs Officer
A teaching hospital, providing a full range of patient care services, with state-of-the-art technology as well as education and research. Comprehensive health care is provided through primary care, tetiary care, and long-term care in areas of medicine, surgery, psychiatry, physical medicine and rehabilitation, neurology, oncology, dentistry, geriatrics, and extended care.

5716 **Shreveport VA Medical Center**
Veterans Health Administration, U S Dept. of V A
510 E Stoner Ave
Shreveport, LA 71101-4295 318-221-8411
800-827-1000
www.shreveport.va.gov
Shirley M. Bealer, Medical Center Director
Todd M. Moore, Assistant Medical Center Director
Erik J. Glover, Associate Medical Center Director
Ruth Davis, DNS, Associate Director for Patient Care Services

Maine

5717 **Maine VA Regional Office**
Veterans Benefits Administration, U S Dept. of V A
1 VA Center
Augusta, ME 4330-6719 207-623-8411
877-421-8263
togus.query@vba.va.gov
www.va.gov
Dale Demers, Director
Scott Karczewski, Manager

5718 **Togus VA Medical Center**
Veterans Health Administration, U S Dept. of V A
1 VA Center
Augusta, ME 04330-6795 207-623-8411
877-421-8263
Fax: 207-623-5792
g.vhacss@forum.va.gov
Scott Karczewski, Regional Office Director
Denise Benson, Veterans Sevice Center Manager
Gregg Morin, Assistant Veterans Service Center Manager
Tracy Sinclair, Support Services Chief

Maryland

5719 **Baltimore Regional Office**
Veterans Benefits Administration, U S Dept. of V A
31 Hopkins Plz
Baltimore, MD 21201-2825 800-827-1000
baltimore.query@vba.va.gov
www.va.gov
Jerry L Calhoun
The Baltimore Regional Office serves 484,013 veterans living in the State of Maryland, 2% of the national veteran population. The Regional Office's jurisdiction includes all counties in the State of Maryland. The Baltimore Regional Office has an assigned staffing of 218. We provide services at the VA Medical Center in Baltimore and Transition Assistance throughout the State. We actively participate in a homeless veterans outreach program based at the Maryland Center for the Veterans Educatio

5720 **Baltimore VA Medical Center**
Veterans Health Administration, U S Dept. of V A
10 N Greene St
Baltimore, MD 21201-1524 410-605-7000
800-463-6295
Fax: 410-605-7901
g.vhacss@forum.va.gov
www.maryland.va.gov
Dennis H. Smith, Director
Nancy Quailey-Giannopoulis, Associate Director for Operations
Frederick P. Soetje, Associate Director for Finance
David O. Barrett, Acting Chief of Staff
The Baltimore Medical Center is nationally recognized for its outstanding patient safety and state-of-the-art technology, the VA Maryland Health Care System is proud of its reputation as a leader in veterans' health care, research and education.

5721 **Fort Howard VA Medical Center**
Veterans Health Administration, U S Dept. of V A
9600 N Point Rd
Fort Howard, MD 21052-3050 410-477-1800
800-351-8387
Fax: 410-477-7177
www.mdva.state.md.us
Thomas Hutchins, Secretary

5722 **Maryland Veterans Centers**
10 N Greene St
Baltimore, MD 21201-1524 410-605-7000
800-463-6295
Fax: 410-605-7901
www.maryland.va.gov
J Y Jacks, Manager
Dennis H Smith, Executive Director
Veterans medical clinic offering disabled veterans medical treatments.

5723 **Perry Point VA Medical Center**
Veterans Health Administration, U S Dept. of V A
Circle Drive
Perry Point, MD 21902 410-642-2411
800-949-1003
Fax: 410-642-1165
g.vhacss@forum.va.gov
www.maryland.va.gov
Dennis H. Smith, Director
Nancy Quailey-Giannopoulis, Associate Director for Operations
Frederick P. Soetje, Associate Director for Finance
David O. Barrett, Acting Chief of Staff
It is nationally recognized for its outstanding patient safety and state-of-the-art technology, the VA Maryland Health Care System is proud of its reputation as a leader in veterans' health care, research and education.

5724 **VA Maryland Health Care System**
10 N Greene St
Baltimore, MD 21201-1524 410-605-7000
800-463-6295
Fax: 410-605-7900
www.maryland.va.gov
Dennis H. Smith, Director
Nancy Quailey-Giannopoulis, Associate Director for Operations
Frederick P. Soetje, Associate Director for Finance
David O. Barrett, Acting Chief of Staff
A dynamic and exciting health care organization that is dedicated to providing quality, compassionate and accessible care and service to Maryland's veterans. As a part of one of the largest health care systems in the United States, the VAMHCS has a reputation as a leader in veterans' health care, reserch and education. Provides comprehensive service to veterans including medical, surgical, rehabilitative, nurological and mental health care on both an inpatient and outpatient basis.

Massachusetts

5725 **Boston VA Regional Office**
Veterans Benefits Administration, U S Dept. of V A
15 New Sudbury Street
JFK Bldg
Boston, MA 2203-9928 617-232-9500
800-827-1000
boston.query@vba.va.gov
www.boston.va.gov
Liza Catucci, Administrative Officer
Michael Lawson, President

5726 **Edith Nourse Rogers Memorial Veterans Hospital**
Veterans Health Administration U S Deptartment of
200 Springs Rd Bldg #23
Bedford, MA 1730-1114 781-687-2000
800-827-1000
Fax: 781-687-3536
g.vhacss@forum.va.gov
www.bedford.va.gov
Michael Mayo-Smith, Manager

5727 **Northampton VA Medical Center**
Veterans Health Administration, U S Dept. of V A
421 N Main St
Leeds, MA 1062
413-584-4040
800-827-1000
g.vhacss@forum.va.gov
Richard Woloss, Manager

5728 **VA Boston Healthcare System: Brockton Division**
Veterans Health Administration, U S Dept. of V A
940 Belmont St
Brockton, MA 02301-5596
508-583-4500
800-865-3384
Fax: 617-323-7700
g.vhacss@forum.va.gov
www.boston.va.gov
Vincent Ng, Acting Director
Susan A. MacKenzie, PhD, Associate Director
Cecilia McVey, BSN, MHA, CAN, Associate Director Nursing & Patient Care Services
VA Boston Healthcare System's consolidated facility consists of the Jamaica Plain campus, located in the heart of Boston's Longwood Medical Community; the West Roxbury campus, located on the Dedham line; and the Brockton campus, located 20 miles south of Boston in the City of Brockton.

5729 **VA Boston Healthcare System: Jamaica Plain Campus**
Veterans Health Administration, U S Dept. of V A
150 S Huntington Ave
Boston, MA 2130-4817
617-232-9500
800-865-3384
Fax: 617-278-4549
g.vhacss@forum.va.gov
www.boston.va.gov
Vincent Ng, Acting Director
Susan A. MacKenzie, PhD, Associate Director
Cecilia McVey, BSN, MHA, CAN, Associate Director Nursing & Patient Care Services
VA Boston Healthcare System's consolidated facility consists of the Jamaica Plain campus, located in the heart of Boston's Longwood Medical Community; the West Roxbury campus, located on the Dedham line; and the Brockton campus, located 20 miles south of Boston in the City of Brockton.

5730 **VA Boston Healthcare System: West Roxbury Division**
Veterans Health Administration, U S Dept. of V A
1400 VFW Pkwy
West Roxbury, MA 2132-4927
617-323-7700
800-865-3384
g.vhacss@forum.va.gov
www.boston.va.gov
Susan A Mac Kenzie, Associate Director
VA Boston Healthcare System's consolidated facility consists of the Jamaica Plain campus, located in the heart of Boston's Longwood Medical Community; the West Roxbury campus, located on the Dedham line; and the Brockton campus, located 20 miles south of Boston in the City of Brockton.

Michigan

5731 **Aleda E Lutz VA Medical Center**
Veterans Health Administration, U S Dept. of V A
1500 Weiss St
Saginaw, MI 48602-5251
989-497-2500
800-827-1000
Fax: 989-791-2428
g.vhacss@forum.va.gov
www.saginaw.va.gov
Jeff Nechanicky, Acting Medical Center Director
Stephanie Young, Associate Director
Penny Holland, R.N., MSN, Associate Director for Patient Care Svcs
Robert W. Dorr, D.O., JD, CHCQM, Chief of Staff
Since 1950, the Aleda E. Lutz VA Medical Center has been improving the health of the men and women who have so proudly served our nation. We consider it our privilege to serve your health care needs in any way we can. Services are available to more than 31,000 veterans living in the Central and Northern 35 counties of Michigan's Lower Peninsula.

5732 **Battle Creek VA Medical Center**
Veterans Health Administration, U S Dept. of V A
5500 Armstrong Rd
Battle Creek, MI 49037-7314
269-966-5600
888-214-1247
888-214-1247
Fax: 269-966-5483
g.vhacss@forum.va.gov
www.battlecreek.va.gov
Mary Beth Skupien, Director
Edward Dornoff, Associate Director
Kay Bower, Associate Director for Patient Care Services
Dr. Shah, Acting Chief of Staff
Since 1924, the Battle Creek, Michigan VA Medical Center has been improving the health of the men and women who have so proudly served our nation. The Battle Creek VA Medical Center consists of 104 medical and psychiatric beds, 32 residential rehabilitation beds, and 103 nursing home care unit beds. In addition, specialized services offered include a Palliative Care Unit, a Substance Abuse Clinic, a Post Traumatic Stress Disorder Program and a Domicilliary.

5733 **Iron Mountain VA Medical Center**
Veterans Health Administration, U S Dept. of V A
325 East H Street
Iron Mountain, MI 49801-4760
906-774-3300
800-827-1000
Fax: 906-779-3114
g.vhacss@forum.va.gov
www.ironmountain.va.gov
James W. Rice, Medical Center Director
William Caron, FACHE, Associate Medical Center Director
Andrea Collins, RN, MSN, Associate Director for Nursing and Patient Care Service
Grace L. Stringfellow, M.D., Chief of Staff
OGJVAMC is a primary and secondary level care facility with 17 acute care beds, 13 in the medical/surgical ward and 4 in the intensive care unit (ICU). The main facility provides limited emergency and acute inpatient care, and collaborates with larger VA Medical Centers in Milwaukee and Madison, WI, to provide higher-level emergency and specialty care services. OGJVAMC also provides rehabilitation and extended care, including palliative and hospice care, in its 40-bed Community Living Center.

5734 **John D Dingell VA Medical Center**
Veterans Health Administration, U S Dept. of V A
4646 John R St
Detroit, MI 48201-1916
313-576-1000
800-827-1000
Fax: 313-576-1112
g.vhacss@forum.va.gov
www.detroit.va.gov
Pamela J. Reeves, M.D., Director
Annette Walker, M.S.H.A., B.S., Associate Director
Ann M. Herm, R.N., B.S.N., M., Associate Director, Patient Care Services
Scott A. Gruber, M.D., Ph.D., Chief of Staff
Our mission is to provide timely, compassionate and high quality care to those we serve by encouraging teamwork, education, research, innovation, and continuous improvement.

5735 **Michigan VA Regional Office**
Veterans Benefits Administration, U S Dept. of V A
477 Michigan Ave
Patrick V McNamara Federal Building
Detroit, MI 48226-1217
800-827-1000
detroit.query@vba.va.gov
www.benefits.va.gov/detroit
David Leonard, Director
Dennis W Paradowski, Assistant Director
The Regional Office Staff are dedicated to providing responsive and timely service to the veterans of Michigan and their families. Their duties include processing and making decisions on claims for disability compensation, and assisting with applications for a wide range of VA benefits.

5736 **VA Ann Arbor Healthcare System**
Veterans Health Administration, U S Dept. of V A
2215 Fuller Rd
Ann Arbor, MI 48105-2303
734-769-7100
800-361-8387
Fax: 734-761-7870
g.vhacss@forum.va.gov
www.annarbor.va.gov

Robert P. McDivitt, FACHE, Director
Randall E. Ritter, Associate Director
Stacey Breedveld, R.N., Associate Director Patient Care
Ginny Creasman, Assistant Director

Since 1953, the VA Ann Arbor Healthcare System (VAAAHS) has provided state-of-the-art healthcare services to the men and women who have so proudly served our nation. We consider it our privilege to serve your healthcare needs in any way we can.

5737 **Vet Center Readjustment Counseling Service**
1940 Eastern Ave SE
Grand Rapids, MI 49507-2771
616-285-5795
800-905-4675
Fax: 616-285-5898
www.va.gov

William Busby, Executive Director
Branden K Lyon, Counselor
Lynn Hall, Clinical Coordinator

Providing a broad range of counseling outreach and referral services to eligible veterans in order to help make readjustments to cilvilian life.

Minnesota

5738 **Minneapolis VA Medical Center**
Veterans Health Administration, U S Dept. of V A
1 Veterans Dr
Minneapolis, MN 55417-2399
612-725-2000
866-414-5058
Fax: 612-725-2049
g.vhacss@forum.va.gov
www.minneapolis.va.gov

Judy Johnson-Mekota, Director
Erik J. Stalhandske, Associate Director
Kent Crossley, Chief of Staff
Helen Pearlman, Nurse Executive

Minneapolis VA Health Care System (VAHCS) is a teaching hospital providing a full range of patient care services with state-of-the-art technology, as well as education and research. Comprehensive health care is provided through primary care, tertiary care and long-term care in areas of medicine, surgery, psychiatry, physical medicine and rehabilitation, neurology, oncology, dentistry, geriatrics and extended care.

5739 **St. Cloud VA Medical Center**
Veterans Health Administration, U S Dept. of V A
4801 Veterans Dr
Saint Cloud, MN 56303-2015
320-252-1670
800-247-1739
Fax: 320-255-6472
g.vhacss@forum.va.gov
www.stcloud.va.gov

Barry I. Bahl, Director
Cheryl Thieschafer, Associate Director
Meri Hauge, BSN, MSN Nurse, Executive/Associate Director for Patient Care Services
Susan Markstrom, MD, Chief of Staff

Specialty care services include audiology, cardiology, dentistry, hematology, oncology, optometry, orthopedics, podiatry, pulmonology, urology and rheumatology. A new Ambulatory Surgery (same-day) Center opened in the fall of 2011 and will provide access to additional outpatient surgical procedures. The medical center offers extensive mental health programming, including acute psychiatric care, Residential Rehabilitation Treatment programs and an outpatient mental health clinic. The programs u

5740 **St. Paul Regional Office**
Veterans Benefits Administration, U S Dept. of V A
1 Federal Dr
Fort Snelling, MN 55111-4080
800-827-1000
stpaul.query@vba.va.gov
www.benefits.va.gov/stpaul

Vincent Crawford, Director

5741 **Vet Center**
405 E Superior St
Ste 160
Duluth, MN 55802-2240
218-722-8654
877-927-8387
Fax: 218-723-8212
www.vetcenter.va.gov

Cynthia Macaulay MEd, Counselor
Rob Evanson, Counselor
Debbie Burt, Office Manager

Counseling, social services and benefits assistance for combat veterans and those sexually traumatized in the military.

Mississippi

5742 **Biloxi/Gulfport VA Medical Center**
Veterans Health Administration, U S Dept. of V A
400 Veterans Ave
Biloxi, MS 39531-2410
228-523-5000
800-296-8872
Fax: 228-563-2898
g.vhacss@forum.va.gov
www.biloxi.va.gov

Anthony L. Dawson, Director
Nancy Weaver, Associate Director
Kenneth Shimon, Chief of Staff
Margaret G Givens, Assciate Director

5743 **Jackson Regional Office**
Veterans Benefits Administration, U S Dept. of V A
1600 E Woodrow Wilson Ave
Jackson, MS 39216-5100
601-364-7000
800-827-1000
Fax: 601-364-7007
jackson.query@vba.va.gov
www.benefits.va.gov/jackson

Neil Anthony Mcphie, Chairman
Barbara Sapin, Vice Chairman

Missouri

5744 **Harry S Truman Memorial Veterans' Hospital**
Veterans Health Administration, U S Dept. of V A
800 Hospital Dr
Columbia, MO 65201-5275
573-814-6000
800-827-1000
Fax: 573-814-6551
g.vhacss@forum.va.gov
www.columbiamo.va.gov

Sallie Houser-Hanfelder, Director
Robert Ritter, Associate Director
Lana Zerrer, Chief of Staff

5745 **John J Pershing VA Medical Center**
Veterans Health Administration, U S Dept. of V A
1500 N Westwood Blvd
Poplar Bluff, MO 63901-3318
573-686-4151
888-557-8262
Fax: 573-778-4156
g.vhacss@forum.va.gov
www.poplarbluff.va.gov

Merk Hedstrom, Medical Center Director
Linda Haga, Research Contact

5746 **Kansas City VA Medical Center**
Veterans Health Administration, U S Dept. of V A
4801 E Linwood Blvd
Kansas City, MO 64128-2226
816-861-4700
800-827-1000
g.vhacss@forum.va.gov
www.kansascity.va.gov
Kenneth Grasing, Research/Development
Ram Sharma, Administrative Officer
Kent Hill, Executive Director
The Kansas City VA Medical Center is a modern, well-equipped teriary care inpatient and outpatient center. As the third largest teaching hospital in the metropolitan area, it maintains educational affiliations with the University of Kansas School of Medicine.

5747 **St. Louis Regional Office**
Veterans Benefits Administration, U S Dept. of V A
400 S 18th St
Saint Louis, MO 63103-2265
800-827-1000
stlouis.query@vba.va.gov
www.stlouis.va.gov

5748 **St. Louis VA Medical Center**
Veterans Health Administration, U S Dept. of V A
915 N Grand Blvd
Saint Louis, MO 63106-1621
314-652-4100
800-228-5459
Fax: 314-289-7009
g.vhacss@forum.va.gov
www.stlouis.va.gov
Dolores Minor, Administrative Officer

Montana

5749 **Montana VA Regional Office**
3633 Veterans Drive
Fort Harrison, MT 59636-188
406-442-7310
800-827-1000
www.va.gov

5750 **V A Montana Healthcare System**
U S Dept. of V A
3687 Veterans Drive
PO Box 1500
Fort Harrison, MT 59636-1500
406-442-6410
877-468-8387
Fax: 406-447-7916
ftharrison.query@vba.va.gov
www.montana.va.gov
Christine Gregory, Director
Vicki Thennis, Interim Associate Director
Trena Bonde, Chief of Staff
Norlynn Nelson, Associate Director for Patient Care
This is a complete, medically reliable dictionary of congenital malformations and disorders. As the authors explain, 'Down syndrome is the only common congenital disorder, the other defects and disorders are rare or very rare, some having been reported fewer than 20 times worlwide.' This dictionary covers them all. Examples: Aagenaes syndrome, Acrocallosal syndrome, and Acrodysostosis

5751 **VA Montana Healthcare System**
Veterans Health Administration, U S Dept. of V A
1892 William St
Fort Harrison, MT 59636
406-447-7945
800-827-1000
Fax: 406-447-7965
g.vhacss@forum.va.gov
www.montana.va.gov
Joseph Underkofel, Executive Director
Gregory Johnson, MD

5752 **Vet Center**
Readjusment Counciling Service Western Mountain Re
2795 Enterprise Ave.
Suite 1
Billings, MT 59102-3238
406-657-6071
Fax: 406-657-6603
www.va.gov
Bob Phillips, Manager
Luanne Anderson, Office Manager
Barry Osgard MS, Counselor
Readjustment counseling service for counseling veterans who are having difficulty adjusting from military service especially those diagnosed with PTSD.

Nebraska

5753 **Grand Island VA Medical System**
Veterans Health Administration, U S Dept. of V A
2201 N Broadwell Ave
Grand Island, NE 68803-2153
308-382-3660
866-580-1810
g.vhacss@forum.va.gov
John Hilbert, Executive Director
Daniel L Parker, Deputy Director

5754 **Lincoln Regional Office**
Veterans Benefits Administration, U S Dept. of V A
3800 Village Dr.
Lincoln, NE 68501-4103
402-471-4444
800-827-1000
Fax: 402-479-5124
lincoln.query@vba.va.gov
www.veteranprograms.com
Bill Gibson, CEO
Daniel Parker, Deputy Director

5755 **Lincoln VA Medical Center**
Veterans Health Administration, U S Dept. of V A
600 S 70th St
Lincoln, NE 68510-2451
402-489-3802
800-827-1000
Fax: 402-486-7860
g.vhacss@forum.va.gov
Ryon L Adams, Research/Development Coordinator

5756 **VA Nebraska-Western Iowa Health Care System**
Veterans Health Administration, U S Dept. of V A
4101 Woolworth Ave
Omaha, NE 68105-1850
402-449-0610
800-451-5796
Fax: 402-449-0684
www.nebraska.va.gov
Marci Mylan, Director
Rowen Zetterman, Chief of Staff

Nevada

5757 **Las Vegas Veterans Center**
1919 S. Jones, Suite A
Las Vegas, NV 89146-905
702-251-7873
Fax: 702-388-6664
www.lasvegas.va.gov
Daryl Harding, Resident Counselor LCSW
Matt Watson, Team Leader MSW
Veterans clinical counseling center for veterans and their dependent individual and group counseling, marital and family counseling, alcohol and drug assessment referral or treatment. Community education and consultation, employment counseling.

5758 **Reno Regional Office**
Veterans Benefits Administration
1000 Locust St
Reno, NV 89502-2597
775-328-1486
800-827-1000
Fax: 775-328-1447
reno.query@vba.va.gov
www.reno.va.gov
Joseph E Dardillo, Administrative Officer

5759 **VA Sierra Nevada Healthcare System**
Veterans Health Administration, U S Dept. of V A
957 Kirman Ave
Reno, NV 89502-2597
775-786-7200
888-838-6256
Fax: 775-328-1816
www.reno.va.gov
Kurt W. Schlegelmich, Director
Michael C. Tadych, Associate Director
Rachel Crossley, Associate Director
Steve E. Brilliant, Chief of Staff

5760 **VA Southern Nevada Healthcare System**
Veterans Health Administration, U S Dept. of V A
6900 North Pecos Rd
Las Vegas, NV 89086
702-791-9000
800-827-1000
Fax: 707-636-3027
g.vhacss@forum.va.gov
www.lasvegas.va.gov
Isabel M. Duff, Acting Director
Ramu Komanduri, Chief of Staff
Sandra L. Solem, Acting Nurse Executive
John L. Stelsel, Assistant Director

New Hampshire

5761 **Manchester Regional Office**
Veterans Benefits Administration, U S Dept. of V A
275 Chestnut St
Manchester, NH 3101-2411
800-827-1000
manchester.query@vba.va.gov
www.va.gov
Jerry Beale, Director

5762 **Manchester VA Medical Center**
Veterans Health Administration, U S Dept. of V A
718 Smyth Rd
Manchester, NH 03104-7007
603-624-4366
800-892-8384
g.vhacss@forum.va.gov
www.manchester.va.gov
Susan MacKenzie, Acting Med Center Director
Tammy A. Krueger, Associate Director
Andrew J. Breuder, Chief of Staff
Carol Williams, Associate Director for Patients

5763 **New Hampshire Veterans Centers**
103 Liberty St
Manchester, NH 3104-3118
603-668-7060
800-562-3127
Fax: 603-666-7404
www.va.gov
Caryl Ahern, Manager
Paulette Landry, Office Manager
Veterans clinic offering combat veterans outpatient counseling

New Jersey

5764 **Disabled American Veterans: Ocean County**
P.O. Box 1806
Toms River, NJ 8754-1806
732-929-0907
Mary Bencivenga, Contact

5765 **East Orange Campus of the VA New Jersey Healthcare System**
385 Tremont Ave
East Orange, NJ 07018-1023
973-676-1000
Fax: 973-676-4226
www.newjersey.va.gov
Kenneth Mizrach, Director
Glen Giaquinto, Associate Director
John A. Griffith, Associate Director
Patrick J. Troy, Nurse Executive

5766 **Lyons Campus of the VA New Jersey Healthcare System**
Veterans Health Administration, U S Dept. of V A
151 Knollcroft Rd
Lyons, NJ 7939-5001
908-647-0180
800-827-1000
Fax: 908-647-3452
g.vhacss@forum.va.gov
www.newjersey.va.gov
James J Farsetta, Director
Donna Henderson, Coordinator

5767 **Newark Regional Office**
Veterans Benefits Administration, U S Dept. of V A
20 Washington Pl
Newark, NJ 07102-3174
973-645-1441
800-827-1000
newark.query@vba.va.gov
www.newjersey.va.gov
Stephen G Abel, Deputy Commissioner for Veterans

New Mexico

5768 **New Mexico State Veterans' Home**
992 South Broadway
Truth or Consequences, NM 87901-927
575-894-4200
800-964-3976
Fax: 575-894-4270
Lori S Montgomery, Administrator
Carol B Wilson, Admission Coordinator
Veterans medical clinic offering disabled veterans medical treatments.

5769 **New Mexico VA Healthcare System**
Veterans Health Administration, US Dept. of VA
1501 San Pedro Dr SE
Albuquerque, NM 87108-5154
505-265-1711
800-465-8262
Fax: 505-256-2855
g.vhacss@forum.va.gov
www.albuquerque.va.gov
George Marnell, Executive Director
Pamela Crowell, Acting Associate Director
Peter Woodbridge, Chief of Staff
Jennifer DeWinne, Acting Assistant Director

New York

5770 **Albany VA Medical Center: Samuel S Stratton**
Veterans Health Administration, U S Dept. of V A
113 Holland Ave
Albany, NY 12208-3410
518-626-5000
800-233-4810
888-838-7890
Fax: 518-626-5500
g.vhacss@forum.va.gov
www.albany.va.gov
Donald W Stuart, Associate Director (Interim)
Linda W Weiss, Director
Laurdes Irzarry, Chief of Staff
Deborah Spath, Associate Director for Patient/N

5771 **Albany Vet Center**
Ste 2
17 Computer Dr W
Albany, NY 12205-1618
518-458-7998
Fax: 518-458-8613
Lloyd Mc Omber, Owner
Melodie Krahula, Team Leader
Provides readjustment counseling for combat veterans and also provides benefits and job counseling for all veterans.

5772 **Bath VA Medical Center**
Veterans Health Administration U S Deptartment of
76 Veterans Avenue
Bath, NY 14810
607-664-4000
877-845-3247
888-823-9659
Fax: 607-664-4000
g.vhacss@forum.va.gov
www.bath.va.gov
Michael Swartz, Medical Center Director
David B. Krueger, Associate Director
Felipe Diaz, Chief of Staff
Shirley A. Pikula, Associate Director for Patient Services

5773 **Bronx VA Medical Center**
Veterans Health Administration, U S Dept. of V A
130 W Kingsbridge Rd
Bronx, NY 10468-9938
718-584-9000
800-877-6976
Fax: 718-733-1223
g.vhacss@forum.va.gov
www.bronx.va.gov
Eric Langhoff, Director
Vincent F Immiti, Associate Director
Kathleen M. Capitulo, Chief of Staff
Kathleen M Capitulo, Associate Director for Patient C

5774 **Brooklyn Campus of the VA NY Harbor Healthcare System**
Veterans Health Administration, U S Dept. of V A
800 Poly Place
Brooklyn, NY 11209-7104
718-836-6600
800-827-1000
g.vhacss@forum.va.gov
www.nyharbor.va.gov
Martina A Parauda, Director
Veronica J Foy, Associate Director, Facilities &
Michael S Simberkoff, Executive Chief of Staff
Elizabeth H Weinshel, Deputy Chief of Staff

5775 **Buffalo Regional Office - Department of Veterans Affairs**
Veterans Benefits Administration
130 South Elmwood Avenue
Buffalo, NY 14202-2465
716-852-3028
800-827-1000
www.va.gov

5776 **Canandiagua VA Medical Center**
Veterans Health Administration, U S Dept. of V A
400 Fort Hill Ave
Canandaigua, NY 14424-1159
585-394-2000
800-204-9917
g.vhacss@forum.va.gov
www.canandaigua.va.gov
Craig S Howard, Medical Center Director
Margaret Owens, Associate Director
Dr. Robert B Babcock, Chief of Staff
Patricia Hryzak Lind, Associate Director for Patient/N

5777 **Castle Point Campus of the VA Hudson Valley Healthcare System**
Veterans Health Administration, U S Dept. of V A
Route 9D
Castle Point, NY 12511
845-831-2000
800-827-1000
Fax: 845-838-5193
g.vhacss@forum.va.gov
www.hudsonvalley.va.gov
Gerald F Culliton, Director
John M. Gary, Associate Director
Patricia A. Burke, Associate Director
Joanne J. Malina, Chief of Staff

5778 **New York City Campus of the VA NY Harbor Healthcare System**
Veterans Health Administration, U S Dept. of V A
423 E 23rd St
New York, NY 10010-5011
212-686-7500
800-827-1000
Fax: 718-567-4082
g.vhacss@forum.va.gov
www.nyharbor.va.gov
Camille R Varacchi, Administrative Officer

5779 **New York Regional Office**
Veterans Benefits Administration, U S Dept. of V A
245 W Houston St
New York, NY 10014-4805
212-714-0699
800-827-1000
Fax: 212-807-4042
newyork.query@vba.va.gov
www.va.gov
Ronna Brown, President

5780 **Northport VA Medical Center**
Veterans Health Administration, U S Dept. of V A
79 Middleville Rd
Northport, NY 11768-2296
631-261-4400
800-827-1000
Fax: 631-266-6710
g.vhacss@forum.va.gov
www.northport.va.gov
Philip C Moschitta, Medical Center Director
Rosie A Chatman, Associate Director for Patient &
Maria Favale, Associate Director
Edward Mack, Chief of Staff

5781 **Syracuse VA Medical Center**
Veterans Health Administration, U S Dept. of V A
800 Irving Ave
Syracuse, NY 13210-2716
315-425-4400
800-792-4334
888-838-7890
g.vhacss@forum.va.gov
www.syracuse.va.gov
James Cody, VA Medical Center Director
Judy Hayman, Associate Medical Center Director
William H Marx, Chief of Staff
Nancy Schmid, Associate Director for Patient/N

5782 **Torah Alliance of Families of Kids with Disabilities**
T AF KI D
1433 Coney Island Ave
Brooklyn, NY 11230-4119
718-252-2236
Fax: 718-252-2216
Juby Shapiro, Manager
Serves over 1k families whose children have a variety of disabilities and special needs. Many of these families are large families in the low socioeconomic level. Offers monthly meetings, guest lectures, parent matching, information of new developments in software, technology and techniques, sibling support groups, pen pal lists, audio and video library, alternative medicine and nutrition information and education on legal awareness and rights of disabled citizens.

5783 **VA Hudson Valley Health Care System**
Veterans Health Administration, U S Department of
2094 Albany Post Road
Montrose, NY 10548-1454
914-737-4400
Fax: 845-788-4244
www.hudsonvalley.va.gov
James J Farsette, Network Director
Michael Sabo, Executive Director

5784 **VA Western NY Healthcare System, Batavia**
Veterans Health Administration, U S Dept. of V A
222 Richmond Ave
Batavia, NY 14020-1227
585-297-1000
800-827-1000
Fax: 585-786-1258
g.vhacss@forum.va.gov
www.va.gov

William F Feeley, Medical Center Director
Miguel Rainstein, Chief of Staff
Jason C Petti, Associate Medical Center Directo
Royce Calhoun, Assistant Director

5785 **VA Western NY Healthcare System, Buffalo**
Veterans Health Administration, U S Dept. of V A
3495 Bailey Ave
Buffalo, NY 14215-1129
716-834-9200
800-532-8387
www.buffalo.va.gov

Brian Stiller, Medical Center Director
Jason C. Petti, Chief of Staff
Royce Calhoun, Associate Medical Center Directo
Miguel Rainstein, Chief of Staff

North Carolina

5786 **Asheville VA Medical Center**
Veterans Health Administration, U S Dept. of V A
1100 Tunnel Rd
Asheville, NC 28805-2043
828-298-7911
800-932-6408
Fax: 828-299-2502
g.vhacss@forum.va.gov
www.asheville.va.gov

Cynthia Beyfogle, Executive Director
David A. Pattillo, Assistant Medical Director
James Wells, Chief of Staff
Dennis J. Mehring, Public Affairs Officer

5787 **Charlotte Vet Center**
2114 Ben Craig Drive
Charlotte, NC 28262-2350
704-549-8025
Fax: 704-549-8261
www.va.gov

Loretta Deaton, Team Leader
Cynthia Algra, Office Manager
Billy Moore, Counselor
Melissa L Saunders, Counsilor

Preadjustment Counseling for Combat Veterans with Post Traumatic Stress Disorder (PTSD).

5788 **Durham VA Medical Center**
Veterans Health Administration, U S Dept. of V A
508 Fulton St
Durham, NC 27705-3875
919-286-0411
800-827-1000
888-878-6890
Fax: 919-286-5944
www.durham.va.gov

Deanne M Seekins, Director
Rudy A Klopfer, Associate Director
John D Shelburne, Chief of Staff
Kathryn Ward-Presson, Associate Director for Nursing P

Since 1953, Durham Veterans Affairs Medical Cetner has been improving the health of the men and women who have so proudly served our nation. We consider it our privilege to serve your health care needs in any way we can. Services are available to more than 200,000 veterans living in a 26-county area of central and eastern North Carolina.

5789 **Fayetteville VA Medical Center**
Veterans Health Administration, U S Dept. of V A
2300 Ramsey St
Fayetteville, NC 28301-3856
910-488-2120
800-771-6106
Fax: 910-822-7926
g.vhacss@forum.va.gov
www.va.gov

Elizabeth Goolsby, Director
James Galkowski, Associate Director, Operations
Jesse Howard III, Acting Chief of Staff
Joyce Alexander-Hines, Associate Director, Patient Care

Since 1940,the Fayetteville VA Medical Center (VAMC) hasimproved the health of the men and women who have so proudly served our nation. We consider it our privilege to serve your health care needs in any way we can. Medical, mental health, women's health careand specialty servicesare available to more than 157,000 veterans living in a 21-county area of North Carolina and South Carolina.

5790 **WG Hefner VA Medical Center - Salisbury**
Vet Health Administration U S Department of VA
1601 Brenner Ave
Salisbury, NC 28144-2515
704-638-9000
800-469-8252
Fax: 704-638-3395
g.vhacss@forum.va.gov
www.salisbury.va.gov

Kaye Green, Director
Linette Barker, Associate Medical Center Directo
Subbarao Pemmaraju, Chief of Staff (Interim)
Michele Hilll, Associate Director for Patient C

Since 1953, Hefner VAMC has been improving the health of the men and women who have so proudly served our nation. We consider it our privilege to serve your health care needs in any way we can. Primary and secondary inpatient health care are available to more than 287,000 veterans living in a 24-county area of the Central Piedmont Region of North Carolina. This includes the Charlotte area with over 100,000 veterans, and the Winston-Salem area with 65,000 veterans.

5791 **Winston-Salem Regional Office**
Veterans Benefits Administration, U S Dept. of V A
251 N Main St
Winston-Salem, NC 27155-2
336-768-5560
800-827-1000
Fax: 336-768-7295
TTY: 800-829-4833
winsalem.query@vba.va.gov
www.va.gov

Glenn Cobb, Executive VP

North Dakota

5792 **Fargo VA Medical Center**
Veterans Health Administration, U S Dept. of V A
2101 North Elm
Fargo, ND 58102-2417
701-232-3241
800-410-9723
Fax: 701-239-7166
g.vhacss@forum.va.gov
www.va.gov

Michael J Murphy, Healthcare Center Director
Dale DeKrey, Associate Director for Operation
J Brian Hancock, Chief of Staff
Julie Bruhn, Associate Director for Patient C

5793 **North Dakota VA Regional Office - Fargo Regional Office**
Veterans Benefits Administration, U S Dept. of V A
2101 Elm St N
Fargo, ND 58102-2417
701-451-4690
800-410-9723
Fax: 701-451-4690
fargo.query@vba.va.gov
www.fargo.va.gov

Thomas Santoro, Director Research Department

Ohio

5794 **Chillicothe VA Medical Center**
Veterans Health Administration, U S Dept. of V A
17273 State Route 104
Chillicothe, OH 45601-9718
740-773-1141
800-358-8262
888-838-6446
Fax: 740-772-7023
g.vhacss@forum.va.gov
www.chillicothe.va.gov

Wendy J. Hepker, Medical Center Director
Keith Sullivan, Associate Medical Center Directo
Deborah M Meesig, Chief of Staff
Ruth Yerardi, Associate Director for Patient C

The Chillicothe VA Medical Center provides acute and chronic mental health services, primary and secondary medical services, a wide range of nursing home care services, specialty medical services as well as specialized women Veterans health clinics. The facility is an active ambulatory care setting and serves as a chronic mental health referral center for VA Medical Center in southern Ohio and parts of West Virginia and Kentucky

5795 **Cincinnati VA Medical Center**
Veterans Health Administration, U S Dept. of V A
3200 Vine St
Cincinnati, OH 45220-2213
513-861-3100
800-827-1000
888-267-7873
Fax: 513-475-6500
g.vhacss@forum.va.gov
www.cincinnati.va.gov

Linda Smith, Director
David Ninneman, Associate Director
Robert Falcone, Chief of Staff
Katheryn Cook, Nurse Executive

5796 **Cleveland Regional Office**
Veterans Benefits Administration, U S Dept. of V A
1240 E 9th St
Cleveland, OH 44199-2068
800-827-1000
Fax: 216-522-8262
cleveland.query@vba.va.gov
www.va.gov

P Hunter Peckham, Director
Robert Ruff, Assistant Director
William Bunkley, Minority Veterans Program Coordi

5797 **Dayton VA Medical Center**
Veterans Health Administration U S Department of V
4100 W 3rd St
Dayton, OH 45428-9000
937-268-6511
800-368-8262
888-838-6446
Fax: 937-262-2170
g.vhacss@forum.va.gov
www.dayton.va.gov

Glenn Costie, Acting Director
Mark Murdock, Associate Director
James T. Hardy, Chief of Staff
Anna Jones, Associate Director, Patient Care

The Dayton VAMC is a state of the art teaching facility that has been serving Veterans for 146 years, having accepted its first patient in 1867. The Dayton VA Medical Center provides a full range of health care through medical, surgical, mental health (inpatient and outpatient), home and community health programs, geriatric (nursing home), physical medicine and therapy services, neurology, oncology, dentistry, and hospice.

5798 **Louis Stokes VA Medical Center - Wade Park Campus**
Veterans Health Administration, U S Dept. of V A
10701 East Blvd
Cleveland, OH 44106-1702
216-791-3800
877-838-8262
888-838-6446
Fax: 440-838-6017
g.vhacss@forum.va.gov
www.cleveland.va.gov

Susan M Fuehrer, Medical Center Director
Darwin Goodspeed, Associate Medical Center Director
Murray D. Altose, Chief of Staff
Inette Sarduy, Associate Director Patient

Oklahoma

5799 **Jack C. Montgomery VA Medical Center**
Veterans Benefits Administration, U S Dept. of V A
1011 Honor Heights Dr
Muskogee, OK 74401-1318
918-577-3000
800-827-1000
muskogee.query@vba.va.gov
www.muskogee.va.gov

Alef Nancy Graham, Manager

5800 **Jack C. Montomery VA Medical Center**
1011 Honor Heights Dr
Muskogee, OK 74401-1318
918-577-3000
800-827-1000
muskogee.query@vba.va.gov
www.muskogee.va.gov

James R. Floyd, Medical Director
Inez Reitz, Acting Associate Director
Thomas D. Schneider, Chief of Staff
Bonnie R Pierce, Associate Director for Patient C

5801 **Oklahoma City VA Medical Center**
Veterans Health Administration, U S Dept. of V A
921 NE 13th St
Oklahoma City, OK 73104-5007
405-456-1000
800-827-1000
Fax: 405-270-1560
www.oklahoma.va.gov

Jimmy A. Murphy, Director
Debra A. Colombe, Associate Director
Mark Huycke, Chief of Staff
Donna DeLise, Associate Director for Patient C

5802 **Oklahoma Veterans Centers Vet Center**
3033 N Walnut Ave
Ste W101
Oklahoma City, OK 73105-2833
405-270-5184
Fax: 405-270-5125

Peter Sharp, Manager
Steve Kenzie, Owner

PTSP counseling for all combat Veterans and victims of sexual trauma/sexual harassment.

Oregon

5803 **Oregon Health Sciences University**
3181 SW Sam Jackson Park Rd
Portland, OR 97239-3098
503-494-8311
ohsu.edu

Joe Robertson, President
James Morgan, Executive Director

5804 **Portland Regional Office**
Veterans Benefits Administration, U S Dept. of V A
100 SW Main St, Floor 2
Portland, OR 97204-2802
503-373-2388
800-827-1000
portland.query@vba.va.gov
www.va.gov

5805 **Portland VA Medical Center**
Veterans Health Administration, U S Dept. of V A
3710 SW U.S. Veterans Hospital Rd.
Portland, OR 97239-2964
503-220-8262
800-949-1004
Fax: 503-273-5319
g.vhacss@forum.va.gov
www.portland.va.gov

John E Patrick, Director
David Stockwell, Deputy Director of Administratio
Tom Anderson, Chief of Staff
Kathleen M Chapman, Deputy Director for Patient Care

The Portland VA Medical Center (PVAMC) is a 303-bed consolidated facility with two main divisions. The medical center serves as the quaternary referral center for Oregon, Southern Washington, and parts of Idaho for the U.S. Department of Veterans Affairs. The Portland VAMC is located atop Marquam Hill on 28.5 acres overlooking the city of Portland. In addition to comprehensive medical and mental health services, the Portland VAMC supports ongoing research and medical education, including nati

5806 **Roseburg VA Medical Center**
Veterans Health Administration, U S Dept. of V A
913 NW Garden Valley Blvd
Roseburg, OR 97471-6523
541-440-1000
800-549-8387
Fax: 541-440-1225
g.vhacss@forum.va.gov
www.roseburg.va.gov

Jim Willis, Director
Mark Traines, MD

5807 **Southern Oregon Rehabilitation Center & Clinics**
Veterans Health Administration, U S Dept. of V A
8495 Crater Lake Hwy
White City, OR 97503
541-826-2111
800-809-8725
Fax: 541-830-3500
g.vhacss@forum.va.gov
www.southernoregon.va.gov

George Andries, Executive Director

Pennsylvania

5808 **Butler VA Medical Center**
Veterans Health Administration, U S Dept. of V A
325 New Castle Rd
Butler, PA 16001-2418
724-282-7171
800-362-8262
Fax: 724-282-7640
g.vhacss@forum.va.gov
www.butler.va.gov

John Gennaro, Director
Rebecca Hubscher, Associate Director
Sharon Parson, Nurse Executive
Timothy Burke, Chief of Staff

VA Butler Healthcare is located in the heart of Butler County, on the bus line, and convenient to community support services for Western Pennsylvania and Eastern Ohio-area Veterans. We have been attending to Veterans' total care since 1947 and are the health care choice for over 18,000 Veterans - providing comprehensive Veteran care including primary, specialty, and mental health care - as well as health maintenance plans, management of chronic conditions and preventative medicine needs.

5809 **Coatesville VA Medical Center**
Veterans Health Administration, U S Dept. of V A
1400 Blackhorse Hill Rd
Coatesville, PA 19320-2040
610-384-7711
800-290-6172
888-558-3812
g.vhacss@forum.va.gov
www.coatesville.va.gov

Gary Devansky, Director
Sheila Chelleppa, Chief of Staff
Nancy Schmid, Associate Director Patient Care
Jonathan Eckman, Associate Director

5810 **Erie VA Medical Center**
Veterans Health Administration, U S Dept. of V A
135 E 38th Street Blvd
Erie, PA 16504-1559
814-868-8661
800-274-8387
888-860-2124
Fax: 814-860-2425
g.vhacss@forum.va.gov
www.erie.va.gov

Michael Adelman, Medical Center Director
Melissa Sundin, Associate Medical Center Directo
Dr. Anthony Behm, Chief of Staff
Dorene Sommers, Associate Director for Patient C

5811 **James E Van Zandt VA Medical Center**
Veterans Health Administration, U S Dept. of V A
2907 Pleasant Valley Blvd
Altoona, PA 16602-4377
814-943-8164
800-827-1000
Fax: 814-940-7898
g.vhacss@forum.va.gov
www.va.gov

Cecil B Hengeveld, Director
Gerald Williams, Executive Director

5812 **Lebanon VA Medical Center**
Veterans Health Administration, U S Dept. of V A
1700 S Lincoln Ave
Lebanon, PA 17042-7597
717-272-6621
800-409-8771
Fax: 717-228-5907
g.vhacss@forum.va.gov
www.lebanon.va.gov

Robert (Bob) Callahan Jr., Director
Robin C. Aube-Warren, Associate Director
Kanan Chatterjee, Chief of Staff
Margaret G Wilson, Associate Director for Patient C

5813 **Pennsylvania Veterans Centers**
Veterans Health Administration, U S Department of
135 E 38th St
Erie, PA 16504
814-868-8661
800-274-8387
Fax: 717-861-8589
www.erie.va.gov

Michael Aldeman, medical Center Director
Melissa Sundin, Associate Director
Anthony Behm, Chief of Staff

Veterans medical clinic offering disabled veterans medical treatments.

5814 **Philadelphia Regional Office and Insurance Center**
Veterans Benefits Administration, U S Dept. of V A
5000 Wissahickon Ave
Philadelphia, PA 19144-4867
215-336-3003
800-827-1000
Fax: 215-336-5542
phillyro.query@vba.va.gov
www.va.gov

Sonny Dicrecchio, Executive Director

5815 **Philadelphia VA Medical Center**
Veterans Health Administration, U S Dept. of V A
3900 Woodland Avenue
Philadelphia, PA 19104
215-823-5800
800-949-1001
g.vhacss@forum.va.gov
www.philadelphia.va.gov

Joseph M Dalpiaz, Director
Ralph Schapira, Chief of Staff
Margaret O'Shea Caplan, Associate Director for Finance
Patricia O'Kane, Acting Associate Director for Cl

5816 **Pittsburgh Regional Office**
Veterans Benefits Administration
1000 Liberty Avenue
Pittsburgh, PA 15222
412-688-6100
800-827-1000
Fax: 412-688-6121
pittsburgh.query@vba.va.gov
www.pittsburgh.va.gov

Micahel E Moreland

5817 **VA Pittsburgh Healthcare System, University Drive Division**
Veterans Health Administration, U S Dept. of V A
University Dr
Pittsburgh, PA 15240-2400
412-688-6000
866-482-7488
Fax: 412-688-6901
g.vhacss@forum.va.gov
www.pittsburgh.va.gov
Timothy Mar Carlos, CEO

5818 **VA Pittsburgh Healthcare System, Highland Drive Division**
Veterans Health Administration, U S Dept. of V A
7180 Highland Dr
Pittsburgh, PA 15206-1206
412-688-6000
800-827-1000
Fax: 412-365-4213
g.vhacss@forum.va.gov
www.pittsburgh.va.gov
Kristin Best, Deputy Adjutant General
Roger Sutton, MD

5819 **Wilkes-Barre VA Medical Center**
Veterans Health Administration, U S Dept. of V A
1111 E End Blvd
Wilkes Barre, PA 18711-30
570-824-3521
877-928-2621
Fax: 570-821-7278
g.vhacss@forum.va.gov
www.wilkes-barre.va.gov
William H Mills, Director (Interim)
Douglas V Paxton Sr., Associate Director
Mirza Z Ali, Chief of Staff
Linda Stout, Associate Director for Nursing S

Rhode Island

5820 **Providence Regional Office**
Veterans Benefits Administration, U S Dept. of V A
380 Westminster St
Providence, RI 2903-3246
401-462-0324
800-827-1000
Fax: 401-254-2320
providence.query@vba.va.gov
www.va.gov
Daniel Evangelista, Acting Associate Director

5821 **Providence VA Medical Center**
Veterans Health Administration, U S Dept. of V A
830 Chalkstone Ave
Providence, RI 02908-4799
401-273-7100
866-363-4486
Fax: 401-457-3360
g.vhacss@forum.va.gov
www.providence.va.gov
Vincent W Ng, Medical Center Director
William J Burney, Medical Center Associate Directo
Gregory M Gillette, Medical Center Chief of Staff
Deborah A Clickner, Medical Center Associate Directo
To fulfill President Lincoln's promise To care for him who shall have borne the battle, and for his widow, and his orphan by serving and honoring the men and women who are America's veterans.

South Carolina

5822 **Columbia Regional Office**
Veterans Benefits Administration, U S Dept. of V A
6437 Garners Ferry Rd
Columbia, SC 29209-2401
803-401-1094
800-827-1000
columbia.query@vba.va.gov
www.va.gov
Jimmie Ruff, Executive Director

5823 **Ralph H Johnson VA Medical Center**
Veterans Health Administration, U S Dept. of V A
109 Bee St
Charleston, SC 29401-5703
843-577-5011
800-827-1000
888-878-6884
Fax: 843-876-5384
g.vhacss@forum.va.gov
www.charleston.va.gov
Carolyn L Adams, Director
Scott Isaacks, Associate Director
Florence N Hutchinson, Chief of Staff
Mary C Fraggos, Associate Director for Patient/N

5824 **William Jennings Bryan Dorn VA Medical Center**
Veterans Health Administration U S Department of V
6439 Garners Ferry Rd
Columbia, SC 29209-1638
803-776-4000
800-293-8262
Fax: 803-695-6739
www.columbiasc.va.gov
Carolyn L Adams, Director
Barbara Temeck, Chief of Staff
David L. Omura, Chief of Staff
Ruth Mustard, Director for Patient Care/Nursin

South Dakota

5825 **Royal C Johnson Veterans Memorial Medical Center**
Veterans Health Administration, U S Dept. of VA
2501 W. 22nd St
Sioux Falls, SD 57105-5046
605-336-3230
800-316-8387
Fax: 605-333-6878
g.vhacss@forum.va.gov
www.siouxfalls.va.gov
Patrick J Kelly, Director
Sara Ackert, Associate Director
Victor Waters, Chief of Staff
Barbara Teal, Associate Director, Patient Care

5826 **Sioux Falls Regional Office**
Veterans Benefits Administration, U S Dept. of V A
2501 W. 22nd St
Sioux Falls, SD 57105-5046
605-336-3230
800-827-1000
Fax: 605-333-5316
siouxfalls.query@vba.va.gov
www.siouxfalls.va.gov

Tennessee

5827 **Alvin C York VA Medical Center**
Veterans Health Administration, U S Dept. of V A
3400 Lebanon Pike
Murfreesboro, TN 37129-1237
615-867-6000
800-876-7093
Fax: 615-867-5768
g.vhacss@forum.va.gov
www.tennesseevalley.va.gov
Juan Morales, Medical System Director
Janice Cobb, Associate Director, Nursing Serv
Emma Metcalf, Chief Operating Officer

5828 **Memphis VA Medical Center**
Veterans Health Administration, U S Dept. of V A
1030 Jefferson Ave
Memphis, TN 38104-2127
901-523-8990
800-636-8262
g.vhacss@forum.va.gov
www.memphis.va.gov
Jay Robinson III, Associate Medical Center Directo
Douglas D Southall, Assistant Medical Center Directo
Margarethe Hagemann, Chief of Staff
Marilyn Kerkhoff, Interim Associate Medical Center

5829 **Mountain Home VA Medical Center - James H Quillen VA Medical Center**
Veterans Health Administration, US Dept. of VA
Corner of Lamont & Veterans Way
Mountain Home, TN 37684
423-926-1171
877-573-3529
g.vhacss@forum.va.gov
www.mountainhome.va.gov

Charlene S Ehret, Medical Center Director
Jimmy H McGlawn, Associate Director
David R Reagan, Chief of Staff
Linda M McConnell, Associate Director, Patient/Nurs

5830 **Nasheville Regional Office**
Veterans Benefits Administration, U S Dept. of V A
110 9th Ave S
Nashville, TN 37203-3817
800-827-1000
nashville.query@vba.va.gov
www.va.gov

Michael R Walsh, Administrative Officer
Donald H Rubin, Research/Development Coordinator

5831 **Nashville VA Medical Center**
Veterans Health Administration, US Dept. of VA
1310 24th Ave S
Nashville, TN 37212-2637
615-327-4751
800-228-4973
Fax: 615-321-6350
g.vhacss@forum.va.gov
www.tennesseevalley.va.gov

Juan Morales, Medical System Director
Michael A Doukas, Chief of Staff
Gary D Trende, Associate Director, Nursing Serv
Gary D Trende, Chief Operating Officer

Texas

5832 **Amarillo VA Healthcare System**
Veterans Health Administration, U S Dept. of V A
6010 Amarillo Blvd West
Amarillo, TX 79106-1991
806-355-9703
800-687-8262
Fax: 806-354-7869
g.vhacss@forum.va.gov
www.amarillo.va.gov

David Welch, Director
Lance Robinson, Associate Director
Grace Stringfelow, Chief of Staff
Louise Anderson, Executive/Chief, Nursing Service

5833 **Amarillo Vet Center**
Department of Veterans Affairs
3414 Olsen Blvd
Suite E
Amarillo, TX 79109-3072
806-351-1104
Fax: 806-351-1104
www.va.gov

Pedro Garcia Jr., Team Leader
Simon Camarillo, Counsilor
William C Santer, Family Therapist
Cathy L Williams, Office Manager

Provides individual, group and family counseling to veterans who served in combat theaters of World War II and Korea, veterans of the Vietnam Era, and veterans of conflicts zones in Lebanon, Grenada, Panama, the Persian Guld and Somalia.

5834 **El Paso VA Healthcare Center**
Veterans Health Administration, U S Dept. of V A
5001 N Piedras
El Paso, TX 79930-4210
915-564-6100
800-672-3782
Fax: 915-564-7920
g.vhacss@forum.va.gov
www.elpaso.va.gov

John A. Mendoza, Director
Elizabeth Lowery, Associate Director
Homer LeMar, Interim Chief of Staff
Timothy McMurry, Associate Director, Patient Care

5835 **Houston Regional Office**
Veterans Benefits Administration, U S Dept. of V A
6900 Almeda Rd
Houston, TX 77030-4200
713-791-1414
800-827-1000
houston.query@vba.va.gov
www.va.gov

Cecil Aultman, Executive Director
Edgar Tucker, Chief Executive Officer

5836 **Michael E. Debakey VA Medical Center**
Veterans Health Administration, U S Dept. of V A
2002 Holcombe Blvd
Houston, TX 77030-4211
713-791-1414
800-553-2278
g.vhacss@forum.va.gov
www.houston.va.gov

Adam C Walmus, Director
J Kalavar, Chief of Staff
Francisco Vazquez, Associate Director
Thelma Grey-Becknell, Associate Director for Patient C

5837 **South Texas Veterans Healthcare System**
Veterans Health Administration, U S Dept. of V A
7400 Merton Minter
San Antonio, TX 78229-4404
210-617-5300
877-469-5300
888-686-6350
g.vhacss@forum.va.gov
www.southtexas.va.gov

Marie L. Wedon, Director
Wade Vlosich, Associate Director
Joe A. Perez, Assistant Director
Julianne Flynne, Chief of Staff

5838 **VA North Texas Health Veterans Affairs Care System: Dallas VA Medical Center**
Veterans Health Administration, U S Dept. of V A
4500 S Lancaster Rd
Dallas, TX 75216-7167
214-742-8387
800-849-3597
Fax: 214-857-1171
www.northtexas.va.gov/index.asp

Jeffrey Milligan, Director
Peter Dancy, Associate Director
Clark R. Gregg, Chief of Staff
Alan Bernstein, Assistant Director

Health care system which serves veterans with medical care and rehabilitation services including spinal cord injury center. For VA benefit inquiries contact 1-800-827-1000. This system has locations in Bonham, Dallas, and Fort Worth.

5839 **Waco Regional Office**
Veterans Benefits Administration, U S Dept. of V A
4800 Memorial Dr
Waco, TX 76711-1
254-752-6581
800-423-1111
TTY: 800-829-4833
waco.query@vba.va.gov
www.centraltexas.va.gov

William F. Harper, Chief of Staff
Russell E. Lloyd, Associate Director of Resources
Karen Spada, Associate Director for Patients
Andrew Garcia, Assistant Director for Operations

Mission is to honor America's Veterans by providing exceptional health care that improves their health and well being.

5840 **West Texas VA Healthcare System**
Veterans Health Administration, U S Dept. of V A
300 Veterans Blvd
Big Spring, TX 79720-5566
432-263-7361
800-472-1365
Fax: 915-264-4834
g.vhacss@forum.va.gov
www.bigspring.va.gov

Andrew M. Welch, Interim Director
Kenneth Allensworth, Associate Director
Raul Zambrano, Chief of Staff
Charles V. Silveri, Associate Director

The West Texas VA Health Care System (WTVAHCS) proudly serves Veterans in 33 counties across 53,000 square miles of rural geography in West Texas and Eastern New Mexico. The George H. O'Brien, Jr. VA Medical Center is located in Big Spring, Texas and the six Community Based Outpatient Clinics (CBOC's) that comprise the remainder of the health care system are located in Abilene, TX, Stamford, TX, San Angelo, TX, Odessa, TX, Fort Stockton, TX, and Hobbs, NM.

Utah

5841 **Utah Division of Veterans Affairs**
Utah Division of Veterans Affairs
550 Foothill Blvd
Ste 202
Salt Lake City, UT 84113-1106
801-582-1565
800-894-9497
Fax: 801-326-2369
www.saltlakecity.va.gov

David J Peifer, Director
Todd Andrews, Assistant to the Director
Karen H. Gribbin, Manager
Our mission is to serve the veteran who served us. The VA Salt Lake City Health Care System is committed to providing our patients with the highest Quality of Care in an environment that is safe. We do this by focusing on Continuous Process Improvement and by supporting a Culture of Safety

5842 **VA Salt Lake City Healthcare System**
Veterans Health Administration, U S Dept. of V A
500 Foothill Drive
Salt Lake City, UT 84148-1
801-582-1565
800-613-4012
Fax: 801-584-1289
www.saltlakecity.va.gov

Steven W Young, Director
Warren E Hill, Associate Director
Karen H. Gribbin, Chief of Staff
Shella Stovall, Associate Director, Patient Care
Our mission is to serve the veteran who served us. The VA Salt Lake City Health Care System is committed to providing our patients with the highest Quality of Care in an environment that is safe. We do this by focusing on Continuous Process Improvement and by supporting a Culture of Safety

Vermont

5843 **Vermont VA Regional Office Center**
Veterans Benefits Administration
215 N Main St
White River Junction, VT 05009-1
802-295-9363
866-687-8387
Fax: 802-290-6354
whiteriver.query@vba.va.gov
www.whiteriver.va.gov

Deborah Amdur, Executive Director
Danielle S. Ocker, Associate Director
Melanie Thompson, Acting Chief of Staff
Laura F. Miraldi, Associate Director for Nursing
The White River Junction VA Medical Center (WRJ VAMC) is responsible for the delivery of health care services to eligible Veterans in Vermont and the 4 contiguous counties of New Hampshire. These services are delivered at the Medical Center's main campus located in White River Junction, Vermont, and at its seven Outpatient Clinics (Bennington, Brattleboro, Colchester, Newport, and Rutland, Vermont; Keene and Littleton, New Hampshire). The White River Junction VA is closely affiliated with the Ge

5844 **Vermont Veterans Centers**
359 Dorset St
South Burlington, VT 05403-6210
802-862-1806
877-927-8387
Fax: 802-865-3319
www.va.gov

Fred Forehand, Team Leader
William Newkirk, Counsilor
George Troutman, Counsilor
Tamara R Thompson, Family Therapist

Veterans medical clinic offering disabled veterans medical treatments.

Virginia

5845 **Hampton VA Medical Center**
Veterans Health Administration, U S Dept. of V A
100 Emancipation Dr
Hampton, VA 23667-1
757-722-9961
800-827-1000
Fax: 757-728-3135
mike.eisenberg@med.va.gov
www.hampton.va.gov

Deanne M Seekins, Medical Center Director
Benita K Stoddard, Associate Director for Operation
G. Arul, Chief of Staff
Shedale Tindall, Associate Director for Patient C

5846 **Hunter Holmes McGuire VA Medical Center**
Veterans Health Administration, U S Dept. of V A
1201 Broad Rock Blvd
Richmond, VA 23249-1
804-675-5000
800-784-8381
Fax: 804-675-5236
g.vhacss@forum.va.gov
www.richmond.va.gov

Charles E Sepich, Director
David P Budinger, Associate Director
Julie Beales, Interim Chief of Staff
Rita A Duval, Associate Director for Patient C

5847 **Roanoke Regional Office**
Veterans Benefits Administration, U S Dept. of V A
116 North Jefferson St
Roanoke, VA 24016-1906
540-362-1999
800-827-1000
Fax: 540-563-4838
www.va.gov

Roger Bohm, Executive
Bert Boyd, COO/Executive Director

5848 **Salem VA Medical Center**
Veterans Health Administration, U S Dept. of V A
1970 Roanoke Blvd
Salem, VA 24153-6478
540-982-2463
800-827-1000
888-982-2463
Fax: 540-983-1096
g.vhacss@forum.va.gov
www.salem.va.gov

Miguel H LaPuz, Director
Carol S Bogedain, Associate Director
Maureen McCarthy, Chief of Staff
Pearl Washington, Nurse Executive

5849 **Virginia Department of Veterans Services**
270 Franklin Rd SW
Roanoke, VA 24011-2204
540-857-7102
Fax: 540-857-6437

Colbert Boyd, Manager

Washington

5850 **Jonathan M Wainwright Memorial VA Medical Center**
Veterans Health Administration, U S Dept. of V A
77 Wainwright Dr
Walla Walla, WA 99362-3975
509-525-5200
888-687-8863
Fax: 509-946-3062
www.va.gov

Michael W Parnicky, R and D Coordinator

5851 **Seattle Regional Office**
Veterans Benefits Administration
915 2nd Ave
Seattle, WA 98174-1060
206-762-1010
800-827-1000
seattle.query@vba.va.gov
www.va.gov

Va Ad Harabanim, Executive Director
Timothy Williams, Chief Executive Officer

5852 **Spokane VA Medical Center**
Veterans Health Administration, U S Dept. of V A
4815 N Assembly St
Spokane, WA 99205-6185
509-434-7000
800-325-7940
Fax: 509-434-7119
g.vhacss@forum.va.gov
www.spokane.va.gov

Alan Prentiss, Chief of Staff
Dirk Minatre, Coordinator
Joseph Manley, Executive Director

5853 **VA Puget Sound Health Care System**
Veterans Health Administration, U S Dept. of V A
1660 S Columbian Way
Seattle, WA 98108-1532
206-762-1010
800-329-8387
g.vhacss@forum.va.gov
www.pugetsound.va.gov

Michael Fisher, Director
Michael Tadych, Deputy Director
Walt Dannenberg, Assistant Director
William Campbell, Chief of Staff

West Virginia

5854 **Huntington Regional Office**
Veterans Benefits Administration, U S Dept. of V A
640 4th Ave
Huntington, WV 25701-1340
304-525-5131
800-827-1000
Fax: 304-399-9344
huntington.query@vba.va.gov
www.va.gov

Mark Bugher, President

5855 **Huntington VA Medical Center**
Veterans Health Administration, U S Dept. of V A
1540 Spring Valley Dr
Huntington, WV 25704-9300
304-429-6741
800-827-8244
Fax: 304-429-6713
www.huntington.va.gov

Edward H Seiler, Director
Suzanne Jene, Associate Director
Jeffery B Breaux, Chief of Staff
Catherine J Locher, Associate Director for Nursing S

5856 **Louis A Johnson VA Medical Center**
Veterans Health Administration, U S Dept. of V A
1 Medical Center Drive
Clarksburg, WV 26301-4155
304-623-3461
800-733-0512
Fax: 304-626-7048
g.vhacss@forum.va.gov
www.clarksburg.va.gov

William E Cox, Director
Jeffrey A Beiler II, Associate Director
Glenn R Snider, Chief of Staff
Theresa J White, Nurse Executive

5857 **Martinsburg VA Medical Center**
Veterans Health Administration, U S Dept. of V A
510 Butler Avenue
Martinsburg, WV 25405-9990
304-263-0811
800-817-3807
Fax: 304-262-7433
www.martinsburg.va.gov

Ann R Brown, Director
Timothy J Cooke, Associate Medical Center Directo
Jonathan E Fierer, Chief of Staff
Susan George, Nursing Programs and Education

5858 **US Department Veterans Affairs Beckley Vet Center**
200 Veterans Ave
Beckley, WV 25801-4301
304-255-2121
877-902-5142
Fax: 304-254-8711
www.beckley.va.gov

Karin L. McGraw, Director

Vet Center services includes individual and group readjustment counseling, referral for benefits assistance, liason with community agencies, marital and family counseling, substance abuse counseling, job counseling and referral, sexual trauma counseling, and community education.

Wisconsin

5859 **Clement J Zablocki VA Medical Center**
Veterans Health Administration U S Department of V
5000 W National Ave
Milwaukee, WI 53295-1
414-384-2000
888-827-1000
888-469-6614
Fax: 414-382-5319
www.milwaukee.va.gov

Robert H Beller, Director
Michael D Erdmann, Chief of Staff
Judith A Murphy, Associate Director for Patient/N

In an effort to improve access to veterans in Milwaukee County, the VAMC has deployed a mobile clinic that provides primary care four days a week to veterans. The Medical Center also assists the Vet Center located in the City of Milwaukee. In addition, this Medical Center participates in a four-way partnership with the WDVA, the Center for Veterans Issues, Ltd., and the Social Development Commission, to operate Vets Place Central, a 72-bed transitional housing program.

5860 **Tomah VA Medical Center**
Veterans Health Administration, U S Dept. of V A
500 E Veterans St
Tomah, WI 54660-3105
608-372-3971
800-872-8662
Fax: 608-372-1224
www.tomah.va.gov

Mario V. DeSanctis, Medical Center Director
David Huffman, Associate Director
David J. Houlihan, Chief of Staff
Judith E. Broad, Associate Director

VAMCTomah has been improving the health of the men and women who have so proudly served our nation. We consider it our privelege to serve your health care needs in any way we can. Services are available to veterans living in a Western/Central area of Wisconsin.

5861 **William S Middleton Memorial VA Hospital Center**
Veterans Health Administration, U S Dept. of V A
2500 Overlook Ter
Madison, WI 53705-2254
608-256-1901
888-478-8321
888-256-1901
Fax: 608-280-7244
www.madison.va.gov

Judy McKee, Director
John Rohrer, Associate Director
Alan J. Bridges, Chief of Staff
Rebecca Kordahl, Associate Director

5862 **Wisconsin VA Regional Office**
Veterans Benefits Administration, U S Dept. of V A
5000 W National Ave
Milwaukee, WI 53295-1
414-384-2000
800-827-1000
Fax: 414-382-5374
milwaukee.query@vba.va.gov
www.milwaukee.va.gov
Philip L Cook, Executive Director
Neil S Mandel, Research/Development Coordinator
Glen Grippen, CEO
In an effort to improve access to veterans in Milwaukee County, the VAMC has deployed a mobile clinic that provides primary care four days a week to veterans. The Medical Center also assists the Vet Center located in the City of Milwaukee. In addition, this Medical Center participates in a four-way partnership with the WDVA, the Center for Veterans Issues, Ltd., and the Social Development Commission, to operate Vets Place Central, a 72-bed transitional housing program.

Wyoming

5863 **Casper Vet Center**
1030 N. Poplar Suite B
Casper, WY 82601-2665
307-261-5355
Fax: 307-261-5439
www.vetcenter.va.gov
James Whipps, Office Manager
Vet Center offering re-adjustment counseling for combat veterans.

5864 **Cheyenne VA Medical Center**
Veterans Health Administration, U S Dept. of V A
2360 E Pershing Blvd
Cheyenne, WY 82001-5356
307-778-7370
877-927-8387
888-483-9127
Fax: 307-638-8923
www.va.gov
Cynthia McCormack, Medical Center Director
Elizabeth Lowery, Associate Director
Jerry Zang, Chief of Staff
Polly Baird, Associate Director

5865 **Sheridan VA Medical Center**
Veterans Health Administration, U S Dept. of V A
1898 Fort Rd
Sheridan, WY 82801-8320
307-672-3473
800-827-1000
866-822-6714
Fax: 307-672-1639
www.sheridan.va.gov/index.asp
Debra L Hirschman, Director
Michele Beach, Director
Wendell Robison, Chief of Staff
Jane Votaw, Nurse Executive

5866 **Wyoming/Colorado VA Regional Office**
Veterans Benefits Administration, U S Dept. of V A
155 Van Gordon St
Lakewood, CO 80228-1709
303-894-7474
800-827-1000
Fax: 303-894-7442
denver.query@vba.va.gov
www.va.gov
E William Belz, Director

Vocational & Employment Programs

Alabama

5867 **ADRS Lakeshore**
Alabama Department Of Rehabilitation Services
3830 Ridgeway Dr.
Birmingham, AL 35259-9127
205-870-5999
800-441-7609
Fax: 205-879-2685
www.rehab.alabama.gov

Stephen G. Kayes, District 1, Mobile
Jimmy Varnado, District 2, Montgomery
Eddie C. Williams, District 5, Huntsville
Charles Wilkinson, District 6, Birmingham

Rehabilitation offering employment services to severely disabled persons. Programs include Adaptive Driving Training, Assistive Technology; Employability Development, and Vocational Evaluation.

5868 **Alabama Goodwill Industries**
2350 Green Springs Highway S
Birmingham, AL 35205
205-323-6331
www.alabamagoodwill.org

David Wells, President & CEO
Ted Springer, Chair
Roger Cartwright, Vice Chair
Tommy Hughley, Treasurer

The mission of Goodwill is to provide rehabilitation services, training, employment, and opportunities for personal growth to the disabled/disadvantaged.

5869 **Arc of Central Alabama**
6001 Crestwood Blvd
Birmingham, AL 35212
205-323-6383
Fax: 205-323-0085
www.arcofcentralalabama.org

Chris B. Stewart, President & CEO
Mike Mitchell, Senior Vice President & COO
Nancy Cook, Vice President, Clinical Services
N. Brooks Greene, Vice President & CFO

The Arc of Central Alabama provides the following services to people with intellectual and developmental disabilities: day programs; residential services; employment services; early intervention; and advocacy.

5870 **Butler Adult Training Center**
South Central Alabama Mental Health
680 Hardscramble Rd.
Greenville, AL 36037
334-382-2353
Fax: 334-382-9518
www.scamhc.org

5871 **Coffee County Training Center**
South Central Alabama Mental Health
801 Aviation Blvd.
Enterprise, AL 36330
334-393-1732
Fax: 334-347-0252
www.scamhc.org

5872 **Easterseals: Achievement Center**
Easterseals of Alabama
510 W Thomason Circle
Opelika, AL 36801-5499
334-745-3501
866-239-2237
Fax: 334-749-5808
info@achievement-center.org
www.achievement-center.org

Star Wray, Executive Director
Randy Burke, Director, Industrial Operations
Clay Dean, Director, Development Services
Danielle Ellis, Director, Vocational Services

Provides vocational development and extended employment programs for physically, mentally, and developmentally disabled individuals and to non-disabled persons who are culturally, socially, or economically disadvantaged.

5873 **Easterseals: Opportunity Center**
6300 McClellan Blvd
Anniston, AL 36206
256-820-9960
Fax: 256-820-9592
smiles@opportunity-center.com
www.opportunity-center.com

5874 **Montgomery Comprehensive Career Center**
1060 East South Blvd.
Montgomery, AL 36116
334-286-1746
Fax: 334-288-7286
montgomery@alcc.alabama.gov
joblink.alabama.gov

5875 **Vocational Rehabilitation Service (VRS)**
Alabama Department Of Rehabilitation Services
602 S Lawrence St.
Montgomery, AL 36104
334-293-7500
800-441-7607
Fax: 334-293-7383
www.rehab.alabama.gov

5876 **Vocational Rehabilitation Service - Opelika**
Alabama Department Of Rehabilitation Services
520 W Thomason Circle
Opelika, AL 36801
334-749-1259
800-671-6835
Fax: 334-749-8753
TTY: 800-499-1816
www.rehab.alabama.gov

5877 **Vocational Rehabilitation Service - Dothan**
Alabama Department Of Rehabilitation Services
795 Ross Clark Circle NE
Ste 2
Dothan, AL 36303
334-699-8600
800-275-0132
Fax: 334-792-1783
TTY: 800-499-1816
www.rehab.alabama.gov

5878 **Vocational Rehabilitation Service - Gadsden**
Alabama Department of Rehabilitation Services
1100 George Wallace Dr.
Gadsden, AL 35903-6501
256-547-6974
800-671-6839
Fax: 256-543-1784
TTY: 800-499-1816
www.rehab.alabama.gov

5879 **Vocational Rehabilitation Service - Homewood**
Alabama Department Of Rehabilitation Services
236 Goodwin Crest Dr.
Birmingham, AL 35209
205-290-4400
800-671-6837
Fax: 205-290-0486
TTY: 800-499-1816
www.rehab.alabama.gov

5880 **Vocational Rehabilitation Service - Huntsville**
Alabama Department Of Rehabilitation Services
3000 Johnson Rd. SW
Huntsville, AL 35805-5847
256-650-1700
800-671-6840
Fax: 256-650-1795
TTY: 800-499-1816
www.rehab.alabama.gov

Eddie C. Williams, Manager

5881 **Vocational Rehabilitation Service - Jackson**
Alabama Department Of Rehabilitation Services
1401 Forest Ave.
PO Box 1005
Jackson, AL 36545
251-246-5708
800-671-6836
Fax: 251-246-5224
TTY: 800-499-1816
www.rehab.alabama.gov

5882 **Vocational Rehabilitation Service - Jasper**
Alabama Department Of Rehabilitation Services
4505 Hwy 78 E
Suite 300
Jasper, AL 35501
205-221-7840
800-671-6841
Fax: 205-221-1062
TTY: 800-499-1816
www.rehab.alabama.gov

5883 **Vocational Rehabilitation Service - Mobile**
Alabama Department Of Rehabilitation Services
2419 Gordon Smith Dr.
Mobile, AL 36617
251-479-8611
800-671-6842
Fax: 251-478-2197
TTY: 800-499-1816
www.rehab.alabama.gov
Stephen G. Kayes, Manger

5884 **Vocational Rehabilitation Service - Muscle Shoals**
Alabama Department Of Rehabilitation Services
1450 E Avalon Ave.
Muscle Shoals, AL 35661
256-381-1110
800-275-0166
Fax: 256-389-3149
TTY: 800-499-1816
www.rehab.alabama.gov

5885 **Vocational Rehabilitation Service - Selma**
Alabama Department Of Rehabilitation Services
722 Alabama Ave.
Selma, AL 36701
334-877-2927
888-761-5995
Fax: 334-877-3796
TTY: 800-499-1816
www.rehab.alabama.gov

5886 **Vocational Rehabilitation Service - Talladega**
Alabama Department Of Rehabilitation Services
31 Arnold St.
Talladega, AL 35160
256-362-1300
800-441-7592
Fax: 256-362-6387
TTY: 800-499-1816
www.rehab.alabama.gov

5887 **Vocational Rehabilitation Service - Troy**
Alabama Department of Rehabilitation Services
1109 Troy Plaza St.
Troy, AL 36081
334-566-2491
800-441-7608
Fax: 334-566-9415
TTY: 800-499-1816
www.rehab.alabama.gov

5888 **Vocational Rehabilitation Service - Tuscaloosa**
Alabama Department of Rehabilitation Services
1305 James I Harrison Jr Parkway E
Suite 300
Tuscaloosa, AL 35405
205-554-1300
800-331-5562
Fax: 205-554-1369
TTY: 800-499-1816
www.rehab.alabama.gov
William Strickland, Manager

5889 **Vocational Rehabilitation Services - Andalusia**
Alabama Department of Rehabilitation Services
1082 Village Square Dr.
Suite 1
Andalusia, AL 36420
334-222-4114
800-671-6833
Fax: 334-427-1216
TTY: 800-499-1816
www.rehab.alabama.gov

5890 **Vocational Rehabilitation Services - Anniston**
Alabama Department of Rehabilitation Services
1910 Coleman Rd.
Anniston, AL 36207
256-240-8800
800-671-6834
Fax: 256-240-6580
TTY: 800-499-1816
www.rehab.alabama.gov

5891 **Vocational and Rehabilitation Service - Decatur**
Alabama Department of Rehabilitation Services
621 Cherry St. NE
Decatur, AL 35602
256-353-2754
800-671-6838
Fax: 256-351-2476
TTY: 800-499-1816
www.rehab.alabama.gov

5892 **Wiregrass Rehabilitation Center, Inc.**
795 Ross Clark Circle
Suitr 1
Dothan, AL 36303
334-792-0022
Fax: 334-712-7632
www.wrcjobs.com
John Brown, Chair
Gloria Daughtry, Vice Chair
Cynthia Green, Director, Development
Trains individuals to become employable and assists them in finding jobs withing their communities. Also assists individuals who have difficulty maintaining employment, those who are on forms of public assistance such as welfare and those who are employable and underemployed.

5893 **Workshops, Inc.**
4244 3rd Ave. S
Birmingham, AL 35222
205-592-9683
www.workshopsinc.org
Susan Crow, Executive Director
Nathalie Brasher, Director, Programs
Kathy Dunn, Director, Operations
Mary Hendley, Director, Development & Marketing
Provides vocational training, sheltered employment and other support services to people with disabilities in central Alabama.

Alaska

5894 **Alaska Division of Vocational Rehabilitation**
Department of Labor & Workforce Development
PO Box 115516
Juneau, AK 99811-5516
907-465-2814
800-478-2815
Fax: 907-465-2856
TTY: 800-478-2815
dol.dvr.info@alaska.gov
www.labor.state.ak.us/dvr
Duane Mayes, Director
Assists individuals with disabilities to obtain and maintain employment.

5895 **Alaska Job Center Network**
Alaska Department of Labor & Workforce Development
PO Box 115509
Juneau, AK 99811-5509
907-465-2712
Fax: 907-465-4537
www.jobs.alaska.gov

5896 **Alaska State Commission for Human Rights**
800 A St
Suite 204
Anchorage, AK 99501-3669
907-276-7474
800-478-4692
Fax: 907-278-8588
humanrights.alaska.gov

Arizona

5897 **Arizona Developmental Disabilities Planning Council (ADDPC)**
3839 North 3rd St.
Suite 306
Phoenix, AZ 85012
602-542-8970
877-665-3176
Fax: 602-542-8978
addpc@azdes.gov
addpc.az.gov

Erica McFadden, Executive Director
Marcella Crane, Grants Manager
Lani St. Cyr, Fiscal Manager

A successor of the Governor's Council on Developmental Disabilities, the ADDPC serves Arizona residents with developmental disabilities and their families through research, education, advocacy, and financial support. The council aims to improve employment, self-advocacy, and community inclusion.

5898 **Beacon Group**
308 W Glenn St.
Tucson, AZ 85705
520-622-4874
Fax: 520-620-6620
www.beacongroup.org

5899 **Business Enterprise Program (BEP)**
Arizona Department of Economic Security
3425 East Van Buren
Suite 102
Phoenix, AZ 85008
602-774-9100
Fax: 602-250-8548
des.az.gov

Nathan Pullen, Manager
Cindy Kerkemeyer, Assistant Program Manager
Arlynn Robertson, Training Coordinator
Audrey Young, Contracts Manager

Provides employment opportunties for legally blind individuals to own merchandising businesses.

5900 **Division of Developmental Disabilities**
Arizona Department of Economic Security
1789 West Jefferson St.
Phoenix, AZ 85007
844-770-9500
Fax: 602-542-6870
DDDCustomerServiceCenter@azdes.gov
des.az.gov

Laura L. Love, Assistant Director/CEO

Provides supports and serivces that help empower individuals with developmental disabilities to exercise their rights, lead independent lives, and be involved in their communities.

5901 **Fair Employment Practice Agency: Arizona**
Arizona Civil Rights Division
2005 N Central Ave.
Phoenix, AZ 85004-2926
602-542-5236
877-491-5742
Fax: 602-542-8885
TTY: 877-624-8090
www.azag.gov

Dawn Northup, Civil Division Chief

Provides legal advice to most state agencies. The office also investigates and prosecutes consumer fraud, white collar crime, organized crime, public corruption, and civil rights.

5902 **Temporary Assistance for Needy Families (TANF)**
1717 W Jefferson St.
Phoenix, AZ 85007
602-542-9935
www.tanf.us/arizona.html

5903 **Vocational Rehabilitation**
Department of Economic Security
1789 W. Jefferson St.
Phoenix, AZ 85007
602-542-4791
Fax: 602-542-2199
des.az.gov

Michael Trailor, Director
Michael Wisehart, Director, Employment & Rehabilitation

This program serves individuals with disabilities seeking jobs and job training by providing them with services that prepare them for entry or rentry into the workforce.

5904 **Yavapai Regional Medical Center-West**
1003 Willow Creek Rd.
Prescott, AZ 86301
928-445-2700
877-843-9762
yrmc.org

Jane Bristol, Chair
Mike Beatty, Vice Chair
Daniel Storvick, Secretary
Tony Ferrulli, Treasurer

Widely recognized for the quality and success of the physical, occupational, and speech therapy programs it offers. Provides a wide range of programs and services that enable patients to reach their maximum level of function and independence and enjoy the highest possible quality of life.

Arkansas

5905 **Arkansas Department of Workforce Services**
Capitol Mall
Suite 2
Little Rock, AR 72201-2981
501-682-2121
855-225-4440
ADWS.Info@arkansas.gov
www.dws.arkansas.gov/

Daryl Bassett, Director
Ron Snead, Deputy Director
Steve Guntharp, Deputy Director
Don Denton, General Counsel

Provides a wide range of services, including unemployment insurance, employment assistance, and Temporary Assistance for Needy Families.

5906 **Arkansas Rehabilitation Services (ARS)**
525 W. Capitol Ave.
Little Rock, AR 72201
501-296-1600
Fax: 501-296-1141
TTY: 501-296-1669
ACECommunications@arkansas.gov
arcareereducation.org

Charisse Childers, Director
Maria Claudio, Chief Financial Officer
Otis Dixon, Chief Information Officer
Charles McAfee, Director of Communications

The Arkansas Rehabilitation Services prepares people with disabilities to work and lead productive, independent lives.

5907 **Easterseals Arkansas**
3920 Woodland Heights Rd.
Little Rock, AR 72212
501-227-3600
info@eastersealsar.com
www.easterseals.com/arkansas

Ron Ekstrand, President & CEO
Stephanie Smith, Chief Operating Officer
Mac Bell, Vice President, Development & Communication
David Ivers, Vice President, External Affairs

Mission is to provide exceptional services to ensure that all people with disabilities or special needs have equal opportunities to live, learn, work, and play in their communities.

5908 **Vocational Rehabilitation Services**
Arkansas Division of Services for the Blind
700 Main St.
Little Rock, AR 72203
501-682-5463
Fax: 501-682-0366
humanservices.arkansas.gov/about-dhs/dsb

Katy Morris, Director
Cassondra Williams, Assistant Director
Jacqueline Plummer, Chief Fiscal Officer
Jim Pearson, Manager, Business and Technology

A comprehensive state program designed to assess the needs of blind or visually impaired individuals, and to plan, develop, and provide them with employment services.

California

5909 **ABLE Industries, Inc.**
8929 W. Goshen Ave.
Visalia, CA 93291
559-651-8150
888-813-2253
Fax: 559-651-0357
www.ableindustries.org

Wende Ayers, Executive Director
Richard Stadtherr, Controller
Kathy Valencia, Human Resource Manager

Committed to improving the lives of people with disabilities by creating opportunities to maximize their independence through job training, employment, life skills education, and community support services.

5910 **AbilityFirst**
1300 East Green St.
Pasadena, CA 91106
626-396-1010
Fax: 626-396-1021
info@abilityfirst.org
www.abilityfirst.org

Lori Gangemi, President/CEO
Sonhui Robilotta, Chief Financial Officer
Keri Castaneda, Chief Program Officer
Josh Chan, Chief Development Officer

Provides programs and services to help children and adults with physical and developmental disabilities reach their full potential throughout their lives. Offers a broad range of employment, recreational, and socialization programs.

5911 **Achievement House & NCI Affiliates**
3003 Cuesta College Rd.
San Luis Obispo, CA 93405
805-543-9383
www.achievementhouse.org

5912 **Anthesis**
4650 Brooks St.
Montclair, CA 91763
909-624-3555
Fax: 909-624-5675
anthesis.us

Mitch Gariador, Executive Director
Kitty DuBois, Director of Human Resources
Terri Perkins, Director of Work Services
Lucy Yamas-Cortez, Program Director

Anthesis seeks to assist adults with disabilities to reach their full potential through services such as vocational training, employment preparation, and placement services.

5913 **Bakersfield ARC**
2240 S. Union Ave.
Bakersfield, CA 93307-4158
661-834-2272
800-834-3160
dkyle@barc-inc.org
www.barc-inc.org

Jim Baldwin, President/CEO
Kenneth Schmitz, Senior Vice President/Chief Financial Officer
Dave Kyle, Senior Vice President/Chief Compliance Officer
Jeffrey Popkin, Senior Vice President/Director of Operations

A nonprofit organization that provides essential job training, employment, and support services for the developmentally disabled and their families.
1949

5914 **California Department of Fair Employment& Housing**
2218 Kausen Dr.
Suite 100
Elk Grove, CA 95758
800-884-1684
TTY: 800-700-2320
contact.center@dfeh.ca.gov
www.dfeh.ca.gov

Kevin Kish, Director
Joan Keegan, Chief Deputy Director
Jannette Wipper, Chief Counsel
Fahizah Alim, Deputy Director of Communications

The Department of Fair Employment and Housing protects Californians from employment, housing, and public accomodation discrimination, as well as hate violence.

5915 **Colton-Redlands-Yucaipa Regional Occupational Program (CRY-ROP)**
1214 Indiana Ct.
Redlands, CA 92374
909-793-3115
Fax: 909-793-6901
www.cryrop.org

Stephanie Houston, Superintendent
Pilar Tabera, President
Patty Holohan, Vice President
Jane Smith, Clerk

Provides hands-on training programs in over 40 high-demand career fields to assist high school students and adults in acquiring marketable job skills. Works in cooperation with local high schools, adult education colleges, and employers to ensure a coordinated integration of academic and career preparation. Support services, career guidance, and services are provided to disabled people.

5916 **Community Employment Services**
Hope Services
30 Las Colinas Ln.
San Jose, CA 95119-1212
408-284-2850
www.hopeservices.org

Brent Kush, Chief Financial Officer/Interim CEO
Sue Bell, Director of Human Resources
Robert Shuck, Vice President of Retail Operations
Dan Orloff, Vice President of Development

Hope Services provides a comprehensive and integrated employment service that provides job training, job placement, and on-the-job training for individuals with developmental disabilities.

5917 **Continuing Education & Employment Development Program**
The Arc San Francisco
1500 Howard St.
San Francisco, CA 94103
415-255-7200
Fax: 415-255-9488
info@thearcsf.org
www.thearcsf.org

Kristen Pedersen, Director

Preparing individuals with disabilities for employment through real-world experiences, trainings, and internships.

5918 **Desert Haven Enterprises**
43437 Copeland Circle
P.O. Box 2110
Lancaster, CA 93535
661-948-8402
Fax: 661-948-1080
www.deserthaven.org

5919 **Employment Development Department**
P.O. Box 826880
MIC 83
Sacramento, CA 94280-0001
916-654-7799
800-758-0398
www.edd.ca.gov

Patrick W. Henning, Director
Sharon Hilliard, Chief Deputy Director
Dennis Petrie, Deputy Director, Workforce Services
Sandra Clifton, General Counsel

Provides job and unemployment listings, disability insurance, and other information for job seekers and employers.

5920 **Feather River Industries**
Work Training Center
1811 Kusel Rd.
Oroville, CA 95966
530-534-1112
866-214-7994
wtcinc.org/

Don Krysakowski, Executive Director
Brett Barker, Chief Operations Officer
Laura Cater, Chief Financial Officer
Karen Oakes, Director of Human Resources

A division of the Work Training Center, Feather River Industries provides vocational training for persons with developmental disabilities provided through wood products fabrication and assembly tasks.

5921 **Fresno City College: Disabled Students Programs and Services**
Fresno City College
1101 E. University Ave.
Fresno, CA 93741
559-442-8237
Fax: 559-499-6038
TTY: 559-442-8237
campusnews@fresnocitycollege.edu
www.fresnocitycollege.edu
Stephanie Crosby, Director
The Disabled Students Programs & Services (DSPS) at Fresno City College provides services for students with physical, learning and/or psychological disabilities to successfully pursue their individual educational, vocational, and personal goals. Some programs offered include basic computer training, adaptive software training, independent living and consumer skills training, note-taking assistance, special classes, and more.

5922 **Heartland Opportunity Center**
323 N.E. St.
Madera, CA 93638
559-674-8828
Fax: 559-674-8857

5923 **INALLIANCE Inc.**
6950 21st Ave.
Sacramento, CA 95820
916-381-1300
Fax: 916-381-9026
info@inallianceinc.com
inallianceinc.com

5924 **Kings Rehabilitation Center**
490 E. Hanford Armona Rd.
Hanford, CA 93230
559-582-9234
www.kingsrehab.com

5925 **Mother Lode Rehabilitation Enterprises, Inc. (MORE)**
399 Placerville Dr.
Placerville, CA 95667
530-622-4848
Fax: 530-622-0204
www.morerehab.org
Susie Davies, Chief Executive Officer
Debi Harlow, Chair
Nancy Cramer, Vice Chair
Christa Campbell, Secretary
A private, nonprofit organization dedicated to supporting persons with disabilities. Established by parents, educators, rehabilitation professionals, and concerned citizens in 1973, MORE now offers training for social, living, and vocational skills.

5926 **Napa Valley PSI Inc.**
651 Trabajo Ln.
P.O. Box 600
Napa, CA 94559-600
707-255-0177
Fax: 707-255-0802
www.napavalleypsi.org
Carol Gonsalves, President
Raymond Ingersoll, Vice President
Eleanor Cullum, Secretary
Debbie Friesen, Treasurer
Provides work training, work opportunities, and job placement services for developmentally disabled adults. Emphasis is on manufacture of quality wood products, primarily wooden office furniture.

5927 **PRIDE Industries**
10030 Foothills Blvd.
Roseville, CA 95747-7102
916-788-2100
800-550-6005
Fax: 916-788-2578
info@prideindustries.com
www.prideindustries.com
Michael Ziegler, President/CEO
Pete Berghuis, Chief Operating Officer
Jeff Dern, Chief Financial Officer
Alan McMillan, Senior Vice President/Chief Information Officer
Provides vocational and employment services that create jobs for people with disabilites; services include career counseling, vocational assessment, work adjustment, work services, job seeking skills, job development, job placement, on-the-job support (coaching), mentoring, independent living skills, transition services, and case management.

5928 **Parents and Friends, Inc**
306 E. Redwood Ave.
P.O. Box 656
Fort Bragg, CA 95437
707-964-4940
Fax: 707-964-8536
rmoon@parentsandfriends.org
www.parentsandfriends.org
Rick Moon, Executive Director
Michael Hall, President
Jacqueline Bazor, Vice Presdient
Sage Statham, Secretary
Serves people with developmental disabilities by providing them with oppotunities to participate in their community.

5929 **PathPoint**
315 W. Haley St.
Suite 202
Santa Barbara, CA 93101
805-966-3310
Fax: 805-966-5582
info@pathpoint.org
www.pathpoint.org
Henry Bruell, President/CEO
Patricia Enger, Chief Operating Officer
Juliette Ugartechea, Chief Financial Officer
Lynn Storey, Vice President of Human Resources
Dedicated to providing comprehensive training and support services that empower people with disabilities or disadvantages to live and work as valued members of the community.

5930 **People Services, Inc**
4195 Lakeshore Blvd.
Lakeport, CA 95453
707-263-3810
Fax: 707-263-0552
idumont@rocketmail.com
www.peopleservices.org
Ilene Dumont, Executive Director
Cindy Ustrud, President
Kathy Windrem, Vice President
Mike Powers, Secretary
Dedicated to serving as the local community agency, providing the delivery of quality services for people with disabilities.

5931 **Porterville Sheltered Workshop**
194 W. Poplar Ave.
Porterville, CA 93257
559-784-1399
Fax: 559-781-5651
pswcares.org/
Don Sowers, Executive Director
Carol Ledbetter, Director of Program Services
Elizabeth Tellez, Director of Finance
Laura Powell, Director of Human Resources
Provides work adjustment and remunerative work programs. Their mission is to assist disabled individuals achieve a more independent and productive life.

5932 **Project Independence**
3505 Cadillac Ave.
Suite O-103
Costa Mesa, CA 92626
714-549-3464
877-444-0144
Fax: 714-549-3559
info@proindependence.org
www.proindependence.org
Debra Marsteller, President/CEO
Robert Watson, Associate Director
Kristen Cook, Director of Human Resources
Todd Eckert, Director of Development
Promotes civil rights for people with developmental disabilities through services which expand independence and choice.

5933 **Projects with Industry (PWI) Program**
Whittier Union High School District
9401 S. Painter Ave.
Whittier, CA 90605
562-698-8121
www.wuhsd.k12.ca.us
Teri Chan, Benefits Coordinator
Ginni Bachtelle, Mentoring Services
The Transitional and Vocational Services Department runs the PWI program, which focuses on career planning, employment preparation, job placement, and career advancement for individuals with mild to significant disabilities.

5934 **Shasta County Opportunity Center**
1265 Redwood Blvd.
Redding, CA 96003 530-225-5781
Fax: 530-225-5751
oppcenter_info@co.shasta.ca.us
www.co.shasta.ca.us
Donnell Ewert, Director, Health and Human Services Agency
An employment training program for people with disabilities in Shasta County. These individuals perform paid work in a number of different work environments and at the same time learn the skills necessary to obtain competetive employment in the local community.

5935 **Social Vocational Services**
3555 Torrance Blvd.
Torrance, CA 90503 310-944-3303
Fax: 310-944-3304
www.socialvocationalservices.org

5936 **South Bay Vocational Center**
20706 Main St.
Carson, CA 90745 310-817-5116
Info@SBVC1.com
www.sbvc1.com
Willie Martin, Supported Employment Program
Viridiana Salazar, Public Relations
Santiago Lindo, Operations Specialist
Kimberly Scanell, Habilitation Services
A not-for-profit organization that has been providing excellent vocational programs and services for individuals with disabilities.

5937 **The Arc Los Angeles and Orange Counties**
12049 Woodruff Ave.
Downey, CA 90241 562-803-4606
Fax: 562-803-6550
www.thearclaoc.org

5938 **Tri-County Independent Living Center**
139 5th St.
Eureka, CA 95501 707-445-8404
Fax: 707-445-9751
aa@tilinet.org
www.tilinet.org
Donalyn Sjostrand, Executive Director
Gail Pascoe, President
Linda Arnold, Vice President
Kevin O'Brien, Treasurer
Aims to provide programs, services, and information for people with disabilities living in Humboldt, Del Norte, and Trinity Counties in northern California in an effort to allow choices for individuals to optimize their independence.

5939 **Unyeway**
11657 Riverside Dr.
Suite 165
Lakside, CA 92040 619-334-6502
Fax: 619-334-6504
www.unyeway.com
Dave Hager, President
Dr. Richard Ferguson, Vice President
Teresa Gillaspy, Secretary/Treasurer
Mike Reaves, Director
A California nonprofit that provides employment opportunities for adults with developmental disabilities such as job placement programs, remunerative work services, and work adjustment training programs.

5940 **Valley Light Industries**
5360 N. Irwindale Ave.
Baldwin Park, CA 91706 626-337-6200
admin@valleylightind.org
www.valleylight.org
Sage Newman, Executive Director
Ivan Campos, Director of Operations
Linda Ma, Finance Manager
Carole Quintana, Interim Chair of the Board
Aims to recognize the unique capacities of individuals with disabilities, and provide them with the same opportunities of employment.

5941 **Work Training Center**
2255 Fair St.
Chico, CA 95928 530-343-7994
866-214-1790
www.wtcinc.org
Don Krysakowski, Executive Director
Brett Barker, Chief Operations Officer
Laura Carter, Chief Financial Officer
Karen Oakes, Director of Human Resources
A nonprofit organization providing work and leisure services to people with disabilities.

Colorado

5942 **Blue Peaks Developmental Services**
703 Fourth St.
Alamosa, CO 81101-2638 719-589-5135
Fax: 719-589-0680
www.bluepeaks.org
Brooke Hayden, Executive Director
Heather Parga, Director of Human Resources
Anita Kinsey, Finance Director
Tyler Chacon, Operation Director
Provides remunerative work for persons with intellectual and developmental disabilities in the San Luis Valley.

5943 **Cheyenne Village**
6275 Lehman Dr.
Colorado Springs, CO 80918 719-592-0200
Fax: 719-548-9947
TTY: 719-592-0224
info@cheyennevillage.org
www.cheyennevillage.org
Ann M. Turner, Executive Director
Jeanne Solze, Business Director
Jeannie Porter, Development Director
Barbara Kitchen, Human Resources Manager
Serves adults with developmental disabilities and intellectual disabilities in El Paso, Teller, and Park Counties.

5944 **Colorado Civil Rights Divsion**
1560 Broadway
Suite 110
Denver, CO 80202 303-894-7855
800-866-7675
DORA_Customercare@state.co.us
www.colorado.gov/pacific/dora/civil-rights
Marguerite Salazar, Executive Director
Chris Myklebust, Deputy Executive Director
Aubrey Elenis, Director of Civil Rights Division
Marisol Larez, Chief Administrative Officer
Embraces the Department's mission of consumer protection and works to protect individuals from discrimination in employment, housing, and at places of public accommodation through enforcement and outreach consistent with the Colorado Civil Rights Laws.

5945 **Developmental Disabilities Resource Center (DDRC)**
11177 West 8th Ave.
Lakewood, CO 80215 303-233-3363
Fax: 303-467-2793
contact@ddrcco.com
ddrcco.com
Beverly Winters, Executive Director
Rob DeHerrera, Deputy Director/Chief Financial Officer
Jane Byron, Director of Human Resources
Pat Jefferson, Director of Access and Community
Residental and employment programs for adults with developmental and intellectual disabilities.

5946 **Division of Vocational Rehabilitation**
Department of Labor and Employment
633 17th St.
Suite 1501
Denver, CO 80202 303-318-8571
www.colorado.gov/dvr
Steve Anton, Director

Assists people with disabilities to succeed at work and living independently.

5947 **Dynamic Dimensions**
567 18th St.
Burlington, CO 80807 719-346-5367
Fax: 719-346-6010
exdir@dynamicdimensions.org
dynamicdimensions.org

Ginny Hallagin, Executive Director
Jolene Lind, Finance Manager
Debbie Lamm, Program Manager
Kristi Staton, Residential Manager
An organization that provides training, advocacy, job placement, and community involvement for individuals with disabilities.

5948 **Eastern Colorado Services for the Developmentally Disabled (ECSDD)**
617 S. 10th Ave.
Sterling, CO 80751 970-522-7121
Fax: 970-522-1173
www.ecsdd.org

Rhonda Roth, Executive Director
Traci Schrade, Finance Director
Dave Fast, Human Resources
Melissa Dassaro, Case Management Director
Assists developmentally disabled individuals by providing vocational opportunities within their communities.

5949 **Hope Center**
3400 Elizabeth St.
Denver, CO 80205-4801 303-388-4801
Fax: 303-388-0249
gghope@comcast.net
www.hopecenterinc.org

Charlse T. Smith, Chairperson
Sid Davidson, Vice Chairperson
John Hanson, Treasurer
Gerie Grimes, President/CEO
Provides educational and vocational opportunities for special-needs and at-risk children and adults from 2-1/2 to adulthood.

5950 **Imagine!**
1400 Dixon Ave.
Lafayette, CO 80026-2790 303-665-7789
www.imaginecolorado.org

Mark Emery, Executive Director
Laura Ball, Director of Human Resources
Jenna Corder, Director of Client Relations
John Nevins, Chief Financial Officer
Provides support services to people of all ages with developmental delays and cognitive disabilities including Autism Spectrum Disorder, Cerebral Palsy, and Down Syndrome.

5951 **Las Animas County Rehabilitation Center**
1205 Congress Dr.
P.O. Box 781
Trinidad, CO 81082-781 719-846-3388
Fax: 719-846-4543
info@scdds.com
www.scdds.com

Duane Roy, Executive Director
Bernice Whalen, Human Resources Manager
Frank Vialpando, Director of Direct Services
Teri Hansford, Finance Director
Provides job placement programs, remunerative work services, and work adjustment training programs.

Connecticut

5952 **Abilities Without Boundaries**
615 W. Johnson Ave.
Cheshire, CT 06410 203-272-5607
Fax: 203-272-4284
www.abilitieswithoutboundaries.org
Julie Rodriguez, Executive Director
Amanda Barnes, Business Manager
John Casey, Financial Controller
Garfield Wellington, Career Services Coordinator
Formerly known as Cheshire Occupational & Career Opportunities (COCO), Abilities Without Boundaries provides opportunities in the community through employment and social experiences for people with developmental disabilities.

5953 **Allied Community Services**
Three Pearson Way
Enfield, CT 06082 860-741-3701
Fax: 860-741-6870
TTY: 860-741-3701
www.alliedgroup.org
Carol Bohnet, President/CEO
Provides individuals with disabilities or other challenges the opportunity to live and enjoy a productive, independent, and fulfilling life.

5954 **Area Cooperative Educational Services (ACES)**
350 State St.
North Haven, CT 06473 203-498-6800
Fax: 203-498-6890
www.aces.org

Thomas M. Danehy, Executive Director
Carol Bunk, Director of Human Resources
Timothy Howes, Assistant Executive Director, Finance & Operations
Evelyn Rossetti-Ryan, Chief, Marketing & Outreach
Offers adult and vocational programs for persons with disabilities.

5955 **Bureau of Rehabilitation Services**
Department of Rehabilitation Services
55 Farmington Ave.
12th Fl.
Hartford, CT 06105 860-424-4844
800-537-2549
Fax: 860-424-4850
TTY: 860-920-7163
dors.brs.contactus@ct.gov
www.ct.gov/brs

David Doukas, Director
Patti Clay, Brueau Chief
Kathleen Marchione, Bureau Chief
A program which aids disabled persons with preparing for, finding, and keeping employment.

5956 **CCARC, Inc.**
950 Slater Rd.
New Britain, CT 06053-1658 860-229-6665
Fax: 860-826-6883
ccarc@ccarc.com
www.ccarc.com

Anne L. Ruwet, CEO
Julie Erickson, Senior Vice President
Maureen Cardone, Chief Operating Officer
Dawn D'Amato, Vice President of Development
Provides support to people with a variety of disabilities by offering day, residential, recreational, and advocacy services.

5957 **CW Resources**
200 Myrtle St.
New Britain, CT 06053 860-229-7700
Fax: 860-229-6847
info@cwresources.org
www.cwresources.org

Ronald H. Buccilli, President
Offers integrated vocational training and employment opportunities for individuals with a variety of different disabilities.

5958 Connecticut Governor's Committee on Employment of People with Disabilities
Connecticut Department of Labor
200 Folly Brook Blvd.
Wethersfield, CT 06109
860-263-6000
dol.webhelp@ct.gov
www.ctdol.state.ct.us
Jonathan Slifka, Chairperson
The Committee promotes the employment of people with disabilities by developing programs and initiatives to increase statewide employment opportunities for disabled individuals.

5959 Fotheringhay Farms
The Caring Community of CT
84 Waterhole Rd.
Colchester, CT 06415
860-267-4463
Fax: 860-267-7628
info@caringcommunityct.org
caringcommunityct.org

5960 George Hegyi Industrial Training Center
5 Coon Hollow Rd.
Derby, CT 06418
203-735-8727
Fax: 203-735-2204
bob.wood@snet.net
www.varcainc.com
Joan Bucci, Executive Director
Robert Wood, President
Cecelia Staiano-Hayes, Program Manager
A private, nonprofit agency that offers work programs to individuals with special needs.

5961 Goodwill of Southern New England
432 Washington Ave.
North Haven, CT 06473
203-777-2000
888-909-8188
www.goodwillsne.org
Jeffrey D. Machado, President/CEO
Justine Beatini, Transitional Resource Specialist
Shirl Berger, Employee Development & Program
Daniel Burgess, Finance Director
Provides training, education and other services which result in employment and expanded opportunities for people with disabilities and other barriers to employment in order to enhance their capacity for independent living, increased quality of life and work.

5962 Kennedy Center
2440 Reservoir Ave.
Trumbull, CT 06611
203-365-8522
Fax: 203-365-8533
info@kennedyctr.org
www.thekennedycenterinc.org
Richar E. Sebastian, Jr., President/CEO
Stuart Gordon, Vice President of Finance
Lynn Pellegrino, Vice President of HR
Marie Kane, HR Generalist
Provides vocational rehabilitation, job training, and job placement services to adults with disabilities.

Delaware

5963 Delaware Division of Vocational Rehabilitation
Delaware Department of Labor
4425 North Market St.
Wilmington, DE 19802
302-761-8275
TTY: 302-761-8275
www.delawareworks.com
Andrea Guest, Director
Ed Tos, Deputy Director
The state's public program that helps people with physical and mental disabilities obtain or retain employment. DVR's commitment is to help people with disabilities increase independence through employment.

5964 Service Source
3030 Bowers St.
Wilmington, DE 19802
302-762-0300
www.servicesource.org
Janet Samuelson, President/CEO
Mark Hall, Executive Vice President/Chief Strategy Officer
David Hodge, Executive Vice President/Chief Financial Officer
Bruce Patterson, Executive Vice President/Chief Operating Officer
ServiceSource is a leading nonprofit disability resource organization with regional offices and programs located in eight states and the District of Columbia.They offer a range of innovative employment, training, habilitation, housing, and other support services. ServiceSource directly employs more than 1,500 individuals on government and commercial affirmative employment contracts.

District of Columbia

5965 District of Columbia Department of Employment Services
4058 Minnesota Ave. NE
Washington, DC 20019
202-724-7000
Fax: 202-673-6993
TTY: 202-698-4817
does@dc.gov
does.dc.gov
Dr. Unique Morris-Hughes, Director
Their mission is to foster economic development and growth in the District of Columbia by providing workforce training, bringing together job seekers and employers, compensating unemployed and injured workers, and promoting safe and healthy workplaces.

5966 Goodwill of Greater Washington
2200 South Dakota Ave. NE
Washington, DC 20018
202-636-4225
888-817-4323
Fax: 202-526-3994
info@dcgoodwill.org
dcgoodwill.org
Catherine Meloy, CEO
Michael Frohm, Chief Operating Officer
Rosa Proctor, Chief Financial Officer
Brendan Hurley, Chief Marketing Officer
Offers vocational training, job training, sheltered employment, and work experience.

5967 Operation Job Match
National Multiple Sclerosis Society
1800 M St. NW
Suite 750
Washington, DC 20006
202-887-0136
Fax: 202-296-3425
info-dcmd@nmss.org
operationjobmatch.org
Cyndi Zagieboylo, President/CEO
Tami Caesar, Chief Financial Officer
Paul Weiss, Chief Operating Officer
Eric Hilty, Chief Legal Officer
Job readiness program for individuals with adult-onset physical disabilities.

5968 Palladium
1331 Pennsylvania Ave. NW
Suite 600
Washington, DC 20004
202-775-9680
thepalladiumgroup.com
Kim Bredhauer, Managing Director/CEO
Residential and employment programs for adults with developmental disabilities.

5969 Rehabilitation Services Administration
400 Maryland Ave. SW
Washington, DC 20202-2800
202-245-7488
www2.ed.gov

5970 **The District of Columbia Office of Human Rights (OHR)**
441 4th St. NW
Suite 570 North
Washington, DC 20001
202-727-4559
Fax: 202-727-9589
TTY: 711
ohr@dc.gov
ohr.dc.gov

Monica Palacio, Director

Upholds local and federal human rights laws, and aims to eradicate discrimination and increase equal opportunity for residents of the District of Columbia.

Florida

5971 **Abilities of Florida: An Affiliate of Service Source**
2735 Whitney Rd.
Clearwater, FL 33760
727-538-7370
servicesource.org

Janet Samuelson, President/CEO
Mark Hall, Executive Vice President/Chief Strategy Officer
David Hodge, Executive Vice President/Chief Financial Officer
Bruce Patterson, Executive Vice President/Chief Operating Officer

Provides a full range of employment services including work evaulation, training, job coaching, job placement, advocacy, and education. Also provides housing assistance and specialized to adults with cystic fibrosis.

5972 **Able Trust, The**
3320 Thomasville Rd.
Suite 200
Tallahassee, FL 32308
850-224-4493
Fax: 850-224-4496
info@abletrust.org
www.abletrust.org

Susanne Homant, President/CEO
Guenevere Crum, Senior Vice President
Allison Chase, Vice President of Youth Services
Michelle Young, Director of Finance

Provides grant funds for employment-related programs for non-profit agencies in Florida. Assists families, individuals, and agencies through educational conferences and youth training programs. Provides businesses free resources for hiring people with disabilities.

5973 **Florida Division of Blind Services**
325 West Gaines St.
Turlington Building, Suite 1114
Tallahassee, FL 32399-0400
850-245-0300
800-342-1828
Fax: 850-245-0363
dbs.myflorida.com

Robert Doyle, Director

An organization that aims to help blind and visually impaired individuals have access to tools, support, and oppotunities in order to live independent lives. Offers a Vocational Rehabilitation program for adults, and a Transition Services program for young adults.

5974 **Florida Division of Vocational Rehabilitation**
4070 Esplanade Way
Tallahassee, FL 32399-7016
800-451-4327
Fax: 850-245-3399
rehabworks.org

5975 **Florida Fair Employment Practice Agency**
Florida Commission on Human Relations
4075 Esplanade Way
Room 110
Tallahassee, FL 32399
850-488-7082
800-342-8170
Fax: 850-487-1007
fchrinfo@fchr.myflorida.com
fchr.state.fl.us

Michelle Wilson, Executive Director

The Commission is the state agency charged with enforcing the state's civil rights laws and serves as a resource on human relations for the people of Florida.

5976 **Goodwill Life Skills Development Program**
Goodwill Industries-Suncoast, Inc.
10596 Gandy Blvd.
St. Petersburg, FL 33702
727-523-1512
888-279-1988
Fax: 727-579-0850
TTY: 727-579-1068
goodwill-suncoast.org

Heather Ceresoli, Chair
Martin W. Gladysz, Senior Vice Chair
Loiuse R. Lopez, Vice Chair
Deborah A. Passerini, President

A training program that enables people with developmental disabilities to gain independence by practicing job skills.

5977 **Goodwill Temporary Staffing**
Goodwill Industries-Suncoast, Inc.
10596 Gandy Blvd.
St. Petersburg, FL 33702
727-523-1512
888-279-1988
Fax: 727-579-0850
TTY: 727-579-1068
goodwill-suncoast.org

Heather Ceresoli, Chair
Martin W. Gladysz, Senior Vice Chair
Loiuse R. Lopez, Vice Chair
Deborah A. Passerini, President

Provides employment links from potential employees, both disabled and non-disabled alike to employers with immediate employment opportunities seeking qualified candidates. Pre-screening on all applicants includes employment history, personal references, law enforcement background checks, and substance screening.

5978 **Goodwill's Community Employment Services**
Goodwill Industries-Suncoast, Inc.
10596 Gandy Blvd.
St. Petersburg, FL 33702
727-523-1512
888-279-1988
Fax: 727-579-0850
TTY: 727-579-1068
goodwill-suncoast.org

Heather Ceresoli, Chair
Martin W. Gladysz, Senior Vice Chair
Louise R. Lopez, Vice Chair
Deborah A. Passerini, President

Provides employment opportunities for people with developmental disabilities. Community Employment Services offer on-the-job training and check ups from a support facilitator.

5979 **Goodwill's Job Connection Center**
Goodwill Industries-Suncoast, Inc.
10596 Gandy Blvd.
St. Petersburg, FL 33702
727-523-1512
888-279-1988
Fax: 727-579-0850
TTY: 727-579-1068
www.goodwill-suncoast.org

Heather Ceresoli, Chair
Martin W. Gladysz, Senior Vice Chair
Louise R. Lopez, Vice Chair
Deborah A. Passerini, President

A local, community-based space where people can search for employment. The center offers carrer planning and exploration, employability workshops, and training.

5980 **Goodwill's JobWorks**
Goodwill Industries-Suncoast, Inc.
10596 Gandy Blvd.
St. Petersburg, FL 33702
727-523-1512
888-279-1988
Fax: 727-579-0850
TTY: 727-579-1068
www.goodwill-suncoast.org

Heather Ceresoli, Chair
Martin W. Gladysz, Senior Vice Chair
Louise R. Lopez, Vice Chair
Deborah A. Passerini, President

A program that provides employment for people with disabilities at MacDill Air Force Base in dining or postal services.

5981 **Lighthouse Central Florida**
215 East New Hampshire St.
Orlando, FL 32804
407-898-2483
lighthousecentralflorida.com
Lee Nasehi, President/CEO
Kyle Johnson, Vice President/Chief Sales & Marketing Officer
Donna Amundson, Vice President/Chief Financial Officer
Kaleb Stunkard, Vice President/Chief Information & Operations Officer
Lighthouse Central Florida (LCF) is the only nonprofit organization offering comprehensive, professional, vision rehabilitation services to Central Floridians of all ages with low vision or blindness.

5982 **One-Stop Service Center**
Goodwill Industries-Suncoast, Inc.
10596 Gandy Blvd.
St. Petersburg, FL 33702
727-523-1512
888-279-1988
Fax: 727-579-0850
TTY: 727-579-1068
goodwill-suncoast.org
Heather Ceresoli, Chair
Martin W. Gladysz, Senior Vice Chair
Louise R. Lopez, Vice Chair
Deborah A. Passerini, President
Provides universal job search and placement related services to any person entering the service center. Each One-Stop Services Center provides on-site representation from a variety of employment-related service providers. All Centers host and/or facilitate local employment fairs and provides access to computerized job postings.

5983 **Palm Beach Habilitation Center**
4522 South Congress Ave.
Palm Springs, FL 33461
561-965-8500
Fax: 561-433-8816
pbhab.com
David Lin, Chief Executive Officer
Jeffrey Chapman, Chief Financial Officer
Jean-Marie Moore, Director of Programs & Services
Jacqueline Nicholson, Director of Development
Providing work evaluation, work adjustment, job placement, employment, residential, and retirement services for mentally, emotionally, and physically disabled adults.

5984 **Primrose Center**
2733 South Ferncreek Ave.
Orlando, FL 32806
407-898-7201
www.primrosecenter.org
Bill McCormac, Chief Executive Officer
Donna Spence, Chief Financial Officer
Leslie North, President/Chair
Vicki Gillett, Secretary
A nonprofit organization that aims to transform the lives of people with developmental disabilities by providing opportunities to achieve their fullest potential. Primrose Center offers an Adult Day Program and an Employment Services Program, which provide opportunities for individuals with intellectual and developmental disabilities to gain employment.

5985 **Project SEARCH**
Goodwill Industries-Suncoast, Inc.
10596 Gandy Blvd.
St. Petersburg, FL 33702
727-523-1512
888-279-1988
Fax: 727-579-0850
TTY: 727-579-1068
www.goodwill-suncoast.org
Heather Ceresoli, Chair
Martin W. Gladysz, Senior Vice Chair
Louise R. Lopez, Vice Chair
Deborah A. Passerini, President
A program for students with disabilities that provides work experience.

5986 **Quest, Inc.**
PO Box 531125
Orlando, FL 32853
407-218-4300
888-807-8378
Fax: 407-218-4301
contact@questinc.org
www.questinc.org
John Gill, President & CEO
Brooke Eakins, Chief Operating Officer
Todd Thrasher, Chief Financial Officer
John Dogaer, Chief Information Officer
Quest helps individuals with developmental disabilities in Central Florida achieve their goals by providing services that increase their capabilities and quality of life. Quest serves more than 1,000 individuals each day in the Orlando and Tampa areas.

5987 **Quest, Inc. - Tampa Area**
3910 US Hwy. 301 N
Tampa, FL 33619
813-423-7700
888-807-8378
Fax: 813-423-7701
contact@questinc.org
www.questinc.org
John Gill, President & CEO
Brooke Eakins, Chief Operating Officer
Todd Thrasher, Chief Financial Officer
John Dogaer, Chief Information Officer
Quest helps individuals with developmental disabilities in Central Florida achieve their goals by providing services that increase their capabilities and quality of life. Quest serves more than 1,000 individuals each day in the Orlando and Tampa areas.

5988 **SCARC, Inc.**
213 West McCollum Ave.
Bushnell, FL 33513
352-793-5156
Fax: 352-793-6545
scarcinc.com

5989 **Seagull Industries for the Disabled**
3879 Byron Dr.
West Palm Beach, FL 33404
561-842-5814
www.seagull.org
Barbara Nurenberg, President/CEO
Linda Moore, Chief Operating Officer
Joyce Hambrick, Director of Program Services
Ellen Hoffacker, Vice President of Finance
Dedicated to improving the quality of life of mentally, physically, and emotionally challenged adults in Palm Beach County, Florida through advocacy and the provision of a variety of social service, vocational training, and residential programs designed to encourage self reliance and independence.

Georgia

5990 **Fair Housing and Equal Employment**
Georgia Commission on Equal Opportunity
7 Martin Luther King, Jr. Dr., SE
3rd Floor-Suite 351
Atlanta, GA 30334
404-463-4706
Fax: 404-656-4399
gceo@gceo.state.ga.us
www.gceo.state.ga.us
Joy Lampley-Fortson, Executive Director/Administrator
Allona L. Cross, Fair Housing Division Director
Ryan Brown, Equal Employment Division Director
The mission of the Commission on Equal Opportunity is to investigate housing and employment discrimination in the state of Georgia.

5991 **Goodwill Career Centers**
Goodwill of North Georgia
2201 Lawrenceville Hwy.
Suite 300
Decatur, GA 30033
404-420-9900
goodwillng.org
Keith T. Parker, President/CEO
Jenny Taylor, Vice President of Career Services
Employment training, assessment, and job placement for people who have disabilities and/or are disadvantaged. The center also

provides access to computers and phones to aid in acquiring employment.

5992 **Griffin Area Resource Center**
931 Hamilton Blvd.
Griffin, GA 30224
770-228-9919
Fax: 770-228-9920
griffinarearesourcecenter.com
Lisa Sassaman, Executive Director
Connie Moody, Director of Support Services
Kim Byrom, Day Support Supervisor
Kim Coggins, Employment Specialist
A CARF (The Rehabilitation Accreditation Commission) accredited Employment and Community Support organization providing daily services to participants with disabilities from 16 years of age and up in a 5 county area.

5993 **IBM National Support Center**
P.O. Box 2150
Atlanta, GA 30301-2150
800-426-2133
TTY: 800-284-9482
www.skepticfiles.org/md001/mobility.htm

5994 **New Ventures**
306 Fort Dr.
LaGrange, GA 30240
706-882-7723
newventures.org
Dave Miller, CEO
Kelly Anderson, Quality Director
Christopher Jarrod Poole, Director of Human Resources
Mike Wilson, Director of Industrial Marketing
A rehabilitation and work training facility for individuals with barriers to employability. The program utilizes community based industrial work of varying levels of difficulty. A return to work conditioning program for the industrially injured is offered which features first-day contact, workers compensation rehabilitation team management, and light-duty work conditioning. A training stipend is paid to defray costs associated with training.

5995 **Vocational and Rehabilitation Agency**
1718 Peachtree St. NW
Suite 376 S.
Atlanta, GA 30309
404-206-6000
844-367-4872
gvs.georgia.gov/
Sean T. Casey, Executive Director
Kevin Harris, Deputy Executive Director
Purpose is to assist eligible individuals with disabilities to become productive members of the Georgia workforce and to live independently.

Hawaii

5996 **Assets School**
One Ohana Nui Way
Honolulu, HI 96818
808-423-1356
Fax: 808-422-1920
info@assets-school.net
assets-school.net
John F. Morton, Chairman
Kristi L. Maynard, Vice Chairman
Kent R. Lau, Secretary
Paul Singer, Head of School
Assets School serves gifted and capable students, specializing in those with dyslexia and other language-based learning differences. They provide a strength-based program, complemented by outreach and training, that empowers students to become effective learners and confident self-advocates.

5997 **Hawaii Fair Employment Practice Agency**
Hawaii Civil Rights Commission
830 Punchbowl St.
Room 411
Honolulu, HI 96813
808-586-8636
Fax: 808-586-8655
TTY: 808-586-8692
DLIR.HCRC.INFOR@hawaii.gov
labor.hawaii.gov/hcrc
William Hoshijo, Executive Director
HCRC enforces state laws prohibiting discrimination in employment.

5998 **Hawaii Vocational Rehabilitation Division**
600 Kapiolani Blvd.
Room 304
Honolulu, HI 96813
808-586-9741
Fax: 808-586-9755
humanservices.hawaii.gov/vocationalrehab/
Maureen Bates, Administrator
Susan Foard, Assistant Administrator
Provides services to Hawaiian residents who experience barriers to employment due to physical or cognitive disabilities.

5999 **Lanakila Rehabilitation Center**
1809 Bachelot St.
Honolulu, HI 96817
808-531-0555
TTY: 808-531-0555
info@lanakilapacific.org
www.lanakilapacific.org
Marian Tsuji, President
Dwayne Masutani, Director of Budget & Finance
Kathleen Racuya-Markrich, Director of Human Resources
Darren Lee, Manager of Information Technology
Lanakila is a private nonprofit organization whose mission is to provide services and supports that assist individuals with physical, mental, or age-related challenges to live as independently as possible within their community. A broad range of services are offered which include meal/senior services, community based adult day programming for individuals with disabilities, work training opportunities, and extended/supported employment for individuals with special needs.

6000 **Services for the Blind Branch**
Division of Vocational Rehabilitation
1901 Bachelot St.
Honolulu, HI 96817
808-586-5275
Fax: 808-586-5361
humanservices.hawaii.gov/vocationalrehab/
Lea Dias, Administrator
Provides employment services to Hawaiian residents who are blind or have visual impairments.

Idaho

6001 **Idaho Commission for the Blind & Visually Impaired**
341 W. Washington St.
P.O. Box 83720
Boise, ID 83720- 0012
208-334-3220
800-542-8688
Fax: 208-334-2963
bcunningham@icbvi.idaho.gov
www.icbvi.state.id.us
Beth Cunningham, Administrator
Bailie Welton, Management Assistant
Mike Walsh, Rehabilitation Services Chief
Jeff Weeks, Vocational Rehabilitation Counselor
A state agency that provides vocational rehabilitation, independent living training, medical intervention, adaptive technology and devices, and employer advocacy.

6002 **Idaho Department of Labor**
317 W. Main St.
Boise, ID 83735
208-332-3570
Fax: 208-334-6300
www@labor.idaho.gov
labor.idaho.gov
Melinda S. Smyser, Director
Provides workforce services and connects job seekers with employers.

6003 **Idaho Division of Vocational Rehabilitation**
650 W. State St.
Room 150
Boise, ID 83720
208-334-3390
Fax: 208-334-5305
vr.idaho.gov
Jane Donnellan, Administrator
Nanna Hanchett, Deputy Administrator

Vocational Rehabilitation assists many individuals with disabilities to go to work. With VR assistance, these individuals have overcome numerous obstacles and disability related barriers to achieve employment.

6004 **Idaho Governor's Committee on Employment of People with Disabilities**
317 W. Main St.
Boise, ID 83735
208-332-3750
Fax: 208-327-7331
www.dol.gov

6005 **Idaho Human Rights Commission**
317 W. Main St.
Boise, ID 83735-0660
208-334-2873
888-249-7025
Fax: 208-334-2664
HRC.inquiry@labor.idaho.gov
humanrights.idaho.gov

Benjamin Earwicker, Administrator
Carmen Barney, Senior Civil Rights Investigator
Rick Rhodes, Senior Civil Rights Investigator
Administers state and federal anti-discrimination laws in Idaho in a manner that is fair, accurate, and timely. Works towards ensuring that all people within the state are treated with dignity and respect in their places of employment, housing, education, and public accomodations.

Illinois

6006 **Ada S. McKinley Community Services, Inc.**
1359 W. Washington Blvd.
Chicago, IL 60607
312-554-0600
Fax: 312-554-0292
info@adasmckinley.org
adasmckinley.org

Jamal Malone, Chief Executive Officer
Peter Greetis, Director of Information Technology
Crystal Officer, Vice President Of Program Operations
Sandor Szajkovics, Chief Financial & Administrator Officer
Mission is to serve those who, because of disabilities or other limiting conditions, need help in finding and pursuing paths leading to healthy, productive, and fulfilling lives.

6007 **Anixter Center**
6610 N. Clark St.
Chicago, IL 60626
773-973-7900
Fax: 773-973-5268
TTY: 773-973-2180
AskAnixter@anixter.org
anixter.org

Rebecca Clark, President/CEO
Eric Gastevich, Chair
Steve Gilson, Treasurer
Tanya Curtis, Secretary
A Chicago-based human services agency that assists people with disabilities to live and work successfully in the community. Anixter Center provides vocational training, employment services, residences, special education, prevention programs, community services, and health care. In addition, Anixter Center offers Illinois' only substance abuse treatment programs specifically for people with disabilities including Addiction Recovery of the Deaf.

6008 **C-4 Work Center**
4740 North Clark St.
Chicago, IL 60640
773-769-0205
888-968-7282
infoc4@c4chicago.org
www.c4chicago.org

Chris Carroll, President/CEO
Kelly Craig Gates, Chief Administrative Officer
Rachel Howland, Director of Human Resources
A social service provider that offers aftercare, case finding, information and referrals, vocational training, and work activities offered to mentally ill persons.

6009 **Clearbrook**
1835 W. Central Rd.
Arlington Heights, IL 60005
847-870-7711
Fax: 847-870-7741
TTY: 847-870-2239
info@clearbrook.org
www.clearbrook.org

Anthony Di Vittorio, President
Don Frick, Vice President of Information Technology
Emma Hershey, Vice President of Finance
Rosa Baez-Lopez, Vice President of Human Resources
A nonprofit organization that offers educational, employment, and residential services to the developmentally disabled children and adults.

6010 **Cornerstone Services**
777 Joyce Rd.
Joliet, IL 60436
815-741-7600
877-444-0304
Fax: 815-723-1177
cornerstoneservices.org

Ben Stortz, President/CEO
Susan Murphy, Vice President/Chief Human Resources Officer
Kim Hudgens, Vice President/Chief Operating Officer
Michelle Allen, Vice President/Chief Development Officer
Cornerstone Services provides progressive, comprehensive services for people with disabilities, promoting choice, dignity, and the opportunity to live and work in the community. Established in 1969, the agency provides developmental, vocational, employment, residential, and behavioral health services at various community-based locations. The nonprofit social service agency helps approximately 750 people each day.

6011 **Fulton County Rehab Center**
500 N. Main St.
Canton, IL 61520
309-647-6510
www.fultoncountyrehabilitationcenter.com

6012 **Glenkirk**
3504 Commercial Ave.
Northbrook, IL 60062
847-272-5111
Fax: 847-272-7350
info@glenkirk.org
glenkirk.org

Arthur G. Fess, Chair
Roger Baron, Vice Chair
Dr. Bruce Bennin, Secretary
A nonprofit organization serving people in north and northwest Chicago that helps infants, children, and adults with developmental disabilities reach higher levels of independence. Glenkirk's residential, vocational, educational, and support programs include services which provide individual evaluation, therapeutic treatment, and training.

6013 **Illinois Life Span Program**
The Arc of Illinois
20901 LaGrange Rd.
Suite 209
Frankfort, IL 60423
800-588-7002
www.illinoislifespan.org

Meg Cooch, Executive Director
Janet Donahue, Director of Development
Deb Fornoff, Life Span Director
A program of The Arc of Illinois that provides resources, advocacy, and services to individuals of all ages with developmental or intellectual disabilities. The program aims to help individuals with disabilities participate fully in their community.

6014 **Jewish Vocational Services**
216 West Jackson Blvd.
Suite 700
Chicago, IL 60606
855-463-6587
info@jvschicago.org
www.jvschicago.org/

Howard Sitron, President/CEO
Wendy Platt Newberger, Vice President/Chief Operating Officer
Vincent Everson, Vice President/Chief Financial Officer
Stacey Show, Vice President/Chief Development Officer
Occupational training and job placement for handicapped persons of all religions.

6015 **Kennedy Job Training Center**
St. Coletta's of Illinois, Inc.
18350 Crossing Dr.
Tinley Park, IL 60487
708-342-5200
Fax: 708-342-2579
www.stcil.org

Andrea Ramirez-Justin, Chairperson
Jeff Kowalis, Board Member
Daniel Michalak, Board Member
Annette Skafgaard, Executive Director

St. Coletta's of Illinois offers vocational evaluation, vocational training work adjustment training, and job placement services for developmentally disabled and hearing impaired persons.

6016 **Knox County Council for Developmental Disabilities**
2015 Windish Dr.
Galesburg, IL 61401
309-344-2600
Fax: 309-344-1754
kccdd.com

Mark Rudolph, Chief Executive Officer
Pam Green, Chief Operating Officer
Jeff Gomer, Chief Financial Officer
Lynndel Messmore, Director of Rehabilitation Services

Offers developmental training, vocational evaluation, work adjustment training, extended training, placement, and supported employment.

6017 **Kreider Services**
500 Anchor Rd.
Dixon, IL 61021-0366
815-288-6691
Fax: 815-288-1636
TTY: 815-288-5931
kreiderservices.org

Mike Hickey, President
Dr. Richard L. Piller, Vice President
Don Vock, Secretary/Treasurer
Cheryl Ebens, Director

A private nonprofit organization that offers day service programs, vocational training programs, job placement, supported employment, respite care, residential and family support for children ages 0-3.

6018 **Lambs Farm**
14245 W. Rockland Rd.
Libertyville, IL 60048
847-362-4636
info@lambsfarm.org
lambsfarm.org

6019 **Land of Lincoln Goodwill Industries**
1220 Outer Park Dr.
Springfield, IL 62704
217-789-0400
info@llgi.org
www.llgi.org

Sharon Durbin, President/CEO
Ron Culves, Vice President of Finance
Brian Durbin, Vice President of Retail Operations
Corey Edens, Vice President of Information Technology

Empowers people with special needs to become self-sufficient through the power of work.

6020 **Orchard Village**
7660 Gross Point Rd.
Skokie, IL 60077
847-967-1800
Fax: 847-967-1801
ov@orchardvillage.org
www.orchardvillage.org

Allison Stark, President/CEO
Erika Vavrik, Director of Development
Jennifer Gentile, Vice President of Programs
Jennifer Burgess, Director of Residential Services

Vocational program and counseling, respite services and community living group homes for the disabled and cognitively impaired. Orchard village also operates a private school especially devoted to teaching young adults independent living and skills necessary to flourish in the community.

6021 **Sertoma Centre**
4343 W. 123rd St.
Alsip, IL 60803
708-371-9700
Fax: 708-371-9747
sertomacentre.org

Gus van den Brink, Executive Director
Paula Phillips, Assistant Executive Director
Robert Straz, President
Frank Tomecek, Vice President

A nationally accredited, not-for-profit agency that provides services to students and adults with developmental disabilities and mental illness. MIssion is to provide opportunities that empower individuals with disabilities to achieve success.

6022 **Shore Training Center**
Shore Community Services
8350 Laramie Ave.
Skokie, IL 60077
847-982-2030
Fax: 847-982-2039
TTY: 847-581-0076
info@shoreservices.org
shoreservices.org

India Alexia Ehioba, CEO

Mission is to improve the quality of life for citizens with developmental disabilities through community based services providing education/training.

6023 **The Workshop**
706 West St.
P.O. Box 6087
Galena, IL 61036-6087
815-777-2211
Fax: 815-777-3386
theworkshopgalena.org

Peg Tonne, Chairperson
Bob Gable, Vice Chairperson
Jean Muchow, Treasurer
Lynn Berning, Executive Director

An organization that provides services to individuals with disabilities in Jo Daviess County such as intake and referral, early intervention for children, vocational evaluation, and work adjustment training services.

6024 **Thresholds**
4101 N Ravenswood Ave.
Chicago, IL 60613
773-572-5500
contact@thresholds.org
www.thresholds.org

Mark Ishaug, Chief Executive Officer
Mark Furlong, Chief Operating Officer
Brent Peterson, Chief Development Officer
Al Shoreibah, Chief Financial Officer

Provider of recovery services for persons with mental illnesses and substance abuse disorders in Illinois. It offers 30 programs at more than 75 locations throughout Chicago and surrounding suburbs and counties. Services include case management, housing, employment, education, psychiatry, primary care, substance use treatment, and research.

6025 **Vocational Rehabilitation Services**
Illinois Department of Human Services
100 South Grand Ave. East
Springfield, IL 62762
800-843-6154
www.dhs.state.il.us

6026 **Washington County Vocational Workshop**
781 E. Holzhauer Dr.
Nashville, IL 62263
618-327-3348

Indiana

6027 ADEC Resources for Independence
19670 State Rd. 120
P.O. Box 398
Bristol, IN 46507
574-848-7451
877-342-8954
info@adecinc.com
adecinc.com

Donna Belusar, President/CEO
Mitch Walorski, Vice President/CFO
Jessica Koscher, Chief Development Officer
Lisa Kendall, Vice President of Human Resources
Serves individuals of all ages with developmental disabilities and delays, as well as visual or physical impairments.

6028 Arc Northwest Indiana
2650 West 35th Ave.
Gary, IN 46408
219-884-1138
Fax: 219-980-7315
btrowbridge@ArcNWI.com
www.arcnwi.com

William Trowbridge, Executive Director
Dan Sutton, Board President
James Brown, Vice President
Joya Williams, Vice President
The Arc Northwest Indiana serves people with intellectual and developmental disabilities and their families by providing programs that aren't adressed by governmental agencies or local providers.

6029 BI-County Services
425 East Harrison St.
Bluffton, IN 46714
260-824-1253
Fax: 260-824-1892
bi-countyservices.com

6030 Carey Services
2724 S. Carey St.
Marion, IN 46953
765-668-8961
Fax: 765-664-6747
info@careyservices.com
www.careyservices.com

James Allbaugh, President/CEO
Yolanda Kincaid, Chief Operations Officer
David Smith, Director of Finance
Bonnie Smith, Director of Human Resources
The mission of Carey Services is to create pathways towards self-sufficiency with personal satisfaction. Carey Services offers employment training and job coaching services.

6031 Evansville Association for the Blind
500 North 2nd Ave.
Evansville, IN 47710
812-422-1181
www.evansvilleblind.org/

Karla Horrell, Executive Director
Prince Samuel, President
Fred Dormeier, Vice President
Dave Emge, Vice President
A nonprofit ogranization that offers employment services to people who are visually impaired.

6032 Four Rivers Resource Services
P.O. Box 249
Hwy. 59 South
Linton, IN 47441
812-847-2231
fourrivers@frrs.org
frrs.org

Kenton Barnes, President
Mary Lou Chapman, Vice President
Ray Hart, Treasurer
Kathy Pennington, Secretary
Employment; community living; connections; follow-along; early intervention; preschool; healthy families; child care resource, referral, and child care voucher program; impact; and transpotation services.

6033 Gateway Services/JCARC
3500 North Morton St.
P.O. Box 216
Franklin, IN 46131
317-738-5500
www.gatewayarc.com

6034 Goodwill of Central & Southern Indiana
1635 W. Michigan St.
Indianapolis, IN 46222
317-524-4313
goodwill@goodwillindy.org
www.goodwillindy.org

Kent A. Kramer, President/CEO
Daniel J. Riley, Senior Vice President/CFO
Cindy L. Graham, Vice President of Marketing
Jay C. Lytle, Vice President/CIO
Offers employment services such as vocational rehabilitation, employer support, and job coaches for individuals with disabilities.

6035 Indiana Civil Rights Commission
100 North Senate Ave.
Room N300
Indianapolis, IN 46204
317-232-2600
800-628-2909
Fax: 317-232-6580
TTY: 800-743-3333
info@icrc.in.gov
www.in.gov/icrc

Gregory L. Wilson, Sr., Executive Director
Doneisha Posey, Deputy Director/General Counsel
Pamella Cook, Chief Financial Officer
Tyler Bracken, Communications Coordinator
Works to develop public policies that ensure equal opportunity in education to all and enforces the civil rights laws of the State of Indiana.

6036 Indiana Disability Employment Initiative
Indiana Department of Workforce Development
10 North Senate Ave.
Indianapolis, IN 46204
800-891-6499
www.in.gov/dwd/2416.htm

6037 New Hope Services
725 Wall St.
Jeffersonville, IN 47130
812-288-8248
info@newhopeservices.org
newhopeservices.org

James A. Bosley, President/CEO
John Broady, Senior Vice President/CFO
Bonnie Long, Senior Vice President/CAO
Jody Reschar, Executive Vice President/COO
Mission is to provide hope through services which are responsive to individual needs. New Hope Services offers a vocational training program for individuals with intellectual or physical disabilities.

6038 New Horizons Rehabilitation
237 Six Pine Ranch Rd.
Batesville, IN 47006
812-934-4528
contact@nhrinc.org
www.nhrinc.org/

Marie Dausch, Executive Director
Darryl Myers, Finance Director
Monica McCory, Director of Adult Services
Provides training and services to children and adults with mental/physical disabilities. The Community Employment services helps individuals ages 14 and up acquire employment.

6039 Noble Of Indiana
Noble, Inc.
7701 East 21st St.
Indianapolis, IN 46219
317-375-2700
Fax: 317-375-2719
www.mynoblelife.org

Julia Huffman, President/CEO
Judy Tidwell, Chief Financial Officer
Erin Hardwick, Director of Pre-Vocational Services
Lorayna Blue, Director of Community Living
Since 1953, Noble of Indiana has been dedicated to its mission: to create opportunities for people with developmental disabilities to live meaningful lives.

6040 **Paladin**
4315 East Michigan Blvd.
Michigan City, IN 46360 219-874-4288
Fax: 219-874-2689
Paladin@paladin.care
www.paladin.care

William S. Trowbridge, President/CEO
Evelyn Marvel, Chief Financial/Operations Officer
Erin Mooneyhan, Development & Marketing Officer
Shalanda Robinson, Corporate Compliance Officer
A nonprofit organization that offers pre-vocational and employment services to individuals with disabilities.

6041 **Putnam County Comprehensive Services**
630 Tennessee St.
Greencastle, IN 46135 765-653-9763
Fax: 765-653-3646
aranck_pccs@yahoo.com
www.pccsinc.org

Andrew Ranck, Executive Director
Terri Hayes, Chief Financial Officer
Teresa Human, Community Living Services Director
Lea Ann Bowman, Human Resource Director
A not-for-profit organization serving individuals with disabilities and similar characteristics in Indiana. Their mission is to provide services to individuals with disabilities in order for them to reach their optimum potential in attitudes, habits, and skills through training and integration, making them contributing members of their community, and to promote community awareness and acceptance of people with different abilities.

6042 **Southern Indiana Resource Solutions**
1579 S. Folsomville Rd.
Boonville, IN 47601 812-897-4840
Fax: 812-897-0123
www.sirs.org

Kelly Mitchell, CEO/President
Adult services including jobs, community connections, and residential and childrens services, including service coordination and all therapies.

6043 **Sycamore Rehabilitation Services**
1001 Sycamore Ln.
P.O. Box 369
Danville, IN 46122-1474 317-745-4715
866-573-0817
Fax: 317-745-8271
info@sycamoreservices.com
sycamoreservices.com

Terry Kessinger, President
Steve Patterson, Vice President
Carol Thralls, Treasurer
Peg Murphy, Secretary
Provides training and services for persons with disabilities that enhance independence in all areas of life.

Iowa

6044 **Access, Inc.**
20 5th St. NW
Hampton, IA 50441 641-456-2532
jennybacker@accessincorporated.org
www.accessincorporated.org

Jenny Backer
A nonprofit organization providing residential and vocational services in Franklin, Butler, and Hardin counties in the state of Iowa. Residential Services include RCF/MR services, Supported Community Living Services, and Community Supervised Apartment Living Arrangement Services. Vocational Services include Work Services and Supported Employment Services. Accredited by the Commission on Accreditation of Rehabilitation Facilities since 1984, and serves individuals with a wide range of needs.

6045 **Iowa Career Connection**
1503 42nd St.
Suite 133
West Des Moines, IA 50266 515-282-5823
contact@iowacareerconnection.com
www.iowacareerconnection.com

L.M. (Al) Fering, President
Tom Cox, Managing Partner
Specializes in accounting and human resources talent acquisition in the Upper-Midwest.

6046 **Iowa Civil Rights Commission**
400 E. 14th St.
Des Moines, IA 50319-0201 515-281-4121
800-457-4416
Fax: 515-242-5840
www.state.ia.us/government/crc

Kristin H. Johnson, Executive Director
A neutral, fact-finding administrative agency that enforces the 'Iowa Civi Rights Act of 1965,' Iowa's anti-discrimination law. The commission doesn not provide legal representation. The commission's vision is a state free of discrimination.

6047 **Iowa Economic Development Authority**
200 East Grand Ave.
Des Moines, IA 50309 515-348-6200
www.iowaeconomicdevelopment.com

Debi Durham, Director
To engender and promote economic development policies and practices which stimulate and sustain Iowa's economic growth and climate and that integrate efforts across public and private sectors.

6048 **Iowa Valley Community College**
3702 S. Center St.
Marshalltown, IA 50158 641-752-4643
800-284-4823
ivinfo@iavalley.edu
www.iavalley.edu/

Christopher Duree, Chancellor
Robin Anctil, Director of Marketing
Jim Wilson, Chief Information Officer
Kathy Pink, Vice Chancellor of District Finance/CFO
Offers two levels of specialized vocational preparatory programming for adults with disabilities. The Career Development Center serves dependent adults. The goal of the program is to maintain or improve skills to enable persons served to enter sheltered or supported employment. The IRP/CBVT programs are non-credit specialized vocational programs for independent adults served by Vocational Rehabilitation and our programs. The goals are for competitive placements in jobs. CARF accredited.

6049 **Iowa Vocational Rehabilitation Services**
510 East 12th St.
Jessie Parker Building
Des Moines, IA 50319-0240 515-281-4211
Fax: 515-281-7645
TTY: 800-532-1486
www.ivrs.iowa.gov/index.html

David Mitchell, Administrator
Kenda Jochimsen, Bureau Chief
Charlie Levine, Assistant Bureau Chief
Iowa Vocational Rehabilitation Services aims to help individuals with disabilities achieve their employment, independence, and economic goals.

6050 **New Focus**
102 W. Washington St.
Centerville, IA 52544 641-437-1722
Peggy Oden, Executive Director
Provides vocational services for adults with disabilities. Includes work activity, supported employment, and supported community living.

Kansas

6051 Kansas Human Rights Commission
900 SW Jackson St.
Suite 568-S
Topeka, KS 66612-1258
785-296-3206
Fax: 785-296-0589
www.khrc.net
Ruth Glover, Executive Director
William Wright, Assistant Director
Mission is to assure equal opportunities in employment, public accommodations, and housing, as well as to prevent discrimination.

6052 Kansas Vocational Rehabilitation Agency
Department for Children & Families
555 S. Kansas
3rd Fl.
Topeka, KS 66603
785-368-7471
866-213-9079
Fax: 785-368-7467
TTY: 785-368-7478
www.dcf.ks.gov
Gina Meier-Hummel, Secretary
Helps people with disabilities achieve employment and self-sufficiency. Also links employers with qualified and productive individuals to meet thier work force needs.

Kentucky

6053 Kentucky Commission on Human Rights
332 West Broadway
Louisville, KY 40202
800-292-5566
kchr.ky.gov/Pages/default.aspx
George W. Stinson, Chair
Robert Asseo, Commissioner
Duane Bonifer, Commissioner
Carol L. Jackson, Commissioner
The state government authority that enforces the Kentucky Civil Rights Act, making it unlawful to discriminate in the areas of employment, financial transactions, housing, and public accommodations.

6054 Kentucky Office for the Blind
275 East Main St.
Frankfort, KY 40621
502-564-4754
800-321-6668
Fax: 502-564-6745
cora.mcnabb@ky.gov
blind.ky.gov
Cora McNabb, Acting Executive Director
Tiffany Smither, Fiscal Administrator
The Office for the Blind offers a wide variety of employment services aimed at providing the skills and opportunities for independence to individuals with visual disabilities.

6055 Kentucky Vocational Rehabilitation Agency
275 East Main St.
Mail Drop 2-EK
Frankfort, KY 40621
502-564-4440
800-372-7172
Fax: 502-564-6745
WFD.VOCREHAB@ky.gov
kcc.ky.gov/Vocational-Rehabilitation/
Becky Cabe, Acting Executive Director
Susie Edwards, Rehabilitation Program Admin
Pat Cruse, CO Administrator
Assists eligible individuals with disabilities achieve their employment goals.

6056 Pioneer Vocational/Industrial Services
150 Corporate Dr.
P.O. Box 1396
Danville, KY 40422
859-236-8413
800-527-4198
Fax: 859-238-7115
TTY: 859-236-1251
pioneer@pioneerservices.org
Mike Pittman, Executive Director
Danny Rigney, Director of Marketing and Operations
Mission is to provide vocational development and extended employment programs to people who are disabled and/or disadvantaged, and to assist them in maximizing independent living skills.

Louisiana

6057 Blind Services
Louisiana Rehabilitation Services
1001 North 23rd St.
P.O. Box 94094
Baton Rouge, LA 70804-9094
225-342-3111
Fax: 225-342-7960
www.laworks.net/
Shannon Joseph, Director, Office of Workforce Development
A section of the Louisiana Rehabilitation Services, Blind Services offers employment opportunities to individuals who are blind or visually impaired.

6058 COEA The Arc of East Ascension
1122 E. Ascension Complex Blvd.
Gonzales, LA 70737
225-621-2000
Fax: 225-621-2022
opportunities@eatel.net
www.coeathearc.com
Norma Dukes, Executive Director
Sharon Morris, Director of Public Relations & Marketing
Gerrie Noto, Human Resources Manager
Niecka Pate, Program Coordinator
Committed to affording individuals the opportunities that reflect and support their choices, dignity, individuality, self-determination, community, coherency, and common sense. The Arc of East Ascension offers educational, employment, community, housing, and recreational services.

6059 Louisiana Rehabilitation Services
Office of Workforce Development
1001 North 23rd St.
P.O. Box 94094
Baton Rouge, LA 70804-9094
225-342-3111
Fax: 225-342-7960
owd@lwc.la.gov
www.laworks.net/WorkforceDev/LRS/LRS_Main.asp
Ava Dejoie, Executive Director
Kenneth A. Burrell, Deputy Executive Director
Rob Roux, Executive Counsel
Bennett Soulier, Chief Financial Officer
Provides services for job seekers and job training programs for individuals with disabilities. Programs include Blind Services and Vocational Rehabilitation.

6060 The Arc Westbank
401 Gretna Blvd.
Gretna, LA 70053
504-361-1131
westbankarc.org/

6061 Vocational Rehabilitation Program
Office of Workforce Development
1001 North 23rd St.
P.O. Box 94094
Baton Rouge, LA 70802-9094
225-342-3111
Fax: 225-342-7960
www.laworks.net
Shannon Joseph, Director, Office of Workforce Development
Offers individuals with disabilities a wide range of services designed to provide them with the skills and resources needed to compete in the interview process, get the job, keep the job, and develop a lifetime career.

Maine

6062 Addison Point Agency
312 Water St.
P.O. Box 207
Addison, ME 04606-0207
207-483-6500
Fax: 207-483-2817
rchartrand@addisonpoint.org
www.addisonpoint.org

Ruth Chartrand, Executive Director of Operations

Provides services to individuals who have intellectual and developmental disabilities, cerebral palsy, autism spectrum disorder, and other disabilities. Provides training services to place these individuals in community employment.

6063 Bangor Veteran Center: Veterans Outreach Center
615 Odlin Rd.
Suite 3
Bangor, ME 04401
207-947-3391
Fax: 207-941-8195
www.maine.va.gov

Kirk Grant, Vet Center Director
George Runnells, Veterans Outreach Specialist
Chad Becker, Office Manager

Readjustment counseling services for veterans of Vietnam, Vietnam Era, Persian Gulf, Panama, Grenada, Lebanon, Somalia, WWII and Korean conflicts, as well as Iraq, Afganistan, and military sexual trauma.

6064 Creative Work Systems
10 Speirs St.
Westbrook, ME 04092
207-879-1140
Fax: 207-879-1146
creativeworksystems.com

Heidi Howard, Executive Director
Edward McGeachey, President
Jim Houle, Vice President
Sam Marcisso, Treasurer

Provides residential, day habilitation, and supported employment services in Central and Southern Maine.

6065 Division for the Blind and Visually Impaired
Bureau of Rehabilitation Services
150 State House Station
Augusta, ME 04333-0150
207-623-6799
Fax: 207-287-5292
www.maine.gov/rehab/dbvi/index.shtml

6066 Maine Commission on Disability & Employment
State Workforce Board
45 Commerce Dr.
Augusta, ME 04330
207-621-5087
SWB.DOL@maine.gov
www.maine.gov

Jennifer Kimble, Chair

Established in 1997, the Commission aims to influence policy related to employment for people with disabilities.

6067 Maine Department Of Labor
54 State House Station
Augusta, ME 04333-0054
207-623-7900
mdol@maine.gov
www.state.me.us/labor

John Butera, Commissioner

Provides a wide range of services such as employment, labor market information, rehabilitation/disability, and others.

6068 Maine Human Rights Commission
Maine Human Rights Commission
51 State House Station
Augusta, ME 04333
207-624-6290
Fax: 207-624-8729
www.maine.gov/mhrc

Amy Sneirson, Executive Director
Barbara Archer Hirsch, Commission Counsel
Alice Neal, Chief Investigator

The State agency with the responsibility of enforcing Maine's anti-discrimination laws. The Commission investigates complaints of unlawful discrimination in employment, housing, education, access to public accommodations, extension of credit, and offensive names.

6069 Northeast Occupational Exchange
29 Franklin St.
Bangor, ME 04401
800-857-0500
Fax: 207-561-4725
TTY: 207-992-2298
www.noemaine.org

Charles O. Tingley, Executive Director
Sharon Greenleaf, Assistant Director

A fully licensed, comprehensive mental health and substance abuse treatment and rehabilitation facility.

Maryland

6070 Ardmore Developmental Center
3000 Lottsford Vista Rd.
Bowie, MD 20721-4001
301-577-2575
Fax: 301-306-9799
grow@ArdmoreEnterprises.org
www.ardmoreenterprises.org

Douglas McQuade, Chief Executive Officer
Jennifer Garofalo, Chief Financial Officer
Bianca Colbert, Director of Human Resources
Heather Deacon, Director of Development & Communications

Offers supported employment programs and vocational education for persons with intellectual and developmental disabilities, as well as residential services and a Day Support program.

6071 Maryland Commission on Civil Rights (FEPA)
6 Saint Paul St.
Suite 900
Baltimore, MD 21202-1631
410-767-8600
800-637-6247
Fax: 410-333-1841
TTY: 410-333-1737
mccr@maryland.gov
www.mccr.maryland.gov

Alvin O. Gillard, Executive Director
Cleveland L. Horton II, Deputy Director
Glendora Hughes, General Counsel
Nicolette Young, Assistant Director

The Maryland Commission on Civil Rights represents the interests of the State of Maryland in ensuring equal opportunity for all individuals in the areas of housing, public accommodations, employment, and state contracts.

6072 Maryland Department of Disabilities
217 E. Redwood St.
Suite 1300
Baltimore, MD 21202
410-767-3660
800-637-4113
info.mdod@maryland.gov
mdod.maryland.gov

Carol Beatty, Secretary
Christian Miele, Deputy Secretary
John Brennan, Assistant Deputy Secretary
Kim McKay, Director, Communications

The Maryland Department of Disabilities is charged with improving services for individuals with disabilities in the areas of housing, employment, community living, technology assistance, trasportation, and more.

6073 Maryland Employment Network
Bel Air, MB
410-803-7184
855-384-2844
Fax: 410-803-8732
www.ticket2workmd.org

Keirstyn Silver, Director
Molly Hall, Program Administrator

A state-wide network of 9 partner agencies that aim to help individuals with disabilities gain quality employment.

6074 **Maryland State Department of Education**
Division of Rehabilitation Services (DORS)
2301 Argonne Dr.
Baltimore, MD 21218 410-554-9442
888-554-0334
TTY: 443-798-2840
dors@maryland.gov
dors.maryland.gov
Suzanne Page, Assistant State Superintendent
Sandy Bowser, Executive Associate
Kimberlee Schultz, Public Affairs Officer
The Division of Rehabilitation Services provides opportunities for individuals with physical and/or mental disabilities that help them gain employment. The Division is composed of the public vocational rehabilitation program, and the Disability Determination Services.

6075 **Melwood**
5606 Dower House Rd.
Upper Marlboro, MD 20772 301-599-8000
Fax: 301-599-0180
services@melwood.org
www.melwood.org
Carol Ann Desantis, President/CEO
Myron Thomas, Chief Operating Officer
Larysa Kautz, Chief of Staff/General Counsel
Romel Buchanan, Vice President of Finance
Melwood is a dynamic nonprofit that creates jobs and opportunities to improve the lives of people with disabilities. Melwood serves more than 2000 people with disabilities each year.

6076 **NFB Career Mentoring**
National Federation of the Blind
200 East Wells St.
Jernigan Place
Baltimore, MD 21230 410-659-9314
Fax: 410-659-5129
nfb@nfb.org
www.nfb.org
John G. Pare, Jr., Executive Director, Advocacy & Policy
A primary initiative of the NFB Jernigan Institute, the Career Mentoring program aims to increase the employment of visually impaired adults. The National Federation of the Blind also offers an employment resource page.

6077 **Office of Fair Practices**
Department of Labor, Licensing & Regulation
1100 North Eutaw St.
Room 613
Baltimore, MD 21202 410-230-6319
Fax: 410-225-3282
TTY: 410-225-7039
dlofp-dllr@maryland.gov
www.dllr.state.md.us/oeope/
Jennifer Dashiell Reed, Director/ADA Officer
Yvette Dickens, EEO Specialist
Aims to ensure qual opportunities for all individuals by enforcing the Equal Employment Opportunity (EEO) Program, the Americans with Disabilities Act, and other equal opportunity programs.

6078 **TLC Speech-Language/Occupational TherapyCamps**
2092 Gaither Rd.
Suite 100
Rockville, MD 20850 301-424-5200
Fax: 301-424-8063
TTY: 301-424-5203
info@ttlc.org
www.ttlc.org
Patricia Ritter, Executive Director
TLC provides small group summer programs for children with special needs. Offers speech-language and occupational therapy summer camps for children ages 3-7.

Massachusetts

6079 **Executive Office of Labor & Workforce Development**
State of Massachusetts
One Ashburton Pl.
Suite 2112
Boston, MA 02108 617-626-7122
Fax: 617-727-1090
www.mass.gov
Charlie Baker, Governor
Karyn Polito, Lt. Governor
Manages the Commonwealth's workforce development and labor departments.

6080 **Gateway Arts Center: Studio, Craft Store& Gallery**
Vinsen Corporation
60-62 Harvard St.
Brookline, MA 02445 617-734-1577
gatewayarts@vinfen.org
www.gatewayarts.org
Rae Edelson, Director
Stephanie Schmidt, Clinical Program Director
Ted Lampe, Program Director
Stephen DeFronzo, Artistic Director
Award winning, nationally recoginized arts based rehabilitation service with over 100 talented adults with disabilities.

6081 **Life-Skills, Inc.**
44 Morris St.
Webster, MA 01570 508-943-0700
Fax: 508-949-6129
info@life-skillsinc.org
life-skillsinc.org
J. Thomas Amick, Chief Executive Officer
Kathy Nolan, Chief Financial Officer
David Kline, Director of Day Habilitation
Eileen Beringer, Director of Human Resources
Accredited through the Commission on Accreditation of Rehabilitation Facilities; offers day, residential, and employment services for individuals with intellectual, developmental, physical, and emotional disabilities.

6082 **Massachusetts Commission Against Discrimination (FEPA)**
1 Ashburton Pl.
Suite 601
Boston, MA 02108 617-994-6000
Fax: 617-994-6024
TTY: 617-994-6196
www.mass.gov
Sunila Thomas-George, Chairman
Monserrate Quinones, Commissioner
Sheila Hubbard, Commissioner
The commission works to eliminate discrimination on a variety of bases and areas, and strives to advance the civil rights of the people of commonwealth through law enforcement, outreach, and training.

6083 **Massachusetts Commission for the Blind**
600 Washington St.
Boston, MA 02111 617-727-5550
800-392-6450
Fax: 617-626-7685
www.mass.gov/eohhs/gov/departments/mcb/
Paul Saner, Commissioner
Provides vocational and social rehabilitation for individuals with visual impairments.

6084 **Massachusetts Governor's Commission on Employment of People with Disabilities**
Department of Employment & Training
19 Standford St.
3rd Fl.
Boston, MA 02114 617-262-5239
Fax: 617-727-0315
www.dol.gov/odep/contact/
Charlie Baker, Governor
State vocational rehabilitation agency.

6085 **Massachusetts Rehabilitation Commission**
600 Washington St.
Boston, MA 02111
617-204-3600
Fax: 617-727-1354
TTY: 800-245-6543
MRC.generalinformation@Massmail.State.MA.US
www.mass.gov
Toni A. Wolf, Commissioner
Helps individuals with disabilities work and live independently. The Commission runs the Vocational Rehabilitation and Community Living programs.

6086 **Viability**
60 Brookdale Dr.
Springfield, MA 01104
413-781-5359
viability.org
Francis Fitzgerald, Chair
Jonathon Dean, Vice Chair
Charlene Smolkowicz, Treasurer
Colleen Holmes, President & CEO
Viability's mission is to help individuals with disabilities achieve their full potential. Services include day programs, employment services, and job training and placements.

6087 **Work Inc.**
25 Beach St.
Dorchester, MA 02122
617-691-1500
info@workinc.org
workinc.org
James Cassetta, President/CEO
Sharon Smith, Chief Operating Officer
Dave Anderson, Chief Financial Officer
Steve Alto, Vice President of Workforce Development
A nationally recognized organization that provides supportive services need to help people with disabilities reach their career goals.

Michigan

6088 **Department of Health & Human Services**
333 S. Grand Ave.
P.O. Box 30195
Lansing, MI 48909
517-373-3740
TTY: 800-649-3777
www.michigan.gov/mdhhs/
Nick Lyon, Director
Nancy Vreibel, Chief Deputy Director
Terrence M. Beurer, Deputy Director, Field Operations Administration
Farah Hanley, Deputy Director, Financial Operations
The DHHS is Michigan's public assistance, child, and family welfare agency. DHS directs the operations of public assistance and service programs through a network of over 100 county department of human service offices around the state.

6089 **Division on Deaf, DeafBlind & Hard of Hearing**
3054 W. Grand Blvd.
Suite 3-600
Detroit, MI 48202
313-437-7035
Fax: 319-456-3721
TTY: 877-499-6232
DODDBHH@Michigan.gov
www.michigan.gov/mdcr/
Anne Urasky, Division Director
Karlee Rose Gruetzner, Rights Representative
Jeanette Johnson, Rights Representative
Alayna Zerlentes, Executive Secretary
A state office with the mission of helping to improve the lives of Michigan citizens who are deaf, deafblind and hard of hearing.

6090 **Michigan Department of Civil Rights**
3054 W. Grand Blvd.
Suite 3-600
Detroit, MI 48202
313-456-3700
800-482-3604
Fax: 313-456-3791
TTY: 877-878-8464
MDCR-INFO@michigan.gov
www.michigan.gov/mdcr
Augustin V. Arbulu, Director
Investigates and resolves discrimination complaints and works to prevent discrimination through educational programs that promote voluntary compliance with civil rights laws.

6091 **Michigan Rehabilitation Services**
Department of Health & Human Services
320 S. Walnut St.
P.O. Box 30010
Lansing, MI 48909
517-373-3390
800-605-6722
Fax: 517-373-0565
TTY: 800-605-6722
www.michigan.gov/mrs
Suzanne Howell, Bureau Director
State vocational rehabilitation agency that provides specialized employment and educational services to teens and adults with disabilities in order to help them find and retain employment.

6092 **Michigan Workforce Development Agency**
201 N. Washington Square
Lansing, MI 48913
517-335-5858
Fax: 517-241-8217
TTY: 888-605-6722
www.michigan.gov/mdcd

6093 **Straits Area Services, Inc.**
1320 W. State St.
Cheboygan, MI 49721
231-627-4319
www.sastogether.org

Minnesota

6094 **Jewish Vocational Service of Jewish Familyand Children's Services**
5905 Golden Valley Rd.
Golden Valley, MN 55422
952-546-0616
Fax: 952-593-1778
jfcs@jfcsmpls.org
www.jfcsmpls.org
Judy Halper, Chief Executive Officer
Lee Friedman, Chief Operating Officer
John Maloy, Chief Financial Officer
Dana Rubin, Development Director
The mission of JVS is to be a recognized leader in delivering employment, training, and career development services that positively impact individuals of all backgrounds, business, and society. JVS offers a vocational rehabilitation program that includes job placement, work adjustment training, and extended employment.

6095 **Minnesota Department of Employment & Economic Development: State Services for the Blind**
2200 University Ave. W.
Suite 240
St. Paul, MN 55114
651-539-2300
800-652-9000
Fax: 651-649-5927
mn.gov/deed/ssb/
Carol Pankow, Director
Offers tools, services, and training for individuals who are blind, DeafBlind, or have a visual impairment and are seeking employment or to live more indepedently.

6096 Minnesota Department of Employment and Economic Development: Vocational Rehab Services
332 Minnesota St.
1st National Bank Bldg., Suite E200
St. Paul, MN 55101
651-259-7114
800-657-3858
DEED.CustomerService@state.mn.us
mn.gov/deed/

Shawntera Hardy, Commissioner
Blake Chaffee, Deputy Commissioner/COO
Jeremy Hanson Willis, Deputy Commissioner of Workforce Development
Kevin McKinnon, Deputy Commissioner of Economic Development

Service for people with disabilities who need skills to prepare for work, or to find and keep a job.

6097 Minnesota Department of Human Rights (FEPA)
Freeman Building
625 Robert St. North
St. Paul, MN 55155
651-539-1100
800-657-3704
Fax: 651-296-9042
TTY: 800-627-3529
Info.MDHR@state.mn.us
mn.gov/mdhr/

Kevin Lindsey, Commissioner
Rowzat Shipchandler, Deputy Commissioner
Peter Zuniga, General Counsel
Christine Dufour, Communications & Community Relations Director

Mission and vision is to make Minnesota discrimination free. The Minnesota Department of Human Rights investigates charges of discrimination, and ensures that businesses comply with equal opportunity requirements.

Mississippi

6098 AbilityWorks
3895 Beasley Rd.
Jackson, MS 39213
601-898-7076
www.mdrs.ms.gov

6099 Mississippi Department of Rehabilitation Services
1281 Highway 51
Madison, MS 39110
601-853-5100
800-443-1000
TTY: 800-443-1000
www.mdrs.ms.gov/

Anita Naik, Office Director, Special Disability Programs
Billy Taylor, Chief of Staff
Dorothy Young, Office Director, Vocational Rehabilitation for the Blind
Lavonda Hart, Office Director, Vocational Rehabilitation

Offers low vision aids and appliances, counseling, social work, educational and professional training, residential services, recreational services, computer training and employment opportunities for Mississippians with disabilities.

6100 Mississippi Employment Secutity Commission
1235 Echelon Prkwy.
P.O. Box 1699
Jackson, MS 39215-1699
601-321-6000
comments@mdes.ms.gov
www.mdes.ms.gov

Mark Henry, Executive Director
Phil Bryant, Governor

A federally funded state agency. The programs of MDES, under direction of the governor of Mississippi, report to the federal government. The goal of the department is to help citizens of Mississippi get jobs.

6101 National Research and Training Center on Blindness and Low Vision
Mississippi State University
108 Herbert-South, Room 150
PO Drawer 6189
Mississippi State, MS 39762-6189
662-325-2001
Fax: 662-325-8989
nrtc@colled.msstate.edu
www.blind.msstate.edu

Michele Capella McDonnall, Research Professor/Director
Douglas Bedsaul, Research & Training Coordinator
Renee Brannon, Business Manager
Sophie Kershaw, Communications Specialist

The NRTC focuses on enhancing the employment and independence of individuals who are blind and visually impaired.

Missouri

6102 Missouri Commission on Human Rights
3315 W. Truman Blvd., Room 212
P.O. Box 1129
Jefferson City, MO 65102-1129
573-751-3325
877-781-4236
Fax: 573-751-2905
TTY: 800-735-2966
mchr@labor.mo.gov
labor.mo.gov/MOHUMANRIGHTS

Dr. Alisa Warren, Executive Director
Anna Crosslin, Commissioner
Ralph Bray, Commissioner
David Thomas, Commissioner

The Missouri Commission on Human Rights enforces the state's anti-discrimination law that prohibits discrimination in housing, employment, and places of public accommodations. It prohibits discrimination due to race, color, religion, national origin, ancestry, sex, disability, age, and familial status. Complaints must be filed within 180 days of the alleged discrimination. If discrimination is found after investigation, the Commission can hold hearings to enforce the law.

6103 Missouri Governor's Council on Disability
301 West High St., Room 840
P.O. Box 1668
Jefferson City, MO 65102-1668
800-877-8249
Fax: 573-526-4109
TTY: 573-751-2600
gcd@oa.mo.gov
disability.mo.gov/gcd/

Yvonne Wright, Commissioner/Chair
Claudia Browner, Executive Director

The Council promotes the full participation of Missouri citizens with disabilities, and provides information about the American with Disabilities Act. They aim to protect persons with disabilities through equal access to services and employment opportunities.

6104 Missouri Vocational Rehabilitation Agency
Department of Elementary & Secondary Education
3024 Dupont Circle
Jefferson City, MO 65109
573-751-3251
877-222-8963
Fax: 573-751-1441
TTY: 573-751-0881
info@vr.dese.mo.gov
dese.mo.gov

C. Jeanne Loyd, Assistant Commissioner

A team of dedicated individuals working for the continuous improvement of education and services for all citizens. Vocational Rehabilitation offers specialized employment and training services for individuals with a physical or mental impairment.

6105 **Vocational Rehabilitation Services for the Blind**
Missouri Department of Social Services
615 Howerton Court
P.O. Box 2320
Jefferson City, MO 65102-2320
573-751-4249
Fax: 573-751-4984
askrsb@dss.mo.gov
dss.mo.gov/fsd/rsb/vr.htm
Patrick Luebbering, Family Support Division Director
Keith Roderick, Deputy Director, Rehabilitation Services for the Blind
A state organization that aims to create employment opportunities for blind and visually impaired persons.

Montana

6106 **Disability Employment & Transitions**
Department of Public Health & Human Services
111 North Last Chance Gulch
P.O. Box 4210
Helena, MT 59604
406-444-2590
Fax: 406-444-3632
dphhs.mt.gov/detd
Nick Domitrovich, Interim Director
Provides services for individuals with disabilities who want to become employed. Focuses on transitions from high school to post-secondary education and work.

6107 **Montana Human Rights Bureau (FEPA)**
P.O. Box 1728
Helena, MT 59624-1728
800-542-0807
Fax: 406-443-3234
www.erd.dli.mt.gov/human-rights
Marieke Beck, Bureau Chief
Enforces state and federal laws prohibiting unlawful discrimination based on age, marital status, disability, race/nationality, color, religion, sex, etc., in the areas of employment, housing, education, and public accommodations.

Nebraska

6108 **Nebraska Department of Labor**
1111 O Street
Suite 222
Lincoln, NE 68508
402-471-4474
ndol.lincolnwfd@nebraska.gov
dol.nebraska.gov
John Albin, Commissioner
Services for individuals with disabilities who want to become employed.

6109 **Nebraska Equal Opportunity Commission (FEPA)**
301 Centennial Mall South, 5th Fl.
P.O. Box 94934
Lincoln, NE 68509-4934
402-471-2024
800-642-6112
Fax: 402-471-4059
www.neoc.ne.gov
Eric Drumheller, Chairperson
Rita Griess, Vice Chairman
Marna Munn, Executive Director
The Nebraska Equal Opportunity Commission is a neutral administrative agency that enforces state policy against discrimination in the areas of employment, housing, and public accommodations.

6110 **Nebraska VR**
Department of Education
PO Box 94987
Lincoln, NE 68509
402-471-3644
877-637-3422
Fax: 402-471-0788
marketingteam.vr@nebraska.gov
www.vr.nebraska.gov
Lindy Foley, Director
An employment program for citizens of Nebraska who experience a disability and are seeking employment.

Nevada

6111 **Bureau of Vocational Rehabilitation**
Rehabilitation Division
3016 W. Charleston
Suite 200
Las Vegas, NV 89102
702-486-5230
TTY: 702-486-1018
detr.state.nv.us
Shelley Hendren, Rehabilitation Administrator
A state and federally funded program that helps people with disabilities find employment, and helps advance the skills of disabled individuals who are already employed.

6112 **Nevada Equal Rights Commission**
1820 East Sahara Ave.
Suite 314
Las Vegas, NV 89104
702-486-7161
800-326-6868
Fax: 702-486-7054
detr.state.nv.us/nerc.htm
Kevin E. Hooks, Commissioner
Sean T. Higgins, Commissioner
Tiffany Young, Commissioner
Ivette Fernandez, Commissioner
Oversees the state's Equal Employment Opportunity program in order to make sure that all citizens of Nebraska recieve the same employment opportunities.

6113 **Nevada Governor's Council on Developmental Disabilities**
896 W. Nye Ln.
Suite 202
Carson City, NV 89703
775-684-8619
Fax: 775-684-8626
elmarquez@dhhs.nv.gov
www.nevadaddcouncil.org
Jodi Thornley, Council Chair
Stephen Schumacher, Council Vice Chair
Kari Horn, Executive Director
Catherine Nielsen, Projects Manager
The Council provides advocacy for individuals with intellectual or developmental disabilities, so that they may live more independent lives and be invovled in the community.

New Hampshire

6114 **New Hampshire Bureau of Vocational Rehabilitation**
New Hampshire Department of Education
101 Pleasant St.
Concord, NH 03301-3860
603-271-3494
Fax: 603-271-1953
info@doe.nh.gov
www.ed.state.nh.us
Lisa Hinson-Hatz, State Director
The Bureau of Vocational Rehabilitation assists citizens of New Hampshire with disabilities secure employment.

6115 **New Hampshire Commission for Human Rights (FEPA)**
2 Industrial Park Dr.
Building 1
Concord, NH 03301
603-271-2767
Fax: 603-271-6339
humanrights@nh.gov
www.nh.gov/hrc
Matt Mayberry, Chair
Sheryl L. Shirley, Commissioner
Harvey Keye, Commissioner
Sylvia E. Gale, Commissioner
Established for the purpose of eliminating discrimination in employment, public accomodations, and the sale or rental of housing or commercial property.

6116 **New Hampshire Employment Security**
45 South Fruit St.
Concord, NH 03301
603-224-3311
800-852-3400
TTY: 800-735-2964
webmaster@nhes.nh.gov
www.nhes.nh.gov

George N. Copadis, Commissioner

Operates a free public employment service and provides assisted and self directed employment and career related services and labor market information for employers and the general public.

New Jersey

6117 **ARC of Hunterdon County, The**
1465 Route 31 South
Annandale, NJ 08801
908-730-7827
www.archunterdon.org

Jessica Lui, Board President
John Samborski, Vice President
Loretta Luzzo, Treasurer

Our mission is to provide support, training, and opportunities to individuals with intellectual and developmental disabilities so that they can achieve the greatest degree of independence and productivity, and become contributing, responsible, and proud members of society.

6118 **ARC of Mercer County**
180 Ewingville Rd.
Ewing, NJ 08638
609-406-0181
Fax: 609-406-9258
arc@arcmercer.org
www.arcmercer.org

Rick Koreyva, Board President
Maria Fischer, 1st Vice President
Steven Cook, Executive Director
Luke Rattan, Assistant Executive Director

Committed to securing for all people with developmental disabilities the opportunity to choose and realize their goals.

6119 **ARC of Monmouth**
1158 Wayside Rd.
Tinton Falls, NJ 07712
732-493-1919
Fax: 732-493-3604
info@arcofmonmouth.org
www.arcofmonmouth.org

Rachel Weiss, President
Janis Swindlehurst, First Vice President
Linda Mayo, Executive Director
Ann Marie McGoldrick, Assistant Executive Director, Workforce Development

A nonprofit organization providing services and supports for individuals who have cognitive and developmental disabilities and their families.

6120 **Abilities Center of New Jersey**
1208 Delsea Dr.
Westville, NJ 08093
856-848-1025
Fax: 856-848-8429
info@abilities4work.com
abilities4work.com

Susan Perron, President/CEO
Sharon Kneubuehl, Vice President
Jack Sheppard, Chairman
Rich Hubler, Vice Chair

A nonprofit organization dedicated to developing employment opportunities for people with disabilities or other disadvantages through education, training, and job placement.

6121 **Abilities of Northwest New Jersey Inc.**
264 Rt 31 North
Washington, NJ 07882
908-689-1118
info@abilitiesnw.com
abilities-nw.com

Cynthia B. Wildermuth, Chief Executive Officer
Sue Zukoski, Chief Development Officer
Michelle Savino, Director of Program Services
Arlene Swanston, Human Resources Manager

Private not-for-profit community rehabilitation program providing vocational training and employment services since 1974 to the disabled and disadvantaged population.

6122 **Alliance Center for Independence (ACI)**
629 Amboy Ave.
First Floor
Edison, NJ 08837
732-738-4388
Fax: 732-738-4416
TTY: 732-738-9644
ctonks@adacil.org
www.adacil.org

Carole Tonks, Executive Director
Luke Koppisch, Deputy Director

ACI is a nonprofit Center for Independent Living that provides information and referral services and develops and implements educational programs and innovative activities that promote activism, peer support, health, wellness, employment, and independent living skills for people with disabilities.

6123 **Arc of Bergen and Passaic Counties**
223 Moore St.
Hackensack, NJ 07601
201-343-0322
Fax: 201-343-0401
arc@arcbp.com
arcbergenpassaic.org

Kathy Walsh, President/CEO
Alice Siegel, Senior Vice President
Catherine Pescatore, Vice President/CFO
Anne Gallucci, Vocational Services Director

A membership organization serving persons with disabilities and their families in Bergen and Passaic Counties, NJ.

6124 **Career Opportunity Development of New Jersey**
901 Atlantic Ave.
Egg Harbor City, NJ 08215-1810
609-965-6871
Fax: 609-965-3099
njcodi.org

Linda L. Carney, President/CEO
Karen Gardner, Chief Financial Officer
Joe Cella, Board Chairperson
Dan Kelly, Vice Chair

A nonprofit organization that provides services to individuals with varying forms of physical, mental, and economic disabilities and disadvantages. Provides services to more than 1,500 unduplicated consumers annually.

6125 **Center for Educational Advancement New Jersey**
11 Minneakoning Rd.
Flemington, NJ 08822
908-782-1480
cea-nj.org/

Michael Skoczek, President/CEO
Philip Ferri, Chair
Andrew Ross, Vice Chair
Michael Collins, Treasurer

A CARF accredited, nonprofit organization that provides opportunities for disbaled individuals to lead productive lives. Programs offered throughout Central New Jersey.

6126 **Easterseals New Jersey**
25 Kennedy Blvd.
Suite 600
East Brunswick, NJ 08816
732-257-6662
Fax: 732-257-7373
www.easterseals.com/nj

Brian Fitzgerald, President & CEO
Helen Drobnis, Chief Advancement Officer & Corporate Secretary
Michael Owen, Chief Human Resources Officer & General Counsel
Aleisha Hart, Chief Financial Officer & Assistant Treasurer

A nonprofit organization that provides opportunities for disabled citizens of New Jersey to be independent and participate in their communities. Easterseals New Jersey serves over 9,000 individuals.

6127 **Eden Autism**
2 Merwick Rd.
Princeton, NJ 08540
609-987-0099
Fax: 609-987-0243
edenautism.org

Michael K. Decker, President/CEO
Jennifer Bizub, Chief Operating Officer
Rachel Tait, Chief Program Officer
Melinda Gorny McAleer, Chief Development Officer
A nonprofit organization that provides a variety of services for chidlren and adults with autism. Services include individualized education, employment training/placement, group residences, and early intervention.

6128 **Edison Sheltered Workshop**
328 Plainfield Ave.
Edison, NJ 08817
732-985-8834
Fax: 732-985-2216
info@eswnj.org
www.eswnj.org

P. Michael Shaffery, Executive Director
Emil Ferlicchi, President
Mark C. Viggiano, Vice President
William Stephens, Treasurer
An organization that provides vocational training and job placement services for disabled individuals who are 16 years old and living in Middlesex County.

6129 **Goodwill Industries of Southern New Jersey**
2835 Route 73
Maple Shade, NJ 08052
856-439-0200
Fax: 856-439-0843
goodwillnj.org

Mark B. Boyd, President/CEO
Michael Shaw, Chief Operating Officer
Stephen Castro, Chief Financial Officer
Tim Reeser, Human Resources Manager
A nonprofit, community-based organization that empowers individuals with special needs by providing them with the opportunity to develop marketable job skills.

6130 **Hudson Community Enterprises**
68-70 Tuers Ave.
Jersey City, NJ 07306
201-434-3303
Fax: 201-434-3660
hce.works

Joseph F. Brown, President
Vocational rehab, transition services and training programs are offered.

6131 **Inroads to Opportunities**
301 Cox St.
Roselle, NJ 07203
908-241-7200
Fax: 908-241-2025
ocuc@inroadsto.com
www.occupationalcenter.org

Letty Esquivel, Director, Mental Health
Nancy Laporte, Director, Assembly Services
Cyndy Walsh Rintzler, Director, Assessment & Vocational Training
Formerly known as the Occupational Center of Union County, the organization offers vocational preparation, transition from school to work, job placement and mental health services to over 500 individuals annually.

6132 **Jersey Cape**
152 Crest Haven Road
Cape May Court House, NJ 08210-1651
609-465-4117
800-599-5232
www.jerseycape.org

Joseph Sittineri, Executive Director
Offers a range of employment programs and services for people with disabilities.

6133 **Jewish Vocational Service (JVS) - East Orange**
7 Glenwood Ave.
Lower Level
East Orange, NJ 07017
973-674-6330
info@jvsnj.org
jvsnj.org

Michael Andreas, Executive Director
Rebecca Shulman, Senior Program Director
Hetal Narciso, Director, Vocational Rehabilitation Services
Meryl Kanner, Director, Career Counseling & Job Placement
Offers vocational rehabilitation services, as well as education and literacy.

6134 **Jewish Vocational Service (JVS) - Livingston**
354 Eisenhower Parkway
Plaza 1, Suite 2150
Livingston, NJ 07039
973-674-6330
info@jvsnj.org
jvsnj.org

Michael Andreas, Executive Director
Rebecca Shulman, Senior Program Director
Hetal Narciso, Director, Vocational Rehabilitation Services
Meryl Kanner, Director, Career Counseling & Job Placement
Houses JVS administration, as well as providing career counseling, job placement and corporate training services.

6135 **Jewish Vocational Service (JVS) - Montclair**
83 Walnut St.
Montclair, NJ 07042
973-744-7733
info@jvsnj.org
jvsnj.org

Michael Andreas, Executive Director
Rebecca Shulman, Senior Program Director
Hetal Narciso, Director, Vocational Rehabilitation Services
Meryl Kanner, Director, Career Counseling & Job Placement
Provides vocational rehabilitation services.

6136 **New Jersey Commission for the Blind and Visually Impaired (CBVI)**
Department of Human Services
153 Halsey St
6th Floor, PO Box 47017
Newark, NJ 07101
973-648-3333
877-685-8878
askcbvi@dhs.state.nj.us
www.state.nj.us/humanservices/cbvi

Bernice Davis, Executive Director
Edward Szajdecki, Chief, Fiscal Services
Ines Matos, Chief, Organizational Logistics
Eva Scott, Director, Blindness Education
The Commission for the Blind and Visually Impaired (CBVI) promotes and provides services in the areas of education, employment, independence and eye health for persons who are blind or visually impaired, their families and the community. It seeks to provide or ensure access to services that will enable consumers to obtain their fullest measure of self-reliance and quality of life and fully integrated into their community.

6137 **New Jersey Division of Vocational Rehabilitation Services (DVRS)**
Department of Labor and Workforce Development
1 John Fitch Plaza
PO Box 110
Trenton, NJ 08625-0110
609-659-9045
Constituent.Relations@dol.nj.gov
careerconnections.nj.gov

Robert Asaro-Angelo, Commissioner
Julie Diaz, Chief of Staff
Caroline M. Stout, Director, Disability Determination Services
Services for individuals with disabilities who want to become employed.

6138 **New Jersey Institute for Disabilities (NJID)**
10A Oak Dr.
Edison, NJ 08837
732-549-6187
www.njid.org

Dominic M. Ursino, President
Robert J. Ferrara, Executive Director
Robert J. Gross, Controller
Debra Gilbert, Director of Human Resources

Dedicated to the provision of comprehensive, superior, multi-faceted programs of service to individuals with developmental and related disabilities.

6139 Occupational Training Center of Burlington County (OTCBC)
2 Manhattan Drive
Burlington, NJ 08016
609-267-6677
Fax: 609-265-8418
info@otcbc.org
otcbc.org

Joseph S Bender, CEO
Mission is to assist individuals with disabilities in reaching their maximum potential.

6140 Occupational Training Center (OTC)
The Arc of Camden County
215 W White Horse Pike
Berlin, NJ 08009
856-768-0845
Fax: 856-767-1378
arcotc@arccamden.org
www.camdencounty.com

Loret McClain, Contact
Provides the following to residents of Camden County: job placement; supported employment; extended employment; vocational evaluation and assessment; work adjustment training; and contract work.

6141 Pathways to Independence, Inc.
60 Kingsland Ave.
Kearny, NJ 07032
201-997-6155
Fax: 201-997-7070
acox@pathwaysnj.org
www.pathwaysnj.org

Alvin Cox, Executive Director
Tessa Farrell, Program Director
Marie Yakabofski, Financial Director
Lisa M. Johnson, Qualilty Assurance Director
Pre-vocational and vocational programming for people with disabilities. Specializing in developmental disabilities, learning disabilities and mental health issues. Serving over 100 people in Hudson, Bergen and Essex Counties. CARF accredited.

6142 Somerset Community Action Program, Inc.
155 Pierce St.
Suite F
Somerset, NJ 08873
732-846-8888
Fax: 732-214-9754
info@somersetcap.org
www.somersetcap.org

Steven Nagel, Executive Director
Mark Harris, Associate Director
Betty Spencer, Education Manager
Provides services for low-income individuals and those with disabilities who want to become employed.

6143 St. John of God Community Services Vocational Rehabilitation
1145 Delsea Dr.
Westville Grove, NJ 08093
856-848-4700
www.sjogcs.org

Denise Murray, Program Manager
Serves Gloucester and Camden Counties providing special education, vocational and habilitative services to residents of southern New Jersey since 1967.

6144 The Arc Gloucester
1555 Gateway Blvd.
West Deptford, NJ 08096
856-848-8648
info@thearcgloucester.org
www.thearcgloucester.org

Lisa Conley, Chief Executive Officer
A nonprofit organization serving people with intellectual and related developmental disabilities and their families through education, advocacy, and direct services.

6145 United Cerebral Palsy Associations of New Jersey
1005 Whitehead Rd. Extension
Suite 1
Ewing, NJ 08638
609-882-4182
888-322-1918
Fax: 609-882-4054
info@advopps.org
cpofnj.org

Jack M. Mudge, Chief Executive Officer
William Curnan, COO & CFO
Karl Craft, Director, Employment Services
Gretchen DiMarco, Director, Community Relations
Dedicated to changing lives and bringing independence to people with all types of disabilities.

New Mexico

6146 Adelante Development Center
3900 Osuna Rd. NE
Albuquerque, NM 87109
505-341-2000
Fax: 505-341-2001
info@GoAdelante.org
www.goadelante.org

Mike Kivitz, President
Bob Walton, Chair
Molly Madden, Secretary
Pamela Sullivan, Treasurer
Serves Albuquerque and Belen.

6147 Goodwill Industries of New Mexico
5000 San Mateo Blvd. NE
Albuquerque, NM 87109
505-881-6401
866-376-0182
Fax: 505-884-3157
goodwillnm.org

Mary Best, President & CEO
Terry Armstrong, Chief Services Officer
Shauna Kastle, Vice President, Operations
Serves Albuquerque, Santa Fe and Rio Rancho.

6148 LifeROOTS
1111 Menaul Blvd. NE
Albuquerque, NM 87107
505-255-5501
StephanieH@LifeROOTSNM.org
www.liferootsnm.org

Kathleen Cates, President & CEO
Dawnita Blackmon-Mosely, Director, Children's Therapy & Services
Angela Ortega, Director, Adult Services
Sylvia Padilla, Director, Quality Assurance
Albuquerque, Rio Rancho and the surrounding area. Mission is to improve the abilities, interests, and choices of children and adults with physical, developmental or behavioral challenges with the goal of achieving their highest levels of self-sufficiency.

6149 New Mexico Commission for the Blind (NMCFTB)
2905 Rodeo Park Dr E
Bldg 4, Suite 100
Santa Fe, NM 87505
505-476-4479
888-513-7968
www.cfb.state.nm.us

Greg Trapp, Executive Director
Offers services for the totally blind, legally blind, visually impaired, and more with health, counseling, educational, recreational, rehabilitation, computer training and professional training services.

6150 New Mexico Division of Vocational Rehabilitation
2935 Rodeo Park Dr. East
Santa Fe, NM 87505
505-954-8500
800-224-7005
Fax: 505-954-8562

Diane Mourning Brown, Executive Director
Purpose is to help people with disabilities achieve a suitable employment outcome.

6151 **New Mexico Workforce Connection**
New Mexico Department of Workforce Solutions
401 Broadway NE
Albuquerque, NM 87102 505-841-8437
Fax: 505-841-8422
www.dws.state.nm.us

6152 **Tohatchi Area of Opportunity & Services**
PO Box 49
Tohatchi, NM 87325 505-722-9287
Fax: 505-722-9189
taos-inc.org
Kimber Crowe, Chief Executive Officer
Gerald Morris, Manager, Program Service
Provides a range of programs for Native Americans with developmental disabilities.

New York

6153 **Adult Career and Continuing Ed Services - Vocational Rehabilitation (ACCESS-VR)**
New York State Education Department
89 Washington Ave.
Albany, NY 12234 518-474-3852
800-222-5627
www.acces.nysed.gov/vr
MaryEllen Elia, Commissioner
Aims to assist people with disabilities with attaining and maintaining employment.

6154 **National Business & Disability Council**
The Viscardi Center
201 I.U. Willets Rd.
Albertson, NY 11507 516-465-1400
info@viscardicenter.org
viscardicenter.org/services/nbdc
John D. Kemp, President & CEO
Sheryl P. Buchel, Executive Vice President & Chief Financial Officer
Michael Caprara, Chief Information Officer
Lauren M. Marzo, Chief Development Officer
The NBDC is a resource for employers seeking to integrate people with disabilities into the workplace and companies seeking to reach them in the consumer marketplace.

6155 **New York State Department of Labor**
Building 12
State Office Campus
Albany, NY 12240 518-457-9000
888-469-7365
TTY: 800-662-1220
www.labor.ny.gov
Roberta Reardon, Commissioner
The mission of the New York State Department of Labor is to help New York work by preparing individuals for the jobs of today and tomorrow. Provides direct job search and counseling services to job seekers, and can refer people who have disabilities for training opportunities. Provides unemployment insurance for those out of work through no fault of their own.

North Carolina

6156 **Division Of Workforce Solutions**
NC Department of Commerce
301 North Wilmington St.
Raleigh, NC 27601-1058 919-814-4600
info@nccommerce.com
www.nccommerce.com/jobs-training
Anthony M. Copeland, Secretary of Commerce
Lockhart Taylor, Assistant Secretary, Employment Security
Linda Cheatham, Assistant Secretary, Workforce
Offers vocational assessment and training, adult developmental activities.

6157 **Division of Vocational Rehabilitation Services (DVRS) Western Regional Office**
200 Enola Rd.
Suite 209
Morganton, NC 28655 828-433-2423
877-472-2729
www.ncdhhs.gov
Chris Egan, Senior Director, Employment Services
Kathie B. Trotter, Director
Services include vocational evaluation, work adjustment, job placement, and an on-site work services program.

6158 **Division of Vocational Rehabilitation Services (DVRS)**
NC Department of Health and Human Services
2001 Mail Service Center
Raleigh, NC 27699-2801 919-855-3500
800-689-9090
TTY: 919-855-3579
www.ncdhhs.gov/divisions/dvrs
Chris Egan, Senior Director, Employment Services
Kathie B. Trotter, Director
Seeks to promote employment and independence for people with disabilities through customer partnership and community leadership.

6159 **LIFESPAN Incorporated**
1511 Shopton Rd.
Suite A
Charlotte, NC 28217 704-944-5100
www.lifespanservices.org
Ken D. Fuquay, President & Chief Ambassador, Empowerment
Christopher White, Chief Operating Officer
Robin Devore, Chief Compliance Officer
Harry Workman, Chief Philanthropy Officer & Ambassador, Generosity
Aims to transform the lives of children and adults with developmental disabilities by providing education, employment, and enrichment programs that promote inclusion, choice, family supports, and other best practices.

6160 **NCWorks Commission**
NC Department of Commerce
301 North Wilmington St.
Raleigh, NC 27601-1058 919-814-4600
NCWorksCommission@nccommerce.com
www.nccommerce.com
Anthony M. Copeland, Secretary of Commerce
Lockhart Taylor, Assistant Secretary, Employment Security
Linda Cheatham, Assistant Secretary, Workforce
Noth Carolina's workforce development board, seeking to prepare workers in the state for the future by increasing access to education and skills training, among other initiatives.

6161 **North Carolina Division of Services for the Blind**
Department of Health and Human Services
2601 Mail Service Center
Raleigh, NC 27699-2601 919-527-6700
800-222-1546
www.ncdhhs.gov/divisions/dsb
Cynthia Speight, Director
Since 1935, the mission of the North Carolina Division of Services for the Blind has been to enable people who are blind or visually impaired to reach their goals of independence and employment.

6162 **Rowan Vocational Opportunities, Inc. (RVO)**
2728 Old Concord Rd.
Salisbury, NC 28146 704-633-6223
www.rowanvocopp.org
Gary Yelton, Executive Director
Skip Kraft, Director, Operations
Glenn McDonald, Director, Sales & Marketing
Wilson Cherry, Director, Community Affairs
Offers vocational assessment and training, adult developmental activities.

6163 Rutherford Vocational Workshop
230 Fairground Rd.
Spindale, NC 28160
828-286-4352
rutherfordlifeservices@gmail.com
rutherfordlifeservices.com

Amanda Freeman, Executive Director
Susan Collins, Director, Finance
John Jarrett, Director, Human Resources

Offers vocational assessment and training, adult developmental activities.

6164 Transylvania Vocational Services (TVS)
11 Mountain Industrial Drive
PO Box 1115
Brevard, NC 28712
828-884-3195
info@tvsinc.org
www.tvsinc.org

Jamie Brandenburg, Chief Executive Officer

A private nonprofit corporation with the mission to provide skills development, career opportunities and related services in a supportive environment for people with barriers to employment.

6165 Webster Enterprises of Jackson County, Inc.
140 Little Savannah Rd.
Sylvia, NC 28779
828-586-8981
Fax: 828-586-8125
grobinson@websterenterprises.org
www.websterenterprises.org

North Dakota

6166 Job Service North Dakota
Job Service North Dakota
PO Box 5507
Bismarck, ND 58506-5507
701-328-2825
Fax: 701-328-4000
TTY: 800-366-6888
www.jobsnd.com

Michelle Kommer, Interim Executive Director

Offers vocational assessment and training, adult developmental activities.

6167 North Dakota Department of Labor, and Human Rights
Dept 406
600 East Boulevard Avenue
Bismarck, ND 58505- 0340
701-328-2660
800-582-8032
800-366-6888
Fax: 701-328-2031
labor@nd.gov
www.nd.gov/labor

Mark Nelson, Manager
Erica Thunder, Labor Commissioner

Through a work-sharing agreement with the Equal Employment Opportunity Commission (EEOC), the North Dakota Department of Labor's Human Rights Division enforces the Americans with Disabilities Act (ADA) as related to employment discrimination.

6168 North Dakota Vocational Rehabilitation Agency
1237 W Divide Ave
Suite 1B
Bismarck, ND 58501-1208
701-328-8950
800-755-2745
Fax: 701-328-8969
dhsvr@nd.gov
www.nd.gov/dhs/dvr/

Russ Cusack, State Director
LouAnn Nider, Chief of Field Services
Patty Wanner, Operations Administrator
Robyn Throlson, Planning & Evaluation Administrator

The North Dakota Vocational Rehabilitation Agency offers services for blind and visually impaired people such as health, counseling, educational, recreational, rehabilitation, computer training and professional training services.

Ohio

6169 Bureau of Vocational Rehabilitation (BVR)
400 East Campus View Blvd.
Columbus, OH 43235
614-438-1200
800-282-4536
susan.pugh@ood.ohio.gov
ood.ohio.gov

Susan Pugh, Deputy Director

State agency that provides vocational rehabilitation services to help people with disabilities become employed and independent.

6170 Greater Cincinnati Behavioral Health Services - Employment Services
1501 Madison Rd.
Cincinnati, OH 45206
513-354-5200
gcbhs.com

Jeff O'Neil, President & CEO
Jeff Kirschner, Chief Operations Officer
Tracey Skale, Chief Medical Officer
Alicia Fine, Vice President, Employment & Recovery Services

Offers the following services: job exploration; job development; job coaching and employment supports; and specizlized programs.

Oklahoma

6171 Office of Disability Concerns
1111 N Lee Ave.
Suite 500
Oklahoma City, OK 73103
405-521-3756
800-522-8224
odc@odc.ok.gov
www.odc.ok.gov

Doug MacMillan, Director
William Ginn, Disability Program Specialist, Client Assistance Program

Mission is to promote the employment of people with disabilities. The vision of the committee is to facilitate partnerships with commitment to full, high quality employment of people with disabilities.

6172 Oklahoma Department of Rehabilitation Services
3535 NW 58th St.
Suite 500
Oklahoma City, OK 73112-4824
405-951-3400
800-845-8476
Fax: 405-951-3529
info@okdrs.gov
www.okrehab.org

Melinda Fruendt, Executive Director

The Oklahoma Department of Rehabilitation Services (DRS) provides assistance to Oklahomans with disabilities through vocational rehabilitation, employment, independent living, residential and outreach programs, and the determination of medical eligibility for disability benefits.

6173 Oklahoma Employment Security Commission (OESC)
PO Box 52003
Oklahoma City, OK 73152-2003
405-557-7100
888-980-9675
TTY: 800-722-0353
OESCHelps@oesc.state.ok.us
www.ok.gov/oesc

Richard McPherson, Executive Director
Teresa Keller, Deputy Director
Jon Eller, Director, Project Management Division
Lisa Graven, Director, Reemployment Services & support

Connects Ohioans with work, as well as enhancing skills and providing unemployment compensation.

Oregon

6174 **Bureau of Labor and Industries (BOLI)**
800 NE Oregon St
Suite 1045
Portland, OR 97232
971-673-0761
Fax: 971-673-0762
mailb@boli.state.or.us
www.oregon.gov/boli

Val Hoyle, Commissioner
Protects Oregonians from unlawful discrimination, defends workers' rights, and provides training to employees and employers.

6175 **Opportunities Foundation of Central Oregon**
PO Box 430
835 E Hwy 126
Redmond, OR 97756
541-548-2611
Fax: 541-548-9573
info@opportunityfound.org
www.opportunityfound.org

David Imig, President
Seth Johnson, Executive Director
Tina DeSouza, Director, Behavior Services
Lew England, Director, Business Relations
Offers supported employment, residential support and behavior consultation services, including employment at three thirft stores.

6176 **Oregon Commission for the Blind**
535 SE 12th Avenue
Portland, OR 97214
971-673-1588
888-202-5463
Fax: 503-234-7468
ocb.mail@state.or.us
www.oregon.gov/Blind

Dacia Johnson, Executive Director
Angel Hale, Director, Rehabilitation Services
Malinda Carlson, Director, Independent Living Services
Eric Morris, Director, Business Enterprise Program
A resource for visually impaired Oregonians, as well as their families, friends, and employers. Nationally recognized programs and staff that make a difference in people's lives every day.

6177 **Oregon Department of Human Services Vocational Rehabilitation (DHS VR)**
500 Summer St. NE
Suite E-15
Salem, OR 97301
503-945-5600
Fax: 503-581-6198
TTY: 503-945-6214
www.oregon.gov/dhs/employment/VR

Fariborz Pakseresht, Director
Ashley Carson Cottingham, Director, Aging & People With Disabilities
Lilia Teninty, Director, Office of Developmental Disabilities Services
Kim Fredlund, Director, Self-Sufficiency Programs
Offers vocational assessments and training, adult developmental activities, and helps remove disability related barriers to employment.

Pennsylvania

6178 **Office of Vocational Rehabilitation (OVR)**
Pennsylvania Department of Labor & Industry
1521 N 6th St.
Harrisburg, PA 17102
717-787-5244
800-442-6351
TTY: 866-830-7327
dli.pa.gov/Individuals/Disability-Services

W. Gerard Oleksiak, Secretary
Helps individuals with disabilities prepare for, obtain, and manage employment, with services provided both directly and through a network of vendors.

6179 **Pennsylvania Department of Labor and Industry (DLI)**
1521 N 6th St.
Harrisburg, PA 17102
www.dli.state.pa.us

W. Gerard Oleksiak, Secretary
Administers benefits to unemployed individuals, oversees the administration of worker's compensation benefits to individuals with job related injuries, and provides vocational rehabilitation to individuals with disabilities.

6180 **Pennsylvania Governor's Cabinet Committee for People With Disabilities**
Department of Human Services
234 Health and Welfare Bldg.
Harrisburg, PA 17105-2675
717-787-3422
800-692-7462
Fax: 717-772-2490
www.dhs.pa.gov

Teresa Miller, Chair
Mission is to assist with disabilities to secure and maintain employment and independence.

6181 **Pennsylvania Human Relations Commission Agency**
Executive Offices
333 Market St.
8th Fl.
Harrisburg, PA 17101-2210
717-787-4410
TTY: 717-787-7279
phrc@pa.gov
phrc.state.pa.us

M. Joel Bolstein, Chair
Raquel O. Yiengst, Vice Chair
Mission is to administer and enforce the PHRAct and the PFEOA of the Commonwealth of Pennsylvania for the identification and elimination of discrimination and the providing of equal opportunity for all persons.

Rhode Island

6182 **Groden Network**
610 Manton Ave.
Providence, RI 02909
401-274-6310
grodennetwork.org

Laurie Vinkavich-Cole, Chief Executive Officer
Grace Toe, Chief Financial Officer
Cooper Woodard, Chief Clinical Officer
Raymond A. Maxwell, Director, Quality Operations
The Groden Network aims to support children & adults with autism, as well as other developmental disailities, by providing educational, therapeutic and other services. The Network also engages in research, and educates families as well. The Network consists of The Groden Center, The Cover Center, and The Halcyon Center.

6183 **Office of Rehabilitation Services**
40 Fountain Street
Providence, RI 02903-1898
401-421-7005
TTY: 401-421-7016
www.ors.ri.gov

Ron Racine, Associate Director
Kathleen Brown, Administrator
Joseph Murphy, Administrator, Vocational Rehabilitation
Laurie DiOrio, Administrator, SBVI
Their goal is to help individuals with physical and mental disabilities prepare for and obtain appropriate employment.

6184 **Rhode Island Services for the Blind and Visually Impaired**
40 Fountain Street
Providence, RI 02903-1898
401-421-7005
TTY: 401-421-7016
www.ors.ri.gov/SBVI.html

Ron Racine, Associate Director
Kathleen Brown, Administrator
Joseph Murphy, Administrator, Vocational Rehabilitation
Laurie DiOrio, Administrator, SBVI
Provides qualifying people with visual impairments opportunities to become self-sustaining members of the community.

South Carolina

6185 **South Carolina Commission for the Blind (SCCB)**
1430 Confederate Ave.
Columbia, SC 29201-79
803-898-8734
publicinfo@sccb.sc.gov
www.sccb.state.sc.us

6186 **South Carolina Department of Employment and Workforce (DEW)**
1550 Gadsden St.
PO Box 995
Columbia, SC 29202
803-737-2400
866-831-1724
Dan Ellzey, Executive Director
Public agency that offers job search assistance, unemployment benefits and a WIA program. Also offered are services for individuals with disabilities.

6187 **South Carolina Governor's Committee on Employment of the Handicapped**
S.C. Vocational Rehabilitation Department
1410 Boston Ave.
West Columbia, SC 29171
803-896-6500
800-832-7526
TTY: 806-896-6553
communications@scvrd.net
www.scvrd.net
Felicia W. Johnson, Commissioner
Goal is to help individuals with physical and mental disabilities prepare for and obtain appropriate employment.

6188 **South Carolina Vocational Rehabilitation Department (SCVRD)**
1410 Boston Ave.
West Columbia, SC 29171
803-896-6500
800-832-7526
TTY: 806-896-6553
communications@scvrd.net
www.scvrd.net
Felicia W. Johnson, Commissioner
The SCVRD's mission is to enable eligible South Carolinians with disabilities to prepare for, achieve and maintain competitive employment.

South Dakota

6189 **South Dakota Department of Human Services**
Hillsview Plaza
3800 E Hwy 34
Pierre, SD 57501
605-773-5990
Fax: 605-773-5483
infodhs@state.sd.us
dlr.sd.gov
Shawnie Rechtenbaugh, Secretary
Provides resources for individuals with developmental disabilities, including rehabilitation services, services for the blind and visually impaired, and long-term services and supports.

6190 **South Dakota Department of Human Services: Div. of Service to the Blind & Visually Impaired**
Hillview Plaza
3800 E Highway 34
Pierre, SD 57501
605-773-3195
Fax: 605-773-5483
dhs.sd.gov/servicetotheblind
Shawnie Rechtenbaugh, Secretary
To provide individualized rehabilitation services that result in optimal employment and independent living outcomes for people with visual impairments.

6191 **South Dakota State Vocational Rehabilitation**
Department of Human Services
3800 E Hwy 34
Hillview Plaza
Pierre, SD 57501
605-773-3195
Fax: 605-773-5483
dhs.sd.gov/rehabservices/vr.aspx
Shawnie Rechtenbaugh, Secretary
Provides employment services to people with significant disabilities.

6192 **South Dakota Workforce Investment Act Training Programs**
123 W Missouri Ave.
Pierre, SD 57501-0405
605-773-3101
Fax: 605-773-3101
dlr.sd.gov/workforce_services/wioa
Marcia Hultman, Department Secretary
Hunter Roberts, Deputy Secretary
Andrew Szilvasi, Contact, Employment Services
Kendra Ringstmeyer, Contact, Workforce Training
Mission is to enhance the South Dakota workforce by providing business with employment-related solutions and helping people with job placement and career transition services

Tennessee

6193 **Tennessee Department Human Services: Vocational Rehabilitation Services**
505 Deaderick St.
Nashville, TN 37243-1403
615-313-4891
Fax: 615-741-6508
TTY: 800-270-1349
www.tn.gov/humanservices
Lee A. Brown, III, Chair, State Rehabilitation Council
Determines eligibility and nature/scope of required VR services, and provides those employment-focused rehabilitation services for individuals with disabilities.

6194 **Tennessee Department of Labor and Workforce Development**
220 French Landing Dr.
Nashville, TN 37243
844-224-5818
www.tn.gov/workforce
Jeff McCord, Commissioner
Steve Hawkins, Deputy Commissioner
Deniece Thomas, Deputy Commissioner
Offers services to employees and employers, including job training and adult education.

6195 **Tennessee Human Rights Commission**
312 Rosa L Parks Ave.
23rd Fl.
Nashville, TN 37243
615-741-5825
800-251-3589
Fax: 615-253-1886
ask.thrc@tn.gov
www.tn.gov/humanrights
Beverly L. Watts, Executive Director
Sabrina Hooper, Deputy Director
Dawn Cummings, General Counsel
Veronica McGraw, Communications Director
An independent state agency charged with preventing and eradicating discrimination in employment, public accomodations, and housing.

Texas

6196 **Ability Connection**
8802 Harry Hines Blvd.
Dallas, TX 75235
214-351-2500
abilityconnection.org
Jim Hanophy, President & CEO
Weslie Brittin, Chief Financial Officer
Tai Green, Chief Development Officer
Brain Petty, Senior Director, Operations

Provides training and support services to children and adults with both physical and intellectual disabilities.

6197 **Concentra**
5080 Spectrum Dr.
Suite 1200W
Addison, TX 75001
866-944-6046
www.concentra.com

Keith Newton, Chair, President & CEO
John Anderson, Executive VP & Chief Medical Officer
John deLorimier, Executive VP, Customer Growth & Experience
Greg Gilbert, Senior VP, Chief Reimbursement & Gov. Relations Officer

Offers employers comprehensive occupational health services and state-of-the-art physical and occupational therapy. Staff works as a team to produce the best possible patient care while delivering cost savings through workers compensation disability management programs.

6198 **Texas Workforce Commission (TWC)**
101 E 15th St.
Austin, TX 78778-0001
512-463-2236
Fax: 512-936-0772
customers@twc.state.tx.us
www.twc.state.tx.us

Ed Serna, Interim Executive Director
Courtney Arbour, Division Director, Workforce Development
Cheryl Fuller, Division Director, Vocational Rehabilitation Services
Aaron S. Demerson, Director, Employer Initiatives

State government agency charged with overseeing and providing workforce development services to employers and job seekers of Texas. Offers career development information, job search resources, training programs, and, as appropriate, unemployment benefits.

6199 **Texas Workforce Commission: Vocational Rehabilitation Services**
101 E 15th St.
Austin, TX 78778-0001
800-628-5115
customers@twc.state.tx.us
twc.texas.gov

Ed Serna, Interim Executive Director
Cheryl Fuller, Division Director, Vocational Rehabilitation Services

Helps people with disabilities prepare for, find and keep jobs. Work related services are individualized and may include counseling, training, medical treatment, assistive devices, jon placement assistance and other services.

Utah

6200 **Utah Department of Human Services: Division of Services for People with Disabilities**
195 North 1950 West
Salt Lake City, UT 84116
801-538-4200
844-275-3773
Fax: 801-538-4279
dhsinfo@utah.gov
dspd.utah.gov

6201 **Utah Employment Services**
2292 South Redwood Rd.
Salt Lake City, UT 84119
801-978-0378
Fax: 801-978-0374
info@utahemploy.com
www.utahemploy.com

6202 **Utah Governor's Committee on Employment for People with Disabilities (GCEPD)**
Utah State Office of Rehabilitation
150 North 1950 West
Salt Lake City, UT 84116
801-238-4560
801-359-5627
leahlobato@utah.gov
jobs.utah.gov/usor

Leah Lobato, Director
Suzy Sanchez, Executive Assistant

Promotes opportunities and provide support for persons with disabilities to lead self-determined lives.

6203 **Utah State Office for Rehabilitation (USOR)**
150 North 1950 West
Salt Lake City, UT 84116
801-238-4560
801-359-5627
UT.DD.Salt.Lake.City@ssa.gov
jobs.utah.gov/usor

Sarah Brenna, Director
Jennifer Roth, Director, Finance
Tara Connolly, Compliance Officer

Provides services for individuals who are blind or visually impaired, deaf or hard of hearing, and those with other disabilities, including vocational rehabilitation.

6204 **Utah State Office of Rehabilition: Vocational Rehabilitation**
150 North 1950 West
Salt Lake City, UT 84116
866-454-8397
jobs.utah.gov/usor/vr

Sarah Brenna, Director
Jennifer Roth, Director, Finance
Tara Connolly, Compliance Officer

Vocational Rehabilitation Services for individuals with disabilities. To assist individuals with disabilities to prepare for and obtain employment and increase their independence.

6205 **Utah State Office of Rehabilition: Services for the Blind and Visually Impaired**
150 North 1950 West
Salt Lake City, UT 84116
866-454-8397
jobs.utah.gov/usor/vr

Sarah Brenna, Director
Jennifer Roth, Director, Finance
Tara Connolly, Compliance Officer

Individuals who are blind or visually impaired receive training, adjustment services, and other assistive aids.

6206 **Veterans Support Center (VSC)**
Union Building
Room 418
Salt Lake City, UT 84112
801-587-7722
veteranscenter.utah.edu

Paul Morgan, Director
Carmen Gold, Career Coach
Alan Heal, VA Benefits Counselor
Aaron Ahern, VA Health Counselor

Readjustment counseling services to veterans.

Vermont

6207 **Vermont Department of Disabilities, Aging and Independent Living (DAIL)**
280 State Dr.
HC2 South
Waterbury, VT 05671-2020
802-241-2401
Fax: 802-241-0386
dail.vermont.gov

Monica Caserta Hutt, Commissioner
Camille George, Deputy Commissioner
Monica White, Director, Operations

Provides programs and services for people with physical and developmental disabilities, as well as those with visual impairments, and those over 60 years of age. Employment services for people with disabilities are also provided.

6208 **Vermont Department of Labor**
5 Green Mountain Dr.
PO Box 488
Montpelier, VT 05601- 0488
802-828-4000
labor.commissioner@vermont.gov
labor.vermont.gov

Lindsay H. Kurrle, Commissioner
Michael A. Harrington, Deputy Commissioner

The primary focus is to help support the efforts to make Vermont a more competitive place to do business and create good jobs.

6209 Vermont Division of Vocational Rehabilitation
280 State Dr.
HC2 South
Waterbury, VT 05671-2040
866-879-6757
Fax: 802-241-0341
vocrehab.vermont.gov

Diane Dalmasse, Division Director
Provides employment services to individuals with physical or developmental disabilities.

Virginia

6210 Campagna Center
418 S Washington St.
Alexandria, VA 22314
703-549-0111
Fax: 703-549-2097
www.campagnacenter.org

Tammy Mann, President & CEO
Richard Galanis, Chief Financial Officer
Edith Hawkins, Chief Program Officer
Joy Myers, Chief Development Officer
Offers social services, on-the-job-training for parents, play therapy, physical therapy, speech therapy and other specialized services.

6211 Didlake
8641 Breeden Ave.
Manassas, VA 20110-8431
703-361-4195
866-361-4195
Fax: 703-369-7141
ask@didlake.org
www.didlake.com

Donna J. Hollis, CEO
Denee McKnight, Vice President, Finance & Administration
Offers situational assessments, work training, employment and job placement services to people with disabilities.

6212 Richmond Research Training Center (RRTC)
PO Box 842011
1314 West Main St.
Richmond, VA 23284-2011
804-828-1851
Fax: 804-828-2193
TTY: 804-828-2494
RRTC@vcu.edu
vcurrtc.org

Paul Wehman, Professor & Director
John Kregel, Associate Director
Katherine Inge, Director, Employment
Susan O'Mara, Director, Social Security Programs
Research and training center report on the supported employment of persons with developmental and other disabilities.

6213 ServiceSource Disability Resource Center
10467 White Granite Dr.
Oakton, VA 22124
703-461-6000
www.servicesource.org

Janet Samuelson, President & CEO
Mark Hall, Executive Vice President & Chief Strategy Officer
David Hodge, Executive Vice President & Chief Financial Officer
Bruce Patterson, Executive Vice President & Chief Operating Officer
Provides training, job placement and employment services in private sector and government contract employment.

6214 SourceAmerica
8401 Old Courthouse Rd.
Vienna, VA 22182
888-411-8424
www.sourceamerica.org

Vincent Loose, President & CEO
Kevin Welch, Chief Financial Officer
Joseph Diaz, Senior Vice President, Operations
Cathy Cooke, Vice President, Programs
SourceAmerica facilitates the Federal AbilityOne Program, which provides employment opportunities for people with disabilities. Provides products and services to government, corporate and nonprofit clients, as well as advocating on behalf of the disabled.

6215 Virginia Department for the Blind and Vision Impaired (DBVI)
401 Azalea Ave.
Richmond, VA 23227
804-371-3151
800-622-2155
www.vdbvi.org

Raymond E. Hopkins, Commissioner
Rick L. Mitchell, Deputy Commissioner, Services
Matt Koch, Deputy Commissioner, Enterprises
Wallica Gaines, Deputy Commissioner, Administration
Offers services for the totally blind, legally blind, visually impaired, and more with health, counseling, educational, recreational, rehabilitation, computer training and professional training services.

Washington

6216 Business Enterprise Program (BEP)
Department of Services for the Blind
PO Box 40959
4565 7th Ave. SE
Olympia, WA 98504-0959
206-906-5500
800-552-7103
info@dsb.wa.gov
dsb.wa.gov

Lou Oma Durand, Executive Director
The Program allows qualified legally-blind individuals to operate food service businesses in government buildings.

6217 Department of Services for the Blind (DSB)
PO Box 40959
4565 7th Ave. SE
Olympia, WA 98504-0959
206-906-5500
800-552-7103
info@dsb.wa.gov
dsb.wa.gov

Lou Oma Durand, Executive Director
Offers a range of services for citizens with viosual impairments, including employment services.

6218 Department of Social & Health Services: Division of Vocational Rehabilitation
Customer Service Center
PO Box 11699
Tacoma, WA 98411-6699
800-637-5627
www1.dshs.wa.gov/dvr

Cheryl Strange, Secretary
Robert Hines, Director
Mission is to empower individuals with disabilities to achieve a greater quality of life by obtaining and maintaining employment.

6219 Department of Social & Health Services: Developmental Disabilities Administration (DDA)
Customer Service Center
PO Box 11699
Tacoma, WA 98411-6699
360-725-3413
800-737-0617
Fax: 360-407-0955
askdshs@dshs.wa.gov
www.dshs.wa.gov/dda

Cheryl Strange, Secretary
Sean Murphy, Assistant Secretary, Behavioral Health
Marybeth Queral, Assistant Secretary, Rehabilitation
David Stillman, Assistant Secretary, Economic Services
Offers persons with developmental disabilities quality supports and services that are individual/family driven, stable and flexible, satisfying to the person and their family, and able to meet individual needs.

6220 SL Start Washington
5709 W Sunset Hwy.
Suite 100
Spokane, WA 99224
509-209-2776
www.slstartwashington.com

Kendra Ellis, Executive Director
Britteny Cornwell, Program Director
Vicki Rozell, State Clinical Director
Amelia PepperDay, Health Services Director

A diversified and innovative human and health services company focused on a wide range of social, employment and long-term services.

West Virginia

6221 **West Virginia Division of Rehabilitation Services (DRS)**
107 Capitol St.
Charleston, WV 25301-2609
304-356-2060
800-642-8207
Fax: 304-766-4905
TTY: 304-766-4809
www.wvdrs.org

6222 **WorkForce West Virginia**
112 California Ave
7th Fl.
Charleston, WV 25305
304-558-2660
800-252-5627
Fax: 304-558-1343
workforcelmi@wv.gov
workforcewv.org

Wisconsin

6223 **Department of Workforce Development: Vocational Rehabilitation**
PO Box 7946
Madison, WI 53707-7946
608-261-0050
800-442-3477
dvr@dwd.wisconsin.gov
dwd.wisconsin.gov/dvr

Caleb Frostman, Secretary
JoAnna Richard, Deputy Secretary
Danielle Williams, Assistant Deputy Secretary
Delora Newton, Administrator, Vocational Rehabilitation

Assists eligible individuals with disabilities with finding employment.

Wyoming

6224 **Department of Workforce Services: Vocational Rehabilitation**
Disability Determination Services
2617 E Lincolnway
Suite B
Cheyenne, WY 82002
307-777-7341
Fax: 800-972-2372
wyomingworkforce.org/workers/vr

Jim Mcintosh, Administrator

Provides services to disabled individuals to enable them to reach vocational goals.

6225 **Wyoming Department of Workforce Services: Unemployment Insurance Division**
PO Box 2760
100 West Midwest
Casper, WY 82602-2760
307-235-3264
Fax: 307-235-3277
wyomingworkforce.org/workers/ui

6226 **Wyoming State Rehabilitation Council (SRC)**
Disability Determination Services
2617 E Lincolnway
Suite B
Cheyenne, WY 82002
307-777-7341
Fax: 800-972-2372
SRCwyoming@gmail.com
wyomingworkforce.org/workers/vr/src

Aleyta Zimmerman, Contact

Assists, empowers and supports people with disabilities to achieve employment, independence and intergration in the workplace and community.

Rehabilitation Facilities, Acute

Alabama

6227 **HealthSouth Lakeshore Rehabilitation Hospital**
3800 Ridgeway Dr
Birmingham, AL 35209-5599 205-868-2000
Fax: 205-868-2029
www.healthsouthlakeshorerehab.com
Vickie Demers, Chief Executive Officer
April Cobb, Chief Nursing Officer
Al Rayburn, Director, Therapy Operations
A 100 bed facility whos key services is physical rehabilitation. Also specialized services (inpatient) infection isolation room. In addition, also has outpatient physical rehabilitation and sports medicine. Patient family support services include patient representative, transportation for elderly/handicapped and patient support groups. Imaging services (diagnostic & theraputic) include ct scanner, diagnostic diagnostic radioisotope facility, MRI, and ultrasound.

6228 **HealthSouth Rehabilitation Hospital of North Alabama**
107 Governors Dr
Huntsville, AL 35801 256-535-2300
Fax: 256-428-2608
www.healthsouthhuntsville.com
Douglas H. Beverly, Chief Executive Officer
Susan Creekmore, Director, Therapy Operations
Risha Hoover, Director, Marketing Operations
Joy McMinn, Director, Nursing
A comprehensive 50 bed rehabilitation hospital serving the need of patients in the North Alabama area. Guides patients with physically disabling conditions along an individualized treatment pathway so they can reach their highest level of physical, social and emotional well-being. A wide range of medical and theraputic services are delivered by qualified and experienced professionals.

6229 **J.L. Bedsole/Rotary Rehabilitation Hospital**
Infirmary Health
5 Mobile Infirmary Circle
Mobile, AL 36607-3513 251-435-3417
www.infirmaryhealth.org
D. Mark Nix, President & CEO
Kenneth C. Brewington, Chief Medical Office, Mobile Infirmary
Jennifer Eslinger, President, Mobile Infirmary
Provides rehabilitation for patients affected by stroke, spinal cord injury, brain injury or other neurological illnesses.

6230 **More Than Just a Job**
Institute On Disability/UCED
60 5th Avenue
Suite 101
New York, NY 10011 212-366-8900
Fax: 603-862-0555
www.forbes.com

6231 **Rocky Mountain Resource & Training Institute**
3630 Sinton Road
Suite 103
Colorado Springs, CO 80907- 5072 719-444-0268
800-949-4262
Fax: 719-444-0269
TTY: 800-949-4232
www.adainformation.org
Jana Copeland, Principal Investigator
Patrick Going, Senior Advisor
Serves people with disabilities and provides training to the agencies that assist them. Facilitates disabled individuals' transition from school to adult life; provides information and resources concerning assistive technology, devices, and services; promotes and ensures compliance with the federal Americans with Disabilities Act (ADA) and other legislation promoting the rights and inclusion of people with disabilities; promotes supported employment, strategic planning and development.

Arkansas

6232 **Central Arkansas Rehab Hospital**
2201 Wildwood Ave
Sherwood, AR 72120-5074 501-834-1800
Fax: 501-834-2227
www.stvincentrehabhospital.com
Lee Frazier, MPH, Dr, CEO
Dr. Sean Foley, Medical Director
Debbie Taylor, Director of Marketing Operations
Stacy Sawyer, Director Of Therapy Operations
A nonprofit hospital licensed for 69 acute care beds with all private rooms. Opened in 1999the hospital offers a full range of outpatient diagnostic services, including MRI,CT,PET along with surgical procedures, cardiology, neurology, neurosurgery, othopedic, rehab and a 24 hour emergency department staffed with board certified emergency room physicians. Includes an outpatient surgery center, rehabilitation hospital, senior health program, diabetic program and physician offices.

6233 **HealthSouth Rehabilitation Hospital**
1401 South J St
Fort Smith, AR 72901-5158 479-785-3300
Fax: 479-785-8599
www.healthsouth.com
Juli Stec, CEO
Provides physical rehabilitation as its key services. Also provides other services such as end-of-life services, pain management and an infection isolation room.

6234 **Northwest Arkansas Rehabilitation Hospital**
153 E Monte Painter Dr
Fayetteville, AR 72703-4002 479-444-2233
Fax: 479-444-2390
www.healthsouthfayetteville.com
Marty Hurlbut, Medical Director
Denise Wilson, Director Of Clinical Services
A 60-bed acute medical rehabilitation hospital that offers comprehensive inpatient and outpatient rehabilitation services.

6235 **Rebsamen Rehabilitation Center**
P.O. Box 159
Jacksonville, AR 72078-159 501-985-7000
Fax: 501-985-7384
www.rebsamenmedicalcenter.com
Mack McAlister, Chairperson
Murice Green, Vice Chairman
Tommy Swaim, Secretary
Mission is to provide personal healthcare for your family. Vision is to develop a family of caregivers to become your community hospital. A 113 bed acute care facility operated by a volunteer Board of Directors made up of community leaders. Rebsamen Medical Center is accredited by the Joint Commission on Accredidation of Healthcare Organizations as well as the Arkansas Department of Health. Through JCAHO we voluntary sumbit to evaluations of our compliance with nationwide hospital standards.

Arizona

6236 **Barrow Neurological Institute Rehab Center**
350 W Thomas Rd
Phoenix, AZ 85013-4409 602-406-3000
Fax: 602-406-4104
www.stjosephs-phx.org
Jackie Aragon, VP Care Management
Linda Hunt, President
Dedicated resources to delivering compassionate, high-quality, affordable health services; serving and advocating for our sisters and brothers who are poor and disenfranchised; and partnering with others in the community to improve the quality of life. Our vision:a growing and diversified health care ministry distinguished by excellent quality and committed to expanding access to those in need.

6237 **HealthSouth Sports Medicine Center**
5111 N Scottsdale Rd
Ste 100
Scottsdale, AZ 85250-7076
480-990-1379
Fax: 480-423-8458
www.healthsouth.com

Troy Meiners, Manager
An out patient facility specialising in sports medicine and treatment of sports injuries.

6238 **Healthsouth Rehab Institute of Tucson**
2650 N Wyatt Dr
Tucson, AZ 85712-6108
520-325-1300
800-333-8628
Fax: 520-327-4045
www.rehabinstituteoftucson.com

Lee Sanford, Plant Manager
Jon Larson, Medical Director
An accredited member of the Joint Commission On Accreditation of Health Care Organizaions (JCAHO) An 80 bed facility specializing in rehabilitation

6239 **Scottsdale Healthcare**
9630 E Shea Blvd
Scottsdale, AZ 85260-6285
480-551-5400
Fax: 480-551-5401
preiley@shc.org

Thomas Sadvary, CEO
Pegg Reiley, Chief Nursing Officer
Kathy Zarubi, Associate VP of Nursing Practice
Lisa Sandoval, Director fo Marketing
A 343 bed full-service hospital providing medical/surgical, critical care, obstetrics, pediatrics, surgery, cardiovascular, and oncology services, as well as the Sleep Disorder Center. All patient rooms are private. Emergency department is a level II Trauma Center. The Radiology Department offers state-of-the-art diagnostic equipment, including MRI, PET/CT scanning, nuclear medicine and ultrasound. Also located are the Piper Surgery Center, Cancer Center, and several medical office plazas.

6240 **St. Joseph Hospital and Medical Center**
350 W Thomas Rd
Phoenix, AZ 85013-4496
602-406-3000
Fax: 602-406-4190
http://hospitals.dignityhealth.org/stjosephs/

Linda Hunt, President
Rehabilitation programs offered by the clinic assists clients with rehabilitation health needs in the comfort of their own home. The home care rehabilitation team of professionals focuses on correcting deficiencies in self-care, mobility skills and communication. Services offered include physical therapy, occupational therapy, speech pathology, rehabilitative nursing and restorative nursing assistants.

California

6241 **Bakersfield Regional Rehabilitation Hospital**
5001 Commerce Dr
Bakersfield, CA 93309-648
661-323-5500
800-288-9829
Fax: 661-633-5254
www.healthsouthbakersfield.com

Chris Yoon, Medical Director
Sandra Hegland, Chief Executive Officer
A specialty hospital that treats an array of physical disabilities. It has 60 beds and offers physical rehabilitation services including support groups and education classes on illnesses such as arthritis, asthma and strokes. No surgery facilities on site.

6242 **Brotman Medical Center: RehabCare Unit**
3828 Delmas Ter
Culver City, CA 90232-6806
310-836-7001
Fax: 310-202-4141

Howard Levine, CEO
The mission of Brotman Medical Center is to deliver innovative, quality health care to our patients and their families in an environment of compassion, respect, patient saftey, education, and fiscal responsibility.

6243 **Casa Colinas Centers for Rehabilitation**
255 E Bonita Ave
Pomona, CA 91767-1923
909-596-7733
866-724-4127
Fax: 909-593-0153
TTY: 909-596-3646
rehab@casacolina.org
www.casacolina.org

Felice Loverso, CEO/President
Steve Norin, Chairman
Stephen W. Graeber, Vice Chairman
Mary Lou Jensen, Secretary
Casa Colina will provide individuals the opportunity to maximize their medical recovery and rehabilitation potential efficiently in an environment that recognizes their uniqueness, dignity and self esteem. The vision is to strategically reposition themselves at the forefront of the post-acute continuum by becoming the center of excellence in the provision of services to persons who can benefit from rehabilitation care.

6244 **Community Hospital of Los Gatos Rehabilitation Services**
815 Pollard Rd
Los Gatos, CA 95032-1400
408-378-6131
Fax: 408-866-4003

Ned Borgstrom, CEO
Rehabilitation Services provide individualized treatment programs for inpatient/outpatient care. The team is supervised by a Physiatrist and may include Nurses, Physical Therapists, Occupational Therapists, Speech/Language Therapists, Psychologists, Case Managers, Dietitians, Respiratory Therapists, Recreation Therapists and/or Prosthetists/Orthotists.

6245 **Garfield Medical Center**
525 N Garfield Ave
Monterey Park, CA 91754-1205
626-573-2222
Fax: 626-571-8972
www.garfieldmedicalcenter.com

Philip Cohen, CEO
Provides quality care to all citizens of all ages. We are foreward looking to meet the changing health care needs of Forsyth and the surrounding area. At the same time, we are a stable organization that is financially sound. We involve all of our medical staff through good communication. We support them by trying to meet their professional needs in training, equipment and services. We emphasize good communication with all county citizens who support us financially and through the use of services

6246 **Grossmont Hospital Rehabilition Center**
5555 Grossmont Center
La Mesa, CA 91942
619-740-6000
800-827-4277
Fax: 619-644-4159
www.sharp.com

Michael Murphy, President/CEO
Daniel Gross, EVP
It is our mission to improve the health of those we serve with a commitment to excellence in all that we do. Our goal is to offer quality care and programs that set community standards, exceed patients' expectations and are provided in a caring, convenient, cost-effective and accessible manner.

6247 **Health South Tustin Rehabilitation Hospita**
14851 Yorba St
Tustin, CA 92780-2925
714-832-9200
Fax: 714-508-4550
www.healthsouth.com

Sandra Yule, CEO

6248 **Holy Cross Comprehensive Rehabilitation Center**
15031 Rinaldi St
Mission Hills, CA 91345-1207
818-365-8051
888-432-5464
Fax: 818-898-4472
www.providence.org

Larry Bowe, CEO
Derek Berz, COO
Known for providing exceptional treatment through its Cancer Centers, Heart Center, Orthopedics, Neurosciences and Rehabilitation Services, as well as Woman's and Children's Services. As a 254-bed, not-for-profit facility, Providence offers a full contin-

uum of health services, from outpatient to inpatient to home health care. Providence operates one of the only round-the-clock trauma centers in the San Fernando Valley and surrounding communities.

6249 Job Hunting Tips for the So-Called Handicapped
Special Needs Project
324 State Street
Suite H
Santa Barbara, CA 93101-2364
818-718-9900
800-333-6867
Fax: 818-349-2027
editor@specialneeds.com
www.specialneeds.com

Hod Gray, Owner
This nifty booklet from the guru of job hunting himself is sincere, useful and brief. *$4.95*

6250 Kentfield Rehabilitation Hospital & Outpatient Center
1125 Sir Francis Drake Blvd
Kentfield, CA 94904-1418
415-456-9680
Fax: 415-485-3563
info@kentfieldrehab.com
www.kentfieldrehab.com

Deborah Doherty, MD
Provides specialized inpatient and outpatient programs. We provide quality services that are patient centered and family-oriented. Under the medical direction of board-certified hospitalists and other physician specialists, our decicated interdisciplinary teams provide a coordinated, comprehensive treatment approach to a wide range of neurological, orthopedic, pulmonary and complex medical problems.

6251 Laurel Grove Hospital: Rehab Care Unit
20103 Lake Chabot Rd
Castro Valley, CA 94546-4093
510-537-1234
Fax: 510-727-2778
nissims@sutterhealth.org
www.edenmedcenter.org

George Bischalaney, CEO & President
Kent Myers, Treasurer
Jeffrey Randall, Secretary
David Davini, CPA Chairman
The mission of Eden Medical Center is carried out by our Board of Directors, employees, physicians and volunteers who are committed to providing our patients and their families with the highest quality medical care and customer service. Creating standards of excellence to ensure quality and value for our patients. Maintaining a financially sound organization through effective clinical and administrative support. Encouraging a culture that supports employees and physicians in development.

6252 Lodi Memorial Hospital West
Lodi Memorial Hospital
975 S Fairmont Ave
Lodi, CA 95240
209-334-3411
800-323-3360
Fax: 209-333-7131

Joseph Harrington, President
Ron Kreutner, Vice President And CFO
Judy Begley RN, MSN, Chief Nursing Officer
Our vision is to provide a system of health-care services which is clinically effective, quality driven and community focused in an environment that supports and encourages excellence. In partnership with our medical staff, we will assume accountability for the health of our community, be responsible for illness and injury prevention and provide care for the ill and injured. We will measure our success on quality outcomes and customer satisfaction.

6253 Long Beach Memorial Medical Center Memorial Rehabilitation Hospital
2801 Atlantic Ave
Long Beach, CA 90806-1701
562-933-2000
Fax: 562-933-9018
www.memorialcare.org

Nissar Syed, Administrator
Barry Arbuckle, President
The hospital offers rehabilitation after catastrophic injury of disabling disease to give patients the opportunity for maximum recovery. The Hospital offers many of the area's finest rehabilitation specialists and most advanced technology, making it one of Southern California's most respected rehabilitation centers.

6254 North Coast Rehabilitation Center
1165 Montgomery Drive
Santa Rosa, CA 95405-4869
707-546-3210
Fax: 707-525-8413

Joyce Cavagnaro, Admissions
Combines state-of-the-art medicine, compassionate care, and the widest array of resources to enhance your health and promote healthy communities. Dedicated to continually introducing new programs and services that help you live life to the fullest.

6255 Northridge Hospital Medical Center
18300 Roscoe Blvd
Northridge, CA 91328
818-885-8500
Fax: 818-885-5435
www.northridgehospital.org

Mike Wall, CEO
dedicating resources to delivering compassionate, high-quality, affordable health services; serving and advocating for our sisters and brothers who are poor and disinfranchised; and partnering with others in the community to improve the quality of life.

6256 PEERS Program
8912 W Olympic Blvd
Beverly Hills, CA 90211-3514
310-553-4833
Fax: 310-553-4833

Paul Berns, Medical Director
Offers a new approach for wheelchair users. PEERS uses a combination of modern physical therapy, the DOUGLAS Reciprocating Gait System and when necessary, functional electrical stimulation to assist selected individuals to walk with recently patented specially made lightweight braces.

6257 PIRS Hotsheet
Placer Independent Resource Services
11768 Atwood Rd
Ste 29
Auburn, CA 95603
530-885-6100
800-833-8453
Fax: 530-885-3032
TTY: 530-885-0326
lbrewer@pirs.org
pirs.org

Susan Miller, Executive Director
Harry Powell, President
Paul Opper, Vice President
Dawn Davidson, Secretary
Monthly newletter to customers and other constituents.
6 pages Monthly

6258 Providence Holy Cross Medical Center
Providence Health System
15031 Rinaldi St
Mission Hills, CA 91345-1285
818-365-8051
818-898-4603
Fax: 818-365-4472
www.providence.org

Kerry Carmody, CEO
Physicains and nurses are among the best and are recoginzed nationally for clinical excellence. We are committed to improving your health and wellness as you journey through life. Our services span beyond the latest advancements in medical procedures, equipment and medication to also include education and wellness services-all provided with compassion and respect. We help our patients understand and use some of the healthiest tools at their disposal, including nutrition & excercise.

6259 Queen of Angels/Hollywood Presbyterian Medical Center
1300 N Vermont Ave
Los Angeles, CA 90027-6005
213-413-3000
Fax: 213-413-3500
www.hollywoodpresbyterian.com

Kathy Wong, Manager
A 434 bed acute-care facility that has been caring for the Hollywood community and surrounding areas since 1924. The hospital is committed to serving local multicultural communities with quality medical and nursing care. With more then 500 physicians representing virtually every speciality. Ready to serve your medi-

cal needs and those of your loved ones and strive to distinguish itself as a leading healthcare provider, recognized for providing quality, innovative care in a compassionate manner.

6260 **Queen of the Valley Hospital**
1000 Trancas St
Napa, CA 94558-2941
707-252-4411
Fax: 707-257-4032
www.thequeen.org

Walt Mickens, President
Vincent Morgese, Vice President
For more then 40 years, Queen of the Valley Hospital has been the premiere medical facility in the Napa Valley. Our long history of providing high quality and caring service is founded on 4 core values:Dignity, Service, Excellence and Justice. These central principals inspire us to reach out to those in need and to help heal the whole person-mind, body and spirit.They are the driving force behind our mission to improve the health and quality of life of people in the community we serve.

6261 **Rancho Los Amigos National Rehabilitation Center**
7601 E Imperial Hwy
Downey, CA 90242-3496
562-401-7111
877-726-2461
888-RAN-CHO1
Fax: 562-401-6690
TTY: 562-401-8450
dhs.lacounty.gov/wps/portal/dhs/rancho

Jorge Orozco, CEO
Mindy Lipson Aisen, Chief Medical Officer
Michelle Sterling, Interim Chief Nursing Officer
Robin Bayus, CFO
Internationally renowned in the field of medical rehabilitation, consistently ranked in the top Rehabilitation Hospitals in the United States by U.S. News and World Report. It is one of the largest comprehensive rehabilitaion centers in the United States. Licensed for 395 beds, providing service through over 20 centers of excellence.

6262 **San Joaquin Valley Rehabilitation Hospital**
7173 N Sharon Ave
Fresno, CA 93720-3329
559-436-3600
Fax: 559-436-3606
sjvrehab.com

Edward Palacios, CEO
Complete comprehensive rehabilitation services from acute rehab, outpatient and community fitness services.

6263 **Santa Clara Valley Medical Center**
County of Santa Clara
751 S Bascom Ave
San Jose, CA 95128-2699
408-885-5000
www.scvmed.org

Paul E. Lorenz, CEO
Jeffrey Arnold, Medical Officer
Trudy Johnson, Director of Patient Care Services & Nursing
Carolyn Brown, Director of Quality & Patient Safety
The mission of the medical center is to provide high-quality, cost-effective medical care to all residence of Santa Clara County regardless of their ability to pay. Make availiable a wide range of inpatient, outpatient, emergency services within resource constraints. Maintain an environment within which the needs of our patients are paramount and where patients, their families and all our visitors are treated in a compassionate, supportive, friendly, and dignified manner.

6264 **Scripps Memorial Hospital at La Jolla**
9888 Genesee Ave
La Jolla, CA 92037-1205
858-626-4123
800-727-4777
Fax: 858-626-6122
www.scripps.org

Sean A Deitch, President/CEO
Gary Fybel, Executive Director/Administrator
One of the county's 6 designated trauma centers, offers a wide range of clinical and surgical services including 24-hour emergency services; intensive care; interventional cardiology and radiology; radiation oncology; cardiothoracic and orthopedic services; neurology; ophthalmology; and mental health and psychology services.

6265 **South Coast Medical Center**
12 Mason
Ste A
Irvine, CA 92618-2733
714-669-4446
Fax: 714-669-4448
info@southcoastmedcenter.com

Leigh Erin Connealy, Manager
Bruce Christian, President
A 208 bed acute care hospital. Services include maternity, surgical, subacute care, psychiatric program, eating disorder treatment, chemical dependency treatment, radiology, ICU/CCU, comprehensive rehabilitation services, bariatric surgery and movement disorders program..

6266 **St. Joseph Rehabilitation Center**
St. Joseph Health System
2200 Harrison Ave
Eureka, CA 95501-3215
707-441-4414
Fax: 707-441-4429
www.stjosepheureka.org

6267 **St. Jude Brain Injury Network**
St. Jude Hospital
130 W Bastanchury Rd
Fullerton, CA 92835-1058
714-446-5626
866-785-8332
Fax: 714-446-5979
ocrcuser@stjoe.org
www.tbioc.org

Jana Gable, Program Coordinator
David Bogdan, Service Coordinator
Lina Marroquin, Servicer Coordinator
Provides comprehensive planning, program referral, assists with funding possibilities, and interagency coordination of services. Areas of emphasis include day treatment, vocational and housing options, and the requirements are adults who have suffered a brain injury from an external force.

6268 **St. Jude Medical Center**
101 E Valencia Mesa Dr
Fullerton, CA 92835-3809
714-871-3280
800-627-8106
Fax: 714-992-3029
stjudemedicalcenter.org

Robert Fraschetti, President
We are one of Southern California's most respected and technologically advanced hospitals, and our four core values: dignity, excellence, service and justice are the guiding principles for everything we do. St. Jude is synonymous with exceptional care that extends beyond good medicine to a commitment to caring for you - mind, body and spirit.

6269 **St. Mary Medical Center**
1050 Linden Ave
Long Beach, CA 90813-3393
562-491-9000
Fax: 562-491-9053
www.stmarymedicalcenter.org

Chris Desicco, CEO

6270 **Sunnyside Nursing Center**
22617 S Vermont Ave
Torrance, CA 90502-2595
310-320-4130
Fax: 310-212-3232
www.sunnysidenursing.com

Shane Dahl, Administrator
Manny Cordero, Director of Nursing
El Sayad, Medical Director
Skilled nursing care facility; residential care facility; intermediate care facility; specialty hospital.

6271 **UCLA Medical Center: Department of Anesthesiology, Acute Pain Services**
U CL A Medical Center
1245 16th Street Medical Plz
Ste 225
Santa Monica, CA 90404
310-794-1841
Fax: 310-794-1511
access@mednet.ucla.edu

Michael Ferrante, Clinical Director
A 337-bed acute-care medical center, has been serving the healthcare needs of West Los Angeles and Santa Monica since

1926. Highly regarded for its primary and specialty care, the medical center features many outstanding clinical programs, including its women's and children's services, emergency services, and family medicine programs.

Colorado

6272 **Children's Hospital Rehabilitation Center**
University of Colorado Health Sciences Center
1056 E 19th Ave
Denver, CO 80218-1007
303-861-8888
800-624-6553
chipteam.org

Lou Blankenship, CEO
Michael J Farrell, Chief Operating Officer
Helen Martinez, Manager

Private not-for-profit pediatric healthcare network, the hospital is 100 percent dedicated to caring for kids of all ages and stages of growth. That dedication is evident in more then 1000 pediatric specialists and more then 2400 employees. It is also our continual dedication that has placed us at the forefront of research in childhood disease with several nationally and internationally recognized medical programs.

6273 **Craig Hospital**
3425 S Clarkson St
Englewood, CO 80113-2899
303-789-8000
Fax: 303-789-8214
khosack@craighospital.org
www.craighospital.org

Michael Fordyce, President
Thomas Balazy, Medical Director
Julie Keegan, VP of Finance
Dona Polonsky, VP of Clinical Services

A 93-bed, private, not-for-profit, free-standing, acute care and rehabilitation hospital that provides a comprehensive system of inpatient and outpatient medical care, rehabilitation, neurosurgical rehabilitative care, an equipment company, and long-term follow up services.

6274 **HealthSouth Rehabilitation Hospital of Colorado Springs**
HealthSouth Corporation
325 S Parkside Dr
Colorado Springs, CO 80910-3134
719-630-8000
Fax: 719-520-0387
www.healthsouthcoloradosprings.com

Steve Schaefer, CEO

A 56 bed rehabilitation hospital, its key services are: cardiology department, physical rehabilitation, and orthopedics department. Accredidted to the Joint Commission on Accreditation of Health Care Organizations (JCAHO)

6275 **Mapleton Center**
North Broadway & Balsam
Boulder, CO 80301-9130
303-440-2273
Fax: 303-441-0536
pr@bch.org
www.bch.org

David Gehant, President/CEO

Comprehensive inpatient and outpatient rehabilitation services for all age groups. Treatment provided by interdisciplinary teams and staff physicians. CARF accredited in brain injury rehabilitation, pediatric rehabilitation, pain management, work hardening and inpatient rehabilitation.

6276 **Mediplex Rehab: Denver**
Vibra Health Care
8451 Pearl St
Thornton, CO 80229-4804
303-288-3000
Fax: 303-496-1120
info@vhdenver.com
www.northvalleyrehab.com

Walter Sacckett, CEO

Encompasses the broadest mix of professional talent, the finest technology and a total commitment by our people to deliver the highest quality care today, and well into the future. The services can be divided into 4 main categories: long term Acute Care and rehab. Skilled nursing facility and residential ventilator program. Outpatient services and pain management. Adult and Geriatric inpatient psychiatric services.

Connecticut

6277 **Mariner Health Care: Connecticut**
23 Liberty Way
Niantic, CT 06357
860-739-4007
Fax: 860-701-2202

District of Columbia

6278 **National Rehabilitation Hospital**
102 Irving St NW
Washington, DC 20010-2949
202-877-1760
Fax: 202-829-2789
www.nrhrehab.org

Edward Healton, Medical Director
Robert Bunning, Associate Medical Director

A private facility dedicated solely to medical rehabilitation. The hospital offers intensive inpatient programs and full-service outpatient programs.

Florida

6279 **Florida Hospital Rehabilitation Center**
601 E Rollins St
Orlando, FL 32803-1248
407-303-1527
855-303-3627
Fax: 407-303-7566
fh.web@flhosp.org

Rex Alleyne, President

Florida Hospital Orlando uses the latest technology to treat over 32,000 inpatients and 53,600 outpatients annually. This 881-bed, acute-carecommunity hospital also serves as a major tertiary facility for much of the Southeast, the Caribbean and South America

6280 **HealthSouth Regional Rehab Center/Florida**
20601 Old Cutler Rd
Miami, FL 33189-2441
305-251-3800
Fax: 305-259-0498
www.healthsouth.com

Murray Rolnick, Medical Director
Elizabeth Izquierdo, Chief Executive Officer

HealthSouth Rehabilitation Hospital of Miami is a member of the HealthSouth Corporation, the nation's largest healthcare services provider. The hospital is accredited by the Joint Commission on Accreditation of Healthcare Organizations (JCAHO) and Commission on Accreditaion of Rehabilitation Facilities (CARF). Services offered include dietary services, occupational therapy, and respitory care.

6281 **HealthSouth Rehab Hospital: Largo**
901 Clearwater Largo Rd N
Largo, FL 33770-4121
727-586-2999
Fax: 727-588-3404
www.healthsouthlargo.com

Elaine Ebaugh, CEO
Linda Russo, Director, Therapies

A specialty hospital devoted to providing comprehensive medical rehabilitation services. The hospital is licensed as a Comprehensive Medical Rehabilitation Hospital by the state of Florida, and accredited by the Joint Commission on Accreditation of Healthcare Organizations (JCAHO). HealthSouth of Largo is the only free standing Rehabilitation Hospital in the Tampa Bay region, and serves patients of all ages. Provides inpatient medical rehabilitation services as well as outpatient programs.

6282 **HealthSouth Sports Medicine & Rehabilitation Center**
3280 Ponce De Leon Blvd
Coral Gables, FL 33134-7252 305-444-0909
Fax: 305-444-5760
www.healthsouth.com

Jay Greeney, President
Ray Jaffet, Administrator

Provides specialized medical and therapeutic services designated to help physically disabled individuals reach their optimum level of independence and function by providing inpatient and outpatient comprehensive medical rehabilitation services.

6283 **HealthSouth Sports Medicine and Rehabilitation Center**
2141 South Highway A1A Alt
Jupiter, FL 33477 561-743-8890
Fax: 561-743-8795

Diane Reiley, Manager

Outpatient orthopedic and sports medicine/physical therapy.

6284 **HealthSouth Treasure Coast Rehabilitation Hospital**
Health South Corporation of Alabama
1600 37th St
Vero Beach, FL 32960-4863 772-778-2100
Fax: 772-567-7041
www.healthsouthtreasurecoast.com

Jimmy Lockhart, Medical Director

HealthSouth Treasure Coast Rehabilitation Hospital is a 90-bed inpatient comprehensive rehabilitation hospital serving Indian River, St. Lucie, Martin and Okeechobee counties. Outpatient services are available at the hospital and at four other clinics. Therapies include physical, occupational, speech and psychology services.

6285 **Manatee Springs Care & Rehabilitation Center**
5627 9th St E
Bradenton, FL 34203-6105 941-753-8941
Fax: 941-739-4409
www.manateespringsrehab.com

Donna Steiermann, Administrator

Skilled rehabilitation facility specializing in PT, OT, speech therapy, aquatic therapy and an indoor pool. Piped oxygen bed for specialized respiratory care. Compassionate end of life care. Some Medicare, private insurance, and Medicaid.

6286 **Perry Health Facility**
207 Marshall Dr
Perry, FL 32347-1897 850-584-6334
Fax: 850-838-1801

Rebkah Hatch, Administrator

Full rehabilitation team available, Physiatrist, DOR, Psychiatrist, Psychologist, RD, Geriatric Nursing, PT/OT/ST/RT, Orthotiet/Prosthetist. Provider for PPO's & HMO's as well as medicare, private insurance and medicare/medicaid.

6287 **Pinecrest Rehabilitation Hospital and Outpatient Centers**
Tenet South Florida
5352 Linton Blvd
Delray Beach, FL 33484-6514 561-498-4440
800-283-8326
Fax: 561-495-3103
www.pinecrestrehab.com

Mark Bryan, CEO

Pinecrest Rehabilitation Hospital is a 90 bed, accredited hospital and is comprised of a Specialty Unit, a Neuro Trauma Unit and Joint Replacement Unit. Additional services at Pincrest include six outpatient rehab centers throughout Palm Beach County. The Outpatient Centers each focus on various specialties such as orthopedic and neurological rehab, pain management, cardiac and pulmonary rehab, occupational medicine, Hearing Institute, dizziness and balance and wellness.

6288 **Rehabilitation Institute of Sarasota**
3251 Proctor Rd
Sarasota, FL 34231-8538 941-921-8796
Fax: 941-922-6228

Stacy Shepherd, Director Clinical Services

a 75-bed hospital that offers individualized medical and theraputic services tailored to patients and clinics for those affected with stroke, multiple sclerosis, Parkinson's, muscular dystrophy and Lou Gehrig's disease (ALS)

6289 **Sea Pines Rehabilitation Hospital**
101 E Florida Ave
Melbourne, FL 32901-8398 321-984-4600
Fax: 321-727-7440
ellen.lyons-olski@healthsouth.com
www.healthsouthseapines.com

Stuart Miller, Medical Director
Donna Bohdal, Director of Therapy Operations
Denise McGrath, Administrator

A 90-bed facility specializing in rehabilitation of brain and spinal injuries.

6290 **Shriners Hospitals for Children: Tampa**
12502 USF Pine Dr
Tampa, FL 33612-9411 813-972-2250
813-281-0300
Fax: 813-975-7125
aargiz-lyons@shrinenet.org
www.shrinershq.org/hospitals/tampa

David Ferrell, FACHE
Maureen Maciel, Chief of Staff
Alicia Argis-Lyons, Develpoment Officer

Recognizing that the family plays a vital role in a child's ability to overcome an illness or injury, Shriners Hospitals helps the family provide the support the child needs by involving the family in all aspects of the child's care and recovery. The purpose of all Shriners Hospitals for Children is to provide care to children with orthopedic problems and burn injuries to help them lead fuller, more productive lives.

6291 **South Miami Hospital**
6200 SW 73rd St
South Miami, FL 33143-4679 786-662-4000
Fax: 786-662-5302
www.baptisthealth.net

Brian E. Keely, CEO

The mission is to improve the health and well-being of individuals, and to promote the sanctity and preservation of life, in the communities we serve. We are committed to maintaining the highest standards of clinical and service excellence, rooted in utmost integrity and moral practice.

6292 **St. Anne's Nursing Center**
11855 Quail Roost Dr
Miami, FL 33177-3956 305-252-4000
Fax: 305-969-6752
www.catholichealthservices.org

Tony Farinella, Executive Director
Francisco Cruz, Medical Director
Julia Shillingford, Director of Nursing

Provides spacious, comfortable accommodations with ample recreational areas in a beautifully landscaped setting.

6293 **St. Anthony's Hospital**
1200 7th Ave N
St Petersburg, FL 33705-1388 727-825-1100
www.stanthonys.com

William Ulbricht, President
James McClint, VP
Ron Colaguori, VP Operations
Mary McNally, VP Mission

A not-for-profit, 395-bed hospital established in 1931. St. Anthony's is dedicated to improving the health of the community through community-owned health care that sets the standard for high-quality, compassionate care.

6294 **St. Anthony's Rehabilitation Hospital**
3487 NW 35th Ave
Lauderdale Lakes, FL 33311-1107 954-485-4023
954-739-6233
www.catholichealthservices.org

Linda Motte, Hospital Administrator
Kathy Torbertsonn, Dir. Rehab.

Provides spacious, comfortable accommodations with ample recreational areas in a beautifully landscaped setting.

6295 **St. Catherine's Rehabilitation Hospital and Villa Maria Nursing Center**
1050 NE 125th St
North Miami, FL 33161-5805
305-357-1735
305-891-3361
www.catholichealthservices.org
Virginia Irving, Hospital Administrator
Jim Reiss, Executive Director
Greg Hartley, Director Rehab
St. Catherine's Rehabilitation Hospital is a CARF accredited, 60 bed facility offering inpatient and outpatient rehabilitation and medical clinics; including physical, occupational, and speech therapy, neurology, neurodiagnostics, wound care, and hyperbaric medicine. Villa Maria Nursing center is a JCAHO accredited, 212 bed skilled nursing center providing short term nursing and rehabilitation, as well as long term care.

6296 **St. John's Nursing Center**
3075 NW 35th Ave
Lauderdale Lakes, FL 33311-1107
954-739-6233
Fax: 954-733-9579
www.catholichealthservices.org
Ralph E. Lawson, Chairman
Elizabeth Worley, Vice Chairman
Thomas Marin, Assistant Secretary
Provides spacious, comfortable accommodations with ample recreational areas in a beautifully landscaped setting.

6297 **Successful Job Accommodation Strategies**
LRP Publications
36- Hiatt Dr
Palm Beach Gardens, FL 33418
561-622-6520
800-341-7874
Fax: 561-622-0757
webmaster@lrp.com
www.lrp.com
Honora McDowell, Product Group Manager
Kenneth Kahn, Chief Executive Officer
This monthly newsletter provides you with quick tips, new accommodation ideas and innovative workplace solutions. You learn the outcomes of the latest cases involving workplace accommodations. *$140.00*
12 pages Monthly

6298 **Tampa General Rehabilitation Center**
1 Tampa General Circle
Tampa, FL 33601-1289
813-844-7000
Fax: 813-844-1477
tgh.org
Ron Hytoff, President/CEO
Devanand Mangar MD, Vice Chief of Staff
Thomas L. Bernasek MD, Chief of Staff
Offers a full range of inpatient and outpatient programs all aimed at helping patients achieve their full potentials. JCAHO and CARF accredited and V.R. designated center. A wide range of inpatient and outpatient programs are available such as Brain and Spinal Cord Injury Programs, Comprehensive Medical Rehabilitation, Pain Management, Cardiac Rehab, Pediatric Therapy Service, Sleep Disorders, Epilepsy, and Wheelchair Seating.Hosts the Florida Alliance for Assistive Services and Technolgy.

6299 **University of Miami: Jackson Memorial Rehabilitation Center**
University of Miami
1611 NW 12th Ave
Miami, FL 33136-1005
305-585-6970
Fax: 305-585-6092
info@jhsmiami.org
www.jhsmiami.org
Michael Butler, Chief Medical Officer
An accredited, non-profit, tertiary care hospital and the major teaching facility for the University of Miami School of Medicine. With more then 1,550 beds, Jackson Memorial is a referral center, a magnet for medical research, and home to the Ryder Trauma Center- the only adult and pediatric level 1 trauma center in Miami-Dade County.

6300 **Winter Park Memorial Hospital**
Florida Hospital
200 N Lakemont Ave
Winter Park, FL 32792-3273
407-646-7000
Fax: 407-646-7639
healthcare@winterparkhospital.com
www.winterparkhospital.com
Ken Bradley, CEO
Offers Acute Rehabilitation.

Georgia

6301 **Candler General Hospital: Rehabilitation Unit**
5353 Reynolds St
Savannah, GA 31405-6015
912-819-6000
Fax: 912-819-8829
www.sjchs.org/body.cfm?id=383
Paul Hinchey, President/CEO
Special Physical Therapy Services at Candler Outpatient Center: Aquatic therapy, pediatric services, outpaitient neurological rehabilitation program, woman's health therapy, orthotics, and spine specialty

6302 **Children's Healthcare of Atlanta at Egleston**
1405 Clifton Rd. NE
Atlanta, GA 30322
www.choa.org
Donna Hyland, President & CEO
Ruth Fowler, Chief Financial Officer
Stephanie M. Jernigan, Campus Director, Egleston
Rehabilitation Center at Egleston accepts children from birth to age 18 with acute or chronic problems. The length of rehab stay varies for each child according to the determined program of care. The center offers inpatient, outpatient and day rehab programs for comprehensive evaluation and treatment.

6303 **Cobb Hospital and Medical Center: Rehab Care Center**
3950 Austell Rd
Austell, GA 30106-1121
770-732-5126
www.wellstar.org
David Anderson, Executive VP
Michael Andrews, Chief Cancer Network Officer
Avril Beckford, Chief Pediatrics Officer
To deliver world class healthcare we equip our healthcare facilities and employees with the best technology, resources and education availiable. To deliver world class healthcare we keep seeking ways to improve the way we deliver care knowing each day holds more miracles, more life, more chances, more compassion, and more opportunities.

6304 **HealthSouth Central Georgia Rehabilitation Hospital**
3351 Northside Dr
Macon, GA 31210-2587
478-201-6500
Fax: 478-471-6536
www.centralgarehab.com

6305 **Specialty Hospital**
Floyd Healthcare Resources
304 Turner McCall Blvd SW
Rome, GA 30165-5621
706-509-5000
Fax: 706-802-4175
contactus@floyd.org
www.floyd.org
Kurt Stuenkel, CEO
Dee Russell, Chief Medical Officer
Our mission is to be responsive to the communities we serve with a comprehensive and technologically advanced heal care system commited to the delivery of care that is characterized by continually improving quality, accessability, affordability and personal dignity.

Hawaii

6306 **Shriners Hospital for Children: Honolulu**
1310 Punahou St
Honolulu, HI 96826-1099
808-941-4466
888-888-6314
Fax: 808-942-8573
jburda@shrinenet.org
www.shrinershospitalsforchildren.org

Kenneth Guidera, Chief Medical Officer
Eugene D'Amore, Vice President
Kathy A. Dean, Vice President Human Resources
Sharon Russell, VP Finance & Accounting

One of 22 hospitals across North America that provide excellent, no-cost medical care to children with orthopedic problems and burn industries.

Idaho

6307 **Pocatello Regional Medical Center**
777 Hospital Way
Pocatello, ID 83201-2797
208-234-6154
Fax: 208-239-3719
robbieo@portmed.org
www.portmed.org

Mark Bukalew, Chairman
John Abreu, VP Finance
Stephen Weeg, Vice-Chairman
David Swindell, Treasurer

Pocatello Regional Medical Center offers 24-hour emergency care, specialized heart services, a dialysis center, a full service rehabilitation unit including transition care, and the Woman's Center For Health including obstetrics.

Illinois

6308 **Builders of Skills**
515 Busse Hwy
Park Ridge, IL 60068-3154
847-318-0870
Fax: 847-292-0873
www.avenuestoindependence.org

Jacqueline Kinmel, Chair
Peg O'herron, Vice Chair
Eric Johnson, Treasurer
Bob Healy, Secretary

Residential setting for hearing-impaired, developmentally disabled adults who are assisted with daily living skills.

6309 **Center for Learning**
National-Louis University
2840 Sheridan Rd
Evanston, IL 60201-1730
847-256-5150
Fax: 845-256-1057

Jerry Dachs, Manager

Psycho-educational evaluations for children, adolescents, and adults. Individualized remedial academic programs, individual counseling

6310 **DBTAC-Great Lakes ADA Center**
1640 W Roosevelt Road
Room 405
Chicago, IL 60608-1316
312-413-1407
800-949-4232
Fax: 312-413-1856
www.adagreatlakes.org

Robin Jones, Project Director
Glenn Fujiura, PhD, Director of Research and Co-Inve
Claudia Diaz, Associate Project Director
Peter Berg, Project Coordinator for Technica

Provides training, technical assistance and consultation on the rights and resposibilities of indiviualsand entities covered by the ADA. Toll free number for technical assistance and materials provided electronically or via mail at no cost.

6311 **Institute of Physical Medicine and Rehabilitation**
6501 N Sheridan Rd
Peoria, IL 61614-2932
309-692-8110
800-957-4767
Fax: 309-692-8673

Lisa Snyder, Medical Director

Comprehensive CARF accredited programs in outpatient medical rehabilitation services. Eight outpatient locations, specialty programs include adult day services, driving evaluations, balance and visual rehabilitation board certified physiatrists.

6312 **LaRabida Children's Hospital and Research Center**
E 65th At Lake Michigan
Chicago, IL 60649
773-363-6700
Fax: 773-363-9554
pr@larabida.org
www.larabida.org

Brenda Wolf, President/CEO

Dedicated to excellence in caring for children with chronic illness, disabilitiesm or who have been abused, allowing them to achieve their fullest potential through expertise and innovation within the health care and academic communities.

6313 **Marianjoy Rehabilitation Hospital and Clinics**
26W171 Roosevelt Rd
Wheaton, IL 60187-6078
630-909-8000
800-462-2366
Fax: 630-909-8001
www.marianjoy.org

Maureen Beal, Chairperson
John Oliverio, Vice Chairman
Kathleen Dvorakk, Treasurer
Thomas A. Keiser, Secretary

Goal at Marianjoy Rehabilitation Hospital is to help you and your family return to the lifestyle you enjoyed before your illness or injury. To meet this goal, we provide you with a dedicated team of experienced professionals to assist you every step of the way.

6314 **Rush Copley Medical Center-Rehab Neuro Physical Unit**
2040 Ogden Ave
Ste 303
Aurora, IL 60504-7222
630-898-3700
866-426-7539
Fax: 630-898-3681
clord@rsh.net
www.rushcopley.com

Barry Finn, CEO
Mary Shilkaitis, VP, Patient Care Services

The mission of the medical center and the medical staff is to work together to serve your healthcare needs through excellence in education, technology and a caring touch. Rush-Copley Medical Center will be the leading healthcare provider of the greater Fox Valley area. At Rush-Copley we pride ourselves on providing everyone with extrodinary service.

Indiana

6315 **ATTAIN**
U S Department of Education/ NI DR R
32 E Washington St
Ste 1400
Indianapolis, IN 46204-3552
317-534-0236
800-528-8246

Gary Hand, Executive Director

The mission of Attain is to create solutions that enable people with functional limitations to live, learn, work and play in the community of their choice. All will have access to assistive devices. We will do this in partnership with people with functional limitations, families and members of the community through training, system change, services and support, research, dissemination and consumer advocacy.

6316 About Special Kids
7172 Graham Rd
Suite 100
Indianapolis, IN 46250-2879
317-257-8683
800-964-4746
Fax: 317-251-7488
FamilyNetw@aboutspecialkids.org
www.aboutspecialkids.org

Joe Brubaker, Executive Director
Jane Scott, Director Of Information
Nancy Stone, Project Director

A Parent to Parent organization that works throughout the state of Indiana to answer questions and provide support, information and resources. We are parents and family members of children with special needs and we help other families and professionals understand the various systems that are encountered related to special needs. Our central office is where parents from the entire state can access information, resources and support.

6317 ArtMix
1505 N. Delaware St.
Indianapolis, IN 46202
317-974-4123
Fax: 317-974-4124
info@artmixindiana.org
www.artmixindiana.org

Gayle Holtman, President/CEO
Linda Wisler, Vice President of Programs
Kathy Pataluch, Vice President of Development
Katy Deadmond, Manager of Community Outreach

Since 1982, ArtMix has been a statewide leader in its mission to transform the lives of people with disabilities through the creation of art. ArtMix programs serve over 6,000 people of all abilities each year, creating opportunities for learning, self-expression, and socialization, as well as increasing community understanding of people with disabilities. ArtMix strives to create a welcoming environment that breaks down barriers, providing an inclusive space for people of all ages and abilities.

6318 Clark Memorial Hospital: RehabCare Unit
1220 Missouri Ave
Jeffersonville, IN 47130-3743
812-282-6631
Fax: 812-283-2656
clarkmemorial.org

Martin Padgett, CEO

The mission of Clark Memorial Hospital is to provide superior health services to the people and communities we serve. The vision of Clark Memorial Hospital is to be the best community healh care provider in the United States. We value each individual and work together to explore new ways to improve the quality of life of all. We persue excellence in all we do. We treat all individuals with the same compassion, dignity, and privacy that we want in ourselves.

6319 Developmental Disabilities Planning Council
402 W Washington St
Indianapolis, IN 46204-2855
317-232-7770
Fax: 317-233-3712
www.state.in.us/gpcpd

Suellen Jackson-Boner, Executive Director
Christine Dahlberg, Associate Director
Jim Geswein, CFO
Betty Jones, Secretary

The mission of the Indiana Governor's Council is to promote public policy which leads to the independence, productivity and inclusion of people with disabilities in all aspects of society. This mission is accomplished through planning, evaluation, collaboration, education, research and advocacy. The Council is consumer-driven and is charged with determining how the service delivery system in both the public and private sectors can be most responsible to the people with disabilities.

6320 Easterseals Crossroads
4740 Kingsway Dr.
Indianapolis, IN 46205
317-466-1000
Fax: 317-466-2000
www.eastersealscrossroads.org

Harold Tenbarge, Chair
Darlisa E. Davis, Treasurer
John Seever, Secretary

Provides services for people with disabilities in central Indiana.

6321 IN-SOURCE
Indiana Resource Center for Families with Special
1703 S Ironwood Dr
South Bend, IN 46613-3414
574-234-7101
800-332-4433
Fax: 574-234-7279
insource@insource.org
insource.org

Richard Burden, Executive Director
Scott Carson, Assistant Director
Dory Lawrence, Project Director
Sally Hamburg, Project Director

The mission of IN*SOURCE is to provide parents, families and service providers in Indiana the information and training necessary to assure effective educational programs and appropriate services for children and young adults with disabilities.

6322 Indiana Congress of Parent and Teachers
2525 N Shadeland Ave
Ste D4
Indianapolis, IN 46219-1770
317-357-5881
Fax: 317-357-3751
www.indianapta.org

Sharon Wise, President
Theresa Distelrath, VP
Job Wise, Secretary
Julie Klingenberger, Treasurer

The mission of the Indiana PTA is three-fold: to support and speak on behalf of children and youth in the schools, community and before governmental agencies and other organizations that make decisions affecting children; to assist parents in developing the skills they need to raise and protect their children; and, to encorage parent and community involvement in the public schools of this state and nation.

6323 Indiana Protection and Advocacy Services Commission
4701 N Keystone Ave
Ste 222
Indianapolis, IN 46205-1561
317-722-5555
800-838-1131
Fax: 317-722-5564
dward@ipas.IN.gov
www.in.gov/ipas

Karen Pedevilla, Education and Training Director

IPAS was created in 1977 by state law to protect and advocate the rights of people with disabilities and its Indiana's federally designated Protection (P&A) system and client assist program. It is an independent state agency, with receives no state funding and is independent from all service providers, as required by federal and state law.

6324 Kokomo Rehabilitation Hospital
829 N Dixon Rd
Kokomo, IN 46901-7709
765-452-6700
Fax: 765-452-7470

Brenda Harry, Admissions Director

a 60 bed facility specializing in rehabilitation services to the people of Indiana.

6325 Memorial Regional Rehabilitation Center
615 N Michigan St
South Bend, IN 46601-1033
574-647-1000

6326 Methodist Hospital Rehabilitation Institute
8701 Broadway
Merrillville, IN 46410-7035
219-738-5500
Fax: 219-755-0448
methodisthospitals.org

Ian McFadden, President/CEO
Matthew Doyle, VP & CFO
Wright Alcorn, VP Operations
Michael Davenport, Vp Medical Affairs

Methodist Hospitals, of all the hospitals in Northwest Indiana, attracts the most complex cases across a range of specialties, including stroke, brain tumor, cancer, trauma and high-risk pregnancy. This is the result of our commitment to providing the expertise and technology needed to offer the most advanced clinical care.

6327 **NAMI Indiana**
P.O. Box 22697
Indianapolis, IN 46222-697 317-925-9399
800-677-6442
Fax: 317-925-9398
info@namiindiana.org
www.namiindiana.org

Marilynn Walker, President
Joshua Sprunger, Executive Director
Linda Williams, Program Coooridnator
Leslie Gay, Office Manager

NAMI Indiana is a non-profit grassroots organization dedicated to improving the lives of people afflicted by serious and persistant mental illness. We are dedicated to helping families through a network of support, education, advocacy, and promotion of research. NAMI's goal is to help establish a system of care that provides community based services for persons with serious mental illness, as well as support for them and their families.

6328 **Parkview Regional Rehabilitation Center**
2200 Randallia Dr
Fort Wayne, IN 46805-4638 260-373-4000
888-480-5151
Fax: 260-373-4288
www.parkview.com

Mike Packnett, President & CEO
Mike Browning, CFO
Rick Henvey, Chief Administrative Officer
Sue Ehinger, President (Parkview & Affiliates)

Provides a full range of inpatient, theraputic services and programs for patients as young as 3 years of age to the very elderly. Our accute care rehabilitation center, is well equipped to care for patients with neurological and orthopedic injuries and diseases.

6329 **Programs for Children with Disabilities: Ages 3 through 5**
Indiana Department of Education
151 W Ohio St
Indianapolis, IN 46204-1905 317-232-0570
877-851-4106
Fax: 317-232-0589
specialed@doe.in.gov
www.doe.in.gov

Heather Neal, Chief of Staff

The division provides leadership and state-level support for public school gifted and talented (grades K-12) programs and for students with disabilities from ages 3-21. The division ensures that Indiana, in its compliance with the federal Individuals With Disabilities Education Act, through monitoring of special education programs, oversight of community and residential programs, provision of mediation and due process rights, and sound fiscal management.

6330 **Programs for Children with Special Health Care Needs**
Indiana State Department of Health
2 N Meridian St
Indianapolis, IN 46204-3021 317-233-1325
www.in.gov/isdh/

Sean Keefer, Chief of Staff

The Children's Special Health Care Services (CSHCS) program provides financial assistance for needed medical treatment to children with serious and chronic medical conditions to reduce complications and promote maximum quality of life.

6331 **Programs for Infants and Toddlers with Disabilities: Ages Birth through 2**
402 W Washington St
Indianapolis, IN 46204-2773 317-232-1144
800-441-7837

6332 **Riley Child Development Center**
705 Riley Hospital Drive
Rm 5837
Indianapolis, IN 46202-5128 317-274-7819
Fax: 317-944-9760
info@child-dev.com

Cristy James, Communication Coordinator

Riley Hospital for Children is Indiana's only comprehensive children's hospital, with pediatric specialists in evry field of medicine and surgery. Riley is committed to providing the highest quality health care to children in a compassionate, family-centered environment. Riley is a national leader in cutting edge research and medical education, ensuring health care excellence for children for generations to come. Riley provides medical care to all children, regardless of family's ability to pay.

6333 **St. Anthony Memorial Hospital: Rehab Unit**
301 W Homer St
Michigan City, IN 46360-4358 219-879-8511
Fax: 219-877-1409
www.saintanthonymemorial.org

Joseph Allegreti, Board of Directors
Calvin Bellamy, Board of Directors

Saint Anthony Memorial is an acute care hospital located in Michigan City, primary serving La Porte and Porter Counties in Indiana as well as Berrien County Michigan.

6334 **State Division of Vocational Rehabilitation**
402 W Washington St
P O Box 7083
Indianapolis, IN 46207-7083 317-233-4475
800-545-7763
Fax: 317-232-6478
vrcommission@fssa.in.gov
www.state.in.us/fssa

Megan Ornellas, Chief of Staff
Susie Howard, Deputy Chief of Staff

Iowa

6335 **Younker Rehabilitation Center of Iowa Methodist Medical Center**
1776 W Lakes Pkwy
Des Moines, IA 50266 515-241-6161
888-584-6311
Fax: 515-241-5137
www.ihs.org

Bill Leaver, President
Kevin Vermeer, EVP
Danny Drake, VP
Kara Dunham, VP Finance

Iowa Health System is the state's first and largest integrated healthcare system. We are physicians, hospitals, civic leaders and local volunteers committed to providing the highest possible quality and the lowest possible cost. We serve over 70 communities in Iowa, Western Illinois, and Eastern Nebraska.

Kansas

6336 **Kansas Rehabilitation Hospital**
1504 SW 8th Ave
Topeka, KS 66606-2714 785-235-6600
Fax: 785-232-8545
www.kansasrehabhospital.com

Mark LeNeave, CEO
Mindy Mitchell, Chief Nursing Officer

A free standing physical rehabilitation hospital located in Topeka Kansas. Designated to provide a barrier-free access to all treatment and patient service areas. This 79-bed facility offers a total rehabilitation environment in a warm, caring setting that encourages patient, family and staff interaction.

6337 **Mid-America Rehabilitation Hospital HealthSouth**
Health South Corporation
5701 W 110th St
Overland Park, KS 66211-2503 913-491-2400
Fax: 913-491-1097
tiffany.kiehl@healthsouth.com
www.midamericarehabhospital.com

Kristen De Hart, CEO
Tiffany Kiehl, Director Marketing/Operations
Paul Matlack, Director Therapy Operations
Damon Parker, Chief Nursing Officer

97 bed Acute Rehab hospital offering full continuum from in-patient, day treatment and outpatient services for individuals with physical limitations due to CVA, TBI, SCI, other traumas, joint replacement, etc.

Kentucky

6338 **Cardinal Hill Rehabilitation Hospital**
2050 Versailles Rd
Lexington, KY 40504-1499 859-254-5701
800-233-3260
Fax: 859-231-1365
webmaster@cardinalhill.org
www.cardinalhill.org

Kerry Gillihan, CEO
William J. Lester, Medical Director
Russell Travis, Assistant Medical Director

CARF-accredited rehab center provides comprehensive inpatient and outpatient services in two locations to people with physical and cognitive disabilities. We provide diagnosis-specific programs to 100 inpatients, outpatient clinics, outpatient therapies, pain management and therapeutic pool services. The Pediatric Center serves children from birth to age 18 years of age.

6339 **HealthSouth Rehabilitation of Louisville**
1227 Goss Ave
Louisville, KY 40217-1287 270-769-3100
Fax: 502-636-0351
www.healthsouth.com

Tim Nichol, Manager
Regina Durbin, Administrator

HealthSouth Rehabilitation Hospitals lead the way, consistently outperforming peers with a unique, intensive approach to rehabilitative care, partnering with every patient to find a treatment plan that works for them. We offer a wide range of comprehensive rehabilitation programsfor a wide variety of diagnoses. At HealthSouth, we provide access to independent private practice physicians, specializing in physical medicine and rehabilitation, who work in conjunction with HealthSouth's highly qual

6340 **Lakeview Rehabilitation Hospital**
134 Heartland Dr
Elizabethtown, KY 42701-2778 270-769-3100
Fax: 270-769-6870
www.healthsouthlakeview.com

Lori Jarboes, CEO
Chris Koford, Medical Director

HealthSouth Rehabilitation Hospitals lead the way, consistently outperforming peers with a unique, intensive approach to rehabilitative care, partnering with every patient to find a treatment plan that works for them. We offer a wide range of comprehensive rehabilitation programsfor a wide variety of diagnoses. At HealthSouth, we provide access to independent private practice physicians, specializing in physical medicine and rehabilitation, who work in conjunction with HealthSouth's highly qual

6341 **Shriners Hospitals for Children, Lexington**
1900 Richmond Rd
Lexington, KY 40502-1204 859-266-2101
800-444-8314
Fax: 859-268-5636
Dwallenius@shrinenet.org
www.shrinershq.org/hospitals/lexington

Warren E. Hopkins, Chairman
Kirk E. Carter, Vice Chairman
Ken R. Dougherty, Treasurer
David E. Hager, Secretary

Shriners Hospitals for Childrenr - Lexington, is a 50-bed pediatric orthopaedic hospital. Our family-centered approach to care is designed to support the whole family during the acute and reconstructive phases of a child's injury. Located in Lexington, Ky., our hospital treats children from all over the country and around the world, and has unique relationships with some of the top hospitals and universities in the world.

Louisiana

6342 **HealthSouth Specialty Hospital Of North Louisiana**
1401 Ezelle St
Ruston, LA 71270-7218 318-251-3126
800-548-9157
Fax: 318-251-1594
mark.rice@lifecare-hospitals.com
www.healthsouth.com

Mark Rice, CEO

A 90-bed specialty hospital offering both inpatient and outpatient services. Acute long term care.

6343 **Our Lady of Lourdes Rehabilitation Center**
4801 Ambassador Caffery Pkwy
Lafayette, LA 70508 337-470-2000
Fax: 318-289-2681
info@lourdesrmc.com
www.lourdesrmc.com

William Barrow, CEO
Gerald R. Boudreaux, Chairman of the Board
D. Wayne Elmore, Secretary

Our Lady of Lourdes outpatient physical medicine and rehabilitation department is compprised of a multi-disciplinary team of physical therapists, oppcuptational therapists and speech languare pathologists.

6344 **Rehabilitation Center of Lake Charles Memorial Hospital**
1701 Oak Park Boulevard
Lake Charles, LA 70601-8911 337-494-3000
Fax: 337-494-2656
webmaster@lcmh.com
www.lcmh.com

Dale Shearer, Director
Larry Graham, President/CEO
Ben F. Thompson, MD, Medical Staff President
Ronald Lewis, Jr., Medical Staff President - Elect

Rehabilitation center offering intensive physical, occupational, speech, neuropsychology, recreational therapies along with rehabilitation nursing.

6345 **Shriners Hospital for Children-Shreveport**
3100 Samford Ave
Shreveport, LA 71103-4239 318-222-5704
Fax: 318-424-7610
jburda@shrinenet.org
www.shrinershospitalsforchildren.org

Richard McCall, Chief of Staff
Phillip Gates, Assistant Chief

An interdisciplinary approach is used in patient care programs to ensure comprehensive care for each patient. The staff includes orthopaedists, pediatricians, nurses, therapists, social workers, child life specialists, and more. The Shreveport Hospital is equipped and staffed to provide care for virtually all pediatric orthopaedic problems, with the exception of acute trauma.

6346 **South Louisiana Rehabilitation Hospital**
715 W Worthy Rd
Gonzales, LA 70737-3844 225-647-8277
Fax: 225-647-2446
sober@powerhouseprograms.com
www.powerhouseprograms.com

Cody Gautreux, Executive Director
Tonja Randolph, President

Power House Programs is a male only facility for the treatment of Chemical Dependency/Dual Diagnosis, located in Gonzales, Louisiana. Applicants must have participated in a primary treatment program for substance abuse prior to acceptance. Our program is divided into 3 phases and is staffed by Board Certified Social Workers and Board Certified Substance Abuse Counselors. We provide individual, group and family therapy; plus 12 step meetings in a community setting.

6347 **St. Frances Cabrini Hospital: Rehab Unit**
St Frances Cabrini Hospital
3330 Masonic Dr
Alexandria, LA 71301-3899 318-487-1122
Fax: 318-448-6822
www.christusstfrancescabrini.org

Curman Gaines, Chairperson
Dallas Hixson, Vice Chairperson

CHRISTUS St. Frances Cabrini Hospital is a 265-bed facility located in Alexandria, Louisiana. Employing approximately 1,400 Associates and with a staff of neary 320 physicians, CHRISTUS St. Frances Cabrini Hospital offers a comprehensive array of services providing the highest quality patient care in a compassionate setting.

6348 **St. Patrick Hospital: Rehab Unit**
524 Doctor Michael Debakey Dr
Lake Charles, LA 70601-5725 337-491-7577
888-722-9355
Fax: 337-430-4284
www.christusstpatrick.org

Ellen Jones, CEO

Committed to providing care and service of the highest quality for children and adults, and to ensuring that the basic human rights of expression, decision making and personal dignity are preseved. We are also committed to treating our patients with respect, understanding and Christian love. We realize that this committment involves much more then attending to your medical needs.

6349 **Thibodaux Regional Medical Center**
602 N Acadia Rd
PO Box 1118
Thibodaux, LA 70301-4847 985-447-5500
800-822-8442
Fax: 985-449-4600
info@thibodaux.com
www.thibodaux.com

Greg Stock, CEO
Jacob Giardina, Chairman
Andrew Hoffman, Chief of Staff

Mission is to provide the highest quality, most cost effective health care services possible to the people of Thibodaux and surrounding areas. The vision is to be the regional medical center of choice for health care services in the southeast Louisiana by recognizing the value of physicians and employees, committing to quality improvement, partnering with other health care providers, and remaining financially viable in a competitive environment.

Maine

6350 **Brewer Rehab and Living Center**
74 Parkway S
Brewer, ME 04412-1628 207-989-7300
800-359-7412
Fax: 207-989-4240

Janet Hope, Executive Director

Brewer Rehab and Living Center accomodates 106 residents. We are located in Brewer, Maine. We have a 24-hour nursing staff and experienced dedicated on-site physical therapists, occupational therapists and speech language pathologists. We have a specialized inpatient program for individuals with brain injury resulting from a traumatic injury or neurological event such as a stroke. We also have a specialized care unit for individuals with Alzheimer's disease and other dementias.

6351 **New England Rehabilitation Hospital of Portland**
335 Brighton Ave
Portland, ME 04102-2363 207-662-8000
Fax: 207-879-8168
www.nerhp.org

Elissa Charbonneau, Medical Director
Amy Morse, CEO

Mission is to provide individuals with guidance, education, support, and motivation while helping them achieve maximum independence and function. Our professionals work with the patient and family through a team approach, to establish and implement an individualized rehabilitation plan designed to meet specific patient goals.

Maryland

6352 **Mt. Washington Pediatric Hospital**
1708 W Rogers Ave
Baltimore, MD 21209-4596 410-578-8600
Fax: 410-466-1715
www.mwph.org

Sheldon Stein, President
Richard Katz, VP, Medical Affairs

Provides inpatient, outpatient and day programs for infants and children with rehabilitation and/or complex medical needs. We are dedicated to maximizing the rehabilitation and development of our patients through the delivery of interdisciplinary services and programs and providing every resource availiable to enable our patients to attain the highest quality of life within their families and their communities.

Massachusetts

6353 **New Bedford Rehabilitation Hospital**
4499 Acushnet Ave
New Bedford, MA 02745-4707 508-995-6900
Fax: 508-998-8131

6354 **New England Rehabilitation Hospital: Massachusetts**
2 Rehabilitation Way
Woburn, MA 01801-6098 781-939-5050
Fax: 781-933-9257
www.newenglandrehab.com

Deniz Ozel, Medical Director

A 168-bed comprehensive inpatient rehabilitation hospital, which includes 2 off-campus satellite units. Offers an array of area outpatient rehabilitation centers. New England Rehabilitation Hospital remains committed to a personal caring approach. The vision is to provide the communities with a complete continuum of acute rehabilitative programs and services.

6355 **Shriners Burns Hospital: Boston**
51 Blossom St
Boston, MA 02114-2623 617-722-3000
800-255-1916
Fax: 617-523-1684
www.shrinershospitalsforchildren.org

Thomas D'Esmond, Administrator
Matthias Donelan, Chief of Staff

Provides treatment for children to their 18th birthday with acute, fresh burns, plastic reconstructive surgery for patients with healed burns, severe scarring and facial deformity. Some non-burn conditions such as Scalded Skin Syndrome, Cleft Lip, Cleft Palate and purpura fulminians are also treated. Call the Hospital for information. All medical treatment is without cost to the patient, parents, or any third party.

6356 **Shriners Hospital Springfield Unit Springfield Unit for Crippled Children**
516 Carew St
Springfield, MA 01104-2330 413-787-2000
800-237-5055
Fax: 413-787-2009
www.shrinershospitalsforchildren.org

Kenneth Guidera, Chief Medical Officer
Eugene D'Amore, Vice President
Kathy A. Dean, Vice President Human Resources
Sharon Russell, VP Finance & Accounting

Shriners Hospital for Children is fully equipped and staffed to provide care for pediatric orthopaedic conditions and disorders.

Michigan

6357 **Covenant Healthcare Rehabilitation Program**
1447 N Harrison
Saginaw, MI 48602-4316
989-583-2930
Fax: 989-583-0000
www.covenanthealthcare.com

Spence Maidlow, President
Juli Martin, Program Director

Offers a broad spectrum of programs and services ranging from obstetrics, neonatal and pediatric care, to acute care including cardiology, oncology, surgery and many other services on the leading edge of medicine. All our programs and services exemplify our commitment to providing quality, compassionate care. As a medical facility with more then 700 beds, and a complete range of medical services, Covenant stands ready to meet the healthcare needs of the 15 counties in Michigan we serve.

6358 **Farmington Health Care Center**
34225 Grand River Ave
Farmington, MI 48335-3440
248-477-7373
Fax: 248-477-2888

Brian Garavaglia, Administrator

Skilled nursing facility specializing in ventilator dependent residents.

6359 **Flint Osteopathic Hospital: RehabCare Unit**
3921 Beecher Rd
Flint, MI 48532-3602
810-606-5000
Fax: 810-762-2153
TTY: 888-633-2368
www.genesys.org

Susan Malone, Program Manager
Joy Finkenbiner, Executive Director

Genesys Health System takes great pride in the fact that we strive to deliver the highest quality health care, in a model healing environment, for the entire continuum of care needed throughout one's life. From birth to the twilight years, and everywhere in between, Genesys is there to get you back to the things you love to do.

6360 **Integrated Health Services of Michigan at Clarkston**
4800 Clintonville Rd
Clarkston, MI 48346-4297
248-674-0903
Fax: 248-674-3359
donna.cook@fundltc.com

Carol Doll, Admissions Director
Margaret Canny, Administrator

At Clarkston Specialty Healthcare Center, our mission is to deliver personalized care to the members of our community at a time when our support is most needed. We strive to maximize and enhance the quality of life in a compassionate and professional environment.

6361 **St. John Hospital: North Shore**
Ascension Health
26755 Ballard St
Harrison Township, MI 48045-2419
586-465-5501
866-501-3627
Fax: 586-466-5352
webcenter@stjohn.org
www.stjohnprovidence.org

David Sessions, CEO

A 96-bed specialty hospital that provides comprehensive physical medicine and rehabilitation, along with a wide range of medical and surgical services. St. John North Shores Hospital also provides emergency and urgent care, extensive outpatient rehabilitation services, and most ancillary diagnostic services.

Minnesota

6362 **Alinna Health**
800 E 28th St
Minneapolis, MN 55407-3798
612-863-4200
866-880-3550
Fax: 612-863-5698
sisterkenny@allina.com
www.allinahealth.org/ahs/ski.nsf/

Helen Kettner, Nurse-Liaison

Courage Kenny Rehabilitation Institute provides a continuum of rehabilitation services for people with short- and long-term conditions and disabilities in communities throughout Minnesota and western Wisconsin. Our goal is to improve health outcomes, make it easier for clients and families to get the right services for their needs, and reduce costs by preventing complications.

Missouri

6363 **Columbia Regional Hospital: RehabCare Unit**
404 N Keene St
Columbia, MO 65201-6698
573-882-2501
Fax: 573-449-7588
www.muhealth.org

James Ross, CEO
Anita Larsen, COO

A medical and physical rehabilitation program serving patients throughout Mid-Missouri with functional deficits due to neurologic, orthopaedic or other medical conditions.

6364 **Jewish Hospital of St. Louis: Department of Rehabilitation**
1 Barnes Jewish Hospital Plz
Saint Louis, MO 63110-1003
314-747-3000
855-925-0631
Fax: 314-454-5277
www.barnesjewish.org

Richard Liedweg, President
Mark Krieger, VP/CFO
John Lynch, Chief Medical Officer
Craig D. Schnuck, Chairman

We take exceptional care of people by providing world-class healthcare, delivering care in a compassionate, respectful and responsive way. By advancing medical knowledge and continously improving our practices. By educating current and future generations of healthcare professionals.

6365 **St. Mary's Regional Rehabilitation Center**
201 NW R D Mize Rd
Blue Springs, MO 64014-2513
816-228-5900
Fax: 816-655-5348

Fleury Yelvington, President/CEO
Amy McKay, Executive Director of Nursing

A 143-bed inpatient physical rehabilitation unit offering PT, OT, ST, recreational therapy, psychiatry and all other ancillary services of a full-service hospital. Specialize in orthopedic and neurologic disabilities.

6366 **Three Rivers Health Care**
2620 N Westwood Blvd
Poplar Bluff, MO 63901-3396
573-785-7721
800-582-9533
Fax: 573-686-5388
info@pbrmc.hma-corp.com
www.poplarbluffregional.com

Charles Stewart, Market CEO
Gerald Faircloth, Administrator
Melissa Samuelson, Chief Nursing Officer
Kevin Fowler, CFO

Poplar Bluff Regional Medical Center is a regional medical center with 2 hospital campuses and more then 100 active physicians. The 423-bed facility is the largest medical center in Southeast Missouri and is located in ButlerCounty. With outreach clinics in Bloomfield, Dexter, Malden, Piedmont, and Puxico, Poplar Bluff Regional Medical Center is committed to serving its 6 county region.

Montana

6367 **St. Vincent Hospital and Health Center**
1233 N 30th St
Billings, MT 59101-165
406-657-7000
Fax: 406-657-8817
www.svhhc.org

Jason Barker, CEO
Steve Loveless, COO
Joan Thullberry, Chief Nursing Officer
Ron Oldfield, VP Finance
Vision is to be recognized for our vitality, best in class performance and providing easy access to compassionate and trust-worthy healthcare. The healthcare we offer is based on community need. We strive to improve the health status of the community, with a special concern for the poor and those who have limited access to healthcare.

Nebraska

6368 **Madonna Rehabilitation Hospital**
5401 South St
Lincoln, NE 68506-2150
402-489-7102
800-676-5448
Fax: 402-483-9406
info@madonna.org
www.madonna.org

Marsha Lommel, CEO
Provides a complete range of inpatient and outpatient rehabilitation for patients of all ages and abilities. Through highly specialized programs and services, Madona offers individualized treatment and support to help every patient.

Nevada

6369 **University Medical Center**
1800 W Charleston Blvd
Las Vegas, NV 89102-2386
702-383-2000
Fax: 702-383-2536
feedback@umcsn.com
www.umcsn.com

Brian Brannman, CEO
Lawrence Barnard, Chief Operating Officer
Joan Brookhyser, Chief Medical Officer
Stephanie Merril, Chief Financial Officer
University Medical Center is dedicated to providing the highest level of health care possible by maintaining its ongoing commitment to personal, individualized care for each patient.Through the latest treatment techniques, comfortable surroundings and a dedicated staff, that commitment is expressed every day, in every area of the hospital.

New Hampshire

6370 **Head Injury Treatment Program at Dover**
307 Plaza Dr
Dover, NH 03820-2455
603-742-2676
Fax: 603-749-5375
www.doverrehab.com

Sue Mills, Program Rep
Jill Bosa, Administrator
A provider of postacute services in the greater New Hampshire Seacost area. We accomodate 112 residents and are licensed by the state of New Hampshire. We employ nearly 150 licensed nurses, therapists, and other healthcare professionals, who strive to provide quality care. The goal of our patient service model is to bridge the gap between hospitalization and home so that recovery and physical functioning are maximized and hospital re-admission is minimized.

6371 **Lakeview NeuroRehabilitation Center**
244 Highwatch Road
Effingham, NH 03882
603-539-7451
800-473-4221
Fax: 603-539-8815
www.lakeviewsystem.com

Anton Merka, Chairman
Carolyn McDermott, President
Christopher Slover, Chief Executive Officer
Tina M. Trudel, PhD, Chief Operating Officer
Residential treatment center serving individuals with neurologic/behavioral disorders. Lakeview serves both children and adults in functionally based program environment. Transistional programs in various group homes also available to clients as they progress in their treatment.

6372 **Northeast Rehabilitation Hospital**
70 Butler St
Salem, NH 03079-3974
603-893-2900
800-825-7292
Fax: 603-893-1638
TTY: 800-439-2370
www.northeastrehab.com

John Prochilo, CEO
NRHN is an organization characterized by the positive and proactive commitment to the delivery of customer centered care. Our employees exemplify our organizational commitment to providing quality rehabilitation services throughout the continuum. NRHN will be prudent with all resources and will take individual and collective responsibility for fiscal health. NRHN will remain a model by which other rehabilitation and post acute networks seek to emulate.

6373 **St. Joseph Hospital Rehabilitation**
172 Kinsley St
Nashua, NH 03060-3688
603-595-3076
800-210-9000
Fax: 603-595-3635
www.stjosephhospital.com

Judy Grilli, Medical Staff Officer
A comprehensive healthcare system that serves the Greater Nashua area, western New Hampshire and Northern Massachusetts. Our hospital is licensed for 208 beds and includes a Level 2 Trauma Center. In addition to the hospital, St. Joseph Healthcare system also includes a satellite emergency center in Milford, 5 family medical centers, a large network of primary care and specialty physician practices.

New Jersey

6374 **Betty Bacharach Rehabilitation Hospital**
61 W Jimmie Leeds Rd
Pomona, NJ 08240-9102
609-652-7000
Fax: 609-652-7487
www.bacharach.org

Philip J. Perskie, Esq., Chairman
Roy Goldberg, Vice Chairman
Craig Anmuth, Medical Director
Ross Berlin, Medical Director
Therapists, nurses and other specialists, led by physiatrists - doctors specially trained in the medical practice of physical medicine and rehabilitation.

6375 **Children's Specialized Hospital**
200 Somerset St.
New Brunswick, NJ 08901
888-244-5373
www.childrens-specialized.org

Warren E. Moore, President & CEO
Charles Chianese, Vice President & Chief Operating Officer
Joseph J. Dobosh Jr., Vice President & Chief Financial Officer
Matthew B. McDonald III, Vice President & Chief Medical Officer
New Jersey's largest comprehensive pediatric rehabilitation hospital, treats children and adolescents from birth through 21 years of age. Programs include spinal dysfunction, brain injury, respiratory, burn, Day Hospital, early intervention, preschool, and cognitive rehabilitation.

6376 **HealthSouth Rehabilitation Hospital**
14 Hospital Dr
Toms River, NJ 08755-6402
732-244-3100
Fax: 732-244-7790
www.rehabnj.com/tomsriver/

Patty Ostaszewski, CEO
Joseph Stillo, Medical Director

A comprehensive 131-bed medical rehabilitation hospital dedicated to treating individuals with a variety of physical disabilities resulting from injury and illness. We serve all of New Jersey, Manhattan, and Philiadelphia. Accredited by the Joint Commission on Accredidation of Healthcare Organizations (JCAHO). The mission of the hospital is to get people back to work, to play, to living.

6377 **JFK Johnson Rehab Institute**
65 James St
Edison, NJ 08820-3947
732-321-7070
Fax: 732-321-0994
www.njrehab.org

Krishna Urs, Physician
David Brown, Physician

JRI has developed programs in such specialties as stroke rehabilitation, orthopedic programs, fitness, cardiac rehabilitation, women's health, pediatrics and brain injury rehabilitation. We also offer the most sophisticated diagnostic services available.

6378 **Kessler Institute for Rehabilitation**
1199 Pleasant Valley Way
West Orange, NJ 07052
973-731-3600
877-322-2580
Fax: 973-243-6819
www.kessler-rehab.com

Sue Kida, President

Provides physical medicine and rehabilitation through the integration of highly specialized care, treatment, technology, education, research, and advocacy.

6379 **Mediplex Rehab: Camden**
1 Cooper Plz
Camden, NJ 08103-1461
856-342-2300
Fax: 856-342-7979
www.cooperhealth.org

John P. Sheridan, Jr. President/CEO
Adrienne Kirby, Phd, President/CEO
Raymond L. Baraldi, Interim Chief Medical Officer
Celeste Johnson, Administrator

Cooper University Hospital is the leading provider of comprehensive health services, medical education and clinical research in Southern New Jersey and the Delaware Valley. With over 550 physicians in over 75 specialties, Cooper is uniquely equipped to provide an almost unlimited number of medical services. The hospital is committed to excellence in medical education, patient care, and research. Offers training programs to medical students, residents, and nurses in a variety of specialties.

6380 **Universal Institute Rehabilitation & Fitness Center**
15 Microlab Rd
Ste 101
Livingston, NJ 07039
973-992-8181
800-468-5440
Fax: 973-992-7178
www.uirehab.com

Adam Steinberg, President
Lisa Lasso, Vice President, Chief Financial Officer

Universal institute is a 15,000 square foot, state of the art rehabilitation facility that specializes in neurological disorders such as brain injuries, spinal cord injury, strokes, etc. Services include PT, OT, speech patholgy, cognitive remediation, aqua therapy and EMG biofeedback.

New Mexico

6381 **HealthSouth Rehabilitation Center: New Mexico**
7000 Jefferson St NE
Albuquerque, NM 87109-4357
505-344-9478
800-293-7226
Fax: 505-345-6722
www.healthsouthnewmexico.com

Sylvia Kelly, CEO
Rocky BigCrane, Director of Plant Operations
Lisa Brower, Director of Therapy Operations
Angela Eaton-Walker, M.D, Medical Director

Our hospital offers highly specialized inpatient rehabilitation services. From hip fractures to joint replacements and stroke to Parkinson's disease - our hospital has the experts, technology and experience to meet your rehabilitation needs.

6382 **St. Joseph Rehabilitation Hospital and Outpatient Center**
Ardence
505 Elm St NE
Albuquerque, NM 87102-2500
505-727-4700
Fax: 505-727-4793

Janelle Raborn, Administrator/CEO
Sherrie Peterson, Director

A member of the four hospital, St. Joseph healthcare system, this facility provides inpatient and outpatient care for those requiring physical medicine and rehabilitation. Specialty programs include brain injury, stroke, spinal cord, orthopedics, occupational and physical therapies, clinical psychology, speech/language pathology, hand clinic and functional capacity evaluations. The only facility in New Mexico accredited in four areas by the commission on accreditation of rehab facilities.

New York

6383 **Burke Rehabilitation Hospital**
785 Mamaroneck Ave
White Plains, NY 10605-2523
914-597-2500
888-99 -URKE
Fax: 914-946-0866
web@burke.org
www.burke.org

John Ryan, Executive Director
Mary Beth Walsh, M.D., Executive Medical Director/CEO
Brett Langley, Physician .

We provide inpatient and outpatient care for a broad range of neurological, musculoskeletal, cardiac, and pulmonary disabilities caused by disease or injury. Burke treats patients who have suffered a stroke, spinal cord injury, brain injury, amputation, joint replacement, complicated fracture, arthritis, cardiac and pulmonary disease, and neurological disorders. Patients are most frequently transferred to Burke from acute care hospitals once their condition is stable and they are able to partici

6384 **Occupational Therapy Strategies and Adaptations for Independent Daily Living**
Haworth Press
10 Alice St
Binghamton, NY 13904-1503
607-722-5857
800-429-6784
Fax: 607-722-6362
orders@haworthpress.com
www.tandf.co.uk

186 pages Softcover
ISBN 0-866563-50-4

6385 **Rusk Institute of Rehabilitation Medicine**
301 East 17th Street
Second Avenue (in the Hospital for
New York, NY 10016-4901
212-263-6034
Fax: 212-263-8510
DevelopmentOffice@nyumc.org
www.med.nyu.edu/rusk

Steven Flanagan, Chairman

Operates under the auspices of the Dept. Of Rehabilitation Medicine of New York University School of Medicine, one of the nations foremost medical schools. The relationship between Rusk and other clinical and research units within the medical center contributes to an environment which provides the optimal rehabilitation setting for patients. Rusk provides patients with access to treatment across a continuum of care depending on their individual medical needs.

6386 **Silvercrest Center for Nursing & Rehabilitation**
144-45 87th Ave
Briarwood, NY 11435-3109
718-480-4000
800-645-9806
Fax: 718-658-2367
admissions@silvercrest.org
www.silvercrest.org

Andrea Gibbon, Clinical Care Coordinator
Penny Blakely, Unit Manager
The Silvercrest Center for Nursing and Rehabilitation has earned a wide-spread reputatiopn for combing the best in clinical care with the best in nursing care and for making available to its communities the broadest menu of services to ease a patients' path to recovery from hospital to home. The Center is for the treatment of medically complex patients beginning their recovery, for the rehabilitation of patients who need restorative therapy before going home and much more.

6387 **Vocational Rehabilitation and Employment**
Books on Special Children
PO Box 305
Congers, NY 10920-305
845-638-1236
Fax: 845-638-0847
www.vba.va.gov/bln/vre/

372 pages Hardcover

North Carolina

6388 **Horizon Rehabilitation Center**
Trans Health Incorporated
3100 Erwin Rd
Durham, NC 27705-4505
919-383-1546
800-541-7750
Fax: 919-383-0862

6389 **Integrated Health Services of Durham**
Duke University Medical Center
3100 Erwin Rd
Durham, NC 27705-4505
919-383-1546
Fax: 919-383-0862

Aaron Lony, Administrator

6390 **Learning Services Corporation**
Corporate Office
10 Speen St
Ste 4
Framingham, MA 01701-4661
508-626-3671
888-419-9955
Fax: 866-491-7396
www.learningservices.com

Susan Snow, Director of Admissions
Deb. Braunling-McMorrow, Ph, President and CEO
A licensed postacute rehabilitation program for adults who have an acquired brain injury. Individuals who are enrolled in the program participate in active, intensive rehabilitation carried out by a team of neuropsychology, speech/language therapy, physical therapy, occupational therapy, vocational services, family services and life skills training. Services include residential rehabilitation, home based treatment, day treatment, subacute rehabilitation and supported living.

Ohio

6391 **Columbus Rehab & Subactute**
44 S Souder Ave
Columbus, OH 43222-1539
614-228-5900
Fax: 614-228-3989
www.columbusrehabskillednursing.com

Kelly Fligor, Administrator
Columbus Rehabilitation and Subacute Institute is a leading provider of long-term skilled nursing care and short-term rehabilitation solutions. Our 120 bed facility offers a full continuum of services and care focused around each individual in today's ever-changing healthcare environment.

6392 **Great Lakes Regional Rehabilitation Center**
3700 Kolbe Rd
Lorain, OH 44053-1611
440-960-3470
Fax: 440-960-4636

Julie Jones, Manager
Provides excellent, innovative and comprehensive rehabilitation programs to people in our community. Committed to a better quality of life for all individuals, the Rehabilitation Center has grown to become a regional resource for individuals needing all types of rehabilitation services.

6393 **HCR Health Care Services**
1 Seagate
Toledo, OH 43604-1541
419-321-5470
800-736-4427
Fax: 419-252-5543

6394 **Heather Hill Rehabilitation Hospital**
Heather Hill
12340 Bass Lake Rd
Chardon, OH 44024-8327
440-285-4040
800-423-2972
Fax: 440-285-0946
info@heatherhill.org

Ed Davis, Operations
Donald Goddard, Chief Medical Officer
Individualized treatment programs for adults and adolescents can participate in and benefit from three-plus hours a day of active therapy.

6395 **Parma Community General Hospital Acute Rehabilitation Center**
7007 Powers Blvd
Parma, OH 44129-5437
440-743-3000
Fax: 440-843-4387
www.parmahospital.org

David Nedrich, Chairman
Thomas P. O'Donnell, First Vice Chairman
Nancy E. Hatgas, Second Assistant Treasurer
Alex I. Koler, First Assistant Treasurer
Parma Hospital offers acute and subacute inpatient care including specialty centers for heart, cancer, robotic surgery, orthopedics, pain management, acute rehabilitation and bariatric care.

6396 **Rehabilitation Institute of Ohio at Miami Valley Hospital**
1 Wyoming St
Dayton, OH 45409-2793
937-208-8000
TTY: 937-208-2006
www.miamivalleyhospital.com

Vanessa Sandarusi, Executive Director
Anita Marie Greer, Program Manager, Acute Therapy Services
Jessica Hallum, Nurse Manager of the Inpatient Rehabilitation Unit
Phillip Boarman, Clinical Coordinator for Acute Care Occupational Therapy and
The Miami Valley Hospital Rehabilitation Institute of Ohio (RIO) is one of the largest and most comprehensive rehabilitation services providers in the United States. RIO offers a full spectrum of specialized rehabilitation programs delivered by the region's most experienced rehabilitation experts.

6397 **Shriners Burn Institute: Cincinnati Unit**
Shriners Hospitals for Children Cincinnati
3229 Burnet Ave
Cincinnati, OH 45229-3095
513-872-6000
800-875-8580
Fax: 513-872-6999
www.shrinershospitalsforchildren.org

Richard Kagan, Chief of Staff
Petra Warner, Assistant Chief of Staff
Tony Lewgood, Interim Administrator
Vanessa Mosley, Development Officer
All the attention and resources are focused on just one kind of patient-the burn-injured child. Shriners combine excellent clinical skill, compassionate care, and innovative research, providing comprehensive pediatric burn care and reconstructive rehabilita-

tion to achieve the best possible outcome for a child that has suffered a burn injury. There is never a charge to the patient or family for any of the medical care or services provided by the Shriners Hospitals throughout North America.

6398 St. Francis Health Care Centre
401 N Broadway St
Green Springs, OH 44836-9653
419-639-2626
800-248-2552
Fax: 419-639-6225

Kim Eicher, CEO
Jane Holmer, Admissions Coordinator
Provides compassionate care for the elderly and physically challenged. We are a healthcare ministry under the sponsorship of the Franciscan Sisters of Our Lady of Perpetual Help. As a Catholic facility. we respectfully offer those we serve, care hope and dignity in a joyful and compassionate manner.

6399 St. Rita's Medical Center Rehabilitation Services
730 W Market St
Lima, OH 45801-4602
419-227-3361
800-232-7762
Fax: 419-226-9750

James Reber, CEO
The St. Rita's Inpatient Acute Care Rehabilitation service provides individualized service to you or your family member 7 days a week, wherever you might stay in the hospital. Acute rehabilitation care includes physical, occupational, and speech therapy services. Our goal is to make you as independent as possible before your discarge to home or, when necessary to extended services in other parts of the hospital.

6400 University of Cincinnati Hospital
Health Alliance
234 Goodman St
Cincinnati, OH 45219-2316
513-584-1000
Fax: 513-584-7712
universityhospital.uchealth.com/

James Kingsbury, President/CEO
University Hospital has an international reputation, bringing thousands of people, from the region and around the world to Cincinnati to receive care from world renowned physicians in state-of-the-art medical facilities.

6401 Upper Valley Medical/Rehab Services
3130 N County Road
25-A
Troy, OH 45373-1309
937-440-4000
Fax: 937-440-7337
info@uvmc.com
www.uvmc.com

Rafay Atiq, Director Rehab Services
A not-for-profit health care system serving the health care needs of Miami County and the surrounding area. The health care system features a state-of-the-art acute care hospital which opened in 1998. Comprehensive inpatient and outpatient services are provided with a full compliment of diagnostic and treatment services and behavioral health care programs.

Oklahoma

6402 Hilcrest Medical Center: Kaiser Rehab Center
1125 S Trenton Ave
Tulsa, OK 74120-5498
918-579-7100
Fax: 918-579-7110
www.hillcrest.com

Perri Craven, Medical Director
Kaiser Rehabilitation Center offers a wide range of services to help people regain functionality and independence after a debilitating injury or illness. Our approach to rehabilitation is a team approach, bringing the expertise of physicians, therapists, nurses and other health professionals together with patient family to achieve the best possible outcome. Each patient is given an individualized treatment plan that stimulates and challenges them to achieve their maximum potential.

6403 Jane Phillips Medical Center
Jane Phillips Medical Center
3500 E Frank Phillips Blvd
Bartlesville, OK 74006-2464
918-333-7200
Fax: 918-331-1360
www.jpmc.org

David Stire, CEO
Mike Moore, CFO
Jane Phillips Health System is sponsored by St. John Health System. This partnership helps our patients by ensuing access to the most sophisticated levels of care availiable in this area. It offers a wide range of services, including general medicine, surgery, cardiopulmonary care, maternal and infant care, cancer treatment, geriatric care, orthopedics, and physical medicine.

6404 Jim Thorpe Rehabilitation Center at Southwest Medical Center
Southwest Medical Center
4100 S. Douglas Ave.
Oklahoma City, OK 73109
405-644-5445
800-677-1238
Fax: 405-644-5384

Al Moorad, Medical Director
Provides inpatient rehabilitation for people with head injuries, spinal cord injuries, orthopedic conditions, pain management, neurological diseases, strokes and a variety of diagnoses that stop individuals from being able to take care of themselves independently. Services available include medical direction, physical therapy, social work, occupational therapy, speech therapy, recreational therapy, and aftercare follow-up.

6405 Mercy Memorial Health Center-Rehab Center
1011 14th Ave NW
Ardmore, OK 73401-1828
580-223-5400
800-572-1182
Fax: 580-220-6463
www.mercy.net

Jan Shores, Manager
Lynn Britton Britton, President/CEO
Randy Combs, Executive Vice President Strategic Growth
Michael McCurry, Executive Vice President/Chief Operating Officer
A full service tertiary hospital with 176 licensed beds, 913 co-workers and 100 physicians. Four primary care clinics

6406 St. Anthony Hospital: Rehabilitation Unit
St. Anthony Hospital
1000 N Lee Ave
Oklahoma City, OK 73102-1036
405-272-7000
800-851-0888
Fax: 405-272-7075
st_anthony@ssmhc.com
www.saintsok.com

S Beaver, President
18 spacious private rooms, each with bathroom, and furnishings designed with patient safety in mind. Horticulture room where patients can work with plants and flowers as part of their rehabilitation. And a residential-style training apartment with fully equipped kitchen, bathroom, and bedroom to make the patient feel more at home.

6407 Valir Health
700 NW 7th St
Oklahoma City, OK 73102-1212
405-609-3600
888-898-2080
Fax: 405-605-8638
info@valir.com
www.valir.com

Dirk O'Hara, Principal
Tonya Purvine, Corporate Compliance Officer
Inpatient Rehab Facility including all therapy services serving people who have been injured and had an illness resulting in a decreased level of independence.

Oregon

6408 **Shriners Hospitals for Children: Portland**
3101 SW Sam Jackson Park Rd
Portland, OR 97239-3095 503-241-5090
800-237-5055
Fax: 503-221-3701
www.shrinershospitalsforchildren.org

Michael Aiona, Chief of Staff
Craig Patchin, Administrator
Mark Thoreson, Development Officer
Joslyn Davidson, M.D, Anesthesiology

Pediatric orthopedic and plastic surgery; inpatient and outpatient services. No charge for any services provided at the Hospital. Diagnosis, rehabilitation, surgery, sports and recreation for ages 0-18 for people with physical disabilities involving bones, muscles or joints or in need of plastic surgery for burn scars or cleft lip/palate.

Pennsylvania

6409 **Allied Services John Heinz Institute of Rehabilitation Medicine**
150 Mundy St
MAC III Building, 1st Floor
Wilkes Barre, PA 18702-6830 570-826-3900
Fax: 570-830-2027
www.allied-services.org

Gerald Franceski, Chairman
Thomas Speicher, Vice-Chairman
William Conaboy, CEO
Gregory Basting, VP Medical Affairs

John Heinz Rehab is one of the foremost providers of rehabilitation in the country. Under the supervision of board-certified psychiatrists, a team of highly qualified professionals provides a broad range of specialized services and therapies for inpatients, with speacialized programs in the areas of brain injury, injured worker recovery and pediatrics. John Heinz Rehab is the only CARF accredited program in northeastern Pennsylvania for treatment of brain injury rehabilitation.

6410 **Allied Services Rehabilitation Hospital**
475 Morgan Hwy
Scranton, PA 18508-2656 570-348-1359
Fax: 570-341-4548
www.allied-services.org

Gerald Franceski, Chairman
Thomas Speicher, Vice-Chairman
William Conaboy, CEO
Gregory Basting, VP Medical Affairs

Committed to help people overcome challenges and reach their greatest potential by providing quality care, people-oriented services and comfort.

6411 **Brighten Place**
131 North Main St
Chalfont, PA 18914-245 215-997-7746
Fax: 215-997-2517
brightenplace@enter.net

William Koffros, CEO

A residential brain injury program with the mission to encourage growth and foster independence on an individual level for each resident. We are CARF accredited and provide additional services which include a day program and respite care.

6412 **Chestnut Hill Rehabilitation Hospital**
8601 Stenton Ave
Wyndmoor, PA 19038-8312 215-233-6200
Fax: 215-233-6879
www.extendedcare.com

Cammi Lubking, Administrator

Chestnut Hill Rehab Hospital is dedicated to meeting patients' physical, emotional, social, and vocational goals. Through innovative programs, sophisticated equipment, and support by specially trained staff members committed to the progress of every patient, Chestnut Hill achieves results.

6413 **Doylestown Hospital Rehabilitation Center**
595 W State St
Doylestown, PA 18901-2597 215-345-2200
Fax: 215-345-2512
www.dh.org

James Brexler, President and Chief Executive Officer
Eleanor Wilson, RN, MSN, MHA, Vice President, Patient Services/Chief Operating Officer
Dan Upton, Vice President, Chief Financial Officer
Scott S. Levy, MD, Vice President, Chief Medical Officer

The mission of Doylestown Hospital is to provide a responsive healing environment for patients and their families, and to improve the quality of life for all members of our community. We combine the creative energies of Medical Staff, Board, Associates and Volunteers to make Doylestown Hospital a place where each patient and family feels healed and whole, even when disease cannot be cured.

6414 **Health Care Solutions**
500 Abbott Dr
Ste B
Broomall, PA 19008-4301 610-544-6023
800-451-1671
Fax: 610-544-6035
www.lincare.com

John Byrnes, CEO
Shawn Schabel, President/COO

Develops unique containment programs, offers equipment set-up, patient instruction, patient assessment and equipment usage. Offers clinical services that include oxygen systems, ventilators, aerosol therapy, suction equipment, T.E.N.S. programs, compression pumps, custom orthotics, enteral feeding.

6415 **HealthSouth Harmarville Rehabilitation Hospital**
P.O. Box 11460
320 Guys Run Road
Pittsburgh, PA 15238-460 412-828-1300
877-937-7342
Fax: 412-828-7705
www.healthsouthharmarville.com

Ken Anthony, Chief Executive Officer
Thomas Franz, M.D., Medical Director
Catherine M. Birk, M.D., Staff Physiatrist
Brian Cicuto, D.O., Staff Physiatrist

A 202-bed facility providing inpatient and outpatient physical medicine and rehabilitation to adults and adolescents in Pennsylvania, West Virginia, Ohio and Maryland.

6416 **HealthSouth Nittany Valley Rehabilitation Hospital**
Health South of Nittany Valley
550 W College Ave
Pleasant Gap, PA 16823-7401 814-359-3421
800-842-6026
Fax: 814-359-5898
www.nittanyvalleyrehab.com

Richard Allatt, Medical Director
Susan Hartman, CEO
Sara Godwin, CNO
Ann Foster, Therapy Operations Director

Comprehensive inpatient and outpatient facilities. Treatment for symptoms relating to: stroke, head injury, pulmonary disease, orthopedic conditions, neurological disorders, cardiac illnesses and spinal cord injuries. Healthsouth Nittany Valley Rehabilitation Hospital is a part of Healthsouth's national network of more than 2,000 facilities in 50 states.

6417 **HealthSouth Rehab Hospital Of Erie**
143 E 2nd St
Erie, PA 16507-1501 814-878-1200
800-234-4574
Fax: 814-878-1399
www.healthsoutherie.com

Douglas Grisier, Medical Director
Shelly Mayes, Director of Therapy Operations

An acute inpatient rehabilitation hospital that was founded in 1986. HealthSouth Erie is one of the only rehabilitation hospitals in the country to hold a triple-certification by the Joint Commission in the areas of Brain Injury, Stroke and Parkinson's disease Rehabilitation.

6418 HealthSouth Rehabilitation Hospital of Altoona
2005 Valley View Blvd
Altoona, PA 16602-4548
814-944-3535
800-873-4220
Fax: 814-944-6160
www.healthsouthaltoona.com
Scott Filler, Chief Executive Officer
Paul Sutton, Director Of Clinical Services
Rakesh (Rock Patel, D.O., Medical Director
Mary Gen Boyles, Director of Nursing Services
Inpatient and outpatient physical rehabilitation programs and services.

6419 Healthsouth Rehabilitation Hospital of Greater Pittsburgh
2380 McGinley Rd
Monroeville, PA 15146-4400
412-856-2400
Fax: 412-856-9320
www.lifecare-hospitals.com
Mary Lee Dadey, Administrator
Rehabilitation and long-term acute care hospital that treats brain injury, stroke, multiple sclerosis, Parkinson's disease, back and spinal cord injuries, cancer, pulmonary disease, cardiac disease, traumatic and work injuries.

6420 Healthsouth Rehabilitation Hospital of Mechanicsburg
175 Lancaster Blvd
Mechanicsburg, PA 17055-3562
717-691-3700
800-933-3831
Fax: 717-697-6524
www.healthsouthpa.com
Mark Freeburn, CEO
Annette Bates, Director of Marketing Operations
Jeff Brandenburg, MPT, Director of Therapy Operations
Michael F. Lupinacci, M.D, Medical Director
HealthSouth provides comprehensive rehabilitation and recovery services to patients with stroke, brain injury, hip fracture, medically complex, pulmonary, wound, spinal cord injury, amputation, and other neuro-muscular, and orthopedic impairments. Our primary goal is to provide individualized treatment programs to people requiring physical rehabilitation and medical recovery in order to help patients get back to work, to play, to living.

6421 Healthsouth Rehabilitation Hospital of York
1850 Normandie Dr
York, PA 17408-1552
717-767-6941
Fax: 717-767-8776
www.healthsouthyork.com
Sally Arthur, Director of Human Resources
Bruce Sicilia, Medical Director
Elaine Charest, Director of Therapy Operations
Daniel C. DeFalcis, M.D., Associate Medical Director
A 120-bed rehabilitation hospital dedicated to providing advanced, comprehensive services to patients who have suffered head injury, spinal cord injury, stroke, burns, amputation, chronic pain and other neurological and musculoskeletal disorders. HRH of York provides outpatient services in seven locations. Healthsouth is located in York, Pennsylvania, approximately 50 miles north of Baltimore and 25 miles south of Harrisburg.

6422 Magee Rehabilitation Hospital
1513 Race St
Philadelphia, PA 19102-1177
215-587-3000
800-966-2433
Fax: 215-568-3736
www.mageerehab.org
Jack Carroll, CEO
A not-for-profit health organization which is the home to the nation's first brain injury rehabilitation program to be accredited by the Commission on the Accreditation of Rehabilitation Facilities (CARF) and is one of 14 federally designated Regional Spinal Cord Injury Centers. Our staff and management are committed to restoring the highest level of independence possible to individuals with disabilities.

6423 Moss Rehabilitation Hospital
1200 W Tabor Rd.
Philadelphia, PA 19141
215-456-9800
Fax: 215-456-9381
www.mossrehab.com
Thomas Smith, Chief Operating Officer
Alberto Esquenazi, Chief Medical Officer
Eileen Hartranft, Program Director
Julie Hensler-Cullen, Director, Quality & Education
An outpatient services center providing rehabilitation services. This 152 bed facility offers comprehensive care to people with broad ranges of conditions, diagnostic laboratories and a multidisciplinary team of rehabilitation professionals.

6424 Shriners Hospitals for Children, Philadelphia
Shrinners Hospitals for Children
3551 N Broad St
Philadelphia, PA 19140-4131
215-430-4000
800-281-4051
Fax: 215-430-4126
www.shrinershq.org
Alan W. Madsen, Chairman of the Board
John A. Cinotto, 1st Vice President
Dale W. Stauss, 2nd Vice President
Ernest Perilli, Administrator
At Shriners Hospitals for Childrenr - Philadelphia, we provide state-of-the-art medical care for children with spinal cord injuries, as well as a host of orthopaedic and neuromusculoskeletal disorders and diseases

6425 Shriners Hospitals for Children, Erie
1645 W 8th St
Erie, PA 16505-5007
814-875-8700
Fax: 814-875-8756
www.shrinershq.org
John Lubahn, Chief of Staff
Charles Walczak, Administrator
The Shriners Hospitals for Children, Erie, is a 30-bed pediatric orthopaedic hospital providing comprehensive orthopaedic care to children at no charge. The hospital is one of 22 Shriners Hospitals throughout North America. The Erie Hospital accepts and treats children with routine and complex orthopaedic and neuromuscular problems, utilizing the latest treatments and technology available in pediatric orthopaedics, resulting in early ambulation and reduced length of stay.

6426 Shriners Hospitals, Philadelphia Unit, for Crippled Children
3551 N Broad St
Philadelphia, PA 19140-4105
215-430-4000
Fax: 215-430-4079
www.shrinershq.org/hospitals/philadelphia
Randal Betz, Chief of Staff
Ernest Perilli, Administrator
Provides comprehensive medical, surgical and rehabilitative care for children with orthopaedic conditions and spinal cord injuries. All services are provided at no charge. The hospital is one of 22 located throughout North America. In addition to treating children with routine and complex orthopaedic problems, the Philadelphia hospital provides a comprehensive and individualized rehabilitation program for children and adolescents who have sustained a traumatic injury to their spine.

South Carolina

6427 Colleton Regional Hospital: RehabCare Unit
501 Robertson Blvd
Walterboro, SC 29488-5714
843-782-2000
Fax: 843-549-7562
www.colletonmedical.com
Mitchell Mongel, CEO
Colleton Medical Center's 8-bed physical and mental rehabilitation department is the oldest in the Lowcountry and has been serving the community for nearly 20 years. Strives to provide patient-centered care in a family atmosphere. The team includes nurses, physical therapists, occupational therapists, speech therapists, and nutritionists. The typical patient requires rehabilita-

tion following a stroke, spinal injury, close head injury, and orthopedic rehabilitation.

6428 **HealthSouth Rehab Hospital: South Carolina**
2935 Colonial Dr
Columbia, SC 29203-6811 803-254-7777
Fax: 803-414-1414
www.healthsouthcolumbia.com

W. Anthony Jackson, CEO
Lydia Carpenter, Director of Therapy Operations
Devin Troyer, M.D., Medical Director
Luanne Burton, Director of Human Resources
Offers a wide range of specialized medical and therapeutic services designed to help physically disabled individuals reach their optimum level of function and independence.

6429 **Shriners Hospitals for Children, Greenville**
950 W Faris Rd
Greenville, SC 29605-4255 864-271-3444
866-459-0013
Fax: 864-271-4471
www.shrinershq.org/hospitals/greenville

Randall Romberger, Administrator
Peter Stasikelis, Chief of Staff
Tracy McReynolds, Development Officer
A 50-bed pediatric orthopaedic hospital providing comprehensive orthopaedic care to children at no charge to their families. The hospital is one of 22 Shriners Hospitals throughout North America. The hospital accepts and treats children with routine and complex orthopaedic problems, utilizing the latest tretments and technology availiable in pediatric orthopaedics, resulting in early ambulatory and reduced length of stay.

Tennessee

6430 **Health South Cane Creek Rehabilitation Center**
Health South Corporation
180 Mount Pelia Rd
Martin, TN 38237-3812 731-587-4231
Fax: 731-588-1454
dayle.unger@healthsouth.com
www.healthsouthcanecreek.com

Eric Garrard, CEO
William Eason, Medical Director
Lindsey Box-Rotger, BSN, RN, C, Director of Quality and Risk Management
Cindy Cooper, RN, Director of Case Management
Offers a wide variety of programs and services for patients in need of acute rehabilitation. Programs and services are availiable through inpatient and outpaitent. Thereapy services availiable are physical, occupational, speech, and respiratory.

6431 **HealthSouth Chattanooga Rehabilitation Hospital**
2412 McCallie Ave
Chattanooga, TN 37404-3398 423-697-9129
800-763-5189
Fax: 423-697-9124
www.healthsouthchattanooga.com

Scott Rowe, CEO
Amjad Munir, Medical Director
Karen Jonakin, Director Clinical Services
Offers orthopaedic rehabilitation, stroke rehabilitation, amputee rehabilitation, brain injury program, pain management, ventilator weaning, carpal tunnel screening, low intensity program, oncology program, aquatic therapy, day treatment, burn program and outpatient services.

6432 **HealthSouth Rehabilitation Cntr/Tennessee**
1282 Union Ave
Memphis, TN 38104-3414 901-722-2000
Fax: 901-729-5171
healthsouthmemphis.com

Tracy Willis, CEO
Toni Wackerfuss, Director of Therapy Operation
An 80-bed acute medical rehabilitation hospital that offers comprehensive inpatient and outpatient rehabilitation services.

6433 **James H And Cecile C Quillen Rehabilitation Hospital**
2511 Wesley St
Johnson City, TN 37601-1723 423-952-1700
800-235-1994
Fax: 423-283-0906
www.msha.com

Tammy Bishop, Manager
A 60-bed, freestanding comprehensive medical rehabilitation hospital. Full range of outpatient and day treatment, 14-bed traumatic brain injury unit, in ground therapeutic pool, transitional living apartment, outdoor ambulation course. All inpatient and outpatient programs utilize an interdisciplinary team approach designed to improve a patient's physical and cognitive functioning.

6434 **Nashville Rehabilitation Hospital**
610 Gallatin Ave
Nashville, TN 37206-3225 615-650-2600
800-227-3108
Fax: 615-650-2562

Alan Miller, CEO
Marc Miller, President
A free-standing physical rehabilitation facility offering services to patients on an inpatient and outpatient basis. Programs include CVA, orthopedic, neuromuscular, traumatic brain injury, spinal cord injury, general rehabilitation and Bridges - geriatric psychiatric unit. Intra-disciplinary team approach is utilized to assist patients in obtaining their maximum fuctional level.

6435 **Patricia Neal Rehab Center : Ft. Sanders Regional Medical Center**
Covenant Health
1901 W Clinch Ave
Knoxville, TN 37916-2307 865-541-1111
800-728-6325
Fax: 865-541-2247
www.patneal.org

J.E. Henry, Co-Chair
David Kugley, Co-Chair
Mary Dillon, M.D., Medical Director, Patricia Neal Rehabilitation Center
Sharon E. Glass, M.D., Stroke Program Director, Patricia Neal Rehabilitation Center
A CARF accredited 73-bed facility, it offers a comprehensive team approach to care. Physical, occupational, recreational, behavioral medicine and speech language therapists work with physiatrists to develop individual plans of care designed to return patients to a normal lifestyle as quickly as possible. In addition, rehabilitation nurses collaborate with specialists to teach self-care techniques and provide education to help patients reach optimal functionality.

6436 **Rehabilitation Center Baptist Hospital**
137 E Blount Ave
Suite 6-B
Knoxville, TN 37920-1643 865-632-5520

6437 **Rehabilitation Center at McFarland Hospital**
University Medical Center
500 Park Ave
Lebanon, TN 37087-3721 615-449-0500
Fax: 615-453-7405
www.universitymedicalcenter.com

Saad Ehtisham, CEO
Matt Caldwell, Chief Executive Officer
Michael Cherry, Chief Financial Officer
Greg Carda, Chief Operating Officer
An Acute Inpatient Rehab, located on the hospital's second floor. The center has 26 patient rooms, three therapy treatment rooms, a patient dining area, and an 'activities of daily living' area which includes a kitchen/laundry area and a patient apartment, for those individuals who will be returning home.

6438 **St. Mary's Medical Center: RehabCare Center**
900 E Oak Hill Ave
Knoxville, TN 37917-4505 865-545-7962
Fax: 865-545-8133
www.tennova.com

Jeffrey Ashin, President
Committed to providing individualized and flexable treatment programs designed for individuals who have been disabled by an

injury or illness. The primary mission of the RehabCare Center is to help patients achieve basic skills that may allow independent living and working.

6439 **Sumner Regional Medical Center**
555 Hartsville Pike
Gallatin, TN 37066-2400 615-328-8888
Fax: 615-328-3903
www.mysumnermedical.com

Susan Peach, BSN, MBA, CEO
Kevin Rinks, Chief Financial Officer
Michael S. Herman, Chief Operating Officer
Anne Melton, RN, MSN, Chief Nursing Officer

SRMC operates as a 155-bed healthcare facility and provides quality Gallatin hospital and medical care services in numerous areas, including cancer treatment, cardiac care, same- day surgery, orthopaedics, diagnostics, women's health and rehabilitation services. As the community grows, SRMC strives to continually improve its services and programs to meet the changing needs of its service area.

Texas

6440 **Bayshore Medical Center: Rehab**
4000 Spencer Hwy
Pasadena, TX 77504-1202 713-359-2000
Fax: 713-359-1283
www.bayshoremedical.com

Dr. Charles Bessire, Board
Jeanna Barnard, FACHE, CEO
Alice Hopkins Adams, Board
Wilfred J. Broussard, Board

A 345-bed facility, providing the award-winning care for which we have been nationally recoginzed. Members are here to care for the physical and emotional well-being of those who arrive at Bayshore Medical Center often frightned, in pain and perhaps even alone. We offer patients solace and security through constant communication and compassionate listening in the midst of their medical emergencies and surgical or diagnostic procedures. Kindness, empathy & quality are triats that patients trust.

6441 **Cecil R Bomhr Rehabilitation Center of Nacogdoches Memorial Hospital**
1204 N Mound St
Nacogdoches, TX 75961-4027 936-564-4611
Fax: 936-564-4616
info@nacmem.org
www.nacmem.org

Jerry Whitaker, Chairperson
Larry Walker, M.D., Vice-Chairperson
Lisa King, Secretary
Walter Scott, Board Member

The goal of Nacogdoches Memorial Hospital's rehabilitation services is to assist patients in attaining their highest potential activity level for independent daily living, thereby reducing the number of necessary hospitalizations. Keeping folks healthy and in their homes lowers healthcare costs for all of us.

6442 **Covenant Health Systems Owens White Outpatient Rehab Center**
9812 Slide Rd
Lubbock, TX 79424-1116 806-725-5627
Fax: 806-723-6009
www.covenanthealth.org

Walt Cathey, Manager

A comprehensive rehabilitation program designed to help patients attain their maximum level of independence following a debilitating stroke, illness or injury. Our fully accredited program features outpatient physical, occupational and speech language therapies, as well as certified athletic trainers and a certified strength and conditioning specialist.

6443 **Gonzales Warm Springs Rehabilitation Hospital**
200 Memorial Dr
Luling, TX 78648-3213 830-875-8400
Fax: 830-875-5029
www.warmsprings.org

Anthony Misitano, President/CEO
Vonnie Cromwell, Operations Manager

Statewide not-for-profit system of inpatient and outpatient rehabilitation speciality centers. Throughout the communities we serve, the Warm Springs Rehabilitation System offers hope and acts as a catalyst for achieving an optimal quality of life by providing comprehensive physical and/or cogenitive care. Investing resources in educational and recreational programs. Supporting research efforts.

6444 **Harris Methodist Fort Worth Hospital Mabee Rehabilitation Center**
1301 Pennsylvania Ave
Fort Worth, TX 76104-2122 817-250-2760
866-847-7342
Fax: 814-250-6846
www.texashealth.org

Lillie Biggins, B.S.N., M.S.N, CEO/President
Elaine Nelson, R.N., M.S.N., Chief Nursing Officer
Joseph Prosser, M.D., M.B.A., Chief Medical Officer

Professionals at the Harris Methodist Fort Worth Hospital's Mabee Rehabilitation Center work closely with each patient to develop a specialzed treatment plan for personal achievement. The center offers highly trained clinical staff members and spacious facilities An incredibly wide range of treatment programs and educational services are provided for both inpatient and outpatient needs.

6445 **HealthSouth Plano Rehabilitation Hospital**
6701 Oakmont Blvd.
Fort Worth, TX 76132-7526 817-370-4700
Fax: 972-423-4293
www.healthsouth.com

Jon F. Hanson, Chairman
John W. Chidsey, Board of director
Donald L. Correll, Board of director
Yvonne M. Curl, Board of director

A 62-bed medical reahabilitation facility serving inpatient and out patient needs in the Northern Dallas area. The team coordinate all aspects of the patient's rehabilitation to maximize results. The overall effort is directed by board-certified physical medicine and rehabilitation physicians who specialize in medical rehabilitation. Whatever the cause of the disability, our services can benefit patients who have functional limitations in such areas as mobility, communication and self care.

6446 **HealthSouth Rehab Hospital Of Arlington**
3200 Matlock Rd
Arlington, TX 76015-2911 817-468-4000
Fax: 817-468-3055
www.healthsouth.com

Jon F. Hanson, Chairman
John W. Chidsey, Board of director
Donald L. Correll, Board of director
Yvonne M. Curl, Board of director

A modern 65-bed hospital dedicated to providng inpatient programs in a general rehabilitation setting for persons recovering for a disabling injury or illness. As part of our continuum of care, we also offer outpatient therapy, a day program, and individual therapy services. Our goal is to help our patients resume a productive and more meaningful life through appropriate rehabilitative care and restorative nursing in a wellness-oriented environment that promotes healing and functional recovery.

6447 **HealthSouth Rehab Hospital Of Austin**
1215 Red River St
Austin, TX 78701-1921 512-474-5700
Fax: 512-479-3765
www.healthsouthaustin.com

Duke Saldiver, CEO
Corey Helm Swartz, Director of Therapy Operations
Maria Arizmendez, M.D., Medical Director
Debbie Belcher, Human Resource Director

A comprehensive 83 bed medical rehabilitation hospital serving the needs of patients in the Central Texas area. The mission is to promote recovery for persons with disabling conditions by providing individualized treatment so they can reach the highest level of physical, social and emotional well-being.

6448 **HealthSouth Rehabilitation Center of Humble Texas**
19002 McKay Blvd
Humble, TX 77338
281-446-6148
Fax: 281-446-5616
www.healthsouthhumble.com

Angie Simmons, CEO
Mikael Simpson, Director of Therapy Operations
Emile Mathurin, Jr., M.D., Medical Director
Christy Dixon, Human Resources Director

Offers comprehensive rehabilitation services for patients with diverse diagnoses. Rehabilitation can be defined as multidisciplinary therapy designed to increase patient's overall functioning to a level that meets or exceeds where the patient was prior to illness or injury or to maximize current level of ability. The benefits of these services to patients and their families is invaluable.

6449 **HealthSouth Rehabilitation Hospital**
6701 Oakmont Blvd
Fort Worth, TX 76132-2957
817-370-4700
Fax: 817-370-4977
www.healthsouthcityview.com

Deborah Hopps, CEO
Mark Bussell, Medical Director
Mark Bussell, M.D., Medical Director
Kenneth Akwar, PharmD, Director of Pharmacy

A 62-bed acute medical rehabilitation hospital that offers comprehensive inpatient and outpatient rehabilitation services.

6450 **HealthSouth Rehabilitation Hospital of Beaumont**
3340 Plaza 10 Dr
Beaumont, TX 77707-2551
409-835-0835
Fax: 409-835-0898

Sam Coco, Director of Therapy Operations
HJ Gaspard, CEO
Linda Smith, M.D., Medical Director
Sam Coco, PT, Director of Therapy Operations

A state of the art freestanding 61-bed comprehensive physical rehabilitation hospital. The hospital is specifically designed to meet the needs of individuals and their families who have experienced a disabling injury or illness or are recovering from a surgery. An experienced team of physicians, nurses, therapists, treat conditions and other disorders.

6451 **HealthSouth Rehabilitation Institute Of San Antonio (RIOSA)**
9119 Cinnamon Hill
San Antonio, TX 78240-5401
210-691-0737
Fax: 210-558-1297
www.hsriosa.com

Scott Butcher, CEO
Richard Senelick, Medical Director
Christine Chesnut, OTR, MPH, Director of Therapy Operations
Linda Hart, LVN, Director of Marketing

HealthSouth Rehabilitation Institute of San Antonio is the largest free-standing physical rehabilitation hospital in San Antonio and is proud to enter our 11th year of delivering quality, comprehensive medical rehabilitation in a pristine environment. HealthSouth annually serves over 1,500 inpatients and more then 20,000 outpatient visits from throughout San Antonio and Mexico. 108-bed hospital has more then 300 personell on staff providing extensive experience.

6452 **Hillcrest Baptist Medical Center: Rehab Care Unit**
100 Hillcrest Medical Blvd
Waco, TX 76712-3239
254-202-2000
Fax: 254-202-8975

Fred Walters, President
Jon Ellis, Secretary

A fully accredited 393-bed acute care facility in Waco including a Level II Trauma Center, Hillcrest Family Health Center, a network of family medicine clinics; and many key services. Hillcrest is a ministry of Texas Baptists and is one of 7 health care institutions affiliated with the Baptist General Convention of Texas.

6453 **Institute for Rehabilitation & Research**
1333 Moursund St
Houston, TX 77030-3405
713-942-6159
800-447-3422
Fax: 713-942-5289
tirr.referrals@memorialhermann.org
www.memorialhermann.org

Jeffrey Berliner, Physician
Michelle Pu, Physician

A national center for information, training, research, and technical assistance in independent living. The goal is to extend the body of knowledge in independent living and to improve the utilization of results of research programs and demonstration projects in this field. It has developed a variety of strategies for collecting, synthesizing, and disseminating information related to the field of independent living.

6454 **Midland Memorial Hospital & Medical Center**
400 Rosalind Redfern Grover Parkway
Midland, TX 79701-9980
432-685-1111
800-833-2916
russell.meyers@midland-memorial.com
www.midland-memorial.com

J.T. Lent Jr., President
Russell Meyers, CEO
Greg Wright, Board of Directors
Pete Hulder, Board of Directors

The Occupational and Physical Therapy Center is a specialzed outpatient clinic. The clinic provides a wide variety of rehabilitation services designed to adequately assist you in returning back to your normal duties. Our highly trained professionals are here to help you with all your rehabilitation needs.

6455 **Navarro Regional Hospital: RehabCare Unit**
Navarro Hospital
3201 W State Highway 22
Corsicana, TX 75110-2469
903-654-6800
Fax: 903-654-6955
www.navarrohospital.com

Xavier Villarreal, CEO
Glenda Teri, Chief Nursing Officer

The rehab unit is located on the 4th floor and is designed for individuals who require intense rehab for an injury or disease process where the goal would be to return home. Our team is committed to helping individuals return to the highest level of functioning. Our team consists of physicians, nurses, physical therapist, occupational therapist, speech therapist, social workers, dieticians and other professionals as needed.

6456 **Rebound: Northeast Methodist Hospital**
12412 Judson Rd
Live Oak, TX 78233-3255
210-757-7000
Fax: 210-757-5072

Joe Hernandez, Manager

Methodist Healthcare provides quality, comprehensive rehabilitation services for children and adults. Working as a team, rehabilitation professionals help patients define and achieve individual goals in restoring function and productivity.

6457 **Rio Vista Rehabilitation Hospital**
1740 Curie Dr
El Paso, TX 79902-2900
915-544-8336
800-999-8392
Fax: 915-544-4838

Gene Miller, Administrator

6458 **San Antonio Warm Springs Rehabilitation Hospital**
5101 Medical Dr
San Antonio, TX 78229-4801
210-595-2380
Fax: 210-614-0649
www.warmsprings.org

Kurt Meyer, SVP Operations
Rick Marek, VP Post Acute Medical

A statewide not-for-profit system of inpatient and outpatient rehabilitation specialty centers. Warm Springs Rehabilitation System offers hope and acts as a catalyst for achieving an optimal quality of life by providing comprehensive physical and/or cognitive rehabilitative care. Invensting resources in educational and recreational programs. Supporting research efforts.

6459 Shannon Medical Center: RehabCare Unit
120 E Harris Ave
San Angelo, TX 76903-5904 325-653-6741
Fax: 325-657-5706
www.shannonhealth.com
Bryan Horner, CEO
Irv Zeitler, VP Medical Affairs
Shane Plymell, Chief financial officer
Gary Gibian, Executive director
Committed to improving the health of our community, using the latest technologies available in the spirit of caring and integrity. Strives to create an environment committed to the values of accountability, service, pride, integrity, respect and excellence. We foster growth toward the highest quality care and customer service and strive for excellent financial performance. We hire and develop the best people to accomplish these tasks.

6460 Shriners Burn Institute: Galveston Unit
815 Market St
Galveston, TX 77550-2725 409-770-6600
Fax: 409-770-6919
www.totalburncare.com
David Herndon, Chief Of Staff
David Ferrell, F.A.C.H.E., Administrator
Providing expert, orthopaedic and burn care to children under 18 regardless of ability to pay.

6461 Shriners Hospitals for Children, Houston
6977 Main St
Houston, TX 77030-3701 713-797-1616
800-853-1240
Fax: 713-797-1029
www.shrinershq.org
David Ferrell, Administrator
Douglas Barnes, Chief of Staff
Melanie Lux, M.D., Director
Gloria Gogola, M.D., Doctor
Shriners Hospitals provides at no charge quality pediatric orthopedic serivces to children ages newborn to 18 years old. These services include both outpatient and inpatient needs. Specialties include cerebrel palsy, spina bifida, scoliosis, hand, hip and feet problems. An application is required and may be completed by phone.

6462 South Arlington Medical Center: Rehab Care Unit
3301 Matlock Rd
Arlington, TX 76015-2908 817-472-4849
Fax: 817-472-4946
mca@hcahealthcare.com
www.medicalcenterarlington.com
Patrice Oliver, Manaager
Above all else, we are committed to the care and improvement of human life. In recognition of this committment, we strive to deliver high-quality, cost-effective healthcare in the communities we serve.

6463 South Texas Rehabilitation Hospital
Ernest Health
425 E Alton Gloor Blvd
Brownsville, TX 78526-3361 956-554-6000
Fax: 956-350-6150
www.strh.ernesthealth.com
Christopher Wilson, Medical Director
Jessie Eason, CEO
Mary Valdez, Director of Marketing
STRH was designed for the provision of specialized rehabilitative care, in the only freestanding acute rehabilitation hospital serving Brownsville and the Rio Grande Valley. The hospital provides rehabilitative services for patients with functional deficits as a result of debilitating illnesses or injuries.

6464 St. David's Rehabilitation Center
St. David s Medical Center
621 Radam Lane
Suite 200
Austin, TX 78745-4237 512-447-1083
Fax: 512-447-1338
www.stdavids.com
Anisa Godinez, Medical Director
Everett Heinze, MD Neurology, Medical Director
Tom Hill, MD, Medical Director
Albert Horn, MD, Medical Director
Mission is to provide exceptional care to every patient every day with a spirit of warmth, friendliness and personal pride. Values are integrity, compassion, accountability, respect and excellence.

6465 Texas NeuroRehab Center
1106 W Dittmar Rd
Austin, TX 78745-6328 512-444-4835
800-252-5151
Fax: 512-462-6749
Alison Crawford Sinsky, Inpatient and Outpatient Manager
Ed Varando, Occupational Therapy Manager
Internationally recognized provider in brain injury/neurobehavioral treatment for children, adolescents, and adults with complex medical, physical and/or behavioral issues. Medical rehabilitation, neurobehavioral, and neuropsychiatric programs combine traditional therapies with education, vocational, substance abuse, and sensory integration services.

6466 Texas Specialty Hospital at Dallas
7955 Harry Hines Blvd
Dallas, TX 75235-3305 214-637-0000
Robin Burns, CEO
66 beds offering active/acute rehabilitation, brain injury day treatment, cognitive rehabilitation, complex care, extended rehabilitation and short term evaluation.

6467 Touchstone Neurorecovery Center
Nexus Health Systems
9297 Wahrenberger Rd
Conroe, TX 77304-2441 936-788-7770
800-414-4824
Fax: 936-788-7785
tncinfo@nhsltd.com
John W. Cassidy, MD, Executive Medical Director
Jude Theriot, MD, Medical Director
Ron Tintner, MD, Associate Clinical Director
Nelson Valena, MD, Director of Physical Medicine and Rehabilitation
Touchstone provides treatment and rehabilitation in a residential environment on a tranquil, wooded 26-acre site just north of Houston in Conroe, TX. Touchstone offers customized treatment programs designed to help individuals with known or suspected brain injury or neurological deficits progress to their highest functional level possible. Touchstone offers both on-campus and off-campus housing in home-like settings for residents based on their needs.

6468 Valley Regional Medical Center: RehabCare Unit
100A E Alton Gloor Blvd
Brownsville, TX 78526-3328 956-350-7000
Fax: 956-350-7111
www.valleyregionalmedicalcenter.com
Billy Bradford Jr., Chair
Francisco Javier Del Castillo, M, Vice Chair
Subramaniam Anandasivam, MD, Board
Christopher Olson, MD, Board
Our mission is to treat our community as family by providing quality compassionate care.

Utah

6469 **HealthSouth Rehab Hospital Of Utah**
8074 S 1300 E
Sandy, UT 84094-743
801-561-3400
801-565-6666
Fax: 801-565-6576
www.healthsouthutah.com

Phil Eaton, CEO
William McNutt, Director of Therapy Operations
Mark Rada, M.D., Interim Medical Director
Richard Ashby, Western Regional Director of Plant Operations/Safety Officer

A full spectrum of services, including inpatient, outpatient, day hospital and home health. Holistic patient care, education and community assimilation are the hallmarks of our programs, and evidence of our leadership in the field of rehabilitation. Working together as a team, we are able to tailor the needs of our patients and provide the highest quality services. We believe that education and involvement of family and friends, will assist them in maintaining independence after discharge.

6470 **LDS Hospital Rehabilitation Center**
8th Ave & C Street
Salt Lake City, UT 84143-0001
801-408-1100
800-527-1118
Fax: 801-408-5610
www.intermountainhealthcare.org

Lizz Daley, Administrator
Jim Sheets, Administrator

Located within a Trauma I Center, this facility provides comprehensive inpatient and outpatient rehabilitation to people with physical disabilities. CARF/JCAHO accredited. Low cost family housing is available and Medicaid/Medicare is accepted.

6471 **Primary Children's Medical Center**
100 Mario Capecchi Dr
Salt Lake City, UT 84113-1100
801-662-1000
Fax: 801-588-2318
www.intermountainhealthcare.org

Scott Parker, President
Kevin Jones, Manager
Ore-Ofe O. Adesina, MD, Ophthalmology
Zeinab A. Afify, MD, Pediatric Hematology Oncology

Primary Children's Medical Center is the pediatric center serving 5 states in the Intermountain West Utah, Idaho, Wyoming, Nevada and Montana. The 289-bed facility is equipped and staffed to treat children with complex illness and injury. PCMC is owned by Intermountain Healthcare, a non-profit health care system. In addition, it is affiliated with the Dept. of Pediatrics, University of Utah, integrating pediatric programs. The hospital is designed to meet the needs of children & their families.

6472 **Shriners Hospitals for Children: Intermountain**
Fairfax Road at Virginia St
Salt Lake City, UT 84103
801-536-3500
800-313-3745
Fax: 801-536-3782
www.shrinershq.org

Kevin Martin, Administrator
Jacques D'Astous, Chief of Staff

One of nineteen hospitals in North America specializing in pediatric orthopedics (plus four hospitals providing pediatric burn treatment). This hospital serves the Intermountain region. All services provided in the hospital are at no cost to family, insurance company, nor state/federal agency regardless of ability to pay.

6473 **Stewart Rehabilitation Center: McKay Dee Hospital**
4401 Harrison Blvd
Ogden, UT 84403-3195
801-387-2080
Fax: 801-387-7720
www.intermountainhealthcare.org

Corey Anden, Nurse Coordinator
Judy Grover, Manager

With 10 affiliated clinics, McKay-Dee serves northern Utah, and portions of southeast Idaho and western Wyoming. A part of Intermountain Healthcare's system of 21 hospitals, McKay-Dee Hospital Center offers nationally ranked programs such as the Heart & Vascular Institute, the Newborn ICU and a new Cancer Treatment Center.

6474 **University Healthcare-Rehabilitation Center**
50 N Medical Dr
Salt Lake City, UT 84132-1
801-587-3422
801-58 -EHAB
Fax: 801-581-2111
www.healthcare.utah.edu/rehab/

David Entwistle, Administrator
Trish Jensen, Program Coordinator

Provides quality, comprehensive, rehabilitation services to persons with complex rehabilitation needs, including spinal cord injuries, head trauma, stroke, and other disabling conditions. Rehabilitation Services has been serving physicians, their patients, and the community since 1965. Rehabilitation Services has been an established leader in comprehensive inpatient, outpatient and home/community rehabilitation programs. Accredited by CARF and JCAHO.

Vermont

6475 **Vermont Achievement Center**
88 Park St
Rutland, VT 05701-4715
802-775-2395
Fax: 802-773-9656
www.vac-rutland.com

Kiki Mc Shane, CEO
Rebecca Wisell, Administrator

Vermont Achievement Center is recognized as a catalyst in building a community where all people are capable of change. Individuals flourish because they are nutured, valued and treated with respect. Education is empowering. The family is the primary influence in a person's life. Children belong in a family. Families are enhanced by support of the community. Children and family services are flexible and responsive to changing needs.

Virginia

6476 **Inova Mount Vernon Hospital Rehabilitation Program**
Inova Rehabilitation Center
2501 Parkers Ln
Alexandria, VA 22306-3209
703-664-7000
800-554-7342
Fax: 703-664-7423
www.inova.com

Barbara Doyle, CEO

Inova Mount Vernon Hospital is a 237-bed hospital offering patients convenience and state-of-the-art care in a community environment. Our hospital sits on 26 acres of beautifully landscaped open space, where patients can find moments of serenity in our specially designed gardens..

6477 **Kluge Children's Rehabilitation Center**
University of Virginia
2270 Ivy Rd
Charlottesville, VA 22903-4977
434-924-5161
800-627-8596
Fax: 434-924-5559
www.healthsystem.virginia.edu

Janet Allaire, Administrator
Richard Stevenson, Research Director

The Kluge Childrens's Rehabilitation Center (KCRC) is a place dedicated to serving children with special needs. Children between the ages of birth and 21 come to the KCRC from all over Virginia, the United States, and even overseas for many reasons. Some need specific therapy or rehabilitation after injuries, accidents, or surgery. Others have chronic illness such as diabetes, and cystic fibrosis. Many families come to find out why their child is experiencing behavior problems.

Washington

6478 Good Samaritan Healthcare Physical Medicine and Rehabilitation
Good Samaritan Hospital
407 14th Ave SE
Puyallup, WA 98372-3770
253-697-4000
Fax: 253-697-5157
info@goodsamhealth.org
www.multicare.org

Glenn Kassman, President
Vince Schmitz, CFO

Good Samaritan is part of the Multi-Care Health System, a non-for-profit medical system serving the growing populations of Pierce and King Counties in the greater Puget Sound region of Washington. Our medical staff includes 1,600 of the regions most respected primary care physicians and specialists.

6479 Northwest Hospital Center for Medical Rehabilitation
1550 N 115th St
Seattle, WA 98133-9733
206-364-0500
Fax: 206-364-0500
TTY: 877-694-4677
www.nwhospital.org

Peter Evans, Chairman
Scott L. Hardman, Vice Chairman
James K. Anderson, Board
C W Schneider, CEO

Provides complete medical and surgical services in both inpatient and outpatient settings. Services across multiple specialties include: 24hr emergency services, critical care, cardiac care, stroke program, cancer care, childbirth center, rehabilitation center, diagnostic imaging and education and wellness services. Mission is to raise the long-term health status of our community by providing personalized, quality care with compassion dignity, and respect.

6480 Providence Medical Center
500 17th Ave
Seattle, WA 98122-5711
206-000-1111
Fax: 206-320-3387
www.providence.org

6481 Providence Rehabilitation Services
Providence Rehabilitation Services
1321 Colby Ave
Everett, WA 98201-1665
425-261-3825
Fax: 425-261-3823
www.providence.org

Jim Phillips, Manager
Leslie Baumgarten, Manager

Continuum of care available: Acute Care, Inpatient Rehabilitation Unit, Transitional Care, Outpatient therapies, and In-home services.

6482 Shriners Hospitals for Children: Spokane
Shriners Hospitals
911 W 5th Ave
Spokane, WA 99204-2901
509-455-7844
Fax: 509-744-1223
www.shrinershq.org/hospitals/spokane

Kristin Monasmith, Public Relations Director
Craig Patchin, Administrator
Paul M. Caskey, M.D., Chief of Staff

Provides pediatric orthopedic services plus burn scar revision to children birth to 18. All services at no charge to the family.

West Virginia

6483 HealthSouth Mountain View Regional Rehab Hospital
1160 Van Voorhis Rd
Morgantown, WV 26505-3437
304-598-1100
800-388-2451
Fax: 304-598-1103
www.healthsouthmountainview.com/

Vicki Demers, Chief Executive Officer
Govind Patel, M.D., Medical Director
Robbin Butler, OTR/L, Director of Therapy Operations
Ginger Dearth, RN, Director of Marketing Operations

A 96-bed inpatient accute rehabilitation hospital. Outpatient services, physical, occupational and speech therapy, and interior therapy pool. Programs include neuro/stroke, brain injury, spinal cord injury and pediatric.

6484 HealthSouth Western Hills Regional Rehab Hospital
3 Western Hills Dr
Parkersburg, WV 26105-8122
304-420-1392
Fax: 304-420-1374
www.healthsouthwesternhills.com

Kalapala Rao, Medical Director
Candace Ross, Director of Human Resources
Greg Holland, Director of Marketing Operations
Michelle Lowers, MS, LSW, Director of Care Management

A 40-bed medical rehabilitation hospital serving inpatient and outpatient needs in the western West Virginia area. Our hospital is accredited by the Joint Commission on Accreditation of Healthcare Organizations (JCAHO) Our mission is to guide patients whtih physically disabling conditions along an individualized treatment pathway so they can reach the highest level of physical, social and emotional well-being. We strive to provide the highest quality care for you and your family.

Wisconsin

6485 Extendicare Health Services, Inc.
3540 South 43rd Street
Milwaukee, WI 53220-2903
414-541-1000
800-395-5000
Fax: 414-541-1942
www.extendicare.com

Timothy Lukenda, CEO
Douglas Harris, SVP
David Pearce, Vice President, General Counsel

Sunrise Care Center is a leading provider of long-term skilled nursing care and short-term rehabilitation solutions. Our 99 bed facility offers a full continuum of services and care focused around each individual in today's ever-changing healthcare environment. Our facility is Medicare and Medicaid certified.

6486 St. Catherine's Hospital
9555 76th St
Pleasant Prairie, WI 53158
262-577-8000
Fax: 262-653-5795
www.uhsi.org

Vicki Lewis, Manager

Committed to living out the healing ministries of the Judeo-Christian faiths by providing exceptional and compassionate healthcare service that promotes the dignity and well-being of the people we serve.

6487 St. Joseph Hospital
611 Saint Joseph Ave
Marshfield, WI 54449-1898
715-387-1713
Fax: 715-389-3939
www.ministryhealth.org

Michael Schmidt, CEO
Catherine Olson, Director

A values-driven healthcare delivery network of aligned hospitals, clinics, long-term care facilities, home care agencies, dialysis centers and many other programs and services in Wisconsin and Minnesota.

Wyoming

6488 **Spalding Rehabilitation Hospital at Memorial Hospital of Laramie**
2301 House Ave
Suite 300
Cheyenne, WY 82001-3748
307-635-4141
800-374-7687
Fax: 307-638-2656
www.imgwy.com

Mitchell Schwarzbach, Executive Director
Tanya Boerkircher, Wyoming Endoscopy Center Manager
Andrea Bailey, Charge Entry Supervisor
Michelle Flanagan, Front Office Supervisor

We are a professional corporation of physicians trained in various medical specialties and subspecialties including Internal Medicine, Gastroenterology and Chest Diseases.It is our mission to provide the highest quality, cost-effective primary and subspecialty medical care, and education to the people of southern Wyoming, western Nebraska, and northern Colorado.

Rehabilitation Facilities, Post-Acute

Alabama

6489 **Alabama Department of Rehabilitation Services**
602 S Lawrence St.
Montgomery, AL 36104
334-293-7500
800-441-7607
Fax: 334-293-7383
www.rehab.alabama.gov
Jane E. Burdeshaw, Commissioner
State agency which provides services and assistance to Alabama's children and adults with disabilities.

6490 **Briarcliff Nursing Home & Rehab Facility**
3201 North Ware Road
McAllen, TX 78501
956-631-5542
Fax: 956-631-5777
http://www.briarcliffnursingcenter.com

6491 **Centers for The Developmentally Disabled - North Central Alabama**
1602 Church St SE
P.O. Box 2091
Decatur, AL 35602
256-350-1458
Fax: 256-350-1485
info@cddnca.org
www.cddnca.org
Earl Brightwell, Executive Director
CDD NCA provides services and programs for individuals who are mentally and/or physically challenged, or developmentally delayed. These services range from early intervention services for infants and toddlers to residential and employment programs for adults. All services are typically provided at no cost to the individual or their family, regardless of income. Funding sources for the CDD NCA include DMH, United Way, and ADRS.

6492 **Cheaha Regional Mental Health Center**
351 W 3rd St
Sylacauga, AL 35150
256-245-1340
Fax: 256-245-1343
Cynthia L. Atkinson, Executive Director
Dr. Shakil Khan, Medical Director
Karen McKinney, Clinical Director, Mental Health Services
Ann Cunningham, Director, Intellectual Disabilities Services
CRMHC provides a continuum of services for persons with intellectual disabilities, serious mental illness and substance abuse in a four county area in east Alabama, which includes Clay, Coosa, Randolph, and Talladega Counties.

6493 **Children's Rehabilitation Service**
Alabama Department of Rehabilitation Services
602 S Lawrence St.
Montgomery, AL 36104
334-293-7500
800-441-7607
Fax: 334-293-7383
www.rehab.alabama.gov
Jane E. Burdeshaw, Commissioner
CRS provides individualized services to children with special health care needs from birth to age 21 and their families at home, school, and in the community. In addition, CRS provides disability services, expertise, and adaptive technology to and for local school systems, assisting teachers, school nurses and other staff in the education of children with disabilities. The CRS Hemophilia Program serves Alabama's children and adults with this life-threatening blood disorder.

6494 **Chilton-Shelby Mental Health Center**
110 Medical Center Dr
Calera, AL 35045
205-755-8800
Fax: 205-668-4957
chiltonshelby.org
Melodie D. Crawford, Chief Executive Officer
Vicki M. Potts, Chief Financial Officer
Kathryn T. Crouthers, Chief Operations Officer
Dena Smitherman, Intellectual Disabilities Division Director
Mental health rehabilitation services and more for the recovery of mentally disabled adults. Serves Chilton and Shelby counties.
Business Office Location

6495 **Darden Rehabilitation Center**
1001 E Broad Street
Ste C
Gadsden, AL 35903-2400
256-547-5751
Fax: 256-547-5761
darden@dardenrehab.org
dardenrehab.org
Lynn Curry, Executive Director
Derek Coburn, Operations Manager
Dana Johnson, Program Coordinator
Lisa Wilson, Executive Assistant
Work adjustment and job placement programs. Serves the counties of Etawah, Marshall, Dekalb, Clair and Cherokee.

6496 **Easterseals Central Alabama**
2185 Normandie Dr.
Montgomery, AL 36111
334-288-0240
Fax: 334-288-7171
info@easterseals ca.org
www.eastersealscentralalabama.org
Lynne Stokley, Chief Executive Officer
Debbie Lynn, Administrator
Serves people with disabilities and their families by providing programs and services.

6497 **Easterseals Northwest Alabama**
1615 Trojan Dr.
Suite 1
Muscle Shoals, AL 35661
256-381-1110
info@eastersealsnwal.org
www.eastersealsnwal.org
Lynne Stokley, Chief Executive Officer
Danny Prince, Administrator
Easterseals provides services for people with disabilities and their families. Services include occupational therapy, physical therapy, speech therapy, and vocational services.

6498 **Easterseals West Alabama**
1110 Dr. Edward Hillard Drive
Tuscaloosa, AL 35401-7446
205-759-1211
800-726-1216
Fax: 205-349-1162
eswa@eswaweb.org
eswaweb.org
Ronny Johnston, Executive Director
Dusty Beam, Administrative Coordinator
Holly Hillard, Director, Development
Leading organization in helping children and adults with disabilities to live with equality, dignity and independence. Rehabilitation services are provided in two divisions: outpatient rehabilitation division (physical therapy, occupational therapy, speech therapy, hearing evaluation, sell and service hearind aids) and vocational division (vocational evaulation and vocational development). Services are rendered regardless of age, race, sex, color, creed, national origin, veteran's status.

6499 **Easterseals West Central Alabama Rehabilitation Center**
2906 Citizens Pkwy
P.O. Box 750
Selma, AL 36702-0750
334-872-8421
800-801-4776
Fax: 334-872-3907
www.eswcarc.us

6500 **Geer Adult Training Center**
P.O. Box 419
83 South Canaan Road
Canaan, CT 06018-419
860-824-7067
Fax: 205-367-8032
geercares.org/content/about-geer
Yvonne Williams, Program Coordinator

6501 **Goodwill Easterseals of the Gulf Coast**
2440 Gordon Smith Dr.
Mobile, AL 36617-2319 251-471-1581
info@al.easterseals.com
www.gesgc.org

Peter D'Olive, Chairman
Frank Harkins, President & CEO
Bill Dillman, Vice President, Marketing & Development

Vocational, medical, pre-school education, day care, recreation and other support services.

6502 **HealthSouth Corporation**
3660 Grandview Parkway
Ste 200
Birmingham, AL 35243-3332 205-967-7116
800-765-4772
Fax: 225-928-0317
healthsouth.com

Jacque Shadle, CEO
Derrick Landreneau, Director of Nursing services

Dedicated to one field of medicine - physical rehabilitation medicine - and are committed to one goal, helping patients achieve the highest level of functioning possible after a debilitating injury or illness.

6503 **Indian Rivers Mental Health Center - Bibb**
2439 Main St
Brent, AL 35034 205-926-4681
Fax: 205-296-6016
www.irmhc.org

6504 **Indian Rivers Mental Health Center - Pickens**
890 Reform St.
Carrollton, AL 35447 205-367-8032
Fax: 205-367-9291
www.irmhc.org

6505 **Indian Rivers Mental Health Center - Tuscaloosa**
2209 - 9th St
Tuscaloosa, AL 35401 205-391-3131
Fax: 205-391-3135
http://www.irmhc.org

Barbara Friedman, President
Elizabeth Rice, First Vice President

Services are available to adults who have serious mental illness resulting in personal, family or work-related problems. Counseling may take place in either individual or group settings, identification, evaluation and treatment services are available to persons who experience problems related to alcohol and drug abuse and counseling services are available for children and adolescents who have a severe emotional disturbance causing discipline problems at home and school.

6506 **Mobile ARC**
2424 Gordon Smith Dr
Mobile, AL 36617-2397 251-479-7409
Fax: 251-473-7649
jzoghby@mobilearc.org
mobilearc.org

Jeff Zoghby, Executive Director
Amy Odom, Public Relations and Development Director

Mobile Arc, Inc. (MARC) offers a wide range of services for persons with intellectual and developmental disabilities.

6507 **Southeastern Blind Rehabilitation Center**
U.S. Department of Veteran Affairs
700 S 19th St
Birmingham, AL 35233-1927 205-558-4706
Fax: 205-933-4484
www.rehab.va.gov/blindrehab/

6508 **UAB Eye Care**
University Of Alabama at Birmingham
1716 University Blvd
Birmingham, AL 35233 205-975-2020
Fax: 205-934-6755
www.uab.edu/optometry/home/eyecare

Rodney W. Nowakowski, Dean
Dr. Marsha Snow, Chief, Low Vision Patient Care
Brittney Bolen, Optometric Technician
Joseph Fleming, D.D., Chief Of Staff

Complete eye services, including low vision services and materials.

6509 **Vaughn-Blumberg Services**
2715 Flynn Rd
P.O. Box 8646
Dothan, AL 36304 334-793-3102
Fax: 334-793-7740
www.vaughnblumbergservices.com

Ed Dorsey, Executive Director
Linda Cunningham, Director of Human Resources
Billy McCarthy, Director of Finance
Karen Amos, Director of Nursing

Provides comprehensive services for people with intellectual disabilities that reside in Houston County as well as assist in facilitating their participation in society to the fullest extent of their individual capabilities. Offers early intervention services for the mentally handicapped adult including diagnosis and evaluation and physical, speech, and occupational therapies. They also offer counseling, day training,employment assistance and residental homes.

Alaska

6510 **Alaska Center for the Blind and Visually Impaired**
3903 Taft Drive
Anchorage, AK 99517-3069 907-248-7770
800-770-7517
Fax: 907-248-7517
info@alaskabvi.org
www.alaskabvi.org

Regan Mattingly, Executive Director
Robert Tasso, Program Manager
Caren Ailleo, Development & Communications Director
Bonnie Lucas, Visually Impaired Senior Coordinator

Services to help the adult residential or community-based student become independent and self-sufficient by offering independent travel, Braille reading and writing, use of assiative technology such as talking computers, manual skills and personal, as well as home management. There is a special program for those 55 years of age and older who are experiencing a vision loss and another program for rural Alaska Native youth who are visually impaired.

Arizona

6511 **Arizona Center for the Blind and Visually Impaired**
3100 E Roosevelt St
Phoenix, AZ 85008-5036 602-273-7411
Fax: 602-273-7410
jlamay@acbvi.org
acbvi.org

James La May, CEO
Frank Vance, Director
Christine Boisen, Chair
Alexia Matek, Secretary

A private, nonprofit organization that provides comprehensive rehabilitation services and more for the blind and visually handicapped. The staff includes 20 instructional and adminstrative professionals.

6512 **Arizona Industries for the Blind**
Suite 130
515 N 51st Avenue
Phoenix, AZ 85043-2711 602-771-9100
Fax: 602-353-5701
DanielMartinez@azdes.gov
www.azdes.gov/aib

Richard Monaco, General Manager
Daniel Martinez, Community Services Liaison

Offers rehabilitation services, vocational/pre-vocational evaluation and training, work adjustment, job development and employment and training opportunties for individuals who are blind.

6513 **Banner Good Samaritan Medical Center**
1111 E McDowell Road
Phoenix, AZ 85006-2666
602-839-2000
Fax: 602-239-5868
www.bannerhealth.com
Steve Narang, MD, Chief Executive Officer
Lorraine Hudspeth, Controller
Letty Cerpa, Senior Accountant
Larry Mann, IT Manager
Nearly 1,700 physicians representing more than 50 specialties work with Banner Good Samaritan staff to care for more then 36,000 inpatients a year. Houses more then 650 licensed patient care beds. A teaching hospital that trains more then 220 physicians annually and a premier medical center in Arizona and the Southwest. Provides a comprehensive foundation of major programs and an equally impressive offering of highly specialized programs not availiable in most hospitals.

6514 **Beacon Group**
308 W Glenn St.
Tucson, AZ 85705
520-622-4874
Fax: 520-620-6620
www.beacongroup.org

6515 **Carondelet Brain Injury Programs and Services (Bridges Now)**
2202 N. Forbes Blvd.
Tucson, AZ 85745-2602
520-872-7324
Fax: 520-873-3743
comments@carondelet.org
carondelet.org
Daisy M Jenkins, Executive VP, Chief HR/Administr
James K Beckmann, President/Chief Executive Officer
Alan Strauss, Executive VP, Finance and Chief Financial Officer
Christen Castellano, MBA, Executive VP and Chief Strategy Officer
Comprehensive outpatient rehabilitation program. PT, OT, ST, Psychology and Rehab Counseling Services.

6516 **Desert Life Rehabilitation & Care Center**
1919 W Medical St
Tucson, AZ 85704-1133
520-369-9620
Fax: 520-867-6612
Amad Nazifi, Executive Director
Accomodates 240 residents. Provides skilled and intermediate nursing with occupational, physical, speech and respiratory therapy services. Offers special programs including an Alzheimer's Unit and a Young Adult program

6517 **Devereux Advanced Behavioral Health Arizona - Scottsdale**
Scottsdale Administrative Office
2025 N 3rd St
Suite 250
Phoenix, AZ 85004
602-283-1573
Fax: 480-443-5587
azadmissions@devereux.org
www.devereuxaz.org
Lane Barker, Executive Director
Yvette Jackson, Director of Operations
Donovan S Carman, MBA, Director of Finance
Janelle Westfall, Clinical Director
Engages in the treatment of behavioral health issues through services such as residential treatment centers, day school, outpatient services, prevention programs, adult foster care, and foster care for children. Also offered are evidence-based interventions to improve lives.

6518 **Devereux Arizona - Tucson**
Tuscon Administrative Office
6141 E Grant Rd
Tucson, AZ 85712
520-296-5551
Fax: 520-296-8244
azadmissions@devereux.org
www.devereuxaz.org
Lane Barker, Executive Director
Yvette Jackson, Director of Operations
Donovan S Carman, MBA, Director of Finance
Janelle Westfall, Clinical Director
Organization offering culturally competent care for individuals with emotional and behavioral health disorders. Some of the programs offered include Adult Foster Care, kinship program, Therapeutic Foster Care Program, Parent Aide and more.

6519 **Freestone Rehabilitation Center**
10617 E Oasis Drive
Mesa, AZ 85208
480-986-1531
Fax: 480-986-1538
Randy Gray, Executive Director
Cherie Vance, Manager

6520 **HealthSouth Valley Of The Sun Rehabilitation Hospital**
13460 N 67th Ave
Glendale, AZ 85304-1000
623-878-8800
Fax: 623-878-5254
healthsouth.com
Beth Bacher, Manager
A 60-bed free-standing hospital that offers acute physical rehabilitation, outpatient therapy services and day hospital treatment. Works in cooperation with local, regional and national managed care organizations and other sources to maximise patient recovery while conserving financial resources.

6521 **Institute for Human Development**
Northern Arizona University
912 Riordan Rd. P.O. Box 5630
Flagstaff, AZ 86011-5630
928-523-4791
Fax: 928-523-9127
TTY: 928-523-1695
ihd@nau.edu
www.nau.edu/ihd
Levi Esguerra, Director
Lisa Andrew, Advisory Commitee
Lynn Black, Advisory Commitee
Maria Bravo, Advisory Commitee
The Institute values and supports the independence, productivity and inclusion of Arizona's citizens with disabilities. Based on the values and beliefs, the Institute conducts training, research and services that further these goals.

6522 **John C Lincoln Hospital North Mountain**
250 E Dunlap Ave
Phoenix, AZ 85020-2871
602-943-2381
Fax: 602-944-8062
webmaster@jcl.com
www.jcl.com/content/northmountain/default.htm
Rhonda Forsyth, President
Bruce Pearson, FACHE, Senior Vice President
Maggi Griffin, RN, MS, Vice President & Chief Executive Officer
Jessica Rivas, RN, MSN, Vice President and Chief Nursing Officer
Mission is to assist each person entrusted to our care to enjoy the fullest gift of health possible, and work with others to build a community where a helping hand is available for our most vulnerable members.

6523 **La Frontera Center**
504 W 29th St
Tucson, AZ 85713-3394
520-884-9920
Fax: 520-792-0654
www.lafronteraaz.org
Kevin Heath, Board Chair
Frank Valenzuela, Vice Chair
Celestino Fernandez, Treasurer
Susan Agrillo, Recording Secretary
A nonprofit community-based behavioral health agency that has been helping southern Arizona children, adults, and families since 1968.

6524 **Manor Care Nursing and Rehab Center: Tucson**
3705 N Swan Rd
Tucson, AZ 85718-6939
520-299-7088
Fax: 520-529-0038
www.hcr-manorcare.com
Clifton J. Porter II, Vice President - Government Rela
Martin Allen, Vice President
A leading provider of short-term post-acute medical care and rehabilitation and long-term skilled nursing care. High quality medical care is provided through registered (RN) and licensed practical (LPN) nurses and certified nursing assistants (CNA) in concert with physical, occupational and speech rehabilitation therapists. Our more then 275 skilled nursing centers are Medicare-and Medicaid-certified.

6525 **Nova Care**
Second Floor
680 American Avenue
King of Prussia, PA 19406-2607
800-331-8840
Fax: 602-256-7292
novacare.com

Scott Lusted, General Manager
Brian Beal, Market Manager

NovaCare Rehabilitation's highly respected clinical team provides preventative and rehabilitative services that maximize functionality and promote well-being. NovaCare Rehabilitation also provides physical therapy and athletic training services to more then 20 professional sports teams and 300 universities, colleges, and highschools thoughout the nation.

6526 **Perry Rehabilitation Center**
3146 E Windsor Avenue
Phoenix, AZ 85008-1199
602-956-0400
Fax: 602-957-7610
perrycenter@qwest.net
www.azafh.com

Diana Casillas, Human Resources Director
Jim Musick, President

Provides services for people with disabilities, cognitive disabilities including residential services, day treatment, job training and job placement.

6527 **Phoenix Veterans Center**
Ste 100
1544 W. Grant St.
Phoenix, AZ 85004-1554
602-358-8494
Fax: 602-379-4130
www.azcremationcenter.com/?

Ken Benckwitz, Manager

Veterans medical clinic offering disabled veterans medical treatments.

6528 **Progress Valley: Phoenix**
10505 North 69th Street
Suite 1100
Paradise Valley, AZ 85253-6106
480-922-9427
Fax: 602-274-5473
recovery@progressvalley.org
alcoholism.about.com

Susanne Lambert, Executive Director
Jennifer White, Director of Programs
Cathie Scott, Sober Housing Manager
Kristine Peltier, Finance Director

Residential aftercare for alcoholism and chemical dependency. Certified chemical dependency counselors provide individual treatment.

6529 **Rehabilitation Services Administration**
Suite 102
3425 East Van Buren
Phoenix, AZ 85008-3202
602-771-9100
800-563-1221
Fax: 602-250-8584
TTY: 855-475-8194
azrsa@azdes.gov

Katharine Levandowsky, Administrator

Provides a variety of specialized services to assist in removing barriers to employment and/or independent living for individuals with physical or mental disabilities. RSA offers 3 major service programs and several specialized programs/services.

6530 **Southern Arizona Association For The Visually Impaired**
3767 East Grant Rd
Tucson, AZ 85716-2935
520-795-1331
Fax: 520-795-1336
reception@saavi.us
www.saavi.us

Michael Gordon, Executive Director
Amy Murillo, Associate Director
Carol Lopez, Finance Director
Lenetta Lefko, Tucson Services Manager

Offers health services, counseling, social work, home and personal management, computer training, low vision aids and more for the visually handicapped 18 years or older.

6531 **Toyei Industries**
Hc 58 Box 55
Ganado, AZ 86505-55
928-736-2417
888-45T-OYEI
Fax: 928-736-2495

Anthony Lincoln, CEO

Serves the needs of developmentally disabled and the severely mentally impaired adult citizens of the Navajo Nation and other Indian Nations. Staff of 60+ serves the needs of all the Navajo adults. Services include day treatment programs, and residential and group home services.

6532 **Yuma Center for the Visually Impaired**
328 W. Spears Street
Yuma, AZ 85365-6580
928-247-8890
Fax: 928-344-1863
https://www.azdes.gov

Calvin Roberts, Executive Director
Kathy Lucero, Store Manager
Dana Clayton, Human Resources Specialist
Lorraine Hudspeth, Controller

A private nonprofit agency offering services for totally blind and legally blind children and adults in the Arizona area.

Arkansas

6533 **Arkansas Lighthouse for the Blind**
P.O. Box 192666
6818 Murray St.
Little Rock, AR 72209- 2666
501-562-2222
Fax: 501-568-5275
info@arkansaslighthouse.org
arkansaslighthouse.org

Bill Johnson, Chief Executive Officer
Danny Novielli, COO
John McAtee, Chief Financial Officer
Ronnie Cates, Director of Communications & Procurement

Manufacturer of textiles, apparel and paper products and employs blind and legally blind individuals.

6534 **Beverly Enterprises Network**
1 Thousand Beverly
Fort Smith, AR 72901-2629
479-201-2000
800-666-9996
Fax: 479-452-5131

Randy Churchey, CEO

Offers a progressive approach to subacute care. The goal of this organization is to assist injured and disabled individuals regain the level of independence to which they have been accustomed. Provides support and training programs, patient and family services and specialty programs for patients.

6535 **Easterseals: Arkansas**
3920 Woodland Heights Rd
Little Rock, AR 72212-2495
501-227-3600
877-533-3700
Fax: 501-227-4021
TTY: 501-227-3686
lrogers@ar.easterseals.com

Sharon Moone-Jochums, President/ CEO
Linda Rogers, VP Programs
Michael E. Stock, Treasurer
Cindy Nash, Secretary

Their mission is to provide exceptional services to ensure that all people with disabilities or special needs have equal opportunities to live, learn, work and play in their communitites.

6536 **HealthSouth Rehabilitation Hospital Of Fort Smith**
1401 South J. Street
Fort Smith, AR 72901-5158
479-785-3300
Fax: 479-785-8599
healthsouth.com

Ryan Cassedy, CEO
Cygnet Schroeder, M.D., Medical Director
Donna Beallis, D.O., Director of Medical Management
Brandi Denham, Director of Human Resources

A free-standing 80-bed comprehensive physical medicine and rehabilitation hospital offering inpatient and outpatient services.

Provides specialized medical and therapy services, designed to assist physically challenged persons to reach their highest level of independent function.

6537 **Lions World Services for the Blind**
2811 Fair Park Blvd
Little Rock, AR 72204-5044
501-664-7100
800-248-0734
Fax: 501-664-2743
training@lwsb.org
www.wsblind.org/

Larry Dickerson, President/ CEO
Tony Woodell, President & Chief Executive Officer
Bill Smith, Director of Development
Melanie Jones, Marketing & Communications Director

Offers services in the areas of health education, recreation, rehabilitation, counseling, employment, computer training and more for all legally blind residents of the U.S. The staff includes 56 full time employees.

6538 **Little Rock Vet Center #0713**
Department of Veterans Affairs of Washington DC
Suite A
201 W Broadway St
North Little Rock, AR 72114- 5505
501-324-6395
877-927-8387
Fax: 501-324-6928

Elizabeth N Ruggiero, Team Leader
Ida L Fogle, Counselor
Van A Hall, Counselor
Darryl A Lasker, Office Manager

Vet Center provides PTSD counseling to veterans of a combat zone. No medical care provided.

6539 **Timber Ridge Ranch NeuroRestorative Services**
4500 W Commerce Dr
North Little Rock, AR 72116
501-758-8799
800-743-6802
Fax: 501-758-8778
neuroinfo@thementornetwork.com
www.neurorestorative.com

Bill Duffy, Chief Operating Officer
Michael E. Hofmeister, MS, MBA, Vice President of Operations
Sean Byrne, MBA, Chief Financial Officer
Roger P. Carrillo, M.Ed, Vice President of Business Development

Comprehensive, individualized services from a transdisciplinary team of licensed professionals assist clients along a course to greater independence. A separate team is dedicated to the needs of children, adolescents, and their families. A clinical team may include professionals from the disciplines of: behavior analysis, neuropsychology, physiatry, psychology, speech-language pathology, occupational therapy, physical therapy, social work, couseling, education, nursing, and case management.

California

6540 **ARC Fresno-Kelso Activity Center**
4567 N Marty Ave
Fresno, CA 93722-7810
559-226-6268
Fax: 559-226-6269
arcfresno@arcfresno.org
arcfresno.org

Lori Ramirez, Executive Director
Catherine Wooliever, Director of Human Resources
Jamie Marrash, Director of Program Services
Pamela Wirth, Director of Finance

The Arc Fresno is a private, non-profit 501 (c) (3) organization who was founded in 1953. They provide services and supports for over 550 individuals with developmental disabilities throughout Fresno County. They currently offer eight (8) programs, and do so with the help of 145 employees.

6541 **ARC Of San Diego-ARROW Center, The**
3030 Market Street
San Diego, CA 92102-3297
619-685-1175
Fax: 619-234-3759
arc-sd.com

Dwight Stratton, Chair
Jerry Wechsler, 1st Vice Chairman
David W. Schneider, President & CEO
Anthony J. DeSalis, Executive Vice President & COO

The ARC of San Diego will be the premier provider of services to persons with disabilities. Arc-SD will be an advocate for diversity of opportunities, enhancing individual life choices as a member of the community. Our values: Everyone will be be treated equally, without prejudice and with respect. Will provide Quality Services and Supports with a well trained and caring staff. State of the art equipment and methods. A willingness to innovate and collaborate.

6542 **ARC Of San Diego-East County Training Center, The**
1374 E Lexington Ave
El Cajon, CA 92019-2312
619-444-9417
Fax: 619-234-3759
arc-sd.com

Dwight Stratton, Chair
Jerry Wechsler, 1st Vice Chairman
David W. Schneider, President & CEO
Anthony J. DeSalis, Executive Vice President & COO

Work adjustment and remunerative work programs.

6543 **ARC Of San Diego-Rex Industries, The**
9575 Aero Dr
San Diego, CA 92123-1803
858-571-4369
800-748-5575
Fax: 858-715-3788
arc-sd.com

Dwight Stratton, Chair
Jerry Wechsler, 1st Vice Chairman
David W. Schneider, President & CEO
Anthony J. DeSalis, Executive Vice President & COO

Offers many different programs including: North County Parent/Infant Program which is an educational program for children, birth to three years who are showing delays in development or who are at risk for developmental delays. The Adult Development Center is a program for adults, eighteen and over, with a developmental disability in the severe to profound range. The program focuses on self-help, communication, daily living and pre-vocational skills. Other programs are available..

6544 **ARC Of San-Diego-South Bay**
1280 Nolan Avenue
Chula Vista, CA 91911-3738
619-427-7524
Fax: 619-427-4657
info@arc-sd.com
www.arc-sd.com/locations

Becky Thaller, Director
Steve Hojsan, Arc Enterprises Director
Michael Bruce, Workshop Manager
David W. Schneider, President & CEO

Provides remunerative work.

6545 **ARC Of Southeast Los Angeles-Southeast Industries**
9501 Washburn Rd
Downey, CA 90242-2913
562-803-1556
Fax: 562-803-4080
www.arcselac.org/

6546 **ARC: VC Community Connections West**
5103 Walker Street
Ventura, CA 93003-7358
805-650-8611
Fax: 805-644-7308
www.arcvc.org

Robert Hogan, President
Gene West, First Vice President
Eve Liebman, Recording Secretary
Kathy Raffaelli, Treasurer

Caring and experienced staff is dedicated to serving participants with a variety of physical, mental and social disabilities who require a higher level of support and supervision. Using a person-centered planning approach, Arc Ventura County promotes self-directed services for all clients and families served. Adult development centers serve individuals with physical and mental disabilities, as well as people with challenging behaviors, who require assistance with basic skills such as self care.

6547 **ARC: VC Ventura**
5103 Walker Street
Ventura, CA 93003-7358
806-650-8611
Fax: 806-644-7308
www.arcvc.org

Robert Hogan, President
Gene West, First Vice President
Eve Liebman, Recording Secretary
Kathy Raffaelli, Treasurer
Arc Ventura County is a private, nonprofit organization that provides educational, vocational and residential services for people with developmental disabilities. Informed decisions, positive changes, and integration in the community are fundamental principals in all programs. As evidence of our programming excellence, Arc Ventura County has been accredited by CARF (The Rehabilitation Accreditation Commission.

6548 **AbilityFirst**
1300 E Green Street
Pasadena, CA 91106-2606
626-396-1010
877-768-4600
Fax: 626-396-1021
info@abilityfirst.org
www.abilityfirst.org

Lori E. Gangemi, President
Steve S. Schultz, Chief Financial Officer
Keri Castaneda, Chief Program Officer
Syed Kazmi, Controller
AbilityFirst serves children and adults with special needs through 24 locations in Southern California.

6549 **Accentcare**
17855 North Dallas Pkwy
Dallas, TX 75287-2468
972-201-3800
800-834-3059
info@accentcare.com
accentcare.com

Mark Pacala, Chairman of the Board and CEO (i
Vincent E. Cook, EVP and Chief Financial Officer
Melvin Warriner, SVP and Chief Culture Officer
Mel Deutsch, General Counsel
Postacute rehabilitation program: home care aides follow through with rehabilitation instructions given by physical, occupational and speech therapists. Other home care services are available, serving special needs for Alzheimer's, blind, brain injury, MS, ostomies, parkinsonism, spinal injury and stroke.

6550 **Anaheim Veterans Center**
859, South Harbor Blvd
Anaheim, CA 92805-4680
714-776-0161
800-225-8387
Fax: 714-776-8904
anaheimvetcenter@yahoo.com
www.longbeach.va.gov/visitors/vet_center.asp

6551 **Azure Acres Recovery Center**
5777 Madison Avenue
Suite 1210
Sacramento, CA 95841-9034
877-977-3755
877-762-3735
Fax: 707-823-8972
info@azureacres.com
azureacres.com

Joe Tinervin, MSW, Executive Director
Michael Roeske, Psy.D., Clinical Director
Christie Splitstone, MA, Counselor/Case Manager
James Canter, CATC, Counselor/Case Manager
Offers rehabilitation services and residential care for the person with an alcohol or drug abuse related problems.

6552 **Back in the Saddle**
2 BITS Trail
P.O. Box 3336
Chelmsford, MA 01824-0936
800-865-2478
877-756-5068
Fax: 800-866-3235
help@BackInTheSaddle.com
www.thesaddle.com

Richard Smith PhD, Owner
Erika Reed, Co-Director
A long term community residential facility for head injured adults. House parents live on-site; and oversee a variety of programs which are individually designed and might include classes in community college, placement in a workshop or on a workstation, volunteer positions and home skills assignments. Recreational outing range from horseback riding to weekend camping. Apartment programs available as set-up. Price: $2800-$3000 per month.

6553 **Ballard Rehabilitation Hospital**
1760 W 16th St
San Bernardino, CA 92411-1150
909-473-1200
800-761-1226
Fax: 909-473-1276
www.ballardrehab.com

Edward C. Palacios, RN,MPH, Administrator
Mary Hunt, Chief Operating Officer
Patty Meinhardt, Director Marketing/Admissions
Ballard Rehab Hospital is a free standing specialty hospital and provides the complete continuum of acute rehabilitation and outpatient rehabilitation, dedicated to providing rehab care to adults and children. The following inpatient and outpatient programs are available: CNA (Stroke) Rehab; Spinal Cord Injury Rehab; Brain Injury Rehab; Pain Management Rehab; Bariatric program, pulmonary program, injured Worker Programs; and Post Amputation Rehab.

6554 **Bayview Nursing and Rehabilitation**
516 Willow Street
Alameda, CA 94501-6132
510-521-5600
Fax: 510-865-6441
TTY: 800-735-2922
http://www.bayviewnursing.com/

Richard S Espinoza, Administrator
Offers a full range of medical services to meet the individual needs of our residents, including short-term rehabilitative services and long termed skilled care. Working with the resident's physician, our staff-including medical specialists, nurses, nutritionists, dietitians, and social workers-establishes a comprehensive treatment plan intended to restore you or your loved one to the highest practicable potential.

6555 **Belden Center**
606 Humboldt St
Santa Rosa, CA 95404-4219
707-579-2735
Fax: 707-579-4145

Casey Harding, Owner
Pamela Fadden, Owner
Postacute rehabilitation program.

6556 **Blind Babies Foundation**
Suite 300
1814 Franklin St
Oakland, CA 94612-3487
510-446-2229
Fax: 510-446-2262
blindbabies.org

Dottie Bridge, President
Aben Hill, 1st Vice President
Clare Friedman, PhD, 2nd Vice President
Beverly Libaire, Treasurer
Mission: when an infant or pre school child is identified as blind or visually impaired, provides family-centered services to support the child's optimal development and access to the world.

6557 Brotman Medical Center: RehabCare Unit
Brotman Medical Center
3828 Delmas Terrace
Culver City, CA 90232-2713
310-836-7000
800-677-1238
Fax: 310-202-4105
phvc.com

Jennifer Cortez, Program Manager
Kevin O'Connor, CEO
Scott Leonard, CTO
Ben Taylor, Senior Editor

Culver City is centrally located within the city of Los Angeles. These are two programs offering inpatient rehabilitation. The acute rehab program is designed for patients who need physical rehabilitation due to injury or medical disability. This program requires patients to participate in 3 hours therapy per day. The sub-acute program is designed especially for patients who need rehab but cannot tolerate the intensity of the acute rehab program..

6558 Build Rehabilitation Industries
12432 Foothill Blvd
Sylmar, CA 91342
818-898-0020
Fax: 818-898-1949
buildindustries.com

6559 California Elwyn
18325 Mt. Baldy Circle
Fountain Valley, CA 92708-6115
714-557-6313
Fax: 714-963-2961
info@elwyn.org
elwyn.org

Charles S. McLister, President & CEO, Elwyn

Provides opportunities for people with disabilities who are 18 or older. Offers Individual Rehabilitation Plans and Supported Employment Services.

6560 California Eye Institute
1360 E Herndon Ave
Fresno, CA 93720-3326
559-449-5000
www.samc.com

Nancy Hollingsworth, President and CEO
Michael W. Martinez, EVP/Chief Operating and Financial Officer
Stephen Soldo, Chief Medical Officer
Christine Sarrico, Chief Financial Officer

A private, nonprofit agency offering services such as health, educational, recreational, rehabilitation and employment counseling to the totally blind, legally blind and visually impaired. The staff includes two full time workers.

6561 Camp Recovery Center
3192 Glen Canyon Rd
Scotts Valley, CA 95066-4916
877-557-6237
Fax: 831-438-2789
camprecovery.com

Michael Johnson, Ph.D, Executive Director
Tim Sinnott, Clinical Director
Zoe R., Case Manager
Jeff Geiger, Clinical Tech Director

A free-standing social model recovery center for chemical dependency located on 25 wooded acres in the Santa Cruz Mountains. The services include: medical detoxification, complete medical evaluation, psychiatric evaluation and counseling, psychological testing, individual counseling and more. Helps the recovery from chemical dependency in a easier, warm and caring environment.

6562 Campobello Chemical Dependency Recovery Center
2448 Guerneville Road
Suite 400
Santa Rosa, CA 95402- 4030
707-546-1547
800-805-1833
Fax: 707-579-1603
campobello.org

6563 Casa Colina Centers for Rehabilitation
P.O. Box 6001
255 East Bonita Avenue
Pomona, CA 91767- 6001
909-596-7733
866-724-4127
Fax: 909-593-0153
TTY: 909-596-3646
casacolina.org

Steve Norin, Chairman
Felice L Loverso, President
Chandrahas Agarwal, Medical Director
Elmer B. Pineda, M.D., Chief Of Medical Staff

Casa Colina, has pioneered effective programs to create opportunity for health, productivity and self-esteem for persons with disability since 1936. Through medical rehabilitation, transitional living, residential, community, and prevention and wellness programs. Casa Colina serves more than 7,000 persons annually. Casa Colina, a non-profit organization, offers a unique spectrum of opportunities, achievement and results to patients and their families.

6564 Casa Colina Padua Village
P.O. Box 6001
255 East Bonita Avenue
Pomona, CA 91767- 6001
909-596-7733
866-724-4127
Fax: 909-593-0153
TTY: 909-596-3646
casacolina.org

Steve Norin, Chairman
Chandrahas Agarwal, Medical Director
Felice L Loverso, President
Elmer B. Pineda, M.D., Chief Of Medical Staff

Long term residential services for adults with developmental disability. Residences include Malmquist House, Woodbend House, and Hillsdale House, all located in Claremont, California.

6565 Casa Colina Residential Services: Rancho Pino Verde
Casa Colina Center for Rehabilitation
P.O. Box 6001
255 East Bonita Avenue
Pomona, CA 91767- 7517
909-596-7733
866-724-4127
Fax: 909-593-0153
TTY: 909-596-3646
www.casacolina.org

Steve Norin, Chairman
Randy Blackman, Vice Chairman
Felice L. Loverso, President
Elmer B. Pineda, M.D., Chief Of Medical Staff

Long term residential services in rural environment for adults with brain injury.

6566 Casa Colina Transitional Living Center
255 East Bonita Avenue
P.O. Box 6001
Pomona, CA 91767- 1923
909-596-7733
866-724-4127
Fax: 909-593-0153
TTY: 909-596-3646
casacolina.org

Steve Norin, Chairman
Felice L Loverso, President
Chandrahas Agarwal, Medical Director
Elmer B. Pineda, M.D., Chief Of Medical Staff

Postacute rehabilitation program.

6567 Casa Colina Transitional Living Center: Pomona
P.O. Box 6001
255 East Bonita Avenue
Pomona, CA 91767- 6001
909-596-7733
866-724-4127
Fax: 909-593-0153
TTY: 909-596-3646
casacolina.org

Steve Norin, Chairman
Felice L Loverso, President
Chandrahas Agarwal, Medical Director
Elmer B. Pineda, M.D., Chief Of Medical Staff

Post acute short term residential program for persons with brain injury. In a home-like setting, therapy promotes successful re-entry to home and community living.

6568 **Cedars of Marin**
PO Box 947
Ross, CA 94957-947 415-454-5310
Fax: 415-454-0573
thecedarsofmarin.org

Jefferson Rice, Board Chair
James Brentano, Board Vice President
Andrew Hinkelman, Board Treasurer
Chuck Greene, Executive Director
The Cedars of Marin has provided residential and day programs for adults with developmental disabilities for over 91 years. Our award-winning programs help our clients to live creative, productive, joyous lives.

6569 **Center for Neuro Skills**
5215 Ashe Rd.
Bakersfield, CA 93313-2988 661-872-3408
800-922-4994
Fax: 661-872-5150
skatomski@neuroskills.com
neuroskills.com

Mark J Ashley, President/CEO and Co-Founder
A comprehensive, post-acute, community based head-injury rehabilitation program serving over 100 clients per year. Since 1980, CNS has effectively treated the entire spectrum of head-injured clients, including those with severe behavioral disorders, cognitive/perceptual impairments, speech/language problems, physical disabilities and post-concussion syndrome.

6570 **Center for the Partially Sighted**
Suite 150
6101 W. Centinela Ave.
Culver City, CA 90230 310-988-1970
Fax: 310-988-1980
low-vision.org

La Donna S. Ringering, Ph.D, President/CEO
Pam Thompson, Director of Psychological Servic
Phyllis Amaral, Clinical Director
Laura Valencia, Psychosocial Services Coordinato
Services for partially sighted and legally blind people include low vision evaluations, the design and prescription of low vision devices and adaptive technology, as well as counseling and rehabilitation training (independent living skills and orientation/mobility training). Special programs include children's program, diabetes and vision loss program, Technology demonstrations. Store carries low vision aids. Catalog available.

6571 **Central Coast Neurobehavioral Center OPTIONS**
P.O. Box 877
800 Quintana Road Suite 2C
Morro Bay, CA 93442-877 805-772-6066
Fax: 805-772-6067

Michael Mamot, CEO
Ole von Frausing-Borch, COO
Serves adults with developmental disabilities, traumatic head injuries, or other neurological impairments. OPTIONS operates two transitional living centers, eight licensed residential facilities, two licensed community integration day programs and a licensed short term stabilization center. Services offered include: supported and independent living services, group and individual vocational services, neuropsychological assessment, occupational therapy, cognitive therapy, speech therapy and more.

6572 **Cerebral Palsy: North County Center**
#209
8525 Gibbs Drive
San Diego, CA 92123-1758 858-571-7803
Fax: 858-571-0919
info@ucpsd.org
www.ucpsd.org

David Carucci, Executive Director
Mary Krieger, Associate Executive Director
Bruce Neufeld, Chief Financial Officer
Sophia Williams, Director of Human Resources
The mission of UCP San Diego County is to advance the independence, productivity and full citizenship of people affected by cerebral palsy and other disabilities. By making solid steps, UCP can build a better community for all in the process.

6573 **Children's Hospital Central California Rehabilitation Center**
9300 Valley Childrens Place
Madera, CA 93636-8762 559-353-3000
www.valleychildrens.org

Todd Suntrapak, President & Chief Executive Officer
David Christensen, MD, SVP Medical Affairs & Chief Medical Officer
Beverly Hayden-Pugh, Vice President & Chief Nursing Officer
Kirk Larson, Vice President & Chief Informati
A 297-bed pediatric medical center on a 50-acre campus. We now have more then 500 doctors practicing in over 40 pediatric subspecialties with clinics and services throughout the state.

6574 **Children's Hospital Los Angeles Rehabilitation Program**
4650 W Sunset Blvd
Los Angeles, CA 90027-6062 323-361-4155
888-631-2452
Fax: 323-361-8101
webmaster@chla.usc.edu
www.childrenshospitalla.org

Richard D. Cordova, President & CEO
Rodney B. Hanners, Senior Vice President and Chief
Henri R. Ford, M.D.
Lawrence L. Foust, J.D., Secretary
Designated as a Level I Pediatric Trauma Canter by the Los Angeles County EMS Agency, the hospital treats more then 1,500 pediatric trauma patients per year. Performs more then 13,900 pediatric surgeries a year, including more complex surgical procedures then any other hospital in Southern California

6575 **Children's Therapy Center**
Ste 120
770 Paseo Camarillo
Camarillo, CA 93010-6092 805-383-1501
Fax: 805-383-1504

Beth Maulhardt, Owner
Provides individual occupational therapy, speech/language therapy, family/child consulting, education services and physical therapy consultation for children. Evaluations and treatment are on an individual basis and special emphasis is placed on a multidisciplinary approach with information sharing, and often team treatment.

6576 **Clausen House**
88 Vernon Street
Oakland, CA 94610-4217 510-839-0050
clausenhouse.org

Deborah Levy, Interim Executive Director
Michael A. Scott, Director of Development
Stan Nicholson, Director of Human Resources
Jaynette Underhill, Director of Program Services
Residential, supported employment, independent and supported living, adult education, and social recreation activities. Serving the developmentally disabled since 1967.

6577 **Community Gatepath**
350 Twin Dolphin Dr
Suite 123
Redwood City, CA 94065 650-259-8500
Fax: 650-697-5010
info@gatepath.org
gatepath.org

Bryan Neider, CEO
Steve D'Eredita, Chief Financial Officer
Tracey Fecher, Vice President of Programs
Erin Montgomery, Vice President of Human Resources
Gatepath is a non-profit organization serving children, youth and adults with special needs and developmental disabilities and their families in the greater San Francisco Bay Area. The organization partners with various local non-profits, businesses, government agencies and third party providers to better serve this community.

6578 Community Hospital and Rehabilitation Center of Los Gatos-Saratoga
815 Pollard Rd
Los Gatos, CA 95032-1438 408-378-6131
Fax: 408-866-4003

Gary Honts, CEO

Offers rehabilitation services, inpatient and outpatient care, physical therapy, occupational therapy and more for the physically challenged adult. We have a commitment to health care excellence. It is in this commitment that we have dedicated ourselves to provide personal and professional service to our patients. Our goal is to work closely with staff, physicians and the community to attain shared goals and positive changes, now and in the future..

6579 Contra Costa ARC
1340 Arnold Drive
Suite 127
Martinez, CA 94553-4189 925-370-1818
Fax: 925-370-2048
www.ContraCostaARC.com

Barbara Maizie, Executive Director
Diana Jorgensen, Program Coordinator
Andrey George, Administrative Coordinator

A private nonprofit membership-based organization dedicated to enhancing the quality of life of individuals with developmental disabilities.

6580 Corona Regional Medical Center- Rehabiltation Center
800 S. Main St.
Corona, CA 92882-3117 951-737-4343
Fax: 951-736-7276
www.coronaregional.com

Diane Mc Donald, Manager
Mark Uffer, Chief Executive Officer
Doreen Dann, Chief Nursing Officer
Douglas Crouse, Chairman of the Board

Offers inpatient and outpatient rehabilitation services. The Center consists of an acute rehab unit, a subacute rehab unit containing modules for long-term ventilator care, respiratory rehab, coma intervention and orthopedics. In addition to inpatient therapies, the Center's outpatient programs include sports and industrial medicine.

6581 Critical Air Medicine
Montgomery Field
8775 Aero Drive
Suite 235
San Diego, CA 92123-1705 858-300-0224
800-247-8326
Fax: 858-300-0228
www.aircharterguide.com

Frank Craven, Publisher of the Air Charter Guide

Offers emergency medical care by air medical transport carriers. These carriers are fully equipped with medical equipment and supplies for cardiovascular emergencies, respiratory supplies, orthopedic supplies and medications..

6582 Crutcher's Serenity House
P.O. Box D
50 Hillcrest Drive
Deer Park, CA 94576-504 707-963-3192
Fax: 707-963-2309

Robert Crutcher, Owner/CEO
Lu Crutcher, Executive Director

A privately owned and operated facility that introduces to residents a new lifestyle free of all chemicals, and a new awareness of their total being. The length of the program is four weeks and is within five minutes of an acute care hospital. The Center is licensed for 19 beds, male and female located in a home-like setting with an emphasis on maintaining a family atmosphere.

6583 Daniel Freeman Rehabilitation Centers
333 N Prairie Ave
PO Box 28990
Santa Ana, CA 92799-4501 714-230-3150
Fax: 714-850-0153
advertising@acupuncturetoday.com
www.acupuncturetoday.com

H Arndt, Associate Administrator
Gabrielle Lindsley, Business Development Manager
Evelyn Petersen, Human Resources / Payroll Manager
Andrea Weeks, Accountant

Comprehensive rehabilitation services which address needs and issues of the physically diabled and their families. We offer accute input rehabilitation, outpatient and short term skilled nursing rehabilitaion. Specialty areas include: brain injury, stroke, spinal chord injury, chronic pain, arthritis..

6584 Delano Regional Medical Center
1401 Garces Highway
Delano, CA 93215-3690 661-725-4800
drmc.com

Bahram Ghaffari, President
Jeremy Klemm, HealthStream Regional Director
Robert A. Frist, HealthStream CEO

Delano Regional Medical Center (DRMC) is proud to be known throughout California & beyond as an innovative regional hospital, deeply rooted in the local communities and committed to providing an exceptional patient experience. A non-profit acute-care facility serving a region of 10 rural central Californiatowns. With over 100 physicians on our active medical staff and additional courtesy or consulting physicians, patients are assured of receiving high-quality care in multiple specialties.

6585 Desert Regional Medical Center
1150 N Indian Canyon Dr
Palm Springs, CA 92262 760-323-6511
800-491-4990
www.desertmedctr.com

Carolyn Caldwell, Chief Executive Officer
Tracey Cowles, Physician Relations Manager
Jeanne Stanton, RN, Chair
Lee Bledsoe, Physician Relations Manager

Our dedicated physicians and caregivers provide a broad array of quality programs and services, including comprehensive cancer care, women's health services, heart care, surgical weight loss reduction and orthopedics.

6586 Devereux Advanced Behavioral Health California
P.O. Box 6784
Santa Barbara, CA 93160 805-968-2525
Fax: 805-968-3247
rpopke@devereux.org
www.devereuxca.org

Amy Evans, Executive Director
Rebecca Popke, Marketing & Admissions Manager
Wendy Cooper, Manager of External Affairs
Veronica Arenas-Soto, Human Resources Director

Serves adults age 18 through 85 who have intellectual and developmental disabilities such as emotional disturbances, neurological impairments, autism, dementia and more. Devereux California currently provides a continuum of services, including on-campus residential, day programs, behavior management and supported living services in the community.

6587 Division of Physical Medicine and Rehabilitation
San Joaquin General Hospital
500 W Hospital Rd
French Camp, CA 95231-9693 209-468-6000
Fax: 209-468-6501

6588 **Dr. Karen H Chao Developmental Optometry Karen H. Chao. O.D.**
Suite A
121 S Del Mar Ave
San Gabriel, CA 91776-1345 626-287-0401
Fax: 626-287-1457
drkhchao@yahoo.com
www.healthgrades.com

Karen Chao, Owner
Karen Chao OD, Owner
Roger C. Holstein, Chief Executive Officer
Jeff Surges, President
Developmental optometrist specializing in the testing and treatment of vision problems and the enhancement of visual performance. Performs visual perceptual testing and training for children and adults. Undetected vision problems interfere with the ability to achieve and are highly correlated with learning difficulties and developmental problems. Provides the opportunity to overcome vision and visual-perceptual dysfunctions..

6589 **Early Childhood Services**
Desert Area Resources and Training
201 E Ridgecrest Blvd
Ridgecrest, CA 93555-3919 760-375-9787
Fax: 760-375-1288
www.dartontarget.org/

Peter V. Berns, Chief Executive Officer
Cris Bridges, Chief of Client Services
Bob Beecroft, Chief Operations Officer
Jeannie Luke, Human Resources Director/Risk Ma
Provides early intervention services to children who have disabilities or are experiencing delays in development. Provides developmental activities to promote the attainment of developmental milestones so that each child may reach his/her maximum potential. The program also provides therapeutic and educational intervention and offers support and guidance to families.

6590 **East Los Angeles Doctors Hospital**
4060 Whittier Boulevard
Los Angeles, CA 90023-2526 323-268-5514
www.elalax.com

Hector Hernandez, Chief Executive Officer
Kamlesh Dhawan, Chief Of Staff
Michael Austerlitz, Vice-Chief Of Staff
Horacio Fleischman, Secretary Treasurer
Postacute rehabilitation program.

6591 **Easterseals Northern California**
2730 Shadelands Dr.
Walnut Creek, CA 94598 925-266-8400
customerservice@esnorcal.org
www.esnorcal.org

Jim Kelleher, Chief Executive Officer
Andrea Pettiford, Vice President, Operations
Creates solutions that change the lives of children and adults with disabilities and special needs, and provides support to family members.

6592 **Easterseals Superior California**
3205 Hurley Way
Sacramento, CA 95864 916-485-6711
Fax: 916-485-2653
info@myeasterseals.org
www.easterseals.com/superior-ca

Gary T. Kasai, President & CEO
Don Nguyen, Chief Financnial Officer
Gary Novak, Chief Marketing & Donor Relations Officer
Karla Odum, Vice President, Human Resources
Dedicated to empowering people with disabilities by providing services, including medical rehabilitation and employment and training services, and promoting independence.

6593 **Exceed: A Division of Valley Resource Center**
P.O. Box 1773
1285 N. Santa Fe
Hemet, CA 92543-1773 951-766-8659
800-423-1227
Fax: 951-929-9758
vrctwohip@aol.com

Pattie Robert, Business Development Specialist
Mary Morse, Marketing Director
Kathy Cooke, Manager
Our vision is an environment where each client is valued as an individual and is provided the opportunity to reach his/her maximum potential. Our mission is to provide service and advocacy, which creates choices and opportunities, for adults with disabilities to reach their maximum potential..

6594 **Eye Medical Center of Fresno**
Eye Medical Center
1360 E. Herndon Avenue
Suite 301 & 210
Fresno, CA 93720-1498 559-486-5000
emcfresno.com

6595 **Fontana Rehabilitation Workshop**
Industrial Support Systems
8333 Almeria Ave
Fontana, CA 92335-3283 909-428-3883
800-755-4755
Fax: 909-428-3835
www.industrial-support.org

Silvia Anderson, Executive Director
U. Jones, CFO
C.Steven Bowen Plant, Operations manager
Bonnie Edwards, Operations Manager
The Fontana Rehabilitation Workshop, Inc., through its business divisions is committed to maintaining a stable environment wherein people with disabilities are provided with those services and supports that enable them to overcome barriers to employment and empower them to maximize their employment potential.

6596 **Foothill Vocational Opportunities**
789 North Fair Oaks Avenue
Pasadena, CA 91103-3045 626-449-0218
Fax: 626-449-0218
info@foothillvoc.org
foothillvoc.org

6597 **Fred Finch Youth Center**
3800 Coolidge Ave
Oakland, CA 94602-3399 510-482-2244
Fax: 510-488-1960
receptionist@fredfinch.org
fredfinch.org

Thomas N. Alexander, President/CEO
FFYC seeks to provide a continuum of high quality programs for the care and treatment of children, youth, young adults, and their families, whose changing needs can best be met by a variety of mental health and support services. The goal is for the program participants to receive the most effective services in the least restrictive environment appropriate to their needs so that they may function at their highest potential.

6598 **Gateway Center of Monterey County**
850 Congress Ave
Pacific Grove, CA 93950-4898 831-372-8002
Fax: 831-372-2411
info@gatewaycenter.org
gatewaycenter.org

Stephanie Lyon, Executive Director
Mike Price, Chief Financial Officer
Desiree Boller, Accounting Assistant
Heidy Welch, Human Resources
Our mission is to be a caring and stimulating environment for the Developmentally Disabled where all people can achieve their individual goals safely and with dignity. Our goal is to continue our programs and to find new and innovative ways of assisting the developmentally disabled to live in our community in surroundings compatable with their ability to live and work at the highest level possible.

6599 **Gateway Industries: Castroville**
7055 Veterans Blvd
Unit A
Burr Ridge, IL 60527
630-321-1333
888-473-3744
Fax: 630-321-1321
www.redshift.com

6600 **Gilroy Workshop**
7471 Monterey Street
Gilroy, CA 95020-3629
408-430-2810
Fax: 408-842-6770
info@leadershipgilroy.org
www.leadershipgilroy.org/

Kristi Alarid, Manager
Sally French, Manager
Denise Martin, Executive Director
Andrea Gamble, Administrative Director
Work adjustment and remunerative work programs..

6601 **Glendale Adventist Medical Center**
1509 Wilson Ter
Glendale, CA 91206-4098
818-409-8000
Fax: 818-546-5609

Kevin Roberts, President/CEO
Warren Tetz, Sr. Vice President and COO
Kelly Turner, Sr. Vice President and CFO
Judy Blair, Sr. Vice President and CNO
Rehabilitative team is made up of physician specialists, as well as professional and certified staff nurses, thereapists and others who meet regularly to ensure tht each patients progress is carefully planned and closely monitored.

6602 **Glendale Memorial Hospital and Health Center Rehabilitation Unit**
Glendale Memorial Hospital and Health Center
1420 South Central Ave
Glendale, CA 91204-2508
818-502-1900
Fax: 818-409-7688
www.glendalememorialhospital.org

Catherine M. Pelley, President
Offers rehabilitation services, occupational therapy, physical therapy, residential services and more for the disabled.

6603 **Goleta Valley Cottage Hospital**
Cottage Health System
351 S Patterson Ave
Santa Barbara, CA 93111-2496
805-967-3411
Fax: 805-681-6437
cverkiak@cottagehealthsystem.org
www.sbch.org

Ronald C. Wreft, President & CEO
Rosemary Bray, Clinical Manager
Diana Gray Miller, Administrator
Betty Jane Petrich, Manager
A 122-bed acute care hospital was founded in 1966 to serve the growing community of Goleta Valley. Today, we admit more then 2,000 patients a year, see more then 17,000 emergency visits, and welcome nearly 400 newborns to our designated 'Baby Friendly' Birth Center each year. We are also recognized for our Level IV trauma designation. We take great pride in fulfilling our goal of providing each patient with comfortable, personalized care.

6604 **HealthSouth Tustin Rehabilitation Hospital**
Health South Corporation
14851 Yorba St
Tustin, CA 92780-2925
714-832-9200
www.tustinrehab.com/

Diana Hanyak, Chief Executive Officer
Rodric Bell, Medical Director
Lindsey Barrett, Director of Case Management
Maryam Jouharzadeh, Pharm.D., Director, Pharmacy
HealthSouth Tustin Rehabilitation Hospital is part of the HealthSouth Corportation, the nation's largest provider of rehabilitative healthcare services, we are the only facility of its kind in Orange County. Fully accredited by the Joint Commission on Accreditation of Healthcare Organizations (JACHO) we provide inpatient and outpatient care designed to meed individual needs of patients and their families.

6605 **Hi-Desert Medical Center**
6601 White Feather Road
Joshua Tree, CA 92252-760
760-366-3711
hdmc.org

Lionel Chadwick, Chief Executive Officer
Tom Duda, Chief Financial Officer
Judy Austin, Chief Operating Officer & Chief
Barbara Staresinic, Director, Human Resources
Postacute rehabilitation program.

6606 **Home of the Guiding Hands**
Suite 200
1825 Gillespie Way
El Cajon, CA 92020-0501
619-938-2850
Fax: 619-938-3055
info@guidinghands.org
guidinghands.org

Mary Miller, President
Debby McNeil, Vice President
Michael Harris, Treasurer
Mark Klaus, Executive Director
The mission of Home og the Guiding Hands is to provide quality services, training and advocacy for people with developmental disabilities, their families, and others who will benefit.

6607 **Hospital of the Good Samaritan Acute Rehabilitation Unit**
1225 Wilshire Blvd
Los Angeles, CA 90017-1901
213-977-2121
800-366-8338
Fax: 213-482-2770
info@goodsam.org
goodsam.org

Andrew B Leeka, President and CEO
Charles T. Munger, Chairman
Physicians, researchers and staff are united by a common mission: to foster growth into one of the most comprehensive medical centers in the West. Services offered include: cardiology and cardiovascular services, neurosciences, movement disorders and Parkinsons disorder, wound care center and transfusion-medicine and surgery center.

6608 **Innovative Rehabilitation Services**
Hacienda La Puente Unified School District
15959 E. Gale Ave
City Of Industry, CA 91745
626-933-1000
Fax: 626-934-2900
info@hlpusd.k12.ca.us
www.hlpusd.k12.ca.us

Matthew Smith, Site Administrator
George Stransky, Counselor
Crystal Ontiveros, Counselor
Provides innovative student-centered learning opportunities and support services to a diverse population that enable individuals to achieve thier goals as lifelong learners, productive workers and effective communicators.

6609 **Janus of Santa Cruz**
Suite 150
200 7th Ave
Santa Cruz, CA 95062-4669
831-462-1060
866-526-8772
janussc.org

Rod Libbey, Executive Director
Bill Morris, Medical Director
Margie Storms, Clinical Director
Chris Storms, Intake Manager
A private not-for-profit corporation, licensed by the state of California. The Janus Clinic has a 3 year accreditation by the Council on Accreditation for Health Care Facilities.

6610 **John Muir Medical Center Rehabilitation Services, Therapy Center**
1601 Ygnacio Valley Rd
Walnut Creek, CA 94598-3122
925-939-3000
Fax: 925-308-8944
www.johnmuirhealth.com

Calvin Knight, President and CEO
Helen Doughty, Librarian
A 324-bed acute care facility that is designated as the only trauma center for Contra Costa County and portions of Solano County.

Recognized as one of the region's premier healthcare providers, areas of specialty include high-and low-risk obstetrics, orthopedics, neurosciences, cardiac care and cancer care. The campus is accredited by the Joint Commission on Accreditation of Healthcare Organizations (JCAHO), a national surveyor of quality patient care.

6611 **Kindred Hospital-La Mirada**
14900 E. Imperial Hwy
La Mirada, CA 90638-2172
562-944-1900
Fax: 562-906-3455
TTY: 800-735-2922
www.kindredlamirada.com
April Myers, Administrator
Adam Darvish, Executive Director
Committed to the delivery of high quality care in a cost-effective manner to enable us to become 'a model of excellence' in Long-Term Acute Care. Committed to treat our patients and families with dignity and respect, in the same manner we would want to be treated.

6612 **King's View Work Experience Center- Atwater**
559 East Bardsley Avenue
P. O. Box 688
Tulare, CA 93275-0688
559-688-7531
Fax: 559-688-3509
info@kingsview.org
www.kingsview.org
Leon Hoover, Chief Executive Officer
Vida Jalali, Chief Financial Officer Interim
Sue Essman, Director of Human Resources
Jeff Gorski, Director of Business Development
The primary mission of the Kings View Work Experience Center (KVWEC) is to serve people who have developmental disabilities. We believe in the dignity and worth of each person and in their right to rehabilitation, education and community integration. It is Kings View's aim to provide quality services to people who need assistance in the development of social, vocational and independent living skills.

6613 **LaPalma Intercommunity Hospital**
7901 Walker St
La Palma, CA 90623-1764
714-670-7400
LPIHInfo@primehealthcare.com
www.lapalmaintercommunityhospital.com
Virg Narbutas, Regional CEO
Sami Shoukair, Chief Medical Officer
Linda Gonzaba, Medical Staff Office Director
Hilda Manzo-Luna, Chief Nursing Officer
Lapalma Intercommunity Hospital endeavors to provide comprehensive, quality healthcare in a convenient, compassionate and cost effective manner. Lapalma is consistenty at the forefront of evolving national healthcare reform. Our organization provides an innovative and integrated healthcare delivery system. We remain ever cognizant of our patient's needs and desires for high quality affordable healthcare.

6614 **Learning Services of Northern California**
131 Langley Drive
Suite B
Lawrenceville, GA 30046-9315
408-848-4379
888-419-9955
Fax: 866-491-7396
www.learningservices.com
Dr. Debra Braunling-McMorrow, President and CEO
Jeanne Mack, Chief Financial Officer and Vice President of Operations
Michael Weaver, Chief Development Officer
Susan Snow, Director of Admissions
Located on 10 acres of ranchland in rural Santa Clara Valley, our Gilroy Program offers treatment, structure, and support in a spacious, campus-based living environment. Sharing living residences are complimented by a treatment and recreation facility for individuals who require intensive support.

6615 **Learning Services: Morgan Hill**
131 Langley Drive
Suite B
Lawrenceville, GA 30046-9315
408-848-4379
888-419-9955
Fax: 866-491-7396
www.learningservices.com
Dr. Debra Braunling-McMorrow, President and CEO
Jeanne Mack, Chief Financial Officer and Vice President of Operations
Michael Weaver, Chief Development Officer
Susan Snow, Director of Admissions
Located in the quaint rural town within walking distance from the old main street of Morgan Hill. Our Morgan Hill program offers the convenience and amenities of small-town living within the supportive community of Morgan Hill.

6616 **Learning Services: Supported Living Programs**
131 Langley Drive
Suite B
Lawrenceville, GA 30046-9315
408-848-4379
888-419-9955
Fax: 866-491-7396
www.learningservices.com
Dr. Debra Braunling-McMorrow, President and CEO
Jeanne Mack, Chief Financial Officer and Vice President of Operations
Michael Weaver, Chief Development Officer
Susan Snow, Director of Admissions
We offer a variety of diverse and stimulating environments for people with different needs, capabilities and personal goals. Within comfortable, homelike, age-appropriate settings we provide the structure and support necessary to ensure the richest possible quality of life. Program offered in both Northern and Southern facilities of California

6617 **Leon S Peters Rehabilitation Center**
2823 Fresno St
Fresno, CA 93721-1324
559-459-6000
www.communitymedical.org
Florence Dunn, Chairwoman
John McGregor, Esquire, Secretary
Tim A. Joslin, President, Chief Executive Officer
Patrick Rafferty, Executive Vice President, Chief Operating Officer
Community's flagship hospital that offers world class specialized critical care with the area's only stroke unit with 24-hour vascular neurology and neurosurgery coverage and a team of specially trained stroke nurses. The world's first G4 CyberKnife. The table Mountain Rancheraia Level 1 Trauma Center. The Leon S. Peters burn center. The region's only perinatology program for high rish pregnancies and deliveries. The Da-Vinci robotic surgical system, and 3 helicopeter landing pads.

6618 **Lion's Blind Center of Diablo Valley, Inc. Lions Center For The Visually Impaired**
175 Alvarado Ave
Pittsburg, CA 94565-4862
925-432-3013
800-750-3937
Fax: 925-432-7014
www.seniorvision.org
Edward Schroth, Executive Director
Barbara Cronin, President
Charles Dunham, First Vice President
Phillis Neitling, Secretary
A private, nonprofit agency offering services such as health, educational, recreational, rehabilitation, employment and counseling to the totally blind, legally blind and visually impaired. The staff includes two full time workers..

6619 **Lion's Blind Center of Oakland**
2115 Broadway
Oakland, CA 94612-2698
510-450-1580
Fax: 510-654-3603
Michelle Taylor Lagunas, Executive Director/ CEO
Christina Easiley, Administrative Manager
Scott Blanks, Director of Rehabilitation Servi
Danette Davis, Orientation & Mobility Instructor
A private nonprofit organization offering services for the totally blind, legally blind, deaf-blind and multihandicapped blind. Services include: professional training, rehabilitation, education,

counseling, social work, self help and more. The staff includes 12 full time and 1 part time worker.

6620 **Living Skills Center for the Visually Impaired**
2430 Road 20
#B112
San Pablo, CA 94806-5005 510-234-4984
Fax: 510-234-4986
info@hcblind.org
www.hcblind.org

Patricia Williams, Executive Director
Patricia Maffei, Program Director
Ronald Hideshima, Adaptive Technology Instructor
Lee Staub, Orientation and Mobility Instruc
A private, nonprofit agency offering services such as independent living skills training, recreational, employment and accessible technology training to the totally blind, legally blind and visually impaired. The staff includes six full time teachers.

6621 **Loma Linda University Orthopedic and Rehabilitation Institute**
25333 Barton Rd
Loma Linda, CA 92354-3123 909-558-1000
Fax: 909-558-0308
www.llu.edu

Richard H. Hart, MD, DrPH, President & Chief Executive Officer
Ronald L. Carter, PhD, Senior Vice President, Educational Affairs
Cari Dominguez, DHS, Senior Vice President, Human Resources
Mark L. Hubbard, Senior Vice President, Risk Management
Offers a full range of clinical programs for both inpatients and outpatient. The specific diagnosis leading to patient admission includes stroke, spinal cord injury, traumatic or anoxic brain damage, amputation, post neurosurgery, chronic neurological disease, Guillain-Barre syndrome, arthritis, multiple trauma or other complex orthopedic problems. The facilities and professional services are comprehensive and ensure that the best care is provided to pediatric and adult patients..

6622 **Manor Care Health Services- Citrus Heights**
7807 Uplands Way
Citrus Heights, CA 95610-7500 916-967-2929
Fax: 916-965-8439
hcr-manorcare.com

Steven M. Cavanaugh, Chief Financial Officer
Paul A. Ormond, Chairman, President and Chief Ex
The nations leader in skilled nursing and rehabilitation care. Our facility has been serving the Sacramento area for more then 12 years. We are known for our beautiful decor, outstanding rehabilitation staff and loving nursing care. We offer short term rehabilitation, long term skilled nursing care, respite care and post hospital surgical care.

6623 **Manor Care Health Services- Palm Desert**
74-350 Country Club Dr
Palm Desert, CA 92260-1608 760-341-0261
Fax: 760-779-1563
hcr-manorcare.com

Steven M. Cavanaugh, Chief Financial Officer
Paul A. Ormond, Chairman, President and Chief Ex
Centrally located in the Coachella Valley, specializing in skilled nursing whith an emphasis on rehabilitation, post surgery recovery, hospice, alzheimer's care and long term care. In addition, we offer 2 unique service options for the discriminating consumer. Our Arcadia unit offers a specialized Alzheimer's care program in a dedicated secure wing. ManorCare offers rehabilitation services including physical, occupational and speech therapies for those recovering from illness injury or surgery.

6624 **Manor Care Health Services-Fountain Valley**
11680 Warner Ave
Fountain Valley, CA 92708-2513 714-241-9800
Fax: 714-966-1654
hcr-manorcare.com

Steven M. Cavanaugh, Chief Financial Officer
Paul A. Ormond, Chairman, President and Chief Ex
Provides 24-hour skilled nursing, rehabilitative therapies and specialized Alzheimer's care. Our in-house therapists provide physical, occupational and speech therapies in our rehabilitation area. Our team is goal oriented and focuses on producing positive outcomes for those recovering from illness, injury or surgery. Our respite care program provides a full range of services for a few days, a week or even a season.

6625 **Manor Care Health Services-Hemet**
1717 W Stetson Ave
Hemet, CA 92545-6882 951-925-9171
Fax: 951-925-8186
hcr-manorcare.com

Steven M. Cavanaugh, Chief Financial Officer
Paul A. Ormond, Chairman, President and Chief Ex
Provides skilled nursing, Rehabilitation services, and specialized Alzheimer's care. In addition we offer short term respite stays for family caregivers that simply need a break from the stress of daily care. Our Arcadia unit staff is specially trained in the care of residents with Alzheimer's disease. The secured unit is designed to provide a soothing and homelike environment while enhancing each resident's remaining abilities.

6626 **Manor Care Health Services-Sunnyvale**
1150 Tilton Dr
Sunnyvale, CA 94087-2440 408-735-7200
Fax: 408-736-8629
hcr-manorcare.com

Steven M. Cavanaugh, Chief Financial Officer
Paul A. Ormond, Chairman, President and Chief Ex
Our in-house therapists provide physical, occupational and speech therapies in our rehabilitation area. Our team is goal oriented and focuses on producing positive outcomes for those recovering from illness, injury or surgery. Our skilled nursing staff works with our therapy department and dietary department to provide positive wound care programs for patients requiring skin management care.

6627 **Manor Care Health Services-Walnut Creek**
1226 Rossmoor Pkwy
Walnut Creek, CA 94595-2538 925-975-5000
Fax: 925-937-1132
hcr-manorcare.com

Steven M. Cavanaugh, Chief Financial Officer
Paul A. Ormond, Chairman, President and Chief Ex
Provides luxurious long term care and rehabilitation services. In house therapists provide, physical, occupational and speech therapies in our rehabilitation area. Our team is goal oriented and focuses on producing positive outcomes for those recovering from illness, injury or surgery. Our years of combined management experience add value to our resident's quality of life.

6628 **Maynord's Chemical Dependency Recovery Centers**
19325 Cherokee Road
Tuolumne, CA 95379-1657 209-928-3737
800-228-8208
Fax: 209-928-1152
maynords.com

James Berry, Director
Maynord's Recovery Centers has always been dedicated to the recovery of good people whose lives are being destroyed by alcohol and drugs. Since 1978, Maynord's residential program has helped thousands of people put their lives back together after addiction has taken its toll. Today, Maynord's offers a treatment system over much of the San Joaquin Valley and the San Francisco Bay Area.

6629 **Maynord's Ranch for Men**
19325 Cherokee Road
Tuolumne, CA 95379-1657 209-928-3737
800-228-8208
Fax: 209-928-1152
maynords.com

James Berry, Director
Provides treatment for chemical dependency problems to men. The treatment addresses their recovery through a comprehensive plan created for their individual needs. Also offers a program for women called the Meadows.

6630 **Meadowbrook Manor**
431 West Remington Boulevard
Bolingbrook, IL 60440 630-759-1112
Fax: 630-759-6925
www.meadowbrookmanor.com

6631 **Meadowview Manor**
41 Crestview Terrace
Bridgeport, WV 26330
304-842-7101
Fax: 304-842-7104

6632 **Memorial Hospital of Gardenia**
1145 West Redondo Beach Blvd
Gardena, CA 90247-3528
310-532-4200
800-782-2288
www.avantihospitals.com
Edward Mirzabegian, Corporate Chief Executive Officer
Postacute rehabilitation program.

6633 **Mercy Medical Group**
Mercy Hospital
3000 Q Street
Sacramento, CA 95816
916-733-3333
www.mymercymedicalgroup.org

6634 **Napa County Mental Health Department**
2344 Old Sonoma Road
Bldg. D
Napa, CA 94559-3708
707-259-8151
800-648-8650
www.countyofnapa.org/MentalHealth/

6635 **Napa Valley Support Systems**
1700 Second Street Suite 212
Napa, CA 94559-1344
707-253-7490
Fax: 707-253-0115
napavalleysupportservices.org
Beth Kahiga, Executive Director
Heather Jump, Administrative Manager
Katy Vanzant, Program Director
Emmy Lesko, Program Supervisor
Work hardening and disciplinary programs.

6636 **North Valley Services**
1040 Washington
Red Bluff, CA 96080-4509
530-527-0407
Fax: 530-527-7091
www.northvalleyservices.org
Joe Brown, President
Larry Donnelley, Vice President
Lynn DeFreece, CEO
Delbert Brownfield, COO
Provides vocational rehabilitation services, such as job counseling, job training, and work experience, to unemployed and underemployed persons, persons with disabilities.

6637 **Northridge Hospital Medical Center Rehabiltation Medicine**
18300 Roscoe Blvd
Northridge, CA 91328-4167
818-885-8500
Fax: 818-701-7367
www.northridgehospital.org/index.htm
Mike L. Wall, President
Thomas L. Hedge, Medical Director
Joel S. Rosen, Associate Medical Director
Alex L. Lin, Managing Director
A full service, comprehensive rehabilitation program suited to treat patients of all ages who have suffered catastrophic or debilitating injury or illness. The goal of the program is to deliver exceptional patient care to maximise each individual's skills and independence.

6638 **Northridge Hospital Medical Center: Centerfor Rehabilitation Medicine**
18300 Roscoe Blvd
Northridge, CA 91328-4167
818-885-8500
Fax: 818-701-7367
www.northridgehospital.com
Mike L. Wall, President
Thomas L. Hedge, Medical Director
Joel S. Rosen, Associate Medical Director
Alex L. Lin, Managing Director
Committed to serving the health needs of our communities with particular attention to the needs of the poor, the disadvantaged, and vulneralbe, and the comfort of the suffering and dying. Catholic Healthcare West has a commitment to quality-quality healthcare services and the promotion of optimal quality of life for all of life.

6639 **Old Adobe Developmental Services**
1301A Rand Street
Suite A
Petaluma, CA 94954-5697
707-763-9807
Fax: 707-763-7708
www.oadsinc.org
Elizabeth Clary, Executive Director
Marie Padgett, Controller
The mission of Old Adobe to provide opportunities for individuals with developmental challenges to reach thier fullest potentials. Our job at OADS is to find ways for these individuals to find full expression in all parts of their lives. We have a partnership with the Adult Education Department of the Petaluma School District in providing services to persons with developmental challenges. We are funded by the Dept. of Rehabilitation and the Dept. Of Developmental services.

6640 **Old Adobe Developmental Services-Rohnert Park Services (Behavioral)**
5401 Snyder Ln.
Rohnert Park, CA 94928-3124
707-584-5859
Fax: 707-664-8057
Elizabeth Clary, Executive Director
Helen Gunderson, Administrative Assistant
The program services are designed to assist individuals who demonstrate basic work skills, to develop social skills and work habits necessary to succeed in supported or competitive employment. Most often individual program services involve working with the client to replace those behavioral excesses that have been a barrier to vocational placement.

6641 **PRIDE Industries**
10030 Foothills Blvd
Roseville, CA 95747-7102
916-788-2100
800-550-6005
Fax: 800-888-0447
info@prideindustries.com
prideindustries.com
Michael Ziegler, President & CEO
Bob Selvester, Vice Chair
Mike Snegg, Treasurer
Tim Yamauchi, Executive Vice President and Chi
To provide opportunities through employment, training, evaluation and placement maximizing community access, independence and quality of life for people with barriers to employment.

6642 **Pacific Hospital Of Long Beach-Neuro Care Unit**
2776 Pacific Ave
Long Beach, CA 90806-2613
562-997-2000
webmaster@phlb.org
Michael D. Drobot, CEO
Clark Todd, President
Teri Plemmons, Administrative Assistant
Our mission is to heal with compassion and to perform with distinction. Our vision: to improve the hospital's orthopedic and Spine Center of Excellence. Achieve exceptional financial performance to enhance hospital services. Improve the vertically integrated ancillary, outpatient and inpatient surgery system. Develop a professionally challenging work environment that reflects an agile, peak performance culture.

6643 **Paradise Vally Hospital-South Bay Rehabilitation Center**
2400 East 4th St
National City, CA 91950-2026
619-470-4321
paradisevalleyhospital.net
Prem Reddy, Chairman
Neerav Jadeja, Administrator
Luis Leon, President
Gemma Rama-Banaag, Chief Nursing Officer
South Bay Rehabilitation Center, offers a complete range of treatment for patients with physical disabilities. Our specialized inpatient and outpatient programs are designed to meet each person's individual needs or injuries, with the goal of restoring as much independence as possible and significantly improving their lives.

6644 **Parents and Friends**
350 South Main Street
Fort Bragg, CA 95437-5408 707-964-4940
parentsandfriends.org

Rick Moon, Executive Director
Jessica Dickey, Administrative Assistant
Kristy Tanguay, Manager
Kathy Connell, Bookkeeper

Parents and Friends provides opportunities for persons with developmental challenges and similar needs to participate fully in our community.

6645 **People Services**
4195 Lakeshore Blvd
Lakeport, CA 95453-6411 707-263-3810
peopleservices.org

Ilene Dumont, Executive Director
Martin Diesman, Director
Vicki Cole, Director
Kathy Ryan, Director

Providing an array of services for adults with developmental disabilities and other people with disabilities. Services include supported employment, work services, supported living, personal, social and community training, transportation, specialized individual services and much more.

6646 **Petaluma Recycling Center**
Old Adobe Developmental Services
315 2nd St
Petaluma, CA 94952-4230 707-763-4761
Fax: 707-763-4921

Elizabeth Clary, Executive Director

Began in 1974; has been one of the major employers of persons with developmental challenges for 26 years; is the primary recycling facility in the growing city of 52,000; accepts over 20 different kinds of recyclables; employs 20-25 persons a day.

6647 **Pomerado Rehabilitation Outpatient Service**
15615 Pomerado Rd
Poway, CA 92064-2405 858-485-6511
Fax: 858-613-4248

Bob Blake, Director Rehab Services
Jonathan Pee, Manager

A 107-bed acute care hospital. In addition to a round-the-clock Emergency Department, Pomerado offers the area's finest outpaitent surgery center and general medical/surgical services. Pomerado Hospital also is home to a world-class Birth Center and a Level II NICU. Fully JCAHO-accredidted, Pomerado is well-known for offering only private rooms, each with a scenic view of the North Countryside, which enhances the healing atmosphere..

6648 **Pride Industries: Grass Valley**
12451 Loma Rica Dr
Grass Valley, CA 95945-9059 530-477-1832
800-550-6005
Fax: 530-477-8038
info@prideindustries.com
www.prideindustries.com

Bob Olsen, Chairman
Bob Selvester, Vice Chairman
Walt Payne, President/CEO
Mike Snegg, Treasurer

Work adjustment and remunerative work programs. We offer an adult day program as well.

6649 **Rancho Adult Day Care Center**
Rancho Los Amigos Medical Center
7601 Imperial Hwy
Downey, CA 90242-3456 562-401-7111
Fax: 562-401-7991
TTY: 562-401-8450
dhs.lacounty.gov/wps/portal/dhs/rancho

Valerie Orange, CEO
Margaret L Campbell, Research Director

Provides personal care, social services and a therapeutic program to older adults in order to improve their quality of life. Offers a Clinical Gerontology Service, an Alzheimer's Disease Diagnostic and Treatment Center and a Geriatric Assessment and Rehabilitation Unit..

6650 **Regional Center for Rehabilitation**
2288 Auburn Blvd
Sacramento, CA 95821-1618 916-421-4167
Fax: 916-925-1586

6651 **Rehabilitation Institute of Santa Barbara**
2415 De La Vina St
Santa Barbara, CA 93105-3819 805-569-8999
Fax: 805-687-3707

Ralph Pollock, President
Scott Silic MBA, Vice President Of Operations
Cheryl Ellis MD, MHA, VP Medical Services

A regional rehabilitation system with an acute care hospital at the center, the Institute provides specialized inpatient and outpatient programs for brain injury, spinal cord injury, stroke, work-related injury, chronic pain, orthopedic problems and more. Offers a 46-bed acute-care rehabilitation hospital, a free-standing outpatient center, the brain injury continuum, chronic pain program..

6652 **Rehabilitation Institute of Southern California**
1800 E La Veta Ave
Orange, CA 92866-2902 714-633-7400
Fax: 714-633-4586
riorehab.org

Praim S. Singh, Executive Director
Carol Reese, Executive Assistant
Grace Lee, Administrative Assistant
Dana Patton, Personnel Officer

Outpatient rehabilitation serving physically and disabled children and adults. Child development programs, adult day care for disabled seniors, child care for disabled and non-disabled children, outpatient therapy, aquatics, adult day healthcare, independent living, vocational services, social services, and housing.

6653 **Rubicon Programs**
2500 Bissell Avenue
Richmond, CA 94804-1815 510-235-1516
Fax: 510-235-2025
www.rubiconprograms.org

Rob Hope, Chief Program Officer
Jane Fischberg, President and Executive Director
Roger Contreras, CFO
Kelly Dunn, General Counsel and Director of Legal Services

Rubicon Programs Inc. helps people and communities build assets to achieve greater independence. Since 1973, Rubicon has built and operated affordable housing and provided employment, job training, mental health, and other supportive services to individuals who have disabilities, are homeless, or are otherwise economically disadvantaged.

6654 **San Bernardino Valley Lighthouse for the Blind**
762 North Sierra Way
San Bernardino, CA 92410-4438 909-884-3121
Fax: 909-884-2964
www.afb.org

Robert Mc Bay, Executive Director
Sandra Wood, Administrative Assistant

Provides training in independent living skills - cooking, mobility and orientation, sewing, Braille and typing. Also, we have classes in macrame, ceramics and basket weaving. Weekly support group and Bible study..

6655 **Santa Clara Valley Blind Center, Inc.**
101 N Bascom Ave
San Jose, CA 95128-1805 408-295-4016
Fax: 408-295-1398
info@visionbeyondsight.org
visionbeyondsight.org

Arnold Chew, President
John Glass, Vice President
Arlene Holmes, Secretary
Sue Szucs, Treasurer

SCVBC's mission is to increase the confidence, independence, and quality of life of the blind and visually impaired through educational, recreational, and rehabilitative programs.

6656 **Scripps Memorial Hospital: Pain Center**
4275 Campus Point Ct.
San Diego, CA 92121-1205 858-626-4123
800-727-4777
clinicalresearch@scrippshealth.com
www.scripps.org
Chris Van Gorder, President and CEO
Richard K Rothberger, Vice President, Chief Financial Officer
Robin B Brown, Chief Executive
Richard R Sheridan, Corporate Senior Vice President
Offers both inpatient and outpatient programs including: physical activity management, individual pain management, group therapy, medication adjustment, pain control classes, occupational therapy, biofeedback training, family counseling, vocational and leisure counseling and recreational therapy.

6657 **Sharp Coronado Hospital**
250 Prospect Place
Coronado, CA 92118-1999 619-522-3600
erica.carlson@sharp.com
sharp.com
Marcia Hall, CEO
Mark Tamsen, Chairman
Tom Smisek, Vice Chairman
Dan Gensler, Secretary
Providing medical and surgical care, intensive care, sub-acute and long-term care, rehabilitation therapies and emergency services in a peaceful setting is part of our live+heal+grow philosophy. We are one of the county's few community-owned hospitals and are proud of our history of providing convenient, award-winning heath care to Coronado and San Diego.

6658 **Shriners Hospitals For Children-Northern California**
2425 Stockton Blvd.
Sacramento, CA 95817 916-453-2000
patientreferrals@shrinenet.org
www.shrinershospitalsforchildren.org
John McCabe, Executive Vice President
Dale W Stauss, Chairman
Jerry G Gantt, 1st Vice President
Chris L Smith, 2nd Vice President
The only hospital in the Shriners system that houses facilities for treatment of all 3 Shriner specialties -spinal cord injuries, orthopaedic, and burns. The hospital features 80 patient beds, 9 parent apartments, 5 state-of-the-art operating rooms, a high-tech Motion Analysis lab, and an entire floor devoted to research.

6659 **Shriners Hospitals for Children: Los Angeles**
3160 Geneva Street
Los Angeles, CA 90020-1199 213-388-3151
patientreferrals@shrinenet.org
www.shrinershospitalsforchildren.org
John McCabe, Executive Vice President
Dale W Stauss, Chairman
Jerry G Gantt, 1st Vice President
Chris L Smith, 2nd Vice President
Shriners Hospitals for Children: Los Angeles, treats children under age 18 with burn scars, orthopedic conditions, cleft lip and palate and limb deficiencies at no cost to the patient or their families.

6660 **Society for the Blind**
1238 S St.
Sacramento, CA 95811-3256 916-452-8271
Fax: 916-492-2483
info@societyfortheblind.org
societyfortheblind.org
Shari Roesler, Executive Director
Shane Snyder, Director of Programs
A private, local nonprofit organization providing blind and visually impaired people with the training supplies and support they need to live independent, productive and fulfilled lives with limited vision. Services include the Low Vision Clinic, Braille classes, computer training, support groups, living skills instruction, mobility training and the Products for Independence Store.

6661 **Solutions at Santa Barbara: Transitional Living Center**
1135 N Patterson Ave
Santa Barbara, CA 93111-1113 805-683-1995
Fax: 805-683-4793
sol1135@aol.com
solutionsatsantabarbara.com
Sue Hannigan, Director
Postacute rehabilitation program. Short-term transitional living program for individuals with traumatic brain injury, stroke, aneurysm and other neurological disorders.

6662 **St. John's Pleasant Valley Hospital Neuro Care Unit**
2309 Antonio Ave
Camarillo, CA 93010-1414 805-389-5800
Jerry Conway, President
Maureen M. Malone, Administrator
Raye Burkhardt, Vice President and Chief Nursing
Houses 82 acute-care beds, a 99-bed extended care unit, and the only hyperbaric medicine unit in Ventura County. Employ's 1,800 people and count 250 active medical staff.

6663 **St. John's Regional Medica Center- Industrial Therapy Center**
1600 North Rose Ave
Oxnard, CA 93030-3723 805-988-2500
www.stjohnshealth.org
Gudrun Moll, Vice President and Chief Nursing
Laurie Harting, President & CEO
Kim Wilson, Vice President
Chris Champlin, Senior Vice President
A non-profit health care facility offering multi-disciplinary programs for pain management and work hardening, as well as physical and occupational therapy.

6664 **Sub-Acute Saratoga Hospital**
13425 Sousa Lane
Saratoga, CA 95070-4663 408-378-8875
Fax: 408-378-7419
subacutesaratoga.com
Jack Stephens, President & CEO
Paul Quintana, Medical Director
Gary Vernon, NHA Administrator
Lindsay Zarcone, Marketing Manager
Dedicated to the fulfillment of human needs, desires, and wishes in illness and in health. The cohesiveness of caring in a family community of staff, patients, and their loved ones. The celebration of each unique life through their therapeutic journey, while preserving their individual spirit. The achievement of advanced medical expertise, knowledge, and skill given with the human touch of caring toward the ultimate goal: enhancing the healing process from acute illness to the joy of going home.

6665 **Synergos Neurological Center: Hayward**
27200 Calaroga Avenue
Hayward, CA 94545-4383 510-264-4000
Fax: 510-264-4007
strosehospital.org
Richard C. Hardwig, Chair
Alan McIntosh, Vice Chair
Lex Reddy, President and CEO
Roger Krissman, Chief Financial Officer
Postacute rehabilitation program.

6666 **Synergos Neurological Center: Mission Hills**
27200 Calaroga Avenue
Hayward, CA 94545-4383 510-264-4000
Fax: 510-264-4007
www.strosehospital.org
Richard C. Hardwig, Chair
Alan McIntosh, Vice Chair
Lex Reddy, President and CEO
Roger Krissman, Chief Financial Officer
For over 30 years, St. Rose Hospital Rehabilitation Services Department has helped thousands of patients recover from illness and injury through the help of our specially trained therapists. These therapists have been trained in specific rehabilitative areas such as physical, occupational, and speech therapies.

6667 **Temple Community Hospital**
235 N Hoover St
Los Angeles, CA 90004-3672
213-382-7252
Fax: 213-382-1874
templecommunityhospital.com

6668 **The Arc of the East Bay**
1101 Walpert St
Hayward, CA 94541-3721
510-582-8151
arcalameda.org

Son Luter, President & CEO

Offers a variety of services and programs for adults and children with intellectual and developmental disabilities.

6669 **Tunnell Center for Rehab**
680 South Fourth Street
Louisville, CA 40202-4807
502-596-7300
Fax: 800-545-0749
web_administrator@kindred.com
kindredhealthcare.com

Mary R., Activities Assistant
Kristen W., Health and Rehabilitation Center

The Tunnell Center for Rehabilitation and Healthcare accomodates 178 residents. We are dedicated to short-term complex medical and rehabilitative care. Using a holistic care management approach we work with residents who have suffered debilitating injury or illness, and who need comprehensive nursing and rehabilitation services to achieve their highest practicable level of functional ability and independence.

6670 **Ukiah Valley Association for Habilitation**
Ukiah, CA 95482-689
707-468-8824
Fax: 707-468-9149
TTY: 800-735-2929
www.uvah.org

Pamela Jensen, Executive Director
Kris Vipond, Business Manager
Sharrae Elston, Director
Suzanne Warner, Employment Training Specialist

Work adjustment and suppoted employment and social and community services.

6671 **Valley Center for the Blind**
2491 W Shaw Avenue
Suite 124
Fresno, CA 93711-3331
559-222-4088
Fax: 559-222-4844

Bud Breslin, Executive Director
Millie Marshall, Marriage Family Therapist
Saramarie Katich, Office Mngr/Program Director
Connie Parrick, Secretary

A private, nonprofit organization that offers educational, health, recreational and professional training services to the totally blind, legally blind or severely visually impaired.

6672 **Villa Esperanza Services**
2060 East Villa Street
Pasadena, CA 91107
626-449-2919
Fax: 626-449-2850
info@villaesperanzaservices.org
www.villaesperanzaservices.org

Candice Rogers, Chairman
Richard Hubinger, President
Vicky Castillo, CFO
Kelly White, Chief Executive Officer

Serving disabled infants to seniors in a school, adult day program, adult work program and residences and adult day health care program and care management program.

6673 **Village Square Nursing And Rehabilitation Center**
Kindred Healthcare, Inc.
1586 West San Marcos Blvd
San Marcos, CA 92078-4019
760-471-2986

6674 **Vista Center for the Blind & Visually Impaired**
2500 El Camino Real,
Suite 100
Palo Alto, CA 94306
650-858-0202
800-660-2009
Fax: 650-858-0214
info@vistacenter.org
www.vistacenter.org

Pam Brandin, Executive Director
Nacole Barth-Ellis, Co-Director of Development
Terry Kurfess, Co-Director of Development
Meg Faville, Administrative Services Manager

Private nonprofit agency that serves the visually impaired in the San Mateo, Santa Clara, San Benito and Santa Cruz Counties with offices in Palo Alto and Santa Cruz. Offers Low Vision Evaluations, mobility training, daily living skills training, social services, counseling, support groups, computer training, other rehabilitation services, and a store.

6675 **Winways at Orange County**
7732 E Santiago Canyon Rd
Orange, CA 92869-1829
714-771-5276
Fax: 714-771-1452
winwaysrehab.com

Pamela Kauss, Director

The program offers clients highly personalized, comprehensive programs to meet the needs of individuals with traumatic brain injury, stroke, tumors, aneurysm, post concussive syndrome or other neurological disorders. Winways also has a special program that provides services to Spanish speaking clients, called Contigo Adelante with materials in Spanish, and Spanish speaking interpreters to assist in the therapy process.

Colorado

6676 **Capron Rehabilitation Center**
Penrose Hospital/ St. Francis Healthcare System
2222 N Nevada Ave
Colorado Springs, CO 80907-6819
719-776-5000
penrosestfrancis.org

Margaret Sabin, President & CEO
Nate Olson, Chief Executive Officer
Jameson Smith, Senior VP & Chief Admnistrative Officer
Gil Porat, Chief Medical Officer

Southern Colorado's most complete inpatient and outpatient rehabilitation center.

6677 **Cerebral Palsy of Colorado**
801 Yosemite Street
Denver, CO 80230
303-691-9339
Fax: 303-691-0846
abilityconnectioncolorado.org

Judith I Ham, CEO
James Reuter, Chairman of the Board
Penfield Tate, Vice Chairman
Kathy Higgins, Treasurer

Provides services for children birth-5 years, employment services for adults, information and referral, donation pickup and cell phone/ink cartridge recycling services.

6678 **Cherry Hills Health Care Center**
Kindred
3575 S Washington St
Englewood, CO 80110-3807
303-789-2265

6679 **Community Hospital Back and Conditioning Clinic**
1060 Orchard Ave
Grand Junction, CO 81501-2997
970-243-3400
800-621-0926
Fax: 970-856-6510

Amy Hibberd, Executive Director
David Scherman, Manager

Post-accute rehabilitation program .

6680 **Devereux Advanced Behavioral Health Colorado**
8405 Church Ranch Blvd.
Westminster, CO 80021 303-466-7391
800-456-2536
www.devereuxco.org

Lisa Gaudia, Interim Clinical Director

A non-profit partner for individuals, families, schools and communities, serving people in the areas of autism, intellectual and developmental disabilities, mental health issues, and child welfare. Programs offered include residential services, community based services, educational programs, employment supports and more.

6681 **Laradon Hall Society for Exceptional Children and Adults**
5100 Lincoln St
Denver, CO 80216-2056 303-296-2400
866-381-2163
Fax: 303-296-4012
laradon.org

William Mitchell, Chair
Suzanne Bradeen, Vice Chair
Jason Adams, Treasurer
Nancy Hodges, Secretary

Laradon provides educational, vocational and residential services to children and adults with developmental disabilities and other special needs. Laradon was founded in 1948. It is among the largest and most comprehensive service providers in Colorado.

6682 **Learning Services: Bear Creek**
7201 W Hampden Ave
Lakewood, CO 80227-5305 303-989-6660
888-419-9955
Fax: 866-491-7396
learningservices.com

Susan Snow, Director of Admissions
Dr. Debra Braunling-McMorrow, President and CEO
Jeanne Mack, Chief Financial Officer
Michael Weaver, Chief Development Officer

Supported living program for persons with acquired brain injury.

6683 **MOSAIC In Colorado Springs**
888 W. Garden of the Gods Road
Ste 100
Colorado Springs, CO 80907-6251 719-380-0451
Fax: 719-380-7055
mosaic_cosprings@mosaicinfo.org
www.mosaicincoloradosprings.org

Tom Maltais, Executive Director

Mosaic in Colorado Springs provides a variety of services to assist adults and families in achieving positive goals. Services to persons with intellectual disabilities include community living options, vocational training and supported employment, spiritual growth and personal development options, and day programs habilitation and community participation.

6684 **Manor Care Nursing and Rehabilitation Center: Boulder**
Manor Care Ohio
2800 Palo Pkwy
Boulder, CO 80301-1540 303-440-9100
Fax: 303-440-9251
www.hcr-manorcare.com

Steven M. Cavanaugh, Chief Financial Officer
Paul A. Ormond, Chairman, President and Chief Ex

150 bed center offers a full spectrum of nursing care and rehabilitation. This includes our Arcadia Special Care Unit for Alzheimer's patients. Specialized unit for post acute skilled nursing care. Physical and massage therapies. And a 48 bed upscale Heritage unit offering additional amenities and furnishings.

6685 **Manor Care Nursing: Denver**
290 S Monaco Pkwy
Denver, CO 80224-1105 303-355-2525
Fax: 303-333-6960
www.hcr-manorcare.com

Steven M. Cavanaugh, Chief Financial Officer
Paul A. Ormond, Chairman, President and Chief Ex

Our center has delveloped a reputation for its luxurious environment, comprehensive rehabilitation service and focus on quality care. A wide range of individual and group activities and many gracious amenities create the finest combination of elegance and professional skilled nursing care. Arcadia, our special care unit for persons with Alzheimer's disease and related memory impairments, promotes independence and preserves dignity within a safe and secure environment.

6686 **Mediplex of Colorado**
8451 Pearl St
Thornton, CO 80229-4804 303-288-3000
Fax: 303-286-5136
info@vhdenver.com

Jan Eyer, Chief Executive Officer

Our programs and services help each patient along the road to recovery toward our ultimate aim; the greatest possible restoration of the individual's self-esteem, ability to set goals, and self-sufficiency. Also offer specialized acute inpatient rehabilitative services, including special programs in Trauma Rehabilitation.

6687 **Platte River Industries**
490 Bryant St
Denver, CO 80204-4808 303-825-0041
Fax: 303-825-0564

Bob Smith, Executive Director

Postacute rehabilitation facility and program..

6688 **Pueblo Diversified Industries**
2828 Granada Blvd
Pueblo, CO 81005-3198 800-466-8393
Fax: 719-564-3407
info@pdipueblo.org
www.pdipueblo.net

Karen K Lillie, President & CEO
Robin Forbes, Director Human Services
Tom Drolshagen, Chief Operating Officer
Tom Denslow, Manager, Human Resources

A place where people can turn limitations into opportunities. People can experience the independence, pride and self worth of securing and maintaining a job.

6689 **SHALOM Denver**
2498 W 2nd Ave
Denver, CO 80223-1007 303-623-0251
Fax: 303-620-9584
shalomdenver.com

Arnie Kover, Disability and Employment Servic
Sara Leeper, Coordinator of Client Services
Vicky Brittain, Mailing Business Manager
Bari Belinsky, Work Services Manager

SHALOM Denver provides employment, training, and job placement opportunities to people with disabilities, resettled immigrants, and people moving from welfare to work.

6690 **SPIN Early Childhood Care & Education Cntr**
1333 Elm Ave
Canon City, CO 81212-4431 719-275-0550
www.starpointco.com/spin

Diane Trujillo, Manager

SPIN center is a fully inclusive non-discriminating community early childhood program, offering a variety of schedule choices for families. The philosophy of the SPIN program is to promote each child's growth and development. Special attention is given to cognitive, physical, speech language and social-emotional growth. Staff is specifically trained to facilitate and prepare environments that promote exploration, key experiences, creativity and self-expression..

6691 **Schaefer Enterprises**
500 26th Street
P.O. Box 200009
Greeley, CO 80631-8427 970-353-0662
Fax: 970-353-2779
www.schaeferenterprises.com

Valorie Randall, Executive Director
Alex Witt, Executive Assistant
Veronica Griego, Production Director

Schaefer Enterprises, Inc., located in Greely, Colorado, is a vaulable community resource that has been fulfilling the outsourcing needs of businesses in Weld County and outlying areas since 1952.

6692 **Spalding Rehab Hospital West Unit**
150 Spring St
Morrison, CO 80465
303-697-4334
Fax: 303-697-0570

A team of rehabilitation and health care professionals offering career development, residential services, supported employment, volunteer services, occupational therapy, day activities and more.

Connecticut

6693 **ACES/ACCESS Inclusion Program**
350 State Street
North Haven, CT 06473-3218
203-498-6800
Fax: 203-234-1369
acesinfo@aces.org
www.aces.org

Thomas M Danehy, Executive Director
Erika Forte, Assistant Executive Director
Evelyn Rossetti, Manager

Provides a person centered planning approach for integrated employment, volunteer community based opportunities for adults who have developmental disabilities..

6694 **Apria Healthcare**
Apira Healthcare Group, Inc.
26220 Enterprise Court
Lake Forest, CA 92630
949-639-2000
800-277-4288
contact_us@apria.com
www.apria.com

Dan Starck, CEO
Debra Morris, CFO
Celina M. Scally, Senior Vice President
Nichola Denney, Executive Vice President, Revenue Management

Provides a broad range of high quality and cost effective specialty infusion therapies and related services to patients in their homes throughout the Northeastern United States. Offer home infusion antibiotic therapy, quality pharmacy services, skilled nursing services and related support services.

6695 **Arc Of Meriden-Wallingford, Inc.**
200 Research Parkway
Meriden, CT 06450
203-237-9975
Fax: 203-639-0946
www.arcmw.org

Pamela Fields, Executive Director
Joseph Palfini, Board President
Becky Blazejowski, Financial Director
Maritza Dell, Director of Program Services

A membership agency that provides comprehensive, full-service, community-based opportunities for people with disabilities. Guided by over 120 community members and an active Board of Directors, the Arc always has its focus on improving the lives of people with disabilities. The Arc of Meriden-Wallingford offers advocacy and assistance to our members along with advocating for the rights and choices of people with disabilities in our community.

6696 **Connecticut Subacute Corporation**
19 Tuttle Pl
Middletown, CT 06457-1881
860-347-6300
Fax: 860-347-2446

Evan K Lyle, Managed Care Director
Cheri Kauset, Corporate Rep.

Specializes in subacute medical and rehabilitation programming. The strength of our system is in its' ability to service a broad range of clinical and psychosocial needs which enable each individual to attain his/her optimal potential. Programming includes neurological and orthopedic rehabilitation, post-surgical and wound care management, intravenous therapy, pulmonary rehabilitation including ventilator services, and long term care..

6697 **Datahr Rehabilitation Institute**
4 Berkshire Blvd
Bethel, CT 06801-1001
203-775-4700
888-8DA-TAHR
Fax: 203-775-4688

Thomas Fanning, CEO

Providers of comprehensive rehabilitation services with a history of nearly 5 decades of service. This institute is recognized as a leading resource in meeting the needs of those disabled by illness, injury or developmental disorders in Connecticut and New York.

6698 **Eastern Blind Rehabilitation Center**
810 Vermont Avenue
Washington, DC 20420
202-461-7600
800-273-8255

Eric K. Shinseki, Secretary of Veterans Affairs
W. Scott Gould, Deputy Secretary of Veterans Aff
Jose D Riojas, Chief of Staff
Richard J Griffin, Acting Inspector General

Provides residential rehabilitation services to eligible legally blind veterans in the Northeast and Middle Atlantic portions of the country. Referral applications by Veterans Administration Medical Centers and Outpatient Clinics in the geographical area served by the Blind Rehabilitation Center.

6699 **FAVRAH Senior Adult Enrichment Program**
23 W Avon Rd
Avon, CT 06001
860-674-8839
Fax: 860-676-0275

Nancy Ralston, Manager

Provides remunerative work. Post acute rehabilitation programs and facility.

6700 **Gaylord Hospital**
Gaylord Farm Road
P.O. Box 400
Wallingford, CT 06492-7048
203-284-2800
866-429-5673
Fax: 203-284-2894
TTY: 203-284-2700
lcrispino@gaylord.org
www.gaylord.org

James Cullen, President

Works to restore ability and build courage. Offers rehabilitation care with one goal in mind: to help patients return to their homes, communities and jobs.

6701 **Hockanum Greenhouse**
Hockanum Industry
290 Middle Tpke
Storrs Mansfield, CT 06268-2908
860-429-6697
Fax: 860-429-7496

Christopher Campbell, Manager
Beth Chaty, Director
Betsy Treiber, Director

A non profit agency that strives to provide gainful employment, training, support and retirement services for developmentally disabled individuals through the dignity of work, community interaction and structured activities.

6702 **Kuhn Employment Oppurtunities**
1630 North Colony Road
P.O. Box 941
Meriden, CT 06450
203-235-2583
860-347-5843
www.kuhngroup.org

Paul O'Sullivan, Chairperson
Mark DuPuis, Vice Chairperson
John J. Ausanka III, Treasurer
James Anderson, Secretary

Kuhn is committed to developing quality skill enhancement programs which provide meaningful employment for persons with disabilities so that they will become independentm gain self-esteem, and be accepted by the community. Our vision is that all individuals have the ability to fully participate in the community through work. Kuhn believes that all participants have a right to integrated community employment.

6703 **Norwalk Hospital Section Of Physical Medicine And Rehabilitation**
34 Maple Street
Norwalk, CT 06856
203-852-2000
Fax: 800-789-4584

Diane M. Allison, Chair
Edward A. Kangas, Vice Chair
Andrew J. Whittingham, Treasurer
Barbara Butler, Secretary

A 25 bed inpatient Rehabilitation Unit. This CARF and JCAHO accredidted rehab unit is located on the 8th floor of Norwalk Hospital. The focus of the rehab unit is to restore lost function and assist patients in returning to the community. Who have recently experienced a life changing medical event. The progam is tailored to meet individual therapy needs and address activities of daily living. Family and caregiver participation in the program is welcomed and encouraged.

6704 **Rehabilitation Associates, Inc.**
1931 Black Rock Tpke
Fairfield, CT 06825-3506 203-384-8681
Fax: 203-384-0956
info@rehabassocinc.com
www.rehabilitationassociatesinc.com
Carol Landsman, Director
A comprehensive outpatient rehabilitation facility offering physical therapy, occupational therapy, speech-language pathology, clinical social work services and nutritional services to all age groups. Facility locations in Fairfield, Stratford, Milford, Shelton and Westport.

6705 **Reliance House**
40 Broadway
Norwich, CT 06360-5702 860-887-6536
Fax: 860-885-1970
reliancehouse.org
Jack Malone, President
Jackie Falman, Vice President
Sam Bliven, Secretary
Raul Walker, Treasurer
A residential vocational and recreational support network. An active and productive clubhouse where people with mental illness can gain skills, strength and self-esteem.

6706 **Yale New Haven Health System-Bridgeport Hospital**
789 Howard Avenue
New Haven, CT 06519 203-384-3000
www.yalenewhavenhealth.org
Marna P. Borgstrom, President and CEO
Richard D'Aquila, Executive Vice President
Peter N. Herbert, MD, Senior VP, Medical Affairs
Kevin Myatt, Senior VP of Human Resources
Medical services are provided by physicians who are specialists in physical medicine and rehabilitation. The physical therapy department provides a variety of services and utilizes sophisticated modalities to restore and reinforce physical abilities.

Delaware

6707 **Alfred I DuPont Hospital for Children**
Division of Rehabilitation
1600 Rockland Road,
PO Box 269
Wilmington, DE 19803-269 302-651-4000
888-533-3543
Fax: 302-651-4055
infodupont@nemours.org
www.nemours.org
William G. Mackenzie, MD, Chair
David J. Bailey, President and Chief Executive Officer
Robert D. Bridges, Executive Vice President, Enterprise Services/Chief Financia
Roy Proujansky, Executive Vice President, Health Operations and Chief Operat
The hospital is a division of Nemours, which operates one of the nations largest subspecialty group practices devoted to pediatric patient care, teaching, and research. A 180-bed hospital that offers all the specialties of pediatric medicine, surgery, and dentistry in a spacious, comfortable, and family focused facility.

6708 **Community Systems Inc.**
2 Penns Way
Suite 301
New Castle, DE 19720 302-325-1500
Fax: 302-325-1505
communitysystems.org
David Paige, Executive Director
Amy Yento, Chair
A 4 state family of non-profit, tax exempt corporations whose mission is helping persons with disabilities to find happiness in their own homes, in their personal relationships, and as contributing members of their community.

6709 **DDDS/Georgetown Center**
5 Academy St
Georgetown, DE 19947-1915 302-856-5366
Fax: 302-856-5305
dhss.delaware.gov/dhss

6710 **Delaware Association for the Blind**
2915 Newport Gap Pike
Landis Lodge Building
Wilmington, DE 19808 302-998-5913
888-777-3925
Fax: 302-691-5810
dabdel.org
Janet L. Berry, Executive Director
Ken Rolph, President
Jennifer Smith, Secretary
Robert Mosch, Treasurer
A private, nonprofit organization that offers adjustment to blindness counseling, recreation activities, summer camps and financial assistance for the legally blind. The staff includes five full time, nine part time and twelve seasonal. Operates a store selling items for the blind.

6711 **Delaware Veterans Center**
810 Vermont Avenue
Washington, DC 20420 302-994-2511
800-273-8255
Fax: 302-633-5591
Slaon D Gibson, Acting Secretary of Veterans Affairs
Jose D Riojas, Chief of Staff
Richard J Griffin, Acting Inspector General
A 60-bed hospital and 60-bed NHCU, both accredited by the Joint Commission on Accreditation of Healthcare Organizations with a VBA Regional Office and 2 Vet Centers (one on campus) offering veterans the unique opportunity to obtain heathcare, benefits services, and Readjustment Counseling at one location. The center provides a wide spectrum of primary and tertiary acute and extended care inpatient and outpatient activities an an academic setting..

6712 **Easterseals Delaware & Maryland's Eastern Shore**
61 Corporate Cir.
New Castle, DE 19720 302-324-4444
Fax: 302-324-4441
www.easterseals.com/de
Kenan J. Sklenar, President & CEO
Pamela Reuther, Chief Operating Officer
Manuel Arencibia, Vice President, Development
Samuel L. Winder, III, Vice President, Finance & Administration
Provides services to ensure that all people with disabilities or special needs and their families have equal opportunities to live, learn, work and play in their communities.

6713 **Edgemoor Day Program**
500 Duncan Rd
Wilmington, DE 19809-2369 302-762-9077
Fax: 302-762-1652
www.dhss.delaware.gov/dhss/main/maps/other/ed
Scott Borino, Executive Director
Carol Koyste, Manager, Finance & Administratio
Brandon Furrowh, Director, Recreation & Youth Pro
Avani Patel, Administrative Assistant
Our mission is providing affordable and accessible services which help improve the quality of life for community members of all ages through a broad range of educational, recreational, self-enrichment, and family support services. ECC is a not-for-profit, community-based, multi-service agency located just north of Wilmington. We provide a broad range of educational, recreational, self-enrichment, and family support services.

6714 **Elwyn Delaware**
321 E 11th St.
Wilmington, DE 19801-3417 302-658-8860
info@elwyn.org
elwyn.org
Charles S. McLister, President & CEO, Elwyn
Provides work training, job placement and supported employment, and elder care services.

6715 **First State Senior Center**
291a N Rehoboth Blvd
Milford, DE 19963-1303 302-422-1510
dhss.delaware.gov/dhss/main/maps/other/dddssr

6716 **Woodside Day Program**
941 Walnut Shade Rd
Dover, DE 19901-7765 302-739-4494
Fax: 302-697-4490
Connie Grace, Supervisor
Joyce Oliver, Manager
.

District of Columbia

6717 **Barbara Chambers Children's Center**
1470 Irving St NW
Washington, DC 20010-2804 202-387-6755
Fax: 202-319-9066
barbarachambers.org
Barbara Chambers, Founder
Mission is to provide comprehensive, quality child care services to the community at large, by offering a variety of opportunities for childrens's intellectual, emotional, social and physical development in a clean, safe, and nurturing environment. Our philosophy is to provide a supportive environment in which children can be children..allowing each child to learn at his/her pace and most of all allowing the child to learn through his/her daily play.

6718 **District of Columbia General Hospital Physical Medicine & Rehab Services**
Room 1358
19th and Mass Ave
Washington, DC 20003 202-727-6055
Fax: 202-675-7819
Dr. Maribel Bieberach, Chairperson PM&R
Dr. Raman Kapur, Staff Physiatrist
Offers comprehensive physical medicine and rehabilitation services including in and outpatient consultations and electrodiagnostic testing; in and outpatient physical and occupational therapy; inpatient recreational therapy, and a multidisciplinary prosthetic clinic which meets once a month..

6719 **George Washington University Medical Center**
George Washington University Medical Center
2150 Pennsylvania Ave NW
Washington, DC 20037-3201 202-741-3000
Fax: 202-741-3183
www.gwdocs.com

6720 **HSC Pediatric Center, The**
1731 Bunker Hill Rd NE
Washington, DC 20017-3026 202-832-4400
800-226-4444
Fax: 202-467-0978
Debbie Zients, CEO
Dr Murry M Pollack, VP, Medical Affairs
Eva Fowler, Media Contact
Provides the highest quality rehabilitative and transitional care for infants, children, adolescents, and young adults with special health care needs and their families in a supportive environment that respects their needs, strengths, vslues and priorities..

6721 **Howard University Child Development Center**
1911 5th St NW
Washington, DC 20001-2314 202-797-8134
Fax: 202-986-6580
Connie Siler, Manager
Offers children with developmental problems diagnosis, treatment, evaluation and follow along visits..

6722 **Psychiatric Institute of Washington**
4228 Wisconsin Ave NW
Washington, DC 20016-2138 202-885-5600
800-369-2273
Fax: 202-885-5614
Ken Courage, Chairman
Carol Desjuns, Chief Operations Officer
Howard Hoffman, Executive Medical Director
Aarti Subramanian, VP/Chief Financial Off
Psychiatric intensive care, crisis intervention, adult day treatment, drug treatment and other services to children and adults who have psychiatric and chemical dependency problems.

6723 **Spina Bifida Program of Children's National Medical Center**
Children's National Medical Center
111 Michigan Ave. NW
Washington, DC 20010 202-476-5000
888-884-2327
childrensnational.org
Kurt Newman, President & CEO
Mark Batshaw, Executive Vice President & Physician-in-Chief
Denice Cora-Bramble, Chief Medical Officer
Aldwin Lindsay, Chief Financial Officer
Provides care and treatment for infants, children and youth with spina bifida of all forms, including spina bifida occulta, meningocele, and myelomeningocele.

Florida

6724 **Bayfront Rehabilitation Center**
Bayfront Medical Center
701 6th St S
St Petersburg, FL 33701-4814 727-823-1234
www.bayfrontstpete.com
Kathryn Gillette, President and CEO
Eric Smith, Chief Financial Officer
Lavah Lowe, Chief Operating Officer
Karen Long, Chief Nursing Executive
Bayfront Medical Center has an Inpatient Rehabilitation Hospital and two outpatient rehabilitation clinics that each provide progressive, comprehensive, individualized treatment. Specialized care in Physiatry (physical medicine), rehab nursing, occupational therapy, speech language pathology, recreational therapy, patient/family services and psychology is tailored to each patient from admission to community and/or school reintegration.

6725 **Brain Injury Rehabilitation Center Dr. P. Phillips Hospital**
Brain Injury Rehabilitation Center Dr. P. Phillips
9400 Turkey Lake Rd
Orlando, FL 32819-8001 407-351-8580
Shannon Elswick, President
Linda Chapin, Chairman
Mark Swanson, Chief Quality Officer
John Hillenmeyer, CEO Emeritus, Orlando Health
Dedicated to restoring brain injured patients with rehabilitation potential to their highest level of functioning. This is accomplished through an interdisciplinary team demonstrating personal responsibility to the patient, their family and each other.

6726 **Brooks Memorial Hospital Rehabilitation Center**
3599 University Blvd. South
Jacksonville, FL 32207-6215 904-858-7600
Fax: 904-858-7619
louise.spierre@brookshealth.org
www.brookshealth.org
Douglas Baer, Chief Executive Officer/ Preside
Holly Morris, Director, Brooks Rehabilitation
Louise Spierre, Medical Director
Floris Singletary, Research Manager, Clinical Resea
An entire care facility featuring five day inpatient evaluation, pre-operative evaluation programs, five week pain management program, referral criteria and treatment goals, therapy services, psychological services and more to the physically challenged.

6727 **Center for Pain Control and Rehabilitation**
Ste 607
2780 Cleveland Ave
Fort Myers, FL 33901-5858 239-337-4332
Mary Bonnette, Owner
.

6728 **Comprehensive Rehabilitation Center at Lee Memorial Hospital**
2776 Cleveland Ave
Fort Myers, FL 33901-5864 239-343-2000
leememorial.org
James R. Nathan, Chief Executive Officer System P
Larry Antonucci, Chief Operating Officer
Jon Cecil, Chief Human Resources Officer
Mike German, Chief Financial Officer
Lee Memorial hospital has achieved national recognition as one of the top 100 hospitals for stroke, orthopedics, and Intensive Care Unit (ICU) It is a 367 bed hospital that provides 24-hour emergency and trauma care, inpatient rehabilitation, orthopedics, neuroscience, trauma, cancer, diabetes, digestive, general surgery, urology, endocrinology, gastroenterology, opthamology, and many others.

6729 **Comprehensive Rehabilitation Center of Naples Community Hospital**
350 7th Street North
Naples, FL 34102 239-436-5000
Fax: 239-436-5250
www.nchmd.org
Allen S. Weiss, CEO
Mariann MacDonald, Chairman
Thomas Gazdic, Chairman/Treasurer
John Lewis, Secretary
Offers rehabilitation services, inpatient and outpatient care at 5 locations in the county and more for the benefit of the disabled.

6730 **Conklin Center for the Blind**
405 White St
Daytona Beach, FL 32114-2999 386-258-3441
Fax: 386-258-1155
info@conklincenter.org
www.conklincenter.org
Robert T Kelly, Executive Director
The Conklin Center's mission is to empower children and adults who are blind and have one or more additional disabilities to develop their potential to be able to obtain competitive employment, live independently and fully participate in community life.

6731 **Davis Center for Rehabilitation Baptist Hospital of Miami**
8900 N Kendall Dr
Miami, FL 33176-2118 786-596-1960
corporatepr@baptisthealth.net
www.baptisthealth.net/bhs
Brian E. Keeley, President and Chief Executive Of
Calvin Babcock, Chairman
A full-service, nonprofit community hospital providing a full range of inpatient and outpatient rehabilitation services. The overall commitment to excellence has extended to this specialized field. Access to medical expertise and services ensures that the best in medical resources are available should an unforeseen medical problem arise.

6732 **Devereux Advanced Behavioral Health Florida - Titusville Campus**
1850 S. Deleon Ave.
Titusville, FL 32780 407-473-5238
800-338-3738
referral@devereux.org
www.devereuxfl.org
Gwendolyn B Skinner, Vice President of Operations
Dave Detro, Human Resource Director
Carlos F Pozzi-Montero, Psy.D, Clinical Director
Lindsey Phillips, Director of External Affairs
The Devereux Florida Titusville Campus offers a variety of residential, foster care and community support services for youth with behavioral and intellectual/developmental disabilities. Services include a residential group home with private rooms and a therapeutic group home.

6733 **Devereux Advanced Behavioral Health - Florida**
Devereux Florida Corporate Office
5850 T.G. Lee Blvd.
Suite 400
Orlando, FL 32822 407-362-9210
800-338-3738
referral@devereux.org
www.devereuxfl.org
Gwendolyn B Skinner, Vice President of Operations
Dave Detro, Human Resource Director
Carlos F Pozzi-Montero, Psy.D, Clinical Director
Lindsey Phillips, Director of External Affairs
Offering care for children with mental health, behavioral, intellectual and developmental disabilities and challenges. Some services offered include a psychiatric program, community based group homes, foster care, counseling centers, case management, abuse and neglect prevention services, community-based care and outreach programs.

6734 **Devereux Florida - Orlando Campus**
Devereux Orlando Campus
6147 Christian Way
Orlando, FL 32808 407-296-5300
800-338-3738
referral@devereux.org
www.devereuxfl.org
Gwendolyn B Skinner, Vice President of Operations
Dave Detro, Human Resource Director
Carlos F Pozzi-Montero, Psy.D, Clinical Director
Lindsey Phillips, Director of External Affairs
The Orlando Campus provides intensive residential services for children and adolescents who suffer from emotional, behavioral and psychological problems. Programs offered include Devereux's Statewide Inpatient Psychiatric Program (SIPP), Residential Group Care and the Residential Treatment Center.

6735 **Devereux Florida - Viera Campus**
Devereux Viera Campus
8000 Devereux Dr.
Viera, FL 32940 321-242-9100
800-338-3738
Fax: 321-259-0786
vischool@devereux.org
www.devereuxfl.org
Gwendolyn B Skinner, Vice President of Operations
Dave Detro, Human Resource Director
Carlos F Pozzi-Montero, Psy.D, Clinical Director
Lindsey Phillips, Director of External Affairs
The campus offers two residential programs for youth with developmental or behavioral challenges: the Intensive Residential Treatment Center (IRTC) and the Intellectual/Developmental Disabilities (I/DD) Program. The Viera Campus also offers six residential units and the Devereux School.

6736 **Devereux Threshold Center for Autism**
Threshold Center For Autism
3550 N Goldenrod Rd
Winter Park, FL 32792 407-671-7060
800-338-3738
Fax: 407-671-6005
referral@devereux.org
www.devereuxfl.org
Gwendolyn B Skinner, Vice President of Operations
Dave Detro, Human Resource Director
Carlos F Pozzi-Montero, Psy.D., Clinical Director
Lindsey Phillips, Director of External Affairs
The Devereux Threshold Center for Autism includes a therapeutic residential program and an adult day treatment program for people with intellectual/developmental disabilities.

6737 **Division of Blind Services**
325 West Gaines Street
Suite 1114
Turlington Building, FL 32399-0400
850-245-0300
800-342-1828
Fax: 850-245-0386
ana.saint-ford@dbs.fldoe.org
dbs.myflorida.com
Aleisa McKinlay, Interim Director
Phyllis Vaughn, Bureau Chief, Administrative Services
William Findley, Bureau Chief, Business Enterprise Program
Edward Hudson, Bureau Chief of the Rehabilitation Center for the Blind and
Serves the totally blind, legally blind, visually impaired, deaf-blind, learning disabled, and more by offering health, counseling, educational, recreational and computer training services.

6738 **Easterseals Northeast Central Florida**
1219 Dunn Ave.
Daytona Beach, FL 32114
386-255-4568
877-255-4568
Fax: 386-258-7677
TTY: 386-310-1157
www.easterseals.com/necfl
Bev Johnson, President & CEO
Melissa Chesley, Vice President, Finance & CFO
Susan B. Moor, Vice President, Philanthropy
Dorothy Lefford, Vice President, Clinical Services
Provides services for individuals with physical, intellectual, and other disabilities.

6739 **Easterseals South Florida**
1475 NW 14th Ave.
Miami, FL 33125
305-325-0470
Fax: 305-325-0578
www.easterseals.com/southflorida
Maurice Woods, President & CEO
Barry R. Vogel, Chief Administrative Officer
Maher Malak, Chief Financial Officer
Marta Quintana, Vice President, Development
The mission of Easterseals South Florida is to provide services to ensure that all children and adults with disabilities or special needs and their families have equal opportunities to live, learn, work and play in their communities.

6740 **Easterseals Southwest Flordia**
Sarasota, FL 34243-2001
941-355-7637
themeadowscup.com

6741 **Easterseals Southwest Florida**
350 Braden Ave.
Sarasota, FL 34243
941-355-7637
Fax: 941-358-3069
www.easterseals-swfl.org
Tom Waters, President & CEO
Patrick Ryan, Chief Operating Officer
George Pfeiffer, Vice President, Government Relations
Linda Poteat-Brown, Director, Human Resources
Provides services to children and adults with physical, neurological and communications disabilities and their families.

6742 **Florida CORF**
Columbia Medical Center: Peninsula
John Feore, Executive VP
Sandra Trovato, Executive Director
Offers Medicare authorized therapy programs for seniors, disabled and others who need rehabilitation. CORF can provide coordinated and extended services in the home after a hospital stay, or when physical status changes. Patients who are treated at CORF, include amputations, arthritis, chronic/acute pain, depression/anxiety, nerve injury, sports injury, stroke and swallowing problems.

6743 **Florida Institute Of Rehabilitation Education (FIRE)**
3071 Highland Oaks Terrace
Tallahassee, FL 32301-4876
850-942-3658
888-827-6033
Fax: 850-942-4518
info@lighthousebigbend.org
Barbara Ross, Executive Director
Evelyn Worley, Assistant Director
Wayne Warner, Vocational Program Director
Toni King, Independent Living Specialist
Provides independent living and vocational rehabilitation services to Florida residents who are legally blind. Services include instruction in orientation and mobility, accessible technology, daily living skills and employability skills. Information, referral and counseling services are also offered. All services are provided without charge.

6744 **Florida Institute for Neurologic Rehabilitation, Inc**
1962 Vandolah Road
P O Box 1348
Wauchula, FL 33873-1348
863-773-2857
800-697-5390
Fax: 863-773-0867
finr.net
John Richards, Administrator
Stephanie Ortiz, RN, Director of Nursing
Kevin E. O'Keefe, Program Director
Dana Lucas, Director of Nursing
A residential rehabilitation facility providing a therapeutic environment in which children, adolescents and adults who have survived head-injury can develop the independence and skills necessary to re-enter the community.

6745 **Fort Lauderdale Veterans Medical Center**
713 NE 3rd Ave
Fort Lauderdale, FL 33304-2619
954-356-7926
Fax: 954-356-7609
www.va.gov/directory/guide/
Robert White, Executive Director
Sloan D Gibson, Acting Secretary
Jose D Riojas, Chief of Staff
Richard J Griffin, Acting Inspector General
Veterans medical clinic offering disabled veterans medical treatments.

6746 **Halifax Hospital Medical Center Eye Clinic Professional Center**
308 Farmington Avenue
Farmington, CT 06032
860-658-4388
888-444-3598
webmaster@evariant.com
www.evariant.com
Bill Moschella, CEO
Rob Grant, Executive Vice President
Michael Clark, Chief Operating Officer
James Orsillo, Chief Financial Officer
Offers services for the totally blind, legally blind, visually impaired, and more with health, counseling, educational, recreational, rehabilitation, computer training and professional training services.

6747 **HealthQuest Subacute and Rehabilitation Programs**
Regenta Park
8700 a C Skinner Pkwy
Jacksonville, FL 32256-836
Fax: 904-641-7896

6748 **HealthSouth Emeral Coast Sports & Rehabilitation Center**
1847 Florida Avenue
Panama City, FL 32405-3730
850-784-4878
Fax: 850-769-7566
www.healthsouthpanamacity.com
Tony Bennett, CEO
Michelle Miller, Manager
Outpatient sports medicine and rehabilitation center providing physical therapy, occupational therapy, industrial rehab, work hardening/work simulation, worksite and ergonomic analysis, FCE's, work assessment and pre-employment goals of returning the clients back to work, and returning to all recreational, sports and functional activities safely..

6749 **HealthSouth Rehabilitation Hospital of Tallahassee**
Healthsouth Corporation
1675 Riggins Rd
Tallahassee, FL 32308-5315 850-656-4800
www.healthsouthtallahassee.com
Heath Phillips, Chief Executive Officer
Robert Robert Rowland, Medical Director
Tom Abbruscato, Controller
Deborah Baird, Director of Quality and Risk Man
North Florida's sole acute rehabilitation hospital between Jacksonville \, Panama City, and Gainesville. With 250 employees providing a full continuum of care form its 70 bed facility, the hospital is accredited by JCAHO, CARF and state designated and certified by Vocational Rehabilitation for traumatic brain injury, as well as a wide variety of other diagnoses. With the addition of our outpatients, the facility has served the greater community by touching the lives of over 50,000 patients.

6750 **HealthSouth Rehabilitation Hospital Of Miami**
20601 Old Cutler Rd
Miami, FL 33189-2441 305-251-3800
www.healthsouthmiami.com
Elizabeth Izquierdo, Chief Executive Officer
Angelo Appio, Director of Marketing Operations
Reyna M. Hernandez, Chief Financial Officer
Paige Keil, Director of Quality and Risk Man
A comprehensive source of medical rehabilitation services for Pinellas County, Florida area residents, their families and their physicians. Offers the people of Florida all the clinical, technical and professional resources of the nation's leading provider of comprehensive rehabilitation care.

6751 **HealthSouth Rehabilitation Hospital of Sarasota**
Health South Corporation in Burmingham Alabama
6400 Edgelake Drive
Sarasota, FL 34240-8813 941-921-8600
866-330-5822
www.healthsouthsarasota.com
Marcus Braz, Chief Executive Officer
Alexander DeJesus, Medical Director
Nancy Arnold, Director of Marketing Operations
Brenda Benner, Director of Human Resources
HealthSouth Rehabilitation Hospital of Sarasota is a 96-bed inpatient rehabilitation hospital that offers comprehensive inpatient rehabilitation services designed to return patients to leading active and independent lives.

6752 **HealthSouth Sea Pines Rehabilitation Hospital**
Sea Pines Rehabilitation Hospital
101 E Florida Ave
Melbourne, FL 32901-8398 321-984-4600
Fax: 321-952-6532
www.healthsouthseapines.com
Stuart Miller, Medical Director
Denise McGrath, Chief Executive Officer
Donna Anderson, Director of Human Resources
Jerry Bishop, Director of Quality and Risk Man
Designed to return patients to leading active, independent lives, HealthSouth Sea Pines Rehabilitation Hospital is a 90-bed rehabilitation hospital that provides a higher level of comprehensive rehabilitation services.

6753 **Holy Cross Hospital**
Catholic Southwest
4725 North Federal Hwy
Fort Lauderdale, FL 33308-4668 954-771-8000
www.holy-cross.com
Patrick Taylor, President & Chief Executive Offi
Luisa Gutman, Senior Vice President & Chief Op
Linda Wilford, Senior Vice President & Chief Fi
Kenneth Homer, Chief Medical Officer & Medical
Holy Cross Hospital in Fort Lauderdale is a full-service, non-profit Catholic hospital, sponsored by the Sisters of Mercy. Holy Cross is a US News & World Report 'Best Hospital' and HealthGrades Distinguished Hospital for Clinical Excellence, 2004 and 2005

6754 **Lee Memorial Hospital**
2776 Cleveland Ave
Fort Myers, FL 33901-5855 239-343-2000
www.leememorial.org
Sanford Cohen, Chairman
Chris Hansen, Vice Chairman
David Collins, Treasurer
Diane Champion, Secretary
Offers a complete inpatient program of intensive rehabilitation designed to restore a patient to a more independent level of functioning. The comprehensive care includes medical rehabilitation and training for spinal cord injury, brain injury, stroke and neurological disorders.

6755 **Lighthouse for the Blind of Palm Beach**
1710 Tiffany Drive East
West Palm Beach, FL 33407-3224 561-586-5600
Fax: 561- 84- 80
lighthousepalmbeaches.org
Marvin A. Tanck, President and CEO
Dont, Mickens, Chair
John R. Banister, Vice Chairman
David B. Cano, MD
A private, non-profit rehabilitation and education agency in its 55th year of service. Offers programs to assist persons who areblind or visually impaired, an on-site Industrial Center, a technology training center, an Aids and appliances Store, special equipment grant programs, outreach services for children and adults, Early Intervention and Preschool Services, and a variety of support groups. These programs provide services and education for blind children and their parents.

6756 **Lighthouse for the Visually Impaired and Blind**
8610 Galen Wilson Blvd
Port Richey, FL 34668-5974 727-815-0303
866-962-5254
Fax: 727-815-0203
lighthouse@lvib.org
www.lvib.org
Sylvia Stinson-Perez, Executive Director
Dr. John Mann, President
Melissa M. Suess, Orientation and Mobility Instruc
Peter James, Business Development Specialist
The Lighthouse offers services for visually impaired or blind adults and children ages 0-5 years old. Counseling, educational services, recreational services, rehabilitation, computer training and support groups.

6757 **MacDonald Training Center**
5420 W Cypress Street
Tampa, FL 33607-1706 813-870-1300
866-948-6184
Fax: 813-872-6010
TTY: 813-873-7631
macdonaldcenter.org
Jim Freyvogel, President/CEO
Judith DeStasio, CFO
Debi Hamilton, Director of Services
Joe Donato, COO
A private, non-profit, community-based human services organization serving adults with disabilities (since 1953). Persons are provided the opportunity to achieve their highest potential through the Center's various programs that include day training, employment, community living and various support services.

6758 **Medicenter of Tampa**
4411 North Habana Avenue
Tampa, FL 33614-7211 813-872-2771
Fax: 813-871-2831
rehabilitationandhealthcarecenteroftampa.com
Dan Davis, President
Mariluz G, Social Services Director
Brenda Pace, Secretary
Hilda B, Medicaid Coordinator
Postacute rehabilitation program. A 174 bed non-profit facility with postacute reahbilitation programs..

6759 Miami Heart Institute Adams Building
4300 Alton Rd
Miami Beach, FL 33140-2997 305-674-2121
www.msmc.com
Steven D. Sonenreich, President/CEO
The mission is to provide high quality health care to our diverse community enhanced through teaching, research, charity care and financial responsibility.

6760 Miami Lighthouse for the Blind
601 SW 8th Ave
Miami, FL 33130-3200 305-856-2288
Fax: 305-285-6967
info@miamilighthouse.com
miamilighthouse.org
Virginia A. Jacko, President & Chief Executive Officer
Sharon Caughill, Special Projects Manager
Jeannie Reinoso, Executive Assistant
Arnie Paniagua, Chief Financial Officer
Offers services for the legally blind and severely visually impaired (including those who are developmentally delayed) of all ages in the areas of counseling and educational, recreational, rehabilitation, computer and vocational training services.

6761 Mount Sinai Medical Center Rehabilitation Unit
4300 Alton Rd
Miami Beach, FL 33140-2997 305-674-2121
www.msmc.com
Steven D. Sonenreich, President/CEO
A comprehensive inpatient and outpatient rehabilitation programs have been helping patients recover for more then 20 years. Fully customized treatment plans based on the needs of each patient is 1 reason why our services are among the best in South Florida. Our team approach takes into account the medical, physical, psychological, social, spiritual, cultural and economic needs of patients and their families.

6762 Neurobehavioral Medicine Center
Ste 1
4821 Us Highway 19
New Port Richey, FL 34652-4259 727-849-2005
Fax: 727-849-2087
Otsenre Matos, Medical Director
Gerard Taylor PhD, Counseling/Stress Management
Donna Taylor RN, Manager
Joyce Park Matos ARNP, Clinical Specialist
A multidisciplinary outpatient program for the evaluation and treatment of chronic pain. Consultation services for hospitalized patients are also provided upon request. Comprehensive treatment of individuals with closed traumatic brain injuries..

6763 North Broward Rehab Unit
North Broward Medical Center
201 E Sample Rd
Deerfield Beach, FL 33064-3596 954-941-8300
www.browardhealth.org
Douglas Ford, Chiefs of Staff
Pauline Grant, Chief Executive Officer
CARF accredited, 30-bed inpatient rehabilitation unit treating adults with brain injuries, spinal cord injuries, stroke, orthopedic and neurologic injuries.

6764 Northwest Medical Center
Health Care Corporation of America
2801 North State Road 7
Margate, FL 33063-5727 954-974-0400
866-256-7720
northwestmed.com
Mark Rader, CEO
Above all else, we are committed to the care and improvement of human life. In recognition of this commitment, we strive to deliver high quality, cost effective healthcare in the communities we serve. We recognize and affirm the unique and intrinsic work of each individual. We treat all those we serve with compassion and kindness. We act with absolute honesty, integrity, and fairness in the way we conduct our business and the way we live our lives.

6765 Pain Institute of Tampa
4178 N Armenia Ave
Tampa, FL 33607-6429 813-875-5913
John E Barsa, Founder & MD
Offers a comprehensive and multidisciplinary approach to pain controll and management. Most services are provided on-site but other services may require you to be referred elswhere. We will monitor and coordinate your care in a manner to provide optimal recovery potential.

6766 Pain Treatment Center, Baptist Hospital of Miami
8900 N Kendall Dr
Miami, FL 33176-2118 786-596-1960
corporatepr@baptisthealth.net
www.baptisthealth.net
Calvin Babcock, Chairman
Brian E. Keeley, President and Chief Executive Of
Since 1960, Baptist Hospital of Miami has been one of the most respected medical centers in South Florida. The hospitals full range of medical and technological services is the natural choice for a growing number of people throughout the world.

6767 Pine Castle
4911 Spring Park Rd
Jacksonville, FL 32207-7496 904-733-2650
Fax: 904-733-2681
info@pinecastle.org
pinecastle.org
Jonathan May, Executive Director
Randall Duncan, Associate Executive Director
Leigh Griffin, Director of Finance
Cliff Evans, Director of Development
Provides remunerative work, training, community employment and community living options for adults with developmental disabilities.

6768 Polk County Association for Handicapped Citizens
1038 Sunshine Dr E
Lakeland, FL 33801-6338 863-858-2252
Fax: 863-665-2330
Kecia Howell, Owner
Anthony J. Senzamici Jr., 1st Vice Chairman
Carol N. Asbill, 2nd Vice Chairman
A private non-profit organization that provides an adult day training program to people with developmental disabilities and is under the direction of a volunteer board of directors. The primary goal for our services is to provide people with knowledge and practical experience to be independent adults so they can become contributing members of their community..

6769 Quest, Inc.
PO Box 531125
Orlando, FL 32853 407-218-4300
888-807-8378
Fax: 407-218-4301
contact@questinc.org
www.questinc.org
John Gill, President & CEO
Brooke Eakins, Chief Operating Officer
Todd Thrasher, Chief Financial Officer
John Dogaer, Chief Information Officer
Quest helps individuals with developmental disabilities in Central Florida achieve their goals by providing services that increase their capabilities and quality of life. Quest serves more than 1,000 individuals each day in the Orlando and Tampa areas.

6770 Quest, Inc. - Tampa Area
3910 US Hwy. 301 N
Tampa, FL 33619 813-423-7700
888-807-8378
Fax: 813-423-7701
contact@questinc.org
www.questinc.org
John Gill, President & CEO
Brooke Eakins, Chief Operating Officer
Todd Thrasher, Chief Financial Officer
John Dogaer, Chief Information Officer
Quest helps individuals with developmental disabilities in Central Florida achieve their goals by providing services that increase their capabilities and quality of life. Quest serves more than 1,000 individuals each day in the Orlando and Tampa areas.

6771 **Rehabilitation Center for Children and Adults**
300 Royal Palm Way
Palm Beach, FL 33480-4305
561-655-7266
Fax: 561-655-3269
info@rcca.org
rcca.org

John C. Whelton, Chairman
Jacob L. Lochner, Co-Chairman
Christopher Adams, MD

A private, nonprofit organization whose purpose is to improve physical function, independence and communication of people with physical disabilities. Any child or adult with a physical or speech disability is eligible for services.

6772 **Renaissance Center**
3599 University Blvd
Suite 604
Jacksonville, FL 32216- 9249
904-399-0905
Fax: 904-743-5109
www.obiplasticsurgery.com/index.php

Lewis Obi, MD

6773 **Rosomoff Comprehensive Pain Center, The**
5200 NE 2nd Avenue
Miami, FL 33137-2706
305-532-7246
Fax: 305-534-3974

Elsayed Abdel-Moty, Director
Hubert Rossomoff, Owner

A state-of-the-art Center of Excellence offering inpatient, outpatient, outpatient rehabilitation services and seniors programs. The Center became an internationally renowned model for the evalutation and treatment of all persons seeking pain relief.

6774 **Sarasota Memorial Hospital/Comprehensive Rehabilitation Unit**
1700 S Tamiami Trail
Sarasota, FL 34239-3509
941-917-9000
Fax: 941-917-2211
www.smh.com

Marguerite G Malone, Chair
Gregory Carter, First Vice Chair
Alex Miller, Second Vice Chair
Joseph J. DeVirgilio, Jt. Treasurer

The goal of the 34-bed Comprehensive Rehabilitation Unit (CRU) is to increase patient functional independence, adjust to illness or disability and successfully return to the community. The unit is dedicated to patients who have experienced conditions such

6775 **Strive Physical Therapy Centers**
2620 SE Maricamp RD
Ocala, FL 34471-4517
352-732-8868
Fax: 352-732-8890
www.striverehab.com

R W Shutes, Owner
Johanna Solbato, Administrator
R.W. Shutes, President and CEO

Certified as an Outpatient Rehabilitation Agency, providing a comprehensive approach to patient evaluation and treatment. Our objective is to return our patients back to a productive life as quickly as possible and safely as possible.

6776 **Sunbridge Care and Rehabilitation**
101 East State Street,
Kennett Square, FL 19348-6105
610-444-6350
Fax: 610-925-4000
info@genesishcc.com
www.genesishcc.com

Dan Hirschfeld, President
George V Hager, Chief Executive Officer
Robert A Reitz, Executive Vice President & Chief Operating Officer
Michael Sherman, Senior VP

A comprehensive medical rehabilitation facility that is committed to helping individuals with disabilities improve their quality of life. This is a 120-bed facility offering a full range of acute and sub-acute inpatient programs as well as community-based

6777 **Tampa Bay Academy**
12012 Boyette Rd
Riverview, FL 33569-5631
813-677-6700
800-678-3838
Fax: 813-671-3145
tlamb@tampahope.org
www.tampahope.org

Renee Scott, Chair
Amy McClure, Vice-Chair
Titania Lamb, Executive Director

A psychiatric residential treatment center and partial hospitalization program for ages 7 to 17.

6778 **Tampa General Rehabilitation Center**
1 Tampa General Circle
P.O. Box 1289
Tampa, FL 33606-3571
813-844-7700
866-844-1411
Fax: 813-844-1477
tgh.org

James R. Burkhart, President & CEO
Bruce Zwiebel, Chief Of Staff
Deana L. Nelson, Chief Operating Officer
Steve Short, Cheif Financial Officer

Offers a full range of programs all aimed at helping patients achieve their full potentials. It is one of three centers in the state that provides Driver Training and Evaluation Programs for persons with disabilities, and also an Assisted Reproduction Pro

6779 **Tampa Lighthouse for the Blind**
1106 West Platt Street
Tampa, FL 33606-2142
813-251-2407
Fax: 813-254-4305
tampalighthouse.org

Sheryl Brown, Executive Director

Offers services for the totally blind, legally blind, visually impaired, and more with health, counseling, educational, recreational, rehabilitation, computer training and professional training services.

6780 **The Arc Tampa Bay**
1501 N Belcher Rd.
Suite 249
Clearwater, FL 33765
727-799-3330
Fax: 727-799-4632
thearctb.org

6781 **Visually Impaired Persons of Southwest Florida**
35 W Mariana Ave
North Fort Myers, FL 33903-5515
239-997-7797
Fax: 239-997-8462

Doug Fowler, Executive Director
Margaret Ruhe Lincoln, Director of operations

Provides training in independent living skills, orientation and mobility, counseling, computer and other communication skills, family support groups, peer counseling, socialization and a low vision clinic. Second location in Charlotte County. Phone: 941-6

6782 **West Florida Hospital: The Rehabilitation Institute**
8383 North Davis Hwy
Pensacola, FL 32514-6039
850-494-4000
800-342-1123
Fax: 850-494-4881
www.westfloridahospital.com

Roman S Bautista, President/CEO
Carol Saxton, Senior VP Patient Care Services

A 58-bed comprehensive rehabilitation facility offering inpatient and outpatient services. JCAHO and CARF accredited and a State designed head and spinal cord injury center. CARF accredited programs include: comprehensive inpatient rehab, spinal cord inju

6783 **West Gables Health Care Center**
2525 SW 75th Ave
Miami, FL 33155-2800
305-262-6800
Fax: 888-453-1928
www.westgablesrehabhospital.com

Jose Vargas, Medical Director
Walter Concepcion, Chief Executive Officer
Cesar Sepulveda, Materials Manager
Zely Santos, Admissions Director

Services provide by West Gables Health Center: activities services are provided onsite to residents. Clinical laboratory services are provided, dental, dietary, housekeeping, mental health services, nursing services, occupational therapy, pharmacy, physic

6784 **Willough at Naples**
9001 Tamiami Trail East
Naples, FL 34113-3397
239-775-4500
800-722-0100
Fax: 239-793-0534
info@thewilloughatnaples.com
thewilloughatnaples.com

James O'Shea, President

A licensed psychiatric hospital in Southwest Florida which provides quality management and treatment for eating disorders and chemical dependency in adults.

Georgia

6785 **Annandale Village**
3500 Annandale Ln
Suwanee, GA 30024-2150
770-945-8381
Fax: 770-945-8693
annandale.org

Adam Pomeranz, Chief Executive Officer
Melissa Burton, Chief Financial Officer
Keith Fenton, Chief Development & Marketing Officer
Nancy Trujillo, Chief Operating Officer

Private nonprofit residential facility for adults with developmental disabilities. Located on 124 acres just north of Atlanta. Annandale provides full program and 24 hour residential services, pay program services, respite care and skilled nursing services.

6786 **Atlanta Institute of Medicine and Rehabilitation**
Ste E
2911 Piedmont Rd NE
Atlanta, GA 30305-2782
404-365-0160
Fax: 404-365-0751

Lawrence E Eppelbaum, Founder
Galina Vayner, MD

One of the most famous medical centers in the state of Georgia. The Institute employs more then 40 highly qualified medical professionals and fully equipped with the latest medical equipment. It has gathered recognition and respect from the people of Atla

6787 **Bobby Dodd Institute (BDI)**
2120 Marietta Blvd NW
Atlanta, GA 30318-2122
678-365-0071
Fax: 678-365-0098
TTY: 678-365-0099
bobbydodd.org

Rodney Hall, Chair
Christopher Rosselli, Vice Chair
Wayne McMillan, President & CEO
John Ralls, Treasurer

BDI annually serves approximately 400 clients in Atlanta, GA. BDI works primarily with people with developmental disabilities such as autism and down syndrome, but includes clients with physical or acquired disabilities.

6788 **Cave Spring Rehabilitation Center**
Georgia Department of Labor
7 Georgia Ave
P.O. Box 303
Cave Spring, GA 30124-2718
706-777-2341
Fax: 706-777-2366
gvra.georgia.gov/cave-spring-center-contacts-

Russell Fleming, Director
Karen Hulsey, Administrative Operations Coordinator
Renee Lambert, Rehabilitation Assistant
Renaultha Houston, Residential Program Supervisor

6789 **Center for the Visually Impaired**
739 West Peachtree St NW
Atlanta, GA 30308-1137
404-875-9011
Fax: 404-607-0062
cviga.org

Susan Hoy, Chair
Fontaine M. Huey, President
Doreen Zaksheske, Vice President of Finance & Operations
Anisio Correia, Vice President for Programs

Offers services to people of all ages who are blind or visually impaired with training in orientation and mobility, computer technology, activities of daily living, communication skills and employment readiness. A so offers two children's programs, a comm

6790 **Devereux Advanced Behavioral Health Georgia**
Devereux Georgia Treatment Network
1291 Stanley Rd.
Kennesaw, GA 30152
770-427-0147
800-342-3357
Fax: 770-427-4030
info@devereux.org
www.devereuxga.org

Gwendolyn B Skinner, Vice President of Operations
Dave Detro, Human Resource Director
Carlos F Pozzi-Montero, Psy.D, Clinical Director
Lindsey Phillips, Director of External Affairs

Facility offering services to youth with emotional and behavioral health challenges. Services include Intensive Residential Treatment, Foster Care Program, Group Homes, and educational programs.

6791 **Easterseals East Georgia**
1500 Wrightsboro Rd.
Augusta, GA 30904
706-667-9695
Fax: 706-667-8831
www.easterseals.com/eastgeorgia

Lynn Smith, Chief Executive Officer

Easterseals East Georgia assists people with disabilities and other special needs to maximize opportunities for employment, independence and full inclusion into society.

6792 **Georgia Industries for the Blind**
700 Faceville Highway
Bainbridge, GA 39819-218
229-248-2666
Fax: 229-248-2669
gvra.georgia.gov/gib/about-us

James Hughes, Executive Director

Offers services for the totally blind, legally blind, visually impaired, and more with health, counseling, educational, recreational, rehabilitation, computer training and professional training services.

6793 **Hillhaven Rehabilitation**
26 Tower Rd NE
Marietta, GA 30060-6947
770-422-8913
800-526-5782
Fax: 770-425-2085

Leslie Ann Marie Parrish, Case Manager
Valerie Hamilton, Administrator

Routine skilled and subacute medical and rehabilitation care including physical therapy, occupational therapy, speech pathology and therapeutic recreation. Programs include stroke and head injury rehab; orthopedic rehab; complex IV therapy; woundcare; can.

6794 **In-Home Medical Care**
Care Master Medical Services
240 Odell Rd
P.O. Box 278
Griffin, GA 30223-4787
770-227-1264
800-542-8889
Fax: 770-412-0014
caremastermedical.com

Nancy Frederick, VP
Eddie Grogan, Chief Executive Officer

Offers the devoted attention of a professional nurse, the use of I.V. therapies, pain management and provision of medical equipment and supplies right where the patient wants to be.

6795 **Learning Services: Harris House Program**
131 Langley Drive
Suite B
Lawrenceville, GA 30046-4446 404-298-0144
888-419-9955
Fax: 866-491-7396
learningservices.com

Dr. Debra Braunling-McMorrow, President and CEO
Susan Snow, Director of Admissions
Michael Weaver, Chief Development Officer
Jeanne Mack, Chief Financial Officer

Situated in the small, historic district of Stone Mountain, just outside of Atlanta, this 6 bed program is designed to encourage independence while providing appropriate support for each individuals needs. Community-based productive activities are customi

6796 **Pain Control & Rehabilitation Institute of Georgia**
Ste 120
2784 N Decatur Rd
Decatur, GA 30033-5993 404-297-1400
Fax: 404-297-1427

Shulim Spektor, CEO
Anna Britman, Office Manager

Provides pain management for chronic and acute pain resulted from injuries, diseases of muscles and nerve, Reflex Sympathetic Dystrophy, perform disabilities and impairment ratings.

6797 **Savannah Association for the Blind**
214 Drayton Street
Savannah, GA 31401-4021 912-236-4473
Fax: 912-234-9286

Gregory Hodges, President
Robert Falligant, Vice-president
Gary Sadowski, Treasurer
Lula Baker, Secretary

Offers services for the totally blind, legally blind, visually impaired, and more with health, counseling, educational, recreational, rehabilitation, computer training and professional training services.

6798 **Shepherd Center for Treatment of Spinal Injuries**
2020 Peachtree Rd NW
Atlanta, GA 30309-1465 404-352-2020
Fax: 404-350-7479
admissions@shepherd.org
www.shepherd.org

Gary R. Ulicny, President & CEO
David F. Apple, Jr., M.D., Medical Director
Angela Beninga, D.O., Staff Physiatrist
ChiChi Berhane, M.D., MBA, Director, Reconstructive Surgery

Dedicated exclusively to the care of patients with spinal cord injuries and other paralyzing spinal disorders. It serves predominately residents of Georgia and neighboring states as one of the only 14 hospitals designated by the U.S. Department of Educati

6799 **Transitional Hospitals Corporation**
Ste 1000
7000 Central Pkwy NE
Atlanta, GA 30328-4592 770-821-5328
800-683-6868
Fax: 770-913-0015
csins.com

Dean Kozee, Owner
Carolyn Norton, Special Projects Consultant/Broker
Amaury Rentas, Event Insurance/Broker

A national network of intensive care hospitals providing care for patients who suffer from a chronic illness and/or catastrophic accident. The mission is founded on providing quality health care to patients who require highly skilled nursing care and acce.

6800 **Walton Rehabilitation Health System**
1355 Independence Dr
Augusta, GA 30901-1037 706-823-8584
866-492-5866
Fax: 706-724-5752
www.waltonfoundation.net

Robert Taylor, Chair
Dennis Skelley, President/CEO
David Dugan, Treasurer
Brent Smith, Secretary

A 58-bed comprehensive physical rehabilitation hospital offering inpatient and outpatient services. Services offered include: stroke recovery, orthopedic injury, pediatrics, head injury, pain management for chronic pain syndrome, TMJ/Craniofacial pain and

Hawaii

6801 **Rehabilitation Hospital of the Pacific**
226 N Kuakini St
Honolulu, HI 96817-2498 808-531-3511
Fax: 808-566-3411
rehabfoundation@rehabhospital.org
www.rehabhospital.org

John Komeiji, Chair
Glenn O. Sexton, Vice Chair
E. Lynne Madden, Secretary/Treasurer
Timothy J. Roe, President & Chief Executive Officer

The only acute care medical rehabilitation organization serving both Hawaii and the Pacific. For over 52 years, the hospital and its 7 outpatient clinics on Oahu, and Maui and Hawaii have been dedicated to providing comprehensive, cost effective rehabilit

Idaho

6802 **Ashton Memorial Nursing Home and Chemical Dependency Center**
700 N 2nd
Ashton, ID 83420 208-652-7461
Fax: 208-652-7595
ashtonmemorial.com

Sheila Kellogg, Administrator

6803 **Idaho Elks Rehabilitation Hospital**
600 N Robbins Rd
Boise, ID 83702 208-489-4444
Fax: 208-344-8883
info@elksrehab.org
www.elksrehab.org

Joseph P. Caroselli, CEO
Doug Lewis, Chief Financial Officer
Mellisa Honsinger, Chief Operating Officer

A nonprofit hospital serving Idaho and the Pacific Northwest. All inpatient and outpatient programs and services are supervised by the hospital's full-time medical directors whose specialty is physical rehabilitative medicine. Services include: occupation

6804 **Portneuf Medical Center Rehabilitation**
777 Hospital Way
Pocatello, ID 83201-4004 208-239-1000
charlesa@portmed.org
www.portmed.org

Mark Buckalew, Chairman
Michael Nosacka, MD
Dan Ordyna, CEO
John Abreu, Vice President

Provides compassionate, quality health care services needed by the people of eastern Idaho in collaboration with other providers and community resources.

Illinois

6805 **Advocate Christ Hospital and Medical Center**
4440 W 95th St
Oak Lawn, IL 60453-2600 708-684-8000
Fax: 708-684-4440
advocatehealth.com

Jim Skogsbergh, CEO
Bill Santulli, COO
Kate K, Director

A 665-bed, not-for-profit teaching, research and referral medical center in Oak Lawn, Illinois. It also is home to the Advocate Hope Childrens's Hospital, one of the most comprehensive providers of pediatric care in the state. The medical center is a lead

6806 Advocate Christ Medical Center & Advocate Hope Children's Hospital
4440 W 95th St
Oak Lawn, IL 60453-2600
708-684-8000
Fax: 708-684-4440
advocatehealth.com

Kenneth Lukhard, CEO
Darcie Brazel, Market Chief Nurse Executive
Jan McCrea, Rehab Services Director
William Adair MD, Medical Director/Rehab Services

The largest fully integrated not-for-profit health care delivery system in metropolitan Chicago and is recognized as one of the top 10 systems in the country. The mission of Advocate Health Care is to serve the health needs of individuals, families and co

6807 Advocate Illinois Masonic Medical Center
836 W Wellington Ave
Chicago, IL 60657-5147
773-975-1600
www.advocatehealth.com/immc

Jim Skogsbergh, CEO
Ajay V. Maker, MD

Consultation, education, family counseling, parent training in behavior modification techniques offered to developmentally disabled adults.

6808 Alexian Brothers Medical Center
800 Biesterfield Rd
Elk Grove Village, IL 60007-3396
847-437-5500
www.alexian.org

Mark Frey, President/CEO
Tracy Rogers, Senior Vice President and Chief Operating Officer
Paul Belter, Senior Vice President and Chief Financial Officer
Patricia Cassidy, Senior Vice President and Chief Strategy Officer

A threefold mission: Works toward maximizing physical function, enhance independent social skills and optimize communication skills consistent with an individual's ability. The Center helps those disabled by accident or illness achieve a new personal best

6809 Back in the Saddle Hippotherapy Program
Corcoran Physical Therapy
4200 W Peterson Ave
Chicago, IL 60646-6074
312-286-2266
847-604-4145
Fax: 847-673-8895

Julie Naughton, Program Coordinator
Maureen Corcoran, Physical Therapist
Tom Corcoran, Owner

A direct medical treatment used by licensed physical therapists who have a strong treatment background in posture and movement, neuromotor function and sensory processing. The benefits of Hippotherapy are available to individuals with just about any disab

6810 Barbara Olson Center of Hope
3206 N Central Ave
Rockford, IL 61101-1797
815-964-9275
Fax: 815-964-9607
info@b-olsoncenterofhope.org
b-olsoncenterofhope.org

Carm Herman, Executive Director
Pam Sondell, Director of Programs and Services
Pam Carey, Director of Human Resources
Mike Marvell, Director of Business Development

We provide vocational employment, educational and social opportunities for adults with developmental disabilities.

6811 Bartolucci Center, The- ILC Enterprises
6415 Stanley Ave
Berwyn, IL 60402-3130
708-745-5277
Fax: 708-698-5090
www.pillarscommunity.org

Zada Clarke, Chairman
Ann Schreiner, President & CEO
Jennifer Hogberg, Vice Chair
Sheila Eswaran, Secretary

A nonprofit tax exempt private social service agency serving suburban Chicago offering day treatment and vocational counseling to individuals who encountered a pattern of job loss due to emotional problems.

6812 Baxter Healthcare Corporation
1 Baxter Pkwy
Deerfield, IL 60015-4625
224-948-2000
800-422-9837
224-948-1812
Fax: 800-568-5020

Phillip L. Batchelor, Corporate Vice President - Quality and Regulatory Affairs
Jean-Luc Butel, Corporate Vice President - President, International
Robert M. Davis, Corporate Vice President - President, Medical Products
Robert Parkinson Jr, Chairman of the Board and Chief Executive Officer

Baxter International Inc. is a global healthcare company that, through its subsidiaries assists healthcare professionals and their patients with treatment of complex medical conditions including hemophelia, immune disorders, kidney disease, cancer, trauma and other conditions. Baxter applies its expertise in medical devices, pharmaceuticals, and biotechnology to make a meaningful difference in patient's lives.

6813 Beacon Therapeutic Diagnostic and Treatment Center
10650 S Longwood Dr
Chicago, IL 60643-2617
773-881-1005
Fax: 773-881-1164

Susan Reyha-Guerrero, President & CEO
Cheryl Thompson, Deputy CEO
Paul Morley, Chief Operating Officer

Offers community day treatment, education, diagnostic services, family counseling, learning disabled, speech and hearing and psychiatric services.

6814 Blind Service Association
17 N State St
Ste 1050
Chicago, IL 60602-3510
312-236-0808
blindserviceassociation.org

Ann Lousin, President
Linda Schwartz, Executive Vice President
Arthur M. Shapiro, Secretary
John Powen, Treasurer

Offers services for the totally blind, legally blind and visually impaired with reading and recording low vision network, social services, referrals and support groups.

6815 Brentwood Subacute Healthcare Center
T HI Brentwood
5400 W 87th St
Burbank, IL 60459-2913
866-300-3257
www.savaseniorcare.com

Audrey Protrowski, Director Business Development
Jill Sattersield, Administrator
John Walton, CEO

Seeks to help patients and their families through what can be a very emotional decision-making process. We provide guidance and consultation on everything from how to properly choose the facility to providing resources that help you cope with the nature of the decision itself.

6816 Caremark Healthcare Services
2211 Sanders Rd
Northbrook, IL 60062-6128
847-559-4700
800-423-1411
Fax: 847-559-3905
www.caremark.com

Larry J. Merlo, President & CEO
Mark Cosby, Executive Vice President

An 80-service-center network providing services anywhere in the U.S. Offers 24 hour access to nursing and pharmacy services, case management resource centers, HIV/AIDS services, women's health services, transplant care services, nutrition support services

6817 **Centegra Northern Illinois Medical Center**
4209 West Shamrock Lane
Suite B
McHenry, IL 60050-8499
815-759-8017
877-236-8347
Fax: 815-759-8062
www.centegra.org

Michael S. Eesley, CEO
Jason Sciarro, President
David L. Tomlinson, Executive Vice President
Kumar Nathan, MD

Providing rehabilitation services in Lake and McHenry Counties, the Rehabilitation Unit is a complete living environment for up to 15 patients after a debilitating illness of trauma. Various locations offering a multitude of services: PT, OT, speech, HT,

6818 **Center for Comprehensive Services**
Mentor Network
P.O. Box 2825
Carbondale, IL 62902-2825
618-457-4008
800-582-4227
Fax: 618-457-5372
dayna.foreman@thementornetwork.com
mentorabi.com

Bill Duffy, Chief Operating Officer
Michael E. Hofmeister, Vice President
Sean Byrne, Chief Financial Officer

Post-acute rehabilitation services for adults and adolescents with acquired brain injuries. Residential, day-treatment and out-patient services tailored to individual needs.

6819 **Center for Rehabilitation at Rush Presbyterian: Johnston R Bowman Health Center**
1653 W Congress Parkway
Chicago, IL 60612-3833
312-942-5000
Fax: 312-942-3601
TTY: 312-942-2207
teri_sommerfeld@rush.edu
www.rush.edu

Larry J. Goodman, CEO

A 613-bed hospital serving adults and children, the John R. Bowman Health Center and Rush University is home to one of the first medical colleges in the Midwest and one of the nation's top-ranked nursing colleges, as well as graduate programs in allied he

6820 **Center for Spine, Sports & Occupational Rehabilitation**
345 E Superior St
Chicago, IL 60611-2654
312-238-7767
800-354-7342
Fax: 312-238-7709
webmaster@ric.org
www.rehabchicago.org

Joanne C. Smith, President & CEO
Edward B. Case, Executive Vice President
M. Jude Reyes, Chair

Offers evaluation and treatment of patients with acute and sub-acute musculoskeletal and sports injuries. RIC offers different levels of care, including inpatient, day rehabilitation, and outpatients services, according to the special needs of each patient

6821 **Children's Home and Aid Society of Illinois**
125 South Wacker Drive
14th Floor
Chicago, IL 60606-4448
312-424-0200
www.childrenshomeandaid.org

Beverley Sibblies, Chairman
Chris Leahy, Vice-Chairman
Mark Tresnowski, Secretary
David Gookin, Treasurer

Private state-wide. Multi-service, racially integrated staff and client populations. Provides educational, placement and community services for children-at-risk and their families. Advocacy, consultation and follow-up services provided according to our ph

6822 **Clinton County Rehabilitation Center**
1665 North Fourth Street
P O Box 157
Breese, IL 62230- 1791
618-526-8800
Fax: 618-526-2021
info@commlink.org
commlink.org

Wesley A. Gozia, President
Judge Joseph L. Heimann, Vice President
John L. Lengerman, Treasurer
Jerry Albers, Secretary

Provides Adult Day Programs (developmental training, work training, job readiness and job placements); Residentail Programs (CILA Intermittent Care, CILA 24 hour care); Infant Programs (early interventions, early head start); Community Services (specializ

6823 **Continucare, A Service of the Rehab Institute of Chicago**
West Suburban Hospital Medical Center
3 Erie Ct
Oak Park, IL 60302-2519
708-383-6200
800-354-7342
Fax: 312-908-1369

Heidi Asbury MD

We respond to the needs of the whole person: body, mind and spirit. We foster a climate of care, hospitality and a spirit of community. We develop systems and structures that attend to the needs of those at risk of discrimination because of age, gender, lifestyle, ethnic background, religious beliefs or socioeconomic status.

6824 **Delta Center**
1400 Commercial Ave
Cairo, IL 62914-1978
618-734-2665
800-471-7213
Fax: 618-734-1999
deltacenter.org

Lisa Tolbert, Executive Director
Lisa Tholbert, Assistant Executive Director

The Delta Center is a non-profit mental health center, substance abuse counseling facility, and also provides various community services to Alexander and Pulaski County, Illinois. The purpose and mission is to promote, encourage, foster and engage exclusi

6825 **Division of Rehabilitation-Education Services, University of Illinois**
Beckwith Hall
201 E. John Street
Champaign, IL 61820- 6901
217-333-4603
Fax: 217-333-0248
disability@uiuc.edu

Ann Fredricksen, Disability Specialist
Jon Gunderson, Coordinator
Pat Malik, Director
Dennis Cable, Accountant

6826 **Easterseals DuPage and Fox Valley**
830 S Addison Ave.
Villa Park, IL 60181-1153
630-620-4433
Fax: 630-620-1148
info@eastersealsdfvr.org
www.easterseals.com/dfv

Theresa Forthofer, President & CEO
Dave Gardner, Chief Financial Officer
Kathy Moreland, Vice President, Development
Maureen Karwowski, Vice President, Clinical Services

The mission of Easterseals DuPage and Fox Valley is to enable infants, children and adults with disabilities to achieve maximum independence and to provide support to their families. Key services provided include physical, occupational, speech-language, nutrition and assistive technology therapies and audiology services for all ages.

6827 **Easterseals Gilchrist Marchman Child Development Center**
1312 S Racine Ave.
Chicago, IL 60608
312-492-7402
Fax: 312-492-9014
www.easterseals.com

Sara Ray Stoelinga, Chief Executive Officer
Ann O'Malley, Contact

An early childhood and education program for children ages 6 weeks to 5 years. Focuses on social and intellectual development through family-centered education.

6828 **Easterseals Jayne Shover Center**
799 S McLean Blvd.
Elgin, IL 60123
847-742-3264
Fax: 847-742-9436
www.easterseals.com/dfv

Theresa Forthofer, President & CEO
Kimberly Garcia, Contact

A free-standing, comprehensive outpatient rehabilitation center serving children and adults with physical and developmental disabilities.

6829 **Easterseals Joliet Region**
212 Barney Dr.
Joliet, IL 60435
815-725-2194
Fax: 815-725-5150
www.easterseals.com/joliet

Deb Condotti, President & CEO
David Gardner, Chief Financial Officer
Vanessa Hunter, Director, Residential & Social Services
Deb Strahanoski, Manager, Development

Services for children and adults with disabilities and their families. Pediatric therapy, residential programs, special home placement, inclusive child care, and early intervention.

6830 **El Valor**
Main Office & Developmental Training Center
1850 W 21st St
Chicago, IL 60608
312-666-4511
Fax: 312-666-6677
TTY: 312-666-3361
info@elvalor.net
elvalor.org

Rafael Malpica, Chairman
Rey B Gonzalez, President & CEO
Carmen Ziegler, Chief Financial Officer
Eduardo Moreno, Director of Employment & Facilities Services

El Valor's mission is to serve people with disabilities and their families, by offering programs in the areas of early childhood education, adult services and parental and community engagement.

6831 **Elgin Training Center**
Association For Individual Development Elgin Area
1135 Bowes Road
Elgin, IL 60123-1321
847-931-6200
Fax: 847-888-6079
www.the-association.org

Chuck Miles, Chairmen
Patrick Flaherty, Vice Chairmen
Walter Dwyer, Treasurer
Lynn O'Shea, Executive Director

Day training services to develop work habits and attitudes while providing training in small product assembly, sorting, packaging, collating, & material handling. Instruction also offered in job related knowledge & in personal, social and independent living skills. There is also an on-site specialized Autism Program. Additionally, residential programs (group homes & apartments) are also available for people with developmental disabilities.

6832 **Family Counseling Center**
PO Box 759
Golconda, IL 62938
618-683-2461
Fax: 618-683-2066
fccinconline.org

Larry Mizell, Executive Director
Connie Duncan, Director
Nora Beth Hacker, Financial Director

Provides counseling, developmental training, evaluations, assisted living services, referrals, psychosocial rehabilitation, and a variety of work services.

6833 **Family Matters**
A RC Community Support Systems
1901 S. 4th St
Ste 209
Effingham, IL 62401-4123
217-347-5428
866-436-7842
Fax: 217-347-5119
deinhorn@arc-css.org
www.fmptic.org

Debbie Einhorn, Executive Director
Debbie Einhorn, Director Family Support
Nancy Mader, Project Coordinator
Barbara Utz, Vice President

Parent Training and Information Center and family support programs for families of children who have disabilities from the ages of birth through 21. Services include: Parent support and training, school advocacy, home visits, information and referral, pa

6834 **Five Star Industries**
1308 Wells Street Road
P O Box 60
Du Quoin, IL 62832-60
618-542-5421
Fax: 618-542-5556
5starind.com

Susan Engelhardt, Executive Director

Incorporated as a private, non-profit corporation under the laws of the State of Illinois, is an equal opportunity employer and provides equal opportunity in compliance with the Civil Rights Act of 1964 and all other appropriate laws, rules and regulation

6835 **HSI Austin Center For Development**
1819 S Kedzie Ave
Chicago, IL 60623-2623
773-854-1676
Fax: 773-854-8300

6836 **Hyde Park-Woodlawn**
950 E 61st St
Chicago, IL 60637-2623
773-324-0280
Fax: 773-324-0285

Clarissa Williams, Manager

6837 **Illinois Center for Autism**
548 South Ruby Lane
Fairview Heights, IL 62208-2614
618-398-7500
Fax: 618-394-9869
info@illinoiscenterforautism.org
illinoiscenterforautism.org

Hardy Ware, Chairperson
Thomas E. Berry, Vice Chairperson
Gary Guthrie, Secretary
Joy Rick, Treasurer

A community-based mental health/educational treatment center dedicated to serving autistic clients.

6838 **Julius and Betty Levinson Center**
1825 K Street NW
Suite 600
Washington, DC 60304-1557
202-776-0406
800-872-5827
Fax: 708-383-9025
www.ucp.org

Woody Connette, Chair
Ian Ridlon, Vice Chair
Mark Boles, Treasurer
Pamela Talkin, Secretary

Houses one of its three adult developmental training programs for substantially physically disabled men and women.

6839 **Lake County Health Department**
18 N. County Street
Waukegan, IL 60085
847-377-2000
Fax: 847-336-1517
www.lakecountyil.gov

Aaron Lawlor, Chairman
Stevenson Mountsier, Vice Chairman
Barry Burton, Administrator

Includes counseling, crisis intervention, emergency management, psychotherapy and chemotherapy management for individuals and families.

6840 Little Friends, Inc.
140 N Wright Street
Naperville, IL 60540-4799
630-355-6533
Fax: 630-355-3176
info@lilfriends.com
www.littlefriendsinc.com

Dan Casey, Chairman
Matt Johanson, Vice Chairman
Michele Calbi, Treasurer
Kathy West, Secretary

Little Friends has been serving children and adults with autism and other developmental disabilities for over 40 years. Based in Naperville, Little Friends operates three schools, vocational training programs, community-based residential services and the

6841 MAP Training Center
7th and Mc Kinley St
Karnak, IL 62956
618-634-9401
Fax: 618-634-9090

Larry Earnhart, President
Cindy Earnhart, Community Liaison

Training, employment, residential and support services, targeted for adults with developmental disabilities.

6842 Macon Resources
2121 Hubbard Ave.
P O Box 2760
Decatur, IL 62524-2760
217-875-1910
Fax: 217-875-8899
TTY: 217-875-8898
maconresources.org

Tom Hill, President
Michael Breheny, Vice President
Barb Nadler, Secretary
Chris Funk, Treasurer

The purpose is to provide a comprehensive array of habilitative/rehabilitative training programs and support services to assist individuals and/or family units of an individual with a developmental disability, mental illness, or other handicapping conditi

6843 Mary Bryant Home for the Blind
2960 Stanton
Springfield, IL 62703-4385
217-529-1611
888-529-1611
Fax: 217-529-6975
mbha@marybryanthome.org
marybryanthome.org

Jerry Curry, Executive Director
Robert E. Maxey, President
Allan J. Rupel, Vice President
Gary Rapaport, Secretary

Supportive living facility for blind or visually impaired adults over the age of 22. A supportive living facility remodeled to foster the move to increased independence for residents. The new apartment style housing combined with personal care and other a

6844 Northern Illinois Special Recreation Association (NISRA)
285 Memorial Drive
Crystal Lake, IL 60014-3650
815-459-0737
Fax: 815-459-0388
info@nisra.org
www.nisra.org

Brian Shahinian, Executive Director
Carol Amoroso, Manager of Finance and Personnel
Kerri Ruddy, Manager of Office Services
Sarah Holcombe, Manager of Communications & Marketing

Leisure and recreation services to those with disabilities who are unable to participate successfully in park district and city recreation programs.

6845 Oak Forest Hospital of Cook County
15900 Cicero Ave
Oak Forest, IL 60452
708-687-7200
Fax: 708-687-7979
TTY: 708-687-4794
http://www.cchil.org

Robert Weinstein, Department Chair
Suja Mathew, Associate Chair

A 654 bed health care center devoted to the diagnosis, rehabilitation and long-term care of adults suffering from chronic illnesses, diseases and physical impairments.

6846 PARC
1913 W. Townline Road
P.O. Box 3418
Peoria, IL 61615-3418
309-691-3800
Fax: 309-689-3613
parcway.org

Pat Kawczynski, Chair
Heyl Royster, Vice Chair
Terry Waters, Treasurer
Alexis Duhon, Secretary

Serves all ages that are diagnosed with developmental and physical disabilities. Programs include early intervention, family support, respite care, vocational training, supported employment, adult day programs and residential.

6847 Peoria Area Blind People's Center
2905 W Garden St
Peoria, IL 61605-1316
309-637-3693
Fax: 309-637-3693
info@cicbvi.org
cicbvi.org

Carol Warren, President
Cora Quinn, Vice President
Prasad Parupalli, Treasurer

Offers services for the totally blind, legally blind, visually impaired, and more with health, counseling, educational, recreational, rehabilitation, computer training and professional training services.

6848 Pioneer Center for Human Services
4031 W Dayton St
McHenry, IL 60050
815-344-1230
Fax: 815-344-3815
TTY: 815-344-6243
gethelp@pioneercenter.org

Dan McCaleb, Chairman
Sam Tenuto, Co-CEO
Frank Samuel, Co-CEO
DJ Newport, MS, Director of Developmental Disability Services

Pioneer Center is a non-profit agency in McHenry County delivering services to more than 4,000 people annually. Pioneer Center provides developmental disability services, youth and family behavioral health services and homeless services (McHenry County PADS).

6849 Prosthetics and Orthotics Center in Blue Island
2310 York St
Blue Island, IL 60406-2411
708-597-2611
800-354-7342
Fax: 800-908-1932
www.rehabchicago.org/about/blue_island.php

6850 RB King Counseling Center
2300 N Edward St
Decatur, IL 62526-4163
217-877-8121
Fax: 217-875-0966

Gordon Cross MD

Offers outpatient, individual, group, divorce and meditation, family and re-adjustment counseling.

6851 REHAB Products and Services
3715 N Vermilion St
Danville, IL 61832-1130
217-446-1146
Fax: 217-446-1191
workse.org

Frank L. Brunacci, President/CEO
Crystal Meece, Vice President Production
Todd Seabaugh, VP Programs
Scott Rudy, VP Operations

janitorial, lawn care, distribution services.

6852 **RIC Northshore**
Rehabilitation Institute of Chicago
345 E Superior St
Chicago, IL 60611-2654
312-238-1000
800-354-7342
webmaster@ric.org
www.rehabchicago.org

Joanne C. Smith, President/CEO
Edward B. Case, Vice President
Provides rehabilitation for sports-related injuries, musculoskeletal conditions, neurological conditions, stroke, arthritis, amputation, burns, and general deconditioning.

6853 **RIC Prosthetics and Orthotics Center**
Rehabilitation Institute of Chicago
345 E. Superior Street
Suite 101
Chicago, IL 60611-4615
312-238-1000
800-345-7342
Fax: 708-957-8353
webmaster@rehabchicago.org
ric.org

Martin Buckner, CPO, Inpatient Coordinator
Nicole T. Soltys, CP, Clinical Coordinator
Robert D. Lipschutz, CP, Director of Prosthetic and Orthotic Education
Walter Afable, CP, Clinical Operations Manager
Offers almost all the prosthetics and orthotics services provided at RIC's main hospital in downtown Chicago, including consultations, fittings and training.

6854 **RIC Windermere House**
5548 S Hyde Park Blvd
Chicago, IL 60637-1909
773-256-5050
800-354-7342
Fax: 773-256-5060
www.rehabchicago.org

Meghan Scalise, Manager
Evaluation, therapeutic services and patient education are offered in the areas of arthritis, multiple sclerosis, musculoskeletal conditions, orthopedics, stroke, spinal cord injury, brain injury and sports medicine.

6855 **Ray Graham Association for People with Disabilities**
901 Warrenville Road
Suite 500
Lisle, IL 60532-1038
630-620-2222
Fax: 630-628-2350
TTY: 630-628-2352
cathyfickerterill@yahoo.com
ray-graham.org

Michael Komoll, Chairperson
Neville Bilimoria, Vice Chairperson
Kim zoeller, President & CEO
Jeff Park, Secretary/Treasurer
Provides developmental services at 15 sites to infants, children and adults with disabilities. Services range from 1 hr/wk respite to full-time residential.

6856 **Reach Rehabilitation Program: Americana Healthcare**
9401 S Kostner Ave
Oak Lawn, IL 60453-2697
708-423-1505
Fax: 708-423-3822

Jean M Roche, Owner
Postacute rehabilitation program.

6857 **Rehabilitation Achievement Center**
345 E Superior St
Chicago, IL 60611-4805
312-238-1000
800-354-7342
www.ric.org

M. Jude Reyes, Chair
Mike P. Krasny, Vice Chair
Joanne C. Smith, President & CEO
Ed Case, Treasurer
Rehabilitation Institute of Chicago (RIC) has aquired the assets of the Rehabilitation Achievement Center (RAC).

6858 **Rehabilitation Institute of Chicago: Alexian Brothers Medical Center**
800 Biesterfield Rd
Elk Grove Village, IL 60007-3361
847-437-5500
866-253-9426
Fax: 847-631-5663
TTY: 847-956-5116
www.alexianbrothershealth.org

Mark Frey, President and Chief Executive Officer
Tracy Rogers, Senior Vice President and Chief Operating Officer
Paul Belter, Senior Vice President and Chief Financial Officer
Janice Jastrowski, Manager
A 32-bed rehabilitation unit under the medical direction and supervision of the Rehabilitation Institute of Chicago.

6859 **Riverside Medical Center**
Mental Health Unit
350 N Wall St
Kankakee, IL 60901-2991
815-933-1671
Fax: 815-935-8160
rhuber@rsh.net
riversidehealthcare.org

Phillip Kambic, CEO
Bill W. Douglas, Vice President
Offers recreation, parenting therapy, emergency services, psychological testing and inpatient treatment programs. Riverside is nationally recognized for its specialty programs in heart care, obstetrics, trauma, oncology, rehabilitation, geriatrics, occupa

6860 **Robert Young Mental Health Center Division of Trinity Regional Haelth System**
Trinity Health Foundation
2701 17th St
Rock Island, IL 61201-5351
309-779-2800
800-322-1431
Fax: 309-779-2027
www.unitypoint.org

Rick Seidler, President & CEO
Jim Hayes, CFO
Tamara Byram, VP, Legal/Compliance
Matt Behrens, Regional VP, UnityPoint Clinic
Services include comprehensive inpatient rehabilitation, chronic pain management programs, outpatient medical rehabilitation, work hardening programs, vocational evaluation, alcohol and other drug dependency rehabilitation programs, Burn Center, and menta

6861 **Sampson-Katz Center**
216 West Jackson Blvd
Suite 700
Chicago, IL 60606-2104
312-673-3400
Fax: 312-553-5544
TTY: 773-761-6672
jvsskc@jvschicago.org
www.jvschicago.org

Andrew M. Glick, Chair
John L. Daniels, Vice Chair
H. Debra Levin, President
Benn Feltheimer, Secretary

6862 **Shelby County Community Services**
160 North Main Street
Memphis, TN 38103-650
901-222-2300
Fax: 912-222-2090
www.shelbycountytn.gov

Dottie Jones, Director
Primary focus is substance abuse treatment.

6863 **Streator Unlimited**
305 N Sterling St
P O Box 706
Streator, IL 61364-2369
815-673-5574
Fax: 815-673-1714
contact@streatorunlimited.org
www.streatorunlimited.org

Jeffrey Dean, Executive Director
Lynn Fukar, Director of Day Services
Julie Caestens, Director Residential Services
Vocational and personal skills training, residential services, client and family support, supported and computerized employ-

ment. Serves adults with intellectual disabilities with the goal of enabling them to reach their fullest potential, live as independ

6864 **Swedish Covenant Hospital Rehabilitation Services**
5145 N California Ave
Chicago, IL 60625-3661
773-878-8200
Fax: 773-561-0490

Mark Newton, President & CEO
Provides acute rehabilitation services, subacute care and outpatient services for many types of disabling injuries and conditions, including amputation, arthritis, brain injury, general deconditioning, multiple sclerosis, musculoskeletal injuries, stroke,

6865 **TCRC Sight Center**
21310 Route 9
Tremont, IL 61568-2558
309-347-7148
Fax: 309-925-4241
info@tcrcorg.com
www.tcrcorg.com

Jamie Durdel, President & CEO
Molly Anderson, Vice President
Offers services for persons who are totally blind, legally blind, partially sighted or visually impaired along with other disabilities. Have support group, rehabilitation classes, orientation and mobility services, counseling services, low vision clinic,

6866 **Tazewell County Resource Center**
Box 12
Rr 1
Tremont, IL 61568
309-347-7148
Fax: 309-925-4241
info@tcrcorg.com
http://www.tcrcorg.com

Jamie Durdel, President & CEO
Molly Anderson, Vice President
A private, nonprofit agency providing programs for the special needs of infants, adults, children and their families residing in Tazewell County. Services offered include: birth-three infant/parent program, adult day care services, family support, residen

6867 **Trumbull Park**
10530 S Oglesby Ave
Chicago, IL 60617-6140
773-375-7022
Fax: 773-375-5528

Gregory Terry, Director
Diana Moore, Site Supervisor
Ada McKinley, Manager
Offers consultation, education, general counseling, recreation, self-help and social services for children and adults.

6868 **University of Illinois Medical Center**
1740 West Taylor Street
Chicago, IL 60612-7232
312-355-4000
866-600-2273
Fax: 312-996-7770
hospital.uillinois.edu

Rajiv Pai, Chief
Marilyn Plomann, Manager
Offers services for the totally blind, legally blind, visually impaired, and more with health, counseling, educational, recreational, rehabilitation, computer training and professional training services.

6869 **VanMatre Rehabilitation Center**
950 S Mulford Rd
Rockford, IL 61108-4274
815-381-8500
866-754-3347
Fax: 815-484-9953
webcontentcoordinator@rhsnet.org
www.vanmatrerehab.com

Gary E. Kaatz, President and Chief Executive Officer
Scott Craig, Medical Director
A CARF-accredited comprehensive rehabilitation center based within the Rockford Memorial Hospital providing inpatient and outpatient services for physically and cognitively challenged persons with debilitating illness and injuries.

6870 **Warren Achievement Center**
1220 E 2nd Ave
Monmouth, IL 61546-2404
309-734-3131
Fax: 309-734-7114
info@warrenachievement.com
warrenachievement.com

Rick Barnhill, President
Jim Kesse, Vice President
Sherry Waite, Chief Operations Officer
Linda Baker, Chief Financial Officer
For developmentally disabled children and adults. Parent-infant education programs are for parents of infants with disabilities or developmental delays; Children's Group Homes which serve children on a fulltime basis and can serve additional children on a

Indiana

6871 **Ball Memorial Hospital**
2401 W University Ave
Muncie, IN 47303-3499
765-747-3111
Fax: 765-747-3313
iuhealth.org/ball-memorial

Mike Haley, CEO
Offers rehabilitation services, occupational therapy, physical therapy and more for the physically challenged child or adult.

6872 **Community Health Network**
1500 N Ritter Ave
Indianapolis, IN 46219-3027
317-355-4275
800-775-7775
Fax: 317-351-7723
www.ecommunity.com

Keith Thompson, Manager
Anita Harden, President
A leading not-for-profit health system offering convenient access to expert physicians, advanced treatments and leading edge technology, all focused on getting patients well and back to their lives. With caring compassion, Community's 5 hospitals and 70+ sites of care continually strive to improve the health and well being of those individuals in central Indiana who entrust care to us.

6873 **Crossroads Industrial Services**
8302 E 33rd Street
Indianapolis, IN 46226
317-897-7320
Fax: 317-897-9763
info@crossroadsindustrialservices.com
www.crossroadsindustrialservices.c om

Anne Shupe, Finance Executive
Curtiss Quirin, CEO
Assisting customers with short-term, seasonal, and long-term outsourcing needs. Many consider Crossroads an extension of their company

6874 **Department of Veterans Affairs Vet Center #418**
302 W. Washington St
Room E120
Indianapolis, IN 46204- 2738
317-232-3910
800-490-4520
Fax: 317-232-7721
www.in.gov/veteran/sso/fac

Charles T. Applegate, Director
Provides readjustment counseling to combat veterans. Onsite assistance for employment problems, vocational rehabilitation and sexual trauma counsel.

6875 **Easterseals Rehabilitation Center**
3701 Bellemeade Ave.
Evansville, IN 47714
812-479-1411
www.easterseals.com/in-sw

Kelly Schneider, President
Guy Davis, Vice President, Administration
Laura Terhune, Vice President, Development
Lisa Fisher, Vice President, Clinical Services
Services include therapy and medical rehabilitation, assistive technology, early intervention, early care and education, and community employment.

6876 **Frasier Rehabilitation Center Division of Clark Memorial Hospital**
2201 Greentree N
Clarksville, IN 47129-8957 812-218-6590
Fax: 812-218-6597
http://www.jhsmh.org/Frazier-Rehab-Institute-
Catherine Lucas Spalding, Administrator
Designed to help patients in their adjustment to a physically limiting condition, both psychologically and physically, by helping to maximize each patient's abilities so he or she can function as independently as possible. The program treats patients whos

6877 **HealthSouth Deaconess Rehabilitation Hospital**
4100 Covert Ave
Evansville, IN 47714-5559 812-476-9983
800-677-3422
Fax: 812-476-4270
www.healthsouthdeaconess.com
Barbara Butler, Chief Executive Officer
Ashok . Dhingra, M.D, Medical Director
Brett Hirt, Director, Therapy Operations
Doron Finn, M.D., Wound Care Program Director
AHealthSouth Deaconess Rehabilitation Hospital is a joint venture partner with Deaconess Health System. Our hospital is an 80-bed inpatient rehabilitation hospital that offers comprehensive inpatient and outpatient rehabilitation services designed to return patients to leading active and independent lives.

6878 **Healthwin Specialized Care**
20531 Darden Rd
South Bend, IN 46637-2999 574-272-0100
Fax: 574-277-3233
info@healthwin.org
healthwin.org
Connie McCahill, President
Lauren Davis, Vice President
John Cergnul, Treasurer
Stephen J. Gazdick, Chief Financial Officer
No other facility in the area has a homelike environment like ours. Its simply part of our culture. Rehabilitation therapy that includes physical, occupational, speech, respiratory and a full time in-house therapist. Other services include a wound special

6879 **Memorial Regional Rehabilitation Center**
615 N Michigan St
South Bend, IN 46601-1033 574-647-1000
877-282-0964
Johan Kuitse, MSA, PT, Outpatient Clinical Manager
Anne Clifford, DPT, Physical Therapists
Shanti Shrestha Dalson, DPT, Physical Therapists
Brandi DeMont, DPT, Physical Therapists
20-bed CARF accredited inpatient rehabilitation, outpatient orthopedic clinic and work performance program, head injury clinic. Outpatient neuro rehab and a driver education and training program are provided.

6880 **Saint Joseph Regional Medical Center- South Bend**
5215 Holy Cross Parkway
Mishawaka, IN 46545-2814 574-335-5000
Fax: 574-237-7312
thefoundation@sjrmc.com
sjmed.com
Albert Gutierrez, President & CEO
Steven Gable, Vice President
Janice Dunn, CFO
Christopher Karam, Chief Operating Officer
Continuum of rehabilitation services offered. Included are: acute rehabilitation, a 26 bed CARF accredited comprehensive inpatient unit, a CARF certified inpatient brain injury program, a CARF outpatient day treatment brain injury program, comprehensive o

Iowa

6881 **Crossroads of Western Iowa**
1 Crossroads Pl
Missouri Valley, IA 51555-6069 712-642-4114
Fax: 712-642-4115
info@cwiowa.org
explorecrossroads.com
Brent Dillinger, CEO
Pat Kocour, President
Steven Van Riper, Vice President
Darci Tierney, Secretary
CWI provides services in Missouri Valley, Onawa and Council Bluffs, Iowa. An array of services for people with mental illness, developmental disabilities and brain injury are provided in each location.

6882 **Des Moines Division-VA Central Iowa Health Care System**
3600 30th St
Des Moines, IA 50310-5753 515-699-5999
800-294-8387
Fax: 515-699-5862
www.centraliowa.va.gov
Judith Johnson-Mekota, Director
Fredrick Bahls, Chief Of Staff
Susan A. Martin, Associate Director
Alton C. Alexander, Associate Director
VA Cental Iowa Health Care System is the result of the 1997 merger of the Des Moines and Knoxville, Iowa, VA Medical Centers. This integrated healthcare system brings 2 previously separate organizational structures, located 40 miles apart, into one cohesi

6883 **Easterseals Iowa**
401 NE 66th Ave.
Des Moines, IA 50313 515-289-1933
Fax: 515-289-1281
TTY: 515-289-4069
www.easterseals.com/ia
Sherri Nielsen, President & CEO
Kevin Small, Chief Financial Officer
Allison Piazza, Chief Development Officer
Provides services to Iowans with disabilities. Services include vocational and employment training, camping recreation and respite services, craft training and sales, home and farm adaptations, and transportation.

6884 **Genesis Regional Rehabilitation Center**
Genesis Health System
1227 E.Rusholme Street
Davenport, IA 52803-3396 563-421-1000
Fax: 563-421-3499
genesishealth.com
Doug Cropper, President & CEO
Kenneth Croken, Vice President
Joseph Lohmuller, Chief Medical Officer
Karen Bolton, Vice President
Serves persons of all ages experiencing a disability, whether acquired at birth or following a serious interdisciplinary service. Rehabilitation programs include acute rehabilitation; adult rehabilitation, pediatric rehabilitation, outpatient orthopaedics

6885 **Homelink**
Van G Miller & Associates
1101 W S Marnan Drive
Waterloo, IA 50701-2817 319-235-7173
866-575-8483
Fax: 319-235-7822
homelinkprivacyofficer@vgm.com
www.vgmhomelink.com
Dave Kazynski, President
Rick Hibben, Coordinator
A national network of home medical equipment, respiratory therapy, rehabilitation and infusion therapy service providers with over 2,500 locations serving all fifty states.

6886 **Iowa Central Industries**
127 Avenue M
Fort Dodge, IA 50501-5797 515-576-2126
Fax: 515-576-2251
Tom Eckman, Executive Director
Services include evaluation and training in pre-vocational and vocational skills, personal behavior management, cognitive skills, communication skills, self-care skills and social skills. Services arranged include: independent living training, medical ser

6887 **Life Skills Laundry Division**
1510 Industrial Rd SW
Le Mars, IA 51031-3009 712-546-4785
Fax: 712-546-4985
Don Nore, Executive Director

6888 **MIW**
909 S 14th Ave
Marshalltown, IA 50158-3610 641-752-3697
Fax: 641-752-1614
Rich Byers, President/CEO
Vocational services for adults with disabilities. Includes organizational employment services, supported employment, job placement.

6889 **Mercy Dubuque Physical Rehabilitation Unit**
250 Mercy Drive
Dubuque, IA 52001-7320 563-589-8000
Fax: 563-589-8162
www.mercydubuque.com
Russel M. Knight, CEO
Provides services which open the door to improved communication, offering the opportunity to enrich the quality of life. Mercy offers many other branches of services including, rehabilitation services for children and a pulmonary rehabilitation program.

6890 **Mercy Medical Center-Pain Services**
1111 6th Ave
Des Moines, IA 50314-2611 515-247-3121
Fax: 515-248-8867
webmaster@mercydesmoines.org
Dana L. Simon, MD
Dave Vellinga, President & CEO
Laurie Conner, Vice President
An outpatient program dedicated to helping people with chronic pain live more productive, satisfying lives. The program is not designed for conditions that are surgically curable, but rather approaches the problem using a comprehensive, holistic treatment.

6891 **Nishna Productions-Shenandoah Work Center**
902 Day Street
Shenandoah, IA 51601-70 712-246-1242
Fax: 712-246-1243
Mary Rolf, President
Sherri Clark, Executive Director
Melissa Mueller, Program Manager
Barb Hammer, Team Leader
Shelter, workshop and job training for the disabled. Some of the services we provide are Work Activity, Adult Day Activity Program, Personal & Social Adjustment, Residential Services, Home & Community Based Services & Employment Resources.

6892 **Northstar Community Services**
3420 University Avenue
Waterloo, IA 50701-2050 319-236-0901
888-879-1365
Fax: 319-236-3701
www.northstarcs.org
Mark Witmar, Executive Director
Jeff Conrey, President
Kathy Folkerts, Vice President
Mary Wankowicz, Director of operations
Provides adult day services, employment services and supported community living so people with disabilities can live and work in the community.

6893 **Options of Linn County**
935 2nd street
SW
Cedar Rapids, IA 52404-3100 319-892-5000
Fax: 319-892-5849
linncounty.org
Joel D. Miller, Auditor
Sharon Gonzalez, Treasurer
Options of Linn County works with community businesses in providing employment services to adults with disabilities. Options is a publicly operated service provider within the Linn County Community Services department.

6894 **RISE**
106 Rainbow Dr
Elkader, IA 52043-9075 563-245-1868
Fax: 563-245-2859
Ed Josten, Manager

6895 **Ragtime Industries**
116 N 2nd St
Albia, IA 52531-1624 641-932-7813
Fax: 641-932-7814
Lisa Glenn, Executive Director
A work-oriented rehabilitation organization which provides training for mentally and physically disabled adults in Monroe County. A variety of programs which help to develop each person's individual potential are offered.

6896 **Sunshine Services**
1106 East 9th St
Spencer, IA 51301-225 712-262-7805
Fax: 712-262-8369
Ann Vandehar, Executive Director

6897 **Tenco Industries**
710 Gateway Dr
Ottumwa, IA 52501-2204 641-682-8114
Fax: 641-684-4223
www.tenco.org
Ben Wright, Executive Director
Dixie Merritt, Vocational Director
Brenda Miller, Marketing and Development DirectoR
Joanie Lundy, Human Resources Director
To advocate and provide opportunities for people with disabilities, or conditions that limit their abilities, to develop and maintain the skills necessary for personal dignity and independence in all areas of life. Provide a wide array of services to individuals with disabilities. By looking at each person as individuals, we are able to work with them to maximize their skills. Residentials services, including HCBS and CSALA are also provided in all communities.

Kansas

6898 **Arrowhead West**
1100 E Wyatt Earp Blvd
Dodge City, KS 67801-5337 620-227-8803
Fax: 620-227-8812
web@arrowheadwest.org
www.arrowheadwest.org
Kelly Mason, Chairperson
Michael Stein, Vice Chairperson
Lori Pendergast, President
Anita Allard, Treasurer
Services and programs offered include: developmental and therapy services for children birth to age 3; adult center-based work services and community integrated employment options; adult life skills and retirement programs; and adult residential services.

6899 **Big Lakes Developmental Center**
1416 Hayes Dr
Manhattan, KS 66502-5066 785-776-9201
Fax: 785-776-9830
biglakes@biglakes.org
biglakes.org
Lori Feldkamp, President
Shawn Funk, Community Education Director

A private nonprofit Community Developmental Disability Organization (CDDO) serving individuals with developmental disabilities in Riley, Geary, Clay and Pottawatome counties in Kansas. Big lakes is supported by county mill levy and federal and state fundi

6900 **Developmental Services of Northwest Kansas**
2703 Hall St
Suite 10
Hays, KS 67601-1964
785-625-5678
800-637-2229
Fax: 785-625-8204

Jerry Michaud, President
Ruth Lang, Administrative Assistant
A private nonprofit organization serving both children and adults with disabilities. Offers services to children ages birth to three years, youth and adults through a network of community-based and outreach programs and inter-agency agreements with other

6901 **ENVISION**
2301 S Water St
Wichita, KS 67213-4819
316-267-2244
Fax: 316-267-4312
Info@envisionus.com
www.envisionus.com

Sam Williams, Chair
Jon Rosell, PhD, Vice-Chair
Michael Monteferrante, President and CEO
Greg Unruh, Vice President, CFO
Provides jobs, job training and vision rehabilitation services to people who are blind or low vision. A private not-for-profit agency uniquely combining employment opportunitites with rehabilitation services and public education.

6902 **Heartspring**
8700 E 29th St N
Wichita, KS 67226-2169
316-634-8700
800-835-1043
Fax: 316-634-0555
kgrover@heartspring.org
www.heartspring.org

Gary W. Singleton, President and CEO
Paul Faber, Executive Vice President, Operations
Katie Grover, Director Of Marketing
David Dorf, CPA, Chief Financial Officer
Heartspring provides outpatient therapies, evaluations and consultations for children with special needs through Heartspring Pediatric Services. The Heartspring School is a residential and day school for children ages 5-21 with multiple disabilities. Children with autism and their families receive resources through the Heartspring CARE program. The Heartspring Hearing Center provides services to individuals of all ages.

6903 **Indian Creek Nursing Center**
6515 W 103rd St
Overland Park, KS 66212-1798
913-633-7000
Fax: 913-642-3982
www.savaseniorcare.com

Randy Sutterfield, Administrator
Postacute rehabilitation program. A 120-bed nursing home facility.

6904 **Johnson County Developmental Supports**
111 South Cherry Street
Olathe, KS 66061-1223
913-715-5000
Fax: 913-715-0800
info@jocogov.org
www.jocogov.org

Ed Eilert, Chairman
Michael Lally, Vice Chair
Scott Tschudy, Treasurer
Jessica Dain, Secretary
JCDS is the community Developmental Disability Organization for Johnson County, Kansas. Provides supports in the form of direct services to people on a daily basis.

6905 **Ketch Industries**
1006 E Waterman St
Wichita, KS 67211-1525
316-383-8700
800-766-3777
Fax: 316-383-8715
webmaster@ketch.org
ketch.org

Fred Badders, Chairman
Carla Bienhoff, Chairman
Loren Anthony, Secretary
Dan Crug, Treasurer
The mission of Ketch is to promote independence for persons with disabilities through innovative learning experiences that support individuals choices for working, living and playing in their community.

6906 **Lakemary Center**
100 Lakemary Dr
Paola, KS 66071-1855
913-557-4000
Fax: 913-557-4910
lakemaryctr.org

William Craig, President
Paul Sokoloff, Chair
Gayle Richardson, Vice Chair
Lydia Marien, Secretary
A private, not-for-profit day and residential training facility which provides for the assessment, education, training, therapy and social development of children and adults, moderate and severe developmental disabilities.

6907 **Northview Developmental Services**
700 E 14th St
Newton, KS 67117-5702
316-283-5170
Fax: 316-283-5196
http://northviewdev.mennonite.net/

Mary Holloway, CEO
The mission is to provide quality supportive and coordinating services to persons with developmental disabilities, assisting them to grow as they integrate into the community. Further, our mission is to improve the quality of their lives by providing acce

Kentucky

6908 **Cardinal Hill Rehabilitation Hospital**
Cadinal Hill Medical Center
2050 Versailles Rd
Lexington, KY 40504-1499
859-254-5701
800-233-3260
Fax: 859-231-1365
www.cardinalhill.org

Gary R. Payne, CEO
Provides occupational health services, therapy services and urgent medical treatment of injured workers.

6909 **Frazier Rehab Institute**
220 Abraham Flexner Way
Louisville, KY 40202-1887
502-582-7400
Fax: 502-582-7477

Jamie Ochsner, Manager
Steve Ahr, VP Frazier Rehab/Neurscience
Frazier Rehab Institute is a regional healthcare system dedicated entirely to rehabilitation. Through an expansive network of inpatient and outpatient facilites in Kentucky and southern Indiana, Frazier offers a wide array of services based on one common

6910 **HealthSouth Northern Kentucky Rehabilitation Hospital**
201 Medical Village Dr
Edgewood, KY 41017-3407
859-341-2044
800-860-6004
Fax: 859-341-2813
www.healthsouthkentucky.com

Richard Evans, CEO
Mary Pfeffer, Director Therapy Operations
Neal Moser, M.D., Medical Director
Mary Beth Bauer, RD, CSG, LD, Director of Quality and Risk Management
Offers all types of inpatient and outpatient rehabilitation services such as occupational therapy, physical therapy, speech therapy.

Respiratory therpay, Psychology, Aquatics, Case Managemenet/Social Work and Nutritional Services.

6911 **King's Daughter's Medical Center's Rehab Unit/Work Hardening Program**
2201 Lexington Ave
Ashland, KY 41101-2843
606-408-4000
888-377-5362
Fax: 606-327-7542
info@kdmc.net
www.kdmc.com

Kristie Whitlatch, President & CEO
Matt Ebaugh, VP / Chief Strategy and Information Officer
Philip Fioret, M.D., VP / Chief Medical Officer
Howard Harrison, Vice President, Facilities

Offers a 27-bed, inpatient rehabilitation services unit treating physical disabilities related to accident or illness. The program provides an interdisciplinary inpatient program designed to restore the individual to the highest level of independence. It

6912 **LifeSkills Industries**
380 Suwannee Trail St
Bowling Green, KY 42103-6499
270-901-5000
800-223-8913
Fax: 270-782-0058
sbell@lifeskills.com
lifeskills.com

Alice Simpson, CEO

LifeSkills will be the reliable advocate, dependable safety net and provider of choice, for high quality, accessable services and supports for the citizens of south-central Kentucky whos lives are affected by mental illness, developmental disablilities or

6913 **Low Vision Services of Kentucky**
120 N. Eagle Creek Drive
Suite 500
Lexington, KY 40509- 1827
859-263-3900
800-627-2020
Fax: 859-977-1136
jvanarsdall@retinaky.com
www.lowvisionky.com

Regina Callihan-May, O.D.
Jeanne Van Arsdall, Co-ordinator
Maryanne Inman, Practice Administrator
William J. Wood, MD, Physician

Offers educational, recreational and rehabilitational services and devices for the visually impaired, legally blind, totally blind.

6914 **Muhlenberg County Opportunity Center**
PO Box 511
Greenville, KY 42345-1416
270-754-5590
Fax: 270-338-5977
muhlon.com

Chuck Hammonds, Manager
Charles Hamonds, Director

Post-acute rehabilitation facility with programs including a workshop with hand packaging of manufactured goods.

6915 **New Vision Enterprises**
1900 Brownsboro Rd
Louisville, KY 40206-2102
502-893-0211
800-405-9135
Fax: 502-893-3885

Larry Sherman, Plant Manager

Offers employment training and services for the blind and legally blind.

6916 **Park DuValle Community Health Center, Inc.**
3015 Wilson Ave
Louisville, KY 40211-1969
502-774-4401
Fax: 502-775-6195
www.pdchc.org

Richard K Jones, President
John Howard MD, Medical Director
Dave Gerwig, CFO
Ann Hagan, Administrator

Offers services for the totally blind, legally blind, visually impaired, and more with health, counseling, educational, recreational, rehabilitation, computer training and professional training services.

Louisiana

6917 **Alliance House**
427 S Foster Drive
Baton Rouge, LA 70806-2723
225-987-0013
Fax: 225-346-0857

6918 **Assumption Activity Center**
4201 Highway 1
Napoleonville, LA 70390-8628
985-369-2907
Fax: 985-369-2657

Warren Gonzales, Manager

A community work center providing prevocational training and extended employment for adults with disabilities. Services include: social services, work activities, specialized training and supported employment.

6919 **Bancroft Rehabilitation Living Centers**
425 Kings Highway East
P.O. Box 20
Haddonfield, NJ 08033-0018
504-482-3075
800-774-5516
Fax: 504-483-2135
lynn.tomaio@bancroft.org
www.bancroft.org

Dr. Robert Voogt, Owner
Toni Pergolin, President & CEO
Cynthia Boyer, Executive Director
Thomas J. Burke, MBA, Chief Financial Officer

Mission is to nurture abilities and independence of people with neurological challenges by providing a broad spectrum of advanced therapeutic and educational programs and by fostering the development of best practices in the field through research and pro

6920 **Deaf Action Center Of Greater New Orleans**
Catholic Charities
1000 Howard Ave
Suite 200
New Orleans, LA 70113-1903
504-523-3755
866-891-2210
Fax: 504-523-2789
TTY: 504-615-4944
www.ccano.org

Tommie A. Vassel, Chairman
Sr.Marjorie Hebert, MSC, President & CEO

This community service and resource center serves deaf, deaf-blind, hard of hearing and speech-impaired persons in the greater New Orleans area regardless of age, religion, race or secondary disability. DAC provides interpreting services, equipment distri

6921 **Donaldsville Area Arc**
1030 Clay St
Donaldsonville, LA 70346-3518
225-473-4516
daarc@eatel.net

6922 **East Jefferson General Hospital Rehab Center**
4200 Houma Blvd
Metairie, LA 70006-2996
504-454-4000
www.ejgh.org

Newell D. Normand, Chairman
Ashton J. Ryan, Jr., Vice Chairman
Mark J, Peters, President & CEO
Judy Brown, CPA, MHA, FACHE, Executive Vice President / Chief Operating Officer

Provides the highest quality, compassionate healthcare to the people we serve. East Jefferson General Hospital will be the region's healthcare leader providing the highest quality care through innovation and collaboration with our team members, medical st

6923 **Family Service Society**
2515 Canal Street
Suite 201
New Orleans, LA 70119-6489 504-822-0800
Fax: 504-822-0831
family@fsgno.org
www.fsgno.org

L. Blake Jones, Chair
Jackie Sullivan, 1st Vice Chair
Kathleen Vogt, 2nd Vice Chair
Ronald P McClain JD, President & CEO
Offers services for the totally blind, legally blind, visually impaired, and more with health, counseling, educational, recreational, rehabilitation, computer training and professional training services.

6924 **Foundation Industries**
9995 Highway 64
Zachary, LA 70791 225-654-6288
Fax: 225-654-3988

Jim Lambert-Oswald, President
Jim Oswald, General Manager
A private, nonprofit sheltered workshop providing extended employment and work activities for the developmentally disabled. Objectives are to build work skills through supervision and develop social interaction.

6925 **Handi-Works Productions**
2700 Lee St
Alexandria, LA 71301-4358 318-442-3377
Fax: 318-473-0858

6926 **Lighthouse for the Blind in New Orleans**
123 State St
New Orleans, LA 70118-5793 504-899-4501
888-792-0163
Fax: 504-895-4162
lighthouselouisiana.org

Curtis Eustis, Chair
Paul Masinter, Chair Elect
Tabatha George, Secretary
Peyton Bush, Treasurer
Offers services for the totally blind, legally blind, visually impaired, and more with health, counseling, educational, recreational, rehabilitation, computer training and professional training services.

6927 **Louisiana Center for the Blind**
101 South Trenton Street
Ruston, LA 71270-4431 318-251-2891
800-234-4166
Fax: 318-251-0109
www.louisianacenter.org

Pam Allen, Executive Director
Neita Ghrigsby, Office Manager
Janette Woodard, Residential Manager
Jack Mendez, Director of Technology
A new kind of orientation and training center for blind persons. The center is privately operated and provides quality instruction in the skills of blindness. Offers employment assistance, computer literacy training, summer training and employment project

6928 **Louisiana State University Eye Center**
Lousiana State University
433 Bolivar Street
New Orleans, LA 70112-2272 504-568-4808
Fax: 504-412-1315
www.lsuhsc.edu

Jayne S. Weiss, Director
Kelli McMichael, Manager
The LSU Eye Center is part of the LSU Medical Center complex in downtown New Orleans. It is in the LSU-Lions Building at 2020 Gravier Street between South Bolivar and South Prieur streets.

6929 **New Orleans Speech and Hearing Center**
1636 Toledano St
New Orleans, LA 70115-4598 504-897-2606
Fax: 504-891-6048

Mary Beth Green, President
Jessica Vinturella, Treasurer
Kindall James, Secretary
This non-residential facility serves male and female clients for purposes of evaluating speech and hearing problems and providing speech therapy, hearing aids and other assistive technology for speech and hearing.

6930 **Port City Enterprises**
836 North Seventh Street
Port Allen, LA 70767-113 225-344-1142
877-344-1142
Fax: 225-344-1192
www.portcityenterprises.org

William Kleinpeter, President
Mark Graffeo, Vice President
L.J. Treuil Jr, Secretary
Philip Bourgoyne, Treasurer
Offers supported employment, sheltered work and supervised programs for the developmentally disabled, ages 22 and over.

6931 **Rehabilitation Center at Thibodeaux Regional**
Rehab Care
602 N Acadia Rd
Thibodaux, LA 70301-4847 985-493-4731
800-822-8442
Fax: 985-449-4600
www.thibodaux.com/centers-services

Jan Torres, Program Manager
Rose Pipes, Clinical Coordinator
Designed to help patients in their adjustment to a physically limiting condition, both physically and psychologically, by helping to maximize each patients abilities so he or she can function as independently as possible.

6932 **St. Patrick RehabCare Unit**
RehabCare
524 Doctor Michael Debakey Dr
Lake Charles, LA 70601-5725 337-491-7590
888-722-9355
Fax: 337-491-7157

Larry A Hauskins, Manager
Ruth Thornton, Admissions
A comprehensive physical and cognitive rehabilitation program designed to help individuals who have experienced a disabling injury or illness.

6933 **The Arc - Iberville**
PO Box 264
Plaquemine, LA 70765-0264 225-687-4062
arciberville@bellsouth.net

6934 **The Arc Caddo-Bossier**
351 Jordan St.
Shreveport, LA 71101 318-221-8392
Janet Parker, Executive Director
Chris Hackler, COO, Program & Services
Nonprofit agency providing services to adults and children with developmental disabilities

6935 **Touro Rehabilitation Center - LCMC (Louisiana Children's Medical Center)**
1401 Foucher St
New Orleans, LA 70115-3515 504-897-8565
Fax: 504-897-8393
www.touro.com/rehab

Jeanette Ray, VP of Rehab and Post Acute Srv
Janet Clark, Director of Inpatient Rehabilitation Programs
Marylee Pontillas, Director of Outpatient Rehab Srv
Lynn Drake, Patient Care Manager
Located in New Orleans' Garden District, Touro Rehabilitation is a comprehensive rehabilitation facility dedicated to the restoration of function and independence for individuals with disabilities. The scope of rehabilitation services is broad, with 3 CARF accreditations for Brain Injury, Spinal Cord Injury and General Rehabilitation. TRC opened in 1984 and offers 69 rehab beds.

TRC is part of Touro Infirmary which has a proud 150 year history as a nonprofit teaching hospital.

6936 **Training, Resource & Assistive-Technology**
2000 Lakeshore Drive
New Orleans, LA 70148-1
504-280-6000
888-514-4275
Fax: 504-280-5707
ggaglian@uno.edu
www.uno.edu

Ken Zangla, Director
Naomi Moore, Assistant Director
Connie Lanier, Coordinator
Peter J. Fos, President
Provides quality services to persons with disabilities, rehabilitation professionals, educators and employers. Built a solid reputation for its innovative training programs and community outreach efforts. The Center is recognized as a valuable resource st

Maine

6937 **Charlotte White Center**
572 Bangor Rd
Dover Foxcroft, ME 04426-3373
207-564-2426
888-440-4158
Fax: 207-564-2404
charlottewhitecenter.com

Richard M. Brown, CEO
Charles G. Clemons, COO
Dale Shaw, CFO
Mary Louis McEwen, President
A nonprofit agency, devoted to assisting adults and children with developmental disabilities, mental health, physical handicaps, and elder age related issues. With headquarters in Dover-Foxcroft Maine, the agency provides multiple levels of social services.

6938 **Iris Network for the Blind**
189 Park Avenue
Portland, ME 04102-2909
207-774-6273
Fax: 207-774-0679
ashah@theiris.org
theiris.org

Leonard Cole, Chairman
Katharine Ray, 1st Vice Chairman
Bruce Roullard, 2nd Vice Chairman
James E. Phipps MBA/JD, Executive Director
A statewide resource and catalyst for people who are visually impaired or blind so they can attain their determined level of independence and integration into the community.

6939 **Roger Randall Center**
45 School St
Houlton, ME 04730-2010
207-532-4068
Fax: 207-532-7334

Rob Moran, Executive Director
Tom Moakler, President
Vicki Moody, Vice President
Peter Crovo, Treasurer
The Roger Randall Cneter is one of five Day Habilitation Programs adminsitered by Community Living Association, a private, non-profit agency. These programs may provide a supportive environment that allows the individual to achieve their maximum growth po

6940 **Sebasticook Farms-Great Bay Foundation**
P.O. Box 65
Saint Albans, ME 04971
207-487-4399
Fax: 207-938-5670

Tom Davis, Executive Director
Pam Erskin, Program Coordinator
Provides residential, educational and vocational services to adults who are developmentally disabled in order to maximize independent living and to provide assistance in obtaining an earned income.

6941 **Social Learning Center**
10 Shelton McMurphey Blvd
Eugene, OR 97401-3363
541-485-2711
877-208-6134
Fax: 541-485-7087
www.oslc.org

Sam Vuchinich, Ph.D, Chair
Gordon Naga Hall, Ph.D., Vice President
Susan Miller, J.D., Secretary/Treasurer
Sally Guyer, Staff Representative
Post accute rehabilitation program.

Maryland

6942 **Blind Industries and Services of Maryland**
3345 Washington Blvd
Baltimore, MD 21227-1602
410-737-2600
888-322-4567
Fax: 410-737-2665
info@bism.org
bism.org

Donald J. Morris, Chairperson
Walter A. Brown, Vice Chairperson
Fredrick J. Puente, President
James R. Berens, Treasurer
Offers a comprehensive residential rehabilitation training program for people who are blind. Areas of instruction: Braille, cane travel, independent living, computer, adjustment and blindness seminars.

6943 **Center for Neuro-Rehabilitation**
2340238 N Cary St
Annapolis, MD 21223
410-263-1704
410-462-4711

Jeanne Fryer
Laurent Pierre-Philippe
Provide community-based inpatient and outpatient acute rehabilitation, vocational services and long-term care. Specializing in treating complex neurological conditions including spinal cord injuries, multiple sclerosis, strokes, and other brain injuries resulting from trauma, anoxia, tumors, genetic malformations and other related conditions. Locations in Annapolis, Bethesda, Frederick, Towson, MD and Fairfax, Va. CNR is licensed, a Medicare provider and CARF accredited.

6944 **Child Find/Early Childhood Disabilities Unit Montgomery County Public Schools**
Ste A4
10731 Saint Margarets Way
Kensington, MD 20895- 2831
301-929-2224
Fax: 301-929-2223

Julie Bader, Supervisor
Offers free developmental screening for children ages 3 years until eligible for kindergarten, evaluation and placement services.

6945 **Greater Baltimore Medical Center**
6701 N Charles St
Baltimore, MD 21204-6881
443-849-2000
800-597-9142
Fax: 443-849-2631
www.gbmc.org

John B. Chessare MD, President & CEO
Harold J. Tucker MD, Chief Of Staff
Eric L. Melchoir, Vice President & CFO
Keith Poisson, Executive VP & COO
Offers services for the visually impaired and blind with low vision exams. Rehabilitation teaching and orientation and mobility in the home or workplace. Also offers a bimonthly newsletter for $12/yr for Hoover patients and monthly share group.

6946 **James Lawrence Kernan Hospital**
2200 Kernan Drive
Baltimore, MD 21207-6697 410-285-6566
888-453-7626
Fax: 410-448-6854
www.umrehabortho.org
Michael Jablonover MD,MBA, President & CEO
John P. Straumanis MD, FAAP, Vice President
W. Walter x Augustin, III, CPA, Vice President of Financial Services
Cheryl D. Lee, RN, MSN, CRRN, Vice President, Patient Care Services
Kernan reigns as Maryland's origional orthopaedic hospital with a staff which consists of a support team of orthopaedic physician assistants and dedicated nurses in the Post Anesthesia Care Unit and on the Medical/Surgical Unit, guaranteeing the highest q

6947 **Levindale Hebrew Geriatric Center**
2401 W Belvedere Ave.
Baltimore, MD 21215-5271 410-601-9355
www.lifebridgehealth.org/Levindale

6948 **Meridan Medical Center For Subacute Care**
770 York Rd
Towson, MD 21204 410-821-5500
Fax: 410-821-6735
Yvette Caldwell, Administrator
Patients receive around-the-clock professional nursing care; physical and occupational, speech and respiratory therapists also assist patients. Each patient's individualized plan of care is reviewed and updated as patient needs change. Careful discharge p.

6949 **Rehabilitation Opportunities**
5100 Philadelphia Way
Lanham, MD 20706-4412 301-731-4242
Fax: 301-731-4191
roiworks.org
Tom Purcell, President
Bruce Shapiro, Vice President
David Fierst, Secretary
Henry Neloms, Treasurer
Organization offering day programs, evaluation, work adjustments and sheltered workshops for persons who are developmentally disabled.

6950 **Rosewood Center**
410-951-5000
888-300-7071
Fax: 410-581-6157
www.dhmh.state.md.us/dda/rosewood
Leslie Smith, Program Director
James Anzalone, Director
Rosewood Center is a State residential Center that supports adults with developmental disabilities from the central Maryland region.

6951 **TLC Speech-Language/Occupational TherapyCamps**
2092 Gaither Rd.
Suite 100
Rockville, MD 20850 301-424-5200
Fax: 301-424-8063
TTY: 301-424-5203
info@ttlc.org
www.ttlc.org
Patricia Ritter, Executive Director
TLC provides small group summer programs for children with special needs. Offers speech-language and occupational therapy summer camps for children ages 3-7.

6952 **Workforce and Technology Center**
Division of Rehabilitation Services
2301 Argonne Drive
Baltimore, MD 21218-1628 410-554-9442
888-554-0334
Fax: 410-554-9112
www.dors.state.md.us
Dan Frye, Chairperson
Josie Thomas, Vice Chairperson
Is one of nine state operated comprehensive rehabilitation facilities in the country providing a wide range of services to individuals with disabilities. The Maryland Division of Rehabilitation Services operates the Workforce and Technology Program. Avail

Massachusetts

6953 **Baroco Corporation**
136 West Street
Northampton, MA 01060-2711 413-534-9978
Fax: 413-585-9019
www.baroco.com
Rick Barnard, President/Owner
Suzanne Darby, Executive Administrator
Julia McLaughlin, Executive Administrator
Janet Lawlor, Executive Administrator
Provides training and therapeutic support for its recipients with developmental disabilities in order to aid them in securing and maintaining placement in a less-restrictive setting.

6954 **Berkshire Meadows**
160 Gould Street
Suite 300
Needham, MA 02494-2300 781-559-4900
Fax: 413-528-0293
lkelly@jri.org
berkshiremeadows.org
Andy Pond, President
Gregory Canfield, Vice President
Deborah Reuman, CFO
Stephen H. Webster, Executive Advisor
Private, non profit school for children, adolescents, young adults who are severely, developmentally disabled. Approved special education learning center, work site program and foster care. Physical therapy, speech and language development, behavioral pro *$8200.00*

6955 **Blueberry Hill Healthcare**
75 Brimbal Ave
Beverly, MA 01915-6009 978-927-2020
Fax: 978-922-5213
admissions@BlueberryHillRehab.com
www.blueberryhillrehab.com
Ralph Epstein, Medical Director
Accomodates 146 residents. We are centrally located close to Route 128 and Route 1A in Beverly Massachusetts. We offer short-term rehab care, long term care and Alzheimer's Special Care Programs. Our interdisciplinary team designs individual care plans fo

6956 **Boston University Hospital Vision Rehabilitation Services**
One Boston Medical Center Place
Boston, MA 02118-2371 617-638-8000
Fax: 617-638-7769
www.bmc.org/rehab.htm
Simona Manasian, Medical Director
Karen Mattie, Director
Jenn Blake, Clinical Outpatient Supervisor
Kara Schworm, Clinical In-patient Supervisor
Offers services for the totally blind, legally blind, visually impaired, and more with health, counseling, educational, recreational, rehabilitation, computer training and professional training services.

6957 **Burbank Rehabilitation Center**
275 Nichols Rd
Fitchburg, MA 01420-1919 978-343-5000
888-840-3627
Fax: 978-343-5342
www.umassmemorialhealthcare.org
David Bennett, Chair
Eric Dickson, President & CEO
The largest community hospital and regional referral center in the area. Offers the most extensive high quality, cost-effective healthcare services in the region. The hospital provides outstanding hospital-based services such as case management of high ri

6958 **Carl and Ruth Shapiro Family National Center for Accessible Media**
WGBH Educational Foundation
1 Guest St.
Boston, MA 02135-2016
617-300-3400
Fax: 617-300-1035
TTY: 617-300-2489
ncam@wgbh.org
ncam.wgbh.org

Donna Danielewski, Director
Madeleine Rothberg, Senior Subject Matter Expert
Geoff Freed, Director of Technology
Bryan Gould, Director of Accessible Learning and Assessment Technologies

The Carl and Ruth Shapiro Family National Center for Accessible Media (NCAM) is a research and development facility dedicated to addressing barriers to media and emerging technologies for people with disabilities in their homes, schools, workplaces, and communities.

6959 **Carroll Center for the Blind**
770 Centre St
Newton, MA 02458-2597
617-969-6200
800-852-3131
Fax: 617-969-6204
www.carroll.org

Josepth Abely, President
Arthur O'Neill, Vice President
Brian Charlson, Director of Computer Training Services
Robert McGillivray, Director of Low Vision Services

Offers services for the totally blind, legally blind, visually impaired, and more with health, counseling, educational, in dependent living, tronell skills, computer traing, recreational, rehabilitation, computer training and professional training services.

6960 **Center for Psychiatric Rehabilitation**
Boston University
940 Commonwealth Ave
West
Boston, MA 02215-1203
617-353-3549
Fax: 617-353-7700
psyrehab@bu.edu
cpr.bu.edu

Kim T. Mueser, Executive Director
Deborah Dolan, Director of operations
Larry Kohn, Director of Development
E. Sally Rogers, Director of Research

The mission of the Center is to increase knowledge, to train treatment personnel, to develop effective rehabilitation programs and to assist in organizing both personnel and programs into efficient and coordinated service delivery systems for people with

6961 **Clark House Nursing Center At Foxhill Village**
Kindred Healthcare
30 Longwood Dr
Westwood, MA 02090-1132
781-326-5652
800-359-7412
Fax: 781-326-4034
www.clarkhousefhv.com

Chris Wasel, Administrator

Clark House At Fox Hill Village accomodates 70 residents. We are part of the Fox Hill Village Assisted Living and Retirement Center campus. Clark House Nursing center has been named a recipient of a 2005 step II quality Award from the American Health Care

6962 **College Internship Program at the Berkshire Center**
18 Park St
Lee, MA 01238-1702
413-243-2576
Fax: 413-243-3351

Lucy Gosselin, Program Director
Laina Hubbard, Admissions Coordinator
Charles D. Houff, Head Therapist

A highly individualized postsecondary program for learning disabled young adults 18-30. Provides job placement services and follow-ups; college support; money management and social skills. Residential students share an apartment and have their own room.

6963 **Devereux Advanced Behavioral Health Massachusetts & Rhode Island**
Devereux School
60 Miles Rd.
P.O. Box 219
Rutland, MA 01543
508-886-4746
800-338-3738
Fax: 508-886-4773
tbeauvai@devereux.org
www.devereuxma.org

Stephen Yerdon, Executive Director
Bonnie Byer, Business Development Director
Evans Chiyombwe, Quality Management Director
Sandy Fleek, Executive Assistant

Serving children and youth with emotional, behavioral, intellectual and developmental disorders. Services include residential treatment, community-based group homes, therapeutic foster care, special needs day school, substance abuse and autism spectrum programs, diagnostic services and in-home services.

6964 **Eagle Pond Rehabilitation and Living Center**
1 Love Lane
P.O. Box 208
South Dennis, MA 02660-3445
508-385-6034
Fax: 508-385-7064
www.eaglepond.com

Paul Marchwat, Executive Director
Ellen Reil, Marketing Director

Eagle Pond accomodates 142 residents. Medicare and Medicaid certified as well as being accredited by the Joint Comission (formerly (JCAHO) which enables us to contract with many insurance companies.

6965 **FOR Community Services**
75 Litwin Ln
Chicopee, MA 01020-4817
413-592-6142
Fax: 413-598-0478
ggolash1@aol.com

Gina Golash, Executive Director

Providing a world of meaning for individuals with developmental disabilities throughout Western Massachusetts since 1967.

6966 **Fairlawn Rehabilitation Hospital**
189 May Street
Worcester, MA 01602-4399
508-791-6351
Fax: 508-831-1277
www.fairlawnrehab.org

Dave Richer, CEO
Peter Bagley MD, Medical Director
Matthew Akulonis, Director Of Support Operations
Judy Chuli, Chief Nursing Officer

Offers comprehensive rehabilitation on both an inpatient and outpatient basis. Specialty programs include: head injury, spinal cord injury, young/senior stroke, oncology, geriatrics and orthopedics.

6967 **Greenery Extended Care Center: Worcester**
59 Acton Street
Worcester, MA 01604-4899
508-791-3147
800-633-0887
Fax: 508-753-6267
worcester@wingatehealthcare.com
wingatehealthcare.com

Scott Schuster, Founder & President
Brian Callahan, CFO
Michael Benjamin, Vice President
Trent Guthrie, Senior Director

173 beds offering complex care, extended rehabilitation and neurobehavioral intervention. Offering life care homes and Nursing home services. Specialties include life events and physical care, long term and home health care, and nursing homes and nursing

6968 **Greenery Rehabilitation & Skilled Nursing Center**
P.O. Box 1330
Middleboro, MA 02346-4330
508-947-9295
Fax: 508-947-7974

6969 Harrington House Nursing And Rehabilitation Center
160 Main Street
Walpole, MA 02081-4037
508-660-3080
Fax: 508-660-1634
www.harringtonrehab.com
Joseph Haron, Medical Director
Accomodates 90 residents. Our state-of-the-art center offers post-accute services including rehabilitation and medical management. Our center also provides a long term care program including hospice services.

6970 HealthSouth Rehabilitation Hospital Of Western Massachusetts
222 State Street
Ludlow, MA 01056-3478
413-308-3300
Fax: 413-547-2738
www.healthsouthrehab.org
Victoria Healy, CEO
Adnan Dahdul, M.D., Medical Director
Deborah Cabanas, Chief Nursing Officer
AnnMaria Elder, M.D., Medical Staff President
A 53-bed acute Rehabilitation Hospital. The facility has been operating for 14 years and has provided rehabilitative care to patients and families in the greater Springfield area with an outstanding reputation for attention to detail and compassion. Becau

6971 Holiday Inn Boxborough Woods
242 Adams Pl
Boxborough, MA 01719-1735
978-263-8701
800-465-4329
Fax: 978-263-0518
box_sales@fine-hotels.com
www.ihg.com/holidayinn
Kevin Murray, Manager
Marcel Girard, Manager
Nancy Ellen Hurley, Chief Marketing Officer
Located on 35 acres of wooded countryside just off I-495 at exit #28. Minutes from the Mass Turnpike, Route 2, 290 and 9. Conference center located on main level with 30,000 square feet of meeting space. Guest rooms feature two-line telephones, voice mail
$129 - $159

6972 Lifeworks Employment Services
1400 Providence Highway
Suite 2300
Norwood, MA 02062- 4551
781-769-3298
Fax: 781-551-0045
www.lifeworksma.org
Dan Burke, President & CEO
Chris Page, Vice President
Brenda Calder, CFO
Mary Hagen, Controller
Providing homes, jobs, education and supportive living for people with developmental disabilities.

6973 Massachusetts Eye and Ear Infirmary & Vision Rehabilitation Center
243 Charles Street
Boston, MA 02114-3002
617-523-7900
Fax: 617-573-4178
TTY: 617-523-5498
www.masseyeandear.org
Wycliffe Grousbeck, Chairman
John Fernandaz, President & CEO
Lily H. Bentas, Secretary
Jonathan Uhrig, Treasurer
Visual rehabilitation encompasses a low vision rehabilitation evaluation, occupational therapy evaluation (with home visit if necessary), and social service evaluation.

6974 New England Center for Children
260 Tremont Street
Boston, MA 02116-2108
617-636-4600
Fax: 617-636-4866
cwelch@necc.org
necc.org
Lisel Macenka, Chair
James C. Burling, Vice Chair
L.Vincent Strully, President
Michael F. Downey, Treasurer
A comprehensive year-round program for students with autism and PDD who require a highly specialized educational and behavior management program. Students are from all over the country and receive intensive, positive, behavioral counseling and social skil

6975 New England Eye Center - Tufts Medical Center
Tufts Medical Center
260 Tremont St
Boston, MA 02116
617-636-4600
800-231-3316
Fax: 617-636-4866
eli_peli@meei.harvard.edu
www.neec.com
Jeannette Spillane, Executive Director
Shana Bellus, Director, Admitting Operations
Linnea Olsson, Special Projects Consultant
ChiHae Kwan, Optometrist
The New England Eye Center offers services for the legally blind and visually impaired, as well as for health care providers. Services include health care, counseling, education, vision research and professional training. Emphasis is on mobility related vision enhancement, including devices for driving and safe walking.

6976 New Medico Rehabilitation and Skilled Nursing Center at Lewis Bay
89 Lewis Bay Rd
Hyannis, MA 02601-5207
508-775-7601
Fax: 508-790-4239
Edmund Steinle, Executive Director
Post acute rehabilitation services.

6977 Protestant Guild Learning Center
411 Waverley Oaks Rd
Suite 104
Waltham, MA 02452-8449
781-893-6000
Fax: 781-893-1171
www.theguildschool.org
Eric H. Rosenberger, President
Thomas P. Corcoran, Vice President & Treasurer
Thomas Belski, Chief Executive Officer
Sandra L. Skinner, Clerk
Offers services for the diagnostically disabled children and adolescents with ages 6-22 years with health, counseling, educational, recreational, rehabilitation, computer training and professional training services.

6978 Shaughnessy-Kaplan Rehabilitation Hospital
1 Dove Ave
Salem, MA 01970
978-745-9000
Fax: 978-740-4730
skrhinfo@partners.org
spauldingrehab.org
Anthony Sciola, CEO
Maureen Banks, RN, MS, MBA, CN, President
Mary Beth DiFilippo, Vice President
Charles Pu, MD, Chief Medical Officer
A 160-bed private, non-profit hospital. We have been providing care for residents of greater North Shore communities since 1975. Shaughnessy has 120 long-term care hospital beds and a 40-bed transitional care unit sometimes referred to as a skilled nursin

6979 Son-Rise Program
2080 South Undermountain Road
Sheffield, MA 01257-9643
413-229-2100
877-766-7473
Fax: 413-229-3202
correspondence@option.org
www.autismtreatmentcenter.org
Barry Neil Kaufman, Co Founder
Samahria Lyte Kaufman, Co Founder

THe Son-Rise Program is a powerful, effective and totally unique treatment for children and adults challengedby Autism, Autuism Spectrum Disorders, Pervasive Developmental Disorder (PDD), Asperger's Syndrome and other developmental difficulties.

6980 **Southern Worcester County Rehabilitation Inc. D/B/A Life-Skills, Inc.**
44 Morris St
Webster, MA 01570-1812
508-943-0700
Fax: 508-949-6129
www.life-skillsinc.org

J Thomas Amick, Executive Director
Kristin Nelson, Board President
Barbara Butrym, Board Vice President
Janice Smith, Board Secretary

Life-Skills, Inc. assists mentally and developmentally challenged adults with meeting their individual needs, and empowering them to take full advantage of meaningful opportunities in their communities. We provide residential, employment, transportation, behavior, and theraputic day habilitation services to 350 adults in MA. We operate thrift & consignment stores, a small cafe, an ice cream shop, mini golf & arcade center, vending and greenhouse businesses, bank courier service, and others.

6981 **Vinfen Corporation**
950 Cambridge Street
Cambridge, MA 02141-1001
617-441-1800
877-284-6336
Fax: 617-441-1858
TTY: 617-225-2000
info@vinfen.org
www.vinfen.org

Philip A. Mason, Ph.D., Chairperson
Bruce L. Bird, Ph.D., CEO/ President
Elizabeth K. Glaser, Chief Operations Officer
Glen Mattera, Chief Financial Officer

A private, nonprofit company, Vinfen Corporation is the largest human services provider in Massachusetts. Vinfen offers clinical, educational, residential and support services to individuals of all ages with mental illness and or developmental disabilities, who also may have another disability (e.g. substance abuse, homelessness, AIDS). The company also trains professionals in the mental health field and helps consumers to learn to live in community-based settings at the highest levels.

6982 **Visiting Nurse Association of North Shore**
5 Federal St
Danvers, MA 01923-3687
508-751-6926
800-728-1862
Fax: 978-777-0308
www.vnacarenetwork.org

Mary Ann O'Connor, CEO/ President
Stephanie Jackman-Havey, Chief Operating Officer/Chief Financial Officer
David Rose, Vice President of Human Resources
Jane Woodbury, Vice President of Fund Development

Home health services including nurses, physical, occupational and speech therapy, home health aides and more. Special programs include nutrition counseling, IV care, pediatric therapy, HIV/AIDS services and wound management. Provides services 7 days a week, 365 days a year and we accept Medicare, Medicaid and most HMO's and health insurers.

6983 **Weldon Center for Rehabilitation**
233 Carew St
Springfield, MA 01104-2377
413-748-6800
Fax: 413-748-6806
mercycares.com

Barbara Haswell, Manager

One of the most vital, necessary health resources in the region by helping thousands of people toward restored health and independence. A comprehensive, integrated, non-profit facility offering inpatient, outpatient, day rehabilitation and pediatric services on one site.

6984 **Youville Hospital & Rehab Center**
1575 Cambridge St
Cambridge, MA 02138-4398
617-876-4344
Fax: 617-547-5501

Michigan

6985 **Botsford Center For Rehabilitation & Health Improvement-Redford**
28050 Grand River Ave.
Farmington Hills, MI 48336-5919
248-471-8000
877-442-7900
Fax: 313-387-3838
www.botsford.org

John Darin, Manager

A 20 bed inpatient physical rehabilitation unit, servicing individuals who have experienced a stroke, amputation, orthopedic fracture, or other neurological impairment.

6986 **Bureau of Services for Blind Persons Training Center**
1541 Oakland Dr
Kalamazoo, MI 49008
269-337-3848
800-292-4200
Fax: 269-337-3872
mossc@michigan.gov

Cheryl Heibeck, Director
Bruce Schultz, Assistant Director

Residential facility that provides instruction to legally blind adults in Braille, computer operation and assistive technology, handwriting, cane travel, cooking, personal management, industrial arts and also crafts. During training students will develop career plans which may include work experience, internships, volunteer opprtunities and even part-time paid employment.

6987 **Chelsea Community Hospital Rehabilitation Unit**
775 South Main Street
Chelsea, MI 48118-1383
734-593-6000
800-231-2211
Fax: 734-475-4191
www.stjoeschelsea.org

Nancy K. Graebner, CEO/ President
Kathy Brubaker, RN, Vice President and Chief Nursing Officer
Randall Forsch, MD, Chief Medical Officer
Barbara Fielder, VP Finance

A private, non-profit, acute care facility that combines the best of small town values with national standards of healthcare excellance. The hospital has a 19-bed acute care inpatient rehabilitation unit with comprehensive outpatient programs, including a coordinated brain injury program.

6988 **Clare Branch**
790 Industrial Dr
Clare, MI 48617-9224
989-386-7707
888-773-7664
Fax: 989-386-2199
mail@mmionline.com
www.mmionline.org

Cris Zeigler, Executive Director

MMI will strive to be the premier provider of person-centered services to people with barriers to employment. We will connect individuals with community resources that provide mutual benefit to them and to the community. MMI will be known for excellence in service provision, ethical business practices, a quality work environment, and for providing services that enhance the dignity and value of the people we serve.

6989 **Clarkston Spec Healthcare Center**
4800 Clintonville Rd
Clarkston, MI 48346-4297
800-454-5909
Margaret Canny, Administrator

120 beds offering active/acute rehabilitation, complex care, day treatment, extended rehabilitation, neurobehavioral intervention and short-term evaluation.

6990 **DMC Health Care Center-Novi**
42005 W 12 Mile Rd
Novi, MI 48377-3113
248-305-7575
Fax: 425-201-1450
novi@patch.com
novi.patch.com

Bud Rosenthal, CEO
Leigh Zareli Lewis, COO
Andreas Turanski, CTO
Melanie Pereira, VP of Finance

The Detroit Medical Center's record of service has provided medical excellence throughout the history of the Metropolitan Detroit area. From the founding of the Children's Hospital in 1886, to the creation of the first mechanical heart at Harpers Hospital 50 years ago, to our compassion for the underdeserved, our legacy of caring is unmatched.

6991 **Eight CAP, Inc. Head Start**
904 Oak Drive
Greenville, MI 48838-9277
616-754-9315
Fax: 616-754-9310
laurelm@8cap.org
www.8cap.org

Ralph Loeschner, Executive Director
Nancy Secor, Contact
Post acute rehabilitation programs.

6992 **Greater Detroit Agency for the Blind and Visually Impaired**
16625 Grand River Ave
Detroit, MI 48227-1419
313-272-3900
Fax: 313-272-6893
gdabvi.org

Frederick J Simpson, Board Chairman
Charles L. Cone, Vice Chairman
Leonard W Robinson, Board Secretary
John W. Rhinesmith, CPA, Board Treasurer
Offers services for seniors 60 and over who are legally blind. Also provides eye health information, counseling, education and rehabilitation services.

6993 **Hope Network Neuro Rehabilitation**
3075 Orchard Vista Dr. SE
PO Box 890
Grand Rapids, MI 49546
616-301-8000
800-695-7273
Fax: 616-301-8010
www.hopenetworkrehab.org

Phil Weaver, President & CEO
Tim Becker, Chief Operating Officer
Andre Pierre, Chief Financial Officer
Kiran Taylor, Chief Medical Officer
Neuro Rehabilitation is a service line of Hope Network, helping those with brain or spinal cord injuries or other neurological conditions recover through treatment techniques and person-centered care.

6994 **Lakeland Center**
26900 Franklin Rd
Southfield, MI 48033-5312
248-350-8070
Fax: 248-350-8078
peggys@thelakelandcenter.net
thelakelandcenter.net

Irving Shapiro, CEO
Santhosh Madhavan, Director Physical Medicine
Gary Yashinsky, Associate Medical Director
Subacute rehabilitation program directed toward those with severe neurologic diagnoses, ie: TBI, cerebral aneurysm, anoxic encephalopathy, CVA and cerebral hemorrhage, orthopedic injuries, and spinal cord injury. Subacute rehabilitation is provided for those who recover slowly and require individualized treatment plans. Residential program available as well.

6995 **Mary Free Bed Rehabilitation Hospital**
235 Wealthy St SE
Grand Rapids, MI 49503-5247
616-493-9657
800-528-8989
Fax: 616-454-3939
info@maryfreebed.com
maryfreebed.com

Kent Riddle, CEO
John Butzer, MD, Medical Director
Randy DeNeff, Vice President of Finance
Founded more than 100 years ago, Mary Free Bed Rehabilitation Hospital is and 80-bed, not-for-profit, acute rehabilitation center. Its mission is to restore hope and freedom through rehabilitation to people with disabilities. Mary Free Bed offers comprehensive inpatient and outpatient rehabilitationfor children and adults using an interdisciplinary approach. Also available are numerous specialty programs designed to increase the quality of life and independence of people with disabilities.

6996 **Michigan Career And Technical Institute**
11611 Pine Lake Rd
Plainwell, MI 49080-9225
269-664-4461
877-901-7360
Fax: 269-664-5850

Dennis Hart, Executive Director
A residential vocational training center for adults with physical, mental or emotional disabilities.

6997 **Mid-Michigan Industries**
2426 Parkway Dr
Mt Pleasant, MI 48858-4723
989-773-6918
888-773-7664
888-773-7664
Fax: 989-773-1317
mmionline.com

Alan Schilling, President
Andrea Christopher, Director Admissions
Linda Wagner, Branch Director
Sheri Alexander, Director of Community Employment
Providing jobs and training for persons with barriers to employment. Services include vocational evaluation, job placement, supported employment, work services, prevocational training and case management

6998 **New Medico Community Re-Entry Service**
216 St Marys Lake Rd
Battle Creek, MI 49017-9710
Fax: 269-962-2241
James Rekshan, Executive Director

6999 **Sanilac County Community Mental Health**
171 Dawson St
Sandusky, MI 48471-1062
810-648-0330
888-225-4447
888-225-4447
Fax: 810-648-0319

Roger Dean, Executive Director
Post-acute rehabilitation facility and programs.

7000 **Special Tree Rehabilitation System**
600 Stephenson Highway
Troy, MI 48083-1110
248-616-0950
800-648-6885
Fax: 248-616-0957
info@specialtree.com
www.specialtree.com

Joseph Richart, CEO
Special Tree exists to provide hope, encouragement, and expertise for people who have experienced life-altering changes. Our team approach to rehabilitation, custom designed for each person's needs and goals, offers these individuals the best opportunity for healing and recovery.

7001 **Thumb Industries**
1263 Sand Beach Rd
Bad Axe, MI 48413-8817
989-269-9229
Fax: 989-269-2587
thumbindustries@hotmail.com
www.thumbindustries.com

Rhonda Wisenbaugh, Executive Director
Provides job training and employment for disabled persons. Vocational rehabilitation agency, manufactures household furnishings, direct mail advertising service.

7002 **Visually Impaired Center**
1422 W Court St
Flint, MI 48503-5008
810-767-4014
Fax: 810-767-0020
www.vicflint.org

a pages

7003 **Welcome Homes Retirement Community for the Visually Impaired**
1953 Monroe Ave NW
Grand Rapids, MI 49505-6242
616-447-7837
888-939-9292
888-939-9292
Fax: 616-447-9891

Beth Lucksted, Manager
Offers services for the totally blind, legally blind, visually impaired, and more with health, counseling, educational, recre-

ational, rehabilitation, computer training and professional training services.

7004 **William H Honor Rehabilitation Center Henry Ford Wyanclotte Hospital**
Henry Ford Health System
2333 Biddle Ave
Wyandotte, MI 48192-4668 734-246-6000
Fax: 734-246-6926
www.henryfordwyandotte.com
Denise Dailing, Administration Leader/rehabilita
James Sexton, Chief Executive Officer
Henry Ford, Owner
Henry Ford Wyandotte Hospital offers an array of educational programs, health screenings, and support groups. The hospital is CARF accredited and has a CARF certified stroke specialty unit.

Minnesota

7005 **Industries: Cambridge**
601 Cleveland St S
Cambridge, MN 55008-1752 763-689-5434
Fax: 763-552-1281
jspicer@industriesinc.org
www.industriesinc.org
Daryl Peterson, Board Chair
Bruce Montgomery, Vice Chair
Marilyn Bachman, Secretary
Kevin Troupe, Treasurer
Nonprofit organization that does vocational assessment and training for people with disabilities.

7006 **Industries: Mora**
500 Walnut St S
Mora, MN 55051-1936 320-679-2354
Fax: 320-679-2355
jspicer@industriesinc.org
www.industriesinc.org
Daryl Peterson, Board Chair
Bruce Montgomery, Vice Chair
Marilyn Bachman, Secretary
Kevin Troupe, Treasurer
Nonprofit organization that does vocational assessment and training for people with disabilities.

7007 **Shriners Hospitals for Children: Twin Cities**
2025 E River Pkwy
Minneapolis, MN 55414-3696 612-596-6100
888-293-2832
888-293-2832
Fax: 612-339-5954
www.shrinershospitalsforchildren.org
Charles C. Lobeck, Administrator
Cary Mielke, M.D, Interim Chief of Staff
Don Engel, Development Officer
Shriners Hospital for Children-Twin Cities offers quality orthopedic medical care regardless of the patients' ability to pay. Shriners Hospitals provide inpatient and outpatient services, surgery, casts, braces, artificial limbs, x-rays and physical and occupational therapy to any child under the age of 18 who may benefit from treatment.

7008 **Vision Loss Resources**
1936 Lyndale Ave S
Minneapolis, MN 55403-3101 612-871-2222
Fax: 612-872-0189
TTY: 612-382-8422
info@vlrw.org
www.visionlossresources.org
Barry Shear, Chair
Lisa David, Vice Chair
Mary McDougall, Secretary
Jackie Peichel, Treasurer
Offers services for the totally blind, legally blind, visually impaired, and more with health, counseling, educational, recreational, rehabilitation, computer training and professional training services.

Mississippi

7009 **Addie McBryde Rehabilitation Center for the Blind**
PO Box 5314
Jackson, MS 39296-5314 601-364-2700
800-443-1000
Fax: 601-364-2677
H. S. McMillan, Executive Director
Shelia Browning, Deputy Director Non-Vocational P
Offers services for the totally blind, legally blind, visually impaired, blind and more with health, counseling, educational, recreational, rehabilitation, computer training services and orientation and mobility.

7010 **Mississippi Methodist Rehabilitation Center**
1350 E Woodrow Wilson Ave
Jackson, MS 39216-5198 601-981-2611
800-223-6672
Fax: 601-364-3571
www.methodistonline.org
Mark A. Adams, President/ CEO
Matthew L. Holleman, III, Chair
Mike P. Sturdivant Jr, Vice Chairman
David L. McMillin, Secretary
Rebuild lives that have been broken by disabilities and impairments from serious illness or severe injury. The challenge is to help patients regain abilities, restore function and movement, and renew emotionally. It features personal rehabilitation treatment plans administered by specialized teams of health care professionals through a variety of outpatient programs, treatments and other services.

Missouri

7011 **Alpine North Nursing and Rehabilitation Center**
4700 NW Cliff View Dr
Kansas City, MO 64150-1237 816-741-5105
Fax: 816-746-1301
Mike Stacks, Executive Director
Bob Richard, Administrator
Postacute rehabilitation program.

7012 **Christian Hospital Northeast**
11133 Dunn Rd
Saint Louis, MO 63136-6119 314-653-5000
877-747-9355
Fax: 314-653-4130
christianhospital.org
Ron McMullen, President
Bryan Hartwick, Vice President Human Resources
Sebastian Rueckert, MD, Vice President and Chief Medical Officer
Jennifer Cordia, Vice President and Chief Nurse Executive
A non-profit organization, a 493 bed acute care facility on 28 acres. Christian Hospital has more then 600 physicians on staff and a diverse workforce of more then 2,5000 health-care professionals who are dedicated to providing the absolute best care with the latest technology and medical advances.

7013 **Easterseals Midwest**
11933 Westline Industrial Dr.
St. Louis, MO 63146 800-200-2119
Fax: 314-394-4007
info@esmw.org
www.easterseals.com/midwest
Wendy Sullivan, Chief Executive Officer
Jeff Arledge, Chief Financial Officer
Tom Barry, Chief Development Officer
Laurel Taylor, Chief Human Resources Officer
Enhances the independence and quality of life of people with disabilities through services, education, outreach and advocacy.

7014 **Integrated Health Services of St. Louis at Gravois**
10954 Kennerly Rd
Saint Louis, MO 63128-2018 314-843-4242
Fax: 314-843-4031
Lisa Niehaus, Administrator

Subacute, skilled and intermediate care; ventilator/tracheostomy management program; wound management program and complex rehabilitation program.

7015 Metropolitan Employment & Rehabilitation Service
M ER S Goodwill
1727 Locust St
Saint Louis, MO 63103-1703
314-241-3464
Fax: 314-241-9348
www.mersgoodwill.org

Lewis C. Chartock, Ph.D., President/ CEO
Dawayne Barnett, CFO
Mark Arens, Executive Vice President, Chief of Program Services
Mark Kahrs, Executive Vice President, Retail Services

Vocational rehabilitation, primarily with the disabled, skills training and placement services.

7016 Poplar Bluff RehabCare Program
Lucy Lee Hospital
2620 N Westwood Blvd
Poplar Bluff, MO 63901-3396
573-785-7721
Fax: 573-686-5987

Jim Martin, Program Manager
Chris Murray, Care Coordinator
Darlene Hill, Care Admissions Coordinator

Provides physical medicine and rehabilitation to individuals with a physically limiting condition. The program is designed to help individuals function as independently as possible by maximizing their strength and abilities.

7017 Shriners Hospitals for Children St. Louis
2001 S Lindbergh Blvd
Saint Louis, MO 63131-3597
314-432-3600
800-850-2960
Fax: 314-432-2930
www.shrinershq.org/hospitals/st.louis

John McCabe, Executive Vice President
Kenneth Guidera, M.D., Chief Medical Officer
Eugene R. D'Amore, Vice President, Hospital Operations
Kathy A. Dean, Vice President, Human Resources

Medical care is provided free of charge for children 18 and under with orthopaedic conditions.

7018 St. Louis Society for the Blind and Visually Impaired
8770 Manchester Rd
Saint Louis, MO 63144-2724
314-960-9000
Fax: 314-968-9003
www.slsbvi.org

David Ekin, President
Chris Pickel, Chair
Ann Shapiro, Vice Chair
Sherine Apte, Secretary

Offers vision rehabilitation services for the totally blind, legally blind, visually impaired, including counseling, educational, recreational, rehabilitation, computer training and professional training services. Low vision aids and appliance available through low vision clinic by appointment.

7019 Truman Medical Center Low Vision Rehabilitation Program
Eye Foundation of Kansas City
2300 Holmes St.
Kansas City, MO 64108
816-404-1780
Fax: 816-404-1786

Nelson R. Sabates, M.D., Chairman
Monika Malecha, MD, Residency Program Director
Abraham Poulose, MD, Director of Clinics

Our program is designed to maximize daily tasks for a person with low vision. We are able to evaluate a person's home and provide recommendations as needed.

7020 Truman Neurological Center
12404 E. US 40 Highway
Independence, MO 64055-1354
816-373-5060
Fax: 816-373-5787
tnccommunity.com

James Landrum, Executive Director
Ann Johnson, Finance Director
Terri Boyce, Office Assistant
Mary Beth Johnson, Compliance Director

A licensed habilitation center established for the purpose of assisting persons with developmental disabilities. The minimum age is 18. Residential care is provided in four group homes in the community licensed by the DMH and CARF accredited.

Montana

7021 Benefis Healthcare
1101 26th St S
Great Falls, MT 59405-5104
406-455-5000
Fax: 406-455-2110
benefis@benefis.org
www.benefis.org

John Goodnow, CEO
Laura Goldhahn-Konen, President
Forrest Ehlinger, Chief Financial & Treasury Officer
Paul Dolan, MD, Chief Medical Information Officer

Benefis Healthcare is a not-for-profit community asses governed by a 15-member local board of directors. Benefis is locally owned and controlled. Benefis is a Level II trauma center- one of only 4 in the state and 107 in the country.

7022 Disability Services Division of Montana
Department of Public Health
Helena, MT 59604
406-444-7734
Fax: 406-444-3465

Keith Messmer, Manager
Sandi Gory, Administrative Assistant
Janice Frisch, Chief Management Operations

Responsible for coordinating, developing and implementing comprehensive programs to assist Montanans with disabilities with activities of daily living, community base services and coordinated programs of habilitation, rehabilitation and independent living.

7023 Easterseals-Goodwill Northern Rocky Mountain
Easterseals National
425 1st Ave. N
Great Falls, MT 59401-2507
406-761-3680
www.esgw.org

Michelle Belknap, President & CEO

Provides services for children and adults with disabilities and other special needs, and support to their families.

Nebraska

7024 Las Vegas Healthcare And Rehabilitation Center
680 South Fourth Street
Louisville, KY 40202
502-596-7300
TTY: 800-545-0749
web_administrator@kindredhealthcare.com
kindredhealthcare.com

Paul J. Diaz, President/ CEO

Accomodates 79 residents. Serving the community for approximately 40 years. Located in close proximity to local hospitals and surrounded by medical complexes, out center offers both short-term rehabilitation and long term.care.

7025 Sierra Pain Institute
265 Golden Ln
Reno, NV 89502-1205
775-323-7092
Fax: 775-323-5259

Lyle Smith, Owner

The program consists of a medically supervised outpatient program managed by an interdisciplinary team with input from specialties of Pain Medicine, Physical Therapy and Occupational Science. The format insures that each patient receives the full range of behavioral techniques in a well-integrated, individually tailored therapeutic regimen.

New Hampshire

7026 **Department of Physical Medicine and Rehabilitation**
Exeter Hospital
5 Alumni Dr
Exeter, NH 03833-2128 603-778-7311
Fax: 603-580-6592
www.exeterhospital.com
Kevin Calahan, President
Offers patient treatment, committed to enhancing the lives of individuals with short and long term physically disabling conditions.

7027 **Farnum Rehabilitation Center**
580 Court St
Keene, NH 03431-1718 603-354-6630
Fax: 603-355-2078
Susan Loughrey, Program Director
Judy Bell, Manager
Offers rehabilitation services, occupational therapy, physical therapy and more for the physically challenged individual.

7028 **Hackett Hill Nursing Center and Integrated Care**
191 Hackett Hill Rd
Manchester, NH 03102-8993 603-668-8161
Fax: 603-622-2584
Daniele Peckham, Administrator
Brett Lennerton, Administrator
A 68-bed certified nursing home.Postacute rehabilitation program.

7029 **Mental Health Center: Riverside Courtyard, The**
3 Twelfth St
Berlin, NH 03570-3860 603-752-7404
Fax: 603-752-5194
Eileen Theriault, Manager
A center to help people that have mental disabilities.

7030 **New Hampshire Rehabilitation and Sports Medicine**
Catholic Medical Center
Ste 201
769 S Main St
Manchester, NH 03102-5166 603-647-1899
800-437-9666
Fax: 603-668-5348
Stuart Draper, Owner
Victor Carbone, Manager
A specialized facility for comprehensive rehabilitation for individuals who have been injured or have a disability.

7031 **New Medico, Highwatch Rehabilitation Center**
Highwatch Rd
Center Ossipee, NH 03814 Fax: 603-539-8888
William Burke, Executive Director
Post-acute rehabilitation service.

7032 **Northern New Hampshire Mental Health and Developmental Services**
87 Washington St
Conway, NH 03818-6044 603-447-3347
Fax: 603-447-8893
www.northernhs.org
Dennis Mackay, CEO
Provides mental health and developmental services to northern New Hampshire, including early intervention, elderly services, residential program, outpatient services, employee assistance programs, inpatient services, etc.

New Jersey

7033 **All Garden State Physical Therapy**
44 Ridge Road
North Arlington, NJ 07031 201-998-6300
Fax: 201-998-6344

7034 **Bancroft**
425 Kings Highway East
PO Box 20
Haddonfield, NJ 08033- 1284 856-429-0010
800-774-5516
Fax: 856-429-1613
TTY: 856-428-2697
inquiry@bancroft.org
www.bancroft.org
Cynthia Boyer, PhD, Executive Director, Brain Injury Services
Toni Pergolin, President and Chief Executive
Clair Rohrer, Med, Executive Director, Programs for Adults
Dennis . Morgan, M.Ed, Executive Director of Bancroft Special Education Programs
Private, not-for-profit organization serving people with disabilities since 1883. Based in Haddonfield, New Jersey, help more than 1000 children and adults with autism, developmental disabilities, brain injuries, and other neurological impairments. Operates more than 140 sites throughout the U.S. and abroad.

7035 **Daughters of Miriam Center/The Gallen Institute**
155 Hazel St
Clifton, NJ 07011-3423 973-772-3700
Fax: 973-253-5389
administration@daughtersofmiriamcenter.org
www.daughtersofmiriamcenter.o rg
Fred Feinstein, Executive Director
Dedicated to providing the highest quality care, the Center has far exceeded a stereotypical nursing home by offering a continuum of care environment, making us a leader in Jewish eldercare.

7036 **Devereux Advanced Behavioral Health New Jersey**
Devereux New Jersey
286 Mantua Grove Rd.
Building 4
West Deptford, NJ 08066 856-599-6400
Fax: 856-423-8916
drenner@devereux.org
www.devereuxnj.org
Brian Hancock, Executive Director
Christine DiGiampaolo, Human Resources Department
Kelly McGhee, Quality Improvement Department
Donna Marie Renner, Development & External Affairs Department
Serves people of all ages who have special needs. Individuals with emotional, behavioral, and developmental disabilities are offered services such as community-based homes and apartments, vocational training programs, family care homes, and consulting services. Devereux New Jersey also has a residential/educational center for individuals with autism.

7037 **Ladacain Network**
Schroth School & Technical Education Center
1701 Kneeley Blvd
Wanamassa, NJ 07712-7622 732-493-5900
Fax: 732-493-5980
ladacin.org
Patricia Carlesimo, Executive Director
Provides an array of services and programs specifically for children and adults with developmental and physical disabilities. Services include approved Department of Education school programs; adult education and training; vocational training, personal care assistance services, in-home and Saturday respite; child care programs, housing opportunities, and more.

7038 **Lourdes Regional Rehabilitation Center**
Our Lady of Lourdes Medical Center
1600 Haddon Ave
Camden, NJ 08103-3101 856-757-3864
856-757-3500
Fax: 856-968-2511
www.lourdesnet.org
Alexander J. Hatala, President
Kimberly D. Barnes, Vice President, Planning and Development
Michael Hammond, Chief Financial Officer
Maureen Hetu, Chief Information Officer
The only comprehensive rehabilitation facility located within an acute care hospital in Southern New Jersey. Patients benefit from the proximity to the full range of state of the art medical and surgical services should the need arise.

7039 Mt. Carmel Guild
1160 Raymond Blvd
Newark, NJ 07102-4168
973-596-4100
Fax: 973-639-6583
Anita Holland, Manager
Offers services for the totally blind, legally blind, visually impaired, and more with health, counseling, educational, recreational, rehabilitation, computer training and professional training services.

7040 Pediatric Rehabilitation Department, JFK Medical Center
65 James St
Edison, NJ 08818-3947
732-321-7362
732-321-7000
Fax: 732-548-7751
www.jfkmc.org
Michael A. Kleiman, DMD, Chair
Douglas A. Nordstrom, Vice Chair
John L. Kolaya, PE, Secretary
Leonard Sendelsky, Treasurer
Comprehensive interdisciplinary, family focused outpatient pediatric rehabilitation services including evaluation and individual and group treatment programs for children birth-21.

7041 REACH Rehabilitation Program: Leader Nursing and Rehabilitation Center
550 Jessup Rd
West Deptford, NJ 08066-1921
856-848-9551
Karen Fattore, Case Manager
Anthony Stenson, Administrator
Postacute rehabilitation program.

7042 REACH Rehabilitation and Catastrophic Long-Term Care
1180 Us Highway 22
Mountainside, NJ 07092-2810
908-654-0020
Fax: 908-654-8661
Allen Swanson, Manager
Archie Ordana, Manager
Postacute rehabilitation program.

7043 Rehabilitation Specialists
18-01 Pollitt Drive
Ste 1A
Fair Lawn, NJ 07410-2815
201-478-4200
800-441-7488
Fax: 201-478-4201
www.rehab-specialists.com
Virgilio Caraballo, President/CEO
Dustin Gordon, Director of Neuropsychological and Clinical Services
Dr. Brian Greenwald, Medical Director
Cindy Dittfield, Director of Marketing & Public Relations
Rehabilitation Specialists, founded in 1983, is a quality, cost effective community re-entry center treating individuals with acquired brain injury. A non clinical environment based in the community is utilized that offers professional services enabling participants to learn skills they need to return to a productive life. Both our Day and Residential programming emphases focus on Functional Life Skills, Work Skills and Learning Skills. Each participant's program is tailored to meet their needs.

7044 Somerset Valley Rehabilitation and Nursing Center
Care-One
11300 Cornell Park Drive
Suite 360
Cincinnati, OH 45242
513-469-7222
Fax: 513-469-7230
info@healthbridge.org
Trudi Matthews, Director of Policy and Public Re
Subacute rehabilitation program, long term care, respite care.

7045 Summit Ridge Center
101 East State Street
Kennett Square, PA 19348
973-736-2000
Fax: 973-736-2764
genesishcc.com

New Mexico

7046 SJR Rehabilitation Hospital
525 S Schwartz Ave
Farmington, NM 87401-5955
505-609-2625
Fax: 505-327-6562
eniemand@sjrmc.net
www.sjrrh.com
Ena M Niemand, Executive Director
Sue Clay, Program Director
Jill Morgan, Nursing Director
Uses a team of professionals to provide a comprehensive rehabilitation program. Accomplishing the best possible physical and cognitive improvement is the aim of the following treatment members: nurses, physical therapists, physicians, speech and occupational therapists, therapeutic recreation specialist. Providing inpatient and out patient services.

7047 Southwest Communication Resource
P.O. Box 788
Bernalillo, NM 87004-788
505-867-3396
Fax: 505-867-3398
info@abrazosnm.org
swcr.org

New York

7048 Aspire of Western New York
2356 N Forest Rd
Getzville, NY 14068-1224
716-838-0047
Fax: 716-894-8257
info@aspirewny.org
aspirewny.org
Thomas A. Sy, Executive Director
Janet Hansen, Chief Operating Officer
Mary Anne Coombe, V.P. of Service Coordination & Fiscal Management Services
Helen Trowbridge Hanes, Vice President of Community Living
Provides comprehensive services to individuals with disabilities from infancy through adulthood. Also serves people with all types of developmental disabilities as well as providing clinical services to persons with other types of disabilities such as: spinal cord injury, head trauma and others. Aspire employs 1500 people.

7049 Bronx Continuing Treatment Day Program
1527 Southern Blvd
Bronx, NY 10460-5619
718-893-1414
Fax: 718-893-0707
Mary Jane Purcell, Manager
Post-acute rehabilitation program.

7050 Brooklyn Bureau of Community Service
285 Schermerhorn St
Brooklyn, NY 11217-1098
718-310-5600
Fax: 718-855-1517
info@WeAreBCS.org
www.wearebcs.org
Marla Simpson, Executive Director
Anthony B. Edwards, MBA, CCF, MFM, CFO
Janelle Farris, Chief Operating Officer
Sonya Shields, Chief Officer for External Relations and Advancement
Offers independent living skills, counseling, work readiness, vocational trianing, job placement and job follow-up services to individuals with disabilities (to include individuals with psychiatric, physical, and developmental disabilities). Special programs to move disabled welfare recipients from welfare to work. Publishes a bi-annual newsletter.

7051 Buffalo Hearing and Speech Center
50 E North St
Buffalo, NY 14203-1002
716-885-8318
Fax: 716-885-4229
askbhsc.org
Frank J. Polino, Chairman
Dennis J. Szefel, First Vice Chairman
Kenneth J. Wilson, Treasurer
Gerald Chiari, Esq., Secretary

Assists individuals with speech, language and/or hearing impairments to achieve maximum communication potential.

7052 **Cora Hoffman Center Day Program**
2324 Forest Ave
Staten Island, NY 10303-1506 718-447-8205
Fax: 718-815-2182

Kevin Kenney, Manager
Post-acute rehabilitation program specializing in Cerebral Palsy. Part of the Cerebral Palsey Association of New York State.

7053 **Devereux Advanced Behavioral Health New York**
Devereux New York
40 Devereux Way
Red Hook, NY 12571 845-758-1899
Fax: 845-758-1817
www.devereuxny.org

John Lopez, Executive Director
Arthur Roberts, Director of Human Resources
Jeffrey Obiekwe, Program Supervisor
Devereux New York provides a wide range of educational, clinical, residential, and community-based programs and services to people of all ages with intellectual disabilities, Autism Spectrum Disorder, and dual diagnoses. Some services include psychotherapy, life skills development, physical therapies, residential programs, case management, self advocacy and more.

7054 **Elmhurst Hospital Center**
7901 Broadway
Elmhurst, NY 11373-1368 718-334-4000
www.nyc.gov/html/hhc/ehc/html/home/home.shtml
Chris D Constantino, Executive Director
Hospital is comprised of 525 beds and is a Level I Trauma Center, and Emergency Heart Care Stattion and a 911 recieving hospital. It is the premiere health care organization for key areas such as Surgery, Cardiology, Women's health, Pediatrics, Rehabilitation Medicine, Renal and Mental Health Services.

7055 **Federation Employment And Guidance Service (F-E-G-S)**
315 Hudson St
New York, NY 10013-1086 212-366-8400
Fax: 212-366-8441
info@fegs.org
www.fegs.org

Gail Magaliff, CEO
Ira Machowsky, Executive Vice President
Thomas M. Higgins, CFO
Kristin M. Woodlock, Chief Operating Officer
The largest and most diversified private, not-for-profit health related and human service organization in the United States. With operations in over 258 facilities, residences, and off-site locations, F-E-G-S has served more then 2 million people since its inception.

7056 **Flushing Hospital**
4500 Parsons Blvd
Flushing, NY 11355-2205 718-670-5000
Fax: 718-670-3082
flushinghospital.org
Robert V. Levine, Executive Vice President and COO
Bruce J. Flanz, President/ CEO
Mounir Doss, Executive Vice President/CFO
Offers services for the totally blind, legally blind, visually impaired, and more with health, counseling, educational, recreational, rehabilitation, computer training and professional training services.

7057 **Gateway Community Industries Inc.,**
1 Amy Kay Pkwy
Kingston, NY 12401-6444 845-331-1261
800-454-9395
Fax: 845-331-4920
info@gatewayindustries.org
gatewayindustries.org

Francoise C. Gunefsky, President/ CEO
Eva Graham, CFO
Ralph Smith, Chief Information Officer
Mary Ann Hildebrandt, Chief Quality and Compliance Officer
Gateway Community Industries, Inc., founded in 1957, is one of the leading independent not-for-profit vocational rehabilitation and training centers for people with mental and/or physical disabilities. The agency provides comprehensive services in vocational evaluation, job training, job placement, vocational work center employment, supported employment, psychiatric rehabilitation, continuing day treatment, and residential habilitation/rehabilitation.

7058 **Henkind Eye Institute Division of Montefiore Hospital**
111 East 210th Street
Bronx, NY 10467-2404 718-920-4321
www.montefiore.org
Philip O. Ozuah, MD, PhD, Executive Vice President/ COO
Steven M. Safyer, MD, President/ CEO
Joel A. Perlman, Executive Vice President, Chief Financial Officer
Alfredo Cabrera, Senior Vice President & Chief Human Resources Officer
Offers services for the totally blind, legally blind, visually impaired, and more with health, counseling, educational, recreational, rehabilitation, computer training and professional training services. Low vision services offered.

7059 **Industries for the Blind of New York State**
194 Washington Ave
Ste 300
Albany, NY 12210-6314 518-456-8671
800-421-9010
Fax: 518-456-3587
customercare@nyspsp.org
www.abilityone.com

Richard Healey, CEO
Offers services for the totally blind, legally blind, visually impaired, and more with health, counseling, educational, recreational, rehabilitation, computer training and professional training services.

7060 **Inpatient Pain Rehabilitation Program**
550 First Avenue
New York, NY 10016 212-263-7300
Fax: 212-598-6468
www.med.nyu.edu

William Pinter Phd, Administrative Director
The Inpatient Rehabilitation Program, established in 1983 specializes in the treatment of chronic pain. Our inpatient program is one of the oldest and well established pain programs in the country. It is the only interdisciplinary inpatient pain program in the tri-state area and one of only 20 pain programs in the entire US to have CARF accreditation. Upon completion of an extensive evaluation, patients are admitted for an 18-day inpatient stay.

7061 **Koicheff Health Care Center**
2324 Forest Ave
Staten Island, NY 10303-1506 718-447-0200
Fax: 718-981-1431

Paul Castello, Clinic Director
Post-accute rehabilitation programs.

7062 **New York-Presbyterian Hospital**
622 W 168th St
New York, NY 10032-3796 212-305-4600
Fax: 212-305-1017
www.nyp.org

Steven J. Corwin, MD, CEO
Robert E. Kelly, MD, President
New York Presbyterian Hospital is internationally recognized for its outstanding comprehensive services. Its medical, surgical, and emergency care services provide each patient with the highest possible level of care. In addition, as part of the Hospital's commitment to the total well-being of each patient, it offers a range of specialized services, as well as special healthcare programs for neighboring communities.

7063 **Norman Marcus Pain Institute**
30 E 40th St
Ste 1100
New York, NY 10016 212-532-7999
Fax: 212-532-5957
support@nmpi.com
backpainusa.com

Norman J Marcus, Medical Director
We focus on muscles as the cause of most common pains, i.e. back, neck, shoulders, and headaches. We make specific muscle

diagnoses and have specific treatments that in many cases will eliminate the need for surgery or relieve the pain. Patients diagnosed with herniated disc, spinal stenosis, rotator cuff tear, impingement syndrome, sciatica, fibromyalgia and headache will generally find relief.

7064 **Pain Alleviation Center**
Comprehensive Pain Management Associates
125 S Service Rd
Jericho, NY 11753-1038 516-997-7246
Fax: 516-997-7281
www.paincenter.com

Alex Weingarten, Director
Phillip Fyman, Director
Marisa French, Manager
One of the first pain clinics to gain national accreditation from the Commission on Accreditation of Rehabilitation Facilities. This is due largely to a patient-centered program based on the latest research.

7065 **Pathfinder Village**
3 Chenango Rd
Edmeston, NY 13335-2314 607-965-8377
Fax: 607-965-8655
info@pathfindervillage.org
www.pathfindervillage.org

Paul Landers, CEO
Caprice S. Eckert, Chief Financial Officer
Kelly A. Meyers, Director of Admissions
Paula B. Schaeffer, Director of Enrichment Programs
Pathfinder Village is a warm, friendly community in the rolling hills of Central New York. Here children and adults with Down Syndrome gain independence, build lasting friendships, become partners in the world and take in all that life has to offer.

7066 **Pilot Industries: Ellenville**
845-331-4300
48 Canal St
Ellenville, NY 12428-1327 845-647-7711
Fax: 845-647-7711

Peter Pierri, Executive Director
Betty Marks, Plant Manager
Post-accute rehabilitation services.

7067 **Skills Unlimited**
405 Locust Ave
Oakdale, NY 11769-1695 631-567-3320
Fax: 631-567-3285
info@skillsunlimited.org
skillsunlimited.org

Richard Kassnove, Executive Director
Our basic goals is to offer persons with disabilities the opportunity to explore and develop their full vocational potential. Our programs are unique in that by offering comprehensive services, individuals are able to deal with many different issues that could potentially affect their vocational success. Any individual that has an impairment that interferes with their ability to work is entitles to the services that we offer.

North Carolina

7068 **Center for Vision Rehabilitation**
Academy Eye Associates
3115 Academy Rd
Durham, NC 27707-2652 919-493-7456
800-942-1499
Fax: 919-493-1718
henry.greene@academyeye.com
academyeye.com

Henry A Greene, Owner
Vision rehabilitation and low-vision care for the visually impaired, post-stroke, head trauma and for neuro-oncology vision complications.

7069 **Diversified Opportunities**
1010 Herring Ave E
Wilson, NC 27893-3311 252-291-0378
Fax: 252-291-1402
www.diversifiedopportunitiesinc.com

Cindy Dixon, Executive Director
Carlton Goff, Business Manager
Ericka Simmons, QP Program Manager
Ken Jones, Chairman
Vocational rehabilitation agency, better outcomes, lower cost, guaranteed performance standards.

7070 **Forsyth Medical Center**
3333 Silas Creek Pkwy
Winston Salem, NC 27103-3090 336-718-5000
Fax: 336-718-9250
www.novanthealth.org

Jeffrey T. Lindsay, President
Denise Mihal, Chief Operating Officer
Stephen J. Motew, MD, Senior Vice President
Bruce D. Walley, MD, Senior Vice President
Provides care that is state-of-the-art and second to none, both because of advanced treatments availiable through our clinical research and technology to the academic excellence-and caring nature-of our doctors and nurses.

7071 **Industries of the Blind**
914-920 W Lee St
Greensboro, NC 27403-2803 336-274-1591
800-909-7086
Fax: 336-544-3739
customerservice@iob-gso.com
industriesoftheblind.com

David Thompson, Chairperson
Scott Thornhill, 1st Vice Chairperson
Ashley S. James, Jr., 2nd Vice Chairperson
Chi Anyansi-Archibong, Secretary
Offers services for the totally blind, legally blind, visually impaired, and more with health, counseling, educational, recreational, rehabilitation, computer training and professional training services.

7072 **Johnston County Industries**
1100 East Preston Street
Selma, NC 27576-3162 919-743-8700
Fax: 919-965-8023
jcindustries.com

John Shallcross, Jr., President
Durwood Woodall, Vice President
Lina Sanders-Johnson, Secretary/Treasurer
JCI is an entrepreneurial not-for-profit corporation dedicated to empowering people with disabilities or disadvantages to succeed through training and employment

7073 **Learning Services: Carolina**
707 Morehead Ave
Durham, NC 27707-1319 919-688-4444
888-419-9955
Fax: 919-419-9966
learningservices.com

Debra Braunling-McMorrow, President and CEO
Jeanne Mack, Chief Financial Officer and Vice President of Operations
Michael Weaver, Chief Development Officer
Terri Dorman, V.P. of Customer Service and Care Management
Located in an historic neighborhood in the heart of Durham, this campus-style setting offers easy access to resources at 3 outstanding facilities: Duke University, The University of North Carolina at Chapel Hill, and Research Triangle Park. This program provides a range of services and activities that draw upon the many resources availiable in the community.

7074 **Lions Club Industries for the Blind**
4500 Emperor Blvd.
Durham, NC 27703 919-596-8277
800-526-1562
Fax: 919-598-1179
inquire@buylci.com

Bill Hudson, President
Offers services for the totally blind, legally blind, visually impaired, and more with health, counseling, educational, recre-

ational, rehabilitation, computer training and professional training services.

7075 **Lions Services Inc.**
5 Penn Plaza
New York, NY 10001 21 -62 -210
lsisale@aol.com

Jimmy R Cranford, President
Jimmy Cranford, President

Offers services for the totally blind, legally blind, visually impaired, and more with health, counseling, educational, recreational, rehabilitation, computer training and professional training services.

7076 **Regional Rehabilitation Center Pitt County Memorial Hospital**
2100 Stantonsburg Rd
Greenville, NC 27834-2818 252-847-4448
Fax: 252-816-7552

Martha M Dixon, VP General Services

An accredited, comprehensive rehabilitation center-part of a statewide network- and we're the largest such facility in eastern North Carolina. Our service area covers 29 counties, and we offer a complete array of rehabilitation services for patients of all ages. Because the Regional Rehabilitation Center is associated with both Pitt County Memorial Hospital And the Brody School of Medicine at East Carolina University, patients have access to a full range of state of the art medical services.

7077 **Rehab Home Care**
2660 Yonkers Rd
Raleigh, NC 27604-3384 800-447-8692
Fax: 919-831-2211

Alan Silver, CEO
Janis Hansen, Chief Operating Officer

A Medicare/Medicaid certified, state-licensed home health agency with emphasis on rehabilitation.

7078 **Thoms Rehabilitation Hospital**
Thoms Rehabilitation Hospital
68 Sweeten Creek Rd
Asheville, NC 28803-2318 828-277-4800
Fax: 828-277-4812
TTY: 800-735-2962
www.carepartners.org

Tracy Buchanan, President & CEO
Gary Bowers, COO

Freestanding physical rehabilitation hospital, founded 1938 - 100 beds, including 90 acute and 10 transitional - JCAHO accredited.

7079 **Winston-Salem Industries for the Blind**
7730 N Point Blvd
Winston Salem, NC 27106-3310 336-759-0551
800-242-7726
Fax: 336-759-0990
info@wsifb.com
www.wsifb.com

Mike Faircloth, Chairman
Karen Carey, Vice Chairman, Secretary
W. Robert Newell, Treasurer
David Horton, Executive Director

Offers services for the totally blind, legally blind, visually impaired, and more with health, counseling, educational, recreational, rehabilitation, computer training and professional training services.

Ohio

7080 **Bellefaire Jewish Children's Bureau**
22001 Fairmount Blvd
Cleveland, OH 44118-4819 216-932-2800
800-879-2522
Fax: 216-932-6704
www.bellefairejcb.org

Adam Jacobs, CEO
Adam G. Jacobs PhD, Executive Vice President

Residential treatment for ages 12 to 17 1/2 at time of admission offering individualized psychotherapy, special education, and group living for severaly emotionally disturbed children and adolescents. Also offers a variety of other programs including specialized and therapuetic foster care, partial hospitilization, outpatient counseling, home-based intensive counseling and adoption services.

7081 **Christ Hospital Rehabilitation Unit**
2139 Auburn Ave
Cincinnati, OH 45219-2906 513-585-2737
Fax: 513-585-4353
www.thechristhospital.com

Mike Keating, President and CEO
Chris Bergman, Vice President and Chief Financial Officer
Berc Gawne, MD, Vice President and Chief Medical Officer
Peter Greis, Vice President and Chief Information Officer

Patients of this 555-bed, not-for-profit acute care facility receive personalized health care provided by trained specialists using the most sophisticated medical technology available, including state-of-the-art intensive care units, surgical facilities, cardiac catheterization labs, three new electrophysiology labs, and the tristates first positron emission tomography (PET) scanning capabilities.

7082 **Cleveland Sight Center**
1909 E 101st St.
Cleveland, OH 44106 216-791-8118
Fax: 216-791-1101
TTY: 216-791-8119
info@clevelandsightcenter.org
www.clevelandsightcenter.org

Larry Benders, President & CEO
Kevin Krencisz, Chief Financial & Administrative Officer
Jassen Tawil, Director, Business Development & Customer Success
Ali Thomas, Director, Human Resources

Social, rehabilitation, education and support services for blind and visually impaired children and adults, early intervention program for children birth to age 6, low vision clinic, aid and appliance shop, Braille and taping transcription, training for rehabilitation, orientation, mobility and computer access, employment services and job placement, recreation program, resident camping, talking books, radio reading services. Free screening.

7083 **Columbus Speech and Hearing Center**
510 E North Broadway St
Columbus, OH 43214-4114 614-263-5151
Fax: 614-263-5365
columbusspeech.org

Dawn Gleason, Au.D., President/ CEO
Karen Deeter, Director of Operations

Serves persons who have speech-language and hearing challenges. Provides vocational rehabilitation services for individuals who are deaf, hard-of-hearing or deaf-blind.

7084 **CommuniCare of Clifton Nursing and Rehabilitation Center**
Communi Care Health Services
4700 Ashwood Drive
Cincinnati, OH 45241 513-489-7100
Fax: 513-281-2559
communicarehealth.com

Stephen L. Rosedale, Founder/ CEO

A long term care facility which specializes in rehabilitation. Offers a full range of rehabilitative services including physical therapy, occupational therapy and speech therapy.

7085 **Doctors Hospital**
5100 W Broad St
Columbus, OH 43228-1672 614-544-1000
800-837-7555
Fax: 614-544-1844
www.ohiohealth.com/homedoctors

David Blom, President/ CEO
Michael Bernstein, Senior Vice President and Chief

We believe our first responsibility is to the patients we serve. We respect the physical, emotional and spiritual needs of our patients and find that compassion is essential to fostering healing and wholeness.

7086 **Dodd Hall at the Ohio State University Hospitals**
410 W 10th Ave
Columbus, OH 43210-1240
614-293-3300
800-293-5123
OSUCareConnection@osumc.edu
www.medicalcenter.osu.edu
Steven G. Gabbe, MD, Senior Vice President / CEO
Larry Anstine, CEO
Gail Marsh, Chief Strategy Officer
Phyllis Teater, Chief Information Officer
Dodd Hall is a full service medical rehabilitation hospital offering comprehensive inpatient and outpatient rehabilitation.

7087 **Easterseals of Mahoning, Trumbull and Columbiana Counties**
299 Edwards St.
Youngstown, OH 44502-1599
330-743-1168
Fax: 330-743-1616
www.easterseals.com/mtc
Maureen Pusch, Chief Executive Officer
Outpatient medical rehabilitation, skill development, vocational support, and transportation services.

7088 **Four Oaks Center**
245 N. Valley Road
Xenia, OH 45385-2605
937-562-6500
Fax: 937-562-6520
www.greenedd.org
Todd McManus, President
Jill A. LaRock, Director
Dr. Vijay Gupta, Vice President
Melinda Mays, Recording Secretary
Starts children on the road to discovery by providing a learning environment rich in opportunities and encouragement. The program was designed to give children with delays or disabilities, or those at-risk the extra help needed to develop fully. Any child under the age of six who exhibits developmental delays, handicapping conditions, or is considered at risk may qualify to participate.

7089 **Genesis Healthcare System**
Rehabilitation Services
800 Forest Ave
Zanesville, OH 43701-2881
740-454-5000
800-322-4762
Fax: 740-455-7527
llynn@genesishcs.org
www.genesishcs.org
Matt Perry, President/ CEO
Paul Masterson, CFO
Richard Helsper, COO
A CARF and JACHO accredited 19-bed rehabilitation facility located within Genesis Healthcare System, a 732 bed, non-profit hospital system, located in Zanesville, Ohio. Freestanding outpatient services, including work hardening, pain management, vocational services, audiology, lymphedema, vestibular rehab, off-the-road driving evals, aquatic therpay, womens health and sports enhancement.

7090 **George A Martin Center**
3603 Washington Ave
Cincinnati, OH 45229-2009
513-221-1017
Fax: 513-221-3817
Karen Doggett, Executive Director
Offers services for the totally blind, legally blind, visually impaired, and more with health, counseling, educational, recreational, rehabilitation, computer training and professional training services.

7091 **Grady Memorial Hospital**
561 W Central Ave
Delaware, OH 43015-1489
740-615-1000
800-487-1115
Fax: 740-368-5114
ohiohealth.com
Bruce Hagen, Regional Executive and President
As a progressive healthcare leader, Grady Memorial Hospital is committed to excellence while providing the Deleware community with comprehensive quality service delivered with compassionate, personal care. Our membership in Ohio's largest healthcare system, Ohio Health, enables us to improve access to a broader range of healthcare services, enhance development of new programs and services, and provide a complete continuum of care for patients in the deleware area.

7092 **Hamilton Adult Center**
3400 Symmes Rd
Hamilton, OH 45015-1359
513-867-5970
Fax: 513-874-2977
Donald Musnuff, Executive Director

7093 **Holzer Clinic**
100 Jackson Pike
Gallipolis, OH 45631-1560
740-446-5000
Fax: 740-446-5532
info@holzer.org
www.holzer.org
T. Wayne Munro, MD, CEO
Brent A. Saunders, Chair
Christopher Meyer, Chief Medical Officer
John Cunningham, Chief Administrative Officer
Serves medical needs of patients in an 8 county area, including counties in Ohio and West Virginia.

7094 **Holzer Clinic Sycamore**
Holzer Medical Center
4th Avenue & Sycamore St
Gallipolis, OH 45631-1560
740-446-5244
Fax: 740-446-5448
info@holzer.org
www.holzer.org
T. Wayne Munro, MD, CEO
Brent A. Saunders, Chair
Christopher Meyer, Chief Medical Officer
John Cunningham, Chief Administrative Officer
Offers an individualized quality comprehensive rehabilitation program for people with disabilities by an interdisciplinary team including physical therapy, occupational, speech, nursing and social services to restore the patient to the highest degree of rehab outcomes attainable.

7095 **IKRON Institute for Rehabilitative and Psychological Services**
2347 Vine St
Cincinnati, OH 45213-1745
513-621-1117
Fax: 513-621-2350
ikron@ikron.org
ikron.org
Randy Strunk, MA, LPCC-S, Executive Director
Ken Carbonell, BBA, Fiscal Director
Melissa Harmeling, MA, PCC-S, Program Director
Jake Striker, President
An accredited mental health facility and a certified rehabilitation center. Through a variety of creative treatment and rehabilitation services, IKRON assists adults with mental health and/or substance abuse problems to attain greater independence, to lead lives of sobriety, to obtain competitive work and live more satisfying lives. IKRON places a strong emphasis on respect and support for persons with problems of adjustment. Special contracts to persons desiring job placement.

7096 **Integrated Health Services at Waterford Commons**
955 Garden Lake Pkwy
Toledo, OH 43614-2777
419-382-2200
Fax: 419-381-8508
Nicole Giesige, Executive Director
A subacute and rehabilitation program specializing in ventilator weaning and management, I.V. therapeutics and pain management, wound management and subacute rehabilitation.

7097 **Lester H Higgins Adult Center**
3041 Cleveland Ave SW
Canton, OH 44707-3625
330-484-4814
Fax: 330-484-9416
http://www.theworkshopsinc.com/
Margalie Belazaire, Manager
Ed Allar, Manager
Post-accute rehabilitation service

7098 **Live Oaks Career Development Campus**
5936 Buckwheat Rd
Milford, OH 45150 513-575-1906
Fax: 513-575-0805

Harold Carr MD, Superintendent
Robin White, President/CEO
Jim Dixon, Principal
Post-accute rehabilitation facility and services.

7099 **Metro Health: St. Luke's Medical Center Pain Management Program**
2500 Metrohealth Dr
Cleveland, OH 44109-1900 216-778-7800
www.metrohealth.org

Mark Moran, President
CARF accredited comprehensive multidisciplinary pain management program.

7100 **MetroHealth Medical Center**
2500 Metrohealth Dr
Cleveland, OH 44109-1900 216-778-7800
www.metrohealth.org

Mark Moran, President
Located on the near west side of Cleveland, is a leader in trauma, emergency, and critical care; women's and childrens's services, including high risk obstetrical care and neonatal intensive care; comprehensive medical and surgical subspecialties.

7101 **Middletown Regional Hospital: Inpatient Rehabilitation Unit**
105 McKnight Dr
Middletown, OH 45044-4838 513-422-1401
800-338-4057
Fax: 513-422-1520
www.middletownhospital.org

C N Reddy, Owner
Douglas McNeill, Chief Executive Officer
Our mission is to serve and help people, improving the status of their health and the quality of thier lives. Our vision is to be the premier integrated delivery system in Southwest Ohio. Our Values are quality, respect, service and teamwork

7102 **Newark Healthcare Center**
680 South Fourth Street
Louisville, KY 40202 502-596-7300
TTY: 800-545-0749
web_administrator@kindred.com
kindredhealthcare.com

Paul J. Diaz, President/ CEO
Accomodates 300 residents. We are located in the heart of Newark, Ohio. Newark Healthcare is a 2004 recipient of the American Health Care Association's Quality Award.

7103 **Parma Community General Hospital Acute Rehabilitation Center**
7007 Powers Blvd
Parma, OH 44129-5495 440-743-3000
Fax: 440-843-4387
www.parmahospital.org

David Nedrich, Chairman
Thomas P. O'Donnell, First Vice Chairman
Alex I. Koler, First Assistant Treasurer
Sharon Martin, Assistant Secretary
The mission of this CARF accredited unit is to provide the most comprehensive, cost-effective, acute rehabilitation program possible in order for every patient and family to adjust to his/her disability and to achieve the maximum potential of independent functioning when returning to community living.

7104 **Peter A Towne Physical Therapy Center**
Ste 10
447 Nilles Rd
Fairfield, OH 45014-2626 513-829-7726
Fax: 513-829-7726

Debbie Wilkerson, Office Manager
Outpatient, private practice physical and occupational therapy. Three other offices in Hamilton, Monroe and West Chester.

7105 **Philomatheon Society of the Blind**
2701 Tuscarawas St W
Canton, OH 44708-4638 330-453-9157
www.philomatheon.com

David Miller, President
Denise Dessecker, Vice President
Angela Randall, Secretary
Paul Williams, Treasurer
Offers services for the totally blind, legally blind, visually impaired, and more with health, counseling, educational, recreational, rehabilitation, computer training and professional training services.

7106 **Providence Hospital Work**
2270 Banning Rd
Cincinnati, OH 45239-6621 513-591-5600
Fax: 513-591-5604

Kay Brogle, Executive Director
Post-acute rehabilitation services.

7107 **Six County, Inc.**
2845 Bell St
Zanesville, OH 43701-1794 740-454-9766
800-344-5818
Fax: 740-588-6452
www.sixcounty.org

John A Creek, President
Tim Llewellyn, Senior VP/Community Intervention
Robert Santos, Ex Vp & Coo
Mary Denoble, Vp Qip
Six County, Inc., is a private, not-for-profit corporation under contract with the Mental Health and Recovery Services Board. Six County, Inc., provides comprehensive community mental health services to people of all ages in each of the six Southeastern Ohio counties served: Coshocton, Guernsey, Morgan, Muskingum, Noble, and Perry. SCI's counseling centers provide a full range of services including outpatient counseling; diagnostic assessment, referrals, and psychological testing.

7108 **Society for Rehabilitation**
9290 Lake Shore Blvd
Mentor, OH 44060-1664 440-352-8993
800-344-3159
Fax: 440-352-6632

Richard Kessler, Executive Director
Vision is to provide individuals with comprehensive services to improve their quality of life. Our mission is to meet the needs of individuals and their families by delivering a wide range of affordable accessible and personalized services, providing treatment by a team of highly qualified, caring professionals. Collaborating with other agencies to meet community needs.

7109 **Southeast Ohio Sight Center**
425 E. Alvarado Street
Suite E
Fallbrook, CA 92028 800-677-4180
www.charityadvantage.com

7110 **St. Francis Rehabilitation Hospital**
401 N Broadway St
Green Springs, OH 44836-9638 419-639-2626
800-248-2552
Fax: 419-639-6225

Kim Eicher, CEO
Dan Schwanke, Chief Executive Officer
Program offers specialized treatment for patients who have suffered a head injury, spinal cord injury, or stroke, or who have an orthopedic injury. The Head Injury Program provides a continuum of care from coma stimulation through transitional living. Their physicians, nurses, counselors and therapists are dedicated to helping our patients develop the motivation, strength and skills needed to overcome or adapt to their disability.

7111 **TAC Enterprises**
2160 Old Selma Rd
Springfield, OH 45505-4600 937-525-7400
Fax: 937-525-7401
info@tacind.com
www.tacind.com

Clifford Meyer, CEO

TAC Enterprises provides employment opportunities for individuals to develop marketable skills by completing contract work in partnership with other industries. Work and self-help skills, social adjustment, and a variety of daily living experiences are offered to the workers by our specialized staff.

Oklahoma

7112 **Dean A McGee Eye Institute**
608 Stanton L Young Blvd
Oklahoma City, OK 73104-5065
405-271-6060
800-787-9012
Fax: 405-271-4442
www.mei.org

Gregory L. Skuta, M.D., President/CEO
Matthew D. Brown, Executive Vice President
Lana G. Ivy, Vice President of Development
Kimberly A. Howard, Chief Financial Officer and Vice President of Finance

Offers services for the totally blind, legally blind, visually impaired, and more with health, counseling, educational, recreational, rehabilitation, computer training and professional training services.

7113 **Jane Phillips Medical Center**
Rehab Care
3500 E Frank Phillips Blvd
Bartlesville, OK 74006-2464
918-333-7200
Fax: 918-333-7801
webmaster@ipmc.org
jpmc.org

David Stire, President/ COO
Mike Moore, Chief Financial Officer/Vice President Fiscal Services
Susan Herron, RN, Vice President Nursing Services
Paul W. McQuillen, MD, Chief Medical Officer

Comprehensive inpatient rehabilitation services are provided to patients with orthopedic, neurologic, and other medical conditions of recent onset or regression, who have experienced a loss of function in activities of daily living, mobility, cognition and communication.

7114 **McAlester Regional Health Center RehabCare Unit**
1 E Clark Bass Blvd
McAlester, OK 74501-4255
918-426-1800
Fax: 918-421-6832
nbrinlee@mrhcok.com
www.mrhcok.com

David Keith, President/ CEO
Cara Bland, Chairman
Evans McBride, Vice-Chairman

A 19-bed inpatient physical rehabilitation unit serving the Southeast Oklahoma area. Offers physical therapy, occupational therapy, social work, speech and psychological services in an interdisciplinary framework.

7115 **Oklahoma League for the Blind**
501 N Douglas Ave
Oklahoma City, OK 73106-5085
405-232-4644
888-522-4644
Fax: 405-236-5438
info@newviewoklahoma.org
www.newviewoklahoma.org

Lauren White, President/ CEO
Carol Campbell, Executive Assistant
John Wilson, Chief Financial Officer
Randy Hearn, Chief Operations Officer

Offers services for the blind and visually impaired, counseling, educational, recreational, rehabilitation, computer training and professional training services.

7116 **Valley View Regional Hospital-RehabCare Unit**
430 N Monte Vista St
Ada, OK 74820-4657
580-332-2323
Fax: 580-421-1395

W. Kent Rogers, President/ CEO

Comprehensive physical medicine and rehabilitation services designed to help patients in their adjustment to a physically limiting condition.

Oregon

7117 **Garten Services**
PO Box 13970
Salem, OR 97309
503-581-1984
Fax: 503-581-4497
garten@garten.org
garten.org

Tim Rocak, CEO
Pamela Best, CFO
Steve Babcock, Mail Services Manager
Stacie Braun, Custodial Services Manager

Garten's mission is to support people with disabilities in their effort to contribute to the community through employment, career, and retirement opportunities. Our actions increase society's awareness of human potential. Garten's vision is to be recognized as an organization positively demonstrating to the community that people with disabilities can be contributing and valued employees of a thriving business.

7118 **Legacy Emanuel Rehabilitation Center**
2801 N. Gantenbein
Portland, OR 97227-1542
503-413-2200
Fax: 503-413-1501
www.legacyhealth.org

Gary Guidetta, Executive Director
Gail Weisgerber, Manager

A non-profit tax-exempt corporation that includes 5 full-service hospitals and a children's hospital. The Legacy system provides an integrated network of healthcare services, including acute and critical care, inpatient and outpatient treatment, community health education and a variety of specialty services.

7119 **Oakcrest Care Center**
2933 Center St NE
Salem, OR 97301-4527
503-585-5850
Fax: 503-585-8781

7120 **Oakhill-Senior Program**
1190 Oakhill Ave SE
Salem, OR 97302-3496
503-364-9086
Fax: 503-365-2879

Jan Dillon, Senior Services Manager

Garten Senior Services provides an adult day service program to seniors with and without developmental disabilities. The program will provide community opportunities, college classes and a wide variety of leisure activities in group and individual settings.

7121 **Pacific Spine and Pain Center**
1801 Highway 99 N
Ashland, OR 97520-9152
541-488-2255
866-482-5515
Fax: 541-482-2433

Janel R Guyette, Manager

7122 **Vision Northwest**
9225 SW Hall Blvd
Portland, OR 97223-6794
503-684-8389
800-448-2232
Fax: 503-684-9359
visionnw.com

Evelyn Maizels, Executive Director

Offers services for the totally blind, legally blind, visually impaired, and more with health, counseling, educational, recreational, rehabilitation, computer training and professional training services.

7123 **Willamette Valley Rehabilitation Center**
1853 W Airway Rd
Lebanon, OR 97355-1233
541-258-8121
Fax: 541-451-1762
wvrc.org

Martin Baughman, Executive Director

Provides the best professional vocational services to those adults in the community who, by virtue of their physical or mental limitations, are negatively impacted by their ability to attain or maintain employment.

Pennsylvania

7124 **Alpine Nursing and Rehabilitation Center of Hershey**
Pennstate
405 Martin Ter
State College, PA 16803-3426 814-865-1710
Fax: 814-863-9423

Melissa A Hardy, Director
Anna Shuey, Administrative Assistant
Postacute rehabilitation program.

7125 **Beechwood Rehabilitation Services A Community Integrated Brain Injury Program**
469 E Maple Ave
Langhorne, PA 19047-1600 215-750-4299
800-782-3299
Fax: 215-750-4327
beechwoodrehab.com

Thomas Felicetti, President
Services include residential, day treatment and community based support services. Individuals with brain injury are served. The facility is Care Accredited.

7126 **Blind & Vision Rehabilitation Services Of Pittsburgh**
1800 West St
Homestead, PA 15120-2578 412-368-4400
800-706-5050
Fax: 412-368-4090
www.bvrspittsburgh.org

Erika M. Arbogast, President
Brian Glass, Director of Information Services and Facilities
Leslie Montgomery, Director of Development and Public Relations
Barbara Peterson, Director of Client Services
Offers services for the totally blind, legally blind, visually impaired, and more with health, counseling, educational, recreational, rehabilitation, computer training and professional training services.

7127 **Bradford Regional Medical Center**
116 Interstate Pkwy
Bradford, PA 16701-1036 814-368-4143
Fax: 814-368-4130
www.brmc.com

Marek Dzionara, Owner
Andrew Lehman, Executive Director
Timothy J. Finan, President and CEO
Offers rehabilitation services to individuals with an alcohol or drug related problem.

7128 **Bryn Mawr Rehabilitation Hospital**
414 Paoli Pike
Malvern, PA 19355-3311 610-251-5400
888-734-2241
888-734-2241
Fax: 610-647-3648

Donna M. Phillips, President
We are dedicated to serving individuals and their families whose lives can be enhanced through physical or cognitive rehabilitation. We continually strive for excellence by providing care and services which are valued by those we serve and by contributing to the community through education, research and prevention of disability.

7129 **Devereux Advanced Behavioral Health - National Office**
National Headquarters
444 Devereux Dr
Villanova, PA 19085 800-345-1292
devereuxhr@devereux.org
www.devereux.org

Samuel G Coppersmith, Esq, Chairman
Robert Q Kreider, President & CEO
Marilyn B Benoit, MD, Senior Vice President, Chief Clinical & Medical Officer
Carl E Clark, Senior Vice President & Chief Operations Officer
Devereux is a behavioral health organization supporting people with autism, intellectual and developmental disabilities, and specialty mental health needs. Some of the services offered by Devereux include diagnostics, special education, professional training, research and advocacy.

7130 **Devereux Pennsylvania**
444 Devereux Dr
Villanova, PA 19085 610-788-6565
800-345-1292
Fax: 610-430-0567
www.devereuxpa.org

Carol Oliver, MS, State Director & Vice President of Operations
Melanie Beidler, MS, Executive Director, Intellectual/Developmental Disabilities
Stephen Bruce, M.Ed, BCBA, Executive Director, Adult Services
Rhea Fernandes, Psy.D., Executive Director, Children's Behavioral Health Services
Devereux Pennsylvania provides educational and residential programs, therapeutic foster care, case management, customized employment and community-based behavioral health programs to children and adults with intellectual and behavioral challenges.

7131 **Fox Subacute Center**
2644 Bristol Rd
Warrington, PA 18976-1404 800-782-2288
James Foulke, CEO
Vic Costenko, COO
Walter Dunsmore, CFO
Fox subacute recognizes the great need for alternative programs for today's medically compromised patients. Fox has developed Models of Care and offers subacute programs fore the management of ventilator-dependent patients. We recognize that the best road to recovery for these patients is an environment with special care in an alternative setting. We believe that setting should be outside the hospital, in facilities where the focus is on the management of individual patients.

7132 **Fox Subacute at Clara Burke**
251 Stenton Ave
Plymouth Meeting, PA 19462-1220 610-828-2272
800-424-7201
Fax: 610-828-7939
admissions@foxsubacute.com
www.foxsubacute.com

Terri Herd, Director of Marketing
Amy Swartley, RN, Director of Admissions
Kathy Palladino, Director of Human Resources
Erik I. Soiferman, DO, FACOI, Chief Medical Officer
Fox Subacute at Clara Burke in Plymouth Meeting, PA offers attentive, nurturing management of ventilator dependent, medically compromised patients in the PA, NJ, DE, Tri-State area. This sixty-bed facility, with its picturesque setting on 16 acres in historic Plymouth Meeting, is ideal for the specialized services and programs offered by Fox. With a team of highly motivated professionals, we offer the discharge alternative to prolonged lengths of stay in more costly acute care settings.

7133 **Good Samaritan Health System**
4th & Walnut Sts
P.O. Box 1281
Lebanon, PA 17042-1281 717-270-7500
www.gshleb.org

Robin Weiler, Manager
Frederick Davis, VP Clinical Services
Offers services for the totally blind, legally blind, visually impaired, and more with health, counseling, educational, recreational, rehabilitation, computer training and professional training services.

7134 **Good Samaritan Hospital-Health System Center**
Good Samaritan Hospital
4th & Walnut Sts
P.O. Box 1281
Lebanon, PA 17042-1281 717-270-7500
www.gshleb.org

June Nafziger-Eberl, Manager
Stuart Hartman, Medical Director
Comprehensive inpatient rehab unit for adults regarding general physical rehabilitation. Specific programs include orthopedic, neurological, stroke, amputee, etc.

7135 **Pediatric Center at Plymouth Meeting Integrated Health Services**
491 Allendale Rd
King of Prussia, PA 19406-1426 610-265-9290
800-220-7337
Fran Currick, Manager
Subacute programs such as intensive respiratory care, stressing ventilator dependent children, pre and post transplant care, total parenteral nutrition, IV therapy, intensive/behavioral oral feeding programs. Provides extensive discharge planning including teaching or review for all the above programs with an emphasis on development and accessing community resources.

7136 **Penn State Milton S. Hershey Medical Center College Of Medicine**
500 University Dr
Hershey, PA 17033-2360 717-531-8521
800-243-1455
Fax: 717-531-4558
www.pennstatehershey.org
Harold L Paz, CEO
Alan L. Brechbill, Executive Director
Wayne Zolko, Associate Vice President for Finance and Business
Andrew S. Resnick, Chief Quality Officer
a non-sectarian, not-for-profit community hospital whose purpose is to provide high quality acute, rehabilitative and preventive health services for the entire community, regardless of creed, race, nationality, or ability to pay.

7137 **Pennsylvania Pain Rehabilitation Center**
Ste 2
252 W Swamp Rd
Doylestown, PA 18901-2465 215-230-9707
Fax: 215-348-5106
Kenneth Lefkowitz, Manager
Post acute rehabilitation facility and programs.

7138 **Rehabilitation & Nursing Center at Greater Pittsburgh, The**
890 Weatherwood Ln
Greensburg, PA 15601-5777 724-837-8076
Fax: 724-837-7456
Nancy Flenner, Administrator
Marsha Echard, Admissions Coordinator
Craig Stepien, Admissions Director
Subacute care, ventilator and pulmonary managment, comprehensive rehabilitation.

Rhode Island

7139 **In-Sight**
43 Jefferson Blvd
Warwick, RI 02888-6400 401-941-3322
Fax: 401-941-3356
cbutler@in-sight.org
in-sight.org
Chris Butler, Executive Director
Lucille Gaboriault, Director of Community Resources
Paul Hopkins, Director of First Impressions
Richard Andrade, Director of Vision Rehabilitation
Offers services for the totally blind, legally blind, visually impaired, and more with health, counseling, educational, recreational, rehabilitation, computer training and professional training services.

7140 **Vanderbilt Rehabilitation Center**
Newport Hospital
167 Point Street
Providence, RI 02903 401-444-3500
www.lifespan.org
Timothy J. Babineau, President/CEO
Kenneth E. Arnold, SVP, General Counsel
Carole M. Cotter, SVP, Chief Information Officer
Cathy Duquette, EVP, Nursing Affairs
The Vanderbilt Rehabilitation Center at Newport Hospital has been providing comprehensive rehabilitation sercices for more than 40 years and is known throughout the region for its unique programs and high-quality, patient focused care.

South Carolina

7141 **Association for the Blind**
One Carriage Lane
Building A
Charleston, SC 29407 843-723-6915
Fax: 843-577-4312
www.abvisc.org
J. Douglas Hazelton, President
Capers A. Grimball, Vice President
Lea B. Kerrison, Secretary
Mary Morrison, Executive Director
Offers services for people who are blind, or are visually impaired with health, counseling, educational, recreational, rehabilitation, computer training and professional training services.

7142 **Hitchcock Rehabilitation Center**
690 Medical Park Dr
Aiken, SC 29801-6348 803-648-8344
800-207-6924
Fax: 803-648-1631
Karen Bowlen, Administrator
Dan Hillman, Case Manager
Carrie Morgan, Finance Director
Comprehensive outpatient rehabilitation for adults, children, geriatrics, pediatric therapy, special needs preschool, sports medicine, home health and hospice.

7143 **Mentor Network, The**
3600 Forest Drive
Suite 100
Columbia, SC 29204-1891 803-799-9025
800-297-8043
Fax: 803-931-8959
thementornetwork.com
Edward Murphy, Executive Chairman
Bruce Nardella, President and CEO
Denis Holler, Chief Financial Officer
Jeffrey Cohen, Chief Information Officer
Mentor provides a full network of individually tailored services for people with development disabilities and their families. Individuals may be served in their homes, shared living home, or in a host home.

Tennessee

7144 **Humana Hospital: Morristown RehabCare**
726 McFarland St
Morristown, TN 37814-3989 423-522-6000
www.lakewayregionalhospital.com
James Perry, Program Director
Designed to help patients in their adjustment to a physically limiting condition by helping to maximize each patient's abilities so he or she can function as independently as possible.

7145 **Opportunity East Rehabilitation Services for the Blind**
758 W Morris Blvd
Morristown, TN 37813-2136 423-586-3922
800-278-6274
Fax: 423-586-1479
volblind.org
Fred Overbay, CEO
Vic Mende, Director Rehabilitation Services
Offers services for the totally blind, legally blind, visually impaired, and more with health, counseling, educational, recreational, rehabilitation, computer training and professional training services.

7146 **Patrick Rehab Wellness Center**
Lincoln County Health System
106 Medical Center Blvd
Fayetteville, TN 37334-2684 931-433-0273
Fax: 931-433-0378
Gloria Meadows, Administrator
Jim Stewart, Principal

Provides rehabilitation services of physical, occupational, and speech therapy. Also, wellness memberships are available to the public.

7147 **PharmaThera**
1785 Nonconnah Blvd
Memphis, TN 38132-2104
901-348-8100
800-767-6714
Fax: 901-348-8270

7148 **Siskin Hospital For Physical Rehabilitation**
1 Siskin Plz
Chattanooga, TN 37403-1306
423-634-1200
info@siskinrehab.org
siskinrehab.org

Bob Main, CEO
Robert P. Main, President
Dedicated exclusively to physical rehabilitation and offers specialized treatment programs in brain injury, amputation, stroke, spinal cord injury, orthopedics, and major multiple trauma. The hospital also provides treatment for neurological disorders and loss of muscle strength and controll following illness or surgery.

7149 **St. Mary's RehabCare Center**
900 E Oak Hill Ave
Knoxville, TN 37917-4556
865-545-7962
Fax: 865-545-8133

Debbie Keeton, Director
Beth Greco, Executive Director
Provides comprehensive rehabilitation services for patients experiencing CVA, head trauma, orthopedic conditions, spinal cord injury or neurological impairment.

Texas

7150 **Alpine Ridge and Brandywood**
444 Devereux Drive
Victoria, TX 19085-2666
361-575-8271
800-345-1292
Fax: 361-575-6520
devereux.org

Robert Q. Kreider, President and CEO
Margaret McGill, SVP, Chief Operations Officer
Robert C. Dunne, SVP & Chief Financial Officer, Treasurer
Marilyn B. Benoit, M.D., SVP, Chief Clinical Officer, Chief Medical Officer

7151 **Amity Lodge**
Devereux Foundation
444 Devereux Drive
Victoria, TX 19085-2666
361-575-8271
800-345-1292
Fax: 361-575-6520
devereux.org

Robert Q. Kreider, President and CEO
Margaret McGill, SVP, Chief Operations Officer
Robert C. Dunne, SVP & Chief Financial Officer, Treasurer
Marilyn B. Benoit, M.D., SVP, Chief Clinical Officer, Chief Medical Officer
Offers residents a continuum of services ranging from minimal care and supervision to total physical and medical care.

7152 **Baylor Institute for Rehabilitation**
3500 Gaston Avenue
Dallas, TX 75246-2017
214-820-9300
800-4BA-YLOR
Fax: 214-841-2679
www.baylorhealth.com

Joel T. Allison, Chief Executive Officer
Gary Brock, President and Chief Operating Officer
LaVone Arthur, Vice President of Business Development
Wm. Stephen Boyd, Chief Legal Officer
A 92-bed specialty hospital offering comprehensive rehabilitation services for persons with spinal cord injury, traumatic brain injury, stroke, amputation, and other orthopedic and neurological disorders.

7153 **Beneto Center**
Devereux Foundation
444 Devereux Drive
Victoria, TX 19085-2666
361-575-8271
800-345-1292
Fax: 361-575-6520
devereux.org

Robert Q. Kreider, President and CEO
Margaret McGill, SVP, Chief Operations Officer
Robert C. Dunne, SVP & Chief Financial Officer, Treasurer
Marilyn B. Benoit, M.D., SVP, Chief Clinical Officer, Chief Medical Officer
Offers a continuum of services for residents requiring services ranging from minimal care and supervision to total physical and medical care.

7154 **CORE Health Care**
E&J Health Care
400 Highway 290
Bldg B, Suite. 205,
Dripping Springs, TX 78620
512-894-0801
866-683-1007
Fax: 512-858-4627

Eric Makowski, CEO
Kristi Jones, Marketing/Admissions Director
Erika Mountz, MBA, OTR/L, Director of Rehabilitation
Annie Freeman, MBA, PHR, Director of Huma Resources
Post acute and transitional rehabilitation, long-term care, community re-entry, for brain injury and complex psychiatric disorders.

7155 **Center for Neuro Skills**
1320 W Walnut Hill Ln
Irving, TX 75038-3007
972-580-8500
800-544-5448
Fax: 972-255-3162
srobinson@neuroskills.com
neuroskills.com

John Schultz, Administrator
Mark J. Ashley, President
Centre for Neuro Skills (CNS) seeks to provide medical rehabilitation programs, lifecare programs, advocacy, and research for people with brain injury in order to achieve a maximum quality of life.

7156 **Dallas Services**
4242 Office Pkwy
Dallas, TX 75204-3629
214-828-9900
Fax: 214-828-9901
www.dallasservices.org

Thomas . Turnage, Ph.D, Executive Director
Clark Thomas, Ph.D., Chair
Melissa Malonson, Vice-Chair
Cynthia O'Brien Robinson, Secretary
Offers four programs:1) an early education for children (6weeks-6yrs)with and without special needs.2)low vision clinic-provides low cost eye examsand glasses to low-income families as well as assistance to individuals who vision problems which cannot be corrected with glasses/surgery.3)mesquite day school- an early head start program for infants and toddlers of low-income families.4)special needs advocacy and inclusion program that offers families of special need children guidance and education.

7157 **Daman Villa**
Devereux Foundation
444 Devereux Drive
Victoria, TX 19085-2666
361-575-8271
800-345-1292
Fax: 361-575-6520
devereux.org

Robert Q. Kreider, President and CEO
Margaret McGill, SVP, Chief Operations Officer
Robert C. Dunne, SVP & Chief Financial Officer, Treasurer
Marilyn B. Benoit, M.D., SVP, Chief Clinical Officer, Chief Medical Officer
Offers residents a continuum of services ranging from minimal care and supervision to total physical and medical care.

7158 **Devereux Advanced Behavioral Health - Texas Victoria Campus**
Texas Victoria Campus
120 David Wade Dr.
P.O. Box 2666
Victoria, TX 77902
361-574-7208
800-383-5000
Fax: 361-575-6250
www.devereuxtx.org

Pam Reed, Executive Director
Offering residential services for people of all ages with emotional, behavioral, developmental, and psychiatric disorders. Services include community based living and vocational programs, residential programs and foster care.

7159 **Devereux Advanced Behavioral Health Texas - League City Campus**
Texas League City Campus
1150 Devereux Dr
League City, TX 77573
281-335-1000
800-373-0011
Fax: 281-554-6290
www.devereuxtx.org

Gail Atkinson, Vice President of Operations & Marketing
Offering long-term hospitalization and intensive residential services for adolescents and young adults with emotional, behavioral, developmental and psychiatric disorders.

7160 **El Paso Lighthouse for the Blind**
200 Washington St
El Paso, TX 79905-3897
915-532-4495
Fax: 915-532-6338
www.lighthouse-elpaso.com

Craig Hays, President
Lea Cochran, Vice President
Lola Dawkins, Secretary
Rusty Hooten, Chief Financial Officer
Enables people of all ages to embody blindness and vision impairment through training, rehabilitation, employment opportunity, advocacy and research. Provides access to opportunities and quality of life so that the blind and visually impaired can reach their fullest potential for self-sufficiency and independence.

7161 **Harris Methodist Fort Worth/Mabee Rehabilitation Center**
612 E. Lamar Boulevard
Arlington, TX 76011-2122
877-847-9355
Fax: 817-882-2753
www.texashealth.org

Louise Baldwin, President
Peggyo Ehrlich, Rehab Manager
Karen Mallett, Executive Director
Douglas D. Hawthorne, Chief Executive Officer
A hospital based inpatient rehab program and outpatient day programs in chronic pain management, work hardening and brain injury transitional services.

7162 **HealthSouth Hospital of Cypress**
13031 Wortham Center Dr
Houston, TX 77065
832-280-2500
feedback@healthsouth.com
healthsouthcypress.com

Jerome Lengel, Executive Officer
Dewitt Hilton, Owner
Offers an individualized approach to the process of rehabilitation for severely injured or disabled individuals. The process begins with a pre-admissions assessment of each referred patient. The Center combines state-of-the-art technology and equipment with multi-disciplinary therapy and education in a cheerful, secure environment.

7163 **Heights Hospital Rehab Unit**
1917 Ashland St
Houston, TX 77008-3994
713-861-6161
Fax: 713-802-8660
www.selectmedical.com

Theresa Davis, CEO
Robert A. Ortenzio, Executive Chairman and Co-Founder
Rocco A. Ortenzio, Vice Chairman and Co-Founder
David S. Chernow, President and Chief Executive Officer
This program is designed to assist patients with physical disabilities achieve their maximum functional abilities.

7164 **Hillcrest Baptist Medical Center**
100 Hillcrest Medical Blvd
Waco, TX 76712
254-202-2000
Fax: 254-202-5105
www.sw.org

Anne Hott Kimberly, Program Director
Ann Gammel, Nurse Manager
Debbie Meurer, Manager
Designed to assist patients in adjustment to a physically limiting condition, utilizing interdisciplinary strategies to maximize each patient's ability and capability.

7165 **Institute for Rehabilitation & Research**
1333 Moursund St
Houston, TX 77030-3405
713-799-5000
800-447-3422
Fax: 713-797-5289
tirr.memorialhermann.org

Carl Josehart, CEO
Jean Herzog, President
Gerard E. Francisco, M.D., Chief Medical Officer
Mary Ann Euliarte, CNO/COO
A national center for information, training, research, and technical assistance in independent living. The goal is to extend the body of knowledge in independent living and to improve the utilization of results of research programs and demonstration projects in this field. It has developed a variety of strategies for collecting, synthesizing, and disseminating information related to the field of independent living.

7166 **Integrated Health Services of Amarillo**
6141 Amarillo Blvd. West
Amarillo, TX 79106
806-356-0488
Fax: 806-356-8074

Mary Bearden, Chairman
Jay L. Barrett, President
Marvin Franz, Executive Director & CEO
Provides acute, post acute, residential and outpatient health care services. IHS of Amarillo is a 153-bed facility with 120 beds licensed by The Texas Department of Health and Human Services, and is accredited by JCAHO. We serve urban and rural populations of over 500,000, drawing from a 5-state region.

7167 **Kanner Center**
Devereax Foundation
444 Devereux Drive
Victoria, TX 19085-2666
361-575-8271
800-345-1292
Fax: 361-575-6520
devereux.org

Robert Q. Kreider, President and CEO
Margaret McGill, SVP, Chief Operations Officer
Robert C. Dunne, SVP & Chief Financial Officer, Treasurer
Marilyn B. Benoit, M.D., SVP, Chief Clinical Officer, Chief Medical Officer
A private nonprofit nationwide network of treatment services for individuals of all ages with emotional and/or developmental disabilities.

7168 **Lighthouse of Houston**
3602 W Dallas St
Houston, TX 77019-1704
713-527-9561
Fax: 713-284-8451
custserv@houstonlighthouse.org
houstonlighthouse.org

Gibson DuTerroil, President
Shelagh Moran, VP/COO
Chelean Zander, VP Community Programs
Serves the blind, visually impaired, deaf-blind and multihandicapped blind. Provides workshops, vocational training and placement, low vision clinic, orientation and mobility, housing, Braille, volunteer services, senior center, visual aid sales, counseling and support, diabetic education and day health activity services and day summer camp, Summer Transition for Youth.

7169 **Mainland Center Hospital RehabCare Unit**
6801 Emmett F Lowry Expy
Texas City, TX 77591-2500 409-938-5000
Fax: 409-938-5501
www.mainlandmedical.com

Michael Ehrat, CEO

The RehabCare program is designed and staffed to assist functionally impaired patients improve to their maximum potential. The opportunities for improvement and adjustments are provided in a pleasant, supportive inpatient environment by therapists from the occupational, physical, recreational and speech therapy disciplines.

7170 **North Texas Rehabilitation Center**
1005 Midwestern Pkwy
Wichita Falls, TX 76302-2211 940-322-0771
Fax: 940-766-4943
ntrehab.org

Mike Castles, President/ CEO

Provides outpatient rehabilitation services to maximize independence or promote development to children and adults with disabilities. Programs include: physical, occupational, speech therapy, closed head injury, infant/child development, support groups, aquatics and wellness program and a child achievement program.

7171 **South Texas Lighthouse for the Blind**
PO BOX 9697
Corpus Christi, TX 78469-3321 361-883-6553
888-255-8011
Fax: 361-883-1041
Customer.service@stlb.net
www.stlb.net

Regis Barber, President
Nicky Ooi, Chief Operations Officer
Alana Manrow, Public Affairs Director

Their mission is to Employ, Educate and Empower their neighbors who are blind and visually impaired. They offer job opportunities in manufacturing, retail and administration, as well as orientation and mobility and adaptive technology training.

7172 **Texas Specialty Hospital at Dallas**
7955 Harry Hines Blvd
Dallas, TX 75235-3305 214-637-0000
Fax: 214-637-6512
Mary.Alexander@fundltc.com

Mary Alexander, CEO
Cathy Campbell, Chief Executive Officer

66 beds offering active/acute rehabilitation, brain injury day treatment, cognitive rehabilitation, complex care, extended rehabilitation and short term evaluation.

7173 **Transitional Learning Center at Gavelston and Lubbock**
1528 Post Office St
Galveston, TX 77550 409-762-6661
Fax: 409-763-3930
www.tlcrehab.org

Brent Masel, MD, President and Medical Director
Gary Seale, Ph.D., VP Clinical Programs
Jim Lovelace, MBA, VP of Operations
Shelley Kessler, CPA, Chief Financial Officer

Specializes solely in post-acute brain injury. A nationally known pioneer in the field and a not for profit with a three fold mission: treatment, research and education. Offers 6 hours of therapy a day from licensed/certified staff, on site physician and nursing services and long-term living for brian injured adults at Tideway on Gavelston Island. Accredited by CARF.

1982

7174 **Treemont Nursing And Rehabilitation Center**
5550 Harvest Hill Rd
Dallas, TX 75230-1684 972-661-1862
Fax: 972-788-1543

Bob Barker, Administrator

Postacute rehabilitation program.

7175 **West Texas Lighthouse for the Blind**
2001 Austin St
San Angelo, TX 76903-8796 325-653-4231
Fax: 325-657-9367
customerservice@lighthousefortheblind.org
www.lighthousefortheblind.org

David Wells, Executive Director
Stephen Horton, Operations Manager
Fonda V. Galindo, Finance & Human Resources Manager
Vickie Sanders, Sales & Marketing Manager

Offers services for the totally blind, legally blind, visually impaired, and more with health, counseling, educational, recreational, rehabilitation, computer training and professional training services.

Utah

7176 **Quincy Rehabilitation Institute of Holy Cross Hospital**
1050 E South Temple
Salt Lake City, UT 84102-1507 801-350-8140
Fax: 801-350-4791

Dave Jenson, President

Postacute rehabilitation program.

7177 **Wasatch Vision Clinic**
849 E 400 S
Salt Lake City, UT 84102-2928 801-328-2020
Fax: 801-363-2201
email@wasatchvision.com
eyeappointment.com

Craig Cutler, Owner
Camron Bateman OD, Doctor

Postacute rehabilitation program.

Vermont

7178 **Rutland Mental Health Services**
78 S Main St
Rutland, VT 05701-4594 802-775-2381
Fax: 802-775-4020
rmhsccn.org

Dan Quinn, President/ CEO
Scott Dikeman, Vice Chairman
Ron Holm, Secretary
Tom Pour, Treasurer

A private, non-profit comprehensive community mental health center. It provides services to individuals and families for mental health and substance abuse related problems and also to persons who are developmentally disabled.

Virginia

7179 **Bay Pine-Virginia Beach**
680 South Fourth Street
Louisville, KY 40202 502-596-7300
TTY: 800-545-0749
web_administrator@kindred.com
kindredhealthcare.com

Paul J. Diaz, President/ CEO

Postacute rehabilitation program.

7180 **Carilion Rehabilitation: New River Valley**
2013 S Jefferson Street
Roanoke, VA 24014 540-981-7377
Fax: 540-981-8233
www.carilionclinic.org

Nancy Howell Agee, President/ CEO
James A. Hartley, Chair
Briggs W. Andrews, Corporate Secretary
G. Robert Vaughan, Jr., Treasurer, SVP

CARF-accredited pain management program, work hardening program and comprehensive outpatient therapy clinic, massage therapy, outpatient programs and more. Program emphasis is on interdisiplinary behavioral rehab based pain management and functional restoration in conjunction with medical treatment. Work hardening is a transdisciplinary work simulation program taylored to the individual. Comprehensive outpatient program is multi-disciplinary with emphasis on manual treatment.

7181 **Faith Mission Home**
3540 Mission Home Ln
Free Union, VA 22940-1505
434-985-2294
Fax: 434-985-7633
www.beachyam.org

Paul Beiler, Manager
Reuben Yoder, Director
A Christian residential center that serves 60 developmentally disabled children, including individuals with Down Syndrome, Cerebral palsy and other similar conditions. Children may be admitted from the time they are ambulatory until they reach 15 years of age. He or she may stay as long as it is in the child's best interests. The training program stresses the following areas: self-care, social, academic, vocational, crafts, speech and physical development.

7182 **ManorCare Health Services-Arlington**
333 N. Summit St.
Toledo, OH 43604
800-366-1232
CareLine@hcr-manorcare.com
hcr-manorcare.com

Marcia K Jarrell, Administrator
Ric Birch, Marketing Director
ManorCare-Arlington offers residents a full Continuum of Care in a caring environment. ManorCare's wide range of services includes subacute medical and rehabilitation programs for short term patients transitioning from hospital to home and Skilled Nursing Care.

7183 **Pines Residential Treatment Center**
825 Crawford Pkwy
Portsmouth, VA 23704-2301
757-393-0061
Fax: 757-393-1029

Lenard J Lexier, Medical Director
Judy Kemp, Admissions Director
A 310-bed residential treatment center in Portsmouth Virginia, providing a therapeutic environment for severely emotionally disturbed children and youth. Five unique programs meet behavioral, educational and emotional needs of males and females, five to twenty-two years of age. Multi-disciplinary teams devise individual service plans to enhance strengths and reverse self-defeating behavior. A highly effective positive reinforcement program with a proven track record.

7184 **Roanoke Memorial Hospital**
Carilion Health System
2013 S Jefferson Street
Roanoke, VA 24014
540-981-7377
Fax: 540-981-8233
www.carilionclinic.org

Nancy Howell Agee, President/ CEO
James A. Hartley, Chair
Briggs W. Andrews, Corporate Secretary
G. Robert Vaughan, Jr., Treasurer, SVP
Carilion Health System exists to improve the health of the communities it serves. The vision is to assure accessible, affordable, high quality healthcare that meets the needs of the community. Motivate and educate individuals to improve their health. Champion community initiatives to reduce health risk

7185 **Southside Virginia Training Center**
P.O. Box 4030
Petersburg, VA 23803-30
804-524-7000
Fax: 804-524-7228
www.svtc.dbhds.virginia.gov

Bob Kaufman, Director, Administrative Service
Offers residential, vocational, occupational, physical, and speech therapies.

7186 **Woodrow Wilson Rehabilitation Center**
P.O. Box 1500
Fishersville, VA 22939-1500
540-332-7000
800-345-9972
Fax: 540-332-7132
www.wwrc.net

Rick Sizemore, Executive Director
Amy Blalock, Admissions and Marketing Director
Comprehensive residential rehabilitation center offering complete medical and vocational rehabilitation services including: vocation evaluation, vocational training, transition from school to work, occupational therapy, physical therapy, speech, language and audiology, assistive technology, rehabilitation engineering, counseling/case management, behavioral health services, nursing and physician services, etc.

Washington

7187 **Arden Rehabilitation And Healthcare Center**
680 South Fourth Street
Louisville, KY 40202
502-596-7300
TTY: 800-545-0749
web_administrator@kindred.com
kindredhealthcare.com

Paul J. Diaz, President/ CEO
Arden can accomodate 90 residents- post-acute/rehabilitation patients as well as long term residents. Medicare certified, the center also takes most managed healthcare insurance plans, as well as VA, respite and hospice patients.

7188 **Bellingham Care Center**
680 South Fourth Street
Louisville, KY 40202
502-596-7300
TTY: 800-545-0749
web_administrator@kindred.com
kindredhealthcare.com

Paul J. Diaz, President/ CEO
Postacute rehabilitation program.

7189 **Division of Vocational Rehabilitation Department of Social and Health Services**
P.O. Box 45130
Olympia, WA 98504-5130
360-704-3560
800-737-0617
Fax: 360-570-6941
krulik@dshs.wa.gov
www1.dshs.wa.gov/dvr

Patrick Raines, Manager
Lynnea Ruttledge, Manager
Information on computers, supported employment, marketing rehabilitation facilities and transition.

7190 **First Hill Care Center**
1334 Terry Ave
Seattle, WA 98101
206-682-2661
Fax: 206-624-0188
www.khseattlefirsthill.com

7191 **Harborview Medical Center, Low Vision Aid Clinic**
Harborview Medical Center
325 9th Ave
Seattle, WA 98104-2499
206-744-3300
TTY: 206-744-3246
comment@u.washington.edu
www.uwmedicine.org

Eileen Whalen, Executive director
J. Richard Goss, M.D., Medical director
Darcy Jaffe, Chief nursing officer and senior associate for patient care
Elise Chayet, Associate administrator, clinical support services and plan
Harborview Medical Center is the only designated Level 1 adult and pediatric trauma and burn center in the state of Washington and serves as the regional trauma and burn referral center for Alaska, Montana and Idaho. UW Medicine physicians and staff based at Harborview provide highly specialized services for vascular, orthopedics, neurosciences, ophthalmology, behavioral health, HIV/AIDS and complex critical care.

7192 Integrated Health Services of Seattle
820 NW 95th St
Seattle, WA 98117-2207
206-783-7649
Fax: 206-781-1448

Jerry Harvey, Administrator
Marlette Basada, Director Nursing
Flavia Lagrange, Director Admissions

Postacute rehabilitation program. IHS provides 24 hour subacute and long-term care. We can handle vent/trach/hemo andritoneal dialysis and provide a full scope of rehabilitation services.

7193 Lakeside Milam Recovery Centers (LMRC)
3315 S. 23rd Street
Ste 102
Tacoma, WA 98405
253-272-2242
800-231-4303
Fax: 253-272-0171
help@lakesidemilam.com
www.lakesidemilam.com

Michael Kinder, Administrator

LMRC was established in 1983 with a single mission, to help victims and families recover from the pain of drug/alcohol addiction. Enlightned by the work of Dr. James Milam in the 1960's and 70's, the founders of LMRC created a treatment system based on a bedrock set of principals.

7194 Lakewood Health Care Center
11411 Bridgeport Way SW
Lakewood, WA 98499-3047
253-581-9002
800-359-7412
Fax: 253-581-7016
www.lakewoodhc.com

Gwynn Rucker, Executive Director
Patty Wood, Administrator
Linda Doll, Social Services
Dr. Mian, Medical Director

Accomodates 80 residents. We offer 24 hour skilled nursing services, long-term care and rehab services which include Physical, Occupational and Speech Therapy.

7195 Manor Care Health Services-Tacoma
5601 S Orchard St
Tacoma, WA 98409-1371
253-474-8421
Fax: 253-471-8857
www.hcr-manorcare.com

Tina Irwin, Administrator

124-bed skilled nursing and rehabilitation center provides services for those seeking long term Skilled Nursing Care, short term subacute care, hospice services, Alzheimer's and respite care. Our Acadia Wing, a specialized Alzheimer's care unit, provides specialized programming and trained staff that truly makes us the leader in Alzheimers Services.

7196 ManorCare Health Services-Lynnwood
3701 188th St SW
Lynnwood, WA 98037-7626
425-775-9222
Fax: 425-712-3685
www.hcr-manorcare.com

Liza Loyet, Administrator

Our in-house therapists provide physical, occupational and speech therapies in our state-of-the-art therapy gym. Our team is goal oriented and focuses on producing positive outcomes for those recovering from illness, injury or surgery.

7197 ManorCare Health Services-Spokane
6025 N Assembly St
Spokane, WA 99205-7674
509-326-8282
Fax: 509-326-4790
www.hcrmanorcare.com

Cheri Kubu, Administrator
Sandra Hayes, Administrator

Provides skilled nursing and respite stays for those needing a break from care giving. We specialize in Rehabilitation Services provided by our in-house occupational, physical and speech therapists.

7198 Northwest Continuum Care Center
Kindred Health Care
128 Old Beacon Hill Dr
Longview, WA 98632-5859
360-423-4060
Fax: 360-636-0958

Steve M. Ross, Executive Director
Tami Wilson, Director of Nursing
Mary R., Activities Assistant
Kristen W., Health and Rehabilitation Center

Accomodates 69 residents. Employs the Angel Care Program designed to address any special needs that may arise during a resident's stay in our facility. The program focuses extra attention on residents and, in some cases, family members. The goal is to meet the special needs of the people we provide care to every day.

7199 Park Manor Convalescent Center
1710 Plaza Way
Walla Walla, WA 99362-4362
509-529-4218
Fax: 509-522-1729
egines@ensigngroup.net
www.parkmanorcare.com

Jed Gines, Administrator
Krista Maiuri, Directr Of Nursing
Sonya Taylor, Director of Rehabilitation
Mike Henckel, Admissions & Marketing Director

Residents of Park Manor enjoy a range of activities, developed to meet their needs, inculding excercise programs, social and recreational activities, arts and crafts, shopping trips and other excursions. We also offer religious services.

7200 Queen Anne Health Care
Queen Anne Health Care
2717 Dexter Ave N
Seattle, WA 98109-1914
206-284-7012
Fax: 206-283-3936
www.queenannehealthcare.com

Heather Eacker, Executive Director
Mary R., Activities Assistant
Kristen W., Health and Rehabilitation Center
Becky D., Activity Director

Our goal is to provide quality, compassionate care. Our cozy building accomodates 120 residents. We offer semi private rooms with space to add items from home for a special personalized touch

7201 Rainier Vista Care Center
920 12th Ave SE
Puyallup, WA 98372-4920
253-841-3422
Fax: 253-848-3937

Linda Larson, Administrator
Nancy L. Erckenbrack, Executive Director
Kristen W., Health and Rehabilitation Center
Becky D., Activity Director

Accomodates 120 residents. We are certified for Medicare and Medicaid and we offer a continuum of healthcare services from short-term or outpatient rehabilitation to long-term care. We offer semi-private and private rooms as well as rehabilitation and hospice suites. Rainier Vista Care Center is a recipient of the American Health Care Association Quality Award.

7202 Rehabilitation Enterprises of Washington
430 E Lauridsen Blvd
Port Angeles, WA 98362-7978
360-452-9789
Fax: 360-452-9700

Brett White, President

REW is the professional trade association representing community rehabilitation programs before government and other publics. These organizations provide a wide array of employment and training services for people with disabilities. The goal is to assist member organizations to provide the highest quality rehabilitative and employment services to their customers.

7203 **Seattle Medical and Rehabilitation Center**
Evergreen Healthcare
12040 NE 128th St
Kirkland, WA 98034-3013
425-899-3000
877-601-2271
TTY: 425-899-2007
evergreenhealthcare.org

Al DeYoung, Chair
Robert H. Malte, Chief Executive Officer
Neil Johnson, RN, MSA, Senior Vice President & Chief Operating Officer
Nancee Hofmeister, Vice President, Chief Nursing Officer

103 beds offering subacute rehabilitation, complex care, subacute treatment and short-term evaluation. Pulmonary unit offering long and short term care for ventilator dependent patients.

7204 **Slingerland Institute for Literacy**
Educators Publishing Service
12729 Northup Way
Suite 1
Bellevue, WA 98005
425-453-1190
Fax: 425-635-7762
mail@slingerland.org
www.slingerland.org

Bonnie Meyer, Executive Director
Elyce Newton, Program Support

A nonprofit public corporation founded in 1977 to carry on the work of Beth H. Slingerland in providing classroom teachers with the techniques, knowledge and understanding necessary for identifying and teaching children with Specific Language Disability. The main objective is to educate teachers in successful methods of identifying, diagnosing and instructing children and adults with SLD and to promote literacy through reading, writing and oral expression.

7205 **Timberland Opportunities Association**
400 W Curtis St
Aberdeen, WA 98520-7698
360-533-5823
Fax: 360-533-5848

Jim Eddy, Executive Director

Provides training and employment for disabled people.

7206 **Vancouver Health and Rehabilitation Center**
400 E 33rd St
Vancouver, WA 98663-2238
360-696-2561
Fax: 360-696-9275
www.vancouverhealthcare.com

Jody Wigen, Human Resources
Joe Joy, Executive Director
Kristen W., Health and Rehabilitation Center
Becky D., Activity Director

Postacute rehabilitation program.

Wisconsin

7207 **Colonial Manor Medical And Rehabilitation Center**
1010 E Wausau Ave
Wausau, WI 54403-3101
715-842-2028
Fax: 715-848-0510
www.colonialmanormrc.com

Ericca Ylitalo, Administrator
Shelley Solberg, Executive Director

Colonial Manor Medical and Rehabilitation Center is part of the Kindred Community and is located in Wausau, Wisconsin. The corporate headquarters are based in Louisville Kentucky. Our facility accomodates 150 residents.

7208 **Waushers Industries**
210 E Chicago Rd
Wautoma, WI 54982-6932
920-787-4696
Fax: 920-787-4698

Richard King, Human Resources

Provides various programming for individuals with disabilities in waushara county.

7209 **Woodstock Health and Rehabilitation Center**
3415 Sheridan Rd
Kenosha, WI 53140-1924
262-657-6175
Fax: 262-657-5756

Debra Lamb, Administrator
Darlene Einerson, Executive Director
Kristen W., Health and Rehabilitation Center
Becky D., Activity Director

Offers a full range of medical services to meet the individual needs of our residents, including short term rehabilitative services and long-tern skilled care.

Rehabilitation Facilities, Sub-Acute

Alabama

7210 **UAB Spain Rehabilitation Center**
1717 6th Ave S
Birmingham, AL 35233-7330 205-934-3450
www.uab.edu/medicine/physicalmedicine/
Tracy L Brewer, Administrative Manager
A 49-bed rehabilitation hospital featuring advanced, individualized care for adolescents and adult patients recovering from a broad variety of health problems. Patient care teams include physiatrists (doctors who specialized in rehabilitation medicine), nurses, nurse practitioners, physical therapists, occupational therapists, speech/language pathologists, psychologists, social workers, rehabilitation professionals and other health care professionals from all areas of the UAB Health System.

Alaska

7211 **Fairbanks Memorial Hospital & Denali Center**
1650 Cowles St
Fairbanks, AK 99701-5998 907-452-8181
Fax: 907-458-5324
www.fmhdc.com
Sheldon Stadnyk, MD, Interim Chief Executive Officer
The Denali Center offers the following rehabilitation services: Physical Therapy, Occupational Therapy, Speech Therapy, Sub-Acute Rehab.

Arizona

7212 **Desert Life Rehabilitation & Care Center**
Kindred Healthcare
1919 W Medical St
Tucson, AZ 85704-1133 520-297-8311
Fax: 520-544-0930
Amad Nazifi, Executive Director
Jane Olmstead, Director of Nursing
Accomodates 240 residents. We provide skilled and intermediate nursing with occupational, physical, speech and respiratory therapy services. We offer special programs including an Alzheimer's Unit and a Young Adult Program, and are located in beautiful Southern Arizona where there is plenty of sunshine, mountains and desert views. Desert Life is a 2005 recipient of the American Health Care Association Quality Award.

7213 **Hacienda Rehabilitation and Care Center**
660 S Coronado Dr
Sierra Vista, AZ 85635-3386 520-459-4900
Fax: 520-458-4082
www.haciendarcc.com
Monica Vandivort, Medical Director
Kristen W., Health and Rehabilitation Center Executive Director
Becky D., Activity Director
Mary R., Activities Assistant
Accomodates 100 residents. We are located in Sierra Vista, near Kartchner Caverns, Fort Huachuca, Coronado National Forest and historic Tombstone. Serving the medical needs of the community since 1983, we strive to provide care with quality, compassion and integrity.

7214 **Kachina Point Health Care & Rehabilitation Center**
505 Jacks Canyon Rd
Sedona, AZ 86351-7856 928-284-1000
Fax: 928-284-0626
Michael Amadei, Medical Director
Accomodates 120 residents. We have met the healthcare needs of the community since 1984. Kachina Point is a 2004 recipient of the American Health Care Association's Quality Award.

7215 **Mayo Clinic Scottsdale**
13400 E Shea Blvd
Scottsdale, AZ 85259-5499 480-301-8000
800-446-2279
Fax: 480-301-9310
www.mayoclinic.org/arizona
Neena S. Abraham, Gastroenterology/ Hepatology
Roberta H. Adams, Hematology/Oncology
Charles H. Adler, Parkinson's Disease and Movement Disorders Center
Neera Agarwal, Hospital Internal Medicine
Mayo clinic is a not-for-profit medical practice dedicated to the diagnosis and treatment of virtually every type of complex illness. Mayo clinic staff members work together to meet your needs. You will see as many doctors, specialists, and other health care professionals as needed to provide comprehensive diagnosis, understandable answers and effective treatment.

7216 **Sonoran Rehabilitation and Care Center**
Kindred
4202 N 20th Ave
Phoenix, AZ 85015-5101 602-264-3824
Fax: 602-279-6234
Jeffrey Barrett, Executive Director
Offers the following rehabilitation services: Respiratory Therapy, Physical Therapy, Speech Therapy, Occupational Therapy, Restorative Therapy, Sub-Acute Rehabilitation, Wound Care.

7217 **Valley Health Care and Rehabilitation Center**
Kindred Health Care Center
5545 E Lee St
Tucson, AZ 85712-4205 520-296-2306
Fax: 520-296-4072
Dale Pelton, Executive Director
Sandra Lewis, Administrator
Offers the following rehabilitation services: Physical Therapy, Occupational Therapy, Speech Therapy, Sub-Acute Rehab.

California

7218 **Alamitos-Belmont Rehab Hospital**
3901 E 4th St
Long Beach, CA 90814-1699 562-434-8421
Fax: 562-433-6732
www.alamitosbelmont.com
John L. Sorensen, Chairman of the Board of Directors.
Jonathan Sloey, Administrator
Offers the following rehabilitation services: Speech Therapy, Occupational Therapy, Physical Therapy, Sub-Acute Rehab.

7219 **Bay View Nursing and Rehabilitation Center**
Kindred Health Care
516 Willow St
Alameda, CA 94501-6132 510-521-5600
Fax: 510-865-9035
www.kindredhealthcare.com
Richard S Espinoza, Administrator
Say Silva, Assistant Executive Director
Accomodates 180 residents. Bay View is a 2004 recipient of the American Health Care Association's Quality Award. We provide short-term rehabilitative care, traditional long-term skilled care and Alzheimer's/dementia special care. Our combination of clinical skill and comprehensive rehabilitation services enables us to care for a variety of complex medical conditions.

7220 **Foothill Nursing and Rehab Center**
401 W Ada Ave
Glendora, CA 91741-4241 626-335-9810
Fax: 626-963-0720
www.foothillnursing.com
Arnie Shafer, Executive Director
Marianne Schultz, Administrator
Offers the following rehabilitation services: Physical Therapy, Occupational Therapy, Speech Therapy, In and Out Patient Rehab.

7221 **Long Beach Memorial Medical Center Memorial Rehabilitation Hospital**
2801 Atlantic Ave
Ground Floor
Long Beach, CA 90806-1701 562-933-9001
Fax: 562-933-9019
www.memorialcare.org/long_beach
Barry Arbuckle, President/CEO
The goal of the MemorialCare Rehabilitation Institute is to help persons with disabilities regain independence and rebuild their lives in an environment where loved ones are involved in the rehabilitation process. We are dedicated to the pursuit of our mission, vision and values.

7222 **Mercy Medical Center Mt. Shasta**
914 Pine St
Mount Shasta, CA 96067-2143 530-926-6111
Fax: 530-926-0517
www.mercymtshasta.org
Greg Lippert, Senior Director of Support and Information Services
Scott Foster, Director of Hospital Finance
Sister Anne Chester, Director of Mission Integration
Joyce Zwanziger, Director Marketing, Community Relations & Volunteer Services
Mercy Medical Center is committed to furthering the healing ministry of Jesus, and to provide high-quality, affordable healthcare to the communities we serve.

7223 **Northridge Hospital Medical Center**
18300 Roscoe Blvd
Northridge, CA 91328-4167 818-885-8500
www.northridgehospital.org
Michael Wall, CEO
Offers the following rehabilitation services: Physical Therapy, Occupational Therapy, Speech Therapy, Sub-Acute Rehab. As a member of the Catholic Heathcare West Northridge Hospital Medical Center is committed to serving the health needs of our communities with particular attention to the needs of the poor, the disadvantaged and vulnerable, and the comfort of the suffering and dying.

7224 **Riverside Community Hospital**
4445 Magnolia Ave
Riverside, CA 92501 951-788-3000
Fax: 630-792-5636
complaint@jointcommission.org
www.riversidecommunityhospital.com
Jaime Wesolowski, President/CEO
Patrick Brilliant, CEO
At Riverside Community Hospital, we are able to provide the healthcare services that you and your family will need through the many stages of your life. Services like Emergency/Trauma, Labor and Delivery, Cardiac Care, Orthopedics and Transplant are among our many Centers of Excellence.

7225 **Saint Jude Medical Center**
101 E Valencia Mesa Dr
Fullerton, CA 92835-3809 714-871-3280
800-870-7537
Fax: 714-992-3029
www.stjudemedicalcenter.org
April De Cou, Wellness Educator
Jane Wang, Wellness Programs Supervisor
Offers the following rehabilitation services: Out-patient Rehab, Sub-Acute Rehab, Occupational Therapy, Physical Therapy, Speech and Audiology Therapy, Pain Management Program.

7226 **South Coast Medical Center**
12 Mason
Suite A
Irvine, CA 92618-2733 714-669-4446
Fax: 714-669-4448
info@southcoastmedcenter.com
www.mission4health.com
Leigh Erin Connealy, Manager
Bruce Christian, President
Offers the following services: physical therapy, occupational therapy, speech therapy, cardica rehabilitation, incontinence program, sub-acute rehabilitation.

7227 **Valley Garden Health Care and Rehabilitation Center**
1517 Knickerbocker Dr
Stockton, CA 95210-3119 209-957-4539
Fax: 209-957-5831
www.valleygardenshealth.com
Dr. Alexande Chan, Medical Director
Accomodates 120 residents. Our center provides short-term nursing and rehabilitative care as well as traditional long-term skilled care. Our combination of clinical skill and comprehensive rehabilitation services enables us to care for a variety of complex medical conditions. Rehabilitative therapies are provided as needed by physical, occupational and speech therapists.

Colorado

7228 **Boulder Community Hospital Mapleton Center**
1100 Balsam
PO Box 9019
Boulder, CO 80301-9019 303-440-2273
info@bch.org
www.bch.org
Lou DellaCava, Chairman
Ric Porreca, Vice Chairman
Jean Dubofsky, Secretary
R. David Hoover, Treasurer
159-bed acute care hospital and 24-hour emergency department.

7229 **Fairacres Manor**
1700 18th Ave
Greeley, CO 80631-5152 970-353-3370
Fax: 970-353-9347
Kathy Gardner, Admissions/Marketing Director
Marla Trujillo, Director of Nursing
Ben Gonzales, Admissions/Marketing Assistant Director
Kathleen Mekelburg, Administrator
Offers the following rehabilitation services: Physical Therapy, Occupational Therapy, Speech Therapy, Restorative Therapy, Skilled Nursing, and Sub-Acute Rehabilitation.

7230 **Rowan Community**
4601 E Asbury Cir
Denver, CO 80222-4722 303-757-1228
Fax: 303-759-3390
Tammy Gleisner, Director/Admissions/Marketing Director
Jeff Jerebker, President/CEO
Bruce Odenthal, VP Operations
John D. Brammeier, CPA, FHFMA, Chief Financial Officer
Rowan is a 70-bed community, small enough to support personal relationships between residents and caregivers. Our residents vary in age, reflecting the diversity of a much larger community. Rowan's focus is on a psycho-social model of care with a dynamic activities and social service program. Our staff is specially trained in behavior management and many are certified Eden AlternativeT associates and certifid Elder Care Specialists.

Connecticut

7231 **Hamilton Rehabilitation and Healthcare Center**
89 Viets St
New London, CT 6320-3355 860-447-1471
Fax: 860-439-0107
Steve Roizen, Executive Director
Offers the following rehabilitation services: Sub-Acute, Occupational Therapy, Speech Therapy, Physical Therapy.

7232 **Hospital For Special Care (HSC)**
2150 Corbin Ave
New Britain, CT 06053-2298 860-223-2761
Fax: 860-827-4849
www.hfsc.org
John J. Votto, President/CEO
Paul J. Scalise, M.D., F.C.C.P, Senior Vice President
Thomas J. Soltis, M.D., M.P.H., Chief of Geriatrics
HSC is a private, not-for-profit 200-bed rehabilitation long-term acute and chronic care hospital, widely-known and respected for its expertise in physical rehabilitation, respiratory care, and med-

ically-complex pediatrics. Special programs for spinal cord injuries, pulmonary rehabilitation, acquired brain injuries, stroke, ventilator management and geriatrics, make HSC an important regional resource for patients with special healthcare needs.

7233 **Masonic Healthcare Center**
MasoniCare Corporation
22 Masonic Ave
PO Box 70
Wallingford, CT 06492-3048
203-679-5900
877-424-3537
Fax: 203-679-6459
info@masonicare.org
www.masonicare.org

Stephen B. McPherson, President
Arthur Santilli, President

The states leading provider of healthcare and retirement living communities for seniors. We are not-for-profit and have more then 100 years of experience behind us. We're recognized for the quality, compassionate care and steadfast support we provide to our residents and patients.

7234 **Stamford Hospital**
30 Shelburne Rd
Stamford, CT 06904-3628
203-276-1000
Fax: 203-325-7905
info@stamhealth.org
www.stamfordhospital.org

Brian Grissler, President/CEO
Kathleen Silard, EVP/Chief Operating Officer
Kevin Gage, Senior Vice President, Finance/Chief Financial Officer
Sharon Kiely, MD, Senior Vice President, Medical Affairs/Chief Medical Officer

A not-for-profit, community teaching hospital that has been serving Stamford and surrounding communities for more then 100 years. We have 305 inpatient beds in medicine, surgery, obstetrics/gynecology, psychiatry, and medical and surgical critical care units and maintain an educational partnership with Columbia University College of Physicians and Surgeons for its teaching program in the internal medicine, family practice, obstetrics/gynecology and surgery

7235 **Windsor Rehabilitation and Healthcare Center**
581 Poquonock Ave
Windsor, CT 06095-2202
860-688-7211
Fax: 860-688-6715
www.windsorrehab.com

Jeffrey Robbins, Medical Director

Accomodates 116 residents. We offer private and semi-private rooms with access to private telephones and cable television. Our goal is to be a comprehensive, leading care center viewed by our community as an excellent resource for patients, families, and professionals.

Delaware

7236 **Arbors at New Castle**
32 Buena Vista Dr
New Castle, DE 19720-4660
302-328-2580
Fax: 302-326-4132
www.extendicareus.com/newcastle

Annette Moore, Administrator

A subacute and rehabilitation center offering skilled medical services, infusion therapies, cardiac recovery services, renal disease services, cancer services and digestive disease services. Skilled rehabilitation services include physical therapy, occupational therapy and speech therapy. Also provides case management and discharge planning, general nursing and restorative care and respite care.

Florida

7237 **Avon Oaks Skilled Care Nursing Facility**
37800 French Creek Rd
Avon, OH 44011-1763
440-934-5204
800-589-5204
jreidy@avonoaks.net
www.avonoaks.net

Natalie McIntyre, Human Resources Director
Stephanie Auvil, RN, BC, Director of Nursing
Joan Reidy, Administrator
Richard J. Reidy, Technologies & Information Manager

Oaks at Avon provides a full range of skilled nursing services including infusion therapy, enteral therapy, wound care, tracheotomy care, and portable diagnostics.

7238 **Boca Raton Rehabilitation Center**
755 Meadows Rd
Boca Raton, FL 33486-2384
561-391-5200
Fax: 561-391-0685

Stanley Mucinic, Administrator
Tracey Dougherty, Administrator

Offers the following rehabilitation services: Occupational Therapy, Speech Therapy, Physical Therapy, Sub-Acute Rehabilitation

7239 **Cape Coral Hospital**
636 Del Prado Blvd
Cape Coral, FL 33990
239-424-2000
Fax: 239-574-1935
www.leememorial.org

Richard Akin, Chairman
Sanford Cohen, MD, Vice Chairman
Marilyn Stout, Treasurer
Diane Champion, Secretary

A 291-bed acute care facility, Cape Coral Hospital features all private rooms. The hospital currently is undergoing a complete renovation, expansion and modernization of the Weigner-Taeni Center for Emergency Services, which will make the emergency department the largest in Lee County.

7240 **Evergreen Woods Health and Rehabilitation Center**
7045 Evergreen Woods Trl
Spring Hill, FL 34608-1306
352-596-8371
Fax: 352-596-8032

Janet Hanciles, Administrator

Offers the following rehabilitation services: Sub-Acute rehabilitation, Occupational therapy, Speech pathology therapy, Physical therapy.

7241 **Healthcare and Rehabilitation Center of Sanford**
950 Mellonville Avenue
Sanford, FL 32771-2237
407-322-8566
Fax: 407-322-0121
www.healthcareandrehabofsanford.com

Dr. S. Joshi, Medical Director
Kate Hilgar, Administrator
Vicky Smith, Director Admissions

We provide post-acute services, rehabilitative services, skilled nursing, short and long term care through Physical, Occupational, and Speech Therapists; Registered and Licensed Practical Nurses; and Certified Nursing Assistants. This is complemented by Social Services, Activities, Nutritional Services, Housekeeping and Laundry Services. With over 224 years of combined experience, our staff of professionals is here to meet the needs of each and every patient and resident.

7242 **Highland Pines Rehabilitation Center**
1111 S Highland Ave
Clearwater, FL 33756-4432
727-446-0581
Fax: 727-442-9425

Paula Anthony, Administrator

Offers the following rehabilitation services: Sub-Acute rehabilitation, Occupational Therapy, Speech Therapy, Physical Therapy.

7243 **Jupiter Medical Center-Pavilion**
1210 S Old Dixie Hwy
Jupiter, FL 33458-7205 561-747-2234
Fax: 561-744-4467
JCouris@jupitermed.com
www.jupitermed.com
John D. Couris, President/Chief Executive Officer
Dale Hocking, Vice President, Finance/Chief Financial Officer
Mike Fehr, Vice President, Information Services/Chief Information Offic
Steven Seeley, Vice President, Chief Operating Officer/Chief Nursing Office
Offers the following rehabilitation services: Sub-Acute Rehabilitation, Occupational Therapy, Speech Therapy, Physical Therapy.

7244 **North Broward Medical Center**
201 E Sample Rd
Deerfield Beach, FL 33064-4441 954-941-8300
Fax: 954-941-4233
www.browardhealth.org
Pauline Grant, CEO
Douglas Ford, Chief of Staff
Offers the following rehabilitation services: Sub-Acute rehabilitation, Physical Therapy, Occupational Therapy, Speech Therapy, Respiratory Therapy.

7245 **Pompano Rehabilitation and Nursing Center**
Senior Health Care Management
51 W Sample Rd
Pompano Beach, FL 33064-3542 954-942-5530
Fax: 954-942-0941
Jeff Nusbusn, Administrator
Offers the following rehabilitation services: Sub-Acute Rehabilitation, Physical Therapy, Occupational Therapy, Speech Therapy

7246 **Rehabilitation Center of Palm Beach**
300 Royal Palm Way
Palm Beach, FL 33480-4385 561-655-7266
Fax: 561-655-3269
info@rcca.org
www.rcca.org
Ellen O'Bannon, Manager
Pamela Henderson, Executive Director
Our mission is to improve the physical function, communication & independence of people with disabilities.

7247 **Rehabilitation and Healthcare Center of Tampa**
4411 N Habana Ave
Tampa, FL 33614-7211 813-872-2771
Fax: 813-871-2831
Dr. Gustavo Barrazuetta, Medical Director
We provide post-acute services, rehabilitative services, skilled nursing, short and long term care through Physical, Occupational, and Speech Therapists; Registered and Licensed Practical Nurses; and Certified Nursing Assistants. This is complemented by Social Services, Activities, Nutritional Services, Housekeeping and Laundry Services. With over 60 years of combined experience, our staff of professionals is here to meet the needs of each and every patient and resident.

7248 **Shands Rehab Hospital**
4101 NW 89th Blvd
Gainesville, FL 32606-3813 352-265-8938
Fax: 352-265-5420
www.ufhealth.org/shands-rehab-hospital
Tim Goldfarb,M.S., Chief Executive Officer
David S. Guzick, M.D., Ph.D., Senior Vice President
Ed . Jimenez, M.B.A, Senior Vice President/Chief Operating Officer
James Roberts, J.D., Senior Vice President/General Counsel
UF Health Shands Rehab Hospital is a 40-bed acute rehab hospital for patients who have suffered strokes, traumatic brain and spinal cord injuries, amputations, burns or major joint replacements.

7249 **St. Anthony's Hospital**
1200 7th Ave N
St Petersburg, FL 33705-1388 727-825-1100
www.stanthonys.com
William Ulbricht, President
Ron Colaguori, VP Operations
James McClintic, M.D., Vice President, Medical Affairs
Sr. Mary McNally, OSF, Vice President, Mission
We offer outstanding diagnostic and treatment options of all types of cancer. Our Susan Sheppard McGillicuddy Breast Center is unmatched in the community in diagnostic services and helping patients navigate their treatment options should they find a cancer diagnosis.

7250 **Winkler Court**
3250 Winkler Avenue Ext
Fort Myers, FL 33916-9414 239-939-4993
Fax: 239-939-1743
www.winklercourt.com
Michael Collier, Medical Director
Michael Stens, Medical Director
We provide post-acute services, rehabilitative services, skilled nursing, short and long term care through Physical, Occupational, and Speech Therapists; Registered and Licensed Practical Nurses; and Certified Nursing Assistants. This is complemented by Social Services, Activities, Nutritional Services, Housekeeping and Laundry Services. With over 100 years of combined experience, our staff of professionals is here to meet the needs of each and every patient and resident.

7251 **Winter Park Memorial Hospital**
Florida Hospital
200 N Lakemont Ave
Winter Park, FL 32792-3273 407-646-7000
Fax: 407-646-7639
healthcare@winterparkhospital.com
www.winterparkhospital.com
Ken Bradley, CEO
Nestled among the oak-shaded, brick-paved streets of one of the most picturesque hometowns in the country, Winter Park Memorial Hospital has continuously served the residents of Winter Park and its surrounding communities for more than 50 years.

Georgia

7252 **Athena Rehab of Clayton**
2055 Rex Rd
Lake City, GA 30260-3944 404-361-5144
Fax: 404-363-6366
Reginald Washington, Administrator
Offers the following rehabilitation services: Sub-Acute rehabilitation, Occupational therapy, Speech therapy, Physical therapy, Restorative care.

7253 **Lafayette Nursing and Rehabilitation Center**
110 Brandywine Blvd
Fayetteville, GA 30214-1500 770-461-2928
Fax: 770-461-8507
www.lafayetterehab.com
Wendy Goza, Medical Director
Lafayette Nursing and Rehab Center accomodates 179 residents. We are Medicare certified and our center also features a 25-bed postacute rehab unit and a 24-bed dementia unit. We have RN's LPN's and CNA's 24 hours a day. We also have physician services availiable seven days a week.

7254 **Savannah Rehabilitation and Nursing Center**
815 E 63rd St
Savannah, GA 31405-4499 912-352-8615
Fax: 912-355-4642
Sandra Casper, Executive Director
At our facility, we provide quality care with modern rehabilitation and restorative nursing techniques. We aim to provide an atmosphere which encourages family involvement in the care-planning process, with the right mix of activities addressing the social, spiritual and intellectual needs of our residents.

7255 **Specialty Hospital**
PO Box 1566
Rome, GA 30162-1566 706-509-4100
Fax: 706-509-4159

7256 **Walton Rehabilitation Health System**
523 13th St.
Augusta, GA 30901-1037 706-823-8505
866-492-5866
Fax: 706-724-5752
Dennis Skelley, President/CEO
Has Centers of Excellence in Stroke Brain Injury, Complex Orthopedics, Spinal Cord Injury and Pain Management. 58-bed nonprofit facility.

7257 **Warner Robins Rehabilitation and Nursing Center**
1601 Elberta Rd
Warner Robins, GA 31093-1393 478-922-2241
Fax: 478-328-1984
www.warnerrobinsrehabilitation.com
Laura Fergason, Administrator
Offers the following rehabilitation services: Sub-Acute rehabilitation, Physical Therapy, Occupational Therapy, Speech Therapy.

Hawaii

7258 **Aloha Nursing and Rehab Center**
45-545 Kamehameha Hwy
Kaneohe, HI 96744-1943 808-247-2220
Fax: 808-235-3676
info@alohanursing.com
alohanursing.com
Charles Harris, Executive Director
Amy Lee, Administrator
Our unique nursing care facility is nestled in the picturesque town of Kaneohe, Oahu, amid the towering Koolau Mountains and the panoramic vistas of Kaneohe Bay. In this tranquil setting, our 141-bed facility offers both long and short term care to residents who meet intermediate or skilled level of care criteria.

Idaho

7259 **Boise Health And Rehabilitation Center**
1001 S Hilton St
Boise, ID 83705-1925 208-345-4464
Fax: 208-345-2998
Jason Ludwig, Medical Director
Aaron Moorhouse, Medical Director
Debbie Mills, Executive Director
Offers the following rehabilitation services: Sub-acute rehabilitation, occupational therapy, speech therapy, physical therapy.

7260 **Eastern Idaho Regional Medical Center**
3100 Channing Way
Idaho Falls, ID 83404-7533 208-529-6111
Fax: 208-529-7021
www.eirmc.com
Cindy Smith-Putnam, Executive Director of Business Development, Marketing & Comm
Lou Fatkin, Executive Director of Risk Management, Physician Relations,
Matt Campbell, Director of Human Resources
Jared Rickabaugh, Director of Quality Management
The largest medical facility in the region, Eastern Idaho Regional Medical Center (EIRMC) is a modern, JCAHO-accredidted, full-service hospital. EIRMC serves as the region's healthcare hub, offering specialty services including open-heart surgery, leading-edge cancer treatment, trauma, neurosurgery, intensive care for adults and infants, and a helicopeter service.

7261 **Kindred Transitional Care and Rehabilitation**
3315 8th St
Lewiston, ID 83501-4966 208-743-9543
Fax: 208-746-8662
www.lewistonrehab.com
Debbie Freeze, Administrator
Lewiston Rehabilitation and Care Center has years of experience providing diversified healthcare services. We have our own staff of physical, occupational and speech therapists. Our therapy gym and rehab kitchen are a lovely atmosphere in which to work toward your therapy goals. We are an Eden Alternative Certified facility.

7262 **Mountain Valley Care and Rehabilitation Center**
601 West Cameron Avenue
PO Box 689
Kellogg, ID 83837- 2004 208-784-1283
Fax: 208-784-0151
www.mountainvalleycare.com
Maryruth Butler, Executive Director
Mountain Valley Care and Rehabilitation Center accomodates 68 residents. We are conveniently located in the heart of Kellogg Idaho. We strive to offer quality care and superior customer service in a home-like environment. Upon admission, you or your loved one is looked after by an assigned staff member. We call this our 'Angel Care' program. Our rehabilitation program focuses on meething the individual needs of the resident so you or your loved one can see how they are going to progress.

7263 **River's Edge Rehabilitation and Healthcare**
Kindred Healthcare
714 N Butte Ave
Emmett, ID 83617-2799 208-365-4425
Fax: 208-365-6989
GDecker@ensigngroup.net
www.riversedgerehab.com
Janis Shields, Executive Director
Steve Balle, MPT, Director of Rehabilitation
Margaret Williams RN, BSN, Director of Nursing
Patty Alsup, Business Office Manager
Emmett Rehab & healthcare accomodates 95 residents. We are located in Emmett, Idaho, a rural community located an easy 30 minute drive from Boise. Emmett Rehab &'healthcare has served the area for more then 40 years by providing healthcare for residents of Gem County.

Illinois

7264 **Chevy Chase Nursing and Rehabilitation Center**
3400 S Indiana Ave
Chicago, IL 60616-3841 312-842-5000
Fax: 312-842-3790
Tony Prather, Administrator
Our approach to care is multidisciplinary; our medical staff members work together as a team in a proactive fashion, challenging residents each and every day, in order to motivate them to rehabilitate and achieve their ultimate potential.

7265 **Glenview Terrace Nursing Center**
1511 Greenwood Rd
Glenview, IL 60026-1513 847-729-9090
Fax: 847-729-9135
www.glenviewterrace.com
Ian Crook, Administrator
We're best known as the industry leader in post-hospital rehabilitation, including orthopedic rehabilitation and stroke recovery. Our highly effective rehabilitation services feature one-on-one physical, occupational, speech and respiratory therapies up to seven days a week.

7266 **Halsted Terrace Nursing Center**
10935 S Halsted St
Chicago, IL 60628-3189 773-928-2000
Fax: 773-928-9154
Ted O'Brien, Administrator
Offers the following rehabilitation services: Sub-acute rehabilitation, physical therapy, occupational therapy, speech therapy, cardiac rehabilitation.

7267 **Harmony Nursing and Rehabilitation Center**
3919 W Foster Ave
Chicago, IL 60625-6056 773-588-9500
Fax: 773-588-9533
www.harmonychicago.com
John Sianghio, Administrator

Offers a friendly healthcare experience. You'll find compassionate experts who provide short-term rehabilitation and therapy, wound care, Alzheimer's and memory loss care, long-term nursing care and more.

7268 **Imperial**
1366 W Fullerton Ave
Chicago, IL 60614-2199 773-248-9300
Fax: 773-935-0036
www.imperialpavilion.com

David Hartman, Administrator
Mary Bangayan, M.D., Pulmonary Care Programme
Sanjay Gill, M.D., Cardiac Management Program
We offer a comprehensive approach to post acute care. One that takes into consideration our guests' unique needs, and utilizes a progressive healthcare model to provide them with a personalized rehabilitation program designed to offer them the fullest possible recovery.

7269 **Jackson Square Nursing and Rehabilitation Center**
5130 W Jackson Blvd
Chicago, IL 60644-4332 773-921-8000
Fax: 773-287-9302
www.jacksonsquarecare.com

Rick Walworth, Administrator
At Jackson Square, there is one primary goal: to help guests regain maximum independence and functioning so that they can safely, comfortably, and happily get their life back. Our physicians, therapists, and nurses use their experience, compassion, and skill-combined with the latest and best technology-to provide comprehensive rehabilitation for a wide range of physical disabilities and medical conditions.

7270 **Renaissance at 87th Street**
2940 W 87th St
Chicago, IL 60652-3832 773-434-8787
Fax: 773-434-8717
www.renaissanceat87.com

Juli Foy, Administrator
At Renaissance at 87th, there is one primary goal: to help guests regain maximum independence and functioning so that they can safely, comfortably, and happily get their life back. Our physicians, therapists, and nurses use their experience, compassion, and skill-combined with the latest and best technology-to provide comprehensive rehabilitation for a wide range of physical disabilities and medical conditions.

7271 **Renaissance at Hillside**
4600 N. Frontage Rd.
Hillside, IL 60162-1761 708-544-9933
Fax: 708-544-9966
www.ariapostacute.com

John Stare, Administrator
Utilizing a progressive healthcare model that takes into account each patient's individual needs, Aria Post Acute Care designs a personalized rehabilitation program offering guests the best chance at the fullest possible recovery.

7272 **Renaissance at Midway**
4437 S Cicero Ave
Chicago, IL 60632-4333 773-884-0484
Fax: 773-884-0485
www.renaissanceatmidway.com

Jeff Baker, Executive Director
At Renaissance at Midway, there is one primary goal: to help guests regain maximum independence and functioning so that they can safely, comfortably, and happily get their life back. Our physicians, therapists, and nurses use their experience, compassion, and skill-combined with the latest and best technology-to provide comprehensive rehabilitation for a wide range of physical disabilities and medical conditions.

7273 **Renaissance at South Shore**
2425 E 71st St
Chicago, IL 60649-2612 773-721-5000
Fax: 773-721-6850
www.rensouthshore.com

Dave Schechter, Administrator
The Renaissance at South Shore is a 248 bed skilled nursing facility with multiple services that include short-term rehabilitation, specialized dementia care and long-term care and hospice care.

Our highly trained nursing professionals provide loving care in a home-like atmosphere.

7274 **Schwab Rehabilitation Hospital**
Mt. Sinai
1401 S California Ave
Chicago, IL 60608-1858 773-522-2010
www.schwabrehab.org

Suzan Rayner, Medical Director
Lisa Thornton, Medical Staff President
Alan Channing, President/ Chief Executive Officer
Anita Halvorsen, Vice President of Schwab Rehabilitation Hospital
Schwab Rehabilitation Hospital is a freestanding, not-for-profit, 102-bed rehabilitation hospital located on Chicago's west side. It offers a therapeutic environment of comprehensive inpatient and outpatient rehabilitation, both for adults and children.

Indiana

7275 **Angel River Health and Rehabilitation**
5233 Rosebud Ln
Newburgh, IN 47630-9283 812-473-4761
Fax: 812-473-5190

Kay Congleton, Executive Director
Our wide array of services enables our patients and residents to receive the medical care they need, the restorative therapy they require, and the support they and their families deserve. We serve many types of patient and resident needs - from short-term rehabilitation to traditional long-term care. Our resident council meets regularly to ensure that our residents' needs are being met to their satisfaction.

7276 **Chalet Village Health and Rehabilitation Center**
Magnolia Health Systems
1065 Parkway St
Berne, IN 46711-2366 260-589-2127
Fax: 260-589-3521
www.chalet-village.net

Vicki Shepherd, Administrator
We provide dedicated, community-centered healthcare which was founded in Indiana, operates in Indiana, for people who live in Indiana.

7277 **Columbus Health and Rehabilitation Center**
2100 Midway St
Columbus, IN 47201-3722 812-372-8447
Fax: 812-375-5117
www.columbushrc.com

Sherry Harrison, Executive Director
William Lustig, Medical Director
Accomodates 235 residents. We offer a continuum of healthcare services. Our center also provides a Special Care Alzheimer's Unit. We are licensed by the Stat of Indiana and are Medicare and Medicaid approved provider. We are proud to offer a friendly home-like atmosphere while providing comprehensive healthcare services. These services include short-term medical and rehabilitation treatment, which is designed to address the individual needs of our residents and patients.

7278 **Harrison Health and Rehabilitation Centre**
150 Beechmont Drive
Corydon, IN 47112-1717 812-738-0550
Fax: 812-738-6273
www.harrisonrehab.com

Sheila Bieker, Executive Director
Bruce Burton, Medical Director
We serve many types of patient and resident needs - from short-term rehabilitation to traditional long-term care. Working with your physician, our staff - including medical specialists, nurses, nutritionists, therapists, dietitians and social workers - establishes a comprehensive treatment plan intended to restore you or your loved one to the fullest practicable potential.

7279 **Indian Creek Health and Rehabilitation Center**
240 Beechmont Dr
Corydon, IN 47112-1718 812-738-8127
877-380-7211
Fax: 812-738-2917
www.indiancreekhrc.com

Bonnie Fallin, Executive Director
Bruce Burton, Medical Director
140 bed facility offering the following rehabilitation services: Sub-Acute rehabilitation, Physical therapy, Occupational Therapy, Speech Therapy, pain management, Wound rehabilitation. Short and long term skilled nursing care certified for Medicare, Medicaid, Private Pay and Private Insurance. Hospice and respite care rated #1 in clinical care in southern Indiana district for 2002.

7280 **Meadowvale Health and Rehabilitation Center**
Kindred Health Care
1529 Lancaster St
Bluffton, IN 46714-1507 260-824-4320
800-743-3333
Fax: 260-824-4689

Todd Beaulieu, Executive Director
Yadagiri Jonna, Medical Director
Working with your physician, our staff - including medical specialists, nurses, nutritionists, therapists, dietitians and social workers - establishes a comprehensive treatment plan intended to restore you or your loved one to the fullest practicable potential.

7281 **Muncie Health Care and Rehabilitation**
680 South Fourth Street
Louisville, KY 40202 502-596-7300
800-545-0749
web_administrator@kindred.com
www.kindredhealthcare.com

Dee Harrold, Executive Director
Dr. Jeffery Hiltz, Medical Director
Offers the following rehabilitation services: Sub-Acute rehabilitation, physical therapy, occupational therapy, speech therapy.

7282 **Rehabilitation Hospital of Indiana**
4141 Shore Dr
Indianapolis, IN 46254-2607 317-329-2000
Fax: 317-329-2104
www.rhin.com

Ian Worden, MHA, MBA, CPA, RHI Board Chair
James G. Terwilliger, MPH, Vice Chair/Secretary
Kyle Netter, MBA, PT, Executive Director of Corporate and Affiliate Relations
Larissa Swan, MS, OTR, Executive Director of Therapies
We approach every patient understanding that every diagnosis, every illness, and every injury are different. It's the collective effort of trained and compassionate team members who value the quality of life of every patient and their caregivers. It's the right kind of treatment- inpatient, outpatient, and follow-up services- provided under the same roof. It's one step closer to home. It's a continuum of care

7283 **Sellersburg Health and Rehabilitation Centre**
7823 Old State Road 60
Sellersburg, IN 47172-1858 812-246-4272
Fax: 812-246-8160
www.sellersburgrehab.com

Dave Powell, Administrator
Chris Hansen, Executive Director
Sellersburg is a modern healthcare center conveniently located on the edge of the community. Our center accomodates 110 residents and includes a rehabilitative program with a goal of returning residents home as quickly as possible. Sellersburg is a 2006 recipient of the American Health Care Association Quality Award.

7284 **Westpark Rehabilitation Center**
1316 N Tibbs Ave
Indianapolis, IN 46222-3024 317-634-8330
Fax: 317-263-9442
www.westparkhealthcare.com

Dave Mc Carroll, Owner
Offers the following rehabilitation services: Sub-acute rehabilitation, occupational therapy, physical therapy, speech therapy, respiratory therapy.

7285 **Westview Nursing and Rehabilitation Center**
1510 Clinic Dr
Bedford, IN 47421-3530 812-279-4494
Fax: 812-275-8313
www.ascseniorcare.com/westview-nursing—rehab

Sholin Montgomery, Executive Director
Mike Spencer, Executive Director
Offers the following rehabilitation services: Sub-acute rehabilitation, physical therapy, occupational therapy, speech therapy.

7286 **Windsor Estates Health and Rehab Center**
429 W Lincoln Rd
Kokomo, IN 46902-3508 765-453-5600
Fax: 765-455-0110
www.kindredkokomo.com

Brenda Alfrey, Administrator
Monica Martin, Executive Director
Our wide array of services enables our patients and residents to receive the medical care they need, the restorative therapy they require, and the support they and their families deserve. We serve many types of patient and resident needs - from short-term rehabilitation to traditional long-term care.

Iowa

7287 **Madison County Rehab Services**
Madison County Hospital
300 W Hutchings St
Winterset, IA 50273-2109 515-462-2373
Fax: 515-462-4492

Marcia Harris, CEO
Panndee Stebbins, Director
Offers the following rehabilitation services: Sub-acute rehabilitation, occupational therapy, physical therapy, speech therapy, home health rehab, wellness programs.

7288 **Mercy Subacute Care**
603 E 12th St
Des Moines, IA 50309-5515 515-247-4400
Fax: 515-643-0945

Bonnie Mc Coy, Manager
Pam Nelson, Intake Coordinator
Offers the following rehabilitation services: Sub-acute rehabilitation, physical therapy, speech therapy, occupational therapy.

Kentucky

7289 **Danville Centre for Health and Rehabilitation**
642 N 3rd St
Danville, KY 40422-1125 859-236-3972
Fax: 859-236-0703
www.danvillecentre.com

Debbie Gibson, Executive Director
We offer short-term rehabilitative care as well as long-term care. Our emphasis is on service excellence - providing quality care in a home-like environment to allow for independence and to enable our patients and residents to receive the medical care they need, the restorative therapy they require, and the support they and their families deserve.

7290 **Fountain Circle Health & Rehabilitation**
Kindred Healthcare
200 Glenway Rd
Winchester, KY 40391 859-744-1800
Fax: 859-744-0285

William Whited, Executive Director
Kathryn Jones, Medical Director
Offers the following rehabilitation services: Sub-acute rehabilitation, speech therapy, physical therapy, occupational therapy.

7291 **Lexington Center for Health and Rehabilitation**
353 Waller Ave
Lexington, KY 40504-2974 859-252-3558
Fax: 859-233-0192

Karole Ward, Administrator

Offers the following rehabilitation services: Sub-acute rehabilitation, speech therapy, occupational therapy, physical therapy.

7292 **Paducah Centre For Health and Rehabilitation**
Wellsouth Health Systems
501 N 3rd St
Paducah, KY 42001-0749 270-444-9661
Fax: 270-443-9407
Jean Glisson, RN, Director of Nursing
Elizabeth Kay Chilton, Admissions Director
Tracy Summers, Rehab/Specialty Program Director
Cathy Ortega, Administrator
Paducah Center is an 86-bed skilled and long-term care facility with a 28-bed Alzheimer's secure unit. This unit has a private courtyard and structured activities throughout the day, and is the only true Alzheimer's secure unit in the area.

7293 **Pathways Brain Injury Program**
4200 Browns Ln
Louisville, KY 40220-1523 502-459-8900
Fax: 502-459-5026
www.hcr-manorcare.com
Pam Pearson, Manager
Offers the following rehabilitation services: Sub-acute rehabilitation, speech therapy, occupational therapy, physical therapy, recreational therapy.

Louisiana

7294 **Guest House of Slidell Sub-Acute and Rehab Center**
1051 Robert Blvd
Slidell, LA 70458-2011 985-643-5630
800-303-9872
Fax: 985-649-6065
Brandy Wheat, Administrator
116 bed healthcare center offering the following subacute services within the skilled nursing setting: physical, occupational, and speech therapies, infusion therapy, respiratory care, wound care, neurological rehabilitation, cardiac reconditioning, pain management, post surgical recovery, orthopedic rehabilitation.

7295 **Irving Place Rehabilitation and Nursing Center**
1736 Irving Pl
Shreveport, LA 71101-4606 318-631-9121
Fax: 318-222-2095
Webster Johnson, Administrator
Offers the following rehabilitation services: sub-acute rehabilitation, speech therapy, occupational therapy, physical therapy

Maine

7296 **Augusta Rehabilitation Center**
188 Eastern Ave
Augusta, ME 04330-5928 207-622-3121
800-457-1220
Fax: 207-623-7666
www.augustarehabcenter.com
Malcolm Dean, Executive Director
Cathleen O'Connor
From intensive short term rehabilitation therapy to longer-term restorative care, our Nursing and Rehabilitation Centers provide a full range of nursing care and social services to treat and support each of our patients and residents. Our clinical capabilities allow us to accept patients with greater medical complexity than a traditional nursing home. This is increasingly important as many patients require transitional care before they are ready to return home.

7297 **Brentwood Rehabilitation and Nursing Center**
370 Portland St
Yarmouth, ME 04096-8101 207-846-9021
800-457-1220
Fax: 207-846-1497
Malcolm Dean, Executive Director
Daniel M. Pierce, Medical Director
Brentwood accomodates 82 residents. We are located at 370 Portland Street in Yarmouth, Maine. We strive to meet the healthcare needs of the greater Yarmouth community, including Portland and Brunswick, which are located within 10 miles of the center. In addition to Brentwood's rehabilitation and skilled nursing services, we also offer Alzheimer's specialty care in a comfortable setting.

7298 **Den-Mar Rehabilitation and Nursing Center**
44 South St
Rockport, MA 01966-1800 978-546-6311
800-439-2370
Fax: 978-546-9185
Christine Marek, Executive Director
Den-Mar nursing and Rehab center accomodates 80 residents. We provide skilled nursing and rehabilitation services as well as long term care. We are certified for Medicare and Medicaid as well as many insurance carriers. We offer semi-private and private rooms, with many common areas for socializing.

7299 **Eastside Rehabilitation and Living Center**
516 Mount Hope Ave
Bangor, ME 04401-4215 207-947-6131
800-457-1220
Fax: 207-942-0884
www.eastsiderehab.com
Ryan Kelley, Executive Director
From intensive short term rehabilitation therapy to longer-term restorative care, our Nursing and Rehabilitation Centers provide a full range of nursing care and social services to treat and support each of our patients and residents. Our clinical capabilities allow us to accept patients with greater medical complexity than a traditional nursing home. This is increasingly important as many patients require transitional care before they are ready to return home.

7300 **Kennebunk Nursing & Rehabilitation Center**
158 Ross Rd
Kennebunk, ME 04043-6532 207-985-7141
800-457-1220
Fax: 207-985-0961
Stephen Alaimo, Executive Director
We treat a variety of conditions and provide an array of services including, but not limited to:Respiratory conditions such as pneumonia and post-acute COPD episodes Cardiac conditions and post surgical care (grafts, valves, stints) Wound Stroke Orthopedic Neurological illnesses Diabetes

7301 **Norway Rehabilitation and Living Center**
29 Marion Ave
Norway, ME 04268-5601 207-743-7075
800-457-1220
Fax: 207-743-9269
Carolyn Farley, Administrator
Norway Rehabilitation and Living Center has been a fixture in the Norway community since 1976. We are a 70-bed facility offering short-term rehabilitation, skilled nursing services, long term care and residential care services. Utilizing an interdisciplinary team led by a physician and consisting of qualified health care specialists, we develop individualized plans of care for each patient that are designed to restore maximum health and optimize functional abilities and independence

7302 **Shore Village Rehabilitation & Nursing Center**
201 Camden St
\, ME 04841-2534 207-596-6423
800-457-1220
Fax: 207-596-7235
Phyllis Nickerson, Administrator
Shore Village accomodates 60 residents and is located in the mid-coast region of the state of Maine. We have a cozy size and a primary goal for the staff is to ensure a home-like atmosphere for all the residents. Shore Village provides skilled nursing and rehabilitation, respite care, and long term care. The facility is dually certified for Medicare and Medicaid and accepts many commercial insurance plans.

Maryland

7303 **Greater Baltimore Medical Center**
6701 N Charles St
Baltimore, MD 21204-6881 443-849-2000
Fax: 443-849-3024
TTY: 800-735-2258
www.gbmc.org

John B. Chessare, M.D., President/Chief Executive Officer
Eric L. Melchior, Executive Vice President/Chief Financial Officer
Keith Poisson, Executive Vice President/Chief Operating Officer
John W. Ellis, Senior Vice President/Corporate Strategy & Business Developm

The 281-bed medical center (acute and sub-acute care) is located on a beautiful suburban campus and handles more than 26,700 in-patient cases and approximately 60,000 emergency room visits annually.

Massachusetts

7304 **Bolton Manor Nursing Home**
400 Bolton St
Marlborough, MA 01752-3912 508-481-6123
800-439-2370
Fax: 508-481-6130

Michele Ricard, Medical Director
Thomas Sullivan, Executive Director

Bolton Manor accomodates 157 residents. We are located in Marlboro, Massachusetts. We provide medical management and long-term care through comprehensive skilled and post-acute nursing services. We also provide physical, occupational, and speech therapy services from an onsite dedicated staff of therapists. The facility is Joint Commission (formerly JCAHO) accredited and has an excellent survey history with the State Department of Public Health.

7305 **Brigham Manor Nursing and Rehabilitation Center**
77 High St
Newburyport, MA 01950-3071 978-462-4221
800-439-2370
Fax: 978-463-3297

Stephen Cynewski, Executive Director

Brigham Manor accomodates 64 residents. We are a Medicare-certified facility offering private, semi-private and multi-bed suites. Our bright, formal dining room, with French doors that open to a shaded courtyard, provides a warm atmosphere for entertaining family and friends. Each resident's personal tastes and medical needs are considered in the planning of our weekly menus.

7306 **Country Gardens Skilled Nursing and Rehabilitation Center**
2045 Grand Army Hwy
Swansea, MA 02777-3932 508-379-9700
800-439-2370
Fax: 508-379-0723

Sandy Sarza, Executive Director

Country Gardens Skilled Nursing and Rehabilitation Center accomodates 86 residents. We are located in a beautiful rural setting conveniently located about 15 minutes east of Providence and 10 minutes west of Fall River. We have provided healthcare service to the greater Swansea area for over 34 years.

7307 **Country Manor Rehabilitation and Nursing Center**
180 Low St
Newburyport, MA 01950-3519 978-465-5361
800-439-2370
Fax: 978-463-9366
www.countryrehab.com

Stephen Doyle, Executive Director

Country Rehabilitation and Nursing Center accomodates 123 residents. We are located in the quaint seaport town of Newburyport, Massachusetts. We provide medical management and long-term care through comprehensive skilled and intermediate nursing services. We also provide physical, occupational, and speech therapy services from an onsite dedicated staff of therapists. The center offers an Alzheimer's special care unit with staff trained in dimentia care and dementia specific programs.

7308 **Franklin Skilled Nursing and Rehabilitation Center**
130 Chestnut St
Franklin, MA 02038-3903 508-528-4600
800-439-2370
Fax: 508-528-7976

Paula Topijan, Executive Director

We treat a variety of conditions and provide an array of services including, but not limited to :Respiratory conditions such as pneumonia and post-acute COPD episodes,Cardiac conditions and post surgical care (grafts, valves, stints),Wound,Stroke,Orthopedic,Neurological illnesses,Diabetes

7309 **Great Barrington Rehabilitation and Nursing Center**
148 Maple Ave
Great Barrington, MA 01230-1906 413-528-3320
800-439-2370
Fax: 413-528-2302
www.greatbarringtonrnc.com

William Kittler, Executive Director
Andrew Potler, Medical Director

Great Barrington Rehabilitation and Nursing Center accomodates 106 residents. As part of a national network of long-term healthcare centers, we have the expertise and resources to provide care appropriate to the individual needs of each and every one of our residents. We provide personal care with minimal daily living assistance to the most skilled treatment for medically complex patients.

7310 **Ledgewood Rehabilitation and Skilled Nursing Center**
87 Herrick St
Beverly, MA 01915-2773 978-921-1392
800-439-2370
Fax: 978-927-8627
www.ledgewoodrehab.com

Frank Silvia, Executive Director

Ledgewood Rehabilitation and Skilled Nursing Center is a unique provider of healthcare services. We are part of a continuum of services that includes acute care services at Beverly Hospital, subacute care at Ledgewood, and care after discharge through Northeast Homecare. We believe this partnership offers the highest quality post-acute services north of Boston.

7311 **Leo P La Chance Center for Rehabilitation and Nursing**
59 Eastwood Cir
Gardner, MA 01440-3901 978-632-8776
Fax: 978-632-5048

Mark Alinger, Administrator
Leo P. LaChance, Founder

A privately owned facility, combines the best of medical technology with the ultimate in healing, compassionate rehabilitation and nursing care. Our goal is to help each client reach that ultimate goal of living life to the fullest.

7312 **Oakwood Rehabilitation and Nursing Center**
11 Pontiac Ave
Webster, MA 01570-1629 508-943-3889
800-439-2370
Fax: 508-949-6125
www.oakwoodrehab.com

Thomas Sullivan, Executive Director

Oakwood Rehabilitation and Nursing Center accomodates 81 residents. We offer 24-hour skilled nursing, inpatient rehabilitation, respite care, and hospice services. Our center has been successfully serving the greater Webster, Massachusetts, community for 35 years. We have a dedicated and caring staff and our common goal is to promote recovery and enhance quality of live whether your needs are short or long term.

7313 **Walden Rehabilitation and Nursing Center**
785 Main St
Concord, MA 01742-3310 978-369-6889
800-439-2370
Fax: 978-369-8392

Ladan Azarm, Executive Director

Walden Rehabilitation and Nursing Center accomodates 123 residents. We are located in the quaint town of Concord, Massachusetts, across the street from Emerson Hospital and a short drive from the town center. Walden provides medical management and long-term care through comprehensive skilled and intermediate nursing services. We also provide physical, occupational, and speech therapy services from an onsite dedicated staff of therapists.

Michigan

7314 **Boulder Park Terrace**
14676 W Upright St
Charlevoix, MI 49720-1201
231-547-1005
Fax: 231-547-1039

Reezie DeVet, President/CEO
Mary-Anne Ponti, COO
A partnership formed with Charlevoix Area Hospital, Boulder Park Terrace is a long-term care facility and Sub-acute Rehabilitation Center located in Chalrevoix near the shores of Lake Michigan. The Sub-acute Rehabilitation Center was created as a transition between an acute care hospital and home. Patients enter into the program to increase their strength, endurance and over-all functioning before returning home.

Minnesota

7315 **Park Health And Rehabilitation Center**
4415 W 36 1/2 St
St Louis Park, MN 55416-4890
952-927-9717
Fax: 952-927-7687
www.extendicare.com

Jennifer Kuhn, Administrator
Park Health & Rehabilitation Center is a leading provider of long-term skilled nursing care and short-term rehabilitation solutions. Our 93 bed facility offers a full continuum of services and care focused around each individual in today's ever-changing healthcare environment.

Missouri

7316 **Barnes-Jewish Hospital Washington University Medical Center**
1 Barnes Jewish Hospital Plz
Saint Louis, MO 63110-1003
314-747-3000
866-867-3627
Fax: 314-362-8877
www.barnesjewish.org

Richard Liekweg, President
John Beatty, Vice President of Human Resources
John Lynch, MD, Chief Medical Officer
David Jaques, MD, Vice President for Surgical Services
Barnes-Jewish Hospital at Washington University Medical Center is the largest hospital in Missouri and the largest private employer in the St. Louis region. An affiliated teaching hospital of Washington University School of Medicine, Barnes-Jewish Hospital has a 1,700 member medical staff with many who are recognized in the 'Best Doctors in America.

Montana

7317 **Parkview Acres Care and Rehabilitation Center**
200 N Oregon St
Dillon, MT 59725-3624
406-683-5105
866-253-4090
Fax: 406-683-6388

Claire Miller, Executive Director
We are Medicare and Medicaid certified skilled nursing facility which accomodates 108 residents serving scenic Dillon and surrounding Montana communities.

Nebraska

7318 **Homestead Healthcare and Rehabilitation Center**
4735 S 54th St
Lincoln, NE 68516-1335
402-488-0977
800-833-0920
Fax: 402-488-4507
www.homesteadrehab.com

Matt Romshek, Executive Director
Gay Bate, RN, Director of Nursing
James Murray, Administrator
James Murray,LPN, Clinical Liaison/Admissions
Homestead Healthcare and Rehabilitation Center is one of the area's oldest providers of skilled nursing and rehabilitation services. We are a 163-bed skilled nursing and rehabilitation center nestled in a lovely, quiet established neighborhood in South Lincoln.

7319 **Madonna Rehabilitation Hospital**
5401 South St
Lincoln, NE 68506-2150
402-413-3000
800-676-5448
Fax: 402-486-5448
info@madonna.org
www.madonna.org

Marsha Lommel, CEO
Tom Stalder, VP Medical Affairs
Madonna provides intensive rehabilitation and expertise for a wide variety of conditions, such as: orthopedic injuries, work injuries, arthritis, amputation, neuromuscular diseases, cardiac conditions, pulmonary disease and conditions including those dependent upon a ventilator, cancer, lymphedema, osteoporosis, wounds, renal disorders, burns, fibromyalgia, multiple scelerosis, parkinson's disease and degenerative diseases.

7320 **Mary Lanning Memorial Hospital**
715 N Saint Joseph Ave
Hastings, NE 68901-4497
402-463-4521
866-460-5884
tanderson@mlmh.org
www.mlmh.org

Beth Schlichtman, Compensation/Benefit Services - Director
Lisa Brandt, Public Relations & Marketing Services - Director
Carrie Edwards, Home Care Services - Director
Chris Page, Ancillary Services - Director
Mary Lanning Healthcare is in its 95th year of providing quality healthcare for residents of the central Nebraska area. We continue to grow and expand, working to provide patient-centered care in a positive environment, while implementing some of the newest technologies available.

Nevada

7321 **Las Vegas Healthcare and Rehabilitation Center**
2832 S Maryland Pkwy
Las Vegas, NV 89109-1502
702-735-5848
800-326-6888
Fax: 702-735-6218
www.lasvegaskindred.com

Randall Fuller, Executive Director
Las Vegas Healthcare accomodates 79 residents. We have been serving the community for approximately 40 years. Located in close proximity to local hospitals and surrounded by medical complexes, our center offers both short-term rehabilitation and long-term care.

New Hampshire

7322 **Dover Rehabilitation and Living Center**
307 Plaza Dr
Dover, NH 03820-2455
603-742-2676
800-735-2964
Fax: 603-749-5375
www.doverrehab.com

Daniel Estee, Executive Director

Dover Rehab is a provider of postacute services in the greater New Hampshire Seacost area. We accomodate 112 residents and are licensed by the state of New Hampshire. We employ nearly 150 licensed nurses, therapists and other healthcare professionals, who strive to provide quality care. The goal of our patient service model is to bridge the gap between hospitalization and home so that recovery and physical functioning are maximized and hospital readmission is minimized.

7323 **Northeast Rehabilitation Clinic**
70 Butler St
Salem, NH 03079-3925
603-893-2900
800-825-7292
Fax: 603-893-1638
TTY: 800-439-2370
www.northeastrehab.com

John Prochilo, CEO/Administrator

Subacute rehabilitation at NRH was designed for people who have experienced an acutely disabling orthopedic, medical, or neurologic condition but who either do not require or are unable to participate in a full acute inpatient program. Impairment groups pertinent to this level of care include brain injury, spinal cord injury (traumatic/non-traumatic), stroke, orthopedic injury, amputation, and neurologic disorder.

New Jersey

7324 **Atlantic Coast Rehabilitation & Healthcare Center**
485 River Ave
Lakewood, NJ 08701-4720
732-364-7100
Fax: 732-364-2442
abby@atlanticcoastrehab.com
www.atlanticcoastrehab.com

Simon Shain, Administrator
Sharon Sckbower, Director of Nursing

Atlantic Coast is family owned and operated. It's a warm, friendly place where caregivers and patients know each other by first name. But it's also an innovative and energetic place, where the most advanced therapies and cutting edge techniques are offered. It's a comprehensive health care center that provides three distinct areas of care:Rehabilitative Therapy & Sub Acute Care, Long Term Care ,Alzheimer's/Memory Impaired Care.

7325 **Crestwood Nursing & Rehabilitation Center**
101 Whippany Rd
Whippany, NJ 7981-1407
973-887-0311
Fax: 973-887-8355

Carol Shepard, Administrator

Sub-acute rehabilitation facility.

7326 **Lakeview Subacute Care Center**
130 Terhune Dr
Wayne, NJ 7470-7104
973-839-4500
87 -UBA-UTE
Fax: 973-839-2729
www.lakeviewsubacute.com

Richard Grosso, Jr, Director
Sue Ahlers, Director of Admission
Kerry Iamurri, Director of Rehab
Nicole Iacolina, Director Social Services

Our comprehensive medical, nursing and rehabilitation services cater to a diverse patient population. In addition to long-term care, we offer exceptional inpatient subacute programs. We're proud to report that our average length of stay for subacute patients is a brief 14 days.

7327 **Merwick Rehabilitation and Sub-Acute Care**
79 Bayard Ln
Princeton, NJ 8540-3045
609-497-3000
Fax: 609-497-3024

Ryan Wismer, Administrator

76-bed skilled nursing and residential center as well as a separate 17-bed comprehensive rehabilitation center. Offers rehabilitation, physiatry, occupational therapy, respite care, speech/hearing therapy, sub-acute care.

7328 **Seacrest Village Nursing Center**
1001 Center St
Little Egg Harbor Twp, NJ 8087-1364
609-296-9292
Fax: 609-296-0508
info@seacrestvillagenj.com
seacrestvillagenj.com

Brian T Holloway, Administrator

Seacrest Village Nursing and Rehabilitation Center has specialized in quality rehabilitation, transitional and restorative care for more then a decade and is a perfect alternative for bridging the gap between hospital and home.

7329 **St. Lawrence Rehabilitation Center**
2381 Lawrenceville Rd
Lawrenceville, NJ 08648-2098
609-896-9500
Fax: 609-895-0242
epiechota@slrc.org
www.slrc.org

Kevin McGuigan, MD, Medical Director
Robyn F. Agri, MD, Doctor
Dr. Madhu Jain, Doctor
Charles Terry MD, Doctor

St. Lawrence Rehabilitation Center, a non-profit facility sponsored by the Roman Catholic Diocese of Trenton, is committed to maximizing the quality of human life by providing comprehensive physical rehabilitation and related programs to meet the healthcare needs of our communities.

7330 **Summit Ridge Center Genesis Eldercare**
20 Summit St
West Orange, NJ 07052-1501
973-736-2000
800-699-1520
Fax: 973-736-2764
info@genesishcc.com
www.genesishcc.com

Michele Cartagena, Director of Admissions
Elizabeth (L Orlando, Rehabilitation Program Director
Tsega Asefaha, LNHA, BS, MHA, Administrator
Elizabeth Martin, Customer Relations Manager

Summit Ridge Center provides skilled nursing, medical and rehabilitative care for patients requiring post-hospital, short stay rehabilitation and for longer term residents. Our Clinical Care Teams are focused on implementing your personalized care program to facilitate your recovery and improve your well-being.

New York

7331 **Beth Abraham Health Services**
612 Allerton Ave
Bronx, NY 10467-7495
718-519-4037
888-238-4223
Fax: 718-547-1366
info@bethabe.org
www.bethabrahamhealthservices.org

Maria Provenzano, Program Director
Yolanda Lester, Director of Admissions
Rosalie Bernard, Director of Nursing Services
Vincent Bonadies, Director of Therapeutic Recreation

Offers the following rehabilitation services: Sub-Acute rehabilitation, brain injury rehabilitation, pain management, post-operative recovery. Home visits and a network of community-based programs help patients and their families with a successful transition home.

7332 **Central Island Healthcare**
825 Old Country Rd
Plainview, NY 11803-4913
516-433-0600
Fax: 516-868-7251

Michael Ostreicher, Administrator

Serving the community for over 33 years, Central Island Healthcare is Long Island's largest and most active sub-acute care provider. We offer comprehensive programs focused on restoring our patients to their maximum potential and returning home. Central Island's 202-bed facility provides top notch professionals and the latest in rehabilitation and therapeutic equipment in a beautiful and comfortable setting.

7333 **Clove Lakes Health Care and Rehabilitation Center**
25 Fanning St
Staten Island, NY 10314-5307
718-289-7900
Fax: 718-761-8701
info@clovelakes.com
www.clovelakes.com

Helene Demisay, CEO

Clove Lakes seeks to rehabilitate those who have sustained injury or illness to the highest level of independence possible and support those with disabling conditions to live meaningful and productive lives.

7334 **Dr. William O Benenson Rehabilitation Pavilion**
36-17 Parsons Blvd
Flushing, NY 11354-5931
718-961-4300
Fax: 718-939-5032

Esther Benenson, Executive Director
Liza Marie Dowd, Director of Nursing
Erika Rossi, Director of Social Services
Diane Marron, Director of Admissions

The Dr. William O Benson Reahbilitation Pavilion is a subacute short-term rehabilitation center committed to the excellence of elevated health care for our patients. Through the use of the most comprehensive and specialized services available, our staff of dedicated professionals are devoted to putting patients back to the road to full recovery 24 hours a day.

7335 **Flushing Manor Nursing and Rehab**
35-15 Parsons Blvd
Flushing, NY 11354-4297
718-961-3500
Fax: 718-461-1784

Esther Benenson, Executive Director
Dr. Ion Oltean, Medical Director
Myung Chung, Director of Nursing
Bridgett Brown, Director of Admissions

At the Flusing Manor Nursing and Rehabilitation, we stress the importance of family involvement because it is the true source of strength and stability in ones life...a tie that brings us all together as a team, enhancing the quality of life of the patients in our care.

7336 **Glengariff Health Care Center**
141 Dosoris Ln
Glen Cove, NY 11542
516-676-1100
Fax: 516-759-0216
www.glenhaven.org

Jean Campo, Director Admissions
Michael Miness, President

Licensed skilled nursing and subacute medical and rehabilitation facility.

7337 **Haym Salomon Home for The Aged**
2340 Cropsey Ave
Brooklyn, NY 11214-5706
718-266-4063
Fax: 718-372-4781

Chain Lipschitz, Administrator

Religious nonmedical health care institution.

7338 **Kings Harbor Multicare Center**
2000 E Gun Hill Rd
Bronx, NY 10469-6016
718-320-0400
Fax: 718-671-5022
info@kingsharbor.com
www.kingsharbor.com

Morris Tenenbaum, Owner
Octavio Marin, Vice President

Kings Harbor Multicare Center provides long-term and short-term skilled nursing care for more then 700 residents. Kings Harbor is located in the Pelham Gardens neighborhood of Northeast Bronx, easily accessible to major highways and near public transportation. A 3 building campus facility with surrounding gardens ensures that residents with similar capabilities are grouped together.

7339 **Northwoods of Cortland**
28 Kellogg Rd
Cortland, NY 13045-3155
607-753-9631
Fax: 607-756-2968

Lawrence Mennig, Administrator

Subacute rehabilitation facility.

7340 **Port Jefferson Health Care Facility**
141 Dosoris Lane
Glen Cove, NY 11542
631-676-1100
Fax: 631-759-0216
www.glengariffcare.com

Ellen Harte, Administrator

Subacute medical and rehabilitative care and long term residential skilled nursing care.

7341 **Rehab Institute at Florence Nightingale Health Center**
1760 3rd Ave
New York, NY 10029-6810
212-410-8760
800-786-8968
Fax: 212-410-8792

7342 **Schnurmacher Center for Rehabilitation and Nursing**
Beth Abraham of Family Health Services
12 Tibbits Ave
White Plains, NY 10606-2438
914-287-7200
888-238-4223
Fax: 914-428-1824
info@schnurmacher.org
www.schnurmacher.org

Linda Murray, Executive Director
Thomas Camisa, Medical Director
Iryn Obaldo Fontanosa, Director of Rehabilitation
Filomena Cristo, Director of Therapeutic Recreation

The environment at Schnurmacher is tailored to the needs of patients who require medical and nursing services but who do not need the complexity of services associated with an acute-care hospital. And Schnurmacher Subacute Medical patients are out of bed more quickly and as often as possible, which helps them maintain functional status while recovery progresses.

7343 **South Shore Healthcare**
275 W Merrick Rd
Freeport, NY 11520-3346
516-623-4000
Fax: 516-223-4599

Winnie Mack, RN, BSN, MPA, Regional Executive Director
Gene Tangney, Senior Vice President/ Regional Executive Director
Michael J. Dowling, President/ CEO
David L. Battinelli, MD, Senior Vice President/Chief Medical Officer

North Shore-LIJ Health System includes 16 award-winning hospitals and nearly 400 physician practice locations throughout New York, including Long Island, Manhattan, Queens and Staten Island. Proudly serving an area of seven million people, North Shore-LIJ delivers world-class services designed for every step of your health and wellness journey.

7344 **St. Camillus Health and Rehabilitation Center**
813 Fay Rd
Syracuse, NY 13219-3009
315-488-2951
Fax: 315-488-3255
info@st-camillus.org
www.st-camillus.org

Aileen Balitz, President
Patrick VanBeveren, PT, DPT, M, Supervisor of Physical Therapy
Nancy, Pirro, RN, Case Manager
Kathy Walsh,PT, DPT, NCS, Designer/Facilitator

Since our founding in 1969, St. Camillus' mission has been to provide high-quality services and facilities emphasizing the rehabilitation of individuals to their maximum potential. The importance of the human spirit drives all we do. We are dedicated to caring for life and helping individuals achieve their highest possible level of independence.

North Carolina

7345 **Chapel Hill Rehabilitation and Healthcare Center**
1602 E Franklin St
Chapel Hill, NC 27514-2892
919-967-1418
800-735-8262
Fax: 919-918-3811

Turner Prichett, Executive Director

Chapel Hill Rehabilitation and Healthcare Center accomodates 120 residents. We are located in downtown Chapel Hill on Franklin Street and we provide roud the clock nursing care 365 days a year. Intensive rehabilitation services are administered by our licensed speech, occupational and physical therapists. Our staff is trained to care for medically complex patients such as those requiring intensive wound care, dialysis, and artificial nutrition.

7346 **Cypress Pointe Rehabilitation and Healthcare Center**
2006 S 16th St
Wilmington, NC 28401-6613
910-763-6271
800-735-8262
Fax: 910-251-9803

Sara Deiter, Executive Director
Dr. Jose Gonzalez, Medical Director
Cypress Pointe offers comprehensive physical, occupational, speech and respiratory therapy services. Following a physician's referral, patients are evaluated to determine their needs. Recommendations are then made for the appropriate interventions and rehabilitation. If therapy is required, a personalized care plan is developed.

7347 **Pettigrew Rehabilitation and Healthcare Center**
1551 W Pettigrew St
Durham, NC 27705-4821
919-286-0751
800-735-8262
Fax: 919-286-5992

La'Ticia Beatty, Executive Director
Pettigrew Rehabilitation and Healthcare Center accomodates 107 residents. Our healthcare center is certified by Medicare and Medicaid. We have experienced staff members who care for our residents. We strive to improve the quality of life our residents experience as a result of the services they receive from our nursing and therapy departments.

7348 **Raleigh Rehabilitation and Healthcare Center**
616 Wade Ave
Raleigh, NC 27605-1237
919-828-6251
800-735-8262
Fax: 919-828-3294
www.raleighrehabhc.com

Steven Jones, Executive Director
Raleigh Rehabilitation and Healthcare Center accomodates 172 residents. We provide short-term rehabilitation-including, physical, occupational, and speech therapies-as well as long-term nursing services. We specialize in neurological disorders, complex diabetes treatment, amputation recovery and pain management. We welcome short stays (respite care). Transportation services are availiable for physician appointments and dialysis treatments.

7349 **Rehabilitation and Healthcare Center of Monroe**
1212 E Sunset Dr
Monroe, NC 28112-4318
704-283-8548
800-735-8262
Fax: 704-283-4664

Judy Olson, Executive Director
We accomodate 159 residents and are certified for Medicare and Medicaid. We specialize in short-term rehabilitation as well as long-term care. Our therapists, wound nurse and dietician work closely to administer wound care. We hav 2 dialysis centers within a 10-block radius and gladly accpet their patients. We have an on-staff medical director as well as a psychiatrist.

7350 **Winston-Salem Rehabilitation and Healthcare Center**
1900 W 1st St
Winston Salem, NC 27104-4220
336-724-2821
800-735-8262
Fax: 336-725-8314

Tom Bauer, Administrator
We accommodate 230 residents and we have approximately 250 employees. Our staffing ratio averages 1 licensed nurse for every 20 residents and 1 Certified Nursing Assistant for every 10 residents. We offer a wide range of services including but not limited to respiratory care, tracheotomy care and gastric tube feeding and we also feature an in house licensed therapy program.

Ohio

7351 **Arbors East Subacute and Rehabilitation Center**
5500 E Broad St
Columbus, OH 43213-1476
614-575-9003
Fax: 614-575-9101

7352 **Arbors at Canton Subacute And Rehabilitation Center**
2714 13th St NW
Canton, OH 44708-3121
330-456-2842
Fax: 330-456-5343
www.laurelsofcanton.com

Amy McDermand, Director of Marketing
Beth Jones, PT, DPT, Rehabilitation Services Director
Cindy Shingler, RN, Director of Nursing
Jennifer Fess, Administrator
We provide individualized, quality care to guests staying short-term for rehabilitation services or long-term for extended care services. The highest level of independence for our guests is the creed of The Laurels of Canton.

7353 **Arbors at Dayton**
320 Albany St
Dayton, OH 45408-1402
937-496-6200
Fax: 937-496-1990
www.extendicareus.com/dayton

Dave Maxwell, Administrator
Carlisa Pedalino, Administrator
Arbors at Dayton is a leading provider of long-term skilled nursing care and short-term rehabilitation solutions. Our 106 bed facility offers a full continuum of services and care focused around each individual in today's ever-changing healthcare environment.

7354 **Arbors at Marietta**
400 N 7th St
Marietta, OH 45750-2024
740-373-3597
Fax: 740-376-0004
www.extendicareus.com/marietta

Joan Florence, Director of Nursing
Kenneth Leopold, Medical Director
Arbors at Marietta is a leading provider of long-term skilled nursing care and short-term rehabilitation solutions. Our 150 bed facility offers a full continuum of services and care focused around each individual in today's ever-changing healthcare environment.

7355 **Arbors at Milford**
5900 Meadow Creek Dr
Milford, OH 45150-5641
513-248-1655
Fax: 513-248-7340
www.extendicareus.com/milford

Bruce Yarwood, President/CEO
Mark Ostendorf, Administrator
Arbors at Milford is a leading provider of long-term skilled nursing care and short-term rehabilitation solutions. Our 139 bed facility offers a full continuum of services and care focused around each individual in today's ever-changing healthcare environment.

7356 **Arbors at Sylvania**
7120 Port Sylvania Dr
Toledo, OH 43617-1158
419-841-2200
Fax: 419-841-2822
www.extendicareus.com/sylvania

Sheril Flowers, Administrator
Graig Hopple, Medical Director
Arbors at Sylvania is a leading provider of long-term skilled nursing care and short-term rehabilitation solutions. Our 79 bed facility offers a full continuum of services and care focused around each individual in today's ever-changing healthcare environment.

7357 **Arbors at Toledo Subacute and Rehab Centre**
2920 Cherry St
Toledo, OH 43608-1716
419-242-7458
Fax: 419-242-6514
www.extendicare.com

Jill Schlievert, Administrator
Subacute rehabilitation services and facility.

7358 **Bridgepark Center for Rehabilitation and Nursing Services**
145 Olive St
Akron, OH 44310-3236
330-762-0901
800-750-0750
Fax: 330-762-0905

Joseph Burick, Medical Director

A skilled nursing and rehabilitation center located in Akron, Ohio, across the street from St. Thomas Hospital with a beautiful view of the Akron skyline. Access to Interstate 77 and State Route 8 is just minutes away. Our entire staff is committed to providing caring, customer-focused skilled nursing and rehabilitation. For your convenience, we accept Medicare, Medicaid and most managed care and private insurance.

7359 **Broadview Multi-Care Center**
5520 Broadview Rd
Parma, OH 44134-1605
216-749-4010
Fax: 216-749-0141
www.broadviewmulticare.com

Harold Shachter, Owner
Mike Flank, VP
Broadview Multi-Care Center is a family run business with more than 40 years of experience providing quality care to the community. We are committed to meeting your needs and providing you with a warm, home-like environment. Our family is on-site and our doors are always open for your suggestions or to drop in and say hello. We always try to take and honor requests, whether it's a favorite food, an exciting activity or a particular room.

7360 **Caprice Care Center**
9184 Market St
North Lima, OH 44452-9558
330-965-9200
Fax: 330-726-6097
www.chcccompanies.com

Lori Crowl, Owner
Becky Berger, Director of Nursin
Stacey Howell, Administrator
Valerie Conzett, Admission Liaison
A 106-bed skilled nursing, subacute and rehabilitation facility. Our goal is to provide comfortable living to all who are in our care. Caprice Health Care Center is a contemporary Medicare and Medicaid approved facility specializing in short-term rehabilitation services. The inpatient/outpatient rehab department includes physical, occupational, speech therapies, indoor aquatic therapy pool, as well as complimentary van transportation for outpatient services.

7361 **Cleveland Clinic**
9500 Euclid Ave
Cleveland, OH 44195-2
216-444-2200
800-801-2273
Fax: 216-444-7021
my.clevelandclinic.org/default.aspx

Gene Altus, Executive Director
Delos M. Cosgrove, MD, Chief Executive Officer, Preside
Joseph F. Hahn, MD, Chief of Staff, Vice Chairman of
David Bronson, MD, Chief Executive Officer, Clevela
A not-for-profit, multispecialty academic medical center that integrates clinical and hospital care with research and education. Cleveland clinic was founded in 1921 by 4 renowned physicians with a vision of providing outstanding patient care based upon the principals of cooperation, compassion and innovation. Today, Cleveland Clinic is one of the largest and most respected hospitals in the country.

7362 **Columbus Rehabilitation And Subacute Institute**
111 West Michigan Street
Milwaukee, WI 53203-2903
800-395-5000
kschaewe@extendicare.com
www.extendicareus.com

Kelly Fligor, Administrator
Jillian Fountain, Secretary
Subacute rehabilitation programs and facility.

7363 **LakeMed Nursing and Rehabilitation Center**
70 Normandy Dr
Painesville, OH 44077-1616
440-357-1311
800-750-0750
Fax: 440-352-9977
www.lakemednursing.com

Connie Eyman, Administrator
Vesta Jones, Executive Director
Our goal is to provide you with quality care and we are known for our successful short-term rehab and care of the clinically complex. We also offer respite services to give caregivers a rest, and hospice services through our local hospice care provider. Our interdisciplinary team works together as they strive to deliver quality care and responsive service to our residents.

7364 **Oregon Nursing And Rehabilitation Center**
904 Isaac Streets Dr
Oregon, OH 43616-3204
419-691-2483
Fax: 419-697-5401
www.extendicareus.com/oregon

Mark Rogers, Administrator
Subacute rehabilitation facility and services.

7365 **Sunset View Castle Nursing Homes Castle Nursing Homes**
434 N Washington St
Millersburg, OH 44654-1188
330-674-0015
Fax: 330-763-2238

Becky Snyder, Admissions Coordinator
Kathy Edwards, Admissions And Marketing
310 licensed, certified beds. Subacute rehabilitation facility and programs.

Oregon

7366 **Care Center East Health & Specialty Care Center**
Expendicare
11325 NE Weidler St
Portland, OR 97220-1950
503-253-1181
Fax: 503-253-1871
www.extendicareus.com

Glydon Kimbrough, Administrator
Subacute rehabilitation facility and programs

7367 **Medford Rehabilitation and Healthcare Center**
Kindred Healthcare
625 Stevens St
Medford, OR 97504-6719
541-779-3551
800-735-1232
Fax: 541-779-3658

Grant Gloor, Administrator
Dane Reeves, Executive Director
Kristen W., Health and Rehabilitation Center
Becky D., Activity Director
We strive to provide quality, compassionate care. Our cozy building accomodates 110 residents. Our smaller size creates an inviting and homelike environment. We offer semi-private rooms with space to add items from home for a special personalized touch.

Pennsylvania

7368 **Dresher Hill Health and Rehabilitation Center**
1390 Camp Hill Rd
Dresher, PA 19034-2805
215-643-0600
Fax: 215-641-0628

Earl Kimble, Administrator
Subacute rehabilitation facility and programs: physical/speech.

7369 **Good Shepherd Rehabilitation**
850 S 5th St
Allentown, PA 18103-3295
610-776-3586
888-447-3422
Fax: 610-776-8336
goodshepherdrehab.org

John Kristel, MBA, MPT, President & CEO
Mike Bonner, MBA, Vice President, Neurosciences
Ronald J. Petula, CPA, Senior Vice President, Finance and Chief Financial Officer
Joseph Shadid, Administrator, Good Shepherd Home-Bethlehem
A world class rehabilitation network, Good Shepherd provides comprehensive inpatient and outpatient services throughout Pennsylvania's Lehigh Valley. Founded in 1908, Good Shepherd has steadily expanded over last 95 years. Good Shepherd is one of the most comprehensive rehabilitation institutes in the world.

7370 **Statesman Health and Rehabilitation Center**
2629 Trenton Rd
Levittown, PA 19056-1428
215-943-7777
Fax: 215-943-1240
www.statesmanskillednursing.com

Jamie Tanner, Administrator
Subacute rehabilitation facility and programs.

7371 **UPMC Braddock**
200 Lothrop St.
Pittsburgh, PA 15213-2582
412-647-8762
800-533-8762
Fax: 412-636-5398
hospitalbill@upmc.edu
upmc.com

Mark Sevco, Administrator
Rodney Jones, Vice President
With a team of more then 43,000 employees, UPMC serves the health needs of more then 4 million people each year, improving lives in western Pennsylvania-and beyond-through redefined models of health care delivery and superb clinical outcomes.

7372 **UPMC McKeesport**
Presby
1500 5th Ave
McKeesport, PA 15132-2422
412-664-2000
Fax: 412-664-2309
fisherpj@upmc.edu
upmc.com

Ronald H Ott, CEO
Offers 56 beds for patients who need skilled nursing care. Offers ongoing rehabilitation and educational programs to patients with cardiac, neurologic, and orthopaedic diagnosis.

7373 **UPMC Passavant**
9100 Babcock Blvd
Pittsburgh, PA 15237-5842
412-367-6700
800-533-8762
gloordc@ph.upmc.edu
upmc.com

William Kristan, Dir Inpatient Physical Therapy
Teresa Petrick, Chief Executive Officer
Patients who have had an acute illness, injury, or exacerbation of a disease and no longer need the intensity of services in the acute care setting, but still require some complex medical care or supervision and rehabilitation services, may be appropriate to be transferred into the Subacute Unit.

Rhode Island

7374 **Kindred Heights Nursing & Rehabilitation Center**
Kindred Healthcare
680 South Fourth Street
Louisville, KY 40202
502-596-7300
800-545-0749
web_administrator@kindred.com
www.kindredheights.com

Sandra Sarza, Manager
Jean Aubin, Director
Kindred Heights Nursing and Rehabilitation Center accomodates 58 residents and serves the needs of elders in the greater East Bay and Providence area. We are conveniently located on Wampanoag Trail in East Providence. Kindred Heights provides skilled nursing, short-term rehab and long-term care in a family environment, but we are large enough to manage the complex nursing and rehab care needs our residents may have.

7375 **Oak Hill Nursing and Rehabilitation Center**
Kindered Health Care
544 Pleasant St
Pawtucket, RI 02860-5776
401-725-8888
800-745-6575
Fax: 401-723-5720
www.oakhillrehab.com

Scott M. Sandborn, Executive Director
Heidi Capela, Director Nursing
Amybeth Almeida, Director Admissions
Aman Nanda, Medical Director
Accomodates 143 residents. Throughout our 40 year history, Oak Hill has developed a reputation as one of the finest healthcare centers in Rhode Island. Our center consists of 3 separate units. A 34-bed post-acute unit provides care to the medically complex and those in need of extensive rehabilitative services. A 20-bed Alzheimer's Special Care Unit provides a unique style of care utilizing habilitative therapy in comfortable, home-like surroundings.

7376 **Southern New England Rehab Center**
200 High Service Avenue
North Providence, RI 02904
401-456-3801
888-456-4501
Fax: 401-456-3784
www.snerc.com

Vivian Hagstrom, Manager
The Center's skilled staff of over 100 professionals provides a full range of coordinated rehabilitative care. Our clinical expertise and compassion make a big difference as we develop first-rate plans of care for the unique needs of each patient. Our medical staff is comprised of physicians board-certified in rehabilitation medicine and internal medicine.

South Carolina

7377 **Tuomey Healthcare System**
129 N Washington St
Sumter, SC 29150-4949
803-774-9000
Fax: 803-774-8737
www.tuomey.com

R Jay Cox, CEO
Here to anticipte the needs of the communities we serve, responding with proactive healthcare initiatives, providing expert rehabilitative services and delivering life-saving acute care.

Tennessee

7378 **Camden Healthcare and Rehabilitation Center**
680 South Fourth Street
Louisville, KY 40202
502-596-7300
800-545-0749
web_administrator@kindred.com
kindredhealthcare.com

Mark Walker, Administrator
Subacute rehabilitation products and services, nursing and life care homes.

7379 **Centennial Medical Center Tri Star Health System**
2300 Patterson St
Nashville, TN 37203-1538
615-342-1000
800-242-5662
Fax: 615-342-1045
Laurel.Haskamp@HCAHealthcare.com
tristarcentennial.com

Thomas L Herron, President/Chief Executive Office
Above all else we are committed to the care and improvement of human life by caring for those we serve with integrity, compassion, a positive attitude, respect and exceptional quality.

7380 **Cordova Rehabilitation and Nursing Center**
955 N Germantown Pkwy
Cordova, TN 38018-6215
901-754-1393
800-848-0299
Fax: 901-754-3332
cdadmi@gracehc.com
www.gracehccordova.com

John Palmer, Administrator
Renee Tutor, Executive Director
Our professional staff can help you make an informed decision. Upon admission, our interdisciplinary team develops a comprehensive care plan to meet not only physical and rehabilitative goals, but also social and emotional needs. We understand the importance of family and resident involvement and encourage participation in the development of a personalized plan of care.

7381 **Erlanger Medical Center Baronness Campus**
975 E 3rd St
Chattanooga, TN 37403-2147 423-778-7000
Fax: 423-778-7615
guestrelations@erlanger.org
www.erlanger.org

Kevin M. Spiegel, FACHE, President and CEO
James Creel, MD, Chief Medical Officer
Gregg T. Gentry, Chief Administrative Officer
Robert M. Brooks, FACHE, Executive Vice President and Chief Operating Officer

Our mission is to improve the health of the people we touch. Our vision is to be recognized locally, regionally, and and nationally, as a premiere healthcare system.

7382 **Huntington Health and Rehabilitation Center**
635 High St
Huntingdon, TN 38344-1703 731-986-8943
Fax: 731-986-3188
huntingdonhealth.com

Heidi Hawkins, Administrator
Windi Summers, Admissions Director

Subacute rehabilitation facility and programs.

7383 **Madison Healthcare and Rehabilitation Center**
431 Larkin Springs Rd
Madison, TN 37115-5005 615-865-8520
800-848-0299
Fax: 615-868-4455

Phyllis Cherry, Executive Director

At our facility, we provide quality care with modern rehabilitation and restorative nursing techniques. We aim to provide an atmosphere which encourages family involvement in the care-planning process, with the right mix of activities addressing the social, spiritual and intellectual needs of our residents.

7384 **Mariner Health of Nashville**
3939 Hillsboro Cir
Nashville, TN 37215-2708 615-297-2100
Fax: 615-297-2197

David Reeves, Administrator
Amy Artrip, Director of Nursing

Religious nonmedical health care institution. 150-bed subacute rehabilitation facility

7385 **Pine Meadows Healthcare and Rehabilitation Center**
700 Nuckolls Rd
Bolivar, TN 38008-1531 731-658-4707
Fax: 731-658-4769
www.pinemeadowshc.com

Larry Shrader, Administrator
Sharon McKeen, Admissions Director

Our goal is to take care of your loved ones. Our professional team works with skilled hands, is directed by creative minds and is guided by compassionate hearts. Upon your admission, our interdisciplinary team develops a comprehensive care plan designed with a goal of meeting not only physical and rehabilitative objectives, but also social and emotional needs. We understand the importance of family and resident involvement and encourage participation in the development of a plan of care.

7386 **Primacy Healthcare and Rehabilitation Center**
Kindred Health Care
6025 Primacy Pkwy
Memphis, TN 38119-5763 901-767-1040
800-848-0299
Fax: 901-685-7362

Donnie Dubert, Executive Director
Dr. Mark Hammond, Medical Director
Kristen W., Health and Rehabilitation Center
Becky D., Activity Director

Upon a resident's admission, our interdisciplinary team develops a comprehensive care plan with a goal of meeting not only physical and rehabilitative objectives but also social and emotional needs. We understand the importance of family and resident involvement and encourage participation in the development of a personalized plan of care.

7387 **Ripley Healthcare and Rehabilitation Center**
118 Halliburton St
Ripley, TN 38063-2011 731-635-5180
Fax: 731-635-0663
www.ripleyhc.com

Johnny Rea, Executive Director
Brandon Whiteside, Executive Director
Jan Hodge, Admissions Directo
Jennifer Pitts, Administrator

Upon admission, our interdisciplinary team develops a comprehensive care plan to meet not only physical and rehabilitative goals, but also social and emotional needs. We understand the importance of family and resident involvement and encourage participation in the development of a personalized care plan. Our goal is to take care of your loved ones.

7388 **Shelby Pines Rehabilitation and Healthcare Center**
3909 Covington Pike
Memphis, TN 38135-2281 901-377-1011
Fax: 901-377-0032

Rene Tutor, Executive Director

Subacute rehabiltation facility and programs.

7389 **Siskin Hospital for Physical Rehabilitation**
1 Siskin Plz
Chattanooga, TN 37403-1306 423-634-1200
Fax: 423-634-4538
TTY: 423-634-1201
info@siskinrehab.org
siskinrehab.org

Robert Main, CEO
Lindsay Wyatt, Media Coordinator, Marketing Co

Dedicated exclusively to physical rehabilitation and offers specialized treatment programs in brain injury, amputation, stroke, spinal cord injury, orthopeadics, and major multiple trauma.

Texas

7390 **North Hills Hospital**
4401 Booth Calloway Rd
North Richland Hills, TX 76180-7399 817-255-1000
Fax: 817-255-1991
northhillshospital.com

Randy Moresi, CEO

North Hills Hospital's services include a wide range of cardiovascular services, surgical services, emergency services, radiology, a rehabilitation unit, a senior health center, therapy services, and women's services.

7391 **Valley Regional Medical Center**
100 E Alton Gloor Blvd
Brownsville, TX 78526-3328 956-350-7000
Fax: 956-350-7111
valleyregionalmedicalcenter.com

Susan Andrews, CEO
Francisco Javier Del Castillo, MD
Subramaniam Anandasivam, MD
Christopher Olson, MD

Above all else, we are committed to the care and improvement of human life. In recognition of this committment, we strive to deliver high quality, cost effective healthcare in the communities we serve. In persuit of our mission, we recognize and affirm the unique and intrinsic worth of each individual. We treat all those we serve with compassion and kindness. We act with absolute honesty and integrity and fairness in the way we conduct our business and the way we live our lives.

Utah

7392 **Crosslands Rehabilitation and Healthcare Center**
680 South Fourth Street
Louisville, KY 40202
502-596-7300
800-545-0749
web_administrator@kindred.com
www.kindredhealthcare.com
John Williams, Executive Director
Lyle Black, Manager
Crossroads Rehabilitation and Healthcare accomodates 120 residents. We are fully Medicare and Medicaid certified. We are proud of our reputation for providing quality, compassionate care. Services availiable include in-house physical, occupational and speech therapies, as well as 24-hour licensed nursing staff coverage. We offer therapeutic recreation, in-house social services and registered dietician services, among many other professional services.

7393 **Federal Heights Rehabilitation and Nursing Center**
Kindred Health Care
680 South Fourth Street
Louisville, KY 40202
502-596-7300
800-545-0749
web_administrator@kindred.com
www.kindredhealthcare.com
Pete Zeigler, Executive Director
Dr. Charles Canfield, Medical Director
Federal Heights accomodates 120 residents. We are located near three major hospitals in the Salt Lake Valley. We specialize in providing nursing services for complex medical and rehabilitation conditions. Our discharge planning works jointly with the family and resident in determining the future needs and goals upon discharge.

7394 **St. George Care and Rehabilitation Center**
Kindred Health Care Publications
1032 E 100 S
Saint George, UT 84770-3005
435-628-0488
800-346-4128
Fax: 435-628-7362
www.stgeorgecare.com
John Larson, Plant Manager
Erin Hammon, Director of Nursing
Derrick Glum, Executive Director
St. George Care and Rehabilitation accomodates 95 residents. We offer a 4,000 square foot rehabilitation gym with an indoor therapy pool for inpatient and outpatient services. Therapy is provided to meet specific needs seven days a week. There is a dietitian on staff for individualized nutritional needs. We offer an Alzheimer's unit with specialized staff. We provide compassionate health services including physicians, nurses, physical therapists, and occupational therapist and licensed aides.

7395 **St. Mark's Hospital**
1200 E 3900 S
Salt Lake City, UT 84124-1390
801-268-7111
Fax: 801-270-3489
www.stmarkshospital.com
Steve B. Bateman, CEO
Above all else we are committed to the care and improvement of human life. In recognition of this commitment, we strive to deliver high quality, cost effective healthcare in the communities we serve. We define quality as 'caring people with the commitment to a continuous process of improvement in the services provided, that will better enable the hospital to meet or exceed our customer's needs and expectations.

7396 **Wasatch Valley Rehabilitation**
Kindred Healthcare
680 South Fourth Street
Louisville, KY 40202
502-596-7300
800-545-0749
web_administrator@kindred.com
www.kindredhealthcare.com
Alex Stevenson, Executive Director
Ric Toomer, Executive Director
Wasatch Valley accomodates 110 residents. We are licensed for Medicare and Medicaid and we are conveniently located in the heart of Salt Lake City with easy access from I-15 and I-215. We are known by the area hospitals as a specialist in wound care and for the care we provide to those with complex medical conditions.

Virginia

7397 **Nansemond Pointe Rehabilitation and Healthcare Center**
200 Constance Rd
Suffolk, VA 23434-4960
757-539-8744
800-828-1140
Fax: 757-539-6128
www.nansemondhc.com
Mel Epelle, Executive Director
Mary R, Activities Assistant
Kristen W., Health and Rehabilitation Center
Becky D., Activity Director
Nansemond Pointe Rehabilitation and Healthcare Center accomodates 160 residents in private and semi-private rooms. We have been serving the needs of Suffolk, Virginia and the surrounding areas for over 38 years. We offer an entire continuum of care from assisted living apartments to skilled nursing to long-term care. Our licensed therapists, working with our dedicated nursing staff, share a common goal- to help our residents improve their level of recovery and independence.

7398 **Rehabilitation and Research Center Virginia Commonwealth University**
1250 East Marshall Street
Richmond, VA 23298
804-828-9000
Fax: 804-828-5074
www.vcuhealth.org
Michael Rao, Ph.D., VCU President & VCUHS President,
Sheldon M. Retchin, M.D., VP Health Sciences & CEO, VCUHS
John Duval, Chief Executive Officer MCV Hosp
Dominic J. Puleo, Executive VP Finance and CFO, VC
The Rehabilitation and Research Center is a collaborative effort between the Department of Physical Medicine and Rehabilitation and the Medical College of Virginia Hospitals. The goals of the Rehabilitation and Research Center at the Medical College of Virginia Hospitals (MCVH) are to provide highly-skilled, interdisciplinary, inpatient rehabilitative care to adults with complex needs; to be an advocate and educator for patients and people with disabilities.

7399 **Warren Memorial Hospital**
1000 N Shenandoah Ave
Front Royal, VA 22630-3598
540-636-0300
800-994-6610
Fax: 540-636-0258
complaint@jointcommission.org
www.valleyhealthlink.com
Mark H. Merrill, President & Chief Executive Officer
Tonya Smith, Vice President of Operations
Pete Gallagher, Senior Vice President & CFO
Joan Roscoe, Vice President of Information Sy
A nonprofit organization of health care providers, Valley Health offers a full spectrum of services in acute care, rehabilitation and extended care facilities, and outpatient and community settings to help the people of the region manage their health and enjoy a high quality of life. Valley Health has the resources to diagnose, treat and help patients manage virtually any medical problem that may be encountered.

7400 **Winchester Rehabilitation Center**
333 W Cork St
Suite 230
Winchester, VA 22601-3870
540-536-5114
800-994-6610
Fax: 540-536-1122
complaint@jointcommission.org
www.valleyhealthlink.com
Mark H. Merrill, President & Chief Executive Officer
Tonya Smith, Vice President of Operations
Pete Gallagher, Senior Vice President & CFO
Joan Roscoe, Vice President of Information Sy
Offers the following rehabilitation services: Sub-Acute inpatient rehabilitation, Speech therapy, Physical therapy, Occupational therapy, Disability evaluations. 30-bed inpatient center.

Washington

7401 Aldercrest Health and Rehabilitation Center
21400 72nd Ave W
Edmonds, WA 98026-7702
425-775-1961
Fax: 425-771-0116
www.aldercrestskillednursing.com
Rick Milsow, Administrator
Aldercrest Health & Rehabilitation Center is a leading provider of long-term skilled nursing care and short-term rehabilitation solutions. Our 124 bed facility offers a full continuum of services and care focused around each individual in today's ever-changing healthcare environment.

7402 Arden Rehabilitation and Healthcare Center
16357 Aurora Ave N
Seattle, WA 98133-5651
206-542-3103
800-833-6384
Fax: 206-542-7192
www.ardenrehab.com
Matthew Preston, Administrator
Ann Zell, Executive Director
Kristen W., Health and Rehabilitation Center
Becky D., Activity Director
Arden Rehabilitation has been an integral part of the Shoreline community since 1953. It is a one-level building set on mature grounds with several beautiful courtyards for the residents to enjoy. Arden can accomodate 90 residents-post acute/rehabilitation patients as well as long-term residents. Medicare certified, the center also takes most managed healthcare insurance plans, as well as VA, respite and hospice patients.

7403 Bellingham Health Care and Rehabilitation Services
1200 Birchwood Ave
Bellingham, WA 98225-1302
360-734-9295
800-833-6384
Fax: 360-671-4368
www.avamererehabofbellingham.com
Melissa Nelson, Executive Director
Dr. Richard McClenahan, Medical Director
Kristen W., Health and Rehabilitation Center
Becky D., Activity Director
At Bellingham Health Care and Rehab, we strive to provide quality, compassionate care. Our cozy building accomodates 84 residents. Our smaller size creates an inviting and homelike environment for your loved one. We offer semi-private rooms with space to add items from home for a special personalized touch. Provides meals served restaurant style in our dinning room overlooking our beautiful grounds.

7404 Bremerton Convalescent and Rehabilitation Center
2701 Clare Ave
Bremerton, WA 98310-3313
360-377-3951
Fax: 360-377-5443
bremertonskillednursing.com
Stephanie Bonanzino, Administrator
Subacute rehabilitation facility and programs.

7405 Edmonds Rehabilitation & Healthcare Centerer
Kindred Healthcare
21008 76th Ave W
Edmonds, WA 98026-7104
425-778-0107
800-833-6384
Fax: 425-776-9532
Jane Davis, Executive Director
At Edmonds Rehabilitation and Healthcare, we strive to provide quality, compassionate care. Our center accomodates 91 residents. Our smaller size creates an inviting and homelike environment. We offer semi-private rooms with space to add items from home for a special personalized touch. Edmonds Rehabilitation and Healthcare provides delicious meals served restaurant style in our dinning room.

7406 Heritage Health and Rehabilitation Center
Kindred Health Care
3605 Y St
Vancouver, WA 98663-2647
360-693-5839
800-833-6384
Fax: 360-693-3991
www.heritagerehab.com
Michael Moses, Executive Director
Su Patchett, Director of Nursing
Heritage Health & Rehabilitation Center is the smallest free-standing healthcare center in southwest Washington with accomodations of 49, enabling more personal care and a more home-like environment. Heritage has licensed nursing staff, restorative aides, and certified nurses assistants, trained and experienced in providing Alzheimer's care, end of life/hospice care, psychiatric care, rehabilitative care, and respite care.

7407 North Auburn Rehabilitation And Health Center
111 West Michigan Street
Milwaukee, WI 53203-2903
800-395-5000
extendicare.com
Allyson Jenkins, Administrator
Subacute rehabilitation facility and programs.

7408 Northwoods Lodge
2321 NW Schold Pl
Silverdale, WA 98383-9504
360-698-3930
Fax: 360-692-2169
www.encorecommunities.com
Leslie Krueger, Owner
Debbie Griffin, Director of Rehab Services
Silverdale Campus, Executive Director
Provides you with a full-range of services from weekly housekeeping and laudry services, to grounds keeping and maintenance. Our monthy fee inculdes utilities and hot, delicious, nutritious meals served table side every day. We offer transportation services, full-time activities directors, and numerous amenities to add to your comfort and enjoyment.

7409 Pacific Specialty & Rehabilitation Center r
1015 N Garrison Rd
Vancouver, WA 98664-1313
360-694-7501
Fax: 360-694-8148
Rebecca Pruett, Administrator
Subacute rehabilitation facility and programs.

7410 Puget Sound Healthcare Center
4001 Capitol Mall Dr SW
Olympia, WA 98502-8657
360-754-9792
Fax: 360-754-2455
www.pugetsoundskillednursing.com
Sheila Oberg, Administrator
Our goal is to provide excellence in patient care, veteran's benefits and customer satisfaction. We have reformed our department internally and are striving for high quality, prompt and seamless service to veterans. Our department employees continue to offer their dedication and commitment to help veterans get the services they have earned.

7411 Vancouver Health & Rhabilitation Center
400 E 33rd St
Vancouver, WA 98663-2238
360-696-2561
800-833-6384
Fax: 360-696-9275
www.vancouverhealthcare.com
Jody Wigen, Human Resources
Joe Joy, Executive Director
Kristen W., Health and Rehabilitation Center
Becky D., Activity Director
At Vancouver Health and Rehab Center we strive to provide quality, compassionate care. Our cozy building accomodates 98 residents. Our smaller size creates an inviting and homelike environment. We offer semi-private rooms with space to add items from home for a special personalized touch. Provides delicious meals served restaurant style in our dining room.

West Virginia

7412 **War Memorial Hospital**
1 Healthy Way
Berkeley Springs, WV 25411-1743 304-258-1234
Fax: 304-258-5618
complaint@jointcommission.org
www.valleyhealthlink.com
Mark H. Merrill, President & Chief Executive Officer
Tonya Smith, Vice President of Operations
Pete Gallagher, Senior Vice President & Chief Financial Officer
Joan Roscoe, Vice President of Information Systems
Offers physical therapy, occupational therapy, speech therapy, social services, and patient/family education for individuals who have experienced a recent physical disability due to disease, dysfunction, or general debilitation. Helps patients to maximize their abilities through activities of daily living, mobility, self-medication, and self-care and restore their ability to return to their previous lifestyle.

Wisconsin

7413 **Cedar Spring Health and Rehabilitation Center**
N27w5707 Lincoln Blvd
Cedarburg, WI 53012-2852 262-376-7676
Fax: 262-376-7808
Mary Wirth, Executive Director
Subacute rehabilitation facility and programs.

7414 **Clearview-Brain Injury Center**
198 Home Rd
Juneau, WI 53039-1401 920-386-3400
877-386-3400
Fax: 920-386-3800
Jane E. Hooper, Administrator
Jacqueline Kuhl, Household Coordinator
Laura Bertagnoli
Kathy Lorenz, AFH Manager
A 30-bed, state certified, subacute neuro-rehabilitation program in Juneau, WI. We are located just 45 minutes northeast of Madison WI and 10 minutes east of Beaver Dam, WI. We are the first and longest standing of only 2 community re-entry programs in the state of Wisconsin providing subacute neuro-rehabilitation to teens and adults who have experienced a brain injury.

7415 **Colonial Manor Medical and Rehabilitation Center**
1010 E Wausau Ave
Wausau, WI 54403-3101 715-842-2028
800-947-6644
Fax: 715-848-0510
Ericca Ylitalo, Administrator
Shelley Solberg, Executive Director
Kristen W., Health and Rehabilitation Center
Becky D., Activity Director
Colonial Manor Medical and Rehabilitation Center is part of the Kindred Community and is located in Wausau, Wisconsin. The corporate headquarters are based in Louisville Kentucky. Our facility accomodates 150 residents.

7416 **Eastview Medical and Rehabilitation Center**
729 Park St
Antigo, WI 54409-2745 715-623-2356
800-947-6644
Fax: 715-623-6345
Wanda Hose, Administrator
Wanda Hose, Executive Director
Kristen W., Health and Rehabilitation Center
Becky D., Activity Director
Eastview Medical Center and Rehabilitation Center accomodates 165 residents. We are Medicare and Medicaid certified, as well as being Joint Commission accredited. Our 'TEAM' approach means specially trained staff work around the clock to assist in meeting rehabilitative goals established by our team of professionals. We encourage family involvement in our rehabilitative process. The support of loved ones is a major key to a speedy recovery.

7417 **Hospitality Nursing Rehabilitation Center**
8633 32nd Ave
Kenosha, WI 53142-5187 262-694-8300
Fax: 262-694-3622
Marla Benson, Administrator
LaRae Nelson, President
Lisa Behling, Secretary
Scott Miller, Treasurer
Subacute rehabilitation facility and programs.

7418 **Kennedy Park Medical Rehabilitation Center**
Kindred Healthcare
6001 Alderson St
Schofield, WI 54476-3614 715-359-4257
800-947-6644
Fax: 715-355-4867
Judy Kowalski, Manager
Jim Torgerson, Executive Director
Kristen W., Health and Rehabilitation Center
Becky D., Activity Director
Kennedy Park Medical & Rehabilitation Center accomodates 154 residents. We are located in Schofield, WI. At Kennedy Park, we specialize in dementia care, with our Reflections and Passages Units. Short-term rehabilitation and sub-acute care are provided in a setting conducive to meeting the individual needs of our residents and patients. We also provide general nursing care for persons with long-term care needs.

7419 **Middleton Village Nursing & Rehabilitation**
Kindred
6201 Elmwood Ave
Middleton, WI 53562-3319 608-831-8300
800-947-6644
Fax: 608-831-4253
www.middletonvillage.com
Nicholas Stamatas, Manager
Ashley Ostrowski, Executive Director
Kristen W., Health and Rehabilitation Center
Becky D., Activity Director
Middleton Village accomodates 97 residents. We specialize in post-surgical and post-acute rehabilitation and long-term care services.

7420 **Mount Carmel Health & Rehabilitation Center**
5700 W Layton Ave
Milwaukee, WI 53220-4099 414-281-7200
Fax: 414-281-4620
Mike Berry, Administrator
Darrin Hull, Executive Director
Kristen W., Health and Rehabilitation Center
Becky D., Activity Director
Subacute rehabilitation facility and programs.

7421 **Mount Carmel Medical and Rehabilitation Center**
680 South Fourth Street
Louisville, KY 40202 502-596-7300
800-545-0749
web_administrator@kindred.com
kindredhealthcare.com
Randy Nitschke, Administrator
Jeanne Piccioni, Executive Director
Mount Carmel Medical and Rehabilitation Center accomodates 155 residents. We are located in Burlington Wisconsin. Mount Carmel Medical and Rehabilitation center is a recipient of the American Health Care Association Quality Award.

7422 **North Ridge Medical and Rehabilitation Center**
1445 N 7th St
Manitowoc, WI 54220-2011 920-682-0314
800-947-6644
Fax: 920-682-0553
Jane Conway, Interim ED
Mary Ann Hamer, Executive Director
North Ridge Medical and Rehabiliation Center accomodates 110 residents. We have been serving the Manitowoc, Wisconsin area for over 25 years. Our goal is to provide services in a warm, homey environment. Many of our staff in all departments have a long history with North Ridge and have worked here for more then 20 years. We also take pride in the fact that we have all in-house staff. Our therapy team is availiable to provide physical, occupational and speech therapy 7 days a week.

7423 **Oshkosh Medical and Rehabilitation Center**
1580 Bowen St
Oshkosh, WI 54901
920-233-4011
Fax: 920-233-5177
Tom Wagner, President
Subacute rehabilitation facility and programs.

7424 **San Luis Medical and Rehabilitation Center**
680 South Fourth Street
Louisville, KY 40202
502-596-7300
800-545-0749
web_administrator@kindred.com
www.kindredhealthcare.com
Heather Dreier, Administrator
Tim Dietzen, Executive Director
Dr. John T. Warren, Medical Director
Kristen W., Health and Rehabilitation Center
San Luis Medical and Rehabilitation Center accomodates 126 residents. We are located in Green bay, WI. At San Luis, we strive to meet the needs of our residents and we specialize in dementia care, with our Reflections Unit. Our goal is to provide short-term rehabilitation and sub-acute care in a setting conducive to assisting the needs of our residents.

7425 **Strawberry Lane Nursing & Rehabilitation Center**
130 Strawberry Lane
Wisconsin Rapids, WI 54494-2156
715-424-1600
Fax: 715-424-4817
Cyndi Glodoski, Admissions Director
Carrie Russert, Administrator
Skilled nursing facility that provides both long term and short term care. Offer Alzheimer's and Dementia care units, as well as Hospice Care. Medicare and Medicaid certified.

Wyoming

7426 **Mountain Towers Healthcare & Rehabilitation Center**
3128 Boxelder Dr
Cheyenne, WY 82001-5808
307-634-7901
800-877-9975
Fax: 307-634-7910
Dan Stackis, Administrator
Toni Wyenn, Director of Nursing
Daniel G. Stackis, Executive Director
Dr. Kent Britton, Medical Director
Mountain Towers Healthcare and Rehabilitation Center accomodates 170 residents, including a 16-bed acute secure unit. We offer a full range of nursing and medical care to meet individual needs. We have a full staff to meet the needs of our residents.

7427 **South Central Wyoming Healthcare and Rehabilitation**
Kindred Healthcare
542 16th St
Rawlins, WY 82301-5241
307-324-2759
800-877-9975
Fax: 307-324-7579
Chris Tanner, Executive Director
Anthony Janusz, Administrator
Kristen W., Health and Rehabilitation Center
Becky D., Activity Director
South Central Wyoming Healthcare and Rehabilitation accomodates 52 residents. We are located in Rawlings, in south central Wyoming. We are Medicare and Medicaid certified by the State of Wyoming. We strive to provide quality personal services, long-term care or short-term rehabilitation to our residents in a comfortable home-like environment.

7428 **Wind River Healthcare and Rehabilitation Center**
Kindred Health Care
1002 Forest Dr
Riverton, WY 82501-2918
307-856-9471
800-877-9975
Fax: 307-856-1665
Jo Ann Aldrich, Executive Director
Amelia Asay, Business Office Manager
Kristen W., Health and Rehabilitation Center
Becky D., Activity Director
Offers a full range of medical services to meet the individual needs of our residents, including short-term rehabilitative services and long-term skilled care. Working with the residents physician, our staff-including medical specialists, nurses, nutritionists, dietitians and social workers-establishes a comprehensive treatment plan intended to restore you or your loved one to the highest practicable potential.

Aging

Associations

7429 **AARP**
601 E Street NW
Washington, DC 20049
202-434-3525
888-687-2277
member@aarp.org
www.aarp.org
Jo Ann Jenkins, CEO
Formerly the American Association of Retired Persons. AARP is a collection of diverse individuals and ideas working as one to influence positive change and improve the lives of those 50 and over. AARP reflects a wide range of attitudes, cultures, lifestyles, and beliefs.
1919

7430 **AARP Alabama**
400 South Union Street
Suite 100
Montgomery, AL 36104
866-542-8167
alaarp@aarp.org
states.aarp.org/region/alabama
Candi Williams, State Director
Lisa Billingsley, Senior Operations Administrator
Provides information, events, news, and resources to Alabamians over 50 years of age, and to a membership of over 430,000.
1920

7431 **AARP Alaska**
3601 C Street
Suite 1420
Anchorage, AK 99503
866-227-7447
Fax: 907-341-2270
ak@aarp.org
states.aarp.org/region/alaska
Ken Helander, Advocacy Director
Ann Secrest, Media Contact
Serves 95,000 members in Alaska, providing information, resources, news, and advocacy on matters relevant to individuals aged 50 years and older.

7432 **AARP Arizona**
7250 N 16th Street
Suite 302
Phoenix, AZ 85020
866-389-5649
aarpaz@aarp.org
states.aarp.org/region/arizona
David Parra, Director, Community Outreach
Alex Suarez, Communications Contact
The chapter seeks to enhance the quality of life for all Arizonans, with an emphasis on individuals 50 years and older.

7433 **AARP Arkansas**
1701 Centerview Drive
Suite 205
Little Rock, AR 72211
866-544-5379
Fax: 501-227-7710
araarp@aarp.org
states.aarp.org/region/arkansas
Charlie Wagener, State President
Seeks to redefine and improve life for Arkansans over the age of 50.

7434 **AARP California: Pasadena**
200 S Los Robles Avenue
Suite 400
Pasadena, CA 91101- 2422
866-448-3614
Fax: 626-583-8500
caaarp@aarp.org
states.aarp.org/region/california
Nancy McPherson, State Director
Joy Hepp, Media Contact, Southern California
Provides news, tools, resources, and research to Californians 50 years and older.

7435 **AARP California: Sacramento**
1415 L Street
Suite 960
Sacramento, CA 95814
866-448-3614
Fax: 916-446-2223
caaarp@aarp.org
states.aarp.org/region/california
Nancy McPherson, State President
Mark Beach, Media Contact, Northern California
Provides news, tools, resources, and research to Californians 50 years and older.

7436 **AARP Colorado**
303 E 17th Avenue
Denver, CO 80203-5012
866-554-5376
Fax: 303-764-5999
coaarp@aarp.org
states.aarp.org/region/colorado
Bob Murphy, State Director
Angela Cortez, Media Contact
The Colorado chapter seeks to keep Coloradans 50 years and older informed, engaged, and active.

7437 **AARP Connecticut**
21 Oak Street
Suite 104
Hartford, CT 06106
866-295-7279
ctaarp@aarp.org
states.aarp.org/region/connecticut
Nora Duncan, State Director
Anna Doroghazi, Assoc. State Dir., Advocacy & Outreach
With nearly 600,000 members, the chapter provides recent news, information, and events for residents of Connecticut who are 50 years and older, as well as advocating for positive social change.

7438 **AARP Delaware**
222 Delaware Avenue
Suite 1630
Wilmington, DE 19801
866-227-7441
kiapalucci@aarp.org
states.aarp.org/region/delaware
Lucretia Young, State Director
Kimberly Iapalucci, Media Contact
Provides news, advocacy, education, and lifestyle information for residents of Delaware who are 50 years and older.

7439 **AARP Florida: Doral**
3750 Nw 87th Avenue
Suite 650
Doral, FL 33178
866-595-7678
Fax: 786-804-4544
flaarp@aarp.org
states.aarp.org/region/florida
Donna L. Ginn, State President
Jeff Johnson, State Director
The chapter provides information, research, and events to 2.7 million members, and Floridians 50 years and older.

7440 **AARP Florida: St. Petersburg**
360 Central Avenue
Suite 1750
St. Petersburg, FL 33701
866-595-7678
Fax: 727-369-5191
flaarp@aarp.org
states.aarp.org/region/florida
Donna L. Ginn, State President
Jeff Johnson, State Director
The chapter provides information, research, and events to 2.7 million members, and Floridians 50 years and older.

7441 **AARP Florida: Tallahassee**
200 West College Avenue
Suite 304
Tallahassee, FL 32301
866-595-7678
Fax: 850-222-8968
flaarp@aarp.org
states.aarp.org/region/florida
Donna L. Ginn, State President
Jeff Johnson, State Director
The chapter provides information, research, and events to 2.7 million members, and Floridians 50 years and older.

7442 **AARP Georgia**
999 Peachtree Street NE
Suite 1110
Atlanta, GA 30309
866-295-7281
Fax: 404-815-7940
gaaarp@aarp.org
states.aarp.org/region/georgia
Debra Tyler-Horton, State Director
Alisa Jackson, Media Contact
The chapter strives to help Georgians 50 years and older.

7443 **AARP Hawaii**
1132 Bishop Street
Suite 1920
Honolulu, HI 96813
866-295-7282
Fax: 808-537-2288
hiaarp@aarp.org
states.aarp.org/region/hawaii
Jessica Wooley, Director, Advocacy
With 150,000 members, the chapter advocates at the state level, and provides information, resources, and volunteer opportunities.

7444 **AARP Idaho**
250 S 5th Street
Suite 800
Boise, ID 83702
866-295-7284
Fax: 208-288-4424
aarpid@aarp.org
states.aarp.org/region/idaho
Lupe Wissel, Idaho AARP State Media Relations
Randy Simon, Media Contact
The chapter advocates for and seeks to improve the lives of residents aged 50 years and older.

7445 **AARP Illinois: Chicago**
222 N LaSalle Street
Suite 710
Chicago, IL 60601
866-448-3613
Fax: 312-372-2204
aarpil@aarp.org
states.aarp.org/region/illinois
Bob Gallo, State Director
Dina Anderson, Media Contact
Advocates for and provides recent news, events, and lifestyle tips to Illinois residents aged 50 years and older.

7446 **AARP Illinois: Springfield**
300 W Edwards Street
3rd Floor
Springfield, IL 62704
866-448-3613
Fax: 217-522-7803
aarpil@aarp.org
states.aarp.org/region/illinois
Bob Gallo, State Director
Dina Anderson, Media Contact
Legislative office of the Illinois chapter.

7447 **AARP Indiana**
One N Capitol Avenue
Suite 1275
Indianapolis, IN 46204- 2025
866-448-3618
Fax: 317-423-2211
inaarp@aarp.org
states.aarp.org/region/indiana
Sarah Waddle, State Director
Jason Tomcsi, Media Contact
The chapter seeks to improve life for residents of Indiana aged 50 years and older.

7448 **AARP Iowa**
600 E Court Avenue
Suite 100
Des Moines, IA 50309
866-554-5378
Fax: 515-244-7767
ia@aarp.org
states.aarp.org/region/iowa
Brad Anderson, State Director
Jeremy Barewin, Media Contact
Provides news, information, and resources to Iowans aged 50 years and older.

7449 **AARP Kansas**
6220 SW 29th Street
Suite 300
Topeka, KS 66614
866-448-3619
Fax: 785-232-1465
ksaarp@aarp.org
states.aarp.org/region/kansas
Maren Turner, Kansas AARP State Media Relations
Mary Tritsch, Media Contact
The chapter provides news, events, and more to Kansans aged 50 years and older.

7450 **AARP Kentucky**
10401 Linn Station Road
Suite 121
Louisville, KY 40223
866-295-7275
kyaarp@aarp.org
states.aarp.org/region/kentucky
Scott Wagenast, Associate State Director
Provides news and resources for Kentuckians over the age of 50.

7451 **AARP Louisiana: Baton Rouge**
301 Main Street
Suite 1012
Baton Rouge, LA 70825
866-448-3620
la@aarp.org
states.aarp.org/region/louisiana
Denise Bottcher, State Director
Andrew Muhl, Director, Advocacy
The office seeks to advocate for and provide resources to residents of Louisiana aged 50 and over.

7452 **AARP Louisiana: New Orleans**
3502 S Carrollton Avenue
Suite C
New Orleans, LA 70118
866-448-3620
la@aarp.org
states.aarp.org/region/louisiana
Denise Bottcher, State Director
Andrew Muhl, Director, Advocacy
AARP Louisiana's Community Resource Center.

7453 **AARP Maine**
53 Baxter Boulevard
Suite 202
Portland, ME 04101
866-554-5380
me@aarp.org
states.aarp.org/region/maine
Lori Parham, State Director
Amy Gallant, Director, Advocacy and Outreach
Seeks to enhance the lives of Mainers aged 50 years and over through advocacy, information sharing, volunteer opportunities, and service. The chapter counts 230,000 members.

7454 **AARP Maryland**
200 St. Paul Place
Suite 2510
Baltimore, MD 21202
866-542-8163
Fax: 410-837-0269
md@aarp.org
states.aarp.org/region/maryland
Jim Campbell, State President
Nancy Carr, Assoc. State Director, Communications
The chapter seeks to enhance the lives of Maryland residents aged 50 and over, as well as caregivers, through resources and a variety of social opportunities.

7455 **AARP Massachusetts**
1 Beacon Street
Suite 2301
Boston, MA 02108
866-448-3621
Fax: 617-723-4224
ma@aarp.org
states.aarp.org/region/massachusetts
Mike Festa, State Director
Cindy Campbell, Director, Communications
Provides news, events, and resources to Massachusetts residents aged 50 and over.

7456 **AARP Michigan**
309 N Washington Square
Suite 110
Lansing, MI 48933
866-227-7448
Fax: 517-482-2794
miaarp@aarp.org
states.aarp.org/region/michigan
Paula D. Cunningham, State Director
The chapter seeks to enhance the quality of life for aging residents of Michigan through information, advocacy, and services.

7457 **AARP Minnesota**
1919 University Avenue
Suite 500
St. Paul, MN 55104
866-554-5381
aarpmn@aarp.org
states.aarp.org/region/minnesota
Will Phillips, State Director
Maro Jo George, Associate State Director, Advocacy
Aims to connect aging residents of Minnesota with financial and other resources to enhance quality of life.

7458 **AARP Mississippi**
141 Township Avenue
Suite 302
Ridgeland, MS 39157
866-554-5382
Fax: 601-898-5429
msaarp@aarp.org
states.aarp.org/region/mississippi
John McDonald, AARP Missouri State Director
Ronda Gooden, Media Contact
Seeks to improve the lives of Mississippians, particularly those over 50 years of age, through events, news, resources, and advocacy.

7459 **AARP Missouri**
9200 Ward Parkway
Suite 350
Kansas City, MO 64114
866-389-5627
Fax: 816-561-3107
aarpmo@aarp.org
states.aarp.org/region/missouri
Craig Eichelman, State Director
Jamayla Long, Media Contact
Provides information to Missourians aged 50 and over on health, finances, and lifestyle, as well as providing advocacy.

7460 **AARP Montana**
30 W 14th Street
Suite 301
Helena, MT 59601
866-295-7278
mtaarp@aarp.org
states.aarp.org/region/montana
Tim Summers, State Director
Stacia Dahl, Media Contact
With 150,000 members, the chapter provides advocacy, education, information, resources, and collaborative projects for Montana residents aged 50 and over.

7461 **AARP Nebraska: Lincoln**
301 S 13th Street
Suite 201
Lincoln, NE 68508
866-389-5651
Fax: 402-323-6908
neaarp@aarp.org
states.aarp.org/region/nebraska
Connie Benjamin, AARP Nebraska State President
Devorah Lanner, Media Contact
Works on behalf of over 200,000 members and their families to provide news, services, information, resources, and advocacy for individuals 50 years and older.

7462 **AARP Nebraska: Omaha**
1941 S 42nd Street
Suite 220
Omaha, NE 68105
402-398-9568
omnebraska@aol.com
states.aarp.org/region/nebraska
Connie Benjamin, AARP Nebraska State President
Devorah Lanner, Media Contact
AARP Nebraska's Information Center.

7463 **AARP Nevada**
5820 S Eastern Avenue
Suite 190
Las Vegas, NV 89119
866-389-5652
aarpnv@aarp.org
states.aarp.org/region/nevada
Maria Dent, State Director
Scott Gulbransen, Media Contact
Provides news, information, and resources to 320,000 members, on matters affecting the lives of individuals aged 50 and over.

7464 **AARP New Hampshire**
45 South Main Street
Suite 202
Concord, NH 03301
866-542-8168
Fax: 603-224-6211
nh@aarp.org
states.aarp.org/region/new-hampshire
Todd Fahey, State Director
Doug McNutt, Associate State Director, Advocacy
Provides information, resources, and advocacy services to 228,000 members, on matters relevant to individuals aged 50 years and older.

7465 **AARP New Jersey**
303 George Street
Suite 505
New Brunswick, NJ 08901
866-542-8165
Fax: 609-987-4634
aarpnJ@aarp.org
states.aarp.org/region/new-jersey
Stephanie Hunsinger, State Director
Jeff Abramo, Media Contact
The chapter seeks to educate and advocate for New Jersey residents aged 50 and over, and their families.

7466 **AARP New Mexico**
535 Cerrillos Road
Suite A
Santa Fe, NM 87501
866-389-5636
Fax: 505-820-2889
aarpnm@aarp.org
states.aarp.org/region/new-mexico
Jennifer Baier, Interim State Director
DeAnza Valencia, Associate State Director, Advocacy
The chapter advocates on behalf of individuals 50 years and older, monitoring seniors' services, utility rates, transportation services, as well as providing financial planning services to members.

7467 **AARP New York: Albany**
1 Commerce Plaza
Suite 706
Albany, NY 12260
866-227-7442
nyaarp@aarp.org
states.aarp.org/region/new-york
Beth Finkel, State President
Erik Kriss, Media Contact
Provides information, resources, news, and advocacy services to residents of New York who are 50 years and older.

7468 **AARP New York: New York City**
750 Third Avenue
31st Floor
New York, NY 10017
866-227-7442
nyaarp@aarp.org
states.aarp.org/region/new-york
Beth Finkel, State President
Erik Kriss, Media Contact
Provides information, resources, news, and advocacy services to residents of New York who are 50 years and older.

7469 **AARP New York: Rochester**
435 E Henrietta Road
Rochester, NY 14620
866-227-7442
nyaarp@aarp.org
states.aarp.org/region/new-york
Beth Finkel, State President
Erik Kriss, Media Contact
Provides information, resources, news, and advocacy services to residents of New York who are 50 years and older.

7470 AARP North Carolina
5511 Capital Center Drive
Suite 400
Raleigh, NC 27606
866-389-5650
ddickerson@aarp.org
states.aarp.org/region/north-carolina
Doug Dickerson, State Director
Michael Oldender, Manager, Outreach and Advocacy
Advocates for community issues such as health care, employment/income security, retirement planning, utilities, and protection from financial abuse, on behalf of a membership 1.1 million strong.

7471 AARP North Dakota
107 W Main Avenue
Suite 125
Bismarck, ND 58501
866-554-5383
Fax: 701-255-2242
aarpnd@aarp.org
states.aarp.org/region/north-dakota
Josh Askvig, State Director
Doreen Redman, Assoc. State Dir., Community Outreach
Provides news, information, resources, events, advocacy, and more to North Dakotans aged 50 and over.

7472 AARP Ohio
17 S High Street
Suite 800
Columbus, OH 43215
866-389-5653
Fax: 614-224-9801
ohaarp@aarp.org
states.aarp.org/region/ohio
Barbara Sykes, State Director
The chapter shares information, advocates, and performs community services for 1.5 million members, 50 years and older, across the state.

7473 AARP Oklahoma
126 N Bryant Avenue
Edmond, OK 73034
866-295-7277
Fax: 405-844-7772
ok@aarp.org
states.aarp.org/region/oklahoma
Sean Voskuhl, State Director
Chad Mullen, Associate State Director, Advocacy
Assists individuals aged 50 and over through advocacy, news, information, resources, and more.

7474 AARP Oregon
9200 SE Sunnybrook Boulevard
Suite 410
Clackamas, OR 97015
866-554-5360
oraarp@aarp.org
states.aarp.org/region/oregon
Ruby Haughton-Pitts, State Director
Joyce DeMonnin, Media Contact
Strives for social change for its 500,000 members, and all individuals 50 years and over, through advocacy and community services.

7475 AARP Pennsylvania: Harrisburg
30 N 3rd Street
Suite 750
Harrisburg, PA 17101
866-389-5654
Fax: 717-236-4078
aarpa@aarp.org
states.aarp.org/region/pennsylvania
Bill Johnston-Walsh, State Director
Steve Gardner, Media Contact
Seeks to enhance the quality of life for 1.8 million members across the state.
1919

7476 AARP Pennsylvania: Philadelphia
1650 Market Street
Suite 675
Philadelphia, PA 19103
866-389-5654
Fax: 215-665-8529
aarpa@aarp.org
states.aarp.org/region/pennsylvania
Bill Johnston-Walsh, State Director
Steve Gardner, Media Contact
Seeks to enhance the quality of life for 1.8 million members across the state.

7477 AARP Rhode Island
10 Orms Street
Suite 200
Providence, RI 02904
866-542-8170
Fax: 401-272-0596
ri@aarp.org
states.aarp.org/region/rhode-island
Kathleen Connell, State Director
John Martin, Director, Communications
Provides news, information, resources, advocacy, and community services to those aged 50 and older in the state.

7478 AARP South Carolina
1201 Main Street
Suite 1720
Columbia, SC 29201
803-765-7381
866-389-5655
scaarp@aarp.org
states.aarp.org/region/south-carolina
Teresa Arnold, State Director
Nikki Hutchison, Associate State Director, Advocacy
Seeks to enhance the quality of life for members and individuals aged 50 and older, through information, resources, education, advocacy, and more.

7479 AARP South Dakota
5101 S Nevada Avenue
Suite 150
Sioux Falls, SD 57108
866-542-8172
sdaarp@aarp.org
states.aarp.org/region/south-dakota
Erik Gaikowski, State Director
Provides news, information, resources, advocacy, and community services to 110,000 members and those aged 50 and older in the state.

7480 AARP Tennessee
150 4th Avenue N
Suite 1350
Nashville, TN 37219
866-295-7274
tnaarp@aarp.org
states.aarp.org/region/tennessee
Rebecca Kelly, State Director
Rob Naylor, Director, Communications
Strives for positive social change for 660,000 members and individuals aged 50 and over.

7481 AARP Texas: Austin
1905 Aldrich Street
Suite 210
Austin, TX 78723
866-227-7443
states.aarp.org/region/texas
Bob Jackson, State Director
Junita Jiminez-Soto, Associate State Director, Communications
The chapter offers news, information, research, and events for individuals aged 50 and over, as well as conducting advocacy on their behalf.

7482 AARP Texas: Dallas
8140 Walnut Hill Lane
Suite 108
Dallas, TX 75231
866-227-7443
states.aarp.org/region/texas
Bob Jackson, State Director
Junita Jiminez-Soto, Associate State Director, Communications
The chapter offers news, information, research, and events for individuals aged 50 and over, as well as conducting advocacy on their behalf.

7483 **AARP Texas: Houston**
2323 S Shepherd Drive
Suite 1100
Houston, TX 77019
866-227-7443
states.aarp.org/region/texas
Bob Jackson, State Director
Junita Jiminez-Soto, Associate State Director, Communications
The chapter offers news, information, research, and events for individuals aged 50 and over, as well as conducting advocacy on their behalf.

7484 **AARP Texas: San Antonio**
1314 Guadalupe Street
Suite 209
San Antonio, TX 78207
866-227-7443
states.aarp.org/region/texas
Bob Jackson, State Director
Junita Jiminez-Soto, Associate State Director, Communications
The chapter offers news, information, research, and events for individuals aged 50 and over, as well as conducting advocacy on their behalf.

7485 **AARP Utah**
6975 Union Park Center
Suite 320
Midvale, UT 84047
866-448-3616
Fax: 801-561-2209
utaarp@aarp.org
states.aarp.org/region/utah
Alan Ormsby, State Director
Danny Harris, Director, Advocacy
Serves 211,000 members in 10 regions across the state, with advocacy, communications, programming, and outreach.

7486 **AARP Vermont**
199 Main Street
Suite 225
Burlington, VT 05401
866-227-7451
Fax: 802-651-9805
vtaarp@aarp.org
states.aarp.org/region/vermont
Greg Marchildon, State Director
Seeks to represent the concerns and interests of Vermonters aged 50 and over.

7487 **AARP Virginia**
707 E Main Street
Suite 910
Richmond, VA 23219
866-542-8164
Fax: 804-819-1923
vaaarp@aarp.org
states.aarp.org/region/virginia
Jim Dau, State Director
Serves Virginians aged 50 and older, and their families, through advocacy, information, resources, and outreach.

7488 **AARP Washington**
18000 International Blvd.
Suite 1020
SeaTac, WA 98188
866-227-7457
Fax: 206-517-9350
waaarp@aarp.org
states.aarp.org/region/washington
Doug Shadel, State Director
Serves 950,000 members through information, advocacy, and a variety of services.

7489 **AARP Washington DC**
100 M Street SE
Suite 650
Washington, DC 20003
866-554-5384
Fax: 202-434-7946
dcaarp@aarp.org
states.aarp.org/region/washington-dc
Louis Davis, Jr., State Director
Peter Rankin, Associate State Director, Advocacy
Provides information, advocacy, and a variety of services to 87,000 members aged 50 and over.

7490 **AARP West Virginia**
300 Summers Street
Suite 400
Charleston, WV 25301
866-227-7458
Fax: 304-344-4633
wvaarp@aarp.org
states.aarp.org/region/west-virginia
Gaylene Miller, State Director
Tom Hunter, Associate State Director, Communications
Provides information, resources, advocacy, and more to individuals aged 50 and over in West Virginia.

7491 **AARP Wisconsin**
222 W Washington Avenue
Suite 600
Madison, WI 53703
866-448-3611
Fax: 608-251-7612
wistate@aarp.org
states.aarp.org/region/wisconsin
Sam Wilson, State Director
Jim Flaherty, Media Contact
The chapter advocates for, and provides a variety of services to, its 840,000 members, aged 50 years and over.

7492 **AARP Wyoming**
2020 Carey Avenue
Mezzanine
Cheyenne, WY 82009
866-663-3290
wyaarp@aarp.org
states.aarp.org/region/wyoming
Sam Shumway, State Director
Tom Lacock, Assoc. State Dir., Advocacy & Comm.
Provides resources, information, and advocates for individuals in Wyoming aged 50 and older, with an emphasis on health care, retirement, and utility issues.

7493 **ABA Commission on Law and Aging**
1050 Connecticut Avenue
Suite 400
Washington, DC 20003
202-662-8690
Fax: 202-662-8698
aging@americanbar.org
www.americanbar.org/aging
Charles P. Sabatino, JD, Director
Erica F. Wood, JD, Assistant Director
The Commission examines the issues that affect the elderly as victims of abuse, dispute resolution, international rights, medicare, voting, health care decision-making and other issues arising from the aging prisons populations.

7494 **ACL Regional Support Center: Region I**
Administration for Community Living
John F. Kennedy Building
Room 2075
Boston, MA 02203
617-565-1158
Fax: 617-565-4511
www.acl.gov
Jennifer Throwe, Regional Administrator
Region I includes CT, MA, ME, NH, RI, and VT.

7495 **ACL Regional Support Center: Region II**
Administration for Community Living
26 Federal Plaza
Room 38-102
New York, NY 10278
212-264-2976
Fax: 212-264-0114
www.acl.gov
Kathleen Otte, Regional Administrator
Region II includes NY, NJ, PR, and VI.

7496 **ACL Regional Support Center: Region III**
Administration for Community Living
801 Market St.
Philadelphia, PA 19107
267-831-2329
www.acl.gov
Rhonda Schwartz, Regional Administrator
Region III includes DC, DE, MD, PA, VA, and WV.

7497 **ACL Regional Support Center: Region IV**
Administration for Community Living
Atlanta Federal Center
61 Forsyth St. SW, Suite 5M69
Atlanta, GA 30303-8909
404-562-7600
Fax: 404-562-7598
www.acl.gov

Costas Miskis, Regional Administrator
Region IV includes AL, FL, GA, KY, MS, NC, SC, and TN.

7498 **ACL Regional Support Center: Region IX**
Administration for Community Living
90 7th St.
T-1800
San Francisco, CA 94103
415-437-8780
Fax: 415-437-8782
www.acl.gov

Fay Gordon, Regional Administrator
Region IX includes CA, NV, AZ, HI, GU, CNMI, and AS.

7499 **ACL Regional Support Center: Region V**
Administration for Community Living
233 N Michigan Ave.
Suite 790
Chicago, IL 60601-5527
312-938-9858
Fax: 312-886-8533
www.acl.gov

Amy Wiatr-Rodriguez, Regional Administrator
Region V includes IL, IN, MI, MN, OH, and WI.

7500 **ACL Regional Support Center: Region VI**
Administration for Community Living
1301 Young St.
Suite 106-850
Dallas, TX 75201
214-767-1865
Fax: 214-767-2951
www.acl.gov

Derek Lee, Regional Administrator
Region VI includes AR, LA, OK, NM, and TX.

7501 **ACL Regional Support Center: Region VII**
Administration for Community Living
601 E 12th St.
Suite S-1801
Kansas City, MO 64106
816-702-4180
www.acl.gov

Lacey Boven, Regional Administrator
Region VII includes IA, KS, MO, and NE.

7502 **ACL Regional Support Center: Region VIII**
Administration for Community Living
1961 Stout St.
Denver, CO 80294-3638
303-844-2951
Fax: 303-844-2943
www.acl.gov

Percy Devine, Regional Administrator
Region VIII includes CO, MT, UT, WY, ND, and SD.

7503 **ACL Regional Support Center: Region X**
Administration for Community Living
701 Fifth Ave., M/S RX-33
Suite 1600
Seattle, WA 98104
206-615-2299
Fax: 206-615-2305
www.acl.gov

Louise Ryan, Regional Administrator
Region X includes AK, ID, OR, and WA.

7504 **AMDA - The Society for Post-Acute andLong-Term Care Medicine**
10500 Little Patuxent Parkway
Suite 210
Columbia, MD 21044
410-740-9743
800-876-2632
Fax: 410-740-4572
info@paltc.org

Arif Nazir, MD, FACP, CMD, President
Karl Steinberg, MD, HMCD, Vice President
The only medical specialty society representing the community of over 50,000 medical directors, physicians, nurse practitioners, physician assistants, and other practitioners working in the various post-acute and long-term care (PA/LTC) settings.
1919

7505 **Academy for Gerontology in HigherEducation**
1220 L Street NW
Suite 901
Washington, DC 20005
202-289-9806
membership@geron.org
www.aghe.org

Judith L. Howe, President
Lisa Hollis-Sawyer, Treasurer
Membership organization comprised of more than 130 colleges and universities that offer education and research program in the field of aging. Affiliated with the Gerontological Society of America.
1919

7506 **Aging Life Care Association**
3275 W Ina Road
Suite 130
Tucson, AZ 85741-2198
520-881-8008
Fax: 520-325-7925
info@aginglifecare.org
www.aginglifecare.org

Julie Wagner, Interim CEO
Amanda Mizell, Member Relations
Julie Wagner, Director of Administration
Joseph Lutovsky, Manager of Technology
A nonprofit association providing geriatric care for aging individuals through sharing of knowledge in 8 areas: health and disability, financial matters, housing, planning, local resources, advocacy, legal and crisis intervention.

7507 **Aging Services of Michigan**
201 North Washington Square
Suite 920
Lansing, MI 48933
517-323-3687
Fax: 517-323-4569
www.leadingagemi.org

David Herbel, President & CEO
Deanna Mitchell, Senior Vice President for Performance & Education
Aging Services of Michigan represents and supports organizations that provide services to the elderly and disabled adults. Types of supports offered by Aging Services include advocacy, education and other programs that enhance an organization's ability to serve their constituencies.

7508 **Aging Services of South Carolina**
2711 Middleburg Dr
Suite 309-A
Columbia, SC 29204
803-988-0005
Fax: 803-988-1017
www.leadingagesc.org

Frazier Jackson, Chair
Vickie Moody, President
Aging Services of South Carolina represents non-profit organizations dedicated to providing high-quality health care, housing and services to the seniors of South Carolina. Supports include public policy initiatives and education.

7509 **Aging Services of Washington**
1102 Broadway
Suite 201
Tacoma, WA 98402
253-964-8870
Fax: 253-964-8876
info@leadingagewa.org
leadingagewa.org

Jay Woolford, Chair
Deb Murphy, CEO
Laura Hofmann, Director, Clinical & Nursing Facility Services
LeighBeth Merrick, Director, Senior Living & Community Services
LeadingAge Washington is a state association supporting non-profit organizations that specialize in housing and long term care for the elderly. Supports offered include advocacy, education and more.

7510 **Aging and Disability Services**
2100 Washington Blvd
4th Floor
Arlington, VA 22204
703-228-1700
TTY: 703-228-1788
arlaaa@arlingtonva.us
aging-disability.arlingtonva.us
Anita Friedman, Director, Department of Human Services
The Aging and Disability Services Division offers care coordination, home care, and supportive services to the aging residents of Arlington. Services are provided to adults over 60, adults with developmental disabilities and their caregivers.

7511 **Aging in America**
2975 Westchester Ave
Suite 301
Purchase, NY 10577
914-205-5030
Fax: 718-824-4242
contact@agingin america.org
aginginamerica.org
Katharine Weiss, Chair
William T Smith, President & CEO
Dina Nejman, Service Coordinator
Kathleen Bufano, Executive Assistant
Non-profit organization providing services for individuals and caregivers to assist them with the challenges of aging. One strategy employed towards this goal is collaboration with other organizations with experience in senior housing and community based services.

7512 **AgingCare**
www.agingcare.com

7513 **Alliance for Aging Research**
1700 K Street NW
Suite 740
Washington, DC 20006
202-293-2856
info@agingresearch.org
www.agingresearch.org
Sue Peschin, President & CEO
Sue Peschin, President & CEO
Kelsey Allcorn, Health Programs Coordinator
Non-profit organization dedicated to supporting and accelerating the pace of medical discoveries to vastly improve the universal human experience of aging and health.

7514 **Alliance for Retired Americans**
815 16th Street NW
4th Floor
Washington, DC 20006
202-637-5399
retiredamericans.org
Robert Roach, Jr., President
Joseph Peters, Jr., Secretary & Treasurer
Joe Etta Brown, Executive Vice President
Liz Shuler, Executive Vice President
National grassroots organization advocates for a progressive political and social agenda that improves the lives of retirees and older Americans.
1920

7515 **American Aging Association**
2885 Sanford Ave SW
Suite 39542
Grandville, MI 49418
contact@americanagingassociation.org
www.americanagingassociation.org
Janko Nikolich-Zugich, Chair & CEO
Christian Sell, President
Dudley Lamming, Secretary
A group of experts dedicated to understanding the basic mechanisms of aging and the development of interventions in age-related diseases to increase human lifespans. This is accomplished through biomedical aging studies and public education.

7516 **American Association for GeriatricPsychiatry**
6728 Old McLean Village Drive
McLean, VA 22101
703-556-9222
Fax: 703-556-8729
main@aagponline.org
www.aagponline.org
Christopher Wood, Executive Director
Information and resources for physician members and affiliates on improving quality of life for older persons with mental disorders. Provides news, facts, tools and expert information for adults coping with mental health issues and aging.
1919

7517 **American Association of Retired Persons**
601 E Street NW
Washington, DC 20049
202-434-3525
888-687-2277
888-687-2277
member@aarp.org
www.aarp.org
Jo Ann Jenkins, Chief Executive Officer
Scott Frisch, Executive Vice-President and COO
Cindy Lewin, Executive Vice President & General Counsel
Karen L Mercer, Senior Vice President & Treasurer
AARP is the nation's leading organization for people age 50 and older. It serves their needs and interests through information and education, advocacy and community services provided by a network of local chapters and experienced volunteers.

7518 **American Disabled for Attendant Programs Today (ADAPT)**
4513 Tyson Ave.
Philadelphia, PA 19135
adapt.org

7519 **American Geriatrics Society**
40 Fulton Street
18th Floor
New York, NY 10038
212-308-1414
Fax: 212-832-8646
info.amger@americangeriatrics.org
www.americangeriatrics.org
Nancy E. Lundebjerg, CEO
Elvy Ickowicz, Senior Vice President of Operations
Alanna Goldstein, Director of Public Affairs & Advocacy
The premier professional organization of healthcare providers dedicated to improving the health and well-being of older adults. With an active membership of over 6,000 health care professionals, the AGS has a long history of affecting change in the provision of healthcare in older adults. The AGS Foundation for Health in Aging (FHA) aims to build a bridge between the research and practice of geriatrics health care professionals and the public.
1919

7520 **American Planning Association**
205 N Michigan Ave
Suite 1200
Chicago, IL 60601
312-431-9100
Fax: 312-786-6700
foundation@planning.org
www.planning.org/ontheradar/aging/
Mary Kay Peck, FAICP, Chair
James Drinan, CEO
Ann Simms, Chief Operating Officer
Harriet Bogdanowicz, Chief Communications Officer
An association supporting planners to develop communities that would be more livable for aging people. The association offers membership, a knowledge center, publications, conferences and meetings, certification, policy and advocacy services, community outreach and more.

7521 **American Public Health Association**
800 I St. NW
Washington, DC 20001
202-777-2742
Fax: 202-777-2534
TTY: 202-777-2500
www.apha.org
Georges C. Benjamin, Executive Director
James Carbo, Chief of Staff
Regina Davis Moss, Associate Executive Director
Kemi Oluwafemi, Chief Financial Officer
The association works to protect all Americans and their communities from preventable, serious health threats.

7522 **American Society for Neurochemistry**
9037 Ron Den Lane
Windermere, FL 34786 407-909-9064
Fax: 407-876-0750
asnmanager@asneurochem.org
asneurochem.org

Sheilah Jewart, Executive Director
Karen Gottlieb, Conference Coordinator
The Society aims to advance and promote cellular and molecular neuroscience knowledge, and to facilitate communication and the dissemination of information within the field and with related disciplines.

7523 **American Society on Aging**
575 Market Street
Suite 2100
San Francisco, CA 94105 415-974-9600
800-537-9728
Fax: 415-974-0300
info@asaging.org
www.asaging.org

Peter Kaldes, President & CEO
Robert R. Lowe, COO
Robert R Lowe, Chief Operating Officer
Carole Anderson, Vice President of Education
Health care and social service professionals, educators, researchers, administrators, businesspersons, students, and senior citizens. Works to enhance the well-being of older individuals and to foster unity among those working with and for the elderly. Offers 25 continuing education programs for professionals in aging-related fields. Publishes 'Aging Today,' a bi-monthly newspaper, and 'Generations, a quarterly journal.
1919

7524 **American Urogynecologic Society**
1100 Wayne Avenue
Suite 825
Silver Spring, MD 20910 301-273-0570
Fax: 301-273-0778
info@augs.org
www.augs.org

Michelle Zinnert, CEO
Colleen Hughes, COO
The leader in female pelvic medicine and reconstructive surgery.
1919

7525 **Argentum**
1650 King Street
Suite 602
Alexandria, VA 22314 703-894-1805
www.alfa.org

James Balda, President & CEO
Maribeth Bersani, COO
Argentum is the leading national association exclusively dedicated to supporting companies operating professionally managed, resident-centered senior living communities and the older adults and families they serve.
1919

7526 **Arizona Center on Aging**
1501 N Campbell
PO Box 245027
Tucson, AZ 85724 520-626-5800
Fax: 520-626-5801
info@aging.arizona.edu
www.aging.arizona.edu

Mindy Fain, MD, Co-Director
Janko Nikolich-Zugish, MD, Co-Director
The mission at Arizona Center of Aging (ACOA) is to promote healthy and functional lives for older adults through comprehensive programs in research, education and training, and clinical care.

7527 **Association for Adult Development andAging**
5999 Stevenson Avenue
Alexandria, VA 22304 www.aadaweb.org
Amber Randolph, President
A division of the American Counseling Association. Individuals holding a master's degree or its equivalent in adult counseling or a related field. Seeks to: improve the competence and skills of ACA and AADA members; expand professional work opportunities in adult development and aging counseling; promote the development of guidelines for professional preparation of counselors. Provides leadership and information to families, legislators, and communities.
1919

7528 **Association for Gerontology in Higher Education**
1220 L St NW
Suite 901
Washington, DC 20005 202-289-9806
Fax: 202-289-9824
geron@geron.org
www.aghe.org

Nina M Silverstein, President
Judith L Howe, President-Elect
Dana B Bradley, Treasurer
Karen Kopera-Frye, Secretary
Membership association of colleges and universities offering gerontology education, training, and research programs on the subject of aging. The association seeks to enhance the knowledge and skills of those who work with older adults and their families.

7529 **Association of Jewish Aging Services**
2519 Connecticut Ave NW
Washington, DC 20008 202-543-7500
Fax: 202-543-4090
info@ajas.org
www.ajas.org

Daniel Reingold, Chair
Don Shulman, President & CEO
Rachel Stevens, Director of Operations
Michael l Sattell, Treasurer
The Association of Jewish Aging Services is a non-profit community-based organization offering support services for the aging population. Inspired by Jewish values, the organization offers resources, conferences, education, professional development and advocacy to its members so they could better serve their communities.

7530 **Association on Aging with Developmental Disabilities**
2385 Hampton Ave.
St. Louis, MO 63139 314-647-8100
Fax: 314-647-8105
agingwithdd@msn.com
agingwithdd.org

Pamela Merkle, Executive Director
Michelle Darden, Program Development Coordinator
Erika Donaldson, Department Director
The organization offers services to accommodate the complex needs of older adults with developmental disabilities such as cerebral palsy, epilepsy, autism, severe learning disabilities and head injuries.

7531 **BrightFocus Foundation**
22512 Gateway Center Drive
Clarksburg, MD 20871 800-437-2423
Fax: 301-258-9454
info@brightfocus.org
www.brightfocus.org

Stacy Pagos Haller, President & CEO
Offers updated and trustworthy information on research, treatments, and resources. Free publications and newsletters.
1919

7532 **Brookdale Center for Healthy Aging**
2180 Third Avenue
8th Floor
New York, NY 10035 212-396-7835
Fax: 212-396-7852
info@brookdale.org
www.brookdale.org

Ruth K. Finkelstein, Executive Director
Jerry Antonatos, Director, Finance/Administration
Brookdale Center for Healthy Aging is one of the country's first university-based gerontology centers. The Center is dedicated to improving the lives of older adults through research, professional development, and advancements in policy and practice. Brookdale works to ensure that aging is framed not as a disease, but as another stage in the life course.
1919

7533 **CARF International**
6951 East Southpoint Rd.
Tucson, AZ 85756-9407
520-325-1044
888-281-6531
Fax: 520-318-1129
TTY: 520-495-7077
info@carf.org
carf.org

Brian J. Boon, President & CEO
Leslie Ellis-Lang, Managing Director, Child & Youth Services
Darren M. Lehrfeld, Chief Accreditation Officer
Di Shen, Chief Research Officer

An independent, nonprofit accreditor of human service providers in the areas of aging services, behavioral health, child and youth services, DMEPOS, employment and community services, medical rehabilitation, and opioid treatment programs.

7534 **Center for Benefits Access**
National Council on Aging
251 18th Street S
Suite 500
Arlington, VA 22202
571-527-3900
centerforbenefits@ncoa.org
www.ncoa.org/centerforbenefits

Leslie Fried, Director

Benefits outreach and enrollment for seniors and younger adults with disabilities.
1919

7535 **Center for Healthy Aging**
National Council on Aging
251 18th Street S
Suite 500
Arlington, VA 22202
571-527-3900
cha@ncoa.org
www.ncoa.org

Binod Suwal, Senior Program Manager

Helping older adults live longer and healthier lives through evidence-based health promotion and disease prevention programs.
1919

7536 **Center for Medicare Advocacy**
PO Box 350
Willimantic, CT 06226
860-456-7790
Fax: 860-456-2614
mshepard@medicareadvocacy.org
www.medicareadvocacy.org

Judith A. Stein, Executive Director
Matthew Shepard, Media Contact

Offers consultation, training, presentation, and materials on an array of topics pertaining to aging.
1919

7537 **Center for Positive Aging**
1440 Dutch Valley Place NE
Suite 120
Atlanta, GA 30324
404-872-9191
Fax: 404-872-1737
www.centerforpositiveaging.org

Ginny Helms, President & CEO
Jacque Thornton, SVP
Jacque Thornton, Sr. Vice President
Susan Watkins, Director of Member Services

The Center for Positive Aging is a partnership of individuals, community organizations and congregations working together to provide health, educational and recreational opportunities for older persons and their families. Through our programs, services, and affiliations, we educate people of all ages and walks of life about living independent and creative lives.
1919

7538 **Children of Aging Parents**
PO Box 167
Richboro, PA 18954-0167
800-227-7294
Fax: 215-945-8720

Louise Fradkin, Co-Founder
Mirca Liberti, Co-Founder

A non-profit clearinghouse for caregivers of the elderly, providing information, referral, educational programs and materials to caregivers.

7539 **Colorado Association of Homes and Services for the Aging**
1888 Sherman St
Suite 610
Denver, CO 80203
303-837-8834
Fax: 303-837-8836
Karen@CAHSA.org
www.cahsa.org

Maureen Hewitt, President
Lynn O'Connor, President-Elect
Laura Landwirth, Executive Director
Karen Simmering, Director of Operations

The association represents nonprofit organizations dedicated to providing health care and housing services to Colorado's elderly. Some services provided by the association include information and education to assist in developing programs for long term care.

7540 **Easter Seals**
40 Holly St.
Suite 401
Toronto, ON, Canada M4S-3C3
416-932-8382
877-376-6362
Fax: 416-932-9844
info@easterseals.ca
www.easterseals.ca

Dave Starrett, President & CEO
Frank Williamson, Director, Finance
Casey Sabawi, Senior Manager, National Corporate Partnerships

Provides services to those with disabilities to help them achieve greater independence, accessibility, and integration.
1919

7541 **Experience Works**
4401 Wilson Boulevard
Suite 220
Arlington, VA 22203
703-522-7272
866-397-9757
www.experienceworks.org

Sally A. Boofer, President & CEO
Rosemary Schmidt, CFO

Helps low income seniors with multiple barriers to employment, get the training they need to find good jobs in their local community.
1919

7542 **Family Caregiver Alliance/National Centeron Caregiving**
101 Montgomery Street
Suite 2150
San Francisco, CA 94104
415-434-3388
800-445-8106
www.caregiver.org

Jacquelyn Kung, PhD, Chief Executive Officer
Wyatt Ritchie, MBA, Managing Director

Caregiver information and assistance via phone or e-mail; fact sheets and publications describing and documenting caregiver needs and services.

7543 **Gerontological Society of America**
1220 L Street NW
Suite 901
Washington, DC 20005
202-842-1275
Fax: 202-842-1150
geron@geron.org
www.geron.org

James Appleby, Chief Executive Officer
Karen Tracy, VP, Strategic Alliances & Communications

Nonprofit professional organization with more than 5,500 members in the field of aging. Provides researchers, educators, practitioners and policy makers with opportunities to understand, advance, integrate and use basic and applied research on aging populations. Also runs the National Adult Vaccination Program (www.navp.org).

7544 **Goodwill Industries International, Inc.**
15810 Indianola Dr.
Rockville, MD 20855
contactus@goodwill.org
www.goodwill.org

Steven C. Preston, President & CEO

Goodwill strives to achieve the full participation in society of disabled persons and other individuals with special needs by expanding their opportunities and occupational capabilities through a network of autonomous, nonprofit, community-based organizations providing services throughout the world in response to local needs.

7545 **Goodwill Industries-Suncoast**
10596 Gandy Boulevard
St. Petersburg, FL 33702
727-523-1512
888-279-1988
www.goodwill-suncoast.org

Heather Ceresoli, CPA, Chair
Deborah A. Passerini, President & CEO
A nonprofit, community-based organization whose mission is to help people achieve self-sufficiency through the dignity and power of work, serving people who are disadvantaged, disabled or elderly. The mission is accomplished through providing independent living skills, affordable housing, and training and placement in community employment.
1919

7546 **Harvey A. Friedman Center for Aging**
Washington University
St. Louis, Campus Box 8217
660 S Euclid
St. Louis, MO 63110
314-747-9212
centerforaging@wustl.edu
publichealth.wustl.edu/aging

Nancy Morrow-Howell, PhD, Director
Natalie Galucia, Center Manager
The Center promotes research, education, policy and service initiatives that enable older adults to remain healthy, active, empowered, contributing and independent for as long as possible.
1919

7547 **Healthy Aging Association**
3500 Coffee Rd
Suite 19
Modesto, CA 95355
209-523-2800
Fax: 209-523-2800
healthy.aging2000@gmail.com
www.healthyagingassociation.org

Mike Mallory, Board President
Dianna L Olsen, Executive Director
Samantha Borba, MA, Fitness Program Manager
Erlinda Bourcier, BA, Health Educator & Senior Coalition Coordinator
A non-profit organization whose mission is to help older Americans live longer, healthier, more independent lives by promoting increased physical activity through fitness programs.

7548 **Heart Touch Project™**
3400 Airport Avenue
Suite 42
Santa Monica, CA 90405
310-391-2558
Fax: 310-391-2168
www.hearttouch.org

Shawnee Isaac Smith, Co-Founder
Rene Russo, Co-Founder
Non-profit, educational and service organization devoted to the delivery of compassionate and healing touch to home or hospital-bound men, women, and children.
1919

7549 **Institute for Life Course and Aging**
246 Bloor Street W.
Room 238
Toronto, Ontario, Canada M5S-1V4
416-978-0377
Fax: 416-978-4771
aging@utoronto.ca
www.grandparentfamily.com

Esme Fuller-Thomson, Director
Susan Murphy, Administration
The Institute is a research center under the auspices of the Faculty of Social Work at the University of Toronto.

7550 **International Federation on Aging**
1 Bridgepoint Drive
Toronto, Ontario, Canada M4M-2B5
416-342-1655
Fax: 416-639-2165
jbarratt@ifa-fiv.org
www.ifa-fiv.org

Greg Shaw, Director, Int'l & Corporate Relations
Dr. Jane Barratt, Secretary General
The IFA seeks to inform, educate and promote policies and practice to improve the quality of life of older persons around the world.
1919

7551 **International Network for the Preventionof Elder Abuse**
The Somers Law Firm
PO Box 368
Nassau, NY 12123
518-281-2777
contactus@inpea.net
www.inpea.net

Susan B. Somers, President
Amanda Phelan, Secretary
Organization for the prevention of elder abuse.
1919

7552 **Jewish Council for the Aging**
12320 Parklawn Drive
Rockville, MD 20852
301-255-4200
senior.helpline@accessjca.org
www.accessjca.org

Norman Goldstein, President
Seeks to assist the elderly of all faiths lead independent lives. Provides transportation, job search assistance, fitness training, computer training and information and referrals. Conducts educational programs and presents an annual productive aging award. Maintains speakers' bureau.
1919

7553 **Jewish Council for the Aging of Greater Washington**
12320 Parklawn Drive
Rockville, MD 20852
301-255-4200
senior.helpline@accessjca.org
www.accessjca.org

Norman Goldstein, President
Seeks to assist the elderly of all faiths lead independent lives. Provides transportation, job search assistance, fitness training, computer training and information and referrals. Conducts educational programs and presents an annual productive aging award. Maintains speakers' bureau.
1919

7554 **Justice in Aging**
1444 Eye St NW
Suite 1100
Washington, DC 20005
202-289-6976
Fax: 202-289-7224
info@justiceinaging.org
www.justiceinaging.org

Phyllis J Holmen, Esq., Chair
Kevin Prindiville, Executive Director
Jennifer Goldberg, Directing Attorney
Tom Smith, Finance & Administration Director
Justice in Aging is a non-profit legal organization whose principal mission is to protect the rights of low-income older adults and vulnerable groups in society. Through advocacy, litigation, and training of local advocates, Justice in Aging seeks to ensure the health and economic security of those they serve.

7555 **Leadership Council of Aging Organizations**
lcao@aarp.org
www.lcao.org

7556 **Leading Age**
2519 Connecticut Avenue NW
Washington, DC 20008-1520
202-783-2242
info@LeadingAge.org
www.leadingage.org

Katie Smith Sloan, President & CEO
Nicole Fallon, Vice President, Health Policy
National association of more than 6,000 nonprofit nursing homes, continuing care retirement communities, independent liv-

ing centers and community service providers serving more than 60,000 older Americans each year.

7557 **LeadingAge**
2519 Connecticut Avenue NW
Washington, DC 20008 202-783-2242
info@leadingage.org
www.leadingage.org

Lea Chambers-Johnson, Executive Team Administrator
Robyn I Stone, Senior Vice President, Research
Cheryl Phillips, Senior Vice President, Public Policy and Health

The work of LeadingAge is focused on advocacy, leadership development, and applied research and promotion of effective services, home health, hospice, community services, senior housing, continuing care communities, nursing homes, as well as technology solutions to seniors and thers with special needs.
1919

7558 **LeadingAge Arizona**
3877 N 7th St
Suite 240
Phoenix, AZ 85014 602-230-0026
Fax: 602-230-0563
pkoester@leadingageaz.org
www.arizonaleadingage.org

Steven Kolnacki, President
Pam Koester, CEO
Donald G Isaacson, Lobbyist
Cheyenne Walsh, Lobbyist

LeadingAge Arizona is a non-profit association representing organizations that provide health care, housing and services to the elderly citizens of Arizona. The association supports these organizations by offering them leadership, education and advocacy services.

7559 **LeadingAge California**
1315 I Street
Suite 100
Sacramento, CA 95814 916-392-5111
Fax: 916-428-4250
info@leadingageca.org

Kathryn Roberts, Chair
Jeannee Parker Martin, President & CEO
Jan Guiliano, Vice President of Education
Felicia Price, Director of Meetings & Events

LeadingAge California advocates for non-profit organizations that provide health care, housing and community services to older adults. Services offered by LeadingAge include advocacy, public education and advertising.

7560 **LeadingAge Connecticut**
110 Barnes Rd
Wallingford, CT 06492 203-678-4477
Fax: 203-678-4650
leadingagect@leadingagect.org
www.leadingagect.org

William Fiocchetta, Chair
Mag Morelli, President
Nurka Carrero, Office Manager
Andrea Bellofiore, Director of Member Programs & Services

LeadingAge Connecticut is a provider of support services to nonprofit organizations serving elderly and chronically ill individuals. Supports include advocacy and information provided to members of skilled nursing facilities, intermediate care facilities, residential care homes, chronic disease hospitals, adult day centers, senior housing communities and more.

7561 **LeadingAge Gulf States**
P.O. Box 1748
Marrero, LA 70073 504-442-0483
Fax: 504-689-3982
kcontrenchis@leadingagegulfstates.org
www.leadingagegulfstates.org

Dennis Adams, Chair
Karen Contrenchis, NFA, CASP, President
Scott Crabtree, Vice Chair
Joe Townsend, Treasurer

Organization offering educational and advocacy supports to long term care organizations working in the areas of senior housing, nursing homes, adult day care, assisted living, retirement communities, Alzheimer programs and home and community based services.

7562 **LeadingAge Illinois**
1001 Warrenville Rd
Suite 150
Lisle, IL 60532 630-325-6170
Fax: 630-325-0749
info@leadingageil.org

Deb Reardanz, Chair
Karen Messer, President & CEO
Angela Schnepf, Executive Vice President
Ruta Prasauskas, Vice President of Health Services

LeadingAge Illinois represents organizations specializing in the field of senior care services, offering them advocacy, networking, public policy and employment resources to help them thrive in their missions.

7563 **LeadingAge Indiana**
PO Box 68829
Indianapolis, IN 46268-0829 317-733-2380
Fax: 317-733-2385
mrinebold@leadingageindiana.org
www.leadingageindiana.org

Mike Rinebold, President
Susan Darwent, Vice President of Operations
Kathy Johnson, RN, WCC, Vice President of Clinical & Regulatory Services
Jennifer Clark, Marketing & Membership

LeadingAge Indiana is an association representing non-profit organizations that provide health care, services and housing for seniors throughout Indiana. LeadingAge offers education, advocacy and networking opportunities to their members.

7564 **LeadingAge Iowa**
4200 University Ave
Suite 305
West Des Moines, IA 50266 515-440-4630
888-440-4630
Fax: 515-440-4631
info@leadingageiowa.org
www.leadingageiowa.org

Bert Vigen, Chair
Shannon Strickler, President & CEO
Matt Blake, Director, Government Relations & Member Services
Liz Davidson, Director of Clinical Services

LeadingAge Iowa serves non-profit and missiondriven organizations dedicated to providing quality housing, health, community, and related services to Iowa's seniors. Supports provided include advocacy, education and collaboration.

7565 **LeadingAge Kentucky**
2501 Nelson Miller Pkwy
Suite 101
Louisville, KY 40223 502-992-4380
Fax: 502-992-4390
info@leadingageky.org
leadingageky.org

Timothy Veno, President & CEO

LeadingAge Kentucky represents non-profit organizations that offer services for the elderly and the disabled. LeadingAge offers advocacy and educational services and resources to their members.

7566 **LeadingAge Maine & New Hampshire**
55 Main St
Suite 316
Newmarket, NH 03857 603-292-6441
lhenderson@leadingagemenh.org
www.leadingagemenh.org

Rebecca Smith, Chair
Deb Riddell, Vice Chair
Lisa Henderson, Executive Director
Katie Sweet, Communications & Education Manager

LeadingAge Maine & New Hampshire aims to promote the interests of its non-profit members which provide healthy, affordable and ethical long-term care to the older citizens of Maine and New Hampshire. LeadingAge offers this support through education, advocacy, representation and collaboration.

7567 **LeadingAge Massachusetts**
246 Walnut St
Suite 203
Newton, MA 02460
617-244-2999
Fax: 617-244-2995
www.leadingagema.org

Jered Stewart, Chairperson
Elissa Sherman, President
Lynn Monaghan, Events & Education Manager
Rita Kostiuk, Member Engagement Manager
LeadingAge Massachusetts represents non-profit providers of health care, housing, and services for seniors in Massachusetts. Some services offered by LeadingAge include education and events, webinars, networking opportunities, technology resources, advocacy and consumer resources.

7568 **LeadingAge Missouri**
3412 Knipp Dr
Suite 102
Jefferson City, MO 65109
573-635-6244
Fax: 573-635-6618
debbiecheshire@leadingagemissouri.org
www.leadingagemissouri.org

Chris Crouch, Chair
Bill Bates, CEO
Nancie McAnaugh, Chief Operating Officer
Debbie Cheshire, Administrative Assistant
LeadingAge Missouri's work is dedicated to assisting its members to be leaders in the delivery of quality long-term health care, housing, and services for older adults in Missouri. Some services provided by LeadingAge include advocacy, public education, consumer resources and more.

7569 **LeadingAge Nebraska**
900 N 90th St
Suite 940
Omaha, NE 68114
402-326-2790
www.leadingagene.org

Julie Sebastian, Board Chair
Jeremy Hohlen, CEO
Cheryl Wichman, Director of Professional Development
Melissa Bergoch, Administrative Support
LeadingAge Nebraska represents the full continuum of mission-driven, non-profit providers of health care, housing and services for older adults in Nebraska. Some supports offered by LeadingAge include educational conferences, webinars, workshops and advocacy.

7570 **LeadingAge New Jersey**
3705 Quakerbridge Rd
Suite 102
Hamilton, NJ 08619
609-452-1161
Fax: 609-452-2907
www.leadingagenj.org

Toni Lynn Davis, Chairperson
Michele M Kent, President & CEO
Diane Borgstrom, Finance Coordinator
Hillary Critelli, Membership & Engagement Specialist
LeadingAge New Jersey represents non-profit nursing homes, assisted living residences, residential health care centers, independent senior housing, and continuing care retirement communities throughout New Jersey. Members are supported through advocacy, education, and fellowship.

7571 **LeadingAge New York**
13 British American Blvd
Suite 2
Latham, NY 12110-1431
518-867-8383
Fax: 518-867-8384
info@leadingageny.org
www.leadingageny.org

James W Clyne, President & CEO
Daniel J Heim, Executive Vice President
Ellen Quinn, SPHR, Vice President of Human Resources
Ami Schnauber, Vice President of Advocacy & Public Policy
LeadingAge New York represents non-profit, mission-driven and public continuing care providers, including nursing homes, senior housing, adult care facilities, continuing care retirement communities, assisted living and community service providers. LeadingAge provides its members with education, publications, conferences and consultation services to help them better serve their communities.

7572 **LeadingAge North Carolina**
222 N Person St
Raleigh, NC 27601
919-571-8333
Fax: 919-571-1297
info@leadingagenc.org
www.leadingagenc.org

Robert Wernet, Chair
Tom Akins, President & CEO
Leslie Roseboro, Vice President
Jennifer Gill, Director of Strategic Communications
LeadingAge North Carolina represents non-profit providers of care, housing, health, community and related services to the elderly. One of its primary goals is to advance policies, practices and research to empower the aging population.

7573 **LeadingAge Ohio**
2233 N Bank Dr
Columbus, OH 43220
614-444-2882
Fax: 614-444-2974
info@leadingageohio.org
www.leadingageohio.org

Judy Budi, Chair
Kenneth Daniel, Vice Chair
Kathryn Brod, President & CEO
Stephanie DeWees, Quality & Regulatory Specialist
LeadingAge Ohio represents long-term care organizations. Service providers supported include those working in the fields of senior housing, adult day care, home- and community-based services, assisted living and nursing. Some supports offered by LeadingAge Ohio include policy advocacy, education, employment support and resources for families.

7574 **LeadingAge Oklahoma**
P.O. Box 1383
El Reno, OK 73036
405-640-8040
inquiry@leadingageok.org
leadingageok.org

Lindsay Fick, President
Mary Brinkley, Executive Director
Mark Gray, Public Policy Congress
Lauren Cantu, Director
LeadingAge Oklahoma represents non-profit organizations that serve the aging people of Oklahoma. LeadingAge assists these organizations through advocacy, consumer services, directories, education, a job bank and more.

7575 **LeadingAge Oregon**
7340 SW Hunziker
Suite 104
Tigard, OR 97223
503-684-3788
Fax: 503-624-0870
info@leadingageoregon.org
www.leadingageoregon.org

Greg Franks, President
Ruth Gulyas, MHA, CEO
Margaret Cervenka, Deputy Director
Denise Wetzel, Manager Membership Services
LeadingAge Oregon represents non-profits that provide housing, health care, community and related services to the elderly and disabled of Oregon. LeadingAge offers its members advocacy, networking events and education to help them succeed in their missions.

7576 **LeadingAge PA**
1100 Bent Creek Blvd
Mechanicsburg, PA 17050
717-763-5724
800-545-2270
Fax: 717-763-1057
info@leadingagepa.org
www.leadingagepa.org

Susan Drabic, Chair
Ronald Barth, President & CEO
Heidie Dolan, Office Manager & Executive Assistant
Brandie Karpew, Manager, Policy Analytics
LeadingAge PA's mission is to promote the interests of its members through education, advocacy, community forums and events. Member organizations include adult day care services, assisted living residences, home care services, skilled nursing facil-

ities and other non-profits that serve the aging population of Pennsylvania.

7577 **LeadingAge RI**
1 Virginia Ave
Providence, RI 02905
401-490-7612
Fax: 401-490-7614
TTY: 401-383-6578
info@leadingageri.org
www.leadingageri.org

Sandra Cullen, President
Stephanie Igoe, Vice President
James Nyberg, MPA, Director
Adderlin Bailey, MPH, Special Projects Assistant
LeadingAge RI seeks to advance excellence in the field of aging services by fostering innovation, collaboration, and ethical leadership through advocacy for public policy, education and professional development.

7578 **LeadingAge Texas**
2205 Hancock Dr
Austin, TX 78756
512-467-2242
Fax: 512-467-2275
info@leadingagetexas.org
www.leadingagetexas.org

Roque Christensen, Chair
George Linial, President & CEO
Melanie Harrison, Director of Education
Alyse Meyer, Director of Public Policy
LeadingAge Texas provides leadership, advocacy, and education for non-profit retirement housing and nursing home communities that serve the needs of Texas retirees.

7579 **LeadingAge Wisconsin**
204 S Hamilton St
Madison, WI 53703
608-255-7060
Fax: 608-255-7064
info@leadingagewi.org
www.leadingagewi.org

Fran Petrick, Chair
John Sauer, President & CEO
Jim Williams, Director of Member Enrichment
Denise May, Director of Business Development
LeadingAge Wisconsin is committed to advancing the fields of long-term care, assisted living and retirement living. Towards this purpose, LeadingAge offers advocacy, education and collaborative strategies to its members so they could better serve aging people.

7580 **LeadingAge Wyoming**
2005 Warren Ave
Cheyenne, WY 82001
307-632-9344
Fax: 307-632-9347
eric@wyohospitals.com
www.leadingagewyoming.org

7581 **Legal Council for Health Justice**
17 N State Street
Suite 900
Chicago, IL 60602
312-427-8990
Fax: 312-427-8419
legalcouncil.org

Tom Yates, Executive Director
Ruth Edwards, Senior Director, Program Services
Provides legal advice and services for persons who are HIV positive or have AIDS, as well as their families. Also serves individuals with disabilities and chronic illnesses, senior citizens, and the homeless.
1919

7582 **LifeSpan Network**
10280 Old Columbia Rd
Suite 220
Columbia, MD 21044
410-381-1176
Fax: 410-381-0240
www.lifespan-network.org

Dennis Hunter, Chair
Kevin Heffner, President
Danna Kauffman, Public Policy Consultant
Kathy Bernetti, CPA, Senior Vice President of Finance
Senior care provider representing more than 330 senior care provider organizations in Maryland and the District of Columbia. Lifespan members include non-profit and proprietary independent living, assisted living, continuing care retirement communities, nursing facilities, subsidized senior housing and community and hospital based services. LifeSpan provides education, advocacy, products and services to its members.

7583 **Medicare Rights Center: New York**
266 W 37th Street
3rd Floor
New York, NY 10018
212-869-3850
Fax: 212-869-3532
info@medicarerights.org
www.medicarerights.org

Frederic Riccardi, President
Seeks to ensure the rights of senior citizens and people with disabilities to quality, affordable health care. Provides counseling services to Medicare beneficiaries with health insurance problems and questions; compiles information on inquiries to detect issues and systemic problems in Medicare claims administration. Educates beneficiaries, advocates, providers, and social workers about developments in Medicare law and how to handle problems.
1919

7584 **Medicare Rights Center: Washington, DC**
1444 I Street NW
Suite 1105
Washington, DC 20005
202-637-0961
Fax: 202-637-0962
info@medicarerights.org
www.medicarerights.org

Frederic Riccardi, President
A consumer service organization that works to ensure access to affordable health care for older adults and peoplw tih disabilities through counseling and advocacy, educational programs, and public policy intiatives.
1919

7585 **National Adult Day Services Association**
11350 Random Hills Road
Suite 800
Fairfax, VA 22030
877-745-1440
info@nadsa.org
www.nadsa.org

Donna Hale, Executive Director
Lance Roberts, Associate Director, Membership
Aims to be the leading voice of the Adult Day Services industry, representing providers, associations of providers, corporations, educators, students, and retired workers.

7586 **National Alliance for Caregiving**
1730 Rhode Island Avenue NW
Suite 812
Washington, DC 20036
202-918-1013
Fax: 202-918-1014
info@caregiving.org
www.caregiving.org

C. Grace Whiting, President & CEO
Coalition of organizations focused on improving the lives of family caregivers.
1919

7587 **National Asian Pacific Center on Aging**
1511 3rd Avenue
Suite 914
Seattle, WA 98101
206-624-1221
Fax: 206-624-1023
napca.org

Joon Bang, President & CEO
Tina Masuda-Draughon, CFO
Advocating for the specific needs of aging Asian Americans and Pacific Islanders.
1919

7588 National Association for Home Care and Hospice
228 Seventh St, SE
Washington, DC 20003
202-547-7424
Fax: 202-547-3540
www.nahc.org

Denise Schrader, Chair
Val J Halamandaris, President
Lucy Andrews, Vice Chair
Karen M Thompson, Secretary
Professional association representing the interests of chronically ill, disabled, and dying Americans and their caregivers. The association offers advocacy services on policy, resources related to hospice and home care, research sponsorships, education for the public on hospice services and more.

7589 National Association of Area Agencies on Aging
1730 Rhode Island Ave, NW
Suite 1200
Washington, DC 20036
202-872-0888
Fax: 202-872-0057
info@n4a.org
www.n4a.org

Kathryn Boles, President
Doug McKenzie, Chief, Finance & Administration
Martin Kleffner, Director of Operations
Joellen Leavelle, Director of Communications
The National Association of Area Agencies on Aging (n4a) is the leading voice on aging issues for Area Agencies on Aging and a champion for Title VI Native American aging programs. n4a provides advocacy, training and technical assistance, employment support and information resources to these agencies.

7590 National Association of Counties
660 N Capitol St NW
Suite 400
Washington, DC 20001
202-393-6226
888-407-6226
Fax: 202-393-2630
nacomeetings@naco.org
www.naco.org

Bryan Desloge, President
Matthew Chase, Executive Director
Deborah Stoutamire, Director of Operations
Alicia Dorsey, Finance Director
NACO brings together elected officials and aging administrators who are interested in providing quality programs and beter policies for their older constituents. NACO members work with Congress, the Administration on Aging, and other federal agencies to ensure that the nation maintains an effective and efficient safety net of services for the elderly and their families.

7591 National Association of Nutrition and Aging Services Programs (NANASP)
1612 K St NW
Suite 200
Washington, DC 20006
202-682-6899
Fax: 202-223-2099
pcarlson@nanasp.org
www.nanasp.org

Tony Sarmiento, Chair
Robert Blancato, Executive Director
Pam Carlson, Membership & Education
Scott Carlson, Finance & Operations
A national membership organization supporting those working to provide older adults with healthy food and nutrition through community-based services. NANASP engages in advocacy on issues such as nutrition, Medicare and Medicaid, elder justice, social security and other retirement security, transportation, and older workers' issues.

7592 National Association of States United for Aging and Disabilities
1201 15th St NW
Suite 350
Washington, DC 20005
202-898-2578
Fax: 202-898-2583
info@nasuad.org
www.nasuad.org

Gary Jessee, President
Martha Roherty, Executive Director
Camille Dobson, Deputy Executive Director
Robert Alonso, Finance Director
The National Association of States United for Aging and Disabilities (NASUAD) represents the nation's agencies serving in the areas of aging and disabilitie. NASUAD supports state leadership as well as national policies that support home and community based services for seniors and individuals with disabilities.

7593 National Center on Elder Abuse
Administration for Community Living
c/o USC Keck School of Medicine
1000 South Fremont Ave., Unit 22
Alhambra, CA 91803
855-500-3537
Fax: 626-470-9978
ncea-info@aoa.hhs.gov
www.ncea.acl.gov

Laura Mosqueda, Director
The NCEA is a national resource center providing up-to-date information on elder abuse, neglect and exploitation to policy makers and the public.
1919

7594 National Clearinghouse on Abuse in Later Life
1400 E Washington Avenue
Suite 227
Madison, WI 53703
608-255-0539
Fax: 608-255-3560
ncall@wcadv.org
www.ncall.us

Bonnie Brandl, Director
Working to end abuse in later life.
1919

7595 National Committee to Preserve SocialSecurity & Medicare
111 K Street NE
Suite 700
Washington, DC 20002
202-216-0420
800-966-1935
Fax: 202-216-0446
webmaster@ncpssm.org
www.ncpssm.org

Max Richtman, President & CEO
An advocacy and education membership organization, works to protect and enhance Federal programs vital to senior's health and economic well-being.
1919

7596 National Council for Aging Care
1200 G Street NW
Washington, DC 20005
877-664-6140
www.aging.com

7597 National Council on Aging
251 18th Street S
Suite 500
Arlington, VA 22202
571-527-3900
membership@ncoa.org
www.ncoa.org

James Knickman, Interim President & CEO
Kristin Kiefer, Cheif Administrative Officer
Donna Whitt, Senior Vice President & Chief Financial Officer
Josh Hodges, Chief Customer Officer
Emphasizes the needs for in-home and community-based health care and social services designed to help older persons remain in or return to their homes and live independently, works to educate and assist voluntary organizations to help develop such services.
1919

7598 **National Falls Prevention Resource Center**
Center for Healthy Aging
251 18th Street S
Suite 500
Arlington, VA 22202
571-527-3900
www.ncoa.org

7599 **National Gerontological Nursing Association**
121 W State St
Geneva, IL 60134
630-748-4616
ngna@affinity-strategies.com
www.ngna.org

Joanne Alderman, President
Sandra Kuebler, Treasurer
Elizabeth Tanner, Secretary
An association providing clinical care for older adults. Their member organizations include clinicians, educators, and researchers specializing in different areas of senior care services.

7600 **National Hispanic Council on Aging**
734 15th St NW
Suite 1050
Washington, DC 20005
202-347-9733
Fax: 202-347-9735
nhcoa@nhcoa.org
www.nhcoa.org

Octavio Martinez, Ph.D, Chair
Yanira Cruz, Ph.D, President & CEO
Maria Eugenia Hernandez-Lane, Vice President
Amina Ferreira, Communications Specialist
The National Hispanic Council on Aging (NHCOA) works to improve quality of life for Hispanic seniors. With a Hispanic Aging Network of community-based organizations across the U.S., the District of Columbia and Puerto Rico, NHCOA aims to provide public education and adovocacy in areas such as economic security, health, and housing.

7601 **National Hospice & Palliative CareOrganization (NHPCO)**
1731 King Street
Suite 100
Alexandria, VA 22314
703-837-1500
800-646-6460
Fax: 703-837-1233
www.nhpco.org

Edo Banach, JD, President & CEO
Hannah Yang Moore, MPH, Chief Advocacy Officer
The organization seeks to improve end-of-life care, widen access to hospice care, and improve quality of life for the dying and their loved ones.
1919

7602 **National Indian Council on Aging, Inc.**
8500 Menaul Blvd. NE
Suite B470
Albuquerque, NM 87112
505-292-2001
Fax: 505-292-1922
info@nicoa.org
www.nicoa.org

Randella Bluehoose, Executive Director
A non-profit organization was founded by members of the National Tribal Chairmen's Association that called for a national organization to advocate for improved, comprehensive health and social services to American Indian and Alaska Native Elders.

7603 **National Institute of Senior Centers**
National Council on Aging
251 18th Street S
Suite 500
Arlington, VA 22202
571-527-3900
www.ncoa.org

1919

7604 **National Institute on Aging**
31 Center Drive, MSC 2292
Building 31 Room 5C27
Bethesda, MD 20892
800-222-2225
niaic@nia.nih.gov
www.nia.nih.gov

Richard J. Hodes MD, Director
Marie A. Bernard, MD, Deputy Director
Seeks to understand the nature of aging, and to extend healthy, active years of life. Free resources are available on topics such as Alzheimer's & dementia, caregiving, cognitive heath, end of life care, and more.

7605 **National Institutes of Health**
9000 Rockville Pike
Bethesda, MD 20892
301-496-4000
nihinfo@od.nih.gov
www.nih.gov

Francis S. Collins, Director
The nation's medical research agency.
1918

7606 **National Older Worker Career Center**
3811 N Fairfax Drive
Suite 900
Arlington, VA 22203
703-558-4200
www.nowcc.org

Cito Vanegas, President & CEO
National non-profit promoting experienced workers as staffing options to government agencies.
1919

7607 **National Resource Center on Nutrition & Aging**
Meals on Wheels America
1550 Crystal Drive
Suite 1004
Arlington, VA 22202
703-548-5558
Fax: 703-548-8024
nutritionandaging.org

Ucheoma Akobundu, Director, Nutrition Strategy
Sharron Corle, Director, Learning & Development
Promoting better nutrition and active healthy aging.
1920

7608 **National Senior Citizens Law Center:Oakland**
1330 Broadway
Suite 525
Oakland, CA 94612
510-663-1055
www.justiceinaging.org

Kevin Prindiville, Executive Director
Advocates nationwide to promote the independence and well-being of low-income elderly individuals, as well as persons with disabilities, with particular emphais on women and racial and ethnic minorities. Advocates through litigation and agency representation and assistance to attotneys and paralegals in field programs.

7609 **National Senior Citizens Law Center: Los Angeles**
3660 Wilshire Boulevard
Suite 718
Los Angeles, CA 90010
213-639-0930
www.justiceinaging.org

Kevin Prindiville, Executive Director
Legal services support center specializing in the legal problems of the elderly poor. Acts as advocate on behalf of elderly, poor clients in litigation and administrative affairs. Sponsors conferences and workshops on areas of the law affecting the elderly. See Legal Resources chapter for specific state resorces.

7610 **National Senior Corps Association**
PO Box 360
Farmington, UT 84025
928-523-6585
sgrove@jfsmetrowest.org
www.nscatogether.org

Erin Kruse, President
Stephanie Grove, Membership Director
Provides service for aging adults.
1919

7611 **National Seniors Council**
1100 North Glebe Road
Suite 1010
Arlington, VA 22201
571-425-4153
nationalseniorscouncil.org

Carole Rhodes, National Director
The council seeks to serve the needs of the new generation of retirees, as an alternative to organizations such as the AARP.

7612 **Office for American Indian, Alaskan Native and Native Hawaiian Elders**
Administration for Community Living
330 C St. SW
Washington, DC 20201
202-401-4634
800-677-1116
olderindians@acl.hhs.gov
olderindians.acl.gov/about

Cynthia LaCounte, Director
Administers the Title VI program by overseeing Title VI funding to programs that provide nutrition, support, and caregiver support services for Native Americans. The Office operates a website that provides technical assistance resources to Title VI directors and serves as a forum for communication between Title VI programs.

7613 **Points of Light: Atlanta**
600 Means Street
Suite 210
Atlanta, GA 30318
404-979-2900
Fax: 404-979-2901
info@pointsoflight.org
www.pointsoflight.org

Natalye Paquin, President & CEO
Robert E. Herrera, CFO
Mobilizing people to take action on the causes they care about.

7614 **Points of Light: Washington, DC**
1400 G Street NW
Washington, DC 20005
404-979-2900
Fax: 404-979-2901
info@pointsoflight.org
www.pointsoflight.org

Natalye Paquin, President & CEO
Robert E. Herrera, CFO
Mobilizing people to take action on the causes they care about.

7615 **Quality Improvement Organizations**
qioprogram.org

1920

7616 **Senior Resource LLC**
questions@seniorresource.com
www.seniorresource.com

1995 pages

7617 **Senior Service America**
8403 Colesville Rd
Suite 200
Silver Spring, MD 20910
301-578-8900
Fax: 301-578-8947
contact@ssa-i.org
www.seniorserviceamerica.org

Spence Limbocker, Chair
Gary A Officer, Executive Director
Donna Satterthwaite, Director, Workforce Development
Lynn Woo, Director of Finance
Senior Service America offers employment programs for seniors in America.

7618 **Society for Neuroscience**
1121 14th Street NW
Suite 1010
Washginton, DC 20005
202-962-4000
marty@sfn.org
sfn.org

Marty Saggese, Executive Director
Melissa Garcia, Associate Executive Director
Large international organization of scientists and physicians devoted to the study of the brain and the nervous system.
1919

7619 **Tennessee Hospital Association**
5201 Virginia Way
Brentwood, TN 37027
615-256-8240
Fax: 615-242-4803
yjames@tha.com
tha.com

Alan Watson, Chairman
Craig Becker, President & CEO
Mary Layne Van Cleave, Executive Vice President & Chief Operating Officer
Beth Atwood, Senior Director, Communications & Marketing
The Tennessee Hospital Association provides education and information to its members in the health care field so that organizations may serve their constituencies more effectively. The association also offers professional development programs in the areas of insurance, administration and operations, project management, financial services and human resources.

7620 **The Gerontological Society of America**
1220 L St NW
Suite 901
Washington, DC 20005
202-842-1275
geron@geron.org
www.geron.org

Barbara Resnick, PhD, CRNP, President
James Appleby, Executive Director & CEO
Patricia M D'Antonio, Senior Director, Professional Affairs & Membership
Judie Lieu, Senior Director, Publications & Marketing
The organization seeks to advance the study of aging by supporting gerontology research. This is accomplished through encourgaging communication among professionals, promoting research publications, expanding gerontology education programs and more.

7621 **US Administration on Aging**
330 C St. SW
Washington, DC 20201
202-401-4634
aclinfo@acl.hhs.gov
acl.gov/about-acl/administration-aging

Edwin Walker, Deputy Assistant Secretary for Aging
The Administration on Aging, an agency in the US Department of Health and Human Services, and under the Administration for Community Living, provides home and community-based care for older persons and their caregivers.

7622 **Unbound**
1 Elmwood Avenue
Kansas City, KS 66103
913-384-6500
800-875-6564
mail@unbound.org
www.unbound.org

Scott Wasserman, President & CEO
Seeks to advance the physical, mental, spiritual, and social welfare of the economically disadvantaged, especially children and aging persons in developing countries. US sponsors provide financial support and correspond with individuals in need; volunteers help provide social services, including medical, educational, and nutritional programs.
1919

7623 **Virginia Center on Aging**
Virginia Commonwealth University
Box 980229
Richmond, VA 23298
804-828-1525
vcoa@vcu.edu
vcoa.chp.vcu.edu

Edward F. Ansello, PhD, Director
Leland Waters, PhD, Associate Director
The Virginia Center on Aging is a statewide agency created by the Virginia General Assembly, with our home at Virginia Commonwealth University. Since 1978, VCoA has worked diligently to protect and improve the quality of life of older Virginians, so that they may remain independent and contributing members in their communities. Our four program areas include: abuse in later life, dementia research, geriatrics education, and lifelong learning.

Books

7624 **Activities in Action**
Routledge (Taylor & Francis Group)
270 Madison Ave
Fl 4 #4
New York, NY 10016-0601
212-695-6599
800-634-7064
Fax: 212-563-2269
www.routledgementalhealth.com
Jeffrey Lim, Director
Francis Chua, Manager
Tamaryn Anderson, Marketing Manager
An invaluable resource which serves as a catalyst for professional and personal growth and provides a national forum on geriatric and activity issues. *$30.00*
116 pages Hardcover
ISBN 1-560241-32-4

7625 **Activities with Developmentally Disabled Elderly and Older Adults**
Routledge (Taylor & Francis Group)
270 Madison Ave
Fl 4 #4
New York, NY 10016-601
212-695-6599
800-637-7064
Fax: 212-563-2269
www.routledgementalhealth.com
Jeffrey Lim, Director
Francis Chua, Manager
Tamaryn Anderson, Marketing Manager
Learn how to effectively plan and deliver activities for a growing number of older people with developmental disabilities. It aims to stimulate interest and continued support for recreation program development and implementation among developmental disability and aging service systems. *$42.00*
164 pages Hardcover
ISBN 1-560241-74-4

7626 **Aging and Developmental Disability: Current Research, Programming, and Practice**
Routledge (Taylor & Francis Group)
270 Madison Ave
Fl 4 #4
New York, NY 10016-601
212-695-6599
800-634-7064
Fax: 212-563-2269
www.routledgementalhealth.com
Joy Hammel, Author
Susan Nochajski, Co-Author
Explores research findings and their implications for practice in relation to normative and disability-related aging experiences and issues. It discusses the effectiveness of specific intervention targeted toward aging adults with developmental disabilities such as Down's Syndrome, cerebral palsy, autism, and epilepsy, and offers suggestions for practice and future research in this area. *$48.00*
112 pages Hardcover
ISBN 0-789010-39-1

7627 **Aging and Family Therapy: Practitioner Perspectives on Golden Pond**
Routledge (Taylor & Francis Group)
270 Madison Ave
Fl 4 #4
New York, NY 10016-601
212-695-6599
800-634-7064
Fax: 212-563-2269
www.routledgementalhealth.com
George Hughston, Author
Victor Christopherson, Co-Author
Marilyn Bojean, Co-Author
Here are creative strategies for use in therapy with older adults and their families. This significant new book provides practitioners with information, insight, reference tools, and other sources that will contribute to more effective intervention with the elderly and their families. *$48.00*
260 pages Hardcover
ISBN 0-866567-78-7

7628 **Aging in Stride**
IlluminAge Communications Partners
2200 1st Ave South
Suite 400
Seattle, WA 98134-1408
206-269-6363
888-620-8816
Fax: 206-269-6350
Dennis Kenny, Owner
Elizabeth N Oettinger, Co-Author
Dennis E Kenny JD, Co-Author
Guide to aging, the special needs of older adults, and the demands of providing care and support. Experts explain potential conflicts, planning opportunities and strategies for success. Six guides. *$24.95*
Paperback

7629 **Aging in the Designed Environment**
Routledge (Taylor & Francis Group)
270 Madison Ave
Fl 4 #4
New York, NY 10016-601
212-216-7800
800-634-7064
Fax: 212-563-2269
www.routledgementalhealth.com
Margaret Christenson, Author
Ellen D Taira, Co-Author
The key sourcebook for physical and occupational therapists developing and implementing environmental designs for the aging. *$30.00*
146 pages Hardcover
ISBN 1-560240-31-0

7630 **Aging with a Disability**
Special Needs Project
324 State Street
Suite H
Santa Barbara, CA 93101-2364
818-718-9900
800-333-6867
Fax: 818-349-2027
editor@specialneeds.com
www.specialneeds.com
Hod Gray, Owner
Laura Mosqueda, Co-Author
Aging with a Disability provides clinicians with a complete guide to the care and treatment of persons aging with a disability. Divided into five parts, this book first addresses the perspective of the person with a disability and his or her family. *$24.95*
328 pages Paperback

7631 **Assistive Technology for Older Persons: A Handbook**
Idaho Assistive Technology Project
University of Idaho
1187 Altiras Dr.
Moscow, ID 83843
208-885-3557
800-432-8324
Fax: 208-885-6102
idahoat@uidaho.edu
www.idahoat.org
Ron Seiler, Project Director
This handbook is designed as a guide for Idaho's older citizens who, as they age, wish to preserve their independence, autonomy, productivity, and dignity. It is intended to provide information about assistive technology, home modifications, and the many service options available to older people in the mcomunities across the state.

7632 **Caring for Those You Love: A Guide to Compassionate Care for the Aged**
Horizon Publishers & Distributors
191 N 650 E
Bountiful, UT 84010-3628
801-295-9451
866-818-6277
Fax: 801-298-1305
www.duanescrowther.com
Duane S. Crowther, Author/President
Jean Crowther, Vice President/Sec
David Crowther, Vice President
This book is a practical guide to coping with special problems of the aged and infirm, and examines the many challenges of caring for the elderly on a personal and family level. *$12.98*
108 pages
ISBN 0-882902-70-9

7633 **Chronically Disabled Elderly in Society**
Greenwood Publishing Group
88 Post Rd W
Westport, CT 06880-4208
203-226-3571
800-225-5800
Fax: 877-231-6980
www.greenwood.com
Merna J Alpert, Author
Lisa Scott, President
Herman Bruggink, CEO
This timely work increases awareness of and knowledge about problems of societal living among the chronically disabled elderly, with implications for policy makers, educational institutions, advocacy groups, families and individuals. *$76.95*
160 pages Hardcover
ISBN 0-313291-09-8

7634 **Coping and Caring: Living with Alzheimer's Disease**
AARP Fulfillment
601 E St NW
Washington, DC 20049
800-687-2277
TTY: 877-434-7589
member@aarp.org
www.aarp.org
Charles Leroux, Author
Steve Cone, Executive Vice President of Inte
Lorraine Cortes-Vazquez, Executive Vice President, Multic
Addresses the questions: What is Alzheimer's? How does the disease progress? How long does it last? How can families cope?
24 pages

7635 **Elder Abuse and Mistreatment**
Routledge (Taylor & Francis Group)
270 Madison Ave
Fl 4 #4
New York, NY 10016-601
212-695-6599
800-634-7064
Fax: 212-563-2269
www.routledgementalhealth.com
Joanna Mellor, Author
Patricia Brownell, Co-Author
Elder Abuse and Mistreatment is a comprehensive overview of current policy issues, new practice models, and up-to-date research on elder abuse and neglect. Experts in the field provide insight into elder abuse with newly examined populations to create an understanding of how to design service plans for victims of abuse and family mistreatment. The book addresses all forms of abuse and neglect, examining the value issues and ethical dilemmas that social workers face in providing service to elderl *$120.00*
284 pages Paperback
ISBN 0-789030-22-1

7636 **Explore Your Options**
Kansas Department on Aging
503 S Kansas Ave
New England Building
Topeka, KS 66603- 3404
785-296-4986
800-432-3535
Fax: 785-296-0256
TTY: 785-291-3167
wwwmail@kdads.ks.gov
www.agingKansas.org
Maria Russo, President
This book will help you through the maze of services available to Kansas seniors. It is designed to help you take an active role in making decisions that affect your health care and living situation.

7637 **Falling in Old Age**
Springer Publishing Company
11 W 42nd St
Fl 15 #15
New York, NY 10036-8002
212-431-4370
877-687-7476
Fax: 212-941-7842
cs@springerpub.com
www.springerjournals.com
Ursula Springer, President
Ted Nardin, CEO
Edie Lambiase, CFO
Presented are practical techniques for the prevention of falls and for determining and correcting the causes. *$60.00*
412 pages Hardcover
ISBN 0-826152-91-6

7638 **Family Intervention Guide to Mental Illness**
New Harbinger Publications
5674 Shattuck Ave
Oakland, CA 94609-1662
510-652-0215
800-748-6273
Fax: 800-652-1613
customerservice@newharbinger.com
www.newharbinger.com
Matthew McKay, Owner
Kim T Mueser, Co-Author
Kirk Johnson, CFO
Bodie Morey, Co-Author
The Family Intervention Guide to Mental Illness outlines the nine fundamental steps to recognizing, managing, and recovering from mental illness. It provides both diagnostic information and details about therapy options and useful medications. With the right advice, determined effort, and a lot of love, you can make a difference. *$17.95*
240 pages
ISBN 1-572245-06-8

7639 **Handbook of Assistive Devices for the Handicapped Elderly**
Routledge (Taylor & Francis Group)
270 Madison Ave
Fl 4 #4
New York, NY 10016-601
212-695-6599
800-634-7064
Fax: 212-563-2269
www.routledgementalhealth.com
Joseph A Breuer, Author
Jeffrey Lin, Director
Francis Chua, Manager
Tamaryn Anderson, Marketing Manager
Concise yet comprehensive reference of assistive devices for handicapped elders. *$42.00*
77 pages Hardcover
ISBN 0-866561-52-5

7640 **Handbook on Ethnicity, Aging and Mental Health**
Greenwood Publishing Group
88 Post Rd W
Westport, CT 6880-4208
203-226-3571
800-225-5800
Fax: 877-231-6980
www.greenwood.com

Deborah K Padgett, Author
Lisa Scott, President
Herman Bruggink, CEO

State-of-the-art reference by leading experts and first book-length appraisal of research, practices and policies concerning mental health needs of the ethnic elderly in America. *$141.95*

376 pages Hardcover
ISBN 0-313282-04-8

7641 **Health Care of the Aged: Needs, Policies, and Services**
Routledge (Taylor & Francis Group)
270 Madison Ave
Fl 4 #4
New York, NY 10016-601
212-695-6599
800-634-7064
Fax: 212-563-2269
www.routledgementalhealth.com

Abraham Monk, Author
Jeffrey Lim, Director
Francis Chua, Manager
Tamaryn Anderson, Marketing Manager

Focusing on the need for developing new service delivery models for the aged, this book examines fiscal, political, and social criteria influencing this challenge of the 1990's. The aged are caught in the sweeping changes currently occurring in the financing, organizing and delivery of human health care services. *$36.00*

800 pages Hardcover
ISBN 1-560240-65-5

7642 **Health Promotion and Disease Prevention in Clinical Practice**
Lippincott, Williams & Wilkins
2001 Market Street
Two Commerce Square
Philadelphia, PA 19103-3603
215-521-8300
800-638-3030
Fax: 215-521-8902
customerservice@lww.com
www.lww.com

Steven H Woolf MD, Co-Author
Steven Jonas MD, Co-Author
Evonne Kaplan-Liss, Co-Author
Rick Perry, CEO

Incorporating the latest guidelines from major organizations, including the U.S. Preventive Services Task Force, this book offers the clinician a complete overview of how to help patients adopt healthy behaviors and to deliver recommended screening tests and immunizations. *$52.95*

218 pages Softcover
ISBN 0-781775-99-1

7643 **Life Planning for Adults with Developmental Disabilities**
New Harbinger Publications
5674 Shattuck Ave
Oakland, CA 94609-1662
510-652-0215
800-748-6273
Fax: 800-652-1613
customerservice@newharbinger.com
www.newharbinger.com

Matthew McKay, Publisher
Kirk Johnson, CFO
Judith Greenbaum PhD, Author

The book begins by assessing the quality of life of the adult with a disability. It offers a wealth of suggestions for making that person's life even better. The book then focuses on long-term planning for the individual with a disability and helps answer the question, Who will take care of my child after I'm gone? *$19.95*

208 pages
ISBN 1-572244-51-1

7644 **Long-Term Care: How to Plan and Pay for It**
NOLO
950 Parker St
Berkeley, CA 94710-2524
510-549-1976
800-728-3555
Fax: 800-645-0895
www.nolo.com

Joseph L Matthews, Author
Ralph Warner, Chariman/CEO
Ann Heron, COO
Bob Dubow, CFO

This book helps you choose a nursing home, or find a viable alternative. Covers how to get the most out of Medicare and other benefit programs.

384 pages Paperback
ISBN 1-413305-21-0

7645 **Mentally Impaired Elderly: Strategies and Interventions to Maintain Function**
Routledge (Taylor & Francis Group)
270 Madison Ave
Fl 4 #4
New York, NY 10016-601
212-695-6599
800-634-7064
Fax: 212-653-2269
www.routledgementalhealth.com

Ellen D Taira, Author
Jeffrey Lim, Director
Francis Chua, Manager
Tamaryn Anderson, Marketing Manager

Provides effective support and sensitive care for the most vulnerable segment of the elderly population, those with mental impairment. *$34.00*

171 pages Hardcover
ISBN 1-560241-68-3

7646 **Mirrored Lives: Aging Children and Elderly Parents**
Praeger Publishers
88 Post Rd W
Westport, CT 06880-4208
203-226-3571
800-225-5800
Fax: 877-231-6980
www.greenwood.com

Tom Koch, Author
Lisa Scott, President
Herman Bruggink, CEO

Discusses geriatric decline connected to nonterminal illness in old age. Koch takes a sensitive but thorough look at the declining years of his father. *$117.95*

240 pages Hardcover
ISBN 0-275936-71-6

7647 **Physical & Mental Issues in Aging Sourcebook**
Omnigraphics
615 Griswold Street
Suite 520
Detroit, MI 48226-3261
610-461-3548
800-234-1340
Fax: 800-875-1340
contact@omnigraphics.com
www.omnigraphics.com

Peter Ruffner, Co-Founder
Fred Ruffner, Co-Founder

Basic information about maintaining health through the post-reproductive years. Includes stats, recommendations for lifestyle modifications, a glossary and resrouce information *$84.00*

660 pages Hard cover
ISBN 0-780802-33-9

7648 **Prescriptions for Independence: Working with Older People Who are Visually Impaired**
American Foundation for the Blind/AFB Press
11 Penn Plz
Suite 300
New York, NY 10001-2006
212-502-7600
800-232-3044
Fax: 212-502-7777
www.afb.org

Carl Augusto, President
Gerda Groff, Co-Author
Richard Obnen, Chairman of the Board
Alan Lindroth, Principal
Easy-to-read manual on how older visually impaired persons can pursue their interests and activities in community residences, senior centers, long-term care facilities and other community settings. Paperback.
99 pages Paperback
ISBN 0-891282-44-0

7649 **Sharing the Burden**
Brookings Institution
1775 Massachusetts Ave NW
Washington, DC 20036-2188
202-797-6000
Fax: 202-797-6004
www.brookings.edu

Joshua N Weiner, Author
Laurel Hixon Illston, Co-Author
Raymond J Hanley, Co-Author
Strobe Talbott, President
The authors examine the cost of public and private initiatives and who would pay for them. Their answers emerge from a large computer simulation model that the authors developed. *$42.95*
342 pages Cloth
ISBN 0-815793-78-2

7650 **Social Security, Medicare, and Government Pensions**
NOLO
950 Parker St
Berkeley, CA 94710-2524
510-549-1976
800-728-3555
Fax: 800-645-0895
www.nolo.com

Joseph L Matthews, Author
Dorothy Matthews Berman, Co-Author
Ralph Warner, Chairman/CEO
Ann Heron, COO
Social Security, Medicare, SSI and more explained in this all-in-one resource that gets you the most out of your retirement benefits. *$24.95*
480 pages Paperback
ISBN 1-413307-53-5

7651 **Successful Models of Community Long Term Care Services for the Elderly**
Routledge (Taylor & Francis Group)
270 Madison Ave
Fl 4 #4
New York, NY 10016-601
212-695-6599
800-637-7064
Fax: 212-563-2269
www.routledgementalhealth.com

Eloise Killeffer, Author
Ruth Bennett, Co-Author
Jeffrey Lim, Director
Francis Chua, Manager
Experienced practitioners provide examples of successful community-based long term care service programs for the elderly. *$72.00*
174 pages Hardcover
ISBN 0-866569-87-3

7652 **Therapeutic Activities with Persons Disabled by Alzheimer's Disease**
Sage Publications
804 Anacapa Stree
Sanat Barbara, CA 93101-2212
805-899-8620
info@sagepub.com
www.sagepub.com

Sara Miller McCune, Founder, Publisher, Chairperson
Blaise Simqu, CEO
Tracey Ozmina, COO
Stephen Barr, Managing Director
A program of functional skills for activities of daily living. Hardcover. *$86.00*
432 pages
ISBN 0-834211-62-9

7653 **Visually Impaired Seniors as Senior Companions: A Reference Guide**
American Foundation for the Blind/AFB Press
11 Penn Plz
Suite 300
New York, NY 10001-2006
212-502-7600
800-232-3044
Fax: 212-502-7777
www.afb.org

Carl Augusto, President
Alan Lindroth, Principal
Richard Obnen, Chairman of the Board
Michael Gilliam, Vice Chairman
This useful guide describes the Senior Companion Program that is intended to broaden opportunities for older persons with disabilities. Appendix includes training materials, evaluation forms, recruitment and public relations information. *$15.00*
108 pages Paperback
ISBN 0-891282-38-6

7654 **Work, Health and Income Among the Elderly**
Brookings Institution
1775 Massachusetts Ave NW
Washington, DC 20036-2188
202-797-6000
Fax: 202-797-6004
www.brookings.edu

Gary Burtless, Author
Strobe Talbott, President
Steven Bennett, Vice President/COO
Stewart Uretsky, Vice President/CFO
Employment, health and financial information for the elderly. *$26.95*
276 pages Cloth
ISBN 0-815711-76-6

Journals

7655 **ATS Journals**
25 Broadway
New York, NY 10004
212-315-8600
atsjournals.org

Marc Moss, President
Polly E. Parsons, President Elect
Juan C. Celed¢N, Secretary/Treasurer
Stephen C. Crane, Executive Director
The American Thoracic Society publishes medical research journals with a focus on respiratory issues. Publications include: Respiratory and Critical Care Medicine, Respiratory Cell and Molecular Biology, and Annals of the American Thoracic Society.

7656 **Gerontology: Abstracts in Social Gerontology**
National Council on the Aging
1901 L St NW
4th Floor
Washington, DC 20036-3506
202-479-1200
Fax: 202-479-0735
TTY: 202-479-6674
info@ncoa.org
www.ncoa.org

James Knickman, Interim President & CEO

Detailed abstracts are provided for recent major journal articles, books, reports and other materials on many facets of aging, including: adult education, demography, family relations, institutional care and work attitudes. Item No. AB100; Journals $114.00; Member Discount: $94.00.
Quarterly

7657 **Journal of the American Academy of Audiology**
American Academy of Audiology
11480 Commerce Park Drive
Suite 220
Reston, VA 20191
703-790-8466
Fax: 703-790-8631
infoaud@audiology.org
www.audiology.org

Gary P. Jacobson, Editor-in-Chief
Devin L. McCaslin, Deputy Editor-in-Chief
The scholarly peer-reviewed journal of the American Academy of Audiology. Publishes articles and clinical reports in all areas of audiology.

7658 **Physical & Occupational Therapy in Geriatrics**
Taylor & Francis Group, LLC
325 Chestnut Street
Suite 800 #800
Philadelphia, PA 19106-2608
215-625-8900
800-354-1420
Fax: 215-625-2940
haworthpress@taylorandfrancis.com
www.tandf.co.uk

Ellen Dunleavey Taira, Editor
Barbara Pucher, CFO
Focuses on current practices and emerging issues in the care of the older client, including long-term care in institutional and community settings, crisis intervention, and innovative programming; the entire range of problems experienced by the elderly; and the current skills needed for working with older clients. *$99.00*
Quarterly

7659 **Research and Practice for Persons with Severe Disabilities**
TASH
1101 15th St. NW
Suite 206
Washington, DC 20005
202-817-3264
Fax: 202-999-4722
info@tash.org
www.tash.org

Stacy Dymond, Editor-in-Chief
Scientific journal publishing articles on special topics in the disability field.
Quarterly

7660 **Research, Advocacy, and Practice for Complex and Chronic Conditions**
Council for Exceptional Children
3100 Clarendon Blvd.
Suite 600
Arlington, VA 22201-5332
888-232-7733
TTY: 866-915-5000
service@exceptionalchildren.org
www.exceptionalchildren.org

Dusty Columbia Embury, Editor
Peer-reviewed journal covering research, issues, and programs relating to the needs of people with physical, health, or multiple disabilities.

Magazines

7661 **A Better Tomorrow**
Thomas Nelson
5301 Wisconsin Avenue NW
Suite 620
Washington, DC 20015
202-364-8000
Fax: 202-364-8910
www.thomasnelson.com/

Bruce Barbour, Publisher
Dale Hanson, Editor
Magazine focusing on issues and concerns of senior citizens.

7662 **AARP Bulletin**
AARP
601 E Street NW
Washington, DC 20049
888-687-2277
www.aarp.org

7663 **AARP Magazine**
American Association of Retired Persons
601 East Street NW
Washington, DC 20049
202-434-3525
888-687-2277
member@aarp.org
www.aarp.org

A Barry Rand, CEO
Steve Cone, Executive Vice President of Integrated Value
Lorraine Cort,s-V zquez, Executive Vice President, Multicultural Markets
Celebrity interviews. Features on health and finance. Movie reviews and more. All with an eye toward the topics and issues you care about most.

7664 **ACE Fitness Matters**
American Council on Exercise (ACE)
4851 Paramount Drive
San Diego, CA 92123
858-576-6500
888-825-3636
Fax: 858-576-6564
support@acefitness.org
www.acefitness.org/

Herb Flentye, Chair
Scott Murdoch, PhD., RD, Vice Chair
Consumer magazine covering health and fitness news. *$25.00*

7665 **AER Report**
Association for Education & Rehabilitation
5680 King Centre Dr.
Suite 600
Alexandria, VA 22315
703-671-4500
Fax: 703-671-6391
www.aerbvi.org

Neva Fairchild, President
Contains organizational news, conference dates and information concerning services to visually impaired people.

7666 **ASN NEURO**
Sage Journals
2455 Teller Road
Thousand Oaks, CA 91320
805-499-9774
journals@sagepub.com
journals.sagepub.com/home/asn

Douglas L. Feinstein, Editor-in-Chief
Sandra J. Hewitt, Deputy Editor-in-Chief
Peer-reviewed open access journal focusing on recent advances in the cellular and molecular neurosciences. It is the official publication of the American Society for Neurochemistry.

7667 **Abstracts in Social Gerontology**
National Council on Aging
1901 L Street NW
4th Floor
Washington, DC 20036
202-479-1200
800-677-1116
Fax: 202-479-0735
TTY: 202-479-6674
info@ncoa.org
www.ncoa.org

James Knickman, Interim President & CEO

Detailed abstracts are provided for recent major journal articles, books, reports and other materials on many facets of aging, including adult education, demography, family relations, institutional care and work attitudes. *$114.00*

7668 **Adapted Physical Activity Quarterly**
Human Kinetics
PO Box 5076
1607 N Market Street
Champaign, IL 61820
217-351-5076
800-747-4457
Fax: 217-351-1549
info@hkusa.com
www.humankinetics.com
Brian Holding, CEO
Rainer Martens, Founder
Journal on the study of physical activity for special populations.

7669 **Aging International**
Transaction Publishers
35 Berrue
New Brunswick, NJ 08901
732-445-1245
888-999-6778
Fax: 732-445-3138
orders@transactionpub.com
www.transactionpub.com/
Mary E. Curtis, Chair
Irving Louis Horowitz, Co-Founder
Journal dedicated to the well-being of older persons worldwide. Explores productive aging, empowerment, life-long learning, health promotion, and services for the elderly, with an emphasis on sharing both common concerns and practical applications. Focuses on social and economic issues, public policies, and use of resources. Published in cooperation with the International Federation on Aging.

7670 **Aging News Alert**
CD Publications
2222 Sedwick Drive
Durham, NC 27713
301-588-6380
855-237-1396
Fax: 800-508-2592
www.cdpublications.com
Michael Gerecht, President
Twice-monthly newsletter reporting on senior programs, funding opportunities and federal actions affecting the elderly.

7671 **Aging Research & Training News**
Business Publishers, Inc.
2222 Sedwick Drive
Durham, NC 27713
800-223-8720
Fax: 800-508-2592
www.bpinews.com
Kimberly Gilbert, Managing Editor
Alexa Chew, Contributing Editor
Compilation of studies of aging populations; reports on innovative programs with aging community; federal funding and laws. *$267.00*
8 pages

7672 **Aging and Society**
Cambridge University Press
32 Avenue of the Americas
New York, NY 10013
212-924-3900
800-221-4512
Fax: 212-691-3239
www.cambridge.org/us/information/contact
Ken Blakemore, Editor
Bill Bythwway, Editor
International journal publishing on topics which further the understanding of human aging. The journal of the Centre for policy on aging and the British Socie for Gerontology.

7673 **American Journal of Geriatric Psychiatry**
Elsevier
1600 John F Kennedy Boulevard
Philadelphia, PA 19103
www.journals.elsevier.com
Charles F. Reynolds III, MD, Editor-in-Chief
Peer-reviewed articles on the rapidly developing field of geriatric psychiatry, including areas such as the diagnosis and classification of psychiatric disorders, epidemiological and biological correlates of mental health of older adults, and psychopharmacology and other somatic treatments. *$582.00*

7674 **American Journal of Speech-LanguagePathology**
American Speech-Language-Hearing Association (ASHA
2200 Research Boulevard
Rockville, MD 20850
301-296-5700
800-638-8255
Fax: 301-296-8580
www.asha.org/
Elizabeth S. McCrea, PhD, CCC-SLP, President
Barbara K. Cone, PhD, CCC-A, Vice President for Academic Affa

7675 **American Legion Magazine**
American Legion National Headquarters
PO Box 1055
700 N. Pennsylvania St.
Indianapolis, IN 46206
317-630-1200
800-433-3318
Fax: 317-630-1223
www.legion.org/
Daniel S. Wheeler, National Adjutant
Philip B. Onderdonk Jr., National Judge Advocate
General interest magazine for veterans. *$152.50*

7676 **American Rehabilitation ServicesAdministration (RSA)**
American Rehabilitation Services Administration (R
400 Maryland Avenue, SW
Washington, DC 20202
202-205-8296
800-USA-LEAR
Fax: 202-205-9874
www2.ed.gov/about/offices/list/osers/rsa
Arne Duncan, Secretary of Education
Jim Shelton, Acting Deputy Secretary
Magazine on rehabilitation of the handicapped. *$9.50*

7677 **Assistive Technology**
RESNA
2025 M St. NW
Suite 800
Arlington, VA 20036
202-367-1121
Fax: 202-367-2121
info@resna.org
www.resna.org
Maureen Linden, President
Journal focusing on assistive technology for persons with disabilities. *$35.00*

7678 **Audecibel**
International Hearing Society
16880 Middlebelt Road
Suite 4
Livonia, MI 48154
734-522-7200
800-521-5247
Fax: 734-522-0200
www.ihsinfo.org/
Kathleen Mennillo, Executive Director
Magazine publishing technical articles and product announcements on hearing aids and hearing. *$25.00*

7679 **Buena Vida**
Casiano Communications
1700 Fern ndez Juncos Avenue
San Juan, PR 00909
787-728-3000
800-468-8167
Fax: 787-268-1001
www.casiano.com/
Manuel A. Casiano, Chairman & CEO
Carlos Rom, Executive Vice President
Health and fitness magazine. *$23.95*

7680 **Challenge Magazine**
Disabled Sports, USA
451 Hungerford Drive
Suite 100
Rockville, MD 20850
301-217-0960
Fax: 301-217-0968
dsusa@dsusa.org
www.disabledsportsusa.org/
Robert Meserve, President
Steven Goodwin, Vice President

Magazine providing information on sports for people with physical disabilities.

7681 **Closing the Gap**
P.O. Box 68
Henderson, MN 56044
507-248-3294
Fax: 507-248-3810
www.closingthegap.com
Dolores Hagen, Co-Founder
Budd Hagen, Co-Founder
Online membership that includes access to the Solutions on-line magazine and archives, archived webinars and the Resource Directory, a guide to over 2,000 products for children and adults with disabilities

7682 **Communication Outlook: Artificial LanguageLaboratory**
Artificial Language Laboratory
405 Computer Center
Michigan State University
Lansing, MI 48824
517-353-0870
Fax: 517-353-4766
www.msu.edu/~artlang/CommOut.html
Dr. John B. Eulenberg, Ph.D., Director
Stephen R. Blosser, B.S.M.E., Technical Director
Magazine reporting on the newest developments in the application of technology for neurologically impaired persons. *$18.00*

7683 **Conscious Choice**
Conscious Communications
920 N Franklin Street
Suite 202
Chicago, IL 60610
312-440-4373
Fax: 312-751-3973
www.consciouscomms.com/
Ross Thompson, Managing Editor
Jim Slama, Publisher
Consumer magazine covering health, nutrition and environmental issues. *$184.00*

7684 **Contemporary Gerontology**
Springer Publishing Company
11 West 42nd Street
15th Floor
New York, NY 10036
212-431-4370
877-687-7476
Fax: 212-941-7842
cs@springerpub.com, journals@springerpub
www.springerpub.com
James C. Costello, Vice President, Journal Publishi
Theodore C. Nardin, Chief Executive Officer & Publis
Scholarly journal covering gerontology.

7685 **Dementia and Geriatric Cognitive Disorders**
S. Karger Publishers, Inc.
26 W Avon Road
P.O. Box 529
Unionville, CT 06085
860-675-7834
800-828-5479
Fax: 860-675-7302
www.karger.com/DEM
Victoria Chan-Pilay, Editor-in-Chief
Open-access journal devoted to the study of cognitive dysfunction in preclinical and clinical studies, concentrating on Alzheimer's and Parkinson's disease, Huntington's chorea and other neurodegenerative diseases.

7686 **Disability Rag's Ragged Edge Magazine**
Advocado Press
PO Box 145
Louisville, KY 40201
502-894-9492
Fax: 502-899-9562
www.advocadopress.org/
Mary Johnson, Mailing Contact/Editor
Magazine of debate on disability rights issues. ISSN# 1095-3949
$17.50
35 pages

7687 **Disability Rights Now**
Disability Rights Education and Defense Fund
3075 Adeline Street
Suite 210
Berkeley, CA 94703
510-644-2555
800-466-4232
Fax: 510-841-8645
info@dredf.org
dredf.org/
Claudia Center, President and Chair
Susan Henderson, Executive Director
Free quarterly publication describing the activities of the Disability Rights Education and Defense Fund, available in alternative formats.

7688 **Disability Statistics Report**
Institute for Health & Aging
2 Koret Way, #N-319X
UCSF Box 0602
San Francisco, CA 94143
415-476-1435
Fax: 415-476-9707
info@nursing.ucsf.edu
nursing.ucsf.edu/iha
David Vlahov, RN, PhD, Dean and Professor
Yolanda Abrea, Fiscal Analyst
Magazine providing statistical data on disability in the US as collected by the Disability Statistics Program.

7689 **Disability Studies Quarterly**
University of Hawaii at Manoa
2500 Campus Road
Honolulu, HI 96822
808-956-8111
Fax: 808-956-3162
manoa.hawaii.edu/
M.R.C. Greenwood, President
Tom Apple, Chief Executive Officer
Scholarly journal containing articles on all aspects of disability.
$3545.00

7690 **Disabled American Veterans Magazines**
Disabled American Veterans National Headquarters
PO Box 14301
Cincinnati, OH 45250
859-441-7300
Fax: 859-441-8056
www.dav.org/
Thomas K Keller, Editor
James Chaney, Mailing Contact
Veterans magazine on disability issues. *$15.00*

7691 **Disabled People as Second Class Citizens**
Springer Publishing Company
11 West 42nd Street
15th Floor
New York, NY 10036
212-431-4370
877-687-7476
Fax: 212-941-7842
cs@springerpub.com, journals@springerpub
www.springerpub.com
James C. Costello, Vice President, Publisher
Theodore C. Nardin, Chief Executive Officer
Disability and legal practice. *$26.95*
320 pages

7692 **Domestic Mistreatment of the Elderly:Towards Prevention**
AARP
601 E Street NW
Washington, DC 20049
202-434-3525
888-687-2277
Fax: 202-434-3443
member@aarp.org
www.aarp.org
Gail E. Aldrich, Board Chair
Robert G. Romasco, President
This comprehensive publication addresses the problem of mistreatment or neglect in the home.
39 pages

7693 Duplex Planet
Duplex Planet
PO Box 1230
Saratoga Springs, NY 12866 518-692-7410
Fax: 518-692-8208
www.duplexplanet.com/
David Greenberger, Editor/ Founder
Consumer journal covering issues of aging and popular culture. *$122.50*

7694 Eating Well Magazine
Eating Well
6221 Shelburne Road
Suite 100
Charlotte, VT 05482 802-985-4500
800-344-3350
Fax: 802-425-3675
www.eatingwell.com
Thomas Witschi, President
Brierley Wright, Managing Editor
Food magazine with emphasis on delicious low-fat cooking and sensible nutrition. *$19.94*

7695 Educational Gerontology
Taylor & Francis
711 3rd Avenue
8th Floor
New York, NY 10017 212-216-7800
800-634-7064
Fax: 212-564-7854
www.taylorandfrancis.com/
D Barry Lumsden, Editor
Kevin Bradley, CEO
Journal publishing original research in the fields of gerontology, adult education, and the social and behavioral sciences.

7696 Elderly Health Services Letter
Health Resources Online
P.O. Box 456
Allenwood, NJ 08720 800-516-4343
Fax: 732-292-1111
Robert K Jenkins, Publisher
An essential tool for senior services professionals. Stays on top of the most current challenges facing senior services professionals, including financing and funding senior services, marketing, positioning senior services for managed care, getting administrative support and more.

7697 Experimental Aging Research
Taylor & Francis
711 3rd Avenue
8th Floor
New York, NY 10017 212-216-7800
800-634-7064
Fax: 212-564-7854
www.taylorandfrancis.com/
Jeffrey Elias, Editor
Kevin Bradley, CEO
International journal devoted to the scientific study of the aging process.

7698 Fitness Diet and Exercise Guide
Family Circle
110 5th Avenue
New York, NY 10011 212-463-1673
800-627-4444
Fax: 212-463-1906
fcfeedback@familycircle.com
www.familycircle.com/
Darcy Jacobs, Executive Editor
Linda Fears, Vice President/Editor in Chief
Magazine suggesting ways to eat healthier and exercise better.

7699 Focus on Geriatric Care and Rehabilitation
Aspen Publishers
7201 McKinney Circle
Frederick, MD 21704 301-644-3599
800-234-1660
Fax: 800-901-9075
www.aspenpublishers.com/
Bob Lemmond, President & CEO
Gustavo Dobles, Vice President & CCO
Monthly journal written for nurses, occupational therapists and administrators in geriatric settings. *$95.00*

7700 Generations
American Society on Aging
575 Market Street
Suite 2100
San Francisco, CA 94105 415-974-9600
800-537-9728
Fax: 415-974-0300
info@asaging.org
www.asaging.org
Peter Kaldest, President & CEO
Robert R. Lowe, COO
Peer-review quarterly journal featuring guest editor. *$30.00*

7701 Geriatrics
ModernMedicine
7500 Old Oak Boulevard
Cleveland, OH 44130 440-891-2769
Fax: 440-891-2635
Don Berman, Director, Business Development
Terry Tetzlaff, Digital Traffic Coordinator
Peer-reviewed, clinical journal for physicians and laypersons relating to medical care of middle-aged and older adults.

7702 Gerontologist
Gerontological Society of America
1220 L Street North West
Washington, DC 20005 202-842-1275
Fax: 202-842-1150
geron@geron.org
www.geron.org
James Appleby, Executive Director and CEO
Linda Krogh Harootyan, Deputy Executive Director
Multidisciplinary peer-reviewed journal presenting new concepts, clinical ideas, and applied research in gerontology. Includes book and audiovisual reviews.

7703 Gerontology
S. Karger Publishers, Inc.
PO Box 529
26 West Avon Road
Unionville, CT 06085 860-675-7834
800-828-5479
Fax: 860-675-7302
karger@snet.net
www.karger.com/
W Meier-Rage, Managing Editor
Monica Brendel, President
Medical journal. *$276.00*

7704 Get Up and Go
Liberty Media Corporation
11551 Forest Central Drive
Suite 305
Dallas, TX 75243 214-341-9429
877-772-1518
Fax: 214-341-9779
www.libertymedia.com/
John C. Malone, Chairman
Gregory B. Maffei, President & CEO
Magazine (tabloid) for people age 50 and over.

7705 **Independent Living Provider**
Equal Opportunity Publications
1160 E Jericho Turnpike
Suite 200
Huntington, NY 11743
516-421-9421
Fax: 516-421-0359
info@eop.com
www.eop.com/
Tamara Flaum-Dreyfuss, President and Publisher
Maureen Gladstone, Account Executive
Business magazine for home health care.

7706 **Informer**
The Simon Foundation for Continence
PO Box 815
Wilmette, IL 60091
847-864-3913
800-23S-mon
Fax: 847-864-9758
info@simonfoundation.org
www.simonfoundation.org
Cheryle Gartley, President and Founder
Elizabeth Tr LaGro, Vice President, Communications a
Magazine for persons with bladder or bowel incontinence.

7707 **Innovations**
National Council on Aging
1901 L Street NW
4th Floor
Washington, DC 20036
202-479-1200
800-677-1116
Fax: 202-479-0735
TTY: 2024796674
info@ncoa.org
www.ncoa.org
James Knickman, Interim President & CEO
Explores significant developments in the field of aging through opinion articles, profiles and research summaries. Features articles on social trends, articles on specific aging programs and information on NCOA's activities. *$50.00*

7708 **Inside MS**
National Multiple Sclerosis Society
733 3rd Avenue
3rd Floor
New York, NY 10017
212-986-3240
800-FIG-HTMS
Fax: 212-986-7981
editor@nmss.org
www.nationalmssociety.org/
Eli Rubenstein, Chairman of the Board
Cynthia Zagieboylo, President & CEO
Magazine for people with multiple sclerosis, their families, attending professionals, and interested donors. Provides information on coping, research, legislation, medical advances and disability rights advocacy. *$2027.00*
80 pages

7709 **International Journal of Aging and Human Development**
Baywood Publishing Company, Inc.
PO Box 337
26 Austin Avenue
Amityville, NY 11701
631-691-1270
800-638-7819
Fax: 631-691-1770
www.baywood.com/
Adult development and aging featuring original research theory, critial reviews.

7710 **International Journal of Technology andAging**
Human Sciences Press
233 Spring Street
New York, NY 10013-1522
212-620-8000
800-221-9369
Fax: 212-463-0742
www.springer.com

7711 **International Psychogeriatrics**
Springer Publishing Company
11 West 42nd Street
15th Floor
New York, NY 10036
212-431-4370
877-687-7476
Fax: 212-941-7842
cs@springerpub.com, journals@springerpub
www.springerpub.com
James C. Costello, Vice President
Theodore C. Nardin, Chief Executive Officer
Scholarly journal covering psychogeriatric practice, research, and education worldwide.

7712 **International Rehabilitation Review**
Rehabilitation International
866 United Nations Plaza
Office 422
New York, NY 10017
212-420-1500
Fax: 212-505-0871
info@riglobal.org
www.riglobal.org
Teuta Rexhepi, Secretary General
Zhang Haidi, President

7713 **JNeurosci**
Society for Neuroscience
1121 14th Street NW
Suite 1010
Washginton, DC 20005
202-962-4000
jn@sfn.org
www.jneurosci.org
Marina R. Picciotto, Editor-in-Chief
Teresa Esch, Features Editor
Official peer-reviewed journal of the Society for Neuroscience, publishing research on a broad range of topics of interest to those working on the nervous system.

7714 **Journal of Aging and Ethnicity**
Springer Publishing Company
11 West 42nd Street
15th Floor
New York, NY 10036
212-431-4370
877-687-7476
Fax: 212-941-7842
www.springerpub.com
James C. Costello, Vice President
Theodore C. Nardin, Chief Executive Officer
Scholarly journal for researchers and professionals in gerontology and geriatrics, emphasizing the ethnic population of North America.

7715 **Journal of Aging and Health**
Sage Publications
2455 Teller Road
Thousand Oaks, CA 91320
805-499-0721
Fax: 805-499-0871
www.sagepub.in/
Kyriakos S Markides, Editor
C Anderson, Circulation Manager
Journal presenting research relative to the social and behavioral factors related to aging and health.

7716 **Journal of Aging and Physical Activity**
Human Kinetics
PO Box 5076
1607 N Market Street
Champaign, IL 61820
217-351-5076
800-747-4457
Fax: 217-351-1549
info@hkusa.com
www.humankinetics.com
Brian Holding, CEO
Rainer Martens, Founder
Journal examining the relationship between physical activity and the aging process.

7717 **Journal of American Aging Association**
American Aging Association
52373 Tyndall Falls Drive
Olmstead Falls, OH 44138
440-793-6565
Fax: 440-793-6598
ameraging@gmail.com
www.americanaging.org

Mitch Harman, Chairperson
LaDora Thompson, President

7718 **Journal of Developmental and PhysicalDisabilities**
Kluwer Academic Publishers
101 Philip Drive
Norwell, MA 02061
212-620-8000
Fax: 212-463-0742
vlib.ustu.ru/storon/kluwer/

Vincent B Hassett, Editor
V Hersen, Advertising Manager
Professional journal.

7719 **Journal of Ethics, Law, and Aging**
Springer Publishing Company
11 West 42nd Street
15th Floor
New York, NY 10036
212-431-4370
877-687-7476
Fax: 212-941-7842
www.springerpub.com

James C. Costello, Vice President, Journal Publishing
Theodore C. Nardin, Chief Executive Officer & Publisher
Scholarly journal covering ethical and legal issues regarding aging for professionals who plan, administer, and provide and finance services to the elderly.

7720 **Journal of Mental Health and Aging**
Springer Publishing Company
11 West 42nd Street
15th Floor
New York, NY 10036
212-431-4370
877-687-7476
Fax: 212-941-7842
www.springerpub.com

James C. Costello, Vice President
Theodore C. Nardin, Chief Executive Officer
Scholarly journal covering aging population for mental health professionals.

7721 **Journal of Nuclear Medicine**
Society of Nuclear Medicine and Molecular Imaging
1850 Samuel Morse Drive
Reston, VA 20190
703-708-9000
800-513-6853
Fax: 703-708-9015
subscriptions@snm.org
jnm.snmjournals.org

Johannes Czernin, MD, Editor-in-Chief
Susan Alexander, Associate Director, Publications
Peer-reviewed journal with clinical investigations, science reports, articles benefitting continuing education, book reviews, employment opportunities, and updates on practice and research. *$58.00*

7722 **Journal of Nuclear Medicine Technology**
Society of Nuclear Medicine and Molecular Imaging
1850 Samuel Morse Drive
Reston, VA 20190
703-708-9000
800-513-6853
Fax: 703-708-9015
subscriptions@snm.org
tech.snmjournals.org

Kathy S. Thomas, MHA, CNMT, PET, Editor-in-Chief
Susan Alexander, Associate Director, Publications
Peer-reviewed journal dedicated to nuclear medicine technology, with information on credentialing, continuing education and licensure requirements, as well as current news and updates on the field. *$58.00*

7723 **Journal of Rehabilitation**
National Rehabilitation Association
PO Box 150235
Alexandria, VA 22315
703-836-0850
888-258-4295
journalofrehab@email.arizona.edu
nationalrehab.org/journal-of-rehabilitation

Wendy Parent-Johnson, Editor
Official journal of the National Rehabilitation Association.
Quarterly

7724 **Journal of Religion, Spirituality & Aging**
www.tandfonline.com

James W. Ellor, Editor
Features articles, research reports and reviews of new books and audiovisual resources on religion and aging.

7725 **Journal of Therapeutic Horticulture**
American Horticultural Therapy Association
610 Freedom Business Center
Suite 110
King of Prussia, PA 19406
610-992-0020
Fax: 301-869-2397
ahta.org/

MaryAnne Millan, HTR, President
Leigh Anne Starling, MS, CRC, HTR, Vice President
Journal containing articles on the therapeutic aspects of gardening and agriculture for persons with disabilities. *$15.00*

7726 **Kaleidoscope: Exploring the Expirence of Disability through Literature/Fine Arts**
United Disability Services
701 S Main Street
Akron, OH 44311
330-762-9755
Fax: 330-762-0912
www.udsakron.org

Karen A. Bozzelli, Chairperson
Bill Choler, Vice Chairperson
Magazine featuring articles on literature and the arts. Disabilitiy related. *$9.00*
64 pages

7727 **Macrobiotics Today**
George Ohsawa Macrobiotic Foundation
PO Box 3998
Chico, CA 95927
530-566-9765
800-232-2372
Fax: 530-566-9768
www.ohsawamacrobiotics.com/

Carl Ferr,, President
Peter Milbury, Director
Magazine covering macrobiotics, health, and nutrition. *$20.00*

7728 **Magazines in Special Media for theHandicapped**
National Library Service for the Blind and Physic
1291 Taylor Street NW
Washington, DC 20011
202-707-5100
800-424-8567
Fax: 202-707-0712
TTY: 202-707-0744
www.loc.gov/nls

Karen Keninger, Director
Isabella Marqu,s de Castilla, Deputy Director
Publication includes: List of over 100 public and private organizations that publish magazines in Braille, on cassette, on disc and computer diskette, or in large print or moon type for visually impaired and physically disabled individuals. Entries include: Name of publisher, address, price. Principal content is a bibliography of periodicals, with brief description, frequency, format, and price of each.

7729 **Massage Therapy Journal**
American Massage Therapy Association
500 Davis St.
Suite 900
Evanston, IL 60201
877-905-2700
info@amtamassage.org
www.amtamassage.org

Steve Albertson, President
Bill Brown, Executive Director
Jeff Flom, Chief Operating Officer

Publication focusing on massage therapy research, techniques, and practices. *$20.00*

7730 **Mature Health**
New York - Haymarket
114 West 26th Street
4th Floor
New York, NY 10001 646-638-6000
Michael Heseltine, Chairman
Kevin Costello, Chief Group Executive
Magazine featuring articles on health aspects of aging, as well as articles on recreation and leisure. *$7.00*

7731 **Mature Years**
United Methodist Publishing House
201 8th Avenue S
PO Box 801
Nashville, TN 37202 615-749-6000
Fax: 615-749-6079
umph.org/
Neil Alexander, President/Publisher
Jeff Barnes, Executive Director
Magazine promoting the physical and spiritual well-being of older adults.

7732 **Men's Health**
Rodale Inc
400 South 10th Street
Emmaus, PA 18098 610-967-5171
800-848-4735
Fax: 610-967-7725
RodaleBooks@cdsfulfillment.com
Maria Rodale, CEO and Chairman
Scott D. Schulman, President
Magazine offering health advice for men.

7733 **Mental Health Report**
Business Publishers, Inc.
2222 Sedwick Drive
Durham, NC 27713 301-495-5570
800-223-8720
Fax: 800-508-2592
www.bpinews.com
Kimberly Gilbert, Managing Editor
Alexa Chew, Contributing Editor
Magazine reporting on legislation affecting the mentally ill and their families. *$325.00*

7734 **Modern Maturity**
AARP
601 E Street NW
Washington, DC 20049-0003 202-434-2277
202-434-3525
Fax: 888-687-2277
member@aarp.org
www.aarp.org
Gail E. Aldrich, Board Chair
Robert G. Romasco, President
Offers news and information of concern to those 50 and older. Features articles on current events, health, recreation, housing, family life, legislation and other issues.

7735 **Molecular Imaging**
Sage Journals
2455 Teller Road
Thousand Oaks, CA 91320 805-499-9774
journals@sagepub.com
journals.sagepub.com/home/mix
Henry F. VanBrocklin, PhD, Editor-in-Chief
Peer-reviewed open access journal focusing on molecular imaging research, including basic science, preclinical studies and human applications. Published in association with the Society of Nuclear Medicine and Molecular Imaging.

7736 **New Living**
New Living Magazine
PO Box 1001
Patchogue, NY 11772 631-751-8819
800-NEW-LIVI
Fax: 631-751-8910
www.newliving.com
Christine Ly Harvey, Publisher and Editor-in-Chief
Features and articles about holistic health and fitness;herbal remedies, preventive medicine, nutrition, mind/body health, spirituality, fitness, recipes, book reviews and more!

7737 **PN**
PVA Publications
2111 E Highland Avenue
Suite 180
Phoenix, AZ 85016 602-224-0500
888-888-2201
Fax: 602-224-0507
www.pn-magazine.com
Richard Hoover, Editor
Sherri Shea, Marketing & Circulation Director
Magazine spotlighting independent living for paraplegics and quadriplegics. *$23.00*

7738 **Prevention**
Rodale Inc
400 South 10th Street
Emmaus, PA 18098 610-967-5171
800-848-4735
Fax: 910-967-8963
RodaleBooks@cdsfulfillment.com
rodaleinc.com/
Maria Rodale, CEO and Chairman
Scott D. Schulman, President
Magazine containing articles on wellness, preventive medicine, self-care, and fitness. *$21.97*

7739 **Remedy**
Rx Remedies
500 Highway 51 North
Suite Q
Ridgeland, MS 39157 601-981-0070
800-826-1197
Fax: 800-729-0167
www.rxremediesms.com/
Joan Montgomery, Publisher
Consumer magazine covering health and wellness for individuals over 50 years in the US. *$183.00*

7740 **Research on Aging**
Sage Publications
2455 Teller Road
Thousand Oaks, CA 91320 805-499-0721
Fax: 805-499-0871
info@sagepub.com
www.sagepub.in/
Angela M O'Rand, Editor
Blaise R Simqu, CEO
Social gerontology journal.

7741 **SELF Magazine**
Cond, Nast
4 Times Square
New York, NY 10036 212-286-2860
800-223-0780
Fax: 212-880-8248
communications@condenast.com
www.condenast.com/
Rochelle Udell, Editor-in-Chief
Larry Burstein, Publisher
Magazine serving as a health sourcebook for contemporary women.

7742 **Secure Retirement, The Newsmagazine for Mature Americans**
The National Committee to Preserve Social Security
111 K Street NE
Suite 700
Washington, DC 20002 202-216-0420
800-966-1935
Fax: 202-216-0446
webmaster@ncpssm.org
www.ncpssm.org
Max Richtman, President & CEO
Magazine for senior citizens and others interested in politics and government and how they affect senior concerns and issues.

7743 **Senior Times Magazine**
Senior Times Magazine
4400 NW 36th Avenue
Gainesville, FL 32601
352-372-5468
Fax: 352-373-9178
www.seniortimesmagazine.com/
Charlie Delatorre, Publisher
Albert Issac, Editor-in-Chief
Magazine devoted to educating senior citizens on recreational, political, health and financial issues. *$15.00*

7744 **Serenity**
Little Sisters of The Poor
601 Maiden Choice Lane
Baltimore, MD 21228
410-744-9367
Fax: 410-788-5614
serenitys@littlesistersofthepoor.org
www.littlesistersofthepoor.org/
S R Marguerite, Publications Coordinator
Saint Jeanne Jugan, Founder
Magazine making known the apostolate of Little Sisters of the Poor and providing a positive view of the elderly and the respect due them.
32 pages

7745 **Society of Nuclear Medicine and MolecularImaging**
1850 Samuel Morse Drive
Reston, VA 20190
703-708-9000
Fax: 703-708-9015
feedback@snmmi.org
www.snmmi.org
Virginia Pappas, CEO
Rebecca Maxey, Director, Communications
The mission of this nonprofit scientific and professional organization is to promote the science, technology and application of nuclear medicine and molecular imaging. Molecular imaging techniques are used to diagnose and manage the treatment of brain disorders such as Alzheimer's and Parkinson's disease, among other conditions.

7746 **Spirit of Change Magazine**
Spirit of Change Magazine
PO Box 405
Uxbridge, MA 01569
508-278-9640
Fax: 508-278-9641
info@spiritofchange.org
www.spiritofchange.org/
Carol Bedrosian, Publisher/Editor
Michella Bedrosian, Advertising Director
Consumer magazine covering holistic health and New Age issues. *$255.00*

7747 **The American Wanderer**
American Volkssport Association (AVA)
1001 Pat Booker Road
Suite 101
Universal City, TX 78148
210-659-2112
Fax: 210-659-1212
AVAHQ@ava.org
www.ava.org
Henry Rosales, Executive Director, AVA
Consumer magazine covering sports and health news. *$20.00*

7748 **Ultrasonic Imaging**
Sage Journals
2455 Teller Road
Thousand Oaks, CA 91320
805-499-9774
journals@sagepub.com
journals.sagepub.com/home/uix
Ernest J. Feleppa, Editor-in-Chief
Roslyn Raskin, Managing Editor
The journal focuses on the rapid publication of original papers on the development and application of ultrasonic techniques, with emphasis on medical diagnosis. Also published are research notes, comments on papers appearing in the journal, book reviews, and occasional review articles.

7749 **VANTAGE**
Signature Group Inc.
15-598 Falconbridge Rd.
Sudbury, ON P3A 5
877-688-1989
Fax: 877-688-0808
www.signaturegroupinc.com/
Paul Misniak, Publisher
Joanie Davies, Mailing Contact
Magazine for active consumers over 55 years of age.

7750 **VFW Auxiliary**
Ladies Auxiliary to the VFW
406 W 34th Street
10th Floor
Kansas City, MO 64111
816-561-8655
Fax: 816-931-4753
info@ladiesauxvfw.org
www.ladiesauxvfw.org/
Armithea "Si Borel, National President
Marilyn Ebersole, Mailing Contact/Editor
VFW auxiliary patriotic services magazine.

7751 **Vegetarian Voice**
North American Vegetarian Society
PO Box 72
Dolgeville, NY 13329
518-568-7970
Fax: 518-568-7979
navs@telenet.net
www.navs-online.org
Maribeth Abrams, Managing Editor
Brian Graff, Executive Manager
Consumer magazine covering vegetarianism, health, cooking, environmental and animal protection issues. *$203.00*
40 pages

7752 **Veggie Life**
EGW.com
4075 Papazian Way
208
Fremont, CA 94538
925-671-9852
Fax: 925-671-0692
www.egw.com/
Shanna Masters, Editor
Rickie Wilson, Advertising Manager
Consumer magazine covering health, nutrition, and vegetarian cooking. *$23.70*
68 pages

7753 **Vim & Vigor Magazine**
McMurry
1010 E. Missouri Ave.
Phoenix, AZ 85014
602-395-5850
800-282-5850
Fax: 602-395-5853
mcmurrytmg.com/
Matthew Peterson, CEO
Fred Petrovsky, COO
Magazine offering articles on health, fitness, and medical research. *$7.00*

7754 **WebMD Magazine**
WebMD, LLC
395 Hudson Street
New York, NY 10014
www.webmd.com/magazine
Vanessa Cognard, Publisher
Kristy Hammam, Editor in Chief

7755 **eNeuro**
Society for Neuroscience
1121 14th Street NW
Suite 1010
Washginton, DC 20005
202-312-7305
eNeuro@sfn.org
www.eneuro.org
Christophe Bernard, Editor-in-Chief
Kelly Newton, Director, Scientific Publications
Open-access journal of the Society for Neuroscience.

Newsletters

7756 **AGRAM**
Assoc of Ohio Philanthropic Homes, Housing/Service
855 S Wall St
Columbus, OH 43206-1921
614-444-2882
Fax: 614-444-2974
www.aopha.org

John Alfano, CEO
Tim White, Executive Director
P Alfano, President/CEO
Weekly

7757 **Aging & Vision News**
Lighthouse International
111 E 59th St
New York, NY 10022-1202
212-821-9216
800-829-0500
Fax: 212-821-9707
info@lighthouse.org
www.lightfair.com

Laurie A Silbersweig, Editorial Director
Intended for professionals engaged in research, education or service delivery in the field of vision and aging.
6-12 pages Newsletter

7758 **Aging News Alert**
C D Publications
8204 Fenton St
Silver Spring, MD 20910-4502
301-588-6380
800-666-6380
Fax: 301-588-6385

Michael Gerecht, President
Ash Gerecht, Co-Owner
Reports on successful senior programs, funding opportunities, and federal actions that effect the elderly. Available in 6, 12 or 24 month subscriptions online and online/print combinations.
$192.00
8 pages Monthly

7759 **CAHSA Connecting**
Colorado Assoc of Homes and Services for the Aging
1888 Sherman St
Suite 610
Denver, CO 80203-1160
303-837-8834
Fax: 303-837-8836
info@cahsa.org
www.leadingagecolorado.org

Laura Landwirth, Executive Director
Elisabeth Borden, Director
Maureen Hewitt, President
Vennita Jenkins, Secretary
CAHSA Connecting is published monthly by the Colorado Association of Homes and Services for the Aging (CAHSA)

7760 **CANPFA-Line**
CT Assoc of Not-for-Profit Providers of the Aging
1340 Wilmington Rdg
Berlin, CT 6037
860-828-2903
Fax: 860-828-8694
leadingagect@leadingagect.org
www.leadingagect.org

Mag Morelli, President
Nurka Carrero, Office Manager
Andrea Bellofiore, Director of Member Programs & Se
Beth Ricker, Finance Manager & Membership Dir
LeadingAge Connecticut promotes and advocates for a vision of the world in which every community offers an integrated and coordinated continuum of high quality, affordable health care, housing and community based services.
Bi-Monthly

7761 **Capitol Focus**
Colorado Assoc of Homes and Services for the Aging
1888 Sherman St
Suite 610
Denver, CO 80203-1160
303-837-8834
Fax: 303-837-8836
info@cahsa.org
www.leadingagecolorado.org

Laura Landwirth, Executive Director
Elisabeth Borden, Director
Maureen Hewitt, President
Vennita Jenkins, Secretary
Capitol Focus is a weekly activities summary of the Colorado Legislature for CAHSA members, provided by staff of the Colorado Association of Homes and Services for the Aging.

7762 **Capsule**
Children of Aging Parents
P.O. Box 167
Richboro, PA 18954-167
215-945-6900
800-227-7294
Fax: 215-945-8720
www.caps4caregivers.org

Karen Rosenberg, Director
An informative newsletter for caregivers.
Quarterly

7763 **Elder Visions Newsletter**
National Indian Council on Aging
8500 Menaul Blvd. NE
Suite B470
Albuquerque, NM 87112
505-292-2001
Fax: 505-292-1922
info@nicoa.org
www.nicoa.org

Randella Bluehouse, Executive Director
Provides information on issues affecting American Indian and Alaska Native Elders.
Quarterly

7764 **Enabling News**
Access II Independent Living Centers
101 Industrial Parkway
Gallatin, MO 64640-1280
660-663-2423
888-663-2423
Fax: 660-663-2517
TTY: 660-663-2663
access@accessii.org
www.accessii.org

Debra Hawman, Executive Director
Gary Matticks, Owner
Debra Hawman, Executive Director
It is a newsletter published by Access II.
8 pages Quarterly

7765 **Independence**
Easterseals
141 W Jackson Blvd.
Suite 1400A
Chicago, IL 60604
312-726-6200
800-221-6827
Fax: 312-726-1494
info@easterseals.com
www.easterseals.com

Angela F. Williams, President & CEO
Glenda Oakley, Chief Financial Officer
Marcy Traxler, Senior Vice President, Network Advancement
John Osterlund, Senior Vice President, Development
Newsletter featuring information on Easterseals services, stories and news from the Office of Public Affairs.
Quarterly

7766 **Innovations**
National Council on Aging
1901 L Street NW
4th Floor
Washington, DC 20036-3506
202-479-1200
Fax: 202-479-0735
TTY: 202-479-6674
info@ncoa.org
www.ncoa.org

James Knickman, Interim President & CEO
Explores significant developments in the field of aging, keeping individuals informed on a broad range of topics.
Quarterly

7767 **Legacy**
Easterseals
141 W Jackson Blvd.
Suite 1400A
Chicago, IL 60604
312-726-6200
800-221-6827
Fax: 312-726-1494
info@easterseals.com
www.easterseals.com

Angela F. Williams, President & CEO
Glenda Oakley, Chief Financial Officer
Marcy Traxler, Senior Vice President, Network Advancement
John Osterlund, Senior Vice President, Development
Newsletter focusing on planned giving and charitable gift annuities for Easterseals.

7768 **NASUA News**
National Association of State Units on Aging
1201 15th Street NW
Suite 350
Washington, DC 20005-2842
202-898-2578
Fax: 202-898-2583
www.nasuad.org

Martha Roherty, Executive Director
Peggie Rice, Director of Policy and Legislative Affairs
Eric Risteen, Chief Operating Officer
Kimberly Fletcher, Conference and Outreach Coordinator
It is the newsletter of the National Association of State Units on Aging
Monthly

7769 **NCOA Week**
National Council on Aging
1901 L Street NW
4th Floor
Washington, DC 20036-3540
202-479-1200
Fax: 202-479-0735
TTY: 202-479-6674
info@ncoa.org
www.ncoa.org

James Knickman, Interim President/CEO
Donna Whitt, SVP/CFO
A concise e-newsletters focused on the issues you care about, including policies that affect funding, grants and awards you can apply for, and best practices you can adapt for your center.
Weekly

7770 **NNEAHSA**
Northn New England Assoc of Homes & Svcs for Aging
PO Box 1428
Standish, ME 04084-1428
207-773-4822
Fax: 207-773-0101
www.agingservicesmenh.org

Sheila Deringis, Editor
Providing healthy, affordable and ethical long-term care to older citizens throughout Maine, New Hampshire and Vermont.

7771 **NSCLC Washington Weekly**
National Senior Citizens Law Center
1444 Eye St NW
Suite 1100
Washington, DC 20005-6547
202-289-6976
Fax: 202-289-7224
www.nsclc.org

Paul Nathanson, Executive Director
Edward King, Executive Director
Edward Spurgeon, Executive Director
Provides the latest case information, administration and congressional developments of importance for the elderly.

7772 **Part B News**
DecisionHealth
9737 Washingtonian Blvd
Two Washingtonian Center, Suite. 20
Gaithersburg, MD 20878-7364
301-287-2682
855-225-5341
Fax: 301-287-2535
customer@decisionhealth.com
www.decisionhealth.com

Scott Kraft, Editor
Scott Kraft, Director, Content Management
Steve Greenberg, President
Tonya Nevin, Vice President, New Business Development
Each week Part B News brings you comprehensive Medicare Part B regulatory coverage, plain-English interpretive guidance, Fee Schedule updates, claims filing strategies, coding, documentation and payment best practices, and the latest on Congressional health care deliberations and how they affect your practice.
$519.00
Yearly

7773 **Post-Polio Health**
Post-Polio Health International
50 Crestwood Executive Ctr.
Suite 440
St. Louis, MO 63126
314-534-0475
Fax: 314-534-5070
editor@post-polio.org
www.post-polio.org

Brian M. Tiburzi, Editor
Post-Polio Health supports Post-Polio Health International's educational, research, and advocacy efforts. Offers information about relevant events.
12 pages Quarterly

7774 **Quality First**
American Assoc of Homes and Services for the Aging
2519 Connecticut Ave NW
Washington, DC 20008-1520
202-783-2242
Fax: 202-783-2255
www.leadingage.org

William L Minnix Jr, President
Features helpful tips for marketing services and earning the public's trust through the web site.
Quarterly

7775 **Senior Focus**
National Council on Aging
1901 L Street
4th Floor
Washington, DC 20036-3540
202-479-1200
Fax: 202-479-0735
TTY: 202-479-6674
info@ncoa.org
www.ncoa.org

James Knickman, Interim President & CEO
Contains health, financial, lifestyle tips written for seniors
Quarterly

7776 **Social Security Bulletin**
US Social Security Administration
2100 M Street NW
Suite 829 #829
Washington, DC 20037- 0002
202-358-6066
800-772-1213
Fax: 202-282-7219
TTY: 800-325-0778
www.ssa.gov/policy

Karyn Tucker, Managing Editor
Richard Balkus, Assoc. Comm. Office Of Dis
Carolyn W. Colvin, Commissioner
James A. Kissko, Chief of Staff
Reports on results of research and analysis pertinent to the Social Security and SSI programs. *$16.00*
Monthly

Support Groups

7777 **Area Agency on Aging of Southwest Arkansas**
600 Columbia Road 11 East
PO Box 1863
Magnolia, AR 71753
870-234-7410
800-272-2127
Fax: 870-234-6804
www.agewithdignity.com

Janet Morrison, Executive Director

The Area Agency on Aging of Southwest Arkansas, Inc. is a non-profit organization serving adults age 60 or older, family caregivers, agencies and organizations working with seniors. It is part of a national network of more than 650 Area Agencies on Aging throughout the United States.

7778 **Area Agency on Aging: Region One**
1366 E Thomas Rd
Suite 108
Phoenix, AZ 85014-5739
602-264-2255
888-783-7500
Fax: 602-230-9132
www.aaaphx.org

Mary Lynn Kasunic, President
Jeannine Berg, Vice Chairman
Bobbie Garland, Vice Chairman
Richard Peitzmeier, Vice Chairman

We have a vast variety of programs and services to enhance the quality of life for residents of Maricopa County, Arizona. If you would like more information about services mentioned within the website please call.

7779 **High Country Council of Governments Area Agency on Aging**
468 New Market Blvd
Boone, NC 28607-1820
828-265-5434
Fax: 828-265-5439
breece@regiond.org
www.regiond.org

Robert L. Johnson, Chairman
Gary D. Blevins, Vice Chair
Brenda Lyerly, Secretary
Danny McIntosh, Treasurer

High Country Council of Governments is the multi-county planning and development agency for the seven northwestern North Carolina counties of Alleghany, Ashe, Avery, Mitchell, Watauga, Wilkes, and Yancey. The High Country region is a voluntary association of towns and counties located in the northern mountains of North Carolina.

7780 **Institute on Aging**
3575 Geary Blvd
San Francisco, CA 94118-3212
415-750-4111
877-750-4111
Fax: 415-750-5337
info@ioaging.org
www.ioaging.org

J. Thomas Briody, MHSc, President
Dustin Harper, Vice President, Community Living Services
Cindy Kauffman, MS, COO
Roxana Tsougarakis, MBA, Chief Financial Officer

Support Services for Elders (SSE) provides care coordination, household management, personal support, bookkeeping, and other assistance to help protect your financial affairs.

7781 **Land-of-Sky Regional Council Area Agency on Aging**
339 New Leicester Hwy
Suite 140
Asheville, NC 28806-2087
828-251-6622
Fax: 828-251-6353
info@landofsky.org
www.landofsky.org

LeeAnne Tucker, Aging & Volunteer Services Director
Terry Albrecht, Program Director
Joan Tuttle, Director
Joe Mc Kinney, Manager

Is the designated regional organization to meet the needs of persons over 60 in Buncombe, Henderson, Madison, and Transylvania counties, by the North Carolina Division of Aging and Adult Services.

7782 **Lumber River Council of Governments Area Agency on Aging**
30 Cj Walker Rd
COMtech Park
Pembroke, NC 28372-7340
910-618-5533
Fax: 910-521-7556
lrcog@mail.lrcog.dst.nc.us
www.lumberrivercog.org

Michelle Gaitley, Nutrition Program Director
Renee Cooper, Nutrition Program Assistant
Kristen Elk Maynor, Aging Program Coordinator
Margaret Lennon, Division Administrator

The Family Caregiver Support Program was created to assist family members, neighbors, and friends who help care for a person over the age of 60, or minor grandchildren being reared by a grandparent over 60.

7783 **Mid-America Regional Council - Aging and Adult Services**
600 Broadway
Suite 200
Kansas City, MO 64105-1659
816-474-4240
Fax: 816-421-7758
marcinfo@marc.org
www.marc.org/Community/Aging/

James Stowe, Director of Aging & Adult Services
Bob Hogan, Manager of Aging Administrative Services
Shannon Halvorsen, Information & Referral Coordinator
Toni Bartram, Administrative Assistant

The Department of Aging and Adult Services offers community-based services to aging people in the Cass, Clay, Jackson, Platte and Ray counties. Services include home care, transportation, legal aid, breaks for caregivers and meal delivery.

7784 **Mid-Carolina Area Agency on Aging**
130 Gillespie Street
3rd Floor, Post Office Drawer 1510
Fayetteville, NC 28301-1510
910-323-4191
Fax: 910-323-9330
gdye@mccog.org
www.mccog.org

James Caldwell, COG Executive Director
Glenda Dye, Aging Director
Lynda Barnett, Aging Care Manager
Carla Smith, Aging Program Specialist

The Mid-Carolina Area Agency on Aging is designated for planning, administration, and advocacy of services for persons aged 60 and older and their spouses who need assistance in order to remain as independent as possible.

7785 **Piedmont Triad Council of Governments Area Agency on Aging**
2216 W Meadowview Rd
Suite 201
Greensboro, NC 27407-3480
336-294-4950
Fax: 336-632-0457
www.ptcog.org

Blair Barton-Percival, Director
Adrienne Calhoun, Assistant Director
Bob Cleveland, Aging Program Planner
Joe Dzugan, Aging Systems Coordinator

Responsible for planning, developing, implementing, and coordinating aging services for seven counties in the Piedmont Triad (Alamance, Caswell, Davidson, Guilford, Montgomery, Randolph, and Rockingham) and their 185,00 residents age 60 and older.

7786 **Southwestern Commission Area Agency on Aging**
125 Bonnie Ln
Sylva, NC 28779-8552
828-586-1962
Fax: 828-586-1968
www.regiona.org

Ryan Sherby, Executive Director
Beth Cook, Workforce Development Director
Janne Mathews, Aging Program Coordinator
Sarajane Melton, Area Agency on Aging Administrator

The Area Agency on Aging (AAA) works on behalf of older adults and their caregivers in the seven southwestern counties of

North Carolina. The Southwestern Commission Area Agency on Aging was established in 1980 as mandated by the 1977 Amendments of the Older Americans Act in order for a Planning and Service Area (PSA) to receive funds from the Act.

7787 **Tompkins County Office for the Aging**
214 W. Martin Luther King Jr./State
Ithaca, NY 14850-4299
607-274-5482
Fax: 607-274-5495
lholmes@tompkins-co.org

Lisa Holmes, Director
Lisa Lunas, Aging Services Planner
Katrina Schickel, Aging Services Specialist
David Stoyell, Aging Services Specialist

We provide objective and unbiased information regarding the array of services available for older adults and their caregivers. Established in 1975, our mission is to assist the senior population of Tompkins County to remain independent in their homes as long as is possible and appropriate, and with a decent quality of life and human dignity.

7788 **Triangle J Council of Governments Area Agency on Aging**
4307 Emperor Blvd
Suite 110
Durham, NC 27703
919-549-0551
Fax: 919-549-9390
ejones@tjcog.org
www.tjaaa.org

Kristen Jackson, Aging Program Coordinator
Mary Warren, Director
Ashley Price, Program Specialist
Jennifer Link, Regional Ombudsman for Long-Term Care

The Triangle J Council of Governments serves to facilitate and support the development of programs addressing the needs of older adults and to support investment in their talents and interests.

7789 **University of California Memory and Aging Center**
675 Nelson Rising Lane
Suite 190
San Francisco, CA 94143-1207
415-353-2057
Fax: 415-476-5591

Bruce L Miller, Director
Mary Koestler, Project Administrator
Carrie Cheung, Clinic Coordinator
Ken Edwards, Administrative Assistant

Provides support for patients and families affected by neurodegenerative diseases. In addition to our established support groups, we continue to develop new support groups.

7790 **Upper Coastal Plain Council of Governments Area Agency on Aging**
PO Box 9
Wilson, NC 27894-9
252-234-5952
Fax: 252-234-5971
www.ucpcog.org

Greg Godard, Executive Director
Jody Riddle, AAA Program Director
Helen Page, Aging Programs Specialist
Abigail W. Harper, Regional Ombudsman

The Upper Coastal Plain Area Agency On Aging is one of 16 Area Agencies on Aging across the state of NC, serving Region L. Counties include Edgecombe, Halifax, Nash, Northampton, and Wilson. The mission of the Area Agency on Aging is to empower senior adults, family caregivers, and individuals with disabilities residing in Edgecombe, Halifax, Nash, Northampton, and Wilson Counties to live independent, meaningful, healthy, and dignified lives.

Blind & Deaf

Audio/Visual

5426 **Getting in Touch**
2612 N Mattis Ave
PO Box 7886
Champaign, IL 61826-1053
217-352-3273
800-519-2707
Fax: 217-352-1221
orders@researchpress.com
www.researchpress.com

Russell Pence, President
David Parkinson, Chairman
Cynthia Martin, Principal
Ann Parkinson, Principal

5438 **Journey**
Landmark Media
3450 Slade Run Dr
Falls Church, VA 22042-3940
703-241-2030
800-342-4336
Fax: 703-536-9540
info@landmarkmedia.com
landmarkmedia.com

Michael Hartogs, President
Richard Hartogs, VP Acquisitions
Peter Hartogs, VP New Business & Development
Eric Miller, Sales Representative

A moving portrayal of the extraordinary journey to Japan of 74-year-old Billie Sinclair, who is deaf, blind and mute. He funds his travels by weaving and selling baskets. In Japan he rides a roller coaster, tries judo and visits a deaf and blind acupuncturist. He demonstrates how it is possible to communicate by touch alone. *$195.00*
Video

Associations

7791 **American Association of the Deaf-Blind**
248 Rainbow Drive
Suite 14864
Livingston, TX 77399-2048
aadb-info@aadb.org
www.aadb.org

Rene Pellerin, President
Mindy Dill, Vice President
Tara Invidiato, Secretary
Sarah Goodwin, Treasurer

The American Association of the Deaf-Blind (AADB) is a non-profit national consumer organization run by and for deaf-blind Americans and their supporters. Deaf-Blind includes all types and degrees of dual vision and hearing loss. The association offers an information clearinghouse, service provider summit, deaf-blind technology summit, research projects, interpretation services, conferences and more.

7792 **American Society for Deaf Children**
PO Box 23
Woodbine, MD 21797
800-942-2732
info@deafchildren.org
deafchildren.org

Alisha Joslyn-Swob, President
Mark Drolsbaugh, Vice President
Rachel Berman, Secretary

The American Society for Deaf Children provides information for the caretakers of deaf children so children can have full communication access in their home, school and community. The society covers areas such as visual language, audiologists, healthcare providers, assistive technology and more.

7793 **Arena Stage**
The Mead Center for American Theater
1101 Sixth St. SW
Washington, DC 20024
202-554-9066
Fax: 202-488-4056
TTY: 202-484-0247
info@arenastage.org
arenastage.org

Edgar Dobie, Executive Director
Molly Smith, Artistic Director
Joseph Berardelli, CFO
Khady Kamara, Managing Director

Arena Stage has played a pioneering role in providing access to all productions for people with disabilities. Access services and programs include wheelchair accessible seating; infrared assistive listening devices; Braille, large print, audio description and sign interpretation at designated performances.

7794 **Association of Late-Deafened Adults**
8038 Macintosh Ln
Suite 2
Rockford, IL 61107-5336
815-332-1515
TTY: 815-332-1515
www.alda.org

Rick Brown, President
Cynthia Moynihan, Vice President
Matt Ferrara, Treasurer
Tina Childress, Secretary

The Association of Late-Deafened Adults supports the empowerment of late-deafened people by offering programs and information resources on a variety of topics: technology, disability laws, airline travel and more.

7795 **Canadian Deafblind Association**
1860 Appleby Line
Unit 14
Burlington, ON, Canada L7L-7H7
905-331-6279
866-229-5832
Fax: 905-319-2027
info@cdbanational.com
www.cdbanational.com

Carolyn Monaco, President
Tom McFadden, National Executive Director

The mission of the Canadian Deafblind Association is to promote and enhance the well-being of people who are deafblind by offering them advocacy, developing and dissemination information, and supporting members and community partners who also serve deafblind people.

7796 **Foundation Fighting Blindness**
7168 Columbia Gateway Dr.
Suite 100
Columbia, MD 21046
410-423-0600
800-683-5555
TTY: 410-363-7139
info@FightBlindness.org
www.blindness.org

Benjamin R. Yerxa, Chief Executive Officer
Jason Menzo, Chief Operating Officer
Todd Durham, VP, Clinical & Outcomes Research

The Foundation Fighting Blindness (FFB) works to promote research in order to prevent, treat and restore vision. FFB is currently the world's leading private funder of retinal disease research, funding over 100 research grants and 150 researchers.

7797 **Future Reflections**
Deaf-Blind Division of the Ntn'l Fed of the Blind
200 E Wells St
Baltimore, MD 21230
410-659-9314
Fax: 410-685-5653
nfbpublications@nfb.org
nfb.org

Deborah Kent Stein, Editor

A magazine for parents and teachers of blind children.

7798 Hearing Loss Association of America
7910 Woodmont Ave
Suite 1200
Bethesda, MD 20814
301-657-2248
Fax: 301-913-9413
inquiry@hearingloss.org
www.hearingloss.org

Barbara Kelley, Executive Director
Lise Hamlin, Director of Public Policy
Carla Beyer-Smolin, National Chapter & Membership Coordinator
Amanda Watson, Meeting Planner

The mission of the Hearing Loss Association of America is to open the world of communication to people with hearing loss by offering information, education, resources, advocacy and training.

7799 Helen Keller National Center for Deaf- Blind Youths and Adults
141 Middle Neck Rd
Sands Point, NY 11050
516-944-8900
TTY: 516-570-3246
hkncinfo@hknc.org
www.helenkeller.org

Kim Zimmer, President & CEO
Marc Feldman, CPA, Chief Financial Officer
Mary Fu, Chief Development Officer
Gary Messina, Chief Facilities Officer

The center serves deafblind people by offering them assistive technology, vocational services, education, case management, interpretation, medical and mental health services, professional training and other supports that would empower them to work and live independently within their communities.

7800 Idaho Commission for the Blind and Visually Impaired
341 W. Washington St
PO Box 83720
Boise, ID 83720-0012
208-334-3220
800-542-8688
Fax: 208-334-2963
bcunningham@icbvi.idaho.gov
www.icbvi.state.id.us

Britt Raubenheimer, Chair
Beth Cunningham, Administrator
Bailie Welton, Management Assistant
Mike Walsh, Rehabilitation Services Chief

The Idaho Commission for the Blind and Visually Impaired works to empower persons who are blind or visually impaired by providing vocational rehabilitation training, skills training and educational opportunities to achieve self fulfillment ang gain employment. The Commission also strives to serve as a resource to families and employers and to expand public awareness regarding the potential of all persons who are blind or visually impaired.

7801 International Hearing Society
16880 Middlebelt Rd
Suite 4
Livonia, MI 48154
734-522-7200
Fax: 734-522-0200
interact@ihsinfo.org
ihsinfo.org

Annette Cross, BC-HIS, President
Kathleen Mennillo, MBA, Executive Director
Fran Vincent, Director, Membership & Marketing
Tara Douglass, Business Development Manager

The International Hearing Society (IHS) represents hearing healthcare professionals worldwide. Members include professionals engaged in the practice of testing human hearing and selecting, fitting and dispensing hearing instruments. IHS offers accreditation programs, advocacy, education and training in support of these services.

7802 Lilac Services for the Blind
1212 N Howard St
Spokane, WA 99201
509-328-9116
800-422-7893
Fax: 509-328-8965
contact@lilacblind.org
lilacblind.org

Eddie Eugenio, President
Cheryl L Martin, Executive Director
Robin Waller, Development Director
Raychel Callary, Certified Orientation & Mobility Specialist

Lilac Services for the Blind provides independent living instruction, adaptive aids, counseling, low-vision evaluations, support groups, Braille transcription services and more for 14 counties in the inland Northwest.

7803 National Center on Deaf-Blindness (NCDB)
Hellen Keller National Center
141 Middle Neck Rd.
Sands Point, NY 11050
541-800-0412
support@nationaldb.org
www.nationaldb.org

Sam Morgan, Director
Julie Durando, Evaluation Coordinator
Peggy Malloy, Information Services & Technology Coordinator

Funded by the federal Department of Education, the Center seeks to improve quality of life for children who are deaf-blind and their families.

7804 National Family Association for Deaf-Blind
PO Box 1667
Sands Point, NY 11050
800-255-0411
Fax: 516-883-9060
nfadb.org

Patti McGowan, President
Diana Griffen, Vice President
Jacqueline Izaguirre, Treasurer
Melanie Knapp, Secretary

The National Family Association for Deaf-Blind (NFADB) is a nonprofit, volunteer-based family association. The association offers advocacy, education and family supports to help create empowerment opportunities for deaf-blind people.

7805 National Federation of the Blind
200 E Wells St.
Baltimore, MD 21230
410-659-9314
Fax: 410-685-5653
nfb@nfb.org
nfb.org

Mark Riccobono, President
John Berggren, Executive Director, Operations
Anil Lewis, Executive Director, Blindness Initiatives
John G. Pare, Jr., Executive Director, Advocacy & Policy

The National Federation of the Blind (NFB) works to help blind people achieve self-confidence, self-respect and self-determination and to achieve complete integration into society on a basis of equality. The Federation provides public educations, information and referral services, scholarships, literature and publications, adaptive equipment, advocacy services, legal services, employment assistance and more.

Camps

7806 Florida Lions Camp
Lions of Multiple District 35
2819 Tiger Lake Road
Lake Wales, FL 33898-9582
863-696-1948
Fax: 863-696-2398
bjcage@hotmail.com
www.lionscampfl.org

Barbara Cage, Executive Director
Liz Cage, Program Director
Carissa Moen, Bookkeeping/Registrar

One-week sessions June-August for youths and adults with visual impairments and other challenging disabilities. Coed, ages 5 and up. A variety of traditional summer camp activities which include: swimming, canoeing, fishing, hiking, camping out and cooking over a fire, games, arts & crafts, singing & dancing, hay-wagon rides, challenge course and much more. Activities are adapted to the age and ability of each camper to ensure maximum participation, safety and fun.

7807 **Florida School for the Deaf and Blind**
207 San Marco Ave
St Augustine, FL 32084-2799
904-827-2200
800-344-3732
Fax: 904-827-2325
www.fsdb.k12.fl.us

Dr. Jeanne Glidden Prickett, EdD, Shelter Administrator
Debbie Schuler, Administrator of Instructional S
Cindy Day, Executive Director of Parent Ser
Terri Wiseman, Administrator of Business Servic

Statewide public boarding school for eligible students who are deaf/hard-of-hearing or blind/visually impaired. FSDB serves children who are pre-k through high school.

Books

7808 **A Handbook for Writing Effective Psychoeducational Reports (2nd Edition)**
PRO-ED Inc.
8700 Shoal Creek Blvd.
Austin, TX 78757-6897
512-451-3246
800-897-3202
Fax: 800-397-7633
general@proedinc.com
www.proedinc.com

Sharon Bradley-Johnson, Author
C. Merle Johnson, Author

This comprehensive book shows how to write useful reports once assessment information has been attained. It is a valuable resource for professionals working in school systems, as well as for those graduate students who are just learning to write reports. *$32.00*
134 pages Paperback
ISBN 1-416401-40-7

7809 **Communicating with People Who Have Trouble Hearing & Seeing: A Primer**
National Association for Visually Handicapped
22 W 21st St
Fl 6
New York, NY 10010-6943
212-255-2804
Fax: 212-727-2931
info@lighthouse.org
www.lighthouse.org

Roger O Goldman, Chairman Of The Board

Line drawings that depict problems for those with both deficiencies. *$2.00*

7810 **Helen and Teacher: The Story of Helen & Anne Sullivan Macy**
American Foundation for the Blind/AFB Press
11 Penn Plz
Suite 300
New York, NY 10001-2006
212-502-7600
800-232-5463
Fax: 212-502-7777
afbinf@afb.net
www.afb.org

Carl Augusto, President
Richard Obnen, Chairman Of The Board
Michael Gilliam, Vice Chairman
Alan Lindroth, Principal

A pictorial biography emphasizing Hellen Keller's accomplishments in public life over a period of more than 60 years. Traces Anne Sullivan's early years and her meeting with Helen Keller, and goes on to recount the joint events of their lives. A definitive biography. $29.95.
Paperback
ISBN 0-891282-89-0

7811 **Independence Without Sight and Sound: Suggestions for Practitioners**
American Foundation for the Blind/AFB Press
11 Penn Plz
Suite 300
New York, NY 10001-2006
212-502-7600
800-232-8463
Fax: 212-502-7777
afbinfo@afb.net
www.afb.org

Carl Augusto, President
Richard Obnen, Chairman Of The Board
Michael Gilliam, Vice Chairman
Alan Lindroth, Principal

This practical guidebook covers the essential aspects of communicating and working with deaf-blind persons. Includes useful information on how to talk with deaf-blind people, and adapt orientation and mobility techniques for deaf-blind travelers. *$39.95*
193 pages Paperback
ISBN 0-891282-46-7

7812 **Reclaiming Independence: Staying in the Drivers Seat When You Are no Longer Drive.**
American Printing House for the Blind
1839 Frankfort Ave
Louisville, KY 40206-3148
502-895-2405
800-223-1839
Fax: 502-899-2274
info@aph.org
www.aph.org

Tuck Tinsley, President
Joseph Paradis, Chairman
Kathleen Huebner, Vice Chairman
Jane Thompson, Executive Director

Useful for both individuals and professionals, this video/resource guide will help you successfuly use rehabilitation and transportation resources. *$60.00*

7813 **Verbal View of the Web & Net**
American Printing House for the Blind
1839 Frankfort Ave
Louisville, KY 40206-3148
502-895-2405
800-223-1839
Fax: 502-899-2274
info@aph.org
www.aph.org

Tuck Tinsley, President
Joseph Paradis, Chairman
Kathleen Huebner, Vice Chairman
Jane Thompson, Executive Director

One of a series of Verbal View titles, Verbal View of the Net & Web explains how to access information on the internet and teaches accessability features of Internet Explorer. *$50.00*

Magazines

7814 **Braille Montior**
National Federation of the Blind
200 E Wells St
Baltimore, MD 21230
410-659-9314
Fax: 410-685-5653
nfbpublications@nfb.org
www.nfb.org

Gary Wunder, Editor

The Braille Monitor is the leading publication of the National Federation of the Blind. It covers the events and activities of the NFB and addresses the many issues and concerns of the blind. *$40.00*
11 times a year

7815 **Deaf-Blind American**
American Association of the Deaf-Blind
248 Rainbow Drive
Suite 14864
Livingston, TX 77399-2048
aadb-info@aadb.org
www.aadb.org

Rene Pellerin, President

The official magazine of the American Association of the Deaf-Blind (AADB).
Quarterly

7816 **Hearing Life Magazine**
Hearing Loss Association of America
7910 Woodmont Ave
Ste 1200
Bethesda, MD 20814-7022
301-657-2248
Fax: 301-913-9413
inquiry@hearingloss.org
www.hearingloss.org

Barbara Kelley, Executive Director
Formerly known as Hearing Loss Magazine, this official publication of the Hearing Loss Association of America helps individuals with hearing loss live a better life.
Bi-Monthly

7817 **Hearing Professional Magazine**
International Hearing Society
Ste 4
16880 Middlebelt Rd
Livonia, MI 48154-3374
734-522-7200
Fax: 734-522-0200
knacarato@ihsinfo.org
www.ihsinfo.org

Kathleen Mennillo, Executive Director
The Hearing Professional magazine is the official publication of the International Hearing Society. This quarterly publication includes industry news, membership highlights and best practices, hearing healthcare legislation, and other information and tools for hearing healthcare professionals.

Newsletters

7818 **AADB E-News**
American Association of the Deaf-Blind
248 Rainbow Drive
Suite 14864
Livingston, TX 77399-2048
aadb-info@aadb.org
www.aadb.org

Rene Pellerin, President
Contains information about the latest events occurring within AADB and in the deaf-blind community.

7819 **ALDA Newsletter**
ALDA
8038 Macintosh Ln
Suite 2
Rockford, IL 61107-5336
815-332-1515
TTY: 815-332-1515
www.alda.org

Rick Brown, President
Articles, stories and poems by and about late-deafened adults.

7820 **Beam**
1850 W Roosevelt Rd
Chicago, IL 60608-1298
312-666-1331
Fax: 312-243-8539
TTY: 312-666-8874
www.chicagolighthouse.org

James Kesteloot, President
Terrence Longo, Assistant Director
Quarterly newsletter of the organization offering progressive programs for the blind, visually impaired, deaf-blind and multi-disabled children and adults, including vocational programs, computer and office skills training, job placement, independent living skills, orientation and mobility training, counseling and a low vision clinic.

7821 **Deaf-Blind Perspective**
National Consortium on Deaf-Blindness
345 Monmouth Ave
Monmouth, OR 97361
503-838-8391
800-438-9376
Fax: 503-838-8150
TTY: 800-854-7013
dbp@wou.edu

John Reiman PhD, Director
Peggy Malloy, Managing Editor
A free publication with articles, essays, and announcements about topics related to people who are deaf-blind. The primary focus is on the education of children and youth with deaf-blindness. Published two times a year (Spring and Fall) by the national consortium on Deaf-blindness at the Teaching Research Institute at Western Oregon University.

7822 **Endeavor Magazine**
American Society for Deaf Children
PO Box 23
Woodbine, MD 21797
800-942-2732
info@deafchildren.org
www.deafchildren.org

Tami Dominguez, Editor
ASDC's qurterly publication featuring committee reports, stories, and fun.
Quarterly

7823 **HKNC Newsletter**
Helen Keller National Center
141 Middle Neck Rd
Sands Point, NY 11050-1218
516-944-8900
Fax: 516-944-7302
TTY: 516-944-8637
hkncinfo@hknc.org
www.hknc.org

Joseph McNulty, Executive Director
Highlights recent activities at the national center.

7824 **InFocus**
7168 Columbia Gateway Dr.
Suite 100
Columbia, MD 21046
410-423-0600
800-683-5555
TTY: 410-363-7139
info@FightBlindness.org
www.blindness.org

Benjamin R. Yerxa, Chief Executive Officer
Presents articles on coping, research updates, and Foundation news.
3x/year

7825 **NAT-CENT**
Helen Keller National Center
141 Middle Neck Rd
Sands Point, NY 11050-1218
516-944-8900
Fax: 516-944-7302
TTY: 516-944-8637
hkncinfo@hknc.org
www.hknc.org

Joseph McNulty, Executive Director
Contains articles on legislation, services, aids and devices, human interest and issues related to deaf-blindness.

7826 **News from Advocates for Deaf-Blind**
National Family Association for Deaf-Blind
PO Box 1667
Sands Point, NY 11050
800-225-0411
Fax: 516-883-9060
www.NFADB.org

Patti McGowan, President
A membership organization which provide resources, education, advocacy, referrals and support for families with children who are deaf-blind; professionals in the field; and individuals who are deaf-blind.
20 pages TriAnnual

Software

7827 **Braille + Mobile Manager**
American Printing House for the Blind
1839 Frankfort Ave
Louisville, KY 40206-0085
502-895-2405
800-223-1839
Fax: 502-899-2284
info@aph.org
aph.org

Tuck Tinsley, President
Joseph Paradis, Chairman
Kathleen Huebner, Vice Chairman
Jane Thompson, Executive Director

Use it like a hand-held PDA or like a laptop. *$1395.00*

7828 **MaximEyes**
American Printing House for the Blind
1839 Frankfort Ave
Louisville, KY 40206-0085
502-895-2405
800-223-1839
Fax: 502-899-2284
info@aph.org
aph.org

Tuck Tinsley, President
Joseph Paradis, Chairman
Kathleen Huebner, Vice Chairman
Jane Thompson, Executive Director

MaximEyes is a plug-in for Internet Explorer that adds a toolbar that allows you to controll the size of website text and images. *$59.95*

Sports

7829 **ASD Athletics**
Alabama Institute for Deaf and Blind
205 South St E
Talladega, AL 35160-2411
256-761-3222
Fax: 256-761-3278
Ripley.Walter@aidb.state.al.us

John Jernigan, Director, Student Development (ASD)
Walter Ripley, Director, Athletics & After-School Programs

Offers students opportunities to participate in a number of organizzed sports including basketball, volleyball, baseball, football, and cheerleading. Student athletes compete at national and international levels.

Support Groups

7830 **Aurora of Central New York**
518 James Street
Suite 100
Syracuse, NY 13203-2282
315-422-7263
Fax: 315-422-4792
TTY: 315-422-9746
auroraofcny.org

John Scala, President
John McCormick, President
Ryan Emery, Treasurer
Leslie Rapson, Secretary

Professional counseling services to assist individuals and their families deal with the trauma of hearing or vision loss.

7831 **Wendell Johnson Speech And Hearing Clinic**
University Of Iowa
250 Hawkins Dr
Iowa City, IA 52242-1025
319-335-8736
Fax: 319-335-8851
kathy-miller@uiowa.edu
www.clas.uiowa.edu/comsci/clinical-services

Linda Souke, Clinic Director
Kathy Miller, Clinic Assistant

The clinic offers assessment and remediation for communication disorders in adults and children. The clinic also offers services during the Summer for school age children needing intervention services because of speech, language, hearing and/or reading problems.

Cognitive

Associations

7832 Academy of Cognitive Therapy
245 N. 15th St
Suite 403
Philadelphia, PA 19102
Fax: 215-537-1789
info@academyofct.org
www.academyofct.org

Lata K McGinn, Ph.D, President
Troy Thompson, Executive Director
Allen Miller, Ph.D, MBA, Treasurer
Elaine Elliott-Moskwa, Ph.D, Secretary

The Academy of Cognitive Therapy is a non-profit organization that supports continuing education and research in cognitive therapy, provides resources for professionals and the public, and offers certification for those skilled in the field.

7833 Adults & Children with Learning & Developmental Disabilities (ACLD)
807 S Oyster Bay Rd.
Bethpage, NY 11714
516-822-0028
www.acld.org

Robert C. Goldsmith, Executive Director
Robert Ciatto, Chief Operating Officer
Aimee C. Keegan, Director, Development & Community Relations
Joel Santana, Director, Regulatory Affairs & Corporate Compliance Officer

Nonprofit serving Long Island by supporting individuals with developmental disabilities and their families.

7834 Albert Ellis Institute
145 East 32nd St.
9th Fl.
New York, NY 10016
212-535-0822
Fax: 212-249-3582
info@albertellis.org
albertellis.org

Kristene A. Doyle, Director

Psychotherapy training Institute focused on the teachings of Albert Ellis, primarily the therapeutic approach known as Rational Emotive Behavior Therapy (REBT).

7835 American Academy of Child & Adolescent Psychiatry
3615 Wisconsin Ave NW
Washington, DC 20016-3007
202-966-7300
Fax: 202-464-0131
communications@aacap.org
www.aacap.org

Gregory K Fritz, MD, President
Heidi B Fordi, CAE, Executive Director
Karen Ferguson, Deputy Director of Clinical Practice
Rob Grant, Communications Director

The American Academy of Child & Adolescent Psychiatry is a non-profit organization engaged in research, education and advocacy specific to child and adolescent psychiatry. The academy's mission is to provide resources and knowledge beneficial to patients, their families and psychiatric professionals.

7836 American Delirium Society
1183 University Dr
Suite 105 - 106
Burlington, NC 27215
410-955-2343
info@americandeliriumsociety.org
www.americandeliriumsociety.org

Rakesh C Arora MD, Ph.D, Director
Noll Campbell, PharmD, MS, Director
John W Devlin, PharmD, Director
Ann Gruber-Baldini, Ph.D, Director

The American Delirium Society fosters research, education, quality improvement, advocacy and science to minimize the impact of delirium on short- and long-term health and well being and the effects of delirium on the health care system as a whole. The organization offers educational resources including videos and publications on the subject.

7837 American Psychiatric Association
1000 Wilson Blvd
Suite 1825
Arlington, VA 22209-3901
703-907-7300
703-907-7300
888-357-7924
Fax: 703-907-1085
apa@psych.org
www.psychiatry.org

Anita Everett, MD, President
Saul M Levin, MD, MPA, CEO & Medical Director
Mark Myers, Director, Administrative Services
Christie Couture, Associate Director of Marketing

The American Psychiatric Association is a medical specialty society with over 37,000 member physicians engaged in the field of psychiatric practice, research, and academia. The association's mission is to ensure humane care and effective treatment of all persons with mental disorders, including substance use disorders. Services offered by them include collegial support, advocacy, publications and more.

7838 Anxiety and Depression Association of America (ADAA)
8701 Georgia Ave.
Suite 412
Silver Spring, MD 20910
240-485-1001
Fax: 240-485-1035
information@adaa.org
adaa.org

Susan K. Gurley, Executive Director
Lise Bram, Deputy Executive Director
Vickie Spielman, Associate Director, Membership & Education
Sasha Sicard, Manager, Membership & Education

The Anxiety and Depression Association of America is an international nonprofit organization and a leader in education, training, and research for anxiety, OCD, PTSD, depression, and related disorders. ADAA encourages the advancement of scientific knowledge about the causes and treatment for mental health issues.

7839 Association for Behavioral and Cognitive Therapies (ABCT)
305 7th Ave
16th Floor
New York, NY 10001
212-647-1890
Fax: 212-647-1865
www.abct.org

Gail Steketee, Ph.D, President
Barbara Kamholz, Ph.D, Convention & Continuing Education Issues
Shireen Rizvi, Ph.D, Academic & Professional Issues
Hilary Vidair, Ph.D, Membership

The ABCT is an organization committed to the advancement of scientific approaches to address the issues of soldiers with PTSD. The association offeres information in a number of areas: combat related stress, military posttraumatic stress disorder, military suicide and veterans' health.

7840 Association for Contextual Behavioral Science
1880 Pinegrove Dr
P.O. Box 655
Jenison, MI 49429
225-302-8688
staff@contextualscience.org
contextualscience.org

Emily Rodrigues, Executive Director
Courtney Zirkle, CMP, Administrative & Social Media Manager

The Association for Contextual Behavioral Science specializes in helping people through research and practice based in contextual behavioral science (including RFT and CBS). The association offers learning resources, training, internships, events, consultations, conferences, continuing education opportunities and more.

7841 Autism National Committee (AUTCOM)
3 Bedford Green
South Burlington, VT 05403
info@autcom.org
www.autcom.org

Anne Bakeman, Membership Coordinator

Seeks to protect and advnce the rights of all individuals with autism, Pervasive Developmental Disorder, and related conditions.

7842 **Autism Network International (ANI)**
PO Box 35448
Syracuse, NY 13235-5448 www.autismnetworkinternational.org
Jim Sinclair, Coordinator
Autistic-run organization offering advocacy and self-help services for autistic people.

7843 **Autism Research Institute**
4182 Adams Ave.
San Diego, CA 92116-2599 866-366-3361
www.autism.com
Stephen Edelson, Ph.D, Executive Director
Anthony Morgali, Producer, ARI Media
Denise Fulton, Administrative Director
Rebecca McKenney, Office Manager
Conducts research on the causes, diagnosis and treatment of autism. The institute also offers a quarterly newsletter that reviews worldwide research, referrals to health care professionals and clinics serving autistic people, advocacy, continuing education and more.

7844 **Autism Services Center**
929 4th Ave.
P.O. Box 507
Huntington, WV 25701-0507 304-525-8014
Fax: 304-525-8026
www.autismservicescenter.org
Ralph N Bentley, President
Jimmie Beirne, Ph.D, CEO
The Autism Services Center assists families and agencies to meet the needs of individuals with autism and other developmental disabilities by offering services such as technical assistance in designing treatment programs, a hotline providing informational packets to callers, supported employment, day programs, residential services and more.

7845 **Autism Society of Minnesota**
Autism Society of Minnesota
2380 Wycliff St.
Suite 102
St. Paul, MN 55114 651-647-1083
Fax: 651-642-1230
info@ausm.org
www.ausm.org
Ellie Wilson, Executive Director
Dawn Brasch, Senior Director, Finance & Operations
Kelly Thomalla, Senior Director, Integration & Advancement
Eric Ringgenberg, Director, Education Programs
The Autism Society of Minnesota (AuSM) is a nonprofit membership organization dedicated to the education, advocacy, and support of individuals and families who have been affected by autism.

7846 **Autism Treatment Center of America**
2080 S Undermountain Rd
Sheffield, MA 01257-9643 413-229-2100
877-766-7473
Fax: 413-229-8931
correspondence@option.org
www.autismtreatmentcenter.org
Barry Neil Kaufman, Founder & CEO
Clyde Haberman, Senior Teacher & Director of Development
Blair Borgeson, Developmental Therapist
Emily Vitale Aronow, Program Advisor & Client Support Coordinator
The Autism Treatment Center of America provides innovative training programs for parents and professionals caring for children challenged by Autism, Autism Spectrum Disorders, Pervasive Developmental Disorders (PDD) and other development difficulties. The center's Son-Rise Program teaches a comprehensive system of treatment and education designed to help families and caregivers enable their children to improve in all areas of learning.

7847 **Autistic Self Advocacy Network (ASAN)**
PO Box 66122
Washington, DC 20035 info@autisticadvocacy.org
autisticadvocacy.org
Julia Bascom, Executive Director
Zoe Gross, Director, Operations
Samantha Crane, Legal Directory & Director, Public Policy
Reid Caplan, Associate Director, Advocacy & Development
Promotes a world in which equal access, rights and opportunities are available to autistic people, through advocacy and empowerment.

7848 **Beck Institute for Cognitive Behavior Therapy**
1 Belmont Ave
Suite 700
Bala Cynwyd, PA 19004 610-664-3020
Fax: 610-709-5336
info@beckinstitute.org
www.beckinstitute.org
Aaron T Beck, Ph.D, President Emeritus
Judith S Beck, Ph.D, President
Lisa Pote, Executive Director
Quethelyn Blake, Finance Manager
The Beck Institute for Cognitive Behavior Therapy serves as a training ground for cognitive therapists and cognitive behavior therapists. The institute provides online resources, training workshops and CBT therapy for the public and mental health professionals.

7849 **Best Buddies**
907-1243 Islington Ave
Toronto, ON, Canada M8X-1Y9 416-531-0003
888-779-0061
Fax: 416-531-0325
info@bestbuddies.ca
bestbuddies.ca
Daniel J Greenglass, Co-Chair
Sarah McCarthy, Program Coordinator
Kimberly Janohan, Program Support
Best Buddies offers programs for people with intellectual or developmental disabilities including those with Down syndrome, autism, cerebral palsy, traumatic brain injury and other undiagnosed disabilities. Programs include schooling, transition programs, sports, scholarships and more.

7850 **Biologically Inspired Cognitive Architectures Society**
4450 Rivanna River Way
Suite 3707
Fairfax, VA 22030-4441 703-910-3014
Fax: 877-532-0197
info@bicasociety.org
bicasociety.org
Alexei V Samsonovich, President-Treasurer
Antonio Chella, Chair
Kamilla R Johannsdottir, Secretary
The Biologically Inspired Cognitive Architectures Society brings together researchers from disjointed fields and communities in order to combine their knowledge into forming a larger, unifying framework for the study of cognitive architectures.

7851 **Brain Injury Alliance of Texas**
9050 N Capital of Texas Hwy
Building 3, Suite 130
Austin, TX 78759 512-326-1212
800-392-0040
Fax: 512-478-3370
www.texasbia.org
Kelly Ramsey, President
Greg Walton, Vice President
Mendi West, Secretary-Treasurer
The Brain Injury Alliance of Texas is a community of people with brain injuries, their families and the professionals that serve them. The alliance offers information, support groups, prevention strategies, educational opportunities, public policy advocacy, a resource library and more.

7852 Brain Injury Association of America (BIAA)
3057 Nutley St.
Suite 805
Fairfax, VA 22031-1931
703-761-0750
Fax: 703-761-0755
info@biausa.org
www.biausa.org

Susan Connors, President & CEO
Mary S. Reitter, Executive Vice President & COO
Robbie Baker, Vice President & CDO
Marianna Abashian, Director, Professional Services

The Brain Injury Association of America is a national organization serving and representing individuals, families and professionals who are touched by a traumatic brain injury (TBI). Its mission is to improve the quality of life for people affected by brain injury through the advancement of research, treatment, education and awareness.
1980

7853 Brain Injury Association of New York State
4 Pine W Plaza
Suite 402
Albany, NY 12205
518-459-7911
800-444-6443
Fax: 518-482-5285
info@bianys.org
bianys.org

Barry Dain, President
Eileen Reardon, Executive Director
Debbie Berenda-Chilandese, Director of Finance & Administration
Victoria Clingan, Director of Engagement & Advocacy

The Brain Injury Association of New York State is a statewide non-profit membership organization that provides education, advocacy and community support services leading to improved outcomes for children and adults with brain injuries and their families. The association also offers chapters and support groups throughout the state, prevention programs, mentoring programs, speakers bureau and publications library.

7854 BroadFutures
National Youth Transitions Center
2013 H St, NW
5th Floor
Washington, DC 20006
202-521-4304
info@broadfutures.org
broadfutures.org

Bradley P Holmes, Chairman
Carolyn K Jeppsen, CEO & President
Diana Eisenstat, Secretary
John Sheffield, Treasurer

BroadFutures offers transitional programs for youth with learning disabilities. The mission of the organization is to assit these youth in overcoming barriers to employment.

7855 Center Academy
6710 86th Ave. N
Pinellas Park, FL 33782
727-541-5716
Fax: 727-544-8186
infopp@centeracademy.com
www.centeracademy.com

Mack R. Hicks, Founder & Chair
Andrew P. Hicks, Chief Executive Officer & Clinical Director
Eric V. Larson, President & Chief Operating Officer
Susan K. Hicks, Vice President

Center Academy assists children with learning disabilities, difficulties in concentration and underdeveloped social skills. Programs offered include high impact learning, community involvement opportunities, ADHD schools, autism and asperger's schools, dyslexia treatment, special education schools and more.

7856 Cerebral Palsy Associations of New York State
Central Office & Metropolitan Services
330 W 34th St
15th Floor
New York, NY 10001-2488
212-947-5770
information@cpofnys.org
www.cpofnys.org

Stephen C Lipinski, Chairman
Susan Constantino, President & CEO
Michael A Alvaro, Executive Vice President
Cheryl Bradway, Office Manager

The Cerebral Palsy Associations of New York is a multi-service organization that provides services and programs for individuals with cerebral palsy and developmental disabilities, as well as resources for families.

7857 Child Neurology Society
1000 W County Rd E
Suite 290
Saint Paul, MN 55126
651-486-9447
Fax: 651-486-9436
nationaloffice@childneurologysociety.org
www.childneurologysociety.org

Kenneth Mack, President
Roger Larson, Executive Director
Sue Hussman, Associate Director
Emily McConnell, Professional Development Manager

The Child Neurology Society is designed for patiens, parents, and professionals alike, with the aim of promoting continued research, providing support, and offering informational resources and guidance on the subject of child neurology. Members include child neurologists and related medical professionals.

7858 Children and Adults with Attention-Deficit Hyperactivity Disorder
CHADD
4601 Presidents Dr
Suite 300
Lanham, MD 20706
301-306-7070
Fax: 301-306-7090
affiliate-services@chadd.org
www.chadd.org

Michael MacKay, President
Leslie Kain, MBA, Executive Director
Robyn Maggio, MSW, Education & Training Coordinator
April Gower, Chief Operating Officer

The Children and Adults with Attention-Deficit/Hyperactivity Disorder (CHADD) is a non-profit organization providing supports to people with ADHD. Some services offered include advocacy, education, employment, a resource directory, training programs, publications on research and more.

7859 Cognitive Neuroscience Society
267 Cousteau Place
Davis, CA 95618
916-850-0837
cnsinfo@cogneurosociety.org
www.cogneurosociety.org

Roberto Cabeza, Ph.D, Board Member
Marta Kutas, Ph.D, Board Member
Kate Tretheway, Executive Director
Sangay Wangmo, Administrative Assistant

The Cognitive Neuroscience Society is committed to investigating the psychological, computational, and neuroscientific bases of cognition through research.

7860 Cognitive Science Society
108 E Dean Keeton
Stop A8000
Austin, TX 78712-1043
512-471-2030
Fax: 512-471-3053
cogsci@austin.utexas.edu
www.cognitivesciencesociety.org

Susan Gelman, Chair
Terry Regier, Chair Elect
Anna Drummey, Executive Officer
Jessica Wong, Conference Officer

The Cognitive Science Society brings together researchers from around the world who desire to understand the workings of the human mind. The society's mission is to promote the study of cognitive science and build connections between researchers in various areas of study (including Artificial Intelligence, Linguistics, Anthropology, Psychology, Neuroscience, Philosophy, and Education).

7861 **Cognitive Science Student Association**
University of California
Berkeley, CA
cssa.berkeley@gmail.com
cssa.berkeley.edu

Timothy Guan, President
Harshali Wadge, Internal Vice President
Connor Brown, Outreach Coordinator
James Wang, Marketing Director

The Cognitive Science Student Association supports and enriches the academic life of anyone interested in the interdisciplinary field of cognitive science. Some programs offered by the association include guest lectures and information sessions, professor-student dinners, academic outreach program and California Cognitive Science Conference.

7862 **Dementia Society of America**
PO Box 600
Doylestown, PA 18901
800-336-3684
knowdementia@dementiasociety.org
www.dementiasociety.org

Kevin Jameson, President & Founder

The Dementia Society of America (DSA) is a nonprofit volunteer-run organization providing resources and information about dementia to individuals, corporations and organizations.

7863 **Depression and Bipolar Support Alliance**
55 E Jackson Blvd
Suite 490
Chicago, IL 60604
800-826-3632
Fax: 312-642-7243
dbsasocial@gmail.com
www.dbsalliance.org

William Gilmer, MD, Chair
Allen Doederlein, President
Cindy Specht, Executive Vice President
Brittany Telander, Development Director

The Depression and Bipolar Support Alliance is a peer-directed national organization dedicated to offering supports to those living with depression or bipolar disorder. Some services they offer include peer support, education, advocacy and research.

7864 **Epilepsy Foundation**
8301 Professional Place E
Suite 200
Landover, MD 20785- 2353
800-332-1000
Fax: 301-459-1569
ContactUs@efa.org
www.epilepsy.com

Robert W Smith, Chair
Phillip M. Gattone, M.Ed, President & CEO
M. Vaneeda Bennett, Chief Development Officer
May J. Liang, Secretary

The Epilepsy Foundation is the national voluntary health agency dedicated to the welfare of people with epilepsy in the U.S. and their families. The organization works to ensure that people with seizures are able to participate in all life experiences; to improve how people with epilepsy are perceived, accepted and valued in society; and to promote research for a cure.

7865 **FOCUS Center for Autism**
126 Dowd Ave.
PO Box 452
Canton, CT 06019
860-693-8809
Fax: 860-693-0141
info@focuscenterforautism.org
www.focuscenterforautism.org

Patricia A. Cables, President
Timothy Grady, Secretary
Donna Swanson, Executive Director
Fred Evans, Associate Director

FOCUS Center for Autism is a nonprofit center to help children and young adults with autism spectrum disorder, and other related disorders, achieve their full potential.

7866 **Geneva Centre for Autism**
112 Merton St.
Toronto, ON, Canada M4S-2Z8
416-322-7877
Fax: 416-322-5894
info@autism.net
www.autism.net

Abe Evreniadis, Chief Executive Officer
Kathy Shaw, Chief Financial Officer
Renita Paranjape, Senior Director, Programs & Services
Kim Takata, Director, Human Resources

The Geneva Centre for Autism's mission is to empower individuals with Autism Spectrum Disorder, and their families, to fully participate in their communities.

7867 **International OCD Foundation**
18 Tremont St
Suite 308
Boston, MA 02108
617-973-5801
Fax: 617-973-5803
info@iocdf.org
iocdf.org

Shannon A Shy, Esq, President
Jeff Szymanski, PhD, Executive Director
Pamela Layne, Director of Operations
Meghan Buco, Communications Manager

The International OCD Foundation aims to provide resources for those living with OCD and their families. The foundation offers a research grant program, public education and a forum for professional networking.

7868 **Lewy Body Dementia Association**
912 Killian Hill Rd, SW
Lilburn, GA 30047
404-975-2322
Fax: 480-422-5434
lbda@lbda.org
www.lbda.org

Christina M Christie, President
Mike Koehler, CEO
Mark Wall, Vice President
Angela Taylor, Director of Programs

The Lewy Body Dementia Association is a non-profit organization dedicated to raising awareness of the Lewy body dementias (LBD). The association offers services and information to people with LBD, their families and caregivers and works to promote research in the area.

7869 **Life Development Institute**
18001 N 79th Ave
Suite B-42
Glendale, AZ 85308
866-736-7811
Fax: 623-773-2788
info@life-development-inst.org
discoverldi.com

Robert Crawford, M.Ed, CEO
Veronica Lieb (Crawford), MA, President
Justin Coller, BS, Director of Operations
Estelle Esposito, Manager of Administrative Services

The Life Development Institute serves older adolescents and adults with learning disabilities, ADD and related disorders. The Institute's mission is to help program participants pursue responsible independent living, enhance academic/workplace literacy skills and facilitate employment or educational placements.

7870 **Life Unlimited**
Life Unlimited, Inc.
2135 Manor Way
Liberty, MO 64068
816-781-4332
www.lifeunlimitedinc.org

Erin Lankford, President
Scott Wingerson, Vice President
Jessie Smith, Secretary
Dan Jurgensen, Treasurer

Life Unlimited is a nonprofit working to provide support and services to individuals with developmental disabilities in the Kansas City Northland. Services include community living, day services, employment services, and recreation programs.

7871 **Mental Health America (MHA)**
500 Montgomery St.
Suite 820
Alexandria, VA 22314
703-684-7722
800-969-6642
Fax: 703-684-5968
info@mhanational.org
www.mhanational.org

Paul Gionfriddo, President & CEO
Mary Giliberti, Executive Vice President, Policy
Jessica Kennedy, Chief of Staff
Theresa Nguyen, Chief Program Officer & Vice President, Research
A nonprofit organization addressing issues related to mental health and mental illness. MHA works to improve the mental health of all Americans, especially individuals with mental disorders, through advocacy, education, research, and service.

7872 **Multiple Sclerosis Association of America**
375 Kings Hwy N
Cherry Hill, NJ 08034
800-532-7667
Fax: 856-661-9797
msaa@mymsaa.org
mymsaa.org

John McCorry, Chair
Gina Murdoch, President & CEO
Lauren Hooper, Northeast Regional Director
Emily MacHenry, Communications Coordinator
The Multiple Sclerosis Association of America is an organization dedicated to providing the most up-to-date resources for those affected by Multiple Sclerosis, including research, publications, assistive equipment, public education, and best practices and policy for professionals working with patients.

7873 **NLP Comprehensive**
PO Box 348
Indian Hills, CO 80454-0348
303-987-2224
800-233-1657
Fax: 303-987-2228
learn@nlpco.com
www.nlpco.com

Tom Dotz, President
Sharon DeBault, Director of Community Relations
Jamie Reaser, PhD, Director of Professional Relations
Christian Miller, Publishing Manager
NLP Comprehensive provides a body of publications by Steve and Connirae Andreas on the subject of NLP (Neuro-linguistic programming), as well as training.

7874 **NLP University - Dynamic Learning Center**
NLP University
PO Box 1112
Ben Lomond, CA 95005
831-336-3457
Fax: 503-738-9546
teresanlp@aol.com
www.nlpu.com

Robert B Dilts, Founder & Director of Training
Teresa Epstein, Coordinator
Deborah Bacon Dilts, Trainer
Judith DeLozier, Trainer
NLP (neuro-lingusitic programming) University seeks to create a context in which professionals of different backgrounds can develop fundamental and advanced NLP skills for applications relevant to their profession. The University provides guidance, training, certification, culture, and community support to those interested in exploring the global potential of Systemic NLP.

7875 **National Alliance on Mental Illness (NAMI)**
3803 N Fairfax Dr
Suite 100
Arlington, VA 22203
703-524-7600
800-950-6264
888-999-6264
Fax: 703-524-9094
info@nami.org
www.nami.org

Steve Pitman, J.D., President
Mary Giliberti, J.D., CEO
Cheri Villa, M.P.A, Chief Operating Officer
David Levy, Chief Financial Officer
NAMI is a grassroots mental health organization working to provide people with mental health issues the technical assistance, tools and referrals to resources they need in order to manage the challenges they face.

7876 **National Association for Developmental Disabilities (NADD)**
12 Hurley Ave.
Kingston, NY 12401
845-331-4336
info@thenadd.org
thenadd.org

Jeanne M. Farr, CEO
Jeffrey Schmunk, Operations Manager
Michelle Jordan, Office Manager
Edward Seliger, Project Coordinator
NADD is a non-profit membership association established for professionals, care providers and families to promote understanding of and services for individuals who have developmental disabilities and mental health needs. The mission of NADD is to advance mental wellness for persons with developmental disabilities through the promotion of excellence in mental health care.

7877 **National Association for Down Syndrome**
1460 Renaissance Dr
Suite 102
Park Ridge, IL 60068
630-325-9112
info@nads.org
www.nads.org

Steve Connors, President
Diane Urhausen, Executive Director
Linda Smarto, Director, Programs and Advocacy
The National Association for Down Syndrome provides services and information to those with Down Syndrome and their families. The association's mission is to maintain a strong network of support systems within their own organization and with medical, educational and school service professionals who work with children and adults with Down Syndrome.

7878 **National Association of Cognitive- Behavioral Therapists**
102 Gilson Ave
Weirton, WV 26062
304-224-2534
800-253-0167
nacbt@nacbt.org
www.nacbt.org

Aldo R Pucci, Ph.D, President
The association's mission is to promote the teaching and practice of cognitive-behavioral psychotherapy and to support those professionals and students seeking to practice it. Some services offered by the association include educational videos, membership, CBT certification, workshops and more.

7879 **National Association of Epilepsy Centers**
600 Maryland Ave SW
Suite 835W
Washington, DC 20024
202-524-6767
888-525-6232
Fax: 202-484-1244
info@naec-epilepsy.org
www.naec-epilepsy.org

Nathan B Fountain, MD, President
Ellen Riker, MHA, Executive Director
Johanna Gray, MPA, Deputy Director
Jennifer McCrindle, MPA, Accreditation & Programs Manager
The National Association of Epilepsy Centers educates public and private policy makers and regulators about appropriate patient care standards, reimbursement and medical services policies. The association is designed to complement the efforts of existing scientific and charitable epilepsy organizations.

7880 **National Ataxia Foundation**
600 Hwy 169 S
Suite 1725
Minneapolis, MN 55426
763-553-0020
Fax: 763-553-0167
naf@ataxia.org
www.ataxia.org

William P Sweeney, President
Charlene Danielson, Treasurer
Joel Sutherland, Executive Director
Susan Hagen, Patient & Research Services Director
The National Ataxia Foundation is a non-profit, membership-supported organization established to help improve the lives

of persons affected by ataxia and their families through support, education, and research.

7881 **National Autism Association**
1 Park Ave
Suite 1
Portsmouth, RI 02871
401-293-5551
877-622-2884
Fax: 401-293-5342
naa@nationalautism.org
nationalautismassociation.org

Lori McIlwain, Board Chairperson
Wendy Fournier, President
Kelly Vanicek, Executive Director
Katie Wright, Vice President

The mission of the National Autism Association is to educate and empower families affected by autism and other neurological disorders, while advocating on behalf of those who cannot fight for their own rights. The association offers programs as well as educational resources.

7882 **National Down Syndrome Congress**
30 Mansell Ct
Suite 108
Roswell, GA 30076
770-604-9500
800-232-6372
Fax: 770-604-9898
info@ndsccenter.org
www.ndsccenter.org

Kishore Vellody, MD, President
David Tolleson, Executive Director
MaryKate Vandemark, Office Manager
Kathy Edwards, Development Director

The National Down Syndrome Congress provides information, advocacy and support concerning all aspects of life for individuals with Down syndrome. It is the purpose of the Congress to create a national climate in which all people will recognize and embrace the value and dignity of people with Down syndrome.

7883 **National Down Syndrome Society**
8 E 41st St
8th Floor
New York, NY 10017
212-460-9330
800-221-4602
Fax: 212-979-2873
info@ndss.org
www.ndss.org

Sara Weir, MS, President
Josh Hill, Executive Assistant
Ashley Helsing, Director of Government Relations
Melissa Robertson, Office Manager

Non-profit organization dedicated to increasing public awareness about Down syndrome as well as engaging in research, education and advocacy. The organization distributes informative materials, encourages and supports the activities of local parent support groups, sponsors conferences and scientific symposiums and undertakes major advocacy efforts.

7884 **National Hydrocephalus Foundation**
12413 Centralia Rd
Lakewood, CA 90715-1653
562-924-6666
888-857-3434
Fax: 562-924-6666
www.nhfonline.org

Michael Fields, President & Treasurer
Debbi Fields, Executive Director
Sarah Dunn, Junior Director
Jaynie Dunn, Secretary

The National Hydrocephalus Foundation assembles and disseminates information pertaining to hydrocephalus, its treatments and outcomes. The foundation also establishes and facilitates a communication network among affected families and individuals.

7885 **Oak-Leyden Developmental Services**
411 Chicago Ave
Oak Park, IL 60302
708-524-1050
Fax: 708-524-2469
info@oak-leyden.org
www.oak-leyden.org

Melissa Wyatt, President
Bertha Magana, Executive Director
Nancy Thomas, Director of Human Resources
Lori Malinski, Director of Fund Development

Oak-Leyden Developmental Services works to help people with developmental disabilities meet life's challenges and reach their highest potential. Services offered by the organization include Early Intervention Program, Vocational Evaluation, Developmental Training Program, Supported Employment Program, Community Integrated Living Arrangements and Multi-disciplinary Clinic.

7886 **Ontario Federation for Cerebral Palsy**
104-1630 Lawrence Ave W
Toronto, ON, Canada M6L-1C5
416-244-9686
877-244-9686
Fax: 416-244-6543
info@ofcp.ca
www.ofcp.ca

Victor Gascon, President
Nilu Alizadeh, Supervisor
Cindy DeGraaff, Planning Services Manager
Deborah Grosdanis, Treasurer

The Ontario Federation for Cerebral Palsy is dedicated to assisting individuals with cerebral palsy through research, financial resources, education, recreation programs, housing and life planning.

7887 **Society for Cognitive Rehabilitation**
668 Exton Commons
Exton, PA 19341
127-647-2369
www.societyforcognitiverehab.org

Kit Malia, President
Rita Carroll, Secretary
Pat Benfield, Treasurer
Ron Savage, Board Member

The Society for Cognitive Rehabilitation is a non-profit organization committed to the advancement of cognitive rehabilitation therapy across the globe.

7888 **St. John Valley Associates**
291 Newberry Dr
Suite 105
Madawaska, ME 04756
207-728-7197
800-339-9502
Fax: 207-728-3825

Robin Jackson-Eldridge, Program Director

A non-profit association with the mission of empowering adult citizens with intellectual disabilities. The association offers center-based community supports and residential supports to help members develop a sense of independence. *$75.00*

7889 **TEACCH Autism Program**
100 Renee Lynne Ct
Carrboro, NC 27510
919-966-2174
Fax: 919-966-4127
teacch@unc.edu
teacch.com

Laura G Klinger, Ph.D, Executive Director
Lauren Turner-Brown, Ph.D, Assistant Director
Rebecca Mabe, Assistant Director, Business & Operations

TEACCH Autism Program offers community-based services, training programs and research to help those with Autism Spectrum Disorder. Some programs offered by TEACCH include clinical evaluations, intervention, consultation and training, living and learning centers, supported employment and more.

7890 **The Arc of North Carolina**
343 E Six Forks Rd
Suite 320
Raleigh, NC 27609
919-782-4632
800-662-8706
Fax: 919-782-4634
info@arcnc.org
www.arcnc.org

John Nash, Executive Director
Melinda Plue, Director of Advocacy & Chapter Development
Nicole Kiefer, Housing Resources Coordinator
Foresa Walker, Director of Human Resources

The Arc of North Carolina is committed to providing services for people with intellectual and developmental disabilities. Services include advocacy, housing, supported employment and other supports.

7891 **The Arc of the United States**
1825 K St NW
Suite 1200
Washington, DC 20006
202-534-3700
800-433-5255
Fax: 202-534-3731
info@thearc.org
www.thearc.org

Peter Berns, Chief Executive Officer
Ruben Rodriguez, Chief Operating Officer
Julie Ward, Senior Executive Officer, Public Policy
Karen Wolf-Branigin, Senior Executive Officer, Chapter Growth & Affiliates

The Arc promotes and protects the rights of people with intellectual and developmental disabilities and actively supports their inclusion and participation in the community throughout their lifetimes. The Arc's clients include people with autism, Down syndrome, Fragile X syndrome, and various other developmental disabilities. Some services offered by The Arc include public policy advocacy, education and vocational services.

7892 **The Hemispherectomy Foundation**
8235 Lethbridge Rd
Millersville, MD 21108
410-987-5221
lynn@hemifoundation.org
hemifoundation.homestead.com

Kristi Hall, President, CEO & Co-Founder
Cris A Hall, Executive Director & Co-Founder
Jane Stefanik, Vice President & Chief Financial Officer
Lindy Shelton, Director of Accounting & Office Manager

The Hemispherectomy Foundation is a non-profit organization dedicated to providing emotional, financial and educational support to individuals and their families who have undergone, or will undergo, a hemispherectomy or similar brain surgery.

7893 **Tourette Association of America**
42-40 Bell Blvd
Suite 205
Bayside, NY 11361
718-224-2999
Fax: 718-279-9596
support@tourette.org
www.tourette.org

Amanda Talty, President & CEO
Tracey Costikyan-Alexander, VP, Resource Development & Chapter Services
Diana Felner, VP, Public Policy
Sonja Mason-Vidal, VP, Finance & Administration

Non-profit organization with the mission of researching and controlling the effects of Tourette syndrome. Some services they offer include seminars, conferences and support groups. The association publishes brochures, flyers, educational materials and papers on treatment and research.

7894 **United Cerebral Palsy**
1825 K St NW
Suite 600
Washington, DC 20006
202-776-0406
800-872-5827
Fax: 202-776-0414
info@ucp.org
ucp.org

Diane Wilush, Chair
Armando Contreras, President & CEO
Ellie Collinson, Chief Program Officer
Tanneka Jones, Director of Finance

United Cerebral Palsy educates, advocates, and provides support services to ensure a life without limits for people with cerebral palsy and other disabilities. Some services offered include networking, educational information, assistive technology information, research, public policy resources and more.

Camps

7895 **Adventure Learning Center at Eagle Village**
4507 170th Ave
Hersey, MI 49639-8785
231-832-2234
800-748-0061
Fax: 231-832-1468
alcinfo@eaglevillage.org
www.eaglevillage.org

Cathey Prudhomme, President/CEO
Jim McCain, Director of Support Services/CFO
Craig Weidner, Director of Advancement

Offers a variety of fun camp experiences with a low staff-to-camper ratio and exciting, challenging activities. This program accepts youth, ages 5-17, who are high risk or special needs - behavioral problems, emotionally unstable or Attention Deficit. The camping experience includes canoeing, hiking, swimming and high adventure activities. Half-week, one-week, and two-week sessions June-August. Coed.

7896 **CNS Camp New Connections**
Mclean Hospital Child/Adolescent Program
115 Mill St
Mailstop115
Belmont, MA 02478-1064
617-855-2000
800-333-0338
Fax: 617-855-2833
mcleaninfo@mclean.harvard.edu
www.mcleanhospital.org

Roya Ostovar PhD, Center Director
Scott L. Rauch, MD., President and Psychiatrist in Ch
Joseph Gold MD, Clinical Director
Cynthia Kaplan, CAP Administrative Director

Four-week summer day camp for children ages 7-17 who have pervasive developmental disorders, Asperger's Syndrome, autism spectrum disorders and non-verbal learning disabilities. The camp is designed to help children develop social skills through fun activities including: communication games, swimming, field trips, drama, and arts and crafts. *$4500.00*

7897 **Camp Baker**
Greater Richmond ARC
7600 Beach Rd
Chesterfield, VA 23838-6513
804-748-4789
Fax: 804-796-6880
richmondarc.org

Robert L. Sommerville, Chair - Officer
Thomas G. Haskins, Vice Chair - Officer
Chriss Mumford, Secretary Officer
Marshall W. Butler Jr., President

An organization created by families, for families that has grown to provide a continuum of programs and services for individuals with developmental disablities acroos the lifespan, helping each person achieve his or her potential and improving the quality of life for everyone in the community.

7898 **Camp Buckskin**
PO Box 389
Ely, MN 55731 763-432-9177
info@campbuckskin.com
www.campbuckskin.com

Tom Bauer, Camp Co-Director
Mary Bauer, Camp Co-Director
Camp is located in Ely, Minnesota. Buckskin helps children with underdeveloped social skills realize their potentials and abilities. Teaches a combination of traditional camp activities, academic activities, and social skills. Ages 6-18.

7899 **Camp Candlelight**
Epilepsy Foundation Arizona
3620 N 4th Ave.
Suite 228
Phoenix, AZ 85013 602-282-3515
800-332-1000
AZ@EFA.org
epilepsyaz.org/events/campcandlelight
Suzanne Matsumori, Executive Director
Min Skivington, Program Manager
Camp Candlelight provides children ages 8 to 17 a unique camp experience that mixes traditional summer camp with special sessions that teach campers about their seizures and gives them resources to manage the challenges that the seizures represent. Staff inclues a neurologist, several nurses, and a school psychologist, in addition to traditional camp staff who are given specialized training in responding appropriately to the needs of kids with epilepsy.

7900 **Camp Civitan**
Civitan Foundation
5008 N Civitan Rd
Williams, AZ 56046 602-953-2944
www.civitanfoundationaz.com
Cody Graham, Camp Director
Dawn Trapp, Executive Director
Camp Civitan offers week long summer camp programs, and weekend programs throughout the year, to children with developmental disabilities. The camp is fully wheelchair accessible, is staffed by medical professionals and there is a 2:1 ratio of campers to staff. Camp Civitan offers campers the experience of traditional camp activities including, swimming, adaptive sports, fishing, music, arts and crafts, and talent shows.

7901 **Camp Evoked Potential**
Alabama's Special Camp for Children and Adults
PO Box 21
5278 Camp Ascca Dr.
Jacksons Gap, AL 36861 256-825-9226
Fax: 256-269-0714
info@campascca.org
www.campascca.org
Matt Rickman, Camp Director
Amber Cotney, Program Director
Jocelyn Jones, Secretary
Camp Evoked Potential is held one week out of the year for children aged 6-18 with epilepsy at Camp ASCCA. Fully funded by The Epilepsy Foundation, persons wishing to attend the camp must apply. The camp provides a barrier free setting situated on 230 acres of wooded land at Lake Martin. The camp is staffed with medical personnel trained to care for children with all types of disabilities and provides a variety of camp activities.

7902 **Camp Horizons**
127 Babcock Hill Rd
PO Box 323
South Windham, CT 06266- 323 860-456-1032
Fax: 860-456-4721
www.camphorizons.org
Adam Milne, Chairman
L. Sanford Rice, Treasurer
Kathleen McNAboe, VP
Deirdhre Delaney, Board Secretary
Bordering Lake Probus, the facilities at the camp are equipped to accomodate a wide range of activities and programs for campers with developmental disabilities, or other challenging emotional and social needs. There is a 5:1 camper-counselor ratio with a schedule of three programs in the morning and four in the afternoon.

7903 **Camp Huntington**
56 Bruceville Rd.
High Falls, NY 12440-5100 845-687-7840
855-707-2267
Fax: 855-707-2267
www.camphuntington.com
Daniel Falk, Executive Director
Dylan Sloan, Program Director
Margaret Short, Health Director
A co-ed residential summer camp specifically designed to focus on adaptive and therapeutic recreation. Campers include those with learning and developmental disabilities, ADD/HD, Autism Spectrum Disorders, Asperger's, PDD, and other special needs. Programs focus on recreation and social skills, independence, and participation.

7904 **Camp Krem**
Camping Unlimited
102 Brook Lane
Boulder Creek, CA 95006 831-338-3210
campkrem@campingunlimited.org
campingunlimited.org
Christina Krem, Camp Director
Kenneth Beebe, Assistant Camp Director
Layla Sharif, Administrator & Mobility Manager
Gail Zigenis, Registrar
Camp Krem - Camping Unlimited offers year-round and summer camping programs for children and adults with developmental disabilities. With a variety of different programs and many facilities on the campground such as a swimming pool, arts and crafts building, amphitheater, music pavilion, and archery range, Camp Krem provides its campers with recreation, education, and adventure opportunities.

7905 **Camp Nissokone**
YMCA Camping Services
1401 Broadway
Suite A
Detroit, MI 48226-8929 313-267-5300
www.ymcadetroit.org
Doug Grimm, Vice President Camping Services
David Marks, Director
A six week summer resident camp program for boys and girls whose learning and behavior styles have made successful participation in the traditional camp program difficult. All camp activities have a special emphasis on building self-esteem and peer relationships. Strong in waterfront, nature, campcrafts and a special arts program.

7906 **Camp Nuhop**
1077 Township Rd. 2916
Perrysville, OH 44864 419-938-7151
www.nuhop.org
Trevor Dunlap, Executive Director & CEO
Chris Clyde, Associate Director
Matt Poland, Director, Outdoor Education
Katelyn Seroka, Director, Summer Camp & Respite Programs
A summer residential program for youth ages 6-18 with learning disabilities, behavioral disorders, or other neuroatypical disorders. Activities include outdoor education and team-building workshops. The staff-to-camper ratio is 3:7 or 3:8.

7907 **Camp Ramapo**
Ramapo for Children
Rt. 52/Salisbury Turnpike
PO Box 266
Rhinebeck, NY 12572 845-876-8403
Fax: 845-876-8414
office@ramapoforchildren.org
www.ramapoforchildren.org
Matthew McKnight, Camp Director
Lenora Sealey, Associate Camp Director
A residential summer camp for youth ages 6-16 with social, emotional, or learning challenges.

7908 **Camp ReCreation**
9272 Madison Ave.
Orangeville, CA 95662 916-988-6835
camprecreation@outlook.com
www.camprecreation.org
Kathi Barber, Camp Director

Camp ReCreation offers residential summer camps and year round programs for children, teens, and adults with developmental disabilities. The summer camp is held at Camp Ronald McDonald in Lassen National Forest. With a 1:1 staff to camper ratio, Camp ReCreation offers wide variety of camp activities, and campers wishing to participate must fill out a camper application.

7909 Camp Royall
250 Bill Ash Rd.
Moncure, NC 27559
919-542-1033
Fax: 919-533-5324
camproyall@autismsociety-nc.org
www.autismsociety-nc.org/camp-royall

Sara Gage, Director

A week-long overnight and day camp for children and adults with autism. Campers participate in traditional camp activities such as swimming, boating, hiking, and arts and crafts. Counselor-to-camper ratio is 1:1 or 1:2, depending on the campers' needs.

7910 Camp Ruggles
PO Box 353
Chepachet, RI 02814
401-567-8914
campruggles@gmail.com
www.campruggles.org

Jim Field, Executive Director
Ethan Roe, Assistant Director

Camp Ruggles is located in Glocester, RI and is a summer day camp for children with emotional and behavioral disabilities. The camp offers 240 hours of supervised therapeutic care for children ages 6-12.

7911 Camp Sisol
Jewish Community Center of Greater Rochester/JCC
1200 Edgewood Ave.
Rochester, NY 14618
585-461-2000
Fax: 585-461-0805
bettertogether@jccrochester.org
www.jccrochester.org

Josh Weinstein, Chief Executive Officer

Coed, ages 5-16. Camp Sisol accommodates children with special needs.

7912 Camp World Light
Florida Baptist Convention
1230 Hendricks Ave
Jacksonville, FL 32207-8619
904-396-2351
800-226-8584
Fax: 904-396-6470
www.campworldlight.com

Anne Wilson, Camp Director
Delicia Garland, Ministry Assistant to Director

Camp is located in Marianna, Florida. One-week sessions June-July for girls with ADD. Ages 3-12. Activities include arts/crafts, challenge/rope courses, clowning, community service, dance, drama, drawing/painting, leadership development, performing arts and sailing.

7913 Camp-A-Lot and Camp-A-Little
The Arc of San Diego
3030 Market Street
San Diego, CA 92102
619-685-1175
Fax: 619-234-3759
info@arc-sd.com
www.arc-sd.com

Anthony J. DeSalis, Esq., President & CEO

Programs of The Arc of San Diego, Camp - A - Lot (ages 18 and up) and Camp - A - Little (ages 5-17) offer recreational summer camp opportunities for individuals with physical and developmental disabilities.

7914 Casowasco Camp, Conference and Retreat Center
158 Casowasco Dr
Moravia, NY 13118-3498
315-364-8756
Fax: 315-364-7636
info@casowasco.org

Mike Huber, Executive Director
Shelly Sherboneau, CRM Coordinating Registrar
Kevin Dunn, Casowasco Assistant Director
Roger Marshall, Property Manager

Camp is located in Moravia, New York. Summer sessions for children with ADD. Coed, ages 6-18 and families.

7915 Center Academy at Pinellas Park
6710 86th Ave. N
Pinellas Park, FL 33782
727-541-5716
Fax: 727-544-8186
infopp@centeracademy.com
www.centeracademy.com

Mack R. Hicks, Founder & Chair
Andrew P. Hicks, Chief Executive Officer & Clinical Director
Eric V. Larson, President & Chief Operating Officer
Susan K. Hicks, Vice President

Specifically designed for the learning disabled child and other children with difficulties in concentration, strategy, social skills, impulsivity, distractibility and study strategies. Programs offered include attention training, visual-motor remediation, socialization skills training, relaxation training, and more.

7916 Dallas Academy
950 Tiffany Way
Dallas, TX 75218
214-324-1481
Fax: 214-327-8537
www.dallas-academy.com

Elizabeth Murski, Head of School

Dallas Academy is a school for children with diagnosed learning differences such as autism, ADD/ADHD, dyslexia, and more. The academy offers a number of summer camps and programs.

7917 Eagle Hill School: Summer Program
242 Old Petersham Road
P.O. Box 116
Hardwick, MA 01037- 0116
413-477-6000
Fax: 413-477-6837
admission@ehs1.org
www.ehs1.org

Peter J. Mc Donald, Headmaster
Marilyn Waller, President
Alden Bianchi, Vice President
Arthur Langhaus, Treasurer

For children ages 9-19 with specific learning (dis)abilities and/or Attention Deficit Disorder, this summer program is designed to remediate academic and social deficits while maintaining progress achieved during the school year. Electives and sports activities are combined with the academic courses to address the needs of the whole person in a camp-like atmosphere.

7918 Englishton Park Academic Remediation
Englishton Park Presbyterian
P.O. Box 228
Lexington, IN 47138-228
812-889-2046
ThomasLisaBarnett@etczone.com
www.englishtonpark.org

Lisa Barnett, Director
Thomas Barnett, Co-Director

Camp is located in Lexington, Indiana. Two-week sessions for children with ADD. Boys and girls, ages 7-12.

7919 Florida Sheriffs Caruth Camp
Florida Sheriffs Youth Ranches
2486 Cecil Webb Place
Boys Ranch, FL 32060
386-842-5501
800-765-3797
Fax: 386-842-2429
fsyr@youthranches.org
www.youthranches.org

Roger Bouchard, President
Bill Frye, Executive Vice President
Janet Bass, Vice President of Operations
Maria Knapp, Vice President of Donor Relation

Camp is located in Inglis, Florida. One-week sessions for children with ADD. Coed, ages 10-15.

7920 Gow School Summer Programs
2491 Emery Rd.
South Wales, NY 14139
716-687-2004
Fax: 716-687-2003
summer@gow.org
www.gow.org

Matthew Fisher, Director

Co-ed summer programs for students ages 8-16 with dyslexia or similar learning disabilities. Offers a blend of morning academics, afternoon/evening traditional camp activities and weekend overnights.

7921 **Hill School of Fort Worth**
4817 Odessa Ave.
Fort Worth, TX 76133
817-923-9482
Fax: 817-923-4894
hillschool@hillschool.org
www.hillschool.org

Roxann Breyer, Head of School
Matt Errico, Dean, Student Success
Jimmy Cessna, Registrar

Provides an alternative learning environment for students with learning differences. Hill School caters to individuals with disabilities by offering smaller class sizes and individualized learning programs. Offers an academic summer program during the month of June.

7922 **Indian Acres Camp for Boys**
1712 Main St
Fryeburg, ME 04037-4327
207-935-2300
Fax: 954-349-7812
geoff@indianacres.com
www.indianacres.com

Michael Burness, Assistant Director
Mary Beth 'Bert' Wiig, Head Counselor, Camp Forest Acre
Lisa Newman, Director
Geoff Newman, Director

Camp is located in Fryeburg, Florida. Four and seven-week sessions June-August for boys with ADD ages 7-16.

7923 **Lab School of Washington**
4759 Reservoir Rd NW
Washington, DC 20007-1921
200-965-6600
www.labschool.org

Katherine Schantz, Head of School
Diana Meltzer, Associate Head of School
Laurelle Sheedy McCready, Associate Head of School for Fin
Bob Lane, Director of Admissions

The Lab School six week summer session includes individualized reading, spelling, writing, study skills and math programs. A multisensory approach addresses the needs of bright learning disabled children. Related services such as speech/language therapy and occupational therapy are integrated into the curriculum. Elementary/Intermediate; Junior High/High School.

7924 **Lions Den Outdoor Learning Center**
600 Kiwanis Dr
Eureka, MO 63025-2212
636-938-5245
Fax: 636-938-5289
www.wymancenter.org

David Hilliard, President
Theresa Mayberry, Executive VP
Kristine Ramsey, Sr. VP
Tony Etzkorn, VP

Varied programs for developmentally disabled children, ages 6 and up, includes daily living, socialization and language skills. Sports, tent camping, crafts, and nature study are also offered. Sliding scale tuition for 2 weeks.

7925 **Maplebrook School**
5142 Route 22
Amenia, NY 12501
845-373-9511
Fax: 845-373-7029
admissions@maplebrookschool.org
www.maplebrookschool.org

Donna Konkolics, Head of School
Roger Fazzone, President
Jennifer Scully, Assistant Head, Postsecondary Studies
Lori Hale, Executive Director

A coeductional boarding school which offers a six week camp for children with learning differences and ADD.

7926 **Marvelwood Summer**
Marvelwood School
476 Skiff Mountain Road
PO Box 3001
Kent, CT 06757-3001
860-927-0047
Fax: 860-927-0021
www.marvelwood.org

Alfred C Brooks, President
Arthur F Goodearl, Jr, Head Of School

The emphasis in this summer program is on diagnosis and remediation of individual reading, spelling, writing, mathematics and study problems. Offered to ages 12-16.

7927 **New Horizons Summer Day Camp**
YMCA of Orange County
13821 Newport Ave.
Suite 150
Tustin, CA 92780
714-508-7635
newhorizons@ymcaoc.org
www.ymcaoc.org/new-horizons

7928 **New Jersey YMHA/YWHA Camps Milford**
21 Plymouth St
Fairfield, NJ 07004-1686
973-575-3333
800-776-5657
Fax: 973-575-4188
info@njycamps.org
www.njycamps.org

Leonard Robinson, President
Bruce Nussman, President

Camp is located in Milford, Pennsylvania. Summer sessions for children with ADD. Coed, ages 6-17 and families.

7929 **Oakland School & Camp**
128 Oakland Farm Way
Troy, VA 22974
434-293-9059
Fax: 434-296-8930
information@oaklandschool.net
www.oaklandschool.net

Carol Williams, Head of School

A highly individualized program that stresses improving reading ability. Subjects taught are reading, English composition, math and word analysis. Recreational activities include horseback riding, sports, swimming, tennis, crafts, archery and camping. For girls and boys, ages 7-13. Students who attend the summer camp often have a variety of learning disabilities, such as ADHD, dyslexia, visual/auditory processing disorders, and more.

7930 **Outside In School Of Experiential Education, Inc.**
PO Box 639
Greensburg, PA 15601
724-837-1518
Fax: 724-837-0801
www.myoutsidein.org

Michael C. Henkel, Executive Director

Camp programs primarily focus on substance abuse, but some services are available for special needs related to school/work. Programs are for boys ages 13-18.

7931 **Phelps School Academic Support Program**
583 Sugartown Rd.
Malvern, PA 19355
610-644-1754
Fax: 610-540-0156
admis@thephelpsschool.org
www.thephelpsschool.org

Charles A. McGeorge, Head of School

The Phelps School is a day and boarding school for grades 6-12. They run an Academic Support Program for English, Reading, Mathematics, and Study Skills for students who have diagnosed learning differences.

7932 **Quest Camp**
907 San Ramon Valley Blvd.
Suite 202
Danville, CA 94526
925-743-2900
800-313-9733
Fax: 925-820-9761
www.questcamps.com

Robert B. Field, PhD., Founder & Executive Director
Debra Forrester-Field, MA, Administrative Director
Aprilyn Artz, MA, Clinical Director
Jodie Knott, Ph.D., Director

Quest Camps are designed using the Quest Camp Therapeutic System developed specifically to help and reduce a campers psychological disability. With locations in San Francisco East Bay, California, Huntington Beach, California, and Pittsburgh, Pennsylvania, camps have a 6:1 camper to staff ratio, with campers receiving sport instruction and participate in physical activity, arts, and games.

7933 **Raven Rock Lutheran Camp**
17912 Harbaugh Valley Road
P.O. Box 136
Sabillasville, MD 21780-136
410-303-2108
800-321-5824

Brenda Minnich, Executive Director
Christ-centered program for youth and developmentally disabled adults.

7934 **Rimland Services for Autistic Citizens**
1265 Hartrey Ave.
Evanston, IL 60202
847-328-4090
Fax: 847-328-8364
TTY: 847-328-4090
www.rimland.org

Lorraine Ganz, President
Barbara Cooper, Secretary
Services include residential living, community day services, and health and wellness programs.

7935 **Rolling Hills Country Day Camp**
P.O. Box 172
Marlboro, NJ 07746
732-308-0405
Fax: 732-780-4726
info@rollinghillsdaycamp.com
www.rollinghillsdaycamp.com

Billy Breitner, Director
Summer sessions for children with ADD. Coed, ages 3-12.

7936 **SOAR Summer Adventures**
226 SOAR Lane
PO Box 388
Balsam, NC 28707
828-456-3435
Fax: 801-820-3050
admissions@soarnc.org
www.soarnc.org

John Willson, Executive Director
A nonprofit adventure program working with disadvantaged youth diagnosed with learning disabilities in an outdoor, challenge-based environment. Focuses on esteem building and social skills development through rock climbing, backpacking, whitewater rafting, mountaineering, sailing, snorkeling, and more. Offers two week, one month, and semester programs. Locations include North Carolina, Florida, Wyoming, California, New York, Belize, Costa Rica, and the Caribbean.

7937 **Sherman Lake YMCA Outdoor Center**
6225 N 39th St
Augusta, MI 49012-9722
269-731-3000
Fax: 269-731-3020
shermanlakeymca@ymcasl.org
www.shermanlakeymca.org

Luke Austenfeld, Executive Director
Jean Henderson, Business Manager
Lorrie Syverson, Director of Camping, Education &
Mark VanDaff, Facility Manager
Summer camping sessions for campers with ADD and spina bifida. Coed, ages 6-15 and families, seniors.

7938 **Squirrel Hollow Summer Camp**
The Bedford School
5665 Milam Rd.
Fairburn, GA 30213
770-774-8001
Fax: 770-774-8005
info@thebedfordschool.org
www.thebedfordschool.org

Betsy Box, Admissions Director
Jeff James, Head of School
Allison Day, Associate Head of School
A remedial summer program for children with academic needs held on the campus of The Bedford School in Fairburn, Georgia. It serves children ages 6-14.

7939 **Summer@Carroll**
Carroll School
25 Baker Bridge Rd.
Lincoln, MA 01773
781-259-8342
summeradmissions@carrollschool.org
www.carrollschool.org

Kristin Curry, Director
Donna Brown, Assistant Director
Summer@Carroll is a unique educational experience designed for children with language-based learning disabilities entering grades 1-9 in the Fall. Carroll's five-week, full-day program provides specialized reading support as well as writing and math classes. Classes are formed according to age and skill level, typically with eight or fewer students in a class.

7940 **Summit Camp**
55 W 38th St.
4th Floor
New York, NY 10018
570-253-4381
info@summitcamp.com
www.summitcamp.com

Shepherd Baum, Director
Leah Love, Assistant Director
Thea Mullis, Travel Director
Maryann Santoro, Admissions Director
The camp is located in Honesdale, Pennsylvania, and is for children ages 8-19 who have a variety of developmental, social, or learning challenges. In addition to traditional camp activities, Summit Camp has a strong focus on social skills development and interpersonal growth.

7941 **Sunnyhill Adventures**
6555 Sunlit Way
Dittmer, MO 63023
636-274-9044
sunnyhilladventures.org

Rob Darroch, Director
Summer camps and year-round programs are offered for youth and adults of all abilities.

7942 **Talisman Summer Camp**
64 Gap Creek Rd.
Zirconia, NC 28790
828-697-6313
info@talismancamps.com
www.talismancamps.com

Linda Tatsapaugh, Operations Director & Owner
Robiyn Mims, Admissions Director & Owner
Cory Greene, Camp Director
Talisman Summer Camp is located 40 minutes south of Asheville, North Carolina. Offers a program of hiking, rafting, climbing, and caving for young people with autism, ADHD and learning disabilities. Coed, ages 6-22.

7943 **Timbertop Camp for Youth with Learning Disabilities**
PO Box 423
Plover, WI 54467
715-869-6262
info@timbertopcamp.org
www.timbertopcamp.org

Pete Matthai, Camp Director
Timbertop Camp is a seven-day outdoor camp for children and youth with learning disabilities. Campers participate in traditional camp activities as well as activities that focus on enhancing cooperative abilities, interpersonal relationships, and self-esteem. The program includes nature exploration, canoeing, arts and crafts, archery, fishing, games, reading instruction, and campfires.

7944 **Triangle Y Ranch YMCA**
YMCA of Southern Arizona
PO Box 1111
Tucson, AZ 85702
520-623-5511
Fax: 520-624-1518
www.tucsonymca.org

Dane Woll, President and CEO
Kerry Dufour, V.P. Chief Development Officer
Cathy Scheirman, Chief Financial Officer
Amanda Thomas, Director of Communications and Special Projects
Summer camp programs for children and young adults ages 6-17. Camp offers horseback riding, sports, story telling, arts & crafts, swimming, archery and nature programs.

7945 **Wendell Johnson Speech And Hearing Clinic**
University Of Iowa
250 Hawkins Dr
Iowa City, IA 52242-1025
319-335-3500
Fax: 319-335-8851
dorothy-albright@uiowa.edu
www.uiowa.edu

Dorothy Albright, Department Administration
Lauren Eldridge, Undergraduate Academic Programs
Mary Jo Yotty, Graduate Programs
Lauren Eldridge, Clinic Appointments

The clinic offers assessment and remediation for communication disorders in adults and children. The clinic also offers a Intensive Summer Residential Clinic for school age children needing intervention services because of speech, language, hearing and/or reading problems.

Books

7946 **A Miracle to Believe In**
Option Indigo Press
2080 S Undermountain Rd
Sheffield, MA 01257-9643
413-229-8727
800-714-2779
Fax: 413-229-8727

Barry Neil Kaufman, Author

A group of people from all walks of life come together and are transformed as they reach out, under the direction of the Kaufmans, to help a little boy the medical world had given up as hopeless. This heartwarming journey of loving a child back to life will not only inspire you, the reader, but presents a compelling new way to deal with life's traumas and difficulties.
379 pages
ISBN 0-449201-08-2

7947 **ADD: Helping Your Child**
Warner Books
1271 Avenue of the Americas
New York, NY 10020-1300
212-522-7200
Fax: 212-522-7989

Barbara Smalley, Author
Bruce Paonessa, Vice President
Elizabeth Nunuz, Manager

The definitive guide to helping children with AD/HD *$12.95*
224 pages Paperback
ISBN 0-446670-13-8

7948 **ADHD Book of Lists: A Practical Guide for Helping Children and Teens with ADDs**
Jossey-Bass
111 River St
Hoboken, NJ 7030-5773
201-748-6000
Fax: 201-748-6008
info@wiley.com
www.wiley.com

Sandra F Rief, Author

Information about Attention Deficit/Hyperactivity Disorder including strategies, supports, and interventions that have been found to be the most effective. For teachers, parents, and counselors. *$29.95*
320 pages
ISBN 0-787965-91-X

7949 **ADHD in the Schools: Assessment and Intervention Strategies**
Guilford Press
72 Spring St
New York, NY 10012-4019
212-431-9800
800-365-7006
Fax: 212-966-6708
info@guilford.com
www.guilford.com

George J DuPaul, Author
Gary Stoner, Co-Author

This landmark volume emphasizes the need for a team effort among parents, community-based professionals, and educators. Provides practical information for educators that is based on empirical findings. Chapters focus on: how to identify and assess students who might have ADHD; the relationship between ADHD and learning disabilities; how to develop and implement classroom-based programs; communication strategies to assist physicians; and the need for community-based treatments. *$36.00*
269 pages Hardcover
ISBN 0-898622-45-X

7950 **ADHD with Comorbid Disorders: Clinical Assessment and Management**
Guilford Press
72 Spring St
New York, NY 10012-4019
212-431-9800
800-365-7006
Fax: 212-966-6708
info@guilford.com
www.guilford.com

Steven R Pliszka, MD, Author
Caryn Leigh Carlson, Co-Author
James M Swanson, Co-Author

$44.00
Cloth
ISBN 1-572304-78-2

7951 **Adolescents with Down Syndrome: Toward a More Fulfilling Life**
Brookes Publishing
P.O. Box 10624
Baltimore, MD 21285-624
410-337-9580
800-638-3775
Fax: 410-337-8539
custserv@brookespublishing.com
www.brookespublishing.com

Maria Sustrova, Author
Lauren Smith, Western Region Sales Representat
Jeannine Blimline, Central Region Sales Representat
Kevin Warg, Northeastern Region Sales Repres

Written for health care professionals, psychologists, other developmental disabilities practitioners, educators, and parents, it covers biomedical concerns; behavioral, psychological, and psychiatric challenges; and education, employment, recreation, community, and legal concerns. *$35.95*
416 pages Paperback
ISBN 1-55766-81-9

7952 **Adult ADD: The Complete Handbook: Everything You Need to Know About How to Cope with ADD**
Prima Publishing
P.O. Box 1260
Rocklin, CA 95677-1260
916-787-7000
800-632-8676
Fax: 916-787-7001

David B Sudderth, Author

In simple and friendly terms, the authors offer help to those leading frustrating lives. They provide coping mechanisms, both psychological and an up-to-date guide to the latest technology *$14.95*
272 pages
ISBN 0-761507-96-5

7953 **All About Attention Deficit Disorders, Revised**
Parent Magic
800 Roosevelt Rd
Glen Ellyn, IL 60137-5839
630-208-0031
800-442-4453
Fax: 630-208-7366
www.parentmagic.com

Thomas Phelan, Owner

A psychologist and expert on ADD outlines the symptoms, diagnosis and treatment of this neurological disorder. *$12.95*
248 pages Paperback
ISBN 1-889140-11-2

7954 Assistive Technology for Individuals with Cognitive Impairments Handbook
Idaho Assistive Technology Project
University of Idaho
1187 Alturas Dr.
Moscow, ID 83843- 2268
208-885-3557
800-432-8324
Fax: 208-885-6102
idahoat@uidaho.edu
www.idahoat.org
Ron Seiler, Project Director
A handbook designed to provide resources and information on finding and acquiring assistive technology for individuals with cognitive impairments.

7955 Attention Deficit Disorder
Sage Publications
2455 Teller Road
Thousand Oaks, CA 91320
800-818-7243
Fax: 800-583-2665
info@sagepub.com
www.sagepub.com
Sara Miller McCune, Founder, Publisher, Chairperson
Blaise R Simqu, President & CEO
A book providing helpful suggestions for both home and classroom management of students with attention deficit disorder.

7956 Attention Deficit Disorder and Learning Disabilities
Books on Special Children
P.O. Box 305
Congers, NY 10920-305
845-638-1236
Fax: 845-638-0847
Barbara Ingersoll, Author
Introduces ADD and learning disabilities. This is an easy reading book. Gives definitions and discusses some effective and controverial medication, dietary, biofeedback, cognitive therapy, and many more issues. *$15.95*
246 pages Softcover
ISBN 0-385469-31-4

7957 Attention Deficit Disorder in Adults Workbook
Taylor Publishing Company
7211 Circle S. Road
Austin, TX 78745-5007
214-637-2800
800-225-3687
Fax: 214-819-8220
Rings@balfour.com
www.balfour.com
Don Percenti, CEO
Workbook for adults with ADD. *$17.99*
192 pages Paperback
ISBN 0-878338-50-0

7958 Attention Deficit Disorder: A Different Perception
Underwood Books
PO Box 1919
Nevada City, CA 95959-1919
800-788-3123
www.underwoodbooks.com
Thorn Hartmann, Author
Supports theory linking ADD to the genetic makeup of men and women who hunted for their food in prehestoric times. Also links second hand smoke to disruptive behavior. *$9.95*
180 pages Paperback
ISBN 0-887331-56-4

7959 Attention Deficit Disorders: Assessment & Teaching
Brooks/Cole Publishing Company
10650 Toebben Drive
Independence, KY 41051
859-525-2230
Fax: 859-282-5700
www.brookscole.com
Janet W Lerner, Author
A handy resource that offers teachers, school psychologists, councelors, social workers, administrators, and parents practical advice for working with children who have attention deficit disorders. *$18.95*
258 pages Paperback
ISBN 0-534250-44-0

7960 Attention-Deficit Hyperactivity Disorder: Symptoms and Suggestons for Treatment
Slosson Educational Publications Inc.
538 Buffalo Rd
East Aurora, NY 14052-280
716-652-0930
888-756-7766
Fax: 800-655-3840
slosson@slosson.com
www.slosson.com
Thomas W Phelan, Author
Steven Slosson, President
John Slosson, Vice President
David Slossan, Vice President
An exhaustive review of current research and decades of experience as practicing school-based professionals, as well as being a parent of an ADHD child, have culminated in this brief, to-the-point, and yet informed ADHD package which has recieved tremendous reviews. Well-grounded answers and suggestions which would facillitate behavior, learning, social-emotional functioning, and other factors in preschool and adolesence are discussed. Answers most commonly asked questions about ADHD/ADD. *$60.00*
61 pages

7961 Attention-Deficit/Hyperactivity Disorder, What Every Parent Wants to Know
Brookes Publishing
P.O. Box 10624
Baltimore, MD 21285-0624
410-337-9580
800-638-3775
Fax: 410-337-8539
custserv@brookespublishing.com
www.brookespublishing.com
Lauren Rohe, Regional Sales Consultant
Jeff Stickler, Educational Sales Representative
Sam Schissler, Educational Sales Representative
Dant Washington, Account Sales Manager
New easy-to-understand, non-technical edition helps teachers and parents get accessible answers to their ADHD. *$21.95*
304 pages Paperback
ISBN 1-557663-98-X

7962 Augmenting Basic Communciation in Natural Contexts
Brookes Publishing
P.O. Box 10624
Baltimore, MD 21285-0624
410-337-9580
800-638-3775
Fax: 410-337-8539
custserv@brookespublishing.com
www.brookespublishing.com
Lauren Rohe, Regional Sales Consultant
Jeff Stickler, Educational Sales Representative
Sam Schissler, Educational Sales Representative
Dant Washington, Account Sales Manager
Here you will find the techniques needed to establish a basic communication system for people of all ages with cognitive disabilities or motor sensory impairments. *$41.95*
304 pages Paperback
ISBN 1-55766 -43-6

7963 Autism 24/7: A Family Guide to Learning at Home & in the Community
Autism Society of North Carolina Bookstore
505 Oberlin Rd
Suite 230
Raleigh, NC 27605-1345
919-743-0204
800-442-2762
Fax: 919-743-0208
info@autismsociety-nc.org
www.autismsociety-nc.org
David Lax, Manager
Martina Ballen, Chair
Beverly Moore, Vice Chair
Elizabeth Phillippi, Secretary
Parents are encouraged to focus on skill sets and behaviors that most negatively affect family functioning, and replacing these behaviors with acceptable alternatives. *$19.95*

7964 **Autism Handbook: Understanding & Treating Autism & Prevention Development**
Oxford University Press
2001 Evans Rd
Cary, NC 27513-2010
919-677-0977
800-445-9714
Fax: 919-677-1303
custserv.us@oup.com
www.oup-usa.org

Thomas Carty, Senior Vice President
Simon Li, Regional Director
Adam Glazer, Director
Thomas McCarty, Manager/VP Operations
$25.00
320 pages
ISBN 0-195076-67-2

7965 **Autism and Learning**
Taylor & Francis
7625 Empire Dr
Florence, KY 41042-2919
212-695-6599
800-634-7064
Fax: 212-563-2269
orders@taylorandfrancis.com
www.taylorandfrancis.com

Rita Jordan, Author
Stuart Powell, Co-Author
This book is about how a cognitive perception on the way in which individuals with autism think and learn may be applied to particular curriculum areas.
160 pages Paperback
ISBN 1-853464-21-X

7966 **Autism in Adolescents and Adults**
Springer Publishing
11 W 42nd St
Floor 15
New York, NY 10036-8002
212-431-4370
Fax: 212-460-1575
service-ny@springer.com
www.springerjournals.com

Eric Schopler, Editor
$63.00
456 pages
ISBN 0-306410-57-5

7967 **Autism...Nature, Diagnosis and Treatment**
Autism Society of North Carolina Bookstore
505 Oberlin Rd
Suite 230
Raleigh, NC 27605-1345
919-743-0204
800-442-2762
Fax: 919-743-0208
jchampion@autismsociety-nc.com
www.autismbookstore.com

David Lax, Manager
Covers perspectives, issues, neurobiological issues and new directions in diagnosis and treatment. *$49.00*

7968 **Autism: Explaining the Enigma**
Wiley Publishers
111 River St
Suite 2000
Hoboken, NJ 7030-5773
201-748-6000
Fax: 201-748-6088
info@wiley.com
www.wiley.com

Uta Firth, Author
Explains the nature of autism. *$27.95*

7969 **Autism: From Tragedy to Triumph**
Branden Books
Po Box 812094
Wellesley, MA 02482
617-734-2045
Fax: 781-790-1056
www.brandenbooks.com

Carol Johnson, Author
Julia Crowder, Co-Author
A new book that deals with the Lovaas method and includes a foreward by Dr. Ivar Lovaas. The book is broken down into two parts — the long road to diagnosis and then treatment. *$12.95*

7970 **Autism: Identification, Education and Treatment**
Routledge (Taylor & Francis Group)
7625 Empire Dr
Florence, KY 41042-2919
212-695-6599
800-634-7064
Fax: 212-563-2269
orders@taylorandfrancis.com
www.routledge.com

Dianne Zager, Editor
Jeffrey Lin, Director
Francis Chua, Manager
Tamaryn Anderson, Marketing Manager
Chapters include medical treatments, early intervention and communication development in autism. *$36.00*
ISBN 0-805820-44-7

7971 **Autism: The Facts**
Oxford University Press
2001 Evans Rd
Cary, NC 27513-2010
919-677-0977
800-445-9714
Fax: 919-677-1303
custserv.us@oup.com
www.oup-usa.org

Simon Cohen, Author
Patrick Bolton, Co-Author
$22.50
128 pages
ISBN 0-192623-27-3

7972 **Autistic Adults at Bittersweet Farms**
Routledge (Taylor & Francis Group)
7625 Empire Dr
Florence, KY 41042-2919
212-695-6599
800-634-7064
Fax: 212-563-2269
orders@taylorandfrancis.com
www.routledge.com

Norman Giddan PhD, Author
Jane Giddan MA, Co-Author
Jefferey Lin, Director
Francis Chua, Manager
A touching view of an inspirational residential care program for autistic adolescents and adults. Also available in softcover. *$94.95*
Hardcover
ISBN 1-560240-42-3

7973 **Be Quiet, Marina!**
Star Bright Books
13 Landsdowne St
Cambridge, MA 02139
617-354-1300
Fax: 617-354-1399
orders@starbrightbooks.com
www.starbrightbooks.com

Kirsten Debear, Author
A noisy little girl with cerebral palsy and a quiet little girl with Down Syndrome learn to play together and eventually become best friends. *$16.95*
40 pages Hardcover
ISBN 1-887734-79-1

7974 **Breakthroughs: How to Reach Students with Autism**
Aquarius Health Care Media
30 Forest Road
PO Box 249
Millis, MA 02054
508-376-1244
Fax: 508-376-1245
aqvideos@tiac.net
www.aquariusproductions.com

Leslie Krussman, President/Producer
Joseph Wellington, Distribution Coordinator
Anne Baker, Billing & Accounting
Jane Hutchinson, Associate Director William Patte
A hands-on, how-to program for reaching students with autism, featuring Karen Sewell, Autism Society of America's teacher of

the year. Here Sewell demonstrates the successful techniques she's developed over a 20-year career. A separate 250 page manual ($59) is also available which covers math, reading, fine motor, self help, social adaptive, vocational and self help skills as well as providing numerous plan reproducibles and an exhaustive listing of equipment and materials resources. Video. *$99.00*

7975 **Bus Girl: Selected Poems**
Brookline Books
8 Trumbull Rd
Suite B-001
Northampton, MA 01060 617-734-6772
800-666-2665
Fax: 617-734-3952
brbooks@yahoo.com
www.brooklinebooks.com
Gretchen Josephson, Author
Lula O Lubchenco, Editor
Poems written over several decades by a young woman with Down Syndrome. *$14.95*
144 pages Paperback
ISBN 1-57129 -41-9

7976 **Change Your Brain, Change Your Life: The Breakthrough Program for Conquering Depression**
Three Rivers Press
3rd Floor
175 Broadway
New York, NY 10019 212-782-9000
Fax: 212-940-7860
www.randomhouse.com
Daniel G Amen MD, Author
Clinical neuroscientist and psychiatrist Amen uses nuclear brain imaging to diagnose and treat behavioral problems. He explains how the brain works, what happens when things go wrong, and how to optimize brain function. Five sections of the brain are discussed, and case studies clearly illustrate possible problems. *$15.00*
352 pages
ISBN 0-812929-98-5

7977 **Child and Adolescent Therapy: Cognitive-Behavioral Procedures, Third Edition**
Guilford Press
72 Spring Street
New York, NY 10012-4019 212-431-9800
800-365-7006
Fax: 212-966-6708
info@guilford.com
www.guilford.com
Chris Jennison, Publisher Emeritus, Education
Seymour Weingarten, Editor-in-Chief
Jody Falco, Managing Editor: Periodicals
Natalie Graham, Editor: School Psychology, Liter
Incorporating significant developments in treatment procedures, theory and clinical research, new chapters in this second edition examine the current status of empirically supported interventions and developmental issues specific to work with adolescents. *$45.00*
432 pages Cloth
ISBN 1-572305-56-8

7978 **Cognitive Behavioral Therapy for Adult Asperger Syndrome**
Autism Society of North Carolina Bookstore
505 Oberlin Rd
Ste 230
Raleigh, NC 27605-1345 919-743-0204
800-442-2762
Fax: 919-743-0208
jchampion@autismsociety-nc.org
www.autismbookstore.com
David Lax, Manager
Text is prepared with case studies and examples from the author's own experiences working as a cognitive-behavioral therapist specializing in adults and adolescents with dual diagnosis, autism spectrum disorders, mood disorders, and anxiety disorders.

7979 **Communication Development in Children with Down Syndrome**
Brookes Publishing
P.O. Box 10624
Baltimore, MD 21285-0624 410-337-9580
800-638-3775
Fax: 410-337-8539
custserv@brookespublishing.com
www.brookespublishing.com
Lauren Rohe, Regional Sales Consultant
Jeff Stickler, Educational Sales Representative
Sam Schissler, Educational Sales Representative
Dant Washington, Account Sales Manager
This book offers an extensive, detailed explanation of communication development in children with Down syndrome relative to their advancing cognitive skills. It introduces a critical framework for assessing and treating hearing, speech, and language problems and provides explicit intervention methods and tested clinical protocols.
Paperback
ISBN 1-55766 -50-5

7980 **Comprehensive Guide to ADD in Adults: Research, Diagnosis & Treatment**
ADD Warehouse
300 NW 70th Ave
Suite 102
Plantation, FL 33317-2360 954-792-8100
800-233-9273
Fax: 954-792-8545
websales@addwarehouse.com
www.addwarehouse.com
Harvey C Parker, Owner
The first to provide broad coverage of the burgeoning field. Written for professionals who diagnose and treat adults with ADD, it provides information from psychologists and physicians on the most current research and treatment issues *$50.95*
426 pages
ISBN 0-876307-60-8

7981 **Concentration Cockpit: Explaining Attention Deficits**
Educators Publishing Service
P.O. Box 9031
Cambridge, MA 02139-9031 617-367-2700
800-225-5750
Fax: 617-547-0412
CustomerService.EPS@schoolspecialty.com
eps.schoolspecialty.com
Rick Holden, President
Melvin D Levine, Author
This eight-page pamphlet explains the administration of The Concentration Cockpit, a newly revised poster that helps children with attention deficits gain insight into their problems and monitor their progress in grappling with these problems. *$64.50*
ISBN 0-838820-59-X

7982 **Coping with ADD/ADHD**
Rosen Publishing Group
29 E 21st St
New York, NY 10010-6209 212-420-1600
800-237-9932
Fax: 888-436-4643
www.rosenpublishing.com
Jaydene Morrison, Author
At least 3.5 million American youngsters suffer from attention deficit disorder. This book defines the syndrome and provides specific information about treatment and counseling. *$16.95*
ISBN 0-823920-70-4

7983 **Count Us In**
Exceptional Parent Library
P.O. Box 1807
Englewood Cliffs, NJ 7632-1207 201-947-6000
800-535-1910
Fax: 201-947-9376
Jason Kingsley, Author
Mitchell Levitz, Co-Author
Offers information on growing up with Downs Syndrome. *$9.95*

7984 **Culture and the Restructuring of Community Mental Health**
Greenwood Publishing Group
130 Cremona Drive
Santa Barbara, CA 93117
805-968-1911
800-368-6868
Fax: 866-270-3856
CustomerService@abc-clio.com
www.greenwood.com
William A Vega, Author
John W Murphy, Co-Author
Michael Millman, Editor, American History
Hilary Clagget, Editor, Business, Economics & Finance
Examines treatment, organizational planning and research issues and offers a critique of the theoretical and programmatic aspects of providing mental health services to traditionally underserved populations. $45.00-$52.95. *$95.00*
168 pages Hardcover
ISBN 0-313268-87-8

7985 **Difficult Child**
Bantam Books
1745 Broadway, 10th Floor
New York, NY 10019
212-782-9000
Fax: 212-302-7985
BBDPublicity@randomhouse.com
www.randomhouse.com/bantamdell
Stanley Turecki, Author
Leslie Tonner, Co-Author
The classic and definitive work on parenting hard-to-raise children with new sections on ADHD and the latest medications for childhood disorders. *$15.95*
302 pages Paperback
ISBN 0-553380-36-2

7986 **Disability Culture Perspective on Early Intervention**
Through the Looking Glass
3075 Adeline Street
Suite 120
Berkeley, CA 94703-2212
510-848-1112
800-644-2666
Fax: 510-848-4445
TTY: 510-848-1005
TLG@lookingglass.org
www.lookingglass.org
Megan Kirshbaum PhD, Author
For parents with physical or cognitive disabilities and their families. Available in Braille, large print or cassette. *$2.00*
12 pages

7987 **Down Syndrome**
Aquarius Health Care Media
30 Forest Road
PO Box 249
Millis, MA 02054-1066
508-376-1244
888-440-2963
Fax: 508-376-1245
www.aquariusproductions.com
Lesile Kussmann, Owner
This is an excellent video for families who have just had a baby with Down Syndrome as well as professionals in the field of genetics and nursing. Through honest and open discussion, parents of children with Down Syndrome express the feelings and concerns they had during the early years of their child's life. Preview option available. *$150.00*
Video

7988 **Driven to Distraction**
Simon & Schuster/Touchstone Publishing
1230 Avenue of the Americas
Fl 11
New York, NY 10020- 1513
212-698-7000
Fax: 212-698-7009
www.simonsays.com
Edward M Hallowell, MD, Author
John J Ratey, MD, Co-Author
A practical book discussing adult as well as child attention deficit disorder (ADD). Non-technical, realistic and optimistic, it is an informative how-to manual for parents and consumers. *$23.00*

7989 **Dyslexia over the Lifespan**
Educators Publishing Service
PO Box 9031
Cambridge, MA 02139-9031
617-367-2700
800-225-5750
Fax: 617-547-0412
eps@schoolspecialty.com
www.epsbooks.com
Margaret B Rawston, Author
Discusses the educational and career development of 56 dyslexic boys from a private school that was one of the first to have a program to detect and treat developmental language disabilities. *$18.00*
224 pages
ISBN 0-838816-70-3

7990 **Embracing the Monster: Overcoming the Challenges of Hidden Disabilities**
Paul H Brookes Publishing Company
PO Box 10624
Baltimore, MD 21285-624
410-337-9580
800-638-3775
Fax: 410-337-8539
www.brookespublishing.com
Veronica Crawford M.A., Author
Larry B Silver, MD, Foreword/Commentary
The author shares her experience of living with LD, ADHD and bipolar disorder to give readers an awareness of the challenges of living with hidden disabilities and what can be done to help *$24.95*
272 pages paperback
ISBN 1-557665-22-2

7991 **Encounters with Autistic States**
Jason Aronson
400 Keystone Industrial Park
Dunmore, PA 18512-1507
800-782-0015
Fax: 201-840-7242
Theodore Mitrani, Author
This book explores and explands the work of the late Frances Tustin, which was devoted to the psychoanalytic understanding of the bewildering elemental world of the autistic child. *$50.00*
448 pages Hardcover
ISBN 0-765700-62-

7992 **Families of Adults With Autism: Stories & Advice For the Next Generation**
Autism Society of North Carolina Bookstore
505 Oberlin Road
Suite 230
Raleigh, NC 27605-1345
919-743-0204
800-442-2762
Fax: 919-743-0208
books@autismsociety-nc.org
www.autismbookstore.com
Tracey Sheriff, Chief Executive Officer
Paul Wendler, Chief Financial Officer
David Laxton, Director of Communications
Kristy White, Director of Development
This book's unique point of view is that of a parent who's been there and done that and is now willing to tell the reader what it was like. *$19.95*

7993 **Family Therapy for ADHD: Treating Children, Adolescents and Adults**
Guilford Press
72 Spring St
New York, NY 10012-4019
800-365-7006
www.guilford.com
Craig A Everett, Author
Sandra Volgy Everett, Co-Author
Presents an innovative approach to assesing and treating ADHD in the family context. *$29.00*
Paperback
ISBN 1-572304-38-3

7994 Fighting for Darla: Challenges for Family Care & Professional Responsibility
Teachers College Press
1234 Amsterdam Ave
New York, NY 10027-6602
212-678-3929
Fax: 212-678-4149
tcpress@tc.columbia.edu

Mary Lynch, Manager
Susan M Klein, Co-Author
Samuel Guskin, Co-Author
Samuel Guskin, Co-Author
Follows the story of Darla, a pregnant adolescent with autism. *$18.95*
161 pages
ISBN 0-807733-56-3

7995 Fragile Success
Brookes Publishing
PO Box 10624
Baltimore, MD 21285-624
410-337-9580
800-638-3775
Fax: 410-337-8539
www.brookespublishing.com

Virginia Walker Sperry, Author
A book about the lives of autistic children, whom the author has followed from their early years at the Elizabeth Ives School in New Haven, CT, through to adulthood. *$27.50*
ISBN 1-557664-58-7

7996 Getting Our Heads Together
Thoms Rehabilitation Hospital
68 Sweeten Creek Rd
Asheville, NC 28803-2318
828-274-2400
Fax: 828-274-9452

Kathi Petersen, Director Planning/Communication
Edgardo Diez MD, Medical Director Brain Injury
Kathy Price, Director Admissions
Chat Norvell, CEO
A handbook for families of head injured patients - available in Spanish as well as English. *$4.00*
40 pages Paperback

7997 Getting a Grip on ADD: A Kid's Guide to Understanding & Coping with ADD
Educational Media Corporation
1443 Old York Rd
Warmister, PA 18794
763-781-0088
800-448-9041
Fax: 215-956-9041
www.educationalmedia.com

Kim Frank Ed.S., Author
Susan Smith-Rex Ed.D., Co-Author
Free catalog of resources.
64 pages Yearly

7998 Getting the Best for Your Child with Autism
Autism Society of North Carolina Bookstore
505 Oberlin Road
Suite 230
Raleigh, NC 27605-1345
919-743-0204
800-442-2762
Fax: 919-743-0208
books@autismsociety-nc.org
www.autismbookstore.com

Tracey Sheriff, Chief Executive Officer
Paul Wendler, Chief Financial Officer
David Laxton, Director of Communications
Kristy White, Director of Development
This treatment guide helps parents navigate the complex and overwhelming world of Autism. *$16.95*

7999 Group Activity for Adults with Brain Injury
Sage Publications
2455 Teller Road
Thousand Oaks, CA 91320
805-499-0721
800-818-7243
Fax: 805-499-0871
info@sagepub.com
www.sagepub.com

Sara Miller McCune, Founder, Publisher, Executive Chairman
Blaise R Simqu, President & CEO
Tracey A. Ozmina, Executive Vice President & Chief Operating Officer
Chris Hickok, Senior Vice President & Chief Financial Officer
This manual addresses attention, memory, reasoning, and language skills in group settings. *$53.00*

8000 Guide to Successful Employment for Individuals with Autism
Brookes Publishing
P.O. Box 10624
Baltimore, MD 21285-0624
410-337-9580
800-638-3775
Fax: 410-337-8539
custserv@brookespublishing.com
www.brookespublishing.com

Marcia Daltow Smith, Author
Ronald G Belcher, Co-Author
Patricia D Juhrs, Co-Author
Lauren Smith, Western Region Sales Representat
Describing all aspects of job placement, this book details strategies for assessing workers, networking for job opportunities, and tailoring job supports to each individual. Also illustrates how to help individuals with autism become productive workers, and with detailed descriptions of specific jobs help provide ideas for employment. *$32.95*
336 pages Paperback
ISBN 1-55766-71-5

8001 Handbook of Autism and Pervasive Developmental Disorders
Autism Society of North Carolina Bookstore
505 Oberlin Road
Suite 230
Raleigh, NC 27605-1345
919-743-0204
800-442-2762
Fax: 919-743-0208
books@autismsociety-nc.org
www.autismbookstore.com

David Laxton, Director of Communications
Paul Wendler, Chief Financial Officer
Tracey Sheriff, Chief Executive Officer
Kristy White, Director of Development
A list of contributors address such topics as characteristics of autistic syndromes and interventions. *$125.00*

8002 Handbook of Career Planning for Students with Special Needs
Pro- Ed Publications
8700 Shoal Creek Boulevard
Austin, TX 78757-6897
512-451-3246
800-897-3202
Fax: 512-451-8542
general@proedinc.com
www.proedinc.com

Donald D Hammill, Owner
Courtney King, Marketing Coordinator
Thomas F. Harrington, Editor
The practitioner's guide will show you how to help special needs adolescents and young adults overcome barriers to employment by identifying goals and problems, assessing interests and aptitudes, involving client families and developing communication skills. *$42.00*
358 pages

8003 **Helping People with Autism Manage Their Behavior**
Indiana Resource Center For Autism
2853 E 10th St
Bloomington, IN 47408-2696
812-855-6508
Fax: 812-855-9630
prattc@indiana.edu
www.iidc.indiana.edu

David Mank, Executive Director
Scott Bellini, Assistant Director
Covers the broad topic of helping people with autism manage their behavior. *$7.00*

8004 **Helping Your Hyperactive: Attention Deficit Child**
Crown Publishing Company (Random House)
1745 Broadway
New York, NY 10019-4305
212-782-9000
800-632-8676
Fax: 212-572-6066
crownpublishing.com

John Taylor, Author
$19.95
ISBN 1-559584-23-8

8005 **Hidden Child: The Linwood Method for Reaching the Autistic Child**
Woodbine House
6510 Bells Mill Road
Bethesda, MD 20817-1636
301-897-3570
800-843-7323
Fax: 301-897-5838
info@woodbinehouse.com
www.woodbinehouse.com

Irv Shapell, Owner
Sabine Oishi, Co-Author
Chronicle of the Linwood Children's Center's successful treatment program for autistic children. *$17.95*
286 pages Paperback
ISBN 0-933149-06-9

8006 **How To Reach and Teach Children and Teens with Dyslexia**
Jossey-Bass
111 River St
Hoboken, NJ 7030-5773
201-748-6000
Fax: 201-748-6008
info@wiley.com
www.wiley.com

Cynthia M Stowe, Author
This practical resource gives educators at all levels essential information, techniques, and tolls for understanding dyslexia and adapting teaching methods in all subject areas to meet the learning style, social, and emotional needs of students who have dyslexia. *$22.95*
340 pages
ISBN 0-130320-18-8

8007 **Hyperactive Child, Adolescent, and Adult: ADD Through the Lifespan**
Oxford University Press
198 Madison Ave
New York, NY 10016-4308
212-726-6000
www.us.oup.com/us

Paul H Wender, Author
Comprehensive general review. Update on previous research by the author, offering a basic text. Published by Cennecticut Association for Children & Adults with Learning Disabilities (CACLD). *$8.75*
162 pages
ISBN 0-195113-49-7

8008 **Identifying and Treating Attention Deficit Hyperactivity Disorder**
Learning Disabilities Association of America
461 Cochran Rd.
Suite 245
Pittsburgh, PA 15228
412-341-1515
Fax: 412-344-0224
info@ldaamerica.org
www.ldaamerica.org

Cindy Cipoletti, Executive Director
Aaron Goldstein, Director, Federal & State Engagement
Nina DelPrato, Administrative Manager
Lauren Closer, Coordinator, Marketing & Development
A resource guide for families and educators on the identification and treatment of Attention Deficit Hyperactivity Disorder (ADHD).

8009 **In Search of Wings: A Journey Back from Traumatic Brain Injury**
Lash & Associates Publishing/Training
100 Boardwalk Drive, Suite 150
Youngsville, NC 27596
919-556-0300
Fax: 919-556-0900
orders@lapublishing.com
www.lapublishing.com

Marilyn Lash, President
Bob Cluett, CEO
Bill Herrin, Director of Graphics & Design
Nick Vidal, Director of IT
The true story of one woman coping with traumatic brain injury after a car accident that affected her cognitive skills and memory
$14.95
233 pages
ISBN 1-882332-00-8

8010 **In Their Own Way**
Alliance for Parental Involvement in Education
375 Hudson Street
New York, NY 10014
212-366-2000
Fax: 212-366-2933
ecommerce@us.penguingroup.com
http://us.penguingroup.com

Thomas Armstrong, Author
John Makinson, Chairman and Chief Executive
Coram Williams, CFO
David Shanks, CEO
For the parents whose children are not thriving in school, Armstrong offers insight into individual learning styles. *$11.95*

8011 **Jumpin' Johnny Get Back to Work, A Child's Guide to ADHD/Hyperactivity**
Ste 15-5
25 Van Zant St
Norwalk, CT 6855-1729
203-838-5010
Fax: 203-866-6108
CACLD@optonline.net
www.CACLD.org

Beryl Kaufman, Executive Director
Written primarily for elementary age youngsters with ADHD to help them understand their disability. Also valuable as an educational tool for parents, siblings, friends and classmates. Includes two pages on medication. *$12.50*
24 pages

8012 **Keys to Parenting a Child with Attention Deficit Disorder**
Barron's Educational Series
250 Wireless Blvd
Hauppauge, NY 11788-3924
631-434-3311
800-645-3476
Fax: 631-434-3723
barrons@barronseduc.com
barronseduc.com

Manuel H Barron, CEO
Francine McNamara MSW CSW, Co/Author
This book shows how to work with the child's school, effectively manage the child's behavior and act as the child's advocate. *$6.95*
160 pages Paperback
ISBN 0-812014-59-6

8013 Keys to Parenting a Child with Downs Syndrome
Barron's Educational Series
250 Wireless Blvd
Hauppauge, NY 11788-3924
631-434-3311
800-645-3476
Fax: 631-434-3723
barrons@barronseduc.com
barronseduc.com

Manuel H Barron, CEO
Lucy Guarino
Down Syndrome poses many challenges for children and their families. This book prepares parents and guardians to raise a child with Down Syndrome by discussing adjustment, advocacy, health and behavior, education and planning for greater independence. *$5.95*
160 pages Paperback
ISBN 0-812014-58-8

8014 Keys to Parenting the Child with Autism
Barron's Educational Series
250 Wireless Blvd
Hauppauge, NY 11788-3924
631-434-3311
800-645-3476
Fax: 631-434-3723
barrons@barronseduc.com
barronseduc.com

Manuel H Barron, CEO
Parents of children with autism will find a solid balance between home and practical information in this book. It explains what autism is and how it is diagnosed, then advises parents on how to adjust to their child and give the best care. *$6.95*
208 pages Paperback
ISBN 0-812016-79-3

8015 LD Child and the ADHD Child: Ways Parents & Professionals Can Help
1406 Plaza Dr
Winston Salem, NC 27103-1470
336-768-1374
800-222-9796
Fax: 336-768-9194
southern@blairpub.com
www.blairpub.com

Carolyn Sakowski, President
Susan H Stevens, Author
Book about learning disabilities available to parents. Stevens cuts through the jargon and complex theories which usually characterize books on the subject to present effective and practical techniques that parents can employ to help their child succeed at home and at school. New edition adds information about ADHD children. *$12.95*
201 pages Paperback
ISBN 0-895871-42-4

8016 Let Community Employment be the Goal for Individuals with Autism
Indiana Resource Center For Autism
2853 E 10th St
Bloomington, IN 47408-2601
812-855-9396
800-825-4733
Fax: 812-855-9630
prattc@indiana.edu
www.iidc.indiana.edu

David Mank, Executive Director
Scott Bellini, Assistant Director
A guide designed for people who are responsible for preparing individuals with autism to enter the work force. *$7.00*

8017 Making the Writing Process Work
Brookline Books
8 Trumbull Rd
Suite B-001
Northampton, MA 01060
617-734-6772
800-666-2665
Fax: 617-734-3952
brbooks@yahoo.com
www.brooklinebooks.com

Karen R Harris, Author
Steve Grahm, Co-Author
Making the Writing Process Work: Strategies for Composition and Self-Regulation is geared toward students who have difficulty organizing their thoughts and developing their writing. The specific strategies teach students how to approach, organize, and produce a final written product. *$24.95*
240 pages Paperback
ISBN 1-57129-10-9

8018 Management of Autistic Behavior
Sage Publications
2455 Teller Road
Thousand Oaks, CA 91320
805-499-0721
800-818-7243
Fax: 800-583-2665
info@sagepub.com
www.sagepub.com

Sara Miller McCune, Founder, Publisher, Executive Chairman
Blaise R Simqu, President & CEO
Tracey A. Ozmina, Executive Vice President & Chief Operating Officer
Stephen Barr, Managing Director/SAGE London
This excellent reference is a comprehensive and practical book that tells what works best with specific problems. *$41.00*
450 pages

8019 Managing Attention Deficit Hyperactivity in Children: A Guide for Practitioners
John Wiley & Sons Inc
111 River St
Hoboken, NJ 07030-5774
201-748-6000
800-825-7550
Fax: 201-748-6088
info@wiley.com
www.wiley.com

Warren J Baker, President
Michael Goldstein, Co-Author
Matthe S Kissner, CEO
Offers information about human personality, structure and dynamics, assessment and adjustment. *$27.50*
214 pages Hardcover
ISBN 0-471121-58-9

8020 Neurobiology of Autism
Johns Hopkins University Press
2715 N Charles St
Baltimore, MD 21218-4363
410-516-6900
Fax: 410-516-6968
www.press.jhu.edu

William Brody, President
Thomas L Kemper, Co-Author
Margaret L Bauman, M.D., Co-Author
Thomas L Kemper, M.D., Co-Author
This book discusses recent advances in scientific research that point to a neurobiological basis for autism and examines the clinical implications of this research. *$28.00*
272 pages
ISBN 0-801880-47-5

8021 Out of the Fog: Treatment Options and Coping Strategies for ADD
Hyperion
1500 Broadway
3rd Floor
New York, NY 10036
212-563-6500
800-331-3761
Fax: 212-456-0176
www.hyperionbooks.com

Robert Miller, President
Suzanne Levert, Co-Author
Discusses the recent recognition of attention deficit disorder as a problem that is not outgrown in adolescence, and cogently summarizes the stumbling blocks this affliction creates in the pursuit of a career or attainment of a healthy family life *$14.95*
300 pages
ISBN 0-786880-87-2

8022 **Overcoming Dyslexia**
Vintage-Random House
3rd Fl
1745 Broadway
New York, NY 10019-4305
212-782-9000
Fax: 212-302-7985
www.randomhouse.com/vintage

Markus Dohle, CEO
Sally Shawitz, M.D., Author
Yale neuroscientist Shaywitz demystifies the roots of dyslexia (a neurologically based reading difficulty affecting one in five children) and offers parents and educators hope that children with reading problems can be helped. *$15.00*
432 pages
ISBN 0-679781-59-5

8023 **Parent Survival Manual**
Springer Publishing Company
11 W 42nd St
15th Floor
New York, NY 10036
212-431-4370
877-687-7476
Fax: 212-941-7842
cs@springerpub.com
www.springerpub.com

Ursula Springer, President
Ted Nardin, CEO
Edie Lambiase, CFO
A guide to crises resolution in autism and related developmental disorders. *$39.95*

8024 **Parent's Guide to Down Syndrome: Toward a Brighter Future**
Brookes Publishing
PO Box 10624
Baltimore, MD 21285-0624
410-337-9580
800-638-3775
Fax: 410-337-8539
custserv@brookespublishing.com
www.brookespublishing.com

Siegfried Pueschel MD PhD, Author
Highlights developmental stages and shows the advances that improve a child's quality of life. Includes discussions on easing the transition from home to school and choosing integration and curricular priorities, as well as guidelines for confronting adolescent and adult issues such as social and sexual needs and independent living and vocational options. *$21.95*
352 pages
ISBN 1-557664-52-8

8025 **Parenting Attention Deficit Disordered Teens**
CACLD
25 Van Zant Street
Norwalk, CT 06855-1729
203-838-5010
Fax: 203-866-6108
CACLD@optonline.net
cacld.org

Beryl Kaufman, Executive Director
Detailed outline of the various problems of adolescents with ADHD. Published by Connecticut Association for Children & Adults with Learning Disabilities (CACLD). *$3.25*
14 pages

8026 **Parents Helping Parents: A Directory of Support Groups for ADD**
Novartis Pharmaceuticals Division
59 State Route 10
East Hanover, NJ 7936-1005
862-778-7500
800-742-2422

Paulo Costa, CEO

8027 **Please Don't Say Hello**
Human Sciences Press
233 Spring St
New York, NY 10013-1522
212-229-2859
800-221-9369
Fax: 212-463-0742
isbndb.com

Charles Stenken, Author
Jaroslav Chobot, Author
Zirul Evany, Author
Bill Feldmaier, Author
With the support and love of his family, and through them the neighborhood children, a nine-year-old autistic boy is able to emerge from his shell. *$10.95*
47 pages Paperback
ISBN 0-89885 -99-8

8028 **Preventable Brain Damage**
Springer Publishing Company
11 W 42nd St
15th Floor
New York, NY 10036
212-431-4370
877-687-7476
Fax: 212-941-7842
cs@springerpub.com
www.springerpub.com

Donald L Templer, Author
Lawrence C Hartlage, Co-Author
Ursula Springer, President
Ted Nardin, CEO
Offers information on brain injuries from motor vehicle accidents, contact sports and injuries of children. *$35.95*
256 pages

8029 **Reading, Writing and Speech Problems in Children**
International Dyslexia Association
40 York Rd.
4th Floor
Baltimore, MD 21204
410-296-0232
Fax: 410-321-5069
info@dyslexiaida.org
dyslexiaida.org

Samuel Torrey Orton, Author
This book provides reading, reading and speech execerises for educating people with dyslexia. *$20.00*
259 pages
ISBN 0-89079 -79-1

8030 **Reality of Dyslexia**
Brookline Books
8 Trumbull Rd
Suite B-001
Northampton, MA 01060
617-734-6772
800-666-2665
Fax: 617-734-3952
brbooks@yahoo.com
www.brooklinebooks.com

John Osmond, Author
An informative and sensitive study of living with dyslexia which affects one in 25. He introduces the reader to the subject by sharing the difficulties of his dyslexic son. He then uses the personal accounts of other children and adult dyslexics, even entire dyslexic families, to illuminate the problems they encounter. *$14.95*
150 pages Paperback
ISBN 1-57129 -17-6

8031 **Relationship Development Intervention with Young Children**
Jessica Kingsley Publishers
400 Market St
Suite 400
Philadelphia, PA 19106
215-922-1161
Fax: 215-992-1417
orders@jkp.com
www.jkp.com

Steven E Gustein, Author
Rachelle Sheely, Co-Author
Social and emotional development activities for Asperger Syndrome, Autism, PDD and NLD. Comprehensive set of activities emphasizes foundation skills for younger children between the

ages of two and eight. Covers skills such as social referencing, regulating behavior, conversational reciprocity, and synchronized actions. For use in therapeutic settings as well as schools and parents. *$22.95*
256 pages
ISBN 1-843107-14-7

8032 Rethinking Attention Deficit Disorder
Brookline Books
8 Trumbull Rd
Suite B-001
Northampton, MA 01060-4533
617-734-6772
800-666-2665
Fax: 617-734-3952
brbooks@yahoo.com
www.brooklinebooks.com
Miriam Cherkes-Julkowski, Author
In contrast to the common focus on behavioral symptoms of attention disorders, this book emphasizes internal factors that make attention regulation difficult. In-depth discussions of social, emotional, and academic consequences and appropriate interventions are provided. *$27.95*
250 pages Paperback
ISBN 1-571290-30-7

8033 Riddle of Autism: A Psychological Analysis
Jason Aronson
4501 Forbes Blvd
Suite 200
Lanham, MD 20706-4346
301-459-3366
800-782-0015
Fax: 301-429-5746
www.rowmanlittlefield.com
Jason Aronson, Author
James Lyons, President/CEO
Stanley Plotnick, Chairman
Dr. Victor examines the myths that cloud an understanding of this disorder and describes the meanings of its specific behavioral symptoms. *$30.00*
356 pages Paperback
ISBN 1-568215-73-8

8034 SCATBI: Scales Of Cognitive Ability for Traumatic Brain Injury
Sage Publications
2455 Teller Road
Thousand Oaks, CA 91320
805-499-0721
800-818-7243
Fax: 805-499-0871
happiness@option.org
www.sagepub.com
Sara Miller McCune, Founder, Publisher, Executive Chairman
Blaise R Simqu, President & CEO
Tracey A. Ozmina, Executive Vice President & Chief Operating Officer
Stephen Barr, Managing Director/SAGE London
Assesses cognitive and linguistic abilities of adolescent and adult parents with head injuries. *$287.00*

8035 Sex Education: Issues for the Person with Autism
Indiana Resource Center For Autism
2853 E 10th St
Bloomington, IN 47408-2696
812-855-6508
800-825-4733
Fax: 812-855-9630
iidc@indiana.edu
www.iidc.indiana.edu
David Mank, Executive Director
Scott Bellini, Assistant Director
Discusses issues of sexuality and provides methods of instruction for people with autism. *$4.00*

8036 Son-Rise: The Miracle Continues
2080 S Undermountain Rd.
Sheffield, MA 01257
413-229-2100
800-562-7171
correspondence@option.org
www.autismtreatmentcenter.org
Barry Neil Kaufman, Founder & CEO
Clyde Haberman, Senior Teacher & Director of Development
Blair Borgeson, Developmental Therapist
Emily Vitale Aronow, Program Advisor & Client Support Coordinator
The center's Son-Rise Program teaches a comprehensive system of treatment and education designed to help families and caregivers enable their children to dramatically improve in all areas of learning. *$12.95*
343 pages
ISBN 0-915811-53-7

8037 Soon Will Come the Light
Future Horizons Inc
721 W Abram St
Arlington, TX 76013-6995
817-277-0727
800-479-0727
Fax: 817-277-2270
www.fhautism.com
Wayne Gilpin, Owner
Jennifer Gilpin, Vice President
Annette Vick, Manager
Offers new perspectives on the perplexing disability of autism. *$19.95*

8038 Successful Job Search Strategies for the Disabled: Understanding the ADA
Wiley Publishing
605 3rd Ave
New York, NY 10158-180
212-850-6000
Fax: 212-850-6088
www.wiley.com
Jeffrey G Allen, Author
Following a concise overview of the Americans with Disabilities Act (ADA), covers such topics as job identification, self-assessment, job leads, resumes, disability disclosure, interviewing, and accommodating specific disabilities. Includes dozen of relevant and instructive situation analyses, case examples, and answers to commonly asked questions. *$165.00*
229 pages

8039 Taking Charge of ADHD Complete Authoritative Guide for Parents
Guilford Press
72 Spring St
New York, NY 10012-4019
212-431-9800
800-365-7006
Fax: 212-966-6708
info@guilford.com
www.guilford.com
Russell A Barkley, Author
Revised and updated to incorporate the most current information on ADHD and its treatment. Provides parents with the knowledge, guidance and confidence they need to ensure that their child receives the best care possible. Also in cloth at $40.00 (ISBN# 1-57230-600-9 *$18.95*
331 pages Paperback
ISBN 1-572305-60-1

8040 Teaching Children with Autism: Strategies for Initiating Positive Interactions
Brookes Publishing
P.O. Box 10624
Baltimore, MD 21285-0624
410-337-9580
800-638-3775
Fax: 410-337-8539
custserv@brookespublishing.com
www.brookespublishing.com
Robert L. Koegel, Author
Lynn Kern Koegel, Co-Author
Robert Miller, Sales Director
Offers strategies for initiating positive interactions and improving learning opportunities. This guide begins with an overview of characteristics and long-term strategies and proceeds through

discussions that detail specific techniques for normalizing environments, reducing disruptive behavior, improving language and social skills, and enhancing generalization. *$39.95*

256 pages Paperback

ISBN 1-557661-80-4

8041 Teaching and Mainstreaming Autistic Children

Love Publishing Company
9101 E Kenyon Ave
Suite 2200
Denver, CO 80237-1854
303-221-7333
Fax: 303-221-7444
www.lovepublishing.com

Stan Love, Owner
Peter Knoblock, Author

Dr. Knoblock advocates a highly organized, structured environment for autistic children, with teachers and parents working together. His premise is that the learning and social needs of autistic children must be analyzed and a daily program designed with interventions that respond to this functional analysis of their behavior. *$24.95*

ISBN 0-89108 -11-9

8042 Techniques for Aphasia Rehab: (TARGET) Generating Effective Treatment

Speech Bin
1965 25th Ave
Vero Beach, FL 32960-3062
772-770-0007
800-477-3324
Fax: 772-770-0006
store.schoolspecialty.com

Mary Jo Santo Pietro, Co-Author
Robert Goldfarb, Co-Author

TARGET is the kind of resource aphasia clinicians beg for. A practical resource that answers not only the what and how questions of treatment, but also the why. It describes dozens of treatment methods and gives you practical exercises and activities to implement each technique. It shows you how to treat all components of the disability, language disorder, overall impairment, communication problems, and the needs of the person with aphasia. *$45.00*

384 pages

ISBN 0-93785 -50-5

8043 Teenagers with ADD

Woodbine House
6510 Bells Mill Rd
Bethesda, MD 20817-1636
301-897-3570
800-843-7323
Fax: 301-897-5838
info@woodbinehouse.com
www.woodbinehouse.com

Irv Shapell, Owner
Chris A Ziegler Dendy, M.S., Author

This best selling guide to understanding and coping with teenagers with attention deficit disorder (ADD) provides complete coverage of the special issues and challenges faced by these teens. Based on current diagnostic criteria and the latest literature and research in the field, the book discusses diagnosis, medical treatment, family and school life, intervention, advocacy, legal rights, and options after high school. Parents find strategies for dealing with their teen's difficult behaviors. *$18.95*

370 pages Paperback

ISBN 0-933149-69-7

8044 Understanding Down Syndrome: An Introduction for Parents

Brookline Books
8 Trumbull Rd
Suite B-001
Northampton, MA 01060-4533
617-734-6772
800-666-2665
Fax: 617-734-3952
brbooks@yahoo.com
www.brooklinebooks.com

Cliff Cunningham, Author

Using positive and readable language, this book helps parents understand Down Syndrome. Medical details are explained in lay terms, and advice is given on working with professionals, obtaining services, and treatment techniques that help the child. Cunningham alerts families to potential problems, the prospects for the child in schooling and the passage to adulthood. Revised 1996. *$14.95*

Softcover

ISBN 1-57129 -09-5

8045 Valley News Dispatch

New York Families For Autistic Children
95-16 Pitkin Avenue
Ozone Park, NY 11417-2834
718-641-3441
Fax: 718-641-2228

Cheryl L. Marsh, Chairperson
Robert Burt, Treasurer

Education, recreation and support services for families and children with developmental disabilities.

8046 Verbal Behavior Approach: How to Teach Children with Autism & Related Disorders

Autism Society of North Carolina Bookstore
505 Oberlin Road
Suite 230
Raleigh, NC 27605-1345
919-743-0204
800-442-2762
Fax: 919-743-0208
books@autismsociety-nc.org
www.autismbookstore.com

David Laxton, Director of Communications
Paul Wendler, Chief Financial Officer
Tracey Sheriff, Chief Executive Officer
Kristy White, Director of Development

Provides full descriptions of how to teach the verbal operants that make up expressive languate which include: manding, tacting, echoing and intraverbal skills. *$19.95*

8047 Without Reason: A Family Copes with two Generations of Autism

Books on Special Children
721 W Abram St
Arlington, TX 76013-6995
817-277-0727
800-489-0727
Fax: 817-277-2270

Wayne Tilton, President

The author discovers his son has autism. He delves into problems of the autistic person and explains reasons for their actions. *$20.95*

292 pages Hardcover

8048 Women with Attention Deficit Disorder: Embracing Disorganization at Home and Work

Underwood-Miller
708 Westover Dr
Lancaster, PA 17601-1242

288 pages

ISBN 1-887424-05-9

8049 You Mean I'm Not Lazy, Stupid or Crazy?!: A Self-Help Book for Adults with ADD

Simon & Schuster
1230 Avenue Of The Americas
11th Floor
New York, NY 10020-1513
212-698-7000
Fax: 212-698-7099
www.simonsays.com

Kate Kelly, Author
Peggy Ramundo, Co-Author

Practical advice on controlling adult ADD, a straightforward guide explains how to get along in groups, become organized, improve memory, and pursue professional help. *$15.00*

464 pages

ISBN 0-684815-31-1

8050 You and Your ADD Child

Nelson Publications
1 Gateway Plz
Port Chester, NY 10573-4674
914-481-5490
Fax: 914-937-8950

Paul Warren MD, Author
Jody Capehart M.Ed., Co-Author

$12.99
252 pages Paperback
ISBN 0-785278-95-8

Journals

8051 **Annals of Dyslexia**
International Dyslexia Association
40 York Road
4th Floor
Baltimore, MD 21204
410-296-0232
Fax: 410-321-5069
info@dyslexiaida.org
dyslexiaida.org/annals-of-dyslexia
Denise Douce, Director, Publications & Resources
IDA is a clearinghouse of scientific data and practice-based information related to dyslexia. Provides community-based referrals and information fact sheets in response to thousands of emails, calls & letters. Our annual conference attracts thousands of outstanding researchers, clinicians, parents, teachers, psychologists, educational therapists and people with dyslexia.
Tri-annual

8052 **Journal of Cognitive Rehabilitation**
Neuroscience Publishers
6555 Carrollton Ave
Indianapolis, IN 46220-1664
317-257-9672
Fax: 317-257-9674
neuroscience.cnter.com
Odie L Bracy, Executive Director
Publication for therapists, family and patient, designed to provide information relevant to the rehabilitation of impairment resulting from brain injury. *$50.00*
36-48 pages Quarterly

Magazines

8053 **AWARE**
National Fibromyalgia Association
1000 Bristol Street North
Suite 17-247
Irvine, CA 92660
714-921-0150
Fax: 714-921-6920
www.fmaware.org
Lynne Matallana, President/Founder
Mark Dobrilovic, Board of Director
John Fry, PhD, Board of Director
Michael Seffinger, DO, FAAFP, Board of Director
Magazine published three times a year with membership only.

8054 **Attention**
Children & Adults with ADHD
8181 Professional Place
Suite 150
Landover, MD 20785- 2264
301-306-7070
800-233-4050
Fax: 301-306-7090
webmaster@chadd.org
www.chadd.org
Bryan Goodman, Director
A bi-monthly publication from CHADD. Free with membership.
Bi-monthly

Newsletters

8055 **ADHD Report**
Guilford Press
72 Spring St
New York, NY 10012-4019
212-431-9800
800-365-7006
Fax: 212-966-6708
info@guilford.com
www.guilford.com
Russell A Barkley PhD, Editor
Presents the most up-to-date information on the evaluation, diagnosis and management of ADHD in children, adolescents and adults. This important newsletter is an invaluable resource for all professionals interested in ADHD. *$49.95*
16 pages BiMonthly
ISSN 1065-8025

8056 **Arc Connection Newsletter**
Arc of Tennessee
151 Athens Way
Suite 100
Nashville, TN 37228
615-248-5878
800-835-7077
Fax: 615-248-5879
info@thearctn.org
thearctn.org
John Lewis, President
John H. Shouse, VP,Planning & Rules committee Chair
Donna Lankford, Secretary
Ann Curl, Treasurer,Budget/Finance Committee Chair
Quarterly publication from the ARC of Tennessee. *$10.00*
12 pages Quarterly

8057 **Arc Light**
Arc of Arizona
5610 S Central Ave
Phoenix, AZ 85040-3090
602-268-6101
800-252-9054
Fax: 602-268-7483
thearcaz@gmail.com
Cindy Waymire, Editor
For people with intellectual and developmental disabilities.
Quarterly

8058 **Autism Research Review International**
Autism Research Institute
4182 Adams Ave
San Diego, CA 92116-2599
619-281-7165
Fax: 619-563-6840
br@autismresearchinstitute.com
autism.com
Steve Edelson, Executive Director
The Autism Research Institute has pubished this quarterly newsletter, Autism Research Review International (ARRI), since 1987. The ARRI has received worldwide praise for it's thoroughness and objectivity in reporting the current developments in biomedical and educational research. The latest findings are gleaned from a computer search of the 25,000 scientific and medical articles published every week. *$18.00*
8 pages Quarterly

8059 **BIATX Newsletter**
Brain Injury Association of Texas
316 W 12th Street
Suite 405
Austin, TX 78701-1845
512-326-1212
800-392-0040
Fax: 512-478-3370
www.texasbia.org
Judith Abner, Director
Penny Phillips, President
Donna Kuhlmann, Chairman
Kelly Ramsay, CFO
A online quarterly e-newsletter, as well as news and updates on the Brain Injury Association of Texas.

8060 **BIAWV Newsletter**
Brain Injury Association of America
PO Box 574
Institute, WV 25112-0574
304-766-4892
800-356-6443
Fax: 304-766-4940
biawv@aol.com
Peggy Brown, Director
Mike Davis, President

8061 **Best Buddies Times**
Best Buddies Times
907-1243 Islington Ave
Toronto, ON, Canada
416-531-0003
888-779-0061
Fax: 416-531-0325
info@bestbuddies.ca
www.bestbuddies.ca

Steven Pinnock, Director
Emily Bolyea-Kyere, Regional Program Manager
Bi-annual newsletter.

8062 **Chadder**
Children & Adults with Attention Deficit Disorder
4601 Presidents Drive
Suite 300
Lanham, MD 20706
301-306-7070
Fax: 301-306-7090
www.chadd.org

Michael MacKay, President
Ruth Hughes, CEO
Susan Buningh, Executive Editor
Christine hoch, Director of Development
Quarterly newsletter
Quarterly

8063 **Cognitive Therapy Today**
Beck Institute for Cognitive Therapy & Research
One Belmont Avenue
Ste 700
Bala Cynwyd, PA 19004-1610
610-664-3020
Fax: 610-709-5336
info@beckinstitute.org
www.beckinstitute.org

Judith S Beck, Director
Aaron T Beck, President
Cognitive Therapy TodayT features articles on a wide range of topics in CBT by leading clinicians from around the world. Articles have addressed evaluating psychotherapies; CBT and special populations, such as soldiers, the elderly, or diagnoses such as schizophrenia; conceptualizing emotions; cross-cultural issues and many other issues of interest to clinicians. You will also find information on workshops, speaking engagements by Beck Institute faculty and more.

8064 **Down Syndrome News**
National Down Syndrome Congress
30 Mansell Court
Suite 108
Roswell, GA 30076
770-604-9500
800-232-6372
Fax: 770-604-9898
info@ndsccenter.org
www.ndsccenter.org

Jim Faber, President
Marilyn Tolbert, 1st VP
Carole J. Guess, 2nd Vice President
Lori Mckee, Treasurer
Must become a member to receive the newsletter.

8065 **Focus Times Newsletter**
Focus Alternative Learning Center
126 Dowd Avenue
PO Box 452
Canton, CT 06019-0452
860-693-8809
Fax: 860-693-0141
info@focuscenterforautism.org
www.focus-alternative.org

Marcia Bok, President
Claudia Godburn, Secretary
Rita Barredo, Treasurer
Monthly online newsletter on autism.

8066 **Imagine!**
Imagine!
1400 Dixon St
Lafayette, CO 80026-2790
303-665-7789
Fax: 303-665-2648
imaginecolorado.org

John Taylor, President
Mark Emery, Executive Director
John Nevins, CFO
Susan LaHoda, Foundation Executive Director
For people of all ages with cognitive, developmental, physical & health related needs, so they may live lives of independence & quality in their homes and communities.
12-16 pages quarterly

8067 **NAMI Advocate**
National Alliance on Mental Illness
3803 N Fairfax Dr
Suite 100
Arlington, VA 22203-3080
703-524-7600
800-950-6264
Fax: 703-524-9094
www.nami.org

Suzanne Vogel-Scibilia, President
Our mission is to provide you with the technical assistance, tools and referrals to resources you need to build organizational capacity and achieve the goals of the NAMI Standards of Excellence.

8068 **NLP News**
NLP Comprehensive
PO.Box 348
Indian Hills, CO 80454-648
303-987-2224
800-233-1657
Fax: 303-987-2228
www.nlpco.com

Christian Miller, Editor
Tom Dotz, President
Tom Hoobyar, Director Of Planning
Sharon DeBault, Director Of Community Relations
An online e-newsletter on Neuro-linguistic programming.

8069 **Pure Facts**
Feingold Association of the US
10955 Windjammer Dr. S
Indianapolis, IN 46256
631-369-9340
help@feingold.org
www.feingold.org

Deborah Lehner, Executive Director
Relationship between foods, food additives and behaviorial or learning challenges.

8070 **REACH**
TEACCH
100 Renee Lynn Ct
Carrboro, NC 27510
919-966-2174
Fax: 919-966-4127
teacch@unc.edu
www.teacch.com

Dr. Laura Klinger, Director
Walter Kelly, Business Officer
Rebecca Mabe, Assistant Director of Business
Mark Klinger, Director of Research
Free online newsletter.

8071 **Rettsyndrome.org**
4600 Devitt Dr
Cincinnati, OH 45246
513-874-3020
800-818-7388
Fax: 513-874-2520
admin@rettsyndrome.org
www.rettsyndrome.org

Peter White, Chair
Gordon Rich, Chief Operating Officer
Steven Kaminsky, Ph.D, Chief Science Officer
Mary Woods, Director of Marketing & Communications
Rettsyndrome.org offers informational resources and programs for those affected by Rett syndrome as well as their families.

8072 **Weekly Wisdom**
Autism Treatment Center of America
2080 S Undermountain Rd
Sheffield, MA 01257-9643
413-229-2100
877-766-7473
Fax: 413-229-3202
www.son-rise.org

Barry Kausman, Owner
Weekly Wisdom is available through a free email subscription.

Audio/Visual

8073 **ADD, Stepping Out of the Dark**
Child Development Media
5632 Van Nuys Blvd
Suite 286
Van Nuys, CA 91401-4602
818-989-7221
800-405-8942
Fax: 818-989-7826

Margie Wagner, Owner
A powerful, effective video, ideal for health professionals, educators and parents providing a visual montage designed to promote an understanding and awareness of attention deficit disorder. Based on actual accounts of those who have ADD, including a neurologist, an office worker, and parents of children with ADD. The DVD allows the viewer to feel the frustration and lack of attention that ADD brings to many. *$52.95*
Video

8074 **ADHD in Adults**
Guilford Press
72 Spring St
New York, NY 10012-4019
212-431-9800
800-365-7006
Fax: 212-966-6708
info@guilford.com
www.guilford.com

Russell A Barkley, Editor
This program integrates information on ADHD with the actual experiences of four adults who suffer from the disorder. Representing a range of professions, from a lawyer to a mother working at home, each candidly discusses the impact of ADHD on his or her daily life. These interviews are augmented by comments from family members and other clinicians who treat adults with ADHD. *$99.00*
DVD 1906
ISBN 0-898629-86-1

8075 **ADHD: What Can We Do?**
Guilford Press
72 Spring St
New York, NY 10012-4019
212-431-9800
800-365-7006
Fax: 212-966-6708
info@guilford.com

Russell A Barkley, Editor
A video program that introduces teachers and parents to a variety of the most effective technologies for managing ADHD in the classroom, at home, and on family outings. *$99.00*
DVD 1906
ISBN 0-898629-72-1

8076 **ADHD: What Do We Know?**
Guilford Press
72 Spring St
New York, NY 10012-4019
212-431-9800
800-365-7006
Fax: 212-966-6708
info@guilford.com
www.guilford.com

Bob Matloff, President
Russell A Barkley, Editor
An introduction for teachers and special education practitioners, school psychologists and parents of ADHD children. Topics outlined in this video include the causes and prevalence of ADHD, ways children with ADHD behave, other conditions that may accompany ADHD and long-term prospects for children with ADHD. *$99.00*
DVD 1906
ISBN 0-898629-71-3

8077 **Around the Clock: Parenting the Delayed AD HD Child**
Guilford Press
72 Spring St
New York, NY 10012-4019
212-431-9800
800-365-7006
Fax: 212-966-6708
info@guilford.com

Joan F Goodman, Editor
Susan Hoban, Editor
This videotape provides both professionals and parents a helpful look at how the difficulties facing parents of ADHD children can be handled. Video. *$150.00*
VHS 1994
ISBN 0-898629-68-3

8078 **Attention Deficit Disorder: Adults**
Aquarius Health Care Media
30 Forest Road
Millis, MA 02054
508-376-1244
888-440-2963
Fax: 508-376-1245
www.aquariusproductions.com

Lesile Kussmann, President/Owner
Joseph Wellington, Distribution Coordinator
Anne Baker, Billing & Accounting
Adults with ADD talk about how the disorder that went undiagnosed for so many years has affected their choice of spouses and work, and what they have found to help them. Biofeedback, which is growing as a treatment, is explained and demonstrated by its founder, Dr. Joel Lubar. Medical treatments like antidepressants and stimulants are also discussed, along with behavioral changes that can help the person with ADD and his or her spouse and family. *$149.00*
Video

8079 **Attention Deficit Disorder: Children**
Aquarius Health Care Media
30 Forest Rd
PO Box 249
Millisrn, MA 02054-7159
508-376-1244
888-440-2963
Fax: 508-376-1245
www.aquariusproductions.com

Lesile Kussmann, President/Owner
Everyone has been impulsive or easily distracted for different periods of time, so these symptoms that are hallmarks of Attention Deficit Disorder (ADD) have also led to criticism that too many people are being diagnosed with this biochemical brain disorder. This program examines who is being diagnosed, and what treatments are working. An innovative private school specializing in alternative education is profiled, and tips on structuring the school and home environment are included. *$149.00*
Video

8080 **Autism: A World Apart**
Fanlight Productions C/O Icarus Films
32 Court Street
Brooklyn, NY 11201-1731
718-488-8900
800-876-1710
Fax: 718-488-8642
info@fanlight.com
www.fanlight.com

Ben Achtenberg, Owner
Nicole Johnson, Publicity Coordinator
Anthony Sweeney, Marketing Director
In this documentary, three families show us what the textbooks and studies cannot: what it's like to live with autism day after day; to raise and love children who may be withdrawn and violent and unable to make personal connections with their families. 29 minutes. *$195.00*
VHS/DVD 1988
ISBN 1-572950-39-0

8081 **Autism: the Unfolding Mystery**
Aquarius Health Care Media
30 Forest Road
PO Box 249
Millis, MA 02054
508-376-1244
Fax: 508-376-1245
www.aquariusproductions.com

Lesile Kussmann, Owner
Explore what it means to be autistic, how you can recognize the signs of autism in your child, and hear about new treatments and programs to help children learn to deal with the disorder. *$145.00*
DVD 1905

8082 **Biology Concepts Through Discovery**
Educational Activities Software
5600 W 83rd Street
Suite 300, 8200 Tower
Bloomington, MN 55437
800-447-5286
Fax: 239-225-9299
info@edmentum.com
http://www.ea-software.com

Vin Riera, President/CEO
Rob Rueckel, CFO
Dave Adams, Chief Academic Officer
Paul Johansen, Chief Technology Officer
These videos, available in English and Spanish versions, encourage learning by presenting interactive problem solving in an effective VISUAL/AUDITORY style. *$89.00*
Video

8083 **Concentration Video**
Learning disAbilities Resources
6 E Eagle Road
Havertown, PA 19083
610-446-6126
800-869-8336
Fax: 610-525-8337
rcooper-ldr@comcast.net

Video

8084 **Educating Inattentive Children**
ADD Warehouse
300 Northwest 70th Avenue
Suite 102
Plantation, FL 33317-2360
954-792-8100
800-233-9273
Fax: 954-792-8545
websales@addwarehouse.com
www.addwarehouse.com

Harvey C Parker, Owner
Ideal for in-service to regular and special educators concerning the problems inattentive, elementarty and secondary students experience. *$49.00*
Video

8085 **Getting Started with Facilitated Communication**
Facilitated Communication Institute, Syracuse Univ
230 Huntington Hal
Syracuse, NY 13244-1
315-443-4752
Fax: 315-443-2258
http://thefci.syr.edu

Annegret Schubert, Director
Describes in detail how to help individuals with autism and/or severe communication difficulties to get started with facilitated communication.
Video

8086 **How to Cope with ADHD: Diagnosis, Treatment & Myths**
Aquarius Health Care Media
30 Forest Road
PO Box 249
Millis, MA 02054
508-376-1244
Fax: 508-376-1245
www.aquariusproductions.com

Lesile Kussmann, President/Owner
Learn how ADHD is diagnosed, clear up some of the myths, explain the treatmens that are availiable, and give you tips on how you can help your child at home. *$145.00*
DVD 1905

8087 **I Just Want My Little Boy Back**
Autism Treatment Center Of America
2080 South Undermountain Road
Sheffield, MA 01257
413-229-2100
800-714-2779
happiness@option.org
www.option.org

Samahria Lyt Kaufman, Co-Founder and Co-Director
Dane Griffith, Director of Administrative Services
Bears Kaufman, Co-Founder and Co-Director
Raun Kaufman, Director of Global Education
A great video for parents and professionals caring for children with special needs. Join one British family and their autistic son before, during and after their journey to America to attend The Son-Rise Program at The Autism Treatment Center of America. This informative, inspirational and deeply moving story not only captures the joy, tears, challenges and triumps of this amazing little boy and his family, but also serves as a powerful introduction to the attitude and principles of the program. *$25.00*

8088 **It's Just Attention Disorder**
Western Psychological Services
625 Alaska Avenue
Torrance, CA 90503-5124
424-201-8800
800-648-8857
Fax: 424-201-6950
customerservice@wpspublish.com
wpspublish.com

Gregg Gillmar, VP
This ground-breaking videotape takes the critical first steps in treating attention-deficit disorder: it enlists the inattentive or hyperactive child as an active participant in his or her treatment. *$99.50*
Video

8089 **Understanding ADHD**
Aquarius Health Care Videos
30 Forest Road
PO Box
Millis, MA 02054
508-376-1244
Fax: 508-376-1245
www.aquariusproductions.com

Leslie Kussmann, President/Owner
A look at some of the controversies surrounding Attention Deficit Hyperactivity Disorder. This video shows how the disorder is diagnosed and presents strategies for living with a child with the disorder. Diverse and candid opinions from teachers, social workers, a behavior specialist, a pediatrician and a parent with ADHD twins. Recommended for child development students, social workers, and caregivers. Preview option available. *$120.00*
Video

8090 **Understanding Attention Deficit Disorder**
CACLD
25 Van Zant Street
Norwalk, CT 6855-1713
203-838-5010
Fax: 203-866-6108
CACLD@optonline.net
www.CACLD.org

Beryl Kaufman, Executive Director
Helen Bosch, President
A video in an interview format for parents and professionals providing the history, symptoms, methods of diagnosis and three approaches used to ease the effects of attention deficit disorder. Published by Connecticut Association for Children & Adults with Learning Disabilities (CACLD). *$20.00*
45 Minutes VHS

8091 **Understanding Autism**
Fanlight Productions C/O Icarus Films
32 Court Street
Brooklyn, NY 11201
718-488-8900
800-876-1710
Fax: 718-488-8642
info@fanlight.com
www.fanlight.com

Ben Achtenberg, Owner
Susan Newman, Editor

Parents of children with autism discuss the nature and symptoms of this lifelong disability and outline a treatment program based on behavior modification principles. 19 minutes *$199.00*
VHS/DVD 1993
ISBN 1-572951-00-1

8092 **We're Not Stupid**
Media Projects Inc
5215 Homer St
Dallas, TX 75206-6623 214-826-3863
Fax: 214-826-3919
mail@mediaprojects.org
www.mediaprojects.org
Fonya Naomi Mondell, Producer
We're Not Stupid is an insightful and very personal video that gives a voice to people who are struggling with learning disabilities. It was made by filmmaker Fonya Naomi Mondell, who is also living with learning differences. The filmmaker camptures the personal stories of young people from all walks of life who discuss what it's like to live with Attention Deficit Disorder and Dyslexia. Their comments are open, honest and direct, and their determination to manage their condition shines through. *$125.00*
Video

8093 **Why Won't My Child Pay Attention?**
ADD Warehouse
300 Northwest 70th Avenue
Suite 102
Plantation, FL 33317-2360 954-792-8100
800-233-9273
Fax: 954-792-8545
www.addwarehouse.com
Sam Goldstein, Ph.D, Author
Michael Goldstein, M.D., Co-Author
Practical and reassuring videotape, noted child psychologist tells parents about two of the most common and complex problems of childhood: inattention and hyperactivity. *$49.50*
224 pages Hardcover 1992
ISBN 0-471530-77-8

Software

8094 **Cogrehab**
Life Science Associates
1 Fenimore Rd
Bayport, NY 11705-2115 631-472-2111
Fax: 631-472-8146
Joann Mandriota, President
Divided into six groups for diagnosis and treatment of attention, memory and perceptual disorders to be used by and under the guidance of a professional. $95.-$1,950

Support Groups

8095 **Autism Society of America**
4340 East-West Highway
Suite 350
Bethesda, MD 20814 301-657-0881
800-328-8476
Fax: 301-657-0869
info@autism-society.org
www.autism-society.org
Scott Badesch, President/CEO
Jennifer Repella, VP Programs
John Dabrowski, CFO
Doreen Allen, Marketing Manager
ASA is the largest and oldest grassroots organization within the autism community, with more than 200 chapters and over 20,000 members and supporters nationwide. ASA is the leading source of education, information and referral about autism and has been the leader in advocacy and legislative initiatives for more than three decades.

8096 **National Autism Hotline**
Autism Services Center
929 4th Ave
PO Box 507
Huntington, WV 25701-1408 304-525-8014
Fax: 304-525-8026
www.autismservicescenter.org
Mike Grady, CEO
Jimmie Beirne, COO
Nathel Lewis, ASC Training Coordinator
Service agency for individuals with autism and developmental disabilities, and their families. Assists families and agencies attempting to meet the needs of individuals with autism and other developmental disabilities. Makes available technical assistance in designing treatment programs and more. The hotline provides informational packets to callers and assists via telephone when possible.

8097 **National Health Information Center**
Office Of Disease Prevention And Health Promotion
P.O. Box 1133
Washington, DC 20013-1133 301-565-4167
800-336-4797
301-468-7394
Fax: 301-984-4256
www.health.gov/nhic
Jessica Rowden, Sec Dept. Health Human Services
William Corr, J.D., Deputy Secretary
National health information center provides information referral and support. NHIC links consumers and health professionals to organizations that are best able to provide reliable health information.

Dexterity

Associations

8098 American Amputee Foundation
1805 Wewoka Dr
North Little Rock, AR 72116
501-835-9290
Fax: 501-835-9292
www.americanamputee.org

Catherine J Walden, Executive Director

Serves primarily as a national information clearinghouse and referral center assisting amputees and their families. The foundation researches and gathers information including studies, product information, services, self-help publications and review articles written within the field.

8099 American Board for Certification in Orthotics, Prosthetics & Pedorthics
330 John Carlyle St
Suite 210
Alexandria, VA 22314
703-836-7114
Fax: 703-836-0838
info@abcop.org
www.abcop.org

Eric Ramcharran, CPO, President
Catherine Carter, Executive Director
Samlane Ketevong, Director, Certification Services
Debbie Ayres, Director, Marketing & Public Relations

The American Board for Certification in Orthotics, Prosthetics and Pedorthics is the national certifying and accrediting body for the orthotic and prosthetic professions.

8100 American Physical Therapy Association
1111 N Fairfax St
Alexandria, VA 22314-1488
703-684-2782
800-999-2782
Fax: 703-684-7343
consumer@apta.org
www.apta.org

Sharon L. Dunn, President
Matthew Hyland, Vice President
Kip Schick, Secretary
Jeanine Gunn, Treasurer

The American Physical Therapy Association fosters advancements in physical therapy practice, research and education. The association offers courses, career counceling, advocacy, publications and more.

8101 American Stroke Association
7272 Greenville Ave
Dallas, TX 75231
888-478-7653
strokeconnection@heart.org
www.strokeassociation.org/STROKEORG

John Warner, Presiednt
James Postl, Chairman
Nancy Brown, Chief Executive Officer
Raymond Vara, Jr., Treasurer

The American Stroke Association offers educational materials, seminars, conferences and transportation for those effected by strokes as well as their families, caregivers and interested professionals.

8102 Charcot-Marie-Tooth Association
PO Box 105
Glenolden, PA 19036
610-499-9264
800-606-2682
Fax: 610-499-9267
info@cmtausa.org
www.cmtausa.org

Gilles Bouchard, Chairman
Amy J Gray, CEO
Kim Magee, Director of Finance
Susan Ruediger, Director of Development

The Charcot-Marie-Tooth Association supports the development of new drugs to treat CMT, to improve the quality of life for people with CMT and to search for a cure. The association also offers a resource center, emotional support group, treatment options, genetic testing, medication and more.

8103 Dyspraxia Foundation USA
1012 Windsor Rd
Highland Park, IL 60035
847-780-3311
foundation@mail.dyspraxiausa.org
www.dyspraxiausa.org

Warren Fried, President & Founder
Theresa A Bidwell, Vice President

Dyspraxia Foundation USA is a non-profit organization centered on understanding, accepting and educating on issues connected to Developmental Dyspraxia.

8104 Epilepsy Foundation
8301 Professional Place E
Suite 200
Landover, MD 20785- 2353
800-332-1000
Fax: 301-459-1569
ContactUs@efa.org
www.epilepsy.com

Robert W Smith, Chair
Philip M Gattone, M.Ed, President & CEO
M. Vaneeda Bennett, Chief Development Officer
Ellen Hobby, Chief Financial Officer & VP, Finance & Administration

The Epilepsy Foundation is the national voluntary agency dedicated to the welfare of people with epilepsy in the U.S. and their families. The organization works to ensure that people with seizures are able to participate in all life experiences and to prevent, control and cure epilepsy through research, education, advocacy and services.

8105 International Parkinson and Movement Disorder Society
555 East Wells Street
Suite 1100
Milwaukee, WI 53202- 3823
414-276-2145
Fax: 414-276-3349
info@movementdisorders.org
www.movementdisorders.org

Christopher Goetz, MD, President
Susan Fox, PhD, Secretary
Victor Fung, MBBS, PhD, FRACP, Treasurer

A professional society of clinicians, scientists, and other healthcare professionals who are interested in Parkinson's disease, related neurodegenerative and neurodevelopmental disorders, hyperkinetic movement disorders, and abnormalities in muscle tone and motor control.

8106 Lewy Body Dementia Association
912 Killian Hill Road S.W.
Lilburn, GA 30047
404-975-2322
Fax: 480-422-5434
www.lbda.org

Mike Koehler, CEO
Shannon McCarty-Caplan, Vice President
Christina M. Christie, President
Angela Taylor, Director of Programs

A nonprofit organization dedicated to raising awareness of the Lewy body dementias (LBD), supporting people with LBD, their families and caregivers and promoting scientific advances.

8107 Multilingual Children's Association
20 Woodside Ave
San Francisco, CA 94127
415-690-0026
Fax: 415-341-1137
www.multilingualchildren.org

8108 National Amputation Foundation
40 Church St
Malverne, NY 11565-1735
516-887-3600
516-887-3600
Fax: 516-887-3667
amps76@aol.com
www.nationalamputation.org

Paul Bernacchio, President
William Sturges, 1st Vice President
Al Pennacchia, 2nd Vice President
Doanld A. Sioss, Executive Secretary

Information & resources for amputees. Scholarship programs for college students with major limb amputation. Free donated durable medical equipment open to anyone in need locally-as items need to be picked up.

Quarterly

8109 **National Commission on Orthotic and Prosthetic Education**
330 John Carlyle Street
Suite 200
Alexandria, VA 22314- 5760 703-836-7114
Fax: 703-836-0838
info@ncope.org
www.ncope.org

Robin C Seabrook, Executive Director
Jonathan D. Day, CPO
Dominique Mungo, Residency Program Manager
Joan M. Dallas, Accreditation Assistant

The mission of NCOPE is to be recognized authority for the development and accreditation of O&P education and residency standards leading to competent patient care in the changing healthcare environment. NCOPE develops, applies, and assures standards for orthotic and prosthetic education through accreditation and approval to promote exemplary patient care.

8110 **National Institute of Neurological Disorders and Stroke**
National Institutes of Health
PO Box 5801
Bethesda, MD 20824 800-352-9424
TTY: 711
www.ninds.nih.gov

Walter J. Koroshetz, Director
Nina Schor, Deputy Director

The mission of the National Institute of Neurological Disorders and Stroke is to reduce the burden of neurological disease by supporting neuroscience research, funding and conducting training and career development programs, and disseminating scientific information on neurological health.

8111 **National Stroke Association**
9707 E Easter Ln
Suite B
Centennial, CO 80112-3754 303-649-9299
800-787-6537
Fax: 303-649-1328
www.stroke.org

James Baranski, CEO
Sharon Jaunchowski, Executive VP
Teran Nash, Customer Relations
Carol Griffin, Development Manager

The only national health organization solely committed to stroke prevention, treatment, rehabilitation and community reintegration. Provides packaged training programs, on-site assistance, physician, patient and family education materials to acute and rehab hospitals. Develops workshops; operates the Stroke Information & Referral Center and produces professional publications such as Stroke: Clinical Updates and the Journal of Stroke and Cerebrovascular Diseases.

8112 **World Chiropractic Alliance**
2950 N Dobson Rd
Suite 3
Chandler, AZ 85224-1819 480-786-9235
800-347-1011
Fax: 480-732-9313
www.worldchiropracticalliance.org

Terry A Rondberg, Founder/CEO
Richard Barwell, President

Dedicated to protecting and strengthening chiropractic around the world. Serving as a watchdog and advocacy organization, we place our emphasis on education and political action.

Books

8113 **Carpal Tunnel Syndrome**
Arthritis Foundation
1330 W Peachtree St
Suite 100
Atlanta, GA 30309 404-872-7100
800-283-7800
Fax: 404-872-0457
help@arthritis.org
www.arthritis.org

John H Klippel, President/CEO
Daniel T. McGowan, Chairman Of The Board
Rowland W. Chang, Vice Chair
Patricia Nov Nelson, Vice Chair

The Arthritis Foundation is committed to raising awareness and reducing the unacceptable impact of arthritis, a disease which must be taken as seriously as other chronic diseases because of its devastatng consequences.

8114 **Don't Feel Sorry for Paul**
Harper Collins Publishing
76 Ninth Ave
New York, NY 10011 800-843-2665
www.barnesandnoble.com

Bernard Wolf, Author
Ann Ledden, Vice President
Lorna Metzler, Manager

Paul is seven but was born with deformities of both hands and feet. Paul must wear a prosthesis on both feet so that he can walk. He has a third prosthesis for his right hand. The third prosthesis has a pair of hooks Paul uses as fingers.

94 pages Hardcover
ISBN 0-39731 -88-0

8115 **Functional Restoration of Adults and Children with Upper Extremity Amputation**
Demos Medical Publishing
11 West 42nd Street
15th Floor
New York, NY 10036-8804 212-683-0072
800-532-8663
Fax: 212-683-0118
www.demosmedpub.com

Robert Meier III, Author
Diane Atkins, OTR, Co-Author

Provides a comprehensive reference to the surgery, prosthetic fitting, and rehabilitation of individuals sustaining an arm amputation. Covers the recent advancements in prosthetics and rehabilitation. *$165.00*

384 pages
ISBN 1-888799-73-0

Magazines

8116 **ABC Mark of Merit Newsletter**
Amer Board for Cert in Otthotics & Prosthetics
330 John Carlyle St
Suite 210
Alexandria, VA 22314-5760 703-836-7114
Fax: 703-836-0838
info@abcop.org
www.abcop.org

Timothy E. Miller, CPO
Curt A. Bertram, President Elect
James H. Wynne, CPO
Donald D. Virostek, CPO/Past President

An online bi-monthly newsletter.

8117 **Active Living Magazine**
American Amputee Foundation
PO Box 94227
North Little Rock, AR 72190 501-835-9290
Fax: 501-835-9292
www.americanamputee.org

Catherine J Walden, Executive Director

A print magazine published four times a year.

8118 **Stroke Connection Magazine**
American Heart Association
7272 Greenville Ave
Dallas, TX 75231-5129
214-373-6300
888-478-7653
Fax: 214-706-5231
www.strokeassociation.org/STROKEORG/

John Caswell, Editor
Debra Lockwood, Chairman
Nancy Brown, CEO
Ralph Sacco, President/Director

Free magazine for stroke survivors and their family caregivers.

Newsletters

8119 **Advocacy Pulse**
American Stroke Association
7272 Greenville Ave
Dallas, TX 75231-5129
214-373-6300
888-478-7653
Fax: 214-706-5231
www.strokeassociation.org/STROKEORG/

Ralph Sacco, President/Director
Debra Lockwood, Chairman
Nancy Brown, CEO

8120 **NINDS Notes**
Ntn'l Institute of Neurological Disorders & Stroke
P.O. Box 5801
Bethesda, MD 20284
301-496-5751
800-352-9424
Fax: 202-944-3295
sbaa@sbaa.org

Caroline Lewis, Executive Officer
Story C. Landis, Director
Denise Dorsey, Chief Administrative Officer
Maryann Sofranko, Deputy Executive Officer

A print newsletter published three times a year.

8121 **Noteworthy Newsletter**
Ntn'l Comm on Orthotic & Prosthetic Education
330 John Carlyle Street
Suite 200
Alexandria, VA 22314- 5760
703-836-7114
Fax: 703-836-0838
info@ncope.org
www.ncope.org

Robin C Seabrook, Executive Director
Jonathan D. Day, CPO
Dominique Mungo, Residency Program Manager
Joan M. Dallas, Accreditation Assistant

The mission of NCOPE is to be recognized authority for the development and accreditation of O&P education and residency standards leading to competent patient care in the changing healthcare environment. NCOPE develops, applies, and assures standards for orthotic and prosthetic education through accreditation and approval to promote exemplary patient care.

8122 **Stroke Smart Magazine**
National Stroke Association
9707 E Easter Ln
Suite B
Centennial, CO 80112-3754
303-649-9299
800-787-6537
Fax: 303-649-1328
www.stroke.org

James Baranski, CEO
Sharon Jaunchowski, Executive VP
Teran Nash, Customer Relations
Carol Griffin, Development Manager

The only national health organization solely committed to stroke prevention, treatment, rehabilitation and community reintegration. Provides packaged training programs, on-site assistance, physician, patient and family education materials to acute and rehab hospitals. Develops workshops; operates the Stroke Information & Referral Center and produces professional publications such as Stroke: Clinical Updates and the Journal of Stroke and Cerebrovascular Diseases.

Hearing

Associations

8123 **Alexander Graham Bell Association for the Deaf and Hard of Hearing**
3417 Volta Pl. NW
Washington, DC 20007
202-337-5220
Fax: 202-337-8314
TTY: 202-337-5221
info@agbell.org
agbell.org

Emilio Alonso-Mendoza, Chief Executive Officer
Lisa Chutjian, Chief Development Officer
Gayla H. Guignard, Chief Strategy Officer
Paul Monarch, Chief Oeprating Officer
The Alexander Graham Bell Association for the Deaf and Hard of Hearing (AG Bell) is the world's oldest and largest membership organization promoting the use of spoken language by children and adults who are hearing impaired. Members include parents of children with hearing loss, adults who are deaf or hard of hearing, educators, audiologists, speech-language pathologists, physicians and other professionals in fields related to hearing loss and deafness.

8124 **American Academy of Audiology (AAA)**
11480 Commerce Park Dr.
Suite 220
Reston, VA 20191
703-790-8466
Fax: 703-790-8631
infoaud@audiology.org
www.audiology.org

Peter E. Gallagher, Executive Director
Kathryn Werner, Vice President, Public Affairs
Amy Miedema, Vice President, Communications & Membership
Dina Santucci, Senior Director, Business Development
The American Academy of Audiology is the world's largest professional organization for audiologists. The Academy is dedicated to providing quality hearing care services through professional development, education, research, and increased public awareness of hearing and balance disorders.

8125 **American Association of People with Disabilities (AAPD)**
2013 H St. NW
5th Floor
Washington, DC 20006
202-521-4316
800-840-8844
communications@aapd.com
www.aapd.com

Maria Town, President & CEO
Jasmin Bailey, Manager, Business Operations
Christine Liao, Manager, Programs
Rachita Singh, Coordinator, Public Relations & Communications
Nonprofit cross-disability member organization dedicated to ensuring economic self-sufficiency and political empowerment for Americans with disabilities. AAPD works in coalition with other disability organizations for the full implementation and enforcement of disability nondiscrimination laws, particularly the Americans With Disabilities Act (ADA) of 1990 and the Rehabilitation Act of 1973.

8126 **American Cochlear Implant Alliance**
P.O. Box 103
McLEAN, VA 22101-103
703-534-6146
info@acialliance.org
www.acialliance.org

Craig A. Buchman, Chair
Teresa A. Zwolan, Vice Chair
Nancy M. Young, Secretary
Jill B. Firszt, Treasurer
A not-for-profit membership organization created with the purpose of eliminating barriers to cochlear implantation by sponsoring research, driving heightened awareness and advocating for improved access to cochlear implants for patients of all ages across the US.

8127 **American Society for Deaf Children**
PO Box 23
Woodbine, MD 21797
800-942-2732
info@deafchildren.org
deafchildren.org

Alisha Joslyn-Swob, President
Mark Drolsbaugh, Vice President
Rachel Berman, Secretary
The American Society for Deaf Children provides information for the caretakers of deaf children so children can have full communication access in their home, school and community. The society covers areas such as visual language, audiologists, healthcare providers, assistive technology and more.

8128 **American Speech-Language-Hearing Association**
2200 Research Blvd
Rockville, MD 20850-3289
301-296-5700
800-638-8255
actioncenter@asha.org
www.asha.org

Gail J. Richard, President
Elise Davis-Mcfaland, President-Elect
Margot L. Beckerman, Chair
Arlene A. Pietranton, CEO
Provides information for both the general public and physicians in an easy-to-access manner. The subjects of focus are speech, hearing and language disorders.

8129 **American Tinnitus Association (ATA)**
PO Box 424049
Washington, DC 20042-4049
800-634-8978
ata.org

Torryn Brazell, Chief Executive Officer
Michael Baker, Development Officer
Joy Onozuka, Tinnitus Research & Communications Officer
ATA is an organization dedicated to finding cures for tinnitus and hyperacusis. ATA's research program focuses on providing seed grants for new areas of tinnitus scientific exploration.

8130 **Association of Adult Musicians with Hearing Loss**
AAMHL, Inc.
P.O. Box 522
Rockville, MD 20848
301-838-0443
info@musicianswithhearingloss.org
www.musicianswithhearingloss.org

Wendy Cheng, President
Jennifer Castellano, Secretary
Janice Rosen, Treasurer
Marshall Chasin, Board Member
The Association of Adult Musicians with Hearing Loss creates a space for adult musicians with hearing loss to discuss the challenges they face in making and listening to music. The association also offers opportunities for public performance.

8131 **Association of Late-Deafened Adults**
8038 Macintosh Ln
Suite 2
Rockford, IL 61107-5336
815-332-1515
TTY: 815-332-1515
www.alda.org

Rick Brown, President
Cynthia Moynihan, Vice President
Matt Ferrara, Treasurer
Tina Childress, Secretary
The Association of Late-Deafened Adults supports the empowerment of late-deafened people by offering programs and information resources on a variety of topics: technology, disability laws, airline travel and more.

8132 **Better Hearing Institute**
1444 I St NW
Suite 700
Washington, DC 20005
202-449-1100
800-327-9355
Fax: 202-216-9646
www.betterhearing.org

Sergei Kochkin, Ph.D, Executive Director
The Better Hearing Institute is a non-profit corporation that educates the public about the neglected problem of hearing loss and what can be done about it. Its mission is to erase the stigma and

end the embarassment that prevents millions of people from seeking help for hearing loss.

8133 **Center for Hearing and Communication**
50 Broadway
6th Floor
New York, NY 10004
917-305-7700
Fax: 917-305-7888
TTY: 917-305-7999
info@chchearing.org
chchearing.org

Laurie Hanin, Executive Director
Ellen Lafargue, Co-Director Speech & Hearing Services
Kshitija Sarpotdar, Director of Finance
Nancy Nadler, Deputy Executive Director & Development Director

The Center for Hearing and Communication provides hearing health services to people of all ages who have hearing loss. Some of its services include free hearing screenings, complete hearing evaluations, pediatric services and more.

8134 **Communication Service for the Deaf**
3520 Gateway Lane
Sioux Falls, SD 57106
866-642-6410
Fax: 605-362-2806
TTY: 866-273-3323
inquiry@c-s-d.org
www.c-s-d.org

Dr. Benjamin Soukup, Founder, Chairman & CEO
Christopher Soukup, President
Brad Hermes, CFO
Ann Marie Mickleson, VP, CSD Interpreting

CSD's mission is to create greater opportunities for Deaf and hard of hearing individuals to reach their full potential. Through global leadership and the development of innovative technologies, CSD provides tools conducive to a positive and fully integrated life.

8135 **Conference of Educational Administrators of Schools and Programs for the Deaf**
PO Box 116
Washington Grove, MD 20880
202-999-2204
TTY: 204-866-6248
ceasd@ceasd.org
www.ceasd.org

Barbara Raimondo, Executive Director
Dr. David Geeslin, President
Stacey Katz Shapiro, Secretary
Mindi Failing, Treasurer

CEASD provides an opportunity for professional educators to work together for the improvement of schools and educational programs for individuals who are deaf or hard of hearing. The organization brings together a rich composite of resources and reaches out to both enhance educational programs and influence educational policy makers.

8136 **Council of American Instructors of the Deaf (CAID)**
PO Box 377
Bedford, TX 76095-0377
817-354-8414
Fax: 817-354-8414
caid@swbell.net
www.caid.org

Keith Mousley, President
Helen Lovato, Office Manager

The CAID continues to follow the tradition begun in 1850 and recognizes the value of bringing fellow teaching professionals together to share experiences and ideas for the purpose of improving learning opportunities for deaf and hard of hearing children, adolescents and young adults.

8137 **Deaf REACH**
3521 12th St NE
Washington, DC 20017-2545
202-832-6681
Fax: 202-832-8454
deaf-reach.org

Sarah E. Brown, Executive Director
Annette Reichman, President
Jonathan Tomar, Vice-President
Myrene Sargent, Director of Administration

The psychosocial rehabilitation approach, ulitzed by all Deaf-REACH programs, provides the solid foundation to member's success. Participants are activly involved in establishing the format and level of highly individualized service delivery that they receive. The concept, which has achieved national acclaim, involves teaching members necessary life skills, thus minimizing the need for assistance from a service professional. This is part of what distinguishes the approach at Deaf-REACH.

8138 **Deaf Women United**
PO Box 61
South Barre, VT 5670
info@dwu.org
www.dwu.org

Alana Beal, President
Keri Darling, Vice President
Caroline Koo, Secretary
Amanda Tuite, Treasurer

It is committed to continuing a community of support of Deaf women from all walks of life.

8139 **Deafness Research Foundation**
363 Seventh Avenue,
10th Floor
New York, NY 10001-3904
212-257-6140
866-454-3924
Fax: 212-257-6139
TTY: 888-435-6104
info@hearinghealthfoundation.org
www.drf.org

Shari Eberts, Chairman
Mark Angelo, President
Robert Boucai, Principal
Judy R. Dubno, Dept. of Otolaryngology-Head and Neck Surgery

Founded in 1958, the Deafness Research Foundation is the leading source of private funding for basic and clinical research in the hearing science. The DRF is committed to making lifelong hearing health a national priority by funding research and implementing education projects in both the government and private sectors.

8140 **Dogs for the Deaf**
10175 Wheeler Rd
Central Point, OR 97502-9360
541-826-9220
800-990-3647
Fax: 541-826-6696
TTY: 541-826-9220
info@dogsforthedeaf.org
dogsforthedeaf.org

Robin Dickson, CEO
Vaughan Maurice, General Manager
Janine Bol, Finance Director
John Drach, Training Dept. Manager

Rescues dogs from shelters and professionally trains them for people with special needs such as: deafness, autism for children, seniors, stroke victims, cerebral palsy, etc.

8141 **Ear Foundation**
1817 Patterson St
Nashville, TN 37203-2110
615-329-7849
800-545-4327
Fax: 615-329-7935
www.earfoundation.org

Suzanne Wyatt, Executive Director

National, nonprofit organization committed to integrating the hearing and balance impaired into the mainstream of society through public awareness and medical education. Also administers The Meniere's Network, a national network of patient support groups providing people with the opportunity to share experiences and coping strategies.

8142 **Georgiana Institute**
736 Harmony Street
New Orleans, LA 70115
203-994-8215
georgianainstitute@snet.net
www.georgianainstitute.org

Annabel Stehli, President

The information source for Auditory Integration Training (AIT)/Digital Auditory Aerobics (DAA).

8143 **HEAR Center**
301 E Del Mar Blvd
Pasadena, CA 91101-2714
626-796-2016
Fax: 626-796-2320
info@hearcenter.org
hearcenter.org

Ellen Simon, Executive Director
Deborah Lorino, Office Manager
Berenice Castro, Accounting Supervisor
Maline Medina, Accounts Receivable/Billing Cle

Auditory and verbal program designed to help hearing impaired children, infants and adults lead normal and productive lives. Seeks to develop auditory techniques to aid people who have communication problems due to deafness. Offers diagnostic evaluations for speech and hearing. Individual auditory, verbal training and speech-language therapy.

8144 **Hearing Education and Awareness for Rockers**
1405 Lyon St
San Francisco, CA 94115-2914
415-409-3277
Fax: 415-409-5683
info@hearnet.com
www.hearnet.com

Kathy Peck, Executive Director
Joseph Monatano, Chief of Audiology
Flash Gordon, Primary Care Physician
John Doyle, Secretary of the Board

H.E.A.R.'s mission is the prevention of hearing loss and tinnitus among musicians and music fans (especially teens) through education awareness and grassroots outreach advocacy.

8145 **Hearing Industries Association**
1444 I Street, N.W.
Suite 700
Washington, DC 20005
202-449-1090
Fax: 202-216-9646
mjones@bostrom.com
www.hearing.org

8146 **Hearing Loss Association of America**
7910 Woodmont Ave
Suite 1200
Bethesda, MD 20814
301-657-2248
Fax: 301-913-9413
inquiry@hearingloss.org
www.hearingloss.org

Barbara Kelley, Executive Director
Lise Hamlin, Director of Public Policy
Carla Beyer-Smolin, National Chapter & Membership Coordinator
Amanda Watson, Meeting Planner

The mission of the Hearing Loss Association of America is to open the world of communication to people with hearing loss by offering information, education, resources, advocacy and training.

8147 **Hearing, Speech and Deafness Center (HSDC)**
1625 19th Ave.
Seattle, WA 98122-2848
206-323-5770
888-222-5036
Fax: 206-328-6871
seattle@hsdc.org
www.hsdc.org

Lindsay Klarman, Execuative Director
Michelle Coleman, Operations Director

Hearing, Speech & Deaf Center (HSDC) is a nonprofit for clients who are deaf, hard of hearing, or who face other communication barriers such as speech challenges. Their mission is to foster inclusive and accessible communities through communication, advocacy, and education.

8148 **House Ear Institute**
2100 W 3rd St
Los Angeles, CA 90057-1944
213-483-4431
800-388-8612
Fax: 213-484-8789
TTY: 213-484-2642
www.hei.org

James Boswell, CEO
John.W House, M.D, President
Daniel. M Graham, Executive Vice President Develop
Neil Segil, Ph.D, Executive Vice President

Offers pediatric hearing tests, otologic and audiologic evaluation and treatment, rehabilitation, hearing aid dispensing, and cochlear implant services. Outreach programs focus on families with hearing impaired children.

8149 **International Catholic Deaf Association**
7202 Buchanan St
Landover Hills, MD 20784-2236
301-429-0697
Fax: 301-429-0698
homeoffice@icda-us.org
icda-us.org

Jean Cox, President
Kate Slosar, Vice President
T.K Hill, Secretary
Jimmy Kelly, Treasurer

An organization of Catholic deaf people and hearing people in the church working with the deaf in the united states of America.

8150 **International Hearing Dog**
5901 E 89th Ave.
Henderson, CO 80640-8315
303-287-3277
Fax: 303-287-3425
info@hearingdog.org
www.hearingdog.org

Valerie Foss-Brugger, President
Robert Cooley, Field Representative
Andrea Paul, Vetinary Technician
Larry Norby, Accounting/HR

Trains and places Hearing dogs with deaf or hard-of-hearing persons, with or without multiple disabilities, nationwide, free of charge to the recipient.

8151 **International Hearing Society**
16880 Middlebelt Rd
Suite 4
Livonia, MI 48154
734-522-7200
Fax: 734-522-0200
interact@ihsinfo.org
ihsinfo.org

Annette Cross, BC-HIS, President
Kathleen Mennillo, MBA, Executive Director
Fran Vincent, Director, Membership & Marketing
Tara Douglass, Business Development Manager

The International Hearing Society (IHS) represents hearing healthcare professionals worldwide. Members include professionals engaged in the practice of testing human hearing and selecting, fitting and dispensing hearing instruments. IHS offers accreditation programs, advocacy, education and training in support of these services.

8152 **League for the Hard of Hearing**
50 Broadway
6th Fl
New York, NY 10004-3810
917-305-7700
TTY: 917-305-7999
www.lhh.org

Laurie Hanin, Executive Director
Ellen Pfeffer Lafargue, Au.D, Director
Dorene Watkins, Coordinator
Anita Stein-Meyers, Au.D, C, Assistant Director

The Center for Hearing and Communication is a leading hearing center offering state-of-the-art hearing testing, hearing aid fitting, speech therapy and full range of services for people of all ages with hearing loss. Visit our offices in New York City and Florida for services that meet all of your hearing and communication needs.

8153 **Lexington School for the Deaf: Center for the Deaf**
30th Avenue and 75th St
Jackson Heights, NY 11370
718-350-3300
Fax: 718-899-9846
TTY: 718-350-3056
generalinfo@lexnyc.org
www.lexnyc.org

Regina Carroll PhD, CEO/Executive Director
Philip W. Bravin, President
Gregory Hlibok, Vice President
Seth Bravin, Treasurer

Offers a comprehensive range of services to deaf, hard of hearing and speech impaired persons from infancy to elderly through its affiliate agencies: The Center for Mental Health Services; The

Lexington Hearing and Speech Center, Lexington Vocational Services, and the Lexington School for the Deaf. The Lexington Center also provides services through its research division which houses the only federally funded Rehabilitation Engineering Center.

8154 **Michigan Association for Deaf and Hard of Hearing**
5236 Dumond Court
Suite C
Lansing, MI 48917-6001
517-487-0066
800-968-7327
Fax: 517-487-0202
www.madhh.org

Nancy Asher, Executive Director
Pat Walton, Office Manager

MADHH is a statewide collaboration agency dedicated to improving the lives of people who are deaf or hard of hearing through leadership in education, advocacy and services.

8155 **Mississippi Speech-Language-Hearing Association**
PO Box 22664
Jackson, MS 39225
800-664-6742
Fax: 601-510-7833
admin@mshausa.org
www.mshausa.org

Claudette Edwards, President
Ricki Garrett, Executive Director

The Mississippi Speech-Language-Hearing Association is the statewide organization supporting audiologists and speech-language pathologists in Mississippi by offering them resources, information, and professional development opportunities so they could better serve their clients.

8156 **National Alliance of Black Interpreters**
P.O. Box 90532
Washington, DC 20090-532
202-810-4451
www.naobidc.org

8157 **National Association of Hearing Officials**
PO Box 4999
Midlothian, VA 23112-17
www.naho.org
Bonny M Fetch CALJ, President

The mission of the National Association of Hearing Officials is to improve the administrative hearing process and thereby benefit hearing officials, their employing agencies, and the individuals they serve through promoting professionalism and by providing traininf, continuing education, a national forum for discussion of issues, and leadership concerning administrative harings.

8158 **National Association of Parents with Children in Special Education**
3642 E Sunnydale Dr.
Chandler Heights, AZ 85142
800-754-4421
Fax: 800-424-0371
contact@napcse.org
www.napcse.org

George Giuliani, President

NAPCSE is a national membership organization dedicated to rendering all possible support and assistance to parents whose children receive special education services, both in and outside of school.

8159 **National Association of Special Education Teachers**
1250 Connecticut Ave., NW
Suite 200
Washington, DC 20036-2643
800-754-4421
Fax: 800-754-4421
contactus@naset.org
www.naset.org

Roger Pierangelo, Executive Director
George Giuliani, Executive Director

The National Association of Special Education Teachers (NASET) is a national membership organization dedicated to rendering all possible support and assistance to those preparing for or teaching in the field of special education. NASET was founded to promote the profession of special education teachers and to provide a national forum for their ideas.

8160 **National Association of the Deaf**
8630 Fenton Street
Suite 820
Silver Spring, MD 20910- 3819
301-587-1788
Fax: 301-587-1791
TTY: 301-587-1789
www.nad.org

Howard A. Rosenblum, CEO
Shane H. Feldman, COO
Marc P. Charmatz, Staff Attorney
Lizzie Sorkin, Director of Communications

Nation's largest organization safeguarding the accessability and civil rights of 28 million deaf and hard of hearing Americans in education, employment, health care, and telecommunications. Focuses on grassroots advocacy and empowerment, captioned media deafness-related information and publications, legal assistance, and policy development.

8161 **National Black Association for Speech Language and Hearing**
P.O. Box 779
Pennsville, NJ 08070
877-936-6235
Fax: 877-936-6235
nbaslh@nbaslh.org
www.nbaslh.org

Cathy Runnels, Interim
Kia N. Johnson, Parliamentarian
Martine Elie, Treasurer

The mission of the National Black Association of Speech-Language and Hearing is to maintain a viable mechanism through which the needs of black professionals, students and individuals with communication disorders can be met.

8162 **National Black Deaf Advocates**
PO Box 32
Frankfort, KY 40602
585-475-2411
800-421-1220
Fax: 585-475-6500
president@nbda.org
www.nbda.org

Benro Ogunyipe, President
Cory Parker, VP
Sharon.D White, Secretary
Betty Henderson, Treasurer

The Mission of the National Black Deaf Advocate is to promote the leadership development, economic and educational opportunities, social equality, and to safeguard the general health and welfare of Black deaf and hard of hearing people.

8163 **National Catholic Office of the Deaf**
7202 Buchanan St
Landover Hills, MD 20784-2299
301-577-1684
Fax: 301-577-1684
TTY: 301-577-4184
info@ncod.org
www.ncod.org

Consuelo Martinez Wild, Executive Director

Helps coordinate efforts of deaf or hard of hearing people who are involved in the ministry, acts as a resource center, assists bishops and pastors become available to the deaf and hard of hearing.

8164 **National Cued Speech Association**
1300 Pennsylvania Ave, NW
Suite 190-713
Washington, DC 20004
917-439-5126
800-459-3529
Fax: 866-269-9877
info@cuedspeech.org
www.cuedspeech.org

Anne Huffman, President
Sarina Roffe, Executive Director
Ben Lachman, Director of Development
Brian Kelly, Treasurer

Champions effective communication, language development and literacy through the use of cued speech.

8165 **National Deaf Women's Bowling Association**
9244 E Mansfield Ave
Denver, CO 80237-1915
303-771-9018
ndwbast@gmail.com

Gayle Willingham, President
Ali Martinez, VP
Holds world Deaf Bowling Torunament annually in July. Also holds Las Vegas Scratch Classic annually in October.

8166 **National Hearing Conservation Association**
3030 W 81st Ave
Westminster, CO 80031
303-224-9022
Fax: 303-458-0002
nhcaoffice@hearingconservation.org
www.hearingconservation.org

Jennifer Tufts, President
Beth Cooper, President Elect
Nancy Wojcik, Secretary/Treasurer
Cory Portnuff, Director of Communications
The mission of the NHCA is to prevent hearing loss due to noise and other environmental factors in all sectors of society.

8167 **National Institute on Deafness and Other Communication Disorders**
31 Center Dr.
MSC 2320
Bethesda, MD 20892-2320
301-827-8183
800-241-1044
Fax: 301-770-8977
TTY: 800-241-1055
nidcdinfo@nidcd.nih.gov
www.nidcd.nih.gov

Debara L. Tucci, Director
Judith A. Cooper, Deputy Director
Timothy J. Wheeles, Executive Officer
Lisa Portnoy, Deputy Executive Officer
The National Institute on Deafness and Other Communication Disorders supports and conducts research to help prevent, detect and diagnose disabilities that affect hearing, balance, taste, smell, voice, speech, and communication.

8168 **National Student Speech Language Hearing Association**
2200 Research Blvd
Suite 450
Rockville, MD 20850-3289
301-296-5650
800-498-2071
Fax: 301-296-8580
TTY: 301-296-5650
nsslha@asha.org
www.nsslha.org

Patricia A. Prelock, PhD, President
Elizabeth S. McCrea, President-Elect
Shelly S. Chabon, Immediate Past President
Donna Fisher Smiley, Vice President for Audiology Practice
The American Speech-Language-Hearing Association is committed to ensuring that all people with speech, language, and hearing disorders receive services to help them communicate effectively.

8169 **Registry of Interpreters for the Deaf**
333 Commerce St
Alexandria, VA 22314-2801
703-838-0030
Fax: 703-838-0454
TTY: 7038380459
ridinfo@rid.org
rid.org

Brenda Walke Prudhomme, President
Kelly L. Flores, VP
Dawn Whitcher, Secretary
Chris Grooms, Treasurer
The Registry of Interpreters for the Deaf, Inc. (RID), a national membership organization, plays a leading role in advocating for excellence in the delivery of interpretation and transliteration services between people who use sign language and people who use spoken language. In collaboration with the Deaf community, RID supports our members and encourages the growth of the profession through the establishment of a national standard for qualified sign language interpreters and transliterators, o

8170 **Sight & Hearing Association**
1246 University Ave. W.,
Suite #226
St. Paul, MN 55104- 4125
651-645-2546
800-992-0424
Fax: 651-645-2742
mail@sightandhearing.org
www.sightandhearing.org

Kathy Webb, Executive Director
Karen Klevar, Screening Director
Bernice Burgy, Program Assistant
Charles F. Barer, President
It is a nonprofit organization with a mission to enable lifetime learning by identifying preventable loss of vision and hearing in children.

8171 **Spring Dell Center**
6040 Radio Station Rd
La Plata, MD 20646-3368
301-934-4561
Fax: 301-870-2439
info@springdellcenter.org
www.springdellcenter.org

Patsy Finch, President
Badgley CPA, Treasurer
Jean Hubbard, Secretary
Donna Rretzlaff, Executive Director
Since 1967, Spring Dell center has been, bridging the gap to enhance the lives of developmentally disabled people. Spring Dell's goal is to empower people in every aspect of their lives through the implementation of two programs, employment/vocational services and residential services including transportation. Spring Dell offers transportation door-to-door for persons with developmental disabilities, including day care programs, supportive environment, residential and any other transportation.

8172 **Starkey Hearing Foundation**
6700 Washington Ave S
Eden Prairie, MN 55344
952-941-6401
866-354-3254
Fax: 952-828-6900
info@starkeyfoundation.org
www.starkeyhearingfoundation.org

Richard S Brown, President
Brady Forseth, Executive Director
Keith Becker, Senior Director of Operations
Bruce Schmaltz, Chief Financial Officer
The Starkey Hearing Foundation works to assist those with hearing impairments by offering hearing aids and aftercare services.

8173 **Telecommunications for the Deaf and Hard of Hearing**
8630 Fenton St
Suite 121
Silver Spring, MD 20910-3803
301-563-9122
Fax: 301-589-3797
TTY: 301-589-3006
tdiforaccess.org

Claude L Stout, Executive Director
James House, Director of Public Relations
John Skjeveland, Business Manager
Promoting equal access to telecommunications and media for people who are deaf, late-deafened, hard of hearing or deaf-blind through consumer education and involvement; technical assistance and consulting; applications of exisiting and emerging technologies; networking and collaboration; uniformity of standards; and national policy development and advocacy.

8174 **The Davis Center**
110 Wesley St.
PO Box 508
Manlius, NY 13104
862-251-4637
Fax: 862-251-4642
ddavis@thedaviscenter.com
www.thedaviscenter.com

Dorinne S. Davis, Director
Offers sound-based therapies supporting positive change in learning, development, and wellness. All ages/all disabilities. Uses The Davis Model of Sound Intervention, an alternative approach.

8175 United States Deaf Ski & Snowboard Association
76 Kings Gate N
Rochester, NY 14617
585-286-2780
info@usdssa.org
usdssa.org

Anthony Di Giovani, Officer

It provides means for deaf people to get together to share their love for skiing and sponsor races for deaf skiers.

8176 Vestibular Disorders Association
5018 NE 15th Ave.
P.O. Box 13305
Portland, OR 97211
503-229-7705
800-837-8428
Fax: 503-229-8064
info@vestibular.org
www.vestibular.org

Sue Hickey, President
Cynthia Ryan, MBA, Executive Director
Kerrie Denner, Outreach Coordinator
Karen Ilari, Administrative Support Coordinator

The mission of the Vestibular Disorders Association is to serve people with vestibular disorders by providing access to information, offering a support network, and elevating awareness of the challenges associated with these disorders. They also aim to support and empower vestibular patients on their journey back to balance.

Camps

8177 ASD Summer Camp
Alabama Institute for Deaf & Blind
205 E South St
P.O. Box 698
Talladega, AL 35160
256-761-3214
Fax: 256-761-3278
TTY: 256-761-3215
wiggins.lavina@aidb.state.al.us
www.aidb.org

Paul Millard, Principal

The Alabama School for the Deaf Summer Enrichment Camp is designed especially for deaf and hard of hearing children ages 6-15. Recreation activities include swimming, skating, outdoor games, horseback riding, field trips, arts and craft. Tuition is free.

8178 Aspen Camp
4862 Snowmass Creek Rd.
Snowmass, CO 81654
970-315-0513
TTY: 970-315-0513
hi@aspencamp.org
www.aspencamp.org

Ryan Commerson, President
Karen Immerson, Vice President
Eric Kaika, Treasurer

Open to the deaf community, including family members and friends as well as those who are deaf, deaf blind, hard of hearing, and late deafened, Camp Aspen provides year round programs for youth and adults.

8179 Camp Alexander Mack
Indiana Deaf Camps Foundation
P.O. Box 158
Milford, IN 46542
574-658-4831
www.campmack.org

Galen Jay, Interim Executive Director
Lauren Carrick, Director of Development/Facility Manager
Amber Barrett, Food Service
Norma Miller, Ordained Minister

Our program is intentionally designed to provide campers with life changing experiences that lead to a formation of personal faith within a safe faith community.

8180 Camp Bishopswood
Diocese of Maine Episcopal
143 State St
Portland, ME 04101
207-772-1953
800-244-6062
Fax: 207-773-0095
mike@bishopswood.org
www.bishopswood.org

Laurie Kazilionis, President
Robert Johnston, VP
Jeff Mansir, Treasurer
Pam Waite, Secretary

Camp is located in Hope, Maine. One to seven-week sessions for hearing impaired children June-August. Coed, ages 7-16.

8181 Camp CaPella
PO Box 552
Holden, ME 04429
207-843-5104
www.campcapella.org

Deb Breindel, Director

Provides summer camp sessions for children with disabilities.

8182 Camp Chris Williams
Lions 11 B-2 and MADHH
5236 Dumond Court
Suite C
Lansing, MI 48917-6001
586-778-4188
Fax: 586-285-1842
TTY: 586-285-1842

Nancy Asher, Executive Director

An exciting summer camp experience for deaf and hard of hearing youth and their siblings ages 8-14.

8183 Camp Comeca & Retreat Center
United Methodist Church
75670 Road 417
Conzad, NE 69130
308-784-2808
www.campcomeca.com

John, Asst. Director

Camp is located in Cozad, Nebraska. Summer sessions for campers with diabetes and hearing impairment. Coed, ages 6-19, families, seniors, single adults.

8184 Camp Emanuel
PO Box 752343
Dayton, OH 45475
937-477-5504
crawford@campemanuel.org
www.campemanuel.weebly.com

Brian Demarke, President
Stephanie Ackner, Vice President
Mary Foreman, Secretary
Nan Crawford, Executive Director

Camp Emanuel is a camp for hearing impaired and hearing youth. There are day sessions for children 5-14 and overnight resident sessions for children and teens 9-17. The camp aims to promote descision making, self-esteem, and acceptance by integrating non-hearing children with hearing children.

8185 Camp Grizzly
NorCal Services For Deaf & Hard Of Hearing
4044 N Freeway Blvd.
Sacramento, CA 95843
916-349-7500
TTY: 916-349-7500
campgrizzly@norcalcenter.org
www.campgrizzly.org

Molly Bowen, Program Leader
Cheryl Bella, Program Leader

A program of NorCal Services for Deaf & Hard of Hearing, Camp Grizzly is a coed camp for children aged 7-18 who have a hearing impairment. Camp Grizzly takes place at the Camp Lodestar campground facilities and offers sporting activities, performing and creative arts, hiking, swimming, playgrounds and campfires.

8186 Camp Isola Bella
410 Twin Lakes Rd.
Salisbury, CT 06079
860-824-5558
Fax: 860-824-4276
TTY: 860-596-0110
ibdirector@asd-1817.org
asd-1817.org/programs/camp-isola-bella

David Guardino, Director

A camp for hearing-impaired children ages 8-17. Qualified deaf and hearing staff members with experience in education, child care and counseling are employed at the camp.

8187 **Camp Joy**
3325 Swamp Creek Rd
Schwenksville, PA 19473-1518 610-754-6878
Fax: 610-754-7880
www.campjoy.com
Angus Murray, Camp Director
A special needs camp for kids and adults (ages 4-80+) with developmental disabilities such as autism, brain injury, neurological disorder, visual and/or hearing impairments, Angelman and Down syndromes, and other developmental disabilities.

8188 **Camp Juliena**
Georgia Center of the Deaf and Hard of Hearing
2296 Henderson Mill Rd.
Suite 115
Atlanta, GA 30345 404-381-8447
888-297-9461
Fax: 404-297-9465
info@gcdhh.org
www.gcdhh.org/camp-juliena
Jimmy Peterson, Executive Director
Andrea Alston, Coordinator, Community Outreach
A week-long residential summer camp for deaf or hard of hearing youth. Activities help campers develop leadership, team-building, social, and communication skills.

8189 **Camp Mark Seven**
Mark Seven Deaf Foundation
144 Mohawk Hotel Rd.
Old Forge, NY 13420 315-207-5706
TTY: 315-357-6089
registrar@campmark7.org
www.campmark7.org
Dave Staehle, Camp Director
A camp program for hard-of-hearing, deaf and hearing people. Coed, open to all ages. The camp is located on the Fourth Lake in the Adirondack Mountains.

8190 **Camp Meadowood Springs**
77650 Meadowood Rd.
Weston, OR 97886 541-276-2752
Fax: 541-276-7227
camp@meadowoodsprings.org
www.meadowoodsprings.org
Michelle Nelson, Camp Director
This camp is designed to help children with communication disorders and learning differences. A full range of activities in recreational and clinical areas is available.

8191 **Camp Pacifica**
California Lions Camp
45895 California Hwy 49
Ahwahnee, CA 93601 559-683-4660
deafcamppacifica@gmail.com
www.camppacifica.org
Angelica Martinez, Camp Director
John Martinez, Assistant Director
Camp Pacifica provides a summer camp experience for children, boys and girls, aged 7-15 who have a hearing impairment. The camp is located in the foothills of Sierra on 52 acres of forested woodland. Activities include, but are not limited to, archery, canoeing, ropes course, swimming, horseback riding, and riflery. The camp costs $360.00 plus a registration fee.

8192 **Camp Ramah in the Poconos**
2100 Arch St.
Philadelphia, PA 19103 215-885-8556
Fax: 215-885-8905
info@ramahpoconos.org
www.ramahpoconos.org
Rabbi Joel Seltzer, Executive Director
Rachel Dobbs Schwartz, Camp Director
Bruce I. Lipton, Director, Finance & Operations
Leah Schatz, Program Director
Camp is located in Lakewood, Pennsylvania. Summer sessions for children with developmental and intellectual disabilities.

8193 **Camp Shocco for the Deaf**
216 North St. E
PO Box 602
Talladega, AL 35161 800-264-1225

8194 **Camp Taloali**
15934 N Santiam Hwy. SE
PO Box 32
Stayton, OR 97383 503-400-6547
campadmin@taloali.org
www.taloali.org
Randall Smith, Camp Administrator
Summer sessions for children who are deaf, hard of hearing, or have a hearing impairment. Camp Taloali emphasizes communication, leadership, and social development.

8195 **Camp Tekoa**
United Methodist Camp Tekoa
PO Box 1793
Flat Rock, NC 28731-1793 828-692-6516
Fax: 828-697-3288
www.camptekoa.org
John Isley, Executive Director
Dave Bollen, Assistant Director
Karen Rohrer, Business Manager
Melisa Coates, Administrative Assistant
Offers special needs camp programs for individuals with developmental disabilities.

8196 **Cochlear Implant Camp**
Listen Foundation
6950 E Belleview Ave.
Suite 203
Greenwood Village, CO 80111 303-781-9440
cochlearimplantcamp@gmail.com
www.listenfoundation.org/cicamp
Allison Biever, President
David Kelsall, MD, Medical Director
Held at the YMCA Rockies Estes Park Center, the camp offers a wide range of activities for children from 3-17 years old with cochlear implants. The camp is 4 days and 3 nights, held during the summer and also offers programs for parents and families. The cost is $700 for a family of four.

8197 **Deaf Kid's Kamp**
Sproul Ranch, Inc.
42263 50th Street West
Suite 610
Quartz Hill, CA 93536 661-675-3323
877-399-5449
www.deafkidskamp.com
Buffy Sproul, Executive Director
Our purpose is to meet the needs of deaf children outside of the classroom setting. These needs, as we have defined them, would include but are not limited to: social contact with peers; contact with the culture of the Deaf Community; educational and recreational programs not available in most school settings.

8198 **Father Drumgoole Connelly Summer Camp**
MIV: Mount Loretto
6581 Hylan Blvd
Staten Island, NY 10309-3830 718-317-2600
Fax: 718-317-2830
www.mountloretto.org
Stephen Rynn, Executive Director
Maryann Virga, Executive Assistant
Loretta Polanish, Executive Secretary
Ed Gani, Facilities Manager
Summer sessions for children with epilepsy, hearing impairment and developmental disabilities. Coed, ages 5-13.

8199 **Lions Camp Crescendo**
1480 Pine Tavern Rd.
PO Box 607
Lebanon Junction, KY 40150 502-264-0120
wibblesb@aol.com
www.lccky.org
Billie J. Flannery, Administrator
Organization dedicated to enhancing quality of life for youths, including those with disabilities, through the delivery of a traditional camping experience.

8200 **Lions Camp Kirby**
1735 Narrows Hill Rd
Upper Black Eddy, PA 18972 610-982-5731
Alice Breon, Camp Director
Offers 2-week camps for deaf and hearing impaired children and their siblings in eastern Pennsylvania.

8201 **Lions Camp Merrick**
PO Box 56
Nanjemoy, MD 20662 301-870-5858
Fax: 301-246-9108
info@lionscampmerrick.org
www.lionscampmerrick.org
Heidi A. Fick, Executive Director
Donna Wadsworth, Office Administrator
This recreational camp for special needs children offers a complete waterfront program including swimming, canoeing and fishing for ages 6-16. Designed for children who are deaf, blind, or have type 1 diabetes. Also helps children to learn to deal with their special conditions.

8202 **Lions Wilderness Camp for Deaf Children, Inc.**
Lions Wilderness Camp Headquarters
PO Box 8
Roseville, CA 95661-9998 campdirector@lionswildcamp.org
www.lionswildcamp.org
David Velasquez, Camp Program Director
Lions Wilderness Camp gives deaf children aged 7-15 an outdoor camp experience helping children to learn outdoor skills and enjoy nature.

8203 **Sandcastle Day Camp**
Children's Beach House
1800 Bay Ave
Lewes, DE 19958 302-645-9184
Fax: 302-645-9467
www.cbhinc.org
Martha P. Tschantz, President
Maryann Helms, Vice President
Linda M. Fischer, Secretary
Charles H. Sterner, Treasurer
Camp is located in Lewes, Delaware. Four-week sessions June-August for Delaware children with hearing impairment or speech/communication impairment. Coed, ages 6-12.

8204 **Sertoma Camp Endeavor**
Sertoma Camp Endeavor
P.O. Box 910
Dundee, FL 33838-0910 863-439-1300
Fax: 863-439-1300
Jeff Nunemaker, Executive Director
The intergration of deaf, hard of hearing and hearing youngsters is a unique characteristic of our camping program. Both hearing, deaf and hard of hearing children have the opportunity to learn about themselves and each other in an informal and empowering setting.

8205 **Texas Lions Camp**
PO Box 290247
Kerrville, TX 78029 830-896-8500
Fax: 830-896-3666
tlc@lionscamp.com
www.lionscamp.com
Stephen S. Mabry, President & CEO
Karen-Anne King, Vice President, Summer Camps
Milton Dare, Director, Development
Joan Dixon, Director, Finance
Texas Lions Camp is a camp dedicated to serving children ages 7-16 in Texas with physical disabilities. While at camp, campers will participate in a variety of activities and be encouraged to become more independent and self-confident.

8206 **YMCA Camp Fitch**
12600 Abels Rd.
North Springfield, PA 16430 814-922-3219
877-863-4824
Fax: 814-922-7000
registrar@campfitchymca.org
campfitchymca.org
Tom Parker, Executive Director
Joe Wolnik, Summer Camp Director
Brandy Duda, Outdoor Education Director
Hannah Kight, Office Manager
Camp is located in North Springfield, Pennsylvania. Camp programs include sessions for children with diabetes or epilepsy.

8207 **Youth Leadership Camp**
National Association of the Deaf
8630 Fenton Street
Suite 820
Silver Spring, MD 20910 301-587-1788
Fax: 301-587-1791
www.nad.org
Christopher Wagnor, President
Melissa S. Draganac-Hawk, VP
Howard A. Rosenblum, CEO
Joshua Beckman, Secretary
Sponsored by the National Association of the Deaf, this camp emphasizes leadership training for deaf teenagers and young adults. In addition to many recreational activities and sports, there are academic offerings and camp projects.

Books

8208 **A Basic Course in American Sign Language**
TJ Publishers
2544 Tarpley Rd
Suite 108
Carrollton, TX 75006-2288 972-416-0800
800-999-1168
Fax: 972-416-0944
customerservice@tjpublishers.com
www.tjpublishers.com
Tom Humphries, Author
Carol Padden, Co-Author
Terrence J O'Rouke, Co-Author
Tanner Beach, Director
The first three DVDs in this series are designed to illustrate and demonstrate each of the exercises and dialogues presented in A Basic Course in American Sign Language. Four Deaf teachers and three hearing students provide a variety of models for the exercises. *$35.95*
288 pages Spiral Bound
ISBN 0-932666-42-6

8209 **A Basic Course in Manual Communication**
National Association of the Deaf
8630 Fenton St.
Suite 820
Silver Spring, MD 20910 301-338-6380
Fax: 301-587-1791
TTY: 301-810-3182
www.nad.org
Terrence J. O'Rourke, Author
Teachers ASL grammar and vocabulary.

8210 **A Basic Vocabulary: American Sign Languagefor Parents and Children**
TJ Publishers
2544 Tarpley Rd
Suite 108
Carrollton, TX 75006-2288 972-416-0800
800-999-1168
Fax: 972-416-0944
customerservice@tjpublishers.com
www.tjpublishers.com
Terrence J O'Rouke, Author
Tanner Beach, Director
Carefully selected words and signs include those that children use every day. Alphabetically organized vocabulary incorporates

developmental lists helpful to both deaf and hearing children and over 1000 clear sign language illustrations. *$9.95*

240 pages Softcover

ISBN 0-932666-00-0

8211 **A Loss for Words**

HarperCollins Publishers
10 E 53rd St
New York, NY 10022-5244
212-207-7901
800-242-7737
Fax: 212-702-2586
spsales@harpercollins.com
www.harpercollins.com

Lou Ann Walker, Author

From the time she was a toddler, Lou Ann Walker was the ears and voice for her deaf parents. Their family life was warm and loving, but outside the home, they faced a world that misunderstood and often rejected them. *$13.00*

224 pages Paperback 1987

ISBN 0-060914-25-4

8212 **Access for All: Integrating Deaf, Hard of Hearing and Hearing Preschoolers**

Gallaudet University Bookstore
800 Florida Avenue NorthEast
Washington, DC 20002-3600
202-651-5530
Fax: 202-651-5489
gupress@gallaudet.edu
http://www.gallaudet.edu

Stephanie Cawthon, Ph.D., Book Review Editor
Peter V. Paul, Ph.D., Editor, Literary Issues
Ye Wang, Ph.D., Senior Associate Editor
Feifei Ye, Ph.D., Associate Editor for Research Methodology

This exciting new 90 minute videotape and manual describes a model program for integrating deaf and hard of hearing children in early education.

169 pages Book & Video

8213 **Advanced Sign Language Vocabulary: A Resource Text for Educators**

Charles C. Thomas
2600 S First St
Springfield, IL 62704-4730
217-789-8980
800-258-8980
Fax: 217-789-9130
books@ccthomas.com
www.ccthomas.com

Michael P. Thomas, President
Elizabeth E Wolf, Co-Author

A resource text for educators, interpreters, parents and sign language instructors. *$53.95*

202 pages Spiral Paper

ISBN 0-398057-22-0

8214 **American Sign Language Handshape Dictionary**

Gallaudet University Press
800 Florida Ave NE
Washington, DC 20002-3600
773-568-1550
800-621-2736
Fax: 773-660-2235
TTY: 888-630-9347
gupress@gallaudet.edu
www.gupress.gallaudet.edu

Richard A Tennant, Author
Marianne Gluszak Brown, Co-Author
Valerie Nelson-Metlay, Illustrator
T. Alan Hurwitz, President

The new DVD shows how each sign is formed from beginning to end. Users can watch a sign at various speeds to learn precisely how to master it themselves. Together, the new edition of The American Sign Language Handshape Dictionary and its accompanying DVD presents students, sign language teachers, and deaf and hearing people alike with the perfect combination for enhancing communication skills in both ASL and English. *$45.00*

408 pages Hardcover

ISBN 1-563680-43-2

8215 **American Sign Language Phrase Book**

TJ Publishers
2544 Tarpley Rd
Suite 108
Carrollton, TX 75006-2288
972-416-0800
800-999-1168
Fax: 972-416-0944
customerservice@tjpublishers.com
www.tjpublishers.com

Lou Fant, Author
Terrence O'Rourke, Principal
Tanner Beach, Director

The author provides interesting, realistic and meaningful situations. Sign language is learned through novel remarks cleverly organized around everyday topics. *$18.95*

362 pages Softcover

ISBN 0-809235-00-5

8216 **American Sign Language: A Look at Its History, Structure & Community**

TJ Publishers
2544 Tarpley Rd
Suite 108
Carrollton, TX 75006-2288
972-416-0800
800-999-1168
Fax: 972-416-0944
customerservice@tjpublishers.com
www.tjpublishers.com

Charlotte Baker-Shenk, Author
Carol Padden, Co-Author
Terrence O'Rourke, Principal
Tanner Beach, Director

Answers basic questions about American Sign Language. What is it? What is its history? Who uses it? What is the Deaf community? Why is ASL important? What are the building blocks of ASL? What is the relationship between ASL and body language? What are examples of ASL -grammar? *$4.95*

22 pages Softcover

ISBN 0-93266 -01-9

8217 **At Home Among Strangers**

Gallaudet University Press
800 Florida Ave NE
Washington, DC 20002-3600
773-568-1550
800-621-2736
Fax: 773-660-2235
TTY: 888-630-9347
gupress@gallaudet.edu
www.gupress.gallaudet.edu

Jerome D Schein, Author
T. Alan Hurwitz, President
Paul Kelly, Vice President Adm And Finance

At Home Among Strangers presents an engrossing portrait of the Deaf community as a complex, nationwide social network that offers unique kinship to deaf people across the country. *$36.95*

264 pages Paperback

ISBN 1-563681-41-2

8218 **BPPV: What You Need to Know**

Vestibular Disorders Association
5018 NE 15th Ave
Portland, OR 97211-5331
503-229-7705
800-837-8428
Fax: 503-229-8064
veda@vestibular.org
www.vestibular.org

P J Haybach, Author
Lisa Haven, Executive Director
Jerry Underwood, Managing Director
Vincente Honrubia, Director

The aim of this book is to present basic information about benign paroxysmal positional vertigo (BPPV) including what it is, causes, how it is diagnosed, various treatments currently in use, and strategies for coping with the symptoms associated with BPPV. *$29.95*

207 pages Hardcover

ISBN 0-963261-14-2

8219 **Ben's Story: A Deaf Child's Right to Sign**
Gallaudet University Bookstore
800 Florida Avenue NorthEast
Washington, DC 20002-3600
202-651-5530
Fax: 202-651-5489
gupress@gallaudet.edu
http://www.gallaudet.edu
Stephanie Cawthon, Ph.D., Book Review Editor
Peter V. Paul, Ph.D., Editor, Literary Issues
Ye Wang, Ph.D., Senior Associate Editor
Feifei Ye, Ph.D., Associate Editor for Research Methodology
This is a mother's story of how she responded to the diagnosis of her son's deafness and how she struggled to have her son educated using sign language.
267 pages Softcover
ISBN 0-930323-47-5

8220 **Book of Name Signs: Naming in American Sign Language**
DawnSign Press
6130 Nancy Ridge Dr
San Diego, CA 92121-3223
858-625-0600
800-549-5350
Fax: 858-625-2336
info@dawnsign.com
www.dawnsign.com
Joe Dannis, President
Sam Supalla, Author
To explain how a name sign is chosen in the Deaf community, professor and researcher Sam Supalla wrote this valuable resource book. Revealing fascinating insights about the origins of ASL name signs, Supalla shows how they serve the same function as given names used in the hearing community. He also details how the history of the name sign system dates back to the early years of deaf education in America. Included for reference is a list of more than 500 name signs available for selection. *$12.95*
120 pages Paperback 1992
ISBN 0-915035-30-4

8221 **Chelsea: The Story of a Signal Dog**
Gallaudet University Bookstore
800 Florida Ave NE
Washington, DC 20002-3600
202-651-5855
866-204-0504
Fax: 773-660-2235
TTY: 202-651-5855
gupress@gallaudet.edu
www.clerccenter.gallaudet.edu
Paul Ogden, Author
T. Alan Hurwitz, President
Paul Kelly, Vice President Adm. And Finance
This is a story of a young deaf couple and their Belgian sheepdog, who acts as their ears. It explains how these dogs are trained and paired with their new owners.
169 pages

8222 **Children of a Lesser God**
Gallaudet University Bookstore
800 Florida Ave NE
Washington, DC 20002-3600
202-651-5855
866-204-0504
Fax: 773-660-2235
TTY: 202-651-5855
gupress@gallaudet.edu
www.clerccenter.gallaudet.edu
Mark Medoff, Author
T. Alan Hurwitz, President
Paul Kelly, Vice President Adm. And Finance
The movie that won the hearts of thousands. This is a story of a deaf woman who refuses to succumb to the hearing people's image of what a deaf person should be.
91 pages Softcover
ISBN 0-822202-03-4

8223 **Choices in Deafness: A Parent's Guide to Communication Options**
Woodbine House
6510 Bells Mill Rd
Bethesda, MD 20817-1636
301-897-3570
800-843-7323
Fax: 301-897-5838
info@woodbinehouse.com
www.woodbinehouse.com
Irv Shapell, Owner
Sue Schwartz, PhD., Editor
A useful aid in choosing the appropriate communication option for a child with a hearing loss. Experts present the following communication options: Auditory-Verbal Approach, Bilingual-Bicultural Approach, Cued Speech, Oral Approach, and Total Communication. This new edition explains medical causes of hearing loss, the diagnostic process, audiological assessment, and cochlear implants. Children and parents also offer their personal experiences. *$24.95*
400 pages Paperback
ISBN 1-890627-73-7

8224 **Cochlear Implants for Kids**
Alexander Graham Bell Association
3417 Volta Pl NW
Washington, DC 20007-2737
202-337-5220
Fax: 202-337-8314
info@agbell.org
Warren Estabrooks MEd, Editor
Alexander T. Graham, Executive Director
Susan Boswell, Director of Communications and Marketing
Judy Harrison, Director of Programs
Designed to educate readers about cochlear implants, including surgery, the importance of rehabilitation and the significance of parents' and professionals' roles. *$12.49*
404 pages Paperback
ISBN 0-882002-08-2

8225 **Cognition, Education and Deafness: Directions for Research and Instruction**
Gallaudet University Press
800 Florida Ave NE
Washington, DC 20002-3600
773-568-1550
800-621-2736
Fax: 773-660-2235
TTY: 888-630-9347
gupress@gallaudet.edu
David S Martin, Editor
T. Alan Hurwitz, President
Paul Kelly, Vice President Adm. And Finance
This groundbreaking book integrates the work of 54 contributors to the 1984 symposium on cognition, education, and deafness. It focuses on cognition and deaf students' growth and development, problem-solving strategies, thinking processes, language development, reading methodology, measurement of potential, and intervention programs. *$50.00*
248 pages Paperback
ISBN 1-563681-49-8

8226 **College and University Programs for Deaf and Hard of Hearing Students**
Gallaudet & NTID
800 Florida Avenue NE
Gallaudet University
Washington, DC 20002
202-651-5000
800-451-8834
Fax: 202-651-5508
www.lulu.com
S. Benaissa, & L. Dunning, Co-Authors
J. DeCaro, M. Karchmer, Co-Authors
J Hochgesang, Co-Author
T. Alan Hurwitz, President
Compiled by Gallaudet University and the National Technical Institute for the Deaf, this publication is a guide to accessibility for deaf and hard of hearing students in American colleges and universities. Available through LuLu Publishing. *$11.50*
240 pages Paperback
ISBN 9-998242-81-9

8227 **Come Sign with Us**
Gallaudet University Press
800 Florida Ave NE
Washington, DC 20002-3600
773-568-1550
800-621-2736
Fax: 773-660-2235
TTY: 888-630-9347
gupress@gallaudet.edu
www.gupress.gallaudet.edu

Jan C Hafer, Author
Robert M Wilson, Co-Author
T. Alan Hurwitz, President
Paul Kelly, Vice President Adm. And Finance

This fun guide for parents and educators on teaching hearing children how to sign has been thoroughly revised with completely new activities that provide contexts for practice. *$39.95*
160 pages Paperback
ISBN 1-563680-51-3

8228 **Comprehensive Reference Manual for Signers and Interpreters**
Charles C. Thomas
2600 S First St
Springfield, IL 62704-4730
217-789-8980
800-258-8980
Fax: 217-789-9130
books@ccthomas.com
www.ccthomas.com

Michael P. Thomas, President
Cheryl M. Hoffman, Author

A classic in sign language literature since its introduction over two decades ago, this updated and expanded sixth edition of Comprehensive Reference Manual for Signers and Interpreters contains almost seven thousand entries, including vocabulary and idioms, with cross-references and sign descriptions. It is intended primarily for interpreters, but it can also be used effectively by signers who have at least a working knowledge of sign language. *$59.95*
404 pages Spiral Paper 1909
ISBN 0-398078-58-4

8229 **Comprehensive Signed English Dictionary**
Gallaudet University Press
800 Florida Ave NE
Washington, DC 20002-3600
773-568-1550
800-621-2736
Fax: 773-660-2235
TTY: 888-630-9347
gupress@gallaudet.edu
www.gupress.gallaudet.edu

Harry Bornstein, Editor
Karen L. Saulnier, Editor
Lillian B. Hamilton, Editor
T. Paul Hurwitz, President

The Comprehensive Signed English Dictionary is the premier volume of the Signed English series. This complete dictionary more than 3,100 signs, including signs reflecting lively, contemporary vocabulary. *$45.00*
464 pages Casebound
ISBN 0-913580-81-3

8230 **Conversational Sign Language II: An Intermediate Advanced Manual**
Gallaudet University Press
800 Florida Ave NE
Washington, DC 20002-3600
773-568-1550
800-621-2736
Fax: 773-660-2235
TTY: 888-630-9347
gupress@gallaudet.edu
www.gupress.gallaudet.edu

William J Madsen, Author
T. Alan Hurwitz, President
Paul Kelly, Vice President Adm. And Finance

This book presents English words and their American Sign Language (ASL) equivalents in 63 lessons. Part one covers 750 words and their signs. Part two deals with the interpretation of 220 English idioms (which have over 300 usages in ASL). Part three presents over 300 ASL idioms and colloquialisms prevalent in informal conversations. *$17.95*
236 pages Paperback
ISBN 0-913580-00-7

8231 **Deaf Empowerment: Emergence, Struggle and Rhetoric**
Gallaudet University Press
800 Florida Ave NE
Washington, DC 20002-3600
773-568-1550
800-621-2736
Fax: 773-660-2235
TTY: 888-630-9347
gupress@gallaudet.edu
www.gupress.gallaudet.edu

Katherine A Jankowski, Author
T. Alan Hurwitz, President
Paul Kelly, Vice President Adm. And Finance

Employing the methodology successfully used to explore other social movements in America, this meticulous study examines the rhetorical foundation that motivated Deaf people to work for social change during the past two centuries. *$49.95*
192 pages Hardcover
ISBN 1-563680-61-0

8232 **Deaf History Unveiled: Interpretations from the New Scholarship**
Gallaudet University Press
800 Florida Ave NE
Washington, DC 20002-3600
773-568-1550
800-621-2736
Fax: 773-660-2235
TTY: 888-630-9347
gupress@gallaudet.edu
www.gallaudet.edu

John Vickrey Van Cleve, Editor
T. Alan Hurwitz, President
Paul Kelly, Vice President Adm. And Finance

Deaf History Unveiled features 16 essays, including work by Harlan Lane, Renate Fischer, Margret Winzer, William McCagg, and other noted historians in this field. Readers will discover the new themes driving Deaf history, including a telling comparison of the similar experiences of Deaf people and African Americans, both minorities with identifying characteristics that cannot be hidden to thwart bias. *$36.95*
316 pages Paperback
ISBN 1-563680-87-4

8233 **Deaf Like Me**
Gallaudet University Press
800 Florida Ave NE
Washington, DC 20002-3600
773-568-1550
800-621-2736
Fax: 773-660-2235
TTY: 888-630-9347
gupress@gallaudet.edu
www.gupress.gallaudet.edu

Thomas S Spradley, Author
James P Spradley, Co-Author
T. Alan Hurwitz, President
Paul Kelly, Vice President Adm. And Finance

Deaf Like Me is the moving account of parents coming to terms with their baby girl's profound deafness. The love, hope, and anxieties of all hearing parents of deaf children are expressed here with power and simplicity. *$16.95*
292 pages Paperback
ISBN 0-930323-11-4

8234 **Deaf Parents and Their Hearing Children**
Through the Looking Glass
3075 Adeline Street
Suite 120
Berkeley, CA 94703
510-848-1112
800-644-2666
Fax: 510-848-4445
tlg@lookingglass.org
www.lookingglass.org

Maureen Block, J.D., President
Thomas Spalding, Treasurer
Alice Nemon, Secretary
Mega Kirshbaum, Author

The focus of this review article is on families with Deaf parents and hearing children. We provide a brief description of the Deaf community, their language, and culture; describe communication patterns and parenting issues in Deaf-parented families, examine the role of the hearing child in a Deaf family and how that experience affects their functioning in the hearing world; and discuss important considerations and resources for families, educators, and health care and service providers. *$2.00*

8 pages

8235 **Deaf in America: Voices from a Culture**

TJ Publishers
2544 Tarpley Rd
Suite 108
Carrollton, TX 75006-2288
972-416-0800
800-999-1168
Fax: 972-416-0944
customerservice@tjpublishers.com
www.tjpublishers.com

Carol Padden, Author
Tom Humphries, Co-Author
Terrence O'Rourke, Principal
Tanner Beach, Director

Now available in paperback, this book opens deaf culture to outsiders, inviting readers to imagine and understand a world of silence. This book shares the joy and satisfaction many people have with their lives and shows that deafness may not be the handicap most hearing people think. *$15.95*

134 pages Softcover
ISBN 0-674194-24-1

8236 **EASE Program: Emergency Access Self Evaluation**

Telecommunications for the Deaf (TDI)
8630 Fenton St
Suite 604
Silver Spring, MD 20910-3822
301-589-3786
Fax: 301-589-3797
tdi-online.org

Claude L Stout, Executive Director
Gloria Carter, Executive Secretary
James House, Public Relations Director
Robert McConnell, Advertising Manager

A complete training, testing, maintenance and self evaluation program that helps emergency service providers prepare for emergency calls from TTY users and to comply with the American with Disabilities Act. *$35.00*

48 pages

8237 **Encyclopedia of Deafness and Hearing Disorders**

Powell's Books
1005 W Burnside St
Portland, OR 97209-3114
503-228-4651
800-873-7323
help@powells.com
www.powells.com

Carol Turkington, Author
Michael Powell, Owner

Presents the most current information on deafness and hearing disorders in an authoritative A-to-Z compendium. *$7.50*

294 pages Hardcover
ISBN 0-816056-15-3

8238 **Expressive and Receptive Fingerspelling for Hearing Adults**

Gallaudet University Bookstore
800 Florida Ave NE
Washington, DC 20002-3600
202-651-5855
866-204-0504
Fax: 773-660-2235
TTY: 202-651-5855
gupress@gallaudet.edu
www.clerccenter.gallaudet.edu

LaVera M Guillory, Author
T. Alan Hurwitz, President
Paul Kelly, Vice President Adm. And Finance

Here is a new and meaningful way for adults to increase their comfort with fingerspelling. The system is based on the principles of phonetics rather than letters of the English alphabet.

42 pages Softcover
ISBN 0-875110-55-X

8239 **Eye-Centered: A Study of Spirituality of Deaf People**

National Catholic Office for the Deaf
7202 Buchanan St
Hyattsville, MD 20784-2236
301-577-1684
Fax: 301-577-1684
info@ncod.org
www.ncod.org

Bill Key, Author
Arvilla Rank, Executive Director
Deacon Patrick Graybill, Vice President
Gregory Schott, Member at Large

The findings of the five-year De Sales Project conducted by The National Catholic Office for the Deaf. *$16.70*

167 pages

8240 **For Hearing People Only**

Harris Communications
15155 Technology Dr
Eden Prairie, MN 55344-2273
952-906-1180
800-825-6758
Fax: 952-906-1099
TTY: 800-825-9187
info@harriscomm.com
www.harriscomm.com

Robert Harris, Owner & President
Kevin Horsky, Business Director
Randall Moore, Manager

For Hearing People Only answers some of the most common questions hearing people ask about Deaf culture and how Deaf people communicate and live. *$35.95*

724 pages Paperback
ISBN 0-963401-63-7

8241 **From Gesture to Language in Hearing and Deaf Children**

Gallaudet University Press
800 Florida Ave NE
Washington, DC 20002-3600
773-568-1550
800-621-2736
Fax: 773-660-2235
TTY: 888-630-9347
gupress@gallaudet.edu
www.gupress.gallaudet.edu

Virginia Volterra, Editor
Carol J. Erting, Editor

In 21 essays on communicative gesturing in the first two years of life, this vital collection demonstrates the importance of gesture in a child's transition to a linguistic system. *$45.95*

358 pages Paperback
ISBN 1-563680-78-5

8242 **From Mime to Sign Package**

TJ Publishers
2544 Tarpley Rd
Suite 108
Carrollton, TX 75006-2288
972-416-0800
800-999-1168
Fax: 972-416-0944
customerservice@tjpublishers.com
www.tjpublishers.com

Gilbert C Eastman, Author
Terrence O'Rourke, Principal
Tanner Beach, Director

More than 1,000 photographs illustrate how natural gestures, mime and facial expressions used every day can become the basis for learning sign language. *$27.95*

183 pages Softcover
ISBN 0-932666-34-5

8243 **GA and SK Etiquette**

Telecommunications for the Deaf
8630 Fenton Street
Suite 604
Silver Spring, MD 20910- 3822
301-589-3786
Fax: 301-589-3797
www.tdi-online.org

Claude L Stout, Executive Director
Keith Cagle, Co-Author
Roy Miller, President
Gloria Carter, Administrator

Promoting equal access to telecommunications and media for people who are deaf, late-deafened, hard-of-hearing or deaf-blind through consumer education and involvement; technical assistance and consulting; applications of exisiting and emerging technologies; networking and collaboration; uniformity of standards; and national policy development and advocacy. *$11.95*

54 pages Paperback
ISBN 0-961462-17-5

8244 Gallaudet Survival Guide to Signing

Gallaudet University Press
800 Florida Ave NE
Washington, DC 20002-3600
773-568-1550
800-621-2736
Fax: 773-660-2235
TTY: 888-630-9347
gupress@gallaudet.edu
www.gallaudet.edu

Jon Mitchiner, Manager
Leonard G. Lane, Author
Jan Skrobisz, Illustrator
T. Alan Hurwitz, President

Features 500 of the most frequently used signs with clear illustrations and descriptions for each one. *$9.95*

218 pages Paperback
ISBN 0-930323-67-X

8245 Goldilocks and the Three Bears: Told in Signed English

Gallaudet University Press
800 Florida Ave NE
Washington, DC 20002-3600
773-568-1550
800-621-2736
Fax: 773-660-2235
TTY: 888-630-9347
gupress@gallaudet.edu
www.gupress.gallaudet.edu

Harry Bornstein, Author
Karen L Saulnier, Co-Author
T. Alan Hurwitz, President
Paul Kelly, Vice President Adm. And Finance

Goldilocks and the Three Bears offers children ages 3 - 8 all of the fun their parents had when they first read about the little girl with the golden curls who turned the Bears' house upside down. *$21.95*

48 pages Hardcover
ISBN 1-563680-57-2

8246 Hearing Impaired Children and Youth with Developmental Disabilities

Gallaudet University Bookstore
800 Florida Ave NE
Washington, DC 20002-3600
202-651-5855
866-204-0504
Fax: 773-660-2235
TTY: 202-651-5855
gupress@gallaudet.edu

Evelyn Cherow, Editor
T. Alan Hurwitz, President
Paul Kelly, Vice President Adm. And Finance

The insights of 24 experts help clarify relationships between hearing impairment and developmental difficulties and propose interdisciplinary cooperation as an approach to the problems created. *$29.95*

394 pages Hardcover
ISBN 0-913580-97-X

8247 Hollywood Speaks: Deafness and the Film Entertainment Industry

University of Illinois Press
1325 S Oak St
MC-566
Champaign, IL 61820-6903
217-333-0950
Fax: 217-244-8082
uipress@uillinois.edu
www.press.uillinois.edu

Willis G. Regier, Director
John S. Schuchman, Author
Kathy O'Neill, Assistant To The Director
Laurie Matheson, Editor-in-Chief

How deafness has been treated in movies and how it provides yet another window onto social history in addition to a fresh angle from which to view Hollywood. *$27.00*

200 pages Paperback 1999
ISBN 0-252068-50-8

8248 I Have a Sister, My Sister is Deaf

HarperCollins Publishers
10 E 53rd St
New York, NY 10022-5244
212-207-7901
800-242-7737
Fax: 212-702-2586
spsales@harpercollins.com
www.harpercollins.com

Jeanne Whitehouse Peterson, Author
Deborah Kogan Ray, Illustrator
Ann Ledden, Vice President
Lorna Metzler, Manager

An emphatic, affirmative look at the relationship between siblings, as a young deaf child is affectionately described by her older sister. This Coretta Scott King Honor Award winner helps young children develop an understanding that deaf children share the same interests as hearing children. *$6.99*

32 pages Paperback 1984
ISBN 0-064430-59-6

8249 Independence Without Sight or Sound

AFB Press
2 Penn Plaza
Suite 1102
New York, NY 10121-2006
212-502-7600
800-232-5463
Fax: 888-545-8331
afbweb@afb.net
www.afb.org

Richard Obnen, Chairman Of The Board
Carl Augusto, President and CEO
Rick Bozeman, Chief Financial Officer
Kelly Bleach, Chief Administrative Officer

This practical guidebook covers the essential aspects of communicating and working with deaf-blind persons. Full of valuable information on subjects such as how to talk with deaf-blind people, adapt orientation and mobility techniques for deaf-blind travelers, and interact with deaf-blind individuals socially, this useful manual also contains a substantial resource section detailing sources of information and adapted equipment. *$39.95*

193 pages Paperback
ISBN 0-891282-46-4

8250 Innovative Practices for Teaching Sign Language Interpreters

Gallaudet University Press
800 Florida Ave NE
Washington, DC 20002-3600
773-568-1550
800-621-2736
Fax: 773-660-2235
TTY: 888-630-9347
gupress@gallaudet.edu
www.gupress.gallaudet.edu

Cynthia B Roy, Editor

Researchers now understand interpreting as an active process between two languages and cultures, with social interaction, sociolinguistics, and discourse analysis as more appropriate theoretical frameworks. Roy's penetrating new book acts upon these new insights by presenting six dynamic teaching practices to help interpreters achieve the highest level of skill. *$45.95*

200 pages Hardcover
ISBN 1-563680-88-2

8251 Intermediate Conversational Sign Language

Gallaudet University Press
800 Florida Ave NE
Washington, DC 20002-3600
773-568-1550
800-621-2736
Fax: 773-660-2235
TTY: 888-630-9347
gupress@gallaudet.edu
www.gupress.gallaudet.edu

Willard J Madsen, Author

This fully illustrated text offers a unique approach to using American Sign Language (ASL) and English in a bilingual setting. Each of the 25 lessons involve sign language conversation using colloquialisms that are prevalent in informal conversations. *$31.50*

400 pages Softcover

ISBN 0-913580-79-1

8252 Interpretation: A Sociolinguistic Model

Sign Media
4020 Blackburn Ln
Burtonsville, MD 20866-1167
301-421-0268
800-475-4756
Fax: 301-421-0270
info@signmedia.com
www.signmedia.com

Verden Ness, President
Dennis Cokely, Author

This text presents a sociolinguistically sensitive model of the interpretation process. The model applies to interpretation in any two languages although this one focuses on ASL and English. *$22.95*

199 pages

ISBN 0-932130-10-0

8253 Interpreting: An Introduction

Registry of Interpreters for the Deaf
333 Commerce St
Alexandria, VA 22314-2801
703-838-0030
Fax: 703-838-0454
TTY: 703-838-0459
ridinfo@rid.org
www.rid.org

Nancy J Frishberg, Author
Shane Feldman, Executive Director
Don Roose, Director
Emil Ladner, Director

This text is written by a practicing interpreter and includes information on history, terminology, research, competence, setting and a comprehensive bibliography. *$24.95*

249 pages Softcover

ISBN 0-916883-07-8

8254 Joy of Signing

Gospel Publishing House
1445 N Boonville Ave
Springfield, MO 65802-1894
417-862-8000
800-641-4310
Fax: 417-862-5881
www.gospelpublishing.com

Lottie L Riekehof, Author

This manual on signing includes illustrations, information on sign origins, practice sentences, and step-by-step descriptions of hand positions and movements. *$23.99*

352 pages Hardcover

ISBN 0-882435-20-5

8255 Joy of Signing Puzzle Book

Harris Communications
15155 Technology Dr
Eden Prairie, MN 55344-2273
952-906-1180
800-825-6758
Fax: 952-906-1099
TTY: 800-825-9187
info@harriscomm.com
www.harriscomm.com

Robert Harris, Owner & President
Kevin Horsky, Business Director
Randall Moore, Manager

Whether one is learning sign language to communicate with a family member, co-worker, student or friend, this puzzle book makes the learning fun and interesting. *$4.50*

57 pages Softcover

ISBN 0-882436-76-7

8256 Kid-Friendly Parenting with Deaf and Hard of Hearing Children

Gallaudet University Press
800 Florida Ave NE
Washington, DC 20002-3600
773-568-1550
800-621-2736
Fax: 773-660-2235
TTY: 888-630-9347
gupress@gallaudet.edu
www.gupress.gallaudet.edu

Daria Medwid, Author
Denise Chapman Weston, Co-Author

At each chapter's beginning, experts (some deaf, some hearing), including I. King Jordan, Jack Gannon, Merv Garretson, and others, offer their insights on the subject discussed. Designed for parents with various styles, Kid-Friendly Parenting is a complete, step-by-step guide and reference to raising a deaf or hard of hearing child. *$35.95*

320 pages Paperback

ISBN 1-563680-31-9

8257 Laurent Clerc: The Story of His Early Years

Gallaudet University Press
800 Florida Ave NE
Washington, DC 20002-3600
773-568-1550
800-621-2736
Fax: 773-660-2235
TTY: 888-630-9347
gupress@gallaudet.edu
www.gupress.gallaudet.edu

Cathryn Carroll, Author
T. Alan Hurwitz, President
Paul Kelly, Vice President Adm. And Finance

In his own voice, Clerc vividly relates the experiences that led to his later progressive teaching methods. Especially influential was his long stay at the Royal National Institute for the Deaf in Paris, where he encountered sharply distinct personalities - the saintly, inspiring deaf teacher Massieu, the vicious Dr. Itard and his heartless experiments on deaf boys, and the Father of the Deaf, Abbe Sicard, who could hardly sign. *$13.95*

208 pages Paperback

ISBN 0-930323-23-8

8258 Linguistics of American Sign Language: An Introduction

Gallaudet University Press
800 Florida Ave NE
Washington, DC 20002-3600
773-568-1550
800-621-2736
Fax: 773-660-2235
TTY: 888-630-9347
gupress@gallaudet.edu
www.gupress.gallaudet.edu

Clayton Valli, Author
Ceil Lucas, Co-Author
Kristin J Mulrooney, Co-Author
Miako Villanueva, President

Completely reorganized to reflect the growing intricacy of the study of ASL linguistics, the 5th edition presents 26 units in seven parts. Part One: Introduction presents a revision of Defining Language and an entirely new unit, Defining Linguistics. Part Two: Phonology has been completely updated with new terminology and examples. *$75.00*

560 pages Hardcover

ISBN 1-563682-83-4

8259 Literacy & Your Deaf Child: What Every Parent Should Know

Gallaudet University Press
800 Florida Ave NE
Washington, DC 20002-3600
773-568-1550
800-621-2736
Fax: 773-660-2235
TTY: 888-630-9347
gupress@gallaudet.edu
www.gupress.gallaudet.edu

David A Stewart, Author
Bryan R Clarke, Co-Author
T. Alan Hurwitz, President
Paul Kelly, Vice President Adm. And Finance

Literacy and Your Deaf Child begins by introducing some common concepts, among them the importance of parental involvement in a deaf child's education. It outlines how children acquire language and describes the auditory and visual links to literacy. *$24.95*

240 pages Paperback
ISBN 1-563681-36-6

8260 Mask of Benevolence: Disabling the Deaf Community, The
DawnSign Press
6130 Nancy Ridge Dr
San Diego, CA 92121-3223
858-625-0600
800-549-5350
Fax: 858-625-2336
info@dawnsign.com
www.dawnsign.com

Joe Dannis, President
Harlan Lane, Author

Dr. Harlan Lane does not view deafness as a handicap but rather a different state from hearing. Deaf people are a societal minority and should be treasured, not eradicated. *$12.95*

360 pages Paperback 1992
ISBN 1-581210-09-5

8261 Mother Father Deaf: Living Between Sound and Silence
Harvard University Press
79 Garden St
Cambridge, MA 02138-1423
617-495-2600
800-405-1619
Fax: 617- 49- 589
contact_hup@harvard.edu
www.hup.harvard.edu

William Sisler, President
Paul Preston, Author

The book explores the intimate intersection of families like his own - families which embody the conflicts and resolutions of two often opposing world views, the Deaf and the Hearing. Although I have normal hearing, both of my parents are profoundly deaf. *$19.50*

278 pages Paperback
ISBN 0-674587-48-0

8262 My First Book of Sign
Gallaudet University Press
800 Florida Ave NE
Washington, DC 20002-3600
773-568-1550
800-621-2736
Fax: 773-660-2235
TTY: 888-630-9347
gupress@gallaudet.edu
www.gupress.gallaudet.edu

Pamela J Baker, Author
Patricia Bellan Gillen, Illustrator
T. Alan Hurwitz, President
Paul Kelly, Vice President Adm. And Finance

Full-color book gives alphabetically grouped signs for 150 words most frequently used by young children. *$22.95*

80 pages Hardcover
ISBN 0-930323-20-3

8263 My Signing Book of Numbers
Gallaudet University Press
800 Florida Ave NE
Washington, DC 20002-3600
773-568-1550
800-621-2736
Fax: 773-660-2235
TTY: 888-630-9347
gupress@gallaudet.edu
www.gupress.gallaudet.edu

Patricia Bellan Gillen, Author

This full-color book helps children learn their numbers in sign language. Each two-page spread of this delightfully illustrated book has the appropriate number of things or creatures for the numbers 0 through 20. *$22.95*

56 pages Hardcover
ISBN 0-930323-37-8

8264 Nursery Rhymes from Mother Goose
Gallaudet University Press
800 Florida Ave NE
Washington, DC 20002-3600
773-568-1550
800-621-2736
Fax: 773-660-2235
TTY: 888-630-9347
gupress@gallaudet.edu
www.gupress.gallaudet.edu

Harry Bornstein, Author
Karen L Saulnier, Co-Author
Patricia Peters, Illustrator
Linda Tom, Illustrator

Young readers, both hearing and deaf, will learn the special charm of rhyme while also discovering new vocabulary and new ways to experience English through signing. As they learn and memorize their favorite verses, children will also strengthen their language skills in a fun, entertaining way. *$21.95*

64 pages Hardcover
ISBN 0-930323-99-8

8265 Outsiders in a Hearing World: A Sociology of Deafness
Sage Publications
2455 Teller Rd
Thousand Oaks, CA 91320-2218
805-499-9774
800-818-7243
Fax: 805-499-0871
www.sagepub.com

Paul C Higgins, Author

An introduction to the social world of deaf people. The author gives a sociologists view of what it's like to be deaf. *$72.95*

208 pages Hardcover 1980
ISBN 0-803914-22-3

8266 Perigee Visual Dictionary of Signing
Harris Communications
15155 Technology Dr
Eden Prairie, MN 55344-2273
952-906-1180
800-825-6758
Fax: 952-906-1099
TTY: 800-825-9187
info@harriscomm.com
www.harriscomm.com

Robert Harris, Owner & President
Kevin Horsky, Business Director
Randall Moore, Manager

An A-to-Z guide to American Sign Language vocabulary. *$15.26*

450 pages Softcover
ISBN 0-399519-52-1

8267 Phone of Our Own: The Deaf Insurrection Against Ma Bell
Gallaudet University Press
800 Florida Ave NE
Washington, DC 20002-3600
773-568-1550
800-621-2736
Fax: 773-660-2235
TTY: 888-630-9347
gupress@gallaudet.edu
www.gupress.gallaudet.edu

Harry G Lang, Author
T. Alan Hurwitz, President
Paul Kelly, Vice President Adm. And Finance

A recount of the history of the teletypewriter, from the three deaf engineers who developed the acoustic coupler that made mass communication on TTY's feasible, through the deaf community's twenty-year struggle against the government and AT&T to have TTY's produced and distributed. *$36.50*

256 pages Hardcover
ISBN 1-563680-90-4

8268 **Place of Their Own: Creating the Deaf Community in America**
Gallaudet University Press
800 Florida Ave NE
Washington, DC 20002-3600
773-568-1550
800-621-2736
Fax: 773-660-2235
TTY: 888-630-9347
gupress@gallaudet.edu
www.gallaudet.edu

John V Van Cleve, Author
Barry A Crouch, Co-Author
T. Alan Hurwitz, President
Paul Kelly, Vice President Adm. And Finance

Traces development of American deaf society to show how deaf people developed a common language and sense of community. Views deafness as the distinguishing characteristic of a distinct culture. *$22.95*

224 pages Paperback
ISBN 0-930323-49-1

8269 **PreReading Strategies**
Gallaudet University Bookstore
800 Florida Ave NE
Washington, DC 20002-3600
202-651-5855
866-204-0504
Fax: 773-660-2235
TTY: 202-651-5855
gupress@gallaudet.edu

David R Schleper, Author
T. Alan Hurwitz, President
Paul Kelly, Vice President Adm. And Finance

Here is a wealth of good advice for preparing students to understand what they read, building comprehension and enjoyment. *$14.95*

65 pages

8270 **Quad City Deaf & Hard of Hearing Youth Group: Tomorrow's Leaders for our Community**
Independent Living Research Utilization ILRU
2323 S Shepherd Dr
Houston, TX 77019-7019
713-520-9058
Fax: 713-520-5785
ilru@ilru.org

Lex Frieden, Director
Rose Sheperd, Manager

IICIL staff see this program as a way to develop young leaders for themovement. Emphasis is given to providing oppportunities for members of the youth group to develop skills in planning and organizing activities.

8271 **Religious Signing: A Comprehensive Guide for All Faiths**
TJ Publishers
P.O. Box 702701
Dallas, TX 75370
972-416-0800
800-999-1168
Fax: 972-416-0944
TTY: 301-585-4440
TJPubinc@aol.com
www.tjpublishers.com

Elaine Costello, Author
Terrence O'Rourke, Principal
Tanner Beach, Director

Contains over 500 religious signs for all denominations and their meanings illustrated by clear upper torso illustrations that show movements of hand, body and face. Includes a section on signing favorite verses, prayers and blessings. *$18.95*

219 pages Softcover
ISBN 0-553342-44-4

8272 **Seeing Voices**
Vintage and Anchor Books
1745 Broadway
3rd Floor
New York, NY 10019
212-782-9000
Fax: 212-572-6066
vintageanchor@randomhouse.com
www.randomhouse.com

Oliver Sacks, Author
Madeline McIntosh, President/Sales/Operations
Markus Dohle, Chairman/CEO
Andrew Weber, SVP Operations And Technology

Well known for his exploration of how people respond to neurological impairments, Dr Sacks explores the world of the deaf and discovers how deaf people respond to their loss of hearing and how they develop language. A highly readable introduction to deaf people, deaf culture and American Sign Language. *$13.95*

240 pages Softcover 2000
ISBN 0-375704-07-8

8273 **Sign Language Interpreting and Interpreter Education**
Oxford University Press
2001 Evans Rd
Cary, NC 27513-2009
919-677-0977
800-445-9714
Fax: 919-677-1303
custserv.us@oup.com
www.oup.com

Marc Marschark, Editor
Rico Peterson, Editor
Elizabeth A Winston, Editor
Patricia Sapere, Contributing Editor

Provides a coherent picture of the field as a whole, including evaluation of the extent to which current practices are supported by validating research. The first comprehensive source, suitable as both a reference book and a textbook for interpreter training programs and a variety of courses on bilingual education, psycholinguistics and translation, and cross-linguistic studies. *$65.00*

328 pages Hardcover
ISBN 0-195176-94-4

8274 **Signed English Starter, The**
Gallaudet University Press
800 Florida Ave NE
Washington, DC 20002-3600
773-568-1550
800-621-2736
Fax: 773-660-2235
TTY: 888-630-9347
gupress@gallaudet.edu
www.gupress.gallaudet.edu

Harry Bornstein, Author
Karen L Saulnier, Co-Author
T. Alan Hurwitz, President
Paul Kelly, Vice President Adm. And Finance

A first course in Signed English for adults and children, the book is fully illustrated (several figures per page), and it is organized in a way that leads to rewarding learning quite rapidly. The authors of this new and exciting text believe firmly that Signed English must be made as easy as possible if it is going to be as useful (and used) as it can and should be. The book explains the rationale for the Signed English system and the conventions used to teach it. *$18.50*

232 pages Paperback
ISBN 0-913580-82-1

8275 **Signing Family: What Every Parent Should Know About Sign Communication, The**
Gallaudet University Press
800 Florida Ave NE
Washington, DC 20002-3600
773-568-1550
800-621-2736
Fax: 773-660-2235
TTY: 888-630-9347
gupress@gallaudet.edu
www.gupress.gallaudet.edu

David A Stewart, Author
Barbara Luetke-Stahlman, Co-Author
T. Alan Hurwitz, President
Paul Kelly, Vice President Adm. And Finance

This reader-friendly book shows parents how to create a set of goals around the communication needs of their deaf child. Describes in even-handed terms the major signing options available, from American Sign Language to Signed English. *$29.95*
192 pages Paperback
ISBN 1-563680-69-6

8276 Signing for Reading Success
Gallaudet University Press
800 Florida Ave NE
Washington, DC 20002-3600
773-568-1550
800-621-2736
Fax: 773-660-2235
TTY: 888-630-9347
gupress@gallaudet.edu
www.gupress.gallaudet.edu

Jan C Hafer, Author
Robert M Wilson, Co-Author
T. Alan Hurwitz, President
Paul Kelly, Vice President Adm. And Finance
This booklet provides summaries of four research students on the usefulness of signing for reading achievement. *$7.95*
24 pages Paperback
ISBN 0-930323-18-1

8277 Signing: How to Speak with Your Hands
TJ Publishers
2427 Bond Street
Suite 108
University Park, IL 60466- 2288
972-416-0800
800-999-1168
Fax: 972-416-0944
customerservice@tjpublishers.com
www.tjpublishers.com

Elaine Costello, Author
Terrence O'Rourke, Principal
Tanner Beach, Director
Presents 1,200 basic signs with clear illustrations in logical topical groupings. Linguistic principles are described at the beginning of each chapter, giving insight into the rules which govern American Sign Language. *$19.95*
248 pages Softcover
ISBN 0-553375-39-3

8278 Signs Across America
Gallaudet University Press
800 Florida Ave NE
Washington, DC 20002-3600
773-568-1550
800-621-2736
Fax: 773-660-2235
TTY: 888-630-9347
gupress@gallaudet.edu
www.gupress.gallaudet.edu

Edgar H Shroyer, Author
Susan P Shroyer, Co-Author
T. Alan Hurwitz, President
Paul Kelly, Vice President Adm. And Finance
A look at regional variations in ASL. Signs for selected words collected from 25 different states. More than 1,200 signs illustrated in the text. *$28.95*
304 pages Paperback
ISBN 0-913580-96-1

8279 Signs for Me: Basic Sign Vocabulary for Children, Parents & Teachers
TJ Publishers
2427 Bond Street
Suite 108
University Park, IL 60466- 2288
972-416-0800
800-999-1168
Fax: 972-416-0944
www.tjpublishers.com

Ben Bahan, Author
Joe Dannis, Co-Author
Terrence O'Rourke, Principal
Tanner Beach, Director
Sign language vocabulary for preschool and elementary school children introduces household items, animals, family members, actions, emotions, safety concerns and other concepts. *$14.95*
112 pages Softcover
ISBN 0-915035-27-8

8280 Signs for Sexuality: A Resource Manual
Planned Parenthood of Western Washington
2001 E Madison St
Seattle, WA 98122-2959
206-328-7715
Fax: 206-328-6810
www.plannedparenthood.org

Marlyn Minken, Author
Laurie Rosen-Ritt, Co-Author
Cecile Richards, President
An important book for those who want to listen to and talk with other people about feelings, loving and caring. *$40.00*
122 pages Softcover

8281 Signs of the Times
Gallaudet University Press
800 Florida Ave NE
Washington, DC 20002-3600
773-568-1550
800-621-2736
Fax: 773-660-2235
TTY: 888-630-9347
gupress@gallaudet.edu
www.gupress.gallaudet.edu

Edgar H Shroyer, Author
Susan P Shroyer, Illustrator
T. Alan Hurwitz, President
Paul Kelly, Vice President Adm. And Finance
An excellent beginner's contact signing book that fills the gap between sign language dictionaries and American Sign Language text. Designed for use as a classroom text. *$34.95*
448 pages Softcover
ISBN 0-913580-76-7

8282 Silent Garden, The
Gallaudet University Press
800 Florida Ave NE
Washington, DC 20002-3600
773-568-1550
800-621-2736
Fax: 773-660-2235
TTY: 888-630-9347
gupress@gallaudet.edu
www.gupress.gallaudet.edu

Paul W Ogden, Author
T. Alan Hurwitz, President
Paul Kelly, Vice President Adm. And Finance
The author explain the broad range of hearing loss types, from minor to profound. Parents also are advised about what type of school their child should attend and what kinds of professional help will be best for the entire family. The book describes all forms of communication, including choices in signing from American Sign Language to the various manual systems based upon English. Technological alternatives are presented also, including when and when not to consider cochler implants. *$34.95*
304 pages
ISBN 1-563680-58-0

8283 Sing Praise Hymnal for the Deaf
LifeWay Christian Resources
1 Lifeway Plz
MSN 146
Nashville, TN 37234-1001
615-251-2000
800-458-2772
Fax: 615-251-3899
www.lifeway.com

Thom Rainer, President/CEO
Jerry Rhyne, CFO/ VP Finance And Buisness
Tim Vineyard, VP Technology And CIO
Designed to be used by interpreters to the deaf, sign-language students, and deaf members of the congregation, this special combinded hymnal edition offers 234 of the most popular hymns. *$12.95*
Hardcover 2000
ISBN 0-767314-09-3

8284 **TDI National Directory & Resource Guide: Blue Book**
Telecommunications for the Deaf
8630 Fenton Street
Suite 604
Silver Spring, MD 20910- 3822
301-589-3786
Fax: 301-589-3797
www.tdi-online.org
Claude L Stout, Executive Director
Promoting Equal Access to Telecommunications and Media for People who are Deaf, Late-Deafened, Hard-of-Hearing or Deaf-Blind. *$20.00*
600 pages Annual

8285 **Theoretical Issues in Sign Language Research**
University of Chicago Press
1427 E 60th St
Chicago, IL 60637-2902
773-702-7700
Fax: 773-702-9756
sales@press.uchicago.edu
www.press.uchicago.edu
Donald A Collins, President
Susan D Fischer, Author
Patricia Siple, Co-Author
These volumes are an outgrowth of a conference held at the University of Rochester in 1986, dealing with the four traditional core areas of phonology, morphology, syntax and semantics. *$29.95*
348 pages Paperback 1990
ISBN 0-226251-52-7

8286 **We CAN Hear and Speak**
Alexander Graham Bell Association
3417 Volta Pl. NW
Washington, DC 20007
202-337-5220
Fax: 202-337-8314
TTY: 202-337-5221
info@agbell.org
agbell.org
Carol Flexer Ph.D, Author
Catherine Richards MA, Co-Author
Written by parents for families of children who are deaf or hard of hearing, this work describes auditory-verbal terminology and approaches and contains personal narratives written by parents and their children who are deaf or hard of hearing. *$6.98*
184 pages Softcover

8287 **Week the World Heard Gallaudet, The**
Gallaudet University Press
800 Florida Ave NE
Washington, DC 20002-3600
202-651-5000
800-621-2736
Fax: 202-651-5508
gupress@gallaudet.edu
www.gupress.gallaudet.edu
Jack R Gannon, Author
T. Alan Hurwitz, President
Paul Kelly, Vice President Adm. And Finance
This day-to-day description of the events surrounding the Deaf President Now movement at Gallaudet University includes full color and black and white photographs and interviews with people involved in the events of that week. *$49.95*
176 pages Hardcover
ISBN 0-930323-54-8

8288 **What is Auditory Processing?**
Abilitations - Speech Bin
P.O. Box 922668
Norcross, GA 30010-2668
770-449-5700
800-850-8602
Fax: 770-510-7290
info@speechbin.com
www.speechbin.com
Susan Bell, Author
What is Auditory Processing? It is and information-packed 16-page booklet created to explain auditory processing and it's disorders and offers practical suggestions for coping with this problem. It describes the listening process and tells how to help children with auditory processing problems. It shows what families and teachers can do to help children who have trouble remembering and understanding what they hear and offers easy-to-use activities and practical suggestions. *$22.69*
16 pages Softcover

8289 **You and Your Deaf Child: A Self-Help Guidefor Parents of Deaf and Hard of Hearing Children**
Gallaudet University Press
800 Florida Ave NE
Washington, DC 20002-3600
773-568-1550
800-621-2736
Fax: 773-660-2235
TTY: 888-630-9347
gupress@gallaudet.edu
www.gupress.gallaudet.edu
John W Adams, Author
T. Alan Hurwitz, President
Paul Kelly, Vice President Adm. And Finance
Eleven chapters focus on such topics as feelings about hearing loss, the importance of communication in the family, and effective behavior management. Many chapters contain practice activities and questions to help parents retain skills taught in the chapter and check their grasp of the material. Four appendices provide references, general resources, and guidelines for evaluating educational programs. *$29.95*
224 pages Paperback
ISBN 1-563680-60-2

Journals

8290 **ADARA**
1022 7th St NE
Washington, DC 20002
301-293-8969
Fax: 301-293-9698
TTY: 301-293-8969
adaraorg@gmail.com
www.adara.org
John Gournaris, Ph.D, President
Kathy Schwabeland, MA, Vice President
Denise Thew Hackett, Ph.D, JADARA Editor
Charles Sterling, MBA, Office Manager
ADARA's mission is to improve service excellence for those who are deaf or hard of hearing. The ADARA Update is a quarterly newsletter published by the association, offering information on events, resources, legislation, employment opportunities and other matters related to the field. JADARA is another publication by them presenting research results, articles on deafness, social services, mental health and other areas of interest.

8291 **American Journal of Audiology**
American Speech-Language-Hearing Association
2200 Research Blvd
Rockville, MD 20850-3289
240-632-2081
800-638-8255
Fax: 301-296-8580
actioncenter@asha.org
www.asha.org
Gary Dunham, Editor-in-Chief
Bridget Murray Law, Managing Editor
Carol Polovoy, Assistant Managing Editor
Kellie Rowden-Racette, Print and Online Writer/Editor
Articles concern screening, assesment, and treatment techniques; prevention; professional issues; supervision; administration. Includes clinical forums, clinical reviews, letters to the editor, or research reports that emphasize clinical practice.
2 x year

8292 **Hearing Professional**
International Hearing Society
16880 Middlebelt Rd
Ste 4
Livonia, MI 48154-3374
734-522-7200
800-521-5247
Fax: 734-522-0200
akovach@ihsinfo.org
www.ihsinfo.org
Kathleen Mennillo, MBA, Executive Director

Provides authoritative technical and business information that will help hearing aid specialists serve the hearing impaired.
bi-monthly

8293 **Journal of Speech, Language and Hearing Research**
American Speech-Language-Hearing Association
2200 Research Blvd
Rockville, MD 20850-3289
301-296-5700
800-638-8255
Fax: 301-296-8580
actioncenter@asha.org
www.asha.org

Gary Dunham, Editor-in-Chief
Bridget Murray Law, Managing Editor
Carol Polovoy, Assistant Managing Editor
Kellie Rowden-Racette, Print and Online Writer/Editor
Pertains broadly to studies of the processess and disorders of hearing, language, and speech diagnosis and treatment of such disorders.

8294 **Journal of the Academy of Rehabilitative Audiology**
Academy of Rehabilitative Audiology
PO Box 2323
Albany, NY 12220-0323
ara@audrehab.org
www.audrehab.org

Anne D. Olsen, Editor
A peer-reviewed journal published annually.

8295 **Literature Journal, The**
Gallaudet University
800 Florida Ave NE
Washington, DC 20002-3695
202-651-5488
800-621-2736
Fax: 202-651-5508
Oluyinka.Fakunle@gallaudet.edu

Charles C Welsh-Charrier, Author
T. Alan Hurwitz, President
Paul Kelly, Vice President Adm. And Finance
This book includes extensive examples of student and teacher entries taken from actual journals of deaf high school students.
$12.95
44 pages Spiral Bound

8296 **Sign Language Studies**
Gallaudet University Press
800 Florida Ave NE
Washington, DC 20002-3695
202-651-5488
800-621-2736
Fax: 202-651-5508
gupress@gallaudet.edu
www.gupress.gallaudet.edu

Ceil Lucas, Editor
T. Alan Hurwitz, President
Paul Kelly, Vice President Adm. And Finance
Presents a unique forum for revolutionary papers on signed languages and other related disciplines, including linguistics, anthropology, semiotics, and deaf studies, history, and literature.
$55.00
Quarterly

8297 **Volta Review**
Alexander Graham Bell Association
3417 Volta Pl. NW
Washington, DC 20007
202-337-5220
Fax: 202-337-8314
TTY: 202-337-5221
vreditor@agbell.org
agbell.org

Emilio Alonso-Mendoza, Chief Executive Officer
Professionally refereed journal that publishes articles and research on education, rehabilitation and communicative development of people who have hearing impairments. Also includes subscription to Volta Voices, up-to-date magazine, bimonthly.
Biannual

Magazines

8298 **Endeavor Magazine**
American Society for Deaf Children
PO Box 23
Woodbine, MD 21797
800-942-2732
info@deafchildren.org
www.deafchildren.org

Tami Dominguez, Editor
ASDC's qurterly publication featuring committee reports, stories, and fun.
Quarterly

8299 **Hearing Health Magazine**
Deafness Research Foundation
363 Seventh Avenue
10th Floor
New York, NY 10001-3904
212-257-6140
866-454-3924
Fax: 212-257-6139
info@drf.org
www.drf.org

Andrea Boidman, Executive Director
Andrea Delbanco, Senior Editor
Yishane Lee, Editor
Julie Grant, Art Director
Serves as a source of quality information and provides the tools and resources to help people seek treatment for and manage hearing loss. Each issue features relevant and timely information on the latest research, articles written by leading authorities in the field, news about the latest technology, and human interest stories about those living with hearing loss.

8300 **Hearing Life Magazine**
Hearing Loss Association of America
7910 Woodmont Ave
Ste 1200
Bethesda, MD 20814-7022
301-657-2248
Fax: 301-913-9413
inquiry@hearingloss.org
www.hearingloss.org

Barbara Kelley, Executive Director
Formerly known as Hearing Loss Magazine, this official publication of the Hearing Loss Association of America helps individuals with hearing loss live a better life.
Bi-Monthly

8301 **Tinnitus Today**
American Tinnitus Association
PO Box 424049
Washington, DC 20042-4049
800-634-8978
ringingears.ata.org

Joy Onozuka, Managing Editor
The magazine contains up-to-date medical and research news, feature articles on urgent tinnitus issues, questions and answers, self-help suggestions and letters to the editor from others with tinnitus. *$35.00*
28 pages 3 x year

Newsletters

8302 **ASHA Leader, The**
American Speech-Language-Hearing Association
2200 Research Blvd
Rockville, MD 20850-3289
301-215-6710
800-638-8255
Fax: 301-296-8580
leader@asha.org
www.asha.org

Gary Dunham, Editor-in-Chief
Bridget Murray Law, Managing Editor
Carol Polovoy, Assistant Managing Editor
Kellie Rowden-Racette, Print and Online Writer/Editor
Association publication containing news, notices of events and activities and information for members on issues facing the profession of audiology and speech-language pathology. *$80.00*
35 pages 2 x month

8303 **American Annals of the Deaf**
Gallaudet University Press
800 Florida Ave NE
Washington, DC 20002-3600
202-651-5000
800-621-2736
Fax: 202-651-5508
paul.3@osu.edu
www.gupress.gallaudet.edu
Peter V. Paul, Editor, Literary Issues
T. Alan Hurwitz, President
Paul Kelly, Vice President Adm. And Finance
Quarterly publication from the Conference of Educational Administrators Serving the Deaf. *$55.00*
Quarterly

8304 **Canine Listener**
Dogs for the Deaf
10175 Wheeler Rd
Central Point, OR 97502
541-826-9220
800-990-3647
800-990-3647
Fax: 541-826-6696
TTY: 541-826-9220
info@dogsforthedeaf.org
dogsforthedeaf.org
Marvin Rhodes, Chair
Susan Bahr, Vice Chair
Kelly Gonzales, Development Director
Janine Bol, Finance Director
Provides information on Hearing Dogs, placements, dog training, and other news about happenings at Dogs for the Deaf.
Quarterly

8305 **Cochlear Implants In Children: Ethics and Choices**
Gallaudet University Press
800 Florida Ave NE
Washington, DC 20002-3600
202-651-5000
800-621-2736
Fax: 202-651-5508
gupress@gallaudet.edu
www.gupress.gallaudet.edu
John B Christiansen, Author
Irene W Leigh, Co-Author
T. Alan Hurwitz, President
Paul Kelly, Vice President Adm. And Finance
Designed to educate readers about cochlear implants, including surgery, the importance of rehabilitation and the significance of parents' and professionals' roles. *$55.00*
340 pages Casebound
ISBN 1-563681-16-1

8306 **Communique**
Michigan Association for Deaf Hard of Hearing
5236 Dumond Court
Suite C
Lansing, MI 48917-6001
517-487-0066
800-968-7327
Fax: 517-487-2586
Nancy Asher, Executive Director
Pat Walton, Office Manager
Provides leadership through advocacy and education. The association conducts leadership training for youth, information and referral services, interpreter referral, legislative advocacy, and a variety of other services.
4-8 pages Bi-annually

8307 **Connect - Commmunity News**
Hearing, Speech & Deafness Center (HSDC)
1625 19th Ave.
Seattle, WA 98122-2848
206-323-5770
888-222-5036
Fax: 206-328-6871
www.hsdc.org
David Delmar, Editor
Connect is the quarterly eNews of the Hearing, Speech & Deafness Center. HSDC is is a nonprofit for clients who are deaf, hard of hearing, or who face other communication barriers such as speech challenges.
8 pages Annual

8308 **Deaf Catholic**
International Catholic Deaf Association
7202 Buchanan St
Landover Hills, MD 20784-2236
301-429-0697
Fax: 301-429-0698
homeoffice@icda-us.org
www.icda-us.org
Jean Cox, President
Kate Slosar, Vice President
TK Hill, Treasurer
Aline Shaw, Secretary
Newsletter reporting the news of the Archdiocese, Deaf Apostolate and each of the Catholic Deaf Organizations. *$20.00*
16 pages Quarterly

8309 **International Hearing Dog, Inc.**
International Hearing Dog
5901 E 89th Ave.
Henderson, CO 80640-8315
303-287-3277
Fax: 303-287-3425
info@hearingdog.org
Valerie Foss-Brugger, Executive Director
Samuel Cheris, Chairman
Matt Bailey, Treasurer
Aspen Matthew, Office Manager
International Hearing Dog, Inc. trains rescued shelter dogs for people who are deaf or hard-of-hearing, with and without disabilities, all at no cost to the recipient. Since 1979, 1300 dogs have been placed throughout all 50 states and Canada.
4-8 pages Quarterly

8310 **League Letter**
Center for Hearing and Communication
50 Broadway
6th Floor
New York, NY 10004-3810
917-305-7700
Fax: 917-305-7888
TTY: 917-305-7999
info@chchearing.org
www.lhh.org
Laurie Hanin, Executive Director
Ellen Lafargue, Au.D., CCC, Director, Hearing Technology
Lois Kam Heymann, M.A., CCC, Director, Communication
Linda Kessler, M.A., CCC-SLP, Assistant Director, Communication
Quarterly

8311 **Listner**
HEAR Center
301 E Del Mar Blvd
Pasadena, CA 91101-2714
626-796-2016
Fax: 626-796-2320
info@hearcenter.org
www.hearcenter.org
Ellen Simon, Executive Director
Berenice Castro, Accounting Supervisro
Debbie Lorino, Office Manager
Chronicals current events, spotlights pediatric and adult clients as well as community outreach events.
Semi-Quarterly

8312 **NAD E-Zine**
National Association of the Deaf
8630 Fenton Street
Suite 820
Silver Spring, MD 20910- 3819
301-587-1788
Fax: 301-587-1791
TTY: 301-587-1789
www.nad.org
Bobbie Beth Scoggins, President
Christopher Wagner, Vice President
Includes up-to-the-minute information about the NAD, including Board news, advocacy, outreach and community activities, as well as NAD Conference and other information.

8313 **NAHO News**
National Association of Hearing Officials
PO Box 4999
Midlothian, VA 23112-17
701-328-3260
www.naho.org
Joy Wezelman, Editor
Janice Deshais, Editor

National Association of Hearing Officials newsletter.

8314 **On the Level**
Vestibular Disorders Association
5018 NE 15th Ave
Portland, OR 97211-5331
503-229-7705
800-837-8428
Fax: 503-229-8064
veda@vestibular.org
www.vestibular.org

Lisa Haven PhD, Executive Director
Jerry Underwood, Director
Vincente Honrubia, Director
Contents of each issue include information about local support groups, a calendar of conferences and training opportunities for health professionals, a list of donors, and special items indexed below. *$5.00*
12 pages Quarterly

8315 **Pinnacle Newsletter**
Academy of Rehabilitative Audiology
PO Box 26532
Minneapolis, MN 55426-532
952-920-0484
Fax: 952-920-6098
sherri.smith@va.gov
www.audrehab.org

John Greer Clark, Editor
Diana Derry, Co-Editor
Sherri Smith, Ph.D., Content Editor
Academy of Rehabilitative Audiology newsletter.

8316 **Soundings Newsletter**
American Hearing Research Foundation
8 South Michigan Avenue
Suite 1205
Chicago, IL 60603- 4539
312-726-9670
Fax: 312-726-9695
www.american-hearing.org

Sharon Parmet, Executive Director
Promote, conduct and furnish financial assistance for medical research into the cause, prevention and cure of deafness, impaired hearing and balance disorders; encourage the collaboration of clinical and laboratory research; encourage and improve teaching in the medical aspects of hearing problems; and disseminate the most reliable scientific knowledge to physicians, hearing professionals and the public.
Quarterly

8317 **Spring Dell Center Newsletter**
Spring Dell Center
6040 Radio Station Rd
La Plata, MD 20646-3368
301-934-4561
Fax: 301-870-2439
www.springdellcenter.org

Donna Retzlaff, Executive Director
Jody Loper, President
Brett Hamorsky, Vice President
Jeff Hubbard, Treasurer
Quarterly

8318 **Vision Magazine**
National Catholic Office of the Deaf
7202 Buchanan St
Hyattsville, MD 20784-2236
301-577-1684
Fax: 301-577-1684
info@ncod.org
www.ncod.org

Arvilla Rank, Editor/Executive Director
Published as a pastoral service for the deaf and hard of hearing. Provides information to members and others working in ministry.
$15.00
Quarterly

Audio/Visual

8319 **Christmas Stories**
Video Learning Library
15838 N 62nd St
Scottsdale, AZ 85254-1988
480-596-9970
800-383-8811
Fax: 480-596-9973
www.videolearning.com

Jim Spencer, Owner
Told by popular deaf story-tellers, the stories included are A Christmas Carol, Night Before Christmas, Story of the First Christmas Tree, Birth of Christ, The Great Walled City, and Little Match Girl. *$29.95*
Video/80 Mins 1986
ISBN 1-882257-02-2

8320 **Fantastic Series Videotape Set**
Gallaudet University Press
800 Florida Ave NE
Washington, DC 20002-3695
202-651-5488
800-621-2736
Fax: 202-651-5489
gupress@gallaudet.edu
www.gupress.gallaudet.edu

Rita Corey, Director
T. Alan Hurwitz, President
Paul Kelly, Vice President Adm. And Finance
These videotapes offer a blend of entertainment and information to both deaf and hearing children ages 6-10. A total of eight tapes in the series. *$254.00*
Video 8 VHS
ISBN 1-563680-12-2

8321 **Fantastic: Colonial Times, Chocolate, and Cars**
Gallaudet University Press
800 Florida Ave NE
Washington, DC 20002-3695
202-651-5488
800-621-2736
Fax: 202-651-5489
gupress@gallaudet.edu
www.gupress.gallaudet.edu

Rita Corey, Director
T. Alan Hurwitz, President
Paul Kelly, Vice President Adm. And Finance
Young viewers visit Colonial Williamsburg in Virginia to see various crafts. Other parts show chocolate being made, and films of old cars. *$39.95*
Video
ISBN 1-563680-06-8

8322 **Fantastic: Dogs at Work and Play**
Gallaudet University Press
800 Florida Ave NE
Washington, DC 20002-3695
202-651-5488
800-621-2736
Fax: 202-651-5489
gupress@gallaudet.edu
www.gupress.gallaudet.edu

Rita Corey, Director
T. Alan Hurwitz, President
Paul Kelly, Vice President Adm. And Finance
See how dogs are trained, including Fantastic's own hearing-ear dog, police dogs, plus puppies, and dogs in space? *$39.95*
Video
ISBN 1-563680-03-3

8323 **Fantastic: Exciting People, Places and Things!**
Gallaudet University Press
800 Florida Ave NE
Washington, DC 20002-3695
202-651-5488
800-621-2736
Fax: 202-651-5489
gupress@gallaudet.edu
www.gupress.gallaudet.edu

Rita Corey, Director
T. Alan Hurwitz, President
Paul Kelly, Vice President Adm. And Finance

Welcomes young viewers for a trip to a crayon factory, a jump rope tournament, and mime by actor Bernard Bragg. *$39.95*
Video
ISBN 1-563680-01-7

8324 **Fantastic: From Post Offices to Dairy Goats**
Gallaudet University Press
800 Florida Ave NE
Washington, DC 20002-3695
202-651-5488
800-621-2736
Fax: 202-651-5489
gupress@gallaudet.edu
www.gupress.gallaudet.edu
Rita Corey, Director
T. Alan Hurwitz, President
Paul Kelly, Vice President Adm. And Finance
In this video children follow the route of a letter from the mailbox through the post office to its final destination. Also, they visit dairy goats and other animals. *$39.95*
Video
ISBN 1-563680-05-X

8325 **Fantastic: Imagination, Actors, and 'Deaf Way'**
Gallaudet University Press
800 Florida Ave NE
Washington, DC 20002-3695
202-651-5488
800-621-2736
202-651-5508
Fax: 202-651-5489
gupress@gallaudet.edu
www.gupress.gallaudet.edu
Rita Corey, Director
T. Alan Hurwitz, President
Paul Kelly, Vice President Adm. And Finance
Deaf clowns, mimes, and actors display the wonders of imagination, along with performances at the international cultural celebration 'Deaf Way.' *$39.95*
Video
ISBN 1-563680-04-1

8326 **Fantastic: Roller Coasters, Maps, and Ice Cream!**
Gallaudet University Press
800 Florida Ave NE
Washington, DC 20002-3695
202-651-5488
800-621-2736
Fax: 202-651-5489
gupress@gallaudet.edu
Rita Corey, Director
T. Alan Hurwitz, President
Paul Kelly, Vice President Adm. And Finance
In this program Mike Montangino leads the way on rides at Kings Dominion, and also to see how maps are drawn, and how ice cream is made. *$39.95*
Video
ISBN 1-563680-07-6

8327 **Fantastic: Skiing, Factories, and Race Hores**
Gallaudet University Press
800 Florida Ave NE
Washington, DC 20002-3695
202-651-5488
800-621-2736
Fax: 202-651-5489
gupress@gallaudet.edu
Rita Corey, Director
T. Alan Hurwitz, President
Paul Kelly, Vice President Adm. And Finance
Snow Skiing starts this program, which continues in a factory where 'who-knows-what' is made. Also, young viewers learn about horse care, and also about the making of Oreos. *$39.95*
Video
ISBN 1-563680-08-4

8328 **Fantastic: Wonderful Worlds of Sports and Travel**
Gallaudet University Press
800 Florida Ave NE
Washington, DC 20002-3695
202-651-5488
800-621-2736
Fax: 202-651-5489
gupress@gallaudet.edu
Rita Corey, Director
T. Alan Hurwitz, President
Paul Kelly, Vice President Adm. And Finance
In this program, young viewers ride on a train, watch deaf athletes compete, and see actor Bernard Bragg perform 'The Lion and the Mouse.' *$39.95*
Video
ISBN 1-563680-02-5

8329 **Fingerspelling: Expressive and Receptive Fluency**
DawnSign Press
6130 Nancy Ridge Dr
San Diego, CA 92121-3223
858-625-0600
800-549-5350
Fax: 858-625-2336
info@dawnsign.com
www.dawnsign.com
Joe Dannis, President
Joyce Linden Groode, Fingerspelling Teacher
Improve your fingerspelling with this new video guide. A 24-page instructional booklet is included with fingerspelling practice suggestions. *$29.95*
120 Minutes
ISBN 1-581210-46-9

8330 **Getting Better**
Vestibular Disorders Association
5018 NE 15th Ave
Portland, OR 97211-5331
503-229-7705
800-837-8428
Fax: 503-229-8064
veda@vestibular.org
www.vestibular.org
Cynthia Ryan MBA, Executive Director
Tony Staser, Development Director
Vicente Honrubia, Director
Joel A. Goebel, MD, FACS, Director, Vestibular & Oculomotor Laboratory
Interviews with physicians, physical therapists, psychologists, social workers, and patients on Managing Symptoms, Diagnosis & Treatment, and Cognitive/Psychological Impacts. *$24.95*
Video

8331 **Helping the Family Understand**
Vestibular Disorders Association
5018 NE 15th Ave
Portland, OR 97211-5331
503-229-7705
800-837-8428
Fax: 503-229-8064
veda@vestibular.org
www.vestibular.org
Cynthia Ryan MBA, Executive Director
Tony Staser, Development Director
Vicente Honrubia, Director
Joel A. Goebel, MD, FACS, Director, Vestibular & Oculomotor Laboratory
Interviews with physicians, physical therapists, psychologists, social workers, and patients on Managing Symptoms, Diagnosis & Treatment and Cognitive/Psychological Impacts. *$24.95*
Video

8332 **Managing Your Symptoms**
Vestibular Disorders Association
5018 NE 15th Ave
Portland, OR 97211-5331
503-229-7705
800-837-8428
Fax: 503-229-8064
veda@vestibular.org
www.vestibular.org

Cynthia Ryan MBA, Executive Director
Tony Staser, Development Director
Vicente Honrubia, Director
Joel A. Goebel, MD, FACS, Director, Vestibular & Oculomotor Laboratory

Interviews with physicians, physical therapists, psychologists, social workers, and patients. on Managing Symptoms, Diagnosis & Treatment, and Cognitive/Psychological Impacts. *$24.95*
Video

Sports

8333 **American Hearing Impaired Hockey Association**
4214 W. 77th Place
Chicago, IL 60652-1618
978-922-0955
Fax: 312-829-2098
kkmm2won@aol.com
www.ahiha.org

Stan Mikita, President
Cheryl Hager, General Manager
Helen Tovey, Registrar, USA Hockey Reg.

The American Hearing Impaired Hockey Association provides deaf and hard of hearing hockey players the opportunity to learn about and improve their hockey skills through our program. We offer these hockey players the opportunity to be coached by a coaching staff with college, national and international experience.

8334 **USA Deaf Sports Federation**
102 N Krohn Pl
PO Box 910338
Lexington, KY 40591-0338
605-367-5760
Fax: 605-782-8441
TTY: 605-367-5761

Jack C Lamberton, President
Mark Apodaca, VP Of Financial Affairs
William J Bowman, VP Of International Affairs
Jeffrey L. Salit?, Vice-President of NSO Affairs

The USA Deaf Sports Federation's purpose was to foster and regulate uniform rules of competition and provide social outlets for deaf members and their friends; serve as a parent organization for regional sports organizations; conduct annual athletic competitions; and assist in the participation of U.S. teams in international competition.

Support Groups

8335 **Dial-a-Hearing Screening Test**
Occupational Hearing Services Inc.
300 S Chester Rd
Suite 301
Swarthmore, PA 19081-1800
610-544-7700
800-622-3277
Fax: 610-543-2802

George Biddle, President/Owner
James Biddle, Vice President
Phyllis Biddle, Treasurer

A national telephone resource providing information about hearing impairments and deafness. Dial-A-Hearing Screening Test: national test number for free telephone hearing test: 1-800-222-EARS, MON-FRI: 9:00 AM to 5:00 PM Eastern time.

Mobility

Associations

8336 **Academy of Spinal Cord Injury Professionals**
206 S. 6th St
Springfield, IL 62701 217-321-2488
Fax: 217-525-1271
www.academyscipro.org
Destiny Nance-Evans, Director Of Memebership Services
Kim Ruff, Director Of Education
An interdisciplinary organization dedicated to advancing the care of people with spinal cord injury/dysfunction, providing resources, research, and insights for SCI/D professionals.

8337 **Academy of Spinal Cord Injury Professionals: Psychologists, Social Workers & Counselors**
Academy of Spinal Cord Injury Professionals
206 S. 6th St.
Springfield, IL 62701 217-321-2488
Fax: 217-525-1271
www.academyscipro.org/
Heather Russell, President, PSWC Section
Lisa Beck, President, Academy of Spinal Cord Injury Professionals
Toby Huston, Vice President
Denny O'Malley, Executive Director
Organizes and operates for scientific and educational purposes to advance and improve the psychosocial care of persons with spinal cord impairment, develops and promotes education and research related to the psychosocial care of persons with spinal cord injury, recognizes psychologists and social workers whose careers are devoted to the problems of spinal cord impairment.

8338 **Acid Maltase Deficiency Association**
P.O. Box 700248
San Antonio, TX 78270-0248 210-494-6144
Fax: 210-490-7161
TiffanyLHouse@aol.com
www.amda-pompe.org
Tiffany House, President
The Acid Maltase Deficiency Association offers resource materials to help raise awareness and provide education and insight into Pompe disease (a.k.a. Acid Maltase Deficiency), a rare genetic disease derived from the family of Lysosomal Storage Disease. The association offers information for patients, their families, as well as medical professionals.

8339 **American Academy of Osteopathy**
The Pyramids
3500 DePauw Blvd.
Suite 1100
Indianapolis, IN 46268-1136 317-879-1881
Fax: 317-879-0563
info@academyofosteopathy.org
www.academyofosteopathy.org
Sherri Quarles, Interim Executive Director & Accountant
Michael P. Rowane, DO, MS, FAOO, President
The mission of the American Academy of Osteopathy is to teach, advocate, and research the science, art and philosophy of osteopathic medicine, emphasizing the integration of osteopathic principles, practice and manipulative treatment in patient care.

8340 **American Association of Neuromuscular & Electrodiagnostic Medicine**
2621 Superior Drive NW
Rochester, MN 55901 507-288-0100
Fax: 507-288-1225
aanem@aanem.org
www.aanem.org
Shirlyn A. Adkins, JD, Executive Director
Scott Gerdes, Finance Director
Lori Nierman, Office Manager
Karen Reilly, Education & Meeting Director
The American Association of Neuromuscular & Electrodiagnostic Medicine (AANEM) is a nonprofit membership association dedicated to the advancement of neuromuscular (NM), musculoskeletal, and electrodiagnostic (EDX) medicine.

8341 **American Back Society**
St. Joseph's Professional Center
2647 E. 14th St.
Suite 401
Oakland, CA 94601 510-536-9929
Fax: 510-536-1812
www.chiroweb.com/hp/abs/index.html
Philip E. Greenman, D.O., FAAO, President
Alexander Hadjipavlou, MD, MSc, 1st Vice President
Stephen Esses, BSc, MD, 2nd Vice President
Aubrey A. Swartz, MD, PharmD, Treasurer/Secretary
The American Back Society is a non-profit organization dedicated to providing an interdisciplinary educational forum for healthcare professionals committed to relieving pain and diminishing impairment in patients suffering from neck and back conditions through proper diagnosis and treatment.

8342 **American Parkinson Disease Association**
135 Parkinson Avenue
Staten Island, NY 10305 800-223-2732
Fax: 718-981-4399
apda@apdaparkinson.org
www.apdaparkinson.org
Leslie A. Chambers, President & CEO
Stephanie Paul, Vice President, Development and Marketing
Robin Kornhaber, MSW, Vice President, Programs and Services
Eloise Caggiano, Senior Director of Development
APDA was founded in 1961 with the dual purpose to find the curefor Parkinson's disease, and to assist Americans living with Parkinson's disease live a quality life.

8343 **American Spinal Injury Association**
9702 Gayton Rd.
Suite 306
Richmond, VA 23238 877-274-2724
asia.office@asia-spinalinjury.org
www.asia-spinalinjury.org
Patty Duncan, Executive Director
Carolyn Moffatt, Association Manager
Kim Ruff, Administrative Assistant
Professional association for physicans and other health professionals working in all aspects of spinal cord injury.

8344 **American Stroke Association**
7272 Greenville Ave
Dallas, TX 75231 888-478-7653
strokeconnection@heart.org
www.strokeassociation.org/STROKEORG
John Warner, President
James Postl, Chairman
Nancy Brown, Chief Executive Officer
Raymond Vara, Jr., Treasurer
The American Stroke Association offers educational materials, seminars, conferences and transportation for those effected by strokes as well as their families, caregivers and interested professionals.

8345 **Amytrophic Lateral Sclerosis Association**
1275 K Street NW
Suite 250
Washington, DC 20005 202-407-8580
Fax: 202-464-8869
alsinfo@alsa-national.org
www.alsa.org
Barbara Newhouse, President/CEO
Calaneet Balas, Executive Vice President, Strategy
Gregory L. Mitchell, Executive Vice President, Finance & Administration
Lance Slaughter, Executive Vice President, Chapter Relations & Governance
The ALS association is the only national not-for-profit health organization dedicated soley to lead the fight against ALS. The Association covers all the bases-research, patient and community services, public education, and advocacy-in providing help and hope to those facing the disease. The mission is to lead the fight to cure and treat ALS through global cutting edge research, and to empower people with Lou Gehrig's disease to live fuller lives & provide them with compassion, care and support.

8346 Arthritis Foundation
1355 Peachtree St NE
6th Floor
Atlanta, GA 30309
404-872-7100
800-283-7800
www.arthritis.org

Laurie Stewart, Secretary/Vice Chair
Rowland W. (Bing) Chang, Chair
Frank Longobardi, Treasurer
Ann M. Palmer, President/CEO

Offers information and referrals regarding educational materials and programs, fund-raising, support groups, seminars and conferences, and aids Americans with arthritis in accessing optimal care.

8347 Association for Neurologically Impaired Brain Injured Children
61-35 220th St
Oakland Gardens, NY 11364
718-423-9550
Fax: 718-423-9838
jdebiase@anibic.org
www.anibic.org

Vincent Tancredi, Chief Financial Officer
John F DeBiase, Executive Director
Rachel Plakstis, MSC Director
Gail Baquero, Residential Director

ANIBIc is a voluntary, multi-service organization that is dedicated to serving individuals with severe learning disabilities, neurological impairments and other developmental disabilities. Services include: residential, vocational, family support services, recreation (children and adults), respite (adult), in home support services, counseling and traumatic brain injury services (adults).

8348 Capital Area Parkinsons Society
PO Box 27565
Austin, TX 78755-2565
512-371-3373
www.capitalareaparkinsons.org

Tereasa Ford, President
Deborah Bryson, Vice President
Donna Hohm, Secretary
Tim Ebest, Treasurer

Founded in 1984, the Capital Area Parkinson's Society addresses the needs for those impacted by Parkinson's disease in central Texas. The organization offers a multitude of support groups, resources, monthly meetings, exercise programs and a community for people afflicted by Parkinson's and their care partners.

8349 Children's Hemiplegia & Stroke Association
4101 W. Green Oaks Blvd
Suite 305-149
Arlington, TX 76016
www.chasa.org

Nancy Atwood, Executive Director & Founder
Jana Smoot White, President
Patti Scrivano, Vice President
Jackie Haley, Treasurer

Founded in 1996, CHASA offers support and information to families of infants, children and young adults who have hemiplegia, hemiparesis or hemiplegic cerebral palsy.

8350 Christopher & Dana Reeve Paralysis Resource Center
636 Morris Turnpike
Suite 3A
Short Hills, NJ 07078
973-467-8270
800-225-0292
InfoSpecialist@ChristopherReeve.org
www.christopherreeve.org

John M Hughes, Chairman
John E McConnell, Vice Chairman
Peter Wilderotter, President & CEO
Matthew Reeve, Vice Chairman, International Development

The Paralysis Resource Center's goal is to provide support and information to those living with paralysis and their caregivers. Some programs offered include financial grants, a family support program, advocay programs, a lending library, rehabilitation centers, a veteran program and a resource guide about paralysis.

8351 Consortium of Multiple Sclerosis Centers
3 University Plaza Dr.
Suite 116
Hackensack, NJ 07601
201-487-1050
Fax: 862-772-7275
www.mscare.org

June Halper, Chief Executive Officer
Gary Cutter, PhD, President
Lisa Skutnik, Chief Operating Officer
Marguerite Herman, Executive Assistant

CMSC provides leadership in clinical research and education; develops vehicles to share information and knowledge among members; disseminates information to the health care community and to persons affected by Multiple Sclerosis; and develops and implements mechanisms to influence health care delivery.

8352 Cure SMA
Cure SMA
925 Busse Rd
Elk Grove Village, IL 60007
800-886-1762
info@curesma.org
www.curesma.org

Jill Jarecki, Chief Scientific Officer
Kenneth Hobby, President
Richard Rubenstein, Chair
Kelly Cole, Secretary

Cure SMA is the largest international organization dedicated solely to eradicating spinal muscular atrophy (SMA) by promoting and supporting research, helping families cope with SMA through informational programs and support, and educating the public and professional community about SMA.

8353 Dystonia Advocacy Network
One East Wacker Drive
Suite 2810
Chicago, IL 60601
dystonia-advocacy.org

8354 Epilepsy Foundation
8301 Professional Place E
Suite 200
Landover, MD 20785- 2353
800-332-1000
Fax: 301-459-1569
ContactUs@efa.org
www.epilepsy.com

Robert W Smith, Chair
Phillip M. Gattone, M.Ed, Preisdent & CEO
M. Vaneeda Bennett, Chief Development Officer
May J. Liang, Secretary

The organization works to ensure that people with epilepsy are able to participate in all life experiences; to improve how people with epilepsy are perceived and treated in society; and to promote research for a cure.

8355 Friends of Disabled Adults and Children
4900 Lewis Rd
Stone Mountain, GA 30083
770-491-9014
866-977-1204
www.fodac.org

Chris Brand, President
Pam Holley, Director of Administration
Betty Felder, DME Office Manager
Ron Hess, Vehicle Modification Coordinator

FODAC's mission is to provide durable medical equipment (DME) at lost cost to the disabled and their families, and to enhance the quality of life for individuals with disabilities or illnesses.

8356 Head Injury Rehabilitation And Referral Service, Inc. (HIRRS)
11 Taft Court
Suite 100
Rockville, MD 20850
301-309-2228
Fax: 301-309-2278
tbi@headinjuryrehab.org
www.headinjuryrehab.org

Maggie Hunter, Director of Admissions and Quality Assurance
Robert Cousland, Director of Rehabilitation
Ricardo Hunter, President
Janet McCloskey, Director of Community Living Services

Head Injury Rehabilitation and Referral Services, Inc. (HIRRS) is a private not-for-profit agency that provides comprehensive brain injury support including long-term living, daily programs, vocational supports and services to individuals that live in the community. The agency is located in Rockville, MD, but serves the DC Metropolitan area.

8357 **International Parkinson and Movement Disorder Society**
555 East Wells St.
Suite 1100
Milwaukee, WI 53202-3823
414-276-2145
Fax: 414-276-3349
info@movementdisorders.org
www.movementdisorders.org

Christopher Goetz, MD, President
Susan Fox, PhD, Secretary
Victor Fung, MBBS, PhD, FRACP, Treasurer

The International Parkinson and Movement Disorder Society (MDS) is a professional society of clinicians, scientists, and other healthcare professionals who are interested in Parkinson's disease, related neurodegenerative and neurodevelopmental disorders, hyperkinetic movement disorders, and abnormalities in muscle tone and motor control.

8358 **Lewy Body Dementia Association**
912 Killian Hill Road S.W.
Lilburn, GA 30047
404-975-2322
Fax: 480-422-5434
www.lbda.org

Christina M. Christie, President
Shannon McCarty-Caplan, Vice President
Mike Koehler, CEO
Angela Taylor, Director of Programs

The Lewy Body Dementia Association (LBDA) is a nonprofit organization dedicated to raising awareness of the Lewy body dementias (LBD), supporting people affected by LBD, and promoting scientific advances.

8359 **Mobility International USA**
132 E Broadway
Suite 343
Eugene, OR 97401
541-343-1284
Fax: 541-343-6812
TTY: 541-343-1284
clearinghouse@miusa.org
www.miusa.org

Susan Sygall, Chief Executive Officer
Cindy Lewis, Director, Programs

A US based national nonprofit organization dedicated to empowering people with disabilities around the world through leadership development, training and international exchange to ensure inclusion of people with disabilities in international exchange and development programs. The National Clearinghouse on Disability & Exchange, a joint project managed by MIUSA, provides free information and referrals.

8360 **Multiple Sclerosis Association of America**
375 Kings Hwy N
Cherry Hill, NJ 08034
800-532-7667
Fax: 856-661-9797
msaa@mymsaa.org
mymsaa.org/

John McCorry, Chair
Monica Derbes Gibson, Vice Chair
Steve Bruneau, Treasurer
Ira M. Levee, Esq., Secretary

MSAA is a national non-profit organization dedicated to enriching the quality of life for evryone affected by Multiple Sclerosis through vital services and support.

8361 **Multiple Sclerosis Foundation**
6520 N. Andrews Ave
Fort Lauderdale, FL 33309-2132
954-776-6805
800-225-6495
Fax: 954-938-8708
admin@msfocus.org
www.msfocus.org

Jules Kuperberg, Executive Director
Alan Segaloff, Co- Executive Director
Kasey Minnis, Director, Operations & Communications
Natalie Blake, Director, Programs & Services

A national, nonprofit organization that provides free support services and public education for persons with Multiple Sclerosis, newsletters, toll-free phone support, information, referrals, home care, assitive technology, and support groups.

8362 **NBIA Disorders Association**
2082 Monaco Ct.
El Cajon, CA 92019-4235
619-588-2315
Fax: 619-588-4093
info@NBIAdisorders.org
www.nbiadisorders.org

Patricia Wood, President
Coleen Lukoff, Development Director
Melissa Woods, Social Media Director
Mike Cohn, Director of Adult Programs

NBIA provides support to families, educates the public and accelerates research with collaborators from around the world.

8363 **National Association for Continence**
P.O. Box 1019
Charleston, SC 29402
800-252-3337
sgregg@nafc.org
www.nafc.org

Katherine F. Jeter, EdD, Founder
Steven G. Gregg, PhD, Executive Director
Donna Deng, Chairperson
Lori Lyons-Willams, Vice Chairperson

NAFC's mission is to educate the public about the causes, diagnosis, categories, treatment options and management alternatives for incontinence, voiding dysfunction and related pelvic floor disorders; to network with other organizations and agencies; to elevate the visibility and priority given to these areas; and to advocate on behalf of consumers who suffer from such symptoms as a result of disease or other illness.

8364 **National Center for Health, Physical Activity and Disability**
4000 Ridgeway Dr.
Birmingham, AL 35209
800-900-8086
Fax: 205-313-7475
email@nchpad.org
www.nchpad.org

James Rimmer, Principal Investigator
Angela Grant, Business Manager
Jeff Underwood, Program Director
Amy Rauworth, Associate Director

NCHPAD Promotes health for people with disability through increased participation in all types of physical and social activities. These include fitness and aquatic activities, recreational and sports programs, adaptive equipment usage, and more.

8365 **National Coalition for Assistive and Rehab Technology**
54 Towhee Court
East Amhurst, NY 14051
716-839-9728
Fax: 716-839-9624
info@ncart.us
www.ncart.us

Don Clayback, Executive Director
Doug Westerdahl, President
Greg Packer, Vice President
Seth Johnson, Secretary/Treasurer

The coalition's mission is to ensure proper and appropriate access to complex rehab and assistive technologies.

8366 **National Council on Independent Living**
2013 H St. NW
6th Floor
Washington, DC 20006
202-207-0334
844-778-7961
Fax: 202-207-0341
TTY: 202-207-0340
ncil@ncil.org
www.ncil.org

Kelly Buckland, Executive Director
Tim Fuchs, Director, Operations
Cara Liebowitz, Coordinator, Development
Eleanor Canter, Coordinator, Communications

A national cross-disability grassroots organization, NCIL advances independent living and the rights of people with disabilities through consumer-driven advocacy.

8367 **National Fibromyalgia Association**
3857 Birch St.
Suite 312
Newport Beach, CA 92660
nfa@fmaware.org
www.fmaware.org

Lynne Matallana, President/Founder
National Fibromyalgia Association's mission is to develop and execute programs dedicated to improving the quality of life for people with fibromyalgia.

8368 **National Mobility Equipment Dealers Association**
3327 West Bearss Ave
Tampa, FL 33618
813-264-2697
866-948-8341
Fax: 813-962-8970
info@nmeda.org
www.nmeda.com

Chad Blake, President
Richard May, Vice President
Bill Koeblitz, Secretary
Jud DeMott, Treasurer
The National Mobility Equipment Dealers Association (NMEDA) is a non-profit trade association dedicated creating and expanding oppotunities of safe transportation for people with disabilities in vehicles modified to fit their specific needs.

8369 **National Spasmodic Dysphonia Association**
300 Park Blvd.
Suite 335
Itasca, IL 60143
800-795-6732
Fax: 630-250-4505
nsda@dysphonia.org
www.dysphonia.org

Charlie Reavis, President
Marcia Sterling, Treasurer
Kimberly Kuman, Executive Director
The National Spasmodic Dysphonia Association (NSDA) is a not-for-profit organization dedicated to advancing medical research into the causes of and treatments for SD, promoting physician and public awareness of the disorder, and providing support to those affected by SD through symposiums, support groups, and on-line resources.

8370 **National Spasmodic Torticollis Association**
9920 Talbert Ave
Fountain Valley, CA 92708
714-378-9837
800-487-8385
NSTAmail@aol.com
www.torticollis.org

Ken Price, President/Treasurer
Diane Truong, Vice President
Janelle Lazzo, Secretary
The mission of the National Spasmodic Torticollis Association is to support the needs and well being of individuals affected by Spasmodic Torticollis; to promote awareness and education; and to advance research for more treatments and a cure.

8371 **Paralyzed Veterans of America**
801 18th St. NW
Washington, DC 20006-3517
800-424-8200
TTY: 800-795-4327
info@pva.org
www.pva.org

David Zurfluh, National President
Charles Brown, National Senior Vice President
Carl Blake, Executive Director
Shaun Castle, Deputy Executive Director
A national organization serving veterans and individuals with spinal cord injury/disorder (SCI/D), as well as their family members and caregivers.

8372 **Parkinson's Disease Research Society**
Northwestern Medicine Central DuPage Hospital
25 N. Winfield Rd
4 North Tower
Winfield, IL 60190
630-933-4384
Fax: 630-933-3077
parkinsonsprogress.org

Carol A. Santi, President
Alex Katz, Vice President
Mitchell King, Treasurer
Cacilia Reich Masover, Secretary
The PDRS mandate is to mount a concerted effort to intensify the research, both in the basic science laboratory as well as with clinical trials, to advance the diagnosis, treatment and prevention of Parkinson's disease.

8373 **Simon Foundation for Continence**
P.O. Box 815
Wilmette, IL 60091
847-864-3913
800-237-4666
Fax: 847-864-9758
webmaster@simonfoundation.org
www.simonfoundation.org

Cheryl B. Gartley, Founder/President
Elizabeth A. LaGro, Vice President, Communications & Education Services
Twila Yednock, Director of Special Events
The Simon Foundation is known throughout the world for its innovative educational projects and tireless efforts on behalf of people with loss of bladder and bowel control. The mission of the foundation is to remove the stigma surrounding incontinence and to provide help for people with incontinence, their families, and the healthcare professionals who provide care for people with incontinence.

8374 **Society for Progressive Supranuclear Palsy**
30 E. Padonia Road,
Suite 201
Timonium, MD 21093
800-457-4777
Fax: 410-785-7009
info@curepsp.org
www.psp.org

Janet Edmunson, Med, Chair
Dan Johnson, Vice-Chair
George S. Jankiewicz, CPA, CFP, Treasurer
John T. Burhoe, Secretary
Members of the Board of Directors of CurePSP accept the major responsibility of implementing the mission of the Foundation for PSP | CBD and Related Brain Diseases. Board members are actively involved in continually defining and redefining the mission and participating in strategic planning to review purposes, programs, priorities, funding needs, and levels of achievement.

8375 **United Spinal Association**
120-34 Queens Blvd
Ste 320
Kew Gardens, NY 11415
718-803-3782
Fax: 718-803-0414
www.unitedspinal.org

8376 **Vermont Back Research Center**
1 S Prospect St
Burlington, VT 05405
802-656-3131
Fax: 802-660-9243
learn@uvm.edu
www.uvm.edu

8377 **World Chiropractic Alliance**
2683 Via De La Valle
Suite G 629
Del Mar, CA 92014
480-786-9235
866-789-8073
Fax: 480-732-9313
www.worldchiropracticalliance.org

Linda Bevel, Manager
Terry A Rondberg DC, Founder/CEO
The World Chiropractic Alliance was founded in 1989 as a non-profit organization dedicated to protecting and strengthening chiropractic around the world. Since its inception, the WCA has played an important role in the global chiropractic community. In 1998, it was granted status as a Non-Governmental Orga-

nization (NGO) associated with the United Nations Department of Public Information.

Camps

8378 **Camp Esperanza**
Southern California Chapter
West 6th Street
Suite 1250
Los Angeles, CA 90017
323-954-5760
800-954-2873
Fax: 213-954-5790
jziegler@arthritis.org
www.arthritis.org

Jennifer Ziegler, Camp Director
Lindsey Gonzales, Regional Director, Human Resources
Manuel Loya, Chief Executive Officer
Teri Lim, Chief Marketing Officer

A one-week camp in August that allows children with arthritis to participate in such activities as horseback riding, swimming, etc. in a fun-filled environment.

8379 **Easterseals Camp Stand by Me**
Easterseals Washington
17809 S Vaughn Rd. NW
PO Box 289
Vaughn, WA 98394
253-884-2722
campadmin@wa.easterseals.com
www.easterseals.com/washington

Cathy Bisaillon, President & CEO
Angela Cox, Camp Director

Camp Stand By Me provides a safe, barrier-free environment for children and adults with any disability to experience all aspects of camp without limitations. Respite weekends offered throughout the year. Activities include campfires, fishing, swimming, sports, archery, and more.

8380 **Hillcroft Services**
501 W Air Park Dr.
Muncie, IN 47303
765-284-4166
www.hillcroft.org

Debbie Bennett, President & CEO
Abby Halstead, Chief Financial Officer
Jessica Hammett, Chief Operations Officer
Dan Wolfert, Vice President, Development & Marketing

Offers a summer camp program for children with autism spectrum disorders.

8381 **Illinois Wheelchair Sport Camps**
University of Illinois
1207 S Oak St.
Champaign, IL 61820
217-333-1970
Fax: 217-244-0014
sportscamp@illinois.edu
www.disability.illinois.edu/camps

8382 **Rising Treetops at Oakhurst**
111 Monmouth Rd.
Oakhurst, NJ 07755
732-531-0215
Fax: 732-531-0292
info@risingtreetops.org
www.risingtreetops.org

Robert Pacenza, Executive Director
Charles Sutherland, Camp Director
Lori Schenck, Assistant Director, Services

A summer and day camp for adults and children with special needs, including autism and physical and intellectual disabilities. Campers experience traditional camp activities while gaining skills for greater independence.

8383 **Twin Lakes Camp**
1451 E Twin Lakes Rd
Hillsboro, IN 47949-8004
765-798-4000
outdoors@twinlakescamp.com
www.twinlakescamp.com

Jon Beight, Executive Director
Duane Bush, Guest Service
Dan Daily, Program Director
Donna Beight, Secretary

Provides a summer camp program for special needs children and young adults. Campers suffer from a wide range of maladies including crippling accidents, Spina Bifida, epilepsy, Cerebral Palsy, Muscular Dystrophy, Quadriplegia, Paraplegia, and other disabling diseases. Campers range in age from 8 to 27.

8384 **YMCA Camp Fitch**
12600 Abels Rd.
North Springfield, PA 16430
814-922-3219
877-863-4824
Fax: 814-922-7000
registrar@campfitchymca.org
campfitchymca.org

Tom Parker, Executive Director
Joe Wolnik, Summer Camp Director
Brandy Duda, Outdoor Education Director
Hannah Kight, Office Manager

Camp is located in North Springfield, Pennsylvania. Camp programs include sessions for children with diabetes or epilepsy.

Books

8385 **Adapted Physical Education and Sport**
Human Kinetics, Inc.
1607 N Market Street
Champaign, IL 61820-2220
217-351-5076
800-747-4457
Fax: 217-351-1549
info@hkusa.com
www.naspem.org

Joseph P Winnick EdD, Author
Scott Kimberly, Owner
Rainer Martens, President/Treasurer
Jill Wikgren, COO

Designed as a resource for both present and future physical education leaders, this book is an exceptional book for teaching exceptional children. It emphasizes the physical education of young people with disabilities. *$68.00*

592 pages Hardcover
ISBN 0-736052-16-X

8386 **Arthritis Bible**
Inner Traditions - Bear & Company
PO Box 388
Rochester, VT 05767-0388
802-767-3174
800-246-8648
Fax: 802-767-3726
customerservice@innertraditions.com
www.innertraditions.com

Craig Weatherby, Author
Leonid Gordin MD, Co-Author

A comprehensive guide to the alternative therapies and conventional treatments for Arthritic diseases including Osteoarthritis, Rheumatoid Arthritis, Gout, Fibromyalgia and more. *$16.95*

272 pages Paperback 1999
ISBN 0-892818-25-5

8387 **Arthritis Helpbook: A Tested Self Management Program for Coping with Arthritis**
Da Capo Press
44 Farnsworth Street,
Boston, MA 02210
617-252-5200
Fax: 617-252-5265
www.dacapopress.com

Kate Lorig, Author
James Fries, Co-Author

The Arthritis Helpbook is the world's leading guide to coping with joint pain, and has been used by more than 600,000 readers over its twenty years in print. It succeeds because of its tested advice, its hundreds of useful hints, and its emphasis on self-management-helping people with arthritis and fibromyalgia to achieve their own health goals. *$18.95*

Paperback
ISBN 0-738210-38-2

8388 Arthritis Sourcebook
McGraw-Hill Professional
7500 Chavenelle Rd
Dubuque, IA 52002-9655
563-584-6000
877-833-5524
Fax: 614-759-3749
www.mhprofessional.com
Earl J Brewer Jr MD, Author
Kathy Cochran Angel, Co-Author
A comprehensive guide to the latest information on treatments, medications, and alternative therapies for arthritis. *$16.95*
272 pages Paperback
ISBN 0-737303-81-6

8389 Arthritis, What Exercises Work: Breakthrough Relief for the Rest of Your Life
MacMillan - St. Martin's Press
175 5th Ave
New York, NY 10010-7703
646-307-5151
Fax: 212-420-9314
press.inquiries@macmillanusa.com
www.us.macmillan.com
Dava Sorbel, Author
Arthur C Klein, Co-Author
What is the most powerful arthritis treatment ever developed to help restore you to a healthy, pain-free, and vigorous life—for the rest of your life? It's exercise. Here are the right exercised for your kind of arthritis, pain-level, age, occupation, and hobbies. *$14.99*
200 pages Paperback 1995
ISBN 0-312130-25-2

8390 Arthritis: A Take Care of Yourself Health Guide
Da Capo Press
44 Farnsworth Street,
Boston, MA 02210
617-252-5200
Fax: 617-252-5265
www.dacapopress.com
James F Fries, Author
Donald M Vickery, Co-Author
In this updated book the author draws on new research to recommend exercises and new pain medications for both arthritis and fibromyalgia. *$18.95*
Paperback 1909
ISBN 0-738202-25-8

8391 Disability and Sport
Human Kinetics, Inc.
1607 N Market Street
Champaign, IL 61820-2220
217-351-5076
800-747-4457
Fax: 217-351-1549
info@hkusa.com
www.naspem.org
Karen P DePauw, Author
Susan J Gavron, Co-Author
Scott Kimberley, Owner
Rainer Martens, President/Treasurer
Provides a comprehensive and practical look at the past, present, and future of disability sport. Topics covered are inclusive of youth through adult participation with in-depth coverage of the essential issues involving athletes with disabilities. This new edition has updated references and new chapter-opening outlines that assist with individual study and class discussions. *$48.00*
408 pages Hardcover
ISBN 0-736046-38-0

8392 Fitness Programming for Physical Disabilities
Human Kinetics, Inc.
1607 N Market Street
Champaign, IL 61820-2220
217-351-5076
800-747-4457
Fax: 217-351-1549
info@hkusa.com
www.naspem.org
Patricia D Miller, Editor
Scott Kimberley, Owner
Rainer Martens, President/Treasurer
Jill Wikgren, COO
A book offering information for developing and conducting exercise programs for groups that included people with physical disabilities. A dozen authorities in exercise science and adapted exercise programming explain how to effectively and safely modify existing programs for individuals with physical disabilities. *$42.00*
232 pages Paperback
ISBN 0-873224-34-5

8393 Freedom from Arthritis Through Nutrition
Tree of Life Publications
PO Box 126
Joshua Tree, CA 92252-0126
760-366-2937
Fax: 760-366-2937
www.treelifebooks.com
Philip J Welsh DDS ND, Author
Bianca Leonardo ND, Co-Author
Reveals the results of 60 years of research on arthritis by noted nutritionist, Dr. Philip J. Welsh, D.D.S. N.D. Here you will find simple, natural, inexpensive, tested ways of coping with the various forms of arthritis, using only nutrition and other natural methods. There are no drugs or gadgets in this program. *$24.95*
255 pages Softcover

8394 Functional Electrical Stimulation for Ambulation by Paraplegics
Krieger Publishing Company
1725 Krieger Drive
PO Box 9542
Malabar, FL 32950
321-724-9542
800-724-0025
Fax: 321-951-3671
info@krieger-publishing.com
www.krieger-publishing.com
Daniel Graupe, Author
Kate H Kohn, Co-Author
FES is employed to enable spinal cord injury patients who are complete paraplegics to stand and ambulate without bracing. The text covers 12 years of amulation experience. *$49.50*
210 pages Paperback 1994
ISBN 0-894648-45-4

8395 Guide to Managing Your Arthritis
Arthritis Foundation
1330 W. Peachtree St
Suite 100
Atlanta, GA 30309
404-872-7100
800-283-7800
Fax: 404-237-8153
AFOrders@pbd.com
www.arthritis.org
Mary Anne Dunkin, Author
John Klippel, President/CEO
Cecile Perich, Chairman
William Brackney, Vice Chair
Expert reviewers answer questions about basic arthritis facts, treatments, research, surgery and more. Also, specific information about six common conditions: rheumatoid arthritis, osteoarthritis, osteoporosis, fibromyalgia, lupus and gout. *$9.95*
193 pages Paperback
ISBN 0-912423-28-5

8396 How to Deal with Back Pain and Rheumatoid Joint Pain: A Preventive and Self Treatment Manua
Global Health Solutions
2146 Kings Garden Way
Falls Church, VA 22043-2593
703-848-2333
800-759-3999
Fax: 703-848-0028
information@watercure.com
www.watercure.com
Fereydoon Batmanghelidj, Author
Xiaopo Batmanjhelidj, President
Kristin Swan, Administrator
The physiology of pain production and its direct relationship to chronic regional dehydration of some joint spaces is explained: Special movements that would create vacuum in the disc spaces

and draw water and the displaced discs into the vertebral joints are demonstrated. *$14.95*

100 pages Paperback

ISBN 0-962994-20-0

8397 Inclusive Games

Human Kinetics
1607 N Market Street
PO Box 5076
Champaign, IL 61825- 5076
217-351-5076
800-747-4457
Fax: 217-351-1549
info@hkusa.com
www.humankinetics.com

Susan L Kasser, Author
Scott Kimberley, Owner
Rainer Martens, President/Treasurer
Jill Wikgren, COO

Features more than 50 games, helpful illustrations, and hundreds of game variations. The book shows how to adapt games so that children of every ability level can practice, play and improve their movement skills together. The game finder makes it easy to locate an appropriate game according to its name, approximate grade level, difficulty within the grade level, skills required/developed, and number of players. *$17.95*

120 pages Paperback

ISBN 0-873226-39-9

8398 Inside The Halo and Beyond: The Anatomy of a Recovery

WW Norton & Company
500 5th Ave
New York, NY 10110-2
212-354-5500
Fax: 212-869-0856
www.wwnorton.com

Maxine Kumin, Author
W Drake McFeely, Chairman/President
Stephen King, VP Finance/CFO
Robert Weil, VP/Executive Editor

A skilled horsewoman and lifelong athlete, poet Kumin was 73 when a riding accident left her with two broken vertebrae in her neck. Kumin survived in the face of overwhelming odds that she would be paralyzed for the rest of her life. Miraculously, however, she was walking again within weeks of the accident; now, though one hand and an arm remain partially immobilized, her life has largely resumed its normal course. Here is the journal of her first nine months of recovery. *$13.95*

192 pages Softcover

ISBN 0-393049-00-0

8399 Life on Wheels: For the Active Wheelchair User

Patient-Centered Guides
1005 Gravenstein Hwy North
Sebastopol, CA 95472-2811
707-827-7000
800-998-9938
Fax: 707-829-0104
order@oreilly.com
www.oreilly.com

Gary Karp, Author

For 1.5 million Americans, life includes a wheelchair for mobility. Life on Wheels is for people who want to take charge of their life experience. Author Gary Karp describes medical issues (paralysis, circulation, rehab, cure research); day-to-day living (exercise, skin, bowel and bladder, sexuality, home access, maintaining a wheelchair); and social issues (self-image, adjustment, friends, family, cultural attitudes, activism). *$24.95*

565 pages Paperback 1999

ISBN 1-565922-53-0

8400 Paralysis Resource Guide

Christopher and Dana Reeve Paralysis Resource Ctr
636 Morris Turnpike
Suite 3A
Short Hills, NJ 07078
973-467-8270
800-539-7309
Fax: 973-912-9433
information@christopherreeve.org
www.paralysis.org

John M. Hughes, Chairman
John E. McConnell, Vice Chair
Matthew Reeve, Vice Chair
Peter T. Wilderotter, President

A comprehensive information tool for people affected by paralysis and for those who care for them. English or Spanish.

336 pages

8401 Primer on the Rheumatic Diseases

Arthritis Foundation
1330 W. Peachtree St
Suite 100
Atlanta, GA 30309-2111
404-872-7100
800-933-7023
Fax: 404-237-8153
AFOrders@pbd.com
www.arthritis.org

Rob Shaw, President
Patience White M.D., Editor
John H. Klippel, Editor

The leading professional book about arthritis and related diseases, the Primer is published by Springer and the Arthritis Foundation. *$79.95*

724 pages Softcover

ISBN 0-387356-64-8

8402 Sport Science Review: Adapted Physical Activity

Human Kinetics
1607 N Market Street
Champaign, IL 61820-2220
217-351-5076
800-747-4457
Fax: 217-351-1549
info@hkusa.com
www.naspem.org

Rainer Martens, President/Treasurer
Scott Kimberley, Owner
Jill Wikgren, COO

This issue of Sport Science Review examines the newly emerging academic discipline of adapted physical activity. Researchers from diverse academic backgrounds and parts of the world review the issues and controversies surrounding inclusion in physical education and sport. *$15.00*

96 pages Paperback

ISBN -073602-07-9

8403 Still Me

Random House
1745 Broadway
3rd Floor
New York, NY 10019-4305
212-782-9000
Fax: 212-572-6066
vintageanchor@randomhouse.com
www.randomhouse.com

Christopher Reeve, Author
Markus Dohle, Chairman/CEO
Madeline McIntosh, President
Andrew Weber, SVP Operations

The man who was Superman begins with his debilitating riding accident, then weaves back and forth between past and present, creating a thorough biography of Reeve's life. *$7.99*

336 pages Paperback 1999

ISBN 0-345432-41-4

8404 **When Your Student Has Arthritis**
Arthritis Foundation
2970 Peachtree Rd NW
PO Box 932915, Ste 200
Atlanta, GA 31193-2915
404-237-8771
800-933-7023
Fax: 404-237-8153
aforders@arthritis.org
www.afstore.org

Rob Shaw, President
An overview of arthritis, including juvenile rhuematoid arthritis and treatment. Also includes a school activities checklist for students, education rights, and how teachers can help.
28 pages

8405 **Yoga for Fibromyalgia: Move, Breathe, and Relax to Improve Your Quality of Life**
Mobility Limited
PO Box 838
Morro Bay, CA 93443-0838
805-772-3560
800-366-6038
Fax: 805-772-4717
shsh@mobilityltd.com
www.mobilityltd.com

Shoosh Lettick Crotzer, Director
The first book devoted exclusively to managing the symptoms of fibromyalgia; the comprehensive program of 26 illustrated poses, breathing techniques, and guided visualization and relaxation sessions can be practiced regardless of age or experience. The Living with Fibromyalgia section discusses lifestyle concerns.
$14.95
128 pages 1908

Journals

8406 **Topics in Spinal Cord Injury Rehabilitation**
American Spinal Injury Association
9702 Gayton Rd.
Suite 306
Richmond, VA 23238
877-274-2724
asia.office@asia-spinalinjury.org
www.asia-spinalinjury.org

Patty Duncan, Executive Director
Carolyn Moffatt, Association Manager
Kim Ruff, Administrative Assistant
Clinical, peer-reviewed information for physiatrists, PTs, OTs, rehabilitation nurses, psychologists, neurologists, orthopedists, and others.

Magazines

8407 **Arthritis Today**
Arthritis Foundation
1330 W. Peachtree St.
Suite 100
Atlanta, GA 30309
404-872-7100
800-933-7023
Fax: 404-237-8153
info.ga@arthritis.org
www.arthritis.org

Dan McGowan, Chairman
Rowland W. Chang, Vice Chair
Ann M. Palmer, President and CEO
Patricia N. Nelson, Secretary
Magazine for patients, physicians, public authorities and others with an interest in the field of arthritis. (Price noted paid for yearly subscription) *$12.95*
Bi-Monthly

8408 **Fibromyalgia AWARE Magazine**
National Fibromyalgia Association
2121 S Towne Centre Pl
suite 30
Orange, CA 92865-6124
714-921-0150
Fax: 714-921-6920
fmaware.org

Lynne Matallana, Editor In Chief
Malina Anderson, CFO
Eroll Landy, Treasurer
Addresses the needs and concerns of people affected by fibromyalgia and overlapping conditions. *$35.00*
3 times a year

8409 **New Mobility**
Leonard Media Group
75-20 Astoria Blvd.
East Elmhurst, NY 11370-2068
215-675-9133
800-404-2898
888-850-0344
Fax: 215-675-9376
jeff@leonardmedia.com
www.newmobility.com

Jean Dobbs, Publisher & Editorial Director
Josie Byzek, Executive Editor
Tim Gilmer, Editor Emeritus
Ian Ruder, Senior Editor
The full-service, full-color lifestyle magazine for the disability community. The award-winning magazine is contemporary, witty and candid. Produced by professional journalists and visual artists, the magazine's voice is uncompromising and unsentimental, yet practical, knowing and friendly. The magazine covers issues that matter to readers: medical news, and cure research; jobs, benefits and civil rights; sports, recreation and travel; product news, technology and innovation. *$27.95*
Monthly

8410 **PALAESTRA: Forum of Sport, Physical Education and Recreation for Those with Disabilities**
Challenge Publications Limited
1807 N. Federal Drive
Urbana, IL 61801
217-359-5940
800-327-5557
Fax: 217-359-5975
www.palaestra.com

David P Beaver EdD, Fonding Editor
Martin.E Block, Editor-in-Chief
Julian U. Stein, Associate Editor
Kathleen Stanton, Asst. Editors
The most comprehensive resource on sport, physical education and recreation for individuals with disabilities, their parents and professionals in the field of adapted physical activity. Published in cooperation with US Paralympics and AAHPERD's Adapted Physical Activity Council. Informative yet entertaining and delivers valuable insights for consumers, families and professionals in the field. Published quarterly.

8411 **PN/Paraplegia News**
PVA Publications
2111 E Highland Ave
Suite 180
Phoenix, AZ 85016-4702
602-224-0500
888-888-2201
Fax: 602-224-0507
www.pn-magazine.com

Richard Hoover, Editor
Ann Santos, Assistant Editor
Packed with timely information on spinal-cord-injury research, new products, legislation that impacts people with disabilities, accessible travel, computer options, car/van adaptations, news for veterans, housing, employment, health care and all issues affecting wheelers and caregivers around the world.

8412 **Spirit Magazine**
Special Olympics International
1133 19th St NW
Washington, DC 20036-3604
202-628-3630
Fax: 202-824-0200
info@specialolympics.org
www.specialolympics.org

Kathy Smallwood, Editor
Timothy P Shriver PhD, Chariman/CEO
J Brady Lum, President/COO

This magazine reflects the power of Special Olympics to build bridges between people with and without intellectual disabilities and spark personal insight, compassion and gratitude for life.
Quarterly

8413 **Strides Magazine**
North American Riding for the Handicapped Assoc
7475 Dakin Street
Suite 600
Denver, CO 80221-6920
303-452-1212
800-369-7433
Fax: 303-252-4610

Carol Nickell, CEO
Sheila Dietrich, Executive Director
William Scebbi, CEO

This engaging magazine is a non-technical, yet accurate journal that focuses on the work of NARHA. Rider profiles, how-to articles, editorials and instructional columns seek to educate a general readership of the diverse aspects of equine facilitated therapy and activities. Each seasonal issue carries a theme.
Quarterly

8414 **Stroke Connection Magazine**
American Stroke Association
7272 Greenville Ave
Dallas, TX 75231-5129
214-373-6300
888-478-7653
Fax: 214-706-1191
www.strokeassociation.org

Ralph Sacco, President/Director
Nancy Brown, CEO
Debra Lockwood, Chairman

From in-depth information on conditions such as aphasia, central pain, high blood pressure and depression, to tips for daily living from healthcare professionals and other stroke survivors. Stroke Connection keeps you abreast of how to cope, how to reduce your risk of stroke and how to make the most of each day.
6 issues

Newsletters

8415 **A World Awaits You**
Mobility International USA
132 E Broadway
Suite 343
Eugene, OR 97401
541-343-1284
Fax: 541-343-6812
TTY: 541-343-1284
clearinghouse@miusa.org
www.miusa.org

Susan Sygall, Chief Executive Officer
Cindy Lewis, Director, Programs

Includes interviews with people with disabilities who have participated in a wide range of international exchange programs.
Annually

8416 **ABS Newsletter**
American Back Society
2648 International Blvd
Suite 502
Oakland, CA 94601-1547
510-536-9929
Fax: 510-536-1812
info@americanbacksoc.org
www.americanbacksoc.org

Scott Haldeman, President
Aubrey Swartz MD, Executive Director

Keeps subscribers current with timely topics on the diagnosis and treatment of a wide spectrum of painful and disabling conditions of the spine.

8417 **Arthritis Foundation Great West Region**
Arthritis Foundation
115 N.E. 100th St
Suite 350
Seattle, WA 98125
206-547-2707
888-391-9389
Fax: 206-547-2805
tzuehl@arthritis.org
www.arthritis.org

Scott Weaver, CEO
Kelsey Birnbaum, Vice President, Development
Deborah Genge, Vice President, Development
Duane Hille, Development Coordinator

Offers regional updates, information on activities and events, resources and medical research for members.
Newsletter

8418 **Arthritis Update**
Arthritis Foundation
1330 W. Peachtree St.
Suite 100
Atlanta, GA 30309
404-872-7100
info.uny@arthritis.org
www.arthritis.org

Dan McGowan, Chairman
Rowland W. Chang, Vice Chair
Ann M. Palmer, President and CEO
Patricia N. Nelson, Secretary

Offers chapter updates, information on activities and events, resources and medical research for members.
Newsletter

8419 **CurePSP Magazine**
Society for Progressive Supranuclear Palsy
2648 International Blvd
Suite 502
Hunt Valley, MD 21031-1002
410-785-7004
800-457-4777
Fax: 410-785-7009
info@curepsp.org
www.psp.org

Richard Gordon Dyne DMin, President
Janet Edmunson, Chair
Dan Johnson, Vice Chair

Informs readers of findings in the area of PSP.

8420 **EpilepsyUSA Magazine**
Epilepsy Foundation of America
8301 Professional Pl
Landover, MD 20785-2237
301-459-3700
Fax: 301-577-2684
www.epilepsyfoundation.org

Brien J Smith Md, Chair
Mark E Nini, Senior Vice Chair
Richard P Denness, President/CEO
Alexandra K Finucane Esq, Executive Vice President

The Epilepsy Foundation's award-winning magazine, epilepsyUSA, is published online four times a year. The magazine is one of the only publications of its kind devoted entirely to news and up-to-the-minute information about epilepsy.

8421 **Exchange**
ALS Association
27001 Agoura Rd
Suite 250
Agoura Hills, CA 91301-5105
818-340-0182
800-782-4747
Fax: 818-880-9006
www.alsa.org

Gary A Leo, CEO
Morton Charlestein, Chairman
Andrew Soffel, Chairman
Julie Sharpe, Executive Director

Covers a broad range of subjects including stories about the lives of ALS patients, special events, research and public policy in the ALS community.
4-6 times/year

8422 **Fibromyalgia Online**
National Fibromyalgia Association
2121 S Towne Centre Pl
suite 300
Ornage, CA 92865-6124
714-921-0150
Fax: 714-921-6920
www.fmaware.org

Lynne Matallana, President/Editor In Chief
Malina Anderson, CFO
Eroll Landy, Treasurer

An educational resource for patients and healthcare professionals that brings the latest news on fibrmyalgia and overlapping conditions.
Monthly

8423 **Focus**
Arthritis Foundation
1330 W. Peachtree St.
Suite 100
Atlanta, GA 30309
404-872-7100
info.coh@arthritis.org
www.arthritis.org

Dan McGowan, Chairman
Rowland W. Chang, Vice Chair
Ann M. Palmer, President and CEO
Patricia N. Nelson, Secretary

Offers chapter updates, information on activities and events, resources and medical research for members.
Newsletter

8424 **Joint Efforts**
Arthritis Foundation
1330 W. Peachtree St.
Suite 100
Atlanta, GA 30309
404-872-7100
800-464-6240
Fax: 415-356-1240
info.nca@arthritis.org
www.arthritis.org

Dan McGowan, Chairman
Rowland W. Chang, Vice Chair
Ann M. Palmer, President and CEO
Patricia N. Nelson, Secretary

Offers chapter updates, information on activities and events, resources and medical research for members.
Newsletter

8425 **MIUSA's Global Impact Newsletter**
Mobility International USA
132 E Broadway
Suite 343
Eugene, OR 97401
541-343-1284
Fax: 541-343-6812
TTY: 541-343-1284
clearinghouse@miusa.org
www.miusa.org

Susan Sygall, Chief Executive Officer
Cindy Lewis, Director, Programs

Each issue features photos, alumni updates, highlights from recent activities, and new publications.
Quarterly

8426 **Motivator**
Multiple Sclerosis Association of America
706 Haddonfield Rd
Cherry Hill, NJ 8002-2652
856-488-4500
800-532-7667
Fax: 856-661-9797
jmasino@mymsaa.org
www.msassociation.org

Andrea L GriesS, Editor
Susan W Courtney, Sr Writer & Creative Director
Amanda Bednar, Contributing Writer

MSAA's 48-plus page magazine highlights and explains many vital issues of importance to our readers affected by MS. These include cover and feature stories about a variety of topics such as depression, assistive technology, the role of pets and service animals, parents with MS, and clinical trials, to name a few.
48 pages Quarterly

8427 **New York Arthritis Reporter**
New York Chapter of the Arthritis Foundation
122 East 42nd Street
New York, NY 10168-1898
212-984-8700
Fax: 212-878-5960
info.ny@arthritis.org
www.arthritis.org

Phyllis Geraghty, Editor
Ross Alfieri, President
Daniel T. McGowan, Chair

Provides public access to current arthritis information and resources on important health issues.
Quarterly

8428 **SCI Psychosocial Process**
American Assoc of Spinal Cord Injury Psych/Soc Wor
75-20 Astoria Blvd
East Elmhurst, NY 11370
718-803-3782
800-404-2898
Fax: 718-803-0414
info@unitedspinal.org
www.unitedspinal.org

David C. Cooper, Chairman
Patrick W. Maher, Vice Chairman
Joseph Gaskins, President and CEO
Denise A. McQuade, Secretary

The purpose of this e journal is disseminating information of value to psychologists, social workers and other psychological caring for spinal cord injured persons.
2 time a year

8429 **SCILIFE**
National Spinal Cord Injury Association
75-20 Astoria Blvd
East Elmhurst, NY 11370
718-803-3782
800-404-2898
Fax: 718-803-0414
info@spinalcord.org
www.unitedspinal.org

David C. Cooper, Chairman
Patrick W. Maher, Vice Chairman
Joseph Gaskins, President and CEO
Denise A. McQuade, Secretary

Filled with issue-driven articles, and news of interest to the SCI community and the larger disability community.
Bi-monthly

Audio/Visual

8430 **A Wheelchair for Petronilia**
Fanlight Productions C/O Icarus Films
32 Court St.
21st Floor
Brooklyn, NY 11201-1731
718-488-8900
800-876-1710
Fax: 718-488-8642
info@fanlight.com
www.fanlight.com

Bob Gliner, Director
Jonathan Miller, President
Meredith Miller, Sales Manager
Anthony Sweeney, Acquisitions

Profiles a program, organized and run by Guatemalans with disabilities, which trains them to manufacture and repair cheap, sturdy wheelchairs designed for conditions in developing countries. 28 Minutes.
VHS/DVD
ISBN 1-572953-98-5

8431 **Beyond the Barriers**
Aquarius Health Care Videos
30 Forest Road
PO Box 249
Millis, MA 02054
508-376-1244
888-440-2963
Fax: 508-376-1245

Mark Wellman, Director
Leslie Kussmann, President/Producer

For too many years, paraplegics, amputees, quadraplegics and the blind have felt trapped by their disabilities. No more! Mark Wellman and other disabled adventurers, rock climb the desert towers of Utah, sail in British Columbia, body-board the big waves of Pipeline and Waimea Bay, scuba dive with sea lions in Mexico and hand glide the California coast. This film delivers the simple message: Don't give up, and never give in. If you can't ever lose, then you can't ever win. Preview option.
Video/47 Mins

8432 **Breathing Lessons: The Life and Work of Mark O'Brien**
Fanlight Productions C/O Icarus Films
32 Court St.
21st Floor
Brooklyn, NY 11201-1731
718-488-8900
800-876-1710
Fax: 718-488-8642
info@fanlight.com
www.fanlight.com
Jessica Yu, Director
Jonathan Miller, President
Meredith Miller, Sales Manager
Anthony Sweeney, Acquisitions
Breathing Lessons breaks down barriers to understanding by presenting an honest and intimate portrait of a complex, intelligent, beautiful and interesting person, who happens to be disabled. *$225.00*
Video/35 Mins 1996
ISBN 1-572958-41-3

8433 **Complete Armchair Fitness**
CC-M Productions
7755 16th St NW
Washington, DC 20012-1460
202-882-7432
800-453-6280
Fax: 202-882-7432
www.armchairfitness.com
Robert Mason, Manager
Armchair Fitness video series. 4 DVDs: Armchair Fitness Aerobic, Armchair Fitness Gentle, Armchair Fitness Strength and Armchair Fitness Yoga. *$120.00*
Video

8434 **How Come You Walk Funny?**
Fanlight Productions C/O Icarus Films
32 Court St.
21st Floor
Brooklyn, NY 11201-1731
718-488-8900
800-876-1710
Fax: 718-488-8642
info@fanlight.com
www.fanlight.com
Tina Hahn, Director
Jonathan Miller, President
Meredith Miller, Sales Manager
Anthony Sweeney, Acquisitions
Profiles a unique experiment in reverse integration: a school where non disabled kids attend a kindergarten designed for children with physical disabilities. The kids and families tackle their differences and discover common ground through finding a way that all can play. *$179.00*
Video/47 Mins 2004
ISBN 1-572958-84-7

8435 **Key Changes: A Portrait of Lisa Thorson**
Fanlight Productions C/O Icarus Films
32 Court St.
21st Floor
Brooklyn, NY 11201-1731
718-488-8900
800-876-1710
Fax: 718-488-8642
info@fanlight.com
www.fanlight.com
Cindy Marshall, Director
Jonathan Miller, President
Meredith Miller, Sales Manager
Anthony Sweeney, Acquisitions
A documentary profiling Lisa Thorson, a gifted vocalist who uses a wheelchair. Ms. Thorson defines herself as a performer first, a person with a disability second, and this thoughtful portrait respects that distinction. Her work as a jazz singer is at the heart of the film, reflecting her philosophy that the biggest contribution that she can make to the struggle for the rights of people with disabilities is doing her art the best way she can. *$149.00*
Video/28 Mins 1993
ISBN 1-572959-30-4

8436 **Wheelchair Bowling**
American Wheelchair Bowling Association
PO Box 69
Clover, VA 24534-69
434-454-2269
Fax: 434-454-6276
garyryan210@gmail.com
www.awba.org
Dick Schaaf, Author
Dave Roberts, Executive Secretary Treasurer
In addition to providing historical background, it includes principles of the game from keeping score through ball drilling for the wheelchair bowler. Through profiles of wheelchair bowlers, the text covers ball delivery, spare making techniques and special equipment that can be used. *$9.95*
96 pages

8437 **Yoga for Arthritis**
Mobility Limited
601 Morro Bay Blvd
Suite E
Morro Bay, CA 93442-2000
805-772-3560
800-366-6038
Fax: 805-772-4717
shsh@mobilityltd.com
www.mobilityltd.com
Shoosh Crotzer, Owner/Executive Director
A yoga-based program with five separate segments, which includes breathing and relaxation techniques, stretching and strengthening routines, and aerobic exercises. This 52-minute program can also be performed seated. Available on DVD or VHS; DVD includes Spanish version. *$19.95*
Video

8438 **Yoga for MS and Related Conditions**
Mobility Limited
601 Morro Bay Blvd
Suite E
Morro Bay, CA 93442-2000
805-772-3560
800-366-6038
Fax: 805-772-4717
shsh@mobilityltd.com
www.mobilityltd.com
Shoosh Crotzer, Owner/Executive Director
A yoga-based program. Shows assisted versions of each exercise for those who require it; is available with an optional Instructional Guidebook with illustrations, alternative positions, and hints. This 48-minute program can also be performed seated. Available on DVD or VHS; DVD includes Spanish version. *$19.95*
Video

Sports

8439 **Access to Sailing**
423 E Shoreline Village Drive
Long Beach, CA 90802
562-901-9999
www.accesstosailing.org
Duncan Milne, Founder/Executive Director
Cliff Larson, Director
Gaile Oslapas, Assistant Director
Provides therapeutic rehabilitation to disabled and disadvantaged children and adults, through interactive sailing outings.

8440 **Achilles Track Club**
42 West 38th Street
Suite 400
New York, NY 10018-6241
212-354-0300
Fax: 212-354-3978
Richard Traum PhD, President/Founder
Mary Bryant, Vice President
Kathleen Bateman, Director

Organization whose goal is to guide disabled athletes into the able-bodied community.

8441 Adaptive Sports Center
PO Box 1639
Crested Butte, CO 81224-1639
970-349-2296
866-349-2296
Fax: 970-349-2077
info@adaptivesports.org
www.adaptivesports.org

Christopher Hensley, Executive Director
Chris Read, CTRS Program Director
Ella Fahrlander, Development Director
Erin English, Marketing/Communications Dir.

Year round adaptive, adventure recreation program located at the base of Crested Butte Mountain Resort, Crested Butte ,CO. The Adaptive Sports Centers provides adaptive downhill and cross country ski lessons, ski rentals and snowboarding lessons in the winter. Offers a variety of wilderness based programs in the summer including multi-day trips into the back country, extensive cycling programs, canoeing, and white water rafting.

8442 American Wheelchair Bowling Association
PO Box 69
Clover, VA 24534-69
434-454-2269
Fax: 434-454-6276
garyryan210@gmail.com
www.awba.org

Joseph L. Fox, Chairman
Wayne Webber, Vice Chairperson
Paul Kenney, Treasurer
Gary Rayan, Secretary

A non-profit organization, composed of wheelchair bowlers, dedicated to encouraging, developing, and regulating wheelchair bowling and wheelchair bowling leagues.

8443 Chesapeake Region Accessible Boating
177 Defense Hwy.
Suite 9
Annapolis, MD 21401
410-266-5722
info@crabsailing.org
crabsailing.org

Brad La Tour, President
Paul Bollinger, Executive Director
Sarah Winchester, Operations Manager
George Pappas, Co-Fleet Director

Chesapeake Region Accessible Boating (CRAB) provides opportunities for the disabled and their friends to sail the Chesapeake Bay. Programs include group sails for organizations representing special guests, sailing clinics and camps, SailFree Sundays for families, and regattas for those who wish to race.

8444 Disabled Sports Program Center
Disabled Sports USA Far West
PO Box 9780
Truckee, CA 96162-7780
530-581-4161
Fax: 530-581-3127

Doug Pringle, President
Marilyn Cummings, Office Manager
Haakon Lang-Ree, Manager

Founded in 1967, Disabled Sports USA Far West is dedicated to innovative programs that provide an environment with positive therapeutic and psychological outcomes. Individuals are empowered to reach their full potential. Our programs allow individuals of all abilities to discover their own strengths and interests.

8445 Disabled Sports USA
451 Hungerford Dr
Suite 100
Rockville, MD 20850-5102
301-217-0960
Fax: 301-217-0968
www.disabledsportsusa.org

Kirk Bauer, Executive Director
Kathy Chandler, Executive Director
Kathy Celo, Operations
Kathy Laffey, Special Projects Manager

Provides year-round sports and recreation opportunities for people with physical disabilities, veterans and non-veterans alike, such as sanctioned regional and national events in alpine and Nordic skiing, cycling, shooting swimming, table tennis, track and field, volleyball, and weightlifiting. The organization handles physical disabilities which restrict mobility, including amputations paraplegia, quadriplegia, cerebral palsy, head injury, mulitple sclerosis, muscular dystrophy, and more.

8446 Disabled Watersports Program
Mission Bay Aquatic Center
1001 Santa Clara Pl
San Diego, CA 92109
858-488-1000
Fax: 858-488-9625
mbac@sdsu.edu
www.missionbayaquaticcenter.com

Kevin Starw, Director
Kevin Waldick, Asst. director
Eric Fehrs, Maintenance Director
Amanda Burgess, Office Supervisor

Devoted to providing accessible water sports and recreational opportunities for individuals with disabilities. Specially designed equipment makes water skiing, wake boarding, keelboat sailing, windsurfing, rowing, surfing, and kayaking possible for people with varying levels of mobility and ability.

8447 Galvin Health and Fitness Center
Rehabilitation Institute of Chicago
345 East Suuperior St.
Chicago, IL 60611
312-238-1000
800-354-7342
800-354-REHA
Fax: 312-238-5017
sports@ric.org
http://www.ric.org

Jude Reyes, Chair
Mike P. Kransy, Vice Chair
Thomas Reynolds III, Vice Chair
Joanne C. Smith, President & CEO

The RIC Sports and Fitness Program offers people with physical disabilities an on-site fitness center, specialized exercise classes and services, and adult and junior competitive and recreational sports opportunities, including the recreational/social Caring for Kids program for youth ages 7-17. Most programs are provided free of charge or for a nominal fee.

8448 Guide to Wheelchair Sports and Recreation
Paralyzed Veterans of America
801 18th St. NW
Washington, DC 20006-3517
800-424-8200
TTY: 800-795-4327
info@pva.org
www.pva.org

David Zurfluh, National President
Charles Brown, National Senior Vice President
Carl Blake, Executive Director
Shaun Castle, Deputy Executive Director

This guide lists descriptions of adaptive sports and recreation, activity and equipment directories, and additional resources for people with disabilities.
28 pages Booklet

8449 Handicapped Scuba Association International
Handicapped Scuba Association
1104 El Prado
San Clemente, CA 92672-4637
949-498-4540
Fax: 949-498-6128
www.hsascuba.com

Jim Gatacre, President
Patricia Derk, Vice President

A nonprofit volunteer organization dedicated to improving the physical and social well being of those with special needs through the exhilarating sport of scuba diving. An educational program for able bodied scuba instructors to learn to teach and certify people with special needs. Accessible travel opportunities.

8450 Lakeshore Foundation
4000 Ridgeway Dr
Birmingham, AL 35209-5563
205-313-7400
Fax: 205-313-7475
information@lakeshore.org
www.lakeshore.org

Jeff Underwood, President & CEO
Beth Curry, Chief Program Officer
Jen Remick, Director, Communications & Membership
Damian Veazey, Associate Director, Communications

Promotes independence for persons with physically disabling conditions and provides opportunities to pursue active, healthy lifestyles.

8451 **National Disability Sports Alliance**
25 W Independence Way
Kingston, RI 02881-1124 401-792-7130
Fax: 401-792-7132
http://nationaldisabilitysportsalliance.webs.
Jerry McCole, Executive Director
Serves to present disabled athletes with the opportunity to perform in many different sports. Participants range from the beginning athlete to the elite, international caliber athlete.

8452 **National Skeet Shooting Association**
5931 Roft Rd
San Antonio, TX 78253-9261 210-688-3371
800-877-5338
Fax: 210-688-3014
nsca@nssa-nsca.com
www.mynssa.com
Michael Hampton, Jr., Executive Director
Royce Graff, NSSA Director
Amber Schwarz, NSC Assistant Director
Linda Mayes, NSSA Director
Offers information on sporting clay targets for the disabled hunter.

8453 **National Sports Center for the Disabled**
33 Parsenn Rd
PO Box 1290
Winter Park, CO 80482 970-726-1518
Fax: 970-726-4112
volunteer@nscd.org
nscd.org
Kim Easton, President & CEO
Diane Eustace, Marketing Director
Beth Fox, Outreach & Education Director
Erica Mays, Human Resources Director
The center's mission is to provide quality outdoor sports and therapeutic recreation programs that positively impact the lives of people with physical, cognitive, emotional, or behavioral challenges. Winter programming includes alpine skiing, snowboarding, ski racing, show shoeing, and cross-country skiing. Summer sports include rafting, sailing, kayaking, camping, hiking, horseback riding, fishing, and rock climbing.
6-8 pages Quarterly

8454 **National Wheelchair Poolplayers Association**
90 Flemons Dr
Somerville, AL 35670 256-778-0449
Fax: 703-817-1215
www.nwpainc.org
Jeffrey Dolezal, President
Bob Calderon, Secretary
Ken Force, Editor
Works together with other groups, organizations, and tournaments to update rules to include wheelchair players.

8455 **Ontario Cerebral Palsy Sports Association**
P.O. Box 60082
Ottawa, ON, Canada K1T-0K9 613-723-1806
866-286-2772
Fax: 613-723-6742
Amanda Fader, Executive Director
Don Sinclair, President
Lorette Dupuis, Vice President
Sue Bartol, Development Director
Organization that provides, promotes and coordinates competitive opportunities as well as encourages individual excellence through sport for athletes within the cerebral palsy family. To that end, OCPSA recruits, develops and supports athletes, coaches and volunteers.

8456 **Professional Association of Therapeutic Horsemanship International (PATH Intl.)**
PO Box 33150
Denver, CO 80233 303-452-1212
800-369-7433
Fax: 303-252-4610
pathintl@pathintl.org
www.pathintl.org
Kathy Alm, Chief Executive Officer
Carrie Garnett, Director, Membership & Operations
Kaye Marks, Director, Marketing & Communications
Bret Maceyak, Director, Credentialing
A national nonprofit equestrian organization dedicated to serving individuals with disabilities by giving disabled individuals the opportunity to ride horses. Establishes safety standards, provides continuing education, and offers networking opportunities for both its individuals and center members. Produces educational materials including fact sheets, brochures, booklets, audio-visual tapes, a directory, and PATH Intl. magazine Strides.

8457 **Special Olympics**
1133 19th St NW
Washington, DC 20036-3604 202-393-1251
Fax: 202-715-1146
info@specialolympics.org
www.specialolympics.org
Timothy P Shriver PhD, Chariman/CEO
J Brady Lum, President/COO
Stephen M Carter, Lead Director/CEO/Vice Chair
A year-round worldwide program that promotes physical fitness, sports training and athletic competition for children and adults with intellectual disabilities.

8458 **Special Olympics International**
1133 19th St NW
Washington, DC 20036-3604 202-393-1251
Fax: 202-715-1146
info@specialolympics.org
www.specialolympics.org
Timothy P Shriver PhD, Chariman/CEO
J Brady Lum, President/COO
Stephen M Carter, Lead Director/CEO/Vice Chair
Provides year-round training and athletic competition in a variety of well-coached, Olympic-type sparts for persons with developmental disabilities. Offers opportunities to develop physical fitness, prepare for entry into school and community sports programs. Athletes express courage, experience joy and participate in gifts, skills and friendship with their families and other Special Olympics athletes. Local information can be provided by regional offices.

8459 **US Paralympics**
United States Olympic Committee
1 Olympic Plaza
Colorado Springs, CO 80909 719-866-2030
888-222-2313
Fax: 719-866-2029
www.teamusa.org/us-paralympics
Scott Blackmun, CEO
Alan Ashley, Chief of Sport Performance
Lisa Baird, Chief Marketing Officer
Morane Kerek, Chief Financial Officer
A division of the US Olympic Committee focused on enhancing programs, funding and opportunities for persons with physical disabilities to participate in Paralympic sports.

8460 **United Foundation for Disabled Archers**
20 NE 9th Ave. Glenwood,
PO Box 251
Glenwood, MN 56334- 251 320-634-3660
info@uffdaclub.com
www.uffdaclub.com
Daniel James Hendricks, President
Russ Kalk, Vice President
Debbie Kalk, Treasurer
It is the mission of the United Foundation for Disabled Archers to promote and provide a means to practice all forms of archery for any physically challenged person.

8461 **Wheelchair Sports, USA**
PO Box 5266
Kendall Park, NJ 08824-5266
732-266-2634
Fax: 732-355-6500

Kelly Behlmann, Owner
Gregg Baumgraten, Chairperson
Denise Hutchins, Vice-Chairperson
Jessica Galli, Secretary

Initiates, stimulates and promotes the growth and development of wheelchair sports.

Support Groups

8462 **Information Hotline**
Arthritis Foundation, Southeast Region Inc
1330 W. Peachtree St.
Suite 100
Atlanta, GA 30309
404-872-7100
800-933-7023
Fax: 404-237-8153
info.ga@arthritis.org
www.arthritis.org

Dan McGowan, Chairman
Rowland W. Chang, Vice Chair
Ann M. Palmer, President and CEO
Patricia N. Nelson, Secretary

The mission of the Arthritis Foundation is to improve lives through leadership in the prevention, control and cure of arthritis and related diseases.

8463 **Kids on the Block Programs**
9385 Gerwig Lane
Suite C
Maryland, MD 21157-2893
410-290-9095
800-368-5437
Fax: 410-290-9358
www.kotb.com

Aric Darroe, President
Jane Thuman, Vice President
Christina Grogan, Marketing Manager

Features life-size puppets in educational programs that enlighten children and adults on the issues of disability awareness, medical and educational differences, and social concerns.

General Disorders

New York

1273 **Camp COAST**
Empowering People's Independence (EPI)
2 Townline Circle
Rochester, NY 14623
585-442-4430
Fax: 585-442-6964
info@epiny.org
www.epiny.org

Michael Radell, Camp Director

Camp COAST is a summer camp for young adults ages 18+ with epilepsy and I/DD.

Associations

8464 **AIDS United**
1424 K Street, N.W.
Ste 200
Washington, DC 20005-1511
202-408-4848
888-234-2437
Fax: 202-408-1818
info@aidsunited.org
www.aidsunited.org

Jesse Milan Jr., JD, Interim President & CEO
Matthew J. Kessler, Vice President, Operations
Cody Barnett, Communications Coordinator
Monique Tula, Vice President, Programs

AIDS United advocates for people living with or affected by HIV/AIDS and the organizations that serve them. AIDS United's mission is to end the AIDS epidemic in the United States through strategic grantmaking, capacity building, policy/advocacy, technical assistance and formative research.

8465 **American Academy for Cerebral Palsy and Developmental Medicine**
555 East Wells
Suite 1100
Milwaukee, WI 53202
414-918-3014
Fax: 414-276-2146
info@aacpdm.org
www.aacpdm.org

Tamara Wagester, Executive Director
Erin Trimmer, Senior Meetings Manager
Heather Schrader, Membership & Administrative Manager
Kay Whalen, Managing Partner

Professional health academy offering multidisciplinary scientific education and promoting excellence in research and services in the area of cerebral palsy and other childhood-onset disabilities.

8466 **American Academy of Allergy, Asthma & Immunology**
555 E Wells St.
Ste 1100
Milwaukee, WI 53202-3823
414-272-6071
Fax: 414-272-6070
info@aaaai.org
www.aaaai.org

Thomas A. Fleisher, M.D.; FAAAAI, President

An association of medical professionals and specialists that places focus on research and treatment for allergic and immunologic diseases, as well as improved patient care.

8467 **American Academy of Otolaryngology - Head and Neck Surgery**
1650 Diagonal Rd
Alexandria, VA 22314-2857
703-836-4444
Fax: 703-683-5100
TTY: 703-519-1585
www.entnet.org

James c. Denneny III, M.D., Executive Vice President & CEO
Sujana S. Chandrasekhar, M.D., President
Carol R. Bradford, Director, Academic
Michael D. Seidman, Director, Academic

The American Academy of Otolaryngology-Head and Neck Surgery (AAO-HNS) is an organization representing specialists who treat the ear, nose, throat, and related structures of the head and neck.

8468 **American Academy of Physical Medicine and Rehabilitation**
9700 W Bryn Mawr Ave
Ste 200
Rosemont, IL 60018-5701
847-737-6000
877-227-6799
Fax: 847-737-6001
info@aapmr.org
www.aapmr.org

Thomas E. Stautzenbach, Executive Director & Chief Executive Officer
Gregory M. Worsowicz, President
Darryl L. Kaelin, Vice President

This national medical specialty society represents more than 6,500 physical medicine and rehabilitation physicians, whose patients include people with physical disabilities and chronic, disabling illnesses. The academy's mission is to maximize quality of life, minimize the incidence and prevalence of impairments and disability, promote societal health and enhance the understanding and development of the specialty. The organization offers information, referrals, and patient materials.

8469 **American Association for Respiratory Care**
9425 N. MacArthur Blvd.
Ste 100
Irving, TX 75063-4706
972-243-2272
Fax: 972-484-2720
info@aarc.org
www.aarc.org

Tom Kallstrom, Executive Director
Steve Bowden, IT, General Inquiries

AARC's mission is to advance the science, technology, ethics and art of respiratory care through research and education for its members and to teach the general public about pulmonary health and disease prevention.

8470 **American Association of Cardiovascular and Pulmonary Rehabilitation**
330 N. Wabash Avenue
Suite 2200
Chicago, IL 60611
312-321-5146
Fax: 312-673-6924
aacvpr@aacvpr.org
www.aacvpr.org

Adam T. deJong, President
Megan Cohen, Executive Director
Jessica Eustice, Director Of Corporate Relations
Abigail Lynn, Operations Senior Manager

The mission of American Association of Cardiovascular and Pulmonary Rehabilitation is to reduce morbidity, mortality, and disability from cardiovascular and pulmonary diseases through education, prevention, rehabilitation, research, and aggressive disease management.

8471 **American Brain Tumor Association**
8550 W. Bryn Mawr Ave
Ste 550
Chicago, IL 60631-4106
773-577-8750
800-886-2282
Fax: 773-577-8738
info@abta.org
www.abta.org

Elizabeth Wilson, President & CEO
Martha Carlos, Chief Communications Officer
Kerri Mink, Chief Operating Officer
Sandy Abraham, Director, Marketing & Communications

A non-profit organization founded in 1973 dedicated to the elimination of brain tumors through research and patient education services.

8472 American Diabetes Association
2451 Crystal Dr.
Suite 900
Arlington, VA 22202
800-342-2383
askada@diabetes.org
www.diabetes.org

Tracey D. Brown, Chief Executive Officer
Charlotte Carter, Chief Financial Officer
Charles Henderson, Chief Development Officer
Kathy Nesbitt, Chief Operating & Strategy Officer

Funds diabetes research, information and advocacy. The mission of the Association is to prevent and cure diabetes and to improve the lives of all people affected by diabetes.

8473 American Group Psychotherapy Association
25 E. 21st St.
6th Floor
New York, NY 10010-6207
212-477-2677
877-668-2472
Fax: 212-979-6627
info@agpa.org
www.agpa.org

Marsha S. Block, Chief Executive Officer
Eleanor F. Counselman, EdD; CGP, President
Nina Brown, Secretary

AGPA serves as the national voice specific to the interests of group psychotherapy. Its 4,100 members and 31 affiliate societies provide a wealth of professional, educational and social support for group psychotherapists in the United States and around the world.

8474 American Head and Neck Society
11300 W. Olympic Blvd
Ste 600
Los Angeles, CA 90064-1663
310-437-0559
Fax: 310-437-0585
www.ahns.info

Dennis Kraus, MD, President
Jonathan Irish, MD, Vice President
Brian B. Burkey, MD; MEd, Secretary
Ehab Hanna, Treasurer

AHNS is a professional organization, formed in 1998 to promote research and education in head and neck oncology. The AHNS offers clinical practice guidelines, details of events, grants, and patient information. It aims to promote and advance the knowledge of prevention, diagnosis, treatment, and rehabilitation of neoplasms and other diseases of the head and neck.

8475 American Lung Association
55 W. Wacker Dr.
Ste 1150
Chicago, IL 60601
312-781-1100
800-548-8252
Fax: 202-452-1085
info@lung.org
www.lung.org

Harold P. Wimmer, President & CEO
Sue . Swan, National Chief Development Officer
Sally Draper, National Vice President, Development
Kim Lacina, National Vice President, Marketing & Communications

The ALA is an organization dedicated to combating tobacco use, eliminating lung diseases, and improving air quality through research, education, and advocacy. The association provides knowledge beneficial to patients, patients' families, and medical professionals and specialists.

8476 American SIDS Institute
528 Raven Way
Naples, FL 34110
239-431-5425
Fax: 239-431-5536
prevent@sids.org
www.sids.org

Marc Peterzell, JD, Chairman
Betty McEntire, PhD, Executive Director & CEO
Nicole Dobson, MD, Board Member
Alfred Steinschneider, MD, President Emeritus

American SIDS Institute is a national nonprofit health care organization that is dedicated to the prevention of sudden infant death and the promotion of infant health through an aggressive, comprehensive nationwide program of research, clinical services, education and family support.

8477 American Sexual Health Association
P.O. Box 13827
Research Triangle Park, NC 27709-3827
919-361-8400
Fax: 919-361-8425
info@ashasexualhealth.org

Lynn Barclay, President & CEO
Deborah Arrindell, Vice President, Health Policy

The American Sexual Health Association is a trusted source of information on sexual health, relationships, and measures to prevent adverse sexual health

8478 American Society of Pediatric Hematology/Oncology
8735 West Higgins Rd.
Ste. 300
Chicago, IL 60631
847-375-4716
Fax: 847-375-6483
info@aspho.org
www.aspho.org

Sally Weir, Executive Director
Steve Biddle, Education Consultant
Jackie Holcomb, Education Manager
Sergio Miranda, Memeber Services

ASPHO is multidisciplinary organization dedicated to promoting optimal care of children and adolescents with blood disorders and cancer by advancing research, education, treatment and professional practice.

8479 American Thoracic Society
25 Broadway
18th Floor
New York, NY 10004-2755
212-315-8600
Fax: 212-315-6498
atsinfo@thoracic.org
www.thoracic.org

Steve Crane, Executive Director
Nicola Black, Associate Director, Governance Activities
Jennifer A. Ian, Director, Member Services & Chapter Relations
Eileen Larsson, Chief Program Officer

The American Thoracic Society is dedicated to research, public health education, and patient care in relation to pulmonary disease, critical illness, and sleep disorders.

8480 Aplastic Anemia and MDS International Foundation
100 Park Ave
Ste 108
Rockville, MD 20850
301-279-7202
800-747-2820
Fax: 301-279-7205
help@aamds.org
www.aamds.org

John Huber, Executive Director
Angie Onofre, Director of Patient Programs and Services
Leigh Clark, Patient Educator
Benita Marcus, Senior Director Of Operations

This organization, formerly known as Aplastic Anemia Foundation of America, provides a resource directory for patient assistance, produces educational material and supports research into AA and MDS.

8481 Arizona Hemophilia Association
826 North 5th Ave
Phoenix, AZ 85003
602-955-3947
info@hemophiliaz.org
www.arizonahemophilia.org

Cindy Komar, Chief Executive Officer
Chelsea Bolyard, Program Director
Yleana Highes, Director, Client Services

The Arizona Hemophilia Association (AHA) is a volunteer based nonprofit organization working to support, educate, and advocate for families affected by bleeding disorders in Arizona.

8482 **CPATH Cerebral Palsy Awareness Transition Hope**
5501A Balcones
Suite 160
Austin, TX 78731
866-742-7284
info@cpathtexas.com
www.cpathtexas.com

Victoria Polega, President
Marielle Deckard, Secretary
Jamie Eppele, Director, Devleopment

CPATH is a non-profit organization whose mission is to provide resources, support, and financial assistance to families and individuals living with cerebral palsy.

8483 **Canadian Cancer Society**
55 St. Clair Avenue W.
Ste 300
Toronto, ON, Canada M4V- 2Y7
416-961-7223
888-939-3333
Fax: 416-961-4189
TTY: 866-786-3934
ccs@cancer.ca
www.cancer.ca

Anne V,zina, Interim President & CEO
Martin Kabat, Chief Executive Officer
Lesley Ring, Vice President, Development & Marketing

A national community-based organization of volunteers whose mission is the eradication of cancer and the enhancement of the quality of life for people living with cancer.

8484 **Canadian Diabetes Association**
1400-522 University Ave
Toronto, ON, Canada M5G-2R5
416-363-3373
800-226-8464
Fax: 416-408-7015
info@diabetes.ca
www.diabetes.ca

Doug Macnamara, President & CEO
Paul Kilbertus, Senior Director, Strategic Communications

The mission of the Canadian Diabetes Association is to promote the health of Canadians through diabetes research, education, service and advocacy.

8485 **Canadian Lung Association**
1750 Courtwood Cres.
Ottawa, ON, Canada K2C-2B5
613-569-6411
888-566-5864
Fax: 613-569-8860
info@lung.ca
www.lung.ca

Terry Dean, President & CEO

The Canadian Lung Association is a non-profit and volunteer-based health charity, dedicated to improving lung health in the Canadian community through research, education, prevention and advocacy.

8486 **Childhood Cancer Canada Foundation**
21 St. Clair Ave E
Ste 801
Toronto, ON, Canada M4T-1L9
416-489-6440
800-363-1062
Fax: 416-489-9812
info@childhoodcancer.ca
www.childhoodcancer.ca

Clare Davenport, President & CEO
Natasha Bowes, Senior Manager, Fund Development
Patricia Zareba, Fund Development Manager
Jessica MacInnis, Manager of Marketing & Communications

A national, volunteer governed, charitable organization dedicated to improving the quality of life for children with cancer. The foundation raises funds to assist with cancer research undertakings across Canada.

8487 **Childhood Leukemia Foundation**
807 Mantoloking Rd
Brick, NJ 08723
732-920-8860
888-253-7109
www.clf4kids.org

Barbara Haramis, Executive Director & Founder
Barb Estelle, Chief Operating Officer
Kim Wetmore, Director, Development
Kate Booth, Program Services Coordinator

The CLF is a national, non-profit organization providing education, information, support, and advocacy for patients of cancer and their families. the foundation works closesly with health professionals, social workers, and specialists to offer a variety of programs that aim to enrich the lives of children living with cancer.

8488 **Emphysema Foundation for Our Right to Survive**
PO Box 20241
Kansas City, MO 64119-0241
866-363-2673
www.emphysema.net

Linda Watson, President
Debbie Snodell, Secretary

EFFORTS is a non-profit organization that takes an active role in promoting research for more effective treatments and perhaps a cure for emphysema and related lung diseases. It also works to further education about the disease and provides a support mailing list for members.

8489 **Environmental Health Center: Dallas**
8345 Walnut Hill Lane
Ste 220
Dallas, TX 75231-4205
214-368-4132
Fax: 214-691-8432
contact@ehcd.com
www.ehcd.com

William J Rea, Director
Chris Rea, Business Manager
Yaqin Pan, M.D., Research Physician
Bertie Griffiths, Ph.D., Microbiologist/Immunologist

Clinic providing patient care in the areas of Immunotherapy, Nutrition, Physical Therapy, Chemical Depuration, Energy Balancing, Electromagnetic Sensitivity Testing, Psychological Support Services, Family Practice Medicine and Internal Medicine. Provides services for individuals whose diseases are caused by environmental factors.

8490 **Epilepsy Foundation of Alabama**
3929 Airport Blvd
Suite 3-310
Mobile, AL 36609-2235
251-341-0170
800-626-1582

Donna Dodson, Executive Director
Paige Norris, Outreach & Program Director
David Toenes, Director, Client Services
Kelly Morris, Board President

The Epilepsy Foundation of Alabama provides health service programs and public education on behalf of people with seizures and epilepsy. Some of their services include emergency medication assistance, information referral, training, employer education, and camping trips.

8491 **Eunice Kennedy Shriver National Institute of Child Health and Human Development (NICHD)**
National Institutes of Health (NIH)
31 Center Dr.
Bldg 31, Rm 2A32
Bethesda, MD 20892-2425
301-496-5097
800-370-2943
Fax: 866-760-5947
TTY: 888-320-6942
nichdinformationresourcecenter@mail.nih.gov
www.nichd.nih.gov

Diana W. Bianchi, Director

The Eunice Kennedy Shriver National Institute of Child Health and Human Development, part of the federal National Institutes of Health, conducts and supports basic, translational, and clinical research in the biomedical, behavioral, and social sciences related to child and maternal health, in medical rehabilitation, and in the reproductive sciences.

8492 **Fragile X Family**
Fanlight Productions
c/o Icarus Films
32 Court Street, 21st Floor
Brooklyn, NY 11201
718-488-8900
800-876-1710
Fax: 718-488-8642
info@fanlight.com
www.fanlight.com

Ben Achtenberg, Founder, Owner
Eric Kutner, Producer

Fragile X Family takes viewers inside the lives of a developmentally disabled family who are affected by Fragile X Syndrome, an inherited chromosomal disorder. *$149.00*
VHS/VIDEO
ISBN 1-572954-14-0

8493 **Herpes Resource Center**
American Social Health Association
P.O. Box 13827
Research Triangle Park, NC 27709-3827
919-361-8400
800-227-8922
Fax: 919-361-8425
customerservice@ashastd.org
www.ashastd.org/stdsstis/herpes/

Lynn Barclay, President & CEO

The Herpes Resource Center (HRC) focuses on increasing education, public awareness, and support to anyone concerned about herpes.

8494 **IKUS Life Enrichment Services**
O-1859 Lake Michigan Dr. NW
Grand Rapids, MI 49534
616-677-5251
Fax: 616-677-2955
info@ikuslife.org
www.ikuslife.org

Scott Blakeney, Executive Director
Amy DeMott, Director, Programs & Services
Nikki Outhier, Director, Development
Lisa Smith, Director, Financial Services

IKUS Life Enrichment Services helps individuals with disabilities learn new skills and experience greater freedom by providing support, recreation and educational services. IKUS also provides respite services to caregivers and families.

8495 **International Academy of Biological Dentistry and Medicine**
19122 Camellia Bend Circle
Suite 101
Spring, TX 77379
281-651-1745
Fax: 281-651-1745
drdawn@drdawn.net
www.iabdm.org

Dr. Dawn Ewing, Executive Director

The IABDM promotes non-toxic diagnostic and therapeutic approaches in dentistry and hosts seminars on biological diagnosis and therapy.

8496 **International Academy of Oral Medicine & Toxicology**
8297 ChampionsGate Blvd
Ste 193
ChampionsGate, FL 33896-8387
863-420-6373
Fax: 863-419-8136
info@iaomt.org
www.iaomt.org

Mark Wisniewski, President
Tammy DeGregorio, Executive Vice President
Kym Smith, Executive Director

A non-profit organization dedicated to funding solid peer-reviewed scientific research in the area of toxic substances used in dentistry as well as providing continuing education and carefully reviewed procedures, protocols, and methodologies to reduce the risk for patients and professionals.

8497 **International Association for Cancer Victors & Friends**
P.O. Box 745
Lakeport, CA 95453
408-834-5300
Fax: 408-264-9659
www.cancervictors.net

a.k.a. Cancer Victors & Friends

8498 **International Association of Hygienic Physicians**
4620 Euclid Blvd
Youngstown, OH 44512-1633
330-788-0526
Fax: 330-788-0093
www.iahp.net

Alec Burton, Co-Founder
Mark A. Huberman, Secretary/Treasurer

The International Association of Hygienic Physicians (IAHP) is a professional association for licensed, primary care physicians (Medical Doctors, Osteopaths, Chiropractors, and Naturopaths) who specialize in Therapeutic Fasting Supervision as an integral part of Hygienic Care.

8499 **International Medical and Dental Hypnotherapy Association**
8852 SR 3001
RR 2
Laceyville, PA 18623-9417
570-869-1021
800-553-6886
Fax: 570-869-1249
www.hypnosisalliance.com/imdha

Linda Otto, Executive Director
Robert Otto, President & CEO
Christie Boecker, Membership Services Coordinator

The association provides and encourages education programs to further, the knowledge, understanding, and application of hypnosis in complementary healthcare; encourages research and scientific publication in the field of hypnosis; and advocates for further recognition and acceptance of hypnosis as an important tool in healthcare and focus for scientific research.

8500 **International Myeloma Foundation**
12650 Riverside Dr
Ste 206
North Hollywood, CA 91607- 3421
818-487-7455
800-452-2873
Fax: 818-487-7454
theimf@myeloma.org
www.myeloma.org

David Girard, Executive Director
Susie Novis, President
Diane Moran, Senior Vice President, Strategic Planning
Selma Plascencia, Director of Operations

The IMF serves myeloma patients, family members, and the medical community, offering a wide range of programs in the areas of Research, Education, Support, and Advocacy.

8501 **International Ventilator Users Network (IVUN)**
50 Crestwood Executive Ctr.
Suite 440
St. Louis, MO 63126-1916
314-534-0475
Fax: 314-534-5070
info@ventusers.org
www.ventnews.org

Saul J. Morse, President & Chair
Daniel J. Wilson, Vice President
Marny K. Eulberg, Secretary
Mike Mrozowicz, Treasurer

To enhance the lives and independence of individuals using ventilators by promoting education, networking and advocacy. IVUN is an affiliate of Post-Polio Health International.

8502 **Leukemia & Lymphoma Society**
3 International Dr
Ste 200
Rye Brook, NY 10573
914-949-5213
800-955-4572
Fax: 914-949-6691
supportservices@lls.org
www.lls.org

Louis DeGennaro, President & CEO
Piper Medcalf, Executive Director
Nancy Hallberg, Chief Marketing Officer
Marcie Klein, Senior Vice President, Communications

The Leukemia and Lymphoma Society is the world's largest voluntary health organization dedicated to funding blood cancer research, education and patient services. The society offers information and support for patients of various blood cancer types, including leukemia, lymphoma, Hodgkin's disease and myeloma. It also offers services and resources to help improve the quality of life of patients and their families.

8503 **Little People of America**
250 El Camino Real
Ste 218
Tustin, CA 92780
714-368-3689
888-572-2001
Fax: 714-368-3367
info@lpaonline.org
www.lpaonline.org

Joanna Campbell, Executive Director
Gary Arnold, President
April Brazier, Senior Vice President
Mark Povinelli, Membership Director

Little People of America is a national non-profit organization that provides support and information to people of short stature and their families. Short stature is generally caused by one of the more than 200 medical conditions known as dwarfism. LPA offers information on employment, education, disability rights, adoption, medical issues, clothing, adaptive products, and the many stages of parenting a short-statured child - from birth to adult.

8504 **Lowe Syndrome Association**
P.O. Box 417
Chicago Ridge, IL 60415
216-630-7723
www.lowesyndrome.org

Lisa Waldbaum, President
Jane Gallery, Treasurer
Tiffany Johnson, Director, Medical & Scientific Affairs

The organization aims to foster communication, provide education, and support research into Lowe Syndrome.

8505 **Lymphoma Canada**
Formerly The Lymphoma Foundation Canada
6860 Century Ave
Ste 202
Mississauga, ON, Canada L5N-2W5
905-858-5967
866-659-5556
info@lymphoma.ca
www.lymphoma.ca

Robin Markowitz, Chief Executive Officer
Lorna Warwick, National Director, Education & Services
Charlene Ragin, Marketing & Communications
Anwar Knight, Director, Mississauga, ON

Lymphoma Canada provides, at no cost and in both official languages: electronic and print materials on the Hodgkin lymphoma, non-Hodgkin lymphoma and CLL, peer and caregiver support groups, educational forums and advocacy on behalf of patients. Lymphoma Canada also funds Canadian research.

8506 **Merrimack Hall Performing Arts Center**
3320 Triana Blvd SW.
Huntsville, AL 35805
256-534-6455
info@merrimackhall.com
www.merrimackhall.com

8507 **Myositis Association**
1940 Duke St.
Suite 200
Alexandria, VA 22314
800-821-7356
tma@myositis.org
www.myositis.org

Bob Goldberg, Executive Director
Theresa Reynolds Curry, Communications Manager
Aisha Morrow, Operations Manager
Charlia Sanchez, Member Services Coordinator

The aim of TMA's programs and services is to provide information, support, advocacy and research for those concerned about myositis, as well as serving those affected by these diseases. Support groups offer members the chance to share and discuss their concerns with people in similar situations.

8508 **National Association for Children of Alcoholics**
10920 Connecticut Ave
Ste 100
Kensington, MD 20895-3007
301-468-0985
888-554-2627
Fax: 301-468-0987
nacoa@nacoa.org
www.nacoa.org

Sis Wenger, President & CEO
Steve Hornberger, Program Director

National non-profit membership and affiliate organization working on behalf of children of alcohol and drug dependent parents to help eliminate the adverse impact of drug use on children through public awareness, policy, advocacy, education, and support.

8509 **National Association for Home Care & Hospice**
228 7th St SE
Washington, DC 20003-4306
202-547-7424
Fax: 202-547-3540
webmaster@nahc.org
www.nahc.org

Val J. Halamandris, President
Lucy Andrews, Vice Chair
Karen Marshall Thompson, Secretary
Thomas Moreland, Treasurer

This is a non-profit trade association representing various home care, hospice and health aid organizations. With services aimed at assiting the chronically ill and disabled, the NAHC offers information on how to choose a home care provider and a zip code driven locator for home care and hospice.

8510 **National Association for Medical Direction of Respiratory Care**
8618 Westwood Center Dr
Ste 210
Vienna, VA 22182-2273
703-752-4359
Fax: 703-752-4360
www.namdrc.org

Phillip Porte, Executive Director
Vickie Parshall, Director, Member Services
Karen Lui, RN, Associate Executive Director

NAMDRC's primary mission is to improve access to quality care for patients with respiratory disease by removing regulatory and legislative barriers to appropriate treatment.

8511 **National Association for Proton Therapy**
1155 15th St NW
Ste 500
Washington, DC 20005
202-495-3133
Fax: 202-530-0659
info@proton-therapy.org
www.proton-therapy.org

Leonard Arzt, Executive Director

The National Association for Proton Therapy (NAPT) is registered as an independent, non-profit, public benefit corporation providing education and awareness for the public, professional and governmental communities. It promotes the therapeutic benefits of proton therapy for cancer treatment in the U.S. and abroad.

8512 **National Association of Anorexia Nervosa and Associated Disorders**
750 E Diehl Road
Ste 127
Naperville, IL 60563
630-577-1333
Fax: 847-433-4632
anadhelp@anad.org
www.anad.org

Laura Zinger, Executive Director
Deb Prinz, Director, Community Relations

A non-profit organization that seeks to alleviate the problems of eating disorders, especially anorexia nervosa and bulimia nervosa, by promoting eating disorder awareness, prevention and recovery through supporting, educating, and connecting individuals, families and professionals.

8513 **National Association of Chronic Disease Diseases**
325 Swanton Way
Decatur, GA 30030
770-458-7400
Fax: 770-458-7401
jrobitscher@chronicdisease.org
www.chronicdisease.org

John W. Robitscher, Chief Executive Officer
Namvar Zohoori, President
John Patton, Director, Communications
Margaret Gillan Ritchie, Communications & Member Services Coordinator

A national public health association founded in 1988 to link the chronic disease program directors of each state and U.S. territory to provide a national forum for chronic disease prevention and control efforts. NACDD aims to mobilize national efforts to reduce chronic diseases and the associated risk factors.

8514 **National Association to Advance Fat Acceptance**
P.O. Box 4662
Foster City, CA 94404-0662
916-558-6880
Fax: 916-558-6881
www.naafaonline.com

8515 **National Cancer Institute**
9609 Medical Center Dr.
Rockville, MD 20850
800-422-6237
TTY: 800-332-8615
nciinfo@nih.gov
www.cancer.gov

Norman E. Sharpless, Director
Douglas R. Lowy, Principal Deputy Director
James Doroshow, Deputy Director, Clinical & Translational Research
Dinah S. Singer, Deputy Director, Scientific Strategy & Development

The National Cancer Institute conducts and supports research, training, health information dissemination, and programs related to cancer, cancer rehabilitation, and the care of cancer patients.

8516 **National Diabetes Information Clearinghouse**
NI of Diabetes and Digestive and Kidney Diseases
31 Center Dr.
Bethesda, MD 20892
800-860-8747
TTY: 866-569-1162
healthinfo@niddk.nih.gov
www.diabetes.niddk.nih.gov

Griffin P. Rodgers, Director
Gregory G. Germino, Deputy Director
Camille Hoover, Executive Officer
Elise Goodwin, Deputy Executive Officer

An information and referral service of the National Institute of Diabetes and Digestive and Kidney Diseases, one of the National Institutes of Health. The clearinghouse responds to written inquiries, develops and distributes publications about diabetes, and provides referrals to diabetes organizations, including support groups. The NDIC maintains a database of patient and professional education materials, from which literature searches are generated.

8517 **National Digestive Diseases Information Clearinghouse**
NI of Diabetes and Digestive and Kidney Diseases
31 Center Dr.
Bethesda, MD 20892
800-860-8747
TTY: 866-569-1162
healthinfo@niddk.nih.gov
www.digestive.niddk.nih.gov

Griffin P. Rodgers, Director
Gregory G. Germino, Deputy Director
Camille Hoover, Executive Officer
Elise Goodwin, Deputy Executive Officer

Information and referral service of the National Institute of Diabetes and Digestive and Kidney Diseases. A central information resource on the prevention and management of digestive diseases, the clearinghouse responds to written inquiries, develops and distributes publications about digestive diseases, provides referrals to digestive disease organizations and support groups, and maintains a database of patient and professional education materials from which literature searches are generated.

8518 **National Fibromyalgia Association**
3857 Birch St.
Suite 312
Newport Beach, CA 92660
nfa@fmaware.org
www.fmaware.org

Lynne Matallana, Founder

National Fibromyalgia Association's mission is to develop and execute programs dedicated to improving the quality of life for people with fibromyalgia.

8519 **National Hemophilia Foundation**
7 Penn Plaza
Suite 1204
New York, NY 10001
212-328-3700
888-463-6643
Fax: 212-328-3777
info@hemophilia.org
www.hemophilia.org

Leonard Valentino, President & CEO
Dawn Rotellini, Chief Operating Officer
Kevin Mills, Chief Scientific Officer
Michelle Rice, Chief External Affairs Officer

The National Hemophilia Foundation is dedicated to finding better treatments and cures for bleeding and clotting disorders and to preventing the complications of these disorders through education, advocacy and research. Established in 1948, the National Hemophilia Foundation has chapters throughout the country.

8520 **National Kidney and Urologic Diseases Information Clearinghouse**
NI of Diabetes and Digestive and Kidney Diseases
31 Center Dr.
Bethesda, MD 20892
800-860-8747
TTY: 866-569-1162
healthinfo@niddk.nih.gov
www.kidney.niddk.nih.gov

Griffin P. Rodgers, Director
Gregory G. Germino, Deputy Director
Camille Hoover, Executive Officer
Elise Goodwin, Deputy Executive Officer

NKUDIC was established in 1987 to increase knowledge and understanding about diseases of the kidneys and urologic system among people with these conditions and their families, health care professionals, and the general public.

8521 **National Organization for Albinism and Hypopigmentation**
P.O. Box 959
East Hampstead, NH 03826-0959
603-887-2310
800-473-2310
Fax: 800-648-2310
info@albinism.org
www.albinism.org

Michael McGowan, Executive Director
Diana McCown, Vice-chair
Kris Baker, Secretary
Kathi O'Donnell, Administration

Organization offering information and support to people with albinism, their families and the professionals who work with them.

8522 **National Organization for Rare Disorders**
55 Kenosia Ave
Danbury, CT 06810
203-744-0100
Fax: 203-263-9938
orphan@rarediseases.org
rarediseases.org

Marshall Summar, MD, Chairman
Peter Saltonstall, President & CEO
Pamela Gavin, Chief Operating Officer
Alexa Moore, Vice President of Business Development

The National Organization for Rare Disorders (NORD) is an organization serving individuals with rare diseases and the organizations that serve them. NORD offers educational programs, advocacy, research and patient services.

8523 **National Organization on Fetal Alcohol Syndrome**
1200 Eton Ct NW
3rd Fl
Washington, DC 20007-3239
202-785-4585
800-666-6327
Fax: 202-466-6456
information@nofas.org
www.nofas.org

Tom Donaldson, President
Kathleen Tavenner Mitchell, Vice President
Andy Kachor, Communications Director
Katelyn Reitz, Development Director

Dedicated to eliminating birth defects caused by alcohol consumption during pregnancy and improving the qualtiy of life for those individuals and families affected.

8524 **Post-Polio Health International**
50 Crestwood Executive Ctr.
Suite 440
St. Louis, MO 63126
314-534-0475
Fax: 314-534-5070
info@post-polio.org
www.post-polio.org

Daniel J. Wilson, President
Mark Mallinger, Vice President
Brian M. Tiburzi, Executive Director
Marny E. Eulberg, Secretary

To enhance the lives and independence of polio survivors, home ventilator users, their caregivers and families, and health professionals through education, networking, and advocacy.

8525 **Prader-Willi Syndrome Association USA**
8588 Potter Park Dr
Ste 500
Sarasota, FL 34238
941-312-0400
800-926-4797
Fax: 941-312-0142
www.pwsausa.org

Ken Smith, Executive Director
Jack Hannings, Development Director
Donny Moore, Development & Communications Specialist

National, nonprofit public charity that works for the benefit of individuals with Prader-Willi syndrome and their families. Dedicated to serving individuals affected by Prader-Willi syndrome (PWS) their families, and interested professionals, providing information, education, and support services to its members.

8526 **Simonton Cancer Center**
P.O. Box 6607
Malibu, CA 90264-6607
818-879-7904
800-459-3424
Fax: 310-457-0421
simontoncancercenter@msn.com
www.simontoncenter.com

Dr. O. Carl Simonton, Founder
Edward Gilbert, MD, Medical Director
Karen Smith Simonton, Executive / Program Director
Jessica Jedvaj, Administrative Assistant

The Simonton Cancer Center is a non-profit organization dedicated to improving the health and lives of cancer patients and their families through psycho-social oncology.

8527 **Special Care Dentistry Association**
330 N. Wabash Avenue
Ste 2000
Chicago, IL 60611-4245
312-527-6764
Fax: 312-673-6663
scda@scdaonline.org
www.scdaonline.org

Kristin Dee, Executive Director
Miriam Robbins, President
Jeffrey Hicks, President-Elect
Sam Zwetchkenbaum, Vice President

The Special Care Dentistry Association serves as a resource to all oral health care professionals who serve or are interested in serving patients with special needs through education and networking to increase access to oral healthcare for patients with special needs.

8528 **Spina Bifida Association**
1600 Wilson Blvd
Ste 800
Arlington, VA 22209
202-944-3285
800-621-3141
Fax: 202-944-3295
sbaa@sbaa.org
www.spinabifidaassociation.org

Sara Struwe, President & CEO
Lee Towns, National Director, Communications & Outreach
Elizabeth Merck, National Director, Development
Nora Beierwaltes, Marketing Coordinator

Non-profit organization whose mission is to promote the prevention of spina bifida and to enhance the lives of all affected. Addresses the specific needs of the spina bifida community and serves as the national representative of almost 60 chapters. Services include Toll free 800 information and referral service, as well as legislative updates.

8529 **Spina Bifida and Hydrocephalus Association of Canada**
167 Lombard Ave
Suite 472
Winnipeg, MB R3B 0T6,
204-925-3650
800-565-9488
Fax: 204-925-3654
info@sbhac.ca
www.sbhac.ca

Susana Scott, President
Linda Randall, Vice President
Bonnie Hidlebaugh, National Manager, Communications & Development Coordinator
Cindy Garofalo, Administrative Assistant

The Spina Bifida and Hydrocephalus Association of Canada has been working on behalf of people with spina bifida and/or hydrocephalus and their families.

8530 **Sunburst Projects**
Sunburst Projects United States Headquarters
2143 Hurley Way
Suite 240
Sacramento, CA 95825
916-440-0889
Fax: 916-440-1208
admin@sunburstprojects.org
www.sunburstprojects.org

Geri DeLaRosa, PhD, Founder & Executive Director
Samantha Voelkel, Camp Director

Sunburst Projects is a international organization that works to keep families together by providing services and support for youth who are infected or affected by HIV/AIDS.

8531 **Taking Control of Your Diabetes (TCOYD)**
990 Highland Dr
Suite 312
Solana Beach, CA 92075
858-755-5683
800-998-2693
Fax: 858-755-6854
info@tcoyd.org
www.tcoyd.org

Steven Edelman, MD, Founder & Director
Sandra Bourdette, Co-Founder & Executive Director Emeritus
Jennifer Braidwood, Director of Marketing & Special Projects
Jill Yapo, Director, Operations

Taking Control of Your Diabetes works to educate and motivate people with diabetes to take a more active role in managing their condition. The organization also offers continuing education programs for medical professionals caring for people with diabetes.

8532 **United Brachial Plexus Network, Inc.**
32 William Rd
Reading, MA 01867
781-315-6161
ubpn@ubpn.org
www.ubpn.org

Richard Looby, President
Dan Aldrich, Co- Vice President & Traumatic BPI Group

The United Brachial Plexus Network, Inc. provides education, information, and assistance for those affected by Brachial Plexus Palsy by offering information, contacts, resources, parent matching, and assistance developing chapters or support groups throughout the United States and the world.

8533 **World Service Office of Overeaters Anonymous**
6075 Zenith Crt NE
Rio Rancho, NM 87144-6424
505-891-2664
Fax: 505-891-4320
info@oa.org
www.oa.org

Sarah Armstrong, Managing Director
OA aims to provide physical, emotional, and practical support for those seeking to improve their dietary habits. OA encourages members to develop a food plan with a health care professional and a sponsor.

Camps

8534 **ADA Camp GranADA**
American Diabetes Association
55 E Monroe St.
Suite 3420
Chicago, IL 60603
312-346-1805
illinoiscamps@diabetes.org
www.diabetes.org

8535 **ADA Camp Needlepoint**
American Diabetes Association
375 Bishops Way
Brookfield, WI 53005
414-778-5500
campsupport@diabetes.org
www.diabetes.org

Becky Barnett, Camp Director
Camp Needlepoint is a summer camp for children who have type 1 diabetes. Coed, ages 8-16. The camp takes place at the YMCA Camp St. Croix in Hudson, Wisconsin.

8536 **ADA Teen Adventure Camp**
American Diabetes Association
55 E Monroe St.
Suite 3420
Chicago, IL 60603
312-346-1805
illinoiscamps@diabetes.org
www.diabetes.org

Paula Williams, Contact
Camping for teenagers with diabetes. Coed, ages 14 to 17. Camp dates are early in August. Located at the YMCA Camp Duncan in Ingleside, Illinois.

8537 **ADA Triangle D Camp**
American Diabetes Association
55 E Monroe St.
Suite 3420
Chicago, IL 60603
312-346-1805
illinoiscamps@diabetes.org
www.diabetes.org

8538 **ASCCA**
Alabama Easter Seal Society
5278 Camp Ascca Dr
P.O. Box 21
Jacksons Gap, AL 36861
256-825-9226
800-843-2267
Fax: 256-825-8332
info@campascca.org
www.campascca.org

John Stephenson, Administrator
Matt Rickman, Camp Director
Dana Rickman, Director, Marketing Communications
Allison Wetherbee, Director, Community Relations
Camp ASCCA is for children and adults with disabilities or health impairements. Camp ASCCA strives to help these individuals achieve equality, independence and dignity in a safe environment.

8539 **Adam's Camp**
6767 South Spruce St.
Suite 102
Centennial, CO 80112
303-563-8290
Contact@AdamsCamp.org
www.adamscampcolorado.org

Lindsay Radford, Executive Director
Lesley Pollard, Director, Communications & Events
Kim Kelleher, Therapy Camp Manager
Rob McIntire, Finance Director
Adam's Camp is a nonprofit organization, with multiple locations across the United States, providing therapeutic programs and recreational camps for children, and the families of children with special needs and developmental delays.

8540 **Adventure Day Camp**
3480 Commission Ct
Lake Ridge, VA 22192
703-491-1444
office@princewilliamacademy.com
www.princewilliamacademy.com

Dr. Samia Harris, Founder & Executive Director
Rebecca Nykwest, Communications Director
Lindsay Chickering, Office Manager
Shiree Slade, Principal
Camping for children with asthma/respiratory ailments and cancer. Coed, ages 2-13.

8541 **Agassiz Village**
238 Bedford St
Suite B
Lexington, MA 02420-3477
781-860-0200
Fax: 781-860-0352
www.agassizvillage.org

Cliff Simmonds, Executive Director
Thomas Semeta, Camp Director
Warren Soar, Facility Director
Warren H Burroughs, Honorary Chairman
Agassiz Village offers a variety of activities for all campers, boys and girls, younger camper and teens, and programs for physically challenged children and teens. By participating in daily activities, campers build a cooperative and positive community of different races, ages, ethnic and cultural backgrounds while enhancing confidence and individuality. Camp is located in Poland, Maine. For ages 8-17.

8542 **Arizona Camp Sunrise**
American Cancer Society
PO Box 27872
Tempe, AZ 85285
602-952-7550
800-865-1582
Fax: 602-404-1118
www.azcampsunrise.org

Barbara Nicholas, Director
Leigh Ansley, Manager
Melissa Lee, Camp Director
Jason Poulter, Technical Media Director
Provides one-week summer camping sessions to children aged 8-16 who have had, or currently have, cancer. The classes range from sports and outdoor games to dance and drama, arts, crafts, and cooking. Other activities planned for the campers include horseback riding, a trip to a lake, a dance, and learning to make friendship bracelets.

8543 **Bearskin Meadow Camp**
Diabetic Youth Families
5167 Clayton Rd
Suite F
Concord, CA 94521
925-680-4994
Fax: 925-680-4863
info@dyf.org
www.dyf.org

Kaylor Glassman, Interim Executive Director
Kaylee Gronau, Camp Director
Christi Rossi, Development, Director
Melissa Clarke-Howard, Development Director
Bearskin Meadow Camp, is a camp program offered by the Diabetes Youth Families organization to children (7-13), teens (14-17), and families who are affected by type 1 diabetes. The camp has traditional camp activities as well as educational opportunities for campers.

8544 **Becket Chimney Corners YMCA Camps and Outdoor Center**
748 Hamilton Rd
Becket, MA 01223 413-623-8991
Fax: 413-623-5890
cburke@bccymca.org
www.bccymca.org
Drew Lipsher, Chair
David Smith, Vice Chair
Christine Kalakay, Chief Financial Officer
Phil Connor, CEO
Half-week and one-week sessions for campers with asthma/respiratory ailments. Coed, ages 3 and up, families, seniors, single adults.

8545 **Breckenridge Outdoor Education Center**
PO Box 697
Breckenridge, CO 80424 970-453-6422
800-383-2632
Fax: 970-453-4676
boec@boec.org
www.boec.org
Sonya Norris, Executive Director
Karen Skruch, Finance Director
Jeff Inouye, Ski Program Director
Jaime Overmyer, Wilderness Program Director
Breckenridge Outdoor Education Center (BOEC) provides year round educational outdoor experiences to individuals with physical and intellectual disabilities. Some programs BOEC offer include, Adaptive Ski and Ride School, Wilderness Programs and adaptive programs for individuals with brain injuries, multiple sclerosis, and Parkinson's Disease.

8546 **Bright Horizons Summer Camp**
Sickle Cell Disease Association of Illinois
8100 S. Western Avenue
Chicago, IL 60620 773-526-5016
866-798-1097
Fax: 773-526-5012
sicklecelldisease-illinois@scdai.org
Darryl H. Armstrong, Chair
TaLana Hughes, Executive Director
Anquineice Brown, Outreach Coordinator
Alana Burke, Case Manager
Camping for children with blood disorders, ages 7-13. The joys of learning include instruction in first aid, swimming and water safety, boating, horseback riding and bowling plus arts and crafts. In addition, there is a traditional menu of camp pleasures, like hayrides, cookouts, nature hikes and sing-a-longs.

8547 **Camp Aldersgate**
2000 Aldersgate Road
Little Rock, AR 72205 501-225-1444
Fax: 501-225-2019
eballew@campaldersgate.net
www.campaldersgate.net
Sonya S. Murphy, Chief Executive Officer
Ali Miller Berry, Director, Programs
Katie Jenkins, Program Coordinator
Kerri Daniels, Director, Development
Camp Aldersgate is a nonprofit organization, offering summer, weekend camps, and year-round social service programs to children, teens and adults with special needs. The camp promotes outdoor recreation and socialization in a completely accessible environment.

8548 **Camp Alpine**
Alpine Alternatives
2518 E. Tudor Road
Ste 105
Anchorage, AK 99507-1105 907-561-6655
800-361-4174
Fax: 907-563-9232
alpinealternatives@arctic.net
www.alpinealternatives.org/programs.html
Margaret Webber, Executive Director
LaVerne Lee, Day Outings Director & Camp Alpine Director
Offers programs aimed at helping disabled youth expand their horizons, master new skills, make new friends, and increase motor coordination. Most importantly, participants experience growth in self-confidence and independence that affects all aspects of an individual's life. Camp services are open to all, regardless of type of disability or age. Activities include canoeing, hiking, swimming, outdoor games, sports, nature identification and much more.

8549 **Camp Anuenue**
250 Williams St. NW
Atlanta, GA 30303 808-595-7500
888-227-2345
Fax: 808-595-7502
www.cancer.org
Pamela K. Meyerhoffer, Chair
Robert E. Youle, Vice Chairman
Douglas K. Kelsey, Board Scientific Officer
Daniel P. Heist, Secretary/Treasurer
(1 week) June, children with or recovered from cancer.

8550 **Camp Beausite NW**
PO Box 1227
Port Hadlock, WA 98339 360-732-7222
campbeausitenw.org
Raina Baker, Executive Director
The camp is located in Chimacum, Washington. Campers range from 7-65 in age and includes those with developmental disabilities, cerebral palsy, autism, Down syndrome, and other physical or mental disabilities. The camp offers five week-long overnight summer camp sessions for adults and children.

8551 **Camp Beyond The Scars**
Burn Institute
8825 Aero Drive
Suite 200
San Diego, CA 92123-2269 858-541-2277
Fax: 858-541-7179
ccoppenrath@burninstitute.org
www.burninstitute.org/camp-beyond-the-scar s
Jess Boles Lohmann, Operations Coordinator
Susan Day, Executive Director
Benjamin Hemmings, Director, Operations
Camp Beyond the Scars, is a weeklong sleepaway summer camp for children aged 8-17 who have survived a burn injury. Staffed by adult burn survivors, healthcare professionals, and off-duty firefighters, the camp provides an inclusive environment for burn survivors to participate in activities including, swimming, basketball, volleyball, archery, golf, and arts and crafts. The camp is free of charge, and is hosted at a camp facility in Romano, California.

8552 **Camp Boggy Creek**
30500 Brantley Branch Rd.
Eustis, FL 32736 352-483-4200
866-462-6449
Fax: 352-483-0589
info@campboggycreek.org
www.boggycreek.org
June Clark, President & CEO
Lisa Hicks, Chief Development Officer
David Mann, Camp Director
Kirstin Cauraugh Youmans, Assistant Camp Director
Year-round sessions for children with a variety of chronic or life-threatening illnesses including cancer, hemophilia, epilepsy, heart defects, HIV, spina bifida and respiratory ailments. Coed, ages 7-16.

8553 **Camp Bon Coeur**
300 Ridge Rd.
Suite K
Lafayette, LA 70506 337-233-8437
Fax: 337-233-4160
info@heartcamp.com
www.heartcamp.com
Susannah Craig, Executive Director
Chelsea Doyle, Summer Program Coordinator
Jessica Becnel, Family Support Group Coordinator
A week-long summer camp program for children ages 7-16 with heart defects. Activities include canoeing, swimming, archery, art, sports, and teambuilding and personal development activities.

8554 **Camp Breathe Easy**
American Lung Association
2452 Spring Rd. SE
Smyrna, GA 30080

8555 **Camp Can Do**
Administrative Office
3 Unami Trail
Chalfont, PA 18914
717-273-6525
campcandoforever.org

Tom Prader, Director, Patient Camp
Stephanie Cole, Director, Patient Camp
Caitlyn McLarnon, Director, Sibling Camp
Camp Can Do is for children ages 8-17 who have been diagnosed with cancer in the last five years. The camp also offers a session for siblings of children with cancer.

8556 **Camp Carefree**
American Diabetes Association
Lions Camp Pride
154 Camp Pride Way
New Durham, NH 03855
campsupport@diabetes.org
www.diabetes.org

Phyllis Woestemeyer, Director
Camp Carefree is a American Diabetes Association summer camp for children with diabetes. The camp is located at Lions Camp Pride in New Durham, New Hampshire.

8557 **Camp Catch-a-Rainbow**
American Cancer Society
250 Williams St. NW
Atlanta, GA 30303
808-595-7500
888-227-2345
Fax: 808-595-7502
www.cancer.org

Pamela K. Meyerhoffer, Chair
Robert E. Youle, Vice Chairman
Douglas K. Kelsey, Board Scientific Officer
Daniel P. Heist, Secretary/Treasurer
Camp Catch-a-Rainbow's programs are available completely free to any child in MI or IN who has or has had cancer, between the ages of 4 and 20, with their doctor's approval. Family Camp is reserved for those campers who have attended camp during that year's summer sessions and their families. Day, week, adult retreat, and family camp are available options.

8558 **Camp Cheerful**
Achievement Centers For Children
15000 Cheerful Lane
Strongsville, OH 44136-5420
440-238-6200
Fax: 440-238-1858
www.achievementcenters.org

Sally Farwell, President & CEO
Scott Peplin, Executive Vice President & CFO
Deborah Osgood, Vice President, Development & Marketing
Maureen Davis, Program Contact
Camp Cheerful provides a number of day and overnight camping options for children and adults who have disabilities. The camp hosts traditional camp activities as well as year-round therapeutic horseback riding sessions and an accessible high ropes challenge course during the summer. The focus of activities is to increase the quality of life while encouraging confidence and independence.

8559 **Camp Christmas Seal**
American Lung Association of Oregon
102 W McDowell Rd
Phoenix, AZ 85003-1213
602-258-7505
Fax: 202-452-1805
info@lungoregon.org
www.lungoregon.org

Kathryn A. Forbes, Chairman
John F. Emanuel, Vice Chair
Harold Wimmer, President/CEO
Penny J. Siewert, Secretary/Treasurer
Camp is located in Sisterhood, Oregon. Sessions for children with asthma/respiratory ailments. Coed, ages 8-15.

8560 **Camp Classen YMCA**
YMCA of Greater Oklahoma City
10840 Main Camp Rd
Davis, OK 73030
580-369-2272
Fax: 580-369-2284
www.itsmycamp.org

Ford C. Price, Chair
Tricia Everest, Vice Chairman
Mike Grady, President & CEO
Don Harris, Vice President & CFO
Camp is located in Davis, Oklahoma. Sessions for children and adults with diabetes. Coed, ages 8-17, families, seniors and single adults.

8561 **Camp Conrad Chinnock**
Diabetes Camping And Educational Services, Inc.
12045 E. Waterfront Dr.
Playa Vista, CA 90094
310-751-3057
Fax: 909-752-5354
info@diabetescamping.org
www.diabetescamping.org

Rocky Wilson, Executive Director
Ryan Martz, Development & Program Director
Dale Lissy, Camp Manager
Melanie Coyne, Director, Camp Operations
Camp Conrad Chinnock offers year round recreational, social, and educational opportunities for children and families with type 1 diabetes.

8562 **Camp Courage North**
True Friends
37569 Courage North Dr.
Lake George, MN 56458
952-852-0101
800-450-8376
Fax: 952-852-0123
info@truefriends.org
www.truefriends.org

John Leblanc, President & CEO
Conor McGrath, Senior Director, Camp & Operations
Jon Salmon, Director, Programs
Camp Courage North provides summer camp sessions for individuals with disabilities.

8563 **Camp Discovery - Illinois**
American Diabetes Association
55 E Monroe St.
Suite 3420
Chicago, IL 60603
312-346-1805
illinoiscamps@diabetes.org
www.diabetes.org

8564 **Camp Discovery Kansas**
American Diabetes Association
608 W Douglas Ave.
Wichita, KS 67203
316-684-6091
campsupport@diabetes.org
www.diabetes.org

8565 **Camp Echoing Hills**
36272 County Rd. 79
Warsaw, OH 43844
740-327-2311
www.ehvi.org

Lauren Unger, Camp Administrator
Summer camp for children and adults with physical, intellectual and developmental disabilities.

8566 **Camp Eden Wood**
True Friends
6350 Indian Chief Rd.
Eden Prairie, MN 55346
952-852-0101
800-450-8376
Fax: 952-852-0123
info@truefriends.org
www.truefriends.org

John Leblanc, President & CEO
Conor McGrath, Senior Director, Camp & Operations
Jon Salmon, Director, Programs
Offers resident camp programs for children, teenagers and adults with developmental, physical or multiple disabilities. Fishing, creative arts, golf, sports and other activities are available. Respite care weekend camps year round for children, teenagers and

adults. Guided vacations for teens and adults with developmental disabilities or other unique needs.

8567 **Camp Floyd Rogers**
PO Box 541058
Omaha, NE 68154 402-885-9022
director@campfloydrogers.com
www.campfloydrogers.com

Dylan Helberg, Camp Director
Carrie Busing, Operations Director

A camp for diabetic children. Coed, ages 8-18. Campers enjoy activities, participate in special events, engage in evening programs, and they meet other children their own age with diabetes.

8568 **Camp Glengarra**
Girl Scouts - Foothills Council
33 Jewett Pl
Utica, NY 13501-4715 315-733-1909
Fax: 315-733-1909

Natalie Brown, Executive Director
Karen Lubecki, Director

Camp Glengarra is located on 500+ acres of fields and forests, about eight miles west of Camden. This Girl Scout Camp hosts a myriad of programs throughout the year as well as summer day and resident camp. Summer sessions for girls 5-17 with ADD or asthma/respiratory ailments.

8569 **Camp Glyndon**
American Diabetes Association
800 Wyman Park Dr
Suite 110
Baltimore, MD 21211-2837 410-265-0075
800-342-2383
Fax: 410-235-4048
askada@diabetes.org
www.childrenwithdiabetes.com

Heather Magoon, Director

Camp is located in Nanjemoy, Maryland. One and two-week sessions July-August for children with diabetes and their families. Coed, ages 8-16.

8570 **Camp H.U.G.**
Arizona Hemophilia Association
826 North 5th Ave
Phoenix, AZ 85003 602-955-3947
888-754-7017
info@arizonahemophilia.org
www.arizonahemophilia.org/camp-programs

Chastity Fermoile, Executive Director
Chelsea Guffy, Business Development Specialist
Yleana Highes, Member Services Supervisor

Camp H.U.G (Hemophilia Uniting Generations) is a weekend camp program of the Arizona Hemophilia Association. The camp is for families who have a member with hemophilia, WWD, and/or other bleeding disorders.

8571 **Camp Harkness**
The Arc Eastern Connecticut
125 Sachem St.
Norwich, CT 06360 860-889-4435
Fax: 860-889-4662
info@thearcect.org
thearcect.org/camp-harkness

Kathleen Stauffer, Chief Executive Officer

A week-long summer camp program for individuals with intellectual and developmental disabilities. The camp is held at Camp Harkness in Waterford, CT.

8572 **Camp Heartland**
One Heartland
26001 Heinz Rd.
Willow River, MN 55795 888-216-2028
Fax: 612-824-6303
helpkids@oneheartland.org
www.oneheartland.org

Patrick Kindler, Executive Director
Katie Donlin, Operations Manager
Katie Bartels, Program Director
Stefanie Tywater-Christiansen, Development Director

A program of One Heartland, a nonprofit organization working to provide camping programs for children with serious illnesses or experiencing social isolation, Camp Heartland is a weeklong summer camp for children, ages 7-15, who are infected or affected by HIV/AIDS. The camp is held in Willow River, Minnesota.

8573 **Camp Hertko Hollow**
4200 University Ave.
Suite 320
Des Moines, IA 50266 515-471-8523
855-502-8500
Fax: 515-288-2531
www.camphertkohollow.com

Jessica Thornton, Executive Director
Deb Holwegner, Camp Director

Camp Hertko Hollow is an educational and recreational summer camp program for children and teens ages 6-17 with diabetes. Campers participate in traditional camp activities and learn about living with diabetes.

8574 **Camp Hickory Hill**
PO Box 1942
Columbia, MO 65205 573-445-9146
camphickoryhill@gmail.com
www.camphickoryhill.com

Jessica Bernhardt, Camp Director

Educates diabetic children concerning diabetes and its care. In addition to daily educational sessions on some aspects of diabetes, campers participate in swimming, sailing, arts and crafts and overnight camping. Coed, ages 7-17.

8575 **Camp Ho Mita Koda**
14040 Auburn Rd.
Newbury, OH 44065 440-739-4095
info@camphomitakoda.org
www.camphomitakoda.org

Ian Roberts, Executive Director
Eric Brown, Camp Director

Camp Ho Mita Koda is a summer camp for children with type 1 diabetes. The camp aims to provide outdoor activities while also educating and building life skills for children with diabetes. Offers overnight camp, family camp, specialty camp, and leadership development programs.

8576 **Camp Hodia**
Idaho Diabetes Youth Programs, Inc.
5439 W Kendall St.
Boise, ID 83706 208-891-1023
info@hodia.org
www.hodia.org

Lisa Gier, Executive Director
Morgan Coenen, Director, Programs
Ciera Miller, Director, Marketing
Sherilyn Robison, Director, Activities

Offers a variety of educational camp programs for children and teens with type 1 diabetes.

8577 **Camp Hollywood HEART**
One Heartland
26001 Heinz Rd.
Willow River, MN 55795 888-216-2028
Fax: 612-824-6303
helpkids@oneheartland.org
www.oneheartland.org

Patrick Kindler, Executive Director
Katie Donlin, Operations Manager
Katie Bartels, Program Director
Stefanie Tywater-Christiansen, Development Director

A program of One Heartland, a nonprofit organization working to provide camping programs for children with serious illnesses or experiencing social isolation. Camp Hollywood HEART is a weeklong summer camp for youths, ages 15-20, who are infected or affected by HIV/AIDS. The camp is held in Malibu, California and is partnership camp between One Heartland and Hollywood Heart.

8578 **Camp Honor**
Arizona Hemophilia Association
826 North 5th Ave
Phoenix, AZ 85003
602-955-3947
888-754-7017
info@arizonahemophilia.org
www.arizonahemophilia.org/camp-programs

Chastity Fermoile, Executive Director
Chelsea Guffy, Business Development Specialist
Yleana Highes, Member Services Supervisor

Camp Honor offers a week long summer camp to children affected by an inherited bleeding disorders. The cost of the camp is $35 for a single camper and $50 dollars for a family (2 or more campers). Camp Honor offers children the chance to partcipate in outdoor activities and educational opportunities. In order to attend the camp there is an application process.

8579 **Camp Independence**
National Kidney Foundation
30 East 33rd Street
New York, NY 10016
770-452-1539
800-622-9010
Fax: 212-689-9261
info@kidney.org
www.kidneyga.org

Gregory W. Scott, Chair
Beth Piraino, President
Bruce Skyer, CEO
Joseph Vassalotti, Chief Medical Officer

Camp Independence is Georgia's a overnight, week-long summer camp providing essential medical care, treatment & fun for kids with kidney disease and transplants. Camp Independence recognizes that campers are normal children but have special needs providing these children with opportunities for development & individual growth, peer support & normal life experiences. Activities include swimming, arts & crafts, fishing and horsebackriding, in addition to archery, games and sports, and ceramics.

8580 **Camp Jened**
United Cerebral Palsy Association New York
P.O. Box 483
Rock Hill, NY 12775-483
845-434-2220
Fax: 845-434-2253

Michael Branam, Executive Director

Camp is located in Rock Hill, New York. Sessions for adults with severe developmental and physical disabilities. Coed, ages 18-99.

8581 **Camp John Warvel**
American Diabetes Association
8604 Allisonville Rd.
Suite 140
Indianapolis, IN 46250
317-352-9226
campsupport@diabetes.org
www.diabetes.org

8582 **Camp Joslin**
The Barton Center for Diabetes Education, Inc.
30 Ennis Rd.
PO Box 356
North Oxford, MA 01537-0356
508-987-2056
Fax: 508-987-2002
info@bartoncenter.org
www.bartoncenter.org

Lynn Butler-Dinunno, Executive Director
Jenna Dufresne, Director, Health Services
Sarah Balko, Director, Camps & Programs
Sadie Vivenzio, Director, Finance

Camp for boys ages 6-16 with diabetes. This program offers active summer sports and activities, supplemented by medical treatment and diabetes education.

8583 **Camp Joy**
3325 Swamp Creek Rd
Schwenksville, PA 19473-1518
610-754-6878
Fax: 610-754-7880
www.campjoy.com

Robert G Griffith, President

A special needs camp for kids and adults (ages 4-80+) with developmental disabilities such as autism, brain injury, neurological disorder, visual and/or hearing impairments, Angelman and Down syndromes, and other developmental disabilities.

8584 **Camp Ko-Man-She**
Diabetes Dayton
2555 S Dixie Dr.
Suite 112
Dayton, OH 45409
937-220-6611
Fax: 937-224-0240
admin@diabetesdayton.org
www.diabetesdaytoncamp.com

Susan McGovern, Executive Director

Camp Ko-Man-She is located in Bellefontaine, Ohio, and is held annually for children with diabetes. The camp's goal is for children to socialize with other children who also have diabetes and to have fun outdoors in a medically supervised setting. Co-ed, ages 8-17.

8585 **Camp Kweebec**
157 Game Farm Rd.
Schwenksville, PA 19473
610-667-2123
Fax: 610-667-6376
info@kweebec.com
www.kweebec.com

Les Weiser, Owner/Director
Maddy Weiser, Owner/Director
Rachel Weiser, Associate Director, Director of
Josh Weiser, Associate Director

Camp is located in Schwenksville, Pennsylvania. Sessions for children and adults with diabetes. Coed, ages 6-16, families, seniors and single adults.

8586 **Camp L-Kee-Ta**
940 Golden Valley Drive
Bettendorf, IA 52722
319-752-3639
800-798-0833
Fax: 319-753-1410
www.gseiwi.org

Teresa Colgan, Chair
Jill Dashner, 1st Vice chiar
Anna Gibney, Development Manager
Ann Hulett, Business Operations Coordinator

Camp is located in Danville, Iowa. Half-week and one-week sessions June-August for children with asthma/respiratory ailments. Girls, ages 7-18 and families.

8587 **Camp Latgawa**
Oregon-Idaho Conference Center
13250 S Fork Little Butte Creek Rd
Eagle Point, OR 97524- 5593
541-826-9699
camplatgawa@hotmail.com
latgawa.gocamping.org/

Eva LaBonty, Director

Camp Latgawa provides year round hospitality for groups up to 90 people. The bunk/dormitory style facilities are heated and have restrooms and showers either in the cabin or nearby.

8588 **Camp Libbey**
Maumee Valley Girl Scout Center
2244 Collingwood Blvd
Toledo, OH 43620-1147
419-243-8216
800-860-4516
Fax: 419-245-5357
www.girlscoutsofwesternohio.org

Jody Wainscott, Chair
Ellen Iobst, 1st Vice Chair
Susan Gantz Matz, 2nd Vice Chair
Jerry Brose, Secretary

Camp for girls 7-18 with asthma/respiratory ailments, diabetes, epilepsy and muscular dystrophy is located in Defiance, Ohio.

8589 **Camp MITIOG**
Share, Inc
7615 N. Platte Purchase Drive
Kansas City, MO 64118
816-221-4450
877-221-4450
Fax: 816-221-1420
midlands@midlandsmc.org
www.midlandsmc.org

Mike Hale, President/Financial Officer
Pam Mathena, Adm. Assistant to MMC Financial Officer
Donna Fletcher, Congregational Consultant
Don McLaughlin, Outreach Coordinator

Camp is located in Excelsior Springs, Missouri. One-week summer sessions for children with spina bifida. Coed, ages 6-16.

8590 **Camp Magruder**
17450 Old Pacific Hwy.
Rockaway Beach, OR 97136
503-355-2310
Fax: 503-355-8701
troy@campmagruder.org
www.campmagruder.org

Troy Taylor, Camp Director
Hope Montgomery, Program Director
Rik Gutzke, Facilities Manager

Camp is located in Rockaway Beach, Oregon. Sessions for teens and adults with developmental disabilities through Camp Hope.

8591 **Camp Nejeda**
Camp Nejeda Foundation
910 Saddlebrook Road
P.O. Box 156
Stillwater, NJ 07875
973-383-2611
Fax: 973-383-9891
info@campnejeda.org

Ernest Post, MD, Secretary
Scott Ross, President
Bill Vierbuchen, Executive Director
Jim Daschbach, Camp Director

For children with diabetes, ages 7-15. Provides an active and safe camping experience which enables the children to learn about and understand diabetes. Activities include boating, swimming, fishing, archery, as well as camping skills.

8592 **Camp Not-A-Wheeze**
2689 E Michelle Way
Gilbert, AZ 85234
602-336-6575
Fax: 602-336-6576
info@campnotawheeze.org
campnotawheeze.org

Alan Crawford, Camp Director

Week-long summer camp for children aged 7-14 with moderate to severe asthma living in Arizona. Campers attending Camp Not-A- Wheeze, participate in a wide range of activities such as, horseback riding, hiking, canoeing, and fishing as well as an asthma education class. Those wishing to attend must fill out and send in a camper application.

8593 **Camp Okizu**
Okizu Foundation
83 Hamilton Dr.
Suite 200
Novato, CA 94949-5755
415-382-9083
Fax: 415-382-8384
info@okizu.org
www.okizu.org

Stuart J. Kaplan, Executive Director
Suzie Randall, Executive Director, Operations
Morgan Santiesteban, Camp Director

Camp Okizu offers a variety of medically supervised, residential camp programs for families who have a child diagnosed with cancer. Programs are offered throughout the year free of charge.

8594 **Camp Paivika**
PO Box 3367
Crestline, CA 92325
909-338-1102
Fax: 909-338-2502
camppaivika@abilityfirst.org
www.abilityfirst.org/camp-paivika

Kelly Kunsek, Camp Director
Lauren Wilson, Program Director
Tina Ronning-Fraynd, Coordinator, Camper Services

As a program of AbilityFirst, Camp Paivika offers overnight summer programs for children, teens and adults with developmental and physical disabilities. The camp is completely accessible and the staff is trained to provide any assistance or personal care a camper needs. Located in San Bernardino National Forest, Camp Paivika provides a traditional summer camp experience in a safe and fun environment.

8595 **Camp Pelican**
PO Box 10235
New Orleans, LA 70181
888-617-1118
Fax: 866-295-3803
camppelican@gmail.com
www.camppelican.org

8596 **Camp Rainbow**
Phoenix Childrens Hospital
1919 E Thomas Rd
Phoenix, AZ 85016
602-933-0157
camprainbow@phoenixchildrens.com
www.phoenixchildrens.org

Emilie Jarboe, Camp Director

Camp Rainbow is for children aged 7-17 who have or had cancer or a chronic blood disorder. The camp is offered for one week during the summer, held at camp Friendly Pines in Prescott, Arizona. Campers must be patients of Phoenix Children's Hospital's Center for Cancer and Blood Disorders, with the camp offering participants the opportunity to experience traditional camp activities including but not limited to, horseback riding, canoeing, fishing, swimming, and archery.

8597 **Camp Reach for the Sky**
The Seany Foundation
3530 Camino del Rio N
Suite 101
San Diego, CA 92108
858-551-0922
www.theseanyfoundation.org

Brian Bonert, Camp Advisory Chair
Benji Quintero, Sib Director
Kerry Whittaker, Roc Camp Director
Pauline Kern, Day Camp Director

Previously run by the American Cancer Society, Camp Reach for the Sky (CR4TS) is now run by The Seany Foundation and provides an opportunity for children with cancer and their siblings to attend a free summer camp. Camp Reach for the Sky offers a multiple programs, including a Resident Oncology Camp, a Sibling Camp and Day Camps.

8598 **Camp Ronald McDonald at Eagle Lake**
2555 49th Street
Sacramento, CA 95817
916-734-4230
Fax: 916-734-4238
mdamos@RMHCNC.org
www.campronald.org

Maria Damos, Camp Director

Camp Ronald McDonald at Eagle Lake collaborates with other nonprofit organizations to provide week long summer camp opportunities for children with special medical needs, financial hardship and/or emotional, developmental or physical disabilities. The camp is fully accessible.

8599 **Camp Ronald McDonald for Good Times**
1250 Lyman Place
Los Angeles, CA 90029
310-268-8488
Fax: 310-473-3338
www.campronaldmcdonald.org

Fatima Djelmane Rodriguez, Executive Director
Brian Crater, Associate Executive Director
Chad Edwards, Program Director
Shannon Edwards, Program Associate

Free year-round residential camping for children with cancer and their families.

8600 **Camp Sawtooth**
Oregon-Idaho Conference Center
P.O. Box 68
Fairfield, ID 83327-68
800-593-7539
sawtooth@gocamping.org
www.gocamping.org

David Hargreaves, Director

Camp located 35 miles north of fairfield, centrally located for all of southern Idaho.

8601 **Camp Seale Harris**
Southeastern Diabetes Education Services
500 Chase Park S.
Ste 104
Birmingham, AL 35244
205-402-0415
Fax: 205-402-0416
info@campsealeharris.org
www.campsealeharris.org

Matthew Munson, Chair
Katie Hester, Vice Chair
Rhonda McDavid, Executive Director
John Latimer, Camp & Community Programs Director

Offering overnight, family, day and community program camps, Camp Seale Harris is a nonprofit organization that offers residential camps for children and teens with diabetes. With multiple programs in Alabama, the volunteer camp counselors are trained adults living with diabetes, to better help the camp attendees gain independence in learning to manage their diabetes. Camp programs run all year round.

8602 **Camp Setebaid**
Setebaid Services, Inc.
PO Box 196
Winfield, PA 17889-0196
570-524-9090
Fax: 570-523-0769
info@setebaidservices.org
www.setebaidservices.org

Mark Moyer, Executive Director

Camping sessions for children with diabetes. The camp also hosts a family day for children with diabetes and their families.

8603 **Camp Smile-A-Mile**
Smile-A-Mile Place
1600 2nd Ave. S.
Birmingham, AL 35233
205-323-8427
Fax: 205-323-6220
info@campsam.org
www.campsam.org

Bruce Hooper, Executive Director
Kellie Reece, Chief Operating Officer
Shannon Rumage, Development Director
Carrie Pomeroy, Camp Director

Camp Smile-A-Mile offers 7 different educational camp opportunities for children and their families who have been affected by childhood cancer in Alabama. The programs run all year long, in a variety of formats.

8604 **Camp Sunburst**
Sunburst Projects United States Headquarters
2143 Hurley Way
Suite 240
Sacramento, CA 95825
916-440-0889
Fax: 916-440-1208
admin@sunburstprojects.org
www.sunburstprojects.org

Geri DeLaRosa, PhD, Founder & Executive Director
Samantha Voelkel, Camp Director

Camp Sunburst is a youth oriented leadership camp that promotes and creates an environment to help youth learn self confidence to change negative social patterns and break cycles of HIV/AIDS infections. Activities campers will participate in include, boating, swimming, art, dance, and sports.

8605 **Camp Sunrise**
Johns Hopkins Hospital
600 North Wolfe Street
CMSC 800
Baltimore, MD 21287-5904
410-955-5311

Sherryce Robinson, Mission Delivery Manager
Kira Elring, Regional Mission Director
Gloria Jetter, Regional Executive Director
Jack Shipkoski, CEO

Week long summer camp in White Hall, MD., for children ages 6-18 who have been diagnosed with or have survived cancer. Camp sunrise also has a 'day camp' program available for children ages 4-5. Camp activities include sports & games, swimming, arts & crafts, and nature hikes.

8606 **Camp Sunshine Dreams**
PO Box 28232
Fresno, CA 93729-8232
pam@campsunshinedreams.org
www.campsunshinedreams.com

Stephanie Scharbach, Contact
Pam Aiello, Contact

Camp Sunshine Dreams provides a summer camp experience to children aged 8-15 with cancer and their siblings.

8607 **Camp Sweeney**
PO Box 918
Gainesville, TX 76241
940-665-2011
Fax: 940-665-9467
info@campsweeney.org
www.campsweeney.org

Ernie Fernandez, Camp Director
Bob Cannon, Program Director
Billie Hood, Business Manager
Kelley King, Registrar

Camp Sweeney teaches self-care and self-reliance to children ages 5-18 with type 1 diabetes. Campers participate in activities such as swimming, fishing, horseback riding and arts and crafts while learning how to self manage their diabetes.

8608 **Camp Tall Turf**
816 Madison SE
Grand Rapids, MI 49507
616-452-7906
Fax: 616-452-7907
info@tallturf.org
www.tallturf.org

Eric Brown, Chair
Ed Van Poolen, Vice Chair
Miriam DeJong, Director of Programs
Victoria P. Gibbs, Interim Executive Director

Camp is located in Walkerville, Michigan. Summer camping sessions for youth with asthma/respiratory ailments and ADD. Coed, ages 8-16.

8609 **Camp Taylor**
Camp Taylor, Inc.
8224 West Grayson Rd.
Modesto, CA 95358-9094
209-545-3853
camp@kidsheartcamp.org
www.kidsheartcamp.org

Kimberlie Gamino, Founder & Executive Director

With several programs, Camp Taylor provides youth, teens, and the families of children with heart disease the opportunity to go to a free medically supervised summer sleepaway camp. Campers are able to enjoy activities such as, swimming, snorkeling, horseback riding, rock-wall, skits, archery, and heart education.

8610 **Camp Vacamas**
256 Macopin Rd
West Milford, NJ 07480
973-838-0942
877-428-8222
www.vacamas.org

Felix A. Urrutia, Executive Director
Kristin Short, Camp Director
Karen Wendolowski, Executive Secretary
Seth Friedman, MPA, Program Director

Disadvantaged children with asthma or sickle cell anemia, ages 8-16, are offered special programs in canoeing, backpacking, camping, music and leadership training. Sliding scale tuition. Year round programs for youth at risk groups. Conference center facility open for group rentals.

8611 **Camp Waziyatah**
530 Mill Hill Rd
Waterford, ME 04088-4011
207-583-2267
Fax: 509-357-2267
info@wazi.com
wazi.com

Gregg Parker, Owner/Director
Mitch Parker, Owner/Director

Camp is located in Waterford, Massachusetts. Three, four and seven-week sessions June-August for campers with cancer and diabetes. Coed, ages 8-15 and families, single adults.

8612 **Camp WheezeAway**
YMCA Camp Chandler
1240 Jordan Dam Rd
Wetumpka, AL 36092
334-229-0035
Fax: 334-649-7516
jikner@ymcamontgomery.org
ymcamontgomery.org/camp/wheezeaway
Jeff Reynolds, Executive Director
Art Mason, Operations Director
For children ages 8-12 with moderate to severe asthma, Camp WheezeAway offers week long summer camp programs that foster confidence building skills. The camp is free and managed by medical professionals. Those with children wishing to attend must apply to the camp and complete a selection process.

8613 **Camp del Corazon**
11615 Hesby St
North Hollywood, CA 91601-3620
818-754-0312
Fax: 818-754-0377
info@campdelcorazon.org
www.campdelcorazon.org
Tiffany Maisonet, Summer Camp Director
Chrissie Endler, Executive Director
Kevin Shannon, MD, President & Medical Director
Kristina Wallace, Director, Development & Operations
Camp del Corazon, is a nonprofit corporation offering a no cost summer camp and other programs to children aged 7-17 living with heart disease. Campers or their guardians must fill out a camp application, with acceptance into the camp dependant upon a nurse review of the parent and cardiology portions of the application.

8614 **Camps for Children & Teens with Diabetes**
Diabetes Society
1165 Lincoln Ave
Suite 300
San Jose, CA 95125-3052
408-287-3785
800-989-1165
Fax: 408-287-2701
info@diabetessociety.org
Sharon Ogbor, Executive Director
Thomas Smith, Director
Since 1974, sponsors up to 20 day camps, family camps and resident camps for children 4 through 17. These camps provide an opportunity for children with diabetes to go to camp, meet other children and gain a better understanding of their diabetes. The total experience can help campers develop more confidence in their abilities to control their diabetes effectively while enjoying the traditional camp experience. Camps are located throughout CA and parts of Nevada.

8615 **Cedar Ridge Camp**
4120 Old Routt Road
Louisville, KY 40299
502-267-5848
Fax: 502-267-0116
info@cedarridgecamp.com
www.cedarridgecamp.com
Andrew Hartmans, Executive Director
Half-week, one and two-week sessions for children with diabetes, developmental disabilities and muscular dystrophy. Coed, ages 6-17.

8616 **Champ Camp**
American Lung Association In Alaska
7420 SW Bridgeport Road
Suite 200
Tigard, OR 97224
503-294-4094
800-586-4872
Fax: 503-294-4120
www.aklung.org
Kathryn A. Forbes, Chairman
John F. Emanuel, Vice Chair
Harold Wimmer, President and CEO
Penny J. Siewert, Secretary/Treasurer
Champ Camp is a week long summer recreation and asthma education program at Camp Kushtaka on the beautiful shores of Kenai Lake. Campers are able to explore their skills in outdoor activities including canoeing, hiking, swimming, archery, and arts and crafts. More importantly, Champ Camp boosts self-confidence and instills a sense of responsibility. It teaches preventive measures to improve asthma management, and avoid asthmatic episodes as well as increases a camper's sense of independence.

8617 **Children's Hospital Burn Camps Program**
13123 E 16th Ave.
PO Box 580
Aurora, CO 80045
720-777-8295
Fax: 720-777-7270
trudy.boulter@childrenscolorado.org
www.noordinarycamps.org
Trudy Boulter, OTH CHT, Program Director
Tim Schuetz, Outreach Coordinator
The Children's Hospital Colorado Burn Camps Program provides rehabilitation and reintegration opportunities for children, teens, adults, and families who have been affected by burn injuries. The Camps Program has partnerships with 7 hospitals across the United States and offers year round programs.

8618 **Clara Barton Camp**
The Barton Center for Diabetes Education, Inc.
30 Ennis Rd.
PO Box 356
North Oxford, MA 01537-0356
508-987-2056
Fax: 508-987-2002
info@bartoncenter.org
www.bartoncenter.org
Lynn Butler-Dinunno, Executive Director
Jenna Dufresne, Director, Health Services
Sarah Balko, Director, Camps & Programs
Sadie Vivenzio, Director, Finance
Camp for girls ages 6-16 with diabetes. Campers participate in traditional camp activities and receive diabetes education. Activities include swimming, boating, sports, dance, music and arts and crafts.

8619 **Diabetes Camp**
Tanager Place
1614 W Mount Vernon Rd.
Mount Vernon, IA 52314
319-363-0681
Fax: 319-365-6411
campmail@tanagerplace.org
www.camptanager.org
Donald Pirrie, Camp Director
Provides recreational activities for children and teens with diabetes. The camp has on-site 24-hour physician and nursing staff. Ages 6-17.

8620 **Dr. Moises Simpser VACC Camp**
Nicklaus Children's Hospital
3200 SW 62nd Ave.
Suite 203
Miami, FL 33155-4076
305-662-8222
Fax: 786-268-1765
bela.florentin@mch.com
www.vacccamp.com
Bela Florentin, Camp Coordinator
Tania Diaz, Camp Clinical Coordinator
VACC Camp is a week-long overnight camp program for ventilation-assisted children and their families. The program includes sailing, swimming, field trips to local attractions, campsite entertainment, structured games, free play, and more. Parents have formal and informal opportunities to network among themselves.

8621 **Dream Street**
Dream Street Foundation
324 S. Beverly Dr.
Suite 500
Beverly Hills, CA 90212
424-333-1371
Fax: 310-388-0302
www.dreamstreetfoundation.org
Patty Grubman, Founder
Run by The Dream Street Foundation, Dream Street Camps provide camping programs for children (aged 4-14) and young adults (18-24) with chronic and life threatening illnesses. The kids program runs in California, with the young adults program running in Arizona. The programs are free of charge, and campers can participate in different activities such as, swimming, arts and crafts, sports, horseback riding, and archery.

8622 **EDI Camp**
Wyman Center
600 Kiwanis Dr
St. Louis, MO 63025-2212
636-938-5245
Fax: 636-938-5289
www.wymancenter.org

David Hilliard, President
Theresa Mayberry, Senior Vice President

Youngsters with diabetes learn how to care for themselves while participating in a wide variety of outdoor activities and trips. The camp, managed and financed by the American Diabetes Association Greater St. Louis Affiliate, offers camperships to children from the Greater St. Louis area, ages 7-16, but nonresidents may also apply.

8623 **Easterseals Camp ASCCA**
PO Box 21
5278 Camp Ascca Dr.
Jacksons Gap, AL 36861
256-825-9226
Fax: 256-269-0714
info@campascca.org
campascca.org

Matt Rickman, Camp Director
John Stephenson, Administrator
Jocelyn Jones, Secretary
Amber Cotney, Program Director

Easterseals Camp ASCCA is Alabama's Special Camp for Children and Adults, offering therapeutic recreation for children and adults with both physical and intellectual disabilities. The camp is located on 260 acres of barrier free woodland on Lake Martin and campers experience a wide variety of educational and recreational activities, including but not limited to: horseback riding, fishing, tubing, swimming, environmental education, arts, canoeing, and zip-lining. 1 week camp fees are $750.00.

8624 **FCYD Camp Utada**
Foundation for Children and Youth with Diabetes
1995 W 9000 S
West Jordan, UT 84088
801-566-6913
www.fcydcamputada.org

Dave Okubo, MD, Co-Founder & Trustee
Elizabeth Elmer, Co-Founder & Trustee
Nathan Gedge, Co-Founder & Trustee

Camping for children with diabetes. Coed, ages 1-18 and families.

8625 **Father Drumgoole Connelly Summer Camp**
MIV Mount Loretto
6581 Hylan Blvd
Staten Island, NY 10309-3830
718-317-2600
Fax: 718-317-2830
www.mountloretto.org

Stephen Rynn, Executive Director
Maryann Virga, Executive Assistant
Loretta Polanish, Executive Secretary
Ed Gani, Facilities Manager

Summer sessions for children with epilepsy, hearing impairment and developmental disabilities. Coed, ages 5-13.

8626 **Florida Diabetes Camp**
Florida Camp for Children & Youth with Diabetes
PO Box 14136
Gainesville, FL 32604-2136
352-334-1321
Fax: 352-334-1326
www.floridadiabetescamp.org

Gary Cornwell, Executive Director
Chris Stakely, Assistant Director
Janet Silverstein, Medical Director

Camp is located in Florida. Offers weekend and summer camps for children with type 1 diabetes.

8627 **Friends Academy Summer Camps**
Duck Pond Rd
Locust Valley, NY 11560
516-393-4207
Fax: 516-465-1720
camp@fa.org
www.fasummercamp.org

Rich Mack, Camp Director

Summer sessions for children with diabetes. Coed, ages 3-14, families.

8628 **God's Camp**
Episcopal Church of Hawaii
68-729 Farrington Hwy
Waialua, HI 96791-9314
808-637-6241
808-637-5505
Fax: 808-637-5505
www.campmokuleia.org

Debbie Alemeda, Manager

Episcopal Church tent camping, 5 nights, July. Church groups, family reunions, weddings, other organizations.

8629 **Growing Together Diabetes Camp**
ETMC
1000 S. Beckham
Tyler, TX 75701
903-597-0351
800-232-8318
info@etmc.org
www.etmc.org

Marty Wiggins, Development Director
Vicki Jowell, Director
Elmer G. Ellis, President
Jerry Massey, Senior Vice President

A summer camp for youths ages 6 to 15 with Type 1 or Type 2 diabetes.

8630 **Happiness Is Camping**
62 Sunset Lake Rd.
Hardwick, NJ 07825
908-362-6733
Fax: 908-362-5197
rich@happinessiscamping.org
www.happinessiscamping.org

Laura San Miguel, President
Julie McMahon, Secretary
Beth Fuchs, Treasurer

Happiness Is Camping is a camp for children with cancer and their siblings, ages 6-16.

8631 **Happy Camp**
Merrimack Hall Performing Arts Center
3320 Triana Blvd SW.
Huntsville, AL 35805
256-534-6455
info@merrimackhall.com
www.merrimackhall.com/happy-headquarters

8632 **Hemophilia Camp**
Tanager Place
1614 W Mount Vernon Rd.
Mount Vernon, IA 52314
319-363-0681
Fax: 319-365-6411
campmail@tanagerplace.org
www.camptanager.org

Donald Pirrie, Camp Director

A six-day camp for children with hemophilia and other bleeding disorders. The camp has onsite 24-hour physician and nursing staff.

8633 **Kiwanis Camp Wyman**
Wyman Center
600 Kiwanis Dr
Eureka, MO 63025-2212
636-938-5245
Fax: 636-938-5289
www.wymancenter.org

Keat Wilkins, Chairman
Dave Hilliard, President/CEO
Tom Etzkorn, VP,Executive Resource Officer
Mindy Sharp, MBA, SVP, Finance & Administration

Summer sessions for youth with diabetes. Coed, ages 8-16, run in conjunction with the American Diabetes Association. Call for program description.

8634 **Kota Camp**
Junior League Of Little Rock
401 South Scott Street
Little Rock, AR 72201
501-375-5557
info@jllr.org
www.jllr.org

Casey Rockwell, President
Jenna Martin, Vice President, Administrative
Lauren Hall, Treasurer
Betsey Mowery, Vice President, Community

Kota Camp is offered to children aged 6-16 with disabilities or medical conditions. Kota derived from a word used by the Quapaw Native American Tribe indigenous to Arkansas, means friend, and reflects the goals of the camp. Children with a disability bring a sibling or friend without a disability, to create a environment of inclusion, participate in camp activities, and promote an understanding of those with special needs. The camp is held at Camp Aldersgate in Little Rock.

8635 **Lions Camp Tatiyee**
5283 W White Mountain Blvd
Lakeside, AZ 85929
480-380-4254
pam@camptatiyee.org
camptatiyee.org

Pamela Swanson, Executive Director

Lions Camp Tatiyee is the only organization in Arizona providing a week long summer camp for individuals with special needs. There is no cost for the camp and all of the programs are adaptable. Some activities that campers can participate in are, go-karting, fishing, art, games, cooking, rock wall, swimming, dances and campfires.

8636 **Makemie Woods Camp**
Presbytery of Eastern Virginia
P.O. Box 39
Barhamsville, VA 23011
757-566-1496
800-566-1496
Fax: 757-566-8803

Mike Burcher, Director
Sherri Egerton, Program Director
Karen Broughman, Office Manager
Anthony Burcher, Storyteller in Residence

Residential Christian camp that tailors each group and individual goals. Counselors serve as teachers, friends and activity leaders. For children 8-18 with diabetes.

8637 **Makemie Woods Camp/Conference Retreat**
Presbytery of Eastern Virginia
P.O. Box 39
Barhamsville, VA 23011
757-566-1496
800-566-1496
Fax: 757-566-8803

Mike Burcher, Director
Sherri Egerton, Program Director
Karen Broughman, Office Manager
Anthony Burcher, Storyteller in Residence

Counselors serve as teachers, friends and activity leaders. The individual is important within the small group. No camper is lost in the crowd, but is an integral partner in the group process. Residential Christian Camp and conference center. Summer camp for children 8-18 and special camp for children with diabetes.

8638 **Marist Brothers Mid-Hudson Valley Camp**
PO Box 197
Esopus, NY 12429
845-384-6620
info@maristbrotherscenter.org

Amy Reinwald-Earle, Camp Director, Special Children
Brother Owen Ormsby, Executive Director
Scott Kuhner, Director of Operations
Mike Trainor, Facilities Director

The camp provides week-long summer sessions for children who have a variety of special needs/illnesses, such as cancer, HIV, deaf or mental disabilities. Each session is specific to the special need/illness.

8639 **MedCamps of Louisiana**
102 Thomas Rd.
Suite 615
West Monroe, LA 71291
318-329-8405
Fax: 318-329-8407
info@medcamps.com
www.medcamps.com

Caleb Seney, Executive Director
Kacie Hobson, Camp Director

Offers camp programs for children with chronic illnesses and physical or developmental disabilities.

8640 **Mountaineer Spina Bifida Camp**
534 New Goff Mountain Rd.
Charleston, WV 25313
info@drewsday.org
www.drewsday.org

Suzie Humphreys, Contact

A summer camp for individuals with spina bifida. Campers can participate in activities such as swimming, wheelchair hockey, baseball, and more.

8641 **Muscular Dystrophy Association Free Camp**
222 S. Riverside Plaza
Suite 1500
Chicago, IL 60606
907-276-2131
800-572-1717
Fax: 907-276-0946
www.mdausa.org

R. Rodney Howell, MD, Chairman
Steven M. Derks, President/CEO
Julie Faber, EVP/CFO
Pete Morgan, EVP/COO

MDA Camp provides a wide range of activities for those who have limited mobility or are in wheelchairs. The camp offers may outdoor sporting activities, art's & crafts and talent shows.

8642 **NeSoDak**
Lutherans Outdoors in South Dakota
2001 S Summit Ave.
Sioux Falls, SD 57197
605-947-4440
800-888-1464
nesodak@losd.org
www.losd.org/nesodak

Vicki Foss, Director

Located in Waubay, South Dakota, NeSoDak provides camp programs for a range of ages. Hosts Camp Gilbert, a summer camp program for children with diabetes.

8643 **Open Hearts Camp**
The Edward J. Madden Open Hearts Camp
250 Monument Valley Rd.
Great Barrington, MA 01230
413-528-2229
hearts@openheartscamp.org
www.openheartscamp.org

David Zaleon, Executive Director

Camp program for children who have had and are fully recovered from open heart surgery or a heart transplant. Four two-week sessions by age group. Small camp - around 15 campers per session.

8644 **Phantom Lake YMCA Camp**
S110W30240 YMCA Camp Rd.
Mukwonago, WI 53149
262-363-4386
office@phantomlakeymca.org
www.phantomlakeymca.org

Karin Mulrooney, Chair
Sara Hacker, Secretary
Bill Canfield, Treasurer

Phantom Lake Camp offers day and residential camping sessions for children ages 3-17. All programs are open to individuals with disabilities.

8645 **Rapahope Children's Retreat Foundation**
2701 Airport Blvd
Mobile, AL 36606
251-476-9880
Fax: 251-476-9495
info@rapahope.org
www.rapahope.org

Melissa McNichol, Executive Director
Roz Dorsett, Assistant Director

Rapahope is an organization that offers a one week long summer camp for children who have, or who have had cancer. For children ages 7-17, the camp offers a wide range of summer camp activities, including but not limited to, swimming, kayaking, horseback riding, and arts. The camp is offered at no cost to campers or their families.

8646 **Roundup River Ranch**
8333 Colorado River Rd.
Gypsum, CO 81637
970-524-2267
Fax: 877-619-0323
info@roundupriverranch.org
www.roundupriverranch.org
Ruth B. Johnson, JD, President & CEO
Sterling Nell Leija, Executive Camp Director
Kendra Perkins, Assustabt Camp Director
Christopher Troxel, Program Coordinator
Roundup River Ranch provides traditional camp experiences for children and their families with chronic and serious illnesses. The Ranch is located in Gypsum, Colorado, with all programs offered free of charge.

8647 **STIX Diabetes Programs**
PO Box 8308
Spokane, WA 99203
509-484-1366
Fax: 509-955-1329
stix@stixdiabetes.org
www.stixdiabetes.org
Tonya Kobluk, Director, Administration & Camps
Cindy Schneider, Director, Community Outreach
Jill Strom, Director, Development
STIX Diabetes Programs is a non-profit organization providing camp experiences for children and teens with diabetes. STIX offers a three-day non-residential day camp for children ages 6-8; a week-long residential camp for youth ages 9-16; and an excursion-based Adventure Camp for teens ages 16-19.

8648 **Shady Oaks Camp**
16300 Parker Rd.
Homer Glen, IL 60491
708-301-0816
Fax: 708-301-5091
soc16300@sbcglobal.net
www.shadyoakscamp.org
Scott Steele, Executive Director
Katie Clark, Camp Director
Gary Schaid, Assistant Director
Shady Oaks Camp provides summer camp programs for children and adults with cerebral palsy and similar disabilities.

8649 **Sherman Lake YMCA Summer Camp**
Sherman Lake YMCA Outdoor Center
6225 N 39th St
Augusta, MI 49012
269-731-3000
Fax: 269-731-3020
shermanlakeymca@ymcasl.org
www.shermanlakeymca.org
Luke Austenfeld, Executive Director
Jean Henderson, Business Manager
Lorrie Syverson, Director,Camping, Education & Retreat Services
Mark VanDaff, Facility Manager
Summer camping sessions for campers with ADD and spina bifida. Coed, ages 6-15 and families, seniors.

8650 **Strength for the Journey**
Oregon-Idaho Conference Center
1505 SW 18th Ave
Portland, OR 97201-2524
503-226-7931
800-593-7539
suttlelake@gocamping.org
www.gocamping.org
Jane Petke, Suttle Lake Camp Director
Geneva Cook, Camping Registrar
Camp is located near Sisters, Oregon at Suttle Lake Camp. Strength for the Journey is a program for adults living with HIV/AIDS.

8651 **Summer Camp for Children with Muscular Dystrophy**
Muscular Dystrophy Association - USA
222 S. Riverside Plaza
Suite 1500
Chicago, IL 60606
520-529-2000
800-572-1717
Fax: 520-529-5300
mda@mdausa.org
www.mdausa.org
R. Rodney Howell, MD, Chairman
Steven M. Derks, President/CEO
Pete Morgan, EVP/COO
Julie Faber, EVP/CFO
Offers a wide range of activities such as adaptive sports, swimming, fishing, archery, scavenger hunts, dances & talent shows, art's & crafts, karaoke, and campfires.

8652 **Suttle Lake Camp**
29551 Suttle Lake Rd.
Sisters, OR 97759
541-595-6663
suttlelake@gocamping.org
suttlelake.gocamping.org
Daniel Petke, Co-Director
Jane Petke, Co-Director
Offers a variety of camp programs, including sessions for individuals with HIV/AIDS.

8653 **TSA CT Kid's Summer Event**
Tourette Syndrome Association of Connecticut (TSA)
c/o Massachusetts Chapter
39 Godfrey Street
Taunton, MA 02780
617-277-7589
www.tsact.org
Tom Meehan, Chairman
Peter Tavolacci, Vice-Chairman
Paul Nazario, Treasurer
TSA of Connecticut sponsors summer events for children with TS/Tourette Syndrome activities of which include minature golf in addition to an Annual Conference. The kids' program at this annual conference provides children who have TS a unique opportunity to meet other children like them who also struggle with TS. Entertainment includes puppeteers, magicians, learning karate from the experts, getting face paintings and more.
uniqu pages

8654 **Texas Lions Camp**
PO Box 290247
Kerrville, TX 78029
830-896-8500
Fax: 830-896-3666
tlc@lionscamp.com
www.lionscamp.com
Stephen S. Mabry, President & CEO
Karen-Anne King, Vice President, Summer Camps
Milton Dare, Director, Development
Joan Dixon, Director, Finance
Texas Lions Camp is a camp dedicated to serving children ages 7-16 in Texas with physical disabilities. While at camp, campers will participate in a variety of activities and be encouraged to become more independent and self-confident.

8655 **The Hole in the Wall Gang Camp**
565 Ashford Center Rd.
Ashford, CT 06278
860-429-3444
info@holeinthewallgang.org
www.holeinthewallgang.org
James H. Canton, Chief Executive Officer
Padraig Barry, Chief Strategy Officer
Kevin Magee, Chief Financial Officer
Hilary Axtmayer, Chief Program Officer
The Hole in the Wall Gang Camp offers summer and weekend camp experiences for children and the siblings of children with serious illnesses. Located in Ashford, Connecticut, campers are able to participate in traditional camp activities in a medically safe environment.

8656 **Twin Lakes Camp**
1451 E Twin Lakes Rd
Hillsboro, IN 47949-8004
765-798-4000
outdoors@twinlakescamp.com
www.twinlakescamp.com

Jon Beight, Executive Director
Dan Daily, Program Director
Duane Bush, Guest Service
Donna Beight, Secretary

Provides a summer camp program for special needs children and young adults. Campers suffer from a wide range of maladies including crippling accidents, Spina Bifida, epilepsy, Cerebral Palsy, Muscular Dystrophy, Quadriplegia, Paraplegia, and other disabling diseases. Campers range in age from 8 to 27.

8657 **Wisconsin Lions Camp**
Wisconsin Lions Foundation
3834 County Rd. A
Rosholt, WI 54473
715-677-4969
877-463-6953
Fax: 715-677-4527
info@wisconsinlionscamp.com
www.wisconsinlionscamp.com

Evett Hartvig, Executive Director
Andrea Yenter, Camp Director
Phillip Potter, Assistant Camp Director
Peter Rekowski, Facility Director

Provides camp programs for youth and adults in Wisconsin with disabilities, including autism, intellectual disabilities, diabetes, epilepsy, visual impairments, and hearing impairments. ACA accredited, located in central Wisconsin, near Stevens Point.

8658 **Y Camp**
YMCA of Greater Des Moines
1192 166th Drive
Boone, IA 50036
515-432-7558
Fax: 515-432-5414
ycamp@dmymca.org
www.y-camp.org

David Sherry, Executive Director
Mike Havlik, Program Director- Environmental
Alex Kretzinger, Program Director- Summer Camp
Amy Joanning, Development Coordinator/Registrar

Camp is located in Boone, Iowa. Year-round one and two-week sessions for boys and girls with cancer, diabetes, asthma, cystic fibrosis, hearing impaired and other disabilities. Coed, ages 6-16 and families.

8659 **YMCA Camp Fitch**
12600 Abels Rd.
North Springfield, PA 16430
814-922-3219
877-863-4824
Fax: 814-922-7000
registrar@campfitchymca.org
campfitchymca.org

Tom Parker, Executive Director
Joe Wolnik, Summer Camp Director
Brandy Duda, Outdoor Education Director
Hannah Kight, Office Manager

Camp is located in North Springfield, Pennsylvania. Camp programs include sessions for children with diabetes or epilepsy.

8660 **YMCA Camp Ihduhapi**
Minneapolis YMCA Camping Services
15200 Hanson Blvd.
Andover, MN 55304
763-230-9622
info@campihduhapi.org
campihduhapi.org

Kerry Pioske, Camp Executive
Josh Cobb, Overnight Camp Director
Devin Hanson, Day Camp Director
Eric Wobschall, Building Superintendent

Camp is located in Loretto, Minnesota. Summer sessions for campers with asthma/respiratory ailments and epilepsy. Coed, ages 7-16.

8661 **YMCA Camp Kitaki**
Lincoln YMCA
570 Fallbrook Blvd.
Suite 210
Lincoln, NE 68521
402-434-9200
Fax: 402-434-9208
info@ymcalincoln.org
www.ymcalincoln.org

Barb Bettin, President/CEO
J.P. Lauterbach, COO
Misty Muff, Chief Administrative Officer
Renee Yost, CFO

Camp is located in Louisville, Nebraska. Summer sessions for children with cystic fibrosis. Coed, ages 7-17 and families.

8662 **YMCA Camp Shady Brook**
YMCA of the Pikes Peak Region (PPYMCA)
316 N. Tejon Street
Colorado Springs, CO 80903
719-329-7227
Fax: 719-272-7026
campinfo@ppymca.org
www.campshadybrook.org

Sonny Adkins, Executive Director
Laura Petersen, Program Director
Patrick Casey, Facility Director
Michaela Eddleston, Conference & Retreat Director

Camp is located in Sedalia, Colorado. One-week sessions for campers with HIV. Boys and girls 7-16. Also families, seniors and single adults.

8663 **YMCA Camp jewell**
YMCA of Greater Hartford
6 Prock Hill Road
P.O. Box 8
Colebrook, CT 06021
860-379-2782
888-412-2267
Fax: 860-379-8715
camp.jewell@ghymca.org
www.ghymca.org

Eric Tucker, Executive Director

Camp is located in Colebrook, Connecticut. Two-week sessions for children with cancer. Coed, ages 8-16. Also families.

8664 **YMCA Camp of Maine**
305 Winthrop Center Rd
P.O. Box 446
Winthrop, ME 04364
207-395-4200
Fax: 207-395-7230
info@maineycamp.org
www.maineycamp.org

Tom Christensen, CVO
Rebecca Henry, Vice CVO
Marty Allen, Treasurer
Heather Priest, Secretary

Activities include arts and crafts, nature study, hiking, and overnight camping, dancing, and singing. Summer session dates run from June through August; for ages 8-16.

8665 **YMCA Outdoor Center Campbell Gard**
4803 Augspurger Road
Hamilton, OH 45011
513-867-0600
Fax: 513-867-0127
camp@gmvymca.org
www.ccgymca.org

Pete Fasano, Executive Director
Katie Depew, Summer Program Director
Tom Andrews, Facilities and Properties Manager
Wendi Moore, Office Manager

Camp is located in Hamilton, Ohio. Camping sessions for children and young adults with developmental disabilities. Runs overnight and day sessions for ages 7-22 and families.

Books

8666 **A Woman's Guide to Living with HIV Infection**
Johns Hopkins University Press
2715 N Charles St
Baltimore, MD 21218-4363
410-516-6900
800-548-1784
Fax: 410-516-6998
jwehmueller@press.jhu.edu
www.press.jhu.edu

Rebecca A Clark M.D., PhD, Author
Robert T Maupin Jr. M.D. FACOG, Co-Author
Jill Hayes Hammer PhD, Co-Author
A resource for women with HIV that discusses coping with the diagnosis, finding a physician, recognizing symptoms, and preventing complications. Explains the latest treatment options and advice on coping with gynecologic infections. *$18.00*
328 pages Hardback

8667 **ABC of Asthma, Allergies & Lupus**
Global Health Solutions
2146 Kings Garden Way
PO Box 3189
Falls Church, VA 22043-2593
703-848-2333
800-759-3999
Fax: 703-848-0028
information@watercure.com
www.watercure.com

Fereydoon Batmanghelidj MD, Author
Xiaopo Batmanghelidj, President
Kristin Swan, Administrator
This book introduces new approaches in preventing and treating asthma, allergies and lupus without toxic chemicals. It also offers new insight on how to prevent and treat children's asthma. *$17.00*
240 pages
ISBN 0-962994-26-x

8668 **AIDS Sourcebook**
Omnigraphics
615 Griswold Street
Suite 520
Detroit, MI 48226
610-461-3548
800-234-1340
Fax: 800-875-1340
contact@omnigraphics.com
www.omnigraphics.com

Peter Ruffner, Co-Founder
Fred Ruffner, Co-Founder
Basic consumer health information about the Human Immunodeficiency Virus (HIV) and Acquired Immunodeficiency Syndrome (AIDS), including facts about its origins, stages, types, transmission, risk factors, and prevention, and featuring details about diagnostic testing, antiretroviral treatments, and co-occurring infections. *$85.00*
600 pages 5th Edition 1911
ISBN 0-780811-47-8

8669 **AIDS and Other Manifestations of HIV Infection**
Elsevier Inc
30 Corporate Dr
Suite 400
Burlington, MA 01803-4252
781-313-4700
800-545-2522
Fax: 800-568-5136
usbkinfo@elsevier.com
www.elsevier.com

Gary Wormser MD, Editor
A comprehensive overview of the biological properties of this etiologic viral agent, its clinicopathological manifestations, the epidemiology of its infection, and present and future therapeutic options. *$249.95*
1000 pages 2004
ISBN 0-127640-51-7

8670 **AIDS in the Twenty-First Century: Disease and Globalization**
Palgrav Macmillan
175 5th Ave
New York, NY 10010-7703
888-330-8477
Fax: 800-672-2054
onlinesupportusa@palgrave.com
www.palgrave-usa.com

Gabriella Georgiades, Editor
Alan Whiteside, Author
Tony Barnett, Co-Author
The authors — exprets in the field for over 15 years — argue that it is vital to not only look at AIDS in terms of prevention and treatment, but to also consider consequences which affect households, communities, companies, governments, and countries. This is a major contribution toward understanding the global public health crisis, as well as the relationship between poverty, inequality, and infectious diseases. *$32.00*
464 pages
ISBN 1-403997-68-5

8671 **Adult Leukemia: A Comprehensive Guide for Patients and Families**
O'Reilly Media Inc
1005 Gravenstein Hwy N
Sebastopol, CA 95472-2811
707-827-7000
800-998-9938
Fax: 707-829-0104
order@oreilly.com
www.oreilly.com

Linda Lamb, Editor
Barb Lackritz, Author
For the tens of thousands of Americans with adult leukemia, Adult Leukemia: A Comprehensive Guide for Patients and Families addresses diagnosis, medical tests, finding a good oncologist, treatments, side effects, getting emotional and other support, resources for further study, and much more. The book includes real-life stories from those who have battled leukemia themselves. *$29.95*
536 pages Paperback
ISBN 0-596500-01-7

8672 **Advanced Breast Cancer: A Guide to Living with Metastic Disease**
O'Reilly Media Inc
1005 Gravenstein Hwy N
Sebastopol, CA 95472-2811
707-827-7000
800-998-9938
Fax: 707-829-0104
order@oreilly.com
www.oreilly.com

Linda Lamb, Editor
Musa Mayer, Author
This is the only book on breast cancer that deals honestly with the realities of living with metastic disease, yet offers hope and comfort. All aspects of facing the disease are covered, including: coping with the shock of recurrence, seeking information and making treatment decisions, communicating effectively with medical personnel finding support, and handling disease progression and end-of-life issues. A comprehensive guide, it also provides updated resources and treatment developments. *$24.95*
532 pages Paperback 1998
ISBN 1-565925-22-X

8673 **Allergies & Asthma: What Every Parent Needs To Know (2nd Edition)**
American Academy of Pediatrics
345 Park Blvd.
Itasca, IL 60143
800-433-9016
Fax: 847-434-8000
mcc@aap.org
www.aap.org

Mark Del Monte, CEO & Executive Vice President
Christine Bork, Chief Development Officer & Sr. Vice President, Development
Roberta Bosak, Chief Administrative Officer & Sr. Vice President, HR
Vera Tait, Chief Medical Officer

Consumer resource for parents who need answers and information about their children's allergies and asthma. Covers advice on identifying allergies and asthma, preventing attacks, minimizing triggers, understanding medications, explaining allergies to young children, and helping children manage symptoms. *$14.95*

174 pages Paperback; eBook available 1910

ISBN 1-581104-45-6

8674 **Allergies Sourcebook**

Omnigraphics
615 Griswold Street
Suite 520
Detroit, MI 48226
610-461-3548
800-234-1340
Fax: 800-875-1340
contact@omnigraphics.com
www.omnigraphics.com

Peter Ruffner, Co-Founder
Fred Ruffner, Co-Founder

Basic comsumer health information about the immune system and allergic disorders, including rhinitis (hay fever), sinusitis, conjunctivitis, asthma, atopic dermatitis, and anaphylaxis, and allergy triggers such as pollen, mold, dust mites, animal dander, chemicals, foods and additives, and medications; along with facts about allergy diagnosis and treatment, tips on avoiding triggers and preventing symptoms, a glossary of related terms, and directories of resources for additional help and info. *$95.00*

608 pages 4th Edition 1911

8675 **Alternative Approach to Allergies**

Harper Collins Publishers
10 E 53rd St
New York, NY 10022-5244
212-207-7901
800-242-7737
Fax: 212-702-2586
spsales@harpercollins.com
www.harpercollins.com

Theron G Randolph M.D., Author
Ralph W Moss PhD, Co-Author

Here is the book that revolutionized the way allergies and other common illnesses were diagnosed and treated.

ISBN 0-060916-93-1

8676 **Alzheimer Disease Sourcebook**

Omnigraphics
615 Griswold Street
Suite 520
Detroit, MI 48226
610-461-3548
800-234-1340
Fax: 800-875-1340
contact@omnigraphics.com
www.omnigraphics.com

Peter Ruffner, Co-Founder
Fred Ruffner, Co-Founder

Alzheimer Disease Sourcebook, Fifth Edition provides updated information about causes, symptoms, and stages of AD and other forms of dementia, including mild cognitive impairment, corticobasal degeneration, dementia with Lewy bodies, frontotemporal dementia, Huntington disease, Parkinson disease, and dementia caused by infections. *$95.00*

600 pages 1911

ISBN 0-780811-50-8

8677 **Alzheimer Disease Sourcebook, 4th Edition**

Omnigraphics
615 Griswold Street
Suite 520
Detroit, MI 48226
610-461-3548
800-234-1340
Fax: 800-875-1340
contact@omnigraphics.com
www.omnigraphics.com

Peter Ruffner, Co-Founder
Fred Ruffner, Co-Founder

Basic consumer health information about alzheimer disease, other dementias, and related disorders, including multi-infarct dementia, dementia with lewy bodies, frontotemporal dementia (pick disease), Wernicke-Korsakoff syndrome (alcohol-related dementia), AIDS dementia complex, Huntington disease, Creutzfeldt-Jacob disease, and delirium. *$84.00*

603 pages

ISBN 0-780810-01-3

8678 **Amyotrophic Lateral Sclerosis: A Guide for Patients and Families**

Demos Medical Publishing
11 West 42nd Street
15th Floor
New York, NY 10036
212-683-0072
800-532-8663
Fax: 212-683-0118
support@demosmedical.com
www.demosmedpub.com

Richard Winters, Executive Editor
Beth Kaufman Barry, Publisher
Noreen Henson, Executive Director of Demos Heal
Reina Santana, Director of Special Sales & Righ

This comprehensive guide covers every aspect of the management of ALS. Beginning with discussions of its clinical features of the disease, diagnosis, and an overview of symptom management, major sections deal with medical and rehabilitative management, living with ALS, managing advanced disease and end-of-life issues, and reources that can provide support and assistance. *$29.95*

470 pages 2001

ISBN 1-888799-28-5

8679 **Arthritis Sourcebook.**

Omnigraphics
615 Griswold Street
Suite 520
Detroit, MI 48226
610-461-3548
800-234-1340
Fax: 800-875-1340
contact@omnigraphics.com
www.omnigraphics.com

Peter Ruffner, Co-Founder
Fred Ruffner, Co-Founder

Basic consumer health information about osteoarthritis, rheumatoid arthritis, other rheumatic disorders, infectious forms of arthritis, and diseases with symptoms linked to arthritis, and facts about diagnosis, pain management, and surgical therapies. *$84.00*

567 pages 2nd Edition

ISBN 0-780806-67-2

8680 **Asthma Sourcebook.**

Omnigraphics
615 Griswold Street
Suite 520
Detroit, MI 48226
610-461-3548
800-234-1340
Fax: 800-875-1340
contact@omnigraphics.com
www.omnigraphics.com

Peter Ruffner, Co-Founder
Fred Ruffner, Co-Founder

Provides information about asthma, including symptoms, remedies and research updates. *$84.00*

581 pages 2nd Edition

ISBN 0-780808-66-9

8681 **Asthma and Allergy Answers: A Patient Education Library**

Asthma and Allergy Foundation of America
8201 Corporate Dr
Suite 1000
Landover, MD 20785
202-466-7643
800-727-8462
Fax: 202-466-8940
info@aafa.org
www.aafa.org

Amy Patterson, Senior Director of Administration & Governance
Jacqui Vok, Director of Programs and Services
William McLin, M.Ed., President/CEO

This resource contains 50 reproducible fact sheets for patients on a variety of popular asthma and allergy topics. Information is written in a patient-friendly question and answer format and packaged in a durable binder for easy storage and use. *$50.00*

8682 **Back & Neck Sourcebook.**

Omnigraphics
615 Griswold Street
Suite 520
Detroit, MI 48226
610-461-3548
800-234-1340
Fax: 800-875-1340
contact@omnigraphics.com
www.omnigraphics.com

Peter Ruffner, Co-Founder
Fred Ruffner, Co-Founder

Basic consumer health information about back and neck pain, spinal cord injuries, and related disorders, such as degenerative disk disease, osteoarthritis, scoliosis, sciatica, spina bifida, and spinal stenosis, and featuring facts about maintaining spinal health, self-care, rehabilitative care, chiropractic care, spinal surgeries, and complementary therapies. *$84.00*

607 pages 2nd Edition
ISBN 0-780807-38-9

8683 **Being Close**

National Jewish Health
1400 Jackson St
Denver, CO 80206-2761
303-398-1002
877-225-5654
Fax: 303-398-1125
allstetterw@njc.org
www.nationaljewish.org

Michael Salem M.D., President/CEO
William Allstetter, Director Media/External Relation

A booklet offering information to patients suffering from a respiratory disorder such as emphysema, asthma or tuberculosis, that discusses sexual problems and feelings.

8684 **Bittersweet Chances: A Personal Journey o f Living and Learning in the Face of Illness**

PublishAmerica
PO Box 151
Frederick, MD 21705-151
301-695-1707
Fax: 301-631-9073
support@publishamerica.com
www.publishamerica.com

Dana Selenke Broehl, Author

Recounts Doug and Dana Broehl's journey of growth through the darkness of cystic fibrosis and the renewed hope of a double lung transplant. *$24.95*

189 pages Softcover
ISBN 1-413713-24-6

8685 **Blood and Circulatory Disorders Sourcebook**

Omnigraphics
615 Griswold Street
Suite 520
Detroit, MI 48226
610-461-3548
800-234-1340
Fax: 800-875-1340
contact@omnigraphics.com
www.omnigraphics.com

Peter Ruffner, Co-Founder
Fred Ruffner, Co-Founder

Blood and Circulatory Disorders Sourcebook, Third Edition offers facts about blood function and composition, the maintenance of a healthy circulatory system, and the types of concerns that arise when processes go awry. It discusses the diagnosis and treatment of many common blood cell disorders, bleeding disorders, and circulatory disorders, including anemia, hemochromatosis, leukemia, lymphoma, hemophilia, hypercoagulation, thrombophilia, atherosclerosis, blood pressure irregularities, coronary *$84.00*

634 pages 2nd Edition
ISBN 0-780807-46-4

8686 **Blooming Where You're Planted: Stories From The Heart**

Meeting Life's Challenges
9042 Aspen Grove Lane
Madison, WI 53717-2700
608-824-0402
Fax: 608-824-0403
help@MeetingLifesChallenges.com
www.makinglifeeasier.com

Shelley Peterman Schwatz, Editor

Author Shelley Peterman Schwarz takes you on her journey of self-discovery and change following her diagnosis of multiple sclerosis in 1979. Her personal stories are warm and humorous, and insightful. This 138-page book will motivate and inspire you to rise above life's challenges and live life to its fullest. *$12.95*

138 pages 1998
ISBN 0-891854-01-1

8687 **Brain Allergies: The Psychonutrient and Magnetic Connections**

McGraw-Hill

William Philpott PhD, Author
Dwight Keating PhD, Author
Linus Pauling PhD, Author

A complete overview of the concept of brain allergies - the theory that exposure to certain foods and other substances triggers mental disorders in people so predisposed, and that such disturbances can be cured by eliminating these substances. *$16.95*

ISBN 0-658003-98-1

8688 **Brain Disorders Sourcebook**

Omnigraphics
615 Griswold Street
Suite 520
Detroit, MI 48226
610-461-3548
800-234-1340
Fax: 800-875-1340
contact@omnigraphics.com
www.omnigraphics.com

Peter Ruffner, Co-Founder
Fred Ruffner, Co-Founder

Brain Disorders Sourcebook, Third Edition provides readers with updated information about brain function, neurological emergencies such as a brain attack (stroke) or seizure, and symptoms of brain disorders. It describes the diagnosis, treatment, and rehabilitation therapies for genetic and congenital brain disorders, brain infections, brain tumors, seizures, traumatic brain injuries, and degenerative neurological disorders such as Alzheimer disease and other dementias, Parkinson disease, and am *$84.00*

600 pages 2nd Edition
ISBN 0-780807-44-0

8689 **Breast Cancer Sourcebook**

Omnigraphics
615 Griswold Street
Suite 520
Detroit, MI 48226
610-461-3548
800-234-1340
Fax: 800-875-1340
contact@omnigraphics.com
www.omnigraphics.com

Peter Ruffner, Co-Founder
Fred Ruffner, Co-Founder

Breast Cancer Sourcebook, Fourth Edition, provides updated information about breast cancer and its causes, risk factors, diagnosis, and treatment. Readers will learn about the types of breast cancer, including ductal carcinoma in situ, lobular carcinoma in situ, invasive carcinoma, and inflammatory breast cancer, as well as common breast cancer treatment complications, such as pain, fatigue, lymphedema, hair loss, and sexuality and fertility issues. Information on preventive therapies, nutrition *$84.00*

600 pages 3rd Edition
ISBN 0-780810-30-3

8690 **Breathe Free**
Lotus Press
P.O. Box 325
Twin Lakes, WI 53181
262-889-8561
800-824-6396
Fax: 262-889-8591
lotuspress@lotuspress.com
www.lotuspress.com

Daniel Gagnon, Author
Amanda Morningstar, Author
An expose on respiratory diseases and their natural treatment. Learn how you can heal and/or manage common colds/flu, earaches/asthma, allergies/hay fever, pleurisy/pneumonia, coughs/sore throats, bronchitis/emphysema, AIDS and ARC related respiration infection. Covers information you wish your doctor would share with you such as what is happening to your body. *$14.95*
179 pages
ISBN 9-780914-95-5

8691 **Cancer Sourcebook**
Omnigraphics
615 Griswold Street
Suite 520
Detroit, MI 48226
610-461-3548
800-234-1340
Fax: 800-875-1340
contact@omnigraphics.com
www.omnigraphics.com

Peter Ruffner, Co-Founder
Fred Ruffner, Co-Founder
Cancer Sourcebook, Sixth Edition provides updated information about common types of cancer affecting the central nervous system, endocrine system, lungs, digestive and urinary tracts, blood cells, immune system, skin, bones, and other body systems. It explains how people can reduce their risk of cancer by addressing issues related to cancer risk and taking advantage of screening exams. *$84.00*
1105 pages 5th Edition
ISBN 0-780809-47-5

8692 **Cancer Sourcebook for Women**
Omnigraphics
615 Griswold Street
Suite 520
Detroit, MI 48226
610-461-3548
800-234-1340
Fax: 800-875-1340
contact@omnigraphics.com
www.omnigraphics.com

Peter Ruffner, Co-Founder
Fred Ruffner, Co-Founder
Cancer Sourcebook for Women, Fourth Edition offers updated information about gynecologic cancers and other cancers of special concern to women, including breast cancer, cancers of the female reproductive organs, and cancers responsible for the highest number of deaths in women. It explains cancer risks-including lifestyle factors, inherited genetic abnormalities, and hormonal medications-and methods used to diagnose and treat cancer. *$84.00*
687 pages 5th Edition
ISBN 0-780808-67-6

8693 **Cardiovascular Diseases and Disorders Sourcebook, 3rd Edition**
Omnigraphics
615 Griswold Street
Suite 520
Detroit, MI 48226
610-461-3548
800-234-1340
Fax: 800-875-1340
contact@omnigraphics.com
www.omnigraphics.com

Peter Ruffner, Co-Founder
Fred Ruffner, Co-Founder
Cardiovascular Diseases and Disorders Sourcebook, Third Edition, provides information about the symptoms, diagnosis, and treatment heart diseases and vascular disorders. It includes demographic and statistical data, an overview of the cardiovascular system, a discussion of risk factors and prevention techniques, a look at cardiovascular concerns specific to women, and a report on current research initiatives. *$84.00*
687 pages Hard cover
ISBN 0-780807-39-6

8694 **Childhood Cancer Survivors: A Practical Guide to Your Future**
O'Reilly Media Inc
1005 Gravenstein Hwy N
Sebastopol, CA 95472-2811
707-827-7000
800-998-9938
Fax: 707-829-0104
order@oreilly.com
www.oreilly.com

Linda Lamb, Editor
Nancy Keene, Author
Wendy Hobbie, Co-Author
Kathy Ruccione, Co-Author
More than 250,000 people have survived childhood cancer - a cause for celebration. Authors Keene, Hobbie, and Ruccione chart the territory of long-term survivorship: relationships; overcoming employment or insurance discrimination; maximizing health; follow-up schedules; medical late effects. The stories of over sixty survivors - their challenges and triumphs - are told. Includes medical history record-keeper. *$27.95*
464 pages Paperback 1906
ISBN 0-596528-51-5

8695 **Childhood Cancer: A Parent's Guide to Solid Tumor Cancers**
O'Reilly Media Inc
1005 Gravenstein Highway North
Sebastopol, CA 95472
707-827-7000
800-889-8969
Fax: 707-829-0104
order@oreilly.com
www.oreilly.com

560 pages Paperback
ISBN 0-596500-14-9

8696 **Childhood Diseases and Disorders Sourcebook, 2nd Edition**
Omnigraphics
615 Griswold Street
Suite 520
Detroit, MI 48226
610-461-3548
800-234-1340
Fax: 800-875-1340
contact@omnigraphics.com
www.omnigraphics.com

Peter Ruffner, Co-Founder
Fred Ruffner, Co-Founder
Basic consumer health information about medical problems often encountered in pre-adolescent children, including respiratory tract ailments, ear infections, sore throats, disorders of the skin and scalp, digestive and genitourinary diseases, infectious diseases, inflammatory disorders, chronic physical and developmental disorders, allergies, and more. *$84.00*
600 pages Hard cover
ISBN 0-780810-31-0

8697 **Childhood Leukemia: A Guide for Families, Friends & Caregivers**
O'Reilly Media Inc
1005 Gravenstein Hwy N
Sebastopol, CA 95472-2811
707-827-7000
800-998-9938
Fax: 707-829-0104
order@oreilly.com
www.oreilly.com

Linda Lamb, Editor
Nancy Keene, Author
The second edition of this comprehensive guide offers detailed and precise medical information for parents that includes day-to-day practical advice on how to cope with procedures, hospitalization, family and friends, school, and social, emotional, and financial issues. It features a wealth of tools for prents and

contains significant updates on treatments and procedures. *$29.95*
528 pages 4th Edition 1910
ISBN 0-596500-15-7

8698 Children with Cerebral Palsy: A Parents' Guide
Woodbine House
6510 Bells Mill Road
Bethesda, MD 20817-1636
301-897-3570
800-843-7323
Fax: 301-897-5838
info@woodbinehouse.com
www.woodbinehouse.com
Irvin Shapell, Owner
Beth Binns, Special Marketing Manager
Sarah Glenner, Office Receptionist;
Fran Marinaccio, Marketing Manager
A classic primer for parents that provides a complete spetrum of information and compassionate advice about cerebral palsy and its effect on their child's development and education. *$18.95*
481 pages
ISBN 0-933149-82-4

8699 Chronic Fatigue Syndrome: Your Natural Gu ide to Healing with Diet, Herbs and Other Methods
Random House Publishing
1745 Broadway
3rd Floor
New York, NY 10019-4305
212-782-9000
Fax: 212-572-6066
ecustomerservice@randomhouse.com
www.randomhouse.com
Susanna Porter, Editor
Michael T Murray N.D.
Explains specific measures sufferers can take to improve stamina, mental energy, and physical abilities. *$15.00*
208 pages
ISBN 1-559584-90-6

8700 Coffee in the Cereal: The First Year with Multiple Sclerosis
Pathfinder Publishing
520-647-0158
800-977-2282
bill@pathfinderpublishing.com
www.pathfinderpublishing.com
96 pages
ISBN 0-934793-07-7

8701 Colon & Rectal Cancer: A Comprehensive Guide for Patients & Families
O'Reilly Media Inc
1005 Gravenstein Hwy N
Sebastopol, CA 95472-2811
707-827-7000
800-998-9938
Fax: 707-829-0104
order@oreilly.com
www.oreilly.com
Linda Lamb, Editor
Lorraine Johnston, Author
The fourth most common cancer, colon and rectal cancer is diagnosed in 130,000 new cases in the United States each year. Patients and families need uo-to-date and in-depth information to participate wisely in treatment decisions (e.g., knowing what sexual and fertility issues to discuss with the doctor before surgery). This book covers coping with tests and treatment side effects, caring for ostomies, finding supportt, and other practical issues. *$24.95*
544 pages Paperback 1999
ISBN 1-565926-33-1

8702 Colon Health: Key to a Vibrant Life
Norwalk Press
P.O. Box 190526
Boise, ID 83719-526
928-445-5567
Fax: 928-445-5567
Norman Walker MD, Editor
Includes complete glossary of terms and index of referrals.

8703 Complementary Alternative Medicine and Multiple Sclerosis
Demos Medical Publishing
11 West 42nd Street
15th Floor
New York, NY 10036
212-683-0072
800-532-8663
Fax: 212-683-0118
support@demosmedical.com
www.demosmedpub.com
Richard Winters, Executive Editor
Beth Kaufman Barry, Publisher
Noreen Henson, Executive Director of Demos Heal
Reina Santana, Director of Special Sales & Righ
Offers reliable information on the relevance, safety, and effectiveness of various alternative therapies that are not typically considered in discussions of MS management, yet are in widespread use. *$24.95*
304 pages
ISBN 1-932603-54-9

8704 Conquering the Darkness: One Story of Recovering from a Brain Injury
Paragon House
1925 Oakcrest Avenue
Suite 7
Saint Paul, MN 55113-2619
651-644-3087
800-447-3709
Fax: 651-644-0997
info@paragonhouse.com
www.paragonhouse.com
Rosemary Yokoi, Publicity Director
Gordon Anderson, Executive Director
Deborah Quinn, Author
The course of recovery from a brain injury by a woman who lived through it. *$15.95*
276 pages 1998
ISBN 1-557787-63-8

8705 Coping with Cerebral Palsy
Rosen Publishing
29 East 21st Street
New York, NY 10010
800-237-9932
Fax: 888-436-4643
www.rosenpublishing.com
Laura Anne Gilman, Author
This second edition book provides parents of children and adults with cerebral palsy the answers to more than 300 questions that have been carefully researched. It represents 40 years of experience by the author and is presented in a highly readable, jargon-free manner. *$31.95*
ISBN 0-823931-50-1

8706 Curing MS: How Science is Solving the Mysteries of Multiple Sclerosis
Random House Publishing
1745 Broadway
3rd Floor
New York, NY 10019-4305
212-782-9000
Fax: 212-572-6066
www.randomhouse.com
Howard L Weiner M.D., Author
Founder-director of the Multiple Sclerosis Center at Mass General Hospital discusses what ends up as a deconstruction of the last 30 years of his own and general MS research and of experience in treating patients with the puzzling disorder. Weiner summarizes what is currently known about treatments and the potential for a cure. *$14.95*
352 pages 1905
ISBN 0-307236-04-8

8707 **Cystic Fibrosis: A Guide for Patient and Family**
Lippincott Williams & Wilkins
16522 Hunters Green Parkway
PO Box 1620
Hagerstown, MD 21741-1620
301-223-2300
800-638-3030
Fax: 301-223-2400
orders@lww.com
www.lww.com

David M Orenstein MD, Author

Text is designed specifically for patients with cystic fibrosis and their families. Explains the disease process, outlines the fundamentals of diagnosing and screening, and addresses the challenges of treatment for those living with CF. Includes new material on carrier testing, infection control, and more. *$51.50*

448 pages 3rd Edition
ISBN 0-781741-52-1

8708 **Diabetes Sourcebook.**
Omnigraphics
615 Griswold Street
Suite 520
Detroit, MI 48226
610-461-3548
800-234-1340
Fax: 800-875-1340
contact@omnigraphics.com
www.omnigraphics.com

Peter Ruffner, Co-Founder
Fred Ruffner, Co-Founder

Diabetes Sourcebook, Fourth Edition contains updated information for people seeking to understand the risk factors, complications, and management of diabetes. It discusses medical interventions, including the use of insulin and oral diabetes medications, self-monitoring of blood glucose, and complementary and alternative therapies. *$84.00*

627 pages 4th Edition
ISBN 0-780810-05-1

8709 **Digestive Diseases & Disorders Sourcebook**
Omnigraphics
615 Griswold Street
Suite 520
Detroit, MI 48226
610-461-3548
800-234-1340
Fax: 800-875-1340
contact@omnigraphics.com
www.omnigraphics.com

Peter Ruffner, Co-Founder
Fred Ruffner, Co-Founder

Digestive Diseases and Disorders Sourcebook provides basic information for the layperson about common disorders of the upper and lower digestive tract. It also includes information about medications and recommendations for maintaining a healthy digestive tract in addition to a glossary of important terms and a directory of digestive diseases organizations are also provided. *$84.00*

323 pages Hard cover
ISBN 0-780803-27-5

8710 **Duchenne Muscular Dystrophy**
Oxford University Press
198 Madison Ave
New York, NY 10016-4308
212-726-6000
800-445-9714
Fax: 919-677-1303
custserv.us@oup.com

William Lamsback, Editor
Alan Emery, Author
Francesco Muntoni, Co-Author

Identification of the genetic defect responsible for Duchenne Muscular Dystrophy and isolation of the protein dystrophin have led to the development of new theories for the disease's pathogenesis. This title incorporates these advances from the field of molecular biology, and describes the resultant opportunities for screening, prenatal diagnosis, genetic counselling and management. *$135.00*

282 pages 3rd Edition 2003
ISBN 0-198515-31-6

8711 **Ear, Nose, and Throat Disorders Sourcebook**
Omnigraphics
615 Griswold Street
Suite 520
Detroit, MI 48226
610-461-3548
800-234-1340
Fax: 800-875-1340
contact@omnigraphics.com
www.omnigraphics.com

Peter Ruffner, Co-Founder
Fred Ruffner, Co-Founder

Ear, Nose and Throat Disorders Sourcebook, Second Edition, provides consumers with updated health information on the most common disorders of the ear, nose, and throat. The book also includes descriptions of current diagnostic tests, discussion of common surgical procedures, including cosmetic surgery on the nose and ears, a glossary of related medical terms, and a directory of sources for further help and information. *$84.00*

631 pages 2nd Edition
ISBN 0-780808-72-0

8712 **Eating Disorders Sourcebook.**
Omnigraphics
615 Griswold Street
Suite 520
Detroit, MI 48226
610-461-3548
800-234-1340
Fax: 800-875-1340
contact@omnigraphics.com
www.omnigraphics.com

Peter Ruffner, Co-Founder
Fred Ruffner, Co-Founder

Provides general imformation, causes and treatments of eating disorders. *$84.00*

557 pages 2nd Edition
ISBN 0-780809-48-2

8713 **Educational Issues Among Children with Spina Bifida**
Spina Bifida Association of America
1600 Wilson Boulevard
Suite 800
Arlington, VA 22209
202-944-3285
800-621-3141
Fax: 202-944-3295
sbaa@sbaa.org
www.sbaa.org

Ana Ximenes, Chair
Sara Struwe, President & CEO
Mark Bohay, National Web Initiatives & Development Manager
Elizabeth Merck, Development Manager

Children with spina bifida/ hydrocephalus often show unique learning strengths and weaknesses that affect their schoolwork. Parents and schools need to work together to help the young people meet their physical, social, emotional, and academic goals.

8714 **Epilepsy, 199 Answers: A Doctor Responds to His Patients' Questions**
Demos Medical Publishing
11 West 42nd Street
15th Floor
New York, NY 10036
212-683-0072
800-532-8663
Fax: 212-683-0118
support@demosmedical.com
www.demosmedpub.com

Richard Winters, Executive Editor
Beth Kaufman Barry, Publisher
Noreen Henson, Executive Director of Demos Heal
Andrew N. Wilner MD, FACP, FAAN, Author

An epilepsy specialist answers questions about the causes, diagnosis, and treatments, and how to live and work with this brain disorder. Includes an epilepsy history timeline, patient health record form, resources, and a glossary. *$19.95*

180 pages
ISBN 1-932603-35-2

8715 Epilepsy: Patient and Family Guide
Demos Medical Publishing
11 West 42nd Street
15th Floor
New York, NY 10036
212-683-0072
800-532-8663
Fax: 212-683-0118
support@demosmedical.com
www.demosmedpub.com

Richard Winters, Executive Editor
Beth Kaufman Barry, Publisher
Noreen Henson, Executive Director of Demos Heal
Orrin Devinsky, MD, Author

A guide for adults with epilepsy and for parents of children with the disorder explains the nature and diversity of seizures, the risks and benefits of the various antiepileptic drugs, and medical and surgical therapies. *$16.95*

408 pages
ISBN 1-932603-41-7

8716 Ethnic Diseases Sourcebook
Omnigraphics
615 Griswold Street
Suite 520
Detroit, MI 48226
610-461-3548
800-234-1340
Fax: 800-875-1340
contact@omnigraphics.com
www.omnigraphics.com

Peter Ruffner, Co-Founder
Fred Ruffner, Co-Founder

Ethnic Diseases Sourcebook provides health information about genetic and chronic diseases that affect ethnic and racial minorities in the United States. Information about mental health services, women's health, and tips for improving health are also included, along with a glossary and a list of resources for additional help and informatio methods, treatment options, and current research initiatives. *$84.00*

648 pages Hard cover
ISBN 0-780803-36-7

8717 From Where I Sit: Making My Way with Cerebral Palsy
Scholastic
557 Broadway
New York, NY 10012-3962
124-484-2800
Fax: 212-343-6934
www.scholastic.com

Dick Robinson, Chairman & CEO
Maureen O'Connell, Executive Vice President, Chief
Kyle Good, Senior Vice President, Corporate
Shelley Nixon, Author

An autobiographical account of a young woman explores how it feels to live with cerebral palsy while struggling to have a full life despite the challenges facing her every day. *$13.00*

136 pages
ISBN 0-590395-84-X

8718 Genetics and Spina Bifida
Spina Bifida Association of America
1600 Wilson Boulevard
Suite 800
Arlington, VA 22209
202-944-3285
800-621-3141
Fax: 202-944-3295
sbaa@sbaa.org
www.sbaa.org

Ana Ximenes, Chair
Sara Struwe, President & CEO
Mark Bohay, National Web Initiatives & Development Manager
Elizabeth Merck, Development Manager

Spina bifida is a birth defect involving incomplete formation of the spine.

8719 Growing Up with Epilepsy: A Pratical Guide for Parents
Demos Medical Publishing
11 West 42nd Street
15th Floor
New York, NY 10036
212-683-0072
800-532-8663
Fax: 212-683-0118
support@demosmedical.com
www.demosmedpub.com

Richard Winters, Executive Editor
Beth Kaufman Barry, Publisher
Noreen Henson, Executive Director of Demos Heal
Lynn Bennett Blackburn, PhD, Author

Developed to help parents with the uniques challenges that this disorder presents *$19.95*

168 pages
ISBN 1-888799-74-9

8720 Guide to Living with HIV Infection: Developed at the Johns Hopkins AIDS Clinic
Johns Hopkins Universty Press
2715 N Charles St
Baltimore, MD 21218-4363
410-516-6900
800-548-1784
Fax: 410-516-6998
webmaster@jhupress.jhu.edu
www.press.jhu.edu

William Brody, President
John G Bartlett, M.D., Author
Ann K Finkbeiner, Co-Author

A handbook and reference for people living with HIV infection and their families, friends, and caregivers. *$19.95*

408 pages 6th Edition
ISBN 0-801884-85-6

8721 Handbook of Chronic Fatigue Syndrome
John Wiley & Sons
1 Wiley Dr.
Somerset, NJ 08875-1272
732-469-4400
800-225-5945
Fax: 732-302-2300
onlinelibrary.wiley.com

Leonard A. Jason, Editor

Discusses diagnosis and treatment as well as the history, phenomenology, symptomatology, assessment, and pediatric and community issues. Introduces phase-based therapy and nutritional approaches. *$110.00*

794 pages 2003
ISBN 0-471415-12-1

8722 Handbook of Epilepsy
Lippincott, Williams & Wilkins
Philadelphia, PA 19106-3713
215-521-8300
800-777-2295
Fax: 301-824-7390

J Lippincott, CEO

Pocket-sized reference provides concise, up-to-date, clinically oriented reviews of each of the major areas of diagnosis and management of epilepsy. *$42.95*

272 pages
ISBN 0-781743-52-4

8723 Healthy Breathing
National Jewish Health
1400 Jackson St
Denver, CO 80206-2761
303-270-2708
877-225-5654
Fax: 303-398-1125
physicianline@njhealth.org
www.nationaljewish.org

Richard A. Schierburg, Chair
Robin Chotin, Vice Chair
Don Silversmith, Vice Chair
Michael Salem, CEO

Offers patients with lung or respiratory disorders information on exercise and healthy breathing.

8724 **Heart of the Mind**
New World Library
14 Pamaron Way
Novato, CA 94949
415-884-2100
800-972-6657
Fax: 415-884-2199
ami@newworldlibrary.com
www.newworldlibrary.com

208 pages
ISBN 1-577311-56-6

8725 **Hepatitis Sourcebook**
Omnigraphics
615 Griswold Street
Suite 520
Detroit, MI 48226
610-461-3548
800-234-1340
Fax: 800-875-1340
contact@omnigraphics.com
www.omnigraphics.com

Peter Ruffner, Co-Founder
Fred Ruffner, Co-Founder

Hepatitis Sourcebook provides basic consumer health information about hepatitis A, hepatitis B, hepatitis C, and other types of hepatitis, including autoimmune hepatitis, alcoholic hepatitis, nonalcoholic steatohepatitis, and toxin-induced hepatitis. It gives the facts about risk factors, prevention, transmission, screening and diagnostic methods, treatment options, and current research initiatives. *$84.00*

570 pages Hard cover
ISBN 0-780807-49-5

8726 **Hip Function & Ambulation**
Spina Bifida Association of America
1600 Wilson Boulevard
Suite 800
Arlington, VA 22209
202-944-3285
800-621-3141
Fax: 202-944-3295
sbaa@sbaa.org
www.sbaa.org

Ana Ximenes, Chair
Sara Struwe, President & CEO
Mark Bohay, National Web Initiatives & Development Manager
Elizabeth Merck, Development Manager

The ability to walk is important in our society, despite recent advances in wheelchair design and wheelchair accessibility. It also is a desire of children with spina bifida.

8727 **Hydrocephalus: A Guide for Patients, Families & Friends**
O'Reilly Media Inc
1005 Gravenstein Hwy N
Sebastopol, CA 95472-2811
707-827-7000
800-998-9938
Fax: 707-829-0104
order@oreilly.com
www.oreilly.com

Linda Lamb, Editor
Chuck Toporek, Author
Kellie Robinson, Author

Hydrocephalus is a life-threatening condition often referred to as, water on the brain, that is treated by surgical placement of a shunt system. Hydrocephalus: A Guide for Patients, Families and Friends educates families so they can select a skilled neurosurgeon, understand treatments, participate in care, know what symptoms need attention, discover where to turn for support, keep records needed for follow-up treatments, and make wise lifestyle choices. *$19.95*

379 pages Paperback 1999
ISBN 1-565924-10-X

8728 **Hypertension Sourcebook**
Omnigraphics
615 Griswold Street
Suite 520
Detroit, MI 48226
610-461-3548
800-234-1340
Fax: 800-875-1340
contact@omnigraphics.com
www.omnigraphics.com

Peter Ruffner, Co-Founder
Fred Ruffner, Co-Founder

This Sourcebook describes the known causes and risk factors associated with essential (or primary) hypertension, secondary hypertension, prehypertension, and other hypertensive disorders. The book also provides information about blood pressure management strategies, including dietary changes, weight loss, exercise, and medications. *$84.00*

588 pages Hard cover
ISBN 0-780806-74-0

8729 **Immune System Disorders Sourcebook.**
Omnigraphics
615 Griswold Street
Suite 520
Detroit, MI 48226
610-461-3548
800-234-1340
Fax: 800-875-1340
contact@omnigraphics.com
www.omnigraphics.com

Peter Ruffner, Co-Founder
Fred Ruffner, Co-Founder

Immune System Disorders Sourcebook provides information about inherited, acquired, and autoimmune diseases including primary immune deficiency, acquired immunodeficiency syndrome (AIDS), lupus, multiple sclerosis, type one diabetes, rheumatoid arthritis, and Graves' disease. Tips for coping with an immune disorder, caregiving, and treatments are presented along with a glossary and directory of additional resourcesories of additional resources. *$84.00*

643 pages 2nd Edition
ISBN 0-780807-48-8

8730 **Informed Touch; A Clinician's Guide To The Evaluation Of Myofascial Disorders**
Inner Traditions/Bear And Company
One Park Street
PO Box 388
Rochester, VT 05767-0388
802-767-3174
800-246-8648
Fax: 802-767-3726
customerservice@innertraditions.com
www.innertraditions.com

Rob Meadows, VP Sales/Marketing
Jessica Arsenault, Sales Associate
Donna Finando, LAc, LMT, Author
Steven Finando, PhD, LAc, Co-Author

A Clinician's guide to the evaluation and treatment of myofascial disorders. *$30.00*

224 pages
ISBN 0-892817-40-5

8731 **Injured Mind, Shattered Dreams: Brian's Survival from a Severe Head Injury**
Brookline Books
8 Trumbull Rd,
Northampton, MA 01060-4533
413-584-0184
800-666-2665
Fax: 413-584-6184
brbooks@yahoo.com
www.brooklinebooks.com

Paperback
ISBN 0-91479 -95-6

8732 **Interdisciplinary Clinical Assessment of Young Children with Developmental Disabilities**
Brookes Publishing
P.O. Box 10624
Baltimore, MD 21285-0624
410-337-9580
800-638-3775
Fax: 410-337-8539
custserv@brookespublishing.com
www.brookespublishing.com
Paul H. Brookes, Chairman
Jeffrey D. Brookes, President
Melissa A. Behm, Executive Vice President
George S. Stamathis, Vice President & Publisher
Offers insight from veteran team members on interdisciplinary team assessments. Professionals organizing a team as well as students preparing for practice will find advice on how practitioners gather information, approach assessment, make decisions, and face the challenges of their individual fields. Includes case studies and appendix of photocopiable questionnaires for clinicians and parents. *$44.95*
796 pages Hardcover
ISBN 1-557664-50-1

8733 **Introduction to Spina Bifida**
Spina Bifida Association of America
1600 Wilson Boulevard
Suite 800
Arlington, VA 22209
202-944-3285
800-621-3141
Fax: 202-944-3295
sbaa@sbaa.org
www.sbaa.org
Ana Ximenes, Chair
Sara Struwe, President & CEO
Mark Bohay, National Web Initiatives & Development Manager
Elizabeth Merck, Development Manager
An aid for parents, family and nonmedical people who care for a child with spina bifida. *$7.00*

8734 **It's All in Your Head: The Link Between Mercury Amalgams and Illness**
Avery Publishing Group
299 W. Houston Street
New York, NY 10014
212-859-1100
Fax: 212-859-1150
info@programexchange.com
208 pages

8735 **Joslin Guide to Diabetes: A Program for Managing Your Treatment**
Joslin Diabetes Center
1 Joslin Pl
Boston, MA 02215-5306
617-732-2400
Fax: 617-732-2452
www.joslin.org
Richard S Beaser, M.D., Author
Amy Campbell,Ms, RD, CDE, Co-Author
Ralph M. James, Chairperson of the Board
John L. Brooks III, President/CEO
Discusses the causes of diabetes, the role of diet and exercise, meal planning and complications. Also provide information on drawing blood, mixing and injecting insulin, special challenges, living with diabetes. *$16.95*
352 pages Revised Edition

8736 **Journey to Well: Learning to Live After Spinal Cord Injury**
Altarfire Publishing
1835 Oak Terrace
Newcastle, CA 95658
Margie Williams, Author
The author's close-up view of what life is like during and after such an incident, including her experience with institutional medicine and insurance companies (for better and for worse), and her determined - and ultimately successful - effort to rehabilitate herself and reconstruct her life. *$15.95*
251 pages
ISBN 0-965555-82-8

8737 **Ketogenic Diet: A Treatment for Children and Others with Epilepsy**
Demos Medical Publishing
11 West 42nd Street
15th Floor
New York, NY 10036
212-683-0072
800-532-8663
Fax: 212-683-0118
support@demosmedical.com
www.demosmedpub.com
Richard Winters, Executive Editor
Beth Kaufman Barry, Publisher
Noreen Henson, Executive Director of Demos Heal
John M. Freeman, MD, Co Author
Patient education reference on the use of the ketogenic diet to conrol epilepsy in children. *$24.95*
328 pages Paperback
ISBN 1-932603-18-2

8738 **Latex Allergy in Spina Bifida Patients**
Spina Bifida Association of America
1600 Wilson Boulevard
Suite 800
Arlington, VA 22209
202-944-3285
800-621-3141
Fax: 202-944-3295
sbaa@sbaa.org
www.sbaa.org
Ana Ximenes, Chair
Sara Struwe, President & CEO
Mark Bohay, National Web Initiatives & Development Manager
Elizabeth Merck, Development Manager
The Spina Bifida Association (SBA) serves adults and children who live with the challenges of Spina Bifida.

8739 **Learning Among Children with Spina Bifida**
Spina Bifida Association of America
1600 Wilson Boulevard
Suite 800
Arlington, VA 22209
202-944-3285
800-621-3141
Fax: 202-944-3295
sbaa@sbaa.org
www.sbaa.org
Ana Ximenes, Chair
Sara Struwe, President & CEO
Mark Bohay, National Web Initiatives & Development Manager
Elizabeth Merck, Development Manager
The Spina Bifida Association (SBA) serves adults and children who live with the challenges of Spina Bifida.

8740 **Let's Talk About Having Asthma**
Rosen Publishing
29 E 21st St
New York, NY 10010-6209
212-420-1600
800-237-9932
Fax: 888-436-4643
www.rosenpublishing.com
Marianna Johnstone, Co-Author
Elizabeth Weitzman, Co-Author
Kelly Chambers, Marketing Assistant
Many kids suffer from asthma, which can overtake them suddenly, causing them terror as they struggle for breath. This book talks about the causes and treatments for asthma, as well as precautions sufferers should take. *$21.95*
ISBN 0-823950-32-8

8741 **Leukemia Sourcebook**
Omnigraphics
615 Griswold Street
Suite 520
Detroit, MI 48226
610-461-3548
800-234-1340
Fax: 800-875-1340
contact@omnigraphics.com
www.omnigraphics.com
Peter Ruffner, Co-Founder
Fred Ruffner, Co-Founder
This Sourcebook provides health information about adult and childhood leukemias focusing on the diagnosis and treatments

for leukemia, including chemotherapy, radiation, drug therapy, and transplantation of peripheral blood stem cells or marrow. Also included are tips for nutrition, pain and fatigue control, and recognizing possible long-term and late effects of leukemia treatment, along with a glossary and directories of additional resources. *$84.00*

564 pages Hard cover

ISBN 0-780806-27-6

8742 **Life After Trauma: A Workbook for Healing**

Guilford Press
72 Spring St
New York, NY 10012-4019
212-431-9800
800-365-7006
Fax: 212-966-6708
info@guilford.com
www.guilford.com

Denaour Rosenbloom, Author
Mary Beth Williams, Co-Author
Barbar E Watkins, Co-Author
Laurie Anne Pearlman, Foreword

A self-help book on how to deal with trauma. *$19.95*

300 pages Paperback 1910

ISBN 1-606236-08-6

8743 **Life Line**

National Hydrocephalus Foundation
12413 Centralia St
Lakewood, CA 90715-1653
562-402-3523
888-857-3434
888-260-1789
Fax: 562-924-6666

Debbi Fields, Executive Director
Michael Fields, President/Treasurer
Jaynie Dunn, Secretary
Sarah Dunn, Junior Director

National Hydrocephalus Foundation quarterly newsletter. *$35.00*

12 pages Quarterly

8744 **Lipomas & Lipomyelomeningocele**

Spina Bifida Association of America
1600 Wilson Boulevard
Suite 800
Arlington, VA 22209
202-944-3285
800-621-3141
Fax: 202-944-3295
sbaa@sbaa.org
www.sbaa.org

Ana Ximenes, Chair
Sara Struwe, President & CEO
Mark Bohay, National Web Initiatives & Development Manager
Elizabeth Merck, Development Manager

The Spina Bifida Association (SBA) serves adults and children who live with the challenges of Spina Bifida.

8745 **Liver Disorders Sourcebook**

Omnigraphics
615 Griswold Street
Suite 520
Detroit, MI 48226
610-461-3548
800-234-1340
Fax: 800-875-1340
contact@omnigraphics.com
www.omnigraphics.com

Peter Ruffner, Co-Founder
Fred Ruffner, Co-Founder

Liver Disorders Sourcebook contains basic consumer health information about the liver, how it works, and how to keep it healthy through diet, vaccination, and other preventive care measures. Readers will learn about the symptoms and treatment options for such diseases as hepatitis, primary biliary cirrhosis, Wilson's disease, hemochromatosis, liver failure, cancer of the liver, and disorders related to drugs and other toxins. *$84.00*

580 pages Hard cover

ISBN 0-780803-83-1

8746 **Living Beyond Multiple Sclerosis: A Woman's Guide**

Hunter House
PO Box 2914
Alameda, CA 94501-914
510-865-5282
800-266-5592
Fax: 510-865-4295
www.hunterhouse.com

Judith Lynn Nichols, Author
Lily Jung, Foreword

This collection of e-mail conversations provides anecdotal and personal information contributed by women with multiple sclerosis. *$14.95*

256 pages

ISBN 0-897932-93-6

8747 **Living Well with Asthma**

Guilford Press
72 Spring St
New York, NY 10012-4019
212-431-9800
800-365-7006
Fax: 212-966-6708
info@guilford.com
www.guilford.com

Cynthia L Divino, Author
Michael R Freedman, Co-Author
Samuel J Rosenberg, Co-Author
James D Crapo, Foreword

Meeting the needs of a growing clinical population, this reader-friendly, practical book offers a lifeline to asthma patients attempting to understand and cope with the psychological ramifications of their illness and its treatment. *$15.95*

213 pages Paperback

ISBN 1-572300-51-4

8748 **Living Well with Chronic Fatigue Syndrome and Fibromyalgia**

Harper Collins Publishers
10 E 53rd St
New York, NY 10022-5244
212-207-7901
800-242-7737
Fax: 212-702-2586
spsales@harpercollins.com
www.harpercollins.com

Mary J Shomon, Author

From the author of Living Well With Hypothyroidism, a comprehensive guide to the diagnosis and treatment of chronic fatigue syndrome and fibromyalgia—vital help for the millions of people suffering from pain, fatigue, and sleep problems. *$14.95*

416 pages 2004

ISBN 0-060521-25-2

8749 **Living Well with HIV and AIDS**

Bull Publishing
PO Box 1377
Boulder, CO 80306-1377
303-545-6350
800-676-2855
Fax: 303-545-6354
www.bullpub.com

David Sobel, MPH, Author
Virginia Gonzalez MPH, Co-Author
Daina Laurent MPH, Co-Author
Kate Lorig RN, Co-Author

New drugs and drug combinations have turned HIV/AIDS into a long-term illness rather than a death sentence. Practical advice on mental adjustments and physical vigilance is outlined. *$18.95*

245 pages 3rd Edition

ISBN 0-923521-52-6

8750 Living With Spinal Cord Injury Series
Fanlight Productions C/O Icarus Films
32 Court St.
21st Floor
Brooklyn, NY 11201
718-488-8900
800-876-1710
Fax: 718-488-8642
info@fanlight.com
www.fanlight.com

Barry Corbet, Producer
Jonathan Miller, President
Meredith Miller, Sales Manager
Anthony Sweeney, Acquisitions

The producer, himself injured in a helicopter crash, brings a unique perspective to this classic three-part series on coming to terms with spinal cord injury. These films offer enduring proof that a tough break doesn't have to mean a ruined life. *$210.00*
VHS 1973

8751 Living with Brain Injury: A Guide for Families
Delmar Cengage Learning
PO Box 6904
Florence, KY 41022-6904
800-354-9706
Fax: 800-487-8488

Richard C Senelick MD, Author
Karla Dougherty, Co-Author

A consumer text to aid people living with brain-injured survivors, includes facts on neuroplasticity, experimental rehabilitation research, and the process of rehabilitation itself. *$19.95*
225 pages Softcover 2001
ISBN 1-891525-09-3

8752 Living with Spina Bifida: A Guide for Families and Professionals
University of North Carolina at Chapel Hill
116 S Boundary St
Chapel Hill, NC 27514-3808
919-966-3561
800-848-6224
Fax: 919-962-2704
uncpress@unc.edu
www.uncpress.unc.edu

Adrian Sandler MD, Author

A handbook that addresses patients' biopsychosocial and developmental needs from birth through adolescence and into adulthood. Sandler's holistic approach encourages families to focus more on the child and less on the disability while providing abundant information about this condition. *$20.95*
296 pages 2004
ISBN 0-807855-47-8

8753 Lung Cancer: Making Sense of Diagnosis, Treatment, and Options
O'Reilly Media Inc
1005 Gravenstein Hwy N
Sebastopol, CA 95472-2811
707-827-7000
800-998-9938
Fax: 707-829-0104
order@oreilly.com
www.oreilly.com

Linda Lamb, Editor
Lorraine Johnston, Author

Straightforward language and the words of patients and their families are the hallmarks of this book on the number one cancer killer in the US. Written by a widely respected author and patient advocate, Lung Cancer: Making Sense of Diagnosis, Treatment, & Options has been meticulously reviewed by top medical experts and physicians. Readers will find medical facts simply explained, advice to ease their daily life, and tools to be strong advocates for themselves or a family member. *$27.95*
530 pages Paperback 2001
ISBN 0-596500-02-5

8754 Lung Disorders Sourcebook
Omnigraphics
615 Griswold Street
Suite 520
Detroit, MI 48226
610-461-3548
800-234-1340
Fax: 800-875-1340
contact@omnigraphics.com
www.omnigraphics.com

Peter Ruffner, Co-Founder
Fred Ruffner, Co-Founder

Lung Disorders Sourcebook offers information about specific types of lung disorders, including diagnosis, treatment, and prevention issues. The book offers advice for preventing some types lung disorder that are acquired by asbestos, radon, and other environmental exposures. *$84.00*
657 pages Hard cover
ISBN 0-780803-39-8

8755 Lupus: Alternative Therapies That Work
Inner Traditions
PO Box 388
Rochester
VT, 05 0388-802-
800-246-8648
802-767-3726
TTY: customerserv
info@innertraditions.com
www.innertraditions.com

Sharon Moore, Author

A comprehensive guise to noninvasive, nontoxic therapies for lupus - written by a lupus survivor. *$14.95*
256 pages 2000
ISBN 0-892818-89-1

8756 MAGIC Touch
MAGIC Foundation for Children's Growth
6645 North Ave
Oak Park, IL 60302-1057
708-383-0808
800-362-4423
Fax: 708-383-0899
mary@magicfoundation.org
www.magicfoundation.org

Mary Andrews, CEO
Dianne Kremidas, Executive Director
Pam Pentaris, Office Manager
Jamie Harvey, Technical Education Teacher

Provides support and education regarding growth disorders in children and related adult disorders, including adult GHD. Dedicated to helping children whose physical growth is affected be a medical problem by assisting families of afflicted children through local support groups, public education/awareness, newsletters, specialty divisions and programs for the children.
36-40 pages Quarterly

8757 Management of Autistic Behavior
Sage Publications
2455 Teller Road
Thousand Oaks, CA 91320
805-499-0721
800-818-7243
Fax: 805-499-0871
info@sagepub.com
www.sagepub.com

Sara Miller McCune, Founder, Publisher, Executive Chairman
Blaise R Simqu, President & CEO
Tracey A. Ozmina, Executive Vice President & Chief Operating Officer
Stephen Barr, Managing Director/SAGE London, President of SAGE Internation

Comprehensive and practical book that tells what works best with specific problems. *$51.00*
450 pages Paperback
ISBN 0-890791-96-1

8758 Management of Genetic Syndromes
John Wiley & Sons
111 River St
Hoboken, NJ 07030-5774
201-748-6000
201-748-6088
info@wiley.com

Suzanne B Cassidy, Editor
Judith E Allanson, Editor

Edited by two of the field's most highly esteemed experts, this landmark volume provides: A precise reference of the physical manifestations of common genetic syndromes, clearly written for professionals and families, Extensive updates, particularly in sections on diagnostic criteria and diagnostic testing, pathogenesis, and management, A tried-and-tested, user-friendly format, with each chapter including information on incidence, etiology and pathogenesis, diagnostic criteria and testing, and d *$204.95*

720 pages 3rd Edition
ISBN 0-470191-41-5

8759 Managing Post Polio: A Guide to Living Well with Post Polio
ABI Professional Publications
PO Box 149
St Petersburg, FL 33731-149
727-556-0950
800-551-7776
Fax: 727-556-2560
www.abipropub.com

Lauro S Halstead MD, Editor

Edited by Lauro S. Halstead, M.D., Managing Post-Polio, 2nd Edition, provides a comprehensive overview dealing with the medical, psychological, vocational, and many other challenges of living with post-polio syndrome. With contributions from over 15 healthcare professionals, the majority of whom are polio survivors themselves, Managing Post-Polio distills and summarizes the wealth of information presented from over the past 20 plus years.

256 pages
ISBN 1-886236-17-8

8760 Meniere's Disease
Vestibular Disorders Association
5018 NE 15th Avenue
Portland, OR 97211
800-837-8428
Fax: 503-229-8064
info@vestibular.org
www.vestibular.org

P. Ashley Wackym, Chair
Cynthia Ryan MBA, Executive Director
Tony Staser, Development Director
Kerrie Denner, Outreach Coordinator

VEDA's website contains a wealth of information on the symptoms, diagnosis and treatment of various types of vestibular disorders. *$5.00*

8761 Menopause without Medicine
Hunter House
PO Box 2914
Alameda, CA 94501-914
510-865-5282
800-266-5592
Fax: 510-865-4295
www.hunterhouse.com

Linda Ojeda PhD, Author

Menopause Without Medicine provides complete information on the symptoms of menopause - hot flashes, fatigue, sexual changes, depression and osteoporosis - and how to alleviate them. *$18.95*

304 pages 5th Edition
ISBN 0-897934-05-3

8762 Movement Disorders Sourcebook
Omnigraphics
615 Griswold Street
Suite 520
Detroit, MI 48226
610-461-3548
800-234-1340
Fax: 800-875-1340
contact@omnigraphics.com
www.omnigraphics.com

Peter Ruffner, Co-Founder
Fred Ruffner, Co-Founder

This Sourcebook provides health information about neurological movement disorders, their symptoms, causes, diagnostic tests, and treatments. Readers will learn about Essential Tremor, Parkinson's Disease, Dystonia, and many other early-onset and adult-onset movement disorders. Information about mobility and assistive technology aids is included, along with a glossary and a listing of additional resources. *$84.00*

600 pages Hard cover
ISBN 0-780810-34-1

8763 Multiple Sclerosis and Having a Baby
Inner Traditions
PO Box 388
Rochester, VT 05767-0388
802-767-3174
800-246-8648
Fax: 802-767-3726
customerservice@innertraditions.com
www.innertraditions.com

Judy Graham, Author

Everything you need to know about conception, pregnancy and parenthood. *$12.95*

160 pages 2001
ISBN 0-892817-88-7

8764 Multiple Sclerosis: 300 Tips for Making Life Easier
Demos Medical Publishing
11 West 42nd Street
15th Floor
New York, NY 10036
212-683-0072
800-532-8663
Fax: 212-683-0118
support@demosmedical.com
www.demosmedpub.com

Richard Winters, Executive Editor
Beth Kaufman Barry, Publisher
Noreen Henson, Executive Director of Demos Heal
Shelley Peterman Schwarz, Author

This latest book in the Making Life Easier series features tip, techniques and shortcuts for conserving time and energy so you can do more of the things you want to do. These tips should help increase the number of good days you have while encouraging you to develop your own techniques for making life easier. *$16.95*

128 pages
ISBN 1-932603-21-2

8765 Multiple Sclerosis: A Guide for Families
Demos Medical Publishing
11 West 42nd Street
15th Floor
New York, NY 10036
212-683-0072
800-532-8663
Fax: 212-683-0118
support@demosmedical.com
www.demosmedpub.com

Richard Winters, Executive Editor
Beth Kaufman Barry, Publisher
Noreen Henson, Executive Director of Demos Heal
Rosalind C. Kalb, Ph.D., Author

Guide for living and coping with multiple sclerosis. *$24.95*

256 pages
ISBN 1-932603-10-7

8766 Multiple Sclerosis: A Guide for the Newly Diagnosed
Demos Medical Publishing
11 West 42nd Street
15th Floor
New York, NY 10036
212-683-0072
800-532-8663
Fax: 212-683-0118
support@demosmedical.com
www.demosmedpub.com

Richard Winters, Executive Editor
Beth Kaufman Barry, Publisher
Noreen Henson, Executive Director of Demos Heal
Nancy J. Holland, RN, EdD, Co Author

A must-have title for anyone who has recently been diagnosed with MS and a good idea for family members and friends. *$19.95*
256 pages
ISBN 1-932603-27-1

8767 Multiple Sclerosis: The Guide to Treatment and Management
Demos Medical Publishing
11 West 42nd Street
15th Floor
New York, NY 10036
212-683-0072
800-532-8663
Fax: 212-683-0118
support@demosmedical.com
www.demosmedpub.com

Richard Winters, Executive Editor
Beth Kaufman Barry, Publisher
Noreen Henson, Executive Director of Demos Heal
Chris H. Polman, MD, FRCP, Co Author

A current guide to modern therapies. *$24.95*
216 pages
ISBN 1-932603-15-4

8768 Muscular Dystrophies
Oxford University Press
198 Madison Avenue
New York, NY 10016
212-726-6000
800-445-9714
Fax: 919-677-1303
custserv.us@oup.com
www.oup.com

Alan E.H. Emery, Author

Describes the opportunities for management of more than 30 types of MD through respiratory care, physiotherapy and surgical correction of contractures, and examines the potential for effective treatment utilizing the new techniques of gene and cell therapy *$165.00*
330 pages
ISBN 0-192632-91-4

8769 Muscular Dystrophy in Children: A Guide for Families
Demos Medical Publishing
11 West 42nd Street
15th Floor
New York, NY 10036
212-683-0072
800-532-8663
Fax: 212-683-0118
support@demosmedical.com

Richard Winters, Executive Editor
Beth Kaufman Barry, Publisher
Noreen Henson, Executive Director of Demos Heal

Defines the available medical options at every stage of the disease and offers guidance even when it may seem that little or nothing can be done. Includes a glossary and suggestions for furhter reading. *$19.95*
144 pages Paperback
ISBN 1-888799-33-1

8770 Muscular Dystrophy: The Facts
Oxford University Press
198 Madison Avenue
New York, NY 10016
212-726-6000
800-445-9714
Fax: 919-677-1303
custserv.us@oup.com
www.oup.com

Peter Harper, Author

A good first book for individuals and families faced with the likelihood or reality of a muscular dystrophy diagnosis. *$22.50*
178 pages
ISBN 0-192632-17-5

8771 My House is Killing Me! The Home Guide for Families with Allergies and Asthma
Johns Hopkins University Press
2175 N Charles St
Baltimore, MD 21218-4363
410-516-6900
800-548-1784
Fax: 410-516-6968
webmaster@jhupress.jhu.edu
www.press.jhu.edu

Jeffrey C May, Author
Jonathan M Samet, M.D., Foreword
Kathleen Keane, Director

Chemical consultant May describes where and how the various parts of a residence can cause temporary or chronic illness for those with allergies or other sensitivities. *$20.95*
352 pages
ISBN 0-801867-30-9

8772 Neuropsychiatry of Epilepsy
Cambridge University Press
100 Brookhill Dr
West Nyack, NY 10994
845-353-7500
845-353-4141
www.cambridge.org

Michael R Trimble, Editor
Bettina Schmitz, Editor

Covers the practical implications of ongoing research, and offers a diagnostic and management perspective. Topics include cognitive aspects, nonepileptic attacks, and clinical aspects. For professionals treating epileptic patients. *$104.00*
232 pages 2nd Edition 1911
ISBN 0-521154-69-7

8773 Nick Joins In
Spina Bifida Association of America
1600 Wilson Boulevard
Suite 800
Arlington, VA 22209
202-944-3285
800-621-3141
Fax: 202-944-3295
sbaa@sbaa.org
www.sbaa.org

Ana Ximenes, Chair
Sara Struwe, President & CEO
Mark Bohay, National Web Initiatives & Development Manager
Elizabeth Merck, Development Manager

When Nick, who is in a wheelchair, enters a regular classroom for the first time, he realizes that he has much to contribute. *$17.00*

8774 No More Allergies
Random House
1745 Broadway
3rd Floor
New York, NY 10019-4305
212-782-9000
Fax: 212-572-6066
www.randomhouse.com

Markus Dohle, CEO
Gary Null PhD, Author

Null redefines a health problem that afflicts 40 million Americans: More than mere hay fever, contemporary allergic reactions include chronic fatigue syndrome, Alzheimer's disease, and even HIV infection. These conditions, he explains, occur when our immune systems break down. This ground-breaking book now prescribes effective solutions. *$23.00*
464 pages 1992
ISBN 0-679743-10-1

8775 **No Time for Jello: One Family's Experience**
Brookline Books
8 Trumbull Rd,
Northampton, MA 01060-4533
413-584-0184
800-666-2665
Fax: 413-584-6184
brbooks@yahoo.com
www.brooklinebooks.com

Softcover
ISBN 0-91479-56-5

8776 **Nocturnal Asthma**
National Jewish Health
1400 Jackson Street
Denver, CO 80206
303-270-2708
877-225-5654
Fax: 303-398-1125
allstetterw@njc.org
nationaljewish.org

Rich Schierburg, Chair
Robin Chotin, Vice Chair
Michael Salem, M.D., President and CEO
Christine Forkner, CFO and Executive Vice President
Offers information to patients about how to understand and manage asthma at night.

8777 **Obesity**
Spina Bifida Association of America
1600 Wilson Boulevard
Suite 800
Arlington, VA 22209
202-944-3285
800-621-3141
Fax: 202-944-3295
sbaa@sbaa.org
www.sbaa.org

Ana Ximenes, Chair
Sara Struwe, President & CEO
Mark Bohay, National Web Initiatives & Development Manager
Elizabeth Merck, Development Manager
The Spina Bifida Association (SBA) serves adults and children who live with the challenges of Spina Bifida. *$8.00*

8778 **Obesity Sourcebook**
Omnigraphics
615 Griswold Street
Suite 520
Detroit, MI 48226
610-461-3548
800-234-1340
Fax: 800-875-1340
contact@omnigraphics.com
www.omnigraphics.com

Peter Ruffner, Co-Founder
Fred Ruffner, Co-Founder
Discusses diseases and other problems associated with obesity.
$78.00
376 pages
ISBN 0-780803-33-6

8779 **Occulta**
Spina Bifida Association of America
1600 Wilson Boulevard
Suite 800
Arlington, VA 22209
202-944-3285
800-621-3141
Fax: 202-944-3295
sbaa@sbaa.org
www.sbaa.org

Ana Ximenes, Chair
Sara Struwe, President & CEO
Mark Bohay, National Web Initiatives & Development Manager
Elizabeth Merck, Development Manager
The Spina Bifida Association (SBA) serves adults and children who live with the challenges of Spina Bifida. *$8.00*

8780 **Official Patient's Sourcebook on Bell's Palsy**
Icon Group International
9606 Tierra Grande Street
Suite 205
San Diego, CA 92126
Fax: 858-635-9414
orders@icongroupbooks.com
www.icongroupbooks.com

ISBN 0-597835-20-9

8781 **Official Patient's Sourcebook on Cystic Fibrosis**
Icon Group International
9606 Tierra Grande Street
Suite 205
San Diego, CA 92126
Fax: 858-635-9414
orders@icongroupbooks.com
icongroupbooks.com

356 pages
ISBN 0-597831-46-7

8782 **Official Patient's Sourcebook on Muscular Dystrophy**
Icon Group International
9606 Tierra Grande Street
Suite 205
San Diego, CA 92126
Fax: 858-635-9414
orders@icongroupbooks.com
icongroupbooks.com

268 pages
ISBN 0-597832-10-2

8783 **Official Patient's Sourcebook on Osteoporosis**
Icon Group International
9606 Tierra Grande Street
Suite 205
San Diego, CA 92126
Fax: 858-635-9414
orders@icongroupbooks.com
icongroupbooks.com

ISBN 0-597833-04-4

8784 **Official Patient's Sourcebook on Post-Polio Syndrome: A Revised and Updated Directory**
Icon Group International
9606 Tierra Grande Street
Suite 205
San Diego, CA 92126
Fax: 858-635-9414
orders@icongroupbooks.com
icongroupbooks.com

124 pages
ISBN 0-597835-31-4

8785 **Official Patient's Sourcebook on Primary Pulmonary Hypertension**
Icon Group International
9606 Tierra Grande Street
Suite 205
San Diego, CA 92126
Fax: 858-635-9414
orders@icongroupbooks.com
icongroupbooks.com

ISBN 0-597831-54-8

8786 **Official Patient's Sourcebook on Pulmonary Fibrosis**
Icon Group International
9606 Tierra Grande Street
Suite 205
San Diego, CA 92126
Fax: 858-635-9414
orders@icongroupbooks.com
icongroupbooks.com

ISBN 0-597831-65-3

8787 **Official Patient's Sourcebook on Scoliosis**
Icon Group International
9606 Tierra Grande Street
Suite 205
San Diego, CA 92126
Fax: 858-635-9414
orders@icongroupbooks.com
icongroupbooks.com

ISBN 0-597829-90-X

8788 **Official Patient's Sourcebook on Sickle Cell Anemia**
Icon Group International
9606 Tierra Grande Street
Suite 205
San Diego, CA 92126
Fax: 858-635-9414
orders@icongroupbooks.com
icongroupbooks.com

ISBN 0-597831-57-2

8789 **Official Patient's Sourcebook on Ulcerative Colitis**
Icon Group International
9606 Tierra Grande Street
Suite 205
San Diego, CA 92126
Fax: 858-635-9414
orders@icongroupbooks.com
icongroupbooks.com

ISBN 0-597834-09-1

8790 **One Day at a Time: Children Living with Leukemia**
Gareth Stevens Publishing
111 East 14th Street
Suite #349
New York, NY 10003
800-542-2595
Fax: 877-542-2596
customerservice@gspub.com
www.garethstevens.com

56 pages Hardcover
ISBN 1-55532 -13-6

8791 **Options: Revolutionary Ideas in the War on Cancer**
People Against Cancer
P.O. Box 10
604 East Street
Otho, IA 50569
515-972-4444
800-662-2623
Fax: 515-972-4415
info@PeopleAgainstCancer.org
www.peopleagainstcancer.com

Frank D. Wiewel, Executive Director/Founder

Publication of People Against Cancer, a nonprofit, grassroots public benefit organization dedicated to 'New Directions in the War on Cancer.' We help people to find the best cancer treatment. We are a democratic organization of people with cancer, their loved ones and citizens working together to protect and enhance medical freedom of choice.

8792 **Osteoporosis Sourcebook**
Omnigraphics
615 Griswold Street
Suite 520
Detroit, MI 48226
610-461-3548
800-234-1340
Fax: 800-875-1340
contact@omnigraphics.com
www.omnigraphics.com

Peter Ruffner, Co-Founder
Fred Ruffner, Co-Founder

Discusses causes, risk factors, treatments and traditional and non-traditional pain management issues concerning osteoporosis. *$84.00*

568 pages Hard cover
ISBN 0-780802-39-1

8793 **Parent's Guide to Allergies and Asthma**
Allergy & Asthma Network Mothers of Asthmatics
Ste 150
PO Box 7474
Fairfax Station, VA 22039-7474
703-323-9170
800-756-5525
Fax: 703-323-9173
custsvc@parent-institute.com
www.parent-institute.com

John H Wherry, Ed.D, President

A up-to-date, easy-to-read resource offering essential information on asthma and allergies.

8794 **Partial Seizure Disorders: A Guide for Patients and Families**
O'Reilly Media Inc
1005 Gravenstein Hwy N
Sebastopol, CA 95472-2811
707-827-7000
800-998-9938
Fax: 707-829-0104
order@oreilly.com
www.oreilly.com

Linda Lamb, Editor
Mitzi Waltz, Author

Partial Seizure Disorders helps patients and families get an accurate diagnosis of this condition, understand medications and their side effects, and learn coping skills and other adjuncts to medication. It walks readers through developmental and school issues for young children; adult issues such as employment and driving; working with an existing health plan; and getting further help through advocacy and support organizations, articles, and online resources. *$19.95*

288 pages Paperback
ISBN 0-596500-03-3

8795 **Penitent, with Roses: An HIV+ Mother Reflects**
University Press of New England
1 Court St
Ste 250
Lebanon, NH 03766-1358
603-448-1533
800-421-1561
Fax: 603-448-7006
www.upne.com

Paula W Peterson, Author

Peterson, a married, middle-class, Jewish mother, was diagnosed with full-blown AIDS four years into her marriage and 11 months after her son was born. In seven poignant autobiographical essays and a collection of letters to her uninfected, four-year-old son, the author maintains an upbeat tone and describes her unsuccessful attempts to find the source of her infection (her husband tested negative), her relationships with her doctors, and her work as an HIV activist. *$26.95*

256 pages 2001
ISBN 1-584651-28-4

8796 **Plan Ahead: Do What You Can**
Spina Bifida Association of America
1600 Wilson Boulevard
Suite 800
Arlington, VA 22209
202-944-3285
800-621-3141
Fax: 202-944-3295
sbaa@sbaa.org
www.sbaa.org

Ana Ximenes, Chair
Sara Struwe, President & CEO
Mark Bohay, National Web Initiatives & Development Manager
Elizabeth Merck, Development Manager

Folic aciid information for women at risk for recurrence. *$15.00*

8797 **Post-Polio Syndrome: A Guide for Polio Survivors and Their Families**
Yale University Press
PO Box 209040
New Haven, CT 6520-9040
203-432-0960
203-432-0948
language.yalepress@yale.edu

Julie K Silver M.D., Author
Laro S Halstead, M.D., Foreword

A guide for polio survivors, their families, and their health care providers offers expert advice on all aspects of post-polio syndrome. Based on the author's experience treating post-polio patients, Silver discusses issues of critical importance, including how to find the best medical care, deal with symptoms, sustain mobility, manage pain, approach insurance issues, and arrange a safe living environment. *$19.50*

304 pages 2002
ISBN 0-300088-08-3

8798 **Prader-Willi Syndrome: Development and Manifestations**
Cambridge University Press
32 Avenue of the Americas
New York, NY 10013-2473
212-924-3900
212-691-3239
www.cambridge.org

Joyce Whittington, Author
Tony Holland, Co-Author
Seeks to identify and provide the latest findings about how best to manage the complex medical, nutritional, psychological, educational, social and therapeutic needs of people with PWS. *$130.00*
230 pages 2004
ISBN 0-521840-29-3

8799 **Preventing Secondary Conditions Associated with Spina Bifida or Cerebral Palsy**
Spina Bifida Association of America
1600 Wilson Boulevard
Suite 800
Arlington, VA 22209
202-944-3285
800-621-3141
Fax: 202-944-3295
sbaa@sbaa.org
www.sbaa.org

Ana Ximenes, Chair
Sara Struwe, President & CEO
Mark Bohay, National Web Initiatives & Development Manager
Elizabeth Merck, Development Manager
This report is for health professionals, parents and teachers. *$3.00*

8800 **Prostate and Urological Disorders Sourcebook**
Omnigraphics
615 Griswold Street
Suite 520
Detroit, MI 48226
610-461-3548
800-234-1340
Fax: 800-875-1340
contact@omnigraphics.com
www.omnigraphics.com

Peter Ruffner, Co-Founder
Fred Ruffner, Co-Founder
Prostate and Urological Disorders Sourcebook provides information about prostate cancer and other prostate problems, such as prostatitis and benign prostatic hyperplasia. A glossary of andrological terms and a directory of resources for additional help and information are also included. *$84.00*
604 pages Hard cover
ISBN 0-780807-97-6

8801 **Protecting Against Latex Allergy**
Spina Bifida Association of America
1600 Wilson Boulevard
Suite 800
Arlington, VA 22209
202-944-3285
800-621-3141
Fax: 202-944-3295
sbaa@sbaa.org
www.sbaa.org

Ana Ximenes, Chair
Sara Struwe, President & CEO
Mark Bohay, National Web Initiatives & Development Manager
Elizabeth Merck, Development Manager
Because awareness and proper action may help prevent an allergic reation, learning about latex allergy is especially important for parents, health care workers and anyone who is exposed to latex regulary. *$20.00*

8802 **Questions and Answers: The ADA and Personswith HIV/AIDS**
US Department of Justice
950 Pennsylvania Ave NW
Washington, DC 20530-9
202-307-0663
800-514-0301
Fax: 202-307-1197
TTY: 800-514-0383
www.ada.gov

Joanne Graham, Manager
Rebecca B. Bond, Chief
Zita Johnson Betts, Deputy Chief
James Bostrom, Deputy Chief
A 16-page publication explaining the requirements for employers, businesses and nonprofit agencies that serve the public, and state and local governments to avoid discriminating against persons with HIV/AIDS.

8803 **Raynaud's Phenomenon**
Arthritis Foundation
1330 W. Peachtree Street
Suite 100
Atlanta, GA 30309
404-872-7100
800-283-7800
Fax: 404-872-0457
arthritis.org

Daniel T. McGowan, Chair
Michael V. Ortman, Vice Chair
Ann M. Palmer, CEO/President
Peter W.C. Barnhart, Treasurer
The Arthritis Foundation is the largest national nonprofit organization that supports the more than 100 types of arthritis and related conditions. Founded in 1948, with headquarters in Atlanta, the Arthritis Foundation has multiple service points located throughout the country.

8804 **Reaching the Autistic Child: A Parent Training Program**
Brookline Books
8 Trumbull Rd,
Northampton, MA 01060-4533
413-584-0184
800-666-2665
Fax: 413-584-6184
brbooks@yahoo.com

Softcover
ISBN 1-571290-56-7

8805 **Respiratory Disorders Sourcebook**
Omnigraphics
615 Griswold Street
Suite 520
Detroit, MI 48226
610-461-3548
800-234-1340
Fax: 800-875-1340
contact@omnigraphics.com
www.omnigraphics.com

Peter Ruffner, Co-Founder
Fred Ruffner, Co-Founder
Respiratory Disorders Sourcebook provides up-to-date information about infectious, inflammatory, occupational, and other types of respiratory disorders. Tips for managing chronic respiratory diseases and suggestions for ways to promote lung health are presented, and the book concludes with a glossary of related terms and a list of additional resources. *$84.00*
638 pages Hard cover
ISBN 0-780810-07-5

8806 **SPINabilities: A Young Person's Guide to Spina Bifida**
Spina Bifida Association of America
1600 Wilson Boulevard
Suite 800
Arlington, VA 22209
202-944-3285
800-621-3141
Fax: 202-944-3295
sbaa@sbaa.org
www.sbaa.org

Ana Ximenes, Chair
Sara Struwe, President & CEO
Mark Bohay, National Web Initiatives & Development Manager
Elizabeth Merck, Development Manager

A cool and practical book for young adults becoming independent. *$22.30*

8807 **Seizures and Epilepsy in Childhood: A Guide**
John Hopkins University Press
2715 N Charles St
Baltimore, MD 21218-4363
410-516-6900
800-548-1784
Fax: 410-516-6998
webmaster@jhupress.jhu.edu
www.press.jhu.edu

Kathleen Keane, Director
Eileen P G Vining MD, Co-Author
Diana J Pillas, Co-Author
John M Freeman, M.D., Co-Author

The award-winning Seizures and Epilepsy in Childhood is the standard resource for parents in need of comprehensive medical information about their child with epilepsy. *$54.00*

432 pages 3rd Edition
ISBN 0-801870-51-4

8808 **Sexuality and the Person with Spina Bifida**
Spina Bifida Association of America
1600 Wilson Boulevard
Suite 800
Arlington, VA 22209
202-944-3285
800-621-3141
Fax: 202-944-3295
sbaa@sbaa.org
www.sbaa.org

Ana Ximenes, Chair
Sara Struwe, President & CEO
Mark Bohay, National Web Initiatives & Development Manager
Elizabeth Merck, Development Manager

Dr Sloan foucuses on sexual development, sexual activity and other important issues. *$11.00*

8809 **Sinus Survival: A Self-help Guide**
Penguin Group
375 Hudson St
New York, NY 10014-3658
212-366-2372
Fax: 212-366-2933
insidesales@penguingroup.com
us.penguingroup.com

Robert S Ivker, Author

Self-help manual for sufferers of bronchitis, sinusitis, allergies, and colds. *$15.95*

336 pages Paperback 2000
ISBN 1-101798-02-6

8810 **Social Development and the Person with Spina Bifida**
Spina Bifida Association of America
1600 Wilson Boulevard
Suite 800
Arlington, VA 22209
202-944-3285
800-621-3141
Fax: 202-944-3295
sbaa@sbaa.org
www.sbaa.org

Ana Ximenes, Chair
Sara Struwe, President & CEO
Mark Bohay, National Web Initiatives & Development Manager
Elizabeth Merck, Development Manager

Examines how spina bifida and hydrocephalus may influence development and learning social skills.

8811 **Solving the Puzzle of Chronic Fatigue**
Essential Science Publishing
1216 S 1580 W
Ste A
Orem, UT 84058-4906
801-224-6228
800-336-6308
Fax: 801-224-6229
info@essentialscience.net
www.essentialsciencepublishing.com

Michael Rosenbaum, Author
Murray Susser, Co-Author

Although primarily a book about CFS, this comprehensive study also provides a detailed overview of candidiasis, including its causes and best approaches for treatment. *$14.95*

190 pages
ISBN 0-943685-11-7

8812 **Son Rise: The Miracle Continues**
New World Library
14 Pamaron Way
Novato, CA 94949
415-884-2100
800-972-6657
Fax: 415-884-2199
ami@newworldlibrary.com
www.newworldlibrary.com

Barry Neil Kaufman, Author

Documents Raun Kaufman's astonishing development from a lifeless, autistic child into a highly verbal, lovable youngster with no traces of his former condition. Details Raun's extraordinary progress from the age of four into young adulthood, also shares moving accounts of five families that successfully used the Son-Rise Program to reach their own special children. *$14.96*

372 pages
ISBN 0-915811-53-7

8813 **Steps to Independence: Teaching Everyday Skills to Children with Special Needs**
Spina Bifida Association of America
1600 Wilson Boulevard
Suite 800
Arlington, VA 22209
202-944-3285
800-621-3141
Fax: 202-944-3295
sbaa@sbaa.org
www.sbaa.org

Ana Ximenes, Chair
Sara Struwe, President & CEO
Mark Bohay, National Web Initiatives & Development Manager
Elizabeth Merck, Development Manager

A guide to help parents teach life skills to their disabled child. *$34.25*

8814 **Stroke Sourcebook**
Omnigraphics
615 Griswold Street
Suite 520
Detroit, MI 48226
610-461-3548
800-234-1340
Fax: 800-875-1340
contact@omnigraphics.com
www.omnigraphics.com

Peter Ruffner, Co-Founder
Fred Ruffner, Co-Founder

Basic Consumer Health Information about Stroke, Including Ischemic, Hemorrhagic, and Mini Strokes, as Well as Risk Factors, Prevention Guidelines, Diagnostic Tests, Medications and Surgical Treatments, and Complications of Stroke.

8815 **Stroke Sourcebook, 2nd Edition**
Omnigraphics
615 Griswold Street
Suite 520
Detroit, MI 48226
610-461-3548
800-234-1340
Fax: 800-875-1340
contact@omnigraphics.com
www.omnigraphics.com

Peter Ruffner, Co-Founder
Fred Ruffner, Co-Founder

Stroke Sourcebook, Second Edition provides updated information about stroke, its causes, risk factors, diagnosis, acute and long-term treatment, and recent innovations in poststroke care. Information on rehabilitation therapies, prevention strategies, and tips on caring for a stroke survivor is also included, along with a glossary of related terms and a directory of organizations that offer additional information to stroke survivors and their families. *$84.00*

626 pages Hard cover
ISBN 0-780810-35-8

8817 **Succeeding With Interventions For Asperger Syndrome Adolescents**
Autsim Society of North Carolina Bookstore
505 Oberlin Road
Suite 230
Raleigh, NC 27605-1345
919-743-0204
800-442-2762
Fax: 919-743-0208
books@autismsociety-nc.org
www.autismbookstore.com
Tracey Sheriff, Chief Executive Officer
David Laxton, Director of Communications
Paul Wendler, Chief Financial Officer
Kristy White, Director of Development
This book includes a very useful outline of all the therapy sessions, which can be used as a template by a practitioner for creating their own interaction therapy intervention for adolescents.

8818 **Symptomatic Chiari Malformation**
Spina Bifida Association of America
1600 Wilson Boulevard
Suite 800
Arlington, VA 22209
202-944-3285
800-621-3141
Fax: 202-944-3295
sbaa@sbaa.org
www.sbaa.org
Ana Ximenes, Chair
Sara Struwe, President & CEO
Mark Bohay, National Web Initiatives & Development Manager
Elizabeth Merck, Development Manager
The Spina Bifida Association (SBA) serves adults and children who live with the challenges of Spina Bifida.

8819 **Taking Charge**
Spina Bifida Association of America
1600 Wilson Boulevard
Suite 800
Arlington, VA 22209
202-944-3285
800-621-3141
Fax: 202-944-3295
sbaa@sbaa.org
Ana Ximenes, Chair
Sara Struwe, President & CEO
Mark Bohay, National Web Initiatives & Development Manager
Elizabeth Merck, Development Manager
Teenagers talk about life and physical disabilities. *$7.95*

8820 **Ten Things I Learned from Bill Porter**
New World Library
14 Pamaron Way
Novato, CA 94949
415-884-2100
800-972-6657
Fax: 415-884-2199
ami@newworldlibrary.com
www.newworldlibrary.com
Shelly Ackerman, Author
Bill Porter worked for the Watkins Corp, selling household products door-to-door in one of Portland's worst neighborhoods. Afflicted with cerebral palsy and burdened with continual pain, Porter was determined not to live on government disability and went on to become Watkin's top-grossing salesman in Portland, the Northwest, and the US. This book was written by the woman who worked as Porter's typist and driver and later became his friend and cospeaker. *$20.00*
192 pages
ISBN 1-577312-03-1

8821 **Thyroid Disorders Sourcebook**
Omnigraphics
615 Griswold Street
Suite 520
Detroit, MI 48226
610-461-3548
800-234-1340
Fax: 800-875-1340
contact@omnigraphics.com
www.omnigraphics.com
Peter Ruffner, Co-Founder
Fred Ruffner, Co-Founder
Thyroid Disorders Sourcebook provides essential information about thyroid and parathyroid function, diseases, and treatments. Also presented are symptoms, risk factors, diagnosis, treatments, thyroid effects on the body, and the impact of environmental conditions on the thyroid. *$84.00*
573 pages Hard cover
ISBN 0-780807-45-7

8822 **Tourette Syndrome: The Facts**
Oxford University Press
198 Madison Avenue
New York, NY 10016
212-726-6000
800-445-9714
Fax: 919-677-1303
custserv.us@oup.com
www.oup.com
Mary Robertson, Co-Editor
Andrea Cavanna, Co-Editor
Johnathan Keats, Author
Jim Cullen, Author
The causes of the syndrome, how it is diagnosed, and the ways in which it can be treated. *$35.00*
122 pages
ISBN 0-198523-98-X

8823 **Tourette's Syndrome: Finding Answers and Getting Help**
O'Reilly Media Inc
1005 Gravenstein Hwy N
Sebastopol, CA 95472-2811
707-827-7019
800-889-8969
Fax: 707-824-8268
order@oreilly.com
www.oreilly.com
416 pages Paperback
ISBN 0-596500-07-6

8824 **Tourette's Syndrome: Tics, Obsessions, Compulsions: Developmental Psychopathology**
John Wiley & Sons
111 River Street
Hoboken, NJ 07030-5774
201-748-6000
Fax: 201-748-6088
www.wiley.com
Peter Booth Wiley, Chairman
Stephen M. Smith, President & CEO
John Kitzmacher, EVP, CFO
Ellis E. Cousens, Executive Vice President, COO
Contains 21 contributions compromising the work of researchers associated with the Yale Child Study Center, which has been at the forefront of research on Tourette's syndrome and associated disorders. *$85.00*
600 pages
ISBN 0-471113-75-1

8825 **Treating Epilepsy Naturally: A Guide to Alternative and Adjunct Therapies**
McGraw-Hill Company
P.O. Box 182605
Columbus, OH 43218
800-338-3987
Fax: 609-308-4480
customer.service@mheducation.com
www.mcgraw-hill.com
David Levin, President and CEO
Patrick Milano, Chief Administrative Officer & CFO
Stephen Laster, Chief Digital Officer
David Stafford, SVP & General Counsel
Offers alternative treatments to replace and to complement traditional therapies and sound advice to find the right health practitioner. *$15.95*
288 pages
ISBN 0-658013-79-3

8826 Understanding Asthma
National Jewish Health
1400 Jackson Street
Denver, CO 80206
303-270-2708
877-225-5654
Fax: 303-398-1125
allstetterw@njc.org
nationaljewish.org

Rich Schierburg, Chair
Robin Chotin, Vice Chair
Michael Salem, M.D., President and CEO
Christine Forkner, CFO and Executive Vice President

Offers a brief introduction to asthma and then goes into the physiology of asthma, the triggers of asthma, and diagnosis and monitoring of asthma.

27 pages

8827 Understanding Asthma: The Blueprint for Breathing
Allergy & Asthma Network Mothers of Asthmatics
8229 Boone Boulevard
Suite 260
Vienna, VA 22182
800-878-4403
Fax: 703-288-5271
www.aanma.org

Michael Amato, Chair
Tonya Winders, President & CEO
Brenda Silvia-Torma, Project Manager
Gary Fitzgerald, Managing Editor

A layman's guide to asthma facts based on a presentation from the first national asthma patient conference.

8828 Understanding Cystic Fibrosis
University Press of Mississippi
3825 Ridgewood Road
Jackson, MS 39211-6492
601-432-6205
800-737-7788
Fax: 601-432-6217
press@ihl.state.ms.us
www.upress.state.ms.us

Leila W. Salisbury, Director
Craig Gill, Assistant Director/Editor-in-Chief
Anne Stascavage, Managing Editor
Vijay Shah, Acquiring Editor

A reference for CF patients and their families. *$14.00*

128 pages
ISBN 0-878059-67-9

8829 Understanding Multiple Sclerosis
University Press of Mississippi
3825 Ridgewood Road
Jackson, MS 39211-6492
601-432-6205
800-737-7788
Fax: 601-432-6217
press@ihl.state.ms.us
www.upress.state.ms.us

Melissa Stauffer, Author
Craig Gill, Assistant Director/Editor-in-Chief
Anne Stascavage, Managing Editor
Vijay Shah, Acquiring Editor

Two psychologists discuss their roles with a member who has multiple sclerosis. Includes chapters on adolescents with multiple sclerosis, employment, and research. *$14.00*

136 pages
ISBN 1-578068-03-7

8830 Urologic Care of the Child with Spina Bifida
Spina Bifida Association of America
1600 Wilson Boulevard
Suite 800
Arlington, VA 22209
202-944-3285
800-621-3141
Fax: 202-944-3295
sbaa@sbaa.org

Ana Ximenes, Chair
Sara Struwe, President & CEO
Mark Bohay, National Web Initiatives & Development Manager
Elizabeth Merck, Development Manager

The Spina Bifida Association (SBA) serves adults and children who live with the challenges of Spina Bifida.

8831 Usher Syndrome
NI on Deafness & Other Communication Disorders
31 Center Dr.
MSC 2320
Bethesda, MD 20892-2320
301-827-8183
800-241-1044
Fax: 301-770-8977
TTY: 800-241-1055
nidcdinfo@nidcd.nih.gov
www.nidcd.nih.gov

Debara L. Tucci, Director
Judith A. Cooper, Deputy Director
Timothy J. Wheeles, Executive Officer
Lisa Portnoy, Deputy Executive Officer

Explains what is Usher Syndrome, who is affected by Usher syndrome, what causes Usher syndrome, how is Usher syndrome treated, and what research is being conducted on Usher syndrome.

8832 What Everyone Needs to Know About Asthma
Allergy & Asthma Network Mothers of Asthmatics
8229 Boone Boulevard
Suite 260
Vienna, VA 22182
800-878-4403
Fax: 703-288-5271
www.aanma.org

Michael Amato, Chair
Tonya Winders, President & CEO
Brenda Silvia-Torma, Project Manager
Gary Fitzgerald, Managing Editor

Offers information and facts on gaining control of asthma, asthma triggers and monitoring asthma disorders.

8833 When the Road Turns: Inspirational Stories About People with MS
Health Communications
3201 SouthWest 15th Street
Deerfield Beach, FL 33442
954-360-0909
800-441-5569
Fax: 954-360-0034

300 pages
ISBN 1-558749-07-1

8834 Young Person's Guide to Spina Bifida
Spina Bifida Association of America
1600 Wilson Boulevard
Suite 800
Arlington, VA 22209
202-944-3285
800-621-3141
Fax: 202-944-3295
sbaa@sbaa.org

Ana Ximenes, Chair
Sara Struwe, President & CEO
Mark Bohay, National Web Initiatives & Development Manager
Elizabeth Merck, Development Manager

Gives practical tips and suggestions for becoming independent and managing your health. *$19.00*

8835 Your Child and Asthma
National Jewish Health
1400 Jackson Street
Denver, CO 80206
303-270-2708
877-225-5654
Fax: 303-398-1125
allstetterw@njc.org
nationaljewish.org

Rich Schierburg, Chair
Robin Chotin, Vice Chair
Michael Salem, M.D., President and CEO
Christine Forkner, CFO and Executive Vice President

A booklet offering information to parents and family about their child with asthma. Offers information on diagnosis, treatments, triggers and family concerns.

8836 **Your Cleft Affected Child**
Hunter House Inc. Publisher
PO Box 2914
Alameda, CA 94501-914
510-865-5282
800-266-5592
Fax: 510-865-4295
www.hunterhouse.com
Carrie T Gruman Trinker, Author
The book also provides in-depth information, guidance, and support on a wide variety of relevant topics, from feeding to surgery to helping a child cope until his/her cleft has been fully corrected. *$16.95*
288 pages Paperback
ISBN 0-897931-85-4

8837 **Your Guide to Bowel Cancer**
Oxford University Press
2001 Evans Road
Cary, NC 27513
919-677-0977
800-445-9714
Fax: 919-677-1303
www.us.oup.com
ISBN 0-340927-46-1

Journals

8838 **AIDS: The Official Journal of the International AIDS Society**
Lippincott Williams & Wilkins
2 Commerce Square
2001 Market St.
Philadelphia, PA 19103
215-521-8300
Fax: 215-521-8902
customerservice@lww.com
lww.com
JA Levy, Co Editor
B. Autran, Co Editor
R. A Coutinho, Co Editor
J. P Phair, Co Editor
The latest groundbreaking research on HIV and AIDS. *$433.00*
18 per year

8839 **American Journal of Orthopsychiatry**
American Psychological Association
750 1st Street NorthEast
Washington, DC 20002-4242
202-336-5500
800-374-2721
Fax: 202-336-5502
TTY: 202-336-6123
www.apa.org
Nadine J. Kaslow, President
Norman B. Anderson, PhD, CEO & EVP
Bonnie Markham, Treasurer
Jennifer F. Kelly, Recording Secretary
Mental health issues from multidisciplinary and interprofessionals perspectives: clinical, research and expository approaches. *$45.00*
160 pages Quarterly

8840 **Annals of Otology, Rhinology and Laryngology**
Annals Publishing Company
4507 Laclede Ave
Saint Louis, MO 63108-2103
314-367-4987
Fax: 314-367-4988
www.annals.com
Ken Cooper, President
Richard J. Smith, Editor
Monica L. Bergers, Editor's Assistant
Jim Cunningham, Advertising Representative
Original, peer-reviewed articles in the fields of otolaryngology - head and neck medicine and surgery, broncho-esophagology, audiology, speech, pathology, allery, and maxillofacial surgery. Official journal of the American Laryngological Association/American Broncho-Esophagological Association. *$170.00*
112 pages Monthly

8841 **Archives of Neurology**
American Medical Association
P.O. Box 10946
Chicago, IL 60654
312-670-7827
800-262-2350
Fax: 312-464-4184
subscriptions@jamanetwork.com
jamanetwork.com
Margaret Vanner, Manager
Mission is to publish scientific information primarily important to those physicians caring for people with neurologic disorders, but also for those interested in the structure and function of the normal and diseased nervous system. *$235.00*
198 pages Monthly

8842 **Cleft Palate-Craniofacial Journal**
American Cleft Palate-Craniofacial Association
2455 Teller Rd.
Thousand Oaks, CA 91320
800-818-7243
Fax: 800-583-2665
journal@acpa-cpf.org
www.cpcjournal.org
Jack C. Yu, Editor
A peer-reviewed, interdisciplinary, international journal dedicated to current research on etiology, prevention, diagnosis, and treatment in all areas pertaining to craniofacial anomalies. Publishes 10 issues a year.

8843 **Developmental Medicine & Childhood Neurology**
American Academy for Cerebral Palsy/Dev. Medicine
555 East Wells
Suite 1100
Milwaukee, WI 53202
414-918-3014
Fax: 414-276-2146
info@aacpdm.org
www.aacpdm.org
Tamara Wagester, Executive Director
Clinical research into the wide range of neurological conditions and disabilities that affect children.

8844 **Journal of Head Trauma Rehabilitation**
Lippincott, Williams & Wilkins
P.O. Box 1620
Hagerstown, MD 21740
301-223-2300
800-638-3030
Fax: 301-223-2400
orders@lww.com
www.lww.com
John D Corrigan PhD, ABPP, Editor
Scholarly journal designed to provide information on clinical management and rehabilitation of the head-injured for the practicing professional. Published bimonthly. *$113.96*

Magazines

8845 **Coping with Cancer Magazine**
Media America
P.O. Box 682268
Franklin, TN 37068-2268
615-790-2400
Fax: 615-794-0179
copingmag.com
53 pages 6 x year

8846 **CurePSP Magazine**
Society for Progressive Supranuclear Palsy
Suite 201
30 E. Padonia Road
Timonium, MD 21093
410-785-7004
800-457-4777
Fax: 410-785-7009
info@curepsp.org
www.psp.org
John T. Burhoe, Chair
Everett R. Cook, Vice Chair
Richard Gordon Zyne, President-CEO
Kathleen Matarazzo Speca, VP,Development & Donor Relations
Quarterly newsletter. The society's mission is to promote and fund research into finding the cause and cure for progressive

supranuclear palsy (PSP). Provides information, support and advocacy to persons diagnosed with PSP, their families and caregivers. Educates physicians and allied health professionals on PSP and how to improve patient care.

8847 **EpilepsyUSA**
Epilepsy Foundation
8301 Professional Place
Landover, MD 20785-2353
301-459-3700
800-332-1000
Fax: 301-459-1569
ContactUs@efa.org
epilepsyfoundation.org

Warren Lammert, Chair
Phil Gattone, President and CEO
May J. Liang, Secretary
Roger Heldman, Treasurer
Magazine reporting on issues of interest to people with epilepsy and their families. *$15.00*
22 pages Bi-Monthly

8848 **MSFOCUS Magazine**
Multiple Sclerosis Foundation
6520 North Andrews Avenue
Fort Lauderdale, FL 33309-2130
954-776-6805
888-673-6287
Fax: 954-351-0630
support@msfocus.org
www.msfocus.org

Jules Kuperberg, Executive Director
Alan Segaloff, Executive Director
Natalie Blake, Program Services Director
Nathalie Sloane, Funds Development Director
Contemporary national, nonprofit organization that provides free support services and public education for persons with Multiple Sclerosis, newsletters, toll-free phone support, information, referrals, home care, assistive technology and support groups.
48 pages Quarterly

8849 **Orthotics and Prosthetics Almanac**
American Orthotic & Prosthetics Association
330 John Carlyle Street
Suite 200
Alexandria, VA 22314
571-431-0876
Fax: 571-431-0899
info@aopanet.org
www.aopanet.org

Anita L. Lampear, President
Charles H. Dankmeyer, Vice President
Thomas F. Fise, JD, Executive Director
Don DeBolt, Chief Operating Officer
Features articles covering current professional, patient care, government, business and National Office activities affecting the orthotics and prosthetics profession and industry. *$40.00*
80 pages Monthly
ISSN 1061-46 1

8850 **PDF News**
Parkinson's Disease Foundation
1359 Broadway
Suite 1509
New York, NY 10018
212-923-4700
800-457-6676
Fax: 212-923-4778
info@pdf.org
www.pdf.org

Howard D. Morgan, Chair
Woodruff Atwell, Ph.D., Vice Chair
Stephen Ackerman, Treasurer
Isobel Robins Konecky, Secretary
8-12 pages Quarterly

8851 **POZ Magazine**
212 W 35th St
New York, NY 10001
212-242-2163
800-973-2376
Fax: 212-675-8505
website@poz.com
poz.com

8852 **SCI Life**
National Spinal Cord Injury Association
11300 Rockville Pike
Suite 803
Rockville, MD 20852
301-468-3902
Fax: 301-468-3904
info@ilcreations.com
ilcreations.com

Quarterly/Free

8853 **Spine**
Lippincott, Williams & Wilkins
530 Walnut St
Philadelphia, PA 19106-3603
215-521-8300
Fax: 215-521-8411
customerservice@lww.com

James N Weinstein DO MSc, Editor
Publishes original papers on theoretical issues and research concerning the spine and spinal cord injuries. *$9.00*
26 Issues Year

Newsletters

8854 **ACPOC News**
Assoc of Children's Prosthetic-Orthotic Clinics
6300 N River Rd
Suite 727
Rosemont, IL 60018-4226
847-698-1637
Fax: 847-823-0536
acpoc@aaos.org
www.acpoc.org

David B. Rotter,CPO, President
Jorge A. Fabregas, Vice President
Hank White,PT,PhD, Secretary-Treasurer
Anna Cuomo, Director
Quarterly publication from the Association of Children's Prosthetic/Orthotic Clinics. Included with membership.
40 pages Quarterly

8855 **AID Bulletin**
Project AID Resource Center
P.O. Box 5190
Kent, OH 44242-0001
330-672-3000
Fax: 330-672-4724
info@kent.edu
www.kent.edu/

Beverly Warren, President
Todd A. Diacon, Provost & SVP
Gregg S. Floyd, Sr. Vice President
Greg Jarvie, Vice President
Has the latest news on upcoming conferences, literature, developments in programs and/or services for disabled persons who are substance abusers. Offers articles on their experiences, ideas and questions of others in this field which includes providers and consumers. *$7.50*

8856 **AIDS Alert**
AHC Media LLC
PO Box 550669
Atlanta, GA 30355
404-262-5436
800-688-2421
Fax: 404-262-5560
www.ahcpub.com/

Joy Daughtery Dickinson, Senior Managing Editor
Source of AIDS news and advice for health care professionals. Covers up-to-the-minute developments and guidance on the entire spectrum of AIDS challenges, including treatment, education, precautions, screening, diagnosis and policy. *$499.00*
Monthly

8857 **Adaptive Tracks**
Adaptive Sports Center
P.O. Box 1639
Crested Butte, CO 81224
970-349-2296
866-349-2296
Fax: 970-349-2077
info@adaptivesports.org
www.adaptivesports.org

Christopher Hensley, Executive Director
Chris Read, CTRS, Program Director
Ella Fahrlander, Development Director
Mike Neustedter, Marketing Director

The Adaptive Sports Center (ASC) of Crested Butte, Colorado is a non-profit organization that provides year-round recreation activities for people with disabilities and their families. The ASC provides adaptive snowboarding downhill skiing, cross country skiing as well as backcountry trips. Summer activities include a variety of wilderness-based programs, multi-day trips into the back country, extensive cycling programs, canoeing, and white water rafting.
6 pages Quarterly

8858 **Arthritis Self-Management**
Rapaport Publishing, Inc.
150 W 22nd St
Ste 800
New York, NY 10011-2421
212-989-0200
Fax: 212-989-4786
ASMcustserv@cdsfulfillment.com
www.arthritisselfmanagement.com

Richard A Rapaport, President
Maryanne Schott Turner, Director of Manufacturing
Richard Boland, Art Director
James Moorehead, Circulation Director

Arthritis Self-Management publishes practical 'how-to' information for the growing number of people with arthritis who want to know more about managing their condition. We focus on the day-to-day and long-term aspects of arthritis in a positive and upbeat style, giving our subscribers up-to-date news, facts, and advice to help them make informed decisions about their health. *$9.97*
BiMonthly

8859 **Breaking Ground**
Tennessee Council on Developmental Disabilities
404 James Robertson Pkwy
Suite 130
Nashville, TN 37243- 0228
615-532-6615
Fax: 615-532-6964
TTY: 615-741-4562
tnddc@tn.gov
www.tn.gov/cdd

Stephanie Brewer cook, Chair
Roger D. Gibbens, Vice Chair
Wanda Willis, Executive Director
Errol Elshtain, Director of Development

Newsletter
20 pages 6 x Year

8860 **Breaking New Ground News Note**
Purdue University
225 West University Street
West Lafayette, IN 47907
765-494-4600
800-825-4264
Fax: 765-496-1356
engineering.purdue.edu/

Paul Jones, Project Manager
Bill Field, Project Director
Denise Heath, Project Asst.
Robert Stuthridge, Project Ergonomist

News, practical ideas and success stories of and for farmers and other agricultural workers with physical disabilities.
2 pages Quarterly

8861 **Diabetes Self-Management**
Rapaport Publishing, Inc.
150 W 22nd St
Ste 800
New York, NY 10011-2421
212-989-0200
Fax: 212-989-4786
www.diabetesselfmanagement.com

Richard A Rapaport, President
Maryanne Schott Turner, Director of Manufacturing
Richard Boland, Art Director
James Moorehead, Circulation Director

Publishes practical how-to information, focusing on the day-to-day and long-term aspects of diabetes in a positive and upbeat style. Gives subscribers up-to-date news, facts and advice to help them maintain their wellness and make informed decisions regarding their health. *$9.97*
BiMonthly

8862 **Directions**
Families of Spinal Muscular Dystrophy
925 Busse Road
Elk Grove Village, IL 60007
847-367-7620
800-886-1762
Fax: 847-367-7623
info@fsma.org
www.fsma.org

Richard Rubenstein, Chair
Kenneth Hobby, President
Sue Kovach, Director of Finance
Megan Lenz, Communications Manager
$35.00
60-70 pages Quarterly

8863 **IAL News**
International Association of Laryngectomees
925B Peachtree Street NE
Suite 316
Atlanta, GA 30309
866-425-3678
www.larynxlink.com

Wade Hampton, President
Susan Reeves, Administrative Manager
Jodi Knott, Director, Voice Institute
Charles Rusky, Treasurer

Focuses on rehabilitation and well-being of persons who have had laryngectomy surgery.

8864 **Informer**
Simon Foundation
P.O. Box 815
Wilmette, IL 60091
847-864-3913
800-237-4666
Fax: 847-864-9758
info@simonfoundation.org
simonfoundation.org

Cheryle Gartley, President and Founder
Elizabeth T. LaGro, VP, Communications & Education
Twila Yednock, Director of Special Events
Monica Liebert, Scientific Liason

Publishes items of interest to people with bladder or bowel incontinence, including medical articles, helpful devices, publications and a pen pal list. Quarterly newsletter.
Quarterly

8865 **Moisture Seekers**
Sjogren's Syndrome Foundation
6707 Democracy Boulevard
Suite 325
Bethesda, MD 20817
301-530-4420
800-475-6473
Fax: 301-530-4415
tms@sjogrens.org
www.sjogrens.org

Kenneth Economou, Chair
Steven Taylor, CEO
Sheriese DeFruscio, VP of Development
Elizabeth Trocchio, Director of Marketing

Newsletter of the organization for lay people and professionals interested in Sjogren's Syndrome. Contains medical news, current research, and essential tips for daily living. *$25.00*
15-16 pages Monthly

8866 **Momentum**
National Multiple Sclerosis Society
Ste 6
421 New Karner Rd
Albany, NY 12205-3838
518-464-0850
800-344-4867
Fax: 518-464-1232
nyr@nmss.org
www.nationalmssociety.org
Eli Rubenstein, Chair
Cynthia Zagieboylo, President & CEO
Sherri Giger, EVP, Marketing
Jennifer Douglas, EVP,Technology
News and information on research progress, medical treatments, patient services, therapeutic claims and activities.

8867 **Options**
People Against Cancer
P.O. Box 10
604 East Street
Otho, IA 50569
515-972-4444
800-662-2623
Fax: 515-972-4415
info@PeopleAgainstCancer.org
www.peopleagainstcancer.com
Frank D. Wiewel, Executive Director/Founder
Publication of People Against Cancer, a nonprofit, grassroots public benefit organization dedicated to 'New Directions in the War on Cancer.' We help people to find the best cancer treatment. We are a democratic organization of people with cancer, their loved ones and citizens working together to protect and enhance medical freedom of choice.
8 pages Quarterly

8868 **PDF Newsletter**
Parkinson's Disease Foundation
1359 Broadway
Suite 1509
New York, NY 10018
212-923-4700
800-457-6676
Fax: 212-923-4778
info@pdf.org
www.pdf.org
Howard D. Morgan, Chair
Woodruff Atwell, Ph.D., Vice Chair
Stephen Ackerman, Treasurer
Isobel Robins Konecky, Secretary
The Parkinson's Disease Foundation (PDF) is a leading national presence in Parkinson's disease research, education and public advocacy.
12-16 pages Quarterly

8869 **Parkinson Report**
National Parkinson Foundation
200 SE 1st Street
Suite 800
Miami, FL 33131
800-473-4636
www.parkinson.org
John L. Lehr, President & CEO
Leilani Pearl, SVP & Chief Communications Officer
Articles, reports and news on Parkinson's disease and the activities of the National Parkinson Foundation.
32 pages Quarterly

8870 **Post-Polio Health**
Post-Polio Health International
50 Crestwood Executive Ctr.
Suite 440
St. Louis, MO 63126
314-534-0475
Fax: 314-534-5070
editor@post-polio.org
www.post-polio.org
Brian M. Tiburzi, Editor
Post-Polio Health supports Post-Polio Health International's educational, research, and advocacy efforts. Offers information about relevant events.
12 pages Quarterly

8871 **Prader-Willi Alliance of New York Newsletter**
244 5th Avenue
Suite D-110
New York, NY 10001
800-442-1655
alliance@prader-willi.org
www.prader-willi.org
Rachel Johnson, Executive Director
The Prader-Willi Foundation is a national, nonprofit public charity that works for the benefit of individuals with Prader-Willi syndrome and their families. *$20.00*
Quarterly

8872 **Quality Care Newsletter**
National Association for Continence
P.O. Box 1019
Charleston, SC 29402-1019
843-352-2559
800-BLA-DER
Fax: 843-352-2563
memberservices@nafc.org
www.nafc.org
Donna Deng, Chairman
Nancy Hicks, Vice Chaiperson
Steven Gregg, Executive Director
Wendy Pokoski, Financial Administrator
Newsletter from NAFC. By donating $25 and becomming a Quality Care donor, you may receive our quarterly newsletter. *$25.00*
14-16 pages Quarterly

8873 **Rasmussen's Syndrome and Hemispherectomy Support Network Newsletter**
55 Kenosia Avenue
Danbury, CT 06810
203-744-0100
Fax: 203-798-2291
http://www.rarediseases.org/rare-disease-info
Ronald J. Bartek, Chair
Sheldon M. Schuster, Vice Chair
Peter L. Saltonstall, President & CEO
Pamela Gavin, COO
National, not-for-profit organization dedicated to providing information and support to individuals affected by Rasmussen's Syndrome and hemispherectomy. Publishes a periodic newsletter and disseminates reprints of medical journal articles concerning Rasmussen's Syndrome and its treatments. Maintains a support network that provides encouragement and information to individuals affected by Rasmussen's Syndrome and their families.

8874 **SCI Psychosocial Process**
Amer Assn of Spinal Cord Injury Psych & Soc Wks
75-20 Astoria Blvd
East Elmhurst, NY 11370
718-803-3782
800-404-2898
Fax: 718-803-0414
info@unitedspinal.org
http://www.unitedspinal.org/
David C. Cooper, Chairman
Patrick W. Maher, Vice Chairman
Joseph Gaskins, President and CEO
Denise A. McQuade, Secretary
Quarterly newsletter.

8875 **Special Care in Dentistry**
Blackwell Publishing
350 Main St
Malden, MA 02148
781-388-0200
Fax: 781-388-8210
www.blackwellpublishing.com
Peter Booth Wiley, Chairman
Stephen M. Smith, President & CEO
John Kitzmacher, EVP, CFO
Ellis E. Cousens, Executive Vice President, COO
$125.00
48 pages BiMonthly

8876 **TSA Newsletter**
Tourette Syndrome Association
42-40 Bell Boulevard
Bayside, NY 11361
718-224-2999
800-237-0717
Fax: 718-279-9596
ts@tsa-usa.org
www.tsa-usa.org

Stephen M. McCall, President

National non-profit membership organization whose mission is to identify the cause of, find the cure for, and control the effects of this disorder. A growing number of local chapters nationwide provide educational materials, seminars, conferences and support groups for over 35,000 members.

Quarterly

8877 **Teens & Asthma**
American Lung Association
530 7th St SE
Washington, DC 20003
202-546-5864
Fax: 202-546-5607
www.epa.gov/

Rolando E Bates Jr, CEO

Tips from other teens with asthma to help those having it get on with the serious business of having fun with the rest of their lives.

Online/Free

8878 **Tethering Cord**
Spina Bifida Association of America
PO Box 5801
Bethesda, MD 20284
301-496-5751
800-352-9424
Fax: 202-944-3295
sbaa@sbaa.org
www.ninds.nih.gov/

Caroline Lewis, Executive Officer
Story C. Landis, Director
Denise Dorsey, Chief Administrative Officer
Maryann Sofranko, Deputy Executive Officer

Tethered spinal cord syndrome is a neurological disorder caused by tissue attachments that limit the movement of the spinal cord within the spinal column. Attachments may occur congenitally at the base of the spinal cord (conus medullaris) or they may develop near the site of an injury to the spinal cord.

8879 **Tourette Syndrome Association Children's Newsletter**
42-40 Bell Boulevard
Bayside, NY 11361
718-224-2999
800-237-0717
Fax: 718-279-9596
ts@tsa-usa.org
tsa-usa.org

Stephen M. McCall, President

National, nonprofit membership organization. Mission is to identify the cause of, find the cure for, and control the effects of this disorder. A growing number of local chapters nationwide provide educational materials, seminars, conferences and support groups for over 35,000 members.

8880 **Ventilator-Assisted Living**
International Ventilator Users Network
50 Crestwood Executive Ctr.
Suite 440
St. Louis, MO 63126-1916
314-534-0475
Fax: 314-534-5070
info@ventusers.org
www.ventnews.org

Brian Tiburzi, Editor

Articles for home mechanical ventilator users, health professionals and industry professionals.

Bi-monthly

8881 **Voice of the Diabetic**
NFB Diabetes Action Network
200 E Wells St.
Baltimore, MD 21230
410-659-9314
Fax: 410-685-5653
nfb@nfb.org
www.nfb.org

Sports

8882 **National Sports Center for the Disabled**
33 Parsenn Rd
PO Box 1290
Winter Park, CO 80482
970-726-1518
Fax: 970-726-4112
volunteer@nscd.org
nscd.org

Kim Easton, President & CEO
Diane Eustace, Marketing Director
Beth Fox, Outreach & Education Director
Erica Mays, Human Resources Director

Organization providing year-round recreation for children and adults with disabilities. Winter programming includes alpine skiing, snowboarding, ski racing, show shoeing, and cross-country skiing. Summer sports include rafting, sailing, kayaking, camping, hiking, horseback riding, fishing, and rock climbing.

8883 **Rehabilitation Institute of Chicago's Virginia Wadsworth Sports Program**
345 East Suuperior St.
Chicago, IL 60611
312-238-1000
800-354-7342
800-354-REHA
Fax: 312-238-5017
sports@ric.org
www.ric.org

Jude Reyes, Chair
mike P. Kransy, Vice Chair
Thomas Reynolds III, Vice Chair
Joanne C. Smith, President & CEO

RIC's Center for Health and Fitness is a full service fitness center for individuals with disablilties and the administrative offices for RIC's Wirtz Sports Program. Eighteen different sport and recreation programs are offered free of charge. The facility is adjacent to RIC's main building and also is the location of a branch of The National Center for Physical Activity and Disability (NCPAD), a joint project operated by the University of Illinois-Chigcago.

8884 **Special Hockey International (SHI)**
93 Bell Farm Rd.
Suite 120B
Barrie, ON, Canada L4M-5G1
specialhockeyinternational.org

Mike Dwyer, President
Bill Weishuhn, Treasurer

The organization has teams throughout North America and Europe, attracting over 70 teams to its annual tournament.

Support Groups

8885 **AAN's Toll-Free Hotline**
Allergy and Asthma Network Mothers of Asthmatics
8229 Boone Boulevard
Suite 260
Vienna, VA 22182
800-878-4403
Fax: 703-288-5271
www.aanma.org

Michael Amato, Chair
Tonya Winders, President & CEO
Brenda Silvia-Torma, Project Manager
Gary Fitzgerald, Managing Editor

Offers answers to questions regarding allergies and asthma, provides referrals and support to assist the patient and his or her family.

8886 **Breaking New Ground Resource Center**
Purdue University
225 S University St
West Lafayette, IN 47907
765-494-5088
800-825-4264
Fax: 765-496-1356
bng@ecn.purdue.edu
engineering.purdue.edu/

Bill Field, Project Director
Paul Jones, Project Manager
Steve Swain, Rural Rehab Specialist
Robert Stuthridge, Project Ergonomist

A resource center devoted to helping farmers and ranchers with physical disabilities. Resource materials and a free newsletter are available to anyone.

8887 **Clearinghouse on Disability Information: Office Special Education & Rehabilitative Service**
U S Department of Education
400 Maryland Ave SW
Washington, DC 20202-1
202-245-7549
800-872-5327
Fax: 202-245-7614
www.ed.gov

Arne Duncan, Secretary Of Education
Tony Miller, Deputy Secretary
Martha Kanter, Under Secretary
Jo Anderson, Senior Advisor

Provides information to people with disabilities or anyone requesting information, by doing research and providing documents in response to inquiries. The information provided includes areas of federal funding for disability-related programs. Information provided may be useful to disabled individuals and their families, schools and universities, teacher's and/or school administrators, and organizations who have persons with disabilities as clients.

8888 **Compassionate Friends, The**
P.O. Box 3696
Oak Brook, IL 60522
630-990-0010
877-969-0010
Fax: 630-990-0246
nationaloffice@compassionatefriends.org
compassionatefriends.org

Patrick O'Donnell, President
Georgia Cockerham, Vice President
Lisa Corrao, COO
Alan Pedersen, Executive Director

Peer support for bereaved parents, grandparents and siblings, offering over 600 chapters in the United States. The organization also offers a quarterly magazine, We Need Not Walk Alone, and TCF resources of brochures, DVDs, and memorial wristbands for the bereaved parent, grandparent and sibling.

8889 **Cornerstone Services**
777 Joyce Rd
Joliet, IL 60436
815-741-7600
Fax: 815-723-1177
cornerstoneservices.org

John R. Rogers, Chair
Vincent A. Benigni, Vice Chairperson
Ben Stortz, President/CEO
Don Hospell, Vice President/COO

Cornerstone Services provides progressive, comprehensive services for people with disabilities, promoting choice, dignity and the opportunity to live and work in the community. Established in 1969, the agency provides developmental, vocational, residential and behavior health services.

8890 **Disability Network**
Ste 54
3600 S Dort Hwy
Flint, MI 48507
810-742-1800
Fax: 810-742-2400
TTY: 810-742-7647
tdn@disnetwork.org
www.disnetwork.org

Bruce Chargo, Chairman
Diane Brown, Treasurer/ Vice Chairman
Mike Zelley, President & CEO
Linda F, Director, Finance, Operations

The Disability Network's mission is to realize consumer empowerment, self determination, full inclusion and participation of all people in the communities through independent living philosophy and the unequivocal implementation of the Americans with Disabilities Act

8891 **Disability and Health: National Center for Birth Defects and Developmental Disabilities**
Centers for Disease Control and Prevention
1600 Clifton Road
Atlanta, GA 30333
404-498-3012
800-232-4636
800-CDC-INFO
Fax: 404-498-3060
cdcinfo@cdc.gov
www.cdc.gov/ncbddd/dh

Dr. Tom Frieden, Director
Sherri A. Berger, COO
Carmen Villar, Chief of Staff
Ileana Arias, Principal Deputy Director

Located within the new CDC, National Center for Birth Defects and Developmental Disabilities, the Disability and Health section, operates a ralatively small program that primarily supports: data collection on the prevalence of people with disabilities & their health status and risk factors for poor health and well-being; research on measures of disability, functioning and health; health promotion intervention studies; and dissemination of health information.

8892 **Easterseals**
141 W Jackson Blvd.
Suite 1400A
Chicago, IL 60604
312-726-6200
800-221-6827
Fax: 312-726-1494
info@easterseals.com
www.easterseals.com

Angela F. Williams, President & CEO
Glenda Oakley, Chief Financial Officer
Marcy Traxler, Senior Vice President, Network Advancement
John Osterlund, Senior Vice President, Development

Easterseals provides services, education, outreach and advocacy for people with disabilities, veterans, senior citizens and their families. Programs include early intervention, workforce development, adult day care, adult services, mental health services, and more.

8893 **Epilepsy Foundation**
8301 Professional Place E
Suite 200
Landover, MD 20785- 2353
800-332-1000
Fax: 301-459-1569
ContactUs@efa.org
www.epilepsy.com

Robert W Smith, Chair
Philip M Gattone, M.Ed, President & CEO
M. Vaneeda Bennett, Chief Development Officer
Ellen Hobby, Chief Financial Officer & VP, Finance & Administration

Offers information, referrals and support groups for those diagnosed with epilepsy.

8894 **Family Support Project for the Developmentally Disabled**
3424 Kossuth Ave
Bronx, NY 10467-2410
718-519-5000
Fax: 718-519-4902
www.nyc.gov/html/hhc/ncbh/home.html

William Walsh, Vice President
Sheldon McLeod, COO

8895 **Head Injury Hotline**
Brain Injury Resource Center
P.O. Box 84151
Seattle, WA 98124-5451
206-621-8558
Fax: 206-329-0912
brain@headinjury.com
www.headinjury.com

Hugh R. MacMahon, Neurology
Constance Miller, Founder
Paul M. Kuroiwa, Performance management consultant
B. Parker Lindner, Communications specialist

Disseminates head injury information and provides referrals to facilitate adjustment to life following head injury. Organizes seminars for professionals, head injury survivors, and their families.

8896 **International Braille and Technology Center for the Blind**
National Federation of the Blind
200 E Wells St.
Baltimore, MD 21230
410-659-9314
Fax: 410-685-5653
nfb@nfb.org
nfb.org/programs-services

John Berggren, Executive Director, Operations

World's largest and most complete evaluation and demonstration center of all assistive technology used by the blind from around the world. Includes all Braille, synthetic speech, print-to-speech scanning, internet and portable devices and programs. Available for tours by appointment to blind persons, employers, technology manufacturers, teachers, parents and those working in the assistive technology field.

8897 **Lung Line Information Service**
National Jewish Health
1400 Jackson Street
Denver, CO 80206
877-225-5654
877-225-5654
Fax: 303-398-1125
allstetterw@njc.org
nationaljewish.org

Rich Schierburg, Chair
Robin Chotin, Vice Chair
Michael Salem, M.D., President & CEO
Christine Forkner, CFO and Executive Vice President

A free information service answering questions, sending literature and giving advice to patients with immunologic or respiratory illnesses. The Line is an educational service and not a substitute for medical care. Diagnosis or suggested treatment will not be provided for a caller's specific condition.

8898 **NCI's Contact Center**
National Cancer Institute
9609 Medical Center Dr.
Rockville, MD 20850
800-422-6237
TTY: 800-332-8615
nciinfo@nih.gov
www.cancer.gov

Norman E. Sharpless, Director
Douglas R. Lowy, Principal Deputy Director
James Doroshow, Deputy Director, Clinical & Translational Research
Dinah S. Singer, Deputy Director, Scientific Strategy & Development

The NCI Contact Center provides accurate, up-to-date information on cancer to patients and their families, health professionals and the general public. The Contact Center can provide specific information in understandable language about particular types of cancer, as well as information on second opinions and the availability of clinical trials.

8899 **National AIDS Hotline**
Centers for Disease Control and Prevention
1600 Clifton Road
Atlanta, GA 30333
404-639-3311
800-232-4636
800-CDC-INFO
Fax: 404-498-3060
www.cdc.gov

Dr. Tom Frieden, Director
Sherri A. Berger, COO
Carmen Villar, Chief of Staff
Ileana Arias, Principal Deputy Director

Offers free confidential information and publications on HIV infection and AIDS.

8900 **PPAL Support Groups**
Parent Professional Advocacy League
77 Rumford Ave.
Waltham, MA 02453
866-815-8122
Fax: 617-542-7832
info@ppal.net
www.ppal.net

Lisa Lambert, Executive Director
Meri Viano, Associate Director
Joel Khattar, Program Manager

The Parent Professional Advocacy League (PPAL) provides family support services and support groups for parents and families of children with emotional, behavioral, and mental health needs.

8901 **PXE International**
Ste 404
4301 Connecticut Ave NW
Washington, DC 20008- 2369
202-362-9599
Fax: 202-966-8553
info@pxe.org
www.pxe.org

Patrick F. Terry, President
Sharon Terry, CEO
Terry M. Dermaid, Executive Director
Ian Terry, Webmaster

Provides support for individuals and families affected by psukdoxanthoma elasticum (PXE), and resources for healthcare professionals. PXE causes select elastic tissue to mineralize, and effects the skin, eyes, cardiovascular, and GI systems.

8902 **Parent Assistance Network**
Good Samaritan Hospital
10 E. 31st Street
Kearney, NE 68847
308-865-7100
800-235-9905
Fax: 308-865-2924
sheilameyer@catholichealth.net

Randy DeFreece, President
Kent Barney, Chairman
Mary Henning, Vice Chairman
Julie Speirs, Secretary

Provides information and emotional support to all parents and especially to parents of children with disabilities in the central Nebraska area. Ongoing activities include parent support group meetings, parent-to-parent networking and referrals and Respite Care provider trainings.

8903 **Post-Polio Support Group**
Adventist Hinsdale Hospital
120 N Oak St
Hinsdale, IL 60521-3829
630-856-9000
Fax: 630-856-6000
www.keepingyouwell.com

David Crane, President

Information and support for polio patients and their families; meets the fourth Wednesday of each month.

8904 Prevent Child Abuse America
288 South Wabash Avenue
10th floor
Chicago, IL 60604
312-663-3520
800-244-5373
800-CHI-DREN
Fax: 312-939-8962
mailbox@preventchildabuse.org
preventchildabuse.org

Fred M. Riley, Chair
David Rudd, Vice Chair
James Hmurovich, President & CEO
Robert Allen, Sr. Director, Administration

Through public education, community partnerships and support services, PCAMW helps everyone play a role in prevention. We share information on prevention stategies and effective parenting at community forums and events and advocate for polices and services that keep children safe. We operate PhoneFriend, a telephone support line for children at home without adult supervision and conduct personal safety workshops in schools, camps and libraries.

8905 Son-Rise Program
2080 S Undermountain Rd.
Sheffield, MA 01257-9643
413-229-2100
877-766-7473
Fax: 413-229-8931
www.autismtreatmentcenter.org

Barry Neil Kaufman, Founder & CEO
Clyde Haberman, Senior Teacher & Director of Development
Blair Borgeson, Developmental Therapist
Emily Vitale Aronow, Program Advisor & Client Support Coordinator

The center's Son-Rise Program teaches a comprehensive system of treatment and education designed to help families and caregivers enable their children to dramatically improve in all areas of learning.

8906 Special Children
1306 Wabash Ave
Belleville, IL 62220-3370
618-234-6876
Fax: 618-234-6150
specialchildren.net

Kathleen Cullen, Administrator

A nonprofit agency serving children with developmental disabilities ages birth to 6 years

8907 Support Works
1607 Dilworth Rd W
Charlotte, NC 28203-5213
704-331-9500
www.supportworks.org

Joel Fisher, Manager

SupportWorks helps people find and form support groups. An 8 page publication Power Tools, clearly walks new group leaders through steps of putting together a healthy self-help group. SupportWorks also has a telephone conference program which allows people with similar diseases or other nonprofit issues to meet by phone conference for free or at very low cost.

8908 Toll-Free Information Line
Asthma and Allergy Foundation of America
8201 Corporate Drive
Suite 1000
Landover, MD 20785
202-466-7643
800-727-8462
800-7 A-THMA
Fax: 202-466-8940
info@aafa.org
aafa.org

Lynn Hanessian, Chair
Yolanda Miller, SVP & COO
Lynda Mitchell, VP, Food Allergies
Nancy Kercher, Secretary

The Asthma and Allergy Foundation of America (AAFA) provides practical information, community based services and support through a national network of chapters and support groups. AAFA develops health education, organizes state and national advocacy efforts and funds research to find better treatments and cures.

8909 Visiting Nurse Association of America
2121 Crystal Drive
Suite 750
Arlington, VA 22202
571-527-1520
888-866-8773
Fax: 571-527-1527
webadmin@vnaa.org
vnaa.org

Mary B. DeVeau, Chair
Linnea Windel, Vice Chair
Tracey Moorhead, President & CEO
Magaret Terry, VP of Quality & Innovation

The VNAA is the official national association for not-for-profit, community based home health organizations known as the Visiting Nurse Associations (VNA's). They created the profession of home health care more then 100 years ag. They have a united mission to bring compassionate, high-quality and cost-effective home care to individuals in their communities.

Speech & Language

Books

8816 **Stuttering**
NI on Deafness & Other Communication Disorders
31 Center Dr.
MSC 2320
Bethesda, MD 20892-2320
301-827-8183
800-241-1044
Fax: 301-770-8977
TTY: 800-241-1055
nidcdinfo@nidcd.nih.gov
www.nidcd.nih.gov

Debara L. Tucci, Director
Judith A. Cooper, Deputy Director
Timothy J. Wheeles, Executive Officer
Lisa Portnoy, Deputy Executive Officer
Describes how speech is produced, treatments for stuttering and research supported by the federal government.

Associations

8910 **Academic Language Therapy Association**
14070 Proton Rd.
Suite 100
Dallas, TX 75244
972-233-9107
Fax: 972-490-4219
office@altaread.org
www.altaread.org

Janna Curry-Dobbs, President
Jo Ann Handy, VP Membership
Susan Louchen, VP Public Relations
Tim Odegard, VP Programs
The Academic Language Therapy Associationr (ALTA) is a non-profit national professional organization with the purpose of establishing, maintaining, and promoting standards of education, practice and professional conduct for Certified Academic Language Therapists. Academic Language Therapy is an educational, structured, comprehensive, phonetic, multisensory approach for the remediation of dyslexia and/or written-language disorders.
1986

8911 **American Speech-Language-Hearing Association**
2200 Research Blvd.
Rockville, MD 20850-3289
301-296-5700
800-638-8255
actioncenter@asha.org
www.asha.org

Gail J. Richard, President
Elise Davis-Mcfaland, President-Elect
Margot L. Beckerman, Chair
Arlene A. Pietranton, Chief Executive Officer
The American Speech-Language Association is the professional, scientific, and credentialing association for members and affiliates who are speech-language pathologists, audiologists, and speech, language, and hearing scientists in the United States and internationally. ASHA provides information for the public, professionals, students, and the research community related to hearing, balance, speech, language and swallowing disorders.

8912 **Aphasia Hope Foundation**
P.O. Box 79701
Houston, TX 77279
855-764-4673
jstradinger@comcast.net
www.aphasiahope.org

Sandy Caudell, Program Diretor
Judi Stradinger, Executive Director
Aphasia Hope Foundation is a nonprofit foundation whose mission is to promote research into the prevention and cure of aphasia and to ensure that all survivors of aphasia and their caregivers are aware of and have access to the best prossible tratments.

8913 **Association of Language Companies**
9707 Key West Ave.
Suite 100
Rockville, MD 20850
240-404-6511
Fax: 301-990-9771
info@alcus.org
www.alcus.org

Christopher Carter, President
Rick Antezana, Vice President
Lenani P. Craig, Treasurer
Susan Amarino, Secretary
The Association of Language Companies (ALC) is a national trade association representing businesses that provide translation, interpretation, localization, and language training services.

8914 **Autism Research Institute**
4182 Adams Ave.
San Diego, CA 92116-2599
866-366-3361
www.autism.com

Stephen Edelson, Executive Director
Rebecca McKenney, Office Manager
Christopher Flynn, Treasurer
Jane Johnson, Secretary
Conducts research on the causes, diagnosis, and treatment of autism and publishes a quarterly newsletter that reviews worldwide research. Literature on causes and treatment available. Refers patients and families to health care professionals and clinics.

8915 **Autism Services Center**
929 4th Ave.
P.O. Box 507
Huntington, WV 25701-0507
304-525-8014
Fax: 304-525-8026
www.autismservicescenter.org

Jimmie Beirne, Chief Executive Officer
Jodi Fields, Director
Barbara Bragg, Director
David Finley, Chief Operations Officer
Provides developmental disabilities services with a specialty in autism. Services include case management, residential, personal care, assessments and evaluations, supported employment, independent living and family support.

8916 **Autism Treatment Center of America**
2080 S Undermountain Rd.
Sheffield, MA 01257-9643
413-229-2100
877-766-7473
Fax: 413-229-8931
correspondence@option.org
www.autismtreatmentcenter.org

Barry Neil Kaufman, Founder & CEO
Clyde Haberman, Senior Teacher & Director of Development
Blair Borgeson, Developmental Therapist
Emily Vitale Aronow, Program Advisor & Client Support Coordinator
The Autism Treatment Center of America provides innovative training programs for parents and professionals caring for children challenged by Autism, Autism Spectrum Disorders, Pervasive Developmental Disorders (PDD) and other development difficulties. The center's Son-Rise Program teaches a comprehensive system of treatment and education designed to help families and caregivers enable their children to dramatically improve in all areas of learning.

8917 **Carl and Ruth Shapiro Family National Center for Accessible Media**
WGBH Educational Foundation
1 Guest St.
Boston, MA 02135-2016
617-300-3400
Fax: 617-300-1035
TTY: 617-300-2489
ncam@wgbh.org
ncam.wgbh.org

Donna Danielewski, Director
Geoff Freed, Director of technology projects and Web media standards
Madeleine Rothberg, Senior Subject Matter Expert
Bryan Gould, Director of Accessible Learning and Assessment Technologies

The Carl and Ruth Shapiro Family National Center for Accessible Media (NCAM) is a research and development facility dedicated to addressing barriers to media and emerging technologies for people with disabilities in their homes, schools, workplaces, and communities.

8918 **Childhood Apraxia of Speech Association**
416 Lincoln Ave.
2nd Fl.
Pittsburgh, PA 15209
412-343-7102
www.apraxia-kids.org
Mary Sturm, President
Michele R. Atkins, Executive Director
Joshua Zellers, Treasurer
Sue Freidurger, Secretary
The Childhood Apraxia of Speech Association is a nonprofit publicly funded charity whose mission is to strengthen the support systems in the lives of children with apraxia so that each child is afforded their best opportunity to develop speech and communication.

8919 **Deafness and Communicative Disorders Branch of Rehab Services Administration Office**
Special Education and Rehab Services
400 Maryland Ave., SW
Washington, DC 20202
800-872-5327
www.ed.gov
Kimberly Richey, Secretary Of Education
Promotes improved rehabilitation services for deaf and hard of hearing people and individuals with speech or language impairments. Provides technical assistance to public and private agencies and individuals.

8920 **Dysphagia Research Society**
2800 West Higgins Rd.
Suite 440
Hoffman Estates, IL 60169
888-775-7361
Fax: 847-885-8393
info@dysphagiaresearch.org
www.dysphagiaresearch.org
Gary H. McCullough, President
Sudarshan R. Jadcherla, President Elect
Susan Langmore, Secretary/Treasurer
Maggie-Lee Huckabee, Councilor
The Dysphagia Research Society is a nonprofit organization with the purpose of enhancing and encouraging research pertinent to normal and disordered swallowing, to promote the dissemination of knowledge related to normal and disordered swallowing, and to provide a multidisciplinary forum for presentation of research into normal and disordered swallowing.

8921 **Hearing, Speech and Deafness Center (HSDC)**
Hearing, Speech & Deafness Center (HSDC)
1625 19th Ave.
Seattle, WA 98122-2848
206-323-5770
888-222-5036
Fax: 206-328-6871
seattle@hsdc.org
www.hsdc.org
Lindsay Klarman, Executive Director
Michelle Coleman, Director of Operations
Hearing, Speech & Deaf Center (HSDC) is a nonprofit for clients who are deaf, hard of hearing, or who face other communication barriers such as speech challenges. Their mission is to foster inclusive and accessible communities through communication, advocacy, and education.

8922 **International Cluttering Association**
705 Tilbury Court
Sun City Center, FL 33573
elanouette@tampabay.rr.com
associations.missouristate.edu/ica
Charley Adams, Ph.D., Chair
Susanne Cook, Chair Elect
Katarzyna Wesierska, Secretary
Dan Hudock, Treasurer
They work to increase awareness of the communication disorder of cluttering worldwide among speech-language therapists/logopedists, healthcare professionals, people with cluttering, and the public.

8923 **International Fluency Association**
Northern Illinois University
Dept. of Communicative Disorders
DeKalb, IL 60115-2899
www.theifa.org
Elaine Kelman, President
Nan Bernstein Ratner, President Elect
Shelly Jo Kraft, Treasurer
Kurt Eggers, Secretary
The International Fluency Association is a not-for-profit, international, interdisciplinary organization devoted to the understanding and management of fluency disorders, and to the improvement in the quality of life for persons with fluency disorders.

8924 **Lindamood-Bell Home Learning Process**
CA
805-541-3836
800-233-1819
www.lindamoodbell.com
Nanci Bell, Founder/Director
Patricia C. Lindamood, Founder/Director
Lindamood-Bell Learning Process is dedicated to enhancing human learning. Lindamood-Belll programs teach children and adults to read, spell, comprehend, and express language.
1986

8925 **Myositis Association**
1940 Duke St.
Suite 200
Alexandria, VA 22314
800-821-7356
tma@myositis.org
www.myositis.org
Bob Goldberg, Executive Director
Linda Kobert, Communications Director
Aisha Morrow, Operations Manager
Ruthann Devine, Program Services Director
The aim of TMA's programs and services is to provide information, support, advocacy and research for those concerned about myositis, as well as serving those affected by these diseases. Support groups offer members the chance to share and discuss their concerns with people in similar situations.

8926 **National Aphasia Association**
P.O. Box 87
Scarsdale, NY 10583
800-922-4622
naa@aphasia.org
www.aphasia.org
Darlene S. Williamson, President
Daniel Martin, Vice President Stretegic Planning
Barbara Kessler, Vice President Community Outreach & Education
The National Aphasia Association (NAA) is a nonprofit organization that promotes public education, research, rehabilitation and support services to assist people with aphasia and their families.

8927 **National Association of Special Education Teachers**
1250 Connecticut Ave., NW
Suite 200
Washington, DC 20036-2643
800-754-4421
Fax: 800-754-4421
contactus@naset.org
www.naset.org
Roger Pierangelo, Executive Director
George Giuliani, Executive Director
The National Association of Special Education Teachers (NASET) is a national membership organization dedicated to rendering all possible support and assistance to those preparing for or teaching in the field of special education. NASET was founded to promote the profession of special education teachers and to provide a national forum for their ideas.

8928 **National Black Association for Speech-Language and Hearing**
P.O. Box 779
Pennsville, NJ 08070
877-936-6235
Fax: 877-936-6235
nbaslh@nbaslh.org
www.nbaslh.org
Cathy Runnels, Interim Chair
Kia N. Johnson, Parliamentarian
Martine Elie, Treasurer

The mission of the National Black Association of Speech-Language and Hearing is to maintain a viable mechanism through which the needs of black professionals, students and individuals with communication disorders can be met.

8929 National Cued Speech Association
1300 Pennsylvania Ave, NW
Suite 190-713
Washington, DC 20004
917-439-5126
800-459-3529
Fax: 866-269-9877
info@cuedspeech.org
www.cuedspeech.org

Anne Huffman, President
Sarina Roffe, Executive Director
Ben Lachman, Director of Development
Brian Kelly, Treasurer

The association champions effective communication, language development and literacy through the use of cued speech. Families are informed about Cued Speech along with other communication options.

8930 National Fragile X Foundation
2100 M St., NW
Suite 170, P.O. Box 302
Washington, DC 20037-1233
800-688-8765
www.fragilex.org

Tony Ferlenda, Chief Executive Officer
Linda Sorensen, Chief Operating Officer
Jayne Dixon Weber, Director of Education & Support Services
Paula Lipford, Volunteer Program Director

Unites the fragile X community to enrich lives through educational and emotional support, promote public and professional awareness and advance research toward improvemed treatments and cure for fragile X syndrome.

8931 National Spasmodic Dysphonia Association
300 Park Blvd.
Suite 335
Itasca, IL 60143
800-795-6732
Fax: 630-250-4505
NSDA@dysphonia.org
www.dysphonia.org

Charlie Reavis, President
Marcia Sterling, Treasurer
Kimberly Kuman, Executive Director

The National Spasmodic Dysphonia Association (NSDA) is a not-for-profit organization dedicated to advancing medical research into the causes of and treatments for SD, promoting physician and public awareness of the disorder, and providing support to those affected by SD through symposiums, support groups, and on-line resources.

8932 National Stuttering Association
119 W. 40th St.
14th Fl.
New York, NY 10018
212-944-4050
800-937-8888
Fax: 212-944-8244
info@westutter.org
www.westutter.org

Gerald Maguire, Chairman
Evan Sherman, Vice Chairman
Bob Wellington, Treasurer
Sarah Onofri, Secretary

A nonprofit organization dedicated to bringing hope, dignity, support, education, and empowerment to children and adults who stutter and their families, and the professionals who serve them.

8933 National Tourette Syndrome Association
42-40 Bell Blvd.
Suite 205
Bayside, NY 11361
888-4TO-URET
www.tsa-usa.org

John Miller, President & CEO
Diana Felner, VP Public Policy
Sonji Mason-Vidal, VP Finance & Administration

The Tourette Association is dedicated to making life better for all people affected by Tourette and Tic Disorders.

8934 Providence Speech and Hearing Center
1301 Providence Ave.
Orange, CA 92868-3892
714-923-1521
855-901-7742
Fax: 714-639-2593
pshc@pshc.org
www.pshc.org

Bruce May, President
Kevin Timone, Vice President - Fund Development
Randy Free, Vice President - Finance
Casey Immel, Treasurer

Mission is to provide the highest quality services available in the identification, diagnosis, treatment and prevention of speech, language and hearing disorders for persons of all ages.

8935 Scottish Rite Center for Childhood Language Disorders
1733 16th St., NW
Washington, DC 20009-3103
202-323-3579
Fax: 202-464-0487
council@scottishrite.org
www.scottishrite.org

Bill Sizemore, Executive Director

Offers speech-language evaluations and treatment, hearing screening and consultations to children ages birth through adolescence. Bilingual services are also available.

8936 Stern Center for Language and Learning
183 Talcott Rd.
Suite 101
Williston, VT 05495-9209
802-878-2332
learning@sterncenter.org
www.sterncenter.org

Blanche Podhajski, President
Michael Shapiro, Chief Operating Officer
Moneer Greenbaum, Director of Development

The Stern Center is a nonprofit learning center dedicated to helping children and adults reach their full potential. Stern Center professionals evaluate and teach all kinds of learners, including those with learning disabilities such as dyslexia or attention deficit disorders.

8937 Stuttering Foundation of America
1805 Moriah Woods Blvd.
Suite 3
Memphis, TN 38117
901-761-0343
800-992-9392
Fax: 901-761-0484
info@stutteringhelp.org
www.stutteringhelp.org

Jane Fraser, President
Dennis Drayna, Director
Joseph R. G. Fulcher, Director
Frances Cook, Director

Provides resources, services, and support to those who stutter and their families, as well as support for research into the causes of stuttering.

8938 Texas Speech-Language-Hearing Association
2025 M St., NW
Suite 800
Washington, DC 20036-2342
855-330-8742
888-729-8742
Fax: 512-463-9468
staff@txsha.org
www.txsha.org

Judy Rudebusch Rich, President
Erin Bellue, VP of Educational & Scientific Affairs
Shannon Butkus, VP of Social & Governmental Policy
Rebecca Linke, VP of Research & Development

Mission is to encourage and promote the role of the speech-language pathologist and audiologist as a professional in the delivery of clinical services to persons with communications disorders. Encourages basic scientific study of processes of individual human communication with reference to speech, hearing and language.

8939 **The Cherab Foundation**
PO Box 1771
Jensen Beach, FL 34958
772-335-5135
help@cherab.org
cherabfoundation.org

Lisa Geng, Founder & President
Jolie Abreu, Vice President

The Cherab Foundation is a world-wide nonprofit organization working to improve the communication skills and education of all children with speech and language delays and disorders. The Cherab Foundation is committed to assisting with the development of new therapeutic approaches, preventions, and cures to neurologically-based speech disorders.

8940 **The Davis Center**
110 Wesley St.
PO Box 508
Manlius, NY 13104
862-251-4637
Fax: 862-251-4642
ddavis@thedaviscenter.com
www.thedaviscenter.com

Dorinne S. Davis, Director

Offers sound-based therapies supporting positive change in learning, development, and wellness. All ages/all disabilities. Uses The Davis Model of Sound Intervention, an alternative approach.

8941 **Wendell Johnson Speech And Hearing Clinic**
University Of Iowa
Iowa City, IA 52242-1025
319-335-8736
Fax: 319-335-8851
TTY: 319-335-8736
speech-path-aud@uiowa.edu
clas.uiowa.edu/comsci/clinical-services

Ann Fennell, Clinical Coordinator

The clinic offers assessment and remediation for communication disorders in adults and children. The clinic also offers a Intensive Summer Residential Clinic for school age children needing intervention services because of speech, language, hearing and/or reading problems.

Camps

8942 **CNS Camp New Connections**
Mclean Hospital Child/Adolescent Program
Mailstop115
115 Mill Street
Belmont, MA 02478
617-855-2000
800-333-0338
Fax: 617-855-2833
mcleaninfo@partners.org
mcleanhospital.org

Scott L. Rauch, MD, President & Chief Psychiatrist
Blaise Aguirre, Clinical Staff
Alan Barry, Clinical Staff
Susan L. Andersen, Research Staff

Four-week summer day camp for children ages 7-17 who have pervasive developmental disorders, Asperger's Syndrome, autism spectrum disorders and non-verbal learning disabilities. The camp is designed to help children develop social skills through fun activities including: communication games, swimming, field trips, drama, and arts and crafts. *$4500.00*

8943 **Camp Meadowood Springs**
77650 Meadowood Rd.
Weston, OR 97886
541-276-2752
Fax: 541-276-7227
camp@meadowoodsprings.org
www.meadowoodsprings.org

Michelle Nelson, Camp Director

This camp is designed to help children with communication disorders and learning differences. A full range of activities in recreational and clinical areas is available.

8944 **Camp Royall**
250 Bill Ash Rd.
Moncure, NC 27559
919-542-1033
Fax: 919-533-5324
camproyall@autismsociety-nc.org
www.autismsociety-nc.org/camp-royall

Sara Gage, Director

A week-long overnight and day camp for children and adults with autism. Campers participate in traditional camp activities such as swimming, boating, hiking, and arts and crafts. Counselor-to-camper ratio is 1:1 or 1:2, depending on the campers' needs.

8945 **Camp Sisol**
Jewish Community Center of Greater Rochester/JCC
1200 Edgewood Ave.
Rochester, NY 14618
585-461-2000
Fax: 585-461-0805
bettertogether@jccrochester.org
www.jccrochester.org

Josh Weinstein, Chief Executive Officer

Coed, ages 5-16. Camp Sisol accommodates children with special needs.

8946 **Childrens Beach House**
100 West 10th Street
Suite 411
Wilmington, DE 19801-1674
302-655-4288
Fax: 302-655-4216
www.cbhinc.org

Martha P. Tschantz, President
Mary Helms, Vice President
Richard T Garrett, Executive Director
Nicholas Imhoff, Business Manager

Camp is located in Lewes, Delaware. Four-week sessions June-August for Delaware children with hearing impairment or speech/communication impairment. Coed, ages 6-12.

8947 **New Horizons Summer Day Camp**
YMCA of Orange County
13821 Newport Ave.
Suite 150
Tustin, CA 92780
714-508-7635
newhorizons@ymcaoc.org
www.ymcaoc.org/new-horizons

8948 **Sequanota Lutheran Conference Center and Camp**
PO Box 245
Jennerstown, PA 15547
814-629-6627
contact@sequanota.com
www.sequanota.com

Rev. Nathan Pile, Executive Director
Angie Pile, Director, Business Management
Ann Ferry, Director, Hospitality
Ron Druist, Director, Facilities

Runs Camp Bethesda, a summer camp for adults with developmental and intellectual disabilities. For ages 18 and up.

8949 **Talisman Summer Camp**
64 Gap Creek Rd.
Zirconia, NC 28790
828-697-6313
info@talismancamps.com
www.talismancamps.com

Linda Tatsapaugh, Operations Director & Owner
Robiyn Mims, Admissions Director & Owner
Cory Greene, Camp Director

Talisman Summer Camp is located 40 minutes south of Asheville, North Carolina. Offers a program of hiking, rafting, climbing, and caving for young people with autism, ADHD and learning disabilities. Coed, ages 6-22.

8950 **Wendell Johnson Speech & Hearing Clinic**
University Of Iowa
250 Hawkins Dr
Iowa City, IA 52242-1025
319-335-8736
Fax: 319-335-8851
kathy-miller@uiowa.edu
www.uiowa.edu

Chuck Wieland, President
Hans Hoerschelman, Vice President
Josh Smith, Budget Officer
Shannon Lizakowski, Secretary

The clinic offers assessment and remediation for communication disorders in adults and children. The clinic also offers a Intensive Summer Residential Clinic for school age children needing intervention services because of speech, language, hearing and/or reading problems.

8951 **YMCA Camp Fitch**
12600 Abels Rd.
North Springfield, PA 16430
814-922-3219
877-863-4824
Fax: 814-922-7000
registrar@campfitchymca.org
campfitchymca.org

Tom Parker, Executive Director
Joe Wolnik, Summer Camp Director
Brandy Duda, Outdoor Education Director
Hannah Kight, Office Manager

Camp is located in North Springfield, Pennsylvania. Camp programs include sessions for children with diabetes or epilepsy.

Books

8952 **Autism 24/7: A Family Guide to Learning at Home & in the Community**
Autism Society of North Carolina Bookstore
Ste 230
505 Oberlin Rd
Raleigh, NC 27605-1345
919-743-0204
800-442-2762
Fax: 919-743-0208
jchampion@autismsociety-nc.org
http://www.autismsociety-nc.org/

Sharon Jeffries-Jones, Chair
Elizabeth Phillippi, Vice Chair
Tracey Sheriff, Chief Executive Officer
Paul Wendler, Chief Financial Officer

Parents are encouraged to focus on skill sets and behaviors that most negatively affect family functioning, and replacing these behaviors with acceptable alternatives. *$19.95*

8953 **Autism Handbook: Understanding & Treating Autism & Prevention Development**
Oxford University Press
2001 Evans Road
Cary, NC 27513
919-677-0977
800-445-9714
Fax: 919-677-1303
http://www.oup.com/us/

320 pages
ISBN 0-195076-67-2

8954 **Autism and Learning**
Taylor & Francis
37-41 Mortimer St
London, UK W1T 3
http://www.informatandm.com
Stuart Powell, Author
Rita Jordan, Editor

This book is about how a cognitive perception on the way in which individuals with autism think and learn may be applied to particular curriculum areas.
160 pages Paperback
ISBN 1-853464-21-X

8955 **Autism in Adolescents and Adults**
Springer Publishing
233 Spring St
New York, NY 10013
877-283-3229
ainy@aveda.com
http://aveda.edu/new-york

Eric Schopler, Editor
Gary B. Mesibov, Editor

This book is a great history lesson in the development of understanding about autism spectrum disorders, and is a testament to how far research and services in the field have come. This book contains lots of information about what general thinking and services used to be like, in an era when still little was understood about these disorders. *$63.00*
456 pages
ISBN 0-306410-57-5

8956 **Autism...Nature, Diagnosis and Treatment**
Autism Society of North Carolina Bookstore
Ste 230
505 Oberlin Rd
Raleigh, NC 27605-1345
919-743-0204
800-442-2762
Fax: 919-743-0208
http://www.autismsociety-nc.org/

Sharon Jeffries-Jones, Chair
Elizabeth Phillippi, Vice Chair
Paul Wendler, Chief Financial Officer
David Laxton, Director of Communications

Covers perspectives, issues, neurobiological issues and new directions in diagnosis and treatment. *$49.00*

8957 **Autism: Explaining the Enigma**
Wiley Publishers
111 River Street
Hoboken, NJ 07030-5774
201-748-6000
Fax: 201-748-6088
http://as.wiley.com

Peter Booth Wiley, Chairman
Stephen M. Smith, President & CEO
John Kitzmacher, EVP, CFO
Ellis E. Cousens, Executive Vice President, COO

Explains the nature of autism. *$27.95*

8958 **Autism: From Tragedy to Triumph**
Branden Publishing Company
17 Station St
Brookline, MA 2445-7995
617-730-5757
http://www.yogainthevillage.com

Karen Wenc, Teaching Staff
Veronica Wolff, Teaching Staff
Annie Hoffman, Teaching Staff
Keith Beasley, Teaching Staff

A new book that deals with the Lovaas method and includes a foreward by Dr. Ivar Lovaas. The book is broken down into two parts — the long road to diagnosis and then treatment. *$12.95*

8959 **Autism: Identification, Education and Treatment**
Routledge (Taylor & Francis Group)
270 Madison Ave
New York, NY 10016-601
212-576-1411
http://books.google.co.in/books/about/Autism.
Dianne Zager, Editor

Chapters include medical treatments, early intervention and communication development in autism. *$36.00*
ISBN 0-805820-44-7

8960 **Autism: The Facts**
Oxford University Press
2001 Evans Road
Cary, NC 27513
919-677-0977
800-445-9714
Fax: 919-677-1303
http://www.oup.com/us/corporate/contact/?view

Simon Baron-Cohen, Co-Author
Patrick Bolton, Co-Author
$22.50
128 pages
ISBN 0-192623-27-3

8961 Autistic Adults at Bittersweet Farms
Routledge (Taylor & Francis Group)
12660 Archbold-Whitehouse Rd.
Whitehouse, OH 43571 419-875-6986
http://www.bittersweetfarms.org/

Robert St. Clair, President
Matt Anderson, VP
Jan Toczynski, Secretary
Jon Ahlberg, Board Member

A touching view of an inspirational residential care program for autistic adolescents and adults. Also available in softcover. *$94.95*
Hardcover
ISBN 1-560240-42-3

8962 Beyond Baby Talk: From Sounds to Sentences, a Parent's Guide to Language Development
Prima Publishing
P.O. Box 1260
Rocklin, CA 95677-1260 916-787-7000
800-632-8676
Fax: 916-787-7001

Fernando Bueno, Editor in Chief
Julie Asbury, Managing Editor
Christopher Buffa, Sr. Editor
Andrea Hill, Community Manager

The authors discuss the best ways to help your child develop the all-important skill of communication and to recognize the signs of language development problems. *$15.95*
224 pages
ISBN 0-761526-47-1

8963 Breaking the Speech Barrier: Language Develpment Through Augmented Means
Brookes Publishing
P.O. Box 10624
Baltimore, MD 21285-0624 410-337-9580
800-638-3775
Fax: 410-337-8539
custserv@brookespublishing.com
readplaylearn.com

Paul Brookes, Owner

This resource describes the creation of the System for Augmenting Language (SAL) for school-age youth with developmental disabilities and offers important insights into the language development of children who are not learning to communicate typically. *$39.95*
224 pages Paperback
ISBN 1-557663-90-0

8964 Breakthroughs: How to Reach Students with Autism
Aquarius Health Care Media
Ste 230
505 Oberlin Rd
Raleigh, NC 27605-1345 919-743-0204
800-442-2762
Fax: 919-743-0208
jchampion@autismsociety-nc.org
www.autismtreatmentcenter.org

Sharon Jeffries-Jones, Chair
Elizabeth Phillippi, Vice Chair
Tracey Sheriff, CEO
Paul Wendler, CFO

A hands-on, how-to program for reaching students with autism, featuring Karen Sewell, Autism Society of America's teacher of the year. Here Sewell demonstrates the successful techniques she's developed over a 20-year career. A separate 250 page manual ($59) is also available which covers math, reading, fine motor, self help, social adaptive, vocational and self help skills as well as providing numerous plan reproducibles and an exhaustive listing of equipment and materials resources. Video. *$99.00*

8965 Childhood Speech, Language & Listening Problems
Wiley Publishing
605 3rd Ave
New York, NY 10158-180 212-850-6000
Fax: 212-850-6088
http://books.google.co.in/books/about/Childho

Patricia McAleer Hamaguchi

Language pathologist Hamaguchi employs her 15 years of experience to show parents how to recognize the most common speech, language, and listening problems. *$16.95*
224 pages Paperback
ISBN 0-471387-53-3

8966 Cognitive Behavioral Therapy for Adult Asperger Syndrome
Autism Society of North Carolina Bookstore
Ste 230
505 Oberlin Rd
Raleigh, NC 27605-1345 919-743-0204
800-442-2762
Fax: 919-743-0208
jchampion@autismsociety-nc.org
http://www.autismsociety-nc.org

Sharon Jeffries-Jones, Chair
Elizabeth Phillippi, Vice Chair
Tracey Sheriff, CEO
Paul Wendler, CFO

Text is prepared with case studies and examples from the author's own experiences working as a cognitive-behavioral therapist specializing in adults and adolescents with dual diagnosis, autism spectrum disorders, mood disorders, and anxiety disorders.

8967 Communication Development and Disorders in African American Children
Brookes Publishing
P.O. Box 10624
Baltimore, MD 21285-0624 410-337-9580
800-638-3775
Fax: 410-337-8539
custserv@brookespublishing.com

Paul Brooks, Owner

Research, Assessment, and Intervention. This text presents research on communication disorders and language development in African American children. Also addresses multicultural aspects of service delivery and intervention and discusses issues in assessing, diagnosing, and treating communication disorders. *$39.00*
400 pages Paperback
ISBN 1-55766 -53-3

8968 Communication Development in Children with Down Syndrome
Brookes Publishing
P.O. Box 10624
Baltimore, MD 21285-0624 410-337-9580
800-638-3775
Fax: 410-337-8539
custserv@brookespublishing.com

Paul Brooks, Owner

This book offers an extensive, detailed explanation of communication development in children with Down syndrome relative to their advancing cognitive skills. It introduces a critical framework for assessing and treating hearing, speech, and language problems and provides explicit intervention methods and tested clinical protocols.
Paperback
ISBN 1-55766 -50-5

8969 Coping for Kids Who Stutter
Speech Bin
P.O. Box 1579
Appleton, WI 54912 419-589-1425
888-388-3224
Fax: 888-388-6344
info@speechbin.com
www.speechbin.com

James R. Henderson, Chairman
Joseph M. Yorio, President & CEO
Rick Holden, EVP, Educators Publishing Service
Patrick T. Collins, EVP, Distribution

Informative book for children and adults about stuttering and how to manage it. *$15.95*
32 pages
ISBN 0-93785 -43-2

8970 **Disorders of Motor Speech: Assessment, Treatment, and Clinical Characterization**
Brookes Publishing
P.O. Box 10624
Baltimore, MD 21285-0624 410-337-9580
800-638-3775
Fax: 410-337-8539
custserv@brookespublishing.com

Paul Brooks, Owner
This book provides a probing examination of normal, dysarthric, and apraxic speech. Great for speech-language pathologists, neurologists, physical or occupational therapists, and physiatrists. *$47.00*
400 pages Hardcover
ISBN 1-55766 -23-1

8971 **Employment for Individuals with Asperger Syndrome or Non-Verbal Learning Disability**
Jessica Kingsley Publishers
400 Market Street
Suite 400
Philadelphia, PA 19106-2513 215-922-1161
866-416-1078
Fax: 215-922-1474
orders@jkp.com
www.jkp.com

Laurie Schlesinger, Vp Of Sales & Marketing
Yvona Fast, Author
Most people with Non-Verbal Learning Disorder (NLD) or Asperger Syndrome (AS) are underemployed. This book sets out to change this. With practical and technical advice on everything from job hunting to interview techniques, from 'fitting in' in the workplace to whether or not to disclose a diagnosis, this book guides people with NLD or AS successfully through the employment mine field. There is also information for employers, agencies and careers counsellors on AS and NLD as 'invisible' disabili *$22.95*
272 pages
ISBN 1-843107-66-X

8972 **Encounters with Autistic States**
Jason Aronson
400 Keystone Industrial Park
Dunmore, PA 18512-1507 800-782-0015
448 pages Hardcover
ISBN 0-765700-62-

8973 **Kitten Who Couldn't Purr**
William Morrow & Company
1350 Avenue of the Americas
New York, NY 10019-4702 212-261-6500
Fax: 212-261-6925
http://www.goodreads.com/book/show/2319648.Th
Otis Chandler, CEO & Co-Founder
Eve Titus, Author
Jonathan the kitten doesn't know how to purr to say thank you, so he sets off to find someone to teach him. *$12.95*
32 pages

8974 **Language Disabilities in Children and Adolescents**
McGraw-Hill School Publishing
PO Box 182605
Columbus, OH 43218 800-338-3987
Fax: 609-308-4480
customer.service@mheducation.com
mcgraw-hill.com

David Levin, President and CEO
Patrick Milano, Chief Administrative Officer & CFO
Stephen Laster, Chief Digital Officer
David Stafford, SVP & General Counsel
A comprehensive review of research in language disabilities.

8975 **Late Talker: What to Do If Your Child Isn' t Talking Yet**
St Martin's Griffin
175 5th Ave
New York, NY 10010-7703 646-307-5151
888-330-8477
Fax: 212-674-6132
customerservice@mpsvirginia.com

Marilyn C Agin, Author
This handbook offers advice on ways to identify the warning signs of a speech disorder, information on how to get the right kind of evaluations and therapy, ways to obtain appropriate services through the school system and health insurance, at-home activities that parents can do with their child to stimulate speech, benefits of nutritional supplementation, and advice from experienced parents who've been there on what to expect and what you can do to be your child's best advocate. *$13.95*
256 pages Paperback
ISBN 0-312309-24-4

8976 **Let Community Employment be the Goal for Individuals with Autism**
Indiana Resource Center For Autism
1905 North Range Road
Bloomington, IN 47408-9801 812-855-6508
800-825-4733
Fax: 812-855-9630
iidc@indiana.edu
www.iidc.indiana.edu/irca

Cathy Pratt, Director
Catherine Davies, Educational Consultant
Pamela Anderson, Outreach/Resource Specialist
Melissa Dubie, Research Associate
A guide designed for people who are responsible for preparing individuals with autism to enter the work force. *$7.00*

8977 **Lollipop Lunch**
Speech Bin-Abilitations
P.O. Box 1579
Appleton, WI 54912-1579 419-589-1425
888-388-3224
Fax: 888-388-6344
info@speechbin.com
www.speechbin.com

James R. Henderson, Chairman
Joseph M. Yorio, President & CEO
Rick Holden, EVP, Educators Publishing Service
Patrick T. Collins, EVP, Distribution
Cleverly illustrated stories and activities for phonological and language development. *$19.95*
128 pages
ISBN 0-937857-54-8

8978 **Management of Autistic Behavior**
Sage Publications
2455 Teller Road
Thousand Oaks, CA 91320 805-499-0721
800-818-7243
Fax: 805-499-0871
info@sagepub.com
www.sagepub.com

Sara Miller McCune, Founder, Publisher, Chairperson
Blaise R Simqu, President & CEO
Tracey A. Ozmina, Executive Vice President & Chief Operating Officer
Stephen Barr, Managing Director/SAGE London, President of SAGE Internation
This excellent reference is a comprehensive and practical book that tells what works best with specific problems. *$41.00*
450 pages

8979 **Motor Speech Disorders**
WB Saunders Company
14 Main Street
Southampton, NY 11968-2822 631-283-5050
800-523-1649
Fax: 631-283-2290
info@saunders.com
www.wbsaunders.com

Joseph R Duffy PhD, Author
Professional text on rehabilitation techniques for motor speech disorders. *$74.00*
592 pages
ISBN 0-323024-52-5

8980 Neurobiology of Autism
Johns Hopkins University Press
National Library of Medicine
Building 38A
Bethesda, MD 20894
410-516-6900
888-346-3656
888-FIN- NLM
Fax: 410-516-6998
info@ncbi.nlm.nih.gov
http://www.ncbi.nlm.nih.gov/pubmed/17919129

Pardo CA, Co-Author
Ebarhat CG, Co-Author

This book discusses recent advances in scientific research that point to a neurobiological basis for autism and examines the clinical implications of this research. *$28.00*

272 pages
ISBN 0-801880-47-5

8981 Nonverbal Learning Disabilities at Home: A Parent's Guide
Jessica Kingsley Publishers
400 Market Street
Suite 400
Philadelphia, PA 19106
215-922-1161
866-416-1078
Fax: 215-922-1474
hello.usa@jkp.com
www.jkp.com

Jessica Kingsley, Chairman & Managing Director
Jemima Kingsley, Director
Octavia Kingsley, Production Director
Lisa Clark, Sr. Commissioning Editor

Explores the variety of daily life problems children with NLD may face, and provides practical strategies for parents to help them cope and grow, from preschool age through their challenging adolescent years. *$19.95*

272 pages Paperback
ISBN 1-853029-40-0

8982 Parent Survival Manual
Springer Publishing Company
11 West 42nd Street
8th Floor
New York, NY 10036
212-355-1501
Fax: 212-355-7370
christieseducation@christies.edu
http://www.christieseducation.com

Craig Lickliter, Manager

A guide to crises resolution in autism and related developmental disorders. *$39.95*

8983 Perspectives: Whole Language Folio
Gallaudet University Bookstore
PO Box 35009
Charlotte, NC 28235-5009
202-651-5750
800-995-0550
Fax: 202-651-5744
www.cpcc.edu/disabilities

Edwin A. Dalrymple, Chairman
Judith N. Allison, Vice Chair
Tony Zeiss, President
Ellen Zaremba, Administrative Assistant to the President

The 19 articles in this collection offer practical help to teachers seeking to emphasize whole language strategies in their classroom. *$9.95*

64 pages

8984 Please Don't Say Hello
Human Sciences Press
233 Spring St
New York, NY 10013
877-283-3229
ainy@aveda.com
aveda.edu/new-york

Phyllis Terri Gold, Author

With the support and love of his family, and through them the neighborhood children, a nine-year-old autistic boy is able to emerge from his shell. *$10.95*

47 pages Paperback
ISBN 0-89885 -99-8

8985 Promoting Communication in Infants and Young Children: 500 Ways to Succeed
Speech Bin-Abilitations
P.O. Box 1579
Appleton, WI 54912-1579
419-589-1425
888-388-3224
Fax: 888-388-6344
info@speechbin.com
www.speechbin.com

James R. Henderson, Chairman
Joseph M. Yorio, President & CEO
Rick Holden, EVP, Educators Publishing Service
Patrick T. Collins, EVP, Distribution

This practical reference for parents, caregivers and professional service providers how to promote communication development in infants and young children. Gives down-to-earth information and activities to help your youngest children succeed. It provides step-by-step suggestions for stimulationg children's speech and language skills. Paperback. *$14.95*

ISBN 0-937857-72-6

8986 Reading, Writing and Speech Problems in Children
International Dyslexia Association
40 York Rd.
4th Floor
Baltimore, MD 21204
410-296-0232
Fax: 410-321-5069
info@dyslexiaida.org
dyslexiaida.org

Samuel Torrey Orton, Author

This book provides reading, reading and speech execerises for educating people with dyslexia. *$20.00*

259 pages
ISBN 0-89079 -79-1

8987 Relationship Development Intervention with Young Children
Taylor & Francis Group
73 Collier St.
London, N1 9BE
44- 0 -0 78
Fax: 44- 0 -0 78
hello.usa@jkp.com
http://www.jkp.com/jkp/distributors.php

Jessica Kingsley, Chairman
Jemima Kingsley, Director
Octavia Kingsley, Production Director
Lisa Clark, Sr. Commissioning Editor

Social and emotional development activities for Asperger Syndrome, Autism, PDD and NLD. Comprehensive set of activities emphasizes foundation skills for younger children between the ages of two and eight. Covers skills such as social referencing, regulating behvior, conversational reciprocity, and synchronized actions. For use in therapeutic settings as well as schools and parents. *$22.95*

256 pages
ISBN 1-843107-14-7

8988 Riddle of Autism: A Psychological Analysis
Jason Aronson
Ste 200
4501 Forbes Blvd
Lanham, MD 20706
301-459-3366
800-462-6420
Fax: 301-429-5746
customercare@nbnbooks.com
http://www.nbnbooks.com

Jason Brockwell, Sales Staff
Michael Sullivan, Sales
Mark Cozy, Sales Staff
Dennis Hayes, Director of Special Markets

Dr. Victor examines the myths that cloud an understanding of this disorder and describes the meanings of its specific behavioral symptoms. *$30.00*

356 pages Paperback
ISBN 1-568215-73-8

8989 **Self-Therapy for the Stutterer**
Stuttering Foundation of America
1805 Moriah Woods Blvd.
Suite 3
Memphis, TN 38117
901-761-0343
800-992-9392
Fax: 901-761-0484
www.stutterhelp.org

Jane Fraser, President
Jean Gruss, Journalist
Robert M. Kurtz, Chairman & CEO
Malcolm Houg Fraser, Founder
A guide to help adults who stutter overcome the problem on their own. *$3.00*
191 pages Paperback
ISBN 0-933388-32-2

8990 **Sex Education: Issues for the Person with Autism**
Indiana Resource Center For Autism
1905 North Range Road
Bloomington, IN 47408-9801
812-855-6508
800-825-4733
Fax: 812-855-9630
www.iidc.indiana.edu/irca

Cathy Pratt, Director
Catherine Davies, Educational Consultant
Pamela Anderson, Outreach/Resource Specialist
Melissa Dubie, Research Associate
Discusses issues of sexuality and provides methods of instruction for people with autism. *$4.00*

8991 **Son-Rise: The Miracle Continues**
2080 South Undermountain Road
Sheffield, MA 01257
413-229-2100
800-714-2779
sonrise@option.org
www.option.org
Samahria Lyt Kaufman, Co-Founder and Co-Director
Dane Griffith, Director of Administrative Services
Bears Kaufman, Co-Founder and Co-Director
Raun Kaufman, Director of Global Education
Part One is the astonishing record of Raun Kaufman's development from an autistic child into a loving, brilliant youngster who shows no traces of his former condition. Part Two follows Raun's development after the age of four, teaching the limitless possibilities of the Son-Rise Program. Part Three shares moving accounts of five other ordinary families who became extraordinary when they used the Son-Rise Program to reach their own unreachable children. *$12.95*
343 pages
ISBN 0-915811-53-7

8992 **Sound Connections for the Adolescent**
Speech Bin
P.O. Box 1579
Appleton, WI 54912-1579
419-589-1425
888-388-3224
Fax: 888-388-6344
info@speechbin.com
www.speechbin.com

James R. Henderson, Chairman
Joseph M. Yorio, President & CEO
Rick Holden, EVP, Educators Publishing Service
Patrick T. Collins, EVP, Distribution
A resource to help older elementary and secondary students understand their sound systems an how it functions. It targets skills critical for academic achievement: phonological awareness, phonemic relationships, phonemic processing, listening and memory and teaches linguistic rules they need to succeed. *$19.95*
Paperback

8993 **Talkable Tales**
Speech Bin-Abilitations
P.O. Box 1579
Appleton, WI 54912-1579
419-589-1425
888-388-3224
Fax: 888-388-6344
www.speechbin.com

James R. Henderson, Chairman
Joseph M. Yorio, President & CEO
Rick Holden, EVP, Educators Publishing Service
Patrick T. Collins, EVP, Distribution
Read-a-rebus stories and pictures targeting most consonant phonemes for K-5 children. *$25.95*
128 pages
ISBN 0-93783 -44-0

8994 **Teaching Children with Autism: Strategies for Initiating Positive Interactions**
Brookes Publishing
P.O. Box 10624
Baltimore, MD 21285-0624
410-337-9585
888-337-8808
Fax: 410-337-8539
custserv@healthpropress.com
http://www.healthpropress.com

Melissa A. Behm, President
Mary Magnus, Director
Stategies for initiating positive interactions and improving learning opportunities. This guide begins with an overview of characteristics and long-term strategies and proceeds through discussions that detail specific techniques for normalizing environments, reducing disruptive behavior, improving language and social skills, and enhancing generalization. *$32.95*
256 pages Paperback
ISBN 1-55766 -80-4

8995 **Teaching and Mainstreaming Autistic Children**
Love Publishing Company
9101 East Kenyon Avenue
Suite 2200
Denver, CO 80237
303-221-7333
Fax: 303-221-7444
http://www.lovepublishing.com/

Peter Knoblock, Author
Dr. Knoblock advocates a highly organized, structured environment for autistic children, with teachers and parents working together. His premise is that the learning and social needs of autistic children must be analyzed and a daily program designed with interventions that respond to this functional analysis of their behavior. *$24.95*
ISBN 0-89108 -11-9

8996 **Techniques for Aphasia Rehab: (TARGET) Generating Effective Treatment**
Speech Bin
P.O. Box 1579
Appleton, WI 54912-1579
419-589-1425
888-388-3224
Fax: 888-388-6344
www.speechbin.com

James R. Henderson, Chairman
Joseph M. Yorio, President & CEO
Rick Holden, EVP, Educators Publishing Service
Patrick T. Collins, EVP, Distribution
Practical treatment manual for use by aphasia clinicians. *$45.00*
384 pages
ISBN 0-93785 -50-5

8997 Understanding & Controlling Stuttering: A Comprehensive New Approach Based on the Valsa Hyp
National Stuttering Association
119 West 40th Street
14th Floor
New York, NY 10018
212-944-4050
800-937-8888
Fax: 212-944-8244
info@westutter.org
www.nsastutter.org
Kenny Koroll, Chair
Tammy Flores, Executive Director
Stephanie Coopen, Family Programs Administrator
Mandy Finstad, Editor/Webmaster
Demonstrates how physical and psychological factors may interact to stimulate and perpetuate stuttering through a Valsalva-Stuttering cycle. *$25.00*
176 pages
ISBN 7-929773-01-3

8998 Verbal Behavior Approach: How to Teach Children with Autism & Related Disorders
Autism Society of North Carolina Bookstore
Ste 230
505 Oberlin Rd
Raleigh, NC 27605-1345
919-743-0204
800-442-2762
Fax: 919-743-0208
http://www.autismsociety-nc.org
Sharon Jeffries-Jones, Chair
Elizabeth Phillippi, Vice Chair
Tracey Sheriff, CEO
Paul Wendler, CFO
Provides full descriptions of how to teach the verbal operants that make up expressive languate which include: manding, tacting, echoing and intraverbal skills. *$19.95*

8999 Without Reason: A Family Copes with two Generations of Autism
Books on Special Children
721 W Abram St
Arlington, TX 76013-6995
817-277-0727
800-489-0727
Fax: 817-277-2270
http://www.fhautism.com/
R. Wayne Gilpin, President
Jennifer Gilpin Yacio, Vice President and Editorial Director
David Reasor, CPA and Administrative Director
Teresa Corey, Conference Administrator
The author discovers his son has autism. He delves into problems of the autistic person and explains reasons for their actions. *$20.95*
292 pages Hardcover

Journals

9000 American Journal of Speech-Language Pathology
American Speech-Language-Hearing Association
2200 Research Boulevard
Rockville, MD 20850-3289
301-296-5700
800-638-8255
Fax: 301-296-8580
nsslha@asha.org
www.asha.org
Elizabeth S. McCrea, PhD, CCC-SLP, President
Barbara K. Cone, PhD, CCC-A, Vice President for Academic Affairs in Audiology
Carolyn W. Higdon, EdD, CCC-SLP, Vice President for Finance
Kaci Roger, Council Member
This is a quarterly journal of clinical practice for speech-language pathologists and language researchers. This journal will be online only beginning January 2010.

9001 Journal of Speech, Language and Hearing Research
American Speech-Language-Hearing Association
2200 Research Boulevard
Rockville, MD 20850-3289
301-296-5700
800-638-8255
Fax: 301-296-8580
nsslha@asha.org
www.asha.org
Elizabeth S. McCrea, PhD, CCC-SLP, President
Barbara K. Cone, PhD, CCC-A, Vice President for Academic Affairs in Audiology
Carolyn W. Higdon, EdD, CCC-SLP, Vice President for Finance
Kaci Roger, Council Member
This bimonthly journal contains basic, as well as applied research in normal and disordered communication processes. It will be available online only beginning January 2010.

9002 Language, Speech, and Hearing Services in Schools
International Fluency Association
Northern Illinois University
Dept. of Communicative Disorders
DeKalb, IL 60115-2899
www.theifa.org
David Shapiro, President
Norimune Kawat, Secretary
Rachel Everard, Treasurer
Shelley Brundage, Membership
This is a quarterly journal focusing on research appropriate to speech-language pathologists and audiologists in schools. The journal will only be available online beginning in January 2010.

Magazines

9003 Communication Outlook
Artificial Language Laboratory
220 Trowbridge Road
East Lansing, MI 48824
517-353-8332
Fax: 517-353-4766
artling@msu.edu
www.msu.edu
Lou Anna K. Simon, President
Satish Udpa, EVP for Administrative Services
Bill Beekman, VP & Secretary
Mark P. Haas, VP for Finance & Treasurer
Communication Outlook (CO) is an international quarterly magazine, which focuses on the techniques and technology of augmentative and alternative communication. CO provides information on technological developments for persons experiencing communication handicaps due to neurological, sensory or neuromuscular conditions. *$18.00*
32 pages Quarterly

Newsletters

9004 Access Academics & Research
American Speech-Language-Hearing Association
2200 Research Boulevard
Rockville, MD 20850-3289
301-296-5700
800-638-8255
Fax: 301-296-8580
nsslha@asha.org
www.asha.org
Elizabeth S. McCrea, PhD, CCC-SLP, President
Barbara K. Cone, PhD, CCC-A, Vice President for Academic Affairs in Audiology
Carolyn W. Higdon, EdD, CCC-SLP, Vice President for Finance
Kaci Roger, Council Member
Dedicated to the specific needs of academic and clinical faculty, PhD students and researchers. The e-newsletter was developed as part of the Focused Initiative on the PhD Shortage in Higher Education.

9005 **Access Audiology**
American Speech-Language-Hearing Association
2200 Research Boulevard
Rockville, MD 20850-3289
301-296-5700
800-638-8255
Fax: 301-296-8580
nsslha@asha.org
www.asha.org

Elizabeth S. McCrea, PhD, CCC-SLP, President
Barbara K. Cone, PhD, CCC-A, Vice President for Academic Affairs in Audiology
Carolyn W. Higdon, EdD, CCC-SLP, Vice President for Finance
Kaci Roger, Council Member

Dedicated to the specific needs of all professionals interested in hearing, balance, and the field of audiology. Each issue spotlights a specific topic of interest and relevance to audiologists.

9006 **Access SLP Health Care**
American Speech-Language-Hearing Association
2200 Research Boulevard
Rockville, MD 20850-3289
301-296-5700
800-638-8255
Fax: 301-296-8580
nsslha@asha.org
www.asha.org

Elizabeth S. McCrea, PhD, CCC-SLP, President
Barbara K. Cone, PhD, CCC-A, Vice President for Academic Affairs in Audiology
Carolyn W. Higdon, EdD, CCC-SLP, Vice President for Finance
Kaci Roger, Council Member

An e-newsletter dedicated to the specific needs of speech-language pathologists in healthcare settings. Each issue of Access SLP Health Care features recent legislative activity impacting SLPs and provides information on clinical issues, continuing education opportunities, and ASHA web-based resources.

9007 **Access Schools**
American Speech-Language-Hearing Association
2200 Research Boulevard
Rockville, MD 20850-3289
301-296-5700
800-638-8255
Fax: 301-296-8580
nsslha@asha.org
www.asha.org

Elizabeth S. McCrea, PhD, CCC-SLP, President
Barbara K. Cone, PhD, CCC-A, Vice President for Academic Affairs in Audiology
Carolyn W. Higdon, EdD, CCC-SLP, Vice President for Finance
Kaci Roger, Council Member

Dedicated to the specific needs of school-based speech-language pathologists. Each Access Schools e-newsletter features recent legislative activity impacting school SLPs and provides information on clinical issues, continuing education opportunities, and ASHA web-based resources.

9008 **Autism Research Review International**
Autism Research Institute
4182 Adams Avenue
San Diego, CA 92116-2599
619-281-7165
866-366-3361
Fax: 619-563-6840
autism.com

Stephen Edelson, Executive Director
Jane Johnson, Managing Director
Valerie Paradiz, Director
Anthony Morgali, Producer

Provides clearly written summaries of articles selected from computer searches. *$18.00*
8 pages Quarterly

9009 **Communicologist**
Texas Speech-Language-Hearing Association
Ste 200
918 Congress Ave
Austin, TX 78701-2342
512-494-1128
888-729-8742
Fax: 512-494-1129

Judith Keller, President
Larry Higdon, Director
Melanie McDonald, President Elect
Tori Gustafson, Vice President

A forum for distributing current information relevant to the practices of speech-language pathology and audiology across the state. Provides TSHA membership with the latest news from the Executive Board and Task Forces, as well as information about regional associations, distinguished service providers, the TSHA Annual Convention, and committee honors and nominations. Also contains advertisements of interest to the field.

9010 **Connect**
Hearing, Speech & Deafness Center (HSDC)
1625 19th Ave.
Seattle, WA 98122
206-323-5770
888-222-5036
Fax: 206-328-6871
seattle@hsdc.org
www.hsdc.org

Lindsay Klarman, Executive Director
Michelle Coleman, Operations Director

A newsletter that addresses concerns of those affected by speech and language disorders. HSDC is a nonprofit for clients who are deaf, hard of hearing, or who face other communication barriers such as speech challenges.
8 pages Quarterly

9011 **NSSLHA Now**
Ntn'l Student Speech Language Hearing Association
2200 Research Boulevard
Rockville, MD 20850-3289
301-296-5700
800-638-8255
Fax: 301-296-8580
nsslha@asha.org
www.asha.org

Elizabeth S. McCrea, PhD, CCC-SLP, President
Barbara K. Cone, PhD, CCC-A, Vice President for Academic Affairs in Audiology
Carolyn W. Higdon, EdD, CCC-SLP, Vice President for Finance
Kaci Roger, Council Member

Published three times per year.

9012 **On Cue**
National Cued Speech Association
1300 Pennsylvania Avenue, NW
Suite 190-713
Washington, DC 20004
301-915-8009
800-459-3529
www.cuedspeech.org

Shannon Howell, President
Penny Hakim, 1st Vice President
John Brubaker, VP Fundraising
Doug Dawson, Treasurer

Published several times a year and mailed to members of the Association.

9013 **Stuttering & Your Child: Help For Parents**
Stuttering Foundation of America
18005 Moriah Woods Blvd
PO Box 11749, Suite 3
Memphis, TN 38111-0749
901-761-0343
800-992-9392
Fax: 901-761-0484
info@stutteringhelp.org
www.StutteringHelp.org

Jane Fraser, President
Dennis Drayna, Director
Joseph R. G. Fulcher, Director
Frances Cook, Director

The Stuttering Foundation provides resources, services and support to those who stutter and their families, as well as support research into the cause of stuttering. The Stuttering Foundation provides a referral list of speech-language pathologists and referrals to other information including research on stuttering, intensive workshops and camps. *$10.00*

9014 **Stuttering Foundation Newsletter**
Stuttering Foundation of America
P.O. Box 11749
Memphis, TN 38111-0749
901-761-0343
800-992-9392
Fax: 901-761-0484
info@stutteringhelp.org
www.stutteringhelp.org

Jane Fraser, President
Jean Gruss, Journalist
Robert M. Kurtz, Chairman & CEO
Malcolm Houg Fraser, Founder

9015 **Voice**
Providence Speech and Hearing Association
1301 Providence Avenue
Orange, CA 92868
714-923-1521
855-901-7742
Fax: 714-744-3841
pshc@pshc.org
www.pshc.org

Lewis Jaffe, President
Bret Rathwick, Vice President - Finance
Casey Immel, Treasurer
Marlene Woodworth, Secretary
People of all ages with speech and hearing problems by providing specialized products and services.

Audio/Visual

9016 **Autism: A World Apart**
Fanlight Productions
c/o Icarus Films
32 Court Street, 21st Floor
Brooklyn, NY 11201
718-488-8900
800-876-1710
Fax: 718-488-8642
info@fanlight.com
www.fanlight.com

Ben Achtenberg, Owner, Founder
Nicole Johnson, Publicity Coordinator
Anthony Sweeney, Marketing Director
In this documentary, three families show us what the textbooks and studies cannot: what it's like to live with autism day after day; to raise and love children who may be withdrawn and violent and unable to make personal connections with their families. 29 minutes.
VHS/DVD
ISBN 1-572950-39-0

9017 **Autism: the Unfolding Mystery**
Aquarius Health Care Media
18 N Main St
Sherborn, MA 1770-1066
508-650-1616
Lesile Kussmann, Owner
Explore what it means to be autistic, how you can recognize the signs of autism in your child, and hear about new treatments and programs to help children learn to deal with the disorder. *$145.00*
DVD

9018 **Getting Started with Facilitated Communication**
Facilitated Communication Institute, Syracuse Univ
370 Huntington Hall
Syracuse, NY 13244-1
315-443-9657
Fax: 315-443-9218

Annegret Schubert, Producer
Describes in detail how to help individuals with autism and/or severe communication difficulties to get started with facilitated communication.
Video

9019 **I Just Want My Little Boy Back**
Autism Treatment Center Of America
2080 South Undermountain Road
Sheffield, MA 01257
413-229-2100
800-714-2779
happiness@option.org
http://www.option.org

Samahria Lyt Kaufman, Co-Founder and Co-Director
Dane Griffith, Director of Administrative Services
Bears Kaufman, Co-Founder and Co-Director
Raun Kaufman, Director of Global Education
A great video for parents and professionals caring for children with special needs. Join one British family and their autistic son before, during and after their journey to America to attend The Son-Rise Program at The Autism Treatment Center of America. This informative, inspirational and deeply moving story not only captures the joy, tears, challenges and triumps of this amazing little boy and his family, but also serves as a powerful introduction to the attitude and principles of the program. *$25.00*

9020 **Understanding Autism**
Fanlight Productions
c/o Icarus Films
32 Court Street, 21st Floor
Brooklyn, NY 11201
718-488-8900
800-876-1710
Fax: 718-488-8642
info@fanlight.com
www.fanlight.com

Ben Achtenberg, Owner, Founder
Nicole Johnson, Publicity Coordinator
Anthony Sweeney, Marketing Director
Parents of children with autism discuss the nature and symptoms of this lifelong disability and outline a treatment program based on behavior modification principles. 19 minutes
VHS/DVD
ISBN 1-572951-00-1

Support Groups

9021 **Autism Society of America**
4340 East West Highway
Suite 350
Bethesda, MD 20814-3067
301-657-0881
800-328-8476
Fax: 301-657-0869
www.autism-society.org

Mary Beth Collins, Director of Programs
Tonia Ferguson, Senior Director of Content
Scott Badesch, President/Chief Executive Officer
John Dabrowski, Chief Financial Officer
ASA is the largest and oldest grassroots organization within the autism community, with a nationwide network of chapters and over 20,000 members and supporters nationwide. ASA is the leading source of education, information and referral about autism and has been the leader in advocacy and legislative initiatives for more than four decades.

9022 **Cherab Foundation**
PO Box 1771
Jensen Beach, FL 34958
772-335-5135
help@cherab.org
cherabfoundation.org

Lisa Geng, Founder & President
Jolie Abreu, Vice President
The Cherab Foundation is a world-wide nonprofit organization working to improve the communication skills and education of all children with speech and language delays and disorders.

9023 **Friends: National Association of Young People who Stutter**
38 S Oyster Bay Rd
Syosset, NY 11791-5033
866-866-8335
lcaggiano@aol.com
www.friendswhostutter.org

Lee Caggiano, President

A national organization created to provide a network of love and support for children and teenagers who stutter, their families, and the professionals who work with them.

9024 **National Health Information Center**
US Department of Health
P.O. Box 1133
Washington, DC 20013-1133
301-565-4167
800-336-4797
301-468-7394
Fax: 301-984-4256
healthypeople@hhs.gov
http://www.healthypeople.gov

Jonathan Fielding, Chair
Shirika Kumanyika, Vice Chair

A health information referral service that puts health professionals and consumers who have health questions in touch with those organizations that are best able to provide answers.

9025 **Speech Pathways**
410 Meadow Creek Drive
Suite 206
Westminster, MD 21158
410-374-0555
800-961-2724
Fax: 410-374-8620
kim.bell@speechpathways.net
speechpathways.net

Kimberly A. Bell, Owner
Karie Hadley, Therapist
Erica Hamilton, Therapist
Julie Kumpar, Therapist

We realize that parent and family support is critical to a child's success, in therapy as well as in life. We offer support at local and regional levels along with traditional speech and language services, and a wide variety of specialized pediatric programs. Our support groups/services are open to the larger community as well as to our clients.

Visual

Associations

9026 American Academy of Ophthalmology
655 Beach St
San Francisco, CA 94109
415-561-8540
866-561-8558
Fax: 415-561-8575
customer_service@aao.org
aao.org

Cynthia Ann Bradford, MD, President
David W Parke II, MD, CEO
Maria M Aaron, MD, Secretary for Annual Meeting
Lynn K Gordon, MD, PhD, Vice Chair, The Council

The American Academy of Ophthalmology is an association of doctors who provide comprehensive eye care, including medical, surgical and optical care. The academy is dedicated to advancing the profession of ophthalmology through programs, public education, courses and advocacy.

9027 American Action Fund for Blind Children and Adults
1800 Johnston St.
Baltimore, MD 21230-4914
410-659-9315
actionfund@actionfund.org
www.actionfund.org

Barbara Loos, President
Ramona Walhof, Vice President
Sandra Halverson, Second Vice President/Medical Transcriptionist
James Omvig, Treasurer

A service agency which specializes in providing to blind people help which is not readily available to them from government programs or other existing service systems. The services are planned especially to meet the needs of blind children, the elderly blind, and the deaf-blind.

9028 American Council of Blind Lions
148 Vernon Ave.
Louisville, KY 40206
502-897-1472
carla40206@gmail.com
www.acb.org/affiliate-ACBL

Carla Ruschival, President

The American Council of Blind Lions (ACBL) works to educate members of local Lions Clubs about the needs and concerns of blind or visually impaired people. The ACBL is open to members from across the United States and encourages blind persons to join their local clubs and participate in civic projects.

9029 American Council of the Blind
1703 N Beauregard St
Suite 420
Alexandria, VA 22311
202-467-5081
800-424-8666
Fax: 703-465-5085
info@acb.org
www.acb.org

Eric Bridges, Executive Director
Tony Stephens, Director, Advocacy & Governmental Affairs

The American Council of the Blind (ACB) is an association working to increase the independence, security, and opportunity for all blind or visually impaired individuals. The Council primarily focuses on developing and maintaining policies to implement the services needed for the blind or visually impaired.

9030 American Council of the Blind Radio Amateurs
19821 Vineyard Ln.
Saratoga, CA 95070
408-257-1034
acbra@acb.org
www.acbhams.org

John Glass, President

A special interest affiliate of the American Council of the Blind, the American Council of the Blind Radio Amateurs (ACBRA) promotes the interest of FCC licensed amaetur radio operators. The ACBRA is made up of legally blind and fully sighted radio amateurs.

9031 American Foundation for the Blind
2 Penn Plaza
Suite 1102
New York, NY 10121
800-232-5463
www.afb.org

Kirk Adams, President & CEO
Darren M. Davis, Executive Administrator Executive Office

The American Foundation for the Blind (AFB) is a national nonprofit that is dedicated to removing barriers, creating solutions, and expanding possibilities for the blind and visually impaired. The AFB is focused on spreading access to technology, elevating the quality of information and tools for professional who serve people with vision loss, and the promotion of independent living for those with vision loss.

9032 American Optometric Association
243 N Lindbergh Blvd
Floor 1
St. Louis, MO 63141-7881
800-365-2219
www.aoa.org

Christopher J. Quinn, O.D, President
Barbara L. Horn, O.D, Vice President
William T. Reynolds, O.D, Secretary-Treasurer

The American Optometric Association (AOA) advocates for improving the quality and availability of eye and vision care. The AOA represents more than 44,000 doctors of optometry, optometric professionals, and optometry students and works to set professional standards, lobby government and organizations on behalf of the profession, and provide research and education leadership.

9033 American Printing House for the Blind
American Printing House for the Blind, Inc.
1839 Frankfort Ave.
Louisville, KY 40206-0085
502-895-2405
800-223-1839
Fax: 502-899-2284
info@aph.org
www.aph.org

9034 Associated Services for the Blind and Visually Impaired
919 Walnut Street
Philadelphia, PA 19107-5237
215-627-0600
Fax: 215-922-0692
asbinfo@asb.org
www.asb.org

Karla S. McCaney, President & CEO
Beth Deering, Director, Human Services
Richard Forsythe, Director, Braille Division & Custom Audio
Joyce Robertson, Director, Finance & Information Technology

Associated Services for the Blind and Visually Impaired (ASB), is a private, nonprofit organization working to provide services, education, training, and resources to promote self-esteem, independence, and self determination in people who are blind or visually impaired. In addition, ASB advocates for the rights of blind and visually impaired persons through community actions and public education.

9035 Association for Education & Rehabilitationof the Blind & Visually Impaired
5680 King Centre Dr.
Suite 600
Alexandria, VA 22315
703-671-4500
Fax: 703-671-6391
aer@aerbvi.org
www.aerbvi.org

Neva Fairchild, President
Sergio Oliva, Secretary
Jennifer Wheeler, Treasurer

The Association for Education and Rehabilitation of the Blind and Visually Impaired (AER) is an international, nonprofit membership organization that supports professionals who provide education and rehabilitation services to people with visual impairments. The AER provides professional development and growth opportunities for its members and advocates to maintain specialized blind services.

9036 **Association for Macular Diseases**
The Association for Macular Diseases, Inc.
210 E 64th St
New York, NY 10065 212-605-3719
association@retinal-research.org
macula.org

Bernard Landou, President

The Association for Macular Diseases provides support and assistance to individuals with macular disease, their caregivers, and professional community.

9037 **Association for Research in Vision and Ophthalmology**
1801 Rockville Pike
Suite 400
Rockville, MD 20852-5622 240-221-2900
Fax: 240-221-0370
arvo@arvo.org
www.arvo.org

9038 **Association for Vision Rehabilitation and Employment**
174 Court St
Binghamton, NY 13901 607-724-2428
Fax: 607-771-8045
avreinfo@avreus.org
www.avreus.org

Ken Fernald, President & CEO
Jenn Small, Chief Operating Officer
Anthony Saccento, Chief Financial Officer
Teri Chamberlin, Director, Health & Rehabilitation Services

The Association for Vision Rehabilitation and Employment, Inc. (AVRE) is a private, nonprofit organization providing rehabilitation and employment services for people who are blind or visually impaired in the Twin Tiers of New York and Pennsylvania. Services include Low Vision, Early Intervention, Orientation and Mobility, Vision Rehabilitation Therapy, and employment preparation and placement.

9039 **Association of Blind Citizens**
PO Box 246
Holbrook, MA 02343 781-961-1023
Fax: 781-961-0004
president@blindcitizens.org
www.blindcitizens.org

9040 **Blind Children's Center**
4120 Marathon St
Los Angeles, CA 90029-3584 323-664-2153
info@blindchildrenscenter.org
www.blindchildrenscenter.org

Sarah E. Orth, Chief Executive Officer
Fernanda Armenta-Schmitt, Director, Education & Family Services

A nonprofit organization working to foster the development and education of children from birth to the 2nd grade who are blind or visually impaired. The Blind Children's Center serves about 100 children a year through a variety of family centered programs including the infant, preschool, and elementary.

9041 **Blind Information Technology Specialists**
8761 E Placita Bolivar
Tucson, AZ 85715-5650 520-232-2100
www.bits-acb.org

Tom L. Jones, President
Earlene Hughes, Vice President
David Tanner, Secretary
Richard Villa, Treasurer

The Blind Information Technology Specialists (BITS) is a nonprofit organization fostering the career development of computer professionals, promoting the use of computer technology and improved information access for people who are blind or visually impaired.

9042 **Blinded Veterans Association**
1001 King St.
Suite 300
Alexandria, VA 22314 800-669-7079
bva@bva.org
www.bva.org

Thomas Zampieri, National President
Joseph D. McNeil, Sr., National Vice President
Donald D. Overton, Jr., Executive Director
Stuart Nelson, Director, Public Relations

The Blinded Veterans Association locates blinded veterans who need assistance, guides them through the rehabilitation process and acts as advocates for them before Congress and the Department of Veterans Affairs in securing the benefits they have earned through their service to the nation. The association also promotes access to technology, practical use of the latest research as well as offering programs for blinded veterans.

9043 **Braille Institute of America**
741 N Vermont Ave.
Los Angeles, CA 90029-3594 323-663-1111
800-272-4553
Fax: 323-663-0867
la@Brailleinstitute.org
www.Brailleinstitute.org

Peter A. Mindnich, President
Gloria Coulston, Vice President, Program Delivery
Nancy N. Neibrugge, Vice President, Program Content

The Braille Institute is a nonprofit organization providing assistance to blind and visually impaired individuals. The institute offers a variety of free programs, classes, and services at 5 regional centers in Southern California.

9044 **California State Library Braille and Talking Book Library**
PO Box 942837
Sacramento, CA 94237-0001 916-654-0640
800-952-5666
btbl@library.ca.gov
www.btbl.ca.gov

9045 **Canine Helpers for the Handicapped**
Canine Helpers for the Handicapped, Inc.
5699 Ridge Rd.
Lockport, NY 14094 716-433-4035
chhdogs@aol.com

Beverly Underwood, Executive Director

A nonprofit organization dedicated to training dogs in order to assist people with disabilities and promote independence.

9046 **Caption Center**
Media Access Group at WGBH
One Guest St.
Boston, MA 02135 617-300-3600
Fax: 617-300-1020
access@wgbh.org

Pat McDonald, Director

The Caption Center was the world's first captioning agency providing access to television for viewers who are visually impaired and/or hard of hearing. The Center develops new solutions and uses closed captioning and descriptive video to promote access to technology .

9047 **Central Association for the Blind & Visually Impaired**
507 Kent St.
Utica, NY 13501 315-797-2233
877-719-9996
www.cabvi.org

Edward P. Welsh, Chair
Kenneth C. Thayer, Vice Chair
Richard Evans, Treasurer
Marie Bord, Secretary

It assists people who are blind or visually impaired to achieve their highest levels of independence.

9048 **Chicago Lighthouse for People who are Blind and Visually Impaired**
1850 W Roosevelt Rd
Chicago, IL 60608-1298 312-666-1331
Fax: 312-243-8539
TTY: 312-666-8874
www.chicagolighthouse.org

Bruce R. Hague, Chairman
Sandra C. Forsythe, Vice Chairman
Janet P. Szlyk, President
David Huber, Treasurer

A non profit agency committed to providing the highest quality educational, clinical, vocational, and rehabilitation services for children, youth and adults who are blind or visually impaired, including deafblind and multi disabled. Also respects personal dignity and partners with individuals to enhance independent living and self sufficiency. This agency is a leader, innovator and advocate for people who are blind or visually impaired, enhancing the quality of life for all individuals.

9049 Clovernook Center for the Blind and Visually Impaired
7000 Hamilton Ave
Cincinnati, OH 45231-5240
513-522-3860
888-234-7156
Fax: 513-728-3946
TTY: 513-522-3860
contact@clovernook.org
www.clovernook.org

Alfred J. Tuchfarber, Chair
Wilbert F. Schwartz, Vice Chair
Mark Jackson, Treasurer
Thomas R. Flottman, Secretary
Mission is to promote independence and foster the highest quality of life for people with visual impairments, including those with additional disabilities. We provide comprehensive program services including training and support for independent living, orientation and mobility instruction, vocational training, job placement, counseling, recreation, and youth services. Meaningful employment opportunities are also provided to individuals who are blind or visually impaired.

9050 Clovernook Printing House, The Clovernook Center for the Blind and Visually Impaired
7000 Hamilton Ave
Cincinnati, OH 45231-5240
513-522-3860
888-234-7156
Fax: 513-728-3946
contact@clovernook.org
www.clovernook.org

Alfred J. Tuchfarber, Chair
Wilbert F. Schwartz, Vice Chair
Mark Jackson, Treasurer
Thomas R. Flottman, Secretary
Clovernook also offers Braille Transcription Services including: Literary Books, Literary Magazines, Religious Materials, Instructional Manuals, ADA Conformance Materials, Literary Textbook Materials, Menus, Braille Alphabet Cards, and Forms. In addition, our Business Operations provide meaningful employment opportunities for individuals who are blind or visually impaired, while at the same time manufacturing high-quality products for customers across the country. *$145.00*
591 pages
ISBN 1-930956-48-7

9051 College of Optometrists in Vision Development
215 W Garfield Rd
Ste 200
Aurora, OH 44202-7884
330-995-0718
888-268-3770
Fax: 330-995-0719
info@covd.org
www.covd.org

David A. Damari, President
Kara Heying, Vice President
Christine Allison, Secretary-Treasurer
Pamela R. Happ, Executive Director
The College of Optometrists in Vision Development (COVD) is an international membership association of eye care professionals including optometrists, optometry students, and vision therapists. Members of COVD provide developmental vision care, vision therapy and vision rehabilitation services for children and adults.

9052 College of Syntonic Optometry
2052 W Morales Dr.
Pueblo West, CO 81007
719-547-8177
877-559-0541
Fax: 719-547-3750
Syntonics@q.com
www.collegeofsyntonicoptometry.com
Hans Lessmann, O.D, FCOVD, President
Robert Fox, O.D, FCOVD, FCSO, Vice President
Larry Wallace, O.D, Ph.D, Education Director
The College of Syntonic Optometry is an international organization dedicated to furthering Phototherapy in the treatment of the visual system. Members of the college include optometrists, and health care professionals.

9053 Columbia Lighthouse for the Blind
1825 K St. NW
Suite 1103
Washington, DC 20006
202-454-6400
Fax: 202-955-6401
info@clb.org
www.clb.org
Tony Cancelosi, President & CEO
Jocelyn Hunter, Senior Director, Communications
Toya Horten, Director, Administrative Operations
Bethany Martin, Manager, Youth & Education Services
Columbia Lighthouse for the Blind (CLB) helps blind and visually impaired individuals in Washington, DC. CLB's services include training and consultation in assistive technology, employment skills, career placement, low vision care, and counseling and rehabilitation services.

9054 DeafBlind Division of the National Federation of the Blind
200 E Wells St.
Baltimore, MD 21230
410-659-9314
Fax: 410-685-5653
nfb@nfb.org
www.nfb.org
Alice Eaddy, Division President
The nation's largest and most influential membership organization of blind persons, with a two-fold purpose: to help blind persons achieve self-confidence and self respect and to act as a vehicle for collective self-expression by the blind. The NFB improves blind people's lives through advocacy, education, research, technology, and programs encouraging independence and self-confidence. It is the leading force in the blindness field today and is the voice of the nations blind.

9055 Desert Blind & Handicapped Association
Desert Blind and Handicapped Association, Inc.
777 E Tahquitz Canyon Way
Suite 200
Palm Springs, CA 92262
760-969-5025
info@desertblind.org
Thomas Samulski, Executive Director
George Holliday, Treasurer
The Desert Blind & Handicapped Association provides free transportation for individuals who are blind or have a disability.

9056 Eye Bank Association of America
1101 17th St NW
Suite 400
Washington, DC 20036
202-775-4999
Fax: 202-429-6036
www.restoresight.org
Kevin P. Corcoran, CAE, President & CEO
Bernie Dellario, Director, Finance
Stacey Gardner, Director, Education
Colleen Bayus, Communications Manager
The Eye Bank Association of America (EBAA) is a nonprofit organization advocating the restoration of sight by advancing donation, transplantation, and research. The EBAA is the oldest transplant association in the United States.

9057 Fidelco Guide Dog Foundation
103 Vision Way
Bloomfield, CT 06002
860-243-5200
Fax: 860-769-0567
admissions@fidelco.org
www.fidelco.org
Karen C. Tripp, Chair
G. Kenneth Bernhard, Esq., Vice Chair
Gregg Barratt, Chief of Staff
Julie Unwin, Chief Operating Officer
The Fidelco Guide Dog Foundation creates increased freedom and independence for men and women who are blind by providing them with guide dogs.

9058 **Fight for Sight**
381 Park Ave S
Suite 809
New York, NY 10016
212-679-6060
Fax: 212-679-4466
Arthur@fightforsight.org
www.fightforsight.org

Arthur Makar, Executive Director
Janice Benson, Associate Director

Fight for Sight is a nonprofit charity working to support eye and vision research through the providing of funds to scientists starting their careers.

9059 **Foundation Fighting Blindness**
7168 Columbia Gateway Dr.
Suite 100
Columbia, MD 21046
410-423-0600
800-683-5555
TTY: 410363713951
info@FightBlindness.org
www.blindness.org

William T. Schmidt, Chief Executive Officer
Valerie Navy-Daniels, Chief Development Officer
Stephen M. Rose, PhD, Chief Research Officer

The Foundation Fighting Blindness (FFB) works to promote research in order to prevent, treat and restore vision. FFB is currently the world's leading private funder of retinal disease research, funding over 100 research grants and 150 researchers.

9060 **Guide Dogs for the Blind**
PO Box 151200
San Rafael, CA 94915
800-295-4050
information@guidedogs.com
www.guidedogs.com

Christine Benninger, Chief Executive Officer & President
Cathy Martin, Chief Financial Officer & Treasurer
Brent Ruppel, Vice President, Community Operations

Guide Dogs for the Blind empowers lives by creating exceptional partnerships between people, dogs, and communities. All of their services provided free of charge of charge to their clients, including personalized training and extensive post-graduation support, plus financial assistance for veterinary care, if needed.

9061 **Guiding Eyes for the Blind**
611 Granite Springs Rd
Yorktown Heights, NY 10598-3499
914-245-4024
800-942-0149
Fax: 914-245-1609
info@guidingeyes.org
www.guidingeyes.org

Thomas Panek, President & Chief Executive Officer

Guiding Eyes for the Blind is a nonprofit organization providing guide dogs for individuals who are blind or visually impaired.

9062 **Horizons for the Blind**
125 Erick St.
A103
Crystal Lake, IL 60014
815-444-8800
800-318-2000
Fax: 815-444-8830
mail@horizons-blind.org
www.horizons-blind.org

Camille Caffarelli, Executive Director
Jeff T. Thorsen, First Vice President & Treasurer
Keith Myers, Second Vice President
Maryann Bartkowski, Secretary

Horizons for the Blind is a nonprofit organization working to improve the quality of life for people who are blind or visually impaired by increasing access to consumer products, services, culture, arts, education, and recreation.

9063 **Independent Visually Impaired Entrepreneurs**
818-238-9321
abazyn@bazyncommunications.com
www.ivie-acb.org

Ardis Bazyn, President

The Independent Visually Impaired Entrepreneurs (IVIE) is a national organization for visually impaired business owners. The IVIE offers an annual convention, planning a program of interest for business owners.

9064 **Institute for Families**
1300 N Vermont Ave.
Suite 1004
Los Angeles, CA 90027
323-361-4649
Fax: 323-665-7869
info@instituteforfamilies.org
instituteforfamilies.org

Gary Huffaker, Chairperson

Institute for Families is a nonprofit organization providing support and information for families of children with vision loss. The Institute provides guidance through a resource and referral network; referring families to organizations specializing in meeting the needs of children with specific vision loss problems.

9065 **International Association of Audio Information Services**
800-280-5325
iaaismember@gmail.com
www.iaais.org

Marjorie Moore, President
Maryfrances Evans, Vice-President

The International Association of Audio Information Services (IAAIS) is a membership organization that works to turn text into speech and providing information through broadcast, telephone or internet. IAAIS connects and supports organizations that deliver equal access information for people with disabilities worldwide.

9066 **Jewish Braille Institute International**
JBI International
110 E 30th St
New York, NY 10016-7393
212-889-2525
800-433-1531
Fax: 212-689-3692
admin@jbilibrary.org
www.jbilibrary.org

Dr. Ellen Isler, President & Cheif Executive Officer
Israel A. Taub, Vice President & Cheif Financil Officer

The Jewish Braille Institute (JBI) International is a nonprofit organization working to meet the Jewish and general cultural needs of the blind and visually impaired.

9067 **Keystone Blind Association**
3056 East State St.
Hermitage, PA 16148
724-347-5501
Fax: 724-347-2204
info@keystoneblind.org
www.keystoneblind.org

Jonathan Fister, President/ CEO
Karen Anderson, Board Member
Sam Bellich, Board Member
Al Boland, Board Member

The Keystone Blind Association works to education, and employ individuals with vision loss. Headquartered in Hermitage, the Association has offices in Meadville and New Castle, Pennsylvania.

9068 **Lighthouse Guild**
250 W 64th St.
New York, NY 10023
212-769-6200
800-284-4422
www.lighthouseguild.org

Calvin W. Roberts, President & CEO
Paul D. Misiti, Chief of Staff
Himanshu R. Shah, Chief Financial Officer
Maura J. Sweeney, Chief Program Officer

Lighthouse Guild is a not-for-profit vision & healthcare organization, addressing the needs of people who are blind or visually impaired, including those with multiple disabilities or chronic medical conditions.

9069 **Lions Clubs International**
300 W 22nd St
Oak Brook, IL 60523-8842
630-571-5466
Fax: 630-571-8890
TTY: 630-571-6533
lions@lionsclubs.org
www.lionsclubs.org

Benedict Ancar, Director
Jui-Tai Chang, Director
Jaime Garcia Cepeda, Director
Kalle Elster, Director

Our 46,000 clubs and 1.35 million members make us the world's largest service club organization. We're also one of the most effective. Our members do whatever is needed to help their local communities. Everywhere we work, we make friends. With children who need eyeglasses, with seniors who don't have enough to eat and with people we may never meet.

9070 Macular Degeneration Foundation
PO Box 531313
Henderson, NV 89053-1313
702-450-2908
888-633-3937
liz@eyesight.org
www.eyesight.org
Liz Trauernicht, President/Director of Communications
Julie Zavala, VP/Asst Director of Operations
David Seftel, M.D., MBA, Executive Vice President/Director of Research Development
Ron Gallemore, Board Of Scientific Advisors
The Macular Degeneration Foundation is dedicated to those who have and will develop macular degeneration. We offer this growing community the latest information, news, hope and encouragement.

9071 National Alliance of Blind Students NABS Liaison
American Council of the Blind
1155 15th St NW
Ste 1004
Washington, DC 20005-2706
202-467-5081
800-424-8666
Fax: 202-467-5085
info@acb.org
www.acb.org
Jill Gaus, President
Lynn Jansen, Vice President
Debby Lieberman, Secretary
Mike Reese, Treasurer
A student affiliate of the American Council of the Blind which is a national organization of blind and visually impaired high school and college students who believe that every blind and visually impaired student has the right to an equal and accessible education. Also encourages blind and visually impaired students to challenge their limits and reach their potential.

9072 National Association for Parents of Children with Visual Impairments (NAPVI)
PO Box 317
Watertown, MA 02471-317
617-972-7441
800-562-6265
Fax: 617-972-7444
spedex.com@gmail.com
www.spedex.com
Susan LaVenture, Executive Director
Julie Urban, President
Venetia Hayden, Vice President
Kim Alfonso, Treasurer
A non profit organization of, by and for parents committed to providing support to the parents of children who have visual impairments . Also a national organization that enables parents to find information and resources for their children who are blind or visually impaired including those with additional disabilities. NAPVI also provides leadership, support, and training to assist parents in helping children reach their potential.

9073 National Association for Visually Handicapped (NAVH)
111 E 59th S
Fl 6
New York, NY 10022-1202
212-889-3141
800-829-0500
Fax: 212-821-9707
TTY: 212-821-9713
info@lighthouse.org
www.lighthouse.org
Alan R. Morse, President & CEO
Lawrence E. Goldschmidt, Deputy Chair & Secretary
Himanshu R. Shah, CFO
Maura J. Sweeney, Senior Vice President, Programs & Services
NAVH is unique in the services it offers to the hard of seeing™ worldwide and is the only non-profit organization solely dedicated to providing assistance to this population. NAVH runs senior support groups, provides individual consultations, informational materials, training in the use of visual aids, and numerous other tools to ensure that the visually impaired can remain independent and lead fulfilling lives.

9074 National Association of Blind Educators
National Federation of the Blind
200 E Wells St.
Baltimore, MD 21230
410-659-9314
Fax: 410-685-5653
nfb@nfb.org
www.nfb.org
Cayte Mendez, Division President
Membership organization of blind teachers, professors and instructors in all levels of education. Provides support and information regarding professional responsibilities, classroom techniques, national testing methods and career obstacles. Publishes The Blind Educator, national magazine specifically for blind educators.

9075 National Association of Blind Lawyers
National Federation of the Blind
200 E Wells St.
Baltimore, MD 21230
303-504-5979
Fax: 303-757-3640
nfb@nfb.org
www.nfb.org
Scott LaBarre, President
Membership organization of blind attorneys, law students, judges and others in the law field. Provides support and information regarding employment, techniques used by the blind, advocacy, laws affecting the blind, current information about the American Bar Association and other issues for blind lawyers.

9076 National Association of Blind Merchants (NABM)
National Federation of the Blind
7450 Chapman Hwy.
Suite 319
Knoxville, TN 37920
888-687-6226
blindmerchants.org
Nicky Gacos, President
Harold Wilson, First Vice President
Ed Birmingham, Second Vice President
Pam Schnurr, Treasurer
Serving as an advocacy and support group, NABM is a membership organization of blind persons employed in self-employment work or the Randolph-Sheppard Vending Program. The organization provides information on issues affecting blind merchants, including rehabilitation, social security, and tax.

9077 National Association of Blind Rehabilitation Professionals
National Federation of the Blind
200 E Wells S.
Baltimore, MD 21230
410-659-9314
Fax: 410-685-5653
nfb@nfb.org
www.nfb.org
Amy Porterfield, Division President
Membership organization

9078 National Association of Blind Students
National Federation of the Blind
200 E Wells St.
Baltimore, MD 21230
410-659-9314
Fax: 410-685-5653
nfb@nfb.org
www.nfb.org
Kathryn Webster, Division President
For over 30 years this national organization of blind students has provided support, information, and encouragement to blind college and university students. NABS leads the way in offering resources in issues such as national testing, accessible textbooks and materials, overcoming negative attitudes about blindness from school personnel, developing new techniques of accomplishing laboratory or field assignments, and many other college experiences.

9079 **National Association of Blind Teachers**
American Council of the Blind
1155 15th St NW
Ste 1004
Washington, DC 20005-2706
202-467-5081
800-424-8666
Fax: 202-467-5085
johnbuckley25@hotmail.com
www.blindteachers.net

Jill Gaus, President
Lynn Jansen, Vice President
Debby Lieberman, Secretary
Mike Reese, Treasurer

Works to advance the teaching profession for blind and visually impaired people, protects the interest of teachers, presents discussions and solutions for special problems encountered by blind teachers and publishes a directory of blind teachers in the US.

9080 **National Association of Blind Veterans**
PO Box 784957
Winter Garden, FL 34778
321-948-1466
president@nabv.org
www.nabv.org

Dwight Sayer, President
Gene Huggins, 1st Vice President
Larry Ball, 2nd Vice President
Patty Sayer, Secretary

A nationwide organization of blind and visually impaired veterans striving to serve fellow veterans who have lost their sight in the service of country or have lost their sight after serving country.

9081 **National Association of Guide Dog Users**
National Federation of the Blind
1003 Papaya Dr
Tampa, FL 33619-4629
813-626-2789
800-558-8261
888-624-3841
president@nagdu.org
www.nagdu.org

Marion Gwizdala, President

Provides information and support for guide dog users and works to secure high standards in guide dog training. Addresses issues of discrimination of guide dog users and offers public education about guide dog use. Biennial newsletter available: Harness Up!

9082 **National Association to Promote the Use of Braille**
National Federation of the Blind
39481 Gallaudet Dr
Apt 127
Fremont, CA 94538
510-248-0100
877-558-6524
Fax: 818-344-7930
mwillows@sbcglobal.net
www.nfbcal.org

Nadine Jacobson, President
Robert Jaquiss, Vice President
Linda Mentink, Second Vice President
Jennifer Dunnam, Secretary

Dedicated to securing improved Braille instruction, increasing the number of Braille materials available to the blind and providing information of Braille in securing independence, education and employment for the blind.

9083 **National Beep Baseball Association**
1501 41st NW
Apt G1
Rochester, MN 55901
866-400-4551
www.nbba.org

Stephen A. Guerra, Secretary

It facilitates and provides the adaptive version of America's favorite pastime for the blind, low vision and legally blind.

9084 **National Braille Association**
95 Allens Creek Rd
Bldg 1 Ste 202
Rochester, NY 14618- 3252
585-427-8260
Fax: 585-427-0263
nbaoffice@nationalBraille.org
www.nationalBraille.org

David Shaffar, Executive Director
Jan Carroll, President
Whitney Gregory-Williams, Vice President
Heidi Lehmann, Secretary

The only national organization dedicated to the professional development of individuals who prepare and produce Braille materials.

9085 **National Braille Press**
88 Saint Stephen St
Boston, MA 02115-4312
617-266-6160
888-965-8965
888-965-8965
Fax: 617-437-0456
contact@nbp.org
www.nbp.org

Brian A. Mac Donald, President
Kimberley Ballard, Vice President
Tony Grima, Vice President of Braille Publications
Diane L. Croft, Publisher

The guiding purposes of National Braille Press are to promote the literacy of blind children through Braille, and to provide access to information that empowers blind people to actively engage in work, family, and commuity affairs.

9086 **National Center for Vision and Child Development**
Lighthouse Guild
250 West 64th Street
New York, NY 10023
646-874-8219
800-284-4422
Fax: 212-821-9707
info@lighthouse.org
www.lighthouseguild.org

Alan R. Morse, President & CEO
Lawrence E. Goldschmidt, Deputy Chair & Secretary
Himanshu R. Shah, CFO
Maura J. Sweeney, Senior Vice President, Programs & Services

The worldwide leader in helping people of all ages who are blind or partially sighted overcome the challenges of vision loss.

9087 **National Diabetes Action Network for the Blind**
National Federation of the Blind
200 E Wells St.
Baltimore, MD 21230
410-659-9314
Fax: 410-685-5653
bernienfb75@gmail.com
www.nfb.org

Bernadette Jacobs, Division President

Leading support and information organization of persons losing vision due to diabetes. Provides personal contact and resource information with other blind diabetics about non-visual techniques of independently managing diabetes, monitoring glucose levels, measuring insulin and other matters concerning diabetes. Publishes Voice of the Diabetic, the leading publication about diabetes and blindness.

9088 **National Eye Institute**
31 Center Drive MSC 2510
Bethesda, MD 20892-2510
301-496-5248
Fax: 301-402-1065
2020@nei.nih.gov
www.nei.nih.gov

Paul A Sieving MD PhD, Director

To conduct and support research for blinding eye diseases, visual disorders, mechanisms of visual function, and the preservation of sight.

9089 **National Federation of the Blind**
200 E Wells St.
Baltimore, MD 21230
410-659-9314
Fax: 410-685-5653
nfb@nfb.org
nfb.org

Mark Riccobono, President
John Berggren, Executive Director, Operations
Anil Lewis, Executive Director, Blindness Initiatives
John G. Pare, Jr., Executive Director, Advocacy & Policy

The National Federation of the Blind (NFB) works to help blind people achieve self-confidence, self-respect and self-determination and to achieve complete integration into society on a basis of equality. The Federation provides public educations, information and referral services, scholarships, literature and publications, adaptive equipment, advocacy services, legal services, employment assistance and more.

9090 **National Industries for the Blind**
1310 Braddock Pl
Alexandria, VA 22314-1691
703-310-0500
Fax: 703-998-8268
info@nib.org
www.nib.org

Gary J. Krump, Chairperson
Ronald Tascarella, Vice Chairperson
Kristin Graham Koehler, Secretary

A nonprofit organization that represents over 100 associated industries serving people who are blind in thirty-six states. These agencies serve people who are blind or visually impaired and help them to reach their full potential. Services include job and family counseling, job skills training, instruction in Braille and other communication skills, children's programs and more.

9091 **National Library Service for the Blind and Physically Handicapped (NLS)**
1291 Taylor St NW
Washington, DC 20011
202-707-5100
800-424-8567
Fax: 202-707-0712
nls@loc.gov
www.loc.gov/nls

Annual

9092 **National Organization of Parents of Blind Children**
National Federation of the Blind
200 E Wells St.
Baltimore, MD 21230
410-659-9314
Fax: 410-685-5653
nfb@nfb.org
nfb.org

Carlton Walker, Division President

Support information and advocacy organization of parents of blind or visually impaired children. Addresses issues ranging from help to parents of a newborn blind infant, mobility and Braille instruction, education, social and community participation, development of self confidence and other vital factors involved in growth of a blind child.

9093 **New Eyes for the Needy**
549 Millburn Avenue
PO Box 332
Short Hills, NJ 07078-332
973-376-4903
Fax: 973-376-3807
neweyesfortheneedy@verizon.net
www.neweyesfortheneedy.org

Susan Dyckman, Executive Director
Marianne Muench Busby, Vice President
Barbara Daney, Treasurer
Suzanne Escousee, Secretary

New Eyes provides new prescription glasses for poor children and adults in the U.S. through a voucher system.

9094 **Prevent Blindness America**
211 W Wacker Drive
Suite 1700
Chicago, IL 60606
312-363-6001
800-331-2020
Fax: 312-363-6052
info@preventblindness.org
www.preventblindness.org

James E. Anderson, Chair
Kira Baldanado, Director
Arzu Bilazer, Creative Director
Mary Bregantini, Senior Director

The nation's leading volunteer eye health and safety organization dedicated to fighting blindness and saving sight. Also touches the lives of millions of people each year through public and professional education, advocacy, certified vision screening training, community and patient service programs and research.

9095 **Seeing Eye, The**
10 Washington Valley Rd
PO Box 375
Morristown, NJ 07963-0375
973-539-4425
Fax: 973-539-0922
info@seeingeye.org
www.seeingeye.org

Peggy Gibbon, Director of Canine Development
James A Kutsch Jr, President/CEO
Dolores Holle, VMD, Director of Canine Medicine & Surgery
Randall Ivens, Director of Human Resources

An organization that concentrates on its mission to enhance the independence, dignity, and self confidence of blind people through the use of seeing eye dogs. The Seeing Eye will be an organization that concentrates on its mission to enhance the independence, dignity, and self confidence of blind people through the use of Seeing Eye dogs, and on improving its ability to fulfill this mission. We will maintain and nuture the spirit of our founders and adhere to the highest standards of respect

9096 **Society for the Blind**
1238 S St.
Sacramento, CA 95811
916-452-8271
Fax: 916-492-2483
info@societyfortheblind.org
societyfortheblind.org

Shari Roeseler, Executive Director
Shane Snyder, Director of Programs

Serving 26 counties in Northern California, Society for the Blind is a full service, nonprofit, agency providing services and programs for people who are blind or have low vision. services include the Low Vision Clinic, Braille Classes, computer training, support groups, living skills instruction, mobility training, and the Products for Independence Store.

9097 **United States Association of Blind Athletes**
1 Olympic Plaza
Colorado Springs, CO 80909-3508
719-866-3224
Fax: 719-866-3400
mlucas@usaba.org
www.usaba.org

Mark A. Lucas, Executive Director
Ryan Ortiz, Assistant Executive Director
John Potts, Goalball High Performance Director
Lacey Markle, Public Relations and Events Coordinator

USABA is a Colorado-based 501 (c) (3) organization that provides life-enriching sports opportunities for every individual with a visual impairment. A member of the U.S. Olympic Committee, USABA provides athletic opportunities in various sports including, but not limited to track and field, nordic and alpine skiing, biathlon, judo, wrestling, swimming, tandem cycling, powerlifting and goalball (a team sport for the blind and visually impaired).

9098 **United States Blind Golfers Association**
125 Gilberts Hill Rd
Lehighton, PA 18235
615-679-9629
info@usblindgolf.com
www.usblindgolf.com

Jim Baker, President
Diane Wilson, Vice President
Tony Schiros, Board Member
Alan Hooper, Board Member

It encourages and enhances opportunities of blind and visually impaired golfers to compete in golf.

9099 **United States Braille Chess Association**
1881 N. Nash St.
Unit 702
Arlington, VA 22209
516-223-8685
www.americanblindchess.org

LA Pietrolungo, President
Alan Dicey, Vice President
Jay Leventhal, Secretary
Alan Schlank, Treasurer

It is dedicated to encourage and assist in the promotion and advancement of correspondence and over-the board chess among chess enthusiasts who are blind or visually impaired.

9100 **Vermont Association for the Blind and Visually Impaired**
60 Kimball Ave
South Burlington, VT 05403
802-863-1358
800-639-5861
Fax: 802-863-1481
general@vabvi.org
www.vabvi.org

James Mooney, President
Thomas Chase, Vice President
Debbie Balserus, Secretary
Patricia Henderson, Treasurer

The Vermont Association for the Blind and Visually Impaired (VABVI), a non-profit organization founded in 1926, is the only private agency to offer free training, services and support to visually impaired Vermonters. Each year we serve hundreds of children from birth to age 22 and adults age 55 and over.

9101 **Vision Forward Association**
912 N. Hawley Road
Milwaukee, WI 53213
414-615-0100
855-878-6056
Fax: 414-256-8748
www.vision-forward.org

Terri Davis, Executive Director
Jacci Borchardt, Program Director
Jacque Cline, Human Resources Director
Dena Fellows, Marketing Director

Its mission is to empower, educate, and enhance the lives of individuals impacted by vision loss through all of life's transitions.

9102 **Vision World Wide**
Apt 302
5707 Brockton Dr
Indianapolis, IN 46220-5481
317-254-1332
800-431-1739
Fax: 317-251-6588
www.visionww.org

Patricia L Prince, President

A non profit organization dedicated to improving the lives of the vision impaired through direct interaction and indirectly through the caregiving community. Also serve both the totally blind and those with various degrees and forms of vision loss.

9103 **Visions Center on Blindness (VCB)**
111 Summit Park Rd.
Spring Valley, NY 10977
845-354-3003
888-245-8333
info@visionsvcb.org
www.visionsvcb.org

Nancy D. Miller, Executive Director & CEO
Natalia S. Young, Chief Operating Officer
Carlos Cabrera, Chief Financial Officer
Ruben Coellar, Chief Program Officer

VISIONS VCB is a 35-acre year round residential rehabilitation and training center in Rockland County, New York. VCB offers comprehensive overnight training and vision rehabilitation facilities.

9104 **Visually Impaired Veterans of America**
American Council of the Blind
1155 15th St NW
Ste 1004
Washington, DC 20005-2706
202-467-5081
800-424-8666
Fax: 202-467-5085
www.acb.org

Jill Gaus, President
Lynn Jansen, Vice President
Debby Lieberman, Secretary
Mike Reese, Treasurer

Maintain, promote and foster the well bring and rehabilitation of all visually Impaired Veterans of the Armed Forces of the United States of America who are eligible to receive from the Veterans Administration; develops and encourages the practice of high standards of personal professional conduct among Visually Impaired Veterans; maintain, promote, and foster public confidence and awareness In Visually Impaired Veterans.

9105 **Washington Ear**
12061 Tech Rd
Ste B
Silver Spring, MD 20904-7826
301-681-6636
Fax: 301-625-1986
information@washear.org
www.washear.org

George Long, Chairman
Neely Oplinger, Executive Director
Freddie L. Peaco, President
Paul D'Addario, President-Elect

A non profit organization providing reading and information services for blind, visually impaired and physically disabled people who cannot effectively read print, see plays, watch television programs and films, or view museum exhibits. Ear free services strive to substitute hearing for seeing, improving the lives of people with limited or no vision by enabling them to be well-informed, fully productive members of their families, their communities and the working world.

Camps

9106 **Camp Barakel**
P.O. Box 159
Fairview, MI 48621-0159
989-848-2279
Fax: 989-848-2280
info@campbarakel.org
www.campbarakel.org

Paul Gardner, Camp Director
Hannah Gardner, Music Coordinator
Jon Ford, Head Lifeguard
Stacy Ford, Adult Program Staff

Five-day Christian camp experience in mid-August for campers ages 18-55 who are physically disabled, visually impaired, upper trainable mentally impaired or educable mentally impaired, bus transportation provided from locations in Lansing, Flint and Bay City, Michigan.

9107 **Camp Bloomfield**
Wayfinder Family Services
5300 Angeles Vista Blvd.
Malibu, CA 90043
323-295-4555
Fax: 323-296-0424
JLucas@WayfinderFamily.org
www.wayfinderfamily.org

Joshua Lucas, MS, Recreation Programs Manager & Camp Director
Miki Jordan, President & Chief Executive Officer
Veronica Arteaga, Chief Program Officer

Camp Bloomfield is a summer camp with week long sessions for children and youth who are blind, visually impaired or multi-disabled. The 45 acre campground offers campers a variety of activities, specifically designed to meet the needs of the children, with campers attending at no cost.

9108 **Camp Challenge**
8914 US Highway 50 East
Bedford, IN 47421
812-834-5159
info@gocampchallenge.com
www.gocampchallenge.com
Maria, Director of Engagement
One and two-week sessions for campers with developmental and or physical disabilities, hearing impairment and the blind/visually impaired. Ages 6-99 and families.

9109 **Camp Lawroweld**
288 West Side Rd.
Weld, ME 04285
207-585-2984
bchase@nnec.org
www.camplawroweld.org
Trevor Schlisner, Director
Camp is located in Weld, Maine. Offers various camp sessions, including a week-long camp for individuals who are blind or visually impaired.

9110 **Camp Lighthouse**
Columbia Lighthouse for the Blind
1825 K St. NW
Suite 1103
Washington, DC 20006
202-454-6400
Fax: 202-955-6401
info@clb.org
www.clb.org
Tony Cancelosi, President & CEO
Jocelyn Hunter, Senior Director, Communications
Toya Horten, Director, Administrative Operations
Bethany Martin, Manager, Youth & Education Services
Camp Lighthouse is a one week day camp program for children ages 6-12 with visual impairments. Activities include games, recreation, arts and crafts, field trips, and Braille activities.

9111 **Camp Lou Henry Hoover**
Girl Scouts of Washington Rock Council
201 East Grove Street
Westfield, NJ 07090
908-518-4400
Fax: 908-232-4508
girlscouts@gshnj.org
www.gshnj.org
Samantha Basek, Field Executive
Susan Brooks, CEO
Camp is located in Middleville, New Jersey. Sessions for girls who are blind/visually impaired, ages 7-18.

9112 **Camp Merrick**
PO Box 56
Nanjemoy, MD 20662
301-870-5858
Fax: 301-246-9108
info@lionscampmerrick.org
www.lionscampmerrick.org
Heidi A. Fick, Executive Director
Donna Wadsworth, Office Administrator
Programs offered April-January for children who are blind/visually impaired, hearing impaired or diabetic. Coed, ages 6-16.

9113 **Camp Winnekeag**
257 Ashby Road
Ashburnham, MA 01430
978-827-4455
Fax: 978-827-4551
sneconference@sneconline.org
www.campwinnekeag.com
Frank Tochterman, Religious Leader
Camp is located in Ashburnham, Massachusetts. Camping sessions for blind/visually impaired children. Coed, ages 8-16.

9114 **Enchanted Hills Camp for the Blind**
Lighthouse for the Blind
1155 Market St.
10th Floor
San Francisco, CA 94103
415-431-1481
afletcher@lighthouse-sf.org
www.lighthouse-sf.org
Tony Fletcher, Director, Enchanted Hills Camp and Retreat
Bryan Bashin, CEO
Enchanted Hills Camp for the Blind is located on 311 acres of land on Mt. Veeder, offering programs for children, teens, adults, deaf-blind, seniors, and families of the blind. The camp gives campers the experience of traditional summer camp but is adapted to meet the needs of the campers.

9115 **Highbrook Lodge**
Cleveland Sight Center
1909 E 101st St.
Cleveland, OH 44106
216-791-8118
Fax: 216-791-1101
TTY: 216-791-8119
info@clevelandsightcenter.org
www.clevelandsightcenter.org
Larry Benders, President & CEO
Kevin Krencisz, Chief Financial & Administrative Officer
Jassen Tawil, Director, Business Development & Customer Success
Ali Thomas, Director, Human Resources
Camp is located in Chardon, Ohio. Summer sessions for children, adults and families who are blind or have low vision. Sessions inclide a wide range of outdoor camp activities. Camp activities focus on gaining independent skills, mobility, orientation and self-confidence in an accessible and traditional camp setting.

9116 **Indian Creek Camp**
Kentucky Tennessee Conference
150 Cabin Circle Drive
Liberty, TN 37095
615-548-4411
Fax: 615-548-4029
www.indiancreekcamp.com
Ken Wetmore, Director
Marty Sutton, Asst. Director
Toni Stephens, Program Director
Stephanie Rufo, Public Relations Director
Camp is located in Liberty, Tennessee. Summer sessions for children and adults who are blind/visually impaired. Coed, ages 7-17, families and seniors.

9117 **Kamp A-Komp-Plish**
9035 Ironsides Rd
Nanjemoy, MD 20662-3432
301-870-3226
301-934-3590
Fax: 301-870-2620
recreation@melwood.org
Jonathan Rondeau, Chief Program Officer
Bekah Carmichael, Director
Doria Fleisher, Associate Director
Marisa Cucuzella, Assistant Director
Camp is located in Nanjemoy, Maryland. Half-week, one-week and two-week sessions for blind/visually impaired children and those with developmental disabilities and mobility limitation. Coed, ages 8-16.

9118 **Kamp Kaleo**
46872 Willow Springs Rd.
Burwell, NE 68823
308-346-5083
kampkaleo@gmail.com
www.kampkaleo.com
David Butz, Camp Administrator
Offers an overnight summer camp for individuals with developmental disabilities. In addition to regular camp activities, there is a strong focus on religious education.

9119 **National Camps for Blind Children**
Christian Record Services
5900 S 58th St.
Suite M
Lincoln, NE 68516
402-488-0981
Fax: 402-488-7582
info@christianrecord.org
www.christianrecord.org
Diane Thurber, President
Lonnie Kreiter, Vice President, Finance
Christian Record Services runs National Camps for Blind Children, summer camps for individuals who are considered legally blind.

9120 **Texas Lions Camp**
PO Box 290247
Kerrville, TX 78029
830-896-8500
Fax: 830-896-3666
tlc@lionscamp.com
www.lionscamp.com

Stephen S. Mabry, President & CEO
Karen-Anne King, Vice President, Summer Camps
Milton Dare, Director, Development
Joan Dixon, Director, Finance

Texas Lions Camp is a camp dedicated to serving children ages 7-16 in Texas with physical disabilities. While at camp, campers will participate in a variety of activities and be encouraged to become more independent and self-confident.

9121 **VISIONS Vacation Camp for the Blind (VCB)**
VISIONS Center on Blindness
111 Summit Park Rd.
Spring Valley, NY 10977
845-354-3003
888-245-8333
info@visionsvcb.org
www.visionsvcb.org

Krystal Findley-Jones, Director

A nonprofit agency that promotes the independence of people of all ages who are blind or visually impaired. Camp offers Braille classes, computers with large print and voice output, support groups, discussions, cooking classes, personal and home management training, and large print and Braille books.

9122 **Wendell Johnson Speech And Hearing Clinic**
University Of Iowa
250 Hawkins Dr
Iowa City, IA 52242-1025
319-335-8736
Fax: 319-335-8851
kathy-miller@uiowa.edu
www.uiowa.edu

Chuck Wieland, President
Hans Hoerschelman, Vice President
Josh Smith, Budget Officer
Shannon Lizakowski, Secretary

The clinic offers assessment and intervention for communication disorders in adults and children as well as an audiology clinic. The clinic also offers several summer programs for children with hearing, speech, language, autism and/or reading disorders, including a summer residential program for teens who stutter.

9123 **YMCA Camp Chingachgook on Lake George**
Capital District YMCA
1872 Pilot Knob Rd.
Kattskill Bay, NY 12844
518-656-9462
Fax: 518-656-9362
chingachgook@cdymca.org
www.lakegeorgecamp.org

Jine Andreozzi, Executive Director
Mike Obermayer, Director, Summer Program
Carol Lewis, Office Manager

Offers sailing programs for people with disabilities.

Books

9124 **A Christian Approach to Overcoming Disability: A Doctor's Story**
Routledge (Taylor & Francis Group)
711 Third Ave.
New York, NY 10017
212-216-7800
Fax: 212-564-7854
orders@taylorandfrancis.com
www.routledge.com

Dr. Elaine Leong Eng, M.D.

A personal account of Dr. Elaine Leong Eng and her career move from obstetrician/gynecologist to full-time mom, as she faces the diagnosis of impending visual impairment. Dr. Eng offers personal experience and faith-based, psychological techniques for coping with disability.

142 pages Hardcover

9125 **AFB Directory of Services for Blind and Visually Impaired Persons in the US and Canada**
American Foundation for the Blind/AFB Press
2 Penn Plaza
Suite 1102
New York, NY 10121
212-502-7600
800-232-5463
Fax: 888-545-8331
afbinfo@afb.net
www.afb.org

Carl Augusto, President & Chief Executive Officer
Rick Bozeman, Finance Director, Chief Financial Officer
Kelly Bleach, Chief Administrative Officer
Stacy Rollins, Executive Administrative Assistant to the President

Comprehensive print resource containing more that 2,500 local, state, regional, and national services throughout the US and Canada for persons who are blind or visually impaired. *$79.95*

624 pages Paperback/onlin
ISBN 0-891288-05-3

9126 **About Children's Eyes**
National Association for Visually Handicapped
111 East 59th Street
New York, NY 10022-1202
212-821-9384
800-829-0500
Fax: 212-821-9707
info@lighthouse.org
lighthouse.org/navh

Mark G. Ackermann, President / CEO

How to identify the child with a visual problem. LightHouse acquired NAVH.

9127 **About Children's Vision: A Guide for Parents**
National Association for Visually Handicapped
111 East 59th Street
New York, NY 10022-1202
212-821-9384
800-829-0500
Fax: 212-821-9707
info@lighthouse.org
lighthouse.org/navh

Mark G. Ackermann, President / CEO

Offers a better understanding of the normal and possible abnormal development of a child's eyesight. LightHouse acquired NAVH. *$.50*

9128 **Access to Art: A Museum Directory for Blind and Visually Impaired People**
American Foundation for the Blind/AFB Press
2 Penn Plaza
Suite 1102
New York, NY 10121
212-502-7600
800-232-5463
Fax: 888-545-8331
afbinfo@afb.net
www.afb.org

Carl R. Augusto, President & Chief Executive Officer
Rick Bozeman, Finance Director, Chief Financial Officer
Kelly Bleach, Chief Administrative Officer
Stacy Rollins, Executive Administrative Assistant to the President

Details the access facilities of over 300 museums, galleries and exhibits in the United States. Also included are organizations offering art-related resources such as, art classes, competitions and traveling exhibits. *$19.95*

144 pages Large Print
ISBN 0-891281-56-8

9129 **African Americans in the Profession of Blindness Services**
Mississippi State University
P.O. Box 6189
Mississippi State, MS 39762
662-325-2001
Fax: 662-325-8989
TTY: 662-325-2694
nrtc@colled.msstate.edu
www.blind.msstate.edu

Jacqui Bybee, Research Associate II
Douglas Bedsaul, Research and Training Coordinator
Anne Carter, Research and Training Coordinator
Brenda Cavenaugh, Ph.D., Research Professor

This study investigated the level of participation by African Americans in vocational rehab. (VR) services to persons who are visually impaired. Using surveys and interviews with all state VR directors, national census data and national RSA data, it was found nationally that African Americans are substantially under-represented in the service provider ranks, yet over-represented as clients. *$20.00*

61 pages Paperback

9130 Age-Related Macular Degeneration

National Association for Visually Handicapped
111 East 59th Street
New York, NY 10022-1202
212-821-9384
800-829-0500
Fax: 212-821-9707
info@lighthouse.org
lighthouse.org/navh

Mark G. Ackermann, President / CEO

A large booklet offering information and up-to-date research on Macular Degeneration. Also available in Russian. Revised in 2007. LightHouse acquired NAVH. *$5.00*

9131 American Anals of the Deaf Reference

800 Florida Ave NE
Washington, DC 20002-3600
202-651-5530
Fax: 202-651-5489
gupress@gallaudet.edu
gupress.gallaudet.edu/annals

Stephanie Cawthon, Ph.D., Book Review Editor
Peter V. Paul, Ph.D., Editor, Literary Issues
Ye Wang, Ph.D., Senior Associate Editor
Feifei Ye, Ph.D., Associate Editor for Research Methodology

The controlled scope of GUPress operations allows the continuance of a highly focused commitment to individual titles that has contributed significantly to its 20 years of leadership in publishing on Deaf issues. Gallaudet University Press brings unmatched experience and knowledge to the marketplace for books on and for the Deaf community, its advocates, and scholars invested in the study of deaf society.

9132 Americans with Disabilities Act Guide for Places of Lodging: Serving Guests Who Are Blind

US Department of Justice
950 Pennsylvania Avenue NorthWest
Washington, DC 20530
202-307-0663
800-574-0301
Fax: 202-307-1197
TTY: 800-514-0383
www.ada.gov

Rebecca B. Bond, Chief
Zita Johnson Betts, Deputy Chief
Sally Conway, Deputy Chief
James Bostrom, Deputy Chief

A 12-page publication explaining what hotels, motels, and other places of transient lodging can do to accommodate guests who are blind or have low vision.

9133 Art and Science of Teaching Orientation and Mobility to Persons with Visual Impairments

American Foundation for the Blind/AFB Press
2 Penn Plaza
Suite 1102
New York, NY 10121
212-502-7600
800-232-5463
Fax: 888-545-8331
afbinfo@afb.net
www.afb.org

Carl R. Augusto, President & Chief Executive Officer
Rick Bozeman, Finance Director, Chief Financial Officer
Kelly Bleach, Chief Administrative Officer
Stacy Rollins, Executive Administrative Assistant to the President

Comprehensive decription of the techniques of teaching orientation and mobility, presented along with considerations and strategies for sensitive and effective teaching. Hardcover. Paperback also available. *$48.00*

200 pages
ISBN 0-891282-45-9

9134 Awareness Training

Landmark Media
3450 Slade Run Drive
Falls Church, VA 22042
703-241-2030
800-342-4336
Fax: 703-536-9540
info@landmarkmedia.com

Michael Hartogs, President
Peter Hartogs, VP New Business & Development
Richard Hartogs, VP Acquisitions
Beverly Weisenberg, Sales Representative

Covers disabilities of various types — vision, hearing, speech disorders, loss of limbs, loss of mobility, or mental/emotional limitations and how to integrate such individuals into various business and educational settings. It is a 4-part series designed to identify and enable others to interact effectively with those suffering such disabilities. *$495.00*

Set of 4

9135 Babycare Assistive Technology

Through the Looking Glass
3075 Adeline Street
Suite 120
Berkeley, CA 94703
510-848-1112
800-644-2666
Fax: 510-848-4445
tlg@lookingglass.org
www.lookingglass.org

Maureen Block, J.D., President
Thomas Spalding, Treasurer
Alice Nemon, Secretary
Mega Kirshbaum, Author

Available in Braille, large print or cassette. Provides an overview of the baby care assistive technology work at Through The Looking Glass including a discussion of TLG's intervention model, the impact of babycare equipment and guidelines for equipment development. *$2.00*

8 pages

9136 Babycare Assistive Technology for Parents with Physical Disabilties

Through the Looking Glass
3075 Adeline Street
Suite 120
Berkeley, CA 94703
510-848-1112
800-644-2666
Fax: 510-848-4445
tlg@lookingglass.org
www.lookingglass.org

Maureen Block, J.D., President
Thomas Spalding, Treasurer
Alice Nemon, Secretary
Mega Kirshbaum, Author

Examines the provision of babycare equipment through the lens of ithe infant/parent relationship, the lens of the family system, and through the lens of culture. Availiable in Braille, large print or cassette. *$2.00*

7 pages

9137 Basic Course in American Sign Language

TJ Publishers
P.O. Box 702701
Dallas, TX 75370
972-416-0800
800-999-1168
Fax: 972-416-0944
TTY: 301-585-4440
TJPubinc@aol.com
www.tjpublishers.com/

Tom Humphries, Author
Carol Padden, Co-Author
Terrance J O'Rourke, Co-Author

Accompanying videotapes and textbooks include voice translations. Hearing students can analyze sound for initial instruction, or opt to turn off the sound to sharpen visual acuity. Package includes the Basic Course in American Sign Language text, Student Study Guide, the original four 1-hour videotapes plus the ABCASI Vocabulary videotape. *$139.95*

280 pages

9138 **Behavioral Vision Approaches for Persons with Physical Disabilities**
Optometric Extension Program Foundation
7754 Braegger Road
Three Lakes, WI 54562
714-250-0176
Info@depf.org
www.depf.org

Kristin R. Jungbluth, President
Eric J. Lindberg, VP
Barbara Kuntz, Secretary
Patricia S. Lindberg, Treasurer
A discussion of the behavioral vision/neuro-motor approach to providing directions for prescriptive and therapeutic services for the visually handicapped child or adult. *$49.50*
197 pages

9139 **Belonging**
Dial Books
375 Hudson St
New York, NY 10014-3657
212-366-2000
Fax: 212-414-3394
www.penguin.com/

Deborah Kent, Author
Meg attended special schools for the blind until she was ready for high school. She decided that she wanted to go to a regular high school. She and her mother practiced her walks to school and studied the layout of the building prior to school starting, but Meg was unprepared for the trip when there were 1,500 students. She adjusted quickly to the crowds and the pace of the new school.
200 pages Hardcover
ISBN 0-80370 -30-1

9140 **Berthold Lowenfeld on Blindness and Blind People**
American Foundation for the Blind/AFB Press
2 Penn Plaza
Suite 1102
New York, NY 10121
212-502-7600
800-232-5463
Fax: 888-545-8331
afbinfo@afb.net
www.afb.org

Carl R. Augusto, President & Chief Executive Officer
Rick Bozeman, Finance Director, Chief Financial Officer
Kelly Bleach, Chief Administrative Officer
Stacy Rollins, Executive Administrative Assistant to the President
These writings of the pioneering educator, author and advocate range over a forty-year period include various ground-breaking papers for the blind educator, a rememberance of Helen Keller and other essays on education, sociology and history. *$21.95*
254 pages Paperback
ISBN 0-891281-01-0

9141 **Blind and Vision-Impaired Individuals**
Mainstream
Ste 830
3 Bethesda Metro Ctr
Bethesda, MD 20814-6301
301-961-9299
800-247-1380
Fax: 301-654-6714

Charles Moster
Mainstreaming blind individuals into the workplace. *$2.50*
12 pages

9142 **Blindness and Early Childhood Development Second Edition**
American Foundation for the Blind/AFB Press
2 Penn Plaza
Suite 1102
New York, NY 10121
212-502-7600
800-232-5463
Fax: 888-545-8331
afbinfo@afb.net
afb.org

Carl R. Augusto, President & Chief Executive Officer
Rick Bozeman, Finance Director, Chief Financial Officer
Kelly Bleach, Chief Administrative Officer
Stacy Rollins, Executive Administrative Assistant to the President
A review of current knowledge on motor and locomotor development, perceptual development, language and cognitive processes, and social, emotional and personality development. Paperback. *$34.95*
384 pages
ISBN 0-891281-23-8

9143 **Blindness: What it is, What it Does and How to Live with it**
American Foundation for the Blind/AFB Press
2 Penn Plaza
Suite 1102
New York, NY 10121
212-502-7600
800-232-5463
Fax: 888-545-8331
afbinfo@afb.net
www.afb.org

Carl R. Augusto, President & Chief Executive Officer
Rick Bozeman, Finance Director, Chief Financial Officer
Kelly Bleach, Chief Administrative Officer
Stacy Rollins, Executive Administrative Assistant to the President
A classic work on how blindness affects self-perception and social interaction and what can be done to restore basic skills, mobility, daily living and an appreciation of life's pleasures. *$15.95*
396 pages Paperback
ISBN 0-891282-05-

9144 **Books are Fun for Everyone**
Nat'l Lib Svc/Blind And Physically Handicapped
1291 Taylor Street North West
Washington, DC 20011
202-707-5100
Fax: 202-707-0712
TTY: 202-707-0744
nls@loc.gov
www.loc.gov/nls

Karen Keninger, Director

9145 **Books for Blind & Physically Handicapped Individuals**
Nat'l Lib Svc/Blind And Physically Handicapped
1291 Taylor Street North West
Washington, DC 20011
202-707-5100
Fax: 202-707-0712
TTY: 202-707-0744
nls@loc.gov
www.loc.gov/nls

Karen Keninger, Director
A free national library program of Braille and recorded materials for blind and physically handicapped persons.

9146 **Books for Blind and Physically Handicapped Individuals**
Nat'l Lib Svc/Blind And Physically Handicapped
1291 Taylor Street North West
Washington, DC 20011
202-707-5100
Fax: 202-707-0712
TTY: 202-707-0744
nls@loc.gov
www.loc.gov/nls

Karen Keninger, Director
A free national library program of Braille and recorded materials for blind and physically handicapped persons is administered by the National Library Service for the Blind and Physically Handicapped Library of Congress.
Annual

9147 **Braille Book Bank, Music Catalog**
National Braille Association
95 Allens Creek Road
Building 1, Suite 202
Rochester, NY 14618
585-427-8260
Fax: 585-427-0263
nbaoffice@nationalBraille.org
www.nationalBraille.org

Jan Carroll, President
Cindi Laurent, Vice President
David Shaffer, Executive Director
Heidi Lehmann, Secretary
Offers hundreds of musical titles in print form, Braille and on cassette.
62 pages

9148 Braille: An Extraordinary Volunteer Opportunity
Nat'l Lib Svc/Blind And Physically Handicapped
1291 Taylor Street North West
Washington, DC 20011
202-707-5100
Fax: 202-707-0712
TTY: 202-707-0744
nls@loc.gov
www.loc.gov/nls

Karen Keninger, Director

9149 Burns Braille Transcription Dictionary
American Foundation for the Blind/AFB Press
2 Penn Plaza
Suite 1102
New York, NY 10121
212-502-7600
800-232-5463
Fax: 888-545-8331
afbinfo@afb.net
afb.org

Carl R. Augusto, President & Chief Executive Officer
Rick Bozeman, Finance Director, Chief Financial Officer
Kelly Bleach, Chief Administrative Officer
Stacy Rollins, Executive Administrative Assistant to the President

A handy, portable guide that is a quick reference for anyone who needs to check print-to-Braille and Braille-to-print meanings and symbols. Paperback. *$21.95*
96 pages 96 pages
ISBN 0-891282-32-7

9150 Can't Your Child See? A Guide for Parents of Visually Impaired Children
Sage Publications
2455 Teller Road
Thousand Oaks, CA 91320
805-499-0721
800-818-7243
Fax: 805-499-0871
info@sagepub.com
www.sagepub.com

Sara Miller McCune, Founder, Publisher, Executive Chairman
Blaise R Simqu, President & CEO
Tracey A. Ozmina, Executive Vice President & Chief Operating Officer
Stephen Barr, Managing Director/SAGE London, President of SAGE Internation

This second edition offers parents optimistic, practical guidelines for helping visually impaired children reach their full potential. *$26.00*
279 pages Paperback

9151 Career Perspectives: Interviews with Blindand Visually Impaired Professionals
American Foundation for the Blind/AFB Press
2 Penn Plaza
Suite 1102
New York, NY 10121
212-502-7600
800-232-5463
Fax: 888-545-8331
afbinfo@afb.net
afb.org

Carl R. Augusto, President & Chief Executive Officer
Rick Bozeman, Finance Director, Chief Financial Officer
Kelly Bleach, Chief Administrative Officer
Stacy Rollins, Executive Administrative Assistant to the President

Profiles of 20 successful archivers who describe in their own words what it takes to pursue and attain professional success in a sighted world. Available in large print, cassette and Braille. *$19.95*
96 pages
ISBN 0-891281-70-2

9152 Careers in Blindness Rehabilitation Services
Mississippi State University
P.O. Box 6189
Mississippi State, MS 39762
662-325-2001
Fax: 662-325-8989
TTY: 662-325-2694
nrtc@colled.msstate.edu
www.blind.msstate.edu

Jacqui Bybee, Research Associate II
Douglas Bedsaul, Research and Training Coordinator
Anne Carter, Research and Training Coordinator
Brenda Cavenaugh, Ph.D., Research Professor

In a follow-up study in a series examining the substantial under-representation of African Americans as professionals in blindness services, researchers questioned college students about their knowledge, opinions and interests in blindness services. *$15.00*
54 pages Paperback

9153 Cataracts
National Association for Visually Handicapped
111 East 59th Street
New York, NY 10022-1202
212-821-9384
800-829-0500
Fax: 212-821-9707
info@lighthouse.org
lighthouse.org/navh

Mark G. Ackermann, President / CEO

A booklet offering information about Cataracts, diagnosis and treatment of this common condition. LightHouse acquired NAVH. *$4.00*

9154 Characteristics, Services, & Outcomes of Rehab. Consumers who are Blind/Visually Impaired
Mississippi State University
P.O. Box 6189
Mississippi State, MS 39762
662-325-2001
Fax: 662-325-8989
TTY: 662-325-2694
nrtc@colled.msstate.edu
www.blind.msstate.edu

Jacqui Bybee, Research Associate II
Douglas Bedsaul, Research and Training Coordinator
Anne Carter, Research and Training Coordinator
Brenda Cavenaugh, Ph.D., Research Professor

Issues regarding the efficacy of separate state agencies providing specialized vocational rehabilitation (VR) services to consumers who are blind have generated spirited discussions within the rehabilitation community throughout the history of the state-federal program. In this monograph, RRTC researches report results of their investigation of services provided to blind consumers in separate and general (combined) rehabilitation agencies. *$20.00*
45 pages Paperback

9155 Childhood Glaucoma: A Reference Guide for Families
NAPVI
1 North Lexington Avenue
White Plains, NY 10601
617-972-7441
800-562-6265
Fax: 617-972-7444
napvi@guildhealth.org
www.napvi.org

Julie Urban, President
Venetia Hayden, Vice President
Susan LaVenture, Executive Director
Randi Sher, Secretary

A vaulable tutorial and resource covering all aspects from genetics through diagnosis, sibling relationships and more.
36 pages

9156 Children with Visual Impairments: A Guide For Parents
American Foundation for the Blind/AFB Press
105 East 22nd Street
New York, NY 10010
212-949-4800
childrensaidsociety.org

William D. Weisberg, Ph.D., President & CEO
Drema Brown, VP of Education
Katherine Eckstein, Chief of Staff
Beverly Colon, VP for Health & Wellness

Written by parents and professional, this book presents a comprehensive overview of the issues that are crucial to the healthy development of children with mild to severe visual impaiments. It also offers insight from parents about coping with the emotional aspects of raising a child with special needs. *$16.95*

416 pages

ISBN 0-933149-36-0

9157 **Classification of Impaired Vision**

National Association for Visually Handicapped
111 East 59th Street
New York, NY 10022-1202
212-821-9384
800-829-0500
Fax: 212-821-9707
info@lighthouse.org
lighthouse.org/navh

Mark G. Ackermann, President / CEO

Designed to provide a foundation for a better understanding of teaching reading, writing, and listning skills to students with visual impairments from preschool age through adult levels. LightHouse acquired NAVH. *$57.95*

322 pages

ISBN 0-398066-93-2

9158 **Communication Skills for Visually Impaired Learners**

Charles C. Thomas
2600 S First St
Springfield, IL 62704-4730
217-789-8980
800-258-8980
Fax: 217-789-9130
books@ccthomas.com
www.ccthomas.com

Michael P. Thomas, President
Randall Harley, Author
Mila Truan, Author
LaRhea Sanford, Author

This book has been designed to provide a foundation for a better understanding of teaching reading, writing, and listening skills to students with visual impairments from preschool age through adult levels. The plan of the book incorporates the latest research findings with the practical experiences learned in the classroom. *$57.95*

322 pages Paperback

ISBN 0-398066-93-2

9159 **Comprehensive Examination of Barriers to Employment Among Persons who are Blind or Impaire**

Mississippi State University
P.O. Box 6189
Mississippi State, MS 39762
662-325-2001
Fax: 662-325-8989
TTY: 662-325-2694
nrtc@colled.msstate.edu
www.blind.msstate.edu

Jacqui Bybee, Research Associate II
Douglas Bedsaul, Research and Training Coordinator
Anne Carter, Research and Training Coordinator
Brenda Cavenaugh, Ph.D., Research Professor

A multi-phase research project designed to: identify barriers to employment; identify and develop innovative successful strategies to overcome these barriers; develop methods for others to utilize these strategies; disseminate this information to rehabilitation providers; replicate the use of selected strategies in other settings. *$20.00*

90 pages Paperback

9160 **Contrasting Characteristics of Blind and Visually Impaired Clients**

Mississippi State University
P.O. Box 6189
Mississippi State, MS 39762
662-325-2001
Fax: 662-325-8989
TTY: 662-325-2694
nrtc@colled.msstate.edu
www.blind.msstate.edu

Jacqui Bybee, Research Associate II
Douglas Bedsaul, Research and Training Coordinator
Anne Carter, Research and Training Coordinator
Brenda Cavenaugh, Ph.D., Research Professor

This report examines cases in the National Blindness and Low Vision Employment Database to identify and profile environmental and personal characteristics of clients who are blind or visually impaired and who were achieving successful and unsuccessful retention of competitive jobs. A total of 787 cases were analyzed. *$15.00*

44 pages Paperback

9161 **Dancing Cheek to Cheek**

Blind Children's Center
4120 Marathon Street
Los Angeles, CA 90029-3584
323-664-2153
info@blindchildrenscenter.org
www.blindchildrenscenter.org

Laura Meyers, Co-Author
Pamela Lansky, Co-Author

Beginning social, play and language interactions. *$10.00*

23 pages

9162 **Development of Social Skills by Blind and Visually Impaired Students**

American Foundation for the Blind/AFB Press
2 Penn Plaza
Suite 1102
New York, NY 10121
212-502-7600
800-232-5463
Fax: 888-545-8331
afbinfo@afb.net
www.afb.org

Carl R. Augusto, President & Chief Executive Officer
Rick Bozeman, Finance Director, Chief Financial Officer
Kelly Bleach, Chief Administrative Officer
Stacy Rollins, Executive Administrative Assistant to the President

Offers an examination of the social interactions of blind and visually impaired children in mainstreamed settings and the community that highlights the need to teach social interaction skills to children and provide them with support. Paperback. *$45.95*

232 pages

ISBN 0-891282-17-4

9163 **Diabetic Retinopathy**

National Association for Visually Handicapped
111 East 59th Street
New York, NY 10022-1202
212-821-9384
800-829-0500
Fax: 212-821-9707
info@lighthouse.org
lighthouse.org/navh

Mark G. Ackermann, President / CEO

A booklet offering information about Diabetic Retinopathy. LightHouse acquired NAVH.

9164 **Diversity and Visual Impairment: The Influence of Race, Gender, Religion and Ethnicity**

American Foundation for the Blind
2 Penn Plaza
Suite 1102
New York, NY 10121
212-502-7600
800-232-5463
Fax: 888-545-8331
afbinfo@afb.net
www.afb.org

Carl R. Augusto, President & Chief Executive Officer
Rick Bozeman, Finance Director, Chief Financial Officer
Kelly Bleach, Chief Administrative Officer
Stacy Rollins, Executive Administrative Assistant to the President

Cultural, social, ethnic, gender, and religious issues can influence the way an individual perceives and copes with a visual impairment. *$45.95*

480 pages

ISBN 0-891283-83-8

9165 Do You Remember the Color Blue: The Questions Children Ask About Blindness
Viking Books
375 Hudson Street
New York, NY 10014-3657
212-366-2000
Fax: 212-366-2933
ecommerce@us.penguingroup.com
www.us.penguingroup.com
John Makinson, Chairman & CEO
The author answers thirteen thought-provoking questions that children have asked her over the years about being blind.
78 pages
ISBN 0-670880-43-4

9166 Don't Lose Sight of Glaucoma
National Eye Institute
2020 Vision Place
Building 31 Room 6a32
Bethesda, MD 20892-3655
301-496-5248
800-869-2020
Fax: 301-402-1065
2020@nei.nih.gov
www.nei.nih.gov

9167 Early Focus: Working with Young Children Who Are Blind or Visually Impaired & Their Families
American Foundation for the Blind/AFB Press
2 Penn Plaza
Suite 1102
New York, NY 10121
212-502-7600
800-232-5463
Fax: 888-545-8331
afbinfo@afb.net
www.afb.org
Carl R. Augusto, President & Chief Executive Officer
Rick Bozeman, Finance Director, Chief Financial Officer
Kelly Bleach, Chief Administrative Officer
Stacy Rollins, Executive Administrative Assistant to the President
Describes early intervention techniques used with blind and visually impaired children and stresses the benefits of family involvement and transdisciplinary teamwork. Paperback. *$32.95*
176 pages
ISBN 0-891282-15-7

9168 Encyclopedia of Blindness and Vision Impairment Second Edition
Facts on File
132 West 31st Street
17th Floor
New York, NY 10001
800-322-8755
Fax: 800-678-3633
CustServ@InfobaseLearning.com
www.factsonfile.com
Jill Sardenga, Author
Susan Shelly, Co-Author
Alan Shelly MD, Co-Author
Scott M Steidl MD, Co-Author
Designed to provide both laymen and professionals with concise, practical information on the second most common disability in the U.S. *$65.00*
340 pages Hardcover
ISBN 0-816042-80-2

9169 Equals in Partnership: Basic Rights for Families of Children with Blindness
NAPVI
1 North Lexington Avenue
White Plains, NY 10601
617-972-7441
800-562-6265
Fax: 617-972-7444
napvi@guildhealth.org
www.napvi.org
Julie Urban, President
Venetia Hayden, Vice President
Susan LaVenture, Executive Director
Randi Sher, Secretary
A comprehensive compilation of educational advocacy materials to help parents better understand the special needs of their children with visual impairments and to assist them in accessing appropriate services for their children.

9170 Eye Research News
Research to Prevent Blindness
645 Madison Avenue
Floor 21
New York, NY 10022-1010
212-752-4333
800-621-0026
Fax: 212-688-6231
www.rpbusa.org
Diane S. Swift, Chair
Brian F. Hofland, PhD, President
David H. Brenner, VP & Secretary
Richard E. Baker, Treasurer & Asst. Secretary
Yearly publication from Research to Prevent Blindness. Free.
4 pages Yearly

9171 Eye and Your Vision
National Association for Visually Handicapped
111 East 59th Street
New York, NY 10022-1202
212-821-9384
800-829-0500
Fax: 212-821-9707
info@lighthouse.org
lighthouse.org/navh
Mark G. Ackermann, President / CEO
A large booklet offering information, with illustrations, on the eye. Includes information on protection of eyesight, how the eye works and vision disorders. Available in Russian and Spanish also. LightHouse acquired NAVH. *$5.00*

9172 Eye-Q Test
National Association for Visually Handicapped
111 East 59th Street
New York, NY 10022-1202
212-821-9384
800-829-0500
Fax: 212-821-9707
info@lighthouse.org
lighthouse.org/navh
Mark G. Ackermann, President / CEO
Five questions and answers to assist in knowing more about vision. Also available in Spanish and Russian. LightHouse acquired NAVH.

9173 Family Context and Disability Culture Reframing: Through the Looking Glass
Through the Looking Glass
3075 Adeline Street
Suite 120
Berkeley, CA 94703
510-848-1112
800-644-2666
Fax: 510-848-4445
tlg@lookingglass.org
www.lookingglass.org
Maureen Block, J.D., President
Thomas Spalding, Treasurer
Alice Nemon, Secretary
Mega Kirshbaum, Author
This article provides an overview of the issues and guiding perspectives underlying 'Through the Lookinglass' eighteen years of work with families. Available in Braille, large print or cassette. *$2.00*
5 pages

9174 Family Guide to Vision Care (FG1)
American Optometric Association
243 North Lindbergh Boulevard
Floor 1
Saint Louis, MO 63141-7881
800-365-2219
aoa.org
David A. Cockrell, OD, President
Andrea P. Thau, OD, Vice President
Barry Barresi, Executive Director
Christopher Quinn, OD, Secretary-Treasurer
Offers information on the early developmental years of your vision, finding a family optometrist and how to take care of your eyesight through the learning years, the working years and the mature years.

9175 **Family Guide: Growth & Development of the Partially Seeing Child**
National Association for Visually Handicapped
111 East 59th Street
New York, NY 10022-1202
212-821-9384
800-829-0500
Fax: 212-821-9707
info@lighthouse.org
lighthouse.org/navh

Mark G. Ackermann, President / CEO
Offers information for parents and guidelines in raising a partially seeing child. LightHouse acquired NAVH. *$.60*

9176 **Fathers: A Common Ground**
Blind Children's Center
4120 Marathon Street
Los Angeles, CA 90029-3584
323-664-2153
info@blindchildrenscenter.org
www.blindchildrenscenter.org

Paula Schmitt, Co-Author
Fernanda Armenta-Schmitt, Co-Author
Exploring the concerns and roles of fathers of children with visual impairments. *$10.00*
50 pages

9177 **Fighting Blindness News**
Foundation Fighting Blindness
7168 Columbia Gateway Drive
Suite 100
Columbia, MD 21046
410-423-0600
800-683-5555
Fax: 410-363-2393
TTY: 800-683-5551
info@FightBlindness.org
www.blindness.org

2x Year

9178 **First Steps**
Blind Children's Center
4120 Marathon Street
Los Angeles, CA 90029-3584
323-664-2153
info@blindchildrenscenter.org
www.blindchildrenscenter.org

Tanni L. Anthony, Co-Author
Fernanda Armenta-Schmitt, Co-Author
A handbook for teaching young children who are visually impaired. Designed to assist students, professionals and parents working with children who are visually impaired. Visit our website for many publications addressing training very young children who are blind or visually impaired. *$35.00*
203 pages

9179 **Foundations of Orientation and Mobility**
American Foundation for the Blind/AFB Press
2 Penn Plaza
Suite 1102
New York, NY 10121
212-502-7600
800-232-5463
Fax: 888-545-8331
afbinfo@afb.net
www.afb.org

Carl R. Augusto, President & Chief Executive Officer
Rick Bozeman, Finance Director, Chief Financial Officer
Kelly Bleach, Chief Administrative Officer
Stacy Rollins, Executive Administrative Assistant to the President
This text has been updated and revised and includes current research from a variety of disciplines, an international perspective, and expanded contents on low vision, aging, multiple disabilities, accessibility, program design and adaptive technology from more that 30 eminent subject experts. *$79.95*
775 pages
ISBN 0-891289-46-3

9180 **Foundations of Rehabilitation Counseling with Persons Who Are Blind or Visually Impaired**
American Foundation for the Blind/AFB Press
2 Penn Plaza
Suite 1102
New York, NY 10121
212-502-7600
800-232-5463
Fax: 888-545-8331
afbinfo@afb.net
www.afb.org

Carl R. Augusto, President & Chief Executive Officer
Rick Bozeman, Finance Director, Chief Financial Officer
Kelly Bleach, Chief Administrative Officer
Stacy Rollins, Executive Administrative Assistant to the President
Rehabilitation professionals have long recognized that the needs of people who are blind or visually impaired are unique and requie a special knowledge and expertise to provide and corrdinate rehabilitation services. *$59.95*
477 pages
ISBN 0-891289-45-3

9181 **General Facts and Figures on Blindness**
Prevent Blindness America
211 West Wacker Drive
Suite 1700
Chicago, IL 60606
800-331-2020
info@preventblindness.org
www.preventblindness.org

Paul G. Howes, Chairman
Hugh R. Parry, President & CEO,Prevent Blindness America
Jerome Desserich, Vice President & Chief Financial Officer
Danielle Disch, Development Manager

9182 **Get a Wiggle On**
American Alliance for Health, Phys. Ed. & Dance
1900 Association Drive
Reston, VA 20191-1598
703-476-3400
800-213-7193
Fax: 703-476-9527
aahperd.org

Dolly D. Lambdin, President
E. Paul Roetert, CEO
Marybell Avery, Director
Frances E. Cleland, Director
Gives teachers and parents practical suggestions for helping blind and visually impaired infants grow and learn like other children. *$5.00*
80 pages
ISBN 0-88314 -77-2

9183 **Gift of Sight**
RP Foundation Fighting Blindness
1401 W Mount Royal Ave
Baltimore, MD 21217-4245
410-225-9409
800-683-5555
Fax: 410-225-3936

9184 **Glaucoma**
Glaucoma Research Foundation
251 Post Street
Suite 600
San Francisco, CA 94108
415-986-3162
800-826-6693
Fax: 415-986-3763
question@glaucoma.org
glaucoma.org

Andrew L. Iwach, MD, Chair
Robert L. Stamper, MD, Vice Chair
Thomas M. Brunner, President and CEO
Bill Stewart, Secretary
Offers information on what glaucoma is, the causes, treatments, types of glaucoma, eye exams and prevention.

9185 **Glaucoma: The Sneak Thief of Sight**
National Association for Visually Handicapped
Fl 6
22 W 21st St
New York, NY 10010-6943
212-242-4438
800-3 C-NCOS
Fax: 631-736-0371
customerservice@cancos.com
cancos.com

Denise Green, Owner
A pamphlet describing the disease, treatment and medications. Also available in Russian and Spanish. Revised in 1999. *$3.50*

9186 **Guidelines and Games for Teaching Efficient Braille Reading**
American Foundation for the Blind/AFB Press
2 Penn Plaza
Suite 1102
New York, NY 10121
212-502-7600
800-232-5463
Fax: 888-545-8331
afbinfo@afb.net
www.afb.org

Carl R. Augusto, President & Chief Executive Officer
Rick Bozeman, Finance Director, Chief Financial Officer
Kelly Bleach, Chief Administrative Officer
Stacy Rollins, Executive Administrative Assistant to the President
Based on research in the areas of rapid reading and precision teaching, these guidelines represent a unique adaptation of a general reading program to the needs of Braille readers. Paperback. *$24.95*
116 pages Paperback
ISBN 0-891281-05-4

9187 **Guidelines for Comprehensive Low Vision Care**
National Association for Visually Handicapped
111 East 59th Street
New York, NY 10022-1202
212-821-9384
800-829-0500
Fax: 212-821-9707
info@lighthouse.org
lighthouse.org/navh

Mark G. Ackermann, President / CEO
A description of the proper method to conduct a low vision evaluation.LightHouse acquired NAVH. *$.50*

9188 **Handbook for Itinerant and Resource Teachers of Blind Students**
National Federation of the Blind
200 East Wells St
Baltimore, MD 21230-4914
410-659-9314
nfb@iamdigex.net

Doris Willoughby, Author
Sharon L Monthei, Co-Author
The Handbook provides help to teachers, school administrators or other school personnel that have experience with blind or visually impaired students. The Handbook devotes 45 pages to Braille and how to teach Braille for parents and teachers. There are other chapters offering information on the law, physical education, fitting in socially, testing and evaluation, home economics, daily living skills and more. *$23.00*
533 pages Softcover
ISBN 0-962412-20-1

9189 **Handbook of Information for Members of the Achromatopsia Network**
P.O. Box 214
Berkeley, CA 94701-214
510-540-4700
Fax: 510-540-4767
www.achromat.org

9190 **Health Care Professionals Who Are Blind or Visually Impaired**
American Foundation for the Blind
2 Penn Plaza
Suite 1102
New York, NY 10121
212-502-7600
800-232-5463
Fax: 888-545-8331
afbinfo@afb.net
afb.org

Carl R. Augusto, President & Chief Executive Officer
Rick Bozeman, Finance Director, Chief Financial Officer
Kelly Bleach, Chief Administrative Officer
Stacy Rollins, Executive Administrative Assistant to the President
This resource is essential reading for older students and young adults who are blind or visually impaired, their families, and the professionals who work with them. *$21.95*
160 pages
ISBN 0-891283-88-9

9191 **Heart to Heart**
Blind Children's Center
4120 Marathon Street
Los Angeles, CA 90029-3584
323-664-2153
info@blindchildrenscenter.org
www.blindchildrenscenter.org

Nancy Chernus-Mansfield, Co-Author
Dori Hayashi, Co-Author
Parents of children who are blind and partially sighted talk about their feelings. *$10.00*
12 pages

9192 **Heartbreak of Being A Little Bit Blind**
National Association for Visually Handicapped
111 East 59th Street
New York, NY 10022-1202
212-821-9384
800-829-0500
Fax: 212-821-9707
info@lighthouse.org
lighthouse.org/navh

Mark G. Ackermann, President / CEO
Summary of what it means to have impaired vision; includes illustrations. LightHouse acquired NAVH.

9193 **Helen Keller National Center Newsletter**
141 Middle Neck Road
Sands Point, NY 11050
516-944-8900
800-225-0411
Fax: 516-944-7302
hkncinfo@hknc.org
www.hknc.org

Joseph McNulty, Executive Director
The center provides evaluation and training in vocational skills, adaptive technology and computer skills, orientation and mobility, independent living, communication, speech-language skills, creative arts, fitness and leisure activities.

9194 **Helping the Visually Impaired Child with Developmental Problems**
Teachers College Press
1234 Amsterdam Avenue
New York, NY 10027
212-678-3929
800-575-6566
Fax: 212-678-4149
tcpress@tc.columbia.edu
www.teacherscollegepress.com

Mary Lynch, Manager
Brian Ellerbeck, Executive Acquisitions Editor
Marie Ellen Larcada, Senior Acquisitions Editor
Emily Spangler, Acquisitions Editor
This book aims to explore the human consequences of severe visual problems combined with other handicaps. The application of child development research to educational interventions, the need for educational and rehabilitative services that serve the human and the special needs of children and their families and the promise of technology in helping to expand communicative possibilities are also discussed. *$18.95*
216 pages Paperback
ISBN 0-807729-02-7

9195 **History and Use of Braille**
American Council of the Blind
2200 Wilson Boulevard
Suite 650
Arlington, VA 22201-3354
202-467-5081
800-424-8666
Fax: 703-465-5085
info@acb.org
acb.org

Kim Charlson, President
Jeff Thom, 1st Vice President
Melanie Brunson, Executive Director

A system of touch reading and writing for blind persons in which raised dots represent the letters of the alphabet.

9196 **How to Thrive, Not Just Survive**
American Foundation for the Blind/AFB Press
2 Penn Plaza
Suite 1102
New York, NY 10121
212-502-7600
800-232-5463
Fax: 888-545-8331
afbinfo@afb.net
www.afb.org

Carl R. Augusto, President & Chief Executive Officer
Rick Bozeman, Finance Director, Chief Financial Officer
Kelly Bleach, Chief Administrative Officer

Practical, hands-on guide for parents, teachers, and everyone involved in helping children develop the skills necessary for socialization, orientations and mobility, and leisure and recreational activities. Some of the subjects covered are eating, dressing, personal hygiene, self-esteem and etiquette. *$24.95*

104 pages Paperback
ISBN 0-89128 -48-7

9197 **Hub**
SPOKES Unlimited
1006 Main Street
Klamath Fals, OR 97601
541-883-7547
Fax: 541-885-2469
spokesunlimited.org

Wendy Howard, Executive Director
Celeste Wolf, Clerical Support Specialist II

Newsletter on rehabilitation, peer counseling, blindness, visual impairments, information and referral.

9198 **If Blindness Comes**
National Federation of the Blind
200 E Wells St
Baltimore, MD 21230
410-659-9314
Fax: 410-685-5653
nfb@nfb.org
www.nfb.org

Kenneth Jerrigan, Editor

An introduction to issues relating to vision loss and provides a positive, supportive philosophy about blindness. It is a general information book which includes answers to many common questions about blindness, information about services and programs for the blind and resource listings. Contact the Materials Center.

9199 **If Blindness Strikes Don't Strike Out**
2600 South 1st Street
Springfield, IL 62704
217-789-8980
800-258-8980
Fax: 217-789-9130
books@ccthomas.com
www.ccthomas.com

Bob Stork, Owner

9200 **Imagining the Possibilities: Creative Approaches to Orientation and Mobility Instructio**
American Foundation for the Blind
2 Penn Plaza
Suite 1102
New York, NY 10121
212-502-7600
800-232-5463
Fax: 888-545-8331
afbinfo@afb.net
afb.org

Carl R. Augusto, President & Chief Executive Officer
Rick Bozeman, Finance Director, Chief Financial Officer
Kelly Bleach, Chief Administrative Officer

Innovative and varied approaches to O&M techniques and teaching and dynamic suggestions on how to analyze learning styles are just some of the important topics included. *$49.95*

378 pages
ISBN 0-891283-82-X

9201 **Increasing Literacy Levels: Final Report**
Mississippi State University
P.O. Box 6189
Mississippi State, MS 39762
662-325-2001
Fax: 662-325-8989
TTY: 662-325-2694
nrtc@colled.msstate.edu
www.blind.msstate.edu

Jacqui Bybee, Research Associate II
Douglas Bedsaul, Research and Training Coordinator
Anne Carter, Research and Training Coordinator
Brenda Cavenaugh, Ph.D., Research Professor

This study is composed of three research projects to identify and analyze the appropriate use of and instruction in Braille, optical devices and other technologies as they relate to literacy and employment of individuals who are blind or visually impaired. *$20.00*

148 pages Paperback

9202 **Information Access Project**
National Federation of the Blind
200 East Wells St
Baltimore, MD 21230-4914
410-659-9314
Fax: 410-685-5653
nfb@nfb.org
nfb.org

Marc Maurer, President

Assists entities covered by the ADA in finding methods for converting visually displayed information, such as flyers, brochures and pamphlets, to formats accessible to individuals who are visually impaired.

9203 **Information on Glaucoma**
Glaucoma Research Foundation
251 Post Street
Suite 600
San Francisco, CA 94108
415-986-3162
800-826-6693
Fax: 415-986-3763
question@glaucoma.org
www.glaucoma.org

Andrew L. Iwach, MD, Chair
Robert L. Stamper, MD, Vice Chair
Thomas M. Brunner, President and CEO
Bill Stewart, Secretary

9204 **Intervention Practices in the Retention of Competitive Employment**
Mississippi State University
P.O. Box 6189
Mississippi State, MS 39762
662-325-2001
Fax: 662-325-8989
TTY: 662-325-2694
nrtc@colled.msstate.edu
www.blind.msstate.edu

Jacqui Bybee, Research Associate II
Douglas Bedsaul, Research and Training Coordinator
Anne Carter, Research and Training Coordinator
Brenda Cavenaugh, Ph.D., Research Professor

This study investigated the methods by which an individual can retain competitive employment after the onset of a significant vi-

sion loss. Interviews were conducted with 89 rehabilitation counselors across the US Strategies that contribute to successful job retention were identified as well as best rehabilitation practices in job retention. *$15.00*
60 pages Paperback

9205 **Know Your Eye**
American Council of the Blind
2200 Wilson Boulevard
Suite 650
Arlington, VA 22201-3354
202-467-5081
800-424-8666
Fax: 703-465-5085
info@acb.org
acb.org

Kim Charlson, President
Jeff Thom, 1st Vice President
Melanie Brunson, Executive Director

9206 **Large Print Loan Library**
National Association for Visually Handicapped
111 East 59th Street
New York, NY 10022-1202
212-821-9384
800-829-0500
Fax: 212-821-9707
info@lighthouse.org
lighthouse.org/navh

Mark G. Ackermann, President / CEO
A huge large print catalog of all the publications, fiction and non-fiction, cassette tapes, books-on-tape and videos available for the visually impaired from the loan library of the National Association for the Visually Handicapped. LightHouse acquired NAVH.

9207 **Large Print Loan Library Catalog**
National Association for Visually Handicapped
111 East 59th Street
New York, NY 10022-1202
212-821-9384
800-829-0500
Fax: 212-821-9707
info@lighthouse.org
lighthouse.org/navh

Mark G. Ackermann, President / CEO
Listing of over 7,000 commercially published and NAVH large print books available through NAVH on a loan basis. Includes a limited selection of titles available for purchase. LightHouse acquired NAVH.

9208 **Large Print Recipies for a Healthy Life**
123601 Wilshire
Los Angeles, CA 90025
310-826-8280
800-481-EYES
Fax: 310-458-8179

Judith Caditz PhD, Author
$21.95
283 pages
ISBN 0-962236-82-9

9209 **Learning to Play**
Blind Children's Center
4120 Marathon Street
Los Angeles, CA 90029-3584
323-664-2153
info@blindchildrenscenter.org
www.blindchildrenscenter.org

Susan L. Recchia, Co-Author
Presenting play activities to the pre-school child who is visually impaired. *$10.00*
12 pages

9210 **Let's Eat**
Blind Children's Center
4120 Marathon Street
Los Angeles, CA 90029-3584
323-664-2153
info@blindchildrenscenter.org
www.blindchildrenscenter.org

Jill Brody, Co-Author
Lynne Webber, Co-Author
Feeding a child with visual impairment. *$10.00*
28 pages

9211 **Library Services for the Blind**
South Carolina State University
300 College Street NorthEast
P.O. Box 7491
Orangeburg, SC 29117
803-536-7045
Fax: 803-536-8902
reference@scsu.edu
library.scsu.edu

Adrienne C. Webber, Dean, Library/Information Services
Ramona S. Evans, Administrative Specialist
Ruth A. Hodges, Reference & Information Specialist
Wanda L. Priester, Library Technical Asst.
News and information on developments in library services for readers who are blind and physically disabled.

9212 **Lifestyles of Employed Legally Blind People**
Mississippi State University
P.O. Box 6189
Mississippi State, MS 39762
662-325-2001
Fax: 662-325-8989
TTY: 662-325-2694
nrtc@colled.msstate.edu
www.blind.msstate.edu

Jacqui Bybee, Research Associate II
Douglas Bedsaul, Research and Training Coordinator
Anne Carter, Research and Training Coordinator
Brenda Cavenaugh, Ph.D., Research Professor
Results from a telephone survey show that visually impaired respondents are involved in a wide variety of activities with little restrictions on their range of activities. Sighted respondents tended to spend more time in child care, obtaining goods and services, attending to self-care activities and engaging in social activities, while visually impaired respondents spent more time in education and passive activities. This report is a study of expenditures and time use. *$10.00*
193 pages Paperback

9213 **Lion**
Lion's Clubs International
300 West 22nd Street
Oak Brook, IL 60523-8842
630-571-5466
Fax: 630-571-8890
TTY: 630-571-6533
www.lionsclubs.org/

Joseph Preston, International President
Jitsuhiro Yamada, 1st Vice President
Robert E. Corlew, 2nd Vice President
Peter Lynch, Executive Director
Publication for the blind.

9214 **Living with Achromatopsia**
P.O. Box 214
Berkeley, CA 94701-214
510-540-4700
Fax: 510-540-4767
www.achromat.org

Frances Futterman, Author
Consists entirely of comments from persons who know firsthand about living with achromatopsia.

9215 **Low Vision Questions and Answers: Definitions, Devices, Services**
American Foundation for the Blind/AFB Press
2 Penn Plaza
Suite 1102
New York, NY 10121
212-502-7600
800-232-5463
Fax: 888-545-8331
afbinfo@afb.net
afb.org

Carl R. Augusto, President & Chief Executive Officer
Rick Bozeman, Chief Financial Officer
Kelly Bleach, Chief Administrative Officer
Stacy Rollins, Executive Administrative Assistant to the President
What does low vision mean? What do low vision services cost? What diseases cause low vision? Answers to these and other questions are presented in a comprehensive format with accompanying photographs. $50.00/pack of 25.
21 pages Pamphlet
ISBN 0-891281-96-7

9216 **Low Vision: Reflections of the Past, Issues for the Future**
American Foundation for the Blind/AFB Press
2 Penn Plaza
Suite 1102
New York, NY 10121
212-502-7600
800-232-5463
Fax: 888-545-8331
afbinfo@afb.net
www.afb.org
Carl R. Augusto, President & Chief Executive Officer
Rick Bozeman, Chief Financial Officer
Kelly Bleach, Chief Administrative Officer
Stacy Rollins, Executive Administrative Assistant to the President
Background papers and a strategies section are used to identify the shifting needs of visually impaired persons and the resources that may be needed to address them. Paperback. *$34.95*
Paperback
ISBN 0-891282-18-1

9217 **Mainstreaming and the American Dream**
American Foundation for the Blind/AFB Press
2 Penn Plaza
Suite 1102
New York, NY 10121
212-502-7600
800-232-5463
Fax: 888-545-8331
afbinfo@afb.net
www.afb.org
Carl R. Augusto, President & Chief Executive Officer
Rick Bozeman, Chief Financial Officer
Kelly Bleach, Chief Administrative Officer
Stacy Rollins, Executive Administrative Assistant to the President
Based on in-depth interviews with parents and professionals, this research monograph presents information on the needs and aspirations of parents of blind and visually impaired children. Paperback. *$34.95*
256 pages Paperback
ISBN 0-891281-91-7

9218 **Mainstreaming the Visually Impaired Child**
NAPVI
1 North Lexington Avenue
White Plains, NY 10601
617-972-7441
800-562-6265
Fax: 617-972-7444
napvi@guildhealth.org
www.napvi.org
Julie Urban, President
Venetia Hayden, Vice President
Susan LaVenture, Executive Director
Randi Sher, Secretary
A unique, informative guide for teachers and educational professionals that work with the visually impaired. *$10.00*
121 pages Paper

9219 **Making Life More Livable**
American Foundation for the Blind
2 Penn Plaza
Suite 1102
New York, NY 10121
212-502-7600
800-232-5463
Fax: 888-545-8331
afbinfo@afb.net
www.afb.org
Carl R. Augusto, President & Chief Executive Officer
Rick Bozeman, Chief Financial Officer
Kelly Bleach, Chief Administrative Officer
Stacy Rollins, Executive Administrative Assistant to the President
Shows how simple adaptations in the home and environment can make a big difference in the lives of blind and visually impaired older persons. The suggestions offered are numerous and specific, ranging from how to mark food cans for greater visibility to how to get out of the shower safley. Large print. *$24.95*
128 pages
ISBN 0-891283-87-0

9220 **Meeting the Needs of People with Vision Loss: Multidisciplinary Perspective**
Resources for Rehabilitation
22 Bonad Road
Winchester, MA 01890
781-368-9080
Fax: 781-368-9096
orders@rfr.org
www.rfr.org
Susan L Greenblatt, Editor
Written by rehabilitation professionals, physicians, and a sociologist, this book discusses how to provide appropriate information and how to serve special populations. Chapters on the role of the family, diabetes and vision loss, special needs of children and adolescents, adults with hearing and vision loss. *$29.95*
ISBN 0-929718-07-0

9221 **Model Program Operation Manual: Business Enterprise Program Supervisors**
Mississippi State University
P.O. Box 6189
Mississippi State, MS 39762
662-325-2001
Fax: 662-325-8989
TTY: 662-325-2694
nrtc@colled.msstate.edu
www.blind.msstate.edu
Jacqui Bybee, Research Associate II
Douglas Bedsaul, Research and Training Coordinator
Anne Carter, Research and Training Coordinator
Brenda Cavenaugh, Ph.D., Research Professor
This monograph serves as a Model Program Operation Manual for Business Enterprise Program Supervisors who administer Randolph-Sheppard vending facilities under the Randolph-Sheppard Act. A wide variety of topics are covered including the role of the State Committee of Blind Venders, the role and responsibilities of the Vending Facility Operator, model qualification, for potential Facility Managers, guidelines for location of vending facilities and policies for closing vending facilities. *$20.00*
199 pages Paperback

9222 **More Alike Than Different: Blind and Visually Impaired Children**
American Foundation for the Blind/AFB Press
2 Penn Plaza
Suite 1102
New York, NY 10121
212-502-7600
800-232-5463
Fax: 888-545-8331
www.afb.org
Carl R. Augusto, President & Chief Executive Officer
Rick Bozeman, Chief Financial Officer
Kelly Bleach, Chief Administrative Officer
Stacy Rollins, Executive Administrative Assistant to the President
Offers photographs of blind and visually impaired children around the world learning to read and write, travel independently and performing basic living skills. Covers the most recent technological advances and demonstrates the universality of educational needs and goals. Paperback. $100.00/pack of 25.
ISBN 0-891281-69-0

9223 **Mothers with Visual Impairments who are Raising Young Children**
American Foundation for the Blind/AFB Press
2 Penn Plaza
Suite 1102
New York, NY 10121
212-502-7600
800-232-5463
Fax: 888-545-8331
afbinfo@afb.net
www.afb.org
Carl R. Augusto, President & Chief Executive Officer
Rick Bozeman, Chief Financial Officer
Kelly Bleach, Chief Administrative Officer
Stacy Rollins, Executive Administrative Assistant to the President
Available in Braille, large print or cassette. *$2.00*
16 pages

9224 Move With Me
Blind Children's Center
4120 Marathon Street
Los Angeles, CA 90029-3584
323-664-2153
info@blindchildrenscenter.org
www.blindchildrenscenter.org

Doris Hug, Co-Author
Nancy Chernus-Mansfield, Co-Author
A parent's guide to movement development for babies who are visually impaired. *$10.00*
12 pages

9225 National Eye Institute
National Institute of Health
31 Center Drive MSC 2510
Bethesda, MD 20892-2510
301-496-5248
Fax: 301-402-1065
www.nei.nih.gov

9226 Orientation and Mobility Primer for Families and Young Children
American Foundation for the Blind/AFB Press
2 Penn Plaza
Suite 1102
New York, NY 10121
212-502-7600
800-232-5463
Fax: 888-545-8331
afbinfo@afb.net
www.afb.org

Carl R. Augusto, President & Chief Executive Officer
Rick Bozeman, Chief Financial Officer
Kelly Bleach, Chief Administrative Officer
Stacy Rollins, Executive Administrative Assistant to the President
Practical information for helping a child learn about his or her environment right from the start. Covers sensory training, concept development and orientation skills. Paperback. *$14.95*
48 pages
ISBN 0-891281-57-6

9227 Out of the Corner of My Eye: Living with Vision Loss in Later Life
American Foundation for the Blind/AFB Press
2 Penn Plaza
Suite 1102
New York, NY 10121
212-502-7600
800-232-5463
Fax: 888-545-8331
www.afb.org

Carl R. Augusto, President & Chief Executive Officer
Rick Bozeman, Chief Financial Officer
Kelly Bleach, Chief Administrative Officer
Stacy Rollins, Executive Administrative Assistant to the President
A personal account of students' vision loss and subsequent adjustment that is full of practical advice and cheerful encouragement, told by an 87 year old retired college teacher who has maintained her independence and zest for life. Available in paperback or on audio cassette. *$23.95*
120 pages
ISBN 0-891281-82-1

9228 Out of the Corner of My Eye: Living with Macular Degeneration
American Foundation for the Blind/AFB Press
2 Penn Plaza
Suite 1102
New York, NY 10121
212-502-7600
800-232-5463
Fax: 888-545-8331
afbinfo@afb.net
www.afb.org

Carl R. Augusto, President & Chief Executive Officer
Rick Bozeman, Chief Financial Officer
Kelly Bleach, Chief Administrative Officer
Stacy Rollins, Executive Administrative Assistant to the President
A personal account of students' vision loss and subsequent adjustment that is full of practical advice and cheerful encouragement, told by an 87 year old retired college teacher who has maintained her independence and zest for life. *$29.95*
168 pages Paperback
ISBN 0-891238-31-2

9229 Pain Erasure: the Bonnie Prudden Way
Ballantine Books
1540 Broadway
New York, NY 10036-4039
212-751-2600
Fax: 212-572-4949

Bonnie Prudden, Author
Revolutionary breakthrough in pain relief involves trigger points-tender areas where muscles have been damaged from falls, childhood ailments, poor posture, and the stresses of daily life.

9230 Patient's Guide to Visual Aids and Illumination
National Association for Visually Handicapped
111 East 59th Street
New York, NY 10022-1202
212-821-9384
800-829-0500
Fax: 212-821-9707
info@lighthouse.org
lighthouse.org/navh

Mark G. Ackermann, President / CEO
A reference booklet offering information on aids for the visually impaired. LightHouse acquired NAVH. *$.75*

9231 Pediatric Visual Diagnosis Fact Sheets
Blind Children's Center
4120 Marathon Street
Los Angeles, CA 90029-3584
323-664-2153
info@blindchildrenscenter.org
blindchildrenscenter.org

Sarah E. Orth, CEO
Collection of fact sheets addressing commonly encountered eye conditions, diagnostic tests and materials. *$10.00*
10 pages

9232 Perkins Activity and Resource Guide: A Handbook for Teachers
Perkins School for the Blind
175 North Beacon Street
Watertown, MA 02472
617-924-3434
Fax: 617-972-7363
info@perkins.org
www.perkins.org

Frederic M. Clifford, Chair of the Board
Philip L. Ladd, Vice Chair of the Board
Leslie Nordon, Secretary
Charles C.J. Platt, Treasurer
This is a comprehensive, two volume guide with over 1,000 pages of activities, resources and instructional strategies for teachers and parents of students with visual and multiple disabilities. *$80.00*

9233 Personal Reader Update
Personal Reader Department
9 Centennial Dr
Peabody, MA 01960-7906
978-977-2000
800-343-0311
Fax: 978-977-2409

9234 Preschool Learning Activities for the Visually Impaired Child
NAPVI
1 North Lexington Avenue
White Plains, NY 10601
617-972-7441
800-562-6265
Fax: 617-972-7444
napvi@guildhealth.org
www.napvi.org

Julie Urban, President
Venetia Hayden, Vice President
Susan LaVenture, Executive Director
Randi Sher, Secretary
This guide for parents offers games and activities to keep visually impaired children active during the preschool years. *$8.00*
91 pages Paperback

9235 Reaching, Crawling, Walking... Let's Get Moving
Blind Children's Center
4120 Marathon Street
Los Angeles, CA 90029-3584
323-664-2153
info@blindchildrenscenter.org
www.blindchildrenscenter.org
Susan S. Simmons, Co-Author
Sharon O'Mara Maida, Co-Author
Orientation and mobility for preschool children who are visually imapired. *$10.00*
24 pages

9236 Reading Is for Everyone
Nat'l Lib Svc/Blind And Physically Handicapped
1291 Taylor Street North West
Washington, DC 20011
202-707-5100
Fax: 202-707-0712
TTY: 202-707-0744
nls@loc.gov
www.loc.gov/nls
Karen Keninger, Director

9237 Reading with Low Vision
Nat'l Lib Svc/Blind And Physically Handicapped
1291 Taylor Street North West
Washington, DC 20011
202-707-5100
Fax: 202-707-0712
TTY: 202-707-0744
nls@loc.gov
www.loc.gov/nls
Karen Keninger, Director

9238 Recording for the Blind & Dyslexic
20 Roszel Road
Princeton, NJ 08540
800-221-4792
Fax: 609-987-8116
Custserv@LearningAlly.org
www.learningally.org/
Brad Grob, Chairman
Harold J. Logan, Vice Chairman
Andrew Friedman, President & CEO
Jim Halliday, Executive Vice President
Provides recorded and computerized textbooks, library services and other educational resources to people who cannot effectively read standard print because of visual impairment, dyslexia or other physical disability. RFB&D is now Learning Ally.

9239 Reference and Information Services From NLS
Nat'l Lib Svc/Blind And Physically Handicapped
1291 Taylor Street North West
Washington, DC 20011
202-707-5100
Fax: 202-707-0712
TTY: 202-707-0744
nls@loc.gov
www.loc.gov/nls
Karen Keninger, Director

9240 Resource List for Persons with Low Vision
American Council of the Blind
2200 Wilson Boulevard
Suite 650
Arlington, VA 22201-3354
202-467-5081
800-424-8666
Fax: 703-465-5085
info@acb.org
acb.org
Kim Charlson, President
Jeff Thom, 1st Vice President
Melanie Brunson, Executive Director

9241 Rose-Colored Glasses
Human Sciences Press
233 Spring St
New York, NY 10013-1522
212-229-2859
800-221-9369
Fax: 212-463-0742
30 pages Hardcover
ISBN 0-87705 -08-8

9242 Say it with Sign
Harris Communications
15155 Technology Drive
Eden Prairie, MN 55344
952-388-2152
800-825-6758
Fax: 952-906-1099
info@harriscomm.com
harriscomm.com
Robert Harris, Owner
Contains both the serious and fun side of signing and provides the basic signs that might be needed in an emergency situation. *$299.50*
10-DVD set

9243 See A Bone
Facts on File
132 West 31st Street
14th Floor
New York, NY 10001
212-967-8800
800-683-5433
Fax: 212-760-0862
info@northernleasing.com
northernleasing.com
Mark Donnell, President
$65.00
352 pages
ISBN 0-816042-80-2

9244 See What I Feel
Britannica Film Company
345 4th Street
San Francisco, CA 94107
415-928-8466
Fax: 415-928-5027
Dave Bekowich, Owner
A blind child tells her friends about her trip to the zoo. Each experience was explained as a blind child would experience it. A teacher's guide comes with this video.
Film

9245 Selecting a Program
Blind Children's Center
4120 Marathon Street
Los Angeles, CA 90029-3584
323-664-2153
info@blindchildrenscenter.org
www.blindchildrenscenter.org
Deborah Chen, Co-Author
Mary Ellen McCann, Co-Author
A free guide for parents of infants and preschoolers with visual impairments.
28 pages

9246 Show Me How: A Manual for Parents of Preschool Blind Children
American Foundation for the Blind/AFB Press
2 Penn Plaza
Suite 1102
New York, NY 10121
212-502-7600
800-232-5463
Fax: 888-545-8331
afbinfo@afb.net
www.afb.org
Carl R. Augusto, President & Chief Executive Officer
Rick Bozeman, Chief Financial Officer
Kelly Bleach, Chief Administrative Officer
Stacy Rollins, Executive Administrative Assistant to the President
A practical guide for parents, teachers and others who help preschool children attain age-related goals. Covers issues on playing precautions, appropriate toys and facilitating relationships with playmates. Paperback. *$12.95*
56 pages
ISBN 0-891281-13-4

9247 **Sign of the Times**
Fanlight Productions
c/o Icarus Films
32 Court Street, 21st Floor
Brooklyn, NY 11201
718-488-8900
800-876-1710
Fax: 718-488-8642
info@fanlight.com
www.fanlight.com

Ben Achtenberg, Owner, Founder
Profiles a public school in the heart of Los Angeles - an American microcosm where over 300 languages are spoken, and where cultures and races collide. Fairfax High, publicized as the site of gang activity and murder, has long been a focus for bad press. But something very right is going on in this school. A Sign of the Times offers a positive example of how the American dream and American education are still alive

9248 **Special Technologies Alternative Resources**
210 McMorran Boulevard
Port Huron, MI 48060
810-987-7323
877-987-READ
star@sccl.lib.mi.us

Arnold H. Larson, Chairman
Kathleen J. Wheelihan, Vice Chairman
Arlene M. Marcetti, Board Member
Stan Arnetti, Director
Addresses the needs of a very unique diverse group of people by offering a full range of library services for people who cannot read standard print. Provides reading material in specialized formats that permit individuals with disabilities to have access to the written word, delivering to customer's mailboxes free of charge. Talking Book Machines, recorded books and magazines, descriptive videos, large print editions and Braille books and magazines.

9249 **Standing on My Own Two Feet**
Blind Children's Center
4120 Marathon Street
Los Angeles, CA 90029-3584
323-664-2153
info@blindchildrenscenter.org
www.blindchildrenscenter.org

Lorie Lynn LaPrelle, Author
A guide to constructing mobility devices for children who are visually impaired. *$10.00*
38 pages

9250 **Starting Points**
Blind Children's Center
4120 Marathon Street
Los Angeles, CA 90029-3584
323-664-2153
info@blindchildrenscenter.org
www.blindchildrenscenter.org

Deborah Chen, Co-Author
Jamie Dote-Kwan, Co-Author
Basic information for the clasroom teacher of 3 to 8 year olds whose multiple disabilities include visual impairment. *$35.00*
157 pages
ISBN 0-891280-61-8

9251 **Step-By-Step Guide to Personal Management for Blind Persons**
American Foundation for the Blind/AFB Press
2 Penn Plaza
Suite 1102
New York, NY 10121
212-502-7600
800-232-5463
Fax: 888-545-8331
afbinfo@afb.net
www.afb.org

Carl R. Augusto, President & Chief Executive Officer
Rick Bozeman, Chief Financial Officer
Kelly Bleach, Chief Administrative Officer
Stacy Rollins, Executive Administrative Assistant to the President
A manual of techniques in the areas of hygiene, grooming, clothing, shopping and child care. *$19.95*
136 pages Spiralbound
ISBN 0-891280-61-8

9252 **Student Teaching Guide for Blind and Visually Impaired College Students**
American Foundation for the Blind/AFB Press
2 Penn Plaza
Suite 1102
New York, NY 10121
212-502-7600
800-232-5463
Fax: 888-545-8331
afbinfo@afb.net
www.afb.org

Carl R. Augusto, President & Chief Executive Officer
Rick Bozeman, Chief Financial Officer
Kelly Bleach, Chief Administrative Officer
Stacy Rollins, Executive Administrative Assistant to the President
A comprehensive resource designed to enable the student to enter the classroom of a university or college with confidence. Large print. *$14.95*
52 pages
ISBN 0-891281-42-8

9253 **Survey of Direct Labor Workers Who Are Blind & Employed by NIB**
Mississippi State University
P.O. Box 6189
Mississippi State, MS 39762
662-325-2001
Fax: 662-325-8989
TTY: 662-325-2694
nrtc@colled.msstate.edu
www.blind.msstate.edu

Jacqui Bybee, Research Associate II
Douglas Bedsaul, Research and Training Coordinator
Anne Carter, Research and Training Coordinator
Brenda Cavenaugh, Ph.D., Research Professor
This report is a follow-up to surveys by National Industries for the Blind in 1983 and 1987 and summarizes the results of a national survey of approximately 500 legally blind direct labor workers. *$10.00*
101 pages Paperback

9254 **Talk to Me**
Blind Children's Center
4120 Marathon Street
Los Angeles, CA 90029-3584
323-664-2153
info@blindchildrenscenter.org
www.blindchildrenscenter.org

Nancy Chernus-Mansfield, Co-Author
Linda Kekelis, Co-Author
A language guide for parents of children who are visually impaired. *$10.00*
11 pages

9255 **Talk to Me II**
Blind Children's Center
4120 Marathon Street
Los Angeles, CA 90029-3584
323-664-2153
Fax: 323-665-3828
info@blindchildrenscenter.org
www.blindchildrenscenter.org

Nancy Chernus-Mansfield, Co-Author
Linda Kekelis, Co-Author
A sequel to Talk to Me *$10.00*
15 pages

9256 **Talking Books & Reading Disabilities**
Nat'l Lib Svc/Blind And Physically Handicapped
1291 Taylor Street North West
Washington, DC 20011
202-707-5100
Fax: 202-707-0712
TTY: 202-707-0744
nls@loc.gov
www.loc.gov/nls

Karen Keninger, Director

9257 **Talking Books for People with Physical Disabilities**
Nat'l Lib Svc/Blind And Physically Handicapped
1291 Taylor Street North West
Washington, DC 20011
202-707-5100
Fax: 202-707-0712
TTY: 202-707-0744
nls@loc.gov
www.loc.gov/nls
Karen Keninger, Director

9258 **Teaching Orientation and Mobility in the Schools: An Instructor's Companion**
American Foundation for the Blind
2 Penn Plaza
Suite 1102
New York, NY 10121
212-502-7600
800-232-5463
Fax: 888-545-8331
afbinfo@afb.net
www.afb.org
Carl R. Augusto, President & Chief Executive Officer
Rick Bozeman, Chief Financial Officer
Kelly Bleach, Chief Administrative Officer
Stacy Rollins, Executive Administrative Assistant to the President
This book, with its useful forms, checklists, and tips, will help O&M instructors and teachers of visually impaired students master the arts of planning schedules, organizing equipment and work routines, working with school personnel and educational team members, and effectively providing instruction to children with diverse needs. *$45.95*
176 pages
ISBN 0-891283-91-1

9259 **Teaching Visually Impaired Children**
Charles C. Thomas
2600 S First St
Springfield, IL 62704-4730
217-789-8980
800-258-8980
Fax: 217-789-9130
books@ccthomas.com
www.ccthomas.com
Michael P. Thomas, President
A comprehensive resource for the classroom teacher who is working with a visually impaired child for the first time, as well as a systematic overview of education for the specialist in visual disabilities. It approaches instructional challenges with clear explanations and practical suggestions, and it addresses common concerns of teachers in a reassuring and positive manner. Also available in cloth. *$49.95*
352 pages Paper 2004
ISBN 0-398074-77-7

9260 **Textbook Catalog**
National Braille Association
95 Allens Creek Road
Building 1, Suite 202
Rochester, NY 14618
585-427-8260
Fax: 585-427-0263
nbaoffice@nationalBraille.org
www.nationalBraille.org
Jan Carroll, President
Cindi Laurent, Vice President
David Shaffer, Executive Director
Heidi Lehmann, Secretary
Lists hundreds of scholarly, college and professional textbooks offered in large print, Braille or on cassette for visually impaired readers.
80 pages

9261 **Three Rivers News**
Carnegie Library of Pitts. Library for the Blind
4724 Baum Boulevard
Pittsburgh, PA 15213
412-687-2440
800-242-0586
Fax: 412-687-2442
Kathleen Kappel, Executive Director
Loans recorded books/magazines and playback equipment, large print books and described videos to western PA residents unable to use standard printed materials due to a visual, physical, or physically-based reading disability.
12 pages Quarterly

9262 **To Love this Life: Quotations by Helen Keller**
American Foundation for the Blind/AFB Press
2 Penn Plaza
Suite 1102
New York, NY 10121
212-502-7600
800-232-5463
Fax: 888-545-8331
www.afb.org
Carl R. Augusto, President & Chief Executive Officer
Rick Bozeman, Chief Financial Officer
Kelly Bleach, Chief Administrative Officer
Stacy Rollins, Executive Administrative Assistant to the President
Inspirational work that offers the penetrating observations of Helen Keller, the beloved deaf-blind champion of the rights of people with disabilities. Also available on cassette at $21.95 (ISBN# 0-89128-348-X) *$21.95*
144 pages Hardcover
ISBN 0-891283-47-1

9263 **Touch the Baby: Blind & Visually Impaired Children As Patients**
American Foundation for the Blind/AFB Press
2 Penn Plaza
Suite 1102
New York, NY 10121
212-502-7600
800-232-5463
Fax: 888-545-8331
afbinfo@afb.net
www.afb.org
Carl R. Augusto, President & Chief Executive Officer
Rick Bozeman, Chief Financial Officer
Kelly Bleach, Chief Administrative Officer
Stacy Rollins, Executive Administrative Assistant to the President
A how-to manual for health care professionals working in hospitals, clinics and doctors' offices. Teaches the special communication and touch-related techniques needed to prevent blind and visually impaired patients from withdrawing from the healthcare workers and the outside world. $25.00/pack of 25.
13 pages
ISBN 0-891281-97-5

9264 **Transition Activity Calendar for Students with Visual Impairments**
Mississippi State University
P.O. Box 6189
Mississippi State, MS 39762
662-325-2001
Fax: 662-325-8989
TTY: 662-325-2694
nrtc@colled.msstate.edu
www.blind.msstate.edu
Jacqui Bybee, Research Associate II
Douglas Bedsaul, Research and Training Coordinator
Anne Carter, Research and Training Coordinator
Brenda Cavenaugh, Ph.D., Research Professor
The Transition Activity Calendar guides the student with a visual disability through the maze of college preparation. Beginning in junior high school, clearly written steps are listed for each grade level. Students planning to enter college after high school graduation can check-off their accomplishments each step of the way. The calendar helps students focus on their goals while providing reminders of tasks yet to be completed. It can be used in a self-directed manner or in a group format. *$4.25*
16 pages Paperback

9265 **Transition to College for Students with Visual Impairments: Report**

Mississippi State University
P.O. Box 6189
Mississippi State, MS 39762
662-325-2001
Fax: 662-325-8989
TTY: 662-325-2694
nrtc@colled.msstate.edu
www.blind.msstate.edu

Jacqui Bybee, Research Associate II
Douglas Bedsaul, Research and Training Coordinator
Anne Carter, Research and Training Coordinator
Brenda Cavenaugh, Ph.D., Research Professor

A report offering results from telephone interviews of college students with visual impairments and mail surveys of college officials which examines the transition experience of successful college students. General domains in the study include demographics, educational history, computers, specialized and adaptive equipment, resources, college preparation, problems adjusting to college and O&M skills. A literature review covers preparing for college, task timelines,and classroom, labs and tests. *$20.00*

151 pages Paperback

9266 **Unseen Minority: A Social History of Blindness in the United States**

American Foundation for the Blind/AFB Press
2 Penn Plaza
Suite 1102
New York, NY 10121
212-502-7600
800-232-5463
Fax: 888-545-8331
abfinfo@abf.org
www.afb.org

Carl R. Augusto, President & Chief Executive Officer
Rick Bozeman, Chief Financial Officer
Kelly Bleach, Chief Administrative Officer
Stacy Rollins, Executive Administrative Assistant to the President

A lively narrative, with anecdotes, that recounts how the blind overcame discrimination to gain full participation in the social, educational, economic and legislative spheres. Hardcover. *$59.95*

573 pages Paperback
ISBN 0-891288-96-1

9267 **Vision Enhancement**

UN Printing
122
1790 E 54th St
Indianapolis, IN 46220-3454
317-254-1332
800-431-1739
Fax: 317-251-6588
www.visionww.org

Patricia L Price, Managing Editor

Designed to encourage and support individuals with vision loss, family members, and caregivers. *$25.00*

72-78 pages Quarterly

9268 **Visual Impairment: An Overview**

American Foundation for the Blind/AFB Press
2 Penn Plaza
Suite 1102
New York, NY 10121
212-502-7600
800-232-5463
Fax: 888-545-8331
afbinfo@afb.net
www.afb.org

Carl R. Augusto, President & Chief Executive Officer
Rick Bozeman, Chief Financial Officer
Kelly Bleach, Chief Administrative Officer
Stacy Rollins, Executive Administrative Assistant to the President

An overall look at the most common forms of vision loss and their impact on the individual. Includes drawings as well as photographs that stimulate how people with vision loss see. Paperback. *$19.95*

56 pages
ISBN 0-891281-74-0

9269 **Visual Impairments And Learning**

Sage Publications
2455 Teller Road
Thousand Oaks, CA 91320
805-499-0721
800-818-7243
Fax: 805-499-0871
info@sagepub.com
www.sagepub.com

Sara Miller McCune, Founder, Publisher, Executive Chairman
Blaise R Simqu, President & CEO
Tracey A. Ozmina, Executive Vice President & Chief Operating Officer
Stephen Barr, Managing Director/SAGE London, President of SAGE Internation

The major focus of this new, third edition is to present a new way of thinking about individuals with visual impairment so that they are viewed as participating members of a seeing world despite their reduced visual functioning. *$40.00*

213 pages
ISBN 0-890798-68-3

9270 **Walking Alone and Marching Together**

National Federation of the Blind
200 E Wells St.
Baltimore, MD 21230
410-659-9314
Fax: 410-685-5653
nfb@nfb.org
nfb.org

Floyd Matson, Author

The history of the organized blind movement, this book spans more than 50 years of civil rights, social issues, attitudes and experiences of the blind. Published in 1990, it has been read by thousands of blind and sighted persons and is used in colleges, libraries and programs across the country as an important tool in understanding blindness and it's impact on both personal lives and the society at large.

9271 **What Do You Do When You See a Blind Person- and What Don't You Do?**

American Foundation for the Blind/AFB Press
2 Penn Plaza
Suite 1102
New York, NY 10121
212-502-7600
800-232-5463
Fax: 888-545-8331
afbinfo@afb.net
afb.org

Carl R. Augusto, President & Chief Executive Officer
Rick Bozeman, Chief Financial Officer
Kelly Bleach, Chief Administrative Officer
Stacy Rollins, Executive Administrative Assistant to the President

Examples of real-life situations that teach sighted persons how to interact effectively with blind persons. Topics covered include how to help someone across the street, how not to distract a guide dog and how to take leave of a blind person. *$25.00*

8 pages
ISBN 0-891281-95-5

9272 **What Museum Guides Need to Know: Access for the Blind and Visually Impaired**

American Foundation for the Blind/AFB Press
2 Penn Plaza
Suite 1102
New York, NY 10121
212-502-7600
800-232-5463
Fax: 888-545-8331
afbinfo@afb.net
www.afb.org

Carl R. Augusto, President & Chief Executive Officer
Rick Bozeman, Chief Financial Officer
Kelly Bleach, Chief Administrative Officer
Stacy Rollins, Executive Administrative Assistant to the President

Explains how blind and visually impaired museum-goers experience art and offers pointers on greeting people, asking if help is needed and teaching about a specific work of art. Contains information on access laws, resources, training guides and guidelines for preparing large print, cassette and Braille materials. *$14.95*

64 pages Paperback
ISBN 0-891281-58-4

9273 **Work Sight**
Lighthouse Guild
250 West 64th Street
New York, NY 10023
646-874-8219
800-284-4422
Fax: 212-821-9707
info@lighthouse.org
www.lighthouseguild.org

Alan R. Morse, President & CEO
Lawrence E. Goldschmidt, Deputy Chair & Secretary
Himanshu R. Shah, CFO
Maura J. Sweeney, Senior Vice President, Programs & Services
Intended for employers and employees who have concerns about vision loss and job performance. *$25.00*

9274 **World Through Their Eyes**
Lighthouse Guild
250 West 64th Street
New York, NY 10023
646-874-8219
800-284-4422
Fax: 212-821-9707
info@lighthouse.org
www.lighthouseguild.org

Alan R. Morse, President & CEO
Lawrence E. Goldschmidt, Deputy Chair & Secretary
Himanshu R. Shah, CFO
Maura J. Sweeney, Senior Vice President, Programs & Services
Intended to help nursing home staff understand how residents with impaired vision perceive the world. Concrete suggestions help staff provide better care to visually impaired residents. *$25.00*

9275 **You Seem Like a Regular Kid to Me**
American Foundation for the Blind/AFB Press
2 Penn Plaza
Suite 1102
New York, NY 10121
212-502-7600
800-232-5463
Fax: 888-545-8331
afbinfo@afb.net
www.afb.org

Carl R. Augusto, President & Chief Executive Officer
Rick Bozeman, Chief Financial Officer
Kelly Bleach, Chief Administrative Officer
Stacy Rollins, Executive Administrative Assistant to the President
An interview with Jane, a blind child, tells other children what it's like to be blind. Jane explains how she gets around, takes care of herself, does her school work, spends her leisure time and even pays for things when she can't see money.
16 pages
ISBN 0-891289-21-6

Journals

9276 **Journal of Visual Impairment and Blindness**
Sheridan Press,
450 Fame Ave
Hanover, PA 17331-1585
717-632-3535
800-352-2210
Fax: 717-633-8929
www.sheridanreprints.com

Sharon Shively, Editor
Published in Braille, regular print and on ASC II disk and cassette, this journal contains a wide variety of subjects including rehabilitation, psychology, education, legislation, medicine, technology, employment, sensory aids and childhood development as they relate to visual impairments. $130 annual individual subscription, $180 annual institutional subscription.
64 pages Monthly
ISSN 0145-48 x

Magazines

9277 **Blind Educator**
National Organization of Blind Educators
200 East Wells Street
Jernigan Place
Baltimore, MD 21230
410-659-9314
Fax: 410-685-5653
nfb@nfb.org
www.nfb.org

Marc Mauer, President
Magazine specifically for blind educators.

9278 **Braille Forum**
American Council of the Blind
2200 Wilson Boulevard
Suite 650
Arlington, VA 22201-3354
202-467-5081
800-424-8666
Fax: 703-465-5085
info@acb.org
www.acb.org

Kim Charlson, President
Jeff Thom, 1st Vice President
Melanie Brunson, Executive Director
Offered in print, Braille, cassette, IBM computer disk and e-mail. $25 per format per year for companies and non-US residents.
48 pages Magazine

9279 **Braille Montior**
National Federation of the Blind
200 E Wells St
Baltimore, MD 21230
410-659-9314
Fax: 410-685-5653
nfbpublications@nfb.org
www.nfb.org

Gary Wunder, Editor
The Braille Monitor is the leading publication of the National Federation of the Blind. It covers the events and activities of the NFB and addresses the many issues and concerns of the blind.
$40.00
11 times a year

9280 **Dialogue Magazine**
Blindskills Inc.
P.O. Box 5181
Salem, OR 97304-0181
503-581-4224
800-860-4224
Fax: 503-581-0178
info@blindskills.com
www.blindskills.com

Marja Byers, Executive Director
B.T. Kimbrough, Editor
Publishes quarterly magazine in Braille, large-type, cassette and email of news items, technology and articles of special interest to visually impaired youth and adults. Annual subscription cost $35 for Braille, large print or cassette, $20 for email. *$35.00*
Quarterly

9281 **Future Reflections**
Deaf-Blind Division of the Ntn'l Fed of the Blind
200 E Wells St
Baltimore, MD 21230
410-659-9314
Fax: 410-685-5653
nfbpublications@nfb.org
nfb.org

Deborah Kent Stein, Editor
A magazine for parents and teachers of blind children.

9282 **Guide Magazine**
The Seeing Eye
P.O. Box 375
10 Washington Valley Road
Morristown, NJ 7963
973-539-4425
Fax: 973-539-0922
info@seeingeye.org
seeingeye.org

James A. Kutsch, Jr., Ph.D., President & CEO
Robert Pudlak, CFO & Director of Administration & Finance
Glenn Cianci, Director of Facilities Management
Jean Thomas, Director of Donor & Public Relations

The Guide offers stories of inspiration from our graduates and news of the latest program developments.

9283 **JBI Voice**
Jewish Braille Institute of America
110 Est 30th Street
New York, NY 10016
212-889-2525
800-433-1531
Fax: 212-689-3692
admin@jbilibrary.org
www.jbilibrary.org

Judy E. Tenney, Chairman
Thomas G. Kahn, Viec Chairman
Dr. Ellen Isler, President and CEO
Israel A Taub, Vice President and CFO

Monthly recorded magazine emphasizing Jewish current events and culture.

9284 **Jewish Braille Review**
Jewish Braille Institute of America
110 Est 30th Street
New York, NY 10016
212-889-2525
800-433-1531
Fax: 212-689-3692
admin@jbilibrary.org
www.jbilibrary.org

Judy E. Tenney, Chairman
Thomas G. Kahn, Viec Chairman
Dr. Ellen Isler, President and CEO
Israel A Taub, Vice President and CFO

The JBI seeks the integration of Jews who are blind, visually impaired and reading disabled into the Jewish community and society in general. More than 20,000 men, women and children in 50 countries receive a broad variety of JBI services.

9285 **Musical Mainstream**
Nat'l Lib Svc/Blind And Physically Handicapped
1291 Taylor Street North West
Washington, DC 20011
202-707-5100
Fax: 202-707-0712
TTY: 202-707-0744
nls@loc.gov
www.loc.gov/nls

Karen Keninger, Director

Articles selected from print music magazines.
Quarterly

9286 **Opportunity**
National Industries for the Blind
1310 Braddock Place
Alexandria, VA 22314-1691
703-310-0500
Fax: 703-998-8268
services@nib.org
www.nib.org

The Honorabl Krump, Esq., Chairman
Louis J. Jablonski, Jr., Vice Chairman
Kevin A. Lynch, President and Chief Executive Officer
James M Kesteloot, Director

Offers information and articles on the newest technology, equipment, services and programs for blind and visually impaired persons.
Quarterly

9287 **Providing Services for People with Vision Loss: Multidisciplinary Perspective**
Resources for Rehabilitation
22 Bonad Road
Winchester, MA 01890-1302
781-368-9080
Fax: 781-368-9096
orders@rfr.org
www.rfr.org

Susan L Greenblatt, Editor

A collection of articles by ophthalmologists and rehabilitation professionals, including chapters on operating a low vision service, starting self-help programs, mental health services, aids and techniques that help people with vision loss. *$19.95*
136 pages
ISBN 0-929718-02-0

Newsletters

9288 **AFB News**
American Foundation for the Blind/AFB Press
2 Penn Plaza
Suite 1102
New York, NY 10121
212-502-7600
800-232-5463
Fax: 888-545-8331
afbinfo@afb.net
www.afb.org

Carl R. Augusto, President & Chief Executive Officer
Rick Bozeman, Chief Financial Officer
Kelly Bleach, Chief Administrative Officer
Stacy Rollins, Executive Administrative Assistant to the President

National newsletter for general readership about blindness and visual impairments featuring people, programs, services and activities.
12 pages Quarterly

9289 **ASB Visions Newsletter**
ASB
919 Walnut Street
Philadelphia, PA 19107-5237
215-627-0600
Fax: 215-922-0692
asbinfo@asb.org
www.asb.org

Karla S. McCaney, President & CEO
Beth Deering, Director, Human Services
Richard Forsythe, Director, Braille Division & Custom Audio
Joyce Robertson, Director, Finance & Information Technology

Newsletter associated services for the blind and visually impaired.

9290 **Adaptive Services Division**
District of Columbia Public Library
901G St NW,
Rm 215
Washington, DC 20001-4531
202-727-2142
Fax: 202-727-0322
TTY: 202-559-5368
lbph.dcpl@dc.gov
www.dclibrary.org

Venetia Demson, Chief, Adaptive Services

DC Regional Library for the blind, deaf and physically handicapped. Provides adaptive technology and training programs.
8 pages Quarterly

9291 **Alumni News**
Guide Dogs for the Blind
P.O. Box 151200
San Rafael, CA 94915-1200
415-499-4000
800-295-4050
Fax: 415-499-4035
guidedogs.com

Bob Burke, Chairman
Stuart Odell, Vice Chairman
Chris Benninger, President and CEO
Jay Harris, Secretary

Restricted to graduates only.

9292 **Annual Report/Newsletter**
National Accreditation Council for Agencies/Blind
Rm 1004
15 E 40th St
New York, NY 10016-401 212-683-5068
Fax: 212-683-4475

Ruth Westman, Executive Director

Provides standards and a program of accreditation for schools and organizations which serve children and adults who are blind or vision impaired.

9293 **Association for Macular Diseases Newsletter**
210 East 64th Street
New York, NY 10065 212-605-3719
Fax: 212-605-3795
association@retinal-research.org
macula.org

Bernard Landou, President
Mary Fern Breheny, Board Member
Patricia Dahl, Board Member
Walter Ross, Editor-In-Chief

Not-for-profit organization promotes education and research in this scarcely explored field. Acts as a nationwide support group for individuals and their families endeavoring to adjust to the restrictions and changes brought about by macular disease. Offers hotline, educational materials, quarterly newsletter, support groups, referrals and seminars for persons and families affected by macular disease.

9294 **Awareness**
NAPVI
1 North Lexington Avenue
White Plains, NY 10601 617-972-7441
800-562-6265
Fax: 617-972-7444
napvi@guildhealth.org
www.napvi.org

Julie Urban, President
Venetia Hayden, Vice President
Susan LaVenture, Executive Director
Randi Sher, Secretary

Newsletter offering regional news, sports and activities, conferences, camps, legislative updates, book reviews, audio reviews, professional question and answer column and more for the visually impaired and their families.

Quarterly

9295 **BTBL News**
Braille and Talking Book Library
P.O. Box 942837
Sacramento, CA 94237-0001 916-654-0261
800-952-5666
Fax: 916-654-1119
btbl@library.ca.gov
www.btbl.ca.gov

Janet Coles, Editor
Christopher Berger, Senior Librarian
Olena Bilyk, Web Developer
Kim Brown, Communications Officer

BTBL News, the quarterly newsletter of the California Braille and Talking Book Library, features articles on topics of interest to library customers, including information about new services, existing services, events, staff and more.

9296 **Canes and Trails**
Guide Dogs for the Blind
P.O. Box 151200
San Rafael, CA 94915-1200 415-499-4000
800-295-4050
Fax: 415-499-4035
guidedogs.com

Bob Burke, Chairman
Stuart Odell, Vice Chairman
Chris Benninger, President and CEO
Jay Harris, Secretary

A quarterly newsletter for orientation and mobility specialists, rehabilitation professionals, teachers, and service providers in the field of blindness and visual impairment.

9297 **Community Connection**
Guide Dogs for the Blind
P.O. Box 151200
San Rafael, CA 94915-1200 415-499-4000
800-295-4050
Fax: 415-499-4035
guidedogs.com

Bob Burke, Chairman
Stuart Odell, Vice Chairman
Chris Benninger, President and CEO
Jay Harris, Secretary

A newsletter produced for our volunteers and other friends of Guide Dogs.

9298 **DVH Quarterly**
University of Arkansas at Little Rock
2801 S University Ave
Little Rock, AR 72204-1000 501-569-3000
Bob Brasher, Editor
Mary Boaz, Manager

Offers information on upcoming events, conferences and workshops on and for visual disabilities. Book reviews, information on the newest resources and technology, educational programs, want ads and more.

Quarterly

9299 **Deaf-Blind Perspective**
National Consortium on Deaf-Blindness
345 North Monmouth Avenue
Monmouth, OR 97361 503-838-8391
800-438-9376
Fax: 503-838-8150
TTY: 800-854-7013

Ingrid Amerson, Child Development Center
Lyn Ayer, Center on Deaf & Blindness
Robert Ayres, Evaluation and Research
Cori Brownell, Center on Early Learning

A free publication with articles, essays, and announcements about topics related to people who are deaf-blind. Published two times a year (Spring and Fall) by the Teaching Research Institute of Western Oregon University, its purpose is to provide information and serve as a forum for discussion and sharing ideas.

9300 **Fidelco**
Fidelco Guide Dog Foundation
103 Vision Way
Bloomfield, CT 06002 860-243-5200
Fax: 860-769-0567
info@fidelco.org
fidelco.org

Karen C. Tripp, Chairman
G. Kenneth Bernhard, Vice Chairman
Eliot D. Matheson, CEO
Diane R. Lindeland, VP, Finance

A newsletter published by Fidelco Guide Dog Foundation.

9301 **Focus**
Visually Impaired Center
1422 W Court St
Flint, MI 48503-5008 810-767-4014
Fax: 810-767-0020

Charles Tommasulo, Executive Director

Newsletter offering information for the visually impaired person in the forms of legislative and law updates, ADA information, support groups, hotlines, and articles on the newest technology in the field.

Quarterly

9302 **Gleams Newsletter**
Glaucoma Research Foundation
2345 Yale Street
2nd Floor
Palo Alto, CA 94306 650-328-3388
800-826-6693
Fax: 415-986-3763
info@glaucoma.org

Tom Brunner, CEO

Offers updated medical & research information on glaucoma. Included are glaucoma treatmant and coping tips, legsilative information, professional articles and book reviews.
6 pages Quarterly

9303 **Guide Dog News**
Guide Dogs for the Blind
P.O. Box 151200
San Rafael, CA 94915-1200
415-499-4000
800-295-4050
Fax: 415-499-4035
guidedogs.com

Bob Burke, Chairman
Stuart Odell, Vice Chairman
Chris Benninger, President and CEO
Jay Harris, Secretary
Read about changes to our teaching techniques, our new Adult Learning Program, vet tips, and find news about our graduates.

9304 **Guideway**
Guide Dog Foundation for the Blind
371 East Jericho Turnpike
Smithtown, NY 11787-2976
631-930-9000
800-548-4337
Fax: 631-930-9009
info@guidedog.org
www.guidedog.org

James C. Bingham, Chairman
Alphonce J. Brown, Jr., Vice Chairman
Wells B. Jones, CEO
Jack Sage, Secretary
Offers updates and information on the foundation's activities and guide dog programs. In print form but is also available on cassette.
Monthly

9305 **Guild Briefs**
Catholic Guild for The Blind
65 East Wacker Place
Suite 1010
Chicago, IL 60601
312-236-8569
Fax: 312-236-8128
www.guildfortheblind.org

Brett Christenson, President
Laura Rounce, Vice President
David Tabak, Executive Director
Toria Emas, Secretary
Monthly publication for individuals who are blind or visually impaired. It contains articles on topics such as service programs, scholarships, education, seniors, research, and government.
12 pages monthly

9306 **IAAIS Report**
Int'l Association of Audio Information Services
3920 Willshire Dr
Lawrence, KS 66049-3673
412-434-6023
800-280-5325
www.iaais.org

Stuart Holland, President
Marjorie Williams, 1st Vice President
Linda Hynson, Secretary
Andrea Pasquale, Treasurer
Newsletter for persons interested in radio reading services. *$7.00*
Quarterly

9307 **Insight**
Eye Bank Association of America
Ste 1010
1015 18th Street NorthWest
Washington, DC 20036
202-775-4999
Fax: 202-429-6036
info@restoresight.org
www.restoresight.org

Colleen Bayus, Communications Manager
An electronic newsletter.

9308 **LampLighter**
Columbia Lighthouse for the Blind
1825 K St. NW
Suite 1103
Washington, DC 20006
202-454-6400
Fax: 202-955-6401
info@clb.org
www.clb.org

Tony Cancelosi, President & CEO
Jocelyn Hunter, Senior Director, Communications
Toya Horten, Director, Administrative Operations
Bethany Martin, Manager, Youth & Education Services
Columbia Lighthouse for the Blind's monthly newsletter. Provides information on community news and events.

9309 **Library Users of America Newsletter**
American Council of the Blind
2200 Wilson Boulevard
Suite 650
Arlington, VA 22201-3354
202-467-5081
800-424-8666
Fax: 703-465-5085
info@acb.org
www.acb.org

Kim Charlson, President
Jeff Thom, 1st Vice President
Melanie Brunson, Executive Director
Published twice yearly, the newsletter contains much information about library services of particular interest to blind and visually impaired patrons, and is available in the following formats: Braille, audiocassette, large print and e-mail.

9310 **Light the Way**
Blind Children's Center
4120 Marathon Street
Los Angeles, CA 90029-3584
323-664-2153
info@blindchildrenscenter.org
blindchildrenscenter.org

Sarah E. Orth, CEO
Newsletter of the Blind Childrens Center, a family-centered agency which serves young children with visual impairments. The center-based and home-based services help the children to acquire skills and build their independence. The center utilizes its expertise and experience to serve families and professionals worldwide through support services, education and research.

9311 **Lighthouse Publication**
Chicago Lighthouse
1850 West Roosevelt Road
Chicago, IL 60608-1298
312-666-1331
Fax: 312-243-8539
TTY: 312-666-8874
publications@chicagolighthouse.org
www.thechicagolighthouse.org

Janet P. Szlyk, Ph.D., President & Chief Executive Officer
Mary Lynne Januszewski, Executive Vice President/CFO
Melanie M. Hennessy, SVP
Terrence J. longo, Executive Vice President/COO

9312 **Lights On**
Fight for Sight
Ste 809
391 Park Ave S
New York, NY 10016-8806
212-679-6060
Fax: 212-679-4466

Mary Prudden, Executive Director
A newsletter published by Fight for Sight.

9313 **Listen Up**
Recording for the Blind & Dyslexic
20 Roszel Rd
Princeton, NJ 8540-6206
609-452-0606
866-732-3585
Fax: 609-520-7990
www.learningally.org

John Kelly, CEO
RFB&D's bi-monthly electronic newsletter for members.

9314 **Long Cane News**
American Foundation for the Blind/AFB Press
2 Penn Plaza
Suite 1102
New York, NY 10121
212-502-7600
800-232-5463
Fax: 888-545-8331
afbinfo@afb.net
www.afb.org
Carl R. Augusto, President & Chief Executive Officer
Rick Bozeman, Chief Financial Officer
Kelly Bleach, Chief Administrative Officer
Stacy Rollins, Executive Administrative Assistant to the President
SemiAnnual

9315 **Magnifier**
Macular Degeneration Foundation
P.O. Box 531313
Henderson, NV 89053
702-450-2908
888-633-3937
liz@eyesight.org
www.eyesight.org
Liz Trauernicht, President & Director of Communications
Julie Zavala, VP & Asst. Director of Operations
David Seftel, EVP & Dircetor, R & D
Ron Gallamore, Board of Scientific Advisors
The Magnifier is the distributed without charge via email and by regular mail to those without access to the Internet. It features breaking news, clinical trails, clarifies recent reports in the media, announces new Internet resources and informs the public of important additions to the web site.

9316 **NAVH Update**
National Association of Visually Handicapped
111 East 59th Street
New York, NY 10022-1202
212-821-9384
800-829-0500
Fax: 212-821-9707
info@lighthouse.org
lighthouse.org/navh
Mark G. Ackermann, President / CEO
A newsletter published by the National Association of Visually Impaired. LightHouse acquired NAVH.

9317 **NBA Bulletin**
National Braille Association
95 Allens Creek Road
Building 1, Suite 202
Rochester, NY 14618
585-427-8260
Fax: 585-427-0263
nbaoffice@nationalBraille.org
www.nationalBraille.org
Jan Carroll, President
Cindi Laurent, Vice President
David Shaffer, Executive Director
Heidi Lehmann, Secretary
Published quarterly and included int he price of the regular and student NBA membership.

9318 **NLS News**
Nat'l Lib Svc/Blind And Physically Handicapped
1291 Taylor Street North West
Washington, DC 20011
202-707-5100
Fax: 202-707-0712
TTY: 202-707-0744
nls@loc.gov
www.loc.gov/nls
Karen Keninger, Director
Newsletter on current program developments.
Quarterly

9319 **NLS Newsletter**
Nat'l Lib Svc/Blind And Physically Handicapped
1291 Taylor Street North West
Washington, DC 20011
202-707-5100
Fax: 202-707-0712
TTY: 202-707-0744
nls@loc.gov
www.loc.gov/nls
Karen Keninger, Director
Newsletter on the service's volunteer activities.
Quarterly

9320 **PBA News**
Prevent Blindness America
211 West Wacker Drive
Suite 1700
Chicago, IL 60606
800-331-2020
info@preventblindness.org
www.preventblindness.org
Paul G. Howes, Chairman
Hugh R. Parry, President & CEO,Prevent Blindness America
Jerome Desserich, Vice President & Chief Financial Officer
Danielle Disch, Development Manager
Newsletter is filled with the information you need to protect your eyes, preserve your sight, and educate yourself about your own eye condition or that of a family member. Publication offered three times yearly.
3 times yearly

9321 **Planned Giving Department of Guide Dogs for the Blind**
Guide Dogs for the Blind
P.O. Box 151200
San Rafael, CA 94915-1200
415-499-4000
800-295-4050
Fax: 415-499-4035
guidedogs.com
Bob Burke, Chairman
Stuart Odell, Vice Chairman
Chris Benninger, President and CEO
Jay Harris, Secretary
A newsletter published by Guide Dogs for the Blind.

9322 **Playback**
Recording for the Blind & Dyslexic
20 Roszel Road
Princeton, NJ 08540
800-221-4792
Fax: 609-987-8116
Custserv@LearningAlly.org
www.learningally.org/
Brad Grob, Chairman
Harold J. Logan, Vice Chairman
Andrew Friedman, President & CEO
Jim Halliday, Executive Vice President
A publication dedicated to our unit's family of members, volunteers, supporters and staff. RFB&D is now Learning Ally.
3x Year

9323 **Quarterly Update**
National Association for Visually Handicapped
111 East 59th Street
New York, NY 10022-1202
212-821-9384
800-829-0500
Fax: 212-821-9707
info@lighthouse.org
lighthouse.org/navh
Mark G. Ackermann, President / CEO
Quarterly newsletter offering information on new products for the visually impaired, advances in medical treatments, new books available in the NAVH large print loan library and any new/updated booklets. Free. LightHouse acquired NAVH.

9324 **RP Messenger**
Texas Association of Retinitis Pigmentosa
P.O. Box 8388
Corpus Christi, TX 78468-8388
361-852-8515
Fax: 361-852-8515
tarp@homebiz101.com
Dorothy Steifel, Executive Director
A bi-annual newsletter offering information on Retinitis Pigmentosa. *$15.00*
Biannual

9325 **SCENE**
Braille Institute
527 North Dale Avenue
Anaheim, CA 92801
714-821-5000
800-272-4553
Fax: 714-527-7621
oc@Brailleinstitute.org
Brailleinstitute.org
Lester M. Sussman, Chairman
Peter A. Mindnich, President
Jon K. Hayashida, OD, FAAO, Vice President, Programs & Services
Rezaur Rehman, Vice President, Finance
Offers information on the organization, question and answer column, articles on the newest technology and more for visually impaired persons.

9326 **STAR**
Special Technologies Alternative Resources
210 McMorran Boulevard
Port Huron, MI 48060
810-987-7323
877-987-READ
star@sccl.lib.mi.us
www.sccl.lib.mi.us
Arnold H. Larson, Chairman
Kathleen J. Wheelihan, Vice Chairman
Arlene M. Marcetti, Board Member
Stan Arnetti, Director
A newsletter published by Special Technologies Alternative Resources.

9327 **Seeing Eye Guide**
The Seeing Eye
P.O. Box 375
10 Washington Valley Road
Morristown, NJ 07963
973-539-4425
Fax: 973-539-0922
info@seeingeye.org
seeingeye.org
James A. Kutsch, Jr., Ph.D., President & CEO
Randall Ivens, Director of Human Resources
Robert Pudlak, CFO & Director of Administration & Finance
David Johnson, Director of Instruction & Training
A quarterly publication from Seeing Eye.
Quarterly

9328 **Shared Visions**
Vista Center for the Blind & Visually Impaired
413 Laurel St
Santa Cruz, CA 95060-4904
831-458-9766
800-705-2970
Fax: 831-426-6233
information@vistacenter.org
Pam Brandin, Executive Director
A quarterly publication for Blind and Visually Impaired individuals from Vista Center for the Blind and Visually Impaired.

9329 **Sharing Solutions: A Newsletter for Support Groups**
Lighthouse Guild
250 West 64th Street
New York, NY 10023
646-874-8219
800-284-4422
Fax: 212-821-9707
info@lighthouse.org
www.lighthouseguild.org
Alan R. Morse, President & CEO
Lawrence E. Goldschmidt, Deputy Chair & Secretary
Himanshu R. Shah, CFO
Maura J. Sweeney, Senior Vice President, Programs & Services
A newsletter for members and leaders of support groups for older adults with impaired vision. The letter provides a forum for support groups members to network and share information, printed in a very large type format.

9330 **Sightings Newsletter**
Schepens Eye Research Institute
20 Staniford Street
Boston, MA 02114
617-912-0100
Fax: 617-912-0110
www.schepens.harvard.edu
Michael Gilmore, Director
Mary E. Leach, Director of Public Affairs
Frances Ng, Director of Human Resources
Ojas P. Mehta, Director, Intellectual Property & Commercial Ventures
Publication of prominent center for research on eye, vision, and blinding diseases; dedicated to research that improves the understanding, management, and prevention of eye diseases and visual deficiencies; fosters collaboration among its faculty members; trains young scientists and clinicians from around the world; promotes communication with scientists in allied fields; leader in the worldwide dispersion of basic scientific knowledge of vision.

9331 **Smith Kettlewell Rehabilitation Engineering Research Center**
2318 Fillmore Street
San Francisco, CA 94115
415-345-2000
Fax: 415-345-8455
rerc@ski.org
ski.org
John Brabyn, Ph.D., CEO/Executive Director
Ruth S. Poole, COO
Arthur Jampolsky, Director
Arthur Jampolsky, M.D., Founder
Reports on technology and devices for persons with visual impairments.

9332 **Student Advocate**
National Alliance of Blind Students NABS Liaison
Ste 1004
1155 15th St NW
Washington, DC 20005-2706
202-467-5081
800-424-8666
Fax: 202-467-5085
www.blindstudents.org
Melanie Brunson, Executive Director
A newsletter created by members of NABS and for any interested parties.

9333 **TBC Focus**
Chicago Public Library Talking Books Center
400 South State Street
Chicago, IL 60605
312-747-4300
800-757-4654
Fax: 312-747-1609
www.chipublib.org
Linda Johnson Rice, President
Christopher Valenti, VP
Christina Benitez, Secretary
Karim Adib, Director
Published quarterly by the Chicago Public Library Talking Book Center. Free of charge.
4 pages Quarterly

9334 **Talking Books Topics**
Nat'l Lib Svc/Blind And Physically Handicapped
1291 Taylor Street North West
Washington, DC 20011
202-707-5100
Fax: 202-707-0712
TTY: 202-707-0744
nls@loc.gov
www.loc.gov/nls
Karen Keninger, Director
New recorded books and program news
Bi-monthly

9335 **Upstate Update**
New York State Talking Book & Braille Library
222 Madison Avenue
Albany, NY 12230-1
518-474-5935
800-342-3688
Fax: 514-474-5786
TTY: 518-474-7121
nyslweb@mail.nysed.gov
www.nysl.nysed.gov

Bernard A. Margolis, State Librarian & Asst. Commissioner for Libraries
Loretta Ebert, Research Library Director
Liza Duncan, Technical Services & Systems

Books on audio cassette, cassette players, Braille books, summer reading programs, Braille writer, magnifiers, closed-circuit T.V., large-print photocopier, cassette books and magazines, children's books on cassette, reference materials on blindness and other handicaps.
4 pages Quarterly

9336 **Visual Aids and Informational Material**
National Association for Visually Handicapped
111 East 59th Street
New York, NY 10022-1202
212-821-9384
800-829-0500
Fax: 212-821-9707
info@lighthouse.org
lighthouse.org/navh

Mark G. Ackermann, President / CEO

A complete listing of the visual aids NAVH carries such as magnifiers, talking clocks, large print playing cards, etc. LightHouse acquired NAVH. *$2.50*
65 pages

9337 **Voice**
Vermont Assn for the Blind & Visually Impaired
60 Kimball Avenue
South Burlington, VT 05403
802-863-1358
800-639-5861
Fax: 802-863-1481
General@vabvi.org
vabvi.org

Thomas Chase, President
Stephen Pouliot, Executive Director
Kathleen Quinlan, Director of Operations
Lori Newsome, Office Manager

The Voice is a newsletter published by Vermont Association for the Blind and Visually Impaired.

9338 **Voice of Vision**
GW Micro
725 Airport North Office Park
Fort Wayne, IN 46825
260-489-3671
Fax: 260-489-2608
www.gwmicro.com

Dan Weirich, Owner

Offers product reviews, product announcements, tips for making systems or applications more accessible, or explanations of concepts of interest to any computer user or would-be computer user. This association newsletter is available in Braille, in large print, on audio cassette and on 3.5 or 5.25 IBM format diskette.
Quarterly

Audio/Visual

9339 **Aging and Vision: Declarations of Independence**
American Foundation for the Blind/AFB Press
2 Penn Plaza
Suite 1102
New York, NY 10121
212-502-7600
800-232-5463
Fax: 888-545-8331
afbinfo@afb.net
www.afb.org

Carl R. Augusto, President & Chief Executive Officer
Rick Bozeman, Chief Financial Officer
Kelly Bleach, Chief Administrative Officer
Stacy Rollins, Executive Administrative Assistant to the President

A very personal look at five older people who have successfully coped with visual impairment and continue to lead active, satisfying lives. Their stories are not only inspirational, but also provide practical, down-to-earth suggestions for adapting to vision loss later in life. 18 minute video tape. Also available in PAL, $52.95, 0-89128-276-9. *$42.95*
VHS
ISBN 0-891282-20-3

9340 **Blindness, A Family Matter**
American Foundation for the Blind/AFB Press
2 Penn Plaza
Suite 1102
New York, NY 10121
212-502-7600
800-232-5463
Fax: 888-545-8331
afbinfo@afb.net
www.afb.org

Carl R. Augusto, President & Chief Executive Officer
Rick Bozeman, Chief Financial Officer
Kelly Bleach, Chief Administrative Officer
Stacy Rollins, Executive Administrative Assistant to the President

A frank exploration of the effects of an individual's visual impairment on other members of the family and how those family members can play a positive role in the rehabilitation process. Features interviews with three families whose 'success stories' provide advice and encouragement, as well as interviews with newly blinded adults currently involved in a rehabilitation program. 23 minute video tape. Also available in PAL, $49.95, 0-89128-271-8. *$43.95*
VHS
ISBN 0-891282-22-X

9341 **Building Blocks: Foundations for Learning for Young Blind and Visually Impaired Children**
American Foundation for the Blind/AFB Press
2 Penn Plaza
Suite 1102
New York, NY 10121
212-502-7600
800-232-5463
Fax: 888-545-8331
afbinfo@afb.net
www.afb.org

Carl R. Augusto, President & Chief Executive Officer
Rick Bozeman, Chief Financial Officer
Kelly Bleach, Chief Administrative Officer
Stacy Rollins, Executive Administrative Assistant to the President

Presents the essential components of a successful early intervention program, including collaboration with family members, positive relationships between parents and professionals, public education, and attention to important programming components such as space exploration, Braille readiness, orientation and mobility, play, cooking and music. Includes interviews with parents. Available in English or Spanish. 10 minute video tape. Also available in PAL, $33.95, 0-89128-268-8. *$26.95*
VHS
ISBN 0-891282-14-9

9342 **Choice Magazine Listening**
85 Channel Drive
Port Washington, NY 11050
516-883-8280
888-724-6423
888-724-6423
Fax: 516-944-5849
choicemag@aol.com
www.choicemagazinelistening.org

Pamela Loeser, Editor in Chief
Ann Schlegel-Kyrkostas, Associate Editor
David Graham Pade, Associate Editor
Michael Tedeschi, Webmaster

A free audio anthology is available bi-monthly to visually impaired/physically disabled or dislexic persons nationwide. Playable on the special free 4-track cassette playback equipment which is provided by the Library of Congress through the National Library Service. Each issue features eight hours of unabridged magazine articles, short stories, poetry and media selections from over 100 sources. College level and older. Bimonthly distribution.
Bi-Monthly

9343 Heart to Heart
Blind Children's Center
4120 Marathon St
Los Angeles, CA 90029-3584 323-664-2153
info@blindchildrenscenter.org
www.blindchildrenscenter.org
Nancy Chernus-Mansfield, Co-Author
Dori Hayashi, Co-Author
Parents of blind and partially sighted children talk about their feelings. *$35.00*
VHS/DVD

9344 Juggler
Beacon Press
24 Farnsworth Street
Boston, MA 02210 617-742-2110
Fax: 617-723-3097
beacon.org
Helene Atwan, Executive Director
Andre was the young son of a wealthy, early Quebec fur trader. Because he was almost totally blind, he was overly protected by his family, and his movement outside his home was very limited.
Film

9345 Let's Eat Video
Blind Children's Center
4120 Marathon Street
Los Angeles, CA 90029-3584 323-664-2153
info@blindchildrenscenter.org
blindchildrenscenter.org
Jill Brody, Co-Author
Lynne Webber, Co-Author
Babies and toddlers with visual impairments lack one major avenue of exploration, and this significantly influences their awareness, perceptions, and anticipation of the food which is presented to them. *$35.00*
VHS/DVD

9346 Look Out for Annie
Lighthouse Guild
250 West 64th Street
New York, NY 10023 646-874-8219
800-284-4422
Fax: 212-821-9707
info@lighthouse.org
www.lighthouseguild.org
Alan R. Morse, President & CEO
Lawrence E. Goldschmidt, Deputy Chair & Secretary
Himanshu R. Shah, CFO
Maura J. Sweeney, Senior Vice President, Programs & Services
Depicts an older woman coping with her vision loss. It focuses on the emotional issues surrounding vision loss and conveys the idea that both the person with the vision disorder and their family and friends will need to make adjustments. *$25.00*
Video

9347 Not Without Sight
American Foundation for the Blind/AFB Press
PO Box 1020
Sewickley, PA 15143-920 412-741-1142
800-232-3044
Fax: 412-741-0609
www.afb.org
Carl R Augusto, President/CEO
Tracy Charlovich, Css
This video describes the major types of visual impairment and their causes and effects on vision, while camera simulations approximate what people with each impairment actually see. Also demonstrates how people with low vision make the best use of the vision they have. 20 minute video tape, $49.95. *$42.95*
VHS 17 min
ISBN 0-891282-27-3

9348 Out of Left Field
American Foundation for the Blind/AFB Press
2 Penn Plaza
Suite 1102
New York, NY 10121 212-502-7600
800-232-5463
Fax: 888-545-8331
afbinfo@afb.net
afb.org
Carl R. Augusto, President & Chief Executive Officer
Rick Bozeman, Chief Financial Officer
Kelly Bleach, Chief Administrative Officer
Stacy Rollins, Executive Administrative Assistant to the President
Illustrates how youngsters who are blind or visually impaired integrated with their sighted peers in a variety of recreational and athletic activities. 17 minute video tape. Also available in PAL, $33.95, 0-89128-270-X. *$29.95*
VHS 17 minutes
ISBN 0-891282-28-0

9349 See What I'm Saying
Fanlight Productions
c/o Icarus Films
32 Court Street, 21st Floor
Brooklyn, NY 11201 718-488-8900
800-876-1710
Fax: 718-488-8642
info@fanlight.com
www.fanlight.com
Ben Achtenberg, Founder, Owner
The documentary follows Patricia, who is deaf and from a Spanish-speaking family, through her first year at the Kendall Demonstration Elementary School of Gallaudet University.
VHS/DVD

9350 See for Yourself
Lighthouse Guild
250 West 64th Street
New York, NY 10023 646-874-8219
800-284-4422
Fax: 212-821-9707
info@lighthouse.org
www.lighthouseguild.org
Alan R. Morse, President & CEO
Lawrence E. Goldschmidt, Deputy Chair & Secretary
Himanshu R. Shah, CFO
Maura J. Sweeney, Senior Vice President, Programs & Services
This video features older adults with impaired vision who have been helped by vision rehabilitation. *$50.00*

9351 Shape Up 'n Sign
Harris Communications
15155 Technology Dr
Eden Prairie, MN 55344-2273 952-906-1180
800-825-6758
Fax: 952-906-1099
info@harriscomm.com
Robert Harris, Owner
An aerobic exercise tape introducing the basic sign language for deaf and hearing children ages six to ten. *$29.95*
30 Minutes DVD

9352 Sight by Touch
Landmark Media
3450 Slade Run Drive
Falls Church, VA 22042 703-241-2030
800-342-4336
Fax: 703-536-9540
info@landmarkmedia.com
Michael Hartogs, President
Peter Hartogs, VP New Business & Development
Beverly Weisenberg, Sales Rep
Richard Hartogs, VP Acquisitions
This video features the life and importance of Louis Braille. Vision-impaired performers and teachers demonstrate how Braille has benefitted their lives, and how improvements are constantly being made. *$195.00*
Video

9353 **Taping for the Blind**
3935 Essex Lane
Houston, TX 77027 713-622-2767
Fax: 713-622-2772
www.afb.org

Carl R. Augusto, President & Chief Executive Officer
Rick Bozeman, Chief Financial Officer
Robin Vogel, VP, Resource Development
Cynthia Fanzetti, Executive Director

An independent non profit educational organization funded by corporations, listeners and individuals, with a mission to turn sight into sound, enriching the lives of individuals with visual, physical and learning disabilities. Founded in 1967 to read materials not availiable through other sources onto standard audio cassettes in our custom recording division. In 1978, Houston Taping For The Blind signed on the air. Reading several dozen popular magazines and best selling books on the air.

9354 **We Can Do it Together!**
American Foundation for the Blind/AFB Press
2 Penn Plaza
Suite 1102
New York, NY 10121 212-502-7600
800-232-5463
Fax: 888-545-8331
afbinfo@afb.net
afb.org

Carl R. Augusto, President & Chief Executive Officer
Rick Bozeman, Chief Financial Officer
Kelly Bleach, Chief Administrative Officer
Stacy Rollins, Executive Administrative Assistant to the President

This video illustrates a transdisciplinary team orientation and mobility program for students with severe visual and multiple impairments, covering both adapted communication systems used to teach mobility skills and basic indoor mobility in the school. For mobility instructors, administrators, teachers of the visually and severely handicapped, occupational, physical and speech therapists and parents. Discussion guide included. 10 minute video tape. Also available in PAL, $33.95, 0-89128-267-X. *$26.95*
VHS
ISBN 0-891282-13-0

Sports

9355 **American Blind Bowling Association**
1209 Somerset Road
Raleigh, NC 27610 919-755-0700
www.abba1951.org

Thomas Lester, President
A.J. Inglesby, 1st Vice President
James Benton, 2nd Vice President
Judy Mandelkow, Tournament Director

Promotes blind bowling throughout the US and Canada by sanctioning blind bowling leagues and conducting a National Tournament. Current membership exceeds 2,000 people in the United States and Canada.

9356 **Basketball: Beeping Foam**
Maxi Aids
42 Executive Blvd.
Farmingdale, NY 11735-4710 631-752-0521
800-522-6294
Fax: 631-752-0689
TTY: 631-752-0738
sales@maxiaids.com
www.maxiaids.com

Elliot Zaretsky, Founder, President & CEO

This sound-making basketball enables the visually impaired to play basketball and other games. *$36.95*

9357 **Blind Outdoor Leisure Development**
P.O. Box 6639
Snowmass Village, CO 81615 970-923-0578
Fax: 970-923-7338
challengeaspen.org

Jimmy Yeager, President
Jack Kennedy, VP
Grayson Stover, Secretary
Kevin Berg, Director

Outdoor recreation for the blind. Winter program of skiing with guides plus numerous summer programs for the visually impaired.

9358 **Challenge Golf**
otivation Media
1245 Milwaukee Ave
Glenview, IL 60025-2400 847-827-9057
Fax: 847-297-6829

Dorothy Bauer, Coordinator

A plain-language video, Challenge Golf is packed with information for beginners or veterans. Peter Longo covers 5 handicaps (one-arm, one-leg, in a seated position, blind, and arthritis) clearly and concisely, on how to play golf with a physical disability. In color, complete with special effects, graphs and real handicapped golfers at play. *$38.95*
Home Edition

9359 **US Association of Blind Athletes**
1 Olympic Plaza
Colorado Springs, CO 80909 719-630-0422
Fax: 719-630-0616
www.usaba.org

Mark A. Lucas, MS, Executive Director
Ryan Ortiz, Assistant Executive Director
John Potts, Goalball High Performance director
Matt Simpson, Membership & Outreach Coordinator

Provides athletic opportunities and training in competitive sports for visually impaired and blind individuals throughout the US Competitions indlcude local, regional and national events, international events, and the Winter and Summer Paralympic Games.

9360 **United States Blind Golf Association**
3094 Shamrock St N
Tallahassee, FL 32309-2735 520-648-1088
info@usblindgolf.com
www.blindgolf.com

Dick Pomo, President

Provides blind and vision impaired gold tournaments to members.

Support Groups

9361 **Braille Institute Orange County Center**
527 North Dale Avenue
Anaheim, CA 92801 714-821-5000
800-272-4553
Fax: 714-527-7621
oc@Brailleinstitute.org
Brailleinstitute.org

Lester M. Sussman, Chairman
Peter A. Mindnich, President
Jon K. Hayashida, OD, FAAO, Vice President, Programs & Services
Rezaur Rehman, Vice President, Finance

Offers services, publications, information and programs free of charge to blind and visually impaired persons of all ages.

9362 **Consumer and Patient Information Hotline**
Prevent Blindness America
211 West Wacker Drive
Suite 1700
Chicago, IL 60606 800-331-2020
info@preventblindness.org
www.preventblindness.org/

Paul G. Howes, Chairman
Hugh R. Parry, President & CEO, Prevent Blindness America
Jerome Desserich, Vice President & Chief Financial Officer
Danielle Disch, Development Manager

A toll-free line offering free information on a broad range of vision, eye health and safety topics including sports eye safety, diabetic retinopathy, glaucoma, cataracts, children's eye disorders and more.

9363 Department of Ophthalmology Information Line

Eye & Ear Infirmary
1855 W Taylor St
Chicago, IL 60612-7242
312-996-6590
Fax: 312-996-7770
eyeweb@uic.edu
www.uic.edu

Jospeh White, President

Offers eye clinic and physician referrals to persons suffering from vision disorders as well as offers emergency information.

9364 Lighthouse International Information and Resource Service

111 East 59th Street
New York, NY 10022-1202
212-821-9384
800-829-0500
Fax: 212-821-9707
info@lighthouse.org
lighthouse.org

Mark G. Ackermann, President / CEO

Provides information about eye diseases, low vision, age-related vision loss, adaptive technology, optical devices, large print and Braille publishers, helps people find low vision services, vision rehabilitation services, and support groups across the U.S.; offers large selection of consumer products.

9365 National Association for Parents of Children with Visual Impairments (NAPVI)

1 North Lexington Avenue
White Plains, NY 10601
617-972-7441
800-562-6265
Fax: 617-972-7444
napvi@guildhealth.org
www.napvi.org

Julie Urban, President
Venetia Hayden, Vice President
Susan LaVenture, Executive Director
Randi Sher, Secretary

In 1979, a group of parents responding to their own needs founded NAPVI, the National Association for Parents of the Visually Impaired, Inc. Never before was there a self-help organization specific to the needs of families of children with visual impairments. Since that time, NAPVI has grown and helped families across the US and in other countries.

9366 VUE: Vision Use in Employment

Carroll Center for the Blind
770 Centre Street
Newton, MA 02458-2597
617-969-6200
800-852-3131
Fax: 617-969-6204
www.carroll.org

Joseph Abely, President
Brian Charlson, Director of Technology
Diane M. Newark, Chief Development Officer
Janet Perry, Human Resources Director

Provides engineering solutions plus training to help people keep jobs despite their vision loss.

9367 Washington Connection

American Council of the Blind
1703 N. Beauregard St
Ste 420
Alexandria, VA 22311
202-467-5081
800-424-8666
Fax: 703-465-5085
info@acb.org
www.acb.org/wc

Kim Charlson, President
Jeff Thom, 1st Vice President
Eric Bridges, Executive Director

Coverage of issues affecting blind people via legislative information, participates in law-making, legislative training seminars and networking of support resources across the US.

2020 Annual Disability Statistics Compendium

List of Tables

Population and Prevalence

Table 1.1 Resident Population—States: 2016 to 2019 . . . 903
Table 1.2 State Resident Population—Projections: 2015 to 2030 . . . 904
Table 1.3 Civilians Living in the Community for the United States and States, by Disability Status: 2019 . . . 905
Table 1.4 Civilians Living in the Community for the United States and States—Hearing Disability: 2019 . . . 906
Table 1.5 Civilians Living in the Community for the United States and States—Vision Disability: 2019 . . . 907
Table 1.6 Civilians Living in the Community for the United States and States—Cognitive Disability: 2019 . . . 908
Table 1.7 Civilians Living in the Community for the United States and States—Ambulatory Disability: 2019 . . . 909
Table 1.8 Civilians Living in the Community for the United States and States—Self-Care Disability: 2019 . . . 910
Table 1.9 Civilians Living in the Community for the United States and States—Independent Living Disability: 2019 . . . 911

Employment

Table 3.1 Employment—Civilians with Disabilities Ages 18 to 64 Years Living in the Community for the United States and States: 2019 . . . 912
Table 3.2 Employment—Civilians without Disabilities Ages 18 to 64 Years Living in the Community for the United States and States: 2019 . . . 913
Table 3.3 Employment—Civilians with Hearing Disabilities Ages 18 to 64 Years Living in the Community for the United States and States: 2019 . . . 914
Table 3.4 Employment—Civilians with Vision Disabilities Ages 18 to 64 Years Living in the Community for the United States and States: 2019 . . . 915
Table 3.5 Employment—Civilians with Cognitive Disabilities Ages 18 to 64 Years Living in the Community for the United States and States: 2019 . . . 916
Table 3.6 Employment—Civilians with Ambulatory Disabilities Ages 18 to 64 Years Living in the Community for the United States and States: 2019 . . . 917
Table 3.7 Employment—Civilians with Self-Care Disabilities Ages 18 to 64 Years Living in the Community for the United States and States: 2019 . . . 918
Table 3.8 Employment—Civilians with Independent Living Disabilities Ages 18 to 64 Years Living in the Community for the United States and States: 2019 . . . 919
Table 3.9 Employment Gap—Civilians Ages 18 to 64 Years Living in the Community for the United States and States, by Disability Status: 2019 . . . 920
Table 3.10 Change in Employment Gap—Civilians Ages 18 to 64 Years Living in the Community for the United States and States, by Disability Status: 2018 to 2019 . . . 921

Table 1.1 Resident Population - States: 2016 to 2019

State	2016	2017	2018	2019
U.S.	323,405,935	325,719,178	327,167,439	328,239,523
AL	4,860,545	4,874,747	4,887,871	4,903,185
AK	741,522	739,795	737,438	731,545
AZ	6,908,642	7,016,270	7,171,646	7,278,717
AR	2,988,231	3,004,279	3,013,825	3,017,804
CA	39,296,476	39,536,653	39,557,045	39,512,223
CO	5,530,105	5,607,154	5,695,564	5,758,736
CT	3,587,685	3,588,184	3,572,665	3,565,287
DE	952,698	961,939	967,171	973,764
DC	684,336	693,972	702,455	705,749
FL	20,656,589	20,984,400	21,299,325	21,477,737
GA	10,313,620	10,429,379	10,519,475	10,617,423
HI	1,428,683	1,427,538	1,420,491	1,415,872
ID	1,680,026	1,716,943	1,754,208	1,787,065
IL	12,835,726	12,802,023	12,741,080	12,671,821
IN	6,634,007	6,666,818	6,691,878	6,732,219
IA	3,130,869	3,145,711	3,156,145	3,155,070
KS	2,907,731	2,913,123	2,911,510	2,913,314
KY	4,436,113	4,454,189	4,468,402	4,467,673
LA	4,686,157	4,684,333	4,659,978	4,648,794
ME	1,330,232	1,335,907	1,338,404	1,344,212
MD	6,024,752	6,052,177	6,042,718	6,045,680
MA	6,823,721	6,859,819	6,902,149	6,892,503
MI	9,933,445	9,962,311	9,995,915	9,986,857
MN	5,525,050	5,576,606	5,611,179	5,639,632
MS	2,985,415	2,984,100	2,986,530	2,976,149

State	2016	2017	2018	2019
MO	6,091,176	6,113,532	6,126,452	6,137,428
MT	1,038,656	1,050,493	1,062,305	1,068,778
NE	1,907,603	1,920,076	1,929,268	1,934,408
NV	2,939,254	2,998,039	3,034,392	3,080,156
NH	1,335,015	1,342,795	1,356,458	1,359,711
NJ	8,978,416	9,005,644	8,908,520	8,882,190
NM	2,085,432	2,088,070	2,095,428	2,096,829
NY	19,836,286	19,849,399	19,542,209	19,453,561
NC	10,156,689	10,273,419	10,383,620	10,488,084
ND	755,548	755,393	760,077	762,062
OH	11,622,554	11,658,609	11,689,442	11,689,100
OK	3,921,207	3,930,864	3,943,079	3,956,971
OR	4,085,989	4,142,776	4,190,713	4,217,737
PA	12,787,085	12,805,537	12,807,060	12,801,989
RI	1,057,566	1,059,639	1,057,315	1,059,361
SC	4,959,822	5,024,369	5,084,127	5,148,714
SD	861,542	869,666	882,235	884,659
TN	6,649,404	6,715,984	6,770,010	6,829,174
TX	27,904,862	28,304,596	28,701,845	28,995,881
UT	3,044,321	3,101,833	3,161,105	3,205,958
VT	623,354	623,657	626,299	623,989
VA	8,414,380	8,470,020	8,517,685	8,535,519
WA	7,280,934	7,405,743	7,535,591	7,614,893
WV	1,828,637	1,815,857	1,805,832	1,792,147
WI	5,772,917	5,795,483	5,813,568	5,822,434
WY	584,910	579,315	577,737	578,759

Citation: Paul, S., Rafal, M., & Houtenville, A. (2020). Annual Disability Statistics Compendium: 2020 (Table 1.1). Durham, NH: University of New Hampshire, Institute on Disability. Note: Authors' calculations using the U.S. Census Bureau, American Community Survey, Public Use Microdata Sample, 2016-2019, which is subject to sampling variation.

Table 1.2 State Resident Population – Projections: 2015 to 2030

State	2015	2020	2025	2030
U.S.	322,365,787	335,804,546	349,439,199	363,584,435
AL	4,663,111	4,728,915	4,800,092	4,874,243
AK	732,544	774,421	820,881	867,674
AZ	7,495,238	8,456,448	9,531,537	10,712,397
AR	2,968,913	3,060,219	3,151,005	3,240,208
CA	40,123,232	42,206,743	44,305,177	46,444,861
CO	5,049,493	5,278,867	5,522,803	5,792,357
CT	3,635,414	3,675,650	3,691,016	3,688,630
DE	927,400	963,209	990,694	1,012,658
DC	506,323	480,540	455,108	433,414
FL	21,204,132	23,406,525	25,912,458	28,685,769
GA	10,230,578	10,843,753	11,438,622	12,017,838
HI	1,385,952	1,412,373	1,438,720	1,466,046
ID	1,630,045	1,741,333	1,852,627	1,969,624
IL	13,097,218	13,236,720	13,340,507	13,432,892
IN	6,517,631	6,627,008	6,721,322	6,810,108
IA	3,026,380	3,020,496	2,993,222	2,955,172
KS	2,852,690	2,890,566	2,919,002	2,940,084
KY	4,351,188	4,424,431	4,489,662	4,554,998
LA	4,673,721	4,719,160	4,762,398	4,802,633
ME	1,388,878	1,408,665	1,414,402	1,411,097
MD	6,208,392	6,497,626	6,762,732	7,022,251
MA	6,758,580	6,855,546	6,938,636	7,012,009
MI	10,599,122	10,695,993	10,713,730	10,694,172
MN	5,668,211	5,900,769	6,108,787	6,306,130
MS	3,014,409	3,044,812	3,069,420	3,092,410

State	2015	2020	2025	2030
MO	6,069,556	6,199,882	6,315,366	6,430,173
MT	999,489	1,022,735	1,037,387	1,044,898
NE	1,788,508	1,802,678	1,812,787	1,820,247
NV	3,058,190	3,452,283	3,863,298	4,282,102
NH	1,456,679	1,524,751	1,586,348	1,646,471
NJ	9,255,769	9,461,635	9,636,644	9,802,440
NM	2,041,539	2,084,341	2,106,584	2,099,708
NY	19,546,699	19,576,920	19,540,179	19,477,429
NC	10,010,770	10,709,289	11,449,153	12,227,739
ND	635,133	630,112	620,777	606,566
OH	11,635,446	11,644,058	11,605,738	11,550,528
OK	3,661,694	3,735,690	3,820,994	3,913,251
OR	4,012,924	4,260,393	4,536,418	4,833,918
PA	12,710,938	12,787,354	12,801,945	12,768,184
RI	1,139,543	1,154,230	1,157,855	1,152,941
SC	4,642,137	4,822,577	4,989,550	5,148,569
SD	796,954	801,939	801,845	800,462
TN	6,502,017	6,780,670	7,073,125	7,380,634
TX	26,585,801	28,634,896	30,865,134	33,317,744
UT	2,783,040	2,990,094	3,225,680	3,485,367
VT	673,169	690,686	703,288	711,867
VA	8,466,864	8,917,395	9,364,304	9,825,019
WA	6,950,610	7,432,136	7,996,400	8,624,801
WV	1,822,758	1,801,112	1,766,435	1,719,959
WI	5,882,760	6,004,954	6,088,374	6,150,764
WY	528,005	530,948	529,031	522,979

Citation: Paul, S., Rafal, M., & Houtenville, A. (2020). Annual Disability Statistics Compendium: 2020 (Table 1.2). Durham, NH: University of New Hampshire, Institute on Disability. Note: Sourced from the U.S. Census Bureau, 2005, Interim State Population Projections, Table 6, which is subject to sampling variation.

Table 1.3 Civilians Living in the Community for the United States and States, by Disability Status: 2019

State	Total	Disability [1]		No Disability	
		Count	%	Count	%
U.S.	323,205,854	41,156,238	12.7	282,049,616	87.3
AL	4,822,516	776,991	16.1	4,045,525	83.9
AK	707,254	81,224	11.5	626,030	88.5
AZ	7,166,899	939,236	13.1	6,227,663	86.9
AR	2,961,735	518,118	17.5	2,443,617	82.5
CA	39,007,866	4,131,700	10.6	34,876,166	89.4
CO	5,664,136	599,443	10.6	5,064,693	89.4
CT	3,516,334	416,285	11.8	3,100,049	88.2
DE	956,549	128,630	13.4	827,919	86.6
DC	696,740	80,506	11.6	616,234	88.4
FL	21,159,836	2,892,429	13.7	18,267,407	86.3
GA	10,424,810	1,315,079	12.6	9,109,731	87.4
HI	1,358,944	160,283	11.8	1,198,661	88.2
ID	1,765,304	244,874	13.9	1,520,430	86.1
IL	12,490,301	1,419,972	11.4	11,070,329	88.6
IN	6,632,029	899,869	13.6	5,732,160	86.4
IA	3,112,602	378,571	12.2	2,734,031	87.8
KS	2,853,285	403,009	14.1	2,450,276	85.9
KY	4,384,951	779,842	17.8	3,605,109	82.2
LA	4,541,927	720,434	15.9	3,821,493	84.1
ME	1,327,745	224,290	16.9	1,103,455	83.1
MD	5,948,457	669,208	11.3	5,279,249	88.7
MA	6,821,140	787,330	11.5	6,033,810	88.5
MI	9,880,650	1,400,651	14.2	8,479,999	85.8
MN	5,581,777	603,101	10.8	4,978,676	89.2
MS	2,905,826	489,036	16.8	2,416,790	83.2

State	Total	Disability [1]		No Disability	
		Count	%	Count	%
MO	6,028,475	888,763	14.7	5,139,712	85.3
MT	1,052,964	139,511	13.2	913,453	86.8
NE	1,905,059	228,223	12.0	1,676,836	88.0
NV	3,043,543	372,627	12.2	2,670,916	87.8
NH	1,343,295	172,882	12.9	1,170,413	87.1
NJ	8,776,794	908,500	10.4	7,868,294	89.6
NM	2,058,682	327,218	15.9	1,731,464	84.1
NY	19,216,347	2,232,990	11.6	16,983,357	88.4
NC	10,286,784	1,371,267	13.3	8,915,517	86.7
ND	745,320	84,400	11.3	660,920	88.7
OH	11,517,862	1,607,396	14.0	9,910,466	86.0
OK	3,873,840	613,031	15.8	3,260,809	84.2
OR	4,175,931	616,150	14.8	3,559,781	85.2
PA	12,593,310	1,795,737	14.3	10,797,573	85.7
RI	1,044,132	135,845	13.0	908,287	87.0
SC	5,056,002	724,298	14.3	4,331,704	85.7
SD	867,844	104,868	12.1	762,976	87.9
TN	6,720,796	1,030,836	15.3	5,689,960	84.7
TX	28,522,360	3,282,543	11.5	25,239,817	88.5
UT	3,180,641	289,731	9.1	2,890,910	90.9
VT	617,798	91,411	14.8	526,387	85.2
VA	8,308,751	1,006,318	12.1	7,302,433	87.9
WA	7,495,588	958,138	12.8	6,537,450	87.2
WV	1,763,441	349,732	19.8	1,413,709	80.2
WI	5,751,698	685,896	11.9	5,065,802	88.1
WY	568,984	77,816	13.7	491,168	86.3

Citation: Paul, S., Rafal, M., & Houtenville, A. (2020). Annual Disability Statistics Compendium: 2020 (Table 1.3). Durham, NH: University of New Hampshire, Institute on Disability. Note: Authors' calculations using the U.S. Census Bureau American Community Survey, Public Use Microdata Sample, 2019, which is subject to sampling variation.

[1] The U.S. Census uses a series of six questions to identify persons with vision, hearing, cognitive, ambulatory, self-care, and independent living disabilities. The cognitive, ambulatory, self-care, and independent living related questions are not asked of individuals less than five years old and the independent living related question is not asked of individuals less than 15 years old. See glossary for more information.

Table 1.4 Civilians Living in the Community for the United States and States – Hearing Disability: 2019

State	Total	Disability	Hearing [1] Count	Hearing [1] % Total	Hearing [1] % Disability
U.S.	323,205,854	41,156,238	11,525,119	3.6	28.0
AL	4,822,516	776,991	209,879	4.4	27.0
AK	707,254	81,224	31,438	4.4	38.7
AZ	7,166,899	939,236	286,214	4.0	30.5
AR	2,961,735	518,118	149,015	5.0	28.8
CA	39,007,866	4,131,700	1,153,006	3.0	27.9
CO	5,664,136	599,443	198,317	3.5	33.1
CT	3,516,334	416,285	104,556	3.0	25.1
DE	956,549	128,630	32,374	3.4	25.2
DC	696,740	80,506	12,924	1.9	16.1
FL	21,159,836	2,892,429	823,749	3.9	28.5
GA	10,424,810	1,315,079	337,948	3.2	25.7
HI	1,358,944	160,283	54,738	4.0	34.2
ID	1,765,304	244,874	83,047	4.7	33.9
IL	12,490,301	1,419,972	375,837	3.0	26.5
IN	6,632,029	899,869	254,783	3.8	28.3
IA	3,112,602	378,571	115,474	3.7	30.5
KS	2,853,285	403,009	126,066	4.4	31.3
KY	4,384,951	779,842	221,141	5.0	28.4
LA	4,541,927	720,434	188,131	4.1	26.1
ME	1,327,745	224,290	71,252	5.4	31.8
MD	5,948,457	669,208	157,080	2.6	23.5
MA	6,821,140	787,330	211,693	3.1	26.9
MI	9,880,650	1,400,651	380,552	3.9	27.2
MN	5,581,777	603,101	191,124	3.4	31.7
MS	2,905,826	489,036	123,801	4.3	25.3

State	Total	Disability	Hearing [1] Count	Hearing [1] % Total	Hearing [1] % Disability
MO	6,028,475	888,763	252,940	4.2	28.5
MT	1,052,964	139,511	51,291	4.9	36.8
NE	1,905,059	228,223	77,410	4.1	33.9
NV	3,043,543	372,627	109,730	3.6	29.4
NH	1,343,295	172,882	46,323	3.4	26.8
NJ	8,776,794	908,500	220,965	2.5	24.3
NM	2,058,682	327,218	103,535	5.0	31.6
NY	19,216,347	2,232,990	527,391	2.7	23.6
NC	10,286,784	1,371,267	371,743	3.6	27.1
ND	745,320	84,400	31,223	4.2	37.0
OH	11,517,862	1,607,396	432,432	3.8	26.9
OK	3,873,840	613,031	192,793	5.0	31.4
OR	4,175,931	616,150	195,582	4.7	31.7
PA	12,593,310	1,795,737	484,373	3.8	27.0
RI	1,044,132	135,845	36,825	3.5	27.1
SC	5,056,002	724,298	194,421	3.8	26.8
SD	867,844	104,868	39,582	4.6	37.7
TN	6,720,796	1,030,836	299,786	4.5	29.1
TX	28,522,360	3,282,543	917,254	3.2	27.9
UT	3,180,641	289,731	87,251	2.7	30.1
VT	617,798	91,411	29,854	4.8	32.7
VA	8,308,751	1,006,318	287,030	3.5	28.5
WA	7,495,588	958,138	288,785	3.9	30.1
WV	1,763,441	349,732	115,631	6.6	33.1
WI	5,751,698	685,896	211,157	3.7	30.8
WY	568,984	77,816	25,673	4.5	33.0

Citation: Paul, S., Rafal, M., & Houtenville, A. (2020). Annual Disability Statistics Compendium: 2020 (Table 1.4). Durham, NH: University of New Hampshire, Institute on Disability. Note: Authors' calculations using the U.S. Census Bureau American Community Survey, Public Use Microdata Sample, 2019, which is subject to sampling variation.

[1] The hearing disability question asks people of all ages, "Is this person deaf or does he/she have serious difficulty hearing?" See glossary for more information.

Table 1.5 Civilians Living in the Community for the United States and States – Vision Disability: 2019

State	Total	Disability	Vision [1] Count	Vision [1] % Total	Vision [1] % Disability	State	Total	Disability	Vision [1] Count	Vision [1] % Total	Vision [1] % Disability
U.S.	323,205,854	41,156,238	7,491,124	2.3	18.2	MO	6,028,475	888,763	157,493	2.6	17.7
AL	4,822,516	776,991	157,503	3.3	20.3	MT	1,052,964	139,511	22,710	2.2	16.3
AK	707,254	81,224	14,867	2.1	18.3	NE	1,905,059	228,223	40,699	2.1	17.8
AZ	7,166,899	939,236	173,175	2.4	18.4	NV	3,043,543	372,627	70,911	2.3	19.0
AR	2,961,735	518,118	101,411	3.4	19.6	NH	1,343,295	172,882	26,677	2.0	15.4
CA	39,007,866	4,131,700	746,326	1.9	18.1	NJ	8,776,794	908,500	170,826	1.9	18.8
CO	5,664,136	599,443	108,260	1.9	18.1	NM	2,058,682	327,218	78,596	3.8	24.0
CT	3,516,334	416,285	66,073	1.9	15.9	NY	19,216,347	2,232,990	385,428	2.0	17.3
DE	956,549	128,630	20,183	2.1	15.7	NC	10,286,784	1,371,267	243,774	2.4	17.8
DC	696,740	80,506	14,243	2.0	17.7	ND	745,320	84,400	14,595	2.0	17.3
FL	21,159,836	2,892,429	541,634	2.6	18.7	OH	11,517,862	1,607,396	264,374	2.3	16.4
GA	10,424,810	1,315,079	255,649	2.5	19.4	OK	3,873,840	613,031	128,862	3.3	21.0
HI	1,358,944	160,283	24,684	1.8	15.4	OR	4,175,931	616,150	102,303	2.4	16.6
ID	1,765,304	244,874	39,069	2.2	16.0	PA	12,593,310	1,795,737	303,469	2.4	16.9
IL	12,490,301	1,419,972	252,901	2.0	17.8	RI	1,044,132	135,845	20,375	2.0	15.0
IN	6,632,029	899,869	158,612	2.4	17.6	SC	5,056,002	724,298	150,224	3.0	20.7
IA	3,112,602	378,571	57,456	1.8	15.2	SD	867,844	104,868	19,651	2.3	18.7
KS	2,853,285	403,009	73,340	2.6	18.2	TN	6,720,796	1,030,836	206,294	3.1	20.0
KY	4,384,951	779,842	156,235	3.6	20.0	TX	28,522,360	3,282,543	694,392	2.4	21.2
LA	4,541,927	720,434	174,603	3.8	24.2	UT	3,180,641	289,731	45,285	1.4	15.6
ME	1,327,745	224,290	26,610	2.0	11.9	VT	617,798	91,411	14,079	2.3	15.4
MD	5,948,457	669,208	111,910	1.9	16.7	VA	8,308,751	1,006,318	186,968	2.3	18.6
MA	6,821,140	787,330	114,074	1.7	14.5	WA	7,495,588	958,138	148,831	2.0	15.5
MI	9,880,650	1,400,651	224,297	2.3	16.0	WV	1,763,441	349,732	69,713	4.0	19.9
MN	5,581,777	603,101	86,010	1.5	14.3	WI	5,751,698	685,896	102,660	1.8	15.0
MS	2,905,826	489,036	106,614	3.7	21.8	WY	568,984	77,816	16,196	2.8	20.8

Citation: Paul, S., Rafal, M., & Houtenville, A. (2020). Annual Disability Statistics Compendium: 2020 (Table 1.5). Durham, NH: University of New Hampshire, Institute on Disability. Note: Authors' calculations using the U.S. Census Bureau American Community Survey, Public Use Microdata Sample, 2019, which is subject to sampling variation.

[1] The vision disability question asks people of all ages, "Is this person blind or does he/she have serious difficulty seeing even when wearing glasses?" See glossary for more information.

Table 1.6 Civilians Living in the Community for the United States and States – Cognitive Disability: 2019

State	Total	Disability	Cognitive [1] Count	Cognitive [1] % Total	Cognitive [1] % Disability
U.S.	323,205,854	41,156,238	15,795,049	4.9	38.4
AL	4,822,516	776,991	285,317	5.9	36.7
AK	707,254	81,224	29,879	4.2	36.8
AZ	7,166,899	939,236	342,165	4.8	36.4
AR	2,961,735	518,118	199,379	6.7	38.5
CA	39,007,866	4,131,700	1,577,238	4.0	38.2
CO	5,664,136	599,443	223,954	4.0	37.4
CT	3,516,334	416,285	171,404	4.9	41.2
DE	956,549	128,630	55,679	5.8	43.3
DC	696,740	80,506	32,376	4.6	40.2
FL	21,159,836	2,892,429	1,071,096	5.1	37.0
GA	10,424,810	1,315,079	521,682	5.0	39.7
HI	1,358,944	160,283	55,201	4.1	34.4
ID	1,765,304	244,874	93,303	5.3	38.1
IL	12,490,301	1,419,972	513,415	4.1	36.2
IN	6,632,029	899,869	343,451	5.2	38.2
IA	3,112,602	378,571	147,074	4.7	38.8
KS	2,853,285	403,009	161,411	5.7	40.1
KY	4,384,951	779,842	311,687	7.1	40.0
LA	4,541,927	720,434	277,712	6.1	38.5
ME	1,327,745	224,290	92,003	6.9	41.0
MD	5,948,457	669,208	264,479	4.4	39.5
MA	6,821,140	787,330	327,060	4.8	41.5
MI	9,880,650	1,400,651	550,263	5.6	39.3
MN	5,581,777	603,101	237,773	4.3	39.4
MS	2,905,826	489,036	176,514	6.1	36.1
MO	6,028,475	888,763	353,181	5.9	39.7
MT	1,052,964	139,511	49,802	4.7	35.7
NE	1,905,059	228,223	79,044	4.1	34.6
NV	3,043,543	372,627	131,504	4.3	35.3
NH	1,343,295	172,882	68,001	5.1	39.3
NJ	8,776,794	908,500	346,364	3.9	38.1
NM	2,058,682	327,218	133,071	6.5	40.7
NY	19,216,347	2,232,990	828,780	4.3	37.1
NC	10,286,784	1,371,267	523,889	5.1	38.2
ND	745,320	84,400	27,971	3.8	33.1
OH	11,517,862	1,607,396	626,668	5.4	39.0
OK	3,873,840	613,031	222,345	5.7	36.3
OR	4,175,931	616,150	255,101	6.1	41.4
PA	12,593,310	1,795,737	735,879	5.8	41.0
RI	1,044,132	135,845	55,833	5.3	41.1
SC	5,056,002	724,298	262,049	5.2	36.2
SD	867,844	104,868	33,329	3.8	31.8
TN	6,720,796	1,030,836	405,596	6.0	39.3
TX	28,522,360	3,282,543	1,269,758	4.5	38.7
UT	3,180,641	289,731	124,144	3.9	42.8
VT	617,798	91,411	36,910	6.0	40.4
VA	8,308,751	1,006,318	366,385	4.4	36.4
WA	7,495,588	958,138	381,831	5.1	39.9
WV	1,763,441	349,732	133,785	7.6	38.3
WI	5,751,698	685,896	257,095	4.5	37.5
WY	568,984	77,816	25,219	4.4	32.4

Citation: Paul, S., Rafal, M., & Houtenville, A. (2020). Annual Disability Statistics Compendium: 2020 (Table 1.6). Durham, NH: University of New Hampshire, Institute on Disability. Note: Authors' calculations using the U.S. Census Bureau American Community Survey, Public Use Microdata Sample, 2019, which is subject to sampling variation.

[1] The cognitive disability question asks people 5 years and older "Because of a physical, mental, or emotional condition, does this person have serious difficulty concentrating, remembering, or making decisions?" See glossary for more information.

Table 1.7 Civilians Living in the Community for the United States and States – Ambulatory Disability: 2019

State	Total	Disability	Ambulatory [1] Count	Ambulatory [1] % Total	Ambulatory [1] % Disability	State	Total	Disability	Ambulatory [1] Count	Ambulatory [1] % Total	Ambulatory [1] % Disability
U.S.	323,205,854	41,156,238	20,869,933	6.5	50.7	MO	6,028,475	888,763	463,202	7.7	52.1
AL	4,822,516	776,991	424,732	8.8	54.7	MT	1,052,964	139,511	67,633	6.4	48.5
AK	707,254	81,224	37,366	5.3	46.0	NE	1,905,059	228,223	108,769	5.7	47.7
AZ	7,166,899	939,236	466,693	6.5	49.7	NV	3,043,543	372,627	196,580	6.5	52.8
AR	2,961,735	518,118	284,795	9.6	55.0	NH	1,343,295	172,882	80,737	6.0	46.7
CA	39,007,866	4,131,700	2,108,334	5.4	51.0	NJ	8,776,794	908,500	473,536	5.4	52.1
CO	5,664,136	599,443	266,974	4.7	44.5	NM	2,058,682	327,218	170,688	8.3	52.2
CT	3,516,334	416,285	199,169	5.7	47.8	NY	19,216,347	2,232,990	1,225,095	6.4	54.9
DE	956,549	128,630	61,742	6.5	48.0	NC	10,286,784	1,371,267	741,020	7.2	54.0
DC	696,740	80,506	42,632	6.1	53.0	ND	745,320	84,400	34,977	4.7	41.4
FL	21,159,836	2,892,429	1,543,979	7.3	53.4	OH	11,517,862	1,607,396	805,970	7.0	50.1
GA	10,424,810	1,315,079	689,580	6.6	52.4	OK	3,873,840	613,031	318,366	8.2	51.9
HI	1,358,944	160,283	79,291	5.8	49.5	OR	4,175,931	616,150	282,818	6.8	45.9
ID	1,765,304	244,874	111,030	6.3	45.3	PA	12,593,310	1,795,737	893,529	7.1	49.8
IL	12,490,301	1,419,972	740,303	5.9	52.1	RI	1,044,132	135,845	66,088	6.3	48.6
IN	6,632,029	899,869	453,213	6.8	50.4	SC	5,056,002	724,298	374,996	7.4	51.8
IA	3,112,602	378,571	170,402	5.5	45.0	SD	867,844	104,868	46,364	5.3	44.2
KS	2,853,285	403,009	192,687	6.8	47.8	TN	6,720,796	1,030,836	535,669	8.0	52.0
KY	4,384,951	779,842	408,316	9.3	52.4	TX	28,522,360	3,282,543	1,636,283	5.7	49.8
LA	4,541,927	720,434	358,915	7.9	49.8	UT	3,180,641	289,731	119,798	3.8	41.3
ME	1,327,745	224,290	102,267	7.7	45.6	VT	617,798	91,411	41,375	6.7	45.3
MD	5,948,457	669,208	337,727	5.7	50.5	VA	8,308,751	1,006,318	496,116	6.0	49.3
MA	6,821,140	787,330	369,112	5.4	46.9	WA	7,495,588	958,138	462,304	6.2	48.3
MI	9,880,650	1,400,651	689,840	7.0	49.3	WV	1,763,441	349,732	193,559	11.0	55.3
MN	5,581,777	603,101	251,936	4.5	41.8	WI	5,751,698	685,896	332,467	5.8	48.5
MS	2,905,826	489,036	277,043	9.5	56.7	WY	568,984	77,816	33,916	6.0	43.6

Citation: Paul, S., Rafal, M., & Houtenville, A. (2020). Annual Disability Statistics Compendium: 2020 (Table 1.7). Durham, NH: University of New Hampshire, Institute on Disability. Note: Authors' calculations using the U.S. Census Bureau American Community Survey, Public Use Microdata Sample, 2019, which is subject to sampling variation.

[1] The ambulatory disability question asks people 5 years old or older, "Does this person have serious difficulty walking or climbing stairs?" See glossary for more information.

Table 1.8 Civilians Living in the Community for the United States and States – Self-Care Disability: 2019

State	Total	Disability	Self-Care [1] Count	Self-Care [1] % Total	Self-Care [1] % Disability
U.S.	323,205,854	41,156,238	7,996,389	2.5	19.4
AL	4,822,516	776,991	145,049	3.0	18.7
AK	707,254	81,224	12,925	1.8	15.9
AZ	7,166,899	939,236	158,689	2.2	16.9
AR	2,961,735	518,118	100,668	3.4	19.4
CA	39,007,866	4,131,700	971,130	2.5	23.5
CO	5,664,136	599,443	95,497	1.7	15.9
CT	3,516,334	416,285	83,526	2.4	20.1
DE	956,549	128,630	23,153	2.4	18.0
DC	696,740	80,506	14,189	2.0	17.6
FL	21,159,836	2,892,429	567,289	2.7	19.6
GA	10,424,810	1,315,079	237,452	2.3	18.1
HI	1,358,944	160,283	29,533	2.2	18.4
ID	1,765,304	244,874	34,831	2.0	14.2
IL	12,490,301	1,419,972	274,119	2.2	19.3
IN	6,632,029	899,869	163,070	2.5	18.1
IA	3,112,602	378,571	62,831	2.0	16.6
KS	2,853,285	403,009	67,100	2.4	16.6
KY	4,384,951	779,842	140,039	3.2	18.0
LA	4,541,927	720,434	138,551	3.1	19.2
ME	1,327,745	224,290	34,354	2.6	15.3
MD	5,948,457	669,208	127,172	2.1	19.0
MA	6,821,140	787,330	157,060	2.3	19.9
MI	9,880,650	1,400,651	268,436	2.7	19.2
MN	5,581,777	603,101	106,179	1.9	17.6
MS	2,905,826	489,036	96,875	3.3	19.8
MO	6,028,475	888,763	165,516	2.7	18.6
MT	1,052,964	139,511	22,031	2.1	15.8
NE	1,905,059	228,223	39,001	2.0	17.1
NV	3,043,543	372,627	71,362	2.3	19.2
NH	1,343,295	172,882	26,571	2.0	15.4
NJ	8,776,794	908,500	196,061	2.2	21.6
NM	2,058,682	327,218	67,096	3.3	20.5
NY	19,216,347	2,232,990	514,437	2.7	23.0
NC	10,286,784	1,371,267	265,383	2.6	19.4
ND	745,320	84,400	13,043	1.7	15.5
OH	11,517,862	1,607,396	282,157	2.4	17.6
OK	3,873,840	613,031	108,401	2.8	17.7
OR	4,175,931	616,150	105,181	2.5	17.1
PA	12,593,310	1,795,737	348,668	2.8	19.4
RI	1,044,132	135,845	27,914	2.7	20.5
SC	5,056,002	724,298	139,968	2.8	19.3
SD	867,844	104,868	15,011	1.7	14.3
TN	6,720,796	1,030,836	180,076	2.7	17.5
TX	28,522,360	3,282,543	665,868	2.3	20.3
UT	3,180,641	289,731	43,924	1.4	15.2
VT	617,798	91,411	13,276	2.1	14.5
VA	8,308,751	1,006,318	191,270	2.3	19.0
WA	7,495,588	958,138	179,596	2.4	18.7
WV	1,763,441	349,732	66,337	3.8	19.0
WI	5,751,698	685,896	130,312	2.3	19.0
WY	568,984	77,816	8,212	1.4	10.6

Citation: Paul, S., Rafal, M., & Houtenville, A. (2020). Annual Disability Statistics Compendium: 2020 (Table 1.8). Durham, NH: University of New Hampshire, Institute on Disability. Note: Authors' calculations using the U.S. Census Bureau American Community Survey, Public Use Microdata Sample, 2019, which is subject to sampling variation.

[1] The self-care disability question asks people 5 years old or older, "Does this person have difficulty dressing or bathing?" See glossary for more information.

Table 1.9 Civilians Living in the Community for the United States and States – Independent Living Disability: 2019

State	Total	Disability	Independent Living [1] Count	% Total	% Disability
U.S.	323,205,854	41,156,238	15,003,428	4.6	36.5
AL	4,822,516	776,991	277,840	5.8	35.8
AK	707,254	81,224	23,347	3.3	28.7
AZ	7,166,899	939,236	322,039	4.5	34.3
AR	2,961,735	518,118	183,789	6.2	35.5
CA	39,007,866	4,131,700	1,672,446	4.3	40.5
CO	5,664,136	599,443	196,506	3.5	32.8
CT	3,516,334	416,285	157,864	4.5	37.9
DE	956,549	128,630	43,096	4.5	33.5
DC	696,740	80,506	31,843	4.6	39.6
FL	21,159,836	2,892,429	1,048,969	5.0	36.3
GA	10,424,810	1,315,079	470,539	4.5	35.8
HI	1,358,944	160,283	65,412	4.8	40.8
ID	1,765,304	244,874	70,476	4.0	28.8
IL	12,490,301	1,419,972	555,878	4.5	39.1
IN	6,632,029	899,869	316,574	4.8	35.2
IA	3,112,602	378,571	127,351	4.1	33.6
KS	2,853,285	403,009	133,477	4.7	33.1
KY	4,384,951	779,842	272,966	6.2	35.0
LA	4,541,927	720,434	247,643	5.5	34.4
ME	1,327,745	224,290	80,900	6.1	36.1
MD	5,948,457	669,208	241,423	4.1	36.1
MA	6,821,140	787,330	296,654	4.3	37.7
MI	9,880,650	1,400,651	508,747	5.1	36.3
MN	5,581,777	603,101	212,076	3.8	35.2
MS	2,905,826	489,036	181,126	6.2	37.0

State	Total	Disability	Independent Living [1] Count	% Total	% Disability
MO	6,028,475	888,763	329,754	5.5	37.1
MT	1,052,964	139,511	46,101	4.4	33.0
NE	1,905,059	228,223	70,890	3.7	31.1
NV	3,043,543	372,627	130,615	4.3	35.1
NH	1,343,295	172,882	57,356	4.3	33.2
NJ	8,776,794	908,500	361,160	4.1	39.8
NM	2,058,682	327,218	116,576	5.7	35.6
NY	19,216,347	2,232,990	894,917	4.7	40.1
NC	10,286,784	1,371,267	496,173	4.8	36.2
ND	745,320	84,400	25,979	3.5	30.8
OH	11,517,862	1,607,396	566,208	4.9	35.2
OK	3,873,840	613,031	212,296	5.5	34.6
OR	4,175,931	616,150	215,230	5.2	34.9
PA	12,593,310	1,795,737	669,154	5.3	37.3
RI	1,044,132	135,845	55,748	5.3	41.0
SC	5,056,002	724,298	264,229	5.2	36.5
SD	867,844	104,868	26,622	3.1	25.4
TN	6,720,796	1,030,836	365,439	5.4	35.5
TX	28,522,360	3,282,543	1,146,186	4.0	34.9
UT	3,180,641	289,731	94,776	3.0	32.7
VT	617,798	91,411	29,214	4.7	32.0
VA	8,308,751	1,006,318	371,692	4.5	36.9
WA	7,495,588	958,138	344,404	4.6	35.9
WV	1,763,441	349,732	128,181	7.3	36.7
WI	5,751,698	685,896	225,126	3.9	32.8
WY	568,984	77,816	20,421	3.6	26.2

Citation: Paul, S., Rafal, M., & Houtenville, A. (2020). Annual Disability Statistics Compendium: 2020 (Table 1.9). Durham, NH: University of New Hampshire, Institute on Disability. Note: Authors' calculations using the U.S. Census Bureau American Community Survey, Public Use Microdata Sample, 2019, which is subject to sampling variation.

[1] The independent living disability question asks people 15 years old or older, "Because of a physical, mental, or emotional condition, does this person have difficulty doing errands alone such as visiting a doctor's office or shopping?" See glossary for more information.

Table 3.1 Employment – Civilians with Disabilities Ages 18-64 Years Living in the Community for the United States and States: 2019

State	Total	Employed		State	Total	Employed	
		Count	% [1]			Count	% [1]
U.S.	20,323,589	7,896,135	38.8	MO	463,213	171,202	36.9
AL	414,279	137,243	33.1	MT	63,386	29,769	46.9
AK	44,762	17,390	38.8	NE	110,657	56,276	50.8
AZ	449,360	176,596	39.2	NV	176,756	69,609	39.3
AR	272,189	89,327	32.8	NH	86,678	38,558	44.4
CA	1,910,288	731,093	38.2	NJ	411,051	163,968	39.8
CO	298,695	141,078	47.2	NM	166,609	59,959	35.9
CT	202,632	87,066	42.9	NY	1,077,425	378,105	35.0
DE	66,055	27,038	40.9	NC	682,617	241,311	35.3
DC	47,171	15,091	31.9	ND	41,314	23,668	57.2
FL	1,264,308	458,703	36.2	OH	821,099	327,428	39.8
GA	688,280	246,055	35.7	OK	324,268	127,799	39.4
HI	62,548	24,343	38.9	OR	303,883	133,723	44.0
ID	122,286	53,536	43.7	PA	900,776	350,024	38.8
IL	696,823	270,467	38.8	RI	71,988	25,284	35.1
IN	464,976	183,853	39.5	SC	362,442	124,370	34.3
IA	181,062	83,081	45.8	SD	51,664	26,949	52.1
KS	208,624	92,388	44.2	TN	533,630	187,900	35.2
KY	433,163	142,106	32.8	TX	1,658,935	695,898	41.9
LA	374,607	130,948	34.9	UT	146,969	73,787	50.2
ME	112,518	40,837	36.2	VT	45,402	18,858	41.5
MD	324,652	141,768	43.6	VA	491,946	213,043	43.3
MA	374,563	155,391	41.4	WA	478,673	201,400	42.0
MI	725,431	263,170	36.2	WV	178,012	55,518	31.1
MN	296,969	142,948	48.1	WI	340,868	148,299	43.5
MS	257,738	81,198	31.5	WY	39,349	20,716	52.6

Citation: Paul, S., Rafal, M., & Houtenville, A. (2020). Annual Disability Statistics Compendium: 2020 (Table 3.1). Durham, NH: University of New Hampshire, Institute on Disability. Note: Authors' calculations using the U.S. Census Bureau American Community Survey, Public Use Microdata Sample, 2019, which is subject to sampling variation.

[1] The percentage of people employed with disabilities.

Table 3.2 Employment – Civilians without Disabilities Ages 18-64 Years Living in the Community for the United States and States: 2019

State	Total	Employed		State	Total	Employed	
		Count	% [1]			Count	% [1]
U.S.	177,316,108	139,393,681	78.6	MO	3,176,346	2,550,253	80.2
AL	2,488,882	1,857,229	74.6	MT	559,261	446,375	79.8
AK	392,728	291,509	74.2	NE	1,019,051	869,067	85.2
AZ	3,787,523	2,889,065	76.2	NV	1,683,963	1,310,320	77.8
AR	1,487,327	1,144,175	76.9	NH	756,201	626,222	82.8
CA	22,491,756	17,204,398	76.4	NJ	5,000,039	3,986,111	79.7
CO	3,283,041	2,681,001	81.6	NM	1,045,595	780,062	74.6
CT	1,976,285	1,579,723	79.9	NY	10,930,067	8,562,645	78.3
DE	501,761	400,833	79.8	NC	5,603,472	4,342,288	77.4
DC	436,843	348,179	79.7	ND	413,290	355,306	85.9
FL	11,247,884	8,738,746	77.6	OH	6,155,190	4,919,321	79.9
GA	5,742,924	4,432,509	77.1	OK	1,989,851	1,531,989	76.9
HI	731,582	586,389	80.1	OR	2,253,208	1,765,057	78.3
ID	911,096	725,365	79.6	PA	6,761,926	5,393,240	79.7
IL	7,000,742	5,575,226	79.6	RI	589,182	479,033	81.3
IN	3,553,964	2,828,357	79.5	SC	2,667,272	2,048,847	76.8
IA	1,680,623	1,401,886	83.4	SD	454,011	380,152	83.7
KS	1,485,630	1,224,075	82.3	TN	3,570,272	2,795,023	78.2
KY	2,221,272	1,708,656	76.9	TX	15,824,988	12,266,009	77.5
LA	2,361,451	1,757,123	74.4	UT	1,745,484	1,417,111	81.1
ME	691,804	570,832	82.5	VT	337,829	277,508	82.1
MD	3,355,722	2,715,711	80.9	VA	4,630,884	3,705,426	80.0
MA	3,962,941	3,241,447	81.7	WA	4,168,654	3,315,806	79.5
MI	5,290,475	4,155,289	78.5	WV	870,742	632,419	72.6
MN	3,091,465	2,638,895	85.3	WI	3,158,103	2,629,052	83.2
MS	1,477,113	1,076,592	72.8	WY	298,393	235,829	79.0

Citation: Paul, S., Rafal, M., & Houtenville, A. (2020). Annual Disability Statistics Compendium: 2020 (Table 3.2). Durham, NH: University of New Hampshire, Institute on Disability. Note: Authors' calculations using the U.S. Census Bureau American Community Survey, Public Use Microdata Sample, 2019, which is subject to sampling variation.

[1] The percentage of people employed without disabilities.

Table 3.3 Employment – Civilians with Hearing Disabilities Ages 18-64 Years Living in the Community for the United States and States: 2019

State	Total	Employed		State	Total	Employed	
		Count	% [1]			Count	% [1]
U.S.	3,883,988	2,130,174	54.8	MO	88,559	48,533	54.8
AL	79,534	38,385	48.2	MT	14,883	8,793	59.0
AK	14,163	7,705	54.4	NE	27,909	18,446	66.0
AZ	86,038	46,259	53.7	NV	37,861	21,236	56.0
AR	53,983	27,266	50.5	NH	16,141	10,336	64.0
CA	359,747	190,086	52.8	NJ	63,911	37,510	58.6
CO	70,605	44,766	63.4	NM	34,995	14,485	41.3
CT	33,200	21,029	63.3	NY	170,869	91,877	53.7
DE	10,282	5,538	53.8	NC	122,600	64,852	52.8
DC	6,369	3,062	48.0	ND	11,050	7,934	71.8
FL	231,116	117,501	50.8	OH	151,790	83,609	55.0
GA	125,561	67,362	53.6	OK	72,290	39,285	54.3
HI	14,605	9,118	62.4	OR	63,271	39,693	62.7
ID	26,744	15,500	57.9	PA	164,450	90,593	55.0
IL	127,006	71,365	56.1	RI	13,145	6,685	50.8
IN	95,774	53,159	55.5	SC	66,140	32,270	48.7
IA	33,939	20,183	59.4	SD	14,828	9,785	65.9
KS	52,201	28,976	55.5	TN	115,779	57,159	49.3
KY	87,768	37,431	42.6	TX	330,974	192,182	58.0
LA	65,203	30,544	46.8	UT	31,333	21,734	69.3
ME	21,477	11,998	55.8	VT	9,768	4,904	50.2
MD	54,324	32,698	60.1	VA	102,531	60,922	59.4
MA	56,221	35,472	63.0	WA	98,662	57,342	58.1
MI	127,991	67,663	52.8	WV	43,619	18,471	42.3
MN	60,093	40,616	67.5	WI	70,290	42,448	60.3
MS	43,893	19,713	44.9	WY	8,503	5,695	66.9

Citation: Paul, S., Rafal, M., & Houtenville, A. (2020). Annual Disability Statistics Compendium: 2020 (Table 3.3). Durham, NH: University of New Hampshire, Institute on Disability. Note: Authors' calculations using the U.S. Census Bureau American Community Survey, Public Use Microdata Sample, 2019, which is subject to sampling variation.

[1] The percentage of people employed with hearing disabilities.

Table 3.4 Employment – Civilians with Vision Disabilities Ages 18-64 Years Living in the Community for the United States and States: 2019

State	Total	Employed Count	Employed % [1]
U.S.	3,785,293	1,743,383	46.0
AL	86,906	37,128	42.7
AK	7,320	2,672	36.5
AZ	87,915	40,641	46.2
AR	53,631	19,444	36.2
CA	358,359	165,555	46.1
CO	56,556	27,775	49.1
CT	32,869	17,235	52.4
DE	10,519	5,252	49.9
DC	8,606	3,411	39.6
FL	243,623	105,905	43.4
GA	135,165	57,783	42.7
HI	10,442	4,899	46.9
ID	21,812	10,579	48.5
IL	129,601	56,859	43.8
IN	84,255	39,363	46.7
IA	24,314	12,123	49.8
KS	39,813	18,277	45.9
KY	90,457	36,189	40.0
LA	94,540	42,565	45.0
ME	11,635	5,429	46.6
MD	51,437	27,729	53.9
MA	51,025	24,641	48.2
MI	117,655	53,941	45.8
MN	40,477	21,657	53.5
MS	59,046	23,796	40.3
MO	83,267	33,618	40.3
MT	9,462	4,627	48.9
NE	18,355	9,469	51.5
NV	32,729	17,431	53.2
NH	14,534	6,809	46.8
NJ	79,697	42,318	53.0
NM	38,732	18,321	47.3
NY	185,726	86,475	46.5
NC	122,592	51,289	41.8
ND	8,216	5,733	69.7
OH	137,279	62,107	45.2
OK	70,526	33,913	48.0
OR	47,807	23,840	49.8
PA	159,644	71,918	45.0
RI	9,526	3,463	36.3
SC	81,561	34,240	41.9
SD	10,768	5,563	51.6
TN	105,674	44,242	41.8
TX	365,735	179,925	49.1
UT	22,025	12,281	55.7
VT	7,708	3,404	44.1
VA	97,497	50,406	51.7
WA	73,579	36,064	49.0
WV	37,290	12,919	34.6
WI	50,168	27,871	55.5
WY	7,218	4,289	59.4

Citation: Paul, S., Rafal, M., & Houtenville, A. (2020). Annual Disability Statistics Compendium: 2020 (Table 3.4). Durham, NH: University of New Hampshire, Institute on Disability. Note: Authors' calculations using the U.S. Census Bureau American Community Survey, Public Use Microdata Sample, 2019, which is subject to sampling variation.

[1] The percentage of people employed with vision disabilities.

Table 3.5 Employment – Civilians with Cognitive Disabilities Ages 18-64 Years Living in the Community for the United States and States: 2019

State	Total	Employed Count	Employed % [1]	State	Total	Employed Count	Employed % [1]
U.S.	9,116,074	2,779,697	30.4	MO	216,406	62,524	28.8
AL	171,759	46,033	26.8	MT	29,204	10,926	37.4
AK	19,696	6,091	30.9	NE	47,026	19,705	41.9
AZ	197,366	60,044	30.4	NV	73,496	21,991	29.9
AR	122,546	27,774	22.6	NH	43,278	17,292	39.9
CA	834,340	228,644	27.4	NJ	188,582	58,119	30.8
CO	137,157	54,021	39.3	NM	78,714	21,016	26.6
CT	100,099	34,078	34.0	NY	476,448	121,729	25.5
DE	34,883	11,865	34.0	NC	302,947	88,153	29.0
DC	22,871	5,359	23.4	ND	16,842	7,882	46.7
FL	546,221	152,817	27.9	OH	377,225	128,428	34.0
GA	305,889	82,328	26.9	OK	134,191	40,005	29.8
HI	26,036	6,276	24.1	OR	155,715	55,081	35.3
ID	57,267	20,592	35.9	PA	440,982	143,804	32.6
IL	298,900	95,314	31.8	RI	35,386	8,911	25.1
IN	209,898	62,521	29.7	SC	148,520	38,993	26.2
IA	87,423	36,793	42.0	SD	21,328	9,942	46.6
KS	99,482	38,364	38.5	TN	238,427	63,358	26.5
KY	193,912	47,188	24.3	TX	703,116	224,978	31.9
LA	162,937	42,008	25.7	UT	75,655	33,119	43.7
ME	56,453	16,048	28.4	VT	22,065	6,632	30.0
MD	147,086	50,333	34.2	VA	204,341	63,375	31.0
MA	191,299	68,741	35.9	WA	221,448	70,991	32.0
MI	335,438	100,171	29.8	WV	76,811	18,912	24.6
MN	150,337	62,479	41.5	WI	157,547	57,229	36.3
MS	105,126	23,058	21.9	WY	15,953	7,662	48.0

Citation: Paul, S., Rafal, M., & Houtenville, A. (2020). Annual Disability Statistics Compendium: 2020 (Table 3.5). Durham, NH: University of New Hampshire, Institute on Disability. Note: Authors' calculations using the U.S. Census Bureau American Community Survey, Public Use Microdata Sample, 2019, which is subject to sampling variation.

[1] The percentage of people employed with cognitive disabilities.

Table 3.6 Employment – Civilians with Ambulatory Disabilities Ages 18-64 Years Living in the Community for the United States and States: 2019

State	Total	Employed Count	Employed % [1]
U.S.	9,260,465	2,426,636	26.2
AL	209,510	42,235	20.1
AK	20,323	4,929	24.2
AZ	202,421	54,987	27.1
AR	144,014	31,402	21.8
CA	836,286	237,973	28.4
CO	116,625	35,894	30.7
CT	81,759	27,186	33.2
DE	26,018	6,565	25.2
DC	21,123	5,069	23.9
FL	610,972	156,187	25.5
GA	338,266	76,920	22.7
HI	28,574	9,142	31.9
ID	53,503	15,469	28.9
IL	315,858	82,245	26.0
IN	215,581	57,885	26.8
IA	72,887	22,054	30.2
KS	87,280	26,143	29.9
KY	215,385	43,736	20.3
LA	170,009	39,119	23.0
ME	48,504	13,119	27.0
MD	140,159	45,265	32.2
MA	148,422	39,664	26.7
MI	328,714	75,723	23.0
MN	104,175	29,349	28.1
MS	136,269	28,060	20.5

State	Total	Employed Count	Employed % [1]
MO	223,834	55,589	24.8
MT	29,768	10,780	36.2
NE	49,318	15,687	31.8
NV	82,424	22,214	26.9
NH	32,795	8,973	27.3
NJ	181,226	49,464	27.2
NM	79,546	21,709	27.2
NY	518,819	129,420	24.9
NC	346,804	81,415	23.4
ND	14,891	5,221	35.0
OH	381,256	101,565	26.6
OK	152,934	42,278	27.6
OR	118,703	34,936	29.4
PA	396,202	95,650	24.1
RI	29,605	7,039	23.7
SC	175,982	41,118	23.3
SD	17,935	5,417	30.2
TN	256,994	56,006	21.7
TX	748,014	219,061	29.2
UT	49,312	16,983	34.4
VT	19,832	6,471	32.6
VA	212,400	64,016	30.1
WA	206,748	63,236	30.5
WV	94,945	20,107	21.1
WI	150,836	41,007	27.1
WY	16,705	4,954	29.6

Citation: Paul, S., Rafal, M., & Houtenville, A. (2020). Annual Disability Statistics Compendium: 2020 (Table 3.6). Durham, NH: University of New Hampshire, Institute on Disability. Note: Authors' calculations using the U.S. Census Bureau American Community Survey, Public Use Microdata Sample, 2019, which is subject to sampling variation.

[1] The percentage of people employed with ambulatory disabilities.

Table 3.7 Employment – Civilians with Self-Care Disabilities Ages 18-64 Years Living in the Community for the United States and States: 2019

State	Total	Employed	
		Count	% [1]
U.S.	3,483,577	572,704	16.4
AL	62,159	8,103	13.0
AK	6,902	569	8.2
AZ	69,414	9,197	13.2
AR	49,001	4,509	9.2
CA	365,006	56,822	15.5
CO	41,968	7,071	16.8
CT	33,329	6,889	20.6
DE	10,845	2,574	23.7
DC	6,325	964	15.2
FL	222,325	36,810	16.5
GA	110,020	11,978	10.8
HI	11,358	1,457	12.8
ID	17,033	2,492	14.6
IL	115,709	17,521	15.1
IN	82,024	14,064	17.1
IA	28,524	6,080	21.3
KS	29,705	4,817	16.2
KY	70,533	7,692	10.9
LA	64,457	10,828	16.7
ME	14,758	1,340	9.0
MD	49,210	10,846	22.0
MA	64,248	11,346	17.6
MI	128,261	17,962	14.0
MN	50,773	12,389	24.4
MS	43,352	5,600	12.9

State	Total	Employed	
		Count	% [1]
MO	80,434	12,291	15.2
MT	8,545	2,741	32.0
NE	19,224	4,405	22.9
NV	27,901	5,397	19.3
NH	10,888	851	7.8
NJ	74,428	12,046	16.1
NM	33,302	6,774	20.3
NY	212,976	36,332	17.0
NC	122,858	21,593	17.5
ND	6,501	1,796	27.6
OH	130,908	24,133	18.4
OK	51,536	10,582	20.5
OR	40,920	5,570	13.6
PA	159,778	26,119	16.3
RI	12,221	1,699	13.9
SC	63,171	9,716	15.3
SD	4,573	1,009	22.0
TN	81,162	12,229	15.0
TX	309,007	54,439	17.6
UT	19,804	3,388	17.1
VT	7,041	648	9.2
VA	82,033	18,087	22.0
WA	78,418	14,439	18.4
WV	30,516	4,423	14.4
WI	63,845	11,036	17.2
WY	4,348	1,041	23.9

Citation: Paul, S., Rafal, M., & Houtenville, A. (2020). Annual Disability Statistics Compendium: 2020 (Table 3.7). Durham, NH: University of New Hampshire, Institute on Disability. Note: Authors' calculations using the U.S. Census Bureau American Community Survey, Public Use Microdata Sample, 2019, which is subject to sampling variation.

[1] The percentage of people employed with self-care disabilities.

Table 3.8 Employment – Civilians with Independent Living Disabilities Ages 18-64 Years Living in the Community for the United States and States: 2019

State	Total	Employed Count	Employed % [1]
U.S.	7,439,051	1,429,321	19.2
AL	140,918	17,345	12.3
AK	13,952	2,091	14.9
AZ	159,171	30,010	18.8
AR	101,104	12,497	12.3
CA	724,978	129,425	17.8
CO	100,857	23,184	22.9
CT	74,715	20,080	26.8
DE	21,617	3,821	17.6
DC	19,571	3,053	15.5
FL	467,005	82,093	17.5
GA	246,518	37,173	15.0
HI	25,201	3,569	14.1
ID	38,518	9,293	24.1
IL	269,452	49,574	18.3
IN	175,812	34,797	19.7
IA	64,031	18,189	28.4
KS	74,550	18,293	24.5
KY	153,155	25,385	16.5
LA	130,486	19,747	15.1
ME	44,708	9,267	20.7
MD	109,900	25,164	22.8
MA	139,311	33,585	24.1
MI	274,370	49,814	18.1
MN	114,249	38,196	33.4
MS	97,224	12,585	12.9
MO	178,218	32,287	18.1
MT	23,653	6,122	25.8
NE	36,548	10,276	28.1
NV	62,300	11,571	18.5
NH	29,664	6,348	21.3
NJ	162,273	30,157	18.5
NM	61,400	9,475	15.4
NY	423,544	67,185	15.8
NC	251,115	46,046	18.3
ND	14,286	4,034	28.2
OH	295,493	67,666	22.8
OK	112,390	22,532	20.0
OR	112,068	26,715	23.8
PA	335,710	68,628	20.4
RI	30,725	5,343	17.3
SC	136,108	24,405	17.9
SD	11,758	3,834	32.6
TN	184,534	26,362	14.2
TX	580,728	111,218	19.1
UT	51,715	13,916	26.9
VT	17,478	3,317	18.9
VA	182,640	42,875	23.4
WA	171,358	36,575	21.3
WV	64,165	10,447	16.2
WI	115,768	29,586	25.5
WY	12,039	4,171	34.6

Citation: Paul, S., Rafal, M., & Houtenville, A. (2020). Annual Disability Statistics Compendium: 2020 (Table 3.8). Durham, NH: University of New Hampshire, Institute on Disability. Note: Authors' calculations using the U.S. Census Bureau American Community Survey, Public Use Microdata Sample, 2019, which is subject to sampling variation.

[1] The percentage of people employed with independent living disabilities.

Table 3.9 Employment Gap – Civilians Ages 18-64 Years Living in the Community for the United States and States, by Disability Status: 2019

State	Disability [1]	No Disability [2]	Gap (% pts) [3]	State	Disability [1]	No Disability [2]	Gap (% pts) [3]
U.S.	38.8	78.6	39.7	MO	36.9	80.2	43.2
AL	33.1	74.6	41.4	MT	46.9	79.8	32.8
AK	38.8	74.2	35.3	NE	50.8	85.2	34.3
AZ	39.2	76.2	36.9	NV	39.3	77.8	38.4
AR	32.8	76.9	44.0	NH	44.4	82.8	38.3
CA	38.2	76.4	38.1	NJ	39.8	79.7	39.8
CO	47.2	81.6	34.3	NM	35.9	74.6	38.6
CT	42.9	79.9	36.9	NY	35.0	78.3	43.2
DE	40.9	79.8	38.8	NC	35.3	77.4	42.0
DC	31.9	79.7	47.7	ND	57.2	85.9	28.6
FL	36.2	77.6	41.3	OH	39.8	79.9	40.0
GA	35.7	77.1	41.3	OK	39.4	76.9	37.4
HI	38.9	80.1	41.1	OR	44.0	78.3	34.2
ID	43.7	79.6	35.8	PA	38.8	79.7	40.8
IL	38.8	79.6	40.7	RI	35.1	81.3	46.1
IN	39.5	79.5	39.9	SC	34.3	76.8	42.4
IA	45.8	83.4	37.5	SD	52.1	83.7	31.5
KS	44.2	82.3	38.0	TN	35.2	78.2	42.9
KY	32.8	76.9	44.0	TX	41.9	77.5	35.5
LA	34.9	74.4	39.4	UT	50.2	81.1	30.8
ME	36.2	82.5	46.2	VT	41.5	82.1	40.5
MD	43.6	80.9	37.2	VA	43.3	80.0	36.6
MA	41.4	81.7	40.2	WA	42.0	79.5	37.4
MI	36.2	78.5	42.2	WV	31.1	72.6	41.4
MN	48.1	85.3	37.1	WI	43.5	83.2	39.6
MS	31.5	72.8	41.2	WY	52.6	79.0	26.3

Citation: Paul, S., Rafal, M., & Houtenville, A. (2020). Annual Disability Statistics Compendium: 2020 (Table 3.9). Durham, NH: University of New Hampshire, Institute on Disability. Note: Authors' calculations using the U.S. Census Bureau American Community Survey, Public Use Microdata Sample, 2019, which is subject to sampling variation.

[1] The percentage of people employed with disabilities.
[2] The percentage of people employed without disabilities.
[3] The difference in percentage points of people employed with and without disabilities.

Table 3.10 Change in Employment Gap – Civilians Ages 18-64 Years Living in the Community for the United States and States, by Disability Status: 2018 to 2019

State	Gap (Between No Disability & Disability)		Gap Change (% pts) [1]
	2018 (%)	2019 (%)	
U.S.	42.0	39.8	-2.0
AL	43.6	41.5	-2.6
AK	28.2	35.4	6.8
AZ	41.9	37.0	-4.9
AR	45.6	44.1	-1.6
CA	41.3	38.2	-3.3
CO	40.2	34.4	-6.2
CT	39.8	37.0	-2.8
DE	41.8	39.0	-2.8
DC	46.1	47.7	1.9
FL	47.1	41.4	-6.1
GA	44.2	41.4	-3.2
HI	35.1	41.2	5.9
ID	41.4	35.8	-5.4
IL	38.9	40.8	2.1
IN	43.8	40.0	-3.8
IA	38.4	37.5	-0.4
KS	35.5	38.1	2.5
KY	44.1	44.1	-0.1
LA	38.4	39.5	0.6
ME	47.7	46.2	-1.7
MD	36.2	37.3	0.8
MA	44.2	40.3	-4.2
MI	41.5	42.3	0.5
MN	37.1	37.2	-0.1
MS	43.8	41.4	-2.8
MO	43.0	43.3	0.0
MT	33.4	32.9	-0.4
NE	34.6	34.4	-0.6
NV	40.7	38.4	-2.7
NH	38.7	38.3	-0.7
NJ	41.6	39.8	-1.6
NM	37.4	38.6	1.6
NY	40.9	43.2	2.1
NC	46.4	42.1	-4.4
ND	29.1	28.7	-0.1
OH	39.9	40.0	0.1
OK	39.3	37.6	-1.3
OR	42.5	34.3	-8.5
PA	39.7	40.9	1.3
RI	41.9	46.2	4.1
SC	45.9	42.5	-3.9
SD	32.6	31.6	-0.6
TN	45.2	43.1	-2.2
TX	42.8	35.6	-6.8
UT	40.3	31.0	-9.3
VT	39.1	40.6	1.9
VA	39.1	36.7	-2.1
WA	44.2	37.5	-7.2
WV	39.9	41.4	1.1
WI	42.2	39.7	-2.2
WY	29.1	26.4	-3.1

Citation: Paul, S., Rafal, M., & Houtenville, A. (2020). Annual Disability Statistics Compendium: 2020 (Table 3.10). Durham, NH: University of New Hampshire, Institute on Disability. Note: Authors' calculations using the U.S. Census Bureau American Community Survey, Public Use Microdata Sample, 2018 & 2019, which is subject to sampling variation.
[1] The difference of the difference in percentage points of people employed with and without disabilities between 2019 and 2018.

Aging

ADHD: What Can We Do?, 8075
ARC Of Southeast Los Angeles-Southeast Industries, 6545
Activities in Action, 7624
Administration on Aging, 3379
Advocacy Centre for the Elderly (ACE), 733
Aging & Vision News, 7757
Aging Brain, 2364
Aging Life Care Association, 7506
Aging News Alert, 7758
Aging Services of Michigan, 7507
Aging Services of South Carolina, 7508
Aging Services of Washington, 7509
Aging and Disability Services, 3919, 7510
Aging and Disability Services Division, 3693
Aging and Disability: Crossing Network Lines, 2365
Aging and Family Therapy: Practitioner Perspectives on Golden Pond, 7627
Aging and Rehabilitation II: The State ofthe Practice, 2366
Aging and Vision: Declarations of Independence, 9339
Aging in America, 7511
Aging in Stride, 7628
Aging in the Designed Environment, 7629
Aging with a Disability, 7630
Alabama Department of Senior Services, 3416
Alabama VA Benefits Regional Office - Montgomery, 5637
Alaska Commission on Aging, 3427
Albany County Department for Aging and Albany Social Services, 3737
Albany VA Medical Center: Samuel S Stratton, 5770
Aleda E Lutz VA Medical Center, 5731
Alexandria VA Medical Center, 5714
Alliance for Aging Research, 7513
Alliance for Retired Americans, 7514
Alvin C York VA Medical Center, 5827
Amarillo VA Healthcare System, 5832
American Aging Association, 7515
American Association of Retired Persons, 7517
American Geriatrics Society, 7519
American Planning Association, 7520
American Society on Aging, 7523
American Wheelchair Bowling Association, 8442
Amyotrophic Lateral Sclerosis: A Guide for Patients and Families, 8678
Area Agency on Aging of Southwest Arkansas, 7777
Area Agency on Aging: Region One, 7778
Arizona Division of Aging and Adult Services, 3439
Arkansas Division of Aging & Adult Services, 3448
Asheville VA Medical Center, 5786
Association for Gerontology in Higher Education, 7528
Association for International Practical Training, 2766
Association of Jewish Aging Services, 7529
Association on Aging with Developmental Disabilities, 7530
Atlanta Regional Office, 5684
Atlanta VA Medical Center, 5685
Attention Getter, 1718
Attention Teens, 1719
Augusta VA Medical Center, 5686
Baltimore Regional Office, 5719
Baltimore VA Medical Center, 5720
Bath VA Medical Center, 5772
Battle Creek VA Medical Center, 5732
Bay Pines VA Medical Center, 5678
Biloxi/Gulfport VA Medical Center, 5742
Blindness, A Family Matter, 9340
Boise Regional Office, 5692
Boise VA Medical Center, 5693
Boston VA Regional Office, 5725
Bronx VA Medical Center, 5773
Brooklyn Campus of the VA NY Harbor Healthcare System, 5774
Buffalo Regional Office - Department of Veterans Affairs, 5775
Building Blocks: Foundations for Learning for Young Blind and Visually Impaired Children, 9341
Butler VA Medical Center, 5808
CARF International, 789, 2079, 7533
California Department of Aging, 3456
Cambia Health Foundation, 790, 3223
Can America Afford to Grow Old?, 4676
Canandiagua VA Medical Center, 5776
Caring for Those You Love: A Guide to Compassionate Care for the Aged, 7632
Carl T Hayden VA Medical Center, 5644
Carl Vinson VA Medical Center, 5687
Castle Point Campus of the VA Hudson Valley Healthcare System, 5777
Center for Disability and Elder Law, Inc., 4651
Center for Positive Aging, 7537
Change Your Brain, Change Your Life: The Breakthrough Program for Conquering Depression, 7976
Cheyenne VA Medical Center, 5864
Children of Aging Parents, 7538
Chillicothe VA Medical Center, 5794
Cincinnati VA Medical Center, 5795
Clement J Zablocki VA Medical Center, 5859
Cleveland Regional Office, 5796
Coatesville VA Medical Center, 5809
Colmery-O'Neil VA Medical Center, 5707
Colorado Association of Homes and Services for the Aging, 7539
Colorado Department of Aging & Adult Services, 3471
Colorado Springs Independence Center, 4070
Colorado/Wyoming VA Medical Center, 5664
Columbia Foundation, 3010
Columbia Regional Office, 5822
Communication Skills for Working with Elders, 2419
Complementary Alternative Medicine and Multiple Sclerosis, 8703
Connecticut Commission on Aging, 3480
Coping and Caring: Living with Alzheimer's Disease, 7634
Court-Related Needs of the Elderly and Persons with Disabilities, 4683
CurePSP Magazine, 8846
DSHS/Aging & Adult Disability Services Administration, 3928
Dayton VA Medical Center, 5797
DeafBlind Division of the National Federation of the Blind, 9054
Delaware Department of Health and Social Services, 3487
Delaware VA Regional Office, 5671
Denver VA Medical Center, 5665
Des Moines VA Medical Center, 5702
Des Moines VA Regional Office, 5703
District of Columbia Office on Aging, 3496
Duchenne Muscular Dystrophy, 8710
Durham VA Medical Center, 5788
Dwight D Eisenhower VA Medical Center, 5708
East Orange Campus of the VA New Jersey Healthcare System, 5765
Edith Nourse Rogers Memorial Veterans Hospital, 5726
Edward Hines Jr Hospital, 5694
Ehrman Medical Library, 4957
El Paso VA Healthcare Center, 5834
Elder Abuse and Mistreatment, 7635
Elder Visions Newsletter, 7763
ElderLawAnswers.com, 4693
Elgin Training Center, 6831
Employment for Individuals with Asperger Syndrome or Non-Verbal Learning Disability, 8971
Enabling News, 7764
Erie VA Medical Center, 5810
Eugene J Towbin Healthcare Center, 5647
Explore Your Options, 7636
Facilitating Self-Care Practices in the Elderly, 2470
Falling in Old Age, 7637
Family Intervention Guide to Mental Illness, 7638
Family-Guided Activity-Based Intervention for Toddlers & Infants, 5422
Fanlight Productions, 24
Fargo VA Medical Center, 5792
Fayetteville VA Medical Center, 5648, 5789
Films & Videos on Aging and Sensory Change, 5425
Florida Adult Services, 3511
Fort Howard VA Medical Center, 5721
Foundations of Orientation and Mobility, 9179
Gainesville Division, North Florida/South Georgia Veterans Healthcare System, 5679
Georgia Department of Aging, 3526
The Gerontological Society of America, 7620
Gerontology: Abstracts in Social Gerontology, 7656
Getting Better, 8330
Golf Xpress, 525
Grand Island VA Medical System, 5753
Grand Junction VA Medical Center, 5666
Hampton VA Medical Center, 5845
Handbook of Assistive Devices for the Handicapped Elderly, 7639
Handbook on Ethnicity, Aging and Mental Health, 7640
Harry S Truman Memorial Veterans' Hospital, 5744
Hartford Regional Office, 5667
Hawaii Executive Office on Aging, 3542
Health Care of the Aged: Needs, Policies, and Services, 7641
Health Promotion and Disease Prevention in Clinical Practice, 7642
Healthy Aging Association, 7547
Helping the Family Understand, 8331
Highlighter and Note Tape, 585
Honolulu VBA Regional Office, 5690
Houston Regional Office, 5835
Hunter Holmes McGuire VA Medical Center, 5846
Huntington Regional Office, 5854
Huntington VA Medical Center, 5855
Idaho Commission on Aging, 3547
Illinois Department on Aging, 3563
Independence Economic Development, 4661
Independent Living Office, 5195
Independent Living Resources, 4505
Indiana Association for Home and Hospice Care (IAHHC), 861
Indianapolis Regional Office, 5698
Innovations, 7766
Institute on Aging, 7780
Insurance Solutions: Plan Well, Live Better, 5198
Interstitial Cystitis Association, 5518
Iowa City VA Medical Center, 5704
Iowa Department on Aging, 3579
Iron Mountain VA Medical Center, 5733
Jack C. Montgomery VA Medical Center, 5799
Jackson Regional Office, 5743
James A Haley VA Medical Center, 5680
James E Van Zandt VA Medical Center, 5811
Jerry L Pettis Memorial VA Medical Center, 5651
John D Dingell VA Medical Center, 5734
John J Pershing VA Medical Center, 5745
John L McClellan Memorial Hospital, 5649
Jonathan M Wainwright Memorial VA Medical Center, 5850
Justice in Aging, 7554
Kansas City VA Medical Center, 5746
Kansas Department on Aging, 3588
Kansas VA Regional Office, 5709
Kentucky Office of Aging Services, 3593
Knoxville VA Medical Center, 5705
Laurel Grove Hospital: Rehab Care Unit, 6251
LeadingAge, 7557
LeadingAge Arizona, 7558
LeadingAge California, 7559
LeadingAge Connecticut, 7560
LeadingAge Gulf States, 7561
LeadingAge Illinois, 7562
LeadingAge Indiana, 7563
LeadingAge Iowa, 7564
LeadingAge Kentucky, 7565
LeadingAge Maine & New Hampshire, 7566

LeadingAge Massachusetts, 7567
LeadingAge Missouri, 7568
LeadingAge Nebraska, 7569
LeadingAge New Jersey, 7570
LeadingAge New York, 7571
LeadingAge North Carolina, 7572
LeadingAge Ohio, 7573
LeadingAge Oklahoma, 7574
LeadingAge Oregon, 7575
LeadingAge PA, 7576
LeadingAge RI, 7577
LeadingAge Texas, 7578
LeadingAge Wisconsin, 7579
LeadingAge Wyoming, 7580
Lebanon VA Medical Center, 5812
Lexington VA Medical Center, 5711
Life Planning for Adults with Developmental Disabilities, 7643
LifeSpan Network, 7582
Lifestyles of Employed Legally Blind People, 9212
Lincoln Regional Office, 5754
Lincoln VA Medical Center, 5755
Long Beach VA Medical Center, 5652
Long-Term Care: How to Plan and Pay for It, 7644
Los Angeles Regional Office, 5653
Louis A Johnson VA Medical Center, 5856
Louis Stokes VA Medical Center - Wade Park Campus, 5798
Louisiana Department of Aging, 3599
Louisville VA Medical Center, 5712
Louisville VA Regional Office, 5713
Lyons Campus of the VA New Jersey Healthcare System, 5766
Maine VA Regional Office, 5717
Making Wise Decisions for Long-Term Care, 5220
Managing Post Polio: A Guide to Living Well with Post Polio, 8759
Managing Your Symptoms, 8332
Manchester Regional Office, 5761
Manchester VA Medical Center, 5762
Marion VA Medical Center, 5695
Martinez Outpatient Clinic, 5654
Martinsburg VA Medical Center, 5857
Maryland Department of Aging, 3616
Math for Successful Living, 1701
MedEscort International, 5594
Memphis VA Medical Center, 5828
Mentally Impaired Elderly: Strategies and Interventions to Maintain Function, 7645
Mercy Medical Group, 6633
Michael E. Debakey VA Medical Center, 5836
Michigan Office of Services to the Aging, 3644
Michigan VA Regional Office, 5735
Mid-America Regional Council - Aging and Adult Services, 7783
Mid-Carolina Area Agency on Aging, 7784
Minneapolis VA Medical Center, 5738
Minnesota Board on Aging, 3651
Mirrored Lives: Aging Children and Elderly Parents, 7646
Mississippi Division of Aging and Adult Services, 3665
Monkeys Jumping on the Bed, 1764
Montana Department of Aging, 3679
Mountain Home VA Medical Center - James H Quillen VA Medical Center, 5829
Muhlenberg County Opportunity Center, 6914
Multiple Sclerosis: 300 Tips for Making Life Easier, 8764
Multiple Sclerosis: The Guide to Treatment and Management, 8767
Muscular Dystrophies, 8768
Muscular Dystrophy in Children: A Guide for Families, 8769
Muscular Dystrophy: The Facts, 8770
Nasheville Regional Office, 5830
Nashville VA Medical Center, 5831
National Association for Home Care & Hospice, 8509
National Association of Area Agencies on Aging, 7589
National Association of Counties, 7590
National Association of Nutrition and Aging Services Programs (NANASP), 7591
National Association of States United for Aging and Disabilities, 7592
National Care Planning Council, 895
National Center on Elder Abuse, 7593
National Council on Aging, 7597
National Council on the Aging Conference, 1915
National Gerontological Nursing Association, 7599
National Hispanic Council on Aging, 7600
National Indian Council on Aging, Inc., 7602
National Institute on Aging, 3397, 4887
Nebraska Department of Health and Human Services, Division of Aging Services, 3688
Nevada Division for Aging: Las Vegas, 3699
New Hampshire Division of Elderly and Adult Services, 3711
New Jersey Department of Aging, 3719
New Mexico Aging and Long-Term Services Department, 3726
New Mexico VA Healthcare System, 5769
New Orleans VA Medical Center, 5715
New York City Campus of the VA NY Harbor Healthcare System, 5778
New York Regional Office, 5779
Newark Regional Office, 5767
North Carolina Division of Aging, 3775
North Chicago VA Medical Center, 5696
North Dakota Department of Human Resources, 3781
North Dakota VA Regional Office - Fargo Regional Office, 5793
North Little Rock Regional Office, 5650
Northampton VA Medical Center, 5727
Northern Arizona VA Health Care System, 5645
Northport VA Medical Center, 5780
Not Without Sight, 9347
Oakland VA Regional Office, 5655
Office for American Indian, Alaskan Native and Native Hawaiian Elders, 7612
Ohio Department of Aging, 3791
Oklahoma City VA Medical Center, 5801
Oklahoma Department of Human Services Aging Services Division, 3801
Options, Resource Center for Independent Living, 1642
Oxford Textbook of Geriatric Medicine, 2547
Pacific Islands Health Care System, 5691
Part B News, 7772
Passion for Justice, 5450
Pennsylvania Department of Aging, 3821
Perry Point VA Medical Center, 5723
Philadelphia Regional Office and Insurance Center, 5814
Philadelphia VA Medical Center, 5815
Physical & Mental Issues in Aging Sourcebook, 7647
Physical & Occupational Therapy in Geriatrics, 7658
Piedmont Triad Council of Governments Area Agency on Aging, 7785
Pittsburgh Regional Office, 5816
Portland Regional Office, 5804
Portland VA Medical Center, 5805
Practicing Rehabilitation with Geriatric Clients, 2559
Prescriptions for Independence: Working with Older People Who are Visually Impaired, 7648
Providence Regional Office, 5820
Providence VA Medical Center, 5821
Ralph H Johnson VA Medical Center, 5823
Reading Rehabilitation Hospital, 4996
Recreation Activities for the Elderly, 2573
Rehabilitation Interventions for the Institutionalized Elderly, 2575
Rehabilitation Research and Development Center, 5656
Reno Regional Office, 5758
Respiratory Disorders Sourcebook, 8805
Retirement Research Foundation, 2976
Rhode Island Department of Elderly Affairs, 3829
Richard L Roudebush VA Medical Center, 5699
Roanoke Regional Office, 5847
Robert J Dole VA Medical Center, 5710
Role Portrayal and Stereotyping on Television, 5259
Roseburg VA Medical Center, 5806
Royal C Johnson Veterans Memorial Medical Center, 5825
Sacramento Medical Center, 5657
Salem VA Medical Center, 5848
San Antonio Area Foundation, 3305
San Diego VA Regional Office, 5658
Seattle Regional Office, 5851
Senior Service America, 7617
Sharing the Burden, 7649
Sheridan VA Medical Center, 5865
Shreveport VA Medical Center, 5716
Sioux Falls Regional Office, 5826
Sister Cities International, 2786
Social Security Bulletin, 7776
Social Security, Medicare, and Government Pensions, 7650
South Dakota Department of Aging, 3852
South Texas Veterans Healthcare System, 5837
Southern Arizona VA Healthcare System, 5646
Southern Oregon Rehabilitation Center & Clinics, 5807
Spokane VA Medical Center, 5852
St. Cloud VA Medical Center, 5739
St. Louis Regional Office, 5747
St. Louis VA Medical Center, 5748
St. Paul Regional Office, 5740
St. Petersburg Regional Office, 5682
Start-to-Finish Library, 1851
Stickybear Typing, 1868
Storybook Maker Deluxe, 1787
Strategies for Teaching Students with Learning and Behavior Problems, 2602
Strides Magazine, 8413
Successful Models of Community Long Term Care Services for the Elderly, 7651
Syracuse VA Medical Center, 5781
Teaching Special Students in Mainstream, 2143
Tennessee Commission on Aging and Disability, 3861
Tennessee Hospital Association, 7619
Texas Department on Aging, 3886
Therapeutic Activities with Persons Disabled by Alzheimer's Disease, 7652
Togus VA Medical Center, 5718
Tomah VA Medical Center, 5860
Tomorrow's Promise: Language Arts, 1857
Tomorrow's Promise: Spelling, 1859
Tompkins County Office for the Aging, 7787
Tourette Syndrome: The Facts, 8822
Triangle J Council of Governments Area Agency on Aging, 7788
US Administration on Aging, 7621
US Department of Veterans Affairs National Headquarters, 5635
University of California Memory and Aging Center, 7789
Utah Department of Aging and Adult Services, 3899
Utah Division of Veterans Affairs, 5841
V A Montana Healthcare System, 5750
VA Ann Arbor Healthcare System, 5736
VA Boston Healthcare System: Brockton Division, 5728
VA Boston Healthcare System: Jamaica Plain Campus, 5729
VA Boston Healthcare System: West Roxbury Division, 5730
VA Central California Health Care System, 5659
VA Connecticut Healthcare System: Newington Division, 5669
VA Connecticut Healthcare System: West Haven, 5670
VA Greater Los Angeles Healthcare System, 5660
VA Illiana Health Care System, 5697
VA Montana Healthcare System, 5751
VA Nebraska-Western Iowa Health Care System, 5756
VA North Indiana Health Care System: Fort Wayne Campus, 5700
VA Northern California Healthcare System, 5661
VA Northern Indiana Health Care System: Marion Campus, 5701

VA Pittsburgh Healthcare System, Highland Drive Division, 5818
VA Pittsburgh Healthcare System, University Drive Division, 5817
VA Puget Sound Health Care System, 5853
VA Salt Lake City Healthcare System, 5842
VA San Diego Healthcare System, 5662
VA Sierra Nevada Healthcare System, 5759
VA Southern Nevada Healthcare System, 5760
VA Western NY Healthcare System, Batavia, 5784
VA Western NY Healthcare System, Buffalo, 5785
Vermont Department of Aging, 3911
Vermont Department of Disabilities, Aging and Independent Living, 3913
Vermont Division of Disability & Aging Services, 3917
Vermont VA Regional Office Center, 5843
Veteran Benefits Administration - Anchorage Regional Office, 5643
Visiting Nurse Association of America, 8909
Visually Impaired Seniors as Senior Companions: A Reference Guide, 7653
WG Hefner VA Medical Center - Salisbury, 5790
Waco Regional Office, 5839
Washington County Disability, Aging and Veteran Services, 3814
Washington DC VA Medical Center, 5677
We Can Do it Together!, 9354
West Palm Beach VA Medical Center, 5683
West Texas VA Healthcare System, 5840
West Virginia Department of Aging, 3944
Wilkes-Barre VA Medical Center, 5819
William Jennings Bryan Dorn VA Medical Center, 5824
William S Middleton Memorial VA Hospital Center, 5861
Wilmington VA Medical Center, 5672
Winston-Salem Regional Office, 5791
Wisconsin Bureau of Aging, 3954
Wisconsin VA Regional Office, 5862
Work, Health and Income Among the Elderly, 7654
Wyoming Department of Aging, 3962
Wyoming/Colorado VA Regional Office, 5866
Yoga for Fibromyalgia: Move, Breathe, and Relax to Improve Your Quality of Life, 8405
Young Person's Guide to Spina Bifida, 8834

AIDS

AHF Federation, 725
AIDS Alert, 8856
AIDS Healthcare Foundation, 726, 2808
AIDS Sourcebook, 8668
AIDS United, 8464
AIDS Vancouver, 727
AIDS and Other Manifestations of HIV Infection, 8669
AIDS in the Twenty-First Century: Disease and Globalization, 8670
AIDS: The Official Journal of the International AIDS Society, 8838
Access & Information Network, 730
Camp Heartland, 1206, 8572
Camp Hollywood HEART, 1005, 8577
Camp Starlight, 1357
Camp Sunburst, 1020, 8604
Caremark Healthcare Services, 6816
Children with Disabilities, 5293
CrescentCare Legal Services, 4654
FC Search, 3357
Glaser Progress Foundation, 3327
Guide to Living with HIV Infection: Developed at the Johns Hopkins AIDS Clinic, 8720
HEAL: Health Education AIDS Liaison, 2100
HIV Infection and Developmental Disabilities, 2482
Harborview Medical Center, Low Vision Aid Clinic, 7191
Health Resources & Services Administration: State Bureau of Health, 3613
Health Resources and Services Administration (HRSA), 3388
Legal Action Center, 4664
Legal Counsel for Health Jusice, 4665
Legislative Network for Nurses, 4710
Levi Strauss Foundation, 2847
Living Well with Chronic Fatigue Syndrome and Fibromyalgia, 8748
Living Well with HIV and AIDS, 8749
A Loving Spoonful, 723
Miami VA Medical Center, 5681
Michigan Association for Deaf, and Hard of Hearing, 3632
Michigan Protection & Advocacy Service, 3645
National AIDS Hotline, 8899
Penitent, with Roses: An HIV+ Mother Reflects, 8795
Questions and Answers: The ADA and Personswith HIV/AIDS, 8802
Ryan White HIV/AIDS Program, 934
Sight by Touch, 9352
Strength for the Journey, 1365, 8650
Sunburst Projects, 8530
Suttle Lake Camp, 1366, 8652
Vinfen Corporation, 6981
Visiting Nurse Association of North Shore, 6982
WORLD, 957

Alternative Therapies

ACNM Foundation, Inc., 3002
Academy for Guided Imagery, 2728
Academy of Integrative Health & Medicine (AIHM), 729
Accreditation Commission for Acupuncture & Oriental Medicine, 731
Accreditation Commission for Midwifery Education (ACME), 732
American Academy of Medical Acupuncture, 738
American Academy of Osteopathy, 8339
American Acupuncture Council, 742
American Association of Acupuncture and Oriental Medicine (AAAOM), 743
American Association of Neuromuscular & Electrodiagnostic Medicine, 8340
American College of Advancement in Medicine (ACAM), 753
American College of Nurse Midwives (ACNM), 754
American Herb Association Newsletter, 5109
American Migraine Foundation, 2075, 3090
American Sexual Health Association, 8477
American Society for the Alexander Technique (AmSAT), 765
American Society of Clinical Hypnosis (ASCH), 766
Aromatherapy Book: Applications and Inhalations, 5116
Aromatherapy for Common Ailments, 5117
Association for Applied Psychophysiology and Biofeedback (AAPB), 773
Ayurvedic Institute, 2733
Bach Flower Therapy: Theory and Practice, 5122
Bastyr Center for Natural Health, 782
Beliefs, Values, and Principles of Self Advocacy, 5124
Brain Allergies: The Psychonutrient and Magnetic Connections, 8687
Center for Mind-Body Medicine, 798
Chinese Herbal Medicine, 5142
Chronic Fatigue Syndrome: Your Natural Gu ide to Healing with Diet, Herbs and Other Methods, 8699
Colon Health: Key to a Vibrant Life, 8702
Council of Colleges of Acupuncture & Oriental Medicine, 810
Creating Wholeness: Self-Healing Workbook Using Dynamic Relaxation, Images and Thoughts, 5150
Curing MS: How Science is Solving the Mysteries of Multiple Sclerosis, 8706
The Davis Center, 945, 8174, 8940
Designing and Using Assistive Technology: The Human Perspective, 2433
Disabled Athlete Sports Association (DASA), 822
Divided Legacy: A History of the Schism in Medical Thought, The Bacteriological Era, 2448
Dr. Ida Rolf Institute (DIRI), 829
Environmental Health Center: Dallas, 8489
Esalen Institute, 835
Everybody's Guide to Homeopathic Medicines, 5169
Feldenkrais Guild of North America (FGNA), 843
Flying Manes Therapeutic Riding, Inc., 844
Handbook of Chronic Fatigue Syndrome, 8721
Healing Herbs, 5183
Health Action, 853
Heart of the Mind, 8724
Herb Research Foundation, 5514
Homeopathic Educational Services, 857
Imagery in Healing Shamanism and Modern Medicine, 5191
Informed Touch; A Clinician's Guide To The Evaluation Of Myofascial Disorders, 8730
International Association of Hygienic Physicians, 8498
International Association of Yoga Therapists (IAYT), 864
International Childbirth Education Association, 2103
International Clinic of Biological Regeneration (ICBR), 867
It's All in Your Head: The Link Between Mercury Amalgams and Illness, 8734
JoanBorysenko.Com, 5519
Journal of Midwifery & Women's Health (JMWH), 2283
Living Beyond Multiple Sclerosis: A Woman's Guide, 8746
Living an Idea: Empowerment and the Evolution of an Alternative School, 2018
Long Beach Department of Health and Human Services, 3464
Los Angeles County Department of Health Services, 3465
Lupus: Alternative Therapies That Work, 8755
National Association for Holistic Aromatherapy (NAHA), 888
National Association to Advance Fat Acceptance, 8514
National Center for Homeopathy, 2113
National Certification Commission for Acupuncture and Oriental Medicine, 901
National Guild of Hypnotists (NGH), 906
National Headache Foundation, 2971
National University of Natural Medicine (NUNM), 911
Nothing is Impossible: Reflections on a New Life, 5233
Nutritional Desk Reference, 5234
Nutritional Influences on Illness:, 5235
Optometric Extension Program Foundation, 3021
Our Own Road, 5448
Pacific Institute of Aromatherapy, 919
Pain Erasure, 5315
Pain Erasure: the Bonnie Prudden Way, 9229
Professional Association of Therapeutic Horsemanship International (PATH Intl.), 929, 8456
Small Wonder, 2050
Solving the Puzzle of Chronic Fatigue, 8811
Structural Integration: The Journal of the Rolf Institute, 2305
Therapeutic Touch International Association (TTIA), 949
Tourette's Syndrome: Tics, Obsessions, Compulsions: Developmental Psychopathology, 8824
United States Trager Association, 952
Upledger Institute International (UII), 954
Weiner's Herbal, 5279

Amputation

American Amputee Foundation, 8098
Amputee Coalition, 769
Baylor Institute for Rehabilitation, 7152
Botsford Center For Rehabilitation & Health Improvement-Redford, 6985
Breaking New Ground Resource Center, 8886
Camp No Limits California, 1008

Camp No Limits Connecticut, 1067
Camp No Limits Florida, 1078
Camp No Limits Idaho, 1105
Camp No Limits Maine, 1162
Camp No Limits Maryland, 1168
Camp No Limits Missouri, 1221
Camp No Limits Texas, 1436
Camp STAR, 1382
Camp sNOw Maine, 1164
Don't Feel Sorry for Paul, 8114
Functional Restoration of Adults and Children with Upper Extremity Amputation, 8115
Hanger, Inc., 852
Healthsouth Rehabilitation Hospital of Mechanicsburg, 6420
Healthsouth Rehabilitation Hospital of York, 6421
International Child Amputee Network, 865
MossRehab ResourceNet, 5526
National Amputation Foundation, 8108
National Commission on Orthotic and Prosthetic Education, 8109
No Limits Foundation, 3000
Northeast Rehabilitation Clinic, 7323
Paddy Rossbach Youth Camp, 1075
Shands Rehab Hospital, 7248
Siskin Hospital For Physical Rehabilitation, 7148
Siskin Hospital for Physical Rehabilitation, 7389
inMotion Magazine, 5387

Amythrophic Lateral Sclerosis

Amytrophic Lateral Sclerosis Association, 8345
Les Turne Amyotrophic Laterial Sclerosis Foundation, 2964

Art & Music Therapies

AbleArts, 1
American Art Therapy Association (AATA), 2
American Association of Cardiovascular and Pulmonary Rehabilitation, 8470
American Brain Tumor Association, 8471
American Music Therapy Association (AMTA), 5
American Thoracic Society, 8479
Art Therapy, 5368
Art Therapy SourceBook, 7
Art and Disabilities, 8
Art and Healing: Using Expressive Art to Heal Your Body, Mind, and Soul, 9
Art for All the Children: Approaches to Art Therapy for Children with Disabilities, 10
Art-Centered Education and Therapy for Children with Disabilities, 2373
Arts Unbound, 11
The Arts of Life, 65
Awakenings Project, The, 13
Canadian Art Therapy Association (CATA), 791
Center for Creative Arts Therapy, 795
Clinical Applications of Music Therapy in Developmental Disability, Pediatrics and Neurolog, 15
Contemporary Art Therapy with Adolescents, 16
Creative Arts Resources Catalog, 17
Creative Arts Therapy Catalogs, 1983
Creative Growth Art Center, 18
Creativity Explored, 19
Deaf West Theatre, 21
Fountain House Gallery, 25
In-Definite Arts Society, 29
Infinity Dance Theater, 30
Interact Center for the Visual and Performing Arts, 32
International Expressive Arts Therapy Association (IEATA), 868
International Journal of Arts Medicine, 2511
Kaleidoscope: Exploring the Experience of Disability through Literature & the Fine Arts, 33
Keshet Dance and Center for the Arts, 34
Mad Hatters: Theatre That Makes a World of Difference, 2745
Manual of Sequential Art Activities for Classified Children and Adolescents, 36
Music Therapy and Leisure for Persons with Disabilities, 39
Music Therapy, Sensory Integration and the Autistic Child, 42
Music for the Hearing Impaired, 44
Music: Physician for Times to Come, 45
NIAD Art Center (Nurturing Independence through Artistic Development), 46
National Arts and Disability Center (NADC), 47
National Endowment for the Arts: Office for AccessAbility, 49
National Library Service for the Blind and Physically Handicapped (NLS), 50, 9091
New Music Therapist's Handbook, 2nd Ed. Berklee School of Music, 53
No Limits, 54
Open Circle Theatre, 57
Pied Piper: Musical Activities to Develop Basic Skills, 58
A Practical Guide to Art Therapy Groups, 5088
Project Onward Gallery, 59
Pure Vision Arts, 60
Special Care in Dentistry, 8875
Survivors Art Foundation, 62
Teaching Basic Guitar Skills to Special Learners, 64
VSA arts, 68
We Are PHAMALY, 69
Your Role in Inclusion Theatre, 5283

Arthritis

American College of Rheumatology, Researchand Education Foundation, 5485
Arthritis Bible, 8386
Arthritis Foundation, 8346
Arthritis Foundation Great West Region, 8417
Arthritis Helpbook: A Tested Self Management Program for Coping with Arthritis, 8387
Arthritis Self-Management, 8858
Arthritis Sourcebook, 8388
Arthritis Sourcebook., 8679
Arthritis Today, 8407
Arthritis Update, 8418
Arthritis, What Exercises Work: Breakthrough Relief for the Rest of Your Life, 8389
Arthritis: A Take Care of Yourself Health Guide, 8390
Back & Neck Sourcebook., 8682
Baptist Health Rehabilitation Institute, 3452
Big Lamp Switch, 463
Body Reflexology: Healing at Your Fingertips, 5128
Boston University Arthritis Center, 4893
Boston University Robert Dawson Evans Memorial Dept. of Clinical Research, 4895
Brigham and Women's Hospital: Robert B Brigham Multipurpose Arthritis Center, 4898
Burke Rehabilitation Hospital, 6383
Camp Esperanza, 8378
Carpal Tunnel Syndrome, 8113
Case Western Reserve University Northeast Ohio Multipurpose Arthritis Center, 4980
Challenge Golf, 9358
Daniel Freeman Rehabilitation Centers, 6583
Freedom from Arthritis Through Nutrition, 8393
Guide to Managing Your Arthritis, 8395
How to Deal with Back Pain and Rheumatoid Joint Pain: A Preventive and Self Treatment Manua, 8396
Indiana University: Multipurpose Arthritis Center, 4850
Information Hotline, 8462
Kids on the Block Programs, 8463
Kuzell Institute for Arthritis and Infectious Diseases, 4772
Loma Linda University Orthopedic and Rehabilitation Institute, 6621
Managing Your Activities, 5223
Managing Your Health Care, 5224
Medical University of South Carolina Arthritis Clinical/Research Center, 4999
National Institute of Arthritis and Musculoskeletal and Skin Diseases, 3393
New York Arthritis Reporter, 8427
Oklahoma Medical Research Foundation, 4987
Playing Card Holders, 5575
Primer on the Rheumatic Diseases, 8401
RIC Northshore, 6852
RIC Windermere House, 6854
Raynaud's Phenomenon, 8803
Swedish Covenant Hospital Rehabilitation Services, 6864
Thumbs Up Cup, 331
University of Michigan: Orthopaedic Research Laboratories, 4921
University of Missouri: Columbia Arthritis Center, 4938
Virginia Chapter of the Arthtitis Foundation, 5030
When Your Student Has Arthritis, 8404
Yoga for Arthritis, 8437
Yoga for MS and Related Conditions, 8438

Asthma

AAN's Toll-Free Hotline, 8885
ABC of Asthma, Allergies & Lupus, 8667
Allergies & Asthma: What Every Parent Needs To Know (2nd Edition), 8673
Allergies Sourcebook, 8674
Allergy & Asthma Today, 5349
American Academy of Allergy, Asthma & Immunology, 8466
Asthma & Allergy Education for Worksite Clinicians, 2730
Asthma & Allergy Essentials for Children's Care Provider, 2731
Asthma Action Cards: Child Care Asthma/Allergy Action Card, 1967
Asthma Action Cards: Student Asthma Action Card, 1968
Asthma Care Training for Kids (ACT), 2732
Asthma Management and Education, 2384
Asthma Sourcebook., 8680
Asthma and Allergy Answers: A Patient Education Library, 8681
Asthma and Allergy Foundation of America, 5492
Bakersfield Regional Rehabilitation Hospital, 6241
Becket Chimney Corners YMCA Camps and Outdoor Center, 8544
Being Close, 8683
Brigham and Women's Hospital: Asthma and Allergic Disease Research Center, 4897
Camp Breathe Easy, 1089, 8554
Camp Christmas Seal, 8559
Camp Glengarra, 8568
Camp L-Kee-Ta, 8586
Camp Not-A-Wheeze, 990, 8592
Camp Tall Turf, 8608
Camp Vacamas, 8610
Camp WheezeAway, 976, 8612
Center for Interdisciplinary Research on Immunologic Diseases, 4900
Champ Camp, 1050, 8616
Hasbro Children's Hospital Asthma Camp, 1401
Johns Hopkins University: Asthma and Allergy Center, 4882
Let's Talk About Having Asthma, 8740
Living Well with Asthma, 8747
MA Report, 2327
Meeting-in-a-Box, 2029
My House is Killing Me! The Home Guide for Families with Allergies and Asthma, 8771
Nocturnal Asthma, 8776
Parent's Guide to Allergies and Asthma, 8793
Power Breathing Program, 2039
Teens & Asthma, 8877
Toll-Free Information Line, 8908
Understanding Asthma, 8826
Understanding Asthma: The Blueprint for Breathing, 8827
What Everyone Needs to Know About Asthma, 8832
YMCA Camp Ihduhapi, 8660
YMCA Camp of Maine, 8664
Your Child and Asthma, 8835

Attention Deficit Disorder

ADD, Stepping Out of the Dark, 8073
ADD: Helping Your Child, 7947
ADDitude Directory, 2123
ADHD Report, 8055
ADHD in Adults, 8074
ADHD in the Classroom: Strategies for Teachers, 2352
ADHD with Comorbid Disorders: Clinical Assessment and Management, 7950
ADHD: What Do We Know?, 8076
ALST: Adolescent Language Screening Test, 2657
Adapted Physical Education for Students with Autism, 2357
Adventure Learning Center at Eagle Village, 7895
All About Attention Deficit Disorders, Revised, 5402, 7953
All Days Are Happy Days Summer Camp, 1412
Around the Clock: Parenting the Delayed AD HD Child, 8077
Attention, 8054
Attention Deficit Disorder, 7955
Attention Deficit Disorder and Learning Disabilities, 7956
Attention Deficit Disorder in Adults Workbook, 7957
Attention Deficit Disorder in Children, 2386
Attention Deficit Disorder: A Different Perception, 7958
Attention Deficit Disorder: Adults, 8078
Attention Deficit Disorder: Children, 8079
Attention Deficit Disorders Association, Southern Region: Annual Conference, 1898
Attention Deficit Disorders: Assessment & Teaching, 7959
Attention-Deficit Hyperactivity Disorder: Symptoms and Suggestons for Treatment, 7960
Attention-Deficit/Hyperactivity Disorder, What Every Parent Wants to Know, 7961
Braille Book Bank, Music Catalog, 9147
Camp World Light, 7912
Casowasco Camp, Conference and Retreat Center, 7914
Chadder, 8062
Clinical Connection, 2256
Clinical Management of Childhood Stuttering, 2nd Edition, 2412
Clinician's Practical Guide to Attention-Deficit/Hyperactivity Disorder, 5370
Cogrehab, 8094
Communication & Language Acquisition: Discoveries from Atypical Development, 2418
Community Signs, 1981
Comprehensive Assessment of Spoken Language (CASL), 1982
Comprehensive Guide to ADD in Adults: Research, Diagnosis & Treatment, 7980
Concentration Cockpit: Explaining Attention Deficits, 7981
Coping for Kids Who Stutter, 8969
Coping with ADD/ADHD, 7982
Counseling Persons with Communication Disorders and Their Families, 2424
Development of Language, 2437
Disorders of Motor Speech: Assessment, Treatment, and Clinical Characterization, 8970
Driven to Distraction, 7988
Educating Inattentive Children, 8084
Englishton Park Academic Remediation, 7918
Family Therapy for ADHD: Treating Children, Adolescents and Adults, 7993
Florida Sheriffs Caruth Camp, 7919
GO-MO Articulation Cards- Second Edition, 1997
Getting a Grip on ADD: A Kid's Guide to Understanding & Coping with ADD, 7997
Gillingham Manaual, 1998
Handbook for Speech Therapy, 2484
Helping Your Hyperactive: Attention Deficit Child, 8004
Hyperactive Child, Adolescent, and Adult: ADD Through the Lifespan, 8007
Identifying and Treating Attention Deficit Hyperactivity Disorder, 8008
Indian Acres Camp for Boys, 7922
It's Just Attention Disorder, 8088
Jumpin' Johnny Get Back to Work, A Child's Guide to ADHD/Hyperactivity, 8011
K-SEALS: Kaufman Survey of Early Academic and Language Skills, 2684
KLST-2: Kindergarten Language Screening Test Edition, 2nd Edition, 2685
Lollipop Lunch, 8977
Managing Attention Deficit Hyperactivity in Children: A Guide for Practitioners, 8019
Maplebrook School, 1295, 7925
Meeting the ADD Challenge: A Practical Guide for Teachers, 2536
Model Program Operation Manual: Business Enterprise Program Supervisors, 9221
New Jersey YMHA/YWHA Camps Milford, 7928
Out of the Corner of My Eye: Living with Macular Degeneration, 9228
Out of the Fog: Treatment Options and Coping Strategies for ADD, 8021
Parenting Attention Deficit Disordered Teens, 8025
Parents Helping Parents: A Directory of Support Groups for ADD, 8026
Readings on Research in Stuttering, 2572
Reference Manual for Communicative Sciences and Disorders, 2574
Rethinking Attention Deficit Disorder, 8032
Rolling Hills Country Day Camp, 7935
Rose-Colored Glasses, 9241
Round Lake Camp, 1263
Sharing Solutions: A Newsletter for Support Groups, 9329
Slingerland Screening Tests, 2710
Solving Language Difficulties, 2051
Speech Bin, 2052, 2712
Speech-Language Pathology and Audiology: An Introduction, 2598
Stuttering & Your Child: Help For Parents, 9013
Stuttering Foundation of America, 8937
Stuttering Severity Instrument for Children and Adults, 2713
Survey of Direct Labor Workers Who Are Blind & Employed by NIB, 9253
Taking Charge of ADHD Complete Authoritative Guide for Parents, 8039
Teenagers with ADD, 8043
Triangle Y Ranch YMCA, 7944
Understanding ADHD, 8089
Understanding Attention Deficit Disorder, 8090
Why Won't My Child Pay Attention?, 8093
Women with Attention Deficit Disorder: Embracing Disorganization at Home and Work, 8048
You Seem Like a Regular Kid to Me, 9275
You and Your ADD Child, 8050

Autism

Aces Adventure Weekend, 1368
Aging and Developmental Disability: Current Research, Programming, and Practice, 7626
Anxiety-Free Kids: An Interactive Guide for Parents and Children, 2371
Arizona Autism Resources, 2801
Aspies For Freedom (AFF), 771, 5490
AuSM Summer Camp, 1200
Autism, 5403
Autism 24/7: A Family Guide to Learning at Home & in the Community, 7963, 8952
Autism Handbook: Understanding & Treating Autism & Prevention Development, 7964, 8953
Autism National Committee (AUTCOM), 7841
Autism Network International (ANI), 7842
Autism New Jersey, 4947
Autism Research Institute, 7843, 8914
Autism Research Review International, 8058, 9008
Autism Services Center, 7844, 8915
Autism Society of America, 8095, 9021
Autism Society of Minnesota, 7845
Autism Summer Respite Program, 1268
Autism Treatment Center of America, 7846, 8916
Autism and Learning, 7965, 8954
Autism in Adolescents and Adults, 7966, 8955
Autism...Nature, Diagnosis and Treatment, 7967, 8956
Autism: A World Apart, 8080, 9016
Autism: Explaining the Enigma, 7968, 8957
Autism: From Tragedy to Triumph, 7969, 8958
Autism: Identification, Education and Treatment, 7970, 8959
Autism: The Facts, 7971, 8960
Autism: the Unfolding Mystery, 8081, 9017
AutismUp: YMCA Summer Social Skills Program, 1269
Autistic Adults at Bittersweet Farms, 7972, 8961
Autistic Self Advocacy Network (ASAN), 7847
Breakthroughs: How to Reach Students with Autism, 7974, 8964
Burger School for the Autistic, 4907
CNS Camp New Connections, 7896, 8942
Camp Baker, 7897
Camp CANOE, 1346
Camp Encourage, 1218
Camp FRIENDship, 1114
Camp Horizons, 1065, 7902
Camp Joy, 1325, 1416, 8187, 8583
Camp Loughridge, 1350
Camp Rising Sun, 1266
Camp Royall, 1310, 7909, 8944
Child With Special Needs: Encouraging Intellectual and Emotional Growth, 5141
Children's Center for Neurodevelopmental Studies, 4751
Cognitive Behavioral Therapy for Adult Asperger Syndrome, 7978, 8966
Communication Unbound, 2420
Courage Center, 4343
Developmental Disabilities: A Handbook for Occupational Therapists, 2439
Division on Autism and Developmental Disabilities (DADD), 2096
Dogs for the Deaf, 8140
Eden Autism, 6127
Emory Autism Resource Center, 4817
Encounters with Autistic States, 7991, 8972
Essential First Steps for Parents of Children with Autism, 5343
Exploring Autism: A Look at the Genetics of Autism, 5507
FOCUS Center for Autism, 7865
Families of Adults With Autism: Stories & Advice For the Next Generation, 7992
Fighting for Darla: Challenges for Family Care & Professional Responsibility, 7994
Filmakers Library: An Imprint Of Alexander Street Press, 5424
Focus Times Newsletter, 8065
Focus on Autism and Other Developmental Disabilities, 2269
Fragile Success, 7995
Friendship 101, 2475
Fundamentals of Autism, 1996
Future Horizons, 27
Geneva Centre for Autism, 7866
Getting Started with Facilitated Communication, 8085, 9018
Going to School with Facilitated Communication, 5179
Guide to Successful Employment for Individuals with Autism, 8000
A Guide to Teaching Students With Autism Spectrum Disorders, 2345
Handbook of Autism and Pervasive Developmental Disorders, 8001
Heartspring, 6902
Helping People with Autism Manage Their Behavior, 8003
Hidden Child: The Linwood Method for Reaching the Autistic Child, 8005
Hillcroft Services, 1138, 8380
Illinois Center for Autism, 6837
Imagery Procedures for People with Special Needs, 5433
Indiana Resource Center for Autism, 4849
Judevine Center for Autism, 4936
Keys to Parenting the Child with Autism, 8014
Kris' Camp, 1086

Let Community Employment be the Goal for Individuals with Autism, 8016, 8976
Little City Foundation, 2965
Little Friends, Inc., 6840
Living with Spina Bifida: A Guide for Families and Professionals, 8752
Louis de la Parte Florida Mental Health Institute Research Library, 4803
Management of Autistic Behavior, 8018, 8757, 8978
Mount Sinai Medical Center, 2924
Music Therapy, 38
National Autism Association, 7881
National Autism Hotline, 8096
Neurobiology of Autism, 8020, 8980
New England Center for Children, 6974
Parent Survival Manual, 8023, 8982
Please Don't Say Hello, 8027, 8984
Prufrock Press, 2171
Reaching the Autistic Child: A Parent Training Program, 8804
Reaching the Child with Autism Through Art, 61
Riddle of Autism: A Psychological Analysis, 8033, 8988
Rimland Services for Autistic Citizens, 1123, 7934
Schools And Services For Children With Autism Spectrum Disorders., 3755
Sex Education: Issues for the Person with Autism, 8035, 8990
Social Skills for Students With Autism Spectrum Disorders and Other Developmental Disorders, 2592
Sometimes You Just Want to Feel Like a Human Being, 5265
Son Rise: The Miracle Continues, 8812
Son-Rise Program, 8905
Son-Rise: The Miracle Continues, 8036, 8991
Soon Will Come the Light, 8037
Special Needs Advocacy Resource Book, 2711
Special Needs Project, 2175
Spokane Center for Independent Living, 4627
TEACCH Autism Program, 7889
Teaching Asperger's Students Social Skills Through Acting, 63
Teaching Children With Autism in the General Classroom, 2611
Teaching Children with Autism: Strategies for Initiating Positive Interactions, 8040, 8994
Teaching Students with Moderate/Severe Disabilities, Including Autism, 2626
Teaching and Mainstreaming Autistic Children, 8041, 8995
Treating Disordered Speech Motor Control, 2640
Uncommon Fathers, 5336
Understanding Autism, 8091, 9020
Valley News Dispatch, 8045
Vanguard School, The, 2758
Virginia Autism Resource Center, 5028
Wendell Johnson Speech And Hearing Clinic, 7831, 7945, 8941, 9122
West Hills Day Camp, 1304
West Virginia Autism Training Center, 5040
Without Reason: A Family Copes with two Generations of Autism, 8047, 8999

Behavioral Disorders

AACRC Annual Conference, 1878
Alternative Teaching Strategies, 2369
American Group Psychotherapy Association, 8473
Association for Contextual Behavioral Science, 7840
Association of Children's Residential Centers (ACRC), 775
Behavior Analysis in Education: Focus on Measurably Superior Instruction, 2388
Behavior Modification, 2389
Behavioral Disorders, 2250
Camp Ruggles, 1399, 7910
Center for Neuro Skills, 6569
Childhood Behavior Disorders: Applied Research & Educational Practice, 2404
Children's Mental Health and EBD E-news, 2309
Creating Positive Classroom Environments: Strategies for Behavior Management, 2426
Devereux Advanced Behavioral Health - National Office, 7129
Devereux Advanced Behavioral Health - Texas Victoria Campus, 7158
Devereux Advanced Behavioral Health Arizona - Scottsdale, 6517
Devereux Advanced Behavioral Health Georgia, 6790
Devereux Advanced Behavioral Health Massachusetts & Rhode Island, 6963
Devereux Advanced Behavioral Health New Jersey, 7036
Devereux Advanced Behavioral Health New York, 7053
Devereux Advanced Behavioral Health Texas - League City Campus, 7159
Devereux Arizona - Tucson, 6518
Devereux Florida - Orlando Campus, 6734
Devereux Florida - Viera Campus, 6735
Devereux Pennsylvania, 7130
Explorer's Club Camp, 1258
Groden Network, 6182
Journal of Emotional and Behavioral Disorders, 2281
Journal of Motor Behavior, 2284
Journal of Vocational Behavior, 2293
Lakeview NeuroRehabilitation Center, 6371
LifeROOTS, 6148
Outside In School Of Experiential Education, Inc., 1392, 7930
Progress Without Punishment: Approaches for Learners with Behavior Problems, 2566
Teaching Students with Learning and Behavior Problems, 2624
ValueOptions, 5547
Volunteers of America (VOA), 956
Working Bibliography on Behavioral and Emotional Disorders, 2648

Birth Defects

BDRC Newsletter, 5494
Baylor College of Medicine Birth Defects Center, 5003
Birth Defect Research for Children (BDRC), 784
Camp Bon Coeur, 1154, 8553
Camp Odayin, 1208
Camp Odayin Family Camp, 1209
Camp Odayin Residential Camp, 1210
Camp Odayin Summer Camp, 1211
Camp Odayin Winter Camp, 1212
Camp Taylor, 1022, 8609
Camp Taylor: Family Camp, 1023, 1103
Camp Taylor: Leadership Camp, 1024
Camp Taylor: Teen Camp, 1025
Camp Taylor: Young Adult Program, 1026
Camp Taylor: Youth Camp, 1027
Camp del Corazon, 1029, 8613
Cornelia de Lange Syndrome Foundation, 2886
Dictionary of Congenital Malformations& Disorders, 5154
Division of Birth Defects and Developmental Disabilities, 3522
Management of Genetic Syndromes, 8758
March of Dimes, 883
National Birth Defect Registry, 5529
National Center on Birth Defects and Developmental Disabilities, 4822
National Fragile X Foundation, 8930
National Organization for Albinism and Hypopigmentation, 8521
National Organization on Fetal Alcohol Syndrome, 8523
Nick & Kelly's Heart Camp, 993
Open Hearts Camp, 1180, 8643
University of Miami: Mailman Center for Child Development, 4811

Blind/Deaf

AADB National Conference, 1879
ASD Athletics, 7829
Alaska Center for the Blind and Visually Impaired, 6510
American Association of the Deaf-Blind, 7791
American Society for Deaf Children, 7792, 8127
Arena Stage, 6, 7793
Association of Late-Deafened Adults, 7794, 8131
Camp Abilities Brockport, 1270
Camp Merrick, 9112
Canadian Deafblind Association, 7795
Communicating with People Who Have Trouble Hearing & Seeing: A Primer, 7809
Deaf-Blind Perspective, 7821, 9299
Florida School for the Deaf and Blind, 7807
A Handbook for Writing Effective Psychoeducational Reports (2nd Edition), 7808
Helen Keller National Center for Deaf- Blind Youths and Adults, 7799
InFocus, 7824
Lions Camp Merrick, 1174, 8201
National Center on Deaf-Blindness (NCDB), 899, 7803
National Family Association for Deaf-Blind, 7804
Silent Call Communications, 195

Brain Injuries

Bancroft, 7034
Before and After Zachariah, 5356
Brain Injury Alliance of Texas, 7851
Brain Injury Association of America (BIAA), 787, 7852
Brain Injury Association of New York State, 7853
Camp Barefoot, 1189
Center for Comprehensive Services, 6818
Center for Neuro-Rehabilitation, 6943
Department of Physical Medicine & Rehabilitation at Sinai Hospital, 813
The Education of Children with Acquired Brain Injury, 2633
The Essential Brain Injury Guide (5th Edition), 5384
Hope Network Neuro Rehabilitation, 858, 6993
Hospital For Special Care (HSC), 7232
Living with Brain Injury: A Guide for Families, 8751
Measure of Cognitive-Linguistic Abilities(MCLA), 2690
National Hydrocephalus Foundation, 7884
Neurobehavioral Medicine Center, 6762
North Broward Rehab Unit, 6763
Occupational Therapy Approaches to Traumatic Brain Injury, 2545
Preventable Brain Damage, 8028
Rasmussen's Syndrome and Hemispherectomy Support Network Newsletter, 8873
Students with Acquired Brain Injury: The School's Response, 2603
Universal Institute Rehabilitation & Fitness Center, 6380
When Billy Broke His Head...and Other, 5472

Cancer

AMC Cancer Research Center, 4778
Adult Leukemia: A Comprehensive Guide for Patients and Families, 8671
Advanced Breast Cancer: A Guide to Living with Metastic Disease, 8672
Adventure Day Camp, 8540
Alexander and Margaret Stewart Trust, 2898
American Society of Pediatric Hematology/Oncology, 8478
Aplastic Anemia and MDS International Foundation, 8480
Arbors at New Castle, 7236
Arizona Camp Sunrise, 8542
Arizona Camp Sunrise & Sidekicks, 983
Association for the Cure of Cancer of the Prostate (CaP CURE)-Prostate Cancer Foundation, 5491
Baxter Healthcare Corporation, 6812
Beliefs: Pathways to Health and Well Being, 5125
Big Sky Kids Cancer Camps, 1228

Breast Cancer Sourcebook, 8689
Camp Adventure, 1271
Camp Anuenue, 1102, 8549
Camp Can Do, 1373, 8555
Camp Catch-A-Rainbow, 1190
Camp Catch-a-Rainbow, 8557
Camp Courage, 1203, 1374, 1404
Camp Debbie Lou, 1405
Camp Dream Street, 1216, 1251
Camp Enchantment, 1265
Camp Firefly, 1092
Camp Good Days and Special Times, 1275
Camp Goodtimes, 1476
Camp Hobe, 1454
Camp Little Red Door, 1131
Camp Mak-A-Dream, 1229
Camp Millennium, 1356
Camp Okizu, 1009, 8593
Camp Okizu: Family Camp, 1010
Camp Okizu: Oncology Camp, 1011
Camp Okizu: SIBS Camp, 1012
Camp Okizu: Teens-N-Twenties Camp, 1013
Camp One Step, 1117
Camp Quality Arkansas, 996
Camp Quality Central Missouri, 1222
Camp Quality Greater Kansas City, 1223
Camp Quality Heartland, 1233
Camp Quality Illinois, 1118
Camp Quality Kansas, 1148
Camp Quality Kentuckiana, 1134, 1150
Camp Quality Louisiana, 1157
Camp Quality New Jersey, 1256
Camp Quality North Michigan, 1194
Camp Quality Northwest Missouri, 1224
Camp Quality Ohio, 1331
Camp Quality Ozarks, 1225
Camp Quality South Michigan, 1195
Camp Quality Texas, 1438
Camp Rainbow, 991, 1439, 8596
Camp Rainbow Gold, 1106
Camp Reach for the Sky, 1017, 8597
Camp Ronald McDonald for Good Times, 1019, 8599
Camp Smile-A-Mile, 968, 8603
Camp Smile-A-Mile: Jr./Sr. Camp, 969
Camp Smile-A-Mile: Off Therapy Family Camp, 970
Camp Smile-A-Mile: On Therapy Family Camp, 971
Camp Smile-A-Mile: Sibling Camp, 972
Camp Smile-A-Mile: Teen Weeklong Camp, 973
Camp Smile-A-Mile: Young Adult Retreat, 974
Camp Smile-A-Mile: Youth Weeklong Camp, 975
Camp SunSibs, 1169
Camp Sunrise, 1170, 8605
Camp Sunshine, 997, 1097, 1163
Camp Sunshine Dreams, 1021, 8606
Camp Ukandu, 1359
Camp Wapiyapi, 1048
Canadian Cancer Society, 8483
Cancer Care, 3121
Cancer Clinical Trials: A Commonsense Guide to Experimental Cancer Therapies and Trials, 5341
Cancer Research Institute, 5496
Cancer Sourcebook, 8691
Cancer Sourcebook for Women, 8692
Candlelighters Childhood Cancer Foundation, 3007
Childhood Cancer Canada Foundation, 8486
Childhood Cancer Survivors: A Practical Guide to Your Future, 8694
Childhood Cancer: A Parent's Guide to Solid Tumor Cancers, 8695
Childhood Leukemia Foundation, 8487
Colon & Rectal Cancer: A Comprehensive Guide for Patients & Families, 8701
Conquering the Darkness: One Story of Recovering from a Brain Injury, 8704
Coping with Cancer Magazine, 8845
Damon Runyon Cancer Research Foundation, 5498
Desert Regional Medical Center, 6585
Double H Ranch, 1289
Eastern Idaho Regional Medical Center, 7260
Fannie E Rippel Foundation, 3097
First Descents, 1060
Foundation for Advancement in Cancer Therapy, 3142
Genetic Nutritioneering, 5178
Happiness Is Camping, 1259, 8630
Healthsouth Rehabilitation Hospital of Greater Pittsburgh, 6419
The Hole in the Wall Gang Camp, 1070, 8655
International Association for Cancer Victors & Friends, 8497
International Myeloma Foundation, 8500
Jane Coffin Childs Memorial Fund for Medical Research, 2892
Jane Phillips Medical Center, 6403
John Muir Medical Center Rehabilitation Services, Therapy Center, 6610
Kids Cancer Alliance, 1151
Leukemia & Lymphoma Society, 8502
Leukemia Sourcebook, 8741
Liver Disorders Sourcebook, 8745
Lung Cancer: Making Sense of Diagnosis, Treatment, and Options, 8753
Lymphoma Canada, 8505
Madonna Rehabilitation Hospital, 7319
Marist Brothers Mid-Hudson Valley Camp, 1296, 8638
Methodist Hospital Rehabilitation Institute, 6326
Multiple Sclerosis National Research Institute, 5527
NCI's Contact Center, 8898
National Association for Proton Therapy, 8511
National Cancer Institute, 3389, 8515
Northwest Hospital Center for Medical Rehabilitation, 6479
One Day at a Time: Children Living with Leukemia, 8790
Options, 8867
Options: Revolutionary Ideas in the War on Cancer, 8791
Parma Community General Hospital Acute Rehabilitation Center, 6395
Prostate and Urological Disorders Sourcebook, 8800
Psychology and Health, 5252
RA Bloch Cancer Foundation, 3078
Rapahope Children's Retreat Foundation, 979, 2797, 8645
Seany Foundation, 2862
Simonton Cancer Center, 8526
Society for Post-Acute and Long-Term Care Medicine (AMDA), 936
St. Anthony's Hospital, 7249
Sumner Regional Medical Center, 6439
V Foundation for Cancer Research, 5546
Victory Junction, 1315
YMCA Camp jewell, 8663
Your Guide to Bowel Cancer, 8837

Cerebral Palsy

American Academy for Cerebral Palsy and Developmental Medicine, 1891, 8465
CPATH Cerebral Palsy Awareness Transition Hope, 8482
Camp CPals, 1429
Cerebral Palsy Associations of New York State, 7856
Cerebral Palsy Foundation (CPF), 799
Cerebral Palsy: North County Center, 6572
Children with Cerebral Palsy: A Parents' Guide, 8698
Coping with Cerebral Palsy, 8705
Developmental Medicine & Childhood Neurology, 8843
From Where I Sit: Making My Way with Cerebral Palsy, 8717
No Time for Jello: One Family's Experience, 8775
Ontario Cerebral Palsy Sports Association, 8455
Ontario Federation for Cerebral Palsy, 7886
Preventing Secondary Conditions Associated with Spina Bifida or Cerebral Palsy, 8799
Ten Things I Learned from Bill Porter, 8820
Treating Cerebral Palsy for Clinicians by Clinicians, 2639
United Cerebral Palsy, 2122, 7894
United Cerebral Palsy of Texas, 3894

Chiropractics

American Chiropractic Association (ACA), 752
International Chiropractors Association (ICA), 866

Chronic Disabilities

Access to Health Care, 2355
Broken Dolls: Gathering the Pieces: Caringfor Chronically Ill Children, 5291
Camp Boggy Creek, 1077, 8552
Camp Discovery, 1063, 1113, 1375, 1415, 1431
Camp Holiday Trails, 1468
Camp Kindle, 1006, 1232
Caring for Children with Chronic Illness, 2397
The Center for Courageous Kids, 1153
Comprehensive Care Coordination for Chronically Ill Adults, 5073
Counseling Parents of Children with Chronic Illness or Disability, 5371
Developing Cross-Cultural Competence:Guideto Working with Young Children & Their Families, 2434
Dream Oaks Camp, 1082
Dream Street, 1032, 8621
Dream Street Foundation, 2828
Family Interventions Throughout Disability, 5304
Flying Horse Farms, 1335
Living with a Brother or Sister with Special Needs: A Book for Sibs, 5308
National Association for Home Care and Hospice, 7588
National Association of Chronic Disease Diseases, 8513
The Painted Turtle, 1042
Roundup River Ranch, 1061, 8646
Screening in Chronic Disease, 5260

Cleft Palate

Camp About Face, 1128
Camp Laughter, 995
Cleft Palate-Craniofacial Journal, 8842
Nasometer, 1819
Your Cleft Affected Child, 8836

Cognitive Disorders

ADHD Book of Lists: A Practical Guide for Helping Children and Teens with ADDs, 7948
ADHD in the Schools: Assessment and Intervention Strategies, 2353, 7949
Academy of Cognitive Therapy, 7832
Adult ADD: The Complete Handbook: Everything You Need to Know About How to Cope with ADD, 7952
Albert Ellis Institute, 7834
American Academy of Child & Adolescent Psychiatry, 7835
American Delirium Society, 7836
Arc Connection Newsletter, 5115, 8056
Arc Light, 8057
Assistive Technology for Individuals with Cognitive Impairments Handbook, 7954
Augmenting Basic Communciation in Natural Contexts, 7962
Be Quiet, Marina!, 7973
Beck Institute for Cognitive Behavior Therapy, 7848
Biologically Inspired Cognitive Architectures Society, 7850
Biology Concepts Through Discovery, 8082
Camp Nissokone, 7905
Child and Adolescent Therapy: Cognitive-Behavioral Procedures, Third Edition, 7977
Children and Adults with Attention-Deficit Hyperactivity Disorder, 7858
Cognitive Neuroscience Society, 7859
Cognitive Science Society, 7860
Cognitive Science Student Association, 7861

Concentration Video, 8083
Count Us In, 7983
Devereux Advanced Behavioral Health California, 6586
Difficult Child, 7985
Disability Culture Perspective on Early Intervention, 7986
Embracing the Monster: Overcoming the Challenges of Hidden Disabilities, 7990
Evaluation and Treatment of the Psychogeriatric Patient, 2467
Getting Our Heads Together, 7996
I Just Want My Little Boy Back, 8087, 9019
Imagine!, 5950, 8066
In Search of Wings: A Journey Back from Traumatic Brain Injury, 8009
In Their Own Way, 8010
Journal of Cognitive Rehabilitation, 8052
Keys to Parenting a Child with Attention Deficit Disorder, 8012
LD Child and the ADHD Child: Ways Parents & Professionals Can Help, 8015
Making the Writing Process Work, 8017
Marvelwood Summer, 7926
A Miracle to Believe In, 7946
NLP Comprehensive, 7873
National Association of Cognitive- Behavioral Therapists, 7878
National Center for PTSD, 5013
Quest Camp, 1040, 7932
Relationship Development Intervention with Young Children, 8031, 8987
Sherman Lake YMCA Outdoor Center, 7937
Society for Cognitive Rehabilitation, 7887
Successful Job Search Strategies for the Disabled: Understanding the ADA, 8038
Techniques for Aphasia Rehab: (TARGET) Generating Effective Treatment, 8042, 8996
You Mean I'm Not Lazy, Stupid or Crazy?!: A Self-Help Book for Adults with ADD, 8049

Cystic Fibrosis

Bittersweet Chances: A Personal Journey o f Living and Learning in the Face of Illness, 8684
Cystic Fibrosis Foundation, 3012
Cystic Fibrosis: Medical Care, 5373
Cystic Fibrosis: A Guide for Patient and Family, 8707
Official Patient's Sourcebook on Cystic Fibrosis, 8781
Understanding Cystic Fibrosis, 8828
YMCA Camp Kitaki, 8661

Dementia

Alzheimer Disease Sourcebook, 8676
Alzheimer Disease Sourcebook, 4th Edition, 8677
Alzheimer's Association, 2945
Bay View Nursing and Rehabilitation Center, 7219
Brain Disorders Sourcebook, 8688
Brewer Rehab and Living Center, 6350
Clinical Alzheimer Rehabilitation, 2411
Country Manor Rehabilitation and Nursing Center, 7307
Dementia Society of America, 7862
Kennedy Park Medical Rehabilitation Center, 7418
Lafayette Nursing and Rehabilitation Center, 7253
Levindale Hebrew Geriatric Center, 6947
Lewy Body Dementia Association, 7868, 8106, 8358
Mississippi Department of Mental Health, 3664
Music Therapy in Dementia Care, 41
Renaissance at South Shore, 7273
San Luis Medical and Rehabilitation Center, 7424

Dental Issues

International Academy of Biological Dentistry and Medicine, 8495
International Academy of Oral Medicine & Toxicology, 8496
International Medical and Dental Hypnotherapy Association, 8499
Special Care Dentistry Association, 8527

Depression

American Foundation for Suicide Prevention (AFSP), 758, 3114
Anxiety and Depression Association of America (ADAA), 770, 7838
Beacon Tree Foundation, 783, 3316
Brain & Behavior Research Foundation, 786, 3119
DAYS: Depression and Anxiety in Youth Scale, 2674
Florida CORF, 6742
Focal Group Psychotherapy, 2473
Freedom from Fear, 845
Hogg Foundation for Mental Health, 856, 3297
Menopause without Medicine, 8761
Motivator, 8426
Phenomenology of Depressive Illness, 2554
Postpartum Support International (PSI), 927
Social Security: Tampa Disability Determination, 3520
The Steve Fund, 948
Stroke Connection Magazine, 8118, 8414
When the Brain Goes Wrong, 5280
World Federation for Mental Health, 960

Developmental Disabilities

AAIDD Annual Meeting, 1880
ACM Lifting Lives Music Camp, 1411
ARC Gateway, 3505
ARC of Hunterdon County, The, 6117
ARC of Mercer County, 6118
ARC of Monmouth, 6119
ARC's Government Report, 5098
Abilities Without Boundaries, 5952
Abilities of Northwest New Jersey Inc., 6121
AbilityWorks, 6098
Activities with Developmentally Disabled Elderly and Older Adults, 7625
Addison Point Agency, 6062
Administration on Disabilities, 3381
Adults & Children with Learning & Developmental Disabilities (ACLD), 7833
Advocate Illinois Masonic Medical Center, 6807
Advocates for Developmental Disabilities, 735
Alliance Center for Independence (ACI), 6122
American Association on Intellectual and Developmental Disabilities (AAIDD), 746
American Journal on Intellectual and Developmental Disabilities (AJIDD), 2249
The Arc Gloucester, 6144
The Arc Los Angeles and Orange Counties, 5937
Arc National Convention, The, 1897
Arc South County Chapter, 3251
Arc of Alaska, 2798
The Arc of Allen County, 2228
Arc of Anderson County, 3265
Arc of Arkansas, 2806
Arc of Blackstone Valley, 3252
Arc of California, 2812
Arc of Colorado, 2875
Arc of Connecticut, 2883
Arc of Davidson County, 3266
Arc of Delaware, 2896
Arc of Dunn County, 3337
Arc of Eau Claire, 3338
Arc of Florida, 2913
Arc of Fox Cities, 3339
Arc of Hamilton County, 3267
Arc of Hawaii, 2939
Arc of Illinois, 2948
Arc of Indiana, 2983
Arc of Iowa, 2987
Arc of Kansas, 2992
Arc of Kentucky, 2995
Arc of Louisiana, 2996
Arc of Maryland, 3005
Arc of Massachusetts, The, 3024
Arc of Michigan, 3040
Arc of Minnesota, 3058
Arc of Mississippi, 3069
Arc of Natrona County, 3351
Arc of Nebraska, 3080
Arc of New Jersey, 3091
The Arc of New Jersey, 2223
Arc of New Mexico, 3105
Arc of North Carolina, 3182
The Arc of North Carolina, 7890
Arc of North Dakota, 3191
Arc of Northern Bristol County, 3025
Arc of Northern Rhode Island, 3253
Arc of Ohio, 3195
Arc of Oregon, 3222
Arc of Pennsylvania, 3228
Arc of Racine County, 3340
Arc of South Carolina, 3262
Arc of Tennessee, 3268
Arc of Texas, The, 3280
Arc of Utah, 3311
Arc of Virginia, 3315
Arc of Washington County, 3269
Arc of Washington State, 3324
Arc of Williamson County, 3270
Arc of Wisconsin Disability Association, 3341
Arc of the District of Columbia, 2900
The Arc of the United States, 5545, 7891
Arc-Dane County, 3342
Arc-Diversified, 3271
Ardmore Developmental Center, 6070
As I Am, 5118
Assessing the Handicaps/Needs of Children, 2374
Assessment in Mental Handicap: A Guide to Assessment Practices & Tests, 2378
The Association for the Gifted (TAG), 2121
Association of University Centers on Disabilities (AUCD), 780, 2148
Bakersfield ARC, 5913
Berkshire Meadows, 6954
Best Buddies, 7849
Blue Peaks Developmental Services, 5942
Breaking Ground, 8859
Breaking the Speech Barrier: Language Develpment Through Augmented Means, 8963
Brooklyn Bureau of Community Service, 7050
Builders of Skills, 6308
COEA The Arc of East Ascension, 6058
California Elwyn, 6559
Camp Abilities Tucson, 985
Camp Achieva, 1370
Camp Anne, 1272
Camp Arye, 1317
Camp Caglewood, 1090
Camp Cheerful, 1318, 8558
Camp Christopher: SumFun Day Camp, 1319
Camp Civitan, 987, 7900
Camp ClapHans, 1347
Camp Confidence, 1202
Camp Dickenson, 1466
Camp Echoing Hills, 1320, 8565
Camp Happiness, 1323
Camp Harkness, 1064, 8571
Camp Hawkins, 1093
Camp Huntington, 1277, 7903
Camp Jaycee, 1252
Camp Jotoni, 1253
Camp Kehilla, 1278
Camp Killoqua, 1477
Camp Krem, 1007, 7904
Camp Lee Mar, 1378
Camp Lotsafun, 1238
Camp Magruder, 1354, 8590
Camp Paradise, 1330
Camp Ramah in the Poconos, 1381, 8192
Camp Ramapo, 1282, 7907
Camp ReCreation, 1016, 7908
Camp Red Leaf, 1119
Camp Sisol, 1284, 7911, 8945
Camp Sun'N Fun, 1257
Camp Tekoa, 1312, 8195
Camp Thunderbird, 1079
Camp Tova, 1285
Camp Whitman on Seneca Lake, 1287
CampCare, 1239

Catalog for Teaching Life Skills to Persons with Development Disability, 1977
Center for Disability Resources, 796, 3263
Change, Inc., 801
Cheyenne Village, 5943
Children's Beach House, 1073
Civitan Foundation, 2804
Clausen House, 6576
Clay Tree Society, 806
Clearbrook, 6009
Colton-Redlands-Yucaipa Regional Occupational Program (CRY-ROP), 5915
Communication Development and Disorders in African American Children, 8967
Communitas Supportive Care Society, 808
Community Employment Services, 5916
Community Gatepath, 6577
Comprehensive Rehabilitation Center of Naples Community Hospital, 6729
Connecticut Office of Protection and Advocacy for Persons with Disabilities, 3483
CranstonArc, 3255
DOCS: Developmental Observation Checklist System, 2675
Datahr Rehabilitation Institute, 6697
Desert Haven Enterprises, 5918
Developmental Disabilities Resource Center (DDRC), 5945
Developmental Disabilities in Infancy and Childhood, 5297
Developmental Disabilities: A Handbook for Interdisciplinary Practice, 2440
Developmental Services Center, 2677
Devereux Advanced Behavioral Health - Florida, 6733
Devereux Advanced Behavioral Health Colorado, 6680
Devereux Advanced Behavioral Health Florida - Titusville Campus, 6732
Devereux Threshold Center for Autism, 6736
Dictionary of Developmental Disabilities Terminology, 5155, 5298
Directory for Exceptional Children, 2131
Directory of Members, 5156
Donaldsville Area Arc, 6921
Dynamic Dimensions, 5947
Dyspraxia Foundation USA, 8103
Eastern Colorado Services for the Developmentally Disabled (ECSDD), 5948
Easterseals, 831, 8892
Easterseals Gilchrist Marchman Child Development Center, 6827
Elwyn, 832
Elwyn Delaware, 4790, 6714
FYI, 2315
Family Support Project for the Developmentally Disabled, 8894
Family-Centered Service Coordination: A Manual for Parents, 5305
Federal Laws of the Mentally Handicapped: Laws, Legislative Histories and Admin. Documents, 4697
Fellow Insider, 2317
Field Notes, 2318
Foundation Industries, 6924
Fragile X Family, 8492
Frank Olean Center, 3257
Gateway Center of Monterey County, 6598
Gateway Industries: Castroville, 6599
Glenkirk, 6012
Goodwill Life Skills Development Program, 5976
Goodwill's Community Employment Services, 5978
Goodwill's JobWorks, 5980
The Guided Tour, Inc., 5619
Handbook of Developmental Education, 2487
Happiness Bag, 1137
Hartford Foundation for Public Giving, 2889
HealthSouth Sports Medicine & Rehabilitation Center, 6282
Hockanum Greenhouse, 6701
Illinois Life Span Program, 6013
Inclusion, 2274
Independence, 7765
Information Services for People with Developmental Disabilities, 5196
Innabah Camps, 1390
Institute for Basic Research in Developmental Disabilities, 4961
Intellectual and Developmental Disabilities (IDD), 2275
James L. Maher Center, 3259
Jersey Cape, 6132
Joseph P Kennedy Jr Foundation, 2906
Kamp Kaleo, 1235, 9118
Katy Isaacson Elaine Gordon Lodge, 1293
Keep the Promise: Managed Care and People with Disabilities, 5206
Kennedy Job Training Center, 6015
Kent County Arc, 3053
Knox County Council for Developmental Disabilities, 6016
Lambs Farm, 6018
Lambton County Developmental Services (LCDS), 876
Legacy, 7767
Life Unlimited, 7870
Life-Span Approach to Nursing Care for Individuals with Developmental Disabilities, 2530
Lifelong Leisure Skills and Lifestyles for Persons with Developmental Disabilities, 5210
Lions Den Outdoor Learning Center, 7924
LoSeCa Foundation, 881
Lutherdale Bible Camp, 1489
MAGIC Foundation for Children's Growth, 2966
MAGIC Touch, 8756
Mainstay Life Services Summer Program, 1391
Match-Sort-Assemble Pictures, 2026
Match-Sort-Assemble SCHEMATICS, 2027
Member Update, 2328
Minnesota Governor's Council on Developmental Disabilities, 3656
Missouri Division Of Developmental Disabilities, 3669
Montgomery County Arc, 3276
Mosholu Day Camp, 1297
Music Therapy for the Developmentally Disabled, 40
NACDD Annual Conference, 1910
Napa Valley PSI Inc., 5926
National Association for Developmental Disabilities (NADD), 7876
National Association of Councils on Developmental Disabilities (NACDD), 891
National Association of State Directors of Developmental Disabilities Services (NASDDDS), 893
National Theatre Workshop of the Handicapped (NTWH), 51
Nevada Governor's Council on Developmental Disabilities, 6113
New Directions For People With Disabilities, 5615
New Directions for People with Disabilities, 2782
New Hampshire Bureau of Developmental Services, 3706
New Hampshire Developmental Disabilities Council, 3710
New Horizons Summer Day Camp, 1039, 7927, 8947
Nuvisions For Disabled Artists, Inc., 56
Oak-Leyden Developmental Services, 7885
Parallels in Time, 5239
Parents and Friends, Inc, 5928
Pioneer Center for Human Services, 6848
Porterville Sheltered Workshop, 5931
President's Committee on People with Intellectual Disabilities, 3404
Prime Time, Inc., 1481
Primrose Center, 5984
Professional Fit Clothing, 1535
Project Independence, 5932
Quest, Inc., 5986, 6769
Quest, Inc. - Tampa Area, 5987, 6770
Raven Rock Lutheran Camp, 7933
Rehabilitation Opportunities, 6949
Relaxation Techniques for People with Special Needs, 5456
Rhode Island Arc, 3260
Richmond Research Training Center (RRTC), 6212
Sebasticook Farms-Great Bay Foundation, 6940
Sequanota Lutheran Conference Center and Camp, 1394, 8948
Sexuality and the Developmentally Handicapped, 5321
Shore Training Center, 6022
Sibpage, 2338
SleepSafe Beds, 170
Social Vocational Services, 5935
Special Services Summer Day Camp, 1299
Spring Dell Center, 8171
St. Francis Camp On The Lake, 1198
St. John Valley Associates, 7888
St. Paul Abilities Network, 939
Steps to Independence: Teaching Everyday Skills to Children with Special Needs, 8813
Summit Camp, 1300, 7940
Sundial Special Vacations, 5618
TERI, 5270
Teacher Education Division (TED), 2119
Tennessee Council on Developmental Disabilities, 3862
Thumb Industries, 7001
Torah Alliance of Families of Kids with Disabilities, 5782
Toyei Industries, 6531
Trips Inc., 5620
United Foundation for Disabled Archers, 8460
Unity Language System, 203
Unyeway, 5939
VBS Special Education Teaching Guide, 2644
Ventures Travel, 5621
Waban Projects, 958
Warren Achievement Center, 6870
Wisconsin Badger Camp, 1492
YAI: National Institute for People with Disabilities, 962
YMCA Outdoor Center Campbell Gard, 1345, 8665
Young Children with Special Needs: A Developmentally Appropriate Approach, 2726

Diabetes

ADA Annual Scientific Sessions, 1883
ADA Camp 180, 1264
ADA Camp Aspire, 1267
ADA Camp GranADA, 1108, 8534
ADA Camp Needlepoint, 8535
ADA Teen Adventure Camp, 1109, 8536
ADA Triangle D Camp, 1110, 8537
American Diabetes Association, 8472
The Barton Center, 1182
The Barton Center Camp Joslin, 1183
The Barton Center Clara Barton Camp, 1184
The Barton Center Danvers Day Camp, 1185
The Barton Center Family Camp, 1186
The Barton Center Worcester Day Camp, 1187
Bearskin Meadow Camp, 999, 8543
Camp AZDA, 984
Camp Adam Fisher, 1403
Camp Buck, 1237
Camp Carefree, 1243, 1306, 8556
Camp Carolina Trails, 1307
Camp Classen YMCA, 8560
Camp Comeca & Retreat Center, 8183
Camp Conrad Chinnock, 1003, 8561
Camp Daypoint, 1484
Camp Discovery - Illinois, 8563
Camp Discovery Kansas, 1146, 8564
Camp Endres, 1348
Camp Floyd Rogers, 1231, 8567
Camp Freedom, 1376
Camp Gilbert, 1409
Camp Glyndon, 8569
Camp Hamwi, 1322
Camp Hertko Hollow, 1143, 8573
Camp Hickory Hill, 1219, 8574
Camp Ho Mita Koda, 1324, 8575
Camp Hodia, 1104, 8576
Camp Hope, 1495
Camp ICANDO, 1455

Camp John Warvel, 1130, 8581
Camp Jordan, 1469
Camp Joslin, 8582
Camp Ko-Man-She, 1326, 8584
Camp Korelitz, 1327
Camp Kudzu, 1096
Camp Kweebec, 8585
Camp Libbey, 8588
Camp Lo-Be-Gon, 1349
Camp Midicha, 1193
Camp Needlepoint, 1487
Camp Nejeda, 1255, 8591
Camp New Horizons North, 1434
Camp New Horizons South, 1435
Camp NoLoHi, 1437
Camp Planet D, 1147
Camp Sandcastle, 1440
Camp Seale Harris, 966, 8601
Camp Setebaid, 1383, 8602
Camp Sioux, 1316
Camp Sugar Falls, 1420
Camp Sweeney, 1443, 8607
Camp Sweet Betes, 1149
Camp Tiponi, 1333
Camp Waziyatah, 8611
Camps for Children & Teens with Diabetes, 1471, 8614
Canadian Diabetes Association, 8484
Cedar Ridge Camp, 8615
Center for the Partially Sighted, 6570
Clara Barton Camp, 8618
Coast to Coast Home Medical, 264
Comprehensive Rehabilitation Center at Lee Memorial Hospital, 6728
Diabetes Camp, 8619
Diabetes Network of East Hawaii, 3534
Diabetes Self-Management, 8861
Diabetes Sourcebook., 8708
EDI Camp, 8622
FCYD Camp Utada, 1459, 8624
Florida Diabetes Camp, 1084, 8626
Friends Academy Summer Camps, 8627
Gales Creek Diabetes Camp, 1362
Growing Together Diabetes Camp, 8629
Immune System Disorders Sourcebook., 8729
JDRF, 873
Joslin Guide to Diabetes: A Program for Managing Your Treatment, 8735
Kids Rock The World Day Camp, 1460
Kiwanis Camp Wyman, 8633
Kluge Children's Rehabilitation Center, 6477
Makemie Woods Camp, 8636
Makemie Woods Camp/Conference Retreat, 8637
Meeting the Needs of People with Vision Loss: Multidisciplinary Perspective, 9220
National Diabetes Action Network for the Blind, 9087
National Institute of Diabetes and Digestive and Kidney Diseases, 3394
NeSoDak, 1410, 8642
No More Allergies, 8774
The Rainbow Club, 1071
Raleigh Rehabilitation and Healthcare Center, 7348
Resources for People with Disabilities and Chronic Conditions, 5258
STIX Diabetes Programs, 1482, 8647
Taking Control of Your Diabetes (TCOYD), 8531
Vermont Overnight Camp, 1465
Voice of the Diabetic, 8881
Y Camp, 8658

Diet & Nutrition

Feingold Association of the US, 842
Genova Diagnostics, 846, 4974
National Association of Anorexia Nervosa and Associated Disorders, 8512
Pure Facts, 8069

Down Syndrome

Adolescents with Down Syndrome: Toward a More Fulfilling Life, 7951
Biomedical Concerns in Persons with Down's Syndrome, 2391
Bobby Dodd Institute (BDI), 6787
Bus Girl: Selected Poems, 7975
Camp Oginali, 1418
Clockworks, 5413
Communication Development in Children with Down Syndrome, 7979, 8968
Down Syndrome, 7987
Down Syndrome Camp, 1214
Down Syndrome News, 8064
Down Syndrome Society of Rhode Island, 3256
Early Communication Skills for Children with Down Syndrome, 2450
Keys to Parenting a Child with Downs Syndrome, 8013
National Association for Down Syndrome, 7877
National Down Syndrome Congress, 7882
National Down Syndrome Society, 7883
Parent's Guide to Down Syndrome: Toward a Brighter Future, 8024
Teaching Children with Down Syndrome about Their Bodies, Boundaries, and Sexuality, 5346
Teaching Reading to Children with Down Syndrome: A Guide for Parents and Teachers, 2619
Understanding Down Syndrome: An Introduction for Parents, 8044

Dyslexia

Annals of Dyslexia, 8051
Annual Conference on Dyslexia and Related Learning Disabilities, 1895
Assets School, 5996
Dyslexia Training Program, 1989
Dyslexia over the Lifespan, 7989
Gow School Summer Programs, 1291, 7920
How To Reach and Teach Children and Teens with Dyslexia, 8006
Individualized Keyboarding, 2004
Instrumental Music for Dyslexics: A Teaching Handbook, 31
International Dyslexia Association, 2104
International Dyslexia Association of DC, 3499
International Dyslexia Association: Arizona Branch, 3443
International Dyslexia Association: Austin Branch, 3874
International Dyslexia Association: Central California Branch, 3463
International Dyslexia Association: Central Ohio Branch, 3787
International Dyslexia Association: Florida Branch, 3516
International Dyslexia Association: Georgia Branch, 3530
International Dyslexia Association: Hawaii Branch, 3544
International Dyslexia Association: Illinois Branch, 3564
International Dyslexia Association: Indiana Branch, 3571
International Dyslexia Association: Iowa Branch, 3573
International Dyslexia Association: Kansas/Missouri Branch, 3584
International Dyslexia Association: Louisiana Branch, 3661
International Dyslexia Association: Maryland Branch, 3614
International Dyslexia Association: New Jersey Branch, 3717
International Dyslexia Association: North Carolina Branch, 3769
International Dyslexia Association: Oregon Branch, 3806
International Dyslexia Association: Pennsylvania Branch, 3816
International Dyslexia Association: Rocky Mountain Branch, 3477
International Dyslexia Association: Tennessee Branch, 3858
International Dyslexia Association: Upper Midwest Branch, 3649
International Dyslexia Association: Virginia Branch, 3920
International Dyslexia Association: Washington State Branch, 3930
International Dyslexia Association: Wisconsin Branch, 3950
Learning Disabilities Sourcebook, 3rd Ed., 35
Let's Write Right: Teacher's Edition, 2528
Louisiana Center for Dyslexia and Related Learning Disorders, 3598
Many Faces of Dyslexia, 2024
Mozart Effect: Tapping the Power of Music to Heal the Body, Strengthen the Mind, 37
Multisensory Teaching of Basic Language Skills: Theory and Practice, 2542
Music and Dyslexia: A Positive Approach, 43
Overcoming Dyslexia, 8022
Overcoming Dyslexia in Children, Adolescents and Adults, 2546
Pre-Reading Screening Procedures, 2703
Reading, Writing and Speech Problems in Children, 8029, 8986
Reality of Dyslexia, 8030
Recording for the Blind & Dyslexic, 9238
Sandhills School, 2750
Southwest Branch of the International Dyslexia Association, 3735
Stern Center for Language and Learning, 8936
TESTS, 2606
Teaching of Reading: A Continuum from Kindergarten through College, The, 2716
To Teach a Dyslexic, 2064
We're Not Stupid, 8092

Education & Counseling

ACA Annual Conference, 1882
ADA National Network, 724
ATIA Conference, 1889
Adapting Early Childhood Curricula for Children with Special Needs (9th Edition), 2358
Advocates for Children of New York (AFC), 734
Alaska Department of Education: Special Education, 2179
American Counseling Association (ACA), 755, 2147
American Disabled for Attendant Programs Today (ADAPT), 757, 7518
American Journal of Occupational Therapy (AJOT), 2248
American Journal of Public Health (AJPH), 5367
American Occupational Therapy Association (AOTA), 761
American Public Health Association, 7521
American Public Health Association (APHA), 763
American Red Cross, 764
Applied Rehabilitation Counseling (Springer Series on Rehabilitation), 2372
Assistive Technology Industry Association (ATIA), 772
Brookline Books, 2150
Building the Healing Partnership: Parents, Professionals and Children with Chronic Illnesses, 2395
Burton Blatt Institute (BBI), 788
Camp Independence, 1094, 8579
Cape Organization for Rights of the Disabled (CORD), 4296
Case Management Society of America (CMSA), 794
Center for Inclusive Design and Innovation, 797, 2081
Center for Workplace Compliance, 4652
Chicago Lawyers' Committee for Civil Rights Under Law, 4653
Childhood Disablity and Family Systems(Routledge Library Editions) (Volume 5), 2405
Children's Specialized Hospital Medical Library - Parent Resource Center, 4948
Choices: A Guide to Sex Counseling with Physically Disabled Adults, 2408

Coalition for Health Funding, 807
Council of Parent Attorneys and Advocates (COPAA), 811
Counseling & Values, 2260
Counseling Today, 2310
Counselor Education & Supervision, 2262
DNA People's Legal Services, 4655
Deciphering the System: A Guide for Families of Young Disabled Children, 2431
Department of Rehabilitation Services & Bureau of Education And Services for the Blind, 2184
Disability Rights Education and Defense Fund, 4658
Disability Rights Texas, 3868, 4659
Dual Relationships in Counseling, 2449
Early Intervention: Implementing Child & Family Services for At-Risk Infants and Toddlers, 2451
Educating Individuals with Disabilities: IDEIA 2004 and Beyond (1st Edition), 2455
Employer Assistance and Resource Network on Disability Inclusion (EARN), 833
Family Engagement, 2316
Family Run Executive Director Leadership Association (FREDLA), 837
Fedcap Rehabilitation Services, 840
Federal Benefits for Veterans and Dependents, 5634
Florida State College at Jacksonville Services for Students with Disabilities, 2192
HEATH Resource Center at the National Youth Transitions Center, 849
High Technology Foundation, 855, 3336
Images of the Disabled, Disabling Images, 2501
Inclusive Play People, 2003
Institute for Educational Leadership (IEL), 862
International Academy of Independent Medical Evaluators, 863
Journal of Addictions & Offender Counseling, 2277
Journal of Counseling & Development, 2279
Journal of Rehabilitation, 2290, 7723
The K&W Guide to Colleges for Studentswith Learning Disabilties (13th Edition), 2635
Lane Community College, 2778
Legislative Handbook for Parents, 4709
Library Manager's Guide to Hiring and Serving Disabled Persons, 2529
Mainstream, 882, 3995
National Bullying Prevention Center Newsletter, 2329
National Business & Disability Council (NBDC), 894
National Center for College Students with Disabilities (NCCSD), 896
National Center on Disability and Journalism (NCDJ), 900
National Collaborative Workforce on Disability (NCWD/Youth), 902
National Diabetes Information Clearinghouse, 8516
National Digestive Diseases Information Clearinghouse, 8517
National Kidney and Urologic Diseases Information Clearinghouse, 8520
National Organization on Disability (NOD), 909, 5532
National Rehabilitation Association (NRA), 910
National Vaccine Information Center (NVIC), 912
Nevada Department of Education: Special Eduction Branch, 2225
OT Practice Magazine, 5394
Partnership on Employment and Acessible Technology (PEAT), 922
Professional Development Programs, 2211
Ramapo Training, 2749
Rehabilitation Technology, 2578
RespectAbility, 932
Sofia University, 937
South Dakota Division of Rehabilitation, 3855
Student Disability Services (SDS), 941
Viability, 955, 6086
Whittier Trust, 2871

Emergency Alert

Cornell Communications, 182
Humanity & Inclusion (HI), 859
MedicAlert Foundation International, 2852
Sidney Stern Memorial Trust, 2863

Environmental Disorders

Alternative Approach to Allergies, 8675
American Academy of Environmental Medicine (AAEM), 737
American Academy of Environmental Medicine Annual Conference, 1893
Protecting Against Latex Allergy, 8801

Epilepsy

Acting Blind, 5399
Boy Inside, The, 5407
Camp COAST, 1273
Camp Candlelight, 986, 7899
Camp EAGR, 1274
Camp Evoked Potential, 965, 7901
Camp Great Rock, 1166
Camp Neuron, 1433
Camp Spike 'n' Wave, 1441
Coelho Epilepsy Youth Summer Camp, 1031
Epilepsy Council of Greater Cincinnati, 3786
Epilepsy Foundation, 7864, 8104, 8354, 8893
Epilepsy Foundation of Alabama, 8490
Epilepsy Foundation of Long Island, 3134
Epilepsy Foundation of Southeast Texas, 3292
Epilepsy Foundation: Central and South Texas, 3293
Epilepsy, 199 Answers: A Doctor Responds to His Patients' Questions, 8714
Epilepsy: Patient and Family Guide, 8715
EpilepsyUSA, 8847
Father Drumgoole Connelly Summer Camp, 8198, 8625
Growing Up with Epilepsy: A Pratical Guide for Parents, 8719
International League Against Epilepsy (ILAE), 869
Kamp Kaleidoscope, 1450
Ketogenic Diet: A Treatment for Children and Others with Epilepsy, 8737
Narcolepsy, 5443
National Association of Epilepsy Centers, 7879
Neuropsychiatry of Epilepsy, 8772
On The Spectrum, 5445
Outsider: The Life and Art of Judith Scott, 5449
Pushin' Forward, 5454
Seizures and Epilepsy in Childhood: A Guide, 8807
Twin Lakes Camp, 8383, 8656
White Cane and Wheels, 5475
YMCA Camp Fitch, 1397, 8206, 8384, 8659, 8951

Head & Neck Injuries

American Academy of Otolaryngology - Head and Neck Surgery, 8467
American Head and Neck Society, 8474
Annals of Otology, Rhinology and Laryngology, 8840
Head Injury Hotline, 8895
Head Injury Rehabilitation: Children, 2489
Health and Rehabilitation Products, 434
IAL News, 8863
Injured Mind, Shattered Dreams: Brian's Survival from a Severe Head Injury, 8731
Journal of Head Trauma Rehabilitation, 8844
Life Line, 8743

Hearing Impairments

ADARA, 8290
The AG Academy for Listening and Spoken Language, 2120
AG Bell Global Listening and Spoken Language Symposium, 1885
ASD Summer Camp, 8177
ASHA Leader, The, 8302
ASSISTECH Special Needs, 162
Academy of Rehabilitative Audiology, 2073
Access for All: Integrating Deaf, Hard of Hearing and Hearing Preschoolers, 8212
Access-USA, 460, 576
Advanced Sign Language Vocabulary: A Resource Text for Educators, 2362, 8213
Alexander Graham Bell Association for the Deaf and Hard of Hearing, 8123
Alternatives in Education for the Hearing Impaired (AEHI), 5482
American Academy of Audiology (AAA), 736, 5483, 8124
American Academy of Audiology Conference, 1892
American Action Fund for Blind Children and Adults, 9027
American Annals of the Deaf, 8303
American Hearing Impaired Hockey Association, 8333
American Journal of Audiology, 8291
American Sign Language Handshape Cards, 1966
American Sign Language Handshape Dictionary, 8214
American Sign Language Phrase Book, 8215
American Sign Language: A Look at Its History, Structure & Community, 8216
American Speech-Language and Hearing Association, 5488
Americans with Disabilities Act: Selected Resources for Deaf, 4673
Amplified Handsets, 176
Amplified Phones, 177
Amplified Portable Phone, 178
Approaching Equality, 4674
Aspen Camp, 1045, 8178
Assessment & Management of Mainstreamed Hearing-Impaired Children, 2375
Association of Adult Musicians with Hearing Loss, 8130
Association of Medical Professionals with Hearing Losses (AMPHL), 778
At Home Among Strangers, 8217
AudiologyOnline, 5493
Auditech: Personal FM Educational System, 1970
Auditech: Personal PA Value Pack System, 285
Auditory-Verbal Therapy for Parents and Professionals, 1971
Aural Habilitation, 2387
Aurora of Central New York, 7830
BPPV: What You Need to Know, 8218
A Basic Course in American Sign Language, 8208
Basic Course in American Sign Language, 9137
Basic Course in American Sign Language(B100) Harris Communications, Inc., 5404
A Basic Course in Manual Communication, 8209
A Basic Vocabulary: American Sign Languagefor Parents and Children, 8210
Battery Device Adapter, 287
Bed Rails, 263
Beginning ASL Video Course, 5405
Belonging, 9139
Ben's Story: A Deaf Child's Right to Sign, 8219
Better Hearing Institute, 8132
Bill Rice Ranch, 1413
Book of Name Signs: Naming in American Sign Language, 8220
Bureau of Services for Blind Persons Training Center, 6986
Camp Alexander Mack, 8179
Camp Bishopswood, 8180
Camp Chris Williams, 1191, 8182
Camp Emanuel, 1321, 8184
Camp Grizzly, 1004, 8185
Camp Isola Bella, 1066, 8186
Camp Juliena, 1095, 8188
Camp Loud And Clear, 1470
Camp Mark Seven, 1280, 8189
Camp Pacifica, 1014, 8191
Camp Sertoma, 1311
Camp Shocco for the Deaf, 967, 8193
Camp Taloali, 1358, 8194

Carl and Ruth Shapiro Family National Center for Accessible Media, 6958, 8917
Center for Hearing and Communication, 8133
Challenge of Educating Together Deaf and Hearing Youth: Making Manistreaming Work, 2400
Chelsea: The Story of a Signal Dog, 8221
Children of a Lesser God, 8222
Choices in Deafness: A Parent's Guide to Communication Options, 8223
Christmas Stories, 8319
Clark-Winchcole Foundation, 3009
Classroom GOALS: Guide for Optimizing Auditory Learning Skills, 1978
Classroom Notetaker: How to Organize a Program Serving Students with Hearing Impairments, 1979
Closed Caption Decoder, 181
Cochlear Implant Camp, 1058, 8196
Cochlear Implants In Children: Ethics and Choices, 8305
Cochlear Implants for Kids, 8224
Cognition, Education and Deafness: Directions for Research and Instruction, 8225
College and University Programs for Deaf and Hard of Hearing Students, 8226
Come Sign with Us, 8227
Communication Service for the Deaf, 8134
Communique, 8306
Comprehensive Reference Manual for Signers and Interpreters, 8228
Comprehensive Signed English Dictionary, 8229
Conference of Educational Administrators of Schools and Programs for the Deaf, 8135
Connect, 9010
Connect - Commmunity News, 8307
Connect Hearing, 421
Conversational Sign Language II: An Intermediate Advanced Manual, 8230
Council of American Instructors of the Deaf (CAID), 8136
Crutches, 610
Custom Earmolds, 289
Deaf Camps, Inc., 1171
Deaf Catholic, 8308
Deaf Children Signers, 5415
Deaf Culture Series, 5416
Deaf Empowerment: Emergence, Struggle and Rhetoric, 8231
Deaf History Unveiled: Interpretations from the New Scholarship, 8232
Deaf Kid's Kamp, 8197
Deaf Like Me, 8233
Deaf Mosaic, 5417
Deaf Parents and Their Hearing Children, 8234
Deaf REACH, 8137
Deaf in America: Voices from a Culture, 8235
Deafness Research Foundation, 8139
Deafness and Communicative Disorders Branch of Rehab Services Administration Office, 8919
Dial-a-Hearing Screening Test, 8335
Digital Hearing Aids, 290
Division for Communication, Language, and Deaf/Hard of Hearing (DCD), 2087
Do You Hear That?, 5418
Door Knock Signaler, 476
Doorbell Signalers, 477
Duracell & Rayovac Hearing Aid Batteries, 291
EASE Program: Emergency Access Self Evaluation, 8236
Ear Foundation, 8141
Education and Auditory Research Foundation, 3274
Education of the Handicapped: Laws, Legislative Histories and Administrative Document, 4692
Educational Audiology for the Limited Hearing Infant and Preschooler, 2458
Effectively Educating Handicapped Students, 2463
Electronic Amplified Stethoscopes, 271
Enchanted Hills Camp for the Blind, 1035, 9114
Encyclopedia of Deafness and Hearing Disorders, 8237
Evaluation and Educational Programming of Students with Deafblindness & Severe Disabilities, 2466
Expressive and Receptive Fingerspelling for Hearing Adults, 8238
Eye-Centered: A Study of Spirituality of Deaf People, 8239
Fantastic Series Videotape Set, 8320
Fantastic: Colonial Times, Chocolate, and Cars, 8321
Fantastic: Dogs at Work and Play, 8322
Fantastic: Exciting People, Places and Things!, 8323
Fantastic: From Post Offices to Dairy Goats, 8324
Fantastic: Imagination, Actors, and 'Deaf Way', 8325
Fantastic: Roller Coasters, Maps, and Ice Cream!, 8326
Fantastic: Skiing, Factories, and Race Hores, 8327
Fantastic: Wonderful Worlds of Sports and Travel, 8328
Fingerspelling: Expressive and Receptive Fluency, 8329
Fold-Down 3-in-1 Commode, 272
For Hearing People Only, 8240
Free Hand: Enfranchising the Education of Deaf Children, 2474
Freedom Three Wheel Walker, 615
From Gesture to Language in Hearing and Deaf Children, 8241
From Mime to Sign Package, 8242
GA and SK Etiquette, 8243
Gallaudet Survival Guide to Signing, 8244
Gallaudet University Press, 2156, 5511
Georgiana Institute, 8142
Global Assistive Devices, Inc., 166
Goldilocks and the Three Bears: Told in Signed English, 8245
HEAR Center, 8143
Harc Mercantile, Ltd., 183
Harris Communications, 292
Healing Dressing for Pressure Sores, 273
Hear You Are, 436
Hearing Aid Batteries, 293
Hearing Aid Battery Testers, 294
Hearing Aid Care Kit, 295
Hearing Education and Awareness for Rockers, 8144
Hearing Health Foundation (HHF), 854, 3147
Hearing Health Magazine, 8299
Hearing Impaired Children and Youth with Developmental Disabilities, 8246
Hearing Loss Association of America, 7798, 8146
Hearing, Speech and Deafness Center (HSDC), 8147, 8921
Helen Keller National Center Newsletter, 9193
Hollywood Speaks: Deafness and the Film Entertainment Industry, 8247
Home Alerting Systems, 485
House Ear Institute, 8148
How to Thrive, Not Just Survive, 9196
I Can't Hear You in the Dark: How to Lean and Teach Lipreading, 2497
I Have a Sister, My Sister is Deaf, 8248
I Heard That!, 2498
I Heard That!2, 2499
Independence Without Sight and Sound: Suggestions for Practitioners, 7811
Independence Without Sight or Sound, 8249
Indiana Deaf Camp, 1140
InfoLoop Induction Receiver, 184
Innovative Practices for Teaching Sign Language Interpreters, 8250
Intermediate Conversational Sign Language, 8251
International Catholic Deaf Association, 8149
International Hearing Dog, 8150
International Hearing Dog, Inc., 8309
International Hearing Society, 7801, 8151
Interpretation: A Sociolinguistic Model, 8252
Interpreting: An Introduction, 8253
Invisible Children, 5437
Jason & Nordic Publishers, Inc., 5203
Journal of the Academy of Rehabilitative Audiology, 8294
Journal of the American Academy of Audiology, 7657
Journey, 5438
Joy of Signing, 8254
Joy of Signing Puzzle Book, 8255
Kid-Friendly Parenting with Deaf and Hard of Hearing Children, 8256
Language Learning Practices with Deaf Children, 2520
Laurent Clerc National Deaf Education Center, 877
Laurent Clerc: The Story of His Early Years, 8257
Learning American Sign Language, 2013
Learning to See: American Sign Language asa Second Language, 2527
Learning to Sign in My Neighborhood, 2015
Legal Right: The Guide for Deaf and Hard of Hearing People, 4707
Lexington School for the Deaf: Center for the Deaf, 8153
Liberty Lightweight Aluminum Stroll Walker, 616
Linguistics of American Sign Language: An Introduction, 8258
Lions Camp Kirby, 8200
Lions Wilderness Camp for Deaf Children, Inc., 1037, 8202
Listen Foundation, 2881
Literacy & Your Deaf Child: What Every Parent Should Know, 8259
Literature Journal, The, 8295
A Loss for Words, 8211
MADAMIST 50/50 PSI Air Compressor, 275
Mainstreaming Deaf and Hard of Hearing Students: Questions and Answers, 2531
Mask of Benevolence: Disabling the Deaf Community, The, 8260
Meniere's Disease, 8760
Michigan Association for Deaf and Hard of Hearing, 3631, 8154
Michigan Commission for the Blind, 3636
Michigan Commission for the Blind - Gaylord, 3635
Michigan Commission for the Blind Training Center, 3637
Michigan Commission for the Blind: Escanaba, 3638
Michigan Commission for the Blind: Flint, 3639
Micro Audiometrics Corporation, 297
Microloop III Basic, 187
Miracle-Ear Children's Foundation, 3019
Mississippi Speech-Language-Hearing Association, 8155
Mother Father Deaf: Living Between Sound and Silence, 8261
Mushroom Inserts, 298
My First Book of Sign, 8262
My Signing Book of Numbers, 8263
MyAlert Body Worn Multifunction Receiver, 188
NAD Broadcaster, 4721
National Association of Blind Educators, 9074
National Association of Blind Lawyers, 9075
National Association of Blind Rehabilitation Professionals, 9077
National Association of Hearing Officials, 8157
National Association of Special Education Teachers, 8159, 8927
National Association of the Deaf, 8160
National Black Association for Speech Language and Hearing, 8161
National Black Association for Speech-Language and Hearing, 8928
National Black Deaf Advocates, 8162
National Catholic Office of the Deaf, 8163
National Deaf Women's Bowling Association, 8165
National Hearing Conservation Association, 8166
National Institute on Deafness and Other Communication Disorders, 3398, 8167
National Student Speech Language Hearing Association, 8168
New Jersey Speech-Language-Hearing Association, 2222
News from Advocates for Deaf-Blind, 7826
Nursery Rhymes from Mother Goose, 8264
On the Level, 8314
Outsiders in a Hearing World: A Sociology of Deafness, 8265
Oval Window Audio, 299

PLA240 Room Loop System, 189
Parents and Teachers, 2550
Patient Transport Chair, 683
Patriot Extra Wide Folding Walkers, 618
Patriot Folding Walker Series, 619
Patriot Reciprocal Folding Walkers, 620
People with Disabilities Who Challenge the System, 5246
Perigee Visual Dictionary of Signing, 8266
Personal FM Systems, 190
Phone Ringers, 191
Phone Strobe Flasher, 192
Phone of Our Own: The Deaf Insurrection Against Ma Bell, 8267
PhoneMax Amplified Telephone, 528
Place of Their Own: Creating the Deaf Community in America, 8268
Pocketalker Personal Amplifier, 193
PreReading Strategies, 8269
Products for People with Disabilities, 452
Quad Canes, 623
Quad City Deaf & Hard of Hearing Youth Group: Tomorrow's Leaders for our Community, 8270
Raising Deaf Kids, 930
Reading and Deafness, 2571
Registry of Interpreters for the Deaf, 8169
Religious Signing: A Comprehensive Guide for All Faiths, 8271
Room Valet Visual-Tactile Alerting System, 503
Say it with Sign, 9242
See What I'm Saying, 9349
Seeing Voices, 8272
Sertoma Camp Endeavor, 1087, 8204
Shape Up 'n Sign, 9351
Show Me How: A Manual for Parents of Preschool Blind Children, 9246
Sign Language Interpreting and Interpreter Education, 8273
Sign Language Studies, 8296
Sign of the Times, 9247
Signaling Wake-Up Devices, 505
Signed English Schoolbook, 2591
Signed English Starter, The, 8274
Signing Family: What Every Parent Should Know About Sign Communication, The, 8275
Signing Naturally Curriculum, 2049
Signing for Reading Success, 8276
Signing: How to Speak with Your Hands, 8277
Signs Across America, 8278
Signs for Me: Basic Sign Vocabulary for Children, Parents & Teachers, 8279
Signs for Sexuality: A Resource Manual, 8280
Signs of the Times, 8281
Silent Garden, The, 8282
Sing Praise Hymnal for the Deaf, 8283
Smoke Detector with Strobe, 506
Sonic Alert, 196
Sonic Alert Bed Shaker, 171
Sound & Fury, 5462
Soundings Newsletter, 8316
Speech Adjust-A-Tone Basic, 197
Speech and the Hearing-Impaired Child, 2597
Standard 3-in-1 Commode, 280
Standard Wheelchair, 693
Starkey Hearing Foundation, 301, 8172
Stick Canes, 629
Store @ HDSC Product Catalog, 456
Strobe Light Signalers, 509
TDI National Directory & Resource Guide: Blue Book, 8284
TTYs: Telephone Device for the Deaf, 199
Telecommunications for the Deaf and Hard of Hearing, 8173
Test of Early Reading Ability Deaf or Hard of Hearing, 2718
Texas School of the Deaf, 2239
Theoretical Issues in Sign Language Research, 8285
There's a Hearing Impaired Child in My Class, 2636
Thinklabs One Stethoscope, 283
To Love this Life: Quotations by Helen Keller, 9262
Toward Effective Public School Program for Deaf Students, 2637
Transfer Bench, 284
USA Deaf Sports Federation, 8334
Ultratec, 302
Usher Syndrome, 8831
Vestibular Disorders Association, 8176
Vision Magazine, 8318
Volta Review, 8297
We CAN Hear and Speak, 8286
Week the World Heard Gallaudet, The, 8287
Weitbrecht Communications, Inc. (WCI), 459
What is Auditory Processing?, 8288
You and Your Deaf Child: A Self-Help Guidefor Parents of Deaf and Hard of Hearing Children, 8289
Youth Leadership Camp, 8207
iLuv SmartShaker 2, 172

Hemophilia

Arizona Hemophilia Association, 8481
Bright Horizons Summer Camp, 8546
Camp Ailihpomeh, 1424
Camp Brave Eagle, 1129
Camp H.U.G., 988, 8570
Camp High Hopes, 1276
Camp Honor, 989, 8578
Camp Hot-to-Clot, 1377
Camp Klotty Pine, 1486
Camp Little Oak, 1279
Hemophilia Camp, 8632
National Hemophilia Foundation, 3160, 8519

Herbal Medicine

American Botanical Council (ABC), 750
American Herbalists Guild (AHG), 759
HerbalEGram, 2323
HerbalGram, 2271

Human Interaction Disabilities

Camp Akeela, 1371
Camp Buckskin, 1201, 7898
Camp Connect, 1244
Eagle Hill School: Summer Program, 1178, 7917
Taking Part: Introducing Social Skills to Young Children, 2715

Immune Deficiencies

IDF National Conference, 1908
Immune Deficiency Foundation, 860, 3017
POZ Magazine, 8851
YMCA Camp Shady Brook, 8662

Incontinence

Adaptive Clothing: Adults, 405, 1498
Adult Absorbent Briefs, 1499
Care Electronics, 466
Duraline Medical Products Inc., 267
Informer, 8864
Kleinert's, 440
MOMS Catalog, 444
National Association for Continence, 8363
Quality Care Newsletter, 8872
Simon Foundation for Continence, 8373
Specialty Care Shoppe, 1545

Language Disorders

Academic Language Therapy Association, 8910
American Speech-Language-Hearing Association, 8128, 8911
Association of Language Companies, 8913
Beyond Baby Talk: From Sounds to Sentences, a Parent's Guide to Language Development, 8962
International Fluency Association, 8923
Language Arts: Detecting Special Needs, 2519
Language Disabilities in Children and Adolescents, 8974
Language and Communication Disorders in Children, 2521
Lindamood-Bell Home Learning Process, 8924
OWLS: Oral and Written Language Scales LC/OE & WE, 2694
PAT-3: Photo Articulation Test, 2695
Peabody Early Experiences Kit (PEEK), 2696
Peabody Language Development Kits (PLDK), 2698
Perspectives: Whole Language Folio, 8983
Preventing Academic Failure - Teachers Handbook, 2562
RULES: Revised, 2706
Receptive-Expressive Emergent-REEL-2 Language Test, 2nd Edition, 2707
Teaching Language-Disabled Children: A Communication/Games Intervention, 2615
Teaching Reading to Disabled and Handicapped Learners, 2620
Test of Language Development: Primary, 2719
Test of Phonological Awareness, 2722
Woodcock Reading Mastery Tests, 2725

Learning Disabilities

AEPS Child Progress Record: For Children Ages Three to Six, 1959
AEPS Child Progress Report: For Children Ages Birth to Three, 2652
AEPS Curriculum for Birth to Three Years, 2354
AEPS Curriculum for Three to Six Years, 1960
AEPS Data Recording Forms: For Children Ages Birth to Three, 2653
AEPS Data Recording Forms: For Children Ages Three to Six, 1961
AEPS Family Interest Survey, 1962
AEPS Family Report: For Children Ages Birth to Three, 5097
AEPS Measurement for Birth to Three Years, 2654
AEPS Measurement for Three to Six Years, 2655
AIR: Assessment of Interpersonal Relations, 2656
AVKO Educational Research Foundation, 2072
Academic Therapy Publications, 2145
Activity-Based Approach to Early Intervention, 2nd Edition, 2356
Adaptive Education Strategies Building on Diversity, 2360
Adaptive Mainstreaming: A Primer for Teachers and Principals, 3rd Edition, 2658
Advanced Language Tool Kit, 1964
Ages & Stages Questionnaires, 2659
All Kinds of Minds, 1965
Alphabetic Phonics Curriculum, 2367
Alternative Educational Delivery Systems, 2368
American College Testing Program, 2660
American School Counselor Association, 2076
Arkansas Department of Special Education, 2180
Assessing Students with Special Needs, 2661
Assessment Log & Developmental Progress Charts for the CCPSN, 2376, 2662
Assessment of Learners with Special Needs, 2663
Assessment: The Special Educator's Role, 2382
Assistive Technology, 179
Association of Educational Therapists (AET), 776
Association on Higher Education & Disability (AHEAD), 781, 2078
BOSC: Directory of Facilities for People with Learning Disabilities, 2124
Beacon Therapeutic Diagnostic and Treatment Center, 6813
Beginning Reasoning and Reading, 1974
Behind Special Education, 2390
Benchmark Measures, 2664
BroadFutures, 7854
Buy!, 1976
CAI, Career Assessment Inventories for the Learning Disabled, 2396
CEC Catalog, 2251
CEC Pioneers Division (CEC-PD), 2080
CREVT: Comprehensive Receptive and Expressive Vocabulary Test, 2666
Camp Nuhop, 1328, 7906

Camp Starfish, 1177
Carolina Curriculum for Infants and Toddlers with Special Needs (3rd Edition), 2398
Carolina Curriculum for Preschoolers with Special Needs, 2399
Catalyst, 2254
Center Academy, 7855
Center Academy at Pinellas Park, 1080, 7915
Charis Hills Camp, 1445
Chemists with Disabilities Committee - American Chemical Society, 5389
Children's Understanding of Disability, 5050
Christian Approach to Overcoming Disability: A Doctor's Story, 5143
Clovernook Printing House, The Clovernook Center for the Blind and Visually Impaired, 9050
Cognitive Approaches to Learning Disabilities, 2413
College Internship Program at the Berkshire Center, 6962
Colorado Department of Education: Special Education Service Unit, 2182
Communicating with Parents of Exceptional Children, 2417
Complete Handbook of Children's Reading Disorders: You Can Prevent or Correct LDs, 2421
Complete Learning Disabilities Resource Guide, 2126
Complete Resource Guide for Pediatric Disorders, 2128
Complete Resource Guide for People with Chronic Illness, 2129
Computer Access/Computer Learning, 2422
Conference of the Association on Higher Education & Disability (AHEAD), 1904, 5145
Council for Educational Diagnostic Services (CEDS), 2083
Council for Exceptional Children (CEC), 809, 2084, 5021
Council for Exceptional Children Annual Convention and Expo, 1905
Critical Voices on Special Education: Problems & Progress Concerning the Mildly Handicapped, 2428
Dallas Academy, 1448, 7916
Department of Public Health Human Services, 2214
Developmental Disabilities of Learning, 2438
Developmental Variation and Learning Disorders, 2441
Disability Matters, 1906
Division for Culturally and Linguistically Diverse Exceptional Learners (DDEL), 2088
Division for Early Childhood of the Council for Exceptional Children, 2090
Division for Learning Disabilities (DLD), 2091
Division on Career Development and Transition (DCDT), 2097
Eagle View Ranch, 1496
Early Childhood Reporter, 2314
Early Intervention, 2266
Educating all Students in the Mainstream, 2457
Educational Care, 2459
Educational Prescriptions, 2461
Educators Resource Guide, 2132
Effective Instruction for Special Education, 2462
Exceptional Children (EC), 2268
Explode the Code, 1993
Feeding Children with Special Needs, 2472
Florida Department of Education: Bureau of Exceptional Education And Student Services, 2191
Focus on Exceptional Children, 2270
Food!, 1994
Frames of Reference for the Assessment of Learning Disabilities, 2678
Graduate Technological Education and the Human Experience of Disability, 2481
Guide to Teaching Phonics, 1999
Handbook for Implementing Workshops for Siblings of Special Children, 2483
Handbook for the Special Education Administrator, 2485
Hawaii Department of Education: Special Needs, 2193
Help Newsletter, 2322
Helping Learning- Disabled Gifted Children Learn Through Compensatory Active Play, 2492
Helping Students Grow, 2493
High Noon Books, 2161
Hill School of Fort Worth, 1449, 7921
How to Teach Spelling/How to Spell, 2495
Howard School, The, 2740
If It Is To Be, It Is Up To Me To Do It!, 2002
If It Is To Be, It Is Up To Us To Help!, 2500
Illinois State Board of Education: Department of Special Education, 2194
Including Students with Special Needs: A Practical Guide for Classroom Teachers, 2505
Indiana Department of Education: Special Education Division, 2195
Infant & Toddler Convection of Fairfield: Falls Church, 2681
Instructional Methods for Students, 2509
Intervention Research in Learning Disabilities, 2513
Intervention in School and Clinic, 2276
Introduction to Learning Disabilities, 2514
Introduction to Special Education: Teaching in an Age of Challenge, 4th Edition, 2515
Issues and Research in Special Education, 2517
Journal of Applied School Psychology, 2278
Journal of Learning Disabilities, 2282
Journal of Postsecondary Education & Disability (JPED), 2287
Journal of Reading, Writing and Learning Disabled International, 2289
Journal of Social Work in Disabilty & Rehabilitation, 5204
Journal of Special Education, 2292
K-BIT: Kaufman Brief Intelligence Test, 2682
K-FAST: Kaufman Functional Academic Skills Test, 2683
Kansas State Board of Education: Special Education Services, 2197
Kaufman Test of Educational Achievement(K-TEA), 2686
Keeping Ahead in School, 2007
Kendall Demonstration Elementary School Curriculum Guides, 2518
Kentucky Department of Education: Divisionof Exceptional Children's Services, 2198
KeyMath Teach and Practice, 2008
Keyboarding by Ability, 1755
LD OnLine - WETA Public Television, 5520
LD Online, 2106
Lab School of Washington, 2189, 7923
Lakeshore Learning Materials, 2009
Learning Disabilities Association of America (LDA), 878
Learning Disabilities Association of New York State (LDANYS), 879
Learning Disabilities Worldwide, 880
Learning Disabilities, Literacy, and Adult Education, 2522
Learning Disabilities: A Contemporary Journal, 2294
Learning Disabilities: A Multidisciplinary Journal, 2295
Learning Disabilities: Concepts and Characteristics, 2523
Learning Disability: Social Class and the Cons of Inequality In American Education, 2524
Learning and Individual Differences, 2525
Life Beyond the Classroom: Transition Strategies for Young People with Disabilities, 5055
Life Centered Career Education: A Contemporary Based Approach, 2689
Life Development Institute, 7869
Literacy Program, 2016
Literature Based Reading, 2017
MTA Readers, 2020
Mainstreaming Exceptional Students: A Guide for Classroom Teachers, 2532
Making School Inclusion Work: A Guide to Everyday Practice, 2021
Making Self-Employment Work for People with Disabilities, 5084
Making the Writing Process Work: Strategies for Composition and Self-Regulation, 2022
Managing Diagnostic Tool of Visual Perception, 2534
Manual Alphabet Poster, 2023
Maryland State Department of Education: Division of Special Education, 2205
Match-Sort-Assemble Job Cards, 2025
Match-Sort-Assemble TOOLS, 2028
McGraw-Hill Company, 2165
Michigan Department of Education: Special Education Services, 2208
Michigan Psychological Association, 2108
Mississippi Department of Education: Office of Special Services, 2213
Missouri Department of Elementary and Secondary Education: Special Education Programs, 2212
More Food!, 2030
More Work!, 2031
Multisensory Teaching Approach, 2032
National Association for Adults with Special Learning Needs, 2109
National Association of Colleges and Employers, 2110
National Association of Parents with Children in Special Education, 2111, 8158
National Association of State Directors of Special Education, 2112
National Center for Learning Disabilities, 2167
National Clearinghouse on Family Support and Children's Mental Health, 2190
National Education Association of the United States, 2115
National Society for Experiential Education, 2116
Nebraska Department of Education: Special Populations Office, 2218
New Hampshire Department of Education: Bureau for Special Education Services, 2220
New Mexico State Department of Education, 2224
New York State Education Department, 2226
North Dakota Department of Education: Special Education, 2217
Oakland School & Camp, 1474, 7929
Ohio Department of Education: Division of Special Education, 2227
Oklahoma State Department of Education, 2229
Oregon Department of Education: Office of Special Education, 2230
Peabody Articulation Decks, 2034
Peabody Individual Achievement Test-Revised Normative Update (PIAT-R-NU), 2697
Pennsylvania Department of Education: Bureau of Special Education, 2231
Peter and Elizabeth C. Tower Foundation, 925, 3166
Phelps School Academic Support Program, 1393, 7931
Phonemic Awareness in Young Children: A Classroom Curriculum, 2035
Phonics for Thought, 2036
Phonological Awareness Training for Reading, 2037
Play!, 2038
Pragmatic Approach, 2560
Preschoolers with Special Needs: Children At-Risk, Children with Disabilities, 2561
Preventing School Dropouts, 2563
Prevocational Assessment, 2564
Primary Phonics, 2040
Promoting Postsecondary Education for Students with Learning Disabilities, 2567
Reading for Content, 2041
Reading from Scratch, 2042
Recipe for Reading, 2043
Remedial and Special Education, 2304
Resource Room, The, 2580
Rewarding Speech, 2044
Rhode Island Department of Education: Office of Special Needs, 2232
SAYdee Posters, 2045
SOAR Summer Adventures, 1313, 7936
Sage Publications, 2174

Semiotics and Dis/ability: Interogating Categories of Difference, 2586
Sequential Spelling: 1-7 with 7 Student Response Books, 2048
Servcies for Students with Disabilities (SSD), 2117
7 Steps for Success, 2344
Social Studies: Detecting and Correcting Special Needs, 2593
South Carolina Department of Education: Office of Exceptional Children, 2234
Special Education Report, 2340
Special Education Today, 2595
Special Education for Today, 2596
Special Siblings: Growing Up With Someone with A Disability, 5269
Spell of Words, 2054
Spellbound, 2055
Spelling Dictionary, 2056
Squirrel Hollow Summer Camp, 1101, 7938
Starting Over, 2057
Strategies for Teaching Learners with Special Needs, 2601
Students with Mild Disabilities in the Secondary School, 2604
Studio 49 Catalog, 2058
Summer@Carroll, 1181, 7939
Syracuse Community-Referenced Curriculum Guide for Students with Disabilties, 2059
Talisman Summer Camp, 1314, 7942, 8949
Teaching Adults with Learning Disabilities, 2610
Teaching Every Child Every Day: Integrated Learning in Diverse Classrooms, 2613
Teaching Exceptional Children (TEC), 2306
Teaching Infants and Preschoolers with Handicaps, 2614
Teaching Learners with Mild Disabilities: Integrating Research and Practice, 2616
Teaching Mathematics to Students with Learning Disabilities, 2617
Teaching Mildly and Moderately Handicapped Students, 2618
Teaching Reading to Handicapped Children, 2621
Teaching Students Ways to Remember, 2061
Teaching Students with Mild and Moderate Learning Problems, 2625
Teaching Students with Special Needs in Inclusive Settings, 2627
Teaching Test-Taking Skills: Helping Students Show What They Know, 2062
Teaching Young Children to Read, 2628
Teaching the Bilingual Special Education Student, 2629
Teaching the Learning Disabled Adolescent: Strategies and Methods, 2630
Tennessee Department of Education, 2236
Test Critiques: Volumes I-X, 2717
Test of Mathematical Abilities, 2nd Edition, 2720
Test of Nonverbal Intelligence, 3rd Edition, 2721
Test of Written Spelling, 3rd Edition, 2723
Texas Education Agency, 2237
Textbooks and the Student Who Can't Read Them: A Guide for Teaching Content, 2632
Timbertop Camp for Youth with Learning Disabilities, 1491, 7943
Tools for Transition, 2065
Topics in Early Childhood Special Education, 2341
Utah State Office of Education: At-Risk and Special Education Service Unit, 2240
VAK Tasks Workbook: Visual, Auditory and Kinesthetic, 2067
Virginia Department of Education: Divisionof Pre & Early Adolescent Education, 2242
West Virginia Department of Education: Office of Special Education, 2244
What School Counselors Need to Know, 2646
Wordly Wise 3000, 2069
Work!, 2070
Working Together & Taking Part, 2071
Worthmore Academy, 2759
Wyoming Department of Education, 2245

Lowe's Syndrome

Lowe Syndrome Association, 8504
Lowe Syndrome Conference, 1909

Lung Disorders

American Lung Association, 8475
BIPAP S/T Ventilatory Support System, 262
Breathe Free, 8690
Canadian Lung Association, 8485
Emphysema Foundation for Our Right to Survive, 8488
Healthy Breathing, 8723
Lung Disorders Sourcebook, 8754
Lung Line Information Service, 8897

Massage Therapy

American Massage Therapy Association (AMTA), 760
American Organization for Bodywork Therapies of Asia (AOBTA), 762
Bonnie Prudden Myotherapy, 785
Massage Therapy Journal, 7729
McKinnon Body Therapy Center, 884

Mental Disabilities

Addictive & Mental Disorders Division, 3674
Agnes M Lindsay Trust, 3088
Ahmanson Foundation, 2809
American Board of Medical Psychotherapists and Psychodiagnosticians, 748
American Psychiatric Association, 7837
Association for Behavioral and Cognitive Therapies (ABCT), 7839
Authoritative Guide to Self- Help Resourcein Mental Health, 5120
Bain, Inc. Center For Independent Living, 4126
Bethy and the Mouse: A Father Remembers His Children with Disabilities, 5357
Blind Services, 6057
C-4 Work Center, 6008
Camp Wesley Woods: Exceptional Persons Camp, 1386
Center for Mental Health Services, 2203
Cheaha Regional Mental Health Center, 6492
Children's Mental Health Network (CMHN), 804
Children's Needs Psychological Perspective, 2407
Chilton-Shelby Mental Health Center, 6494
Colorado Division of Mental Health, 3473
Complete Mental Health Resource Guide, 2127
Consulting Psychologists Press, 2423
Cornerstone Services, 6010, 8889
Counseling Psychologist, 2261
Criminal Law Handbook on Psychiatric & Psychological Evidence & Testimony, 4684
Culture and the Restructuring of Community Mental Health, 7984
Department Of Health & Social Services - Division Of Behaviorial Health, 3431
Department of Behavioral Healthcare, Developmental Disabilities and Hospitals, 3827
Depression and Bipolar Support Alliance, 7863
Developmental Disability Services Section, 3768
Dimensions of State Mental Health Policy, 4686
DisAbility LINK, 814, 4127
Division of Mental Health and Substance Abuse, 3778
Eating Disorders Sourcebook., 8712
Ecology of Troubled Children, 2452
Emotional Problems of Childhood and Adolescence, 2464
Favarh ARC, 839
Florida Department of Mental Health and Rehabilitative Services, 3513
Fred Finch Youth Center, 6597
Georgia Division of Mental Health, Developmental Disabilities & Addictive Diseases, 3528
Giant Food Foundation, 3015
Haldimand-Norfolk Resource Education and Counseling, 851
Handbook on Supported Education for Peoplewith Mental Illness, 2488
Hawaii Department of Health, Adult Mental Health Division, 3538
Home Health Care Provider: A Guide to Essential Skills, 2494
Idaho Mental Health Center, 3552
Illinois Department of Mental Health and Developmental Disabilities, 3561
Inroads to Opportunities, 6131
International Handbook on Mental Health Policy, 4703
Invisible Disabilities Association (IDA), 872
Judge David L Bazelon Center for Mental Health Law, 4663
Law Center Newsletter, 4705
Louisiana Department of Health - Mental Health Services, 3600
Louisiana Rehabilitation Services, 6059
Maine Department of Health and Human Services, 3607
Maryland Division of Mental Health, 3619
Massachusetts Department of Mental Health, 3626
Mental & Physical Disability Law Digest, 2537
Mental Disabilities and the Americans with Disabilities Act, 4715
Mental Disability Law, Evidence and Testimony, 4716
Mental Health America (MHA), 885, 7871
Mental Health Association in Pennysylvania, 3817
Mental Health Concepts and Techniques for the Occupational Therapy Assistant, 2538
Mental Health Law Reporter, 4717
Mental Health and Mental Illness, 2539
Mentally Ill Individuals, 2540
MindFreedom International (MFI), 886
Minnesota Department of Human Services: Behavioral Health Division, 3653
NASW-NYS Chapter, 1912
National Alliance on Mental Illness (NAMI), 7875
National Alliance on Mental Illness (Texas), 3875
National Association for the Dually Diagnosed Conferences, 1914
National Association of School Psychologists, 2166
National Institute of Mental Health, 3395
Nebraska Department of Mental Health, 3689
Nevada Division of Mental Health and Developmental Services, 3700
New Hampshire Department of Mental Health, 3709
New Jersey Division of Mental Health Services, 3721
New State Office of Mental Health Agency, 3743
New York State Office of Mental Health, 3750
North Hastings Community Integration Association, 915
Office of Rehabilitation Services, 4540, 6183
Ohio Department of Mental Health, 3792
Oklahoma Department of Mental Health & Substance Abuse Services, 3803
Orchard Village, 6020
Oregon Department of Mental Health, 3810
Parental Concerns in College Student Mental Health, 2549
People First of Canada, 924
Personality and Emotional Disturbance, 2553
Providing Services for People with Vision Loss: Multidisciplinary Perspective, 9287
Psychiatric Mental Health Nursing, 2568
Psychiatric Staffing Crisis in Community Mental Health, 2300
Psycho-Educational Assessment of Preschool Children, 2705
Psychological and Social Impact of Illness and Disability, 2570
Readings: A Journal of Reviews and Commentary in Mental Health, 2302
Rhode Island Department of Mental Health, 3830
Rhode Island Services for the Blind and Visually Impaired, 3835, 6184
SAMHSA News, 2336
Seagull Industries for the Disabled, 5989
Services for the Seriously Mentally Ill: A Survey of Mental Health Centers, 2588

Social and Emotional Development of Exceptional Students: Handicapped, 2594
South Carolina Department of Mental Health, 3845
South Dakota Department of Social Services Division of Behavioral Health, 3854
State Mental Health Representative for Children and Youth, 3760
Substance Abuse and Mental Health Services Administration (SAMHSA), 3407
Sunnyhill, Inc., 4384
Teaching Disturbed and Disturbing Students: An Integrative Approach, 2612
Tennessee Department of Mental Health, 3864
Texas Federation of Families for Children's Mental Health, 3887
Texas Health and Human Services (HHS), 3889
Thresholds, 950, 6024
Treating Families of Brain Injury Survivors, 2641
Understanding and Teaching Emotionally Disturbed Children & Adolescents, 2642
Utah Division Of Substance Abuse & Mental Health, 3901
VA Maryland Health Care System, 5724
Virginia Department of Mental Health, 3922
WY Department of Health: Mental Health and Substance Abuse Service Division, 3959
We Can Speak for Ourselves: Self Advocacy by Mentally Handicapped People, 5337
Well Mind Association of Greater Washington, 3503
Youth MOVE National, 963

Multiple Disabilities

ACL Regional Support Center: Region I, 7494
ACL Regional Support Center: Region II, 7495
ACL Regional Support Center: Region III, 7496
ACL Regional Support Center: Region IV, 7497
ACL Regional Support Center: Region IX, 7498
ACL Regional Support Center: Region V, 7499
ACL Regional Support Center: Region VI, 7500
ACL Regional Support Center: Region VII, 7501
ACL Regional Support Center: Region VIII, 7502
ACL Regional Support Center: Region X, 7503
APSE National Conference, 1886
Abilities Expo, 1890
Ability Center, 72, 537, 658, 4425
Ability Center of Greater Toledo, 1659, 4486
Ability Center of Greater Toledo: Bryan, 4487
AbleData, 1607, 5479
Access Pass, 5605
Accessible Home of Your Own, 1940
Adam's Camp, 1043, 8539
Adam's Camp: Alaska, 980
Adam's Camp: Colorado, 1044
Adam's Camp: New England, 1241
The Adaptive Sports Foundation, 3176
Administration for Community Living, 2186
Adventures Without Limits, 1352
Alternative Work Concepts, 2074
American Association of People with Disabilities (AAPD), 744, 5484, 8125
American Therapeutic Recreation Association, 767
Americans with Disabilities Act Information and Technical Assistance, 3382
Anderson Woods, 1126
Anthesis, 5912
Arc of Bergen and Passaic Counties, 6123
Association of People Supporting Employment First (APSE), 779
B'nai B'rith Camp: Kehila Program, 1353
BRiDGES, 4440
Blood and Circulatory Disorders Sourcebook, 8685
Blowitz-Ridgeway Foundation, 2950
Bothin Foundation, 2817
Breckenridge Outdoor Education Center, 1046, 8545
The Bridge Center, 1188
Buck and Buck Clothing, 1510
Burns-Dunphy Foundation, 2819
CQL Accreditation, 1901
CW Resources, 5957
California Community Foundation, 2820
Camp AIM, 1369
Camp Albrecht Acres, 1141
Camp Aldersgate, 994, 8547
Camp Allen, 1242
Camp Alpine, 982, 8548
Camp Amp, 1372
Camp Aranzazu, 1425
Camp Barnabas, 1217
Camp Be An Angel, 1426
Camp Beausite NW, 1475, 8550
Camp Blessing, 1427
Camp CAMP, 1428
Camp CaPella, 1160, 8181
Camp Callahan, 1112
Camp Christian Berets, 1002
Camp Conquest, 1414
Camp Courage North, 1204, 8562
Camp Courageous of Iowa, 1142
Camp Deeny Riback, 1250
Camp Dream, 1091
Camp Easterseals UCP, 1467
Camp Eden Wood, 1205, 8566
Camp Friendship, 1408
Camp Giddy-Up, 1453
Camp Grace Bentley, 1192
Camp Howe, 1175
Camp Jabberwocky, 1176
Camp John Marc, 1432
Camp Kee-B-Waw, 1485
Camp Knutson, 1207
Camp Koinonia, 1417
Camp Korey, 1478
Camp Kostopulos, 1456
Camp Lily Lehigh Valley, 1379
Camp Little Giant, 1115
Camp Merry Heart, 1254
Camp Millhouse, 1132
Camp Orchard Hill, 1380
Camp Oty'Okwa, 1329
Camp Pa-Qua-Tuck, 1281
Camp Paivika, 1015, 8594
Camp Perfect Wings, 1351
Camp Red Cedar, 1135
Camp Reece, 1283
Camp Rocky Mountain Village, 1047
Camp Ronald McDonald at Eagle Lake, 1018, 8598
Camp Sealth, 1479
Camp Sno Mo, 1246
Camp Spearhead, 1407
Camp Spencer Superstars, 1384
Camp Stepping Stone, 1332
Camp Summit, 1442
Camp Sunnyside, 1144
Camp Tanager, 1145
Camp Thorpe, 1463
Camp Tuolumne Trails, 1028
Camp Twin Lakes, 1098
Camp Twin Lakes: Rutledge, 1099
Camp Twin Lakes: Will-A-Way, 1100
Camp Venture, Inc., 1286
Camp Victory, 1385
Camp Wediko, 1247
Camp Wonder, 1421
Camp Woodlands, 1387
Camp Yavneh: Yedidut Program, 1248
Camp for All, 1444
Camp-A-Lot and Camp-A-Little, 1030, 7913
Canonicus Camp & Conference Center, 1400
Cardiovascular Diseases and Disorders Sourcebook, 3rd Edition, 8693
Center for Independence of the Disabled, 4007
Center for Independence of the Disabled- Daly City, 4008
Center for Independent Living: Oakland, 4011
Center for Parent Information and Resources, 2735
Center on Human Policy: School of Education, 4955
Centers for Medicare and Medicaid Services, 3383
Challenge Aspen, 1049
Chesapeake Region Accessible Boating, 8443
Childhood Diseases and Disorders Sourcebook, 2nd Edition, 8696
Children's Fresh Air Society Fund, 3008
Children's Healthcare of Atlanta at Egleston, 6302
Children's Specialized Hospital, 6375
City of Lakewood Recreation and Inclusion Services for Everyone (R.I.S.E.), 1057
Civil Rights Division/Disability Rights Section, 3384
Civitan Acres, 1472
Closing the Gap's Annual Conference, 1903
Clover Patch Camp, 1288
Clovernook Center for the Blind and Visually Impaired, 9049
Colorado Lions Camp, 1059
Community Resources for Independence: Mendocino/Lake Branch, 4026
Connecticut State Independent Living Council, 4083
Courage Kenny Rehabilitation Institute, 2738
Courageous Acres, 1334
Creating Memories, 1360
Creative Designs, 1516
Cristo Vive International: Idaho Camp, 1107
Cristo Vive International: Minnesota Camp, 1213
Cristo Vive International: Texas Camp Conroe, 1446
Cristo Vive International: Texas Camp Rio Grande Valley, 1447
Cultural Diversity, Families and the Special Education System, 2429
Cunard Line, 5609
Danmar Products, 422
Deutsch Foundation, 2827
Digestive Diseases & Disorders Sourcebook, 8709
Disability Analysis Handbook: Tools for Independent Practice, 5375
Disability Determination Services, 3857
Disability Research and Dissemination Center, 816, 2086
Disability Rights Advocates, 4657
Disability Rights of Pennsylvania (DRP), 3815
Disability and Communication Access Board, 3535
Disability and Health: National Center for Birth Defects and Developmental Disabilities, 8891
Discovery Camp, 1458
Dragonfly Forest Summer Camp, 1388
Dvorak Raft Kayak & Fishing Expeditions, 5611
Ear, Nose, and Throat Disorders Sourcebook, 8711
Easter Seal Camp Wawbeek, 1488
Easter Seals, 7540
Eastern Colorado Services for the Disabled, 3476
Easterseals Arkansas, 5907
Easterseals Camp, 1033
Easterseals Camp ASCCA, 977, 8623
Easterseals Camp Challenge, 1083
Easterseals Camp Fairlee, 1172
Easterseals Camp Harmon, 1034
Easterseals Camp Hemlocks, 1068
Easterseals Camp Stand by Me, 1480, 8379
Easterseals Central Alabama, 6496
Easterseals Central Texas, 3870
Easterseals Crossroads, 6320
Easterseals Delaware & Maryland's Eastern Shore, 6712
Easterseals DuPage and Fox Valley, 6826
Easterseals East Georgia, 6791
Easterseals Iowa, 6883
Easterseals Jayne Shover Center, 6828
Easterseals Joliet Region, 6829
Easterseals Midwest, 4372, 7013
Easterseals Nebraska Camp, 1234
Easterseals New Jersey, 6126
Easterseals New York, 3131
Easterseals North Texas, 3871
Easterseals Northeast Central Florida, 6738
Easterseals Northern California, 6591
Easterseals Northwest Alabama, 6497
Easterseals Oregon Summer Camp, 1361
Easterseals Rehabilitation Center, 6875
Easterseals South Florida, 6739
Easterseals Southwest Florida, 6741
Easterseals Superior California, 6592
Easterseals Tennessee Camping Program, 1422
Easterseals of Mahoning, Trumbull and Columbiana Counties, 7087
Easterseals-Goodwill Northern Rocky Mountain, 7023

Educating Children with Multiple Disabilities: A Transdisciplinary Approach, 2454
Educating Students Who Have Visual Impairments with Other Disabilities, 2456
El Valor, 6830
Enhancing Everyday Communication for Children with Disabilities, 5376
Equal Opportunity Employment Commission, 3386
Equalizer 5000 Home Gym, 640
Ethnic Diseases Sourcebook, 8716
Eugene and Agnes E Meyer Foundation, 2901
Eunice Kennedy Shriver National Institute of Child Health and Human Development (NICHD), 8491
Federal Communications Commission, 3387
Financial Aid for the Disabled and Their Families, 2832, 3364
Firemans Fund Foundation, 2833
Florida Fair Employment Practice Agency, 5975
Florida Lions Camp, 7806
Friends of Disabled Adults and Children, 8355
Friendship Circle Day Camp, 1290
Gallo Foundation, 2835
Gateway Arts Center: Studio, Craft Store& Gallery, 6080
Goodwill Industries International, 847
Goodwill Industries International, Inc., 7544
HWH Foundation, 3206
Habilitation Benefits Coalition, 850
Hammill Institute on Disabilities, 2159
Handi Camp, 1389
Happy Camp, 978, 8631
Harbor Haven Summer Program, 1260
HealthyWomen, 5513
Henry W Bull Foundation, 2839
Hepatitis Sourcebook, 8725
Hyams Foundation, 3034
Hypertension Sourcebook, 8728
IBM National Support Center, 5993
IKUS Life Enrichment Services, 8494
Incight, 2101
Including All of Us: An Early Childhood Curriculum About Disability, 2503
Independence Now: The Center for Independent Living, 4289
Independent Living, 4451
Independent Living Approach to Disability Policy Studies, 2507
Indian Trails Camp, 1197
Inspiring Possibilities, 2325
Institute for Human Centered Design, 1929
Interdisciplinary Clinical Assessment of Young Children with Developmental Disabilities, 8732
International Center for the Disabled, 1629
Iowa Compass, 3576
John W Anderson Foundation, 2986
Joni and Friends (JAF), 875
Just Like Everyone Else, 5205
Kamp Kiwanis, 1292
Kamp for Kids at Camp Togowauk, 1179
Kansas Commission on Disability Concerns, 3587
Kenneth T and Eileen L Norris Foundation, 2842
Kota Camp, 998, 8634
League at Camp Greentop, 1173
Lions Camp Crescendo, 1152, 8199
Lions Camp Tatiyee, 992, 8635
Longwood Foundation, 2897
Loudoun County Adaptive Recreation Camps, 1473
Louisiana Lions Camp, 1158
M&M Health Care Apparel Company, 1528
Making a Difference: A Wise Approach, 5222
Mane Stream, 1261
Mayor of the West Side, 5056
MedCamps of Louisiana, 1159, 8639
Merrimack Hall Performing Arts Center, 8506
Moss Rehabilitation Hospital, 6423
Mt Hood Kiwanis Camp, 1364
Nantahala Outdoor Center, 5596
National Association for Parents of Children with Visual Impairments (NAPVI), 9072, 9365
National Association of City and County health Officials, 890
National Center for Health, Physical Activity and Disability, 898, 8364
National Council on Disability, 3391
National Council on Independent Living, 4095, 8366
National Council on Independent Living (NCIL), 903
National Disability Rights Network (NDRN), 904
National Health Council, 907
National Institute on Disability, Independent Living, and Rehabilitation Research (NIDILRR), 908, 3399, 4794
National Sports Center for the Disabled, 8453, 8882
New Hampshire Bureau of Vocational Rehabilitation, 6114
North Dakota Department of Labor, and Human Rights, 6167
Nothern Suburban Special Recreation Association Day Camps, 1122
Office of Disability Employment Policy, 3400
Office of Fair Housing and Equal Opportunity, 3401
Office of Retirement and Disability Policy (ORDP), 3402
Office of Special Education Programs, 3403
Official Patient's Sourcebook on Bell's Palsy, 8780
Official Patient's Sourcebook on Osteoporosis, 8783
Official Patient's Sourcebook on Sickle Cell Anemia, 8788
Official Patient's Sourcebook on Ulcerative Colitis, 8789
Overnight Camps, 1461
PACER Center (Parent Advocacy Coalition for Educational Rights), 917
PACER E-News, 2333
PACER Partners, 2334
PACESETTER, 2335
Pacific Rim International Conference on Disability And Diversity, 1918
Palm Beach Habilitation Center, 5983
Partnership to Improve Patient Care, 923
Perkins Activity and Resource Guide: A Handbook for Teachers, 9232
Phantom Lake YMCA Camp, 1490, 8644
Physical Management of Multiple Handicaps: A Professional's Guide, 2557
Pine Tree Camp, 1165
Placer Independent Resource Services, 4054
Primary Care Collaborative, 928
Protection & Advocacy System: Alaska, 3434
Recreation Unlimited: Day Camp, 1338
Recreation Unlimited: Residential Camp, 1339
Recreation Unlimited: Respite Weekend Camp, 1340
Recreation Unlimited: Specialty Camp, 1341
Rehabilitation Services Administration, 3405
Rhode Island Disability Law Center, 3832
Rising Treetops at Oakhurst, 1262, 8382
Rotary Camp, 1342
Senior Program for Teens and Young Adults with Special Needs, 2751
SeriousFun Children's Network, 1069
Shady Oaks Camp, 1124, 8648
Silver Towers Camp, 1464
Social Security Administration, 3406, 3517
Social Security: Baltimore Disability Determination, 3621
Social Security: Maine Disability Determination, 3612
Society for Disability Studies, 2118
Southwest Conference On Disability, 1921
Southwestern Center for Independent Living, 4354
Special Camp For Special Kids, 1041
St. Augustine Rainbow Camp, 1343
Starting Points, 9250
Steelcase Foundation, 3057
Stepping Stones: Camp Allyn, 1344
Summaries of Legal Precedents & Law Review, 4728
Sunnyhill Adventures, 1226, 7941
Sunshine Campus, 1301
Tennessee Division of Rehabilitation, 3865
Texas Lions Camp, 1451, 8205, 8654, 9120
Texas Speech-Language-Hearing Association, 8938
That All May Worship: An Interfaith Welcome to People with Disabilities, 5271
Thyroid Disorders Sourcebook, 8821
Timber Pointe Outdoor Center, 1125
To Live with Grace and Dignity, 5273
True Friends, 1215
US Department of Education: Office for Civil Rights, 3408
US Department of Labor: Office of Federal Contract Compliance Programs, 3409
US Department of Veterans Affairs, 3411
US Office of Personnel Management, 3412
US Role in International Disability Activities: A History, 5275
The Ultimate Guide to Sex and Disability, 5272
United States Department of the Interior National Park Service, 5586
United States Disabled Golf Association (USDGA), 951
Upward Bound Camp, 1367
Utah Labor Commission, 3904
Variety Club Camp and Developmental Center, 1395
Wage and Hour Division of the Employment Standards Administration, 3501
Wagon Road Camp, 1303
Weyerhaeuser Company Foundation, 3333
Wilderness Inquiry, 5603, 5622
Wisconsin Elks/Easterseals Respite Camp, 1493
Wisconsin Lions Camp, 1494, 8657
Wonderland Camp, 1227
World Institute on Disability (WID), 961
YMCA Camp Chingachgook on Lake George, 1305, 9123

Multiple Sclerosis

Blooming Where You're Planted: Stories From The Heart, 8686
Coffee in the Cereal: The First Year with Multiple Sclerosis, 8700
Consortium of Multiple Sclerosis Centers, 8351
Dressing Tips and Clothing Resources for Making Life Easier, 426
MSFOCUS Magazine, 8848
Momentum, 8866
Multiple Sclerosis Association of America, 7872, 8360
Multiple Sclerosis Foundation, 8361
Multiple Sclerosis and Having a Baby, 8763
Multiple Sclerosis: A Guide for Families, 8765
Multiple Sclerosis: A Guide for the Newly Diagnosed, 8766
Understanding Multiple Sclerosis, 8829
When the Road Turns: Inspirational Stories About People with MS, 8833

Muscular Dystrophy

MDA Summer Camp, 1121
MDA/ALS Newsmagazine, 2297
Muscular Dystrophy Association Free Camp, 8641
Muscular Dystrophy Association USA (MDA), 887
Official Patient's Sourcebook on Muscular Dystrophy, 8782
Quest Magazine, 2301
Summer Camp for Children with Muscular Dystrophy, 8651

Neurological Impairments

Aerie Experiences, 1088
Archives of Neurology, 8841
Association for Neurologically Impaired Brain Injured Children, 8347
Child Neurology Society, 7857
Digest of Neurology and Psychiatry, 2442
Dystonia Advocacy Network, 8353
NLP University - Dynamic Learning Center, 7874
National Institute of Neurological Disorders and Stroke, 3396, 8110

National Spasmodic Torticollis Association, 8370
Pervasive Developmental Disorders: Findinga Diagnosis and Getting Help, 5345
Rehabilitation Nursing for the Neurological Patient, 2576

Obesity

The Obesity Medicine Association (OMA), 947
Obesity Sourcebook, 8778
World Service Office of Overeaters Anonymous, 8533

Obsessive Compulsive Disorders

International OCD Foundation, 7867

Orthopedical Disabilities

American Board for Certification in Orthotics, Prosthetics & Pedorthics, 8099
American Journal of Orthopsychiatry, 8839
Camp Manito & Camp Lenape, 1072
Doing Things Together, 5419
Orthotics and Prosthetics Almanac, 8849
Osteoporosis Sourcebook, 8792
Sun-Mate Seat Cushions, 249

Pain Management

AMI, 260
American Academy of Pain Medicine (AAPM), 739
American Academy of Pain Medicine Foundation, 740, 2912
Foot Snugglers, 1523
TRU-Mold Shoes, 1548

Parkinson Disease

Allen P & Josephine B Green Foundation, 3070
American Parkinson Disease Association, 8342
Capital Area Parkinsons Society, 8348
Centers of Excellence Leadership Conference, 1902
International Parkinson and Movement Disorder Society, 8105, 8357
Movement Disorders Sourcebook, 8762
National Parkinson Foundation, 2925
PDF News, 8850
PDF Newsletter, 8868
Parkinson Report, 8869
Parkinson's Disease Foundation, 2973, 3165
Parkinson's Disease Research Society, 8372
Young Onset Parkinson Conference, 1923

Pediatric Issues

AEPS Family Report: Birth to Three Years, 5284
Administration on Children, Youth and Families, 3380
American Academy of Pediatrics (AAP), 741
American Camp Association (ACA), 751
American SIDS Institute, 8476
Assessment of Children and Youth, 2379
Association of Independent Camps, 777
Camp Okawehna, 1419
Child and Parent Resource Institute (CPRI), 802
Child with Disabling Illness, 2403
Childcare and the ADA, 4677
Children's Alliance, 803
Children's National Medical Center, 805
Choosing Options and Accommodations for Children, 2409
Commonly Asked Questions About Child Care Centers and the Americans with Disabilities Act, 4679
Disabilities Sourcebook, 424
Disabled Children's Fund (DCF), 824
Division of Special Education, 3869
Family Resource Center on Disabilities, 836
Family Voices, 838
Federation for Children with Special Needs, 841
Formed Families: Adoption of Children with Handicaps, 4698
Handbook of Epilepsy, 8722
Human Exceptionality: School, Community,and Family (12th Edition), 2496, 5075
LeBonheur Cardiac Kids Camp, 1423
Maternal and Child Health Bureau - Health Resources and Services Administration, 3620
National Association for Children of Alcoholics, 8508
National Center for Education in Maternal and Child Health (NCEMCH), 897
National Federation of Families for Children's Mental Health (NFFCMH), 905
Newsline, 5313
PEAK Parent Center, 918, 2168, 5238
PPAL In Print, 4725
PPAL Support Groups, 8900
Parent Professional Advocacy League (PPAL), 920
Parents Helping Parents (PHP), 921
Pediatric Early Elementary (PEEX II) Examination, 2699
Pediatric Exam of Educational-PEERAMID Readiness at Middle Childhood, 2700
Pediatric Examination of Educational Readiness, 2701
Pediatric Extended Examination at-PEET Three, 2702
Ronald McDonald House Charities (RMHC), 933
Universal Pediatrics, 953

Phenylketonuria

Cristine M. Trahms Program for Phenylketonuria, 2427
A Teacher's Guide to PKU, 2348

Physical Disabilities

ACPOC News, 8854
ADA In Details: Interpreting the 2010 Americans with Disabilities Act Stands, 4670
ASCCA, 8538
AUT Secondary Control, 70
AUTone, 71
Abilities, Inc., 728
Able Trek Tours, 5604
AbleApparel - Affordable Adaptive Clothing and Accessories, 5478
Accelerator Shield, 73
Accelerator/Brake Foot Control, 74
Accelerator/Brake Hand Control, 75
Accent on Living Magazine, 5100
Access Control Systems: NHX Nurse Call System, 174
Access Design Services: CILs as Experts, 5101
Access To Independence Inc., 5102
Access Unlimited, 5480
Access to Recreation, 403
Accessibility Lift, 335
Accessible Journeys, 5606
Accessible Vans Of America, 5623
Achievement Products, 404
Achieving Diversity and Independence, 5104
Achilles Track Club, 8440
Action Products, 225
Action X-Treme Camp, 1452
Ad Lib Drop-In Center: Consumer Management, Ownership and Empowerment, 5106
Adapted Physical Activity, 5286
Adapted Physical Activity Programs, 2246
Adapted Physical Education and Sport, 8385
Adaptive Sports Center, 8441
Adaptive Tracks, 8857
Address Book, 577
Adjustable Bath Seat, 133
Adjustable Chair, 205
Adjustable Clear Acrylic Tray, 206
Adjustable Incline Board, 336
Adjustable Raised Toilet Seat & Guard, 134
Adjustable Rigid Chair, 207
Adjustable Tee Stool, 208
Adjustable Wedge, 226
Advantage Wheelchair & Walker Bags, 635
Aerospace Compadre, 538
Alante, 539
Albany Vet Center, 5771
Alert, 2308
Alexian Brothers Medical Center, 6808
AlumiRamp, 337
Aluminum Crutches, 607
Aluminum Kiddie Canes, 608
Aluminum Walking Canes, 609
American Academy of Physical Medicine and Rehabilitation, 8468
American Airlines, 5588
American Association on Health and Disability (AAHD), 745
American Back Society, 8341
American Board of Disability Analysts (ABDA), 747
American Board of Disability Analysts Annual Conference, 1894
American Board of Professional Disability Consultants, 749
American Disabled Golfers Association (ADGA), 756
American Discount Medical, 410
American Hotel and Lodging Association, 5589
American Hotel and Lodging Association Foundation, 2899
American Mobility: Personal Mobility Solutions, 5487
American Physical Therapy Association, 8100
Amigo Mobility International, 540
Amigo Mobility International Inc., 541
Amtrak, 5590
Anglo California Travel Service, 5607
Applied Kinesiology: Muscle Response in Diagnosis, Therapy and Preventive Medicine, 5114
Apria Healthcare, 411
Area Access, 338
Arizona Department of Economic Security, 3437
ArjoHuntleigh, 135
Armstrong Medical, 412
Arthur C. Luf Children's Burn Camp, 1062
Assistive Technology Sourcebook, 414
Association for Driver Rehabilitation Specialists, 2077
Association of Assistive Technology Act Programs (ATAP), 774
Association of Mouth and Foot Painting Artists (AMPFA), 12
Automatic Card Shuffler, 5557
Automobile Lifts for Scooters, Wheelchairs and Powerchairs, 76
Avis Rent A Car System, LLC, 5624
Back-Huggar Pillow, 227
Back-Saver, 339
BackSaver, 209
Backyards and Butterflies: Ways to Include Children with Disabilities in Outdoor Activities, 5289
Bagel Holder, 304
Bailey, 415
Bariatric Wheelchairs Regency FL, 659
Barrier Free Travel: A Nuts and Bolts Guide for Wheelers and Slow Walkers (3rd Edition), 5123
Basement Motorhome Lift, 340
Bath Fixtures, 136
Bath Products, 137
Bath Shower & Commode Chair, 138
Bath and Shower Bench 3301B, 139
Bathroom Transfer Systems, 140
Bathtub Safety Rail, 141
Battery Operated Cushion, 637
BeOK Key Lever, 462
Beach Center on Families and Disability, 3583
Behavioral Vision Approaches for Persons with Physical Disabilities, 9138
Beyond the Barriers, 8431
Big Lifter, 341
Big Red Switch, 180
Bookholder: Roberts, 464
Boulder Vet Center, 5663

Bounder Plus Power Wheelchair, 708
Bounder Power Wheelchair, 709
Box Top Opener, 306
BraunAbility, 77, 342
Bravo! + Three-Wheel Scooter, 542
Breaking New Ground News Note, 8860
Breez 1025, 710
Breezy, 660
Bruno Independent Living Aids, 343
Building Bridges: Including People with Disabilities in International Programs, 2770
Burnt Gin Camp, 1402
Butlers Wheelchair Lifts, 344
Button Aid, 251
Bye-Bye Decubiti (BBD), 228
Bye-Bye Decubiti Air Mattress Overlay, 163
COM Hand Control, 78
Camp "I Am Me", 1111
Camp Amigo, 1076
Camp Beyond The Scars, 1000, 8551
Camp Nah-Nah-Mah, 1457
Camp Riley, 1136
Canine Companions for Independence (CCI), 792
Capscrew, 308
Car Cane, 79
Carendo, 210
Carex Health Brands, 418
Center for Independent Living, 4009
Center for Libraries and Educational Improvement, 5138
Century Bath System, 211
Challenged Athletes Foundation (CAF), 800
Champion 1000, 661
Champion 2000, 662
Champion 3000, 663
Chariot, 345
Charles Campbell Childrens Camp, 1230
Charlotte Vet Center, 5787
Child Convertible Balance Beam Set, 467
Child Variable Balance Beam, 468
Child's Mobility Crawler, 469
Childhood Leukemia: A Guide for Families, Friends & Caregivers, 8697
Children's Hospital Burn Camps Program, 1051, 8617
Children's Hospital Burn Camps Program: England Exchange Program Burn Camp, 1052
Children's Hospital Burn Camps Program: Family Burn Camp, 1053
Children's Hospital Burn Camps Program: Summer Burn Camp, 1054
Children's Hospital Burn Camps Program: Winter Burn Camp, 1055
Children's Hospital Burn Camps Program: Young Adult Retreat, 1056
Choice Switch Latch and Timer, 470
Choosing a Wheelchair: A Guide for Optimal Independence, 664
Clarke Healthcare Products, Inc., 143
Classique, 346
Clearway, 347
Client Assistance Program (CAP), 3554
Clip Board Notebook, 582
Columbus McKinnon Corporation, 348
Combination File/Reference Carousel, 518
Commode, 144
Communication Aids for Children and Adults, 420
Commuter & Kid's Commuter, 698
Compass Health, 265
Complete Armchair Fitness, 8433
Computer Workstation and Activity Table, 519
Convaid, 665, 699
Convert-Able Table, 212
Cordless Big Red Switch, 471
Cordless Receiver, 309
Council for Children with Behavioral Disorders (CCBD), 2082
Council of Administrators of Special Education (CASE), 2085
Council of State Administrators of Vocational Rehabilitation (CSAVR), 812
Courier Travel, 5608
The Creative Mobility Group, LLC, 5627
Crescent Porter Hale Foundation, 2825
Cruiser Bus Buggy 4MB, 543
Curb-Sider, 349
Curb-Sider Super XL, 350
Cursive Writing Skills, 1984
Custom, 666
Custom Durable, 667
Custom Lift Residential Elevators, 351
DEUCE Environmental Control Unit, 472
DW Auto & Home Mobility, 80
Damaco D90, 711
Dancing from the Inside Out, 20
Dayspring Associates, Inc., 423
Deluxe Bath Bench with Adjustable Legs, 145
Deluxe Convertible Exercise Staircase, 352
Deluxe Nova Wheeled Walker & Avant Wheeled Walker, 611
Deluxe Roller Knife, 310
Deluxe Signature Guide, 583
Deluxe Sock and Stocking Aid, 252
Deluxe Standard Wood Cane, 612
Demand Response Transportation Through a Rural ILC, 5152
Department of Insurance/OSFM, 1928
Department of Veterans Affairs Regional Office - Vocational Rehab Division, 5631
Department of Veterans Benefits, 5632
Developing Organized Coalitions and Strategic Plans, 5153
Dialysis at Sea Cruises, 5610
Digi-Flex, 474
Digital Shifter, 81
Disability Bookshop Catalog, 425
Disability Funders Network (DFN), 815
Disability Law Colorado, 4656
Disability Rights Bar Association (DBRA), 817
Disability Rights Florida, 818, 3509
Disability Rights International (DRI), 819
Disability Rights Louisiana, 820
Disability and Health Journal, 2265
Disability and Sport, 8391
Disability:IN, 821
DisabilityAdvisor.com, 2154, 5501
DisabilityResources.org, 5502
Disabled American Veterans, 5674
Disabled American Veterans Headquarters, 5633
Disabled Businesspersons Association (DBA), 823
Disabled Drummers Association (DDA), 825
Disabled In Action (DIA), 826
Disabled Peoples' International (DPI), 827
Disabled Sports Program Center, 8444
Disabled Sports USA, 8445
Disabled Watersports Program, 8446
Disabled and Alone: Life Services for the Handicapped, Inc., 828
Division for Early Childhood (DEC), 2089
Division for Physical, Health & Multiple Disabilities: Complex and Chronic Conditions, 2092
Division for Research (CEC-DR), 2093
Division of International Special Education and Services (DISES), 2094
Division of Visual and Performing Arts Education (DARTS), 2095
Dormakaba USA Inc., 478
Dressing Stick, 253
Drew Karol Industries, 266
Drive Master Company, 82
Driving Systems Inc., 83
Dual Brake Control, 84
Dual Brush with Suction Base, 311
Dual Security Bed Rail, 164
Dual Switch Latch and Timer, 479
Dual-Mode Charger, 638
Duro-Med Industries, 268
Dynamic Living, 5504
Dynamic Systems, Inc., 229
E-Wheels Electric Senior Mobility Scooter, 544
Eagle Sportschairs, LLC, 720
Early Childhood Technical Assistance Center (ETCA), 830
East Penn Manufacturing Company, 721
Easterseals Project Action Consulting, 5591
Easy Access Travel, 5612
Easy Pivot Transfer Machine, 353
Easy Stand, 354
Easy Things to Make Things Simple: Do It Yourself Modifications for Disabled Persons, 5165
Economical Liberty, 355
Edge, 668
Elan Stair Lift, 356
Elastic Shoelaces, 254
Electric Can Opener & Knife Sharpener, 312
Electric Leg Bag Emptier and Tub Slide Shower Chair, 146
Electric Mobility Corporation, 545
Elite Curved Stair Lift, 357
Elite Stair Lift, 358
Emerging Leaders, 5420
Enable America Inc., 834
Enhancer Cushion, 230
Enrichments Catalog, 427
Entervan, 85
Environmental Traveling Companions, 5613
Equalizer 1000 Series, 639
Equipment Shop, 428
Essential Medical Supply, Inc., 429
Etac USA: F3 Wheelchair, 669
Europa Superior Folding Cane, 614
Evac + Chair Emergency Evacuation Chair, 214
Evacu-Trac, 670
Everest & Jennings, 430
Explorer+ 4-Wheel Scooter, 546
Express Medical Supply, 431
Expressive Arts for the Very Disabled and Handicapped of All Ages, 23
Extensions for Independence, 522
Fairway Spirit Adaptive Golf Car: Model4852, 523
Featherspring Shoe Inserts, 641
Featherweight Reachers, 255
Fitness Programming for Physical Disabilities, 8392
FlagHouse, Inc., 432
Florence C and Harry L English Memorial Fund, 2930
Foam Decubitus Bed Pads, 165
Folding Chair with a Rigid Feel, 671
Folding Lightweight Power Wheelchair, 712
Folding Pot Stabilizer, 313
Foot Inversion Tread, 481
Foot Placement Ladder, 482
Foot Steering Systems, 86
Formula Series Active Mobility Wheelchairs, 672
Four Way Switches, 87
Four-Ingredient Cookbook, 5175
Freedom Bath, 147
Freedom Motors USA, Inc., 88
Freedom Ryder Handcycles, 524
Freedom Wheels, 359
Freestyle II, 673
Frequently Asked Questions About Multiple Chemical Sensitivity, 5176
Functional Forms, 231
GEICO Philanthropic Foundation, 2903
Gadabout Wheelchairs, 674
Galvin Health and Fitness Center, 8447
Gas and Brake Pedal Guard, 89
Gear Shift Adaptor, 90
Gear Shift Extension, 91
Gem Wheelchair & Scooter Service: Mobility & Homecare, 642, 675, 713
Gendron, 676
General Motors Mobility Program for Persons with Disabilities, 5592
Geo-Matt for High Risk Patients, 232
Geronimo, 714
Getting Around Town, 2478
Glendale Memorial Hospital and Health Center Rehabilitation Unit, 6602
Global Perspectives on Disability: A Curriculum, 2479
Golden Technologies, 215
Good Grips Cutlery, 314
Grand Lodge of the International Association of Machinists and Aerospace Workers, 848
Gresham Driving Aids, 92
Guardianship Services Associates, 4660
Guide Service of Washington, 5614

A Guide to International Educational Exchange, 2760
Guidelines on Disability, 5181
H.E.L.P. Knife, 315
Hand Brake Control Only, 93
Hand Camp, 1085
Hand Control Multi-Function Buttons, 94
Hand Gas & Brake Control, 95
Hand Parking Brake, 96
HandBrake, 97
Handi Holder, 316
Handi Home Lift, 360
Handi Lift, 361
Handi Prolift, 362
Handi-Ramp, 363
Handicapped Scuba Association International, 8449
Handicaps, Inc., 98
Hands-Free Controller, 5572
Handy-Helper Cutting Board, 317
Hard Manufacturing Company, 167
Hartford Vet Center, 5668
Headlight Dimmer Switch, 99
HealthCare Solutions, 435
HealthCraft SuperPole, 483
HealthSouth Rehab Hospital: South Carolina, 6428
HiRider, 677
Hig's Manufacturing, 437
High Profile Single Compartment Cushion, 233
High-Low Chair, 216
Hip Function & Ambulation, 8726
Home Bed Side Helper, 169
Home is in the Heart: Accommodating Peoplewith Disabilities in the Homestay Experience, 5429
Homemade Battery-Powered Toys, 2000
Homewaiter, 364
Hoosier Burn Camp, 1139
Horcher Lifting Systems, 365
Horizontal Steering Systems, 100
Horn Control Switch, 101
Hospital Environmental Control System, 486
Hostelling North America, 5584
Houston Center for Independent Living (HCIL), 4569
How Come You Walk Funny?, 8434
How We Play, 5431
Huntleigh Healthcare, 438
Hydrocephalus: A Guide for Patients, Families & Friends, 8727
I'm Not Disabled, 5432
Ideas for Kids on the Go, 5188
Identity Group, 487
Illinois Wheelchair Sport Camps, 1120, 8381
Imp Tricycle, 700
Inclinette, 366
Inclusive Games, 8397
Independent Living Centers and Managed Care: Results of an ILRU Study on Involvement, 5193
Independent Living Challenges the Blues, 5194
Independent Living Research Utilization, 4662
Independent Living for Persons with Disabilities and Elderly People, 5077
Inflatable Back Pillow, 234
Innerlip Plates, 318
Innovations in Special Education Technology Division (ISET), 2102
Innovative Products, 678
Innovative Programs: An Example of How CILs Can Put Their Work in Context, 5197
Inside The Halo and Beyond: The Anatomy of a Recovery, 8398
International Rehabilitation Review, 7712
Invacare Corporation, 274, 439
Invacare Fulfillment Center, 548
Invacare Top End, 722
Issues in Independent Living, 5200
It isn't Fair!: Siblings of Children with Disabilities, 5054
Job Accommodation Network, 2105
Job Accommodation Network (JAN), 874
Jobri, 235
Joey Interior Platform Lift, 368
John Edward Fowler Memorial Foundation, 2905
Joint Efforts, 8424
Journal of Musculoskeletal Pain, 2285
Journal of Prosthetics and Orthotics, 2288
JoySpinner, 102
Julius and Betty Levinson Center, 6838
Kersey Mobility, 103
Kessler Institute for Rehabilitation, 104, 2742, 6378
Key Changes: A Portrait of Lisa Thorson, 8435
Kid's Custom, 701
Kid's Edge, 702
Kid's Liberty, 703
Kid-Friendly Chairs, 704
KlearVue, 369
Koala Miniflex, 705
Koret Foundation, 2843
Ladybug Corner Chair, 217
Lakeshore Foundation, 8450
Land of Lincoln Goodwill Industries, 6019
Lectra-Lift, 370
Left Foot Gas Pedal, 105
Left Foot Gas Pedal, The, 106
Leg Elevation Board, 489
Leisure Lift, 549
Letter Writing Guide, 586
Lettering Guide Value Pack, 587
Leveron Door Lever, 490
Liberty, 679
Liberty LT, 371
Life on Wheels: For the Active Wheelchair User, 8399
LifeLines, 5209, 5307
Lift-All, 372
Lifter, 373
Lifts for Swimming Pools and Spas, 374
Lightweight Breezy, 680
Lisa Beth Gerstman Camp, 1294
Little People of America, 8503
Living in the Community, 5213
Long Handled Bath Sponges, 148
Long Oven Mitts, 319
Longreach Reacher, 491
Loop Scissors, 492
Loud, Proud and Passionate, 5214
Low Tech Assistive Devices: A Handbook for the School Setting, 2019
Lumex Cushions and Mattresses, 236
Lumex Recliner, 218
MIUSA's Global Impact Newsletter, 8425
MVP+ 3-Wheel Scooter, 550
Mac's Lift Gate, 375
Maddak Inc., 445
Majors Medical Equipment, 681
Making Informed Medical Decisions: Where to Look and How to Use What You Find, 5219
Marriott International, 5593
Maryland State Department of Education, 6074
Massena Independent Living Center, 4453
Maxi Aids, 446
MedDev Corporation, 276
Medi-Grip, 277
Medpro Static Air Chair Cushion, 237
Medpro Static Air Mattress Overlay, 238
Meeting the Needs of Employees with Disabilities, 5226
Mental and Physical Disability Law Reporter, 4718
Midland Treatment Furniture, 2541
Mini-Max Cushion, 239
Mirror Go Lightly, 256
Mobility International USA, 8359
MobilityWorks, 107
Modular Wall Grab Bars, 149
Molded Sock and Stocking Aid, 257
MossRehab Travel Resources, 5595
Motorhome Lift, 377
Multi-Function Spinner Knobs, 108
NADR Conference, 1911
NCDE Survival Strategies for Overseas Living for People with Disabilities, 5228
NEXT Conference & Exposition, 1913
NEXUS Wheelchair Cushioning System, 240
National Association of Disability Representatives (NADR), 892
National Business & Disability Council, 6154
National Car Rental System, 5625
National Coalition of Federal Aviation Employees with Disabilities, 3390
National Council of Architectural Registration Boards (NCARB), 1932
National Council on Rehabilitation Education (NCRE), 2114
National Disability Sports Alliance, 8451
National Foundation for Facial Reconstruction, 3159
National Foundation of Wheelchair Tennis, 2854
National Health Law Program (NHeLP), 4666
National Hookup, 5229
National Mobility Equipment Dealers Association, 8368
National Right to Work Legal Defense Foundation, 3320, 4667
National Skeet Shooting Association, 8452
National Wheelchair Poolplayers Association, 8454
Native American Disability Law Center, 914
Natural Access, 682
New Hampshire Veterans Centers, 5763
New Mobility, 8409
Nick Joins In, 8773
No Barriers, 5444
North Carolina Client Assistance Program, 3773
Northwest Limousine Service, 5626
Norwegian Cruise Line, 5616
Nosey Cup, 321
O&P Almanac, 2330
Official Patient's Sourcebook on Scoliosis, 8787
One Thousand FS, 644, 715
Open for Business, 5446
Open to the Public, 5447
Operation Job Match, 5967
Oregon Talking Book & Braille Services, 4990
Organ Transplants: Making the Most of Your Gift of Life, 5237
Out-N-About American Walker, 617
Out-Sider III, 379
Out-Sider Meridian, 380
Outdoor Independence, 552
P.T. Rail, 150
PALAESTRA: Forum of Sport, Physical Education and Recreation for Those with Disabilities, 8410
PVA Architecture, 1935
Pac-All Wheelchair Carrier, 645
Pace Saver Plus II, 553
Pain Centers: A Revolution in Health Care, 2548
Palmer Independence, 554
Palmer Twosome, 555
Parent Centers and Independent Living Centers: Collectively We're Stronger, 5316
Paring Boards, 322
Park Brake Extension, 109
Parker Bath, 381
Parking Brake Extension, 110
Partial Seizure Disorders: A Guide for Patients and Families, 8794
Partnering with Public Health: Funding& Advocacy Opportunities for CILs and SILCs, 5241
Pathfinders Camp, 1462
Patient Lifting & Injury Prevention, 382
Pediatric Seating System, 241
Peer Counseling: Roles, Functions, Boundaries, 5242
Peer Mentor Volunteers: Empowering People for Change, 5243
Pencil/Pen Weighted Holders, 526
People with Disabilities & Abuse: Implications for Center for Independent Living, 5245
Performance Health, 323
Performance Health Enrichments Catalog, 450
Permobil, 646
Permobil Max 90, 716
Permobil Super 90, 717
Personal Perspectives on Personal Assistance Services, 5248
Physical Disabilities and Health Impairments: An Introduction, 2555
Physical Education and Sports for Exceptional Students, 2556
Physically Handicapped in Society, 2558
Plastic Card Holder, 496

Polaris Trail Blazer, 556
Portable Hand Controls by Handicaps, Inc., 111
Portable Shampoo Bowl, 151
Portable Wheelchair Ramp, 383
Posture-Glide Lounger, 684
Power Door, 497
Power Transfer Seat Base (6-Way), 112
Power Wheelchairs, 718
Power for Off-Pavement, 719
PowerLink 2 Control Unit, 324
Prairie Cruiser, 685
Prelude, 152
Prime Engineering, 219
Prone Support Walker, 621
ProtectaCap, ProtectaCap+PLUS, ProtectaChin Guard and ProtectaHip, 498
Protection & Advocacy for People with Disabilities, 3839
Public Technology Institute, 3500
Push Pull Hand Controls, 113
Push Rock Hand Controls, 114
Push-Button Quad Cane, 622
Quad Commander, 499
Quadtro Cushion, 242
Quickie 2, 557
REACH/Resource Centers on Independent Living, 4669
RESNA Annual Conference, 1919
ROW Adventures, 5617
Ragtime Industries, 6895
Raised Line Drawing Kit, 529
Ramplette Telescoping Ramp, 384
Rampvan, 115
Rand-Scot, 624
Rascal 3-Wheeler, 558
Rascal Convertable, 559
Redman Apache, 687
Redman Crow Line, 688
Reduced Effort Steering, 116
Regent, 560
Rehabiliation Engineering Research Center on Accessible Public Transportation, 5598
Rehabilitation Engineering and AssistiveTechnology Society of North America (RESNA), 453, 1645
Rehabilitation Institute of Chicago's Virginia Wadsworth Sports Program, 8883
Rehabilitation Institute of Southern California, 6652
Rehabilitation International, 931
Rehabilitation International World Congress, 1920
Research, Advocacy, and Practice for Complex and Chronic Conditions, 7660
Resources for Independent Living, 4618
Ricon Classic, 386
Ricon Corporation, 387
Right Angle Hand Controls, 117
Right Hand Gas and Brake Control, 118
Rock-King Wheelchair Kit, 689
Rocker Balance Square, 502
Roll Chair, 221
Rollators, 625
Rolls 2000 Series, 690
SWAB Steering Wheel, 119
Safari Scooter, 562
Safari Tilt, 222
Safe Path Products, 454
Safety Deck II, 647
Scoota Bug, 563
Scooter & Wheelchair Battery Fuel Gauges and Motor Speed Controllers, 648
Seven Fifty-Five FS, 706
Sexual Adjustment, 5261
Sexuality and Disabilities: A Guide for Human Service Practitioners, 5262
Shilo Inns & Resorts, 5599
Shoe Horn and Sock Remover, 259
Shower Bathtub Mat, 154
Shower and Commode Chair, 155
Sierra 3000/4000, 564
Signature and Address Self-Inking Stamps, 532
Silicone Padding, 243
Skyway, 691
Slicing Aid, 325
Small Appliance Receiver, 326
Smart Leg, 388
SmartScoot Lightweight Travel Scooter, 565
Smooth Mover, 389
Socialization Games for Persons with Disabilities, 5264, 5579
Society for Progressive Supranuclear Palsy, 8374
Soft-Touch Convertible Flotation Mattress, 244
Soft-Touch Gel Flotation Cushion, 245
Softfoot Ergomatta, 649
Solo Scooter, 566
SoloRider Industries, 567
Southampton Fresh Air Home, 1298
Space-Saver, 390
Spatial Tilt Custom Chair, 223
Spec-L Clothing Solutions, 1542
Special Children, 8906
Special Clothes for Children, 5544
Special Needs Trust Handbook, 5268
Special Olympics, 8457
Special Olympics International, 8458
SpectraLift, 391
Spectrum Products Catalog, 393
Spenco Medical Group, 246
Spider Network Systems, 120
Spinner Knobs, 121
Spirit Magazine, 8412
Sport Science Review: Adapted Physical Activity, 8402
Sportaid, 455
St. Clair County Library Special Technologies Alternative Resources (S.T.A.R.), 4920
StairClimber, 627
StairLIFT SC & SL, 394
Stand-Up Wheelchairs, 692
Standing Aid Frame with Rear Entry, 628
Starbridge, 940
Steady Write, 533
Steel Food Bumper, 327
Steering Device, 122
Steering Wheel Devices, 123
Still Me, 8403
Stop-Leak Gel Flotation Mattress, 247
Stove Knob Turner, 328
Stryker, 248
Super Grade IV Hand Controls, 124
Superarm Lift for Vans, 395
SureHands Lift & Care Systems, 396
Suregrip Bathtub Rail, 156
Surf Chair, 694
Systems 2000, 569
TIDI Products, LLC, 630
TMX Tricycle, 707
TV & VCR Remote, 510
Talking Bathroom Scale, 157
TapGear, 125
Teaching Individuals with Physical and Multiple Disabilities, 2060
Technology and Handicapped People, 2631
Television Remote Controls with Large Numbers, 535
Terra-Jet: Utility Vehicle, 570
Terrier Tricycle, 571
Terry-Wash Mitt: Medium Size, 158
Texas Governor's Committee on People with Disabilities, 3888
Therapy Putty, 513
They Don't Come with Manuals, 5333
Thick-n-Easy, 330
Three Rivers News, 9261
Thyssen Krupp Access Solutions, 397
Tilt-N-Table, 650
Tim's Trim, 126
Touch/Ability Connects People with Disabilities & Alternative Health Care Pract., 5274
Tourette's Syndrome: Finding Answers and Getting Help, 8823
Transfer Bench with Back, 224
Transfer Tub Bench, 159
Transportation Equipment for People with Disabilities, 127
Travelers Aid International, 5600
Treating Adults with Physical Disabilities: Access and Communication, 2638
Treating Epilepsy Naturally: A Guide to Alternative and Adjunct Therapies, 8825
Tri-Grip Bathtub Rail, 160
Tri-Lo's, 573
Triumph 3000/4000, 574
Triumph Scooter, 575
Tub Slide Shower Chair, 161
Tulsa City-County Library System: Outreach Services, 4988
Turn Signal Cross-Over, 128
Twin-Rest Seat Cushion & Glamour Pillow, 250
21st Century Scientific, Inc. - Bounder Power Wheelchair, 657
U-Step Walking Stabilizer: Walker, 631
US Department Veterans Affairs Beckley Vet Center, 5858
US Department of Transportation, 3410
US Paralympics, 8459
US Servas, 5601
Undercounter Lid Opener, 332
Understanding and Accommodating Physical Disabilities: Desk Reference, 5276
Uni-Turner, 333
United Access, 129
Universal Hand Cuff, 334
Uppertone, 514
Vangater, Vangater II, Mini-Vangater, 398
Vantage Mobility International, 130
Vehicle Access Remote Control, 131
Ventura Enterprises, 632
Vermont Back Research Center, 8376
Versatrainer, 399
Vestibular Board, 400
Veterans Support Center (VSC), 6206
Vista Wheelchair, 695
WA Department of Services for the Blind, 3932
WCIB Heavy-Duty Folding Cane, 633
Walgreens Home Medical Center, 457
Walker Leg Support, 634
Wardrobe Wagon: The Special Needs Clothing Store, 5548
West Penn Burn Camp, 1396
Wheel Life News, 651
Wheelchair Accessories, 652
Wheelchair Aide, 653
Wheelchair Back Pack and Tote Bag, 654
Wheelchair Bowling, 8436
Wheelchair Carrier, 401
Wheelchair Getaways, 5628
Wheelchair Sports, USA, 8461
Wheelchair Work Table, 656
A Wheelchair for Petronilia, 8430
Wheelchair with Shock Absorbers, 696
WheelchairNet, 5552
Wheelchairs and Transport Chairs, 697
Wheelers Accessible Van Rentals, 132, 5602, 5629
Wheelin Around e-Guide, 5587
Williams Lift Company, 402
Window-Ease, 515
Work in the Context of Disability Culture, 5282
A World Awaits You, 5089, 5583, 8415
World Chiropractic Alliance, 8112, 8377
World of Options, 2792
Youth as Self Advocates (YASA), 964
Youville Hospital & Rehab Center, 6984

Polio

Official Patient's Sourcebook on Post-Polio Syndrome: A Revised and Updated Directory, 8784
Post-Polio Health, 7773, 8870
Post-Polio Health International, 926, 8524
Post-Polio Support Group, 8903
Post-Polio Syndrome: A Guide for Polio Survivors and Their Families, 8797

Prader-Willi Syndrome

PWSA (USA) Conference, 1917
Prader-Willi Alliance of New York Newsletter, 8871
Prader-Willi Syndrome Association USA, 8525

Prader-Willi Syndrome: Development and Manifestations, 8798

Rare Disabilities

Acid Maltase Deficiency Association, 8338
Alternating Hemiplegia of Childhood Foundation, 2811
Brachial Plexus Palsy Foundation, 3230
Charcot-Marie-Tooth Association, 8102
Children's Tumor Foundation, 3122
The Hemispherectomy Foundation, 7892
NBIA Disorders Association, 8362
National Ataxia Foundation, 7880
National Organization for Rare Disorders, 8522
Rettsyndrome.org, 8071
A Teacher's Guide to Isovaleric Acidemia, 2346
A Teacher's Guide to Methylmalonic Acidemia, 2347
United Brachial Plexus Network, Inc., 8532

Respiratory Disorders

ATS Journals, 7655
Advances in Cardiac and Pulmonary Rehabilitation, 2363
American Association for Respiratory Care, 8469
CHAMP Camp, 1127
Camp Luv-A-Lung, 1406
Camp Pelican, 1156, 8595
Dr. Moises Simpser VACC Camp, 1081, 8620
International Ventilator Users Network (IVUN), 870, 8501
National Association for Medical Direction of Respiratory Care, 8510
Official Patient's Sourcebook on Primary Pulmonary Hypertension, 8785
Official Patient's Sourcebook on Pulmonary Fibrosis, 8786
Sinus Survival: A Self-help Guide, 8809
Trail's Edge Camp, 1199
Ventilator-Assisted Living, 8880

Severe Disabilites

Annual TASH Conference, 1896
Assessment of Individuals with Severe Disabilities, 2380
Bodie, Dolina, Smith & Hobbs, P.C., 5127
Camp Jened, 8580
Camp New Hope, 1116, 1309
Collaborative Teams for Students with Severe Disabilities, 2416
Curriculum Decision Making for Students with Severe Handicaps, 2430
Including Students with Severe and Multiple Disabilites in Typical Classrooms, 2504
Instruction of Persons with Severe Handicaps, 2005
Life After Trauma: A Workbook for Healing, 8742
Not Dead Yet, 916
Research and Practice for Persons with Severe Disabilities, 7659
TASH, 942
TASH Connections, 4729

Sexual Abuse & Related Conditions

Herpes Resource Center, 8493
Prevent Child Abuse America, 8904
Shining Bright: Head Start Inclusion, 5459
Wilmington Vet Center, 5673

Sjogren's Syndrome

Moisture Seekers, 8865
Sjogren's Syndrome Foundation, 3022

Speech Disorders

ASHA Convention, 1887
Accent 1400, 173
Adaptive Technology Catalog, 406
American Journal of Speech-Language Pathology, 9000
Aphasia Hope Foundation, 8912
Assessment and Remediation of Articulatoryand Phonological Disorders, 2377
Awareness Training, 9134
Camp Chatterbox, 1249
Camp Littlefoot, 1167
Camp Meadowood Springs, 1355, 8190, 8943
Cherab Foundation, 9022
The Cherab Foundation, 944, 2927, 8939
Childhood Apraxia of Speech Association, 8918
Childhood Speech, Language & Listening Problems, 8965
Childrens Beach House, 8946
Communication Outlook, 9003
Dysphagia Research Society, 8920
The Hanen Centre, 946
International Cluttering Association, 8922
Journal of Speech, Language and Hearing Research, 8293, 9001
Kitten Who Couldn't Purr, 8973
Language Parts Catalog, 2010
Language Tool Kit, 2011
Language, Speech and Hearing Services in School, 2012
Language, Speech, and Hearing Services in Schools, 9002
Late Talker: What to Do If Your Child Isn' t Talking Yet, 8975
Luminaud, Inc., 443
Motor Speech Disorders, 8979
Myositis Association, 8925
National Aphasia Association, 8926
National Cued Speech Association, 8164, 8929
National Spasmodic Dysphonia Association, 8369, 8931
National Stuttering Association, 8932
National Tourette Syndrome Association, 8933
Nonverbal Learning Disabilities at Home: A Parent's Guide, 8981
Prentke Romich Company, 194
Prentke Romich Company Product Catalog, 451
Promoting Communication in Infants and Young Children: 500 Ways to Succeed, 8985
Providence Speech and Hearing Center, 8934
Sandcastle Day Camp, 8203
Scottish Rite Center for Childhood Language Disorders, 8935
Sound Connections for the Adolescent, 8992
Spartan Stuttering Laboratory, 938
Step-by-Step Communicator, 198
Stuttering, 8816
TLC Speech-Language/Occupational TherapyCamps, 2714, 6078, 6951
Take a Chance, 5581
TalkTrac Wearable Communicator, 200
Talkable Tales, 8993
Understanding & Controlling Stuttering: A Comprehensive New Approach Based on the Valsa Hyp, 8997
Voice Amplified Handsets, 204
Wendell Johnson Speech & Hearing Clinic, 8950

Spina Bifida

Agassiz Village, 8541
Camp MITIOG, 1220, 8589
Educational Issues Among Children with Spina Bifida, 8713
Genetics and Spina Bifida, 8718
In the Middle, 5434
Introduction to Spina Bifida, 8733
Latex Allergy in Spina Bifida Patients, 8738
Learning Among Children with Spina Bifida, 8739
Lipomas & Lipomyelomeningocele, 8744
Mountaineer Spina Bifida Camp, 1483, 8640
Obesity, 8777
Occulta, 8779
Plan Ahead: Do What You Can, 8796
SPINabilities: A Young Person's Guide to Spina Bifida, 8806
Sexuality and the Person with Spina Bifida, 8808
Sherman Lake YMCA Summer Camp, 8649
Social Development and the Person with Spina Bifida, 8810
Spina Bifida Association, 8528
Spina Bifida Program of Children's National Medical Center, 6723
Spina Bifida and Hydrocephalus Association of Canada, 8529
Symptomatic Chiari Malformation, 8818
Taking Charge, 8819
Urologic Care of the Child with Spina Bifida, 8830

Spinal Cord Injuries

ASIA Annual Scientific Meeting, 1888
Academy of Spinal Cord Injury Professionals, 8336
Academy of Spinal Cord Injury Professionals: Psychologists, Social Workers & Counselors, 8337
American Spinal Injury Association, 8343
Camp PossAbility, 1133
Christopher & Dana Reeve Foundation, 4949
Christopher & Dana Reeve Paralysis Resource Center, 8350
Cure SMA, 8352
Directions, 8862
Functional Electrical Stimulation for Ambulation by Paraplegics, 8394
Guide to Wheelchair Sports and Recreation, 8448
Head Injury Rehabilitation And Referral Service, Inc. (HIRRS), 8356
Journey to Well: Learning to Live After Spinal Cord Injury, 8736
Living With Spinal Cord Injury Series, 8750
National Coalition for Assistive and Rehab Technology, 8365
National Fibromyalgia Association, 8367, 8518
NeuroControl Corporation, 5536
PVA Adaptive Sports, 5675
PVA Summit & Expo, 1916
Paralysis Resource Guide, 8400
Paralyzed Veterans of America, 5597, 8371
SCI Life, 8852
SCI Psychosocial Process, 8874
Shirley Ryan AbilityLab, 935
Southeastern Paralyzed Veterans of America, 5688
Spinal Cord Dysfunction, 2599
Spine, 8853
Sports n' Spokes Magazine, 5585
Tethering Cord, 8878
Topics in Spinal Cord Injury Rehabilitation, 8406
United Spinal Association, 8375
VA North Texas Health Veterans Affairs Care System: Dallas VA Medical Center, 5838

Stroke

American Stroke Association, 8101, 8344
Children's Hemiplegia & Stroke Association, 8349
National Stroke Association, 8111
Pedal-in-Place Exerciser, 494
Stroke Sourcebook, 2nd Edition, 8815

Theater & Dance Therapies

American Dance Therapy Association (ADTA), 4
Disability and Social Performance: Using Drama to Achieve Successful Acts, 22
National Association for Drama Therapy, 48
National Theatre of the Deaf, 52
Non-Traditional Casting Project, 55
Phoenix Dance, 5451

Tinnitus

American Tinnitus Association (ATA), 768, 8129
Tinnitus Today, 8301

Tourette Syndrome

TSA CT Kid's Summer Event, 8653
TSA Newsletter, 8876
Tourette Association of America, 7893

Tourette Association of America National Education Conference, 1922
Tourette Syndrome Association Children's Newsletter, 8879
Twitch and Shout, 5467

Visual Impairments

AAO Annual Meeting, 1881
AER Annual International Conference, 1884
AFB Center on Vision Loss, 3109
AFB Directory of Services for Blind and Visually Impaired Persons in the US and Canada, 9125
AFB News, 9288
AFB Press, 2144
About Children's Eyes, 9126
About Children's Vision: A Guide for Parents, 9127
Access to Art: A Museum Directory for Blind and Visually Impaired People, 9128
Adaptek Systems, 175
Adaptive Services Division, 9290
Adjustable Folding Support Cane for the Blind, 589
African Americans in the Profession of Blindness Services, 9129
Age-Related Macular Degeneration, 9130
Ai Squared, 5481
All Terrain Cane, 590
American Academy of Ophthalmology, 9026
American Anals of the Deaf Reference, 9131
American Blind Bowling Association, 9355
American Council of Blind Lions, 9028
American Council of the Blind, 3, 9029
American Council of the Blind Radio Amateurs, 9030
American Foundation for the Blind, 3115, 9031
American Optometric Association, 9032
American Printing House for the Blind, 9033
Americans with Disabilities Act Guide for Places of Lodging: Serving Guests Who Are Blind, 9132
Amerock Corporation, 2947
Annual Report/Newsletter, 9292
Arizona Rehabilitation State Services for the Blind and Visually Impaired, 3440
Arkenstone: The Benetech Initiative, 1559
Art and Science of Teaching Orientation and Mobility to Persons with Visual Impairments, 9133
Assemblies of God Center for the Blind, 4934
Associated Services for the Blind and Visually Impaired, 4992, 9034
Association for Education & Rehabilitationof the Blind & Visually Impaired, 9035
Association for Macular Diseases, 9036
Association for Macular Diseases Newsletter, 9293
Association for Research in Vision and Ophthalmology, 9037
Association for Vision Rehabilitation and Employment, 9038
Association of Blind Citizens, 9039
Awareness, 9294
Babycare Assistive Technology, 9135
Babycare Assistive Technology for Parents with Physical Disabilties, 9136
Backgammon Set: Deluxe, 5558
Basketball: Beeping Foam, 9356
Beam, 7820
Berthold Lowenfeld on Blindness and Blind People, 9140
Beyond Sight, Inc., 592
Big Number Pocket Sized Calculator, 593
Big and Bold Low Vision Timer, 305
Blind Babies Foundation, 2816
Blind Children's Center, 9040
Blind Children's Center Annual Meeting, 1899
Blind Children's Fund, 3042
Blind Educator, 9277
Blind Information Technology Specialists, 9041
Blind Outdoor Leisure Development, 9357
Blind and Vision-Impaired Individuals, 9141
Blinded Veterans Association, 9042
Blinded Veterans Association National Convention, 1900
Blindness, 5406
Blindness and Early Childhood Development Second Edition, 9142
Blindness: What it is, What it Does and How to Live with it, 9143
Board Games: Peg Solitaire, 5559
Board Games: Snakes and Ladders, 5560
Bold Line Paper, 578
Books are Fun for Everyone, 9144
Books for Blind and Physically Handicapped Individuals, 9146
Braille Calendar, 579
Braille Documents, 5408
Braille Elevator Plates, 594
Braille Forum, 9278
Braille Institute Orange County Center, 9361
Braille Institute of America, 9043
Braille Notebook, 580
Braille Paper, 1595
Braille Playing Cards, 5561
Braille Timer, 307
Braille Touch-Time Watches, 595
Braille: An Extraordinary Volunteer Opportunity, 9148
Braille: Bingo Cards, Boards and Call Numbers, 5562
Braille: Greeting Cards, 581
Braille: Rook Cards, 5563
Brailon Plastic Sheets, 1596
Bureau Of Exceptional Education And Student Services, 3507
Burns Braille Transcription Dictionary, 9149
California Department of Education: Special Education Division, 2181
California State Library Braille and Talking Book Library, 4766, 9044
Camp Abilities, 981
Camp Barakel, 9106
Camp Bloomfield, 1001, 9107
Camp Can-Do, 1430
Camp Challenge, 1155, 9108
Camp Dogwood, 1308
Camp Inter-Actions, 1245
Camp Lawroweld, 1161, 9109
Camp Lighthouse, 1074, 9110
Camp Lou Henry Hoover, 9111
Camp Mauchatea, 1398
Camp Winnekeag, 9113
Can't Your Child See? A Guide for Parents of Visually Impaired Children, 9150
Can-Do Products Catalog, 142
Canine Helpers for the Handicapped, 793, 9045
Caption Center, 4899, 9046
Cards: Musical, 5564
Cards: UNO, 5565
Career Perspectives: Interviews with Blindand Visually Impaired Professionals, 9151
Careers in Blindness Rehabilitation Services, 9152
Carolyn's Low Vision Products, 419, 1513
Cataracts, 9153
Characteristics, Services, & Outcomes of Rehab. Consumers who are Blind/Visually Impaired, 9154
Chess Set: Deluxe, 5566
Chicago Lighthouse for People who are Blind and Visually Impaired, 9048
Childhood Glaucoma: A Reference Guide for Families, 9155
Children with Visual Impairments: A Guide For Parents, 9156
Choice Magazine Listening, 9342
A Christian Approach to Overcoming Disability: A Doctor's Story, 9124
Circline Illuminated Magnifer, 596
Classification of Impaired Vision, 9157
Cleveland Sight Center, 7082
College of Optometrists in Vision Development, 9051
College of Syntonic Optometry, 9052
Columbia Lighthouse for the Blind, 9053
Committee for Purchase from People Who Are Blind or Severely Disabled, 3385
Communication Skills for Visually Impaired Learners, 9158
Community Services for the Blind and Partially Sighted Store: Sight Connection, 1980
Comprehensive Examination of Barriers to Employment Among Persons who are Blind or Impaire, 9159
Connecticut Board of Education and Servicefor the Blind, 3479
Consumer and Patient Information Hotline, 9362
Contrasting Characteristics of Blind and Visually Impaired Clients, 9160
DVH Quarterly, 9298
Dancing Cheek to Cheek, 9161
Dazor Lighting Technology, 473
Defining Rehabilitation Agency Types, 2432
Delaware Division for the Visually Impaired, 3490
Department of Medicine and Surgery Veterans Administration, 5630
Department of Ophthalmology Information Line, 9363
Department of Workforce Development: Vocational Rehabilitation, 6223
Department of Workforce Services: Vocational Rehabilitation, 6224
Desert Blind & Handicapped Association, 9055
Desk-Top Talking Calculator, 520
Development of Social Skills by Blind and Visually Impaired Students, 9162
Diabetic Retinopathy, 9163
Dialogue Magazine, 9280
Dice: Jumbo Size, 5567
Digital Talking Compass, 475
Discovery Day Camp, 1240
Diversity and Visual Impairment: The Influence of Race, Gender, Religion and Ethnicity, 9164
The Division for the Visually Impaired, 3494
Division of Blind Services, 6737
Division of Vocational Rehabilitation Services (DVRS), 6158
Division on Visual Impairments and Deafblindness (DVIDB), 2098
Do You Remember the Color Blue: The Questions Children Ask About Blindness, 9165
Dominoes with Raised Dots, 5568
Don't Lose Sight of Glaucoma, 9166
Early Focus: Working with Young Children Who Are Blind or Visually Impaired & Their Families, 9167
Echo Grove Camp, 1196
Encyclopedia of Blindness and Vision Impairment Second Edition, 9168
Equals in Partnership: Basic Rights for Families of Children with Blindness, 9169
Evansville Association for the Blind, 6031
Exceptional Teaching Inc, 1992
Eye Bank Association of America, 9056
Eye Bank Association of America Annual Meeting, 1907
Eye Research News, 9170
Eye and Your Vision, 9171
Eye-Q Test, 9172
Family Context and Disability Culture Reframing: Through the Looking Glass, 9173
Family Guide to Vision Care (FG1), 9174
Family Guide: Growth & Development of the Partially Seeing Child, 9175
Fathers: A Common Ground, 9176
Fidelco Guide Dog Foundation, 2887, 9057
Fight for Sight, 9058
Fighting Blindness News, 9177
Filomen M. D'Agostino Greenberg Music School, 2099
First Steps, 9178
Focus, 8423, 9301
Foundation Fighting Blindness, 3013, 5509, 7796, 9059
Foundations of Rehabilitation Counseling with Persons Who Are Blind or Visually Impaired, 9180
Four in a Row Game: Tactile, 5571
Freedom Scientific, 5510
General Facts and Figures on Blindness, 9181
Get a Wiggle On, 9182

Giant Print Address Book, 584
Gift of Sight, 9183
Glaucoma, 9184
Glaucoma Research Foundation, 2836, 5512
Glaucoma: The Sneak Thief of Sight, 9185
Gleams Newsletter, 9302
Guide Dog Foundation for the Blind, 3146
Guide Dogs for the Blind, 9060
Guidelines and Games for Teaching Efficient Braille Reading, 9186
Guidelines for Comprehensive Low Vision Care, 9187
Guideway, 9304
Guiding Eyes for the Blind, 9061
Guild Briefs, 9305
Handbook for Itinerant and Resource Teachers of Blind Students, 9188
Handbook of Information for Members of the Achromatopsia Network, 9189
Hawaii Department of Human Services, 3539
Health Care Professionals Who Are Blind or Visually Impaired, 9190
Heart to Heart, 5427, 9191, 9343
Heartbreak of Being A Little Bit Blind, 9192
Helen and Teacher: The Story of Helen & Anne Sullivan Macy, 7810
Helping the Visually Impaired Child with Developmental Problems, 9194
Highbrook Lodge, 1336, 9115
History and Use of Braille, 9195
Horizons for the Blind, 4835, 9062
Hub, 9197
Hull Park and Retreat Center, 1363
Humanware, 1602
Huntsville Subregional Library for the Blind & Physically Handicapped, 4745
IAAIS Report, 9306
Idaho Commission for the Blind & Visually Impaired, 6001
Idaho Commission for the Blind and Visually Impaired, 7800
If Blindness Comes, 9198
Imagining the Possibilities: Creative Approaches to Orientation and Mobility Instructio, 9200
Increasing Literacy Levels: Final Report, 9201
Independent Visually Impaired Entrepreneurs, 9063
Indian Creek Camp, 9116
Information & Referral Center, 2508
Information Access Project, 9202
Information on Glaucoma, 9203
Insight Horse Camp, 1337
Institute for Families, 9064
International Association of Audio Information Services, 9065
International Braille and Technology Center for the Blind, 8896
International Directory of Libraries for the Disabled, 5199
Intervention Practices in the Retention of Competitive Employment, 9204
Iowa Department for the Blind, 3577
JBI Voice, 9283
Jewish Braille Institute International, 9066
Jewish Braille Review, 9284
Journal of Visual Impairment and Blindness, 9276
Juggler, 9344
Kamp A-Komp-Plish, 9117
Kentucky Office for the Blind, 3592, 6054
Know Your Eye, 9205
LS&S, 441
Labeling Kits, 488
LampLighter, 9308
Large Button Speaker Phone, 185
Large Display Alarm Clock, 597
Large Print Loan Library, 9206
Large Print Loan Library Catalog, 9207
Large Print Recipies for a Healthy Life, 9208
Learning to Play, 9209
Let's Eat, 9210
Let's Eat Video, 5439, 9345
Library Services for the Blind, 9211
Library Users of America Newsletter, 9309
Light the Way, 9310
Lighthouse Central Florida, 5981
Lighthouse Guild, 2107, 5521, 9068
Lighthouse International Information and Resource Service, 9364
Lighthouse Low Vision Products, 442
Lilac Services for the Blind, 7802
Lion, 9213
Lions Clubs International, 2779, 9069
Living with Achromatopsia, 9214
Long Cane News, 9314
Long Ring Low Vision Timers, 320
Look Out for Annie, 9346
Louis R Lurie Foundation, 2848
Low Vision Questions and Answers: Definitions, Devices, Services, 9215
Low Vision Telephones, 598
Low Vision Watches & Clocks, 599
Low Vision: Reflections of the Past, Issues for the Future, 9216
Macular Degeneration Foundation, 9070
Magni-Cam & Primer, 600
Maine Division for the Blind and Visually Impaired, 3609
Mainstreaming and the American Dream, 9217
Mainstreaming the Visually Impaired Child, 9218
Making Life More Livable, 9219
Man's Low-Vision Quartz Watches, 602
Massachusetts Commission for the Blind, 6083
Metropolitan Washington Ear, 186
Miami-Dade County Disability Services and Independent Living (DSAIL), 4117
Michigan Commission for the Blind: Grand Rapids, 3640
Michigan Council of the Blind and Visually Impaired (MCBVI), 3641
Michigan Library for the Blind and Physically Handicapped, 4914
Mideastern Michigan Library Co-op, 4916
Minnesota Department of Employment & Economic Development: State Services for the Blind, 6095
Minnesota State Services for the Blind, 3659
Missouri Rehabilitation Services for the Blind, 3671
MonoMouse Electronic Magnifiers, 603
More Alike Than Different: Blind and Visually Impaired Children, 9222
Mothers with Visual Impairments who are Raising Young Children, 9223
Move With Me, 9224
Musical Mainstream, 9285
NFB Career Mentoring, 6076
NLS News, 9318
NLS Newsletter, 9319
NanoPac, 1769
National Alliance of Blind Students NABS Liaison, 9071
National Association for Visually Handicapped (NAVH), 9073
National Association of Blind Merchants (NABM), 889, 9076
National Association of Blind Students, 9078
National Association of Blind Teachers, 9079
National Association of Guide Dog Users, 9081
National Association to Promote the Use of Braille, 9082
National Braille Association, 9084
National Braille Press, 9085
National Camps for Blind Children, 1236, 9119
National Center for Vision and Child Development, 9086
National Eye Institute, 3392, 9088, 9225
National Eye Research Foundation, 2969
National Federation of the Blind, 3020, 7805, 9089
National Industries for the Blind, 9090
National Organization of Parents of Blind Children, 9092
Nebraska Commission for the Blind & Visually Impaired, 3686
Nevada Bureau of Vocational Rehabilitation, 3695
New England Eye Center - Tufts Medical Center, 6975
New Eyes for the Needy, 9093
New Jersey Commission for the Blind and Visually Impaired (CBVI), 3718, 6136
New Mexico Commission for the Blind (NMCFTB), 3728, 6149
New Vision Store, 447
New York State Commission for the Blind, 3746
North Carolina Division of Services for the Blind, 6161
North Dakota Vocational Rehabilitation Agency, 6168
North Georgia Talking Book Center, 4823
Oklahoma Department of Rehabilitation Services, 3804, 6172
Opportunity, 9286
Oregon Health Sciences University, 5803
Orientation and Mobility Primer for Families and Young Children, 9226
Out of Left Field, 9348
Out of the Corner of My Eye: Living with Vision Loss in Later Life, 9227
PBA News, 9320
PXE International, 8901
Patient's Guide to Visual Aids and Illumination, 9230
Pearle Vision Foundation, 3304
Pediatric Visual Diagnosis Fact Sheets, 9231
Pennsylvania Bureau of Blindness & Visual Services, 3819
Perkins Brailler, 527
Personal Reader Update, 9233
Pet Partners, 495
Playback, 9322
Preschool Learning Activities for the Visually Impaired Child, 9234
Prevent Blindness America, 9094
Psychoeducational Assessment of Visually Impaired and Blind Students, 2569
Quantum Technologies, 5540
Quarterly Update, 9323
RP Messenger, 9324
Reaching, Crawling, Walking... Let's Get Moving, 9235
Reading Is for Everyone, 9236
Reading with Low Vision, 9237
Reference and Information Services From NLS, 9239
Rehabilitation Resource Manual: VISION, 2577
Reizen Braille Labeler, 530
Research to Prevent Blindness, 3168
Resource List for Persons with Low Vision, 9240
Robert Ellis Simon Foundation, 2859
SCENE, 9325
Say What Clothing Identifier, 258
See A Bone, 9243
See What I Feel, 9244
See for Yourself, 9350
Seeing Eye Guide, 9327
Seeing Eye, The, 9095
Selecting a Program, 9245
Self-Therapy for the Stutterer, 8989
Services for the Blind Branch, 6000
Services for the Blind and Visually Impaired, 3836
Shared Visions, 9328
Sharp Calculator with Illuminated Numbers, 531
Sightings Newsletter, 9330
Smith Kettlewell Rehabilitation Engineering Research Center, 9331
Society for the Blind, 9096
SourceAmerica, 6214
Special Technologies Alternative Resources, 9248
Standing on My Own Two Feet, 9249
State Library of Kansas, 4863
State Library of Ohio: Talking Book Program, 4985
Step-By-Step Guide to Personal Management for Blind Persons, 9251
Stretch-View Wide-View Rectangular Illuminated Magnifier, 604
Student Teaching Guide for Blind and Visually Impaired College Students, 9252
TBC Focus, 9333
Tactile Braille Signs, 511
Tactile Checkers Set, 5580
Tactile Thermostat, 512

Talk to Me, 9254
Talk to Me II, 9255
Talking Calculators, 201
Talking Digital Thermometer, 281
Talking Food Cans, 329
Talking Thermometers, 282
Talking Watches, 202
Taping for the Blind, 9353
Teaching Orientation and Mobility in the Schools: An Instructor's Companion, 9258
Teaching Visually Impaired Children, 9259
Technology Assistance for Special Consumers, 1654
Technology for the Disabled, 5464
Texas Commission for the Blind, 3882
Texas Workforce Commission: Vocational Rehabilitation Services, 6199
Textbook Catalog, 9260
Tic Tac Toe, 5582
Timex Easy Reader, 605
Touch the Baby: Blind & Visually Impaired Children As Patients, 9263
Touch-Dots, 536
Transition Activity Calendar for Students with Visual Impairments, 9264
Transition to College for Students with Visual Impairments: Report, 9265
US Association of Blind Athletes, 9359
Unisex Low Vision Watch, 606
United States Association of Blind Athletes, 9097
United States Blind Golf Association, 9360
Unseen Minority: A Social History of Blindness in the United States, 9266
Upstate Update, 9335
Utah Division of Services for the Disabled, 3902
Utah State Library Division: Program for the Blind and Disabled, 5012
VIP Newsletter, 2343
VISIONS Vacation Camp for the Blind (VCB), 1302, 9121
VUE: Vision Use in Employment, 9366
Vermont Association for the Blind and Visually Impaired, 9100
Vermont Division for the Blind & Visually Impaired, 3916
Veteran's Voices Writing Project, 5636
Virginia Department for the Blind and Vision Impaired (DBVI), 3921, 6215
Vision Enhancement, 9267
Vision Foundation, 3038
Vision World Wide, 9102
Visions Center on Blindness (VCB), 9103
Vista Center for the Blind & Visually Impaired, 6674
Visual Aids and Informational Material, 9336
Visual Impairment: An Overview, 9268
Visual Impairments And Learning, 9269
Visually Impaired Veterans of America, 9104
Vocational Rehabilitation Agency: Oregon Commission for the Blind, 3813
Vocational Rehabilitation Services for the Blind, 6105
Voice of Vision, 9338
Volunteer Transcribing Services, 2068
WP and HB White Foundation, 2980
Walking Alone and Marching Together, 9270
Washington Connection, 9367
Washington Ear, 9105
Wayfinder Family Services, 2870
What Do You Do When You See a Blind Person-and What Don't You Do?, 9271
What Museum Guides Need to Know: Access for the Blind and Visually Impaired, 9272
When You Have a Visually Impaired Student in Your Classroom: A Guide for Teachers, 2647
Work Sight, 9273
Working with Visually Impaired Young Students: A Curriculum Guide for 3 to 5 Year Olds, 2650
World Through Their Eyes, 9274

Women

The Advocacy Centre, 943
International Women's Health Coalition (IWHC), 871
National Women's Health Network (NWHN), 913
A Woman's Guide to Living with HIV Infection, 8666
Women to Women Healthcare, 959
Women with Visible & Invisible Disabilitiees: Multiple Intersections, Issues, Therapies, 5386

Alabama

ADRS Lakeshore, 5867
Alabama Goodwill Industries, 5868
Alabama Institute for Deaf and Blind Library and Resource Center, 4741
Alabama Power Foundation, 2794
Alabama Radio Reading Service Network (ARRS), 4742
Alabama Regional Library for the Blind and Physically Handicapped, 4743
Alabama VA Benefits Regional Office - Montgomery, 5637
Alabama VA Medical Center - Birmingham, 5638
Andalusia Health Services, 2795
Arc Of Alabama, The, 2796
Arc of Central Alabama, 5869
Birdie Thornton Center, 3965
Butler Adult Training Center, 5870
Camp Evoked Potential, 965
Camp Seale Harris, 966
Camp Shocco for the Deaf, 967
Camp Smile-A-Mile, 968
Camp Smile-A-Mile: Jr./Sr. Camp, 969
Camp Smile-A-Mile: Off Therapy Family Camp, 970
Camp Smile-A-Mile: On Therapy Family Camp, 971
Camp Smile-A-Mile: Sibling Camp, 972
Camp Smile-A-Mile: Teen Weeklong Camp, 973
Camp Smile-A-Mile: Young Adult Retreat, 974
Camp Smile-A-Mile: Youth Weeklong Camp, 975
Camp WheezeAway, 976
Central Alabama Veterans Healthcare System, 5639
Coffee County Training Center, 5871
Dothan Houston County Library System, 4744
Easterseals Camp ASCCA, 977
Easterseals: Achievement Center, 5872
Easterseals: Opportunity Center, 5873
Happy Camp, 978
Huntsville Subregional Library for the Blind & Physically Handicapped, 4745
Independent Living Center of Mobile, 3966
Independent Living Resources Of Greater Bi rmingham: Alabaster, 3967
Independent Living Resources of Greater Birmingham: Jasper, 3968
Independent Living Resources of Greater Bi rmingham, 3969
Montgomery Center for Independent Living, 3970
Montgomery Comprehensive Career Center, 5874
National Center for Health, Physical Activ ity and Disability, 898
Public Library Of Anniston-Calhoun County, 4746
Rapahope Children's Retreat Foundation, 979, 2797
State of Alabama Independent Living/Homebo und Service (SAIL), 3971
Technology Assistance for Special Consumers, 4747
Tuscaloosa VA Medical Center, 5640
Vocational Rehabilitation Service (VRS), 5875
Vocational Rehabilitation Service - Opelika, 5876
Vocational Rehabilitation Service - Dothan, 5877
Vocational Rehabilitation Service - Gadsde n, 5878
Vocational Rehabilitation Service - Homewo od, 5879
Vocational Rehabilitation Service - Huntsv ille, 5880
Vocational Rehabilitation Service - Jackso n, 5881
Vocational Rehabilitation Service - Jasper, 5882
Vocational Rehabilitation Service - Mobile, 5883
Vocational Rehabilitation Service - Muscle Shoals, 5884
Vocational Rehabilitation Service - Selma, 5885
Vocational Rehabilitation Service - Tallad ega, 5886
Vocational Rehabilitation Service - Troy, 5887
Vocational Rehabilitation Service - Tuscal oosa, 5888
Vocational Rehabilitation Services - Andal usia, 5889
Vocational Rehabilitation Services - Annis ton, 5890
Vocational and Rehabilitation Service - Decatur, 5891
Wiregrass Rehabilitation Center, Inc., 5892
Workshops, Inc., 5893

Alaska

Access Alaska: ADA Partners Project, 3972
Access Alaska: Fairbanks, 3973
Access Alaska: Mat-Su, 3974
Adam's Camp: Alaska, 980
Alaska Division of Vocational Rehabilitati on, 5894
Alaska Job Center Network, 5895
Alaska SILC, 3975
Alaska State Commission for Human Rights, 5896
Alaska State Library Talking Book Center, 4748
Alaska VA Healthcare System - Anchorage, 5641
Arc of Alaska, 2798
Arctic Access, 3976
Camp Abilities, 981
Camp Alpine, 982
DAV Department of Alaska, 5642
Hope Community Resources, 3977
Kenai Peninsula Independent Living Center, 3978
Kenai Peninsula Independent Living Center: Seward, 3979
Keni Peninsula Independent Living Center: Central Peninsula, 3980
Rasmuson Foundation, 2799
Southeast Alaska Independent Living, 3981
Southeast Alaska Independent Living: Ketch ikan, 3982
Southeast Alaska Independent Living: Sitka, 3983
Veteran Benefits Administration - Anchorage Regional Office, 5643

Arizona

ASSIST! to Independence, 3984
American Foundation Corporation, 2800
Arizona Autism Resources, 2801
Arizona Braille and Talking Book Library, 4749
Arizona Bridge to Independent Living, 3985
Arizona Bridge to Independent Living: Phoenix, 3986
Arizona Bridge to Independent Living: Mesa, 3987
Arizona Camp Sunrise & Sidekicks, 983
Arizona Community Foundation, 2802
Arizona Developmental Disabilities Plannin g Council (ADDPC), 5897
Arizona Instructional Resource Center for Students who are Blind or Visually Impaired, The, 2803
Beacon Group, 5898
Bonnie Prudden Myotherapy, 785
Books for the Blind of Arizona, 4750
CARF International, 789
Camp AZDA, 984
Camp Abilities Tucson, 985
Camp Candlelight, 986
Camp Civitan, 987
Camp H.U.G., 988
Camp Honor, 989
Camp Not-A-Wheeze, 990
Carl T Hayden VA Medical Center, 5644
Children's Center for Neurodevelopmental Studies, 4751
Civitan Foundation, 2804
Community Outreach Program for the Deaf, 3988
DIRECT Center for Independence, 3989
Division of Developmental Disabilities, 5900
Fair Employment Practice Agency: Arizona, 5901
Flagstaff City-Coconino County Public Library, 4752
Fountain Hills Lioness Braille Service, 4753
International Child Amputee Network, 865
Lions Camp Tatiyee, 992
Margaret T Morris Foundation, 2805
National Center on Disability and Journalism (NCDJ), 900
New Horizons Independent Living Center: Prescott Valley, 3990
Nick & Kelly's Heart Camp, 993
Northern Arizona VA Health Care System, 5645
Prescott Public Library, 4754
Services Maximizing Independent Living and Empowerment (SMILE), 3991
Southern Arizona VA Healthcare System, 5646
Special Needs Center/Phoenix Public Library, 4755
Sterling Ranch: Residence for Special Women, 3992
Temporary Assistance for Needy Families (TANF), 5902
Vocational Rehabilitation, 5903
Wheelers Accessible Van Rentals, 5629
World Research Foundation, 4756
Yavapai Regional Medical Center-West, 5904

Arkansas

Arc of Arkansas, 2806
Arkansas Department of Workforce Services, 5905
Arkansas Independent Living Council, 3993
Arkansas Regional Library for the Blind and Physically Handicapped, 4757
Arkansas Rehabilitation Services (ARS), 5906
Arkansas School for the Blind, 4758
Camp Aldersgate, 994
Camp Laughter, 995
Camp Quality Arkansas, 996
Delta Resource Center for Independent Living, 3994
Easterseals Arkansas, 5907
Educational Services for the Visually Impaired, 4759
Eugene J Towbin Healthcare Center, 5647
International Association of Yoga Therapists (IAYT), 864
John L McClellan Memorial Hospital, 5649
Kota Camp, 998
Library for the Blind and Physically Handi capped SW Region of Arkansas, 4760
Mainstream, 882, 3995
North Little Rock Regional Office, 5650
Northwest Ozarks Regional Library for the Blind and Handicapped, 4761
Sources for Community IL Services, 3997
Spa Area Independent Living Services, 3998
Winthrop Rockefeller Foundation, 2807

California

AAO Annual Meeting, 1881
ABLE Industries, Inc., 5909
AHF Federation, 725
AIDS Healthcare Foundation, 726, 2808
Abilities Expo, 1890
Ability 1st, 4096
AbilityFirst, 5910
Academy of Integrative Health & Medicine (AIHM), 729
Access Center of San Diego, 3999
Access to Independence, 4000
Access to Independence of Imperial Valley, 4001
Access to Independence of North County, 4002
Achievement House & NCI Affiliates, 5911
Ahmanson Foundation, 2809
Alice Tweed Touhy Foundation, 2810
American Academy of Medical Acupuncture, 738
American Acupuncture Council, 742
Anglo California Travel Service, 5607
Anthesis, 5912
Arc of California, 2812
Atkinson Foundation, 2813
Baker Commodities Corporate Giving Program, 2814
Bakersfield ARC, 5913
Bank of America Foundation, 2815
Bearskin Meadow Camp, 999
Beaumont Senior Center: Community Access Center, 4003
Blind Babies Foundation, 2816

Blind Children's Center Annual Meeting, 1899
Bothin Foundation, 2817
Braille Institute Library, 4762
Braille Institute Santa Barbara Center, 4763
Braille Institute Sight Center, 4764
Braille and Talking Book Library: California, 4765
Briggs Foundation, 2818
Burns-Dunphy Foundation, 2819
California Community Foundation, 2820
California Department of Fair Employment & Housing, 5914
California Endowment, 2821
California Foundation For Independent Living Centers, 4004
California Foundation for Independent Living Centers, 4005
California State Independent Living Counci l (SILC), 4006
California State Library Braille and Talki ng Book Library, 4766
Camp Beyond The Scars, 1000
Camp Bloomfield, 1001
Camp Christian Berets, 1002
Camp Conrad Chinnock, 1003
Camp Firefly, 1092
Camp Grizzly, 1004
Camp Krem, 1007
Camp No Limits California, 1008
Camp Okizu, 1009
Camp Okizu: Family Camp, 1010
Camp Okizu: Oncology Camp, 1011
Camp Okizu: SIBS Camp, 1012
Camp Okizu: Teens-N-Twenties Camp, 1013
Camp Pacifica, 1014
Camp Paivika, 1015
Camp ReCreation, 1016
Camp Reach for the Sky, 1017
Camp Ronald McDonald at Eagle Lake, 1018
Camp Ronald McDonald for Good Times, 1019
Camp Sunburst, 1020
Camp Sunshine Dreams, 1021
Camp Taylor, 1022
Camp Taylor: Leadership Camp, 1024
Camp Taylor: Teen Camp, 1025
Camp Taylor: Young Adult Program, 1026
Camp Taylor: Youth Camp, 1027
Camp Tuolumne Trails, 1028
Camp del Corazon, 1029
Camp-A-Lot and Camp-A-Little, 1030
Canine Companions for Independence (CCI), 792
Carrie Estelle Doheny Foundation, 2822
Center for Independence of the Disabled, 4007
Center for Independence of the Disabled- Daly City, 4008
Center for Independent Living, 4009
Center for Independent Living: East Oakland, 4010
Center for Independent Living: Oakland, 4011
Center for Independent Living: Tri-County, 4012
Center for Independent Living:Fresno, 4013
Center for Independent Living; Oakland, 4014
Center of Independent Living: Visalia, 4015
Central Coast Center for IL: San Benito, 4016
Central Coast Center for Independent Living, 4017
Central Coast Center: Independent Living - Santa Cruz Office, 4018
Central Coast for Independent Living, 4019
Central Coast for Independent Living: Watsonville, 4020
Challenged Athletes Foundation (CAF), 800
Clearinghouse for Specialized Media and Translations, 4767
Coelho Epilepsy Youth Summer Camp, 1031
Coeta and Donald Barker Foundation, 2823
College Student's Guide to Merit and Other No-Need Funding, 3353
Colton-Redlands-Yucaipa Regional Occupational Program (CRY-ROP), 5915
Communities Actively Living Independent and Free, 4021
Community Access Center, 4022
Community Access Center: Indio Branch, 4023
Community Access Center: Perris, 4024
Community Employment Services, 5916
Community Rehabilitation Services, 4025
Community Resources for Independence: Mendocino/Lake Branch, 4026
Community Resources for Independence: Napa, 4027
Community Resources for Independent Living: Hayward, 4028
Community Resources for Independent Living, 4029
Conrad N Hilton Foundation, 2824
Continuing Education & Employment Developm ent Program, 5917
Crescent Porter Hale Foundation, 2825
Cunard Line, 5609
DRAIL (Disability Resource Agency for Independent Living), 4030
David and Lucile Packard Foundation, 2826
Dayle McIntosh Center: Laguna Niguel, 4031
Desert Haven Enterprises, 5918
Deutsch Foundation, 2827
Directory of Financial Aids for Women, 3355
Disability Resource Agency for Independent Living: Modesto, 4032
Disability Services & Legal Center, 4033
Disabled Businesspersons Association (DBA), 823
Disabled Resources Center, 4034
Dream Street, 1032
Dream Street Foundation, 2828
East Bay Community Foundation, 2829
Easterseals Camp, 1033
Easterseals Camp Harmon, 1034
Employment Development Department, 5919
Enchanted Hills Camp for the Blind, 1035
Environmental Traveling Companions, 5613
Esalen Institute, 835
Evelyn and Walter Hans Jr, 2830
FREED Center for Independent Living, 4035
FREED Center for Independent Living: Marys ville, 4036
Family Caregiver Alliance, 2831
Feather River Industries, 5920
Financial Aid for Asian Americans, 3359
Financial Aid for Hispanic Americans, 3360
Financial Aid for Native Americans, 3361
Financial Aid for Research and Creative Ac tivities Abroad, 3362
Financial Aid for Veterans, Military Personnel and their Dependents, 3363
Financial Aid for the Disabled and Their F amilies, 2832, 3364
Firefighters Kids Camp, 1036
Firemans Fund Foundation, 2833
First Step Independent Living, 4037
Fred Gellert Foundation, 2834
Fresno City College: Disabled Students Programs and Services, 5921
Fresno County Free Library Blind and Handicapped Services, 4769
Gallo Foundation, 2835
Glaucoma Research Foundation, 2836, 4770
Harden Foundation, 2837
Health Action, 853
Heartland Opportunity Center, 5922
Henry J Kaiser Family Foundation, 2838
Henry W Bull Foundation, 2839
Herrick Health Sciences Library, 4771
High School Senior's Guide to Merit and Ot her No-Need Funding, 3373
Homeopathic Educational Services, 857
How to Pay for Your Degree in Business & Related Fields, 3374
How to Pay for Your Degree in Education & Related Fields, 3375
INALLIANCE Inc., 5923
Independent Living Center of Kern County, 4038
Independent Living Center of Lancaster, 4039
Independent Living Resource Center: Santa Barbara, 4041
Independent Living Resource Center: San Fr ancisco, 4042
Independent Living Resource Center: Santa Maria Office, 4043
Independent Living Resource Center: Ventur a, 4044
Independent Living Resource of Contra Coast, 4045
Independent Living Resource of Fairfield, 4046
Independent Living Resource: Antioch, 4047
Independent Living Resource: Concord, 4048
Independent Living Resources (ILR), 4049
Independent Living Service Northern California: Redding Office, 4050
Independent Living Services of Northern California, 4051
International Expressive Arts Therapy Association (IEATA), 868
Irvine Health Foundation, 2840
Jerry L Pettis Memorial VA Medical Center, 5651
Joni and Friends (JAF), 875
Joseph Drown Foundation, 2841
Kenneth T and Eileen L Norris Foundation, 2842
Kings Rehabilitation Center, 5924
Koret Foundation, 2843
Kuzell Institute for Arthritis and Infectious Diseases, 4772
LA84 Foundation, 2844
LJ Skaggs and Mary C Skaggs Foundation, 2845
Legler Benbough Foundation, 2846
Levi Strauss Foundation, 2847
Lions Wilderness Camp for Deaf Children, Inc., 1037
Little Heroes Preschool Burn Camp, 1038
Long Beach VA Medical Center, 5652
Los Angeles Regional Office, 5653
Louis R Lurie Foundation, 2848
Luke B Hancock Foundation, 2849
Marin Center for Independent Living, 4052
Marin Community Foundation, 2850
Martinez Outpatient Clinic, 5654
Mary A Crocker Trust, 2851
McKinnon Body Therapy Center, 884
MedicAlert Foundation International, 2852
Mother Lode Independent Living Center (DRAIL: Disability Resource Agency for Independent, 4053
Mother Lode Rehabilitation Enterprises, In c. (MORE), 5925
Napa Valley PSI Inc., 5926
National Center on Caregiving at Family Caregiver Alliance (FCA), 2853
National Foundation of Wheelchair Tennis, 2854
New Beginnings: The Blind Children's Center, 4773
New Directions For People With Disabilitie s, 5615
New Directions for People with Disabilities, 2782
New Horizons Summer Day Camp, 1039
Oakland VA Regional Office, 5655
Our Way: The Cottage Apt Homes, 3996
PRIDE Industries, 5927
Pacific Institute of Aromatherapy, 919
Parents Helping Parents (PHP), 921
Parents and Friends, Inc, 5928
Parker Foundation, 2855
Pasadena Foundation, 2856
PathPoint, 5929
People Services, Inc, 5930
Placer Independent Resource Services, 4054
Porterville Sheltered Workshop, 5931
Project Independence, 5932
Projects with Industry (PWI) Program, 5933
Quest Camp, 1040
RC Baker Foundation, 2857
Ralph M Parsons Foundation, 2858
Research & Training Center on Mental Health for Hard of Hearing Persons, 4774
Robert Ellis Simon Foundation, 2859
Rolling Start, 4056
Rolling Start: Victorville, 4057
Rosalind Russell Medical Research Center for Arthritis, 4775
Sacramento Medical Center, 5657
San Diego VA Regional Office, 5658
San Francisco Foundation, 2860
San Francisco Public Library for the Blind and Print Handicapped, 4776
San Jose State University Library, 4777

Santa Barbara Foundation, 2861
Seany Foundation, 2862
Services Center For Independent Living, 4058
Shasta County Opportunity Center, 5934
Sidney Stern Memorial Trust, 2863
Sierra Health Foundation, 2864
Silicon Valley Community Foundation, 2865
Silicon Valley Independent Living Center, 4059
Silicon Valley Independent Living Center: South County Branch, 4060
Social Vocational Services, 5935
Sofia University, 937
Sonora Area Foundation, 2866
South Bay Vocational Center, 5936
Southern California Rehabilitation Service s, 4061
Special Camp For Special Kids, 1041
Stella B Gross Charitable Trust C/O Bank of The West Trust Department, 2867
Teichert Foundation, 2868
The Arc Los Angeles and Orange Counties, 5937
The Painted Turtle, 1042
Through the Looking Glass, 4062
Tri-County Independent Living Center, 4063, 4591, 5938, 5938
Unyeway, 5939
VA Central California Health Care System, 5659
VA Greater Los Angeles Healthcare System, 5660
VA Northern California Healthcare System, 5661
VA San Diego Healthcare System, 5662
Valley Light Industries, 5940
WM Keck Foundation, 2869
WORLD, 957
Wayfinder Family Services, 2870
Westside Center for Independent Living, 4064
Whittier Trust, 2871
Willam G Gilmore Foundation, 2872
Work Training Center, 5941
World Experience Teenage Exchange Program, 2791
World Institute on Disability (WID), 961

Canada

A Loving Spoonful, 723
AIDS Vancouver, 727
Advocacy Centre for the Elderly (ACE), 733
Canadian Art Therapy Association (CATA), 791
Child and Parent Resource Institute (CPRI), 802
Clay Tree Society, 806
Communitas Supportive Care Society, 808
Disabled Peoples' International (DPI), 827
Haldimand-Norfolk Resource Education and C ounseling, 851
Lambton County Developmental Services (LCDS), 876
LoSeCa Foundation, 881
North Hastings Community Integration Assoc iation, 915
People First of Canada, 924
St. Paul Abilities Network, 939
The Advocacy Centre, 943
The Hanen Centre, 946

Colorado

AMC Cancer Research Center, 4778
AV Hunter Trust, 2873
Adam's Camp, 1043
Adam's Camp: Colorado, 1044
Adolph Coors Foundation, 2874
American Universities International Programs, 2762
Arc of Colorado, 2875
Aspen Camp, 1045
Atlantis Community, 4065
Blue Peaks Developmental Services, 5942
Bonfils-Stanton Foundation, 2876
Boulder Public Library, 4779
Boulder Vet Center, 5663
Breckenridge Outdoor Education Center, 1046
Camp Rocky Mountain Village, 1047
Camp Wapiyapi, 1048
Center for Independence, 4066
Center for People with Disabilities, 4067
Center for People with Disabilities: Pueblo, 4068
Center for People with Disabilities: Bould er, 4069
Challenge Aspen, 1049
Champ Camp, 1050
Cheyenne Village, 5943
Children's Hospital Burn Camps Program, 1051
Children's Hospital Burn Camps Program: En gland Exchange Program Burn Camp, 1052
Children's Hospital Burn Camps Program: Fa mily Burn Camp, 1053
Children's Hospital Burn Camps Program: Su mmer Burn Camp, 1054
Children's Hospital Burn Camps Program: Wi nter Burn Camp, 1055
Children's Hospital Burn Camps Program: Yo ung Adult Retreat, 1056
City of Lakewood Recreation and Inclusion Services for Everyone (R.I.S.E.), 1057
Cochlear Implant Camp, 1058
Colorado Civil Rights Divsion, 5944
Colorado Lions Camp, 1059
Colorado Springs Independence Center, 4070
Colorado Talking Book Library, 4780
Colorado/Wyoming VA Medical Center, 5664
Comprecare Foundation, 2877
Connections for Independent Living, 4071
Denver CIL, 4072
Denver Foundation, 2878
Denver VA Medical Center, 5665
Developmental Disabilities Resource Center (DDRC), 5945
Disability Center for Independent Living, 4073
Disabled Resource Services, 4074
Disbled Resource Services, 4075
Division of Vocational Rehabilitation, 5946
Dr. Ida Rolf Institute (DIRI), 829
Dvorak Raft Kayak & Fishing Expeditions, 5611
Dynamic Dimensions, 5947
Eastern Colorado Services for the Developm entally Disabled (ECSDD), 5948
El Pomar Foundation, 2879
First Descents, 1060
Grand Junction VA Medical Center, 5666
Greeley Center for Independence, 4076
Helen K and Arthur E Johnson Foundation, 2880
Hope Center, 5949
Imagine!, 5950
Independent Life Center, 4077
Invisible Disabilities Association (IDA), 872
Las Animas County Rehabilitation Center, 5951
Listen Foundation, 2881
National Jewish Medical & Research Center, 4781
PEAK Parent Center, 918
Professional Association of Therapeutic Ho rsemanship International (PATH Intl.), 929
Roundup River Ranch, 1061
Southwest Center for Independence, 4078
Southwest Center for Independence: Cortez, 4079
The Obesity Medicine Association (OMA), 947
Wyoming/Colorado VA Regional Office, 5866

Connecticut

Abilities Without Boundaries, 5952
Aetna Foundation, 2882
Allied Community Services, 5953
American Institute for Foreign Study, 2761
Arc of Connecticut, 2883
Area Cooperative Educational Services (ACES), 5954
Arthur C. Luf Children's Burn Camp, 1062
Bureau of Rehabilitation Services, 5955
CCARC, Inc., 5956
CW Resources, 5957
Camp Harkness, 1064
Camp Horizons, 1065
Camp Isola Bella, 1066
Camp No Limits Connecticut, 1067
Center for Disability Rights, 4080
Center for Independent Living SC, 4081
Chapel Haven, 4082
Community Foundation of Southeastern Connecticut, 2884
Connecticut Braille Association, 4782
Connecticut Governor's Committee on Employment of People with Disabilities, 5958
Connecticut Library for the Blind and Phys ically Handicapped, 4783
Connecticut Mutual Life Foundation, 2885
Connecticut State Independent Living Council, 4083
Connecticut State Library, 4784
Connecticut Tech Act Project: Connecticut Department of Social Services, 4785
Cornelia de Lange Syndrome Foundation, 2886
Disabilities Network of Eastern Connecticu t, 4084
Disability Resource Center of Fairfield County, 4085
Easterseals Camp Hemlocks, 1068
Favarh ARC, 839
Fidelco Guide Dog Foundation, 2887
Fotheringhay Farms, 5959
GE Foundation, 2888
George Hegyi Industrial Training Center, 5960
Goodwill of Southern New England, 5961
Hartford Foundation for Public Giving, 2889
Hartford Insurance Group, 2890
Hartford Regional Office, 5667
Hartford Vet Center, 5668
Henry Nias Foundation, 2891
Independence Northwest Center for Independent Living, 4086
Jane Coffin Childs Memorial Fund for Medical Research, 2892
Kennedy Center, 5962
New Horizons Village, 4087
Prevent Blindness Connecticut, 4786
Rich Foundation, 2937
Scheuer Associates Foundation, 2894
SeriousFun Children's Network, 1069
The Hole in the Wall Gang Camp, 1070
VA Connecticut Healthcare System: Newington Division, 5669
VA Connecticut Healthcare System: West Haven, 5670
Yale University: Vision Research Center, 4787

Delaware

Arc of Delaware, 2896
Arc of Utah, 3311
Camp Manito & Camp Lenape, 1072
Children's Beach House, 1073
Delaware Assistive Technology Initiative (DATI), 4788
Delaware Division of Vocational Rehabilita tion, 5963
Delaware Library for the Blind and Physically Handicapped, 4789
Delaware VA Regional Office, 5671
Elwyn Delaware, 4790
Freedom Center for Independent Living, 4088
Independent Resource Georgetown, 4090
Independent Resources: Dover, 4091
Independent Resources: Wilmington, 4092
Longwood Foundation, 2897
Service Source, 5964
Wilmington VA Medical Center, 5672
Wilmington Vet Center, 5673

District of Columbia

AG Bell Global Listening and Spoken Langua ge Symposium, 1885
Access Pass, 5605
Alexander and Margaret Stewart Trust, 2898
American Association of Acupuncture and Or iental Medicine (AAAOM), 743
American Association of People with Disabilities (AAPD), 744
American Hotel and Lodging Association Fou ndation, 2899
American Public Health Association (APHA), 763
American Red Cross, 764
American Tinnitus Association (ATA), 768
Amputee Coalition, 769

Annual TASH Conference, 1896
Arc National Convention, The, 1897
Arc of the District of Columbia, 2900
Association of Assistive Technology Act Pr ograms (ATAP), 774
Camp Lighthouse, 1074
Center for Mind-Body Medicine, 798
Children's National Medical Center, 805
Chronicle Guide to Grants, 3352
Coalition for Health Funding, 807
Department of Medicine and Surgery Veterans Administration, 5630
Department of Veterans Affairs Regional Office - Vocational Rehab Division, 5631
Department of Veterans Benefits, 5632
Disability Rights International (DRI), 819
Disabled American Veterans, 5674
District of Columbia Center for Independen t Living, 4094
District of Columbia Department of Employment Services, 5965
District of Columbia Public Library: Services for the Deaf Community, 4791
District of Columbia Regional Library for the Blind and Physically Handicapped, 4792
Eugene and Agnes E Meyer Foundation, 2901
Eye Bank Association of America Annual Meeting, 1907
Federal Benefits for Veterans and Dependents, 5634
Federal Student Aid Information Center, 2902
GEICO Philanthropic Foundation, 2903
Georgetown University Center for Child and Human Development, 4793
Goodwill of Greater Washington, 5966
Guide Service of Washington, 5614
HEATH Resource Center at the National Youth Transitions Center, 849
Habilitation Benefits Coalition, 850
Institute for Educational Leadership (IEL), 862
Jacob and Charlotte Lehrman Foundation, 2904
Joseph P Kennedy Jr Foundation, 2906
Kiplinger Foundation, 2907
Laurent Clerc National Deaf Education Cent er, 877
Montgomery County Arc, 3276
Morris and Gwendolyn Cafritz Foundation, 2908
NACDD Annual Conference, 1910
National Association of City and County he alth Officials, 890
National Association of Councils on Develo pmental Disabilities (NACDD), 891
National Center for Education in Maternal and Child Health (NCEMCH), 897
National Certification Commission for Acup uncture and Oriental Medicine, 901
National Collaborative Workforce on Disability (NCWD/Youth), 902
National Council on Independent Living, 4095
National Council on Independent Living (NCIL), 903
National Disability Rights Network (NDRN), 904
National Health Council, 907
National Institute on Disability, Independ ent Living, and Rehabilitation Research (NIDILRR), 908, 4794
National Women's Health Network (NWHN), 913
Operation Job Match, 5967
PVA Adaptive Sports, 5675
PVA Summit & Expo, 1916
Paddy Rossbach Youth Camp, 1075
Palladium, 5968
Partnership to Improve Patient Care, 923
Paul and Annetta Himmelfarb Foundation, 2909
Primary Care Collaborative, 928
Public Welfare Foundation, 2910
Rehabilitation Research and Development Center, 5656
Rehabilitation Services Administration, 5969
Sister Cities International, 2786
Student Guide, 3378
TASH, 942
The District of Columbia Office of Human Rights (OHR), 5970
US Department of Veterans Affairs National Headquarters, 5635
VA Medical Center, Washington DC, 5676
Washington DC VA Medical Center, 5677

Florida

Abilities of Florida: An Affiliate of Service Source, 5971
Able Trust, 2911
Able Trust, The, 5972
Adult Day Training, 4097
Alpha One: Bangar, 4280
American Academy of Pain Medicine (AAPM), 739
American Academy of Pain Medicine Foundati on, 740, 2912
American Disabled Golfers Association (ADGA), 756
Arc of Florida, 2913
Bank of America Client Foundation, 2914
Barron Collier Jr Foundation, 2915
Bay Pines VA Medical Center, 5678
Birth Defect Research for Children (BDRC), 784
Brevard County Talking Books Library, 4795
Broward County Talking Book Library, 4796
CIL of Central Florida, 4098
Camiccia-Arnautou Charitable Foundation, 2916
Camp Amigo, 1076
Camp Boggy Creek, 1077
Camp No Limits Florida, 1078
Camp Thunderbird, 1079
Caring and Sharing Center for Independent Living, 4099
Caring and Sharing Center: Pasco County, 4100
Center Academy at Pinellas Park, 1080
Center for Independent Living in Central Florida, 4101
Center for Independent Living of Broward, 4102
Center for Independent Living of Florida Keys, 4103
Center for Independent Living of N Florida, 4104
Center for Independent Living of NW Florid a, 4105
Center for Independent Living of North Central Florida, 4106
Center for Independent Living of North Cen tral Florida, 4107
Center for Independent Living of S Florida, 4108
Center for Independent Living of SW Florida, 4109
Centers of Excellence Leadership Conferenc e, 1902
Chatlos Foundation, 2917
Coalition for Independent Living Options: Okeechobee, 4110
Coalition for Independent Living Options: Fort Pierce, 4111
Coalition for Independent Living Options, 4112
Coalition for Independent Living Options: Stuart, 4113
Dade County Talking Book Library, 4797
Dialysis at Sea Cruises, 5610
Disability Matters, 1906
Disability Rights Florida, 818
Disabled Drummers Association (DDA), 825
Dr. Moises Simpser VACC Camp, 1081
Dream Oaks Camp, 1082
Easterseals Camp Challenge, 1083
Edyth Bush Charitable Foundation, 2918
Enable America Inc., 834
FPL Group Foundation, 2919
Federal Grants & Contracts Weekly, 3358
Florida Diabetes Camp, 1084
Florida Division of Blind Services, 4798, 5973
Florida Division of Vocational Rehabilitation, 5974
Florida Fair Employment Practice Agency, 5975
Florida Instructional Materials Center for the Visually Impaired (FIMC-VI), 4799
Foundation & Corporate Grants Alert, 3365
Gainesville Division, North Florida/South Georgia Veterans Healthcare System, 5679
Goodwill Life Skills Development Program, 5976
Goodwill Temporary Staffing, 5977
Goodwill's Community Employment Services, 5978
Goodwill's Job Connection Center, 5979
Goodwill's JobWorks, 5980
Hand Camp, 1085
Hillsborough County Talking Book Library Tampa-Hillsborough County Public Library, 4800
Jacksonville Public Library: Talking Books /Special Needs, 4801
James A Haley VA Medical Center, 5680
Jefferson Lee Ford III Memorial Foundation, 2920
Jessie Ball duPont Fund, 2921
Kris' Camp, 1086
Lakeland Adult Day Training, 4115
Lee County Library System: Talking Books Library, 4802
Lighthouse Central Florida, 4116, 5981
Lost Tree Village Charitable Foundation, 2922
Louis de la Parte Florida Mental Health Institute Research Library, 4803
Miami Foundation, The, 2923
Miami VA Medical Center, 5681
Miami-Dade County Disability Services and Independent Living (DSAIL), 4117
Mount Sinai Medical Center, 2924
National Parkinson Foundation, 2925
Norwegian Cruise Line, 5616
Ocala Adult Day Training, 4118
One-Stop Service Center, 5982
Orange County Library System: Audio-Visual Department, 4804
Palm Beach Habilitation Center, 5983
Pearlman Biomedical Research Institute, 4805
Pinellas Park Adult Day Training, 4119
Pinellas Talking Book Library for the Blind and Physically Handicapped, 4806
Primrose Center, 5984
Project SEARCH, 5985
Publix Super Markets Charities, 2926
Quest, Inc., 5986
Quest, Inc. - Tampa Area, 5987
SCARC, Inc., 5988
SCCIL at Titusville, 4120
Seagull Industries for the Disabled, 5989
Self Reliance, 4121
Sertoma Camp Endeavor, 1087
Space Coast Center for Independent Living, 4122
St. Petersburg Regional Office, 5682
Suncoast Center for Independent Living, Inc., 4123
Talking Book Service: Mantatee County Central Library, 4807
Talking Books Library for the Blind and Physically Handicapped, 4808
Talking Books/Homebound Services, 4809
The Cherab Foundation, 944, 2927
University of Miami: Bascom Palmer Eye Institute, 4810
University of Miami: Mailman Center for Child Development, 4811
Upledger Institute International (UII), 954
West Florida Regional Library, 4812
West Palm Beach VA Medical Center, 5683
Young Onset Parkinson Conference, 1923
disAbility Solutions for Independent Livin g, 4124

Georgia

Aerie Experiences, 1088
Arc Of Georgia, 2928
Arms Wide Open, 4125
Athens Talking Book Center-Athens-Clarke County Regional Library, 4813
Atlanta Regional Office, 5684
Atlanta VA Medical Center, 5685
Augusta Talking Book Center, 4814
Augusta VA Medical Center, 5686
Bain, Inc. Center For Independent Living, 4126
Bainbridge Subregional Library for the Blind & Physically Handicapped, 4815
Camp Breathe Easy, 1089
Camp Caglewood, 1090

Camp Dream, 1091
Camp Hawkins, 1093
Camp Independence, 1094
Camp Juliena, 1095
Camp Kudzu, 1096
Camp Twin Lakes, 1098
Camp Twin Lakes: Rutledge, 1099
Camp Twin Lakes: Will-A-Way, 1100
Carl Vinson VA Medical Center, 5687
Center for Inclusive Design and Innovation, 797
Columbus Subregional Library For The Blind And Physically Handicapped, 4816
Community Foundation for Greater Atlanta, 2929
DisAbility LINK, 814, 4127
Disability Connections, 4128
Emory Autism Resource Center, 4817
Emory University Laboratory for Ophthalmic Research, 4818
Fair Housing and Equal Employment, 5990
Florence C and Harry L English Memorial Fund, 2930
Georgia Library for the Blind and Physically Handicapped, 4819
Georgia Power, 2931
Goodwill Career Centers, 5991
Griffin Area Resource Center, 5992
Hall County Library: East Hall Branch and Special Needs Library, 4820
Harriet McDaniel Marshall Trust in Memory of Sanders McDaniel, 2933
IBM National Support Center, 5993
John H and Wilhelmina D Harland Charitable Foundation, 2935
Lettie Pate Whitehead Foundation, 2936
Living Independence for Everyone (LIFE), 4130
Macon Library for the Blind and Physically Handicapped, 4821
Multiple Choices Center for Independent Living, 4131
National Center on Birth Defects and Developmental Disabilities, 4822
New Ventures, 5994
North District Independent Living Program, 4132
North Georgia Talking Book Center, 4823
Oconee Regional Library, 4824
Rome Subregional Library for the Blind and Physically Handicapped, 4825
South Georgia Regional Library-Valdosta Talking Book Center, 4826
Southeastern Paralyzed Veterans of America, 5688
Southwest District Independent Living Program, 4133
Squirrel Hollow Summer Camp, 1101
Statewide Independent Living Council of Ge orgia, 4134
SunTrust Bank, Atlanta Foundation, 2938
Talking Book Center Brunswick-Glynn County Regional Library, 4827
Vocational and Rehabilitation Agency, 5995
Walton Options for Independent Living, 4135

Hawaii

Arc of Hawaii, 2939
Assets School, 5996
Assistive Technology Resource Centers of Hawaii (ATRC), 4828
Atherton Family Foundation, 2940
Camp Anuenue, 1102
Camp Taylor: Family Camp, 1023, 1103
Center For Independent Living- Kauai, 4136
GN Wilcox Trust, 2941
Hawaii Center For Independent Living, 4137
Hawaii Center for Independent Living-Maui, 4138
Hawaii Centers for Independent Living, 4139
Hawaii Community Foundation, 2942
Hawaii Fair Employment Practice Agency, 5997
Hawaii State Library for the Blind and Physically Handicapped, 4829
Hawaii Vocational Rehabilitation Division, 5998
Hilo Vet Center, 5689
Honolulu VBA Regional Office, 5690
Kauai Center for Independent Living, 4140
Lanakila Rehabilitation Center, 5999
McInerny Foundation Bank Of Hawaii, Corporate Trustee, 2943
Pacific Islands Health Care System, 5691
Pacific Rim International Conference on Disability And Diversity, 1918
Services for the Blind Branch, 6000
Sophie Russell Testamentary Trust Bank Of Hawaii, 2944

Idaho

American Falls Office: Living Independently for Everyone (LIFE), 4141
Boise Regional Office, 5692
Boise VA Medical Center, 5693
Camp Hodia, 1104
Camp No Limits Idaho, 1105
Camp Rainbow Gold, 1106
Cristo Vive International: Idaho Camp, 1107
Dawn Enterprises, 4142
Disability Action Center NW, 4143
Disability Action Center NW: Coeur D'Alene, 4144
Disability Action Center NW: Lewiston, 4145
Idaho Assistive Technology Project, 4830
Idaho Commission for Libraries: Talking Book Service, 4831
Idaho Commission for the Blind & Visually Impaired, 6001
Idaho Department of Labor, 6002
Idaho Division of Vocational Rehabilitatio n, 6003
Idaho Falls Office: Living Independently for Everyone (LIFE), 4146
Idaho Governor's Committee on Employment of People with Disabilities, 6004
Idaho Human Rights Commission, 6005
Living Independence Network Corporation, 4148
Living Independence Network Corporation: Twin Falls, 4149
Living Independence Network Corporation: C aldwell, 4150
Living Independent for Everyone (LIFE): Pocatello Office, 4151
Living Independently for Everyone (LIFE): Blackfoot Office, 4152
Living Independently for Everyone: Burley, 4153
National Association for Holistic Aromatherapy (NAHA), 888
ROW Adventures, 5617
Southwestern Idaho Housing Authority, 4154

Illinois

ADA Camp GranADA, 1108
ADA Teen Adventure Camp, 1109
ADA Triangle D Camp, 1110
ATIA Conference, 1889
Access Living of Metropolitan Chicago, 4155
Ada S. McKinley Community Services, Inc., 6006
Alzheimer's Association, 2945
American Academy of Pediatrics (AAP), 741
American Massage Therapy Association (AMTA), 760
Amerock Corporation, 2947
Anixter Center, 6007
Arc of Illinois, 2948
Assistive Technology Industry Association (ATIA), 772
Benjamin Benedict Green-Field Foundation, 2949
Blowitz-Ridgeway Foundation, 2950
C-4 Work Center, 6008
Camp "I Am Me", 1111
Camp Callahan, 1112
Camp Discovery, 1063, 1113, 1375, 1375, 1415, 1431
Camp FRIENDship, 1114
Camp Little Giant, 1115
Camp One Step, 1117
Camp Quality Illinois, 1118
Camp Red Leaf, 1119
Center for Creative Arts Therapy, 795
Center on Deafness, 4156
Chaddick Institute for Metropolitan Development, 2951
Chicago Community Trust, 2952
Chicago Community Trust and Affiliates, 2953
Chicago Public Library Talking Book Center, 4832
Clearbrook, 6009
Community Foundation of Champaign County, 2954
Community Residential Alternative, 4157
Cornerstone Services, 6010
Courier Travel, 5608
Department of Ophthalmology and Visual Science, 4833
Division of Rehabilitation Services, 4129, 4158
Dr Scholl Foundation, 2955
DuPage Center for Independent Living, 4159
Duchossois Foundation, 2956
Easterseals, 831
Edward Hines Jr Hospital, 5694
Evenston Community Foundation, 2957
Family Resource Center on Disabilities, 836
Field Foundation of Illinois, 2958
Fite Center for Independent Living, 4160
Francis Beidler Charitable Trust, 2959
Fred J Brunner Foundation, 2960
Fulton County Rehab Center, 6011
George M Eisenberg Foundation for Charities, 2961
Glenkirk, 6012
Grover Hermann Foundation, 2962
Guild for the Blind, 4834
Horizons for the Blind, 4835
Illinois Department of Rehab Services, 4161
Illinois Early Childhood Intervention Clearinghouse, 4836
Illinois Life Span Program, 6013
Illinois Machine Sub-Lending Agency, 4837
Illinois Regional Library for the Blind and Physically Handicapped, 4838
Illinois Valley Center for Independent Living, 4162
Illinois Wheelchair Sport Camps, 1120
Illinois and Iowa Center for Independent L iving, 4163
Impact Center for Independent Living, 4164
International Academy of Independent Medical Evaluators, 863
Jacksonville Area CIL: Havana, 4165
Jacksonville Area Center for Independent Living, 4166
Jewish Vocational Services, 6014
John D and Catherine T MacArthur Foundation, 2963
Kennedy Job Training Center, 6015
Knox County Council for Developmental Disabilities, 6016
Kreider Services, 6017
LIFE Center for Independent Living, 4167
LINC-Monroe Randolph Center, 4168
Lake County Center for Independent Living, 4169
Lambs Farm, 6018
Land of Lincoln Goodwill Industries, 6019
Les Turne Amyotrophic Laterial Sclerosis Foundation, 2964
Life Center for Independent Living: Pontia c, 4170
Lions Clubs International, 2779
Little City Foundation, 2965
Living Independently Now Center (LINC), 4171
Living Independently Now Center: Sparta, 4172
Living Independently Now Center: Waterloo, 4173
Lowe Syndrome Conference, 1909
MAGIC Foundation for Children's Growth, 2966
MDA Summer Camp, 1121
Marion VA Medical Center, 5695
McDonald's Corporation Contributions Program, 2967
Michael Reese Health Trust, 2968
Mid-Illinois Talking Book Center, 4839
Muscular Dystrophy Association USA (MDA), 887
National Eye Research Foundation, 2969
National Eye Research Foundation (NERF), 4840
National Foundation for Ectodermal Dysplasias, 2970
National Headache Foundation, 2971

National Lekotek Center, 4841
North Chicago VA Medical Center, 5696
Northwestern University Multipurpose Arthritis & Musculoskeletal Center, 4842
Nothern Suburban Special Recreation Associ ation Day Camps, 1122
OMRON Foundation OMRON Electronics, 2972
Opportunities for Access: A Center for Independent Living, 4175
Options Center for Independent Living: Bou rbonnais, 4176
Options Center for Independent Living: Wat seka, 4177
Orchard Village, 6020
PACE Center for Independent Living, 4178
Peoria Area Community Foundation, 2974
Polk Brothers Foundation, 2975
Progress Center for Independent Living, 4179
Progress Center for Independent Living: Bl ue Island, 4180
Regional Access & Mobilization Project, 4181
Regional Access & Mobilization Project: Be lvidere, 4182
Regional Access & Mobilization Project: De Kalb, 4183
Regional Access & Mobilization Project: Fr eeport, 4184
Retirement Research Foundation, 2976
Rimland Services for Autistic Citizens, 1123
Ronald McDonald House Charities (RMHC), 933
Rotary Youth Exchange, 2784
Sears-Roebuck Foundation, 2977
Sertoma Centre, 6021
Shady Oaks Camp, 1124
Shirley Ryan AbilityLab, 935
Shore Training Center, 6022
Siragusa Foundation, 2978
Skokie Accessible Library Services, 4843
Soyland Access to Independent Living (SAIL), 4185
Soyland Access to Independent Living: Char leston, 4186
Soyland Access to Independent Living: Shel byville, 4187
Soyland Access to Independent Living: Sull ivan, 4188
Springfield Center for Independent Living, 4189
Square D Foundation, 2979
Stone-Hayes Center for Independent Living, 4190
The Workshop, 6023
Thresholds, 950, 6024
Timber Pointe Outdoor Center, 1125
University of Illinois at Chicago: Lions of Illinois Eye Research Institute, 4844
VA Illiana Health Care System, 5697
Vocational Rehabilitation Services, 5908, 6025
Voices of Vision Talking Book Center at DuPage Library System, 4845
WP and HB White Foundation, 2980
Washington County Vocational Workshop, 6026
Washington Square Health Foundation, 2981
West Central Illinois Center for Independent Living, 4191
West Central Illinois Center for Independe nt Living: Macomb, 4192
Wheat Ridge Ministries, 2982
Will Grundy Center for Independent Living, 4193

Indiana

ADEC Resources for Independence, 6027
Allen County Public Library, 4846
American Camp Association (ACA), 751
Anderson Woods, 1126
Arc Northwest Indiana, 6028
Arc of Indiana, 2983
Assistive Technology Training and Informat ion Center (ATTIC), 4194
Association of Independent Camps, 777
BI-County Services, 6029
Ball Brothers Foundation, 2984
Bartholomew County Public Library, 4847
CHAMP Camp, 1127
Camp About Face, 1128
Camp Brave Eagle, 1129
Camp John Warvel, 1130
Camp Little Red Door, 1131
Camp Millhouse, 1132
Camp PossAbility, 1133
Camp Red Cedar, 1135
Camp Riley, 1136
Carey Services, 6030
Community Foundation of Boone County, 2985
DAMAR Services, 4195
Elkhart Public Library for the Blind and Physically Handicapped, 4848
Evansville Association for the Blind, 6031
Everybody Counts Center for Independent Living, 4196
Feingold Association of the US, 842
Four Rivers Resource Services, 4197, 6032
Future Choices Independent Living Center, 4198
Gateway Services/JCARC, 6033
Goodwill of Central & Southern Indiana, 6034
Happiness Bag, 1137
Hillcroft Services, 1138
Hoosier Burn Camp, 1139
Independent Living Center of Eastern Indiana (ILCEIN), 4199
Indiana Association for Home and Hospice Care (IAHHC), 861
Indiana Civil Rights Commission, 6035
Indiana Deaf Camp, 1140
Indiana Disability Employment Initiative, 6036
Indiana Resource Center for Autism, 4849
Indiana University: Multipurpose Arthritis Center, 4850
Indianapolis Regional Office, 5698
Indianapolis Resource Center for Independe nt Living, 4200
John W Anderson Foundation, 2986
Lake County Public Library Talking Books Service, 4851
League for the Blind and Disabled, 4201
Martin Luther Homes of Indiana, 4202
New Hope Services, 6037
New Horizons Rehabilitation, 6038
Noble Of Indiana, 6039
Paladin, 6040
Putnam County Comprehensive Services, 6041
Richard L Roudebush VA Medical Center, 5699
Ruben Center for Independent Living, 4203
SILC, Indiana Council on Independent Livin g (ICOIL), 4204
Southern Indiana Center for Independent Living, 4205
Southern Indiana Resource Solutions, 6042
Special Services Division: Indiana State Library, 4852
St. Joseph Hospital Rehabilitation Center, 4853
Sycamore Rehabilitation Services, 6043
Talking Books Service Evansville Vanderburgh County Public Library, 4854
VA North Indiana Health Care System: Fort Wayne Campus, 5700
VA Northern Indiana Health Care System: Marion Campus, 5701
Wabash Independent Living Center & Learning Center (WILL), 4206

Iowa

Access, Inc., 6044
Arc of Iowa, 2987
Black Hawk Center for Independent Living, 4207
Camp Albrecht Acres, 1141
Camp Courageous of Iowa, 1142
Camp Hertko Hollow, 1143
Camp Sunnyside, 1144
Camp Tanager, 1145
Central Iowa Center for Independent Living, 4208
Des Moines VA Medical Center, 5702
Des Moines VA Regional Office, 5703
Evert Conner Rights & Resources CIL, 4209
Hall-Perrine Foundation, 2988
Hope Haven, 4210
Iowa Career Connection, 6045
Iowa City VA Medical Center, 5704
Iowa Civil Rights Commission, 6046
Iowa Department for the Blind Library, 4855
Iowa Economic Development Authority, 6047
Iowa Registry for Congenital and Inherited Disorders, 4856
Iowa Valley Community College, 6048
Iowa Vocational Rehabilitation Services, 6049
Knoxville VA Medical Center, 5705
League of Human Dignity, Center for Indepe ndent Living, 4211
Library Commission for the Blind, 4857
Mid-Iowa Health Foundation, 2989
New Focus, 6050
Principal Financial Group Foundation, 2990
Siouxland Community Foundation, 2991
South Central Iowa Center for Independent Living, 4213
Universal Pediatrics, 953
VA Central Iowa Health Care System, 5706
Youth MOVE National, 963

Kansas

Advocates for Better Living For Everyone (A.B.L.E.), 4215
Arc of Kansas, 2992
Association for Applied Psychophysiology and Biofeedback (AAPB), 773
Camp Discovery Kansas, 1146
Camp Planet D, 1147
Camp Quality Kansas, 1148
Camp Sweet Betes, 1149
Center for Independent Living SW Kansas: L iberal, 4216
Center for Independent Living Southwest Kansas, 4217
Center for Independent Living Southwest Ka nsas: Dodge City, 4218
Center for the Improvement of Human Functioning, 4858
Central Kansas Library Systems Headquarter s (CSLS), 4859
Coalition for Independence, 4219
Colmery-O'Neil VA Medical Center, 5707
Cowley County Developmental Services, 4220
Dwight D Eisenhower VA Medical Center, 5708
Hutchinson Community Foundation, 2993
Independence, 4221
Independent Connection, 4222
Independent Connection: Abilene, 4223
Independent Connection: Beloit, 4224
Independent Connection: Concordia, 4225
Independent Living Resource Center, 4040, 4226
Kansas Human Rights Commission, 6051
Kansas Services for the Blind & Visually Impaired, 4227
Kansas VA Regional Office, 5709
Kansas Vocational Rehabilitation Agency, 6052
LINK: Colby, 4228
Living Independently in Northwest Kansas: Hays, 4229
Manhattan Public Library, 4860
Northwest Kansas Library System Talking Books, 4861
Prairie IL Resource Center, 4230
Prairie Independent Living Resource Center, 4231
Resource Center for Independent Living: Emporia, 4234
Resource Center for Independent Living: Ar kansas City, 4235
Resource Center for Independent Living: Bu rlington, 4236
Resource Center for Independent Living: Co ffeyville, 4237
Resource Center for Independent Living: El Dorado, 4238
Resource Center for Independent Living: Ft Scott, 4239
Resource Center for Independent Living: Ot tawa, 4240
Resource Center for Independent Living: Ov erland Park, 4241
Resource Center for Independent Living: To peka, 4242

Richard W Higgins Charitable Foundation, 2994
Robert J Dole VA Medical Center, 5710
South Central Kansas Library System, 4862
Southeast Kansas Independent Living (SKIL), 4243
Southeast Kansas Independent Living: Independence, 4244
Southeast Kansas Independent Living: Chanu te, 4245
Southeast Kansas Independent Living: Colum bus, 4246
Southeast Kansas Independent Living: Fredo nia, 4247
Southeast Kansas Independent Living: Hays, 4248
Southeast Kansas Independent Living: Pitts burg, 4249
Southeast Kansas Independent Living: Sedan, 4250
Southeast Kansas Independent Living: Yates Center, 4251
State Library of Kansas, 4863
Three Rivers Independent Living Center, 4252
Three Rivers Independent Living Center: Clay, 4253
Three Rivers Independent Living Center: Ma nhattan, 4254
Three Rivers Independent Living Center: Se neca, 4255
Three Rivers Independent Living Center: To peka, 4256
Topeka & Shawnee County Public Library Talking Books Service, 4864
Topeka Independent Living Resource Center, 4257
Whole Person: Nortonville, 4258
Whole Person: Nortonville, The, 4259
Whole Person: Prairie Village, 4260
Whole Person: Prairie Village, The, 4261
Whole Person: Tonganoxie, 4262
Wichita Public Library/Talking Book Service, 4865
Wichita Public Library/Talking Book Servic e, 4866

Kentucky

Arc of Kentucky, 2995
Camp Quality Kentuckiana, 1134, 1150
Center for Accessible Living, 4263
Center for Accessible Living: Murray, 4264
Center for Independent Living: Kentucky Department for the Blind, 4265
Children's Alliance, 803
Disability Coalition of Northern Kentucky, 4266
Disability Resource Initiative, 4267
Disabled American Veterans Headquarters, 5633
EnTech: Enabling Technologies of Kentuckiana, 4867
Independence Place, 4268
Kentucky Commission on Human Rights, 6053
Kentucky Office for the Blind, 6054
Kentucky Talking Book Library - Kentucky Dept. for Libraries and Archives, 4868
Kentucky Vocational Rehabilitation Agency, 6055
Kids Cancer Alliance, 1151
Lexington VA Medical Center, 5711
Lions Camp Crescendo, 1152
Louisville Free Public Library, 4869
Louisville VA Medical Center, 5712
Louisville VA Regional Office, 5713
Pathfinders for Independent Living, 4269
Pioneer Vocational/Industrial Services, 6056
SILC Department of Vocational Rehabilitation, 4270
The Center for Courageous Kids, 1153

Louisiana

Alexandria VA Medical Center, 5714
Arc of Louisiana, 2996
Baton Rouge Area Foundation, 2997
Blind Services, 6057
COEA The Arc of East Ascension, 6058
Camp Bon Coeur, 1154
Camp Challenge, 1155
Camp Pelican, 1156
Camp Quality Louisiana, 1157
Central Louisiana State Hospital Medical and Professional Library, 4870
Community Foundation of Shreveport-Bossier, 2998
Disability Rights Louisiana, 820
Louisiana Lions Camp, 1158
Louisiana Rehabilitation Services, 6059
Louisiana State Library, 4871
Louisiana State University Genetics Sectio n of Pediatrics, 4872
MedCamps of Louisiana, 1159
New Horizons: Central Louisiana, 4271
New Horizons: Northeast Louisiana, 4272
New Horizons: Northwest Louisiana, 4273
New Orleans VA Medical Center, 5715
Resources for Independent Living: Baton Rouge, 4274
Resources for Independent Living: Metairie, 4275
Shreveport VA Medical Center, 5716
Southwest Louisiana Independence Center: L ake Charles, 4276
Southwest Louisians Independence Center: Lafayette, 4277
State Library of Louisiana: Services for the Blind and Physically Handicapped, 4873
The Arc Westbank, 6060
Vocational Rehabilitation Program, 6061
Volunteers of America of Greater New Orlea ns, 4278
W Troy Cole Independent Living Specialist, 4279

Maine

Addison Point Agency, 6062
Alpha One: South Portland, 4281
BCR Foundation, 2999
Bangor Public Library, 4874
Bangor Veteran Center: Veterans Outreach Center, 6063
Camp CaPella, 1160
Camp Lawroweld, 1161
Camp No Limits Maine, 1162
Camp Sunshine, 997, 1097, 1163, 1163
Camp sNOw Maine, 1164
Cary Library, 4875
Creative Work Systems, 6064
Division for the Blind and Visually Impair ed, 6065
High School Students Guide to Study, Travel, and Adventure Abroad, 2772
Lewiston Public Library, 4876
Maine Commission on Disability & Employmen t, 6066
Maine Department Of Labor, 6067
Maine Human Rights Commission, 6068
Maine State Library, 4877
Maine VA Regional Office, 5717
Motivational Services, 4282
No Limits Foundation, 3000
Northeast Occupational Exchange, 6069
Pine Tree Camp, 1165
Portland Public Library, 4879
Shalom House, 4283
Togus VA Medical Center, 5718
UNUM Charitable Foundation, 3001
Waban Projects, 958
Waterville Public Library, 4880
Women to Women Healthcare, 959

Maryland

AAIDD Annual Meeting, 1880
ACNM Foundation, Inc., 3002
APSE National Conference, 1886
ASHA Convention, 1887
Accreditation Commission for Midwifery Education (ACME), 732
American Association on Health and Disabil ity (AAHD), 745
American Association on Intellectual and Developmental Disabilities (AAIDD), 746
American College of Nurse Midwives (ACNM), 754
American Health Assistance Foundation, 3003
American Occupational Therapy Association (AOTA), 761
American Occupational Therapy Foundation, 3004
American Society of Clinical Hypnosis (ASCH), 766
Anxiety and Depression Association of Amer ica (ADAA), 770
Arc of Maryland, 3005
Ardmore Developmental Center, 6070
Association for International Practical Training, 2766
Association of People Supporting Employmen t First (APSE), 779
Association of University Centers on Disabilities (AUCD), 780
Baltimore Community Foundation, 3006
Baltimore Regional Office, 5719
Baltimore VA Medical Center, 5720
Broadmead, 4284
CASA Inc., 4426
CQL Accreditation, 1901
Camp Great Rock, 1166
Camp Littlefoot, 1167
Camp No Limits Maryland, 1168
Camp SunSibs, 1169
Camp Sunrise, 1170
Candlelighters Childhood Cancer Foundation, 3007
Change, Inc., 801
Children's Fresh Air Society Fund, 3008
Clark-Winchcole Foundation, 3009
Columbia Foundation, 3010
Community Health Funding Report, 3354
Corporate Giving Program, 3011
Council of Colleges of Acupuncture & Orien tal Medicine, 810
Council of Parent Attorneys and Advocates (COPAA), 811
Council of State Administrators of Vocational Rehabilitation (CSAVR), 812
Cystic Fibrosis Foundation, 3012
Deaf Camps, Inc., 1171
Department of Physical Medicine & Rehabilitation at Sinai Hospital, 813
Disability Funding News, 3356
Disabled Children's Fund (DCF), 824
Eastern Shore Center for Independent Living, 4285
Easterseals Camp Fairlee, 1172
Family Run Executive Director Leadership Association (FREDLA), 837
Fort Howard VA Medical Center, 5721
Foundation Fighting Blindness, 3013
Freedom Center, 4286
George Wasserman Family Foundation, 3014
Giant Food Foundation, 3015
Goodwill Industries International, 847
Grand Lodge of the International Association of Machinists and Aerospace Workers, 848
Harry and Jeanette Weinberg Foundation, 3016
Housing Unlimited, 4287
Humanity & Inclusion (HI), 859
IDF National Conference, 1908
Immune Deficiency Foundation, 860, 3017
Independence Now, 4288
Independence Now: The Center for Independent Living, 4289
Johns Hopkins University Dana Center for Preventive Ophthalmology, 4881
Johns Hopkins University: Asthma and Allergy Center, 4882
Kennedy Krieger Institute, 3018
League at Camp Greentop, 1173
Lions Camp Merrick, 1174
Making Choices for Independent Living, 4290
Maryland Commission on Civil Rights (FEPA), 6071
Maryland Department of Disabilities, 6072
Maryland State Department of Education, 6074
Maryland State Library for the Blind and Physically Handicapped, 4883
Maryland Veterans Centers, 5722

Melwood, 6075
Montgomery County Department of Public Libraries/Special Needs Library, 4884
NFB Career Mentoring, 6076
National 4-H Council, 2781
National Epilepsy Library (NEL), 4885
National Federation of Families for Children's Mental Health (NFFCMH), 905
National Federation of the Blind, 3020
National Federation of the Blind Jernigan Institute, 4886
National Institute on Aging, 4887
National Rehabilitation Information Center (NARIC), 4888
Office of Fair Practices, 6077
Optometric Extension Program Foundation, 3021
Perry Point VA Medical Center, 5723
Red Notebook, 4889
Resources for Independence, 4291
RespectAbility, 932
Ryan White HIV/AIDS Program, 934
Sjogren's Syndrome Foundation, 3022
Social Security Library, 4890
Society for Post-Acute and Long-Term Care Medicine (AMDA), 936
Southern Maryland Center for LIFE, 4292
TLC Speech-Language/Occupational Therapy Camps, 6078
Trace Research and Development Center, 4891
VA Maryland Health Care System, 5724
Warren Grant Magnuson Clinical Center, 4892
Youth for Understanding International Exchange, 2793

Massachusetts

Abbot and Dorothy H Stevens Foundation, 3023
Adlib, 4293
Arc of Cape Cod, 4294
Arc of Massachusetts, The, 3024
Arc of Northern Bristol County, 3025
Boston Center for Independent Living, 4295
Boston Foundation, 3026
Boston Globe Foundation, 3027
Boston University Arthritis Center, 4893
Boston University Center for Human Genetics, 4894
Boston University Robert Dawson Evans Memorial Dept. of Clinical Research, 4895
Boston VA Regional Office, 5725
Braille and Talking Book Library, Perkins School for the Blind, 4896
Brigham and Women's Hospital: Asthma and Allergic Disease Research Center, 4897
Brigham and Women's Hospital: Robert B Brigham Multipurpose Arthritis Center, 4898
Bushrod H Campbell and Ada F Hall Charity Fund, 3028
Camp Howe, 1175
Camp Jabberwocky, 1176
Camp Starfish, 1177
Cape Organization for Rights of the Disabled (CORD), 4296
Caption Center, 4899
Center for Interdisciplinary Research on Immunologic Diseases, 4900
Center for Living & Working: Fitchburg, 4297
Center for Living & Working: Framingham, 4298
Center for Living & Working: Worcester, 4299
Clipper Ship Foundation, 3029
Community Foundation of Western Massachusetts, 3030
Developmental Evaluation and Adjustment Fa cilities, 4300
Eagle Hill School: Summer Program, 1178
Edith Nourse Rogers Memorial Veterans Hospital, 5726
Executive Office of Labor & Workforce Deve lopment, 6079
Family Voices, 838
Federation for Children with Special Needs, 841
Feldenkrais Guild of North America (FGNA), 843
Frank R and Elizabeth Simoni Foundation, 3031
Friendly Ice Cream Corp Contributions Prog ram, 3032
Gateway Arts Center: Studio, Craft Store & Gallery, 6080
Greater Worcester Community Foundation, 3033
Harvard University Howe Laboratory of Ophthalmology, 4901
Hyams Foundation, 3034
Independence Associates, 4301
Independent Living Center of Stavros: Gree nfield, 4302
Independent Living Center of Stavros: Spri ngfield, 4303
Independent Living Center of the North Sho re & Cape Ann, 4304
Kamp for Kids at Camp Togowauk, 1179
Laboure College Library, 4902
Learning Disabilities Worldwide, 880
Life-Skills, Inc., 6081
Massachusetts Commission Against Discrimin ation (FEPA), 6082
Massachusetts Commission for the Blind, 6083
Massachusetts Governor's Commission on Employment of People with Disabilities, 6084
Massachusetts Rehabilitation Commission, 4903, 6085
MetroWest Center for Independent Living, 4305
Multi-Cultural Independent Living Center of Boston, 4306
New England Regional Genetics Group, 4878
Northampton VA Medical Center, 5727
Northeast Independent Living Program, 4307
Open Hearts Camp, 1180
Parent Professional Advocacy League (PPAL), 920
Raytheon Company Contributions Program, 3035
Renaissance Clubhouse, 4308
Scandinavian Exchange, 2785
Schepens Eye Research Institute, 4904
Southeast Center for Independent Living, 4309
Student Independent Living Experience Massachusetts Hospital School, 4310
Summer@Carroll, 1181
TJX Foundation, 3036
Talking Book Library at Worcester Public Library, 4905
The Barton Center, 1182
The Barton Center Camp Joslin, 1183
The Barton Center Clara Barton Camp, 1184
The Barton Center Danvers Day Camp, 1185
The Barton Center Family Camp, 1186
The Barton Center Worcester Day Camp, 1187
The Beveridge Family Foundation, Inc., 3037
The Bridge Center, 1188
The Rainbow Club, 1071
VA Boston Healthcare System: Brockton Division, 5728
VA Boston Healthcare System: Jamaica Plain Campus, 5729
VA Boston Healthcare System: West Roxbury Division, 5730
Vermont Overnight Camp, 1465
Viability, 955, 6086
Work Inc., 6087
Youth as Self Advocates (YASA), 964

Michigan

Aleda E Lutz VA Medical Center, 5731
Alternating Hemiplegia of Childhood Foundation, 2811
Ann Arbor Area Community Foundation, 3039
Ann Arbor Center for Independent Living, 4311
Arc Michigan, 4312
Arc of Michigan, 3040
Arc/Muskegon, 4313
Artificial Language Laboratory, 4906
Bad Axe: Blue Water Center for Independent Living, 4314
Battle Creek VA Medical Center, 5732
Bay Area Coalition for Independent Living, 4315
Berrien Community Foundation, 3041
Blind Children's Fund, 3042
Burger School for the Autistic, 4907
Camp Barefoot, 1189
Camp Catch-A-Rainbow, 1190
Camp Chris Williams, 1191
Camp Grace Bentley, 1192
Camp Midicha, 1193
Camp Quality North Michigan, 1194
Camp Quality South Michigan, 1195
Capital Area Center for Independent Living, 4316
Caro: Blue Water Center for Independent Li ving, 4317
Center for Independent Living of Mid-Michigan, 4318
Chi Medical Library, 4908
Community Connections of Southwest Michigan, 4319
Community Foundation of Monroe County, 3043
Cowan Slavin Foundation, 3044
Cristo Rey Handicappers Program, 4320
Daimler Chrysler, 3045
Department of Health & Human Services, 6088
Detroit Center for Independent Living, 4321
Disability Advocates of Kent County, 4322
Disability Connection, 4323
Disability Network Southwest Michigan, 4324
Disability Network of Mid-Michigan, 4325
Disability Network of Oakland & Macomb, 4326
Disability Network/Lakeshore, 4327
Division on Deaf, DeafBlind & Hard of Hear ing, 6089
Echo Grove Camp, 1196
Frank & Mollie S VanDervoort Memorial Foun dation, 3046
Fremont Area Community Foundation, 3047
Glaucoma Laser Trial, 4909
Grand Rapids Foundation, 3048
Grand Traverse Area Community Living Management Corporation, 4328
Grand Traverse Area Library for the Blind and Physically Handicapped, 4910
Granger Foundation, 3049
Great Lakes/Macomb Rehabilitation Group, 4329
Harvey Randall Wickes Foundation, 3050
Havirmill Foundation, 3051
Hope Network Neuro Rehabilitation, 858
Indian Trails Camp, 1197
Iron Mountain VA Medical Center, 5733
JARC, 4330
John D Dingell VA Medical Center, 5734
Kelly Services Foundation, 3052
Kent County Arc, 3053
Kent District Library for the Blind and Physically Handicapped, 4911
Kresge Foundation, 3054
Lanting Foundation, 3055
Lapeer: Blue Water Center for Independent Living, 4331
Livingston Center for Independent Living, 4332
Macomb Library for the Blind & Physically Handicapped, 4912
Michigan Braille and Talking Book Library, 4913
Michigan Commission for the Blind: Independent Living Rehabilitation Program, 4333
Michigan Commission for the Blind: Detroit, 4334
Michigan Department of Civil Rights, 6090
Michigan Library for the Blind and Physically Handicapped, 4914
Michigan Rehabilitation Services, 6091
Michigan VA Regional Office, 5735
Michigan Workforce Development Agency, 6092
Michigan's Assistive Technology Resource, 4915
Mideastern Michigan Library Co-op, 4916
Monroe Center for Independent Living, 4335
Muskegon Area District Library for the Bli nd and Physically Handicapped, 4917
Northland Library Cooperative, 4918
Oakland County Library for the Visually & Physically Impaired, 4919
Port Huron: Blue Water Center for Independ ent Living, 4336
Rollin M Gerstacker Foundation, 3056
Sandusky: Blue Water Center for Independen t Living, 4337
Southeastern Michigan Commission for the Blind, 4338
Spartan Stuttering Laboratory, 938

St. Clair County Library Special Technologies Alternative Resources (S.T.A.R.), 4920
St. Francis Camp On The Lake, 1198
Steelcase Foundation, 3057
Straits Area Services, Inc., 6093
Student Disability Services (SDS), 941
Superior Alliance for Independent Living (SAIL), 4339
The Creative Mobility Group, LLC, 5627
Trail's Edge Camp, 1199
University of Michigan: Orthopaedic Research Laboratories, 4921
Upper Peninsula Library for the Blind, 4922
VA Ann Arbor Healthcare System, 5736
Vet Center Readjustment Counseling Service, 5737
Washtenaw County Library for the Blind & Physically Handicapped, 4923
Wayne County Regional Library for the Blind, 4924
Wayne State University: CS Mott Center for Human Genetics and Development, 4925
disAbility Connections, 4340

Minnesota

Access North Center for Independent Living of Northeastern MN, 4341
Accessible Space, Inc., 4342
Accreditation Commission for Acupuncture & Oriental Medicine, 731
Advocates for Developmental Disabilities, 735
Arc of Minnesota, 3058
AuSM Summer Camp, 1200
Burnett Foundation, 3059
Camp Buckskin, 1201
Camp Confidence, 1202
Camp Courage North, 1204
Camp Eden Wood, 1205
Camp Heartland, 1206
Camp Hollywood HEART, 1005
Camp Knutson, 1207
Camp Odayin, 1208
Camp Odayin Family Camp, 1209
Camp Odayin Residential Camp, 1210
Camp Odayin Summer Camp, 1211
Camp Odayin Winter Camp, 1212
Century College, 4926
Closing the Gap's Annual Conference, 1903
Communication Center/Minnesota State Services for the Blind, 4927
Courage Center, 4343
Cristo Vive International: Minnesota Camp, 1213
Deluxe Corporation Foundation, 3060
Down Syndrome Camp, 1214
Duluth Public Library, 4928
Freedom Resource Center for Independent Living: Fergus Falls, 4344
General Mills Foundation, 3061
Hugh J Andersen Foundation, 3062
Independent Life Styles, 4570
James R Thorpe Foundation, 3063
Jay and Rose Phillips Family Foundation, 3064
Jewish Vocational Service of Jewish Family and Children's Services, 6094
Metropolitan Center for Independent Living, 4345
Minneapolis Foundation, 3065
Minneapolis VA Medical Center, 5738
Minnesota Association of Centers for Independent Living, 4346
Minnesota Department of Employment & Econo mic Development: State Services for the Blind, 6095
Minnesota Department of Employment and Economic Development: Vocational Rehab Services, 6096
Minnesota Department of Human Rights (FEPA), 6097
Minnesota Library for the Blind and Physically Handicapped, 4929
Miracle-Ear Children's Foundation, 3019
OPTIONS, 4347
Options Interstate Resource Center for Independent Living, 4348
Ordean Foundation, 3066
Otto Bremer Foundation, 3067
PACER Center (Parent Advocacy Coalition for Educational Rights), 917
Perry River Home Care, 4349
Rochester Area Foundation, 3068
SMILES, 4350
SMILES: Mankato, 4351
Southeastern Minnesota Center for Independent Living: Red Wing, 4352
Southeastern Minnesota Center for Independent Living: Rochester, 4353
Special U, 4930
St. Cloud VA Medical Center, 5739
St. Paul Regional Office, 5740
True Friends, 1215
University of Minnesota at Crookston, 2788
Ventures Travel, 5621
Vinland Center Lake Independence, 4355
Wilderness Inquiry, 5622

Mississippi

AbilityWorks, 6098
Alpha Home Royal Maid Association for the Blind, 4356
Arc of Mississippi, 3069
Biloxi/Gulfport VA Medical Center, 5742
Blind and Physically Handicapped Library Services, 4931
Gulf Coast Independent Living Center, 4357
Jackson Regional Office, 5743
LIFE of Mississippi, 4359
LIFE of Mississippi: Biloxi, 4360
LIFE of Mississippi: Greenwood, 4361
LIFE of Mississippi: Hattiesburg, 4362
LIFE of Mississippi: McComb, 4363
LIFE of Mississippi: Meridian, 4364
LIFE of Mississippi: Oxford, 4365
LIFE of Mississippi: Tupelo, 4366
Mississippi Department of Rehabilitation Services, 6099
Mississippi Employment Secutity Commission, 6100
Mississippi Library Commission, 4932
Mississippi Library Commission\Talking Book and Braille Services, 4933
National Research and Training Center on Blindness and Low Vision, 6101

Missouri

Access II Independent Living Center, 4367
Allen P & Josephine B Green Foundation, 3070
American Academy of Environmental Medicine (AAEM), 737
American Academy of Environmental Medicine Annual Conference, 1893
Anheuser-Busch, 3071
Arc of the US Missouri Chapter, 3072
Assemblies of God Center for the Blind, 4934
Bootheel Area Independent Living Services, 4368
Camp Barnabas, 1217
Camp Encourage, 1218
Camp Hickory Hill, 1219
Camp MITIOG, 1220
Camp No Limits Missouri, 1221
Camp Quality Central Missouri, 1222
Camp Quality Greater Kansas City, 1223
Camp Quality Northwest Missouri, 1224
Camp Quality Ozarks, 1225
Church of the Nazarene, 4935
Coalition for Independence: Missouri Branc h Office, 4369
Delta Center for Independent Living, 4370
Disability Resource Association, 4371
Disabled Athlete Sports Association (DASA), 822
Easterseals Midwest, 4372
Greater Kansas City Community Foundation & Affiliated Trusts, 3073
Greater St Louis Community Foundation, 3074
H&R Block Foundation, 3075
Harry S Truman Memorial Veterans' Hospital, 5744
Independent Living Center of Southeast Missouri, 4373
International Clinic of Biological Regeneration (ICBR), 867
International Ventilator Users Network (IVUN), 870
James S McDonnell Foundation, 3076
John J Pershing VA Medical Center, 5745
Judevine Center for Autism, 4936
Kansas City VA Medical Center, 5746
Lutheran Blind Mission, 4937
Lutheran Charities Foundation of St Louis, 3077
Midland Empire Resources for Independent Living (MERIL), 4374
Missouri Commission on Human Rights, 6102
Missouri Governor's Council on Disability, 6103
Missouri Vocational Rehabilitation Agency, 6104
National Car Rental System, 5625
Northeast Independent Living Services, 4375
On My Own, 4376
Ozark Independent Living, 4377
Paraquad, 4378
People to People International, 2783
Places for People, 4379
Post-Polio Health International, 926
RA Bloch Cancer Foundation, 3078
RAIL, 4380
SEMO Alliance for Disability Independence, 4381
Southwest Center for Independent Living (S CIL), 4383
Southwestern Center for Independent Living, 4354
St. Louis Regional Office, 5747
St. Louis VA Medical Center, 5748
Sunnyhill Adventures, 1226
Sunnyhill, Inc., 4384
Tri-County Center for Independent Living, 4385
University of Missouri: Columbia Arthritis Center, 4938
Veteran's Voices Writing Project, 5636
Victor E Speas Foundation, 3079
Vocational Rehabilitation Services for the Blind, 6105
West Central Independent Living Solutions, 4386
Whole Person, The, 4387
Whole Person: Kansas City, 4388
Wolfner Talking Book & Braille Library, 4939
Wonderland Camp, 1227

Montana

American College of Advancement in Medicine (ACAM), 753
Big Sky Kids Cancer Camps, 1228
Camp Mak-A-Dream, 1229
Charles Campbell Childrens Camp, 1230
Disability Employment & Transitions, 6106
Living Independently for Today and Tomorro w, 4389
MonTECH, 4940
Montana Human Rights Bureau (FEPA), 6107
Montana Independent Living Project, Inc., 4390
Montana State Library-Talking Book Library, 4941
Montana VA Regional Office, 5749
North Central Independent Living Services, 4391
Summit Independent Living Center: Kalipsell, 4392
Summit Independent Living Center: Hamilton, 4393
Summit Independent Living Center: Missoula, 4394
Summit Independent Living Center: Ronan, 4395
V A Montana Healthcare System, 5750
VA Montana Healthcare System, 5751
Vet Center, 5741, 5752

Nebraska

Arc of Nebraska, 3080
Camp Floyd Rogers, 1231
Camp Kindle, 1006, 1232
Camp Quality Heartland, 1233
Center for Independent Living of Central Nebraska, 4396

Cooper Foundation, 3081
Easterseals Nebraska Camp, 1234
Grand Island VA Medical System, 5753
Kamp Kaleo, 1235
League of Human Dignity: Lincoln, 4397
League of Human Dignity: Norfolk, 4398
League of Human Dignity: Omaha, 4399
Lincoln Regional Office, 5754
Lincoln VA Medical Center, 5755
Mosaic, 3082
Mosaic Of De, 4093
Mosaic of Axtell Bethpage Village, 4400
Mosaic of Beatrice, 4401
Mosaic: Pontiac, 4174
Mosiac: York, 4402
National Camps for Blind Children, 1236
Nebraska Assistive Technology Partnership Nebraska Department of Education, 4942
Nebraska Department of Labor, 6108
Nebraska Equal Opportunity Commission (FEPA), 6109
Nebraska Library Commission: Talking Book and Braille Service (TBBS), 4943
Nebraska VR, 6110
Slosburg Family Charitable Trust, 3083
Union Pacific Foundation, 3084
VA Nebraska-Western Iowa Health Care System, 5756

Nevada

Bureau of Vocational Rehabilitation, 6111
Camp Buck, 1237
Camp Lotsafun, 1238
CampCare, 1239
Carson City Center for Independent Living, 4403
Discovery Day Camp, 1240
EL Wiegand Foundation, 3085
Las Vegas Veterans Center, 5757
Las Vegas-Clark County Library District, 4944
Nell J Redfield Foundation, 3086
Nevada Equal Rights Commission, 6112
Nevada Governor's Council on Developmental Disabilities, 6113
Nevada State Library and Archives, 4945
Northern Nevada Center for Independent Liv ing: Fallon, 4404
Reno Regional Office, 5758
Rural Center for Independent Living, 4405
Southern Nevada Center for Independent Living: North Las Vegas, 4406
Southern Nevada Center for Independent Living: Las Vegas, 4407
VA Sierra Nevada Healthcare System, 5759
VA Southern Nevada Healthcare System, 5760
William N Pennington Foundation, 3087

New Hampshire

Adam's Camp: New England, 1241
Agnes M Lindsay Trust, 3088
Camp Allen, 1242
Camp Connect, 1244
Camp Inter-Actions, 1245
Camp Sno Mo, 1246
Camp Wediko, 1247
Camp Yavneh: Yedidut Program, 1248
Foundation for Seacoast Health, 3089
Granite State Independent Living Foundation, 4408
Manchester Regional Office, 5761
Manchester VA Medical Center, 5762
National Guild of Hypnotists (NGH), 906
New Hampshire Bureau of Vocational Rehabil itation, 6114
New Hampshire Commission for Human Rights (FEPA), 6115
New Hampshire Employment Security, 6116
New Hampshire State Library: Talking Book Services, 4946
New Hampshire Veterans Centers, 5763

New Jersey

ARC of Hunterdon County, The, 6117
ARC of Mercer County, 6118
ARC of Monmouth, 6119
Abilities Center of New Jersey, 6120
Abilities of Northwest New Jersey Inc., 6121
Alliance Center for Independance, 4409
Alliance Center for Independence (ACI), 6122
American Migraine Foundation, 3090
Arc of Bergen and Passaic Counties, 6123
Arc of New Jersey, 3091
Arnold A Schwartz Foundation, 3092
Autism New Jersey, 4947
Avis Rent A Car System, LLC, 5624
Camden City Independent Living Center, 4410
Camp Chatterbox, 1249
Camp Deeny Riback, 1250
Camp Dream Street, 1216, 1251
Camp Jaycee, 1252
Camp Jotoni, 1253
Camp Merry Heart, 1254
Camp Nejeda, 1255
Camp Quality New Jersey, 1256
Camp Sun'N Fun, 1257
Campbell Soup Foundation, 3093
Career Opportunity Development of New Jersey, 6124
Center for Educational Advancement New Jersey, 6125
Center for Independent Living: Long Branch, 4411
Center for Independent Living: South Jersey, 4412
Children's Hopes & Dreams Wish Fulfillment Foundation, 3094
Children's Specialized Hospital Medical Library - Parent Resource Center, 4948
Christopher & Dana Reeve Foundation, 4949
Community Foundation of New Jersey, 3095
DAWN Center for Independent Living, 4413
Dial: Disabled Information Awareness & Liv ing, 4414
Disability Rights New Jersey, 4415
Disabled American Veterans: Ocean County, 5764
East Orange Campus of the VA New Jersey Healthcare System, 5765
Easterseals New Jersey, 6126
Eden Autism, 6127
Edison Sheltered Workshop, 6128
Explorer's Club Camp, 1258
Eye Institute of New Jersey, 4950
FM Kirby Foundation, 3096
Family Resource Associates, 4416
Fannie E Rippel Foundation, 3097
Fund for New Jersey, 3098
Goodwill Industries of Southern New Jersey, 6129
Happiness Is Camping, 1259
Harbor Haven Summer Program, 1260
Heightened Independence and Progress: Hack ensack, 4417
Heightened Independence and Progress: Jers ey City, 4418
Hudson Community Enterprises, 6130
Inroads to Opportunities, 6131
Jersey Cape, 6132
Jewish Vocational Service (JVS) - East Orange, 6133
Jewish Vocational Service (JVS) - Livingst on, 6134
Jewish Vocational Service (JVS) - Montclai r, 6135
Lyons Campus of the VA New Jersey Healthcare System, 5766
Mane Stream, 1261
Martin Luther Homes of Iowa, 4212
Merck Company Foundation, 3099
Mycoclonus Research Foundation, 4951
Nabisco Foundation, 3100
New Jersey Commission for the Blind and Visually Impaired (CBVI), 6136
New Jersey Division of Vocational Rehabilitation Services (DVRS), 6137
New Jersey Institute for Disabilities (NJID), 6138
New Jersey Library for the Blind and Handicapped, 4952
Newark Regional Office, 5767
Occupational Training Center of Burlington County (OTCBC), 6139
Occuptational Training Center (OTC), 6140
Ostberg Foundation, 3101
Pathways to Independence, Inc., 6141
Progressive Center for Independent Living, 4419
Progressive Center for Independent Living: Flemington, 4420
Project Freedom, 4421
Project Freedom: Hamilton, 4422
Project Freedom: Lawrence, 4423
Prudential Foundation, 3102
Rising Treetops at Oakhurst, 1262
Robert Wood Johnson Foundation, 3103
Round Lake Camp, 1263
Somerset Community Action Program, Inc., 6142
St. John of God Community Services Vocational Rehabilitation, 6143
The Arc Gloucester, 6144
Total Living Center, 4424
United Cerebral Palsy Associations of New Jersey, 6145
Verizon Foundation, 3179
Victoria Foundation, 3104

New Mexico

ADA Camp 180, 1264
Ability Center, 4425
Adelante Development Center, 6146
Arc of New Mexico, 3105
CHOICES Center for Independent Living, 4427
Camp Enchantment, 1265
Camp Rising Sun, 1266
Dental Amalgam Syndrome (DAMS) Newsletter, 4768
Frost Foundation, 3106
Goodwill Industries of New Mexico, 6147
LifeROOTS, 6148
McCune Charitable Foundation, 3107
Native American Disability Law Center, 914
New Mexico Commission for the Blind (NMCFTB), 6149
New Mexico Division of Vocational Rehabilitation, 6150
New Mexico State Library for the Blind and Physically Handicapped, 4953
New Mexico State Veterans' Home, 5768
New Mexico Technology Assistance Program, 4428
New Mexico VA Healthcare System, 5769
New Mexico Workforce Connection, 6151
New Vistas, 4429
San Juan Center for Independence, 4430
Santa Fe Community Foundation, 3108
Southwest Conference On Disability, 1921
Tohatchi Area of Opportunity & Services, 6152

New York

ADA Camp Aspire, 1267
AFB Center on Vision Loss, 3109
AIM Independent Living Center: Corning, 4431
AIM Independent Living Center: Elmira, 4432
ARISE, 4433
ARISE: Oneida, 4434
ARISE: Oswego, 4435
ARISE: Pulaski, 4436
AT&T Foundation, 3110
Abilities, Inc., 728
Access to Independence of Cortland County , Inc., 4437
Action Toward Independence: Middletown, 4438
Action Toward Independence: Monticello, 4439
Adult Career and Continuing Ed Services - Vocational Rehabilitation (ACCESS-VR), 6153
Advocates for Children of New York (AFC), 734
Albany VA Medical Center: Samuel S Stratton, 5770
Albany Vet Center, 5771
Altman Foundation, 3111
Ambrose Monell Foundation, 3112
American Chai Trust, 3113

American Foundation for Suicide Prevention (AFSP), 758, 3114
American Foundation for the Blind, 3115
American-Scandinavian Foundation, 2763
Andrew Heiskell Braille and Talking Book Library, 4954
Annual Conference on Dyslexia and Related Learning Disabilities, 1895
Arthur Ross Foundation, 3116
Artists Fellowship, 3117
Autism Summer Respite Program, 1268
AutismUp: YMCA Summer Social Skills Program, 1269
BRiDGES, 4440
Basic Facts on Study Abroad, 2767
Bath VA Medical Center, 5772
Bodman Foundation, 3118
Brain & Behavior Research Foundation, 786, 3119
Bronx Independent Living Services, 4441
Bronx VA Medical Center, 5773
Brooklyn Campus of the VA NY Harbor Healthcare System, 5774
Brooklyn Center for Independence of the Disabled, 4442
Brooklyn Home for Aged Men, 3120
Buffalo Regional Office - Department of Veterans Affairs, 5775
Buffalo State (SUNY), 2769
Burton Blatt Institute (BBI), 788
Camp Abilities Brockport, 1270
Camp Adventure, 1271
Camp Anne, 1272
Camp EAGR, 1274
Camp Good Days and Special Times, 1275
Camp High Hopes, 1276
Camp Huntington, 1277
Camp Kehilla, 1278
Camp Little Oak, 1279
Camp Mark Seven, 1280
Camp Pa-Qua-Tuck, 1281
Camp Ramapo, 1282
Camp Reece, 1283
Camp Sisol, 1284
Camp Tova, 1285
Camp Venture, Inc., 1286
Camp Whitman on Seneca Lake, 1287
Canandiagua VA Medical Center, 5776
Cancer Care, 3121
Canine Helpers for the Handicapped, 793
Capital District Center for Independence, 4443
Castle Point Campus of the VA Hudson Valley Healthcare System, 5777
Catskill Center for Independence, 4444
Center for Community Alternatives, 4445
Center for Independence of the Disabled of New York, 4446
Center for Independence of the Disabled of New York, 4447
Center on Human Policy: School of Education, 4955
Cerebral Palsy Foundation (CPF), 799
Children's Tumor Foundation, 3122
Clover Patch Camp, 1288
Commonwealth Fund, 3123
Community Foundation for Greater Buffalo, 3124
Community Foundation of Herkimer & Oneida Counties, 3125
Community Foundation of the Capitol Region, 3126
Comsearch: Broad Topics, 3127
DD Center/St Lukes: Roosevelt Hospital Center, 4448
DE French Foundation, 3128
Dana Foundation, 3129
David J Green Foundation, 3130
Disability Rights Bar Association (DBRA), 817
Disabled In Action (DIA), 826
Disabled and Alone: Life Services for the Handicapped, Inc., 828
Double H Ranch, 1289
Easterseals New York, 3131
Edna McConnel Clark Foundation, 3132
Edward John Noble Foundation, 3133
Ehrman Medical Library, 4957
Employer Assistance and Resource Network on Disability Inclusion (EARN), 833
Epilepsy Foundation of Long Island, 3134
Episcopal Charities, 3135
Esther A & Joseph Klingenstein Fund, 3136
FC Search, 3357
Fay J Lindner Foundation, 3137
Fedcap Rehabilitation Services, 840
Finger Lakes Developmental Disabilities Service Office, 4958
Finger Lakes Independence Center, 4449
Flying Manes Therapeutic Riding, Inc., 844
Ford Foundation, 3138
Fortis Foundation, 3139
Foundation 1000, 3366
Foundation Center, 3140
Foundation Center Library Services, 3141
Foundation Directories, 3367
Foundation Grants to Individuals, 3368
Foundation for Advancement in Cancer Therapy, 3142
Freedom from Fear, 845
Friendship Circle Day Camp, 1290
Gebbie Foundation, 3143
Gladys Brooks Foundation, 3144
Glickenhaus Foundation, 3145
Gow School Summer Programs, 1291
Grant Guides, 3370
Guide Dog Foundation for the Blind, 3146
Guide to Funding for International and Foreign Programs, 3371
Guide to US Foundations their Trustees, Officers and Donors, 3372
Harlem Independent Living Center, 4450
Hearing Health Foundation (HHF), 854, 3147
Hearst Foundations, 3148
Helen Keller International, 4959
Helen Keller National Center for Deaf - Blind Youths And Adults, 4960
Henry and Lucy Moses Fund, 3149
Herman Goldman Foundation, 3150
IBM Corporation, 2934
Independent Living, 4089, 4451
Institute for Basic Research in Developmental Disabilities, 4961
Institute for Visual Sciences, 4962
International Christian Youth Exchange, 2774
International Women's Health Coalition (IWHC), 871
JDRF, 873
JGB Cassette Library International, 4963
John Edward Fowler Memorial Foundation, 2905
John H and Ethel G Nobel Charitable Trust, 2893
Kamp Kiwanis, 1292
Katy Isaacson Elaine Gordon Lodge, 1293
Kenneth & Evelyn Lipper Foundation, 3151
Learning Disabilities Association of New York State (LDANYS), 879
Lisa Beth Gerstman Camp, 1294
Long Island Alzheimer's Foundation, 3152
Long Island Center for Independent Living, 4452
Louis and Anne Abrons Foundation, 3153
Maplebrook School, 1295
Margaret L Wendt Foundation, 3154
Marist Brothers Mid-Hudson Valley Camp, 1296
Massena Independent Living Center, 4453
Merrill Lynch & Company Foundation, 3155
Metzger-Price Fund, 3156
Milbank Foundation for Rehabilitation, 3157
Morgan Stanley Foundation, 3158
Mosholu Day Camp, 1297
NASW-NYS Chapter, 1912
NYS Independent Living Council, 4454
Nassau County Office for the Physically Challenged, 4455
Nassau Library System, 4964
National Association for the Dually Diagno sed Conferences, 1914
National Braille Association, 4965
National Business & Disability Council, 6154
National Business & Disability Council (NBDC), 894
National Center on Deaf-Blindness (NCDB), 899
National Directory of Corporate Giving, 3376
National Foundation for Facial Reconstruction, 3159
National Hemophilia Foundation, 3160
National Organization on Disability (NOD), 909
Neisloss Family Foundation, 3161
New York City Campus of the VA NY Harbor Healthcare System, 5778
New York Community Trust, 3162
New York Foundation, 3163
New York Regional Office, 5779
New York State Department of Labor, 6155
New York State Talking Book & Braille Library, 4966
North Country Center for Independent Livin g, 4456
Northern New York Community Foundation, 3164
Northern Regional Center for Independent Living: Watertown, 4457
Northern Regional Center for Independent L iving: Lowville, 4458
Northport VA Medical Center, 5780
Northwest Limousine Service, 5626
Not Dead Yet, 916
Options for Independence: Auburn, 4459
PWSA (USA) Conference, 1917
Parkinson's Disease Foundation, 2973, 3165
Peter and Elizabeth C. Tower Foundation, 925, 3166
Postgraduate Center for Mental Health, 4967
Putnam Independent Living Services, 4460
Reader's Digest Foundation, 3167
Regional Center for Independent Living, 4461
Rehabilitation International, 931
Rehabilitation International World Congress, 1920
Rehabilitation Research Library, 4968
Research to Prevent Blindness, 3168
Resource Center for Accessible Living, 4462
Resource Center for Independent Living, 4232, 4463
Resource Center for Independent Living, In c. (RCIL), 4233
Rita J and Stanley H Kaplan Foundation, 3169
Robert Sterling Clark Foundation, 3170
Skadden Fellowship Foundation, 3171
Southampton Fresh Air Home, 1298
Southern Adirondack Independent Living, 4464
Southern Adirondack Independent Living Cen ter, 4465
Southern Tier Independence Center, 4466
Southwestern Independent Living Center, 4467
Special Services Summer Day Camp, 1299
St George's Society of New York, 3172
Stanley W Metcalf Foundation, 3173
Starbridge, 940
State University of New York, 2787
State University of New York Health Sciences Center, 4969
Staten Island Center for Independent Living, Inc., 4468
Stonewall Community Foundation, 3174
Suffolk Cooperative Library System: Long Island Talking Book Library, 4970
Suffolk Independent Living Organization (SILO), 4469
Summit Camp, 1300
Sunshine Campus, 1301
Surdna Foundation, 3175
Syracuse VA Medical Center, 5781
Taconic Resources for Independence, 4470
The Adaptive Sports Foundation, 3176
The Davis Center, 945
Therapeutic Touch International Association (TTIA), 949
Tisch Foundation, 3177
Torah Alliance of Families of Kids with Disabilities, 5782
Tourette Association of America National E ducation Conference, 1922
United Spinal Association, 4971
VA Hudson Valley Health Care System, 5783
VA Western NY Healthcare System, Batavia, 5784
VA Western NY Healthcare System, Buffalo, 5785
VISIONS Vacation Camp for the Blind (VCB), 1302

Van Ameringen Foundation, 3178
Wagon Road Camp, 1303
Wallace Memorial Library, 4972
West Hills Day Camp, 1304
Westchester Disabled on the Move, 4471
Westchester Independent Living Center, 4472
Western New York Foundation, 3180
William T Grant Foundation, 3181
Xavier Society for the Blind, 4973
YAI: National Institute for People with Disabilities, 962
YMCA Camp Chingachgook on Lake George, 1305

North Carolina

American Herbalists Guild (AHG), 759
Arc of North Carolina, 3182
Asheville VA Medical Center, 5786
Association on Higher Education & Disability (AHEAD), 781
Bob & Kay Timberlake Foundation, 3183
Camp Carefree, 1243, 1306
Camp Carolina Trails, 1307
Camp Dogwood, 1308
Camp New Hope, 1116, 1309
Camp Royall, 1310
Camp Sertoma, 1311
Camp Tekoa, 1312
Charlotte Vet Center, 5787
Children's Mental Health Network (CMHN), 804
Conference of the Association on Higher Education & Disability (AHEAD), 1904
Davidson College, Office of Study Abroad, 2771
Disability Awareness Network, 4473
Disability Rights & Resources, 4474
Division Of Workforce Solutions, 6156
Division of Vocational Rehabilitation Services (DVRS) Western Regional Office, 6157
Division of Vocational Rehabilitation Serv ices (DVRS), 6158
Duke Endowment, 3184
Durham VA Medical Center, 5788
Early Childhood Technical Assistance Center (ETCA), 830
Fayetteville VA Medical Center, 5648, 5789
First Union Foundation, 3185
Foundation for the Carolinas, 3186
Genova Diagnostics, 846, 4974
Grayson Foundation, 2932
Joy: A Shabazz Center for Independent Living, 4475
Kate B Reynolds Charitable Trust, 3187
LIFESPAN Incorporated, 6159
Live Independently Networking Center, 4476
Live Independently Networking Center: Hickory, 4477
Mary Reynolds Babcock Foundation, 3188
NCWorks Commission, 6160
National Center for College Students with Disabilities (NCCSD), 896
North Carolina Division of Services for the Blind, 6161
North Carolina Library for the Blind and Physically Handicapped, 4975
Older Americans Report, 3377
Pathways for the Future Center for Indepen dent Living, 4478
Pediatric Rheumatology Clinic, 4976
Rowan Vocational Opportunities, Inc. (RVO), 6162
Rutherford Vocational Workshop, 6163
SOAR Summer Adventures, 1313
Talisman Summer Camp, 1314
Transylvania Vocational Services (TVS), 6164
Triangle Community Foundation, 3189
United States Disabled Golf Association (USDGA), 951
University of North Carolina at Chapel Hill: Neuroscience Research Building, 4977
Victory Junction, 1315
WG Hefner VA Medical Center - Salisbury, 5790
Webster Enterprises of Jackson County, Inc., 6165
Western Alliance Center for Independent Living, 4479
Western Alliance for Independent Living, 4480
Winston-Salem Regional Office, 5791

North Dakota

Alex Stern Family Foundation, 3190
Arc of North Dakota, 3191
Camp Sioux, 1316
Dakota Center for Independent Living: Dickinson, 4481
Dakota Center for Independent Living: Bism arck, 4482
Fargo VA Medical Center, 5792
Fraser, 4483
Freedom Resource Center for Independent Li ving: Fargo, 4484
Job Service North Dakota, 6166
North Dakota Community Foundation, 3192
North Dakota Department of Labor, and Human Rights, 6167
North Dakota State Library Talking Book Services, 4978
North Dakota VA Regional Office - Fargo Regional Office, 5793
North Dakota Vocational Rehabilitation Agency, 6168
Resource Center for Independent Living: Minot, 4485

Ohio

Ability Center of Greater Toledo, 4486
Ability Center of Greater Toledo: Bryan, 4487
Access Center for Independent Living, 4488
Akron Community Foundation, 3193
Albert G and Olive H Schlink Foundation, 3194
American Society for the Alexander Technique (AmSAT), 765
Antioch College, 2764
Arc of Ohio, 3195
Bahmann Foundation, 3196
Bureau of Vocational Rehabilitation (BVR), 6169
Camp Arye, 1317
Camp Cheerful, 1318
Camp Christopher: SumFun Day Camp, 1319
Camp Echoing Hills, 1320
Camp Emanuel, 1321
Camp Hamwi, 1322
Camp Happiness, 1323
Camp Ho Mita Koda, 1324
Camp Ko-Man-She, 1326
Camp Korelitz, 1327
Camp Nuhop, 1328
Camp Oty'Okwa, 1329
Camp Paradise, 1330
Camp Quality Ohio, 1331
Camp Stepping Stone, 1332
Camp Tiponi, 1333
Case Western Reserve University, 4979
Case Western Reserve University Northeast Ohio Multipurpose Arthritis Center, 4980
Center for Independent Living Options, 4489
Chillicothe VA Medical Center, 5794
Cincinnati Children's Hospital Medical Center, 4981
Cincinnati VA Medical Center, 5795
Cleveland FES Center, 4982
Cleveland Foundation, 3197
Cleveland Public Library, 4983
Cleveland Regional Office, 5796
Columbus Foundation and Affiliated Organizations, 3198
Courageous Acres, 1334
Dayton VA Medical Center, 5797
Eleanora CU Alms Trust, 3199
Eva L And Joseph M Bruening Foundation, 3200
Fairfield Center for Disabilities and Cerebral Palsy, 4490
Flying Horse Farms, 1335
Fred & Lillian Deeks Memorial Foundation, 3201
GAR Foundation, 3202
George Gund Foundation, 3203
Greater Cincinnati Behavioral Health Services - Employment Services, 6170
Greater Cincinnati Foundation, 3204
HCR Manor Care Foundation, 3205
HWH Foundation, 3206
Harry C Moores Foundation, 3207
Helen Steiner Rice Foundation, 3208
Highbrook Lodge, 1336
Insight Horse Camp, 1337
Lake Erie College, 2777
Linking Employment, Abilities and Potentia l, 4491
Louis Stokes VA Medical Center - Wade Park Campus, 5798
Mid-Ohio Board for an Independent Living Environment (MOBILE), 4492
Nationwide Foundation, 3209
Nordson Corporate Giving Program, 3210
Ohio Regional Library for the Blind and Physically Handicapped, 4984
Ohio Statewide Independent Living Council, 4493
Parker-Hannifin Foundation, 3211
Recreation Unlimited: Day Camp, 1338
Recreation Unlimited: Residential Camp, 1339
Recreation Unlimited: Respite Weekend Camp, 1340
Recreation Unlimited: Specialty Camp, 1341
Rehabilitation Service of North Central Oh io, 4494
Reinberger Foundation, 3212
Robert Campeau Family Foundation, 3213
Rotary Camp, 1342
Samuel W Bell Home for Sightless, 4495
Services for Independent Living, 4382, 4496
Sisler McFawn Foundation, 3214
Society for Equal Access: Independent Living Center, 4497
St. Augustine Rainbow Camp, 1343
Stark Community Foundation, 3215
State Library of Ohio: Talking Book Program, 4985
Stepping Stones: Camp Allyn, 1344
Stocker Foundation, 3216
Toledo Community Foundation, 3217
United States Trager Association, 952
William J and Dorothy K O'Neill Foundation, 3218
YMCA Outdoor Center Campbell Gard, 1345
Youngstown Foundation, 3219

Oklahoma

Ability Resources, 4498
Anne and Henry Zarrow Foundation, 3220
Camp CANOE, 1346
Camp ClapHans, 1347
Camp Endres, 1348
Camp Lo-Be-Gon, 1349
Camp Loughridge, 1350
Camp Perfect Wings, 1351
Green County Independent Living Resource Center, 4499
Jack C. Montgomery VA Medical Center, 5799
Jack C. Montomery VA Medical Center, 5800
Office of Disability Concerns, 6171
Oklahoma City VA Medical Center, 5801
Oklahoma Department of Rehabilitation Services, 6172
Oklahoma Employment Security Commission (OESC), 6173
Oklahoma Library for the Blind & Physically Handicapped, 4986
Oklahoma Medical Research Foundation, 4987
Oklahoma Veterans Centers Vet Center, 5802
Oklahomans for Independent Living, 4500
Progressive Independence, 4501
Sarkeys Foundation, 3221
Tulsa City-County Library System: Outreach Services, 4988

Oregon

A Guide to International Educational Exchange, 2760
Abilitree, 4502
Adventures Without Limits, 1352
Arc of Oregon, 3222
B'nai B'rith Camp: Kehila Program, 1353
Building Bridges: Including People with Disabilities in International Programs, 2770
Bureau of Labor and Industries (BOLI), 6174
Cambia Health Foundation, 790, 3223
Camp Magruder, 1354
Camp Meadowood Springs, 1355
Camp Millennium, 1356
Camp Starlight, 1357
Camp Taloali, 1358
Camp Ukandu, 1359
Creating Memories, 1360
Eastern Oregon Center for Independent Living, 4503
Easterseals Oregon Summer Camp, 1361
Gales Creek Diabetes Camp, 1362
HASL Independent Abilities Center, 4504
Hull Park and Retreat Center, 1363
IPSL Institute of Global Learning, 2773
Independent Living Resources, 4505
Jackson Foundation, 3225
Lane Community College, 2778
Laurel Hill Center, 4506
Leslie G Ehmann Trust, 3226
MindFreedom International (MFI), 886
Mt Hood Kiwanis Camp, 1364
National University of Natural Medicine (NUNM), 911
Opportunities Foundation of Central Oregon, 6175
Oregon Commission for the Blind, 6176
Oregon Department of Human Services Vocational Rehabilitation (DHS VR), 6177
Oregon Health Sciences University, 5803
Oregon Health Sciences University, Elks' Children's Eye Clinic, 4989
Oregon Talking Book & Braille Services, 4990
Portland Regional Office, 5804
Portland VA Medical Center, 5805
Postpartum Support International (PSI), 927
Progressive Options, 4507
Roseburg VA Medical Center, 5806
SPOKES Unlimited, 4508
Southern Oregon Rehabilitation Center & Cl inics, 5807
Strength for the Journey, 1365
Sundial Special Vacations, 5618
Suttle Lake Camp, 1366
Swindells Charitable Foundation Trust, 2895
Talking Book & Braille Services Oregon State Library, 4991
Trips Inc., 5620
Umpqua Valley Disabilities Network, 4509
University of Oregon, 2789
Upward Bound Camp, 1367
World of Options, 2792

Pennsylvania

Abilities in Motion, 4510
Accessible Journeys, 5606
Aces Adventure Weekend, 1368
Air Products Foundation, 3227
American Disabled for Attendant Programs Today (ADAPT), 757
American Organization for Bodywork Therapies of Asia (AOBTA), 762
Anthracite Region Center for Independent Living, 4511
Arc of Pennsylvania, 3228
Arcadia Foundation, 3229
Associated Services for the Blind and Visu ally Impaired, 4992
Beaver College, 2768
Brachial Plexus Palsy Foundation, 3230
Brian's House, 4512
Butler VA Medical Center, 5808
Camp AIM, 1369
Camp Achieva, 1370
Camp Akeela, 1371
Camp Amp, 1372
Camp Can Do, 1373
Camp Freedom, 1376
Camp Hot-to-Clot, 1377
Camp Lee Mar, 1378
Camp Lily Lehigh Valley, 1379
Camp Orchard Hill, 1380
Camp Ramah in the Poconos, 1381
Camp STAR, 1382
Camp Setebaid, 1383
Camp Spencer Superstars, 1384
Camp Victory, 1385
Camp Wesley Woods: Exceptional Persons Camp, 1386
Camp Woodlands, 1387
Carnegie Library of Pittsburgh Library for the Blind & Physically Handicapped, 4993
Coatesville VA Medical Center, 5809
Columbia Gas of Pennsylvania Corporate Giv ing, 3231
Community Resources for Independence, 4513
Community Resources for Independence, Inc., Bradford, 4514
Community Resources for Independence: Lewistown, 4515
Community Resources for Independence: Alto ona, 4516
Community Resources for Independence: Clar ion, 4517
Community Resources for Independence: Clea rfield, 4518
Community Resources for Independence: Herm itage, 4519
Community Resources for Independence: Lewi sburg, 4520
Community Resources for Independence: Oil City, 4521
Community Resources for Independence: Warr en, 4522
Community Resources for Independence: Well sboro, 4523
Connelly Foundation, 3232
Dolfinger-McMahon Foundation, 3233
Dragonfly Forest Summer Camp, 1388
Elwyn, 832
Erie VA Medical Center, 5810
Free Library of Philadelphia: Library for the Blind and Physically Handicapped, 4994
Freedom Valley Disability Center, 4524
Handi Camp, 1389
Heinz Endowments, 3234
Henry L Hillman Foundation, 3235
Innabah Camps, 1390
Institute on Disabilities At Temple Univ., 4525
International University Partnerships, 2776
James E Van Zandt VA Medical Center, 5811
Jewish Healthcare Foundation of Pittsburgh, 3236
Juliet L Hillman Simonds Foundation, 3237
Learning Disabilities Association of Ameri ca (LDA), 878
Lebanon VA Medical Center, 5812
Lehigh Valley Center for Independent Living, 4526
Liberty Resources, 4527
Life and Independence for Today, 4528
Mainstay Life Services Summer Program, 1391
Northeastern Pennsylvania Center for Independent Living, 4529
Oberkotter Foundation, 3238
Office of Vocational Rehabilitation (OVR), 6178
Outside In School Of Experiential Education, Inc., 1392
PECO Energy Company Contributions Program, 3239
PNC Bank Foundation, 3240
Pennsylvania College of Optometry Eye Institute, 4995
Pennsylvania Department of Labor and Industry (DLI), 6179
Pennsylvania Governor's Cabinet Committee for People With Disabilities, 6180
Pennsylvania Human Relations Commission Agency, 6181
Pennsylvania Veterans Centers, 5813
Phelps School Academic Support Program, 1393
Philadelphia Foundation, 3241
Philadelphia Regional Office and Insurance Center, 5814
Philadelphia VA Medical Center, 5815
Pittsburgh Foundation, 3242
Pittsburgh Regional Office, 5816
Raising Deaf Kids, 930
Reading Rehabilitation Hospital, 4996
Sequanota Lutheran Conference Center and Camp, 1394
Shenango Valley Foundation, 3243
South Central Pennsylvania Center for Inde pendence Living, 4530
Staunton Farm Foundation, 3244
Stewart Huston Charitable Trust, 3245
Teleflex Foundation, 3246
The Guided Tour, Inc., 5619
Three Rivers Center for Independent Living: New Castle, 4531
Three Rivers Center for Independent Livi ng: Washington, 4532
Three Rivers Center for Independent Living, 4214, 4533
Tri-County Patriots for Independent Living, 4534
USX Foundation, 3247
VA Pittsburgh Healthcare System, University Drive Division, 5817
VA Pittsburgh Healthcare System, Highland Drive Division, 5818
Variety Club Camp and Developmental Center, 1395
Voices for Independence, 4535
West Penn Burn Camp, 1396
Wilkes-Barre VA Medical Center, 5819
William B Dietrich Foundation, 3248
William Talbott Hillman Foundation, 3249
William V and Catherine A McKinney Charitable Foundation, 3250
YMCA Camp Fitch, 1397

Rhode Island

Arc South County Chapter, 3251
Arc of Blackstone, 4536
Arc of Blackstone Valley, 3252
Arc of Northern Rhode Island, 3253
Camp Mauchatea, 1398
Camp Ruggles, 1399
Canonicus Camp & Conference Center, 1400
Champlin Foundations, 3254
CranstonArc, 3255
Down Syndrome Society of Rhode Island, 3256
Frank Olean Center, 3257
Franklin Court Assisted Living, 4537
Groden Network, 6182
Hasbro Children's Hospital Asthma Camp, 1401
Horace A Kimball and S Ella Kimball Foundation, 3258
IN-SIGHT Independent Living, 4538
James L. Maher Center, 3259
Ocean State Center for Independent Living, 4539
Office Of Library & Information Services for the Blind and Physically Handicapped, 4997
Office of Rehabilitation Services, 4540, 6183
PARI Independent Living Center, 4541
Providence Regional Office, 5820
Providence VA Medical Center, 5821
Rhode Island Arc, 3260
Rhode Island Foundation, 3261
Rhode Island Services for the Blind and Visually Impaired, 6184
Talking Books Plus, 4998
The Steve Fund, 948

South Carolina

Arc of South Carolina, 3262
Burnt Gin Camp, 1402
Camp Adam Fisher, 1403

Camp Courage, 1203, 1374, 1404, 1404
Camp Debbie Lou, 1405
Camp Luv-A-Lung, 1406
Camp Spearhead, 1407
Center for Disability Resources, 796, 3263
Colonial Life and Accident Insurance Company Contributions Program, 3264
Columbia Disability Action Center, 4542
Columbia Regional Office, 5822
DREAMMS for Kids, 4956
Disability Action Center, 4543
Disability Research and Dissemination Cent er, 816
Graham Street Community Resources, 4544
Medical University of South Carolina Arthritis Clinical/Research Center, 4999
Ralph H Johnson VA Medical Center, 5823
South Carolina Commission for the Blind (SCCB), 6185
South Carolina Department of Employment and Workforce (DEW), 6186
South Carolina Governor's Committee on Employment of the Handicapped, 6187
South Carolina Independent Living Council, 4545
South Carolina State Library, 5000
South Carolina Vocational Rehabilitation Department (SCVRD), 6188
Walton Options for Independent Living: Nor th Augusta, 4546
William Jennings Bryan Dorn VA Medical Center, 5824

South Dakota

Adjustment Training Center, 4547
Black Hills Workshop & Training Center, 4548
Camp Friendship, 1408
Camp Gilbert, 1409
Native American Advocacy Program for Perso ns with Disabilities, 4550
NeSoDak, 1410
Prairie Freedom Center for Independent Living: Sioux Falls, 4551
Prairie Freedom Center for Independent Li ving: Madison, 4552
Prairie Freedom Center for Independent Liv ing: Yankton, 4553
Royal C Johnson Veterans Memorial Medical Center, 5825
Sioux Falls Regional Office, 5826
South Dakota Assistive Technology Project: DakotaLink, 4554
South Dakota Department of Human Services, 6189
South Dakota Department of Human Services: Div. of Service to the Blind & Visually Impaired, 6190
South Dakota State Library, 5001
South Dakota State Vocational Rehabilitati on, 6191
South Dakota Workforce Investment Act Training Programs, 6192
Western Resources for dis-ABLED Independence, 4555

Tennessee

ACM Lifting Lives Music Camp, 1411
All Days Are Happy Days Summer Camp, 1412
Alvin C York VA Medical Center, 5827
American Board of Disability Analysts (ABDA), 747
American Board of Disability Analysts Annual Conference, 1894
American Board of Medical Psychotherapists and Psychodiagnosticians, 748
American Board of Professional Disability Consultants, 749
American Therapeutic Recreation Associatio n, 767
Arc of Anderson County, 3265
Arc of Davidson County, 3266
Arc of Hamilton County, 3267
Arc of Tennessee, 3268
Arc of Washington County, 3269
Arc of Williamson County, 3270
Arc-Diversified, 3271
Benwood Foundation, 3272
Bill Rice Ranch, 1413
Camp Conquest, 1414
Camp Joy, 1325, 1416
Camp Koinonia, 1417
Camp Oginali, 1418
Camp Okawehna, 1419
Camp Sugar Falls, 1420
Camp Wonder, 1421
Case Management Society of America (CMSA), 794
Center for Independent Living of Middle Tennessee, 4556
Community Foundation of Greater Chattanooga, 3273
DisAbility Resource Center: Knoxville, 4557
Easterseals Tennessee Camping Program, 1422
Education and Auditory Research Foundation, 3274
International Paper Company Foundation, 3275
Jackson Center for Independent Living, 4558
Jackson Independent Living Center, 4358
LeBonheur Cardiac Kids Camp, 1423
Memphis Center for Independent Living, 4559
Memphis VA Medical Center, 5828
Mountain Home VA Medical Center - James H Quillen VA Medical Center, 5829
Nasheville Regional Office, 5830
Nashville VA Medical Center, 5831
National Association of Blind Merchants (NABM), 889
Tennessee Department Human Services: Vocational Rehabilitation Services, 6193
Tennessee Department of Labor and Workforc e Development, 6194
Tennessee Human Rights Commission, 6195
Tennessee Library for the Blind and Physically Handicapped, 5002
Tennessee Technology Access Program (TTAP), 4560
Tri-State Resource and Advocacy Corporation, 4561
Vision Foundation, 3038

Texas

AADB National Conference, 1879
ABLE Center for Independent Living, 4562
Abell-Hangar Foundation, 3277
Ability Connection, 6196
Access & Information Network, 730
Albert & Bessie Mae Kronkosky Charitable Foundation, 3278
Amarillo VA Healthcare System, 5832
Amarillo Vet Center, 5833
American Botanical Council (ABC), 750
American Express Foundation, 3279
Arc of Texas, The, 3280
Army and Air Force Exchange Services, 2765
Attention Deficit Disorders Association, Southern Region: Annual Conference, 1898
Austin Resource Center for Independent Living, 4563
Austin Resource Center: Round Rock, 4564
Austin Resource Center: San Marcos, 4565
BA and Elinor Steinhagen Benevolent Trust, 3281
Baylor College of Medicine Birth Defects Center, 5003
Baylor College of Medicine: Cullen Eye Institute, 5004
Brazoria County Center For Independent Living, 4566
Brown Foundation, 3282
Brown-Heatly Library, 5005
CH Foundation, 3283
Camp Ailihpomeh, 1424
Camp Aranzazu, 1425
Camp Be An Angel, 1426
Camp Blessing, 1427
Camp CAMP, 1428
Camp CPals, 1429
Camp Can-Do, 1430
Camp John Marc, 1432
Camp Neuron, 1433
Camp New Horizons North, 1434
Camp New Horizons South, 1435
Camp No Limits Texas, 1436
Camp NoLoHi, 1437
Camp Quality Texas, 1438
Camp Rainbow, 991, 1439
Camp Sandcastle, 1440
Camp Spike 'n' Wave, 1441
Camp Summit, 1442
Camp Sweeney, 1443
Camp for All, 1444
Center for Research on Women with Disabilities, 5006
Centre, The, 4567
Charis Hills Camp, 1445
Christian Education for the Blind, 5007
Cockrell Foundation, 3284
Communication Service for the Deaf: Rapid City, 4549
Communities Foundation of Texas, 3285
Community Foundation of North Texas, 3286
Concentra, 6197
Cristo Vive International: Texas Camp Conr oe, 1446
Cristo Vive International: Texas Camp Rio Grande Valley, 1447
Crockett Resource Center for Independent Living, 4568
Cullen Foundation, 3287
Curtis & Doris K Hankamer Foundation, 3288
Dallas Academy, 1448
Dallas Foundation, 3289
David D & Nona S Payne Foundation, 3290
Easy Access Travel, 5612
El Paso Natural Gas Foundation, 3291
El Paso VA Healthcare Center, 5834
Epilepsy Foundation of Southeast Texas, 3292
Epilepsy Foundation: Central and South Texas, 3293
Hanger, Inc., 852
Harris and Eliza Kempner Fund, 3294
Hill School of Fort Worth, 1449
Hillcrest Foundation, 3295
Hoblitzelle Foundation, 3296
Hogg Foundation for Mental Health, 856, 3297
Houston Center for Independent Living (HCIL), 4569
Houston Endowment, 3298
Houston Public Library: Access Center, 5008
Houston Regional Office, 5835
Independent Living Research Utilization Project, 4571
International League Against Epilepsy (ILAE), 869
John G & Marie Stella Kennedy Memorial Foundation, 3299
John S Dunn Research Foundation, 3300
Kamp Kaleidoscope, 1450
LIFE/ Run Centers for Independent Living, 4572
LIFE: Fort Hall, 4147
Lisle, 2780
Lola Wright Foundation, 3301
Meadows Foundation, 3302
Michael E. Debakey VA Medical Center, 5836
Moody Foundation, 3303
NADR Conference, 1911
National Association of Disability Represe ntatives (NADR), 892
Office for Students with Disabilities, University of Texas at Arlington, 4573
Palestine Resource Center for Independent Living, 4574
Panhandle Action Center for Independent Living Skills, 4575
Pearle Vision Foundation, 3304
REACH of Dallas Resource Center on Independent Living, 4576
REACH of Denton Resource Center on Independent Living, 4577
REACH of Fort Worth Resource Center on Ind ependent Living, 4578

RISE-Resource: Information, Support and Empowerment, 4579
SAILS, 4580
San Antonio Area Foundation, 3305
Shell Oil Company Foundation, 3306
South Texas Charitable Foundation, 3307
South Texas Veterans Healthcare System, 5837
Sterling-Turner Foundation, 3308
TLL Temple Foundation, 3309
Talking Book Program/Texas State Library, 5009
Texas Department of Assistive and Rehabili tative Services, 4581
Texas Lions Camp, 1451
Texas Workforce Commission (TWC), 6198
Texas Workforce Commission: Vocational Rehabilitation Services, 6199
University of Texas Southwestern Medical Center/Allergy & Immunology, 5010
University of Texas at Austin Library, 5011
VA North Texas Health Veterans Affairs Car e System: Dallas VA Medical Center, 5838
VOLAR Center for Independent Living, 4582
Valley Association for Independent Living (VAIL), 4583
Valley Association for Independent Living: Harlingen, 4584
Waco Regional Office, 5839
West Texas VA Healthcare System, 5840
William Stamps Farish Fund, 3310
World Federation for Mental Health, 960

Utah

Action X-Treme Camp, 1452
Active Re-Entry, 4585
Active Re-Entry: Vernal, 4586
Camp Giddy-Up, 1453
Camp Hobe, 1454
Camp ICANDO, 1455
Camp Kostopulos, 1456
Camp Nah-Nah-Mah, 1457
Central Utah Independent Living Center, 4587
Discovery Camp, 1458
FCYD Camp Utada, 1459
Kids Rock The World Day Camp, 1460
Marriner S Eccles Foundation, 3312
National Care Planning Council, 895
OPTIONS for Independence, 4588
OPTIONS for Independence: Brigham Satellit e, 4589
Overnight Camps, 1461
Pathfinders Camp, 1462
Questar Corporation Contributions Program, 3313
Red Rock Center for Independence, 4590
Utah Assistive Technology Program (UTAP) Utah State University, 4592
Utah Department of Human Services: Division of Services for People with Disabilities, 6200
Utah Division of Veterans Affairs, 5841
Utah Employment Services, 6201
Utah Governor's Committee on Employment for People with Disabilities (GCEPD), 6202
Utah Independent Living Center, 4593
Utah Independent Living Center: Minersville, 4594
Utah Independent Living Center: Tooele, 4595
Utah State Library Division: Program for the Blind and Disabled, 5012
Utah State Office for Rehabilitation (USOR), 6203
Utah State Office of Rehabilition: Vocational Rehabilitation, 6204
Utah State Office of Rehabilition: Service s for the Blind and Visually Impaired, 6205
VA Salt Lake City Healthcare System, 5842
Veterans Support Center (VSC), 6206

Vermont

Camp Thorpe, 1463
National Center for PTSD, 5013
Silver Towers Camp, 1464
Vermont Assistive Technology Program, 4596
Vermont Center for Independent Living: Ben nington, 4597
Vermont Center for Independent Living: Chi ttenden, 4598
Vermont Center for Independent Living: Mon tpelier, 4599
Vermont Community Foundation, 3314
Vermont Department of Disabilities, Aging and Independent Living (DAIL), 6207
Vermont Department of Labor, 6208
Vermont Department of Libraries - Special Services Unit, 5014
Vermont Department of Libraries -Special Services Unit, 5015
Vermont Division of Vocational Rehabilitat ion, 6209
Vermont VA Regional Office Center, 5843
Vermont Veterans Centers, 5844

Virginia

ACA Annual Conference, 1882
ADA Annual Scientific Sessions, 1883
AER Annual International Conference, 1884
ASIA Annual Scientific Meeting, 1888
Access Independence, 4600
Access Services, 5016
Alexandria Library Talking Book Service, 5017
American Academy of Audiology (AAA), 736
American Academy of Audiology Conference, 1892
American Chiropractic Association (ACA), 752
American Counseling Association (ACA), 755
American National Bank and Trust Company, 2946
Appalachian Independence Center, 4601
Arc of Virginia, 3315
Arlington County Department of Libraries, 5018
Beacon Tree Foundation, 783, 3316
Blinded Veterans Association National Convention, 1900
Blue Ridge Independent Living Center, 4602
Blue Ridge Independent Living Center: Christianburg, 4603
Blue Ridge Independent Living Center: Low Moor, 4604
Braille Circulating Library for the Blind, 5019
Brain Injury Association of America (BIAA), 787
Camp Dickenson, 1466
Camp Easterseals UCP, 1467
Camp Foundation, 3317
Camp Holiday Trails, 1468
Camp Jordan, 1469
Camp Loud And Clear, 1470
Campagna Center, 6210
Camps for Children & Teens with Diabetes, 1471
Central Rappahannock Regional Library, 5020
Civitan Acres, 1472
Clinch Independent Living Services, 4605
Community Foundation of Richmond & Central Virginia, 3318
Council for Exceptional Children (CEC), 809, 5021
Council for Exceptional Children Annual Convention and Expo, 1905
Didlake, 6211
Disability Funders Network (DFN), 815
Disability Resource Center, 4114, 4606
Disability:IN, 821
ENDependence Center of Northern Virginia, 4607
Equal Access Center for Independence, 4608
From the State Capitals: Public Health, 3369
Hampton VA Medical Center, 5845
Hunter Holmes McGuire VA Medical Center, 5846
Independence Empowerment Center, 4609
Independence Resource Center, 4610
Independent Living Center Network: Department of the Visually Handicapped, 4611
International Chiropractors Association (ICA), 866
International Student Exchange Programs (I SEP), 2775
James Branch Cabell Library, 5022
John Randolph Foundation, 3319
Junction Center for Independent Living, 4612
Junction Center for Independent Living: Du ffield, 4613
Loudoun County Adaptive Recreation Camps, 1473
Lynchburg Area Center for Independent Living, 4614
March of Dimes, 883
Mental Health America (MHA), 885
NEXT Conference & Exposition, 1913
National Association of State Directors of Developmental Disabilities Services (NASDDDS), 893
National Council on the Aging Conference, 1915
National Rehabilitation Association (NRA), 910
National Right to Work Legal Defense Foundation, 3320
National Vaccine Information Center (NVIC), 912
Newport News Public Library System, 5023
Norfolk Foundation, 3321
Northern Virginia Resource Center for Deaf and Hard of Hearing Persons, 5024
Oakland School & Camp, 1474
Peidmont Independent Living Center, 4615
Peninsula Center for Independent Living, 4616
Piedmont Independent Living Center, 4617
RESNA Annual Conference, 1919
Resources for Independent Living, 4055, 4618
Richmond Research Training Center (RRTC), 6212
Roanoke City Public Library System, 5025
Roanoke Regional Office, 5847
Robey W Estes Family Foundation, 3322
Salem VA Medical Center, 5848
ServiceSource Disability Resource Center, 6213
SourceAmerica, 6214
Staunton Public Library Talking Book Center, 5026
University of Virginia Health System General Clinical Research Group, 5027
Valley Associates for Independent Living (VAIL), 4619
Valley Associates for Independent Living: Lexington, 4620
Virginia Autism Resource Center, 5028
Virginia Beach Foundation, 3323
Virginia Beach Public Library Special Services Library, 5029
Virginia Chapter of the Arthtitis Foundation, 5030
Virginia Department for the Blind and Vision Impaired (DBVI), 6215
Virginia Department of Veterans Services, 5849
Virginia State Library for the Visually and Physically Handicapped, 5031
Volunteers of America (VOA), 956
Woodrow Wilson Rehabilitation Center Training Program, 4621

Washington

ADA National Network, 724
Alliance for People with Disabilities: Sea ttle, 4622
Alliance of People with Disabilities: Redmond, 4623
Arc of Washington State, 3324
Bastyr Center for Natural Health, 782
Ben B Cheney Foundation, 3325
Business Enterprise Program (BEP), 5899, 6216
Camp Beausite NW, 1475
Camp Goodtimes, 1476
Camp Killoqua, 1477
Camp Korey, 1478
Camp Sealth, 1479
Community Foundation of North Central Washington, 3326
Community Services for the Blind and Parti ally Sighted Store: Sight Connection, 4624
Department of Services for the Blind (DSB), 6217
Department of Social & Health Services: Division of Vocational Rehabilitation, 6218
Department of Social & Health Services: Developmental Disabilities Administration (DDA), 6219
DisAbility Resource Connection: Everett, 4625
Easterseals Camp Stand by Me, 1480
Glaser Progress Foundation, 3327
Greater Tacoma Community Foundation, 3328
Inland Northwest Community Foundation, 3329

Jonathan M Wainwright Memorial VA Medical Center, 5850
Kitsap Community Resources, 4626
Medina Foundation, 3330
Meridian Valley Clinical Laboratory, 5032
Norcliffe Foundation, 3331
Ophthalmic Research Laboratory Eye Institute/First Hill Campus, 5033
Prime Time, Inc., 1481
SL Start Washington, 6220
STIX Diabetes Programs, 1482
Seattle Regional Office, 5851
Spokane Center for Independent Living, 4627
Spokane VA Medical Center, 5852
Stewardship Foundation, 3332
Tacoma Area Coalition of Individuals with Disabilities, 4628
VA Puget Sound Health Care System, 5853
Washington Talking Book and Braille Library, 5034
Western Washington University, 2790
Weyerhaeuser Company Foundation, 3333
Wheelchair Getaways, 5628

West Virginia

Appalachian Center for Independent Living, 4629
Appalachian Center for Independent Living: Spencer, 4630
Arc Of West Virginia, The, 3334
Bernard McDonough Foundation, 3335
Cabell County Public Library/Talking Book Department/Subregional Library for the Blind, 5035
Division of Rehabilitation Services: Staff Library, 5036
High Technology Foundation, 855, 3336
Huntington Regional Office, 5854
Huntington VA Medical Center, 5855
Job Accommodation Network (JAN), 874
Kanawha County Public Library, 5037
Louis A Johnson VA Medical Center, 5856
Martinsburg VA Medical Center, 5857
Mountain State Center for Independent Living, 4631
Mountain State Center for Independent Living, 4632
Mountaineer Spina Bifida Camp, 1483
Northern West Virginia Center for Independent Living, 4633
Ohio County Public Library Services for the Blind and Physically Handicapped, 5038
Talking Book Department, Parkersburg and Wood County Public Library, 5039
US Department Veterans Affairs Beckley Vet Center, 5858
West Virginia Autism Training Center, 5040
West Virginia Division of Rehabilitation Services (DRS), 6221
West Virginia Library Commission, 5041
West Virginia School for the Blind Library, 5042
WorkForce West Virginia, 6222

Wisconsin

AACRC Annual Conference, 1878
Able Trek Tours, 5604
American Academy for Cerebral Palsy and Developmental Medicine Annual Conference, 1891
Arc of Dunn County, 3337
Arc of Eau Claire, 3338
Arc of Fox Cities, 3339
Arc of Racine County, 3340
Arc of Wisconsin Disability Association, 3341
Arc-Dane County, 3342
Association of Children's Residential Centers (ACRC), 775
Association of Educational Therapists (AET), 776
Brown County Library, 5043
Camp Daypoint, 1484
Camp Kee-B-Waw, 1485
Camp Klotty Pine, 1486
Camp Needlepoint, 1487
Center for Independent Living of Western Wisconsin, 4634
Clement J Zablocki VA Medical Center, 5859
Department of Workforce Development: Vocational Rehabilitation, 6223
Easter Seal Camp Wawbeek, 1488
Eye Institute of the Medical College of Wisconsin and Froedtert Clinic, 5044
Faye McBeath Foundation, 3343
Helen Bader Foundation, 3344
Independence First, 4635
Independence First: West Bend, 4636
Inspiration Ministries, 4637
Johnson Controls Foundation, 3345
Lutherdale Bible Camp, 1489
Lynde and Harry Bradley Foundation, 3346
Mid-State Independent Living Consultants: Wausau, 4638
Mid-state Independent Living Consultants: Stevens Point, 4639
Milwaukee Foundation, 3347
North Country Independent Living, 4640
North Country Independent Living: Ashland, 4641
Northwestern Mutual Life Foundation, 3348
Options for Independent Living, 4642
Options for Independent Living: Fox Valley, 4643
Phantom Lake YMCA Camp, 1490
SB Waterman & E Blade Charitable Foundation, 3350
Society's Assets: Elkhorn, 4644
Society's Assets: Kenosha, 4645
Society's Assets: Racine, 4646
Timbertop Camp for Youth with Learning Dis abilities, 1491
Tomah VA Medical Center, 5860
William S Middleton Memorial VA Hospital Center, 5861
Wisconsin Badger Camp, 1492
Wisconsin Elks/Easterseals Respite Camp, 1493
Wisconsin Lions Camp, 1494
Wisconsin Regional Library for the Blind & Physically Handicapped, 5045
Wisconsin VA Regional Office, 5862

Wyoming

Arc of Natrona County, 3351
Camp Hope, 1495
Casper Vet Center, 5863
Cheyenne VA Medical Center, 5864
Department of Workforce Services: Vocational Rehabilitation, 6224
Eagle View Ranch, 1496
RENEW: Gillette, 4647
RENEW: Rehabilitation Enterprises of North Eastern Wyoming, 4648
Rehabilitation Enterprises of North Easter n Wyoming: Newcastle, 4649
Sheridan VA Medical Center, 5865
Wyoming Department of Workforce Services: Unemployment Insurance Division, 6225
Wyoming Services for Independent Living, 4650
Wyoming Services for the Visually Impaired, 5046
Wyoming State Rehabilitation Council (SRC), 6226
Wyoming's New Options in Technology (WYNOT) - University of Wyoming, 5047

A

A-Solution, 515
A4 Tech (USA) Corporation, 1657
AACRAO, 2257
AACRC Annual Conference, 1878
AADB E-News, 7818
AADB National Conference, 1879
AAIDD, 2249, 2274, 2275, 2315, 2317, 2318, 2328
AAIDD Annual Meeting, 1880
AAMHL, Inc., 8130
AAN's Toll-Free Hotline, 8885
AAO Annual Meeting, 1881
AARP, 7429, 2273, 7662, 7692, 7734
AARP Alabama, 7430
AARP Alaska, 7431
AARP Arizona, 7432
AARP Arkansas, 7433
AARP Bulletin, 7662
AARP California: Pasadena, 7434
AARP California: Sacramento, 7435
AARP Colorado, 7436
AARP Connecticut, 7437
AARP Delaware, 7438
AARP Florida: Doral, 7439
AARP Florida: St. Petersburg, 7440
AARP Florida: Tallahassee, 7441
AARP Fulfillment, 4704
AARP Fulfillment, 1947, 5189, 5220, 5306, 7634
AARP Georgia, 7442
AARP Hawaii, 7443
AARP Idaho, 7444
AARP Illinois: Chicago, 7445
AARP Illinois: Springfield, 7446
AARP Indiana, 7447
AARP Iowa, 7448
AARP Kansas, 7449
AARP Kentucky, 7450
AARP Louisiana: Baton Rouge, 7451
AARP Louisiana: New Orleans, 7452
AARP Magazine, 7663
AARP Maine, 7453
AARP Maryland, 7454
AARP Massachusetts, 7455
AARP Michigan, 7456
AARP Minnesota, 7457
AARP Mississippi, 7458
AARP Missouri, 7459
AARP Montana, 7460
AARP Nebraska: Lincoln, 7461
AARP Nebraska: Omaha, 7462
AARP Nevada, 7463
AARP New Hampshire, 7464
AARP New Jersey, 7465
AARP New Mexico, 7466
AARP New York: Albany, 7467
AARP New York: New York City, 7468
AARP New York: Rochester, 7469
AARP North Carolina, 7470
AARP North Dakota, 7471
AARP Ohio, 7472
AARP Oklahoma, 7473
AARP Oregon, 7474
AARP Pennsylvania: Harrisburg, 7475
AARP Pennsylvania: Philadelphia, 7476
AARP Rhode Island, 7477
AARP South Carolina, 7478
AARP South Dakota, 7479
AARP Tennessee, 7480
AARP Texas: Austin, 7481
AARP Texas: Dallas, 7482
AARP Texas: Houston, 7483
AARP Texas: San Antonio, 7484
AARP Utah, 7485
AARP Vermont, 7486
AARP Virginia, 7487
AARP Washington, 7488
AARP Washington DC, 7489
AARP West Virginia, 7490
AARP Wisconsin, 7491
AARP Wyoming, 7492
ABA Commission on Law and Aging, 7493
ABA Commission on Mental & Physical Disability Law, 4688, 4716
ABA Commission on Mental and Physical Disability, 2537
Abacus, 1658
Abbot and Dorothy H Stevens Foundation, 3023
ABC Mark of Merit Newsletter, 8116
ABC of Asthma, Allergies & Lupus, 8667
ABC-CLIO, 2501
Abell-Hangar Foundation, 3277
ABI Professional Publications, 8759
Abilitations, 2052
Abilitations - Speech Bin, 8288
Abilities Center of New Jersey, 6120
Abilities Expo, 1890
Abilities in Motion, 4510
Abilities of Florida: An Affiliate of Service Source, 5971
Abilities of Northwest New Jersey Inc., 6121
Abilities Without Boundaries, 5952
Abilities, Inc., 728
Abilitree, 4502
Ability 1st, 4096
Ability Center, 72, 537, 658, 4425
Ability Center of Greater Toledo, 1659, 4486
Ability Center of Greater Toledo: Bryan, 4487
Ability Connection, 6196
Ability Jobs, 5477
Ability Magazine, 5388, 5477
Ability Research, 1555
Ability Resources, 4498
AbilityFirst, 5910, 6548
AbilityWorks, 6098
Abingdon Press, 5358
ABLE Center for Independent Living, 4562
ABLE Industries, Inc., 5909
ABLE Program MCC-Longview, 2727
Able to Laugh, 5398
Able Trek Tours, 5604
Able Trust, 2911
Able Trust, The, 5972
AbleApparel - Affordable Adaptive Clothing and Accessories, 5478
AbleArts, 1
AbleData, 1607, 5479
AbleNet, Inc., 180, 198, 200, 256, 287, 309, 324, 326, 470, 471, 479, 504, 510, 1562, 1571, 1581, 1591, 1685, 1995, 2392, 5555, 5578
Ablex Publishing Corporation, 2629
About Children's Eyes, 9126
About Children's Vision: A Guide for Parents, 9127
About Special Kids, 6316
ABS Newsletter, 8416
Abstracts in Social Gerontology, 7667
ACA Annual Conference, 1882
Academic Language Therapy Association, 8910
Academic Press, Journals Division, 2293
Academic Software, 1558, 1579, 1592, 1732, 1745, 1766
Academic Software Inc, 1556
Academic Therapy Publications, 2145, 2396
Academic Therapy Publications / High Noon Books, 2145, 2161
Academy Eye Associates, 7068
Academy for Gerontology in Higher Education, 7505
Academy for Guided Imagery, 2728
Academy of Cognitive Therapy, 7832
Academy of Integrative Health & Medicine (AIHM), 729
Academy of Rehabilitative Audiology, 2073, 8294, 8315
Academy of Spinal Cord Injury Professionals, 8336
Academy of Spinal Cord Injury Professional s: Psychologists, Social Workers & Counselors, 8337
Academy of Spinal Cord Injury Professionals, 8337
Accelerator Shield, 73
Accelerator/Brake Foot Control, 74
Accelerator/Brake Hand Control, 75
Accent 1400, 173
Accent Books & Products, 1951, 5187, 5188, 5190, 5215, 5230, 5250, 5261, 5318
Accent on Living Magazine, 5100
Accent Special Publications, 1940
Accentcare, 6549
Access & Information Network, 730
Access Academics & Research, 9004
Access Alaska: ADA Partners Project, 3972
Access Alaska: Fairbanks, 3973
Access Alaska: Mat-Su, 3974
Access Audiology, 9005
Access Center for Independent Living, 4488
Access Center of San Diego, 3999
Access Control Systems: NHX Nurse Call System, 174
Access Currents, 1937
Access Design Services: CILs as Experts, 5101
Access Equals Opportunity, 1938
Access for 911 and Telephone Emergency Services, 5103
Access for All, 1939
Access for All: Integrating Deaf, Hard of Hearing and Hearing Preschoolers, 8212
Access II Independent Living Center, 4367
Access II Independent Living Centers, 7764
Access Independence, 4600
Access Living of Metropolitan Chicago, 4155
Access North Center for Independent Living of Northeastern MN, 4341
Access Pass, 5605
Access Schools, 9007
Access Services, 5016
Access SLP Health Care, 9006
Access to Art: A Museum Directory for Blind and Visually Impaired People, 9128
Access to Health Care, 2355
Access to Independence, 4000, 5102
Access To Independence Inc., 5102
Access to Independence of Cortland County , Inc., 4437
Access to Independence of Imperial Valley, 4001
Access to Independence of North County, 4002
Access To Recreation, 403, 613, 655
Access to Recreation, 403, 385
Access to Sailing, 8439
Access Unlimited, 5480
Access Utah Network, 3895
Access with Ease, 308
Access, Inc., 6044
Access-USA, 460, 576
Access-USA: Transcription Services, 461
Accessibility Lift, 335
Accessible Home of Your Own, 1940
Accessible Journeys, 5606
Accessible Space, Inc., 4342
Accessible Vans Of America, 5623
AccessText Network, 2146
Accreditation Commission for Acupuncture & Oriental Medicine, 731
Accreditation Commission for Midwifery Education (ACME), 732
ACE Fitness Matters, 7664
Ace Mobility, LLC, 70, 71, 74, 75, 78, 81, 97, 102, 119, 120, 121, 125, 131
Aces Adventure Weekend, 1368
ACES/ACCESS Inclusion Program, 6693
Achievement Centers For Children, 1318, 8558
Achievement House & NCI Affiliates, 5911
Achievement Products, 404
Achieving Diversity and Independence, 5104
Achilles Track Club, 8440
Acid Maltase Deficiency Association, 8338
ACL Regional Support Center: Region I, 7494
ACL Regional Support Center: Region II, 7495
ACL Regional Support Center: Region III, 7496
ACL Regional Support Center: Region IV, 7497
ACL Regional Support Center: Region IX, 7498
ACL Regional Support Center: Region V, 7499
ACL Regional Support Center: Region VI, 7500
ACL Regional Support Center: Region VII, 7501
ACL Regional Support Center: Region VIII, 7502
ACL Regional Support Center: Region X, 7503
ACM Lifting Lives Music Camp, 1411
ACNM Foundation, Inc., 3002
ACPOC News, 8854
Acrontech International, 1810
ACT Assessment Test Preparation Reference Manual, 1958
Acting Blind, 5399

Action Products, 225
Action Toward Independence: Middletown, 4438
Action Toward Independence: Monticello, 4439
Action X-Treme Camp, 1452
Active Citizenship and Disability: Impleme nting the Personalization of Support, 5070
Active Living Magazine, 8117
Active Re-Entry, 4585
Active Re-Entry: Vernal, 4586
Activities in Action, 7624
Activities with Developmentally Disabled Elderly and Older Adults, 7625
Activity-Based Approach to Early Intervention, 2nd Edition, 2356
Activity-Based Intervention: 2nd Edition, 5105
Ad Lib Drop-In Center: Consumer Management, Ownership and Empowerment, 5106
AD/HD and the College Student: The Everyth ing Guide to Your Most Urgent Questions, 2349
ADA and City Governments: Common Problems, 5095
ADA Annual Scientific Sessions, 1883
ADA Camp 180, 1264
ADA Camp Aspire, 1267
ADA Camp GranADA, 1108, 8534
ADA Camp Needlepoint, 8535
ADA Guide for Small Businesses, 5090
ADA In Details: Interpreting the 2010 Amer icans with Disabilities Act Stands, 4670
ADA Information Services, 5091
ADA Knowledge Translation Center, 724
ADA National Network, 724
ADA Pipeline, 5092
ADA Questions and Answers, 5093, 5476
Ada S. McKinley Community Services, Inc., 6006
ADA Tax Incentive Packet for Business, 5094
ADA Technical Assistance Program, 3521
ADA Teen Adventure Camp, 1109, 8536
ADA Triangle D Camp, 1110, 8537
ADA-TA: A Technical Assistance Update from the Department of Justice, 5096
Adam's Camp, 1043, 8539, 1044
Adam's Camp: Alaska, 980
Adam's Camp: Colorado, 1044
Adam's Camp: New England, 1241
Adams Media, 5053
Adaptable Housing: A Technical Manual for Implementing Adaptable Dwelling, 1941
Adaptations by Adrian, 1497
Adapted Physical Activity, 5286
Adapted Physical Activity Programs, 2246
Adapted Physical Activity Quarterly, 7668
Adapted Physical Education and Sport, 8385
Adapted Physical Education for Students with Autism, 2357
Adaptek Systems, 175
Adapting Early Childhood Curricula for Children with Special Needs (9th Edition), 2358
Adapting Instruction for the Mainstream: A Sequential Approach to Teaching, 2359
Adaptivation, 1557
Adaptive Baby Care, 5400
Adaptive Baby Care Equipment Video and Book Through the Looking Glass, 5401
Adaptive Clothing: Adults, 405, 1498
Adaptive Education Strategies Building on Diversity, 2360
Adaptive Environments Center, 1924
Adaptive Mainstreaming: A Primer for Teachers and Principals, 3rd Edition, 2658
Adaptive Services Division, 9290
Adaptive Sports Center, 8441, 8857
The Adaptive Sports Foundation, 3176
Adaptive Technology Catalog, 406
Adaptive Tracks, 8857
Adaptivemall.com, 1963
ADARA, 8290
ADD Challenge: A Practical Guide for Teachers, 2350
ADD Warehouse, 7980, 8084, 8093
ADD, Stepping Out of the Dark, 8073
ADD-SOI Center, The, 2651
ADD: Helping Your Child, 7947
Addictive & Mental Disorders Division, 3674
Addie McBryde Rehabilitation Center for the Blind, 7009
Addison Point Agency, 6062
Addison-Wesley Publishing Company, 5141
ADDitude Directory, 2123
Address Book, 577
ADEC Resources for Independence, 6027
Adelante Development Center, 6146
ADHD Book of Lists: A Practical Guide for Helping Children and Teens with ADDs, 7948
ADHD Coaching: A Guide for Mental Health P rofessionals, 2351
ADHD in Adults, 8074
ADHD in the Classroom: Strategies for Teachers, 2352
ADHD in the Schools: Assessment and Intervention Strategies, 2353, 7949
ADHD Report, 8055
ADHD with Comorbid Disorders: Clinical Assessment and Management, 7950
ADHD: What Can We Do?, 8075
ADHD: What Do We Know?, 8076
Adjustable Bath Seat, 133
Adjustable Chair, 205
Adjustable Clear Acrylic Tray, 206
Adjustable Folding Support Cane for the Blind, 589
Adjustable Incline Board, 336
Adjustable Raised Toilet Seat & Guard, 134
Adjustable Rigid Chair, 207
Adjustable Tee Stool, 208
Adjustable Wedge, 226
AdjustaCart, 516
Adjustment Training Center, 4547
Adlib, 4293
Administration Building D HS S Campus, 3487
Administration for Community Living, 2186, 908, 3379, 3381, 3399, 3404, 4794, 7494, 7495, 7496, 7497, 7498, 7499, 7500, 7501, 7502, 7503, 7593, 7612
Administration on Aging, 3379
Administration on Children, Youth and Families, 3380
Administration on Disabilities, 3381
Administrative Office, 1373, 8555
Adobe News, 5107
Adolescents and Adults with Learning Disab ilities and ADHD, 2361
Adolescents with Down Syndrome: Toward a More Fulfilling Life, 7951
Adolph Coors Foundation, 2874
ADRS Lakeshore, 5867
Adult Absorbent Briefs, 1499
Adult ADD: The Complete Handbook: Everyt hing You Need to Know About How to Cope with ADD, 7952
Adult Career and Continuing Ed Services - Vocational Rehabilitation (ACCESS-VR), 6153
Adult Day Training, 4097
Adult Lap Shoulder Bodysuit, 1500
Adult Leukemia: A Comprehensive Guide for Patients and Families, 8671
Adult Long Jumpsuit with Feet, 407
Adult Short Jumpsuit, 408, 1501
Adult Sleeveless Bodysuit, 1502
Adult Swim Diaper, 1503
Adult Tee Shoulder Bodysuit, 1504
Adult Waterproof Overpant, 1505
Adults & Children with Learning & Developm ental Disabilities (ACLD), 7833
Advance for Providers of Post-Acute Care, 2247
Advanced Breast Cancer: A Guide to Living with Metastic Disease, 8672
Advanced Language Tool Kit, 1964
Advanced Sign Language Vocabulary: A Resource Text for Educators, 8213
Advanced Sign Language Vocabulary: A Resource Text for Educators, 2362
Advances in Cardiac and Pulmonary Rehabilitation, 2363
Advantage Bag Company, 635
Advantage Wheelchair & Walker Bags, 635
Adventist HealthCare, 2729
Adventist Hinsdale Hospital, 8903
Adventure Day Camp, 8540
Adventure Learning Center at Eagle Village, 7895
Adventures in Musicland, 1713
Adventures Without Limits, 1352
The Advocacy Centre, 943
Advocacy Centre for the Elderly (ACE), 733
Advocacy Pulse, 8119
Advocacy Services of Alaska, 3435
Advocado Press, 4712, 7686
The Advocado Press, 5083
Advocate, 5108
Advocate Christ Hospital and Medical Center, 6805
Advocate Christ Medical Center & Advocate Hope Children's Hospital, 6806
Advocate Illinois Masonic Medical Center, 6807
Advocates for Better Living For Everyone (A.B.L.E.), 4215
Advocates for Children of New York (AFC), 734
Advocates for Developmental Disabilities, 735
AEPS Child Progress Record: For Children Ages Three to Six, 1959
AEPS Child Progress Report: For Children Ages Birth to Three, 2652
AEPS Curriculum for Birth to Three Years, 2354
AEPS Curriculum for Three to Six Years, 1960
AEPS Data Recording Forms: For Children Ages Birth to Three, 2653
AEPS Data Recording Forms: For Children Ages Three to Six, 1961
AEPS Family Interest Survey, 1962
AEPS Family Report: Birth to Three Years, 5284
AEPS Family Report: For Children Ages Birth to Three, 5097
AEPS Family Report: For Children Ages Three to Six, 5285
AEPS Measurement for Birth to Three Years, 2654
AEPS Measurement for Three to Six Years, 2655
AER Annual International Conference, 1884
AER Report, 7665
Aerie Experiences, 1088
Aerospace America, Inc., 538
Aerospace Compadre, 538
Aetna Foundation, 2882
AFB Center on Vision Loss, 3109
AFB Directory of Services for Blind and Visually Impaired Persons in the US and Canada, 9125
AFB News, 9288
AFB Press, 2144, 8249
African Americans in the Profession of Blindness Services, 9129
The AG Academy for Listening and Spoken Language, 2120
AG Bell Global Listening and Spoken Langua ge Symposium, 1885
Agassiz Village, 8541
Age Appropriate Puzzles, 5554
Age-Related Macular Degeneration, 9130
Agency for Healthcare Research and Quality, 2202
Agency of Human Services, 1656
Agency of Human Svcs Dept Disabilities, Aging & IL, 3916
Ages & Stages Questionnaires, 2659
Aging & Vision News, 7757
Aging and Developmental Disability: Current Research, Programming, and Practice, 7626
Aging and Disabilities, 3913
Aging and Disability Services, 3919, 7510
Aging and Disability Services Division, 3693
Aging and Disability: Crossing Network Lin es, 2365
Aging and Family Therapy: Practitioner Perspectives on Golden Pond, 7627
Aging and Rehabilitation II: The State of the Practice, 2366
Aging and Society, 7672
Aging and Vision: Declarations of Independence, 9339
Aging Brain, 2364
Aging in America, 7511
Aging in Stride, 7628
Aging in the Designed Environment, 7629
Aging International, 7669

Aging Life Care Association, 7506
Aging News Alert, 7670, 7758
Aging Research & Training News, 7671
Aging Services of Michigan, 7507
Aging Services of South Carolina, 7508
Aging Services of Washington, 7509
Aging with a Disability, 7630
AgingCare, 7512
Agnes M Lindsay Trust, 3088
AGRAM, 7756
AGS, 1982, 2008, 2034, 2050, 2065, 2682, 2683, 2684, 2686, 2694, 2696, 2697, 2698, 2715
AHC Media LLC, 8856
AHEAD, 2287
AHF Federation, 725
Ahmanson Foundation, 2809
AHRC New York City, 1272, 1293
A I Squared, 1679
AI Squared, 1677
Ai Squared, 1714, 5481
AID Bulletin, 8855
AIDS Alert, 8856
AIDS and Other Manifestations of HIV Infec tion, 8669
AIDS Healthcare Foundation, 726, 2808, 725
AIDS in the Twenty-First Century: Disease and Globalization, 8670
AIDS Sourcebook, 8668
AIDS Treatment Data Network, 2342
AIDS United, 8464
AIDS Vancouver, 727
AIDS: The Official Journal of the Internat ional AIDS Society, 8838
AIM Independent Living Center: Corning, 4431
AIM Independent Living Center: Elmira, 4432
AIMS Multimedia, 1691
Aiphone Corporation, 174
Air Products Foundation, 3227
AIR: Assessment of Interpersonal Relations, 2656
AJ Pappanikou Center, 2337, 2338
Akron Community Foundation, 3193
Alabama Council For Developmental Disabilities, 3413
Alabama Department of Education: Division of Special Education Services, 2178
Alabama Department of Public Health, 3414
Alabama Department of Rehabilitation Services, 3415, 6489
Alabama Department Of Rehabilitation Services, 5867, 5875, 5876, 5877, 5879, 5880, 5881, 5882, 5883, 5884, 5885, 5886
Alabama Department of Rehabilitation Services, 3971, 5878, 5887, 5888, 5889, 5890, 5891, 6493
Alabama Department of Senior Services, 3416
Alabama Disabilities Advocacy Program, 3417
Alabama Division of Rehabilitation and Crippled Children, 3418
Alabama Easter Seal Society, 8538
Alabama Goodwill Industries, 5868
Alabama Governor's Committee on Employment of Persons with Disabilities, 3419
Alabama Institute for Deaf & Blind, 8177
Alabama Institute for Deaf and Blind, 7829
Alabama Institute for Deaf and Blind Library and Resource Center, 4741
Alabama Power Foundation, 2794
Alabama Public Library Service, 4743
Alabama Radio Reading Service Network (ARRS), 4742
Alabama Regional Library for the Blind and Physically Handicapped, 4743
Alabama State Department of Human Resources, 3420
Alabama VA Benefits Regional Office - Montgomery, 5637
Alabama VA Medical Center - Birmingham, 5638
Alabama's Special Camp for Children and Adults, 965, 7901
Alamitos-Belmont Rehab Hospital, 7218
Alante, 539
Alaska Center for the Blind and Visually Impaired, 6510
Alaska Commission on Aging, 3427
Alaska Department of Education: Special Education, 2179
Alaska Department of Handicapped Children, 3428
Alaska Department of Labor & Workforce Development, 5895
Alaska Division of Vocational Rehabilitati on, 5894
Alaska Division of Vocational Rehabilitati on:, 3429
Alaska Job Center Network, 5895
Alaska SILC, 3975
Alaska State Commission for Human Rights, 5896
Alaska State Library Talking Book Center, 4748
Alaska VA Healthcare System - Anchorage, 5641
Albany County Department for Aging and Alb any Social Services, 3737
Albany VA Medical Center: Samuel S Stratton, 5770
Albany Vet Center, 5771
Albert & Bessie Mae Kronkosky Charitable Foundation, 3278
Albert Ellis Institute, 7834
Albert G and Olive H Schlink Foundation, 3194
ALDA, 7819
ALDA Newsletter, 7819
Aldercrest Health and Rehabilitation Center, 7401
Aldersgate Camp & Retreat Center, 1279
Aleda E Lutz VA Medical Center, 5731
Alert, 2308
Alex Stern Family Foundation, 3190
Alexander and Margaret Stewart Trust, 2898
Alexander Graham Bell Association, 1885, 1971, 1978, 1979, 2120, 2387, 2499, 2550, 2597, 5418, 8224, 8286, 8297
Alexander Graham Bell Association for the Deaf and Hard of Hearing, 8123
Alexandria Library Talking Book Service, 5017
Alexandria VA Medical Center, 5714
Alexian Brothers Medical Center, 6808
Alfred I DuPont Hospital for Children, 6707
Alfred I. duPont Hospital for Children, 4788
Alice Tweed Touhy Foundation, 2810
AliMed, 409
AliMed, Inc., 133, 141
Alimed, Inc., 409
Alinna Health, 6362
All About Attention Deficit Disorders, Revised, 7953
All About Attention Deficit Disorders, Rev ised, 5402
All About You: Appropriate Special Interactions and Self-Esteem, 1715
All Days Are Happy Days Summer Camp, 1412
All Garden State Physical Therapy, 7033
All Kinds of Minds, 1965
All Star Review, 1716
All Terrain Cane, 590
All-Turn-It Spinner, 5555
Allegheny Health Network, 1396
Allen County Public Library, 4846
Allen P & Josephine B Green Foundation, 3070
Allergies & Asthma: What Every Parent Need s To Know (2nd Edition), 8673
Allergies Sourcebook, 8674
Allergy & Asthma Network, 5349
Allergy & Asthma Network Mothers of Asthmatics, 8793, 8827, 8832
Allergy & Asthma Today, 5349
Allergy and Asthma Network Mothers of Asthmatics, 8885
Alliance Center for Independance, 4409
Alliance Center for Independence (ACI), 6122
Alliance for Aging Research, 7513
Alliance for Disabled in Action, 4409
Alliance for Parental Involvement in Education, 5335, 8010
Alliance for People with Disabilities: Sea ttle, 4622
Alliance for Retired Americans, 7514
Alliance House, 6917
Alliance of People with Disabilities: Redmond, 4623
Allied Community Services, 5953
Allied Services John Heinz Institute of Rehabilitation Medicine, 6409
Allied Services Rehabilitation Hospital, 6410
Allina Health, 2738
Allyn & Bacon, 1692, 2505, 2509, 2514, 2515, 2519, 2532, 2561, 2593, 2596, 2602, 2618, 2627, 2663, 2726
Allyn & Bacon Longman College Faculty, 2625
Aloha Nursing and Rehab Center, 7258
Aloha Special Technology Access Center, 1608
Alpha Home Royal Maid Association for the Blind, 4356
Alpha One: Bangar, 4280
Alpha One: South Portland, 4281
Alphabetic Phonics Curriculum, 2367
Alpine Alternatives, 981, 982, 8548
Alpine North Nursing and Rehabilitation Center, 7011
Alpine Nursing and Rehabilitation Center of Hershey, 7124
Alpine Ridge and Brandywood, 7150
ALS Association, 8421
ALST: Adolescent Language Screening Test, 2657
Alta Bates Medical Center, 4771
Altarfire Publishing, 8736
Alternating Hemiplegia of Childhood Foundation, 2811
Alternative Approach to Allergies, 8675
Alternative Educational Delivery Systems, 2368
Alternative Teaching Strategies, 2369
Alternative Work Concepts, 2074
Alternatives in Education for the Hearing Impaired (AEHI), 5482
Altimate Medical, 354
Altman Foundation, 3111
Aluminum Crutches, 607
Aluminum Kiddie Canes, 608
Aluminum Walking Canes, 609
AlumiRamp, 337
AlumiRamp, Inc., 337
Alumni News, 9291
Alvin C York VA Medical Center, 5827
Alzheimer Disease Sourcebook, 8676
Alzheimer Disease Sourcebook, 4th Edition, 8677
Alzheimer's Association, 2945
Alzheimer's Store, 636
Amarillo VA Healthcare System, 5832
Amarillo Vet Center, 5833
Ambrose Monell Foundation, 3112
AMC Cancer Research Center, 4778
AMDA - The Society for Post-Acute and Long-Term Care Medicine, 7504
Amer Assn of Spinal Cord Injury Psych & Soc Wks, 8874
Amer Board for Cert in Otthotics & Prosthetics, 8116
American Academy for Cerebral Palsy and Developmental Medicine, 1891, 8465
American Academy for Cerebral Palsy/Dev. Medicine, 8843
American Academy of Allergy, Asthma & Immu nology, 8466
American Academy of Audiology, 1892, 7657
American Academy of Audiology (AAA), 736, 5483, 8124
American Academy of Audiology Conference, 1892
American Academy of Child & Adolescent Psychiatry, 7835
American Academy of Dermatology, 1063, 1113, 1375, 1431
American Academy of Environmental Medicine (AAEM), 737
American Academy of Environmental Medicine Annual Conference, 1893
American Academy of Medical Acupuncture, 738
American Academy of Ophthalmology, 9026
American Academy Of Opthamology, 1881
American Academy of Osteopathy, 8339
American Academy of Otolaryngology - Head and Neck Surgery, 8467
American Academy of Pain Medicine, 740, 2912
American Academy of Pain Medicine (AAPM), 739
American Academy of Pain Medicine Foundati on, 740, 2912
American Academy of Pediatrics, 8673
American Academy of Pediatrics (AAP), 741

American Academy of Physical Medicine & Rehab, 5379
American Academy of Physical Medicine and Rehabilitation, 8468
American Action Fund for Blind Children and Adults, 9027
American Acupuncture Council, 742
American Advertising Dist of Northern Virginia, 2256
American Aging Association, 7515, 7717
American Airlines, 5588
American Alliance for Health, Phys. Ed. & Dance, 9182
American Amputee Foundation, 8098, 8117
American Anals of the Deaf Reference, 9131
American Annals of the Deaf, 8303
American Art Therapy Association, 5368
American Art Therapy Association (AATA), 2
American Assn on Intellecutal/Devel. Disabilities, 1880
American Assoc of Homes and Services for the Aging, 7774
American Assoc of Spinal Cord Injury Psych/Soc Wor, 8428
American Association for Geriatric Psychiatry, 7516
American Association for Respiratory Care, 8469
American Association of Acupuncture and Or iental Medicine (AAAOM), 743
American Association of Cardiovascular and Pulmonary Rehabilitation, 8470
American Association of Neuromuscular & El ectrodiagnostic Medicine, 8340
American Association of People with Disabilities (AAPD), 744, 5484, 8125
American Association of People with Disabilities, 5271
American Association of Retired Persons, 7517, 7663
American Association of the Deaf-Blind, 7791, 1879, 7815, 7818
American Association on Health and Disabiity, 2265
American Association on Health and Disabil ity (AAHD), 745
American Association on Intellectual and Developmental Disabilities (AAIDD), 746
American Back Society, 8341, 8416
American Bar Association, 4714, 4718, 4724
American Blind Bowling Association, 9355
American Board for Certification in Orthotics, Prosthetics & Pedorthics, 8099
American Board of Disability Analysts, 748, 749, 5375
American Board of Disability Analysts (ABDA), 747
American Board of Disability Analysts Annual Conference, 1894
American Board of Medical Psychotherapists and Psychodiagnosticians, 748
American Board of Professional Disability Consultants, 749
American Botanical Council, 2271, 2323
American Botanical Council (ABC), 750
American Brain Tumor Association, 8471
American Camp Association, 777
American Camp Association (ACA), 751
American Cancer Society, 8542, 8557
American Chai Trust, 3113
American Chemical Society, 5389
American Chiropractic Association (ACA), 752
American Cleft Palate-Craniofacial Association, 8842
American Cochlear Implant Alliance, 8126
American College of Advancement in Medicine (ACAM), 753
American College of Nurse Midwives, 732, 2283, 3002
American College of Nurse Midwives (ACNM), 754
American College of Rheumatology, Research and Education Foundation, 5485
American College Testing Program, 2660, 1958, 2493, 2704
American Council of Blind Lions, 9028
American Council of the Blind, 3, 9029, 9071, 9079, 9104, 9195, 9205, 9240, 9278, 9309, 9367
American Council of the Blind Radio Amateu rs, 9030
American Council on Exercise (ACE), 7664
American Counseling Association, 1882, 2260, 2262, 2277, 2279, 2310, 2449
American Counseling Association (ACA), 755, 2147
American Counselling Association, 2076
American Dance Therapy Association (ADTA), 4
American Delirium Society, 7836
American Diabetes Association, 8472, 984, 1108, 1109, 1110, 1130, 1146, 1147, 1149, 1193, 1243, 1264, 1267, 1307, 1316, 1327, 1349, 1374, 1376, 1420, 1434, 1435, 1437, 1439, 1440, 1455, 1471, 1484, 1487, 1883, 8534, 8536, 8537, 8556, 8563, 8564, 8569, 8581
American Disabled for Attendant Programs Today (ADAPT), 757
American Disabled for Attendant Programs T oday (ADAPT), 7518
American Disabled Golfers Association (ADGA), 756
American Discount Medical, 410, 410
American Express Foundation, 3279
American Falls Office: Living Independently for Everyone (LIFE), 4141
American Foundation Corporation, 2800
American Foundation for Suicide Prevention (AFSP), 758, 3114
American Foundation for the Blind, 3115, 9031, 2647, 3109, 9164, 9190, 9200, 9219, 9258
American Foundation for the Blind / AFB Press, 2144
American Foundation for the Blind/ AF B Press, 1637
American Foundation for the Blind/AFB Press, 7648, 7653, 7810, 7811, 9125, 9128, 9133, 9140, 9142, 9143, 9149, 9151, 9156, 9162, 9167, 9179, 9180, 9186, 9196, 9215, 9216, 9217, 9222, 9223, 9226, 9227, 9228, 9246, 9251, 9252, 9262, 9266, 9268, 9271, 9272, 9275, 9288, 9314, 9339, 9340, 9341, 9347, 9348, 9354
American Geriatrics Society, 7519
American Group Psychotherapy Association, 8473
American Head and Neck Society, 8474
American Health Assistance Foundation, 3003
American Health Care Association, 5380
American Hearing Impaired Hockey Associati on, 8333
American Hearing Research Foundation, 8316
American Heart Association, 8118
American Herb Association Newsletter, 5109
American Herbalists Guild (AHG), 759
American Horticultural Therapy Association, 7725
American Hotel and Lodging Association, 5589
American Hotel and Lodging Association Fou ndation, 2899
American Institute for Foreign Study, 2761
American Institute of Architects, 1925
American Journal of Audiology, 8291
American Journal of Geriatric Psychiatry, 7673
American Journal of Occupational Therapy (AJOT), 2248
American Journal of Orthopsychiatry, 8839
American Journal of Physical Medicine & Rehabilitation, 5365
American Journal of Psychiatry, 5366
American Journal of Public Health (AJPH), 5367
American Journal of Speech-Language Pathology, 9000
American Journal of Speech-Language Pathology, 7674
American Journal on Intellectual and Devel opmental Disabilities (AJIDD), 2249
American Legion Magazine, 7675
American Legion National Headquarters, 7675
American Liver Foundation, 5486
American Lung Association, 8475, 1089, 8554, 8877
American Lung Association In Alaska, 8616
American Lung Association of Oregon, 8559
American Massage Therapy Association, 7729
American Massage Therapy Association (AMTA), 760
American Medical Association, 5201, 8841
American Medical Industries, 261
American Medical Industries, Inc., 412
American Migraine Foundation, 2075, 3090
American Mobility: Personal Mobility Solutions, 5487
American Music Therapy Association (AMTA), 5
American National Bank and Trust Company, 2946
American Network of Community Options & Resource, 5206
American Network of Community Options & Resources, 5156
American Occupational Therapy Association, 2248, 5394
American Occupational Therapy Association (AOTA), 761
American Occupational Therapy Foundation, 3004
American Optometric Association, 9032, 9174
American Organization for Bodywork Therapies of Asia (AOBTA), 762
American Orthopsychiatric Association, 2302
American Orthotic & Prosthetic Association, 2330
American Orthotic & Prosthetics Association, 8849
American Parkinson Disease Association, 8342
American Physical Therapy Association, 8100, 1913
American Planning Association, 7520
American Printing House for the Blind, 9033, 7812, 7813, 7827, 7828
American Printing House for the Blind, Inc., 9033
American Psychiatric Association, 7837, 5366
American Psychological Association, 2261, 8839
American Public Health Association, 7521, 5367
American Public Health Association (APHA), 763
American Red Cross, 764
American Rehabilitation Services Administration (R, 7676, 7676
American School Counselor Association, 2076
American Sexual Health Association, 8477
American SIDS Institute, 8476
American Sign Language Handshape Dictionary, 8214
American Sign Language Handshape Cards, 1966
American Sign Language Phrase Book, 8215
American Sign Language: A Look at Its Hist ory, Structure & Community, 8216
American Social Health Association, 8493
American Society for Deaf Children, 7792, 8127, 7822, 8298
American Society for Neurochemistry, 7522
American Society for the Alexander Technique (AmSAT), 765
American Society of Clinical Hypnosis (ASCH), 766
American Society of Landscape Architects, 1926, 1952
American Society of Pediatric Hematology/O ncology, 8478
American Society on Aging, 7523, 7700
American Speech-Language and Hearing Association, 5488
American Speech-Language-Hearing Association, 8128, 8911
American Speech-Language-Hearing Association, 1887, 2012, 8291, 8293, 8302, 9000, 9001, 9004, 9005, 9006, 9007
American Speech-Language-Hearing Association (ASHA, 7674
American Spinal Injury Association, 8343, 1888, 8406
American Stroke Association, 8101, 8344, 8119, 8414
American Therapeutic Recreation Associatio n, 767
American Thermoform Corporation, 1597
American Thoracic Society, 8479
American Tinnitus Association, 8301
American Tinnitus Association (ATA), 768, 8129
American Universities International Programs, 2762
American Urogynecologic Society, 7524

American Volkssport Association (AVA), 7747
The American Wanderer, 7747
American Wheelchair Bowling Association, 8442, 8436
American-Scandinavian Foundation, 2763
Americans with Disabilities Act Information and Technical Assistance, 3382
Americans With Disabilities Act Annotated: Legislative History, Regulations & Commentary, 4671
Americans with Disabilities Act Checklist for New Lodging Facilities, 5110
Americans with Disabilities Act Guide for Places of Lodging: Serving Guests Who Are Blind, 9132
Americans with Disabilities Act Handbook, 5111
Americans with Disabilities Act Manual, 4672
Americans with Disabilities Act: ADA Home Page, 5489
Americans with Disabilities Act: Selected Resources for Deaf, 4673
Amerock Corporation, 2947
AMI, 260
Amigo Mobility International, 540, 372, 378, 540
Amigo Mobility International Inc., 541
Amity Lodge, 7151
Amplified Handsets, 176
Amplified Phones, 177
Amplified Portable Phone, 178
Amplify Life, 1238
Amputee Coalition, 769, 1075, 5387
Amtrak, 5590
Amyotrophic Lateral Sclerosis: A Guide for Patients and Families, 8678
Amytrophic Lateral Sclerosis Association, 8345
Anaheim Veterans Center, 6550
Analog Switch Pad, 1558
Andalusia Health Services, 2795
Anderson Woods, 1126
Andrew Heiskell Braille and Talking Book Library, 4954
Angel River Health and Rehabilitation, 7275
Anglo California Travel Service, 5607
Anheuser-Busch, 3071
Anixter Center, 6007
Ann Arbor Area Community Foundation, 3039
Ann Arbor Center for Independent Living, 4311
Annals of Dyslexia, 8051
Annals of Otology, Rhinology and Laryngolo gy, 8840
Annals Publishing Company, 8840
Annandale Village, 6785
Anne and Henry Zarrow Foundation, 3220
Annual Conference on Dyslexia and Related Learning Disabilities, 1895
Annual Report Sarkeys Foundation, 5113
Annual Report/Newsletter, 9292
Annual TASH Conference, 1896
Antecedent Control: Innovative Approaches to Behavioral Support, 2370
Anthesis, 5912
Anthony Brothers Manufacturing, 5556
Anthracite Region Center for Independent Living, 4511
Antioch College, 2764
Anxiety and Depression Association of Amer ica (ADAA), 770, 7838
Anxiety-Free Kids: An Interactive Guide for Parents and Children, 2371
APA Access, 2307
Aphasia Hope Foundation, 8912
Apira Healthcare Group, Inc., 6694
Aplastic Anemia and MDS International Foundation, 8480
Appalachian Center for Independent Living, 4629
Appalachian Center for Independent Living: Spencer, 4630
Appalachian Independence Center, 4601
Applied Kinesiology: Muscle Response in Diagnosis, Therapy and Preventive Medicine, 5114
Applied Rehabilitation Counseling (Springe r Series on Rehabilitation), 2372
Approaching Equality, 4674
Apria Healthcare, 411, 6694
Apria Healthcare Group, Inc., 411
APSE, 1886
APSE National Conference, 1886
APT Technology, 472
Aqua Massage International, 260
Aquarius Health Care Media, 5403, 7974, 7987, 8078, 8079, 8081, 8086, 8964, 9017
Aquarius Health Care Videos, 5171, 5334, 5440, 5441, 5442, 5444, 5447, 5448, 5457, 5460, 5462, 5466, 5468, 8089, 8431
Aquatic Access, 374
Arbors at Canton Subacute And Rehabilitation Center, 7352
Arbors at Dayton, 7353
Arbors at Marietta, 7354
Arbors at Milford, 7355
Arbors at New Castle, 7236
Arbors at Sylvania, 7356
Arbors at Toledo Subacute and Rehab Centre, 7357
Arbors East Subacute and Rehabilitation Center, 7351
The Arc, 1897
The Arc - Iberville, 6933
The Arc Caddo-Bossier, 6934
ARC Community Support Systems, 6833
Arc Connection Newsletter, 5115, 8056
The Arc Eastern Connecticut, 1064, 8571
ARC Fresno-Kelso Activity Center, 6540
ARC Gateway, 3505
The Arc Gloucester, 6144, 1257
Arc Light, 8057
The Arc Los Angeles and Orange Counties, 5937
Arc Massachusetts, 5108
Arc Michigan, 4312
Arc National Convention, The, 1897
Arc Northwest Indiana, 6028
Arc Of Alabama, The, 2796
Arc of Alaska, 2798
The Arc of Allen County, 2228
The Arc of Anchorage, 2798
Arc of Anderson County, 3265
Arc of Arizona, 8057
The Arc of Arizona, 2801
Arc of Arkansas, 2806
Arc of Bergen and Passaic Counties, 6123
Arc of Blackstone, 4536
Arc of Blackstone Valley, 3252
Arc of California, 2812
The Arc of Camden County, 6140
Arc of Cape Cod, 4294
Arc of Central Alabama, 5869
Arc of Colorado, 2875
Arc of Connecticut, 2883
Arc of Davidson County, 3266
Arc of Delaware, 2896, 3491
Arc of Dunn County, 3337
Arc of Eau Claire, 3338
Arc of Florida, 2913
Arc of Fox Cities, 3339
Arc Of Georgia, 2928
Arc of Hamilton County, 3267
Arc of Hawaii, 2939
ARC of Hunterdon County, The, 6117
Arc of Illinois, 2948
The Arc of Illinois, 6013
Arc of Indiana, 2983
Arc of Iowa, 2987
Arc of Kansas, 2992
Arc of Kentucky, 2995
Arc of Louisiana, 2996
Arc of Maryland, 3005
Arc of Massachusetts, The, 3024
ARC of Mercer County, 6118
Arc Of Meriden-Wallingford, Inc., 6695
Arc of Michigan, 3040
Arc of Minnesota, 3058
Arc of Mississippi, 3069
ARC of Monmouth, 6119
Arc of Natrona County, 3351
Arc of Nebraska, 3080
Arc of New Jersey, 3091
The Arc of New Jersey, 2223
Arc of New Mexico, 3105
Arc of North Carolina, 3182
The Arc of North Carolina, 7890
Arc of North Dakota, 3191
Arc of Northern Bristol County, 3025
Arc of Northern Rhode Island, 3253
Arc of Ohio, 3195
Arc of Oregon, 3222
Arc of Pennsylvania, 3228
Arc of Racine County, 3340
The Arc of San Diego, 1030, 7913
ARC Of San Diego-ARROW Center, The, 6541
ARC Of San Diego-East County Training Center, The, 6542
ARC Of San Diego-Rex Industries, The, 6543
ARC Of San-Diego-South Bay, 6544
Arc of South Carolina, 3262
ARC Of Southeast Los Angeles-Southeast Industries, 6545
Arc of Tennessee, 3268, 5115, 8056
Arc of Texas, The, 3280
Arc of the District of Columbia, 2900, 5098
The Arc of the East Bay, 6668
The Arc of the United States, 5545, 7891
Arc of the US Missouri Chapter, 3072
Arc of Utah, 3311
Arc of Virginia, 3315
Arc of Washington County, 3269
Arc of Washington State, 3324
Arc Of West Virginia, The, 3334
Arc of Williamson County, 3270
Arc of Wisconsin Disability Association, 3341
The Arc San Francisco, 5917
Arc South County Chapter, 3251
The Arc Tampa Bay, 6780
The Arc Westbank, 6060
ARC's Government Report, 5098
Arc-Dane County, 3342
Arc-Diversified, 3271
Arc/Muskegon, 4313
ARC: VC Community Connections West, 6546
ARC: VC Ventura, 6547
ARCA - Dakota County Technical College, 5099
ARCA Newsletter, 5099
Arcadia Foundation, 3229
Arcadia University, 2768
Architect Magazine, 1942
Archives of Neurology, 8841
Arctic Access, 3976
Arden Rehabilitation And Healthcare Center, 7187
Arden Rehabilitation and Healthcare Center, 7402
Ardence, 6382
Ardmore Developmental Center, 6070
Area Access, 338, 338
Area Agency on Aging of Southwest Arkansas, 7777
Area Agency on Aging: Region One, 7778
Area Cooperative Educational Services (ACES), 5954
Arena Stage, 6, 7793
Argentum, 7525
ARISE, 4433
ARISE: Oneida, 4434
ARISE: Oswego, 4435
ARISE: Pulaski, 4436
Arista Surgical Supply Company, 607
Arista Surgical Supply Company/AliMed, 159, 612, 622, 695
Arizona State Department of Health Services, 2347
Arizona Autism Resources, 2801
Arizona Braille and Talking Book Library, 4749
Arizona Bridge to Independent Living, 3985, 5131
Arizona Bridge to Independent Living: Phoenix, 3986
Arizona Bridge to Independent Living: Mesa, 3987
Arizona Camp Sunrise, 8542
Arizona Camp Sunrise & Sidekicks, 983
Arizona Center for Disability Law, 3444
Arizona Center for the Blind and Visually Impaired, 6511
Arizona Center on Aging, 7526
Arizona Civil Rights Division, 5901
Arizona Community Foundation, 2802
Arizona Department of Economic Security, 3437, 5899, 5900
Arizona Department of Health Services, 3438, 2348, 2472

Arizona Developmental Disabilities Plannin g Council (ADDPC), 5897
Arizona Division of Aging and Adult Services, 3439
Arizona Hemophilia Association, 8481, 988, 989, 8570, 8578
Arizona Industries for the Blind, 6512
Arizona Instructional Resource Center for Students who are Blind or Visually Impaired, The, 2803
Arizona Rehabilitation State Services for the Blind and Visually Impaired, 3440
Arizona State Library, 4749
Arjo Inc, 210, 211, 376, 381, 382
ArjoHuntleigh, 135, 135, 147, 152
Arkansas Assistive Technology Projects, 3447
Arkansas Children's Neuroscience Center, 995
Arkansas Department of Special Education, 2180
Arkansas Department of Workforce Services, 5905
Arkansas Division of Aging & Adult Services, 3448
Arkansas Division of Developmental Disabilities Services, 3449
Arkansas Division of Services for the Blind, 3450
Arkansas Division of Services for the Blind, 5908
Arkansas Governor's Developmental Disabili ties Council, 3451
Arkansas Independent Living Council, 3993
Arkansas Lighthouse for the Blind, 6533
Arkansas Regional Library for the Blind and Physically Handicapped, 4757
Arkansas Rehabilitation Services (ARS), 5906
Arkansas School for the Blind, 4758
Arkenstone: The Benetech Initiative, 1559
Arlington County Department of Libraries, 5018
Arlington County Library, 5018
Arms Wide Open, 4125
Armstrong Medical, 412
Army and Air Force Exchange Services, 2765
Arnold A Schwartz Foundation, 3092
Arnold School of Public Health, USC, 816, 2086
Aromatherapy Book: Applications and Inhalations, 5116
Aromatherapy for Common Ailments, 5117
Around the Clock: Parenting the Delayed AD HD Child, 8077
Arrowhead West, 6898
Art and Disabilities, 8
Art and Healing: Using Expressive Art to Heal Your Body, Mind, and Soul, 9
Art and Science of Teaching Orientation and Mobility to Persons with Visual Impairments, 9133
Art for All the Children: Approaches to Art Therapy for Children with Disabilities, 10
Art Therapy, 5368
Art Therapy SourceBook, 7
Art-Centered Education and Therapy for Children with Disabilities, 2373
Arthritis Bible, 8386
Arthritis Foundation, 8346, 5223, 5224, 8113, 8395, 8401, 8404, 8407, 8417, 8418, 8423, 8424, 8803
Arthritis Foundation Distribution Center, 5452
Arthritis Foundation Great West Region, 8417
Arthritis Foundation, Southeast Region Inc, 8462
Arthritis Helpbook: A Tested Self Manageme nt Program for Coping with Arthritis, 8387
Arthritis Self-Management, 8858
Arthritis Sourcebook, 8388
Arthritis Sourcebook., 8679
Arthritis Today, 8407
Arthritis Update, 8418
Arthritis, What Exercises Work: Breakthrou gh Relief for the Rest of Your Life, 8389
Arthritis: A Take Care of Yourself Health Guide, 8390
Arthur C. Luf Children's Burn Camp, 1062
Arthur Ross Foundation, 3116
Artic Business Vision (for DOS) and Artic WinVision (for Windows 95), 1680
Artic Technologies, 1680
Artificial Language Laboratory, 4906, 7682, 9003
Artists Fellowship, 3117
ArtMix, 6317
The Arts of Life, 65
Arts Unbound, 11
As I Am, 5118
ASB, 447, 512, 577, 578, 581, 582, 4992, 5564, 5567, 9289
ASB Visions Newsletter, 9289
ASCCA, 8538
Ascension Health, 6361
ASD Athletics, 7829
ASD Summer Camp, 8177
ASHA Convention, 1887
ASHA Leader, The, 8302
Asheville VA Medical Center, 5786
Ashton Memorial Nursing Home and Chemical Dependency Center, 6802
ASIA Annual Scientific Meeting, 1888
ASN NEURO, 7666
Aspen Camp, 1045, 8178
Aspen Publishers, 5111, 5268, 7699
Aspies For Freedom (AFF), 771, 5490
Aspire of Western New York, 7048
Assemblies of God Center for the Blind, 4934
Assessing Students with Special Needs, 2661
Assessing the Handicaps/Needs of Children, 2374
Assessment & Management of Mainstreamed Hearing-Impaired Children, 2375
Assessment and Remediation of Articulatory and Phonological Disorders, 2377
Assessment in Mental Handicap: A Guide to Assessment Practices & Tests, 2378
Assessment Log & Developmental Progress Charts for the CCPSN, 2376, 2662
Assessment of Children and Youth, 2379
Assessment of Individuals with Severe Disabilities, 2380
Assessment of Learners with Special Needs, 2663
Assessment of the Feasibility of Contracting with a Nominee Agency, 4675
Assessment of the Technology Needs of Vending Facilitiy Managers In Tennessee, 2381
Assessment: The Special Educator's Role, 2382
Assets School, 5996
ASSIST! to Independence, 3984
ASSISTECH, 171, 172, 201
Assistech, 528
ASSISTECH Special Needs, 162
Assistive Technology, 179, 7677, 153
Assistive Technology Educational Network of Florida, 3506
Assistive Technology for Individuals with Cognitive Impairments Handbook, 7954
Assistive Technology for Infants and Toddl ers with Disabilities Handbook, 5048
Assistive Technology for Older Persons: A Handbook, 7631
Assistive Technology for Parents with Disa bilities Handbook, 5287
Assistive Technology for School-Age Children with Disabilities - Handbook, 5049
Assistive Technology in the Schools: A Guide for Idaho Educators, 2383
Assistive Technology Industry Association, 1889
Assistive Technology Industry Association (ATIA), 772
Assistive Technology Journal, 413
Assistive Technology Resource Centers of Hawaii (ATRC), 4828
Assistive Technology Resource Centers of Hawaii, 3533
Assistive Technology Sourcebook, 414
Assistive Technology Training and Informat ion Center (ATTIC), 4194
Assoc of Children's Prosthetic-Orthotic Clinics, 8854
Assoc of Ohio Philanthropic Homes, Housing/Service, 7756
Assoc. for Educ. & Rehab of the Blind/Vis. Imp., 1884
Assoc. on Handicapped Student Service Program, 5133
Associated Services for the Blind and Visu ally Impaired, 4992, 9034
Association for Adult Development and Aging, 7527
Association for Applied Psychophysiology and Biofeedback (AAPB), 773
Association for Behavioral and Cognitive Therapies (ABCT), 7839
Association for Contextual Behavioral Science, 7840
Association for Driver Rehabilitation Spec ialists, 2077
Association for Education & Rehabilitation, 7665
Association for Education & Rehabilitation of the Blind & Visually Impaired, 9035
Association for Gerontology in Higher Education, 7528
Association For Individual Development Elgin Area, 6831
Association for International Practical Training, 2766
Association for Macular Diseases, 9036
Association for Macular Diseases Newsletter, 9293
The Association for Macular Diseases, Inc., 9036
Association for Neurologically Impaired Brain Injured Children, 8347
Association for Research in Vision and Oph thalmology, 9037
Association for the Blind, 7141
Association for the Cure of Cancer of the Prostate (CaP CURE)-Prostate Cancer Foundation, 5491
The Association for the Gifted (TAG), 2121
Association for Vision Rehabilitation and Employment, 9038
Association of Adult Musicians with Hearing Loss, 8130
Association of Assistive Technology Act Pr ograms (ATAP), 774
Association of Blind Citizens, 9039
Association of Children's Residential Centers (ACRC), 775
Association of Children's Residential Centers, 1878
Association of Educational Therapists (AET), 776
Association of Independent Camps, 777
Association of Jewish Aging Services, 7529
Association of Language Companies, 8913
Association of Late-Deafened Adults, 7794, 8131
Association of Medical Professionals with Hearing Losses (AMPHL), 778
Association of Mouth and Foot Painting Art ists (AMPFA), 12
Association of People Supporting Employmen t First (APSE), 779
Association of Schools & Programs of Public Health, 5381
Association of University Centers on Disabilities (AUCD), 780, 2148
Association on Aging with Developmental Disabilities, 7530
Association on Handicapped Student Service Program, 2308
Association on Higher Education & Disability (AHEAD), 781, 2078
Assumption Activity Center, 6918
Asthma & Allergy Education for Worksite Clinicians, 2730
Asthma & Allergy Essentials for Children's Care Provider, 2731
Asthma Action Cards: Child Care Asthma/Allergy Action Card, 1967
Asthma Action Cards: Student Asthma Action Card, 1968
Asthma and Allergy Answers: A Patient Educ ation Library, 8681
Asthma and Allergy Foundation of America, 5492, 1967, 1968, 2029, 2039, 2384, 2730, 2731, 2732, 8681, 8908
Asthma Care Training for Kids (ACT), 2732
Asthma Management and Education, 2384
Asthma Sourcebook., 8680
Aston-Patterning, 2385
At Home Among Strangers, 8217
AT&T Foundation, 3110
Athena Rehab of Clayton, 7252

Athens Talking Book Center-Athens-Clarke County Regional Library, 4813
Atherton Family Foundation, 2940
ATIA Conference, 1889
Atkinson Foundation, 2813
ATLA, 3426
Atlanta Institute of Medicine and Rehabilitation, 6786
Atlanta Regional Office, 5684
Atlanta VA Medical Center, 5685
Atlantic Coast Rehabilitation & Healthcare Center, 7324
Atlantis Community, 4065
ATS Journals, 7655
ATTAIN, 1606, 6315
Attainment Company, 1717, 426
Attention, 8054
Attention Deficit Disorder, 7955
Attention Deficit Disorder and Learning Disabilities, 7956
Attention Deficit Disorder in Adults Workbook, 7957
Attention Deficit Disorder in Children, 2386
Attention Deficit Disorder: A Different Perception, 7958
Attention Deficit Disorder: Adults, 8078
Attention Deficit Disorder: Children, 8079
Attention Deficit Disorders Association, Southern Region: Annual Conference, 1898
Attention Deficit Disorders: Assessment & Teaching, 7959
Attention Getter, 1718
Attention Teens, 1719
Attention-Deficit Hyperactivity Disorder: Symptoms and Suggestons for Treatment, 7960
Attention-Deficit/Hyperactivity Disorder, What Every Parent Wants to Know, 7961
Attitudes Toward Persons with Disabilities, 5119
Attorney General's Office: Disability Rights Bureau & Health Care Bureau, 3553
ATV Solutions, 561, 568, 572
AUCD, 2148
Audecibel, 7678
Audio Book Contractors, 591
AudiologyOnline, 5493
Auditech, 285, 286, 1969, 1970
Auditech: Classroom Amplification System Focus CFM802, 1969
Auditech: Personal FM Educational System, 1970
Auditech: Personal PA Value Pack System, 285
Auditech: Pocketalker Pro, 286
Auditory-Verbal Therapy for Parents and Professionals, 1971
Augmentative Communication Systems (AAC), 1560
Augmenting Basic Communciation in Natural Contexts, 7962
Augusta Rehabilitation Center, 7296
Augusta Talking Book Center, 4814
Augusta VA Medical Center, 5686
Aural Habilitation, 2387
Aurora of Central New York, 7830
AuSM Summer Camp, 1200
Austin Resource Center for Independent Living, 4563
Austin Resource Center: Round Rock, 4564
Austin Resource Center: San Marcos, 4565
AUT Secondary Control, 70
Authoritative Guide to Self- Help Resource in Mental Health, 5120
Autism, 5403
Autism 24/7: A Family Guide to Learning at Home & in the Community, 7963, 8952
Autism and Learning, 7965, 8954
Autism Community Store, 1972
Autism Handbook: Understanding & Treating Autism & Prevention Development, 7964, 8953
Autism in Adolescents and Adults, 7966, 8955
Autism National Committee (AUTCOM), 7841
Autism Network International (ANI), 7842
Autism New Jersey, 4947
Autism Research Institute, 7843, 8914, 8058, 9008
Autism Research Review International, 8058, 9008
Autism Services Center, 7844, 8915, 8096
Autism Society of America, 8095, 9021
Autism Society of Minnesota, 7845, 1200, 7845
Autism Society of North Carolina Bookstore, 7963, 7967, 7978, 7992, 7998, 8001, 8046, 8952, 8956, 8966, 8998
Autism Summer Respite Program, 1268
Autism Treatment Center Of America, 8087, 9019
Autism Treatment Center of America, 7846, 8916, 8072
Autism-Products.com, 1973
Autism...Nature, Diagnosis and Treatment, 7967, 8956
Autism: A World Apart, 8080, 9016
Autism: Explaining the Enigma, 7968, 8957
Autism: From Tragedy to Triumph, 7969, 8958
Autism: Identification, Education and Treatment, 7970, 8959
Autism: The Facts, 7971, 8960
Autism: the Unfolding Mystery, 8081, 9017
AutismUp, 1269
AutismUp: YMCA Summer Social Skills Program, 1269
Autistic Adults at Bittersweet Farms, 7972, 8961
Autistic Self Advocacy Network (ASAN), 7847
Automatic Card Shuffler, 5557
Automatic Wheelchair Anti-Rollback Device, 636
Automobile Lifts for Scooters, Wheelchairs and Powerchairs, 76
Automobility Program, 3045
AUTone, 71
Autsim Society of North Carolina Bookstore, 8817
AV Hunter Trust, 2873
Avery Publishing Group, 8734
Avis Rent A Car System, LLC, 5624
AVKO Educational Research Foundation, 2072, 2002, 2004, 2048, 2064, 2500, 2528, 2716
Avon Oaks Skilled Care Nursing Facility, 7237
Awakenings Project, The, 13
AWARE, 8053
Awareness, 9294
Awareness Training, 9134
AwareNews, 5121
Away We Ride, 1720
Away We Ride IntelliKeys Overlay, 1561
Ayer Company Publishers, 2558
Ayurvedic Institute, 2733
Azure Acres Recovery Center, 6551

B

B'nai B'rith Camp: Kehila Program, 1353
BA and Elinor Steinhagen Benevolent Trust, 3281
Babycare Assistive Technology, 9135
Babycare Assistive Technology for Parents with Physical Disabilties, 9136
Babyface: A Story of Heart and Bones, 5288
Bach Flower Therapy: Theory and Practice, 5122
Back & Neck Sourcebook., 8682
Back in the Saddle, 6552
Back in the Saddle Hippotherapy Program, 6809
Back-Huggar Pillow, 227
Back-Saver, 339
Backgammon Set: Deluxe, 5558
BackSaver, 209
BackSaver Products Company, 209
Backyards and Butterflies: Ways to Include Children with Disabilities in Outdoor Activities, 5289
Bad Axe: Blue Water Center for Independent Living, 4314
Bagel Holder, 304
Bahmann Foundation, 3196
Bailey, 415
Bailey Manufacturing Company, 205, 206, 208, 221, 226, 336, 400, 415, 467, 468, 469, 481, 482, 489, 502, 656
Bain, Inc. Center For Independent Living, 4126
Bainbridge Subregional Library for the Blind & Physically Handicapped, 4815
Baker Commodities Corporate Giving Program, 2814
Bakersfield ARC, 5913
Bakersfield Regional Rehabilitation Hospital, 6241
Ball Brothers Foundation, 2984
Ball Memorial Hospital, 6871
Ballantine Books, 5233, 9229
Ballard Rehabilitation Hospital, 6553
Baltimore Community Foundation, 3006, 3008
Baltimore Regional Office, 5719
Baltimore VA Medical Center, 5720
Bancroft, 7034
Bancroft Rehabilitation Living Centers, 6919
Bangor Public Library, 4874
Bangor Veteran Center: Veterans Outreach Center, 6063
Bank of America, 3295
Bank of America Client Foundation, 2914
Bank of America Foundation, 2815
Bank of Hawaii, 2941
Bankers Trust Company, 2893
Banner Good Samaritan Medical Center, 6513
Bantam Books, 5263, 7985
Baptist General Convention of Oklahoma, 1351
Baptist Health Rehabilitation Institute, 3452
Baptist Heath, 3452
Barbara Chambers Children's Center, 6717
Barbara Olson Center of Hope, 6810
Bariatric Wheelchairs Regency FL, 659
Barnes-Jewish Hospital Washington University Medical Center, 7316
Baroco Corporation, 6953
Barrier Free Travel: A Nuts and Bolts Guid e for Wheelers and Slow Walkers (3rd Edition), 5123
Barron Collier Jr Foundation, 2915
Barron's Educational Series, 5052, 8012, 8013, 8014
Barrow Neurological Institute Rehab Center, 6236
Bartholomew County Public Library, 4847
Bartolucci Center, The- ILC Enterprises, 6811
The Barton Center, 1182
The Barton Center Camp Joslin, 1183
The Barton Center Clara Barton Camp, 1184
The Barton Center Danvers Day Camp, 1185
The Barton Center Family Camp, 1186
The Barton Center for Diabetes Education, Inc., 1071, 1182, 1183, 1184, 1185, 1186, 1187, 1465, 8582, 8618
The Barton Center Worcester Day Camp, 1187
Baruch College, 1619
Basement Motorhome Lift, 340
A Basic Course in American Sign Language, 8208
Basic Course in American Sign Language, 9137
Basic Course in American Sign Language (B100) Harris Communications, Inc., 5404
A Basic Course in Manual Communication, 8209
Basic Facts on Study Abroad, 2767
Basic Math: Detecting Special Needs, 1692
Basic Rear Closure Sweat Top, 1506
A Basic Vocabulary: American Sign Language for Parents and Children, 8210
Basketball: Beeping Foam, 9356
Bastyr Center for Natural Health, 782
BAT Personal Keyboard, 517
Bath and Shower Bench 3301B, 139
Bath Fixtures, 136
Bath Products, 137
Bath Shower & Commode Chair, 138
Bath VA Medical Center, 5772
Bathroom Transfer Systems, 140
Bathtub Safety Rail, 141
Baton Rouge Area Foundation, 2997
Battenberg & Associates, 1721
Battery Device Adapter, 287
Battery Operated Cushion, 637
Battle Creek VA Medical Center, 5732
Baxter Healthcare Corporation, 6812, 273
Bay Area Coalition for Independent Living, 4315
Bay Pine-Virginia Beach, 7179
Bay Pines VA Medical Center, 5678
Bay View Nursing and Rehabilitation Center, 7219
Bayfront Medical Center, 6724
Bayfront Rehabilitation Center, 6724
Baylor College of Medicine, 5004, 5006
Baylor College of Medicine Birth Defects Center, 5003
Baylor College of Medicine: Cullen Eye Institute, 5004
Baylor Institute for Rehabilitation, 7152
Bayshore Medical Center: Rehab, 6440

Bayview Nursing and Rehabilitation, 6554
Baywood Publishing Company, Inc., 7709
BCR Foundation, 2999
BDRC Newsletter, 5494
Be Quiet, Marina!, 7973
Beach Center on Families and Disability, 3583
Beacon Group, 5898, 6514
Beacon Press, 9344
Beacon Therapeutic Diagnostic and Treatment Center, 6813
Beacon Tree Foundation, 783, 3316
Beam, 7820
Bearskin Meadow Camp, 999, 8543
Beaumont Senior Center: Community Access Center, 4003
Beaver College, 2768
Beck Institute for Cognitive Behavior Therapy, 7848
Beck Institute for Cognitive Therapy & Research, 8063
Becket Chimney Corners YMCA Camps and Outdoor Center, 8544
Bed Rails, 263
The Bedford School, 1101, 7938
Beechwood Rehabilitation Services A Community Integrated Brain Injury Program, 7125
Before and After Zachariah, 5356
Beginning ASL Video Course, 5405
Beginning Reasoning and Reading, 1974
Behavior Analysis in Education: Focus on Measurably Superior Instruction, 2388
Behavior Modification, 2389
Behavior Skills: Learning How People Should Act, 1722
Behavioral Disorders, 2250
Behavioral Health Network Inc., 1179
Behavioral Vision Approaches for Persons with Physical Disabilities, 9138
Behind Special Education, 2390
Being Close, 8683
Belden Center, 6555
Beliefs, Values, and Principles of Self Advocacy, 5124
Beliefs: Pathways to Health and Well Being, 5125
Bellefaire Jewish Children's Bureau, 7080
Bellingham Care Center, 7188
Bellingham Health Care and Rehabilitation Services, 7403
Belonging, 9139
Ben B Cheney Foundation, 3325
Ben's Story: A Deaf Child's Right to Sign, 8219
Bench Marks, 5126
Benchmark Measures, 2664
Benefis Healthcare, 7021
Beneto Center, 7153
Benjamin Benedict Green-Field Foundation, 2949
Benwood Foundation, 3272
BeOK Key Lever, 462
Berklee Press Publications, 53
Berkley Publishing Group, 5328
Berkshire Meadows, 6954
Bernard McDonough Foundation, 3335
Berrien Community Foundation, 3041
Berthold Lowenfeld on Blindness and Blind People, 9140
Best Buddies, 7849
Best Buddies Times, 8061, 8061
Beth Abraham Health Services, 7331
Beth Abraham of Family Health Services, 7342
Bethany House Publishers (Baker Publishing Group), 5355
Bethy and the Mouse: A Father Remembers His Children with Disabilities, 5357
Better Hearing Institute, 8132
Better Sleep, 250
A Better Tomorrow, 7661
Betty Bacharach Rehabilitation Hospital, 6374
The Beveridge Family Foundation, Inc., 3037
Beverly Enterprises Network, 6534
Beyond Baby Talk: From Sounds to Sentence s, a Parent's Guide to Language Development, 8962
Beyond Sight, Inc., 592
Beyond Tears: Living After Losing a Child, 5290
Beyond the Barriers, 8431
BI-County Services, 6029
BIATX Newsletter, 8059
BIAWV Newsletter, 8060
Big and Bold Low Vision Timer, 305
Big Lakes Developmental Center, 6899
Big Lamp Switch, 463
Big Lifter, 341
Big Number Pocket Sized Calculator, 593
Big Red Switch, 180
Big Sky Kids Cancer Camps, 1228
BIGmack Communication Aid, 1562
Bill Rice Ranch, 1413
Biloxi/Gulfport VA Medical Center, 5742
Biologically Inspired Cognitive Architectures Society, 7850
Biology Concepts Through Discovery, 8082
Biomedical Concerns in Persons with Down's Syndrome, 2391
BioMedical Life Systems, 269, 569
BIPAP S/T Ventilatory Support System, 262
Birdie Thornton Center, 3965
Birmingham Alliance for Technology Access Center, 1609
Birmingham Independent Living Center, 1609
Birth Defect Research for Children, 5494, 5529
Birth Defect Research for Children (BDRC), 784
Bittersweet Chances: A Personal Journey o f Living and Learning in the Face of Illness, 8684
Black Hawk Center for Independent Living, 4207
Black Hills Workshop, 4548
Black Hills Workshop & Training Center, 4548
Blackwell Publishing, 8875
Blind & Vision Rehabilitation Services Of Pittsburgh, 7126
Blind and Physically Handicapped Library Services, 4931
Blind and Vision-Impaired Individuals, 9141
Blind Babies Foundation, 2816, 6556
Blind Children's Center, 9040, 1899, 5427, 5439, 9161, 9176, 9178, 9191, 9209, 9210, 9224, 9231, 9235, 9245, 9249, 9250, 9254, 9255, 9310, 9343, 9345
Blind Children's Center Annual Meeting, 1899
Blind Children's Fund, 3042, 2343
Blind Educator, 9277
Blind Industries and Services of Maryland, 6942
Blind Information Technology Specialists, 9041
Blind Outdoor Leisure Development, 9357
Blind Service Association, 6814
Blind Services, 6057
Blinded Veterans Association, 9042, 1900
Blinded Veterans Association National Convention, 1900
Blindness, 5406
Blindness and Early Childhood Development Second Edition, 9142
Blindness, A Family Matter, 9340
Blindness: What it is, What it Does and How to Live with it, 9143
Blindskills Inc., 9280
Blocks in Motion, 1723
Blood and Circulatory Disorders Sourcebook, 8685
Blooming Where You're Planted: Stories Fro m The Heart, 8686
Blowitz-Ridgeway Foundation, 2950
Blue Chip II, 435
Blue Peaks Developmental Services, 5942
Blue Ridge Independent Living Center, 4602
Blue Ridge Independent Living Center: Christianburg, 4603
Blue Ridge Independent Living Center: Low Moor, 4604
Blue Skies: A Complete Multi-Media Curricu lum on the Cloud, 1975
Blueberry Hill Healthcare, 6955
Bluegrass Technology Center, 1610
Board Games: Peg Solitaire, 5559
Board Games: Snakes and Ladders, 5560
Bob & Kay Timberlake Foundation, 3183
Bobby Dodd Institute (BDI), 6787
Boca Raton Rehabilitation Center, 7238
Bodie, Dolina, Smith & Hobbs, P.C., 5127
Bodman Foundation, 3118
Body of Knowledge/Hellerwork, 5130
Body Reflexology: Healing at Your Fingertips, 5128
Body Silent: The Different World of the Disabled, 5129
Body Suits, 416, 1507
Bodyline Comfort Systems, 227
Boise Health And Rehabilitation Center, 7259
Boise Regional Office, 5692
Boise VA Medical Center, 5693
Bold Line Paper, 578
Bolton Manor Nursing Home, 7304
BOMA Magazine, 1943
Bonfils-Stanton Foundation, 2876
Bonnie Prudden Myotherapy, 785
Book of Name Signs: Naming in American Sig n Language, 8220
Bookholder: Roberts, 464
Books are Fun for Everyone, 9144
Books for Blind & Physically Handicapped Individuals, 9145
Books for Blind and Physically Handicapped Individuals, 9146
Books for the Blind of Arizona, 4750
Books on Special Children, 2124, 2143, 2374, 6387, 7956, 8047, 8999
Bootheel Area Independent Living Services, 4368
Booties with Non-Skid Soles, 1508
BOSC: Directory of Facilities for People with Learning Disabilities, 2124
Boston Center for Independent Living, 4295
Boston Foundation, 3026
Boston Globe Foundation, 3027
Boston University, 4893, 6960
Boston University Arthritis Center, 4893
Boston University Center for Human Genetics, 4894
Boston University Hospital Vision Rehabilitation Services, 6956
Boston University Robert Dawson Evans Memorial Dept. of Clinical Research, 4895
Boston VA Regional Office, 5725
Bothin Foundation, 2817
Botsford Center For Rehabilitation & Health Improvement-Redford, 6985
Boulder Community Hospital Mapleton Center, 7228
Boulder Park Terrace, 7314
Boulder Public Library, 4779
Boulder Vet Center, 5663
Bounder Plus Power Wheelchair, 708
Bounder Power Wheelchair, 709
Box Top Opener, 306
Boxlight, 1675
Boxlight Corporation, 1675
Boy Inside, The, 5407
BPPV: What You Need to Know, 8218
Brachial Plexus Palsy Foundation, 3230
Bradford Regional Medical Center, 7127
Braille + Mobile Manager, 7827
Braille and Audio Reading Download (BARD), 5495
Braille and Talking Book Library, 9295
Braille and Talking Book Library, Perkins School for the Blind, 4896
Braille and Talking Book Library: California, 4765
Braille Book Bank, Music Catalog, 9147
Braille Calendar, 579
Braille Circulating Library for the Blind, 5019
Braille Documents, 5408
Braille Elevator Plates, 594
Braille Forum, 9278
Braille Institute, 9325
Braille Institute Library, 4762
Braille Institute of America, 9043
Braille Institute Orange County Center, 9361
Braille Institute Santa Barbara Center, 4763
Braille Institute Sight Center, 4764
Braille Keyboard Labels, 1594
Braille Montior, 7814, 9279
Braille Notebook, 580
Braille Paper, 1595
Braille Playing Cards, 5561
Braille Timer, 307

Braille Touch-Time Watches, 595
Braille: An Extraordinary Volunteer Opportunity, 9148
Braille: Bingo Cards, Boards and Call Numbers, 5562
Braille: Greeting Cards, 581
Braille: Rook Cards, 5563
Brailon Plastic Sheets, 1596
Brailon Thermoform Duplicator, 1597
Brain & Behavior Research Foundation, 786, 3119
Brain Allergies: The Psychonutrient and Magnetic Connections, 8687
Brain Clinic, The, 2665
Brain Disorders Sourcebook, 8688
Brain Injury Alliance of Texas, 7851
Brain Injury Association of America, 5384, 8060
Brain Injury Association of America (BIAA), 787, 7852
Brain Injury Association of New York State, 7853
Brain Injury Association of Texas, 8059
Brain Injury Rehabilitation Center Dr. P. Phillips Hospital, 6725
Brain Injury Rehabilitation Center Dr. P. Phillips, 6725
Brain Injury Resource Center, 8895
Brainy Camps, Children's National, 1166
Branden Books, 7969
Branden Publishing Company, 8958
Brandt Industries, 465
BraunAbility, 77, 342, 85, 115, 398
Bravo! + Three-Wheel Scooter, 542
Brawner Building, 2898
Brazoria County Center For Independent Living, 4566
Breaking Barriers, 2392
Breaking Ground, 8859
Breaking New Ground News Note, 8860
Breaking New Ground Resource Center, 8886
Breaking the Speech Barrier: Language Develpment Through Augmented Means, 8963
Breakthroughs: How to Reach Students with Autism, 7974, 8964
Breast Cancer Sourcebook, 8689
Breathe Free, 8690
Breathing Lessons: The Life and Work of Mark O'Brien, 8432
Breckenridge Outdoor Education Center, 1046, 8545
Breez 1025, 710
Breezy, 660
Bremerton Convalescent and Rehabilitation Center, 7404
Brentwood Rehabilitation and Nursing Cente r, 7297
Brentwood Subacute Healthcare Center, 6815
Brevard County Libraries, 4795
Brevard County Library System, 4809
Brevard County Talking Books Library, 4795
Brewer Rehab and Living Center, 6350
Brian's House, 4512
Briarcliff Nursing Home & Rehab Facility, 6490
The Bridge Center, 1188
Bridge Newsletter, 5131
Bridgepark Center for Rehabilitation and Nursing Services, 7358
Bridgeport Art Center, 59
BRiDGES, 4440
Bridging the Gap: A National Directory of Services for Women & Girls with Disabilities, 5132
Briefs, 1509
Briggs Foundation, 2818
Brigham and Women s Hospital, 4898
Brigham and Women's Hospital: Asthma and Allergic Disease Research Center, 4897
Brigham and Women's Hospital: Robert B Brigham Multipurpose Arthritis Center, 4898
Brigham Manor Nursing and Rehabilitation Center, 7305
Bright Horizons Summer Camp, 8546
Brighten Place, 6411
BrightFocus Foundation, 7531
Brike International, 524
Bringing Out the Best, 5409
Britannica Film Company, 5419, 5473, 9244
BroadFutures, 7854
Broadmead, 4284
Broadview Multi-Care Center, 7359
Broken Dolls: Gathering the Pieces: Caring for Chronically Ill Children, 5291
Bronx Continuing Treatment Day Program, 7049
Bronx Independent Living Services, 4441
Bronx VA Medical Center, 5773
Brookdale Center for Healthy Aging, 7532
Brooke Publishing, 2616
Brookes Publishing, 1959, 1960, 1961, 1962, 2035, 2059, 2354, 2356, 2370, 2376, 2398, 2399, 2402, 2406, 2409, 2416, 2418, 2433, 2434, 2436, 2453, 2454, 2456, 2471, 2482, 2488, 2504, 2506, 2522, 2530, 2542, 2583, 2603, 2607, 2622, 2645, 2652, 2653, 2654, 2655, 2659, 2662, 2667, 2678, 2680, 5055, 5084, 5086, 5097, 5105, , 5149, 5155, 5168, 5170, 5210, 5246, 5265, 5269, 5284, 5285, 5293, 5296, 5297, 5298, 5314, 5324, 5330, 5340, 5350, 5351, 5370, 5376, 5392, 5393, 5422, 5459, 5465, 7951, 7961, 7962, 7979, 7995, 8000, 8000, 8024
Brookes Publishing Company, 2149, 2360, 2380, 2382, 2388, 2415, 2457, 2491, 2557, 2649
Brookings Institution, 4676, 7649, 7654
Brookline Books, 14, 2150, 8, 22, 2018, 2021, 2022, 2061, 2062, 2378, 2395, 2414, 2431, 2435, 2440, 2465, 2502, 2584, 2587, 2605, 2608, 2613, 2615, 2628, 2632, 5124, 5160, 5165, 5212, 5216, 5218, 5254, 5289, 5292, 5295, 5305, 5320, 5337, 5354, 5357, 7975, 8017, 8030, 8032, 8044, 8731, 8775, 8804
Brookline Books Publications, 2452
Brooklyn Bureau of Community Service, 7050
Brooklyn Campus of the VA NY Harbor Healthcare System, 5774
Brooklyn Center for Independence of the Disabled, 4442
Brooklyn Home for Aged Men, 3120
Brooks / Cole Publishing Company, 2426
Brooks Memorial Hospital Rehabilitation Center, 6726
Brooks Rehabilitation Hospital, 2734
Brooks/Cole Publishing Company, 2151, 7959
Brotman Medical Center, 6557
Brotman Medical Center: RehabCare Unit, 6242, 6557
Broward County Talking Book Library, 4796
Brown County Library, 5043
Brown Foundation, 3282
Brown-Heatly Building, 3889
Brown-Heatly Library, 5005
Bruno Independent Living Aids, 343
Bruno Independent Living Aids, Inc., 76, 339, 341, 343, 345, 349, 350, 356, 357, 358, 368, 373, 379, 380, 390
Bryn Mawr Rehabilitation Hospital, 7128
BTBL News, 9295
Buck & Buck, 1506, 1508, 1511, 1512, 1514, 1515, 1517, 1518, 1520, 1521, 1522, 1523, 1527, 1529, 1530, 1531, 1532, 1533, 1534, 1536, 1537, 1538, 1539, 1540, 1541, 1546, 1549, 1550, 1551, 1552, 1553
Buck and Buck Clothing, 1510
Budget Cotton/Poly Open Back Gown, 1511
Budget Flannel Open Back Gown, 1512
Buena Vida, 7679
Buffalo Hearing and Speech Center, 7051
Buffalo Regional Office - Department of Veterans Affairs, 5775
Buffalo State (SUNY), 2769
Build Rehabilitation Industries, 6558
Builders of Skills, 6308
Building Blocks: Foundations for Learning for Young Blind and Visually Impaired Children, 9341
Building Bridges: Including People with Disabilities in International Programs, 2770
Building Owners & Managers Association, 1943
Building Owners and Managers Association International, 1927
Building Skills for Independence in the Ma instream, 2393
Building Skills for Success in the Fast-Pa ced Classroom, 2394
Building the Healing Partnership: Parents, Professionals and Children, 2395, 5292
Bull Publishing, 8749
Bulletin of the Association on the Handicapped, 5133
Burbank Rehabilitation Center, 6957
Bureau of Elderly & Adult Services, 3711
Bureau of Employment Programs Division of Workers' Compensation, 3939
Bureau Of Exceptional Education And Student Services, 3507
Bureau of Labor and Industries (BOLI), 6174
Bureau of Rehabilitation Services, 5955, 6065
Bureau of Rehabilitations Services, 4785
Bureau of Services for Blind Persons Train ing Center, 6986
Bureau of Vocational Rehabilitation, 6111
Bureau of Vocational Rehabilitation (BVR), 6169
Burger School for the Autistic, 4907
Burke Rehabilitation Hospital, 6383
Burn Institute, 1000, 8551
Burn Program at Arkansas Children's, 997
Burnett Foundation, 3059
Burns Braille Transcription Dictionary, 9149
Burns-Dunphy Foundation, 2819
BurnsBooks Publishing, 2152
Burnt Gin Camp, 1402
Burton Blatt Institute (BBI), 788
Bus Girl: Selected Poems, 7975
Bushrod H Campbell and Ada F Hall Charity Fund, 3028
Business as Usual, 5410
Business Enterprise Program (BEP), 5899, 6216
Business Publishers, 3377, 4710, 4717
Business Publishers, Inc., 7671, 7733
Butler Adult Training Center, 5870
Butler Mobility Products, 344
Butler VA Medical Center, 5808
Butlers Wheelchair Lifts, 344
Button Aid, 251
Buy!, 1976
Buying Time: The Media Role in Health Care, 5411
Bye-Bye Decubiti (BBD), 228
Bye-Bye Decubiti Air Mattress Overlay, 163

C

C D Publications, 7758
C&C Software, 1698
C-4 Work Center, 6008
CA Health and Human Services Agency Dept of Rehab, 3462
Cabell County Public Library/Talking Book Department/Subregional Library for the Blind, 5035
Cabinet for Health Services, 3593
CACLD, 5430, 8025, 8090
Cadinal Hill Medical Center, 6908
Caglewood, Inc., 1090
Cahaba Media Group, 2272
CAHSA Connecting, 7759
CAI, Career Assessment Inventories for the Learning Disabled, 2396
California Community Care News, 5071
California Community Foundation, 2820
California Department of Aging, 3456
California Department of Education: Special Education Division, 2181
California Department of Fair Employment & Housing, 5914, 4690, 4691, 4694
California Department of Handicapped Children, 3457
California Department of Rehabilitation, 3458
California Elwyn, 6559
California Endowment, 2821
California Eye Institute, 6560
California Financial Power of Attorney, 5135
California Foundation For Independent Living Centers, 4004
California Foundation for Independent Living Centers, 4005

California Governor's Committee on Employment of People with Disabilities, 3459
California Lions Camp, 1014, 8191
California Protection & Advocacy: (PAI) A Nonprofit Organization, 3460
California School of Professional Psychology, 4774
California State Council on Developmental Disabilities, 3461
California State Independent Living Counci l (SILC), 4006
California State Library Braille and Talki ng Book Library, 4766, 9044
Cambia Health Foundation, 790, 3223
Cambridge Career Products Catalog, 417
Cambridge Educational, 417, 1773
Cambridge University Press, 5070, 7672, 8772, 8798
Camden City Independent Living Center, 4410
Camden Healthcare and Rehabilitation Center, 7378
Camiccia-Arnautou Charitable Foundation, 2916
Camp "I Am Me", 1111
Camp Abilities, 981
Camp Abilities Brockport, 1270
Camp Abilities Tucson, 985
Camp About Face, 1128
Camp Achieva, 1370
Camp Adam Fisher, 1403
Camp Adventure, 1271
Camp Ailihpomeh, 1424
Camp AIM, 1369
Camp Akeela, 1371
Camp Akeela Winter Address, 1371
Camp Albrecht Acres, 1141
Camp Aldersgate, 994, 8547
Camp Alexander Mack, 8179
Camp Allen, 1242
Camp Alpine, 982, 8548
Camp Amigo, 1076
Camp Amp, 1372
Camp Anne, 1272
Camp Anuenue, 1102, 8549
Camp Aranzazu, 1425
Camp Arye, 1317
Camp AZDA, 984
Camp Baker, 7897
Camp Barakel, 9106
Camp Barefoot, 1189
Camp Barnabas, 1217
Camp Be An Angel, 1426
Camp Beausite NW, 1475, 8550
Camp Beyond The Scars, 1000, 8551
Camp Bishopswood, 8180
Camp Blessing, 1427
Camp Bloomfield, 1001, 9107
Camp Boggy Creek, 1077, 8552
Camp Bon Coeur, 1154, 8553
Camp Brave Eagle, 1129
Camp Breathe Easy, 1089, 8554
Camp Buck, 1237
Camp Buckskin, 1201, 7898
Camp Caglewood, 1090
Camp Callahan, 1112
Camp Callahan, Inc., 1112
Camp CAMP, 1428
Camp Can Do, 1373, 8555
Camp Can-Do, 1430
Camp Candlelight, 986, 7899
Camp CANOE, 1346
Camp CaPella, 1160, 8181
Camp Carefree, 1243, 1306, 8556
Camp Carolina Trails, 1307
Camp Catch-A-Rainbow, 1190
Camp Catch-a-Rainbow, 8557
Camp Challenge, 1155, 9108
Camp Chatterbox, 1249
Camp Cheerful, 1318, 8558
Camp Chris Williams, 1191, 8182
Camp Christian Berets, 1002
Camp Christmas Seal, 8559
Camp Christopher: SumFun Day Camp, 1319
Camp Civitan, 987, 7900
Camp ClapHans, 1347
Camp Classen YMCA, 8560
Camp COAST, 1273
Camp Comeca & Retreat Center, 8183
Camp Confidence, 1202
Camp Connect, 1244
Camp Conquest, 1414
Camp Conrad Chinnock, 1003, 8561
Camp Courage, 1203, 1374, 1404
Camp Courage North, 1204, 8562
Camp Courageous of Iowa, 1142
Camp CPals, 1429
Camp Daypoint, 1484
Camp Debbie Lou, 1405
Camp Deeny Riback, 1250
Camp del Corazon, 1029, 8613
Camp Dickenson, 1466
Camp Discovery, 1063, 1113, 1375, 1415, 1431
Camp Discovery - Illinois, 8563
Camp Discovery Kansas, 1146, 8564
Camp Dogwood, 1308
Camp Dream, 1091
Camp Dream Foundation, 1091
Camp Dream Street, 1216, 1251
Camp EAGR, 1274
Camp Easterseals UCP, 1467
Camp Echoing Hills, 1320, 8565
Camp Eden Wood, 1205, 8566
Camp Emanuel, 1321, 8184
Camp Enchantment, 1265
Camp Encourage, 1218
Camp Endres, 1348
Camp Esperanza, 8378
Camp Evoked Potential, 965, 7901
Camp Fire Heart of Oklahoma, 1346
Camp Firefly, 1092
Camp Floyd Rogers, 1231, 8567
Camp for All, 1444
Camp Foundation, 3317
Camp Freedom, 1376
Camp FRIENDship, 1114
Camp Friendship, 1408
Camp Giddy-Up, 1453
Camp Gilbert, 1409
Camp Gilbert, Inc., 1409
Camp Glengarra, 8568
Camp Glyndon, 8569
Camp Good Days and Special Times, 1275
Camp Goodtimes, 1476
Camp Grace Bentley, 1192
Camp Great Rock, 1166
Camp Grizzly, 1004, 8185
Camp H.U.G., 988, 8570
Camp Hamwi, 1322
Camp Hanover, 1469
Camp Happiness, 1323
Camp Harkness, 1064, 8571
Camp Hawkins, 1093
Camp Heartland, 1206, 8572
Camp Hebron, 1368
Camp Hertko Hollow, 1143, 8573
Camp Hickory Hill, 1219, 8574
Camp High Hopes, 1276
Camp Ho Mita Koda, 1324, 8575
Camp Hobe, 1454
Camp Hodia, 1104, 8576
Camp Holiday Trails, 1468
Camp Hollywood HEART, 1005, 8577
Camp Honor, 989, 8578
Camp Hope, 1495
Camp Horizons, 1065, 7902
Camp Hot-to-Clot, 1377
Camp Howe, 1175
Camp Huntington, 1277, 7903
Camp ICANDO, 1455
Camp Independence, 1094, 8579
Camp Inter-Actions, 1245
Camp Isola Bella, 1066, 8186
Camp J CC, 2751
Camp Jabberwocky, 1176
Camp Jaycee, 1252
Camp Jaycee Administrative Office, 1252
Camp Jened, 8580
Camp John Marc, 1432
Camp John Warvel, 1130, 8581
Camp Jordan, 1469
Camp Joslin, 8582
Camp Jotoni, 1253
Camp Joy, 1325, 1416, 8187, 8583
Camp Juliena, 1095, 8188
Camp Kee-B-Waw, 1485
Camp Kehilla, 1278
Camp Killoqua, 1477
Camp Kindle, 1006, 1232
Camp Klotty Pine, 1486
Camp Knutson, 1207
Camp Ko-Man-She, 1326, 8584
Camp Koinonia, 1417
Camp Korelitz, 1327
Camp Korey, 1478
Camp Kostopulos, 1456
Camp Krem, 1007, 7904
Camp Kudzu, 1096
Camp Kudzu, Inc., 1096
Camp Kweebec, 8585
Camp L-Kee-Ta, 8586
Camp Latgawa, 8587
Camp Laughter, 995
Camp Lawroweld, 1161, 9109
Camp Lee Mar, 1378
Camp Libbey, 8588
Camp Lighthouse, 1074, 9110
Camp Lily Lehigh Valley, 1379
Camp Little Giant, 1115
Camp Little Oak, 1279
Camp Little Red Door, 1131
Camp Littlefoot, 1167
Camp Lo-Be-Gon, 1349
Camp Lotsafun, 1238
Camp Lou Henry Hoover, 9111
Camp Loud And Clear, 1470
Camp Loughridge, 1350
Camp Luv-A-Lung, 1406
Camp Magruder, 1354, 8590
Camp Mak-A-Dream, 1229
Camp Manito & Camp Lenape, 1072
Camp Mark Seven, 1280, 8189
Camp Mauchatea, 1398
Camp Meadowood Springs, 1355, 8190, 8943
Camp Merrick, 9112
Camp Merry Heart, 1254
Camp Midicha, 1193
Camp Millennium, 1356
Camp Millhouse, 1132
Camp MITIOG, 1220, 8589
Camp Nah-Nah-Mah, 1457
Camp Needlepoint, 1487
Camp Nejeda, 1255, 8591
Camp Nejeda Foundation, 1255, 8591
Camp Neuron, 1433
Camp New Hope, 1116, 1309
Camp New Horizons North, 1434
Camp New Horizons South, 1435
Camp Nissokone, 7905
Camp No Limits California, 1008
Camp No Limits Connecticut, 1067
Camp No Limits Florida, 1078
Camp No Limits Idaho, 1105
Camp No Limits Maine, 1162
Camp No Limits Maryland, 1168
Camp No Limits Missouri, 1221
Camp No Limits Texas, 1436
Camp NoLoHi, 1437
Camp Not-A-Wheeze, 990, 8592
Camp Nuhop, 1328, 7906
Camp Odayin, 1208, 1208, 1209, 1210, 1211, 1212
Camp Odayin Family Camp, 1209
Camp Odayin Residential Camp, 1210
Camp Odayin Summer Camp, 1211
Camp Odayin Winter Camp, 1212
Camp Oginali, 1418
Camp Okawehna, 1419
Camp Okizu, 1009, 8593
Camp Okizu: Family Camp, 1010
Camp Okizu: Oncology Camp, 1011
Camp Okizu: SIBS Camp, 1012
Camp Okizu: Teens-N-Twenties Camp, 1013
Camp One Step, 1117
Camp Orchard Hill, 1380

Camp Oty'Okwa, 1329
Camp Pa-Qua-Tuck, 1281
Camp Pacifica, 1014, 8191
Camp Paivika, 1015, 8594
Camp Paradise, 1330
Camp Pelican, 1156, 8595
Camp Perfect Wings, 1351
Camp Planet D, 1147
Camp PossAbility, 1133
Camp PossAbility, Inc., 1133
Camp Quality Arkansas, 996
Camp Quality Central Missouri, 1222
Camp Quality Greater Kansas City, 1223
Camp Quality Heartland, 1233
Camp Quality Illinois, 1118
Camp Quality Kansas, 1148
Camp Quality Kentuckiana, 1134, 1150
Camp Quality Louisiana, 1157
Camp Quality New Jersey, 1256
Camp Quality North Michigan, 1194
Camp Quality Northwest Missouri, 1224
Camp Quality Ohio, 1331
Camp Quality Ozarks, 1225
Camp Quality South Michigan, 1195
Camp Quality Texas, 1438
Camp Rainbow, 991, 1439, 8596
Camp Rainbow Gold, 1106
Camp Ramah in the Poconos, 1381, 8192
Camp Ramapo, 1282, 7907
Camp Reach for the Sky, 1017, 8597
Camp Recovery Center, 6561
Camp ReCreation, 1016, 7908
Camp Red Cedar, 1135
Camp Red Leaf, 1119
Camp Reece, 1283
Camp Riley, 1136
Camp Rising Sun, 1266
Camp Rocky Mountain Village, 1047
Camp Ronald McDonald at Eagle Lake, 1018, 8598
Camp Ronald McDonald for Good Times, 1019, 8599
Camp Royall, 1310, 7909, 8944
Camp Ruggles, 1399, 7910
Camp Sandcastle, 1440
Camp Sawtooth, 8600
Camp Seale Harris, 966, 8601
Camp Sealth, 1479
Camp Sertoma, 1311
Camp Setebaid, 1383, 8602
Camp Shocco for the Deaf, 967, 8193
Camp Sioux, 1316
Camp Sisol, 1284, 7911, 8945
Camp Smile-A-Mile, 968, 8603
Camp Smile-A-Mile: Jr./Sr. Camp, 969
Camp Smile-A-Mile: Off Therapy Family Camp, 970
Camp Smile-A-Mile: On Therapy Family Camp, 971
Camp Smile-A-Mile: Sibling Camp, 972
Camp Smile-A-Mile: Teen Weeklong Camp, 973
Camp Smile-A-Mile: Young Adult Retreat, 974
Camp Smile-A-Mile: Youth Weeklong Camp, 975
Camp Sno Mo, 1246
Camp sNOw Maine, 1164
Camp Spearhead, 1407
Camp Spencer Superstars, 1384
Camp Spike 'n' Wave, 1441
Camp STAR, 1382
Camp Starfish, 1177
Camp Starlight, 1357
Camp Stepping Stone, 1332
Camp Sugar Falls, 1420
Camp Summit, 1442
Camp Sun'N Fun, 1257
Camp Sunburst, 1020, 8604
Camp Sunnyside, 1144
Camp Sunrise, 1170, 8605
Camp Sunshine, 997, 1097, 1163
Camp Sunshine Dreams, 1021, 8606
Camp SunSibs, 1169
Camp Sweeney, 1443, 8607
Camp Sweet Betes, 1149
Camp Tall Turf, 8608
Camp Taloali, 1358, 8194
Camp Tanager, 1145
Camp Taylor, 1022, 8609
Camp Taylor, Inc., 1022, 1023, 1024, 1025, 1026, 1027, 1103, 8609
Camp Taylor: Family Camp, 1023, 1103
Camp Taylor: Leadership Camp, 1024
Camp Taylor: Teen Camp, 1025
Camp Taylor: Young Adult Program, 1026
Camp Taylor: Youth Camp, 1027
Camp Tekoa, 1312, 8195
Camp Thorpe, 1463
Camp Thunderbird, 1079
Camp Tiponi, 1333
Camp Tova, 1285
Camp Tuolumne Trails, 1028
Camp Twin Lakes, 1098, 1094
Camp Twin Lakes: Rutledge, 1099
Camp Twin Lakes: Will-A-Way, 1100
Camp Ukandu, 1359
Camp Vacamas, 8610
Camp Venture, Inc., 1286
Camp Victory, 1385
Camp Wapiyapi, 1048
Camp Waziyatah, 8611
Camp Wediko, 1247
Camp Wesley Woods: Exceptional Persons Camp, 1386
Camp WheezeAway, 976, 8612
Camp Whitman on Seneca Lake, 1287
Camp Winnekeag, 9113
Camp Wonder, 1421
Camp Woodlands, 1387
Camp World Light, 7912
Camp Yavneh: Yedidut Program, 1248
Camp-A-Lot and Camp-A-Little, 1030, 7913
Campagna Center, 6210
Campaign Math, 1693
Campbell Soup Foundation, 3093
CampCare, 1239
Camping Unlimited, 1007, 7904
Campobello Chemical Dependency Recovery Center, 6562
Camps for Children & Teens with Diabetes, 1471, 8614
Can America Afford to Grow Old?, 4676
Can't Your Child See? A Guide for Parents of Visually Impaired Children, 9150
Can-Do Products Catalog, 142
Canadian Art Therapy Association (CATA), 791
Canadian Cancer Society, 8483
Canadian Deafblind Association, 7795
Canadian Diabetes Association, 8484
Canadian Lung Association, 8485
Canandiagua VA Medical Center, 5776
Cancer Care, 3121
Cancer Clinical Trials: A Commonsense Guide to Experimental Cancer Therapies and Trials, 5341
Cancer Research Institute, 5496
Cancer Sourcebook, 8691
Cancer Sourcebook for Women, 8692
Candlelighters Childhood Cancer Foundation, 3007
Candler General Hospital: Rehabilitation Unit, 6301
Canes and Trails, 9296
Canine Companions for Independence (CCI), 792
Canine Helpers for the Handicapped, 793, 9045
Canine Helpers for the Handicapped, Inc., 793, 9045
Canine Listener, 8304
Canonicus Camp & Conference Center, 1400
CANPFA-Line, 7760
CAPCO Capability Corporation, 1815
Cape Coral Hospital, 7239
Cape Organization for Rights of the Disabled (CORD), 4296
Capital Area Center for Independent Living, 4316
Capital Area Parkinsons Society, 8348
Capital District Center for Independence, 4443
Capital District YMCA, 1305, 9123
Capitol Focus, 7761
Caprice Care Center, 7360
Capron Rehabilitation Center, 6676
Capscrew, 308
Capsule, 7762
Caption Center, 4899, 9046
Captus Press, 5079
Car Builder Deluxe, 1724
Car Cane, 79
Cardinal Hill Rehabilitation Hospital, 6338, 6908
Cardiovascular Diseases and Disorders Sourcebook, 3rd Edition, 8693
Cards: Musical, 5564
Cards: UNO, 5565
Care Center East Health & Specialty Care Center, 7366
Care Electronics, 466
Care Master Medical Services, 6794
Care-One, 7044
Career Development and Transition for Exceptional Individuals, 2252
Career Opportunity Development of New Jersey, 6124
Career Perspectives: Interviews with Blind and Visually Impaired Professionals, 9151
Career Success for Disabled High-Flyers, 5081
CAREERS & the disABLED Magazine, 5369
Careers in Blindness Rehabilitation Services, 9152
Caremark Healthcare Services, 6816
Carendo, 210
Carex Health Brands, 418, 418
Carey Services, 6030
CARF International, 789, 2079, 7533
Carilion Health System, 7184
Carilion Rehabilitation: New River Valley, 7180
Caring and Sharing Center for Independent Living, 4099
Caring and Sharing Center: Pasco County, 4100
The Caring Community of CT, 5959
Caring for America's Heroes, 5136
Caring for Children with Chronic Illness, 2397
Caring for Persons with Developmental Disabilities, 5412
Caring for Those You Love: A Guide to Compassionate Care for the Aged, 7632
Carl and Ruth Shapiro Family National Center for Accessible Media, 6958, 8917
Carl T Hayden VA Medical Center, 5644
Carl Vinson VA Medical Center, 5687
Carnegie Library of Pitts. Library for the Blind, 9261
Carnegie Library of Pittsburgh Library for the Blind & Physically Handicapped, 4993
Caro: Blue Water Center for Independent Living, 4317
Carolina Computer Access Center, 1612
Carolina Curriculum for Infants and Toddlers with Special Needs (3rd Edition), 2398, 5350
Carolina Curriculum for Preschoolers with Special Needs, 2399, 2667
Carolyn's Low Vision Products, 419, 1513
Carondelet Brain Injury Programs and Services (Bridges Now), 6515
Carpal Tunnel Syndrome, 8113
Carrie Estelle Doheny Foundation, 2822
Carroll Center for the Blind, 6959, 9366
Carroll School, 1181, 7939
Carson City Center for Independent Living, 4403
Cary Library, 4875
Casa Colina Center for Rehabilitation, 6565
Casa Colina Centers for Rehabilitation, 6563
Casa Colina Padua Village, 6564
Casa Colina Residential Services: Rancho Pino Verde, 6565
Casa Colina Transitional Living Center, 6566
Casa Colina Transitional Living Center: Pomona, 6567
Casa Colinas Centers for Rehabilitation, 6243
CASA Inc., 4426
Case Management Society of America (CMSA), 794
Case Manager Magazine, 2253
Case Western Reserve University, 4979
Case Western Reserve University Northeast Ohio Multipurpose Arthritis Center, 4980
Casey Eye Institute, 4989
Casiano Communications, 7679
Casowasco Camp, Conference and Retreat Center, 7914
Casper Vet Center, 5863

Castle Point Campus of the VA Hudson Valley Healthcare System, 5777
Catalog for Teaching Life Skills to Persons with Development Disability, 1977
Catalyst, 2254
The Catalyst, 2254
Cataracts, 9153
Catholic Charities, 6920
Catholic Charities Disability Services, 1319, 1323
Catholic Guild for The Blind, 9305
Catholic Medical Center, 7030
Catholic Southwest, 6753
Catskill Center for Independence, 4444
Cave Spring Rehabilitation Center, 6788
CC-M Productions, 8433
CCARC, Inc., 5956
CD Publications, 3354, 7670
CDR Reports, 5134
CEC Catalog, 2251
CEC Pioneers Division (CEC-PD), 2080
Cecil R Bomhr Rehabilitation Center of Nacogdoches Memorial Hospital, 6441
Cedar Ridge Camp, 8615
Cedar Spring Health and Rehabilitation Cen ter, 7413
Cedars of Marin, 6568
Cengage Learning, 2496, 5075
Centegra Northern Illinois Medical Center, 6817
Centennial Medical Center Tri Star Health System, 7379
Center Academy, 7855
Center Academy at Pinellas Park, 1080, 7915
Center for Accessible Living, 4263
Center for Accessible Living: Murray, 4264
Center for Accessible Technology, 1613
Center for Applied Special Technology, 1614
Center for Assistive Technology & Inclusive Education Studies, 1615
Center for Benefits Access, 7534
Center for Best Practices in Early Childhood, 1725
Center for Community Alternatives, 4445
Center for Comprehensive Services, 6818
The Center for Courageous Kids, 1153
Center for Creative Arts Therapy, 795
Center for Development and Disability, 1266
Center for Disabilities & Development, 3576
Center for Disabilities Studies, 3891
Center for Disability and Elder Law, Inc., 4651
Center for Disability Resources, 796, 3263, 2233
Center for Disability Rights, 4080
Center for Disability Services, 1288
Center for Educational Advancement New Jersey, 6125
Center for Health Research: Eastern Washin gton University, 5137
Center for Healthy Aging, 7535, 7598
Center for Hearing and Communication, 8133, 8310
Center for Human Potential, 2669
Center for Inclusive Design and Innovation, 797, 2081
Center for Independence, 4066
Center for Independence of the Disabled, 4007
Center for Independence of the Disabled of New York, 4446
Center for Independence of the Disabled of New York, 4447
Center for Independence of the Disabled- Daly City, 4008
Center for Independent Living, 4009
Center for Independent Living in Central Florida, 4101
Center for Independent Living of Mid-Michigan, 4318
Center for Independent Living of Broward, 4102
Center for Independent Living of Central Nebraska, 4396
Center for Independent Living of Florida Keys, 4103
Center for Independent Living of Middle Tennessee, 4556
Center for Independent Living of N Florida, 4104
Center for Independent Living of North Central Florida, 4106
Center for Independent Living of North Cen tral Florida, 4107
Center for Independent Living of NW Florid a, 4105
Center for Independent Living of S Florida, 4108
Center for Independent Living of SW Florida, 4109
Center for Independent Living of Western Wisconsin, 4634
Center for Independent Living Options, 4489
Center for Independent Living SC, 4081
Center for Independent Living Southwest Kansas, 4217
Center for Independent Living Southwest Ka nsas: Dodge City, 4218
Center for Independent Living SW Kansas: L iberal, 4216
Center For Independent Living- Kauai, 4136
Center for Independent Living: East Oakland, 4010
Center for Independent Living: Kentucky Department for the Blind, 4265
Center for Independent Living: Long Branch, 4411
Center for Independent Living: Oakland, 4011
Center for Independent Living: South Jersey, 4412
Center for Independent Living: Tri-County, 4012
Center for Independent Living:Fresno, 4013
Center for Independent Living; Oakland, 4014
Center for Interdisciplinary Research on Immunologic Diseases, 4900
Center for Learning, 6309
Center for Libraries and Educational Improvement, 5138
Center for Living & Working: Fitchburg, 4297
Center for Living & Working: Framingham, 4298
Center for Living & Working: Worcester, 4299
Center for Medicare Advocacy, 7536
Center for Mental Health Services, 2203
Center for Mind-Body Medicine, 798
Center for Neuro Skills, 6569, 7155
Center for Neuro-Rehabilitation, 6943
Center for Neuropsychology, Learning & Dev elopment, 2670
Center for Pain Control and Rehabilitation, 6727
Center for Parent Information and Resources, 2735
Center for People with Disabilities, 4067
Center for People with Disabilities: Pueblo, 4068
Center for People with Disabilities: Bould er, 4069
Center For Personal Development, 2668
Center for Positive Aging, 7537
Center for Psychiatric Rehabilitation, 6960
Center for Public Representation, 3623, 4726
Center for Rehabilitation at Rush Presbyterian: Johnston R Bowman Health Center, 6819
Center for Rehabilitation Technology, 518
Center for Research on Women with Disabilities, 5006
Center for Spinal Cord Injury Recovery, 2736
Center for Spine, Sports & Occupational Rehabilitation, 6820
Center for Student Health and Counseling, 2671
Center for the Improvement of Human Functioning, 4858
Center for the Partially Sighted, 6570
Center for the Visually Impaired, 6789
Center for Vision Rehabilitation, 7068
Center for Workplace Compliance, 4652
Center of Independent Living: Visalia, 4015
Center on Deafness, 4156
Center on Disability Studies, 1918
Center on Evaluation of Assistive Technology, 1616
Center on Human Policy: School of Education, 4955
Center on the Social & Emotional Foundations for Early Learning (CSEFEL), 5497
Centering Corporation, 5180, 5309
Centering Corporation Grief Resources, 5139
Centers for Disease Control and Prevention, 5140, 4822, 8891, 8899
Centers for Medicare & Medicaid Services, 2204
Centers for Medicare and Medicaid Services, 3383
Centers for The Developmentally Disabled - North Central Alabama, 6491
Centers of Excellence Leadership Conferenc e, 1902
Central Alabama Veterans Healthcare System, 5639
Central Arkansas Rehab Hospital, 6232
Central Association for the Blind & Visual ly Impaired, 9047
Central Coast Center for IL: San Benito, 4016
Central Coast Center for Independent Living, 4017
Central Coast Center: Independent Living - Santa Cruz Office, 4018
Central Coast for Independent Living, 4019
Central Coast for Independent Living: Watsonville, 4020
Central Coast Neurobehavioral Center OPTIONS, 6571
Central Iowa Center for Independent Living, 4208, 5157
Central Island Healthcare, 7332
Central Kansas Library Systems Headquarter s (CSLS), 4859
Central Library Downtown, 5043
Central Louisiana State Hospital Medical and Professional Library, 4870
Central Office & Metropolitan Services, 7856
Central Rappahannock Regional Library, 5020
Central Utah Independent Living Center, 4587
Centre, The, 4567
Century Bath System, 211
Century College, 4926
Cerebral Palsy Associations of New York State, 7856
Cerebral Palsy Foundation (CPF), 799
Cerebral Palsy of Colorado, 6677
Cerebral Palsy: North County Center, 6572
Ceres Press, 1955
CH Foundation, 3283
CHADD, 7858
Chadder, 8062
Chaddick Institute for Metropolitan Development, 2951
Chalet Village Health and Rehabilitation C enter, 7276
Challenge Aspen, 1049
Challenge Golf, 9358
Challenge Magazine, 2255, 7680
Challenge of Educating Together Deaf and Hearing Youth: Making Manistreaming Work, 2400
Challenge Publications Limited, 8410
Challenged Athletes Foundation (CAF), 800
Challenged Scientists: Disabilities and the Triumph of Excellence, 2401
Chamberlain Group, 2956
CHAMP Camp, 1127
Champ Camp, 1050, 8616
Champion 1000, 661
Champion 2000, 662
Champion 3000, 663
Champlin Foundations, 3254
Change Your Brain, Change Your Life: The Breakthrough Program for Conquering Depression, 7976
Change, Inc., 801
Chapel Haven, 4082
Chapel Hill Rehabilitation and Healthcare Center, 7345
Characteristics, Services, & Outcomes of Rehab. Consumers who are Blind/Visually Impaired, 9154
Charcot-Marie-Tooth Association, 8102
Chariot, 345
Charis Hills Camp, 1445
Charles C Thomas Publisher LTD, 2153
Charles C. Thomas, 10, 23, 36, 2357, 2362, 2373, 2386, 2400, 2410, 2425, 2458, 2460, 2466, 2490, 2492, 2497, 2594, 2620, 2626, 2650, 5264, 5310, 5325, 5377, 5382, 5579, 8213, 8228, 9158, 9259
Charles Campbell Childrens Camp, 1230
Charlotte Vet Center, 5787
Charlotte White Center, 6937
Chase Bank of Texas, 3281
Chatlos Foundation, 2917

Cheaha Regional Mental Health Center, 6492
Cheever Publishing, 5100
Chelsea Community Hospital Rehabilitation Unit, 6987
Chelsea: The Story of a Signal Dog, 8221
Chemists with Disabilities Committee - American Chemical Society, 5389
Cherab Foundation, 9022
The Cherab Foundation, 944, 2927, 8939
Cherry Hills Health Care Center, 6678
Chesapeake Region Accessible Boating, 8443
Chess Set: Deluxe, 5566
Chestnut Hill Rehabilitation Hospital, 6412
Chevy Chase Nursing and Rehabilitation Cen ter, 7264
Cheyenne VA Medical Center, 5864
Cheyenne Village, 5943
Chi Medical Library, 4908
Chicago Community Trust, 2952
Chicago Community Trust and Affiliates, 2953
Chicago Lawyers' Committee for Civil Rights Under Law, 4653
Chicago Lighthouse, 9311
Chicago Lighthouse for People who are Blind and Visually Impaired, 9048
Chicago Public Library Talking Book Center, 4832
Chicago Public Library Talking Books Center, 9333
Chicago Review Press, 5356
Child and Adolescent Therapy: Cognitive-Be havioral Procedures, Third Edition, 7977
Child and Parent Resource Institute (CPRI), 802
Child Care and the ADA: A Handbook for Inclusive Programs, 2402
Child Convertible Balance Beam Set, 467
Child Development Media, 8073
Child Find/Early Childhood Disabilities Unit Montgomery County Public Schools, 6944
Child Neurology Society, 7857
Child Variable Balance Beam, 468
Child with Disabling Illness, 2403
Child With Special Needs: Encouraging Inte llectual and Emotional Growth, 5141
Child's Mobility Crawler, 469
Childcare and the ADA, 4677
Childcare Services Division, 3420
Childhood Apraxia of Speech Association, 8918
Childhood Behavior Disorders: Applied Research & Educational Practice, 2404
Childhood Cancer Canada Foundation, 8486
Childhood Cancer Guides/O'Reilly Media, 5348
Childhood Cancer Survivors: A Practical Guide to Your Future, 8694
Childhood Cancer: A Parent's Guide to Solid Tumor Cancers, 8695
Childhood Disablity and Family Systems (Routledge Library Editions) (Volume 5), 2405
Childhood Diseases and Disorders Sourceboo k, 2nd Edition, 8696
Childhood Glaucoma: A Reference Guide for Families, 9155
Childhood Leukemia Foundation, 8487
Childhood Leukemia: A Guide for Families, Friends & Caregivers, 8697
Childhood Speech, Language & Listening Pro blems, 8965
Children & Adults with ADHD, 8054
Children & Adults with Attention Deficit Disorder, 8062
Children and Adults with Attention-Deficit Hyperactivity Disorder, 7858
Children and Youth Assisted by Medical Technology in Educational Settings, 2nd Edition, 2406
Children of a Lesser God, 8222
Children of Aging Parents, 7538, 7762
Children s Hospital Boston, 3624
Children s Medical Program, 3666
Children with Cerebral Palsy: A Parents' G uide, 8698
Children with Disabilities, 5293
Children with Special Health Care Needs, 3945
Children with Visual Impairments: A Guide For Parents, 9156
Children's Aid Society, 1303
Children's Alliance, 803
Children's Assessment Center, The, 2672
Children's Association for Maximum Potential, 1428
Children's Beach House, 1073, 8203
Children's Burn Camp Of North Florida, Inc., 1076
Children's Center for Neurodevelopmental Studies, 4751
Children's Fresh Air Society Fund, 3008
Children's Healthcare of Atlanta at Egleston, 6302
Children's Hemiplegia & Stroke Association, 8349
Children's Home and Aid Society of Illinois, 6821
Children's Hopes & Dreams Wish Fulfillment Foundation, 3094
Children's Hospital Burn Camps Program, 1051, 8617
Children's Hospital Burn Camps Program: En gland Exchange Program Burn Camp, 1052
Children's Hospital Burn Camps Program: Fa mily Burn Camp, 1053
Children's Hospital Burn Camps Program: Su mmer Burn Camp, 1054
Children's Hospital Burn Camps Program: Wi nter Burn Camp, 1055
Children's Hospital Burn Camps Program: Yo ung Adult Retreat, 1056
Children's Hospital Central California Reh abilitation Center, 6573
Children's Hospital Los Angeles Rehabilitation Program, 6574
Children's Hospital Rehabilitation Center, 6272
Children's Medical Services, 3453
Children's Mental Health and EBD E-news, 2309
Children's Mental Health Network (CMHN), 804
Children's National Medical Center, 805, 6723
Children's Needs Psychological Perspective, 2407
Children's Oncology Services Inc., 1117
Children's Press, 5158
Children's Rehabilitation Service, 6493
Children's Special Health Services Program, 3848
Children's Specialized Hospital, 6375, 1249
Children's Specialized Hospital Medical Library - Parent Resource Center, 4948
Children's Therapy Center, 6575
Children's Tumor Foundation, 3122
Children's Understanding of Disability, 5050
Childrens Beach House, 8946
Childrens Hospital Medical Center, 4900
Chiles Foundation, 3224
Chillicothe VA Medical Center, 5794
Chilton-Shelby Mental Health Center, 6494
Chinese Herbal Medicine, 5142
Choice Magazine Listening, 9342
Choice Switch Latch and Timer, 470
CHOICES Center for Independent Living, 4427
Choices in Deafness: A Parent's Guide to C ommunication Options, 8223
Choices, Choices 5.0, 1825
Choices: A Guide to Sex Counseling with Physically Disabled Adults, 2408
Choosing a Wheelchair: A Guide for Optimal Independence, 664
Choosing Options and Accommodations for Children, 2409
Choosing Outcomes and Accommodations for Children (COACH) (2nd Edition), 5351
Christ Hospital Rehabilitation Unit, 7081
A Christian Approach to Overcoming Disability: A Doctor's Story, 9124
Christian Approach to Overcoming Disabilit y: A Doctor's Story, 5143
Christian Education for the Blind, 5007
Christian Hospital Northeast, 7012
Christian Record Services, 1236, 9119
Christmas Stories, 8319
Christopher & Dana Reeve Foundation, 4949
Christopher & Dana Reeve Paralysis Resource Center, 8350
Christopher and Dana Reeve Paralysis Resource Ctr, 8400
Chronic Fatigue Syndrome: Your Natural Gu ide to Healing with Diet, Herbs and Other Methods, 8699
Chronically Disabled Elderly in Society, 7633
Chronicle Guide to Grants, 3352
Church of the Nazarene, 4935
CIL of Central Florida, 4098
Cincinnati Children's Hospital Medical Center, 4981
Cincinnati VA Medical Center, 5795
Circline Illuminated Magnifer, 596
Cirriculum Development for Students with Mild Disabilities, 2410
CITE: Lighthouse for Central Florida, 1611
City Of Lakewood, 1057
City of Lakewood Recreation and Inclusion Services for Everyone (R.I.S.E.), 1057
Civil Rights Division/Disability Rights Se ction, 3384
Civitan Acres, 1472
Civitan Foundation, 2804, 987, 7900
Clara Barton Camp, 8618
Clare Branch, 6988
Clark Health Care Products, 138
Clark House Nursing Center At Foxhill Village, 6961
Clark Memorial Hospital: RehabCare Unit, 6318
Clark-Winchcole Foundation, 3009
Clarke Healthcare Products, Inc., 143
Clarkston Spec Healthcare Center, 6989
Classification of Impaired Vision, 9157
Classique, 346
Classroom GOALS: Guide for Optimizing Auditory Learning Skills, 1978
Classroom Notetaker: How to Organize a Program Serving Students with Hearing Impairments, 1979
Clausen House, 6576
Clay Tree Society, 806
Clearbrook, 6009
Clearinghouse for Specialized Media and Translations, 4767
Clearinghouse on Disability Information: Office Special Education & Rehabilitative Service, 8887
Clearview-Brain Injury Center, 7414
Clearway, 347
Cleft Palate-Craniofacial Journal, 8842
Clement J Zablocki VA Medical Center, 5859
Cleveland Clinic, 7361
Cleveland FES Center, 4982
Cleveland Foundation, 3197
Cleveland Public Library, 4983
Cleveland Regional Office, 5796
Cleveland Sight Center, 7082, 1336, 9115
Client Assistance Program (CAP), 3554
Client Assistance Program: Alabama, 3421
Client Assistance Program: Alaska, 3430
Client Assistance Program: California, 3462
Clinch Independent Living Services, 4605
Clinical Alzheimer Rehabilitation, 2411
Clinical Applications of Music Therapy in Developmental Disability, Pediatrics and Neurolog, 15
Clinical Connection, 2256
Clinical Management of Childhood Stuttering, 2nd Edition, 2412
Clinician's Practical Guide to Attention-Deficit/Hyperactivity Disorder, 5370
Clinton County Rehabilitation Center, 6822
Clip Board Notebook, 582
Clipper Ship Foundation, 3029
Clock, 1726
Clockworks, 5413
Close Encounters of the Disabling Kind, 5414
Close-Up 6.5, 1563
Closed Caption Decoder, 181
Closing the Gap, 5144, 7681
Closing the Gap's Annual Conference, 1903
Clove Lakes Health Care and Rehabilitation Center, 7333
Clover Patch Camp, 1288
Clovernook Center for the Blind and Visually Impaired, 9049
Clovernook Printing House, The Clovernook Center for the Blind and Visually Impaired, 9050
CNS Camp New Connections, 7896, 8942
Co: Writer, 1826
Coalition for Health Funding, 807
Coalition for Independence, 4219

Coalition for Independence: Missouri Branc h Office, 4369
Coalition for Independent Living Options: Okeechobee, 4110
Coalition for Independent Living Options: Fort Pierce, 4111
Coalition for Independent Living Options, 4112
Coalition for Independent Living Options: Stuart, 4113
Coalition for the Education of Disabled Children, 5173
Coast to Coast Home Medical, 264, 264
Coatesville VA Medical Center, 5809
Cobb Hospital and Medical Center: Rehab Ca re Center, 6303
Cochlear, 288
Cochlear Implant Camp, 1058, 8196
Cochlear Implants for Kids, 8224
Cochlear Implants In Children: Ethics and Choices, 8305
Cockrell Foundation, 3284
COEA The Arc of East Ascension, 6058
Coelho Epilepsy Youth Summer Camp, 1031
Coeta and Donald Barker Foundation, 2823
Coffee County Training Center, 5871
Coffee in the Cereal: The First Year with Multiple Sclerosis, 8700
Cognition, Education and Deafness: Directi ons for Research and Instruction, 8225
Cognitive Approaches to Learning Disabilities, 2413
Cognitive Behavioral Therapy for Adult Asperger Syndrome, 7978, 8966
Cognitive Neuroscience Society, 7859
Cognitive Science Society, 7860
Cognitive Science Student Association, 7861
Cognitive Solutions Learning Center, 2673
Cognitive Strategy Instruction That Really Improves Children's Academic Skills, 2414
Cognitive Therapy Today, 8063
Cogrehab, 8094
Coleman Tri- County Services, 4157
Collaborating for Comprehensive Services for Young Children and Families, 2415
Collaborative Teams for Students with Severe Disabilities, 2416
College and University, 2257
College and University Programs for Deaf and Hard of Hearing Students, 8226
The College at Brockport, State Univ of New York, 1270
College Board, 2117
College Internship Program at the Berkshire Center, 6962
College of Optometrists in Vision Development, 9051
College of Syntonic Optometry, 9052
College Student's Guide to Merit and Other No-Need Funding, 3353
Colleton Regional Hospital: RehabCare Unit, 6427
Colmery-O'Neil VA Medical Center, 5707
Colon & Rectal Cancer: A Comprehensive Guide for Patients & Families, 8701
Colon Health: Key to a Vibrant Life, 8702
Colonial Life and Accident Insurance Company Contributions Program, 3264
Colonial Manor Medical And Rehabilitation Center, 7207
Colonial Manor Medical and Rehabilitation Center, 7415
Colorado Assoc of Homes and Services for the Aging, 7759, 7761
Colorado Association of Homes and Services for the Aging, 7539
Colorado Civil Rights Divsion, 5944
Colorado Department of Aging & Adult Servi ces, 3471
Colorado Department of Education, 2182
Colorado Department of Education: Special Education Service Unit, 2182
Colorado Developmental Disabilities Council, 3472
Colorado Division of Mental Health, 3473
Colorado Health Care Program for Children with Special Needs, 3474
Colorado Lions Camp, 1059
Colorado Springs Independence Center, 4070
Colorado Talking Book Library, 4780
Colorado/Wyoming VA Medical Center, 5664
Colton-Redlands-Yucaipa Regional Occupational Program (CRY-ROP), 5915
Columbia Disability Action Center, 4542
Columbia Foundation, 3010
Columbia Gas of Pennsylvania Corporate Giv ing, 3231
Columbia Lighthouse for the Blind, 9053, 1074, 9110, 9308
Columbia Medical Center: Peninsula, 6742
Columbia Regional Hospital: RehabCare Unit, 6363
Columbia Regional Office, 5822
Columbus Foundation and Affiliated Organizations, 3198
Columbus Health and Rehabilitation Center, 7277
Columbus McKinnon Corporation, 348
Columbus Mckinnon Corporation, 348
Columbus Rehab & Subactute, 6391
Columbus Rehabilitation And Subacute Institute, 7362
Columbus Speech and Hearing Center, 7083
Columbus Subregional Library For The Blind And Physically Handicapped, 4816
COM Hand Control, 78
Combination File/Reference Carousel, 518
Come Sign with Us, 8227
Committee for Purchase from People Who Are Blind or Severely Disabled, 3385
Commode, 144
Common ADA Errors and Omissions in New Construction and Alterations, 4678
Commonly Asked Questions About Child Care Centers and the Americans with Disabilities Act, 4679
Commonly Asked Questions About the ADA and Law Enforcement, 4681
Commonly Asked Questions About Title III of the ADA, 4680
Commonpoint Queens, 1268, 1299
Commonwealth Fund, 3123
Communi Care Health Services, 7084
CommuniCare of Clifton Nursing and Rehabilitation Center, 7084
Communicating with Parents of Exceptional Children, 2417
Communicating with People Who Have Trouble Hearing & Seeing: A Primer, 7809
Communication & Language Acquisition: Discoveries from Atypical Development, 2418
Communication Aids for Children and Adults, 420
Communication Center/Minnesota State Services for the Blind, 4927
Communication Development and Disorders in African American Children, 8967
Communication Development in Children with Down Syndrome, 7979, 8968
Communication Disorders Quarterly, 2258
Communication Outlook, 9003
Communication Outlook: Artificial Language Laboratory, 7682
Communication Service for the Deaf, 8134
Communication Service for the Deaf: Rapid City, 4549
Communication Skills for Visually Impaired Learners, 9158
Communication Skills for Working with Elders, 2419
Communication Unbound, 2420
Communicologist, 9009
Communique, 8306
Communitas Supportive Care Society, 808
Communities Actively Living Independent and Free, 4021
Communities Foundation of Texas, 3285
Community Access Center, 4022
Community Access Center: Indio Branch, 4023
Community Access Center: Perris, 4024
Community Connection, 9297
Community Connections of Southwest Michigan, 4319
Community Disability Services: An Evidence -Based Approach to Practice, 5072
Community Employment Services, 5916
Community Exploration, 1827
Community Foundation for Greater Buffalo, 3124
Community Foundation for Greater Atlanta, 2929
Community Foundation of Boone County, 2985
Community Foundation of Champaign County, 2954
Community Foundation of Greater Chattanooga, 3273
Community Foundation of Herkimer & Oneida Counties, 3125
Community Foundation of Monroe County, 3043
Community Foundation of New Jersey, 3095
Community Foundation of North Central Washington, 3326
Community Foundation of North Texas, 3286
Community Foundation of Richmond & Central Virginia, 3318
Community Foundation of Shreveport-Bossier, 2998
Community Foundation of Southeastern Connecticut, 2884
Community Foundation of the Capitol Region, 3126
Community Foundation of Western Massachusetts, 3030
Community Gatepath, 6577
Community Health Funding Report, 3354
Community Health Network, 6872
Community Hospital and Rehabilitation Center of Los Gatos-Saratoga, 6578
Community Hospital Back and Conditioning Clinic, 6679
Community Hospital of Los Gatos Rehabilitation Services, 6244
Community Outreach Program for the Deaf, 3988
Community Rehabilitation Services, 4025
Community Residential Alternative, 4157
Community Residential Care Association of CA, 5071
Community Resource Directory, 2125
Community Resources for Independence, 4513
Community Resources for Independence, Inc., Bradford, 4514
Community Resources for Independence: Lewistown, 4515
Community Resources for Independence: Mendocino/Lake Branch, 4026
Community Resources for Independence: Alto ona, 4516
Community Resources for Independence: Clar ion, 4517
Community Resources for Independence: Clea rfield, 4518
Community Resources for Independence: Herm itage, 4519
Community Resources for Independence: Lewi sburg, 4520
Community Resources for Independence: Napa, 4027
Community Resources for Independence: Oil City, 4521
Community Resources for Independence: Warr en, 4522
Community Resources for Independence: Well sboro, 4523
Community Resources for Independent Living: Hayward, 4028
Community Resources for Independent Living, 4029
Community Services for the Blind and Partially Sighted Store: Sight Connection, 1980
Community Services for the Blind and Parti ally Sighted Store: Sight Connection, 4624
Community Signs, 1981
Community Skills: Learning to Function in Your Neighborhood, 1727
Community Supports for People with Disabilities (CSP), 2210
Community Systems Inc., 6708

Commuter & Kid's Commuter, 698
Companion Activities, 1728
Compass Health, 265
Compass Learning, 1712, 1726, 1762, 1787, 1799, 1800, 1801, 1805, 1827, 1833, 1857, 1858, 1859
Compassionate Friends, The, 8888
Complementary Alternative Medicine and Mul tiple Sclerosis, 8703
Complete Armchair Fitness, 8433
The Complete Guide to Creating a Special Needs Life Plan, 5332
Complete Handbook of Children's Reading Disorders: You Can Prevent or Correct LDs, 2421
Complete IEP Guide: How to Advocate for Yo ur Special Ed Child (8th Edition), 5051, 5352
Complete Learning Disabilities Resource Gu ide, 2126
Complete Mental Health Resource Guide, 2127
Complete Resource Guide for Pediatric Diso rders, 2128
Complete Resource Guide for People with Ch ronic Illness, 2129
Complying with the Americans with Disabili s Act, 4682
Comprecare Foundation, 2877
Comprehensive Assessment of Spoken Language (CASL), 1982
Comprehensive Care Coordination for Chroni cally Ill Adults, 5073
Comprehensive Examination of Barriers to Employment Among Persons who are Blind or Impaire, 9159
Comprehensive Guide to ADD in Adults: Research, Diagnosis & Treatment, 7980
Comprehensive Pain Management Associates, 7064
Comprehensive Reference Manual for Signers and Interpreters, 8228
Comprehensive Rehabilitation Center at Lee Memorial Hospital, 6728
Comprehensive Rehabilitation Center of Naples Community Hospital, 6729
Comprehensive Signed English Dictionary, 8229
Compuserve: Handicapped Users' Database, 1617
Computer Access Center, 1618
Computer Access/Computer Learning, 2422
Computer Center for Visually Impaired People: Division of Continuing Studies, 1619
Computer Resources for People with Disabilities, 1620
Computer Workstation and Activity Table, 519
Computer-Enabling Drafting for People with Physical Disabilities, 1621
Computerized Speech Lab, 1681
Comsearch: Broad Topics, 3127
Concentra, 6197
Concentration Cockpit: Explaining Attention Deficits, 7981
Concentration Video, 8083
Concepts on the Move Advanced Overlay CD, 1564
Concepts on the Move Advanced Preacademics, 1729
Concepts on the Move Basic Overlay CD, 1565
Conditional Love: Parents' Attitudes Toward Handicapped Children, 5294
Cond, Nast, 7741
Conference of Educational Administrators o f Schools and Programs for the Deaf, 8135
Conference of the Association on Higher Education & Disability (AHEAD), 1904, 5145
Confidence Learning Center, 1202
Conklin Center for the Blind, 6730
Connect, 9010
Connect - Commmunity News, 8307
Connect Hearing, 421
Connecticut Board of Education and Service for the Blind, 3479
Connecticut Braille Association, 4782
Connecticut Burns Care Foundation, 1062
Connecticut Commission on Aging, 3480
Connecticut Department of Children and Youth Services, 3481
Connecticut Department of Education: Bureau of Special Education, 2183
Connecticut Department of Labor, 5958
Connecticut Developmental Disabilities Council, 3482
Connecticut Governor's Committee on Employment of People with Disabilities, 5958
Connecticut Library for the Blind and Phys ically Handicapped, 4783
Connecticut Mutual Life Foundation, 2885
Connecticut Office of Protection and Advocacy for Persons with Disabilities, 3483
Connecticut State Government, 4784
Connecticut State Independent Living Council, 4083
Connecticut State Library, 4784
Connecticut Subacute Corporation, 6696
Connecticut Tech Act Project: Connecticut Department of Social Services, 4785
Connections for Independent Living, 4071
Connelly Foundation, 3232
Conover Company, 1863, 1865
Conquering the Darkness: One Story of Recovering from a Brain Injury, 8704
Conrad N Hilton Foundation, 2824
Conscious Choice, 7683
Conscious Communications, 7683
Consortium of Multiple Sclerosis Centers, 8351
Constellations, 5146
Consulting Psychologists Press, 2423
Consumer and Patient Information Hotline, 9362
Consumer Care Products, 231
Consumer Care Products, LLC, 621, 628
Consumer's Guide to Home Adaptation, 1944
Contemporary Art Therapy with Adolescents, 16
Contemporary Gerontology, 7684
Continucare, A Service of the Rehab Institute of Chicago, 6823
Continuing Care, 2259
Continuing Education & Employment Developm ent Program, 5917
Contra Costa ARC, 6579
Contrasting Characteristics of Blind and Visually Impaired Clients, 9160
Convaid, 665, 699, 222, 543
Conversational Sign Language II: An Interm ediate Advanced Manual, 8230
Conversations, 1828
Convert-Able Table, 212
Convert-O-Bike, 5556
Cooking Class: Learning About Food Preparation, 1730
Cooper Foundation, 3081
Coordinacion De Servicios Centrado En La Familia, 5295
Coping and Caring: Living with Alzheimer's Disease, 7634
Coping for Kids Who Stutter, 8969
Coping with ADD/ADHD, 7982
Coping with Cancer Magazine, 8845
Coping with Cerebral Palsy, 8705
Coping+Plus: Dimensions of Disability, 5147
Cora Hoffman Center Day Program, 7052
Corcoran Physical Therapy, 6809
Cordless Big Red Switch, 471
Cordless Receiver, 309
Cordova Rehabilitation and Nursing Center, 7380
CORE Health Care, 7154
Core-Reading and Vocabulary Development, 1829
Corflex Inc., 234
Cornelia de Lange Syndrome Foundation, 2886
Cornell Communications, 182
Cornell University, ILR School, 833
Cornerstone Services, 6010, 8889
Cornucopia Software, 1861
Corona Regional Medical Center- Rehabiltation Center, 6580
Corporate Giving Program, 3011
Corporate Office, 6390
Corwin Press Inc., 2634
Cottage Health System, 6603
Cottage Rehabilitation Hospital, 2737
Cotton Full-Back Vest, 1514
Cotton/Poly House Dress, 1515
Council for Children with Behavioral Disorders (CCBD), 2082
Council for Disability Rights, 5134
Council for Educational Diagnostic Services (CEDS), 2083
Council for Exceptional Children, 2090, 2250, 2251, 2268, 2306, 2344, 2345, 2475, 2478, 2592, 2646, 2689, 5021, 7660
Council for Exceptional Children (CEC), 809, 2084, 5021, 2080, 2082, 2083, 2087, 2088, 2091, 2092, 2093, 2094, 2095, 2096, 2097, 2098, 2102, 2119, 2121
Council for Exceptional Children Annual Convention and Expo, 1905
Council News, 5148
Council of Administrators of Special Education (CASE), 2085
Council of American Instructors of the Dea f (CAID), 8136
Council of B BB s Foundation, 1938
Council of Colleges of Acupuncture & Orien tal Medicine, 810
Council of Parent Attorneys and Advocates (COPAA), 811
Council of State Administrators of Vocational Rehabilitation (CSAVR), 812
Council on Quality and Leadership, 1901
Counseling & Values, 2260
Counseling in Terminal Care & Bereavement, 5149
Counseling in the Rehabilitation Process, 2425
Counseling Parents of Children with Chronic Illness or Disability, 5371
Counseling Persons with Communication Disorders and Their Families, 2424
Counseling Psychologist, 2261
Counseling Today, 2310
Counselor Education & Supervision, 2262
Count Us In, 7983
Country Gardens Skilled Nursing and Rehabilitation Center, 7306
Country Manor Rehabilitation and Nursing C enter, 7307
County College of Morris, 1621
County of Santa Clara, 6263
Courage Center, 4343
Courage Kenny Rehabilitation Institute, 2738
Courageous Acres, 1334
Courageous Community Services, 1334
Courier Travel, 5608
Court-Related Needs of the Elderly and Persons with Disabilities, 4683
Covenant Health, 6435
Covenant Health Systems Owens White Outpatient Rehab Center, 6442
Covenant Healthcare Rehabilitation Program, 6357
Cowan Slavin Foundation, 3044
Cowley County Developmental Services, 4220
CPATH Cerebral Palsy Awareness Transition Hope, 8482
CQL Accreditation, 1901
Craig Hospital, 6273
CranstonArc, 3255
CRC Press, 2578
CreateSpace, an Amazon Company, 5359
Creating Memories, 1360
Creating Memories for Disabled Children, 1360
Creating Options for Family Recovery: A Pr ovider's Guide to Promoting Parental Mental Health, 5372
Creating Positive Classroom Environments: Strategies for Behavior Management, 2426
Creating Wholeness: Self-Healing Workbook Using Dynamic Relaxation, Images and Thoughts, 5150
Creative Arts Resources Catalog, 17
Creative Arts Therapy Catalogs, 1983
Creative Designs, 1516
Creative Growth Art Center, 18
The Creative Mobility Group, LLC, 5627
Creative Work Systems, 6064
Creativity Explored, 19
Crescent Porter Hale Foundation, 2825
CrescentCare Legal Services, 4654
Crestwood Communication Aids, 420
Crestwood Nursing & Rehabilitation Center, 7325

CREVT: Comprehensive Receptive and Expressive Vocabulary Test, 2666
Criminal Law Handbook on Psychiatric & Psychological Evidence & Testimony, 4684
Cristine M. Trahms Program for Phenylketonuria, 2427
Cristo Rey Handicappers Program, 4320
Cristo Vive International: Idaho Camp, 1107
Cristo Vive International: Minnesota Camp, 1213
Cristo Vive International: Texas Camp Conr oe, 1446
Cristo Vive International: Texas Camp Rio Grande Valley, 1447
Critical Air Medicine, 6581
Critical Voices on Special Education: Prob lems & Progress Concerning the Mildly Handicapped, 2428
Crockett Resource Center for Independent Living, 4568
Crosslands Rehabilitation and Healthcare Center, 7392
Crossroads Industrial Services, 6873
Crossroads of Western Iowa, 6881
Crown Publishing Company (Random House), 8004
Cruiser Bus Buggy 4MB, 543
Crutcher's Serenity House, 6582
Crutches, 610
CT Assoc of Not-for-Profit Providers of the Aging, 7760
Cullen Foundation, 3287
Cultural Diversity, Families and the Special Education System, 2429
Culture, 5197
Culture and the Restructuring of Community Mental Health, 7984
Cunard Line, 5609
Curb-Sider, 349
Curb-Sider Super XL, 350
Cure SMA, 8352, 8352
CurePSP Magazine, 8419, 8846
Curing MS: How Science is Solving the Myst eries of Multiple Sclerosis, 8706
Curriculum Decision Making for Students with Severe Handicaps, 2430
Cursive Writing Skills, 1984
Curtis & Doris K Hankamer Foundation, 3288
Curtis Instruments, Inc., 648
Custom, 666
Custom Durable, 667
Custom Earmolds, 289
Custom Lift Residential Elevators, 351
Customer Service Center, 6218, 6219
CV Mosby Company, 2321
CW Resources, 5957
Cypress Pointe Rehabilitation and Healthca re Center, 7346
Cystic Fibrosis Foundation, 3012
Cystic Fibrosis: Medical Care, 5373
Cystic Fibrosis: A Guide for Patient and F amily, 8707

D

D AR S, 3883
D C General Hospital, 3495
Da Capo Press, 8387, 8390
Da Capo Press/ Perseus Books Group, 5067
DA Schulman, 637
Dade County Talking Book Library, 4797
Daimler Chrysler, 3045
Dakota Center for Independent Living: Dickinson, 4481
Dakota Center for Independent Living: Bism arck, 4482
Dallas Academy, 1448, 7916
Dallas Foundation, 3289
Dallas Services, 7156
Damaco, 711
Damaco D90, 711
Daman Villa, 7157
DAMAR Services, 4195
Damon Runyon Cancer Research Foundation, 5498
Dana Alliance for Brain Initiatives, 3129
Dana Foundation, 3129
Dancing Cheek to Cheek, 9161
Dancing from the Inside Out, 20
Daniel Freeman Rehabilitation Centers, 6583
Daniels and Fisher Tower, 2876
Danmar Products, 422
Danville Centre for Health and Rehabilitat ion, 7289
DARCI, 1871
Darci Too, 1566
Darden Rehabilitation Center, 6495
Datahr Rehabilitation Institute, 6697
Daughters of Miriam Center/The Gallen Institute, 7035
DAV Department of Alaska, 5642
David and Lucile Packard Foundation, 2826
David D & Nona S Payne Foundation, 3290
David Fulton Publishers (Routledge), 2633
David J Green Foundation, 3130
Davidson College, 2771
Davidson College, Office of Study Abroad, 2771
The Davis Center, 945, 8174, 8940
Davis Center for Rehabilitation Baptist Hospital of Miami, 6731
DAWN Center for Independent Living, 4413
Dawn Enterprises, 4142
DawnSign Press, 8220, 8260, 8329
Dayle McIntosh Center: Laguna Niguel, 4031
DAYS: Depression and Anxiety in Youth Scale, 2674
Dayspring Associates, Inc., 423
Dayton VA Medical Center, 5797
Dazor Lighting Technology, 473, 596, 604
DBTAC-Great Lakes ADA Center, 6310
DD Center/St Lukes: Roosevelt Hospital Center, 4448
DDDS/Georgetown Center, 6709
DE French Foundation, 3128
Deaf Action Center Of Greater New Orleans, 6920
Deaf Camps, Inc., 1171
Deaf Catholic, 8308
Deaf Children Signers, 5415
Deaf Culture Series, 5416
Deaf Empowerment: Emergence, Struggle and Rhetoric, 8231
Deaf History Unveiled: Interpretations from the New Scholarship, 8232
Deaf in America: Voices from a Culture, 8235
Deaf Kid's Kamp, 8197
Deaf Like Me, 8233
Deaf Mosaic, 5417
Deaf Parents and Their Hearing Children, 8234
Deaf REACH, 8137
Deaf West Theatre, 21
Deaf Women United, 8138
Deaf-Blind American, 7815
Deaf-Blind Division of the Ntn'l Fed of the Blind, 7797, 9281
Deaf-Blind Perspective, 7821, 9299
DeafBlind Division of the National Federat ion of the Blind, 9054
Deafness and Communicative Disorders Branch of Rehab Services Administration Office, 8919
Deafness Research Foundation, 8139, 8299
Dean A McGee Eye Institute, 7112
Deciphering the System: A Guide for Families of Young Disabled Children, 2431
DecisionHealth, 7772
Defining Rehabilitation Agency Types, 2432
Delano Regional Medical Center, 6584
Delaware Assistive Technology Initiative (DATI), 4788
Delaware Assistive Technology Initiative (DATI), 3485
Delaware Association for the Blind, 6710
Delaware Client Assistance Program, 3486
Delaware Department of Health and Social Services, 3487
Delaware Department of Labor, 5963
Delaware Department of Public Instructing, 3488
Delaware Developmental Disability Council, 3489
Delaware Division for the Visually Impaire d, 3490
Delaware Division of Vocational Rehabilita tion, 5963
Delaware Library for the Blind and Physically Handicapped, 4789
Delaware Protection & Advocacy for Persons with Disabilities, 3491
Delaware VA Regional Office, 5671
Delaware Veterans Center, 6711
Delaware Workers Compensation Board, 3492
Delmar Cengage Learning, 8751
Delta Center, 6824
Delta Center for Independent Living, 4370
Delta Resource Center for Independent Living, 3994
Delta Society National Service Dog Center, 495
Deluxe Bath Bench with Adjustable Legs, 145
Deluxe Convertible Exercise Staircase, 352
Deluxe Corporation, 3060
Deluxe Corporation Foundation, 3060
Deluxe Nova Wheeled Walker & Avant Wheeled Walker, 611
Deluxe Roller Knife, 310
Deluxe Signature Guide, 583
Deluxe Sock and Stocking Aid, 252
Deluxe Standard Wood Cane, 612
Demand Response Transportation Through a Rural ILC, 5152
Dementia and Geriatric Cognitive Disorders, 7685
Dementia Society of America, 7862
Demos Health Publishing, 5123
Demos Medical Publishing, 5198, 8115, 8678, 8703, 8714, 8715, 8719, 8737, 8764, 8765, 8766, 8767, 8769
Demystifying Job Development: Field-Based Approaches to Job Development for the Disabled, 5390
Den-Mar Rehabilitation and Nursing Center, 7298
Dennis Developmental Center, 2676
Dental Amalgam Syndrome (DAMS) Newsletter, 4768
Denver CIL, 4072
Denver Foundation, 2878
Denver VA Medical Center, 5665
Department for Children & Families, 6052
Department Human Services, 3721
Department of Heath Education, 3745
Department of Aging and Independent Living, 4596
Department of Behavioral Healthcare, Developmental Disabilities and Hospitals, 3827
Department of Blind Rehabilitation, 3630
Department of Economic Security, 5903
Department of Education, 2185, 3692, 3705, 4929, 6110
Department of Elementary & Secondary Education, 6104
Department of Employment & Training, 6084
Department of Health, 3537
Department of Health & Human Services, 6088, 6091
Department of Health & Rehabilitative Services, 3508
Department Of Health & Social Services - Division Of Behaviorial Health, 3431
Department Of Health and Human Services, 3450
Department of Health and Human Services, 3690, 3706, 6161
Department of Housing & Urban Development (HUD), 5195
Department of Human Rights, 3575
Department of Human Services, 3448, 4158, 4161, 6136, 6180, 6191
Department of Insurance/OSFM, 1928
Department of Justice ADA Mediation Program, 4685
Department of Labor, 3799, 3918
Department of Labor & Workforce Development, 3436, 5894
Department of Labor and Employment, 5946
Department of Labor and Industrial Realtions, 3673
Department of Labor and Workforce Development, 6137
Department of Labor, Licensing & Regulation, 6077
Department of Medicine and Surgery Veterans Administration, 5630

Department Of Ophthalmalogy, 4810
Department of Ophthalmology and Visual Science, 4833
Department of Ophthalmology Information Line, 9363
Department of Pennsylvania, 3819
Department of Physical Medicine & Rehabilitation at Sinai Hospital, 813
Department of Physical Medicine and Rehabilitation, 7026
Department of Public Health & Human Services, 6106
Department of Public Health Human Services, 2214
Department of Public Instruction: Exceptional Children & Special Programs Division, 2185
Department of Rehabilitation Services, 5955
Department of Rehabilitation Services & Bureau of Education And Services for the Blind, 2184
Department of Services for the Blind, 6216
Department of Services for the Blind (DSB), 6217
Department of Social & Health Services: Division of Vocational Rehabilitation, 6218
Department of Social & Health Services: Developmental Disabilities Administration (DDA), 6219
Department of Social Services, 3603
Department of Veteran s Affairs, 5656
Department of Veterans Affairs, 5714, 5833
Department of Veterans Affairs Vet Center #418, 6874
Department of Veterans Affairs of Washington DC, 6538
Department of Veterans Affairs Regional Office - Vocational Rehab Division, 5631
Department of Veterans Benefits, 5632
Department of Workforce Development: Vocational Rehabilitation, 6223
Department of Workforce Services: Vocational Rehabilitation, 6224
Depression and Bipolar Support Alliance, 7863
Dept of Labor & Workforce Development, 3866
Des Moines Division-VA Central Iowa Health Care System, 6882
Des Moines VA Medical Center, 5702
Des Moines VA Regional Office, 5703
Descriptive Language Arts Development, 1812
Desert Area Resources and Training, 6589
Desert Blind & Handicapped Association, 9055
Desert Blind and Handicapped Association, Inc., 9055
Desert Haven Enterprises, 5918
Desert Life Rehabilitation & Care Center, 6516, 7212
Desert Regional Medical Center, 6585
Design for Acessibility, 1945
Designing and Using Assistive Technology: The Human Perspective, 2433
Designs for Comfort, 1524
Desk-Top Talking Calculator, 520
Detroit Center for Independent Living, 4321
DEUCE Environmental Control Unit, 472
Deutsch Foundation, 2827
Developing Cross-Cultural Competence:Guide to Working with Young Children & Their Families, 2434
Developing Individualized Family Support Plans: A Training Manual, 2435
Developing Organized Coalitions and Strategic Plans, 5153
Developing Personal Safety Skills in Children with Disabilities, 5296
Developing Staff Competencies for Supporting People with Disabilities, 2436
Development of Language, 2437
Development of Social Skills by Blind and Visually Impaired Students, 9162
Developmental Disabilities Council, 1623
Developmental Disabilities in Infancy and Childhood, 5297
Developmental Disabilities of Learning, 2438
Developmental Disabilities Planning Council, 6319
Developmental Disabilities Resource Center (DDRC), 5945
Developmental Disabilities: A Handbook for Occupational Therapists, 2439
Developmental Disabilities: A Handbook for Interdisciplinary Practice, 2440
Developmental Disability Council: Arizona, 3441
Developmental Disability Services Section, 3768
Developmental Evaluation and Adjustment Fa cilities, 4300
Developmental Medicine & Childhood Neurolo gy, 8843
Developmental Services Center, 2677
Developmental Services of Northwest Kansas, 6900
Developmental Variation and Learning Disorders, 2441
Devereax Foundation, 7167
Devereux Advanced Behavioral Health - Texas Victoria Campus, 7158
Devereux Advanced Behavioral Health Arizona - Scottsdale, 6517
Devereux Advanced Behavioral Health California, 6586
Devereux Advanced Behavioral Health Colorado, 6680
Devereux Advanced Behavioral Health Florida - Titusville Campus, 6732
Devereux Advanced Behavioral Health Georgia, 6790
Devereux Advanced Behavioral Health Massachusetts & Rhode Island, 6963
Devereux Advanced Behavioral Health - Florida, 6733
Devereux Advanced Behavioral Health - National Office, 7129
Devereux Advanced Behavioral Health Connecticut, 2755
Devereux Advanced Behavioral Health New Jersey, 7036
Devereux Advanced Behavioral Health New York, 7053
Devereux Advanced Behavioral Health Texas - League City Campus, 7159
Devereux Arizona - Tucson, 6518
Devereux Florida - Orlando Campus, 6734
Devereux Florida - Viera Campus, 6735
Devereux Florida Corporate Office, 6733
Devereux Foundation, 7151, 7153, 7157
Devereux Georgia Treatment Network, 6790
Devereux New Jersey, 7036
Devereux New York, 7053
Devereux Orlando Campus, 6734
Devereux Pennsylvania, 7130
Devereux School, 6963
Devereux Threshold Center for Autism, 6736
Devereux Viera Campus, 6735
Diabetes Camp, 8619
Diabetes Camping And Educational Services, Inc., 1003, 8561
Diabetes Dayton, 1326, 1333, 8584
Diabetes Network of East Hawaii, 3534
Diabetes Self-Management, 8861
Diabetes Society, 8614
Diabetes Solutions of Oklahoma, Inc., 1348
Diabetes Sourcebook., 8708
Diabetic Retinopathy, 9163
Diabetic Youth Families, 999, 8543
Diagnostic Report Writer, 1813
Dial Books, 9139
Dial-a-Hearing Screening Test, 8335
Dial: Disabled Information Awareness & Liv ing, 4414
Dialog Corporation, 1632
Dialogue Magazine, 9280
Dialysis at Sea Cruises, 5610
Dialysis Clinic, Inc., 1419
DiaMedica Inc., 5341
Dice: Jumbo Size, 5567
Dictionary of Congenital Malformations & Disorders, 5154
Dictionary of Developmental Disabilities Terminology, 5155, 5298
Didlake, 6211
Diestco Manufacturing Company, 652
Different Dream Parenting: A Practical Guide to Raising a Child with Special Needs, 5342
Different Roads to Learning, 1985
Difficult Child, 7985
Digest of Neurology and Psychiatry, 2442
Digestive Diseases & Disorders Sourcebook, 8709
Digi-Flex, 474
Digital Hearing Aids, 290
Digital Shifter, 81
Digital Talking Compass, 475
Dilemma, 1731
Dimensions of State Mental Health Policy, 4686
Dino-Games, 1732
Diocese of Maine Episcopal, 8180
DIRECT Center for Independence, 3989
Directions, 8862
Directions: Technology in Special Education, 1733
Directory for Exceptional Children, 2131
Directory of Accessible Building Products, 1946
Directory of Financial Aids for Women, 3355
Directory of Members, 5156
Directory Of Services For People With Disa bilities, 2130
DIRLINE, 1622
Disabilities Network of Eastern Connecticu t, 4084
Disabilities Rights Center, Inc, 3713
Disabilities Sourcebook, 424
Disability & Rehabilitation Journal, 5374
Disability & Society, 2263
Disability Action Center, 4543
Disability Action Center NW, 4143
Disability Action Center NW: Coeur D'Alene, 4144
Disability Action Center NW: Lewiston, 4145
Disability Advocates of Kent County, 4322
Disability Analysis Handbook: Tools for Independent Practice, 5375
Disability and Communication Access Board, 3535
Disability and Health Journal, 2265
Disability and Health: National Center for Birth Defects and Developmental Disabilities, 8891
Disability and Rehabilitation, 2445
Disability and Social Performance: Using Drama to Achieve Successful Acts, 22
Disability and Sport, 8391
Disability Awareness Guide, 5157
Disability Awareness Network, 4473
Disability Bookshop Catalog, 425
Disability Center for Independent Living, 4073
Disability Coalition of Northern Kentucky, 4266
Disability Compliance for Higher Education, 2311, 4687
Disability Connection, 4323
Disability Connections, 4128
disAbility Connections, 4340
Disability Culture Perspective on Early Intervention, 7986
Disability Determination Section, 3940
Disability Determination Service: Birmingham, 3422
Disability Determination Services, 3857, 6224, 6226
Disability Discrimination Law, Evidence an d Testimony, 4688
Disability Employment & Transitions, 6106
Disability Funders Network (DFN), 815
Disability Funding News, 2443, 3356
DisAbility Information and Resources, 5499
Disability Law Center, 3905
Disability Law Center of Alaska, 3434
Disability Law Colorado, 4656
Disability Law in the United States, 4689
Disability Law Project, 3906
DisAbility LINK, 814, 4127
Disability Matters, 1906
Disability Ministries at St. Augustine Parish, 1343
Disability Network, 8890
Disability Network of Mid-Michigan, 4325
Disability Network of Oakland & Macomb, 4326
Disability Network Southwest Michigan, 4324
Disability Network/Lakeshore, 4327
Disability Policy Consortium, 3867
Disability Pride Newsletter, 2312
Disability Rag's Ragged Edge Magazine, 7686
Disability Research and Dissemination Cent er, 816, 2086

Disability Resource Agency for Independent Living: Modesto, 4032
Disability Resource Association, 4371
Disability Resource Center, 4114, 4606
Disability Resource Center of Fairfield County, 4085
DisAbility Resource Center: Knoxville, 4557
DisAbility Resource Connection: Everett, 4625
Disability Resource Initiative, 4267
Disability Resources, 2313
Disability Resources Monthly, 2313
Disability Rights & Resources, 4474
Disability Rights Activist, 5500
Disability Rights Advocates, 4657
Disability Rights Bar Association (DBRA), 817
Disability Rights Center of Kansas, 3589
Disability Rights Education and Defense Fund, 4658
Disability Rights Education and Defense Fund, 4671, 4727, 5446, 7687
Disability Rights Florida, 818, 3509
Disability Rights International (DRI), 819
Disability Rights Louisiana, 820
Disability Rights Montana, 3675
Disability Rights Movement, 5158
Disability Rights New Jersey, 4415
Disability Rights Now, 7687
Disability Rights of Pennsylvania (DRP), 3815
Disability Rights Texas, 3868, 4659
Disability Rights Vermont, 3907
Disability Rights Wisconsin: Milwaukee Office, 3949
Disability Rights: Washington, 3929
Disability Services & Legal Center, 4033
Disability Services Division of Montana, 7022
disAbility Solutions for Independent Livin g, 4124
Disability Statistics Report, 7688
Disability Studies and the Inclusive Class room, 2444
Disability Studies Quarterly, 2264, 7689
Disability Under the Fair Employment & Housing Act: What You Should Know About the Law, 4690
Disability, Sport and Society, 2446
Disability:IN, 821
DisabilityAdvisor.com, 2154, 5501
DisabilityResources.org, 5502
Disabled & Alone/Life Services for the Handicapped, 5209, 5307
Disabled American Veterans, 5674
Disabled American Veterans Headquarters, 5633
Disabled American Veterans Magazines, 7690
Disabled American Veterans National Headquarters, 7690
Disabled American Veterans: Ocean County, 5764
Disabled and Alone: Life Services for the Handicapped, Inc., 828
Disabled Athlete Sports Association (DASA), 822
Disabled Businesspersons Association (DBA), 823
Disabled Children's Fund (DCF), 824
Disabled Drummers Association (DDA), 825
Disabled God: Toward a Liberatory Theology of Disability, 5358
Disabled In Action (DIA), 826
Disabled People as Second Class Citizens, 7691
Disabled People's International Fifth World Assembly as Reported by Two US Participants, 5159
Disabled Peoples' International (DPI), 827
Disabled Resource Services, 4074, 5151
Disabled Resources Center, 4034
Disabled Rights: American Disability Polic y and the Fight for Equality, 2447
Disabled Sports Program Center, 8444
Disabled Sports USA, 8445
Disabled Sports USA Far West, 8444
Disabled Sports, USA, 7680
Disabled Watersports Program, 8446
Disabled We Stand, 5160
Disabled, the Media, and the Information Age, 5161
Disbled Resource Services, 4075
Discount School Supply, 1986
Discover Technology, 5503
Discovery Camp, 1458
Discovery Day Camp, 1240
Discovery Education, 1691
Discovery House Publishers, 5342
Discovery Newsletter, 5162
Discrimination is Against the Law, 4691
Disorders of Motor Speech: Assessment, Treatment, and Clinical Characterization, 8970
District of Columbia Center for Independen t Living, 4094
District of Columbia Department of Employment Services, 5965
District of Columbia Department of Handicapped Children, 3495
District of Columbia General Hospital Physical Medicine & Rehab Services, 6718
The District of Columbia Office of Human Rights (OHR), 5970
District of Columbia Office on Aging, 3496
District of Columbia Public Library, 4791, 9290
District of Columbia Public Library: Services for the Deaf Community, 4791
District of Columbia Public Schools: Special Education Division, 2187
District of Columbia Regional Library for the Blind and Physically Handicapped, 4792
Diversified Opportunities, 7069
Diversity and Visual Impairment: The Influ ence of Race, Gender, Religion and Ethnicity, 9164
Divided Legacy: A History of the Schism in Medical Thought, The Bacteriological Era, 2448
Division for Communication, Language, and Deaf/Hard of Hearing (DCD), 2087
Division for Culturally and Linguistically Diverse Exceptional Learners (DDEL), 2088
Division for Early Childhood (DEC), 2089
Division for Early Childhood of the Counci l for Exceptional Children, 2090
Division for Learning Disabilities (DLD), 2091
Division for Physical, Health & Multiple Disabilities: Complex and Chronic Conditions, 2092
Division for Research (CEC-DR), 2093
Division for the Blind and Visually Impair ed, 6065
The Division for the Visually Impaired, 3494
Division of Birth Defects and Developmental Disabilities, 3522
Division of Blind Services, 6737
Division of Developmental Disabilities, 3716, 5900
Division of Disability Aging & Rehab Services, 1606
Division of Graham-Field, 430
Division of International Special Education and Services (DISES), 2094
Division of Labor and Management, 3849
Division of Mental Health and Substance Abuse, 3778
Division of Physical Medicine and Rehabilitation, 6587
Division of Rehabilitation, 6707
Division of Rehabilitation Services, 4129, 4158, 3524, 6952
Division of Rehabilitation Services (DORS), 6074
Division of Rehabilitation Services: Staff Library, 5036
Division of Rehabilitation-Education Services, University of Illinois, 6825
Division of Special Education, 3869
Division of Visual and Performing Arts Education (DARTS), 2095
Division of Vocational Rehabilitation, 5946, 6000
Division of Vocational Rehabilitation Department of Social and Health Services, 7189
Division of Vocational Rehabilitation Services (DVRS) Western Regional Office, 6157
Division of Vocational Rehabilitation (DVR), 3432
Division of Vocational Rehabilitation Serv ices (DVRS), 6158
Division of Workers Compensation, 3510
Division of Workers' Compensation Department of Labor & Employment, 3475
Division Of Workforce Solutions, 6156
Division on Autism and Developmental Disabilities (DADD), 2096
Division on Career Development and Transition (DCDT), 2097
Division on Deaf, DeafBlind & Hard of Hear ing, 6089
Division on Visual Impairments and Deafblindness (DVIDB), 2098
Dixie EMS, 389
DMC Health Care Center-Novi, 6990
DNA People's Legal Services, 4655
Do You Hear That?, 5418
Do You Remember the Color Blue: The Questi ons Children Ask About Blindness, 9165
Do-Able Renewable Home, 1947
Do2learn, 1987
DOCS: Developmental Observation Checklist System, 2675
Doctors Hospital, 7085
Dodd Hall at the Ohio State University Hospitals, 7086
Dogs for the Deaf, 8140, 8304
Doing Things Together, 5419
Dolfinger-McMahon Foundation, 3233
Dolphin Computer Access, 2155
Domestic Mistreatment of the Elderly: Towards Prevention, 7692
Dominoes with Raised Dots, 5568
Don Johnston, 521, 1988, 1723, 1750, 1790, 1807, 1808, 1814, 1822, 1826, 1836, 1845, 1848, 1851, 1852, 1877
Don't Call Me Special: A First Look at Dis ability, 5052
Don't Feel Sorry for Paul, 8114
Don't Lose Sight of Glaucoma, 9166
Donaldsville Area Arc, 6921
Door Knock Signaler, 476
Doorbell Signalers, 477
Dormakaba USA Inc., 478
Dothan Houston County Library System, 4744
Double H Ranch, 1289
Dover Rehabilitation and Living Center, 7322
Down Syndrome, 7987
Down Syndrome Camp, 1214
Down Syndrome Foundation, 1214
Down Syndrome News, 8064
Down Syndrome Society of Rhode Island, 3256
Doylestown Hospital Rehabilitation Center, 6413
DPS with BCP, 1811
Dr Scholl Foundation, 2955
Dr. Ida Rolf Institute (DIRI), 829
Dr. Karen H Chao Developmental Optometry Karen H. Chao. O.D., 6588
Dr. Moises Simpser VACC Camp, 1081, 8620
Dr. William O Benenson Rehabilitation Pavilion, 7334
Draft: Builder, 1814
Dragonfly Forest Summer Camp, 1388
DRAIL (Disability Resource Agency for Independent Living), 4030
Dream Oaks Camp, 1082
Dream Street, 1032, 8621
Dream Street Foundation, 2828, 1032, 8621
Dreamer, 1660
DREAMMS for Kids, 4956, 1733
Dresher Hill Health and Rehabilitation Cen ter, 7368
Dressing Stick, 253
Dressing Tips and Clothing Resources for Making Life Easier, 426
Drew Karol Industries, 266, 266
Drive DeVilbiss Healthcare, 213
Drive Master Company, 82, 86, 100, 116, 123
Driven to Distraction, 7988
Driving Systems Inc., 83
DRS Connection, 5151
DRTAC: Southeast ADA Center, 5092
DSHS/Aging & Adult Disability Services Administration, 3928
Dual Brake Control, 84
Dual Brush with Suction Base, 311
Dual Relationships in Counseling, 2449
Dual Security Bed Rail, 164
Dual Switch Latch and Timer, 479
Dual-Mode Charger, 638
Duane Morrs Llt, 3248

Duchenne Muscular Dystrophy, 8710
Duchossois Foundation, 2956
Duke Endowment, 3184
Duke Medical Center, 4976
Duke University Medical Center, 6389
Duluth Public Library, 4928
DuPage Center for Independent Living, 4159
Duplex Planet, 7693, 7693
Duracell & Rayovac Hearing Aid Batteries, 291
Duraline Medical Products Inc., 267, 267
Durham VA Medical Center, 5788
Duro-Med Industries, 268, 268
Dusters, 1517
Dutch Neck T-Shirt, 1518
Duxbury Braille Translator, 1598
Duxbury Systems, 1598
Duxbury Systems Incorporated, 1604
DVH Quarterly, 9298
Dvorak Raft Kayak & Fishing Expeditions, 5611
DW Auto & Home Mobility, 80
Dwight D Eisenhower VA Medical Center, 5708
Dyna Vox Technologies, 1682
Dynamic Dimensions, 5947
Dynamic Living, 5504
Dynamic Systems, Inc., 229, 229, 249
DynaVox Technologies Speech Communication Devices, 1682
Dyslexia over the Lifespan, 7989
Dyslexia Training Program, 1989
Dysphagia Research Society, 8920
Dyspraxia Foundation USA, 8103
Dystonia Advocacy Network, 8353

E

E VA S, 1688
E&J Health Care, 7154
E-Wheels Electric Senior Mobility Scooter, 544
Eagle Hill School, 1178
Eagle Hill School: Summer Program, 1178, 7917
Eagle Mount Bozeman, 1228
Eagle Pond Rehabilitation and Living Cente r, 6964
Eagle Sportschairs, LLC, 720
Eagle View Ranch, 1496
Ear Foundation, 8141
Ear, Nose, and Throat Disorders Sourcebook, 8711
Early Childhood Intervention Clearinghouse, 2266
Early Childhood Reporter, 2314
Early Childhood Services, 6589
Early Childhood Technical Assistance Center (ETCA), 830
Early Communication Skills for Children wi th Down Syndrome, 2450
Early Focus: Working with Young Children W ho Are Blind or Visually Impaired & Their Families, 9167
Early Games for Young Children, 1736
Early Intervention, 2266
Early Intervention: Implementing Child & Family Services for At-Risk Infants and Toddlers, 2451
Early Learning 1, 5569
Early Music Skills, 1737
EASE Program: Emergency Access Self Evalua tion, 8236
East Bay Community Foundation, 2829
East Jefferson General Hospital Rehab Center, 6922
East King County Office, 4623
East Los Angeles Doctors Hospital, 6590
East Orange Campus of the VA New Jersey Healthcare System, 5765
East Penn Manufacturing Company, 721, 721
Easter Seal Camp Wawbeek, 1488
Easter Seals, 7540
Eastern Blind Rehabilitation Center, 6698
Eastern Colorado Services for the Developm entally Disabled (ECSDD), 5948
Eastern Colorado Services for the Disabled, 3476
Eastern Idaho Regional Medical Center, 7260
Eastern Oregon Center for Independent Living, 4503
Eastern Shore Center for Independent Living, 4285
Eastern Shore Center for Independent Living, 5164
Eastern Washington University, 4677
Easterseals, 831, 8892, 5192, 5222, 5240, 7765, 7767
Easterseals Arkansas, 5907
Easterseals Camp, 1033
Easterseals Camp ASCCA, 977, 8623
Easterseals Camp Challenge, 1083
Easterseals Camp Fairlee, 1172
Easterseals Camp Harmon, 1034
Easterseals Camp Hemlocks, 1068
Easterseals Camp Stand by Me, 1480, 8379
Easterseals Central Alabama, 6496
Easterseals Central Illinois, 1125
Easterseals Central Texas, 3870
Easterseals Chicagoland & Greater Rockford, 1114
Easterseals Colorado, 1047
Easterseals Crossroads, 6320
Easterseals Delaware & Maryland's Eastern Shore, 6712
Easterseals Delaware & Maryland's Eastern Shore, 1172
Easterseals DuPage and Fox Valley, 6826
Easterseals East Georgia, 6791
Easterseals Eastern Pennsylvania, 1379
Easterseals Florida, 1083
Easterseals Gilchrist Marchman Child Devel opment Center, 6827
Easterseals Iowa, 6883, 1144
Easterseals Jayne Shover Center, 6828
Easterseals Joliet Region, 6829
Easterseals Midwest, 4372, 7013
Easterseals National, 7023
Easterseals Nebraska, 1234
Easterseals Nebraska Camp, 1234
Easterseals New Hampshire, 1244, 1246
Easterseals New Jersey, 6126, 1254
Easterseals New York, 3131
Easterseals North Texas, 3871
Easterseals Northeast Central Florida, 6738
Easterseals Northern California, 6591
Easterseals Northwest Alabama, 6497
Easterseals Oak Hill, 1068
Easterseals of Alabama, 5872
Easterseals of Mahoning, Trumbull and Colu mbiana Counties, 7087
Easterseals Oregon, 1361
Easterseals Oregon Summer Camp, 1361
Easterseals Project Action Consulting, 5591
Easterseals Rehabilitation Center, 6875
Easterseals South Florida, 6739
Easterseals Southern California, 1033
Easterseals Southwest Flordia, 6740
Easterseals Southwest Florida, 6741
Easterseals Superior California, 6592
Easterseals Tennessee, 1422
Easterseals Tennessee Camping Program, 1422
Easterseals UCP North Carolina & Virginia, 1467
Easterseals Washington, 1480, 8379
Easterseals West Alabama, 6498
Easterseals West Central Alabama Rehabilit ation Center, 6499
Easterseals Western & Central Pennsylvania, York, 1372
Easterseals Wisconsin, 1485, 1488, 1493
Easterseals-Goodwill Northern Rocky Mountain, 7023
Easterseals: Achievement Center, 5872
Easterseals: Arkansas, 6535
Easterseals: Opportunity Center, 5873
Eastside Rehabilitation and Living Center, 7299
Eastview Medical and Rehabilitation Center, 7416
Easy Access Travel, 5612
Easy Pivot Transfer Machine, 353
Easy Ply, 269
Easy Stand, 354
Easy Things to Make Things Simple: Do It Yourself Modifications for Disabled Persons, 5165
EasyStand 6000 Glider, 613
Eating Disorders Sourcebook., 8712
Eating Skills: Learning Basic Table Manners, 1738
Eating Well, 7694
Eating Well Magazine, 7694
Echo Grove Camp, 1196
ECHO Housing: Recommended Construction and Installation Standards, 1948
Ecology of Troubled Children, 2452
Economical Liberty, 355
Eden Autism, 6127
Edge, 668
Edgemoor Day Program, 6713
EDI Camp, 8622
Edison Sheltered Workshop, 6128
Edith Nourse Rogers Memorial Veterans Hospital, 5726
Edmonds Rehabilitation & Healthcare Center er, 7405
Edna McConnel Clark Foundation, 3132
Educating all Students in the Mainstream, 2457
Educating Children with Disabilities: A Transdisciplinary Approach, 2453
Educating Children with Multiple Disabilities: A Transdisciplinary Approach, 2454
Educating Inattentive Children, 8084
Educating Individuals with Disabilities: IDEIA 2004 and Beyond (1st Edition), 2455
Educating Students Who Have Visual Impairments with Other Disabilities, 2456
Education and Auditory Research Foundation, 3274
The Education of Children with Acquired Brain Injury, 2633
Education of the Handicapped: Laws, Legislative Histories and Administrative Document, 4692
Educational Activities, 1829
Educational Activities Software, 1694, 1700, 1731, 1747, 1812, 1828, 1831, 1843, 1849, 1867, 8082
Educational Audiology for the Limited Hearing Infant and Preschooler, 2458
Educational Care, 2459
Educational Equity Concepts, 2003, 2503, 5132
Educational Gerontology, 7695
Educational Intervention for the Student, 2460
Educational Issues Among Children with Spi na Bifida, 8713
Educational Media Corporation, 7997
Educational Prescriptions, 2461
Educational Productions, 5397, 5461, 5471
Educational Services for the Visually Impaired, 4759
Educational Software Institute, 1734
Educational Tutorial Consortium, 2067
Educators Publishing Service, 2007, 2020, 2032, 2036, 2042, 2367, 2441, 2459, 2461, 2495, 2560, 2562, 2664, 2699, 2700, 2701, 2702, 2703, 2710, 7204, 7981, 7989
Educators Resource Guide, 2132
Edward Hines Jr Hospital, 5694
The Edward J. Madden Open Hearts Camp, 1180, 8643
Edward John Noble Foundation, 3133
Edwin Mellen Press, 2485, 5321
Edyth Bush Charitable Foundation, 2918
Effective Instruction for Special Education, 2462
Effectively Educating Handicapped Students, 2463
Eggleston Services, 1472
EGW.com, 7752
Ehrman Medical Library, 4957
Eight CAP, Inc. Head Start, 6991
Ekso Bionics, 270
El Paso Lighthouse for the Blind, 7160
El Paso Natural Gas Foundation, 3291
El Paso VA Healthcare Center, 5834
El Pomar Foundation, 2879
El Valle Community Parent Resource Center, 3872
El Valor, 6830
EL Wiegand Foundation, 3085
Elan Stair Lift, 356
Elastic Shoelaces, 254
Elder Abuse and Mistreatment, 7635
Elder Visions Newsletter, 7763
ElderLawAnswers.com, 4693, 5506
Elderly Health Services Letter, 7696
Eleanora CU Alms Trust, 3199
Electric Can Opener & Knife Sharpener, 312
Electric Leg Bag Emptier and Tub Slide Shower Chair, 146
Electric Mobility Corporation, 545

Electro Kinetic Technologies, 542, 546, 550, 564, 574, 575, 710
Electronic Amplified Stethoscopes, 271
Electronic Courseware Systems, 1739, 1713, 1737, 1753, 1754, 1788
Electronic House, 1949
Electronic House: Enhanced Lifestyles with Electronics, 1949
Electronic Speech Assistance Devices, 1683
Elgin Training Center, 6831
Elite Curved Stair Lift, 357
Elite Stair Lift, 358
Elkhart Public Library for the Blind and Physically Handicapped, 4848
Elmhurst Hospital Center, 7054
Elsevier, 7673
Elsevier Health, 2253
Elsevier Inc, 8669
Elwyn, 832
Elwyn Delaware, 4790, 6714
Embracing the Monster: Overcoming the Cha llenges of Hidden Disabilities, 7990
Emerging Horizon, 2267
Emerging Leaders, 5420
Emory Autism Resource Center, 4817
Emory University, 4817
Emory University Laboratory for Ophthalmic Research, 4818
Emotional Problems of Childhood and Adolescence, 2464
Emotorsports, 525
Emphysema Foundation for Our Right to Survive, 8488
Employer Assistance and Resource Network on Disability Inclusion (EARN), 833
Employment Development Department, 5919, 3459
Employment Discrimination Based on Disability, 4694
Employment for Individuals with Asperger S yndrome or Non-Verbal Learning Disability, 8971
Employment Options Inc., 5372
Employment Resources Program, 1624
Employment Standards Administration Department of Labor (ESA), 4695
Empowering People's Independence (EPI), 1273, 1274
Enable America Inc., 834
Enabling & Empowering Families: Principles & Guidelines for Practice, 2465
Enabling Devices, 480, 5570
Enabling News, 7764
Enabling Romance: A Guide to Love, Sex & Relationships for the Disabled, 5166
Enabling Technologies Company, 1599
Enchanted Hills Camp for the Blind, 1035, 9114
Encounters with Autistic States, 7991, 8972
Encyclopedia of Basic Employment and Daily Living Skills, 1991
Encyclopedia of Blindness and Vision Impairment Second Edition, 9168
Encyclopedia of Deafness and Hearing Disorders, 8237
Encyclopedia of Disability, 5167
Encyclopedia of Genetic Disorders & Birth Defects, 5299
Endeavor Magazine, 7822, 8298
ENDependence Center of Northern Virginia, 4607
eNeuro, 7755
Enforcing the ADA: A Status Report from the Department of Justice, 4696
Englishton Park Academic Remediation, 7918
Englishton Park Presbyterian, 7918
Enhancer Cushion, 230
Enhancing Everyday Communication for Child ren with Disabilities, 5376
Enrichments Catalog, 427
EnTech: Enabling Technologies of Kentuckiana, 4867
Entervan, 85
Environmental Health Center: Dallas, 8489
Environmental Traveling Companions, 5613
ENVISION, 6901
EP Resource Guide, 5163
Epilepsy Council of Greater Cincinnati, 3786
Epilepsy Foundation, 7864, 8104, 8354, 8893, 4885, 8847
Epilepsy Foundation Arizona, 986, 7899
Epilepsy Foundation of Alabama, 8490
Epilepsy Foundation of America, 8420
Epilepsy Foundation of Long Island, 3134
Epilepsy Foundation Of Northern California, 1031
Epilepsy Foundation of Southeast Texas, 3292
Epilepsy Foundation Texas, 1433, 1441, 1450
Epilepsy Foundation: Central and South Texas, 3293
Epilepsy, 199 Answers: A Doctor Responds t o His Patients' Questions, 8714
Epilepsy: Patient and Family Guide, 8715
EpilepsyUSA, 8847
EpilepsyUSA Magazine, 8420
Episcopal Charities, 3135
Episcopal Church of Hawaii, 8628
Equal Access Center for Independence, 4608
Equal Opportunity Employment Commission, 3386
Equal Opportunity Publications, 5369, 7705
Equalizer 1000 Series, 639
Equalizer 5000 Home Gym, 640
Equals in Partnership: Basic Rights for Families of Children with Blindness, 9169
Equip for Equality, 3555
Equip for Equality - Carbondale Office, 3556
Equip for Equality - Moline Office, 3557
Equip for Equality - Springfield Office, 3558
Equipment Shop, 428
ERIC Clearinghouse on Disabilities and Gifted Education, 5505
Erie VA Medical Center, 5810
Erlanger Medical Center Baronness Campus, 7381
Ernest Health, 6463
Esalen Institute, 835
ESCIL Update Newsletter, 5164
ESI Master Resource Guide, 1734
ESpecial Needs, 1990
The Essential Brain Injury Guide (5th Edit ion), 5384
Essential First Steps for Parents of Child ren with Autism, 5343
Essential Medical Supply, Inc., 429
Essential Science Publishing, 8811
Esther A & Joseph Klingenstein Fund, 3136
Esu Memorial Union, 4863
Etac USA: F3 Wheelchair, 669
Ethical Issues In Home Health Care (2nd Edition), 5377
Ethnic Diseases Sourcebook, 8716
ETMC, 8629
Eugene and Agnes E Meyer Foundation, 2901
Eugene J Towbin Healthcare Center, 5647
Eunice Kennedy Shriver National Institute of Child Health and Human Development (NICHD), 8491
Europa Superior Folding Cane, 614
Eva L And Joseph M Bruening Foundation, 3200
Evac + Chair Emergency Evacuation Chair, 214
Evac + Chair North America LLC, 214
Evacu-Trac, 670
Evaluation and Educational Programming of Students with Deafblindness & Severe Disabilities, 2466
Evaluation and Treatment of the Psychogeriatric Patient, 2467
Evansville Association for the Blind, 6031
Evelyn and Walter Hans Jr, 2830
Evenston Community Foundation, 2957
Everest & Jennings, 430, 672
Evergreen Healthcare, 7203
Evergreen Woods Health and Rehabilitation Center, 7240
Evert Conner Rights & Resources CIL, 4209
Everybody Counts Center for Independent Living, 4196
EveryBody's Different: Understanding and Changing Our Reactions to Disabilities, 5168
Everybody's Guide to Homeopathic Medicines, 5169
Everyday Social Interaction: A Program for People with Disabilities, 5170
Everything Parent's Guide to Special Educa tion, 5053
Evio Plastics, 316
Exceed: A Division of Valley Resource Cent er, 6593
Exceptional Children (EC), 2268
Exceptional Children in Focus, 2468
Exceptional Education, 2025, 2026, 2027, 2028, 2564
Exceptional Lives: Special Education in T oday's Schools, 4th Edition, 2469
Exceptional Parent Library, 4711, 5163, 5326, 5329, 5331, 5435, 5453, 7983
Exceptional Parent Magazine, 5300
Exceptional Student in the Regular Classroom (6th Edition), 5353
Exceptional Teaching Inc, 1992, 1992
Exchange, 8421
Executive Office of Labor & Workforce Deve lopment, 6079
Executive Offices, 6181
Exeter Hospital, 7026
Expendicare, 7366
Experience Works, 7541
Experimental Aging Research, 7697
Explode the Code, 1993
Explore Your Options, 7636
Explorer's Club Camp, 1258
Explorer+ 4-Wheel Scooter, 546
Exploring Autism: A Look at the Genetics of Autism, 5507
Express Medical Supply, 431
Expressive and Receptive Fingerspelling fo r Hearing Adults, 8238
Expressive Arts for the Very Disabled and Handicapped of All Ages, 23
Exquisite Egronomic Protective Wear, 1519
Extendicare Health Services, Inc., 6485
Extensions for Independence, 522
Eye & Ear Infirmary, 9363
Eye and Your Vision, 9171
Eye Bank Association of America, 9056, 1907, 9307
Eye Bank Association of America Annual Meeting, 1907
Eye Foundation of Kansas City, 7019
Eye Institute of New Jersey, 4950
Eye Institute of the Medical College of Wisconsin and Froedtert Clinic, 5044
Eye Medical Center, 6594
Eye Medical Center of Fresno, 6594
Eye Relief Word Processing Software, 1872
Eye Research News, 9170
Eye-Centered: A Study of Spirituality of Deaf People, 8239
Eye-Q Test, 9172
Eyegaze Computer System, 1567
EZ Dot, 1815
EZ Healthcare, 261
EZ Keys, 1735
EZ Keys for Windows, 1816

F

Face First, 5421
Face of Inclusion, 5301
Facilitated Communication Institute, Syracuse Univ, 8085, 9018
Facilitating Self-Care Practices in the Elderly, 2470
Facts on File, 5299, 9168, 9243
Fair Employment Practice Agency: Arizona, 5901
Fair Housing and Equal Employment, 5990
Fair Housing Design Guide for Accessibility, 1950
Fairacres Manor, 7229
Fairbanks Memorial Hospital & Denali Center, 7211
Fairfax County Public Library, 5016
Fairfield Center for Disabilities and Cerebral Palsy, 4490
Fairlawn Rehabilitation Hospital, 6966
Fairway Golf Cars, 523
Fairway Spirit Adaptive Golf Car: Model 4852, 523

Faith Mission Home, 7181
Fall Fun, 1740
Falling in Old Age, 7637
Families Magazine, 5302
Families of Adults With Autism: Stories & Advice For the Next Generation, 7992
Families of Spinal Muscular Dystrophy, 8862
Families, Illness & Disability, 5303
Family Caregiver Alliance, 2831
Family Caregiver Alliance/National Center on Caregiving, 7542
Family Challenges: Parenting with a Disability, 5171
Family Circle, 7698
Family Context and Disability Culture Reframing: Through the Looking Glass, 9173
Family Counseling Center, 6832
Family Engagement, 2316
Family Guide to Vision Care (FG1), 9174
Family Guide: Growth & Development of the Partially Seeing Child, 9175
Family Intervention Guide to Mental Illness, 7638
Family Interventions Throughout Disability, 5304
Family Matters, 6833
Family Resource Associates, 4416, 5060
Family Resource Center on Disabilities, 836
Family Run Executive Director Leadership Association (FREDLA), 837
Family Service Society, 6923
Family Support Project for the Developmentally Disabled, 8894
Family Therapy for ADHD: Treating Children, Adolescents and Adults, 7993
Family Voices, 838, 964
Family-Centered Early Intervention with Infants and Toddlers, 2471
Family-Centered Service Coordination: A Manual for Parents, 5305
Family-Guided Activity-Based Intervention for Toddlers & Infants, 5422
Fanlight Productions, 24, 20, 69, 5056, 5118, 5280, 5333, 5398, 5399, 5407, 5410, 5411, 5421, 5428, 5431, 5434, 5443, 5445, 5449, 5450, 5451, 5454, 5467, 5470, 5472, 5474, 5475, 8492, 9016, 9020, 9247,
Fanlight Productions C/O Icarus Films, 8080, 8091, 8430, 8432, 8434, 8435, 8750
Fannie E Rippel Foundation, 3097
Fantastic Series Videotape Set, 8320
Fantastic: Colonial Times, Chocolate, and Cars, 8321
Fantastic: Dogs at Work and Play, 8322
Fantastic: Exciting People, Places and Thi ngs!, 8323
Fantastic: From Post Offices to Dairy Goat s, 8324
Fantastic: Imagination, Actors, and 'Deaf Way', 8325
Fantastic: Roller Coasters, Maps, and Ice Cream!, 8326
Fantastic: Skiing, Factories, and Race Hor es, 8327
Fantastic: Wonderful Worlds of Sports and Travel, 8328
Farewell, My Forever Child, 5359
Fargo VA Medical Center, 5792
Farmington Health Care Center, 6358
Farnum Rehabilitation Center, 7027
Fashion Collection, 1528
Father Drumgoole Connelly Summer Camp, 8198, 8625
Fathers: A Common Ground, 9176
Favarh ARC, 839
FAVRAH Senior Adult Enrichment Program, 6699
Fay J Lindner Foundation, 3137
Faye McBeath Foundation, 3343
Fayetteville VA Medical Center, 5648, 5789
FC Search, 3357
FCYD Camp Utada, 1459, 8624
FDR Series of Low Vision Reading Aids, 1676
Feather River Industries, 5920
Featherlite, 547
Featherspring Shoe Inserts, 641
Featherweight Reachers, 255
Fedcap Rehabilitation Services, 840
Federal Aviation Administration, 3390
Federal Benefits for Veterans and Dependents, 5634
Federal Communications Commission, 3387
Federal Emergency Management Agency, 2188
Federal Grants & Contracts Weekly, 3358
Federal Heights Rehabilitation and Nursing Center, 7393
Federal Laws of the Mentally Handicapped: Laws, Legislative Histories and Admin. Documents, 4697
Federal Student Aid Information Center, 2902
Federation Employment And Guidance Service (F-E-G-S), 7055
Federation for Children with Special Needs, 841, 5313
Feeding Children with Special Needs, 2472
Feingold Association of the US, 842, 8069
Feldenkrais Guild of North America (FGNA), 843
Fellow Insider, 2317
FHI 360, 5508
Fiat Products, 136
Fibromyalgia AWARE Magazine, 8408
Fibromyalgia Online, 8422
Fidelco, 9300
Fidelco Guide Dog Foundation, 2887, 9057, 9300
Field Foundation of Illinois, 2958
Field Notes, 2318
Fifth Third Bank, 3199
Fight for Sight, 9058, 9312
Fighting Blindness News, 9177
Fighting for Darla: Challenges for Family Care & Professional Responsibility, 7994
Filmakers Library, 5423
Filmakers Library: An Imprint Of Alexander Street Press, 5424
Films & Videos on Aging and Sensory Change, 5425
Films Media Group, 1862, 5455
Filomen M. D'Agostino Greenberg Music Scho ol, 2099
Final Report: Challenges and Strategies of Disabled Parents: Findings from a Survey (1997), 5344
Financial Aid for Asian Americans, 3359
Financial Aid for Hispanic Americans, 3360
Financial Aid for Native Americans, 3361
Financial Aid for Research and Creative Ac tivities Abroad, 3362
Financial Aid for the Disabled and Their F amilies, 2832, 3364
Financial Aid for Veterans, Military Personnel and their Dependents, 3363
Finger Lakes Developmental Disabilities Service Office, 4958
Finger Lakes Independence Center, 4449
Fingerspelling: Expressive and Receptive Fluency, 8329
Firefighters Burn Institute, 1036, 1038
Firefighters Kids Camp, 1036
The Firefly Foundation, 1092
Firemans Fund Foundation, 2833
Firemans Fund Insurance Companies, 2833
First Descents, 1060
First Hill Care Center, 7190
First Manhattan Company, 3153
First State Senior Center, 6715
First Step Independent Living, 4037
First Steps, 9178
First Union Foundation, 3185
Fite Center for Independent Living, 4160
Fitness Diet and Exercise Guide, 7698
Fitness Programming for Physical Disabilit ies, 8392
Five Green & Speckled Frogs, 1741
Five Green & Speckled Frogs IntelliKeys Overlay, 1568
Five Star Industries, 6834
FlagHouse, Inc., 432
Flagstaff City-Coconino County Public Library, 4752
Flannel Gowns, 1520
Flannel Pajamas, 1521
FlexShield Keyboard Protectors, 1661
Flint Osteopathic Hospital: RehabCare Unit, 6359
Float Dress, 1522
Florence C and Harry L English Memorial Fund, 2930
Florida Adult Services, 3511
Florida Baptist Convention, 7912
Florida Camp for Children & Youth with Diabetes, 1084, 8626
Florida Commission on Human Relations, 5975
Florida CORF, 6742
Florida Department of Education: Bureau of Exceptional Education And Student Services, 2191
Florida Department of Handicapped Children, 3512
Florida Department of Mental Health and Rehabilitative Services, 3513
Florida Developmental Disabilities Council, 3514
Florida Diabetes Camp, 1084, 8626
Florida Division of Blind Services, 4798, 5973
Florida Division of Vocational Rehabilitation, 3515, 5974
Florida Fair Employment Practice Agency, 5975
Florida Hospital, 6300, 7251
Florida Hospital Rehabilitation Center, 6279
Florida Institute for Neurologic Rehabilitation, Inc, 6744
Florida Institute Of Rehabilitation Education (FIRE), 6743
Florida Instructional Materials Center for the Visually Impaired (FIMC-VI), 4799
Florida Lions Camp, 7806
Florida School for the Deaf and Blind, 7807
Florida Sheriffs Caruth Camp, 7919
Florida Sheriffs Youth Ranches, 7919
Florida State College at Jacksonville Services for Students with Disabilities, 2192
Floyd Healthcare Resources, 6305
Flushing Hospital, 7056
Flushing Manor Nursing and Rehab, 7335
Flying Horse Farms, 1335
Flying Manes Therapeutic Riding, Inc., 844
FM Kirby Foundation, 3096
Foam Decubitus Bed Pads, 165
Focal Group Psychotherapy, 2473
Focus, 8423, 9301
Focus Alternative Learning Center, 8065
FOCUS Center for Autism, 7865
Focus on Autism and Other Developmental Disabilities, 2269
Focus on Exceptional Children, 2270
Focus on Geriatric Care and Rehabilitation, 7699
Focus Times Newsletter, 8065
Fold-Down 3-in-1 Commode, 272
Folding Chair with a Rigid Feel, 671
Folding Lightweight Power Wheelchair, 712
Folding Pot Stabilizer, 313
Fontana Rehabilitation Workshop, 6595
Food!, 1994
Foot Inversion Tread, 481
Foot Placement Ladder, 482
Foot Snugglers, 1523
Foot Steering Systems, 86
Foothill Nursing and Rehab Center, 7220
Foothill Vocational Opportunities, 6596
FOR Community Services, 6965
For Hearing People Only, 8240
Force A Miracle, 5172
Ford Foundation, 3138
Formed Families: Adoption of Children with Handicaps, 4698
Formerly Adaptive Environments, 1929
Formerly Houston-Love Memorial Library, 4744
Formerly Resources for Children with Special Needs, 5516
Formerly The Lymphoma Foundation Canada, 8505
Formula Series Active Mobility Wheelchairs, 672
Forsyth Medical Center, 7070
Fort Howard VA Medical Center, 5721
Fort Lauderdale Veterans Medical Center, 6745
Fort Mason Center, 5613
Fortis Foundation, 3139
Fortress, 644, 666, 668, 673, 679, 698, 701, 702, 703, 706, 715
Forum, 5173
Fotheringhay Farms, 5959

Foundation & Corporate Grants Alert, 3365
Foundation 1000, 3366
Foundation Center, 3140, 3127, 3141, 3357, 3366, 3367, 3368, 3370, 3372, 3376, 5174
Foundation Center Library Services, 3141
Foundation Directories, 3367
Foundation Fighting Blindness, 3013, 5509, 7796, 9059, 9177
Foundation for Advancement in Cancer Therapy, 3142
Foundation For Blind Children, 2803
Foundation for Children and Youth with Diabetes, 1459, 8624
Foundation For Dreams, Inc., 1082
Foundation for Seacoast Health, 3089
Foundation for the Carolinas, 3186
Foundation Fundamentals for Nonprofit Organizations, 5174
Foundation Grants to Individuals, 3368
Foundation Industries, 6924
Foundation Management Services, 3200
Foundations of Orientation and Mobility, 9179
Foundations of Rehabilitation Counseling with Persons Who Are Blind or Visually Impaired, 9180
Fountain Circle Health & Rehabilitation, 7290
Fountain Hills Lioness Braille Service, 4753
Fountain House Gallery, 25
Four in a Row Game: Tactile, 5571
Four Oaks Center, 7088
Four Rivers Resource Services, 4197, 6032
Four Way Switches, 87
Four-Ingredient Cookbook, 5175
The Fowler Center for Outdoor Learning, 1189
Fox Subacute at Clara Burke, 7132
Fox Subacute Center, 7131
FPL Group Foundation, 2919
Fraction Factory, 1695
Fragile Success, 7995
Fragile X Family, 8492
Frames of Reference for the Assessment of Learning Disabilities, 2678
Francis Beidler Charitable Trust, 2959
Frank & Mollie S VanDervoort Memorial Foun dation, 3046
Frank Olean Center, 3257
Frank R and Elizabeth Simoni Foundation, 3031
Franklin Court Assisted Living, 4537
Franklin Skilled Nursing and Rehabilitation Center, 7308
Fraser, 4483
Frasier Rehabilitation Center Division of Clark Memorial Hospital, 6876
Frazier Rehab Institute, 6909
Fred & Lillian Deeks Memorial Foundation, 3201
Fred Finch Youth Center, 6597
Fred Gellert Foundation, 2834
Fred J Brunner Foundation, 2960
Free and User Supported Software for the IBM PC: A Resource Guide, 1742
Free Appropriate Public Education: The Law and Children with Disabilities, 4699
Free Hand: Enfranchising the Education of Deaf Children, 2474
Free Library of Philadelphia: Library for the Blind and Physically Handicapped, 4994
FREED Center for Independent Living, 4035
FREED Center for Independent Living: Marys ville, 4036
Freedom Bath, 147
Freedom Center, 4286
Freedom Center for Independent Living, 4088
Freedom from Arthritis Through Nutrition, 8393
Freedom from Fear, 845
Freedom Motors USA, Inc., 88
Freedom Resource Center for Independent Living: Fergus Falls, 4344
Freedom Resource Center for Independent Li ving: Fargo, 4484
Freedom Rider, 433, 433
Freedom Ryder Handcycles, 524
Freedom Scientific, 5510, 1837
Freedom Scientific Blind/Low Vision Group, 1600
Freedom Three Wheel Walker, 615
Freedom Valley Disability Center, 4524
Freedom Wheels, 359, 359
Freestone Rehabilitation Center, 6519
Freestyle II, 673
Fremont Area Community Foundation, 3047
Frequently Asked Questions About Multiple Chemical Sensitivity, 5176
Fresno City College, 5921
Fresno City College: Disabled Students Programs and Services, 5921
Fresno County Free Library Blind and Handicapped Services, 4769
Friday Afternoon, 1830
Friendly Ice Cream Corp Contributions Prog ram, 3032
Friends Academy Summer Camps, 8627
Friends In Art (FIA), 26
Friends of Disabled Adults and Children, 8355
Friends of Libraries for Deaf Action, 4889
Friends: National Association of Young Peo ple who Stutter, 9023
Friendship 101, 2475
Friendship Circle Day Camp, 1290
Friendship Circle Upper East Side, 1290
Friendship Press, 5068
From Gesture to Language in Hearing and Deaf Children, 8241
From Mime to Sign Package, 8242
From the State Capitals: Public Health, 3369
From Where I Sit: Making My Way with Cereb ral Palsy, 8717
Frost Foundation, 3106
FSSI, 2679
Fulton County Rehab Center, 6011
Fun for Everyone, 1995
Functional Assessment Inventory Manual, 2476
Functional Electrical Stimulation for Ambu lation by Paraplegics, 8394
Functional Forms, 231
Functional Literacy System, 1863
Functional Resources, 1625
Functional Restoration of Adults and Child ren with Upper Extremity Amputation, 8115
Functional Skills Screening Inventory, 1625
Fund for New Jersey, 3098
Fundamentals of Autism, 1996
The Fundamentals of Special Education: A Practical Guide for Every Teacher, 2634
Future Choices Independent Living Center, 4198
Future Horizons, 27
Future Horizons Inc, 8037
Future Horizons, Inc., 38, 61, 63
Future Reflections, 7797, 9281
FYI, 2315

G

G W Micro, 1690
GA and SK Etiquette, 8243
GA Baptist Children's Homes & Family Ministries, 1093
Gadabout Wheelchairs, 674, 674
Gainesville Division, North Florida/South Georgia Veterans Healthcare System, 5679
Gales Creek Camp Foundation, 1362
Gales Creek Diabetes Camp, 1362
Gallaudet & NTID, 8226
Gallaudet Survival Guide to Signing, 8244
Gallaudet University, 8295
Gallaudet University Bookstore, 2518, 2531, 2636, 4673, 8212, 8219, 8221, 8222, 8238, 8246, 8269, 8983
Gallaudet University Press, 2156, 5511, 2527, 2591, 8214, 8217, 8225, 8227, 8229, 8230, 8231, 8232, 8233, 8241, 8244, 8245, 8250, 8251, 8256, 8257, 8258, 8259, 8262, 8263, 8264, 8267, 8268, 8274, 8275, 8276, 8278, 8282, 8287, 8289, 8296, 8303, 8305, 8320, 8321, 8322, 8323, 8324, 8325, 8326, 8327, 8328
Gallery Bookshop, 2421, 2438, 2513, 2534
Gallo Foundation, 2835
Galvin Health and Fitness Center, 8447
GAR Foundation, 3202
Garaventa Canada, 670
Gareth Stevens Publishing, 8790
Garfield Medical Center, 6245
Garten Services, 7117
Gas and Brake Pedal Guard, 89
Gateway Arts Center: Studio, Craft Store & Gallery, 6080
Gateway Center of Monterey County, 6598
Gateway Community Industries Inc.,, 7057
Gateway Industries: Castroville, 6599
Gateway Services/JCARC, 6033
Gaylord Hospital, 6700
GE Foundation, 2888
Gear Shift Adaptor, 90
Gear Shift Extension, 91
Gebbie Foundation, 3143
Geer Adult Training Center, 6500
GEICO Philanthropic Foundation, 2903
Gem Wheelchair & Scooter Service: Mobility & Homecare, 642, 675, 713
Gendron, 676, 659
General Electric Company, 2888
General Facts and Figures on Blindness, 9181
General Mills Foundation, 3061
General Motors Mobility Program for Persons with Disabilities, 5592
Generations, 7700
Genesee District Library, 4914
Genesis Health System, 6884
Genesis Healthcare System, 7089
Genesis Regional Rehabilitation Center, 6884
Genetic Disorders Sourcebook, 5177
Genetic Nutritioneering, 5178
Genetics and Spina Bifida, 8718
Geneva Centre for Autism, 7866
Genova Diagnostics, 846, 4974
Geo-Matt for High Risk Patients, 232
George A Martin Center, 7090
George Gund Foundation, 3203
George Hegyi Industrial Training Center, 5960
George M Eisenberg Foundation for Charities, 2961
George Ohsawa Macrobiotic Foundation, 7727
George Washington University, 849
George Washington University Medical Center, 6719
George Washington University Medical Center, 6719
George Wasserman Family Foundation, 3014
Georgetown University, 897
Georgetown University Center for Child and Human Development, 4793
Georgia Advocacy Office, 3523
Georgia Center of the Deaf and Hard of Hearing, 1095, 8188
Georgia Client Assistance Program, 3524
Georgia Commission on Equal Opportunity, 5990
Georgia Council On Developmental Disabilities, 3525
Georgia Council On Developmental Disabilities, 5221
Georgia Department of Aging, 3526
Georgia Department of Handicapped Children, 3527
Georgia Department of Labor, 4129, 6788
Georgia Division of Mental Health, Developmental Disabilities & Addictive Diseases, 3528
Georgia Industries for the Blind, 6792
Georgia Library for the Blind and Physically Handicapped, 4819
Georgia Power, 2931
Georgia Public Library, 4819
Georgia State Board of Workers' Compensation, 3529
Georgiana Institute, 8142
Geriatrics, 7701
Geronimo, 714
Gerontological Society of America, 7543, 7702
The Gerontological Society of America, 7620
Gerontologist, 7702
Gerontology, 7703
Gerontology: Abstracts in Social Gerontology, 7656
Get a Wiggle On, 9182

Get Ready for Jetty!: My Journal About ADH D and Me, 2477
Get Up and Go, 7704
Getting a Grip on ADD: A Kid's Guide to Understanding & Coping with ADD, 7997
Getting Around Town, 2478
Getting Better, 8330
Getting in Touch, 5426
Getting Our Heads Together, 7996
Getting Ready for the Outside World (G.R.O.W.), 2200
Getting Started with Facilitated Communication, 8085, 9018
Getting the Best for Your Child with Autism, 7998
Giant Food Foundation, 3015
Giant Print Address Book, 584
Gift of Sight, 9183
Gillingham Manaual, 1998
Gilroy Workshop, 6600
Girl Scouts - Foothills Council, 8568
Girl Scouts of Washington Rock Council, 9111
Gladys Brooks Foundation, 3144
Glaser Progress Foundation, 3327
Glaucoma, 9184
Glaucoma Laser Trial, 4909
Glaucoma Research Foundation, 2836, 4770, 5512, 9184, 9203, 9302
Glaucoma: The Sneak Thief of Sight, 9185
Gleams Newsletter, 9302
Glendale Adventist Medical Center, 6601
Glendale Memorial Hospital and Health Center Rehabilitation Unit, 6602
Glendale Memorial Hospital and Health Center, 6602
Glengariff Health Care Center, 7336
The Glenholme School, 2755
Glenkirk, 6012
Glenview Terrace Nursing Center, 7265
Glickenhaus Foundation, 3145
Global Assistive Devices, Inc., 166
Global Health Solutions, 8396, 8667
Global Perspectives on Disability: A Curriculum, 2479
Glossary of Terminology for Vocational Assessment/Evaluation/Work, 2480
GM Mobility Program, 5592
GN Wilcox Trust, 2941
GO-MO Articulation Cards- Second Edition, 1997
Goals and Objectives, 1817
Goals and Objectives IEP Program Curriculum Associates LLC, 1818
GoalView: Special Education and RTI Studen t Management Information System, 1743
God's Camp, 8628
Going to School with Facilitated Communication, 5179
Gold Violin, Inc., 626
Golden Technologies, 215, 539, 560, 563
Goldilocks and the Three Bears: Told in Signed English, 8245
Goleta Valley Cottage Hospital, 6603
Golf Xpress, 525
Gonzales Warm Springs Rehabilitation Hospital, 6443
A Good and Perfect Gift: Faith, Expectatio ns, and a Little Girl Named Penny, 5355
Good Grips Cutlery, 314
Good Samaritan Health System, 7133
Good Samaritan Healthcare Physical Medicine and Rehabilitation, 6478
Good Samaritan Hospital, 6478, 7134, 8902
Good Samaritan Hospital-Health System Center, 7134
Good Shepherd Rehabilitation, 7369
The Goodtimes Project, 1476
Goodwill Career Centers, 5991
Goodwill Easterseals of the Gulf Coast, 6501
Goodwill Industries - Suncoast, 4097
Goodwill Industries International, 847
Goodwill Industries International, Inc., 7544
Goodwill Industries of New Mexico, 6147
Goodwill Industries of Southern New Jersey, 6129
Goodwill Industries-Suncoast, 7545
Goodwill Industries-Suncoast, Inc., 5976, 5977, 5978, 5979, 5980, 5982, 5985
Goodwill Life Skills Development Program, 5976
Goodwill of Central & Southern Indiana, 6034
Goodwill of Greater Washington, 5966
Goodwill of North Georgia, 5991
Goodwill of Southern New England, 5961
Goodwill Temporary Staffing, 5977
Goodwill's Community Employment Services, 5978
Goodwill's Job Connection Center, 5979
Goodwill's JobWorks, 5980
Gospel Publishing House, 8254
Govennor's Council on Developmental Disabilities, 5126
Government, 4789
Governor's Committee on Employment and Rehabilitation of People with Disabilities, 3432
Governor's Council on Developmental Disabilities, 3442
Governor's Council on Disabilities and Spe cial Education, 3433
Governor's Developmental Disability Council, 3572
Governor's Office oe Executive Policy & Programs, 3842
Gow School Summer Programs, 1291, 7920
GPK Inc., 499, 514
Graduate Technological Education and the Human Experience of Disability, 2481
Grady Memorial Hospital, 7091
Graham Street Community Resources, 4544
Graham-Field, 653
Graham-Field Health Products, 218, 236, 384, 684
Gram Newsletter, The, 2319
Grand Island VA Medical System, 5753
Grand Junction VA Medical Center, 5666
Grand Lodge of the International Association of Machinists and Aerospace Workers, 848
Grand Rapids Foundation, 3048
Grand Traverse Area Community Living Management Corporation, 4328
Grand Traverse Area Library for the Blind and Physically Handicapped, 4910
Granger Foundation, 3049
Granite State Independent Living Foundation, 4408
Grant Guides, 3370
Grassroots Consortium, 3873
Grayson Foundation, 2932
Great Barrington Rehabilitation and Nursing Center, 7309
Great Lakes Hemophilia Foundation, 1486
Great Lakes Regional Rehabilitation Center, 6392
Great Lakes/Macomb Rehabilitation Group, 4329
Greater Baltimore Medical Center, 6945, 7303
Greater Cincinnati Behavioral Health Services - Employment Services, 6170
Greater Cincinnati Foundation, 3204
Greater Detroit Agency for the Blind and Visually Impaired, 6992
Greater Kansas City Community Foundation & Affiliated Trusts, 3073
Greater Milwaukee Area Health Care Guide f or Older Adults, 2133
Greater Milwaukee Area Senior Housing Opti ons, 2134
Greater Richmond ARC, 7897
Greater St Louis Community Foundation, 3074
Greater Tacoma Community Foundation, 3328
Greater Worcester Community Foundation, 3033
Greeley Center for Independence, 4076
Green County Independent Living Resource Center, 4499
Greenery Extended Care Center: Worcester, 6967
Greenery Rehabilitation & Skilled Nursing Center, 6968
Greenroots Consortium, 3873
Greenville County Recreation District, 1407
Greenwood Publishing Group, 2157, 2401, 2487, 2524, 4682, 4686, 4702, 4703, 4715, 4722, 5147, 5161, 5182, 5196, 5259, 5276, 5294, 5317, 5322, 7633, 7640, 7984
Gresham Driving Aids, 92, 87, 89, 91, 94, 108, 110, 113, 114, 117, 118, 127, 128
Grey House Publishing, 2158, 2126, 2129, 2132
Grief: What it is and What You Can Do, 5180
Griffin Area Resource Center, 5992
Groden Network, 6182
Grossberg Company, 3014
Grossmont Hospital Rehabilition Center, 6246
Group Activity for Adults with Brain Injury, 7999
Grover Hermann Foundation, 2962
Growing Readers, 2320
Growing Together Diabetes Camp, 8629
Growing Up with Epilepsy: A Pratical Guide for Parents, 8719
Guardianship Services Associates, 4660
Guest House of Slidell Sub-Acute and Rehab Center, 7294
Guide Dog Foundation for the Blind, 3146, 9304
Guide Dog News, 9303
Guide Dogs for the Blind, 9060, 9291, 9296, 9297, 9303, 9321
Guide Magazine, 9282
Guide Service of Washington, 5614
A Guide to Disability Rights Laws, 5087
Guide to Funding for International and Foreign Programs, 3371
A Guide to International Educational Excha nge, 2760
Guide to Living with HIV Infection: Develo ped at the Johns Hopkins AIDS Clinic, 8720
Guide to Managing Your Arthritis, 8395
Guide to Successful Employment for Individuals with Autism, 8000
Guide to Teaching Phonics, 1999
A Guide to Teaching Students With Autism S pectrum Disorders, 2345
Guide to the Selection of Musical Instruments, 28
Guide to US Foundations their Trustees, Officers and Donors, 3372
Guide to Wheelchair Sports and Recreation, 8448
The Guided Tour, Inc., 5619
Guidelines and Games for Teaching Efficient Braille Reading, 9186
Guidelines for Comprehensive Low Vision Care, 9187
Guidelines on Disability, 5181
Guideway, 9304
Guiding Eyes for the Blind, 9061
Guild Briefs, 9305
Guild for the Blind, 4834
Guilford Press, 5120, 5385, 7949, 7950, 7977, 7993, 8039, 8055, 8074, 8075, 8076, 8077, 8742, 8747
Guilford Publication, 2352
Gulf Coast Independent Living Center, 4357
GW Micro, 1569, 9338

H

H UD U SE R, 1941
H&R Block Foundation, 3075
H.E.L.P. Knife, 315
Habilitation Benefits Coalition, 850
Hacienda La Puente Unified School District, 6608
Hacienda Rehabilitation and Care Center, 7213
Hackett Hill Nursing Center and Integrated Care, 7028
Haldimand-Norfolk Resource Education and C ounseling, 851
Halifax Hospital Medical Center Eye Clinic Professional Center, 6746
Hall County Library: East Hall Branch and Special Needs Library, 4820
Hall-Perrine Foundation, 2988
Hallmarks and Features of High-Quality Com munity-Based Services, 5074
Halsted Terrace Nursing Center, 7266
Hamilton Adult Center, 7092
Hamilton Rehabilitation and Healthcare Cen ter, 7231
Hammill Institute on Disabilities, 2159
Hampton VA Medical Center, 5845
Hand Brake Control Only, 93
Hand Camp, 1085
Hand Control Multi-Function Buttons, 94
Hand Gas & Brake Control, 95
Hand Parking Brake, 96
Handbook About Care in the Home, 5306

Handbook for Implementing Workshops for Siblings of Special Children, 2483
Handbook for Itinerant and Resource Teachers of Blind Students, 9188
Handbook for Speech Therapy, 2484
Handbook for the Special Education Administrator, 2485
A Handbook for Writing Effective Psychoedu cational Reports (2nd Edition), 7808
Handbook of Acoustic Accessibility, 2486
Handbook of Adaptive Switches and Augmentative Communication Devices, 1745
Handbook of Assistive Devices for the Handicapped Elderly, 7639
Handbook of Autism and Pervasive Developmental Disorders, 8001
Handbook of Career Planning for Students with Special Needs, 8002
Handbook of Chronic Fatigue Syndrome, 8721
Handbook of Developmental Education, 2487
Handbook of Epilepsy, 8722
Handbook of Information for Members of the Achromatopsia Network, 9189
Handbook of Services for the Handicapped, 5182
Handbook on Ethnicity, Aging and Mental Health, 7640
Handbook on Supported Education for People with Mental Illness, 2488
HandBrake, 97
Handi Camp, 1389
Handi Holder, 316
Handi Home Lift, 360
Handi Lift, 361
Handi Prolift, 362
Handi Vangelism Ministries International, 1389
Handi-Lift, 346, 355, 360, 361, 362, 371
Handi-Ramp, 363, 363
Handi-Works Productions, 6925
Handicapped Scuba Association, 8449
Handicapped Scuba Association International, 8449
Handicaps, Inc., 98, 73, 90, 106, 109, 111, 122, 124, 340, 377, 395
HandiWARE, 1746
Hands to Love, 1085
Hands-Free Controller, 5572
Handy-Helper Cutting Board, 317
The Hanen Centre, 946
Hanger, Inc., 852
Hanley Wood Media Inc., 1942
Happiness Bag, 1137
Happiness Bag, Inc., 1137
Happiness Is Camping, 1259, 8630
Happy Camp, 978, 8631
Harbor Haven Summer Program, 1260
Harbor House Law Press, 2160
Harborview Medical Center, 7191
Harborview Medical Center, Low Vision Aid Clinic, 7191
HARC Mercantile, 176, 177, 178, 181, 183, 184, 185, 187, 188, 189, 190, 191, 193, 199, 204, 271, 283, 293, 294, 295, 476, 477, 485, 503, 505, 506, 509, 597
Harc Mercantile, Ltd., 183
Hard Manufacturing Company, 167
Harden Foundation, 2837
Harlem Independent Living Center, 4450
Harmony Nursing and Rehabilitation Center, 7267
Harper Collins Publishers, 37, 8675, 8748
Harper Collins Publishers/Basic Books, 5185
Harper Collins Publishing, 8114
HarperCollins Publishers, 8211, 8248
Harriet & Robert Heilbrunn Guild School, 2739
Harriet McDaniel Marshall Trust in Memory of Sanders McDaniel, 2933
Harrington House Nursing And Rehabilitation Center, 6969
Harris and Eliza Kempner Fund, 3294
Harris Communications, 292, 196, 292, 2013, 2049, 5404, 5405, 5415, 5416, 5417, 8240, 8255, 8266, 9242, 9351
Harris Methodist Fort Worth Hospital Mabee Rehabilitation Center, 6444
Harris Methodist Fort Worth/Mabee Rehabilitation Center, 7161
Harrisburg Office, 3815
Harrison Health and Rehabilitation Centre, 7278
Harry and Jeanette Weinberg Foundation, 3016
Harry C Moores Foundation, 3207
Harry S Truman Memorial Veterans' Hospital, 5744
Hartford Foundation for Public Giving, 2889
Hartford Insurance Group, 2890
Hartford Regional Office, 5667
Hartford Vet Center, 5668
Harvard University Howe Laboratory of Ophthalmology, 4901
Harvard University Press, 8261
Harvey A. Friedman Center for Aging, 7546
Harvey Randall Wickes Foundation, 3050
Hasbro Children's Hospital Asthma Camp, 1401
HASL Independent Abilities Center, 4504
Hausmann Industries, 168
Havirmill Foundation, 3051
Hawaii Assistive Technology Training and, 3536
Hawaii Center For Independent Living, 4137
Hawaii Center for Independent Living-Maui, 4138
Hawaii Centers for Independent Living, 4139
Hawaii Civil Rights Commission, 5997
Hawaii Community Foundation, 2942
Hawaii Department for Children With Special Needs, 3537
Hawaii Department of Education, 2193
Hawaii Department of Education: Special Needs, 2193
Hawaii Department of Health, Adult Mental Health Division, 3538
Hawaii Department of Human Serv, 3539
Hawaii Department of Human Services, 3539
Hawaii Disability Compensation Division Department of Labor and Industrial Relations, 3540
Hawaii Disability Rights Center, 3541
Hawaii Executive Office on Aging, 3542
Hawaii Fair Employment Practice Agency, 5997
Hawaii State Council on Developmental Disabilities, 3543
Hawaii State Library for the Blind and Physically Handicapped, 4829
Hawaii Vocational Rehabilitation Division, 5998
Haworth Press, 2278, 2285, 2331, 2363, 2439, 2467, 2470, 2481, 2544, 2549, 2575, 4698, 5143, 5204, 5262, 6384
Haym Salomon Home for The Aged, 7337
The Hazard Building, 3827
HCR Health Care Services, 6393
HCR Manor Care Foundation, 3205
Head Injury Hotline, 8895
Head Injury Rehabilitation And Referral Service, Inc. (HIRRS), 8356
Head Injury Rehabilitation: Children, 2489
Head Injury Treatment Program at Dover, 6370
Headlight Dimmer Switch, 99
Headliner Hats, 1524
HEAL: Health Education AIDS Liaison, 2100
Healing Dressing for Pressure Sores, 273
Healing Herbs, 5183
Health Action, 853
Health Alliance, 6400
Health and Rehabilitation Products, 434
Health and Wellfare, 3548
Health Care Corporation of America, 6764
Health Care for Students with Disabilities, 2491
Health Care Management in Physical Therapy, 2490
Health Care of the Aged: Needs, Policies, and Services, 7641
Health Care Professionals Who Are Blind or Visually Impaired, 9190
Health Care Quality Improvement Act of 1986, 4700
Health Care Solutions, 6414
Health Communications, 8833
Health KiCC, 3850
Health Promotion and Disease Prevention in Clinical Practice, 7642
Health Resources & Services Administration, 934
Health Resources & Services Administration : State Bureau of Health, 3613
Health Resources and Services Administrati on (HRSA), 3388
Health Resources Online, 7696
Health South Cane Creek Rehabilitation Center, 6430
Health South Corporation, 6337, 6430, 6604
Health South Corporation in Burmingham Alabama, 6751
Health South Corporation of Alabama, 6284
Health South of Nittany Valley, 6416
Health South Tustin Rehabilitation Hospita, 6247
Healthcare and Rehabilitation Center of Sanford, 7241
HealthCare Solutions, 435
HealthCraft SuperPole, 483
Healthline, 2321
HealthQuest Subacute and Rehabilitation Programs, 6747
HealthSouth Central Georgia Rehabilitation Hospital, 6304
HealthSouth Chattanooga Rehabilitation Hospital, 6431
HealthSouth Corporation, 6502, 6274
Healthsouth Corporation, 6749
HealthSouth Deaconess Rehabilitation Hospital, 6877
HealthSouth Emeral Coast Sports & Rehabilitation Center, 6748
HealthSouth Harmarville Rehabilitation Hospital, 6415
HealthSouth Hospital of Cypress, 7162
HealthSouth Lakeshore Rehabilitation Hospi tal, 6227
HealthSouth Mountain View Regional Rehab Hospital, 6483
HealthSouth Nittany Valley Rehabilitation Hospital, 6416
HealthSouth Northern Kentucky Rehabilitation Hospital, 6910
HealthSouth Plano Rehabilitation Hospital, 6445
HealthSouth Regional Rehab Center/Florida, 6280
HealthSouth Rehab Hospital Of Arlington, 6446
HealthSouth Rehab Hospital Of Austin, 6447
HealthSouth Rehab Hospital Of Erie, 6417
HealthSouth Rehab Hospital Of Utah, 6469
HealthSouth Rehab Hospital: Largo, 6281
HealthSouth Rehab Hospital: South Carolina, 6428
Healthsouth Rehab Institute of Tucson, 6238
Healthsouth Rehabilitation Hospital of Greater Pittsburgh, 6419
HealthSouth Rehabilitation Center of Humble Texas, 6448
HealthSouth Rehabilitation Center: New Mexico, 6381
HealthSouth Rehabilitation Cntr/Tennessee, 6432
HealthSouth Rehabilitation Hospital, 6233, 6376, 6449
Healthsouth Rehabilitation Hospital of Mechanicsburg, 6420
HealthSouth Rehabilitation Hospital of Tallahassee, 6749
HealthSouth Rehabilitation Hospital of Altoona, 6418
HealthSouth Rehabilitation Hospital of Beaumont, 6450
HealthSouth Rehabilitation Hospital of Colorado Springs, 6274
HealthSouth Rehabilitation Hospital Of Fort Smith, 6536
HealthSouth Rehabilitation Hospital Of Miami, 6750
HealthSouth Rehabilitation Hospital of North Alabama, 6228
HealthSouth Rehabilitation Hospital of Sarasota, 6751
HealthSouth Rehabilitation Hospital Of Western Massachusetts, 6970
Healthsouth Rehabilitation Hospital of York, 6421
HealthSouth Rehabilitation Institute Of San Antonio (RIOSA), 6451
HealthSouth Rehabilitation of Louisville, 6339

HealthSouth Sea Pines Rehabilitation Hospital, 6752
HealthSouth Specialty Hospital Of North Louisiana, 6342
HealthSouth Sports Medicine & Rehabilitation Center, 6282
HealthSouth Sports Medicine and Rehabilitation Center, 6283
HealthSouth Sports Medicine Center, 6237
HealthSouth Treasure Coast Rehabilitation Hospital, 6284
HealthSouth Tustin Rehabilitation Hospital, 6604
HealthSouth Valley Of The Sun Rehabilitation Hospital, 6520
HealthSouth Western Hills Regional Rehab Hospital, 6484
Healthwin Specialized Care, 6878
Healthy Aging Association, 7547
Healthy Breathing, 8723
HealthyWomen, 5513
HEAR Center, 8143, 8311
Hear You Are, 436
Hearing Aid Batteries, 293
Hearing Aid Battery Testers, 294
Hearing Aid Care Kit, 295
Hearing Center, 421
Hearing Education and Awareness for Rocker s, 8144
Hearing Health Foundation (HHF), 854, 3147
Hearing Health Magazine, 8299
Hearing Impaired Children and Youth with Developmental Disabilities, 8246
Hearing Industries Association, 8145
Hearing Life Magazine, 7816, 8300
Hearing Loss Association of America, 7798, 8146, 7816, 8300
Hearing Professional, 8292
Hearing Professional Magazine, 7817
Hearing, Speech & Deafness Center (HDSC), 456
Hearing, Speech & Deafness Center (HSDC), 8307, 8921, 9010
Hearing, Speech and Deafness Center (HSDC), 8147, 8921
Hearst Foundations, 3148
Heart of the Mind, 8724
Heart to Heart, 5427, 9191, 9343
Heart Touch Project™, 7548
Heartbreak of Being A Little Bit Blind, 9192
Heartland Opportunity Center, 5922
Heartspring, 6902
HEATH Resource Center at the National Youth Transitions Center, 849
Heather Hill, 6394
Heather Hill Rehabilitation Hospital, 6394
Heightened Independence and Progress: Hack ensack, 4417
Heightened Independence and Progress: Jers ey City, 4418
Heights Hospital Rehab Unit, 7163
Heinz Endowments, 3234
Heldref Publications, 2284
Helen and Teacher: The Story of Helen & Anne Sullivan Macy, 7810
Helen Bader Foundation, 3344
Helen K and Arthur E Johnson Foundation, 2880
Helen Keller International, 4959
Helen Keller National Center, 7823, 7825
Helen Keller National Center for Deaf - Blind Youths And Adults, 4960
Helen Keller National Center for Deaf- Blind Youths and Adults, 5184, 7799
Helen Keller National Center Newsletter, 9193
Helen Steiner Rice Foundation, 3208
Hellen Keller National Center, 899, 7803
Helm Distributing, 639, 640
HELP, 1744
Help Newsletter, 2322
Helping Hands, 5428
Helping Learning- Disabled Gifted Children Learn Through Compensatory Active Play, 2492
Helping People with Autism Manage Their Behavior, 8003
Helping Students Grow, 2493
Helping the Family Understand, 8331
Helping the Visually Impaired Child with Developmental Problems, 9194
Helping Your Hyperactive: Attention Deficit Child, 8004
Hemisphere Publishing Corporation, 2289
The Hemispherectomy Foundation, 7892
Hemophilia Camp, 8632
Henkind Eye Institute Division of Montefiore Hospital, 7058
Henry and Lucy Moses Fund, 3149
Henry Ford Health System, 7004
Henry J Kaiser Family Foundation, 2838
Henry Kaufmann Campgrounds, 1278
Henry L Hillman Foundation, 3235
Henry Nias Foundation, 2891
Henry W Bull Foundation, 2839
Hepatitis Sourcebook, 8725
Herb Research Foundation, 5514
HerbalEGram, 2323
HerbalGram, 2271
Heritage Health and Rehabilitation Center, 7406
Herman Goldman Foundation, 3150
Herman M. Holloway, Sr. Campus, 3494
Herpes Resource Center, 8493
Herrick Health Sciences Library, 4771
Hi-Desert Medical Center, 6605
Hidden Child: The Linwood Method for Reaching the Autistic Child, 8005
Hig's Manufacturing, 437
High Country Council of Governments Area A gency on Aging, 7779
High Noon Books, 2161
High Profile Single Compartment Cushion, 233
High School Senior's Guide to Merit and Ot her No-Need Funding, 3373
High School Students Guide to Study, Travel, and Adventure Abroad, 2772
High Tech Center, 1626
High Technology Foundation, 855, 3336
High-Low Chair, 216
Highbrook Lodge, 1336, 9115
Highland Pines Rehabilitation Center, 7242
Highlighter and Note Tape, 585
Hilcrest Medical Center: Kaiser Rehab Cent er, 6402
Hill School of Fort Worth, 1449, 7921
Hillcrest Baptist Medical Center, 7164
Hillcrest Baptist Medical Center: Rehab Care Unit, 6452
Hillcrest Foundation, 3295
Hillcroft Services, 1138, 8380
Hillhaven Rehabilitation, 6793
Hillsborough County Talking Book Library Tampa-Hillsborough County Public Library, 4800
Hillsview Plaza, 3853, 6189
Hillview Plaza, 6190
Hilo Vet Center, 5689
Hip Function & Ambulation, 8726
HiRider, 677
Hiring Idahoans with Disabilities, 5391
His & Hers, 1525
History and Use of Braille, 9195
Hitchcock Rehabilitation Center, 7142
HIV Infection and Developmental Disabilities, 2482
HKNC Newsletter, 7823
Hoblitzelle Foundation, 3296
Hockanum Greenhouse, 6701
Hockanum Industry, 6701
Hocoma AG, 484
Hoffmann + Krippner Inc., 1684
Hogg Foundation for Mental Health, 856, 3297
The Hole in the Wall Gang Camp, 1070, 8655
Holiday Inn Boxborough Woods, 6971
Holiday Lake 4-H Educational Center, 1470
Hollywood Speaks: Deafness and the Film En tertainment Industry, 8247
Holston Conference of United Methodist Church, 1466
Holt Paperbacks (Macmillan Publishers), 5364
Holy Cross Comprehensive Rehabilitation Center, 6248
Holy Cross Hospital, 6753
Holzer Clinic, 7093
Holzer Clinic Sycamore, 7094
Holzer Medical Center, 7094
Home Alerting Systems, 485
Home Bed Side Helper, 169
Home Delivery Incontinent Supplies, 444
Home Health Care Provider: A Guide to Esse ntial Skills, 2494
Home is in the Heart: Accommodating People with Disabilities in the Homestay Experience, 5429
Home of the Guiding Hands, 6606
HomeCare Magazine, 2272
Homelink, 6885
Homemade Battery-Powered Toys, 2000
Homeopathic Educational Services, 857
The Homestead Group Administrative Offices, 3253
Homestead Healthcare and Rehabilitation Ce nter, 7318
Homewaiter, 364
Honolulu VBA Regional Office, 5690
Hooleon Corp, 1572
Hooleon Corporation, 1601, 1594, 1605, 1661
Hoosier Burn Camp, 1139
Hope Center, 5949
Hope Community Resources, 3977
Hope Haven, 4210
Hope Network Neuro Rehabilitation, 858, 6993
Hope Services, 5916
Horace A Kimball and S Ella Kimball Foundation, 3258
Horcher Lifting Systems, 365
Horcher Medical Systems, 365
Horizon Publishers & Distributors, 7632
Horizon Rehabilitation Center, 6388
Horizons for the Blind, 4835, 9062
Horizontal Steering Systems, 100
Horn Control Switch, 101
Hospice Alternative, 5185
Hospital Audiences, 1939
Hospital Environmental Control System, 486
Hospital For Special Care (HSC), 7232
Hospital of the Good Samaritan Acute Rehabilitation Unit, 6607
Hospitality Nursing Rehabilitation Center, 7417
Hostelling International, 5584
Hostelling North America, 5584
House Ear Institute, 8148
Housing and Transportation of the Handicapped, 4701
Housing Unlimited, 4287
Houston Center for Independent Living (HCIL), 4569
Houston Endowment, 3298
Houston Public Library: Access Center, 5008
Houston Regional Office, 5835
How Come You Walk Funny?, 8434
How Difficult Can This Be ? (Fat City) - Rick Lavoie, 5430
How to Conduct an Assessment, 2679
How to Cope with ADHD: Diagnosis, Treatment & Myths, 8086
How to Deal with Back Pain and Rheumatoid Joint Pain: A Preventive and Self Treatment Manua, 8396
How to File a Title III Complaint, 5186
How to Live Longer with a Disability, 5187
How to Pay for Your Degree in Business & Related Fields, 3374
How to Pay for Your Degree in Education & Related Fields, 3375
How To Reach and Teach Children and Teens with Dyslexia, 8006
How to Read for Everyday Living, 1831
How to Teach Spelling/How to Spell, 2495
How to Thrive, Not Just Survive, 9196
How to Write for Everyday Living, 1747
How We Play, 5431
Howard Heinz Endowment, 3234
Howard School, The, 2740
Howard University Child Development Center, 6721
HSC Pediatric Center, The, 6720
HSI Austin Center For Development, 6835
Hub, 9197
Hudson Community Enterprises, 6130

Hugh J Andersen Foundation, 3062
Hull Park and Retreat Center, 1363
Human Exceptionality: School, Community, and Family (12th Edition), 2496, 5075
Human Kinetics, 2246, 5286, 7668, 7716, 8397, 8402
Human Kinetics, Inc., 8385, 8391, 8392
Human Resource Management and the Americans with Disabilities Act, 4702
Human Sciences Press, 2554, 7710, 8027, 8984, 9241
Human Ware, 1678
Humana Hospital: Morristown RehabCare, 7144
Humanity & Inclusion (HI), 859
Humanware, 1602
Hunter Holmes McGuire VA Medical Center, 5846
Hunter House, 8746, 8761
Hunter House Inc. Publisher, 8836
Hunter House Publishers, Inc, 1620
Huntington Health and Rehabilitation Cente r, 7382
Huntington Regional Office, 5854
Huntington VA Medical Center, 5855
Huntleigh Healthcare, 438
Huntsville Subregional Library for the Blind & Physically Handicapped, 4745
Huntsville-Madison County Public Library, 4745
Hutchinson Community Foundation, 2993
HWH Foundation, 3206
Hyams Foundation, 3034
Hyde Park-Woodlawn, 6836
Hydrocephalus: A Guide for Patients, Families & Friends, 8727
Hyperactive Child, Adolescent, and Adult: ADD Through the Lifespan, 8007
Hyperion, 8021
Hypertension Sourcebook, 8728
Hypokalemic Periodic Paralysis Resource Page, 5515

I

I Can't Hear You in the Dark: How to Lean and Teach Lipreading, 2497
I ET Resources, 1717
I Have a Sister, My Sister is Deaf, 8248
I Heard That!, 2498
I Heard That!2, 2499
I Just Want My Little Boy Back, 8087, 9019
I KNOW American History, 1748
I KNOW American History Overlay CD, 1749
I Wonder Who Else Can Help, 2273
I'm Not Disabled, 5432
IAAIS Report, 9306
IAL News, 8863
IBM Corporation, 2934
IBM National Support Center, 5993
Icon Group International, 8780, 8781, 8782, 8783, 8784, 8785, 8786, 8787, 8788, 8789
Idaho Assistive Technology Project, 1627, 2001, 4830, 2383, 5048, 5049, 5287, 5391, 7631, 7954
Idaho Commission for Libraries: Talking Book Service, 4831
Idaho Commission for the Blind & Visually Impaired, 6001
Idaho Commission for the Blind and Visually Impaired, 7800
Idaho Commission on Aging, 3547
Idaho Council on Developmental Disabilities, 3548
Idaho Council on Developmental Disabilities, 5278
Idaho Department of Handicapped Children, 3549
Idaho Department of Labor, 6002
Idaho Diabetes Youth Programs, Inc., 1104, 8576
Idaho Disability Determinations Service, 3550
Idaho Division of Vocational Rehabilitatio n, 6003
Idaho Elks Rehabilitation Hospital, 6803
Idaho Falls Office: Living Independently for Everyone (LIFE), 4146
Idaho Governor's Committee on Employment of People with Disabilities, 6004
Idaho Human Rights Commission, 6005
Idaho Industrial Commission, 3551
Idaho Mental Health Center, 3552
Ideas for Kids on the Go, 5188
Ideas for Making Your Home Accessible, 1951
Identifying and Treating Attention Deficit Hyperactivity Disorder, 8008
Identity Group, 487
IDF National Conference, 1908
If Blindness Comes, 9198
If Blindness Strikes Don't Strike Out, 9199
If I Only Knew What to Say or Do, 5189
If It Is To Be, It Is Up To Me To Do It!, 2002
If It Is To Be, It Is Up To Us To Help!, 2500
If it Weren't for the Honor: I'd Rather Have Walked, 5190
IKRON Institute for Rehabilitative and Psychological Services, 7095
IKUS Life Enrichment Services, 8494, 1197
Illinois and Iowa Center for Independent L iving, 4163
Illinois Assistive Technology Project, 3559
Illinois Center for Autism, 6837
Illinois Council on Developmental Disability, 3560
Illinois Department of Human Services, 6025
Illinois Department of Mental Health and Developmental Disabilities, 3561
Illinois Department of Rehab Services, 4161
Illinois Department of Rehabilitation, 3562
Illinois Department on Aging, 3563
Illinois Early Childhood Intervention Clearinghouse, 4836
Illinois Fire Safety Alliance, 1111
Illinois Life Span Program, 6013
The Illinois Life Span Project, 2948
Illinois Machine Sub-Lending Agency, 4837
Illinois Regional Library for the Blind and Physically Handicapped, 4838
Illinois State Board of Education, 3554
Illinois State Board of Education: Department of Special Education, 2194
Illinois Valley Center for Independent Living, 4162
Illinois Wheelchair Sport Camps, 1120, 8381
IlluminAge Communications Partners, 7628
iLuv SmartShaker 2, 172
Imagery in Healing Shamanism and Modern Medicine, 5191
Imagery Procedures for People with Special Needs, 5433
Images of the Disabled, Disabling Images, 2501
Imagine!, 5950, 8066, 8066
Imagining the Possibilities: Creative Approaches to Orientation and Mobility Instructio, 9200
Immune Deficiency Foundation, 860, 3017, 1908
Immune System Disorders Sourcebook., 8729
Imp Tricycle, 700
Impact Center for Independent Living, 4164
Imperial, 7268
Implementing Family-Centered Services in Early Intervention, 2502
In Search of Wings: A Journey Back from T raumatic Brain Injury, 8009
In the Middle, 5434
In Their Own Way, 8010
In Time and with Love: Caring for the Spec ial Needs Infant and Toddler, 5360
In Touch Systems, 1667, 1668
In-Definite Arts Society, 29
In-Home Medical Care, 6794
In-Sight, 7139
IN-SIGHT Independent Living, 4538
IN-SOURCE, 6321
INALLIANCE Inc., 5923
Incight, 2101
Incite Learning Series, 1750
Inclinator Company of America, 335, 364, 366, 391, 394
Inclinette, 366
Include Us, 5435
INCLUDEnyc, 5516
Including All of Us: An Early Childhood Curriculum About Disability, 2503
Including Students with Severe and Multiple Disabilites in Typical Classrooms, 2504
Including Students with Special Needs: A Practical Guide for Classroom Teachers, 2505
Inclusion, 2274
Inclusive & Heterogeneous Schooling: Assessment, Curriculum, and Instruction, 2506, 2680
Inclusive Games, 8397
Inclusive Leisure Services (3rd Edition), 5076
Inclusive Play People, 2003
Increasing Capabilities Access, 3447
Increasing Capabilities Access Network, 1628
Increasing Literacy Levels: Final Report, 9201
Independence, 4221, 5192, 7765
Independence Associates, 4301
Independence CIL, 5247
Independence Economic Development, 4661
Independence Empowerment Center, 4609
Independence First, 4635
Independence First: West Bend, 4636
Independence Northwest Center for Independent Living, 4086
Independence Now, 4288
Independence Now: The Center for Independent Living, 4289
Independence Place, 4268
Independence Resource Center, 4610
Independence Without Sight and Sound: Suggestions for Practitioners, 7811
Independence Without Sight or Sound, 8249
Independent Connection, 4222
Independent Connection: Abilene, 4223
Independent Connection: Beloit, 4224
Independent Connection: Concordia, 4225
Independent Driving Systems, 367, 367
Independent Life Center, 4077
Independent Life Styles, 4570
Independent Living, 4089, 4451
Independent Living Aids, 142, 157, 192, 531, 532, 534, 535, 586, 587, 593, 595, 602, 605, 606
Independent Living Approach to Disability Policy Studies, 2507
Independent Living Center Network: Department of the Visually Handicapped, 4611
Independent Living Center of Eastern Indiana (ILCEIN), 4199
Independent Living Center of Kern County, 4038
Independent Living Center of Lancaster, 4039
Independent Living Center of Mobile, 3966
Independent Living Center of Southeast Missouri, 4373
Independent Living Center of Stavros: Gree nfield, 4302
Independent Living Center of Stavros: Spri ngfield, 4303
Independent Living Center of the North Sho re & Cape Ann, 4304
Independent Living Centers and Managed Care: Results of an ILRU Study on Involvement, 5193
Independent Living Challenges the Blues, 5194
Independent Living for Persons with Disabi lities and Elderly People, 5077
Independent Living for Physically Disabled People, 5078
Independent Living Office, 5195, 4265
Independent Living Provider, 7705
Independent Living Research Utilization, 4662, 5200
Independent Living Research Utilization Project, 4571
Independent Living Research Utilization (ILRU), 5074
Independent Living Research Utilization ILRU, 5101, 5104, 5106, 5152, 5153, 5159, 5176, 5193, 5194, 5213, 5241, 5242, 5243, 5245, 5274, 5282, 5316, 8270
Independent Living Resource Center, 4040, 4226
Independent Living Resource Center: Santa Barbara, 4041
Independent Living Resource Center: San Fr ancisco, 4042
Independent Living Resource Center: Santa Maria Office, 4043
Independent Living Resource Center: Ventur a, 4044
Independent Living Resource of Contra Coast, 4045

Independent Living Resource of Fairfield, 4046
Independent Living Resource: Antioch, 4047
Independent Living Resource: Concord, 4048
Independent Living Resources, 4505
Independent Living Resources (ILR), 4049
Independent Living Resources of Greater Birmingham: Jasper, 3968
Independent Living Resources of Greater Bi rmingham, 3969
Independent Living Resources Of Greater Bi rmingham: Alabaster, 3967
Independent Living Service Northern California: Redding Office, 4050
Independent Living Services of Northern California, 4051
Independent Resource Georgetown, 4090
Independent Resources: Dover, 4091
Independent Resources: Wilmington, 4092
Independent Visually Impaired Entrepreneur s, 9063
Indian Acres Camp for Boys, 7922
Indian Creek Camp, 9116
Indian Creek Health and Rehabilitation Center, 7279
Indian Creek Nursing Center, 6903
Indian Rivers Mental Health Center - Bibb, 6503
Indian Rivers Mental Health Center - Picke ns, 6504
Indian Rivers Mental Health Center - Tusca loosa, 6505
Indian Trails Camp, 1197
Indiana Association for Home and Hospice Care (IAHHC), 861
Indiana Civil Rights Commission, 6035
Indiana Client Assistance Program, 3567
Indiana Congress of Parent and Teachers, 6322
Indiana Deaf Camp, 1140
Indiana Deaf Camps Foundation, 8179
Indiana Department of Education, 2195, 6329
Indiana Department of Education: Special Education Division, 2195
Indiana Department of Workforce Development, 6036
Indiana Developmental Disability Council, 3568
Indiana Directory of Disability Resources, 2135
Indiana Disability Employment Initiative, 6036
Indiana Hemophilia & Thrombosis Center, 1129
Indiana Protection & Advocacy Services Commission, 3569
Indiana Protection and Advocacy Services Commission, 6323
Indiana Resource Center For Autism, 8003, 8016, 8035, 8976, 8990
Indiana Resource Center for Autism, 4849
Indiana Resource Center for Families with Special, 6321
Indiana State Commission for the Handicapped, 3570
Indiana State Department of Health, 6330
Indiana University: Multipurpose Arthritis Center, 4850
Indianapolis Regional Office, 5698
Indianapolis Resource Center for Independe nt Living, 4200
Individualized Keyboarding, 2004
Industrial Accident Board de dept, 3492
Industrial Support Systems, 6595
Industries for the Blind of New York State, 7059
Industries of the Blind, 7071
Industries: Cambridge, 7005
Industries: Mora, 7006
Infant & Toddler Convection of Fairfield: Falls Church, 2681
Infinity Dance Theater, 30
Infirmary Health, 6229
Inflatable Back Pillow, 234
Infobase Publishing, 1862
InFocus, 1677, 7824
Infogrip, 516, 517, 1603, 1665, 1666, 1669
InfoLoop Induction Receiver, 184
Informa Healthcare, 5154
Information & Referral Center, 2508
Information & Referral Services, 1696
Information + Referral Services, 1696
Information Access Project, 9202
Information from HEATH Resource Center, 2162
Information Hotline, 8462
Information on Glaucoma, 9203
Information Services for People with Developmental Disabilities, 5196
Information, Protection & Advocacy for Persons with Disabilities, 3497
Information, Protection and Advocacy Center for Handicapped Individuals, 3498
Informed Touch; A Clinician's Guide To The Evaluation Of Myofascial Disorders, 8730
Informer, 7706, 8864
Ingham Regional Medical Center, 4908
Injured Mind, Shattered Dreams: Brian's Survival from a Severe Head Injury, 8731
Inland Northwest Community Foundation, 3329
inMotion Magazine, 5387
Innabah Camps, 1390
Inner Traditions, 5114, 5122, 8755, 8763
Inner Traditions - Bear & Company, 8386
Inner Traditions/Bear And Company, 8730
Innerlip Plates, 318
Innovation Management Group, 1751, 5517
Innovations, 7707, 7766
Innovations in Special Education Technology Division (ISET), 2102
Innovative Practices for Teaching Sign Language Interpreters, 8250
Innovative Products, 678
Innovative Programs: An Example of How CILs Can Put Their Work in Context, 5197
Innovative Rehabilitation Services, 6608
Innoventions, 600
Inova Mount Vernon Hospital Rehabilitation Program, 6476
Inova Rehabilitation Center, 6476
Inpatient Pain Rehabilitation Program, 7060
Inroads to Opportunities, 6131
Inside MS, 7708
Inside The Halo and Beyond: The Anatomy o f a Recovery, 8398
Insight, 9307
Insight Horse Camp, 1337
Insights, 2324
Inspiration Ministries, 4637
Inspired By Drive, 140
Inspiring Possibilities, 2325
Institute for Basic Research in Developmental Disabilities, 4961
Institute for Educational Leadership (IEL), 862
Institute for Families, 9064
Institute for Health & Aging, 7688
Institute for Human Centered Design, 1929, 1944
Institute for Human Development, 3668, 6521
Institute for Life Course and Aging, 7549
Institute For Rehabilitation & Research, 4571
Institute for Rehabilitation & Research, 6453, 7165
Institute for Visual Sciences, 4962
Institute of Living: Hartford Hospital, 2442
Institute of Physical Medicine and Rehabilitation, 6311
Institute on Aging, 7780
Institute on Disabilities At Temple Univ., 4525
Institute on Disability, 2219
Institute On Disability/UCED, 6230
Instruction of Persons with Severe Handicaps, 2005
Instructional Methods for Students, 2509
Instrumental Music for Dyslexics: A Teachi ng Handbook, 31
Insurance Solutions: Plan Well, Live Better, 5198
Int'l Association of Audio Information Services, 9306
Integrated Health Services at Waterford Commons, 7096
Integrated Health Services of Amarillo, 7166
Integrated Health Services of Durham, 6389
Integrated Health Services of Michigan at Clarkston, 6360
Integrated Health Services of Seattle, 7192
Integrated Health Services of St. Louis at Gravois, 7014
Intellectual and Developmental Disabilitie s (IDD), 2275
Intelli Tools, 1662, 1663, 1671, 1752, 1873, 1876
IntelliKeys, 1662
IntelliKeys USB, 1663
IntelliPics Studio 3, 1752
IntelliTalk, 1873
Intensive Early Intervention and Beyond, 5436
Inter-Actions, 1245
Interact Center, 32
Interact Center for the Visual and Perform ing Arts, 32
Interactions: Collaboration Skills for School Professionals, 2510
Interdisciplinary Clinical Assessment of Young Children with Developmental Disabilities, 8732
An Interdisciplinary Journal for the Socia l Study of Health, Illness and Medicine, 5112
Intermediate Conversational Sign Language, 8251
International Academy of Biological Dentistry and Medicine, 8495
International Academy of Independent Medical Evaluators, 863
International Academy of Oral Medicine & Toxicology, 8496
International Association for Cancer Victors & Friends, 8497
International Association of Audio Informa tion Services, 9065
International Association of Hygienic Phys icians, 8498
International Association of Laryngectomees, 8863
International Association of Yoga Therapists (IAYT), 864
International Braille and Technology Center for the Blind, 8896
International Catholic Deaf Association, 8149, 8308
International Center for the Disabled, 1629
International Child Amputee Network, 865
International Childbirth Education Association, 2103
International Chiropractors Association (ICA), 866
International Christian Youth Exchange, 2774
International Clinic of Biological Regeneration (ICBR), 867
International Cluttering Association, 8922
International Directory of Libraries for the Disabled, 5199
International Dyslexia Association, 2104, 2024, 3614, 3649, 3735, 3806, 8029, 8051, 8986
International Dyslexia Association of DC, 3499
International Dyslexia Association: Arizona Branch, 3443
International Dyslexia Association: Austin Branch, 3874
International Dyslexia Association: Central California Branch, 3463
International Dyslexia Association: Central Ohio Branch, 3787
International Dyslexia Association: Florida Branch, 3516
International Dyslexia Association: Georgia Branch, 3530
International Dyslexia Association: Hawaii Branch, 3544
International Dyslexia Association: Illinois Branch, 3564
International Dyslexia Association: Indiana Branch, 3571
International Dyslexia Association: Kansas/Missouri Branch, 3584
International Dyslexia Association: Louisiana Branch, 3661
International Dyslexia Association: Maryland Branch, 3614
International Dyslexia Association: Oregon Branch, 3806
International Dyslexia Association: Pennsylvania Branch, 3816
International Dyslexia Association: Rocky Mountain Branch, 3477
International Dyslexia Association: Tennessee Branch, 3858
International Dyslexia Association: Upper Midwest Branch, 3649
International Dyslexia Association: Virginia Branch, 3920

International Dyslexia Association: Washington State Branch, 3930
International Dyslexia Association: Wisconsin Branch, 3950
International Dyslexia Association: Iowa Branch, 3573
International Dyslexia Association: New Jersey Branch, 3717
International Dyslexia Association: North Carolina Branch, 3769
International Education, 2767
International Expressive Arts Therapy Association (IEATA), 868
International Federation on Aging, 7550
International Fluency Association, 8923, 9002
International Handbook on Mental Health Policy, 4703
International Hearing Dog, 8150, 8309
International Hearing Dog, Inc., 8309
International Hearing Society, 7801, 8151, 7678, 7817, 8292
International Journal of Aging and Human Development, 7709
International Journal of Arts Medicine, 2511
International Journal of Technology and Aging, 7710
International League Against Epilepsy (ILAE), 869
International Medical and Dental Hypnotherapy Association, 8499
International Myeloma Foundation, 8500
International Network for the Prevention of Elder Abuse, 7551
International OCD Foundation, 7867
International Paper Company Foundation, 3275
International Parkinson and Movement Disor der Society, 8105, 8357
International Psychogeriatrics, 7711
International Rehabilitation Review, 7712
International Student Exchange Programs (I SEP), 2775
International University Partnerships, 2776
International Ventilator Users Network, 8880
International Ventilator Users Network (IVUN), 870, 8501
International Women's Health Coalition (IWHC), 871
Interpretation: A Sociolinguistic Model, 8252
Interpreting Disability: A Qualitative Reader, 2512
Interpreting: An Introduction, 8253
Interstitial Cystitis Association, 5518
Intervention in School and Clinic, 2276
Intervention Practices in the Retention of Competitive Employment, 9204
Intervention Research in Learning Disabilities, 2513
Introduction to Learning Disabilities, 2514
Introduction to Special Education: Teaching in an Age of Challenge, 4th Edition, 2515
Introduction to Spina Bifida, 8733
Introduction to the Profession of Counseling, 2516
Invacare, 134, 149, 156, 224, 274, 388, 548, 690, 722
Invacare Corporation, 274, 439
Invacare Fulfillment Center, 548
Invacare Top End, 722
Invisible Children, 5437
Invisible Disabilities Association (IDA), 872
InvoTek, Inc., 1570
IOS Press, 5077, 5085
Iowa Career Connection, 6045
Iowa Central Industries, 6886
Iowa Child Health Specialty Clinics, 3574
Iowa City VA Medical Center, 5704
Iowa Civil Rights Commission, 6046
Iowa Commission of Persons with Disabilities, 3575
Iowa Compass, 3576
Iowa Department for the Blind, 3577
Iowa Department for the Blind Library, 4855
Iowa Department of Human Services, 3578
Iowa Department of Public Instruction: Bureau of Special Education, 2196
Iowa Department on Aging, 3579
Iowa Economic Development Authority, 6047
Iowa Protection & Advocacy for the Disabled, 3580
Iowa Registry for Congenital and Inherited Disorders, 4856
Iowa Valley Community College, 6048
Iowa Vocational Rehabilitation Services, 6049
IPACHI, 3497
IPSL Institute of Global Learning, 2773
Iris Network for the Blind, 6938
Iron Horse Productions, 696
Iron Mountain VA Medical Center, 5733
Ironwood Springs Christian Ranch, 1213
Irvine Health Foundation, 2840
Irving Place Rehabilitation and Nursing Ce nter, 7295
ISC, 5229
Issues and Research in Special Education, 2517
Issues in Independent Living, 5200
It isn't Fair!: Siblings of Children with Disabilities, 5054
It's All in Your Head: The Link Between Mercury Amalgams and Illness, 8734
It's Just Attention Disorder, 8088

J

J E Stewart Teaching Tools, 2031
J.D. McCarty Center, 1347
J.L. Bedsole/Rotary Rehabilitation Hospita l, 6229
Jack C. Montgomery VA Medical Center, 5799
Jack C. Montomery VA Medical Center, 5800
Jackson Center for Independent Living, 4558, 5202
Jackson Foundation, 3225
Jackson Independent Living Center, 4358
Jackson Regional Office, 5743
Jackson Square Nursing and Rehabilitation Center, 7269
Jacksonville Area Center for Independent Living, 4166
Jacksonville Area CIL: Havana, 4165
Jacksonville Public Library: Talking Books /Special Needs, 4801
Jacob and Charlotte Lehrman Foundation, 2904
JAMA: The Journal of the American Medical Association, 5201
James A Haley VA Medical Center, 5680
James Branch Cabell Library, 5022
James E Van Zandt VA Medical Center, 5811
James H And Cecile C Quillen Rehabilitation Hospital, 6433
James L. Maher Center, 3259
James Lawrence Kernan Hospital, 6946
James R Thorpe Foundation, 3063
James S McDonnell Foundation, 3076
Jane Coffin Childs Memorial Fund for Medical Research, 2892
Jane Phillips Medical Center, 6403, 7113, 6403
Janus of Santa Cruz, 6609
JARC, 4330
Jason & Nordic Publishers, Inc., 5203
Jason Aronson, 7991, 8033, 8972, 8988
Jawonio, 3738
Jawonio Vocational Center, 3739
Jay and Rose Phillips Family Foundation, 3064
JBI International, 9066
JBI Voice, 9283
JCIL Advocate Times, 5202
JDRF, 873
JE Stewart Teaching Tools, 1817, 1976, 1981, 1994, 2030, 2038, 2070
Jefferson Industries, 247
Jefferson Lee Ford III Memorial Foundation, 2920
Jelly Bean Switch, 1571
Jennifer Roberts Building, 4051
Jeremy P Tarcher, 5169
Jerry L Pettis Memorial VA Medical Center, 5651
Jersey Cape, 6132
Jessica Kingsley Publishers, 41, 42, 58, 5080, 5081, 5082, 5332, 8031, 8971, 8981
Jessie Ball duPont Fund, 2921
Jewish Braille Institute International, 9066
Jewish Braille Institute of America, 9283, 9284
Jewish Braille Review, 9284
Jewish Community Center of Greater Columbus, 1317
Jewish Community Center of Greater Rochester/JCC, 1284, 7911, 8945
Jewish Council for the Aging, 7552
Jewish Council for the Aging of Greater Washington, 7553
Jewish Healthcare Foundation of Pittsburgh, 3236
Jewish Hospital of St. Louis: Department of Rehabilitation, 6364
Jewish Vocational Service (JVS) - East Orange, 6133
Jewish Vocational Service (JVS) - Livingst on, 6134
Jewish Vocational Service (JVS) - Montclai r, 6135
Jewish Vocational Service of Jewish Family and Children's Services, 6094
Jewish Vocational Services, 6014
JFK Johnson Rehab Institute, 6377
JGB Audio Library for the Blind, 2739
JGB Cassette Library International, 4963
Jim Thorpe Rehabilitation Center at Southwest Medical Center, 6404
JK Designs, 151
JNeurosci, 7713
JoanBorysenko.Com, 5519
Job Accommodation Network, 2105
Job Accommodation Network (JAN), 874
The Job Developer's Handbook: Practical Ta ctics for Customized Employment, 5086
Job Hunting Tips for the So-Called Handicapped, 6249
Job Service North Dakota, 6166, 6166
Job Success for Persons with Developmental Disabilities, 5082
Jobri, 235, 235
Joey Interior Platform Lift, 368
John C Lincoln Hospital North Mountain, 6522
John D and Catherine T MacArthur Foundation, 2963
John D Dingell VA Medical Center, 5734
John Edward Fowler Memorial Foundation, 2905
John G & Marie Stella Kennedy Memorial Foundation, 3299
John H and Ethel G Nobel Charitable Trust, 2893
John H and Wilhelmina D Harland Charitable Foundation, 2935
John Hopkins University Press, 8807
John J Pershing VA Medical Center, 5745
John L McClellan Memorial Hospital, 5649
John Muir Medical Center Rehabilitation Services, Therapy Center, 6610
John O Pastore Center, 3833
John Randolph Foundation, 3319
John S Dunn Research Foundation, 3300
John W Anderson Foundation, 2986
John Wiley & Sons, 8721, 8758, 8824
John Wiley & Sons Inc, 8019
Johns Hopkins Children's Center, 1169, 1170
Johns Hopkins Hospital, 8605
Johns Hopkins University Dana Center for Preventive Ophthalmology, 4881
Johns Hopkins University Press, 5383, 8020, 8666, 8771, 8980
Johns Hopkins University: Asthma and Allergy Center, 4882
Johns Hopkins Universty Press, 8720
Johnson Controls Foundation, 3345
Johnson County Developmental Supports, 6904
Johnston County Industries, 7072
Joint Efforts, 8424
Jonathan M Wainwright Memorial VA Medical Center, 5850
Joni and Friends (JAF), 875
Joseph Drown Foundation, 2841
Joseph P Kennedy Jr Foundation, 2906
Joseph Willard Health Center, 2681
Joslin Diabetes Center, 8735
Joslin Guide to Diabetes: A Program for Managing Your Treatment, 8735
Jossey-Bass, 7948, 8006
Journal of Addictions & Offender Counselin g, 2277
Journal of Aging and Ethnicity, 7714

Journal of Aging and Health, 7715
Journal of Aging and Physical Activity, 7716
Journal of American Aging Association, 7717
Journal of Applied School Psychology, 2278
Journal of Cognitive Rehabilitation, 8052
Journal of Counseling & Development, 2279
Journal of Developmental and Physical Disabilities, 7718
Journal of Disability & Religion, 5361
Journal of Disability Policy Studies, 2280
Journal of Emotional and Behavioral Disorders, 2281
Journal of Ethics, Law, and Aging, 7719
Journal of Head Trauma Rehabilitation, 8844
Journal of Learning Disabilities, 2282
Journal of Mental Health and Aging, 7720
Journal of Midwifery & Women's Health (JMWH), 2283
Journal of Motor Behavior, 2284
Journal of Musculoskeletal Pain, 2285
Journal of Nuclear Medicine, 7721
Journal of Nuclear Medicine Technology, 7722
Journal of Positive Behavior Interventions, 2286
Journal of Postsecondary Education & Disability (JPED), 2287
Journal of Prosthetics and Orthotics, 2288
Journal of Public Health, 5378
Journal of Reading, Writing and Learning Disabled International, 2289
Journal of Rehabilitation, 2290, 7723
Journal of Religion, Spirituality & Aging, 7724
Journal of School Health Association, 2291
Journal of Social Work in Disabilty & Rehabilitation, 5204
Journal of Special Education, 2292
Journal of Speech, Language and Hearing Re search, 8293, 9001
Journal of the Academy of Rehabilitative A udiology, 8294
Journal of the American Academy of Audiolo gy, 7657
Journal of Therapeutic Horticulture, 7725
Journal of Visual Impairment and Blindness, 9276
Journal of Vocational Behavior, 2293
Journey, 5438
Journey to Well: Learning to Live After S pinal Cord Injury, 8736
Joy of Signing, 8254
Joy of Signing Puzzle Book, 8255
Joy: A Shabazz Center for Independent Living, 4475
JoySpinner, 102
Judevine Center for Autism, 4936
Judge David L Bazelon Center for Mental Health Law, 4663
Judson Press, 5363
Juggler, 9344
Juliet L Hillman Simonds Foundation, 3237
Julius and Betty Levinson Center, 6838
Jumpin' Johnny Get Back to Work, A Child's Guide to ADHD/Hyperactivity, 8011
Jumpsuits, 1526
Junction Center for Independent Living, 4612
Junction Center for Independent Living: Du ffield, 4613
Junior League Of Little Rock, 998, 8634
Jupiter Medical Center-Pavilion, 7243
Just Like Everyone Else, 5205
Justice in Aging, 7554

K

The K&W Guide to Colleges for Students with Learning Disabilties (13th Edition), 2635
K-BIT: Kaufman Brief Intelligence Test, 2682
K-FAST: Kaufman Functional Academic Skills Test, 2683
K-SEALS: Kaufman Survey of Early Academic and Language Skills, 2684
Kachina Point Health Care & Rehabilitation Center, 7214
Kaleidoscope: Exploring the Experience of Disability through Literature & the Fine Arts, 33
Kaleidoscope: Exploring the Expirence of Disability through Literature/Fine Arts, 7726
Kamp A-Komp-Plish, 9117
Kamp for Kids at Camp Togowauk, 1179
Kamp Kaleidoscope, 1450
Kamp Kaleo, 1235, 9118
Kamp Kiwanis, 1292
Kanawha County Public Library, 5037
Kanner Center, 7167
Kansas Advocacy and Protective Services, 3585
Kansas City VA Medical Center, 5746
Kansas Client Assistance Program, 3586
Kansas Commission on Disability Concerns, 3587
Kansas Department on Aging, 3588, 7636
Kansas Developmental Disability Council, 3589
Kansas Human Rights Commission, 6051
Kansas Rehabilitation Hospital, 6336
Kansas Services for the Blind & Visually Impaired, 4227
Kansas State Board of Education: Special Education Services, 2197
Kansas VA Regional Office, 5709
Kansas Vocational Rehabilitation Agency, 6052
Kaplan Early Learning Company, 2006
Kaplen JCC on the Palisades, 1251
Kate B Reynolds Charitable Trust, 3187
Katy Isaacson Elaine Gordon Lodge, 1293
Kauai Center for Independent Living, 4140
Kaufman Test of Educational Achievement (K-TEA), 2686
Kay Elemetrics Corporation, 1681, 1819
Kayelemetrics Corporation, 1824
Keats Publishing, 5234
Keep the Promise: Managed Care and People with Disabilities, 5206
Keeping Ahead in School, 2007
Keeping Our Families Together, 5207
Kelly Services Foundation, 3052
Kenai Peninsula Independent Living Center, 3978
Kenai Peninsula Independent Living Center: Seward, 3979
Kendall Demonstration Elementary School Curriculum Guides, 2518
Keni Peninsula Independent Living Center: Central Peninsula, 3980
Kennebunk Nursing & Rehabilitation Center, 7300
Kennedy Center, 5962
Kennedy Job Training Center, 6015
Kennedy Krieger Institute, 2741, 3018
Kennedy Park Medical Rehabilitation Center, 7418
Kenneth & Evelyn Lipper Foundation, 3151
Kenneth T and Eileen L Norris Foundation, 2842
Kensington Publishing, 5339
Kent County Arc, 3053
Kent District Library for the Blind and Physically Handicapped, 4911
Kentfield Rehabilitation Hospital & Outpatient Center, 6250
Kentucky Assistive Technology Service Network, 1630
Kentucky Cabinet for Health and Family Services, 3590
Kentucky Commission on Human Rights, 6053
Kentucky Council on Developmental Disability, 3591
Kentucky Department of Education: Division of Exceptional Children's Services, 2198
Kentucky Office for the Blind, 3592, 6054
Kentucky Office of Aging Services, 3593
Kentucky Protection & Advocacy, 3594
Kentucky Talking Book Library - Kentucky Dept. for Libraries and Archives, 4868
Kentucky Tennessee Conference, 9116
Kentucky Vocational Rehabilitation Agency, 6055
Kersey Mobility, 103
Keshet Dance and Center for the Arts, 34
Kessler Institute for Rehabilitation, 104, 2742, 6378
Ketch Industries, 6905
Ketogenic Diet: A Treatment for Children and Others with Epilepsy, 8737
Key Changes: A Portrait of Lisa Thorson, 8435
Key Tronic KB 5153 Touch Pad Keyboard, 1664
Keyboard Tutor, Music Software, 1754
Keyboarding by Ability, 1755
Keyboarding for the Physically Handicapped, 1756
Keyboarding with One Hand, 1757
KeyMath Teach and Practice, 2008
Keys to Parenting a Child with Attention Deficit Disorder, 8012
Keys to Parenting a Child with Downs Syndrome, 8013
Keys to Parenting the Child with Autism, 8014
Keystone Blind Association, 9067
The Keystone Group, 3255
KeyTronic, 1664
Keywi, 1684
KG Saur/Division of RR Bowker, 5199
Kid's Custom, 701
Kid's Edge, 702
Kid's Liberty, 703
Kid-Friendly Chairs, 704
Kid-Friendly Parenting with Deaf and Hard of Hearing Children, 8256
KIDS (Keyboard Introductory Development Series), 1753
Kids Cancer Alliance, 1151
KiDS NEED MoRE, 1271
Kids on the Block Programs, 8463
Kids Rock The World Day Camp, 1460
Kindered Health Care, 7375
Kindred, 6678, 7216, 7419
Kindred Health Care, 7198, 7219, 7280, 7386, 7393, 7406, 7428
Kindred Health Care Center, 7217
Kindred Health Care Publications, 7394
Kindred Healthcare, 6961, 7212, 7263, 7290, 7367, 7374, 7396, 7405, 7418, 7427
Kindred Healthcare, Inc., 6673
Kindred Heights Nursing & Rehabilitation Center, 7374
Kindred Hospital-La Mirada, 6611
Kindred Transitional Care and Rehabilitati on, 7261
King Keyboard, 1665
King's Daughter's Medical Center's Rehab Unit/Work Hardening Program, 6911
King's Rule, 1697
King's View Work Experience Center- Atwater, 6612
Kings Harbor Multicare Center, 7338
Kings Rehabilitation Center, 5924
Kiplinger Foundation, 2907
Kitsap Community Resources, 4626
Kitten Who Couldn't Purr, 8973
Kiwanis Camp Wyman, 8633
KlearVue, 369
Kleinert's, 440
KLST-2: Kindergarten Language Screening Test Edition, 2nd Edition, 2685
Kluge Children's Rehabilitation Center, 6477
Kluwer Academic Publishers, 7718
Knee Socks, 1527
Know Your Eye, 9205
Knowing Your Rights, 4704
Knox County Council for Developmental Disabilities, 6016
Knoxville VA Medical Center, 5705
Koala Miniflex, 705
Koicheff Health Care Center, 7061
Koinonia Foundation of Tennessee, 1417, 1418
Kokomo Rehabilitation Hospital, 6324
Koret Foundation, 2843
Kostopulos Dream Foundation, 1456
Kota Camp, 998, 8634
Kreider Services, 6017
Kresge Foundation, 3054
Krieger Publishing Company, 2408, 2610, 8394
Kris' Camp, 1086
Kris' Camp/Therapy Intensive Programs, Inc., 1086
Kroepke Kontrols, 84, 93, 95, 96, 99, 101, 105
Kuhn Employment Oppurtunities, 6702
Kuschall of America, 661, 662, 663, 671
Kuschall USA/Invacare, 207
Kuzell Institute for Arthritis and Infectious Diseases, 4772

L

La Frontera Center, 6523
La-Z-Boy, 370
LA84 Foundation, 2844
Lab School of Washington, 2189, 7923
LaBac Systems, 718
Labeling Kits, 488
Laboure College Library, 4902
Ladacain Network, 7037
Ladies Auxiliary to the VFW, 7750
Ladybug Corner Chair, 217
Lafayette Nursing and Rehabilitation Center, 7253
LaFayette-Walker Public Library, 4823
Lake County Center for Independent Living, 4169
Lake County Health Department, 6839
Lake County Public Library Talking Books Service, 4851
Lake Erie College, 2777
Lake Michigan Academy, 2743
Lakeland Adult Day Training, 4115
Lakeland Center, 6994
Lakemary Center, 6906
LakeMed Nursing and Rehabilitation Center, 7363
Lakeshore Camp and Retreat Center, 1416, 1421
Lakeshore Foundation, 8450
Lakeshore Learning Materials, 2009
Lakeside Milam Recovery Centers (LMRC), 7193
Lakeview NeuroRehabilitation Center, 6371
Lakeview Rehabilitation Hospital, 6340
Lakeview Subacute Care Center, 7326
Lakewood Health Care Center, 7194
Lambs Farm, 6018
Lambton County Developmental Services (LCDS), 876
LampLighter, 9308
Lanakila Rehabilitation Center, 5999
Land of Lincoln Goodwill Industries, 6019
Land-of-Sky Regional Council Area Agency o n Aging, 7781
Landmark Media, 5406, 5432, 5438, 5464, 9134, 9352
Landscape Architecture Magazine, 1952
Lane Community College, 2778
Language and Communication Disorders in Children, 2521
Language Arts: Detecting Special Needs, 2519
Language Disabilities in Children and Adolescents, 8974
Language Learning Practices with Deaf Children, 2520
Language Parts Catalog, 2010
Language Tool Kit, 2011
Language, Speech and Hearing Services in School, 2012
Language, Speech, and Hearing Services in Schools, 9002
Lanting Foundation, 3055
LaPalma Intercommunity Hospital, 6613
Lapeer: Blue Water Center for Independent Living, 4331
LaRabida Children's Hospital and Research Center, 6312
Laradon Hall Society for Exceptional Children and Adults, 6681
Large Button Speaker Phone, 185
Large Display Alarm Clock, 597
Large Print DOS, 1759
Large Print Keyboard, 1666
Large Print Keyboard Labels, 1572
Large Print Loan Library, 9206
Large Print Loan Library Catalog, 9207
Large Print Recipies for a Healthy Life, 9208
Large Print/Braille Keyboard Labels, 1603
Large Type, 1874
Las Animas County Rehabilitation Center, 5951
Las Vegas Healthcare And Rehabilitation Center, 7024
Las Vegas Healthcare and Rehabilitation Ce nter, 7321
Las Vegas Veterans Center, 5757
Las Vegas-Clark County Library District, 4944
Lash & Associates Publishing/Training, 8009
Late Talker: What to Do If Your Child Isn' t Talking Yet, 8975
Latex Allergy in Spina Bifida Patients, 8738
Laureate Learning Systems, 1760
Laurel Designs, 5175
Laurel Grove Hospital: Rehab Care Unit, 6251
Laurel Hill Center, 4506
Laurent Clerc National Deaf Education Cent er, 877
Laurent Clerc: The Story of His Early Year s, 8257
Law Center Newsletter, 4705
LC Technologies Inc, 1567
LD Child and the ADHD Child: Ways Parents & Professionals Can Help, 8015
LD Monthly Report, 2326
LD Online, 2106, 2320, 2326
LD OnLine - WETA Public Television, 5520
LDS Hospital Rehabilitation Center, 6470
Leadership Council of Aging Organizations, 7555
Leading Age, 7556
LeadingAge, 7557
LeadingAge Arizona, 7558
LeadingAge California, 7559
LeadingAge Connecticut, 7560
LeadingAge Gulf States, 7561
LeadingAge Illinois, 7562
LeadingAge Indiana, 7563
LeadingAge Iowa, 7564
LeadingAge Kentucky, 7565
LeadingAge Maine & New Hampshire, 7566
LeadingAge Massachusetts, 7567
LeadingAge Missouri, 7568
LeadingAge Nebraska, 7569
LeadingAge New Jersey, 7570
LeadingAge New York, 7571
LeadingAge North Carolina, 7572
LeadingAge Ohio, 7573
LeadingAge Oklahoma, 7574
LeadingAge Oregon, 7575
LeadingAge PA, 7576
LeadingAge RI, 7577
LeadingAge Texas, 7578
LeadingAge Wisconsin, 7579
LeadingAge Wyoming, 7580
League at Camp Greentop, 1173
The League for People with Disabilities, Inc., 1173
League for the Blind and Disabled, 4201
League for the Hard of Hearing, 8152
League Letter, 8310
League of Human Dignity, Center for Indepe ndent Living, 4211
League of Human Dignity: Lincoln, 4397
League of Human Dignity: Norfolk, 4398
League of Human Dignity: Omaha, 4399
Learn About the ADA in Your Local Library, 5208
Learning About Numbers, 1698
Learning Activity Packets, 1864
Learning American Sign Language, 2013
Learning Among Children with Spina Bifida, 8739
Learning and Individual Differences, 2525
Learning Company, 1761, 1699, 1846
Learning Corporation of America, 5413, 5437
Learning Disabilities Association of Ameri ca (LDA), 878
Learning Disabilities Association of America, 2295, 8008
Learning Disabilities Association of Arkansas, 2322
Learning Disabilities Association of New York State (LDANYS), 879
Learning disAbilities Resources, 8083
Learning Disabilities Sourcebook, 3rd Ed., 35
Learning Disabilities Worldwide, 880
Learning Disabilities, Literacy, and Adult Education, 2522
Learning Disabilities: A Contemporary Jour nal, 2294
Learning Disabilities: A Multidisciplinary Journal, 2295
Learning Disabilities: Concepts and Characteristics, 2523
Learning Disability Quarterly, 2296
Learning Disability: Social Class and the Cons of Inequality In American Education, 2524
Learning English: Primary, 1832
Learning English: Rhyme Time, 1833
Learning House, 2687
Learning Independence Through Computers, 1631
Learning Resources, 2014
Learning Services Corporation, 6390
Learning Services of Northern California, 6614
Learning Services: Bear Creek, 6682
Learning Services: Carolina, 7073
Learning Services: Harris House Program, 6795
Learning Services: Morgan Hill, 6615
Learning Services: Supported Living Programs, 6616
Learning to Feel Good and Stay Cool: Emoti onal Regulation Tools for Kids With AD/HD, 2526
Learning to Play, 9209
Learning to See: American Sign Language as a Second Language, 2527
Learning to Sign in My Neighborhood, 2015
Learning Tools International, 1743
LearningRx, 2688
Lebanon VA Medical Center, 5812
LeBonheur Cardiac Kids Camp, 1423
LeBonheur Children's Hospital, 1423
Lectra-Lift, 370
Ledgewood Rehabilitation and Skilled Nursing Center, 7310
Lee County Library System: Talking Books Library, 4802
Lee Memorial Hospital, 6754
Left Foot Gas Pedal, 105
Left Foot Gas Pedal, The, 106
Leg Elevation Board, 489
Legacy, 7767
Legacy Emanuel Rehabilitation Center, 7118
Legal Action Center, 4664
Legal Center for People with Disabilities & Older People, 3478, 4706
Legal Council for Health Justice, 7581
Legal Counsel for Health Jusice, 4665
Legal Right: The Guide for Deaf and Hard of Hearing People, 4707
Legal Rights of Persons with Disabilities, 4708
Legislative Handbook for Parents, 4709
Legislative HQ, 5674
Legislative Network for Nurses, 4710
Legler Benbough Foundation, 2846
Lehigh Valley Center for Independent Living, 4526
Lehigh Valley Center for Independent Living, 5211
Leisure Lift, 549
Leo P La Chance Center for Rehabilitation and Nursing, 7311
Leon S Peters Rehabilitation Center, 6617
Leonard Media Group, 8409
Les Turne Amyotrophic Laterial Sclerosis Foundation, 2964
Leslie G Ehmann Trust, 3226
Lester Electrical, 638
Lester H Higgins Adult Center, 7097
Let Community Employment be the Goal for Individuals with Autism, 8016, 8976
Let's Eat, 9210
Let's Eat Video, 5439, 9345
Let's Talk About Having Asthma, 8740
Let's Write Right: Teacher's Edition, 2528
Letter Writing Guide, 586
Lettering Guide Value Pack, 587
Lettie Pate Whitehead Foundation, 2936
Leukemia & Lymphoma Society, 8502
Leukemia Sourcebook, 8741
Levenger, 601
Leveron Door Lever, 490
Levi Strauss Foundation, 2847
Levindale Hebrew Geriatric Center, 6947
Levinson Medical Center, 2744
Lewiston Public Library, 4876
Lewy Body Dementia Association, 7868, 8106, 8358
Lexia I, II and III Reading Series, 1834
Lexia Learning Systems, 1834, 1842
Lexington Center for Health and Rehabilita tion, 7291

Lexington School for the Deaf: Center for the Deaf, 8153
Lexington VA Medical Center, 5711
Liberty, 679
Liberty Lightweight Aluminum Stroll Walker, 616
Liberty LT, 371
Liberty Media Corporation, 7704
Liberty Resources, 4527
Library Commission for the Blind, 4857
Library Cooperative/ Library for the blind, 4918
Library for the Blind & Physically Handicapped, 4998
Library for the Blind and Physically Handi capped SW Region of Arkansas, 4760
Library Manager's Guide to Hiring and Serving Disabled Persons, 2529
Library Services for the Blind, 9211
Library Users of America Newsletter, 9309
Life After Trauma: A Workbook for Healing, 8742
Life and Independence for Today, 4528
Life Beyond the Classroom: Transition Strategies for Young People with Disabilities, 5055
Life Beyond the Classroom: Transition Str ategies for Young People with Disabilities, 5392
LIFE Center for Independent Living, 4167
Life Center for Independent Living: Pontia c, 4170
Life Centered Career Education: A Contemporary Based Approach, 2689
Life Development Institute, 7869
Life Line, 8743
LIFE of Mississippi, 4359
LIFE of Mississippi: Biloxi, 4360
LIFE of Mississippi: Greenwood, 4361
LIFE of Mississippi: Hattiesburg, 4362
LIFE of Mississippi: McComb, 4363
LIFE of Mississippi: Meridian, 4364
LIFE of Mississippi: Oxford, 4365
LIFE of Mississippi: Tupelo, 4366
Life on Wheels: For the Active Wheelchair User, 8399
Life Planning for Adults with Developmental Disabilities, 7643
Life Science Associates, 8094
Life Skills Laundry Division, 6887
Life Unlimited, 7870
Life Unlimited, Inc., 7870
Life Way Christian Resources Southern Baptist Conv, 2644
Life-Skills, Inc., 6081
Life-Span Approach to Nursing Care for Individuals with Developmental Disabilities, 2530
LIFE/ Run Centers for Independent Living, 4572
LIFE: Fort Hall, 4147
LifeBridge Health, 813
LifeCare Alliance - Central Ohio Diabetes Assoc., 1322
LifeLines, 5209, 5307
Lifelong Leisure Skills and Lifestyles for Persons with Developmental Disabilities, 5210
LifeROOTS, 6148
LifeSkills Industries, 6912
LIFESPAN Incorporated, 6159
LifeSpan Network, 7582
Lifestand, 692
Lifestyles of Employed Legally Blind People, 9212
LifeWay Christian Resources, 8283
LifeWay Christian Resources Southern Baptist Conv., 2595
Lifeworks Employment Services, 6972
Lift-All, 372
Lifter, 373
Lifts for Swimming Pools and Spas, 374
Light the Way, 9310
Lighthouse Central Florida, 4116, 5981
Lighthouse for the Blind, 1035, 9114
Lighthouse for the Blind in New Orleans, 6926
Lighthouse for the Blind of Palm Beach, 6755
Lighthouse for the Visually Impaired and Blind, 6756
Lighthouse Guild, 2107, 5521, 9068, 442, 9086, 9273, 9274, 9329, 9346, 9350
Lighthouse International, 5425, 7757
Lighthouse International Information and Resource Service, 9364
Lighthouse Low Vision Products, 442
Lighthouse of Houston, 7168
Lighthouse Publication, 9311
Lights On, 9312
Lightweight Breezy, 680
Lilac Services for the Blind, 7802
LINC-Monroe Randolph Center, 4168
Lincoln County Health System, 7146
Lincoln Regional Office, 5754
Lincoln VA Medical Center, 5755
Lincoln YMCA, 8661
Lindamood-Bell Home Learning Process, 8924
Lindustries, 490
Linguistics of American Sign Language: An Introduction, 8258
LINK: Colby, 4228
Linking Employment, Abilities and Potentia l, 4491
Lion, 9213
Lion's Blind Center of Diablo Valley, Inc. Lions Center For The Visually Impaired, 6618
Lion's Blind Center of Oakland, 6619
Lion's Clubs International, 9213
Lions 11 B-2 and MADHH, 8182
Lions Camp Crescendo, 1152, 8199
Lions Camp Kirby, 8200
Lions Camp Merrick, 1174, 8201
Lions Camp Tatiyee, 992, 8635
Lions Club Industries for the Blind, 7074
Lions Clubs International, 2779, 9069
Lions Den Outdoor Learning Center, 7924
Lions of Multiple District 35, 7806
Lions Services Inc., 7075
Lions Wilderness Camp for Deaf Children, Inc., 1037, 8202
Lions Wilderness Camp Headquarters, 1037, 8202
Lions World Services for the Blind, 6537
Lipomas & Lipomyelomeningocele, 8744
Lippincott Williams And Wilkins, 2548
Lippincott Williams & Wilkins, 8707, 8838
Lippincott, Williams & Wilkins, 2403, 2535, 2538, 2539, 2568, 5365, 5373, 7642, 8722, 8844, 8853
Lisa Beth Gerstman Camp, 1294
Lisa Beth Gerstman Foundation, 1294
Lisle, 2780
Listen Foundation, 2881, 1058, 8196
Listen Up, 9313
Listner, 8311
Literacy & Your Deaf Child: What Every Pa rent Should Know, 8259
Literacy Program, 2016
Literature Based Reading, 2017
Literature Journal, The, 8295
Little City Foundation, 2965
Little Friends, Inc., 6840
Little Heroes Preschool Burn Camp, 1038
Little Mack Communicator, 1685
Little People of America, 8503
Little Red Door Cancer Agency, 1131
Little Red Hen, 1762
Little Rock Vet Center #0713, 6538
Little Sisters of The Poor, 7744
Live Independently Networking Center, 4476
Live Independently Networking Center: Hickory, 4477
Live Oaks Career Development Campus, 7098
Liver Disorders Sourcebook, 8745
Livin', 5211
Living an Idea: Empowerment and the Evolution of an Alternative School, 2018
Living Beyond Multiple Sclerosis: A Woman 's Guide, 8746
Living in a State of Stuck, 5212
Living in the Community, 5213
Living Independence for Everyone (LIFE), 4130
Living Independence Network Corporation, 4148
Living Independence Network Corporation: Twin Falls, 4149
Living Independence Network Corporation: C aldwell, 4150
Living Independent for Everyone (LIFE): Pocatello Office, 4151
Living Independently for Everyone (LIFE): Blackfoot Office, 4152
Living Independently for Everyone (LIFE): Pocate, 4152
Living Independently for Everyone: Burley, 4153
Living Independently for Today and Tomorro w, 4389
Living Independently in Northwest Kansas: Hays, 4229
Living Independently Now Center (LINC), 4171
Living Independently Now Center: Sparta, 4172
Living Independently Now Center: Waterloo, 4173
Living Skills Center for the Visually Impaired, 6620
Living Well with Asthma, 8747
Living Well with Chronic Fatigue Syndrome and Fibromyalgia, 8748
Living Well with HIV and AIDS, 8749
Living with a Brother or Sister with Speci al Needs: A Book for Sibs, 5308
Living with Achromatopsia, 9214
Living with Brain Injury: A Guide for Fami lies, 8751
Living with Spina Bifida: A Guide for Fami lies and Professionals, 8752
Living With Spinal Cord Injury Series, 8750
Livingston Center for Independent Living, 4332
LJ Skaggs and Mary C Skaggs Foundation, 2845
Lloyd Hearing Aid Corporation, 289, 290, 291, 298
Lodi Memorial Hospital, 6252
Lodi Memorial Hospital West, 6252
Lola Wright Foundation, 3301
Lollipop Lunch, 8977
Loma Linda University Orthopedic and Rehabilitation Institute, 6621
Long Beach Department of Health and Human Services, 3464
Long Beach Memorial Medical Center Memorial Rehabilitation Hospital, 6253, 7221
Long Beach VA Medical Center, 5652
Long Cane News, 9314
Long Handled Bath Sponges, 148
Long Island Alzheimer's Foundation, 3152
Long Island Center for Independent Living, 4452
Long Island Talking Book Library System, 4970
Long Oven Mitts, 319
Long Ring Low Vision Timers, 320
Long-Term Care: How to Plan and Pay for It, 7644
Longman Education/Addison Wesley, 2379, 2510
Longman Group, 2604
Longman Publishing Group, 2463, 2572, 2658, 2661
Longreach Reacher, 491
Longwood Foundation, 2897
Look Out for Annie, 9346
Look Who's Laughing, 5440
Looking Good: Learning to Improve Your Appearance, 1763
Loop Scissors, 492
Los Angeles County Department of Health Services, 3465
Los Angeles Regional Office, 5653
LoSeCa Foundation, 881
A Loss for Words, 8211
Lost Tree Village Charitable Foundation, 2922
Lotus Press, 8690
Loud, Proud and Passionate, 5214
Loudoun County Adaptive Recreation Camps, 1473
Loudoun County Parks, Recreation & Community Svcs, 1473
Louis A Johnson VA Medical Center, 5856
Louis and Anne Abrons Foundation, 3153
Louis de la Parte Florida Mental Health Institute Research Library, 4803
Louis R Lurie Foundation, 2848
Louis Stokes VA Medical Center - Wade Park Campus, 5798
Louisiana Assistive Technology Access Network, 3597
Louisiana Center for Dyslexia and Related Learning Disorders, 3598
Louisiana Center for the Blind, 6927
Louisiana Department of Aging, 3599
Louisiana Department of Education, 2199

Louisiana Department of Education: Office of Special Education Services, 2199
Louisiana Department of Health - Mental Health Services, 3600
Louisiana Developmental Disability Council, 3601
Louisiana Learning Resources System, 3602
Louisiana Lions Camp, 1158
Louisiana Rehabilitation Services, 6059, 6057
Louisiana State Library, 4871
Louisiana State University Eye Center, 6928
Louisiana State University Genetics Sectio n of Pediatrics, 4872
Louisville Free Public Library, 4869
Louisville VA Medical Center, 5712
Louisville VA Regional Office, 5713
Lourdes Regional Rehabilitation Center, 7038
Lousiana State University, 6928
Love Publishing Company, 2270, 2390, 2417, 2621, 2630, 4699, 8041, 8995
Love: Where to Find It, How to Keep It, 5215
Loving & Letting Go, 5309
Loving Justice, 4711
A Loving Spoonful, 723
Low Tech Assistive Devices: A Handbook for the School Setting, 2019
Low Vision Questions and Answers: Definitions, Devices, Services, 9215
Low Vision Services of Kentucky, 6913
Low Vision Telephones, 598
Low Vision Watches & Clocks, 599
Low Vision: Reflections of the Past, Issues for the Future, 9216
Lowe Syndrome Association, 8504, 1909
Lowe Syndrome Conference, 1909
Loyola Press, 5362
LPDOS Deluxe, 1758
LRP Publications, 2311, 2314, 2340, 3358, 3365, 4687, 4708, 5062, 5273, 6297
LS&S, 441, 452
Lucy Lee Hospital, 7016
Luke B Hancock Foundation, 2849
Lumber River Council of Governments Area A gency on Aging, 7782
Lumex Cushions and Mattresses, 236
Lumex Recliner, 218
Luminaud, Inc., 443, 434, 1683
Lung Cancer: Making Sense of Diagnosis, Treatment, and Options, 8753
Lung Disorders Sourcebook, 8754
Lung Line Information Service, 8897
Lupus: Alternative Therapies That Work, 8755
Lutheran Blind Mission, 4937
Lutheran Charities Foundation of St Louis, 3077
Lutherans Outdoors in South Dakota, 1410, 8642
Lutherdale Bible Camp, 1489
Lutherdale Ministries, 1489
Luxis International, Inc., 641
Lyme Disease Foundation, 5522
Lymphoma Canada, 8505
Lynchburg Area Center for Independent Living, 4614
Lynde and Harry Bradley Foundation, 3346
Lynne Rienner Publishers, 2163
Lyons Campus of the VA New Jersey Healthcare System, 5766

M

M ER S Goodwill, 7015
M Evans and Company, 5315
M&M Health Care Apparel Company, 1528
MA Report, 2327
Mac's Lift Gate, 375
Mac's Lift Gate, Inc., 375
MacDonald Training Center, 6757
MacMillan - St. Martin's Press, 8389
Macomb Library for the Blind & Physically Handicapped, 4912
Macon Library for the Blind and Physically Handicapped, 4821
Macon Resources, 6842
Macrobiotics Today, 7727
Macular Degeneration Foundation, 9070, 9315
Mad Hatters: Theatre That Makes a World of Difference, 2745
Mada Medical Products, 139, 263, 272, 275, 280, 284, 610, 615, 616, 618, 619, 620, 623, 629, 683, 693
MADAMIST 50/50 PSI Air Compressor, 275
Maddak Inc., 445
Madison County Hospital, 7287
Madison County Rehab Services, 7287
Madison Healthcare and Rehabilitation Cent er, 7383
Madonna Rehabilitation Hospital, 6368, 7319
Magazines in Special Media for the Handicapped, 7728
Magee Rehabilitation Hospital, 6422
MAGIC Foundation for Children's Growth, 2966, 8756
MAGIC Touch, 8756
Magic Wand Keyboard, 1667
Magni-Cam & Primer, 600
Magnifier, 9315
Magnifier Bookweight, 601
Magnolia Health Systems, 7276
Main Office & Developmental Training Center, 6830
Maine Assistive Technology Projects, 3605
Maine Association of Non Profits, 3001
Maine Bureau of Elder and Adult Services, 3606
Maine CITE, 1633
Maine Commission on Disability & Employmen t, 6066
Maine Department of Health and Human Services, 3607
Maine Department Of Labor, 6067
Maine Developmental Disabilities Council, 3608
Maine Division for the Blind and Visually Impaired, 3609
Maine Human Rights Commission, 6068, 6068
Maine Office of Elder Services, 3610
Maine State, 4877
Maine State Library, 4877
Maine VA Regional Office, 5717
Maine Workers' Compensation Board, 3611
Mainland Center Hospital RehabCare Unit, 7169
Mainstay Life Services, 1391
Mainstay Life Services Summer Program, 1391
Mainstream, 882, 3995, 2540, 5414, 9141
Mainstream Living, 5523
Mainstream Magazine, 5217
Mainstream Online Magazine of the Able-Disabled, 5524
Mainstreaming and the American Dream, 9217
Mainstreaming Deaf and Hard of Hearing Students: Questions and Answers, 2531
Mainstreaming Exceptional Students: A Guide for Classroom Teachers, 2532
Mainstreaming the Visually Impaired Child, 9218
Mainstreaming: A Practical Approach for Teachers, 2533
Majors Medical Equipment, 681
Makemie Woods Camp, 8636
Makemie Woods Camp/Conference Retreat, 8637
Making a Difference, 5221
Making a Difference: A Wise Approach, 5222
Making Changes: Family Voices on Living Disabilities, 5218
Making Choices for Independent Living, 4290
Making Informed Medical Decisions: Where to Look and How to Use What You Find, 5219
Making Life More Livable, 9219
Making News: How to Get News Coverage of Disability Rights Issues, 4712, 5083
Making School Inclusion Work: A Guide to Everyday Practice, 2021
Making Self-Employment Work for People wit h Disabilities, 5084
Making the Writing Process Work, 8017
Making the Writing Process Work: Strategie s for Composition and Self-Regulation, 2022
Making Wise Decisions for Long-Term Care, 5220
Man's Low-Vision Quartz Watches, 602
Management of Autistic Behavior, 8018, 8757, 8978
Management of Genetic Syndromes, 8758
Managing Attention Deficit Hyperactivity in Children: A Guide for Practitioners, 8019
Managing Diagnostic Tool of Visual Perception, 2534
Managing Post Polio: A Guide to Living Well with Post Polio, 8759
Managing Your Activities, 5223
Managing Your Health Care, 5224
Managing Your Symptoms, 8332
Manatee Springs Care & Rehabilitation Center, 6285
Manchester Regional Office, 5761
Manchester VA Medical Center, 5762
Mane Stream, 1261
Manhattan Public Library, 4860
Manidokan Outdoor Ministry Center, 1171
Manor Care Health Services- Citrus Heights, 6622
Manor Care Health Services- Palm Desert, 6623
Manor Care Health Services-Fountain Valley, 6624
Manor Care Health Services-Hemet, 6625
Manor Care Health Services-Sunnyvale, 6626
Manor Care Health Services-Tacoma, 7195
Manor Care Health Services-Walnut Creek, 6627
Manor Care Nursing and Rehab Center: Tucson, 6524
Manor Care Nursing and Rehabilitation Center: Boulder, 6684
Manor Care Nursing: Denver, 6685
Manor Care Ohio, 6684
ManorCare Health Services-Arlington, 7182
ManorCare Health Services-Lynnwood, 7196
ManorCare Health Services-Spokane, 7197
Manual Alphabet Poster, 2023
Manual of Sequential Art Activities for Classified Children and Adolescents, 36
Many Faces of Dyslexia, 2024
MAP Training Center, 6841
MAPCON Technologies, 2164
Maplebrook School, 1295, 7925
Mapleton Center, 6275
MarbleSoft, 5569, 5577
March of Dimes, 883
Margaret L Wendt Foundation, 3154
Margaret T Morris Foundation, 2805
Marianjoy Rehabilitation Hospital and Clinics, 6313
Marin Center for Independent Living, 4052
Marin Community Foundation, 2850
Mariner Health Care: Connecticut, 6277
Mariner Health of Nashville, 7384
Marion VA Medical Center, 5695
Marist Brothers Mid-Hudson Valley Camp, 1296, 8638
Mark Elmore Associates Architects, 1930
Mark Seven Deaf Foundation, 1280, 8189
Marmon Valley, 1337
Marriner S Eccles Foundation, 3312
Marriott International, 5593
Marshall & Ilsley Trust Company, 3350
Marshall & Ilsley Trust of Florida, 2994
Marshall University College Of Educational & Human, 5040
Martin Luther Homes of Indiana, 4202
Martin Luther Homes of Iowa, 4212
Martin Technology, 627
Martinez Outpatient Clinic, 5654
Martinsburg VA Medical Center, 5857
Marvelwood School, 7926
Marvelwood Summer, 7926
Mary A Crocker Trust, 2851
Mary Bryant Home for the Blind, 6843
Mary Free Bed Rehabilitation Hospital, 6995
Mary Lanning Memorial Hospital, 7320
Mary Reynolds Babcock Foundation, 3188
Maryland Client Assistance Program Division of Rehabilitation Services, 3615
Maryland Commission on Civil Rights (FEPA), 6071
Maryland Department of Aging, 3616
Maryland Department of Disabilities, 6072, 1634
Maryland Department of Handicapped Children, 3617
Maryland Developmental Disabilities Council, 3618

Maryland Division of Mental Health, 3619
Maryland Employment Network, 6073
Maryland State Department of Education, 6074, 4883
Maryland State Department of Education: Division of Special Education, 2205
Maryland State Library for the Blind and Physically Handicapped, 4883
Maryland Technology Assistance Program, 1634
Maryland Veterans Centers, 5722
Mask of Benevolence: Disabling the Deaf Community, The, 8260
Masonic Healthcare Center, 7233
MasoniCare Corporation, 7233
Massachusetts Assistive Technology Partnership, 3624
Massachusetts Client Assistance Program, 3625
Massachusetts Commission Against Discrimin ation (FEPA), 6082
Massachusetts Commission for the Blind, 6083
Massachusetts Department of Education, 2201
Massachusetts Department of Education: Program Quality Assurance, 2201
Massachusetts Department of Mental Health, 3626
Massachusetts Developmental Disabilities Council, 3627
Massachusetts Eye & Ear Infirmary, 4901
Massachusetts Eye and Ear Infirmary & Vision Rehabilitation Center, 6973
Massachusetts Governor's Commission on Employment of People with Disabilities, 6084
Massachusetts Office on Disability, 3625
Massachusetts Rehabilitation Commission, 4903, 6085
Massage Therapy Journal, 7729
Massena Independent Living Center, 4453
MAT Factory, Inc., 643, 647, 649
Match-Sort-Assemble Job Cards, 2025
Match-Sort-Assemble Pictures, 2026
Match-Sort-Assemble SCHEMATICS, 2027
Match-Sort-Assemble TOOLS, 2028
Maternal and Child Health Bureau - Health Resources and Services Administration, 3620
Math for Everyday Living, 1700
Math for Successful Living, 1701
Math Rabbit, 1699
Mature Health, 7730
Mature Years, 7731
Maumee Valley Girl Scout Center, 8588
Maxi Aids, 446, 79, 144, 145, 150, 154, 155, 160, 164, 169, 197, 202, 251, 253, 258, 259, 281, 282, 304, 305, 307, 312, 313, 315, 317, 320, 327, 328, 329, 383, 446, 475, 483, 488, 511, 519, 520, 527, 529, 530, 533, 536, 544, 565, 579, 580, 583, 584, 589, 590, , 594, 599, 603, 608, 609, 614, 625, 631, 633, 689, 697, 712, 1595, 1596, 5557, 5558, 5559, 5560, 5561, 5562, 5563, 5565, 5566, 5568, 5571, 5575, 5580, 5582, 9356
MaximEyes, 7828
Maynord's Chemical Dependency Recovery Centers, 6628
Maynord's Ranch for Men, 6629
Mayo Clinic Scottsdale, 7215
Mayor of the West Side, 5056
Mc Graw- Hill, School Publishing, 2614
McAlester Regional Health Center RehabCare Unit, 7114
McCune Charitable Foundation, 3107
McDonald's Corporation Contributions Program, 2967
McFarland & Company, 1742, 2529
McGraw-Hill, 8687
McGraw-Hill Company, 2165, 7, 2556, 5178, 8825
McGraw-Hill Professional, 8388
McGraw-Hill School Publishing, 2005, 2359, 2377, 2464, 2468, 2516, 2523, 2533, 2555, 2598, 2601, 2623, 8974
McGraw-Hill School Publishn, 2521
McGraw-Hill, School Publishing, 2060, 2437
McInerny Foundation Bank Of Hawaii, Corporate Trustee, 2943
McKey Mouse, 1668
McKinnon Body Therapy Center, 884
Mclean Hospital Child/Adolescent Program, 7896, 8942
McMurry, 7753
MDA Summer Camp, 1121
MDA/ALS Newsmagazine, 2297
The Mead Center for American Theater, 6, 7793
Meadowbrook Manor, 6630
Meadows Foundation, 3302
Meadowvale Health and Rehabilitation Cente r, 7280
Meadowview Manor, 6631
Meals on Wheels America, 7607
Measure of Cognitive-Linguistic Abilities (MCLA), 2690
Mecalift Sling Lifter, 376
Med Covers, 654
MED-EL Corporation, USA, 296
MedCamps of Louisiana, 1159, 8639
MedDev Corporation, 276, 276
MedEscort International, 5594
Medford Rehabilitation and Healthcare Cent er, 7367
Medi-Grip, 277
Media Access Group at WGBH, 4899, 9046
Media America, 8845
Media Projects Inc, 8092
Medical Aspects of Disability: A Handbook For The Rehabilitation Professional, 5225
Medical Rehabilitation, 2535
Medical Research Institute Of San Francisco, 4772
Medical University of South Carolina Arthritis Clinical/Research Center, 4999
MedicAlert Foundation International, 2852
Medicare and Medicaid Patient and Program Protection Act of 1987, 4713
Medicare Rights Center: New York, 7583
Medicare Rights Center: Washington, DC, 7584
Medicenter of Tampa, 6758
Medina Foundation, 3330
Mediplex of Colorado, 6686
Mediplex Rehab: Camden, 6379
Mediplex Rehab: Denver, 6276
MEDLINE, 1632
Medpro, 237, 238, 244, 245
Medpro Static Air Chair Cushion, 237
Medpro Static Air Mattress Overlay, 238
MedStar National Rehabilitation Network, 2746
Meeting Life's Challenges, 8686
Meeting the ADD Challenge: A Practical Guide for Teachers, 2536
Meeting the Needs of Employees with Disabilities, 5226
Meeting the Needs of People with Vision Loss: Multidisciplinary Perspective, 9220
Meeting-in-a-Box, 2029
Mega Wolf Communication Device, 1686
Melwood, 6075
Member Update, 2328
Memorial Hospital of Gardenia, 6632
Memorial Regional Rehabilitation Center, 6325, 6879
Memory Castle, 1835
Memphis Center for Independent Living, 4559
Memphis VA Medical Center, 5828
Men's Health, 7732
Meniere's Disease, 8760
Menopause without Medicine, 8761
Mental & Physical Disability Law Reporter, 4714
Mental & Physical Disability Law Digest, 2537
Mental and Physical Disability Law Reporter, 4718
Mental Disabilities and the Americans with Disabilities Act, 4715
Mental Disability Law, Evidence and Testimony, 4716
Mental Health America (MHA), 885, 7871
Mental Health and Mental Illness, 2539
Mental Health Association in Pennsylvania, 3817
Mental Health Center: Riverside Courtyard, The, 7029
Mental Health Commission, 4683
Mental Health Concepts and Techniques for the Occupational Therapy Assistant, 2538
Mental Health Law Reporter, 4717
Mental Health Report, 7733
Mental Health Unit, 6859
Mentally Disabled and the Law, 4719
Mentally Ill Individuals, 2540
Mentally Impaired Elderly: Strategies and Interventions to Maintain Function, 7645
Mentor Network, 6818
Mentor Network, The, 7143
Merck Company Foundation, 3099
Mercy Dubuque Physical Rehabilitation Unit, 6889
Mercy Hospital, 6633
Mercy Medical Center Mt. Shasta, 7222
Mercy Medical Center-Pain Services, 6890
Mercy Medical Group, 6633
Mercy Memorial Health Center-Rehab Center, 6405
Mercy Subacute Care, 7288
Meridan Medical Center For Subacute Care, 6948
Meridian Valley Clinical Laboratory, 5032
Merion Publications, 2247
Merrill Lynch & Company Foundation, 3155
Merrimack Hall Performing Arts Center, 8506, 978, 8631
Merwick Rehabilitation and Sub-Acute Care, 7327
MessageMate, 1573
Metamorphous Press, 5125
Methodist Hospital Rehabilitation Institute, 6326
Metro Health: St. Luke's Medical Center Pain Management Program, 7099
MetroHealth Medical Center, 7100
Metrolina Association for the Blind, 5408
Metropolitan Center for Independent Living, 4345
Metropolitan Employment & Rehabilitation Service, 7015
Metropolitan Washington Ear, 186
MetroWest Center for Independent Living, 4305
Metzger-Price Fund, 3156
The Meyer Foundation, 2901
MI Coalition for Deaf & Hard of Hearing People, 1191
Miami Dade Public Library System, 4797
Miami Foundation, The, 2923
Miami Heart Institute Adams Building, 6759
Miami Lighthouse for the Blind, 6760
Miami VA Medical Center, 5681
Miami-Dade County Disability Services and Independent Living (DSAIL), 4117
Michael E. Debakey VA Medical Center, 5836
Michael Reese Health Trust, 2968
Michigan Association for Deaf and Hard of Hearing, 3631, 8154
Michigan Association for Deaf Hard of Hearing, 8306
Michigan Association for Deaf, and Hard of Hearing, 3632
Michigan Braille and Talking Book Library, 4913
Michigan Career And Technical Institute, 6996
Michigan Client Assistance Program, 3633
Michigan Coalition for Staff Development and School Improvement, 3634
Michigan Commission for the Blind - Gaylord, 3635
Michigan Commission for the Blind, 3636
Michigan Commission for the Blind Training Center, 3637
Michigan Commission for the Blind: Independent Living Rehabilitation Program, 4333
Michigan Commission for the Blind: Detroit, 4334
Michigan Commission for the Blind: Escanab a, 3638
Michigan Commission for the Blind: Flint, 3639
Michigan Commission for the Blind: Grand Rapids, 3640
Michigan Council of the Blind and Visually Impaired (MCBVI), 3641
Michigan Department of Civil Rights, 6090
Michigan Department of Education: Special Education Services, 2208
Michigan Department of Handicapped Children, 3642
Michigan Dept Of Energy, Labor & Economic Growth, 3636
Michigan Developmental Disabilies Council, 3643
Michigan Library for the Blind and Physically Handicapped, 4914
Michigan Office of Services to the Aging, 3644
Michigan Protection & Advocacy Service, 3645
Michigan Psychological Association, 2108

Michigan Rehabilitation Services, 3646, 6091
Michigan State University, 938, 4906
Michigan VA Regional Office, 5735
Michigan Workforce Development Agency, 6092
Michigan's Assistive Technology Resource, 4915
Micro Audiometrics, 297
Micro Audiometrics Corporation, 297
Microcomputer Evaluation of Careers & Academics (MECA), 1865
Microloop III Basic, 187
Microsoft Accessibility Technology for Everyone, 5525
Microsystems Software, 1746
Mid-America Regional Council - Aging and Adult Services, 7783
Mid-America Rehabilitation Hospital HealthSouth, 6337
Mid-Carolina Area Agency on Aging, 7784
Mid-Illinois Talking Book Center, 4839
Mid-Iowa Health Foundation, 2989
Mid-Michigan Industries, 6997
Mid-Ohio Board for an Independent Living Environment (MOBILE), 4492
Mid-state Independent Living Consultants: Stevens Point, 4639
Mid-State Independent Living Consultants: Wausau, 4638
Middleton Village Nursing & Rehabilitation, 7419
Middletown Regional Hospital: Inpatient Rehabilitation Unit, 7101
Mideastern Michigan Library Co-op, 4916
Midland Empire Resources for Independent Living (MERIL), 4374
Midland Memorial Hospital & Medical Center, 6454
Midland Treatment Furniture, 2541
Milbank Foundation for Rehabilitation, 3157
Millstone 4-H Center, 1311
Milwaukee Foundation, 3347
MindFreedom International (MFI), 886
Mindplay, 1693, 1844
Mini-Max Cushion, 239
Minneapolis Foundation, 3065
Minneapolis VA Medical Center, 5738
Minneapolis YMCA Camping Services, 8660
Minnesota Assistive Technology Project, 3650
Minnesota Association of Centers for Independent Living, 4346
Minnesota Board on Aging, 3651
Minnesota Children with Special Needs, Minnesota Department of Health, 3652
Minnesota Department of Employment & Econo mic Development: State Services for the Blind, 6095
Minnesota Department of Employment and Economic Development: Vocational Rehab Services, 6096
Minnesota Department of Human Rights (FEPA), 6097
Minnesota Department of Human Services: Behavioral Health Division, 3653
Minnesota Department of Labor & Industry Workers Compensation Division, 3654
Minnesota Disability Law Center, 3655, 3657
Minnesota Governor's Council on Developmental Disabilities, 3656
Minnesota Library for the Blind and Physically Handicapped, 4929
Minnesota Protection & Advocacy for Persons with Disabilities, 3657
Minnesota STAR Program, 1635, 5146
Minnesota State Council on Disability (MSCOD), 3658
Minnesota State Services for the Blind, 3659
A Miracle to Believe In, 7946
Miracle-Ear Children's Foundation, 3019
Miriam, 2691
Mirror Go Lightly, 256
Mirrored Lives: Aging Children and Elderly Parents, 7646
Mission Bay Aquatic Center, 8446
Mississippi Assistive Technology Division, 3662
Mississippi Client Assistance Program, 3663
Mississippi Department of Education: Office of Special Services, 2213
Mississippi Department Of Human Services, 3665
Mississippi Department of Mental Health, 3664
Mississippi Department of Rehabilitation Services, 6099
Mississippi Department of Rehabilitation Services, 3663
Mississippi Division of Aging and Adult Services, 3665
Mississippi Employment Secutity Commission, 6100
Mississippi Library Commission, 4932, 4931
Mississippi Library Commission\Talking Book and Braille Services, 4933
Mississippi Methodist Rehabilitation Center, 7010
Mississippi Project START, 1636
Mississippi Speech-Language-Hearing Association, 8155
Mississippi State Department of Health, 3666
Mississippi State University, 2381, 2432, 2508, 4675, 6101, 9129, 9152, 9154, 9159, 9160, 9201, 9204, 9212, 9221, 9253, 9264, 9265
Mississippi: Workers Compensation Commission, 3667
Missouri Commission on Human Rights, 6102
Missouri Department of Elementary and Secondary Education: Special Education Programs, 2212
Missouri Department Of Mental Health, 3669
Missouri Department of Social Services, 6105
Missouri Division Of Developmental Disabilities, 3669
Missouri Governor's Council on Disability, 6103
Missouri Protection & Advocacy Services, 3670
Missouri Rehabilitation Center, 2747
Missouri Rehabilitation Services for the Blind, 3671
Missouri Vocational Rehabilitation Agency, 6104
MIUSA's Global Impact Newsletter, 8425
MIV Mount Loretto, 8625
MIV: Mount Loretto, 8198
MIW, 6888
MMB Music, 17, 28, 44, 64, 1983, 2058, 2511
MN Governor's Council on Development Disabilities, 5239
Mobile ARC, 6506
Mobility International USA, 8359, 2479, 2760, 2770, 2792, 5089, 5214, 5228, 5420, 5429, 5583, 8415, 8425
Mobility Limited, 8405, 8437, 8438
Mobility Parts and Service, 558, 559
Mobility Training for People with Disabilities, 5310
MobilityWorks, 107
Model Program Operation Manual: Business Enterprise Program Supervisors, 9221
Modern Maturity, 7734
ModernMedicine, 7701
Modular Wall Grab Bars, 149
Moisture Seekers, 8865
Molded Sock and Stocking Aid, 257
Molecular Imaging, 7735
Momentum, 8866
MOMS Catalog, 444
Monkeys Jumping on the Bed, 1764
MonoMouse Electronic Magnifiers, 603
Monroe Center for Independent Living, 4335
Montana Blind & Low Vision Services, 3677
Montana Council on Developmental Disabilit ies, 3678
Montana Department of Aging, 3679
Montana Department of Handicapped Children, 3680
Montana Human Rights Bureau (FEPA), 6107
Montana Independent Living Project, Inc., 4390
Montana Protection & Advocacy for Persons with Disabilities, 3681
Montana State Fund, 3682
Montana State Library-Talking Book Library, 4941
Montana VA Regional Office, 5749
MonTECH, 3676, 4940
Montgomery Center for Independent Living, 3970
Montgomery Comprehensive Career Center, 5874
Montgomery County Arc, 3276
Montgomery County Department of Public Libraries/Special Needs Library, 4884
Montgomery Field, 6581
Moody Foundation, 3303
MOOSE: A Very Special Person, 5216
More Alike Than Different: Blind and Visually Impaired Children, 9222
More Food!, 2030
More Than a Job: Securing Satisfying Caree rs for People with Disabilities, 5393
More Than Just a Job, 6230
More Work!, 2031
Morgan Stanley Foundation, 3158
Morris and Gwendolyn Cafritz Foundation, 2908
Morse Code WSKE, 1765
Mosaic, 3082, 4202
MOSAIC In Colorado Springs, 6683
Mosaic of Axtell Bethpage Village, 4400
Mosaic of Beatrice, 4401
Mosaic Of De, 4093
Mosaic: Pontiac, 4174
Mosholu Day Camp, 1297
Mosholu Montefiore Community Center, 1297
Mosiac: York, 4402
Moss Rehabilitation Hospital, 6423, 5595
MossRehab ResourceNet, 5526
MossRehab Travel Resources, 5595
Mother Father Deaf: Living Between Sound a nd Silence, 8261
Mother Lode Independent Living Center (DRAIL: Disability Resource Agency for Independent, 4053
Mother Lode Rehabilitation Enterprises, In c. (MORE), 5925
Mother to Be, 5311
Mothers with Visual Impairments who are Raising Young Children, 9223
Motivational Services, 4282
Motivator, 8426
Motor Speech Disorders, 8979
Motorhome Lift, 377
Mount Carmel Health & Rehabilitation Center, 7420
Mount Carmel Medical and Rehabilitation Center, 7421
Mount Sinai Medical Center, 2924
Mount Sinai Medical Center Rehabilitation Unit, 6761
Mountain Home VA Medical Center - James H Quillen VA Medical Center, 5829
Mountain State Center for Independent Living, 4631
Mountain State Center for Independent Living, 4632
Mountain Towers Healthcare & Rehabilitation Center, 7426
Mountain Valley Care and Rehabilitation Ce nter, 7262
Mountaineer Spina Bifida Camp, 1483, 8640
Mouthsticks, 1574
Move With Me, 9224
Movement Disorders, 2298
Movement Disorders Sourcebook, 8762
Moxie, 551
Mozart Effect: Tapping the Power of Music to Heal the Body, Strengthen the Mind, 37
MSFOCUS Magazine, 8848
Mt Hood Kiwanis Camp, 1364
Mt Sinai Medical Center, 4805
Mt. Carmel Guild, 7039
Mt. Sinai, 7274
Mt. Washington Pediatric Hospital, 6352
MTA Readers, 2020
Muhlenberg County Opportunity Center, 6914
Multi-Cultural Independent Living Center of Boston, 4306
Multi-Function Spinner Knobs, 108
Multi-Scan Single Switch Activity Center, 1766
Multilingual Children's Association, 8107
Multiple Choices Center for Independent Living, 4131
Multiple Sclerosis and Having a Baby, 8763

Multiple Sclerosis Association of America, 7872, 8360, 8426
Multiple Sclerosis Foundation, 8361, 8848
Multiple Sclerosis National Research Institute, 5527
Multiple Sclerosis: 300 Tips for Making Life Easier, 8764
Multiple Sclerosis: A Guide for Families, 8765
Multiple Sclerosis: A Guide for the Newly Diagnosed, 8766
Multiple Sclerosis: The Guide to Treatment and Management, 8767
Multisensory Teaching Approach, 2032
Multisensory Teaching of Basic Language Skills: Theory and Practice, 2542
Muncie Health Care and Rehabilitation, 7281
Muppet Learning Keys, 1767
Muscular Dystrophies, 8768
Muscular Dystrophy Association, 2297, 2301
Muscular Dystrophy Association - USA, 8651
Muscular Dystrophy Association Free Camp, 8641
Muscular Dystrophy Association National Office, 1121
Muscular Dystrophy Association USA (MDA), 887
Muscular Dystrophy in Children: A Guide fo r Families, 8769
Muscular Dystrophy: The Facts, 8770
Mushroom Inserts, 298
Music and Dyslexia: A Positive Approach, 43
Music for the Hearing Impaired, 44
Music Therapy, 38
Music Therapy and Leisure for Persons with Disabilities, 39
Music Therapy for the Developmentally Disa bled, 40
Music Therapy in Dementia Care, 41
Music Therapy, Sensory Integration and the Autistic Child, 42
Music, Disability, and Society, 2543
Music: Physician for Times to Come, 45
Musical Mainstream, 9285
Muskegon Area District Library for the Bli nd and Physically Handicapped, 4917
Muu Muu, 1529
MVP+ 3-Wheel Scooter, 550
My Body is Not Who I Am, 5441
My Country, 5442
My First Book of Sign, 8262
My House is Killing Me! The Home Guide for Families with Allergies and Asthma, 8771
My Own Pain, 1768
My Signing Book of Numbers, 8263
MyAlert Body Worn Multifunction Receiver, 188
Mycoclonus Research Foundation, 4951
Myositis Association, 8507, 8925
Myths and Facts, 4720

N

N AH B Research Center, 1946
Nabisco Foundation, 3100
NACDD Annual Conference, 1910
NAD Broadcaster, 4721
NAD E-Zine, 8312
NADR Conference, 1911
NAHO News, 8313
NAMI Advocate, 8067
NAMI Indiana, 6327
NanoPac, 1769
Nansemond Pointe Rehabilitation and Health care Center, 7397
Nantahala Outdoor Center, 5596
Napa County Mental Health Department, 6634
Napa Valley PSI Inc., 5926
Napa Valley Support Systems, 6635
NAPVI, 4709, 9155, 9169, 9218, 9234, 9294
Narcolepsy, 5443
Nasheville Regional Office, 5830
Nashville Rehabilitation Hospital, 6434
Nashville VA Medical Center, 5831
Nasometer, 1819
Nassau County Office for the Physically Challenged, 4455
Nassau Library System, 4964
NASUA News, 7768
NASW, 1912
NASW-NYS Chapter, 1912
Nat l Council for Community Behavioral Healthcare, 2300
Nat'l Council for Community Behavioral Healthcare, 2588
Nat'l Lib Svc/Blind And Physically Handicapped, 9144, 9145, 9146, 9148, 9236, 9237, 9239, 9256, 9257, 9285, 9318, 9319, 9334
NAT-CENT, 7825
National 4-H Council, 2781
National Ability Center, 1452, 1453, 1458, 1460, 1461, 1462
National Accreditation Council for Agencies/Blind, 9292
National Adult Day Services Association, 7585
National AIDS Hotline, 8899
National Allergy and Asthma Network, 2327
National Alliance for Caregiving, 7586
National Alliance of Black Interpreters, 8156
National Alliance of Blind Students NABS Liaison, 9071
National Alliance of Blind Students NABS Liaison, 9332
National Alliance of the Disabled (NAOTD), 5528
National Alliance on Mental Illness, 8067
National Alliance on Mental Illness (NAMI), 7875
National Alliance on Mental Illness (Texas), 3875
National Alliance on Mental Illness of New York State, 3742
National Amputation Foundation, 8108
National Aphasia Association, 8926
National Arts and Disability Center (NADC), 47
National Asian Pacific Center on Aging, 7587
National Assoc of State Directors of DD Services, 5249
National Association for Adults with Speci al Learning Needs, 2109
National Association for Children of Alcoholics, 8508
National Association for Continence, 8363, 8872
National Association for Developmental Disabilities (NADD), 7876
National Association for Down Syndrome, 7877
National Association for Drama Therapy, 48
National Association for Holistic Aromatherapy (NAHA), 888
National Association for Home Care & Hospice, 8509
National Association for Home Care and Hospice, 7588
National Association for Medical Direction of Respiratory Care, 8510
National Association for Parents of Children with Visual Impairments (NAPVI), 9072, 9365
National Association for Proton Therapy, 8511
National Association for the Dually Diagno sed Conferences, 1914
National Association for Visually Handicapped (NAVH), 9073
National Association for Visually Handicapped, 7809, 9126, 9127, 9130, 9153, 9157, 9163, 9171, 9172, 9175, 9185, 9187, 9192, 9206, 9207, 9230, 9323, 9336
National Association of Anorexia Nervosa and Associated Disorders, 8512
National Association of Area Agencies on Aging, 7589
National Association of Blind Educators, 9074
National Association of Blind Lawyers, 9075
National Association of Blind Merchants (NABM), 889, 9076
National Association of Blind Rehabilitati on Professionals, 9077
National Association of Blind Students, 9078
National Association of Blind Teachers, 9079
National Association of Blind Veterans, 9080
National Association of Chronic Disease Di seases, 8513
National Association of City and County he alth Officials, 890
National Association of Cognitive- Behavioral Therapists, 7878
National Association of Colleges and Employers, 2110
National Association of Councils on Develo pmental Disabilities (NACDD), 891
National Association of Counties, 7590
National Association of Disability Represe ntatives (NADR), 892
National Association of Disability Representatives, 1911
National Association of Epilepsy Centers, 7879
National Association of Guide Dog Users, 9081
National Association of Hearing Officials, 8157, 8313
National Association of Nutrition and Aging Services Programs (NANASP), 7591
National Association of Parents with Child ren in Special Education, 2111, 8158
National Association of School Psychologists, 2166
National Association of School Psychologists, 2368, 2407, 2525, 2705
National Association of Special Education Teachers, 8159, 8927
National Association of State Directors of Developmental Disabilities Services (NASDDDS), 893
National Association of State Directors of Special Education, 2112
National Association of State Units on Aging, 7768
National Association of States United for Aging and Disabilities, 7592
National Association of the Deaf, 8160, 4707, 4721, 8207, 8209, 8312
National Association of Visually Handicapped, 9316
National Association to Advance Fat Acceptance, 8514
National Association to Promote the Use of Braille, 9082
National Ataxia Foundation, 7880
National Autism Association, 7881
National Autism Hotline, 8096
National Autism Resources, 2033
National Beep Baseball Association, 9083
National Birth Defect Registry, 5529
National Black Association for Speech Language and Hearing, 8161
National Black Association for Speech-Lang uage and Hearing, 8928
National Black Deaf Advocates, 8162
National Braille Association, 4965, 9084, 9147, 9260, 9317
National Braille Press, 9085
National Brain Tumor Foundation - National Brain Tumor Society, 5530
National Bullying Prevention Center Newsle tter, 2329
National Business & Disability Council, 5531, 6154
National Business & Disability Council (NBDC), 894
National Camps for Blind Children, 1236, 9119
National Cancer Institute, 3389, 8515, 8898
National Car Rental System, 5625
National Care Planning Council, 895
National Catholic Office for the Deaf, 8239
National Catholic Office of the Deaf, 8163, 8318
National Center for College Students with Disabilities (NCCSD), 896
National Center for Education in Maternal and Child Health (NCEMCH), 897
National Center for Health, Physical Activ ity and Disability, 898, 8364
National Center for Homeopathy, 2113
National Center for Learning Disabilities, 2167
National Center for PTSD, 5013
National Center for Vision and Child Development, 9086
National Center on Birth Defects and Developmental Disabilities, 4822
National Center on Caregiving at Family Caregiver Alliance (FCA), 2853
National Center on Deaf-Blindness (NCDB), 899, 7803

National Center on Disability and Journalism (NCDJ), 900
National Center on Elder Abuse, 7593
National Cerebral Palsy of American, 3894
National Certification Commission for Acup uncture and Oriental Medicine, 901
National Clearinghouse on Abuse in Later Life, 7594
National Clearinghouse on Family Support and Children's Mental Health, 2190
National Clearinghouse on Postsecondary Education, 2162
National Coalition for Assistive and Rehab Technology, 8365
National Coalition of Federal Aviation Employees with Disabilities, 3390
National Collaborative Workforce on Disability (NCWD/Youth), 902
National Commission on Orthotic and Prosth etic Education, 8109
The National Committee to Preserve Social Security, 7742
National Committee to Preserve Social Security & Medicare, 7595
National Conference on Building Codes and Standards, 1931
National Consortium on Deaf-Blindness, 7821, 9299
National Council for Aging Care, 7596
National Council of Architectural Registration Boards (NCARB), 1932
National Council on Aging, 7597, 7534, 7535, 7603, 7667, 7707, 7766, 7769, 7775
National Council on Disability, 3391, 4734, 5227
National Council on Independent Living, 4095, 8366
National Council on Independent Living (NCIL), 903
National Council on Multifamily Housing Industry, 1950
National Council on Rehabilitation Education (NCRE), 2114
National Council on the Aging, 7656
National Council on the Aging Conference, 1915
National Cued Speech Association, 8164, 8929, 9012
National Deaf Women's Bowling Association, 8165
National Diabetes Action Network for the Blind, 9087
National Diabetes Information Clearinghouse, 8516
National Digestive Diseases Information Clearinghouse, 8517
National Directory of Corporate Giving, 3376
National Disability Rights Network (NDRN), 904
National Disability Sports Alliance, 8451
National Down Syndrome Congress, 7882, 8064
National Down Syndrome Society, 7883
National Education Association of the United States, 2115
National Endowment for the Arts Office, 1945
National Endowment for the Arts: Office for AccessAbility, 49
National Epilepsy Library (NEL), 4885
National Eye Institute, 3392, 9088, 9225, 9166
National Eye Research Foundation, 2969
National Eye Research Foundation (NERF), 4840
National Falls Prevention Resource Center, 7598
National Family Association for Deaf-Blind, 7804, 7826
National Federation of Families for Children's Mental Health (NFFCMH), 905
National Federation of the Blind, 3020, 7805, 9089, 889, 6076, 7814, 8896, 9074, 9075, 9076, 9077, 9078, 9081, 9082, 9087, 9092, 9188, 9198, 9202, 9270, 9279
National Federation of the Blind Jernigan Institute, 4886
National Fibromyalgia Association, 8367, 8518, 8053, 8408, 8422
National Foundation for Ectodermal Dysplasias, 2970
National Foundation for Facial Reconstruction, 3159
National Foundation of Wheelchair Tennis, 2854
National Fragile X Foundation, 8930
National Gerontological Nursing Association, 7599
National Guild of Hypnotists (NGH), 906
National Headache Foundation, 2971
National Headquarters, 7129
National Health Council, 907
National Health Information Center, 8097, 9024
National Health Law Program (NHeLP), 4666
National Hearing Conservation Association, 8166
National Hemophilia Foundation, 3160, 8519
National Hemophilia Foundation - Western PA, 1377
National Hispanic Council on Aging, 7600
National Hookup, 5229
National Hospice & Palliative Care Organization (NHPCO), 7601
National Human Genome Research Institute, 2206
National Hydrocephalus Foundation, 7884, 8743
National Indian Council on Aging, 7763
National Indian Council on Aging, Inc., 7602
National Industries for the Blind, 9090, 9286
National Institue Health, 4892
National Institute of Arthritis and Muscul oskeletal and Skin Diseases, 3393
National Institute of Building Sciences, 1933, 1953, 1957
National Institute of Diabetes and Digesti ve and Kidney Diseases, 3394
National Institute of Environmental Health Sciences, 2215
National Institute of General Medical Scie nces, 2207
National Institute of Health, 9225
National Institute of Mental Health, 3395
National Institute of Neurological Disorders and Stroke, 3396, 8110
National Institute of Senior Centers, 7603
National Institute on Aging, 3397, 4887, 7604
National Institute on Deafness and Other Communication Disorders, 3398, 8167
National Institute on Disability, Independ ent Living, and Rehabilitation Research (NIDILRR), 908, 3399, 4794
National Institutes of Health, 7605, 2206, 3392, 3393, 3394, 3395, 3396, 3398, 8110
National Institutes of Health (NIH), 8491
National Jewish Health, 8683, 8723, 8776, 8826, 8835, 8897
National Jewish Medical & Research Center, 4781
National Kidney and Urologic Diseases Information Clearinghouse, 8520
National Kidney Foundation, 8579
National Lekotek Center, 4841, 5573
National Library of Medicine, 1622
National Library Office, 4984
National Library Service, 5495
National Library Service for the Blind and Physic, 7728
National Library Service for the Blind and Physically Handicapped (NLS), 50, 9091
National Library Service in Washington, 4985
National Mobility Equipment Dealers Associ ation, 8368
National Multiple Sclerosis Society, 5967, 7708, 8866
National Older Worker Career Center, 7606
National Organization for Albinism and Hypopigmentation, 8521
National Organization for Rare Disorders, 8522
National Organization of Blind Educators, 9277
National Organization of Parents of Blind Children, 9092
National Organization on Disability (NOD), 909, 5532
National Organization on Fetal Alcohol Syndrome, 8523
National Park Service, 5605
National Parkinson Foundation, 2925, 1902, 8869
National Parkinson Foundation & ADPF, 1923
National Rehabilitation Association, 7723
National Rehabilitation Association (NRA), 910, 2290
National Rehabilitation Hospital, 6278, 1616
National Rehabilitation Information Center (NARIC), 4888, 5533
National Research and Training Center on Blindness and Low Vision, 6101
National Resource Center on Nutrition & Aging, 7607
National Right to Work Legal Defense Foundation, 3320, 4667
National Science Foundation, 2241
National Senior Citizens Law Center, 7771
National Senior Citizens Law Center: Los Angeles, 7609
National Senior Citizens Law Center: Oakland, 7608
National Senior Corps Association, 7610
National Seniors Council, 7611
National Skeet Shooting Association, 8452
National Society for Experiential Education, 2116
National Spasmodic Dysphonia Association, 8369, 8931
National Spasmodic Torticollis Association, 8370
National Spinal Cord Injury Association, 8429, 8852
National Sports Center for the Disabled, 8453, 8882
National Stroke Association, 8111, 8122
National Student Speech Language Hearing A ssociation, 8168
National Stuttering Association, 8932, 8997
National Technology Database, 1637
National Theatre of the Deaf, 52
National Theatre Workshop of the Handicapp ed (NTWH), 51
National Tourette Syndrome Association, 8933
National University of Natural Medicine (NUNM), 911
National Vaccine Information Center (NVIC), 912
National Wheelchair Poolplayers Association, 8454
National Women's Health Network (NWHN), 913
National Youth Leadership Network Youth Leader Blog (NYLN), 5534
National Youth Transitions Center, 7854
National-Louis University, 6309
Nationwide Foundation, 3209
Native American Advocacy Program for Perso ns with Disabilities, 4550
Native American Disability Law Center, 914
Natl. Clearinghouse for Alcohol & Drug Information, 2648
Natural Access, 682
Navarro Hospital, 6455
Navarro Regional Hospital: RehabCare Unit, 6455
NAVH Update, 9316
Nazarene Publishing House, 4935
NBA Bulletin, 9317
NBIA Disorders Association, 8362
NC Department of Commerce, 6156, 6160
NC Department of Health and Human Services, 6158
NCD Bulletin, 5227
NCDE Survival Strategies for Overseas Livi ng for People with Disabilities, 5228
NCI's Contact Center, 8898
NCOA Week, 7769
NCWorks Commission, 6160
Neal Freeling, 3641
Nebraska Advocacy Services, 3684
Nebraska Assistive Technology Partnership Nebraska Department of Education, 4942
Nebraska Client Assistance Program, 3685
Nebraska Commission for the Blind & Visually Impaired, 3686
Nebraska Department of Education: Special Populations Office, 2218
Nebraska Department of Health & Human Services of Medically Handicapped Children's Prgm, 3687
Nebraska Department of Health and Human Services, Division of Aging Services, 3688
Nebraska Department of Labor, 6108

Nebraska Department of Mental Health, 3689
Nebraska Equal Opportunity Commission (FEPA), 6109
Nebraska Library Commission: Talking Book and Braille Service (TBBS), 4943, 5535
Nebraska Planning Council on Developmental Disabilities, 3690
Nebraska VR, 6110
Nebraska Workers' Compensation Court, 3691
Neisloss Family Foundation, 3161
Nell J Redfield Foundation, 3086
Nelson Publications, 8050
NeSoDak, 1410, 8642
Neurobehavioral Medicine Center, 6762
Neurobiology of Autism, 8020, 8980
NeuroControl Corporation, 5536
Neuropsychiatry of Epilepsy, 8772
Neuropsychology Assessment Center, 2692
Neuroscience Publishers, 8052
Neuroxcel, 2748
Nevada Assistive Technology Project, 3694
Nevada Blind Children's Foundation, 1240
Nevada Bureau of Vocational Rehabilitation, 3695
Nevada Community Enrichment Program (NCEP), 3696
Nevada Department of Education: Special Eduction Branch, 2225
Nevada Developmental Disability Council, 3697
Nevada Diabetes Association, 1237
Nevada Disability Advocacy and Law Center -Sparks/Reno Office, 3698
Nevada Division for Aging: Las Vegas, 3699
Nevada Division of Mental Health and Devel opmental Services, 3700
Nevada Equal Rights Commission, 6112
Nevada Governor's Council on Developmental Disabilities, 6113
Nevada State Library and Archives, 4945
Nevada's Care Connection, 2136
New Bedford Rehabilitation Hospital, 6353
New Beginnings: The Blind Children's Center, 4773
New Behavioural Network, 1258
New Directions for People with Disabilities, 2782
New Directions For People With Disabilitie s, 5615
New England Center for Children, 6974
New England Eye Center - Tufts Medical Center, 6975
New England Regional Genetics Group, 4878
New England Rehabilitation Hospital of Portland, 6351
New England Rehabilitation Hospital: Massachusetts, 6354
New Eyes for the Needy, 9093
New Focus, 6050
New Hampshire Workers Compensation Board, 3704
New Hampshire Assistive Technology Partnership Project, 3705
New Hampshire Bureau of Developmental Services, 3706
New Hampshire Bureau of Vocational Rehabil itation, 6114
New Hampshire Client Assistance Program, 3707
New Hampshire Commission for Human Rights, 3708
New Hampshire Commission for Human Rights (FEPA), 6115
New Hampshire Department of Education, 6114
New Hampshire Department of Education: Bureau for Special Education Services, 2220
New Hampshire Department of Mental Health, 3709
New Hampshire Developmental Disabilities Council, 3710
New Hampshire Division of Elderly and Adult Services, 3711
New Hampshire Employment Security, 6116
New Hampshire Governor's Commission on Disability, 3712
New Hampshire Protection & Advocacy for Persons with Disabilities, 3713
New Hampshire Rehabilitation and Sports Medicine, 7030
New Hampshire State Library: Talking Book Services, 4946
New Hampshire Veterans Centers, 5763
New Harbinger Publications, 2473, 7638, 7643
New Hope Services, 6037
New Horizons in Sexuality, 5230
New Horizons Independent Living Center, 5057
New Horizons Independent Living Center: Prescott Valley, 3990
New Horizons Rehabilitation, 6038
New Horizons Summer Day Camp, 1039, 7927, 8947
New Horizons Village, 4087
New Horizons: Central Louisiana, 4271
New Horizons: Northeast Louisiana, 4272
New Horizons: Northwest Louisiana, 4273
New Jersey Commission for the Blind and Visually Impaired (CBVI), 3718, 6136
New Jersey Council on Developmental Disabilities, 5244
New Jersey Department of Aging, 3719
New Jersey Department of Education, 2221
New Jersey Department of Education: Office of Special Education Program, 2221
New Jersey Department of Health and Senior Service, 3720
New Jersey Department of Health/Special Child Health Services, 3720
New Jersey Department of Labor & Workforce Development, 1638
New Jersey Developmental Disabilities Council, 5302
New Jersey Division of Mental Health Services, 3721
New Jersey Division of Vocational Rehabilitation Services (DVRS), 6137
New Jersey Governor's Liaison to the Office of Disability Employment Policy, 3722
New Jersey Institute for Disabilities (NJID), 6138
New Jersey Library for the Blind and Handicapped, 4952
New Jersey Medical School, 4950
New Jersey Protection & Advocacy for Persons with Disabilities, 3723
New Jersey Protection and Advocacy, 4415
New Jersey Speech-Language-Hearing Association, 2222
New Jersey YMHA/YWHA Camps Milford, 7928
New Language of Toys: Teaching Communicati on Skills to Children with Special Needs, 5312, 5574
New Living, 7736
New Living Magazine, 7736
New Medico Community Re-Entry Service, 6998
New Medico Rehabilitation and Skilled Nursing Center at Lewis Bay, 6976
New Medico, Highwatch Rehabilitation Center, 7031
New Mexico Aging and Long-Term Services Department, 3726
New Mexico Client Assistance Program, 3727
New Mexico Commission for the Blind (NMCFTB), 3728, 6149
New Mexico Department of Health: Children's Medical Services, 3729
New Mexico Department of Workforce Solutions, 6151
New Mexico Division of Vocational Rehabilitation, 6150
New Mexico Governor's Committee on Concerns of the Handicapped, 3730
New Mexico Protection & Advocacy for Persons with Disabilities, 3731
New Mexico State Department of Education, 2224
New Mexico State Library for the Blind and Physically Handicapped, 4953
New Mexico State Veterans' Home, 5768
New Mexico Technology Assistance Program, 1639, 3732, 4428
New Mexico VA Healthcare System, 5769
New Mexico Workers Compensation Administration, 3733
New Mexico Workforce Connection, 6151
New Mobility, 8409
New Music Therapist's Handbook, 2nd Ed. Berklee School of Music, 53
New Orleans Resources for Independent Living, 4274
New Orleans Speech and Hearing Center, 6929
New Orleans VA Medical Center, 5715
New State Office of Mental Health Agency, 3743
New Ventures, 5994
New Vision Enterprises, 6915
New Vision Store, 447
New Vistas, 4429
New Voices: Self Advocacy By People with Disabilities, 5231
New World Library, 8724, 8812, 8820
New York - Haymarket, 7730
New York Arthritis Reporter, 8427
New York Branch International Dyslexia Association, 1895
New York Chapter of the Arthritis Foundation, 8427
New York City Bar, 4684
New York City Campus of the VA NY Harbor Healthcare System, 5778
New York Client Assistance Program, 3744
New York Community Trust, 3162
New York Department of Handicapped Children, 3745
New York District Kiwanis Foundation, 1292
New York Families For Autistic Children, 8045
New York Foundation, 3163
New York Public Library, 4954
New York Regional Office, 5779
New York State Commisionon Qualityof Careand Advoc, 3751
New York State Commission for the Blind, 3746
New York State Commission on Quality of Care, 3747
New York State Congress of Parents and Teachers, 3748
New York State Department of Labor, 6155
New York State Education Department, 2226, 3764, 6153
New York State Library and Education, 4966
New York State Office of Advocates for Persons with Disabilities, 3749
New York State Office of Mental Health, 3750
New York State Talking Book & Braille Library, 4966
New York State Talking Book & Braille Library, 9335
New York State Talking Book and Braille Library, 5063
New York State TRAID Project, 3751
New York University Medical Center, 4957
New York-Presbyterian Hospital, 7062
Newark Healthcare Center, 7102
Newark Regional Office, 5767
Newport Hospital, 7140
Newport News Public Library System, 5023
News from Advocates for Deaf-Blind, 7826
Newsletter of PA's AT Lending Library, 5537
Newsline, 5313
NEXT Conference & Exposition, 1913
Nexus Health Systems, 6467
NEXUS Wheelchair Cushioning System, 240
NFB Career Mentoring, 6076
NFB Diabetes Action Network, 8881
NI of Diabetes and Digestive and Kidney Diseases, 8516, 8517, 8520
NI on Deafness & Other Communication Disorders, 8816, 8831
NIAD Art Center (Nurturing Independence through Artistic Development), 46
Nick & Kelly Children's Fund, 993
Nick & Kelly's Heart Camp, 993
Nick Joins In, 8773
Nicklaus Children's Hospital, 1081, 8620
Nightshirts, 1530
NINDS Notes, 8120
Nintendo, 5572
Nishna Productions-Shenandoah Work Center, 6891
NJY Camps, 1263
NLP Comprehensive, 7873, 8068
NLP News, 8068

NLP University, 7874
NLP University - Dynamic Learning Center, 7874
NLS News, 9318
NLS Newsletter, 9319
NNEAHSA, 7770
No Barriers, 5444
No Boundaries, 547, 551
No Limits, 54
No Limits Communications & New Mobility, 507
No Limits Foundation, 3000, 1008, 1067, 1078, 1105, 1162, 1164, 1168, 1221, 1436
No Longer Disabled: the Federal Courts & the Politics of Social Security Disability, 4722
No More Allergies, 8774
No Time for Jello: One Family's Experience, 8775
Noble Of Indiana, 6039
Noble, Inc., 6039
Nocturnal Asthma, 8776
NOLO, 4723, 5135, 7644, 7650
NOLO (Internet Brands), 5051, 5352
Nolo's Guide to Social Security Disability Getting and Keeping Your Benefits, 4723
Non-Traditional Casting Project, 55
Nonverbal Learning Disabilities at Home: A Parent's Guide, 8981
NorCal Services For Deaf & Hard Of Hearing, 1004, 8185
Norcliffe Foundation, 3331
Nordson Corporate Giving Program, 3210
Norfolk Foundation, 3321
Norman Marcus Pain Institute, 7063
North American Riding for the Handicapped Assoc, 8413
North American Vegetarian Society, 7751
North Atlantic Books, 2448
North Auburn Rehabilitation And Health Center, 7407
North Broward Medical Center, 7244, 6763
North Broward Rehab Unit, 6763
North Carolina Workers Compensation Board, 3770
North Carolina Assistive Technology Project, 3771
North Carolina Children & Youth Branch, 3772
North Carolina Client Assistance Program, 3773
North Carolina Department of Insurance, 1928
North Carolina Department of Public Instruction: Exceptional Children Division, 2216
North Carolina Developmental Disabilities, 3774
North Carolina Division of Aging, 3775
North Carolina Division of Services for the Blind, 6161
North Carolina Industrial Commission, 3776
North Carolina Library for the Blind and Physically Handicapped, 4975
North Carolina Publc of Health, 3772
North Central Independent Living Services, 4391
North Chicago VA Medical Center, 5696
North Coast Rehabilitation Center, 6254
North Country Center for Independent Livin g, 4456
North Country Independent Living, 4640
North Country Independent Living: Ashland, 4641
North Dakota Workers Compensation Board, 3779
North Dakota Client Assistance Program, 3780
North Dakota Community Foundation, 3192
North Dakota Department of Education: Special Education, 2217
North Dakota Department of Human Resources, 3781
North Dakota Department of Human Services, 3782
North Dakota Department of Labor, and Human Rights, 6167
North Dakota State Library Talking Book Services, 4978
North Dakota State Library Talking Book Services, 5162
North Dakota VA Regional Office - Fargo Regional Office, 5793
North Dakota Vocational Rehabilitation Agency, 6168
North District Independent Living Program, 4132
North Georgia Talking Book Center, 4823
North Hastings Community Integration Assoc iation, 915
North Hills Hospital, 7390
North Little Rock Regional Office, 5650
North Ridge Medical and Rehabilitation Cen ter, 7422
North Star Community Services, 5232
North Texas Rehabilitation Center, 7170
North Valley Services, 6636
Northampton VA Medical Center, 5727
Northeast Independent Living Program, 4307
Northeast Independent Living Services, 4375
Northeast Occupational Exchange, 6069
Northeast Rehabilitation Clinic, 7323
Northeast Rehabilitation Hospital, 6372
Northeast Wisconsin Directory of Services for Older Adults, 2137
Northeastern Pennsylvania Center for Independent Living, 4529
Northern Arizona University, 6521
Northern Arizona VA Health Care System, 5645
Northern Illinois Center for Adaptive Technology, 1640
Northern Illinois Special Recreation Association (NISRA), 6844
Northern Nevada Center for Independent Liv ing: Fallon, 4404
Northern Nevada Center for Independent Living, 5148
Northern New Hampshire Mental Health and Developmental Services, 7032
Northern New York Community Foundation, 3164
Northern Regional Center for Independent Living: Watertown, 4457
Northern Regional Center for Independent L iving: Lowville, 4458
Northern Utah Center for Independent Living, 4588
Northern Virginia Resource Center for Deaf and Hard of Hearing Persons, 5024
Northern West Virginia Center for Independent Living, 4633
Northland Library Cooperative, 4918
Northn New England Assoc of Homes & Svcs for Aging, 7770
Northport VA Medical Center, 5780
Northridge Hospital Medical Center, 6255, 7223
Northridge Hospital Medical Center Rehabiltation Medicine, 6637
Northridge Hospital Medical Center: Center for Rehabilitation Medicine, 6638
Northstar Community Services, 6892
Northview Developmental Services, 6907
Northwest Arkansas Rehabilitation Hospital, 6234
Northwest Continuum Care Center, 7198
Northwest Hospital Center for Medical Rehabilitation, 6479
Northwest Kansas Library System Talking Books, 4861
Northwest Limousine Service, 5626
Northwest Medical Center, 6764
Northwest Ozarks Regional Library for the Blind and Handicapped, 4761
Northwestern Medicine Central DuPage Hospital, 8372
Northwestern Mutual Life Foundation, 3348
Northwestern University Multipurpose Arthritis & Musculoskeletal Center, 4842
Northwoods Lodge, 7408
Northwoods of Cortland, 7339
Norton- Lambert Corporation, 1563
Norwalk Hospital Section Of Physical Medicine And Rehabilitation, 6703
Norwalk Press, 8702
Norway Rehabilitation and Living Center, 7301
Norwegian Cruise Line, 5616
Nosey Cup, 321
Not Dead Yet, 916
Not Without Sight, 9347
Noteworthy Newsletter, 8121
Nothern Suburban Special Recreation Associ ation Day Camps, 1122
Nothing is Impossible: Reflections on a N ew Life, 5233
Nova Care, 6525
Novartis Pharmaceuticals Division, 8026
NSCLC Washington Weekly, 7771
NSSLHA Now, 9011
Ntn'l Comm on Orthotic & Prosthetic Education, 8121
Ntn'l Institute of Neurological Disorders & Stroke, 8120
Ntn'l Student Speech Language Hearing Association, 9011
Nursery Rhymes from Mother Goose, 8264
Nutritional Desk Reference, 5234
Nutritional Influences on Illness:, 5235
Nuvisions For Disabled Artists, Inc., 56
NYS Commission on Quality of Care & Advocacy for Persons with Disabilities, 3740
NYS Independent Living Council, 4454
NYSARC, 3741

O

O&P Almanac, 2330
O'Reilly Media Inc, 8671, 8672, 8694, 8695, 8697, 8701, 8727, 8753, 8794, 8823
Oak Forest Hospital of Cook County, 6845
Oak Hill Nursing and Rehabilitation Center, 7375
Oak-Leyden Developmental Services, 7885
Oakcrest Care Center, 7119
Oakhill-Senior Program, 7120
Oakland County Library for the Visually & Physically Impaired, 4919
Oakland School & Camp, 1474, 7929
Oakland VA Regional Office, 5655
Oakwood Rehabilitation and Nursing Center, 7312
OASYS, 1866
Oberkotter Foundation, 3238
Obesity, 8777
The Obesity Medicine Association (OMA), 947
Obesity Sourcebook, 8778
Ocala Adult Day Training, 4118
OCCK, 1641
Occulta, 8779
Occupational Hearing Services Inc., 8335
Occupational Therapy Across Cultural Boundaries, 2544
Occupational Therapy and Vocational Rehabi litation, 5395
Occupational Therapy Approaches to Traumatic Brain Injury, 2545
Occupational Therapy in Health Care, 2331
Occupational Therapy Strategies and Adaptations for Independent Daily Living, 6384
Occupational Training Center of Burlington County (OTCBC), 6139
Occuptational Training Center (OTC), 6140
Ocean State Center for Independent Living, 4539
Oconee Regional Library, 4824
ODHH Directory of Resources and Services, 2138
Office for American Indian, Alaskan Native and Native Hawaiian Elders, 7612
Office for Students with Disabilities, University of Texas at Arlington, 4573
Office of Administration, 3845
Office of Disability Concerns, 6171
Office of Disability Employment Policy, 3400
Office Of Disease Prevention And Health Promotion, 8097
Office of Elderly Affairs, 3599
Office of Fair Housing and Equal Opportuni ty, 3401
Office of Fair Practices, 6077
Office of Grants Management, 2963
Office of Juvenile Justice and Delinquency Prevention, 5538
Office Of Library & Information Services for the Blind and Physically Handicapped, 4997
Office of Mental Health, 3743
Office of Rehabilitation Services, 4540, 6183
Office of Retirement and Disability Policy (ORDP), 3402
Office of Special Education Programs, 3403
Office of the Commissioner, 1638
Office of the Governor, 3846
Office of Vocational Rehabilitation (OVR), 6178

Office of Vocational Rehabilitation Servic es (OVRS), 3807
Office of Workforce Development, 6059, 6061
Official Patient's Sourcebook on Bell's Pa lsy, 8780
Official Patient's Sourcebook on Cystic Fi brosis, 8781
Official Patient's Sourcebook on Muscular Dystrophy, 8782
Official Patient's Sourcebook on Osteoporo sis, 8783
Official Patient's Sourcebook on Post-Poli o Syndrome: A Revised and Updated Directory, 8784
Official Patient's Sourcebook on Primary Pulmonary Hypertension, 8785
Official Patient's Sourcebook on Pulmonary Fibrosis, 8786
Official Patient's Sourcebook on Scoliosis, 8787
Official Patient's Sourcebook on Sickle Ce ll Anemia, 8788
Official Patient's Sourcebook on Ulcerativ e Colitis, 8789
Ohio Bureau for Children with Medical Hand icaps, 3788
Ohio Bureau of Worker's Compensation, 3789
Ohio Civil Rights Commission (OCRC), 4668
Ohio Client Assistance Program, 3790
Ohio Coalition for the Education of Children with Disabilities, 2332
Ohio County Public Library Services for the Blind and Physically Handicapped, 5038
Ohio Department of Aging, 3791
Ohio Department of Education, 2227
Ohio Department of Education: Division of Special Education, 2227
Ohio Department of Health, 3788
Ohio Department of Mental Health, 3792
Ohio Developmental Disabilities Council, 3793
Ohio Developmental Disability Council (ODD C), 3794
Ohio Governor's Council on People with Disabilities, 3795
Ohio Regional Library for the Blind and Physically Handicapped, 4984
Ohio Rehabilitation Services Commission, 3796
Ohio Statewide Independent Living Council, 4493
Ohio Women, Infants, & Children Program - Ohio Department of Health, 3797
Okizu Foundation, 1009, 1010, 1011, 1012, 1013, 8593
Oklahoma Workers Compensation Board, 3799
Oklahoma City VA Medical Center, 5801, 5136
Oklahoma Client Assistance Program/Office of Disability Concerns, 3800
Oklahoma Department of Human Services Aging Services Division, 3801
Oklahoma Department of Labor, 3802
Oklahoma Department of Mental Health & Substance Abuse Services, 3803
Oklahoma Department of Rehabilitation Services, 3804, 6172
Oklahoma Employment Security Commission (OESC), 6173
Oklahoma League for the Blind, 7115
Oklahoma Library for the Blind & Physically Handicapped, 4986
Oklahoma Medical Research Foundation, 4987
Oklahoma State Department of Education, 2229
Oklahoma Veterans Centers Vet Center, 5802
Oklahomans for Independent Living, 4500
Old Adobe Developmental Services, 6639, 6646
Old Adobe Developmental Services-Rohnert Park Services (Behavioral), 6640
Old MacDonald's Farm Deluxe, 1770
Old MacDonald's Farm IntelliKeys Overlay, 1575
Older Americans Report, 3377
Omnigraphics, 35, 424, 5177, 7647, 8668, 8674, 8676, 8677, 8679, 8680, 8682, 8685, 8688, 8689, 8691, 8692, 8693, 8696, 8708, 8709, 8711, 8712, 8716, 8725, 8728, 8729, 8741, 8745, 8754, 8762, 8778, 8800, 8805, 8814, 8815, 8821
OMRON Foundation OMRON Electronics, 2972
On a Green Bus: A UKanDu Little Book, 1836
On Cue, 9012
On My Own, 4376
On the Level, 8314
On the Road to Autonomy: Promoting Self-Competence in Children & Youth with Disabilities, 5314
On The Spectrum, 5445
One Day at a Time: Children Living with Leukemia, 8790
One for All Lift All, 378
One Heartland, 1005, 1206, 8572, 8577
One Thousand FS, 644, 715
One-Stop Service Center, 5982
ONLINE, 2693
OnScreen, 1669
Ontario Cerebral Palsy Sports Association, 8455
Ontario Federation for Cerebral Palsy, 7886
Open Back Nightgowns, 1531
Open Book, 1837
Open Circle Theatre, 57
Open for Business, 5446
Open Hearts Camp, 1180, 8643
Open to the Public, 5447
Opening the Courthouse Door: An ADA Access Guide for State Courts, 4724
Operation Job Match, 5967
Ophthalmic Research Laboratory Eye Institute/First Hill Campus, 5033
Opportunities for Access: A Center for Independent Living, 4175
Opportunities Foundation of Central Oregon, 6175
Opportunity, 9286
Opportunity East Rehabilitation Services for the Blind, 7145
Optelec U S, 1676, 1758, 1759
Optimum Resource, 1706, 1707, 1708, 1709, 1710, 1711, 1724, 1771, 1782, 1783, 1784, 1785, 1786, 1839, 1841, 1847, 1850, 1853, 1854, 1855, 1856, 1860, 1868
Optimum Resource Educational Software, 1771
Optimum Resource Software, 1838
Optimum Resources/Stickybear Software, 1772
Option Indigo Press, 5463, 7946
OPTIONS, 4347
Options, 8867
Options Center for Independent Living: Bou rbonnais, 4176
Options Center for Independent Living: Wat seka, 4177
OPTIONS for Independence, 4588
Options for Independence: Auburn, 4459
OPTIONS for Independence: Brigham Satellit e, 4589
Options for Independent Living, 4642
Options for Independent Living: Fox Valley, 4643
Options Interstate Resource Center for Independent Living, 4348
Options of Linn County, 6893
Options, Resource Center for Independent Living, 1642
Options: Revolutionary Ideas in the War on Cancer, 8791
Optometric Extension Program Foundation, 3021, 9138
Oral Hull Foundation for the Blind, 1363
Orange County Library System: Audio-Visual Department, 4804
Orchard Village, 6020
Ordean Foundation, 3066
Oregon Advocacy Center, 3808
Oregon Client Assistance Program, 3809
Oregon Commission for the Blind, 6176
Oregon Council on Developmental Disabilities, 5236
Oregon Department of Education:, 2230
Oregon Department of Education: Office of Special Education, 2230
Oregon Department of Human Services Vocational Rehabilitation (DHS VR), 6177
Oregon Department of Mental Health, 3810
Oregon Health Sciences University, 5803
Oregon Health Sciences University, Elks' Children's Eye Clinic, 4989
Oregon Nursing And Rehabilitation Center, 7364
Oregon Perspectives, 5236
Oregon Talking Book & Braille Services, 4990
Oregon Technology Access for Life, 3811
Oregon-Idaho Conference Center, 8587, 8600, 8650
Oregon-Idaho Conference UMC - Camp Registrar, 1365
Organ Transplants: Making the Most of Your Gift of Life, 5237
Orientation and Mobility Primer for Families and Young Children, 9226
Origin Instruments Corporation, 1576
Orthotics and Prosthetics Almanac, 8849
Oryx Press, 2017
Osborn Medical Corporation, 278, 278
Oshkosh Medical and Rehabilitation Center, 7423
Osigian Office Center, 2085
Ostberg Foundation, 3101
Osteogenesis Imperfecta Foundation, 5539
Osteoporosis Sourcebook, 8792
Osterguard Enterprises c/o Jim's Shop, 650
OT Practice Magazine, 5394
Otto Bremer Foundation, 3067
Ottobock, 588
Our Lady of Lourdes Medical Center, 7038
Our Lady of Lourdes Rehabilitation Center, 6343
Our Own Road, 5448
Our Way: The Cottage Apt Homes, 3996
Out of Left Field, 9348
Out of the Corner of My Eye: Living with Vision Loss in Later Life, 9227
Out of the Corner of My Eye: Living with Macular Degeneration, 9228
Out of the Fog: Treatment Options and Cop ing Strategies for ADD, 8021
Out-N-About American Walker, 617
Out-Sider III, 379
Out-Sider Meridian, 380
Outdoor Independence, 552
Outside In School Of Experiential Education, Inc., 1392, 7930
Outsider: The Life and Art of Judith Scott, 5449
Outsiders in a Hearing World: A Sociology of Deafness, 8265
Oval Window Audio, 299
Overcoming Dyslexia, 8022
Overcoming Dyslexia in Children, Adolescents and Adults, 2546
Overcoming Mobility Barriers International, 1934
Overnight Camps, 1461
OWLS: Oral and Written Language Scales LC/OE & WE, 2694
Oxford Journals, Oxford University Press, 5378
Oxford Textbook of Geriatric Medicine, 2547
Oxford University Press, 2547, 2585, 2599, 5260, 7964, 7971, 8007, 8273, 8710, 8768, 8770, 8822, 8837, 8953, 8960
Ozark Independent Living, 4377

P

P CI Educational Publishing, 1715
P.T. Rail, 150
Pac-All Carriers, 645
Pac-All Wheelchair Carrier, 645
PACE Center for Independent Living, 4178
Pace Saver, 549, 553
Pace Saver Plus II, 553
PACER Center, 2309, 2316, 2325, 2329, 2333, 2334, 2335
PACER Center (Parent Advocacy Coalition for Educational Rights), 917
PACER E-News, 2333
PACER Partners, 2334
PACESETTER, 2335
Pacific Hospital Of Long Beach-Neuro Care Unit, 6642
Pacific Institute of Aromatherapy, 919
Pacific Islands Health Care System, 5691
Pacific Rehab, Inc., 493
Pacific Rim International Conference on Disability And Diversity, 1918
Pacific Specialty & Rehabilitation Center r, 7409
Pacific Spine and Pain Center, 7121
Paddy Rossbach Youth Camp, 1075

Paducah Centre For Health and Rehabilitati on, 7292
Pain Alleviation Center, 7064
Pain Centers: A Revolution in Health Care, 2548
Pain Control & Rehabilitation Institute of Georgia, 6796
Pain Erasure, 5315
Pain Erasure: the Bonnie Prudden Way, 9229
Pain Institute of Tampa, 6765
Pain Treatment Center, Baptist Hospital of Miami, 6766
The Painted Turtle, 1042
Paladin, 6040
PALAESTRA: Forum of Sport, Physical Educat ion and Recreation for Those with Disabilities, 8410
Palestine Resource Center for Independent Living, 4574
Palgrav Macmillan, 8670
Palladium, 5968
Palm Beach County Library, 4808
Palm Beach Habilitation Center, 5983
Palmer & Dodge, 3028
Palmer Independence, 554
Palmer Industries, 552, 554, 555
Palmer Twosome, 555
Panhandle Action Center for Independent Living Skills, 4575
Panties, 1532
Paradise Vally Hospital-South Bay Rehabilitation Center, 6643
Paragon House, 8704
Parallels in Time, 5239
Paralysis Resource Guide, 8400
Paralyzed Veterans of America, 5597, 8371, 1916, 1935, 5585, 5675, 8448
Paraquad, 4378
PARC, 6846
Parent Assistance Network, 8902
Parent Centers and Independent Living Centers: Collectively We're Stronger, 5316
Parent Connection, 3876
Parent Magic, 5402, 7953
Parent Professional Advocacy League, 4725, 8900
Parent Professional Advocacy League (PPAL), 920
Parent Survival Manual, 8023, 8982
Parent to Parent of New York State, 3752
Parent's Guide to Allergies and Asthma, 8793
Parent's Guide to Down Syndrome: Toward a Brighter Future, 8024
Parent-Child Interaction and Developmental Disabilities, 5317
Parental Concerns in College Student Mental Health, 2549
Parenting, 5318
Parenting Attention Deficit Disordered Teens, 8025
Parenting with a Disability, 5319
Parents and Friends, 6644
Parents and Friends, Inc, 5928
Parents and Teachers, 2550
Parents Helping Parents (PHP), 921
Parents Helping Parents: A Directory of Support Groups for ADD, 8026
Parents Supporting Parents Network, 3877
Parents, Let's Unite for Kids, 1643
PARI Independent Living Center, 4541
Paring Boards, 322
Park Brake Extension, 109
Park DuValle Community Health Center, Inc., 6916
Park Health And Rehabilitation Center, 7315
Park Manor Convalescent Center, 7199
Parker Bath, 381
Parker Foundation, 2855
Parker Publishing Company, 5128
Parker-Hannifin Foundation, 3211
Parking Brake Extension, 110
Parkinson Report, 8869
Parkinson's Disease Foundation, 2973, 3165, 8850, 8868
Parkinson's Disease Research Society, 8372
Parkview Acres Care and Rehabilitation Cen ter, 7317
Parkview Regional Rehabilitation Center, 6328
Parma Community General Hospital Acute Rehabilitation Center, 6395, 7103
Parrot Easy Language Simple Anaylsis, 1821
Parrot Software, 1813, 1821, 1840
Part B News, 7772
Part of the Team, 5240
Partial Seizure Disorders: A Guide for Patients and Families, 8794
Partnering with Public Health: Funding & Advocacy Opportunities for CILs and SILCs, 5241
Partners Resource Network, 3878
Partnership on Employment and Acessible Technology (PEAT), 922
Partnership to Improve Patient Care, 923
Parts of Speech, 1839
Pasadena Foundation, 2856
Passion for Justice, 5450
PAT-3: Photo Articulation Test, 2695
Pathfinder Publishing, 8700
Pathfinder Village, 7065
Pathfinders Camp, 1462
Pathfinders for Independent Living, 4269
PathPoint, 5929
Pathways Brain Injury Program, 7293
Pathways for the Future Center for Indepen dent Living, 4478
Pathways To Inclusion (2nd Edition), 5079
Pathways to Independence, Inc., 6141
Patient and Family Education, 2551
Patient Lifting & Injury Prevention, 382
Patient Transport Chair, 683
Patient's Guide to Visual Aids and Illumination, 9230
Patient-Centered Guides, 664, 5219, 5237, 8399
Patient-Centered Guides/O'Reilly Media, 5345
Patricia Neal Rehab Center : Ft. Sanders R egional Medical Center, 6435
Patrick and Anna M Cudahy Fund, 3349
Patrick Rehab Wellness Center, 7146
Patriot Extra Wide Folding Walkers, 618
Patriot Folding Walker Series, 619
Patriot Reciprocal Folding Walkers, 620
Paul and Annetta Himmelfarb Foundation, 2909
Paul H Brookes Publishing Company, 2391, 2552, 7990
PBA News, 9320
PCI, 5576
PCI Education Publishing, 1722, 1738, 1977
PDF News, 8850
PDF Newsletter, 8868
Peabody Articulation Decks, 2034
Peabody Early Experiences Kit (PEEK), 2696
Peabody Individual Achievement Test-Revised Normative Update (PIAT-R-NU), 2697
Peabody Language Development Kits (PLDK), 2698
PEAK Parent Center, 918, 2168, 5238
Pearle Vision Foundation, 3304
Pearlman Biomedical Research Institute, 4805
Pearson, 2725, 5353
Pearson Education, 2469
Pearson Higher Education, 2358
Pearson Performance Solutions, 448
PECO Energy Company Contributions Program, 3239
Pedal-in-Place Exerciser, 494
Pediatric Center at Plymouth Meeting Integrated Health Services, 7135
Pediatric Early Elementary (PEEX II) Examination, 2699
Pediatric Exam of Educational-PEERAMID Readiness at Middle Childhood, 2700
Pediatric Examination of Educational Readiness, 2701
Pediatric Extended Examination at-PEET Three, 2702
Pediatric Rehabilitation Department, JFK Medical Center, 7040
Pediatric Rheumatology Clinic, 4976
Pediatric Seating System, 241
Pediatric Visual Diagnosis Fact Sheets, 9231
Peer Counseling: Roles, Functions, Boundaries, 5242
Peer Mentor Volunteers: Empowering People for Change, 5243
PEERS Program, 6256
Pegasus LITE, 1875
Peidmont Independent Living Center, 4615
Pencil/Pen Weighted Holders, 526
Penguin Books USA, 5288
Penguin Group, 8809
Peninsula Center for Independent Living, 4616
Penitent, with Roses: An HIV+ Mother Refle cts, 8795
Penn State Milton S. Hershey Medical Center College Of Medicine, 7136
Pennstate, 7124
Pennsylvania Workers Compensation Board, 3818
Pennsylvania Bureau of Blindness & Visual Services, 3819
Pennsylvania Client Assistance Program, 3820
Pennsylvania College of Optometry Eye Institute, 4995
Pennsylvania Council on Independent Living, 4511
Pennsylvania Department of Aging, 3821
Pennsylvania Department of Children with Disabilities, 3822
Pennsylvania Department of Education: Bureau of Special Education, 2231
Pennsylvania Department of Labor & Industry, 6178
Pennsylvania Department of Labor and Industry (DLI), 6179
Pennsylvania Developmental Disabilities Council, 3823
Pennsylvania Governor's Cabinet Committee for People With Disabilities, 6180
Pennsylvania Human Relations Commission Agency, 6181
Pennsylvania Pain Rehabilitation Center, 7137
Pennsylvania Veterans Centers, 5813
Pennsylvania's Initiative on Assistive Technology, 1644
Penrose Hospital/ St. Francis Healthcare System, 6676
People & Families, 2299
People Against Cancer, 8791, 8867
People and Families, 5244
People First of Canada, 924
People Services, 6645
People Services, Inc, 5930
People to People International, 2783
People with Disabilities & Abuse: Implications for Center for Independent Living, 5245
People With Disabilities Press (iUniverse), 5078
People with Disabilities Who Challenge the System, 5246
People's Voice, 5247
Peoria Area Blind People's Center, 6847
Peoria Area Community Foundation, 2974
Perfect Solutions, 1577
Performance Health, 323, 449, 306, 310, 311, 319, 323, 332, 333, 352, 427, 450, 462, 611, 634, 1574, 2541
Performance Health Enrichments Catalog, 450
Perigee Visual Dictionary of Signing, 8266
Perkins Activity and Resource Guide: A Handbook for Teachers, 9232
Perkins Brailler, 527
Perkins School for the Blind, 9232
Permobil, 646, 716, 717
Permobil Max 90, 716
Permobil Super 90, 717
Permobil USA, 705
Perry Health Facility, 6286
Perry Point VA Medical Center, 5723
Perry Rehabilitation Center, 6526
Perry River Home Care, 4349
Person to Person: Guide for Professionals Working with the Disabled, 2552
Personal FM Systems, 190
Personal Perspectives on Personal Assistance Services, 5248
Personal Reader Department, 9233
Personal Reader Update, 9233

Personality and Emotional Disturbance, 2553
Perspectives, 5249
Perspectives on a Parent Movement, 5320
Perspectives: Whole Language Folio, 8983
Pervasive Developmental Disorders: Finding a Diagnosis and Getting Help, 5345
Pet Partners, 495
Petaluma Recycling Center, 6646
Peter A Towne Physical Therapy Center, 7104
Peter and Elizabeth C. Tower Foundation, 925, 3166
Pettigrew Rehabilitation and Healthcare Center, 7347
Peytral Publications, 2170
Phantom Lake YMCA Camp, 1490, 8644
PharmaThera, 7147
Phelps School Academic Support Program, 1393, 7931
Phenomenology of Depressive Illness, 2554
Philadelphia Foundation, 3241
Philadelphia Regional Office and Insurance Center, 5814
Philadelphia VA Medical Center, 5815
Phillip Roy, Inc., 1578, 1975, 1991
Philomatheon Society of the Blind, 7105
Phoenix Childrens Hospital, 991, 8596
Phoenix Dance, 5451
Phoenix Veterans Center, 6527
Phonak, 300
Phone of Our Own: The Deaf Insurrection Against Ma Bell, 8267
Phone Ringers, 191
Phone Strobe Flasher, 192
PhoneMax Amplified Telephone, 528
Phonemic Awareness in Young Children: A Classroom Curriculum, 2035
Phonics for Thought, 2036
Phonological Awareness Training for Reading, 2037
Physical & Mental Issues in Aging Sourcebo ok, 7647
Physical & Occupational Therapy in Geriatr ics, 7658
Physical Disabilities and Health Impairments: An Introduction, 2555
Physical Education and Sports for Exceptional Students, 2556
Physical Management of Multiple Handicaps: A Professional's Guide, 2557
Physically Handicapped in Society, 2558
Physically Impaired Association of Michigan, 4915
Piece of Cake Math, 1702
Pied Piper: Musical Activities to Develop Basic Skills, 58
Piedmont Independent Living Center, 4617
Piedmont Living Center, 4615
Piedmont Triad Council of Governments Area Agency on Aging, 7785
Pilot Industries: Ellenville, 7066
Pine Castle, 6767
Pine Meadows Healthcare and Rehabilitation Center, 7385
Pine Tree Camp, 1165
Pine Tree Society, 1165
Pinecrest Rehabilitation Hospital and Outpatient Centers, 6287
Pinellas Park Adult Day Training, 4119
Pinellas Talking Book Library for the Blind and Physically Handicapped, 4806
Pines Residential Treatment Center, 7183
Pinnacle Newsletter, 8315
Pioneer Center for Human Services, 6848
Pioneer Vocational/Industrial Services, 6056
PIRS Hotsheet, 6257
Pittsburgh Foundation, 3242
Pittsburgh Regional Office, 5816
PLA240 Room Loop System, 189
A Place for Me, 5397
Place of Their Own: Creating the Deaf Community in America, 8268
Place to Live, 5250
Placer Independent Resource Services, 4054, 6257
Places for People, 4379
Plan Ahead: Do What You Can, 8796
Planned Giving Department of Guide Dogs fo r the Blind, 9321
Planned Parenthood of Western Washington, 8280
Plastic Card Holder, 496
Platte River Industries, 6687
Play!, 2038
Playback, 9322
Playing Card Holders, 5575
Please Don't Say Hello, 8027, 8984
Please Understand Me: Software Program and Books, 1773
Plenum Publishing Corporation, 5150
Plum Enterprises, 498, 1519
PM&R Journal, 5379
PN, 7737
PN/Paraplegia News, 8411
PNC Bank Foundation, 3240
Pocatello Regional Medical Center, 6307
Pocketalker Personal Amplifier, 193
Points of Light: Atlanta, 7613
Points of Light: Washington, DC, 7614
Polaris Industries, 556
Polaris Trail Blazer, 556
Polk Brothers Foundation, 2975
Polk County Association for Handicapped Citizens, 6768
Polyester House Dress, 1533
Pomerado Rehabilitation Outpatient Service, 6647
Pompano Rehabilitation and Nursing Center, 7245
Pond, 1774
Pool Exercise Program - Arthritis Water Exercise / Arthritis Foundation, 5452
Poplar Bluff RehabCare Program, 7016
Port City Enterprises, 6930
Port Huron: Blue Water Center for Independ ent Living, 4336
Port Jefferson Health Care Facility, 7340
Portable Hand Controls by Handicaps, Inc., 111
Portable Large Print Computer, 1678
Portable Shampoo Bowl, 151
Portable Wheelchair Ramp, 383
PortaPower Plus, 1670
Porterville Sheltered Workshop, 5931
Portland Public Library, 4879
Portland Regional Office, 5804
Portland VA Medical Center, 5805
Portneuf Medical Center Rehabilitation, 6804
Post-Polio Health, 7773, 8870
Post-Polio Health International, 926, 8524, 7773, 8870
Post-Polio Support Group, 8903
Post-Polio Syndrome: A Guide for Polio Sur vivors and Their Families, 8797
Postgraduate Center for Mental Health, 4967
Postpartum Support International (PSI), 927
Posture-Glide Lounger, 684
Potty Learning for Children who Experience Delay, 5453
Powell's Books, 8237
Power Breathing Program, 2039
Power Door, 497
Power for Off-Pavement, 719
Power of Attorney for Health Care, 4726
Power Transfer Seat Base (6-Way), 112
Power Wheelchairs, 718
PowerLink 2 Control Unit, 324
POZ Magazine, 8851
PPAL In Print, 4725
PPAL Support Groups, 8900
A Practical Guide to Art Therapy Groups, 5088
Practicing Rehabilitation with Geriatric Clients, 2559
Prader-Willi Alliance Of New York, 1917
Prader-Willi Alliance of New York Newslett er, 8871
Prader-Willi Syndrome Association USA, 8525
Prader-Willi Syndrome: Development and Manifestations, 8798
Praeger - ABC-CLIO, 5054
Praeger Publishers, 7646
Pragmatic Approach, 2560
Prairie Cruiser, 685
Prairie Freedom Center for Independent Living: Sioux Falls, 4551
Prairie Freedom Center for Independent Li ving: Madison, 4552
Prairie Freedom Center for Independent Liv ing: Yankton, 4553
Prairie IL Resource Center, 4230
Prairie Independent Living Resource Center, 4231
Pre-Reading Screening Procedures, 2703
Prelude, 152
Prentke Romich Company, 194, 173, 203, 486, 1806
Prentke Romich Company Product Catalog, 451
Preparing for ACT Assessment, 2704
PreReading Strategies, 8269
Presby, 7372
Presbytery of Eastern Virginia, 8636, 8637
Preschool Learning Activities for the Visually Impaired Child, 9234
Preschoolers with Special Needs: Children At-Risk, Children with Disabilities, 2561
Prescott Public Library, 4754
Prescriptions for Independence: Working with Older People Who are Visually Impaired, 7648
President's Committee on People with Disabilities: Arkansas, 3454
President's Committee on People with Intellectual Disabilities, 3404
Prevent Blindness America, 9094, 9181, 9320, 9362
Prevent Blindness Connecticut, 4786
Prevent Child Abuse America, 8904
Preventable Brain Damage, 8028
Preventing Academic Failure - Teachers Handbook, 2562
Preventing School Dropouts, 2563
Preventing Secondary Conditions Associated with Spina Bifida or Cerebral Palsy, 8799
Prevention, 7738
Prevocational Assessment, 2564
PRIDE Industries, 5927, 6641
Pride Industries: Grass Valley, 6648
Pride Mobility, 686
Prima Publishing, 7952, 8962
Primacy Healthcare and Rehabilitation Cent er, 7386
Primary Care Collaborative, 928
Primary Children's Medical Center, 6471
Primary Phonics, 2040
Primary Special Needs and the National Cur riculum, 2565
Prime Engineering, 219, 219
Prime Time, Inc., 1481
Primer on the Rheumatic Diseases, 8401
Primrose Center, 5984
The Princeton Review - Penguin Random House, 2635
Principal Financial Group Foundation, 2990
Print, Play & Learn #1 Old Mac's Farm, 1775
Print, Play & Learn #7: Sampler, 1776
Printed Rear Closure Sweat Top, 1534
Prisma Health Children's Hospital, 1404, 1406
Pro- Ed Publications, 2574, 2675, 2718, 2723, 8002
Pro- Max/ Division Of Bow- Flex Of America, 399
PRO-ED, 2169
PRO-ED Inc., 2451, 5396, 7808
Products for People with Disabilities, 452
Professional Association of Therapeutic Ho rsemanship International (PATH Intl.), 929, 8456
Professional Development Programs, 2211
Professional Fit Clothing, 1535
Profex Medical Products, 165
Programming Concepts, 1727, 1730, 1763, 1809, 1870
Programs for Aphasia and Cognitive Disorders, 1840
Programs for Children with Disabilities: Ages 3 through 5, 6329
Programs for Children with Special Health Care Needs, 6330
Programs for Infants and Toddlers with Disabilities: Ages Birth through 2, 6331
Progress Center for Independent Living, 4179
Progress Center for Independent Living: Bl ue Island, 4180

Progress Valley: Phoenix, 6528
Progress Without Punishment: Approaches for Learners with Behavior Problems, 2566
Progressive Center for Independent Living, 4419
Progressive Center for Independent Living: Flemington, 4420
Progressive Independence, 4501
Progressive Options, 4507
Project AID Resource Center, 8855
Project Freedom, 4421
Project Freedom: Hamilton, 4422
Project Freedom: Lawrence, 4423
Project Independence, 5932
Project Kindle, 1006, 1232
Project Onward Gallery, 59
Project SEARCH, 5985
Projects with Industry (PWI) Program, 5933
Promoting Communication in Infants and Young Children: 500 Ways to Succeed, 8985
Promoting Postsecondary Education for Students with Learning Disabilities, 2567
Prone Support Walker, 621
Propet Leather Walking Shoes, 1536
Prorter Sargent, 2131
Prostate and Urological Disorders Sourcebo ok, 8800
Prosthetics and Orthotics Center in Blue Island, 6849
ProtectaCap, ProtectaCap+PLUS, ProtectaChin Guard and ProtectaHip, 498
Protecting Against Latex Allergy, 8801
Protection & Advocacy for People with Disabilities, 3839
Protection & Advocacy for Persons with Developmental Disabilities: Alaska, 3435
Protection & Advocacy for Persons with Disabilities: Arizona, 3444
Protection & Advocacy Project, 3783
Protection & Advocacy System: Alaska, 3434
Protection and Advocacy (PA I), 3460
Protection and Advocacy Agency of NY, 3753
Protection and Advocacy System, 3961
Protestant Guild Learning Center, 6977
Providence Health System, 6258
Providence Holy Cross Medical Center, 6258
Providence Hospital Work, 7106
Providence Medical Center, 6480
Providence Regional Office, 5820
Providence Rehabilitation Services, 6481, 6481
Providence Speech and Hearing Association, 9015
Providence Speech and Hearing Center, 8934
Providence VA Medical Center, 5821
Provider Magazine, 5380
Providing Services for People with Vision Loss: Multidisciplinary Perspective, 9287
Prudential Financial, 3102
Prudential Foundation, 3102
Prufrock Press, 2171, 2371, 2611, 2711
PSS CogRehab Software, 1820
Psy-Ed Corporation, 5300
Psychiatric Institute of Washington, 6722
Psychiatric Mental Health Nursing, 2568
Psychiatric Staffing Crisis in Community Mental Health, 2300
Psycho-Educational Assessment of Preschool Children, 2705
Psychoeducational Assessment of Visually Impaired and Blind Students, 2569
Psychological & Educational Publications, 2484, 2713
Psychological & Social Impact of Disabilit y, 5251
Psychological and Social Impact of Illness and Disability, 2570
Psychological Software Services, 1820
Psychology and Health, 5252
Psychology of Disability, 5253
Public Health Reports, 5381
Public Interest Law Center of Philadelphia, 3824, 4705
Public Library Of Anniston-Calhoun County, 4746
Public Radio WBHM 90.3 FM, 4742
Public Technology Institute, 3500
Public Welfare Foundation, 2910
PublishAmerica, 8684
Publix Super Market Corporation Office, 2926
Publix Super Markets Charities, 2926
Pueblo Diversified Industries, 6688
Puget Sound Healthcare Center, 7410
Punctuation Rules, 1841
Purdue University, 8860, 8886
Purdue University Press, 5072
Pure Facts, 8069
Pure Vision Arts, 60
Push Pull Hand Controls, 113
Push Rock Hand Controls, 114
Push-Button Quad Cane, 622
Pushin' Forward, 5454
Putnam County Comprehensive Services, 6041
Putnam Independent Living Services, 4460
Puzzle Games: Cooking, Eating, Community and Grooming, 5576
Puzzle Power: Sampler, 1777
Puzzle Power: Zoo & School Days, 1778
Puzzle Tanks, 1703
PVA Adaptive Sports, 5675
PVA Architecture, 1935
PVA Publications, 7737, 8411
PVA Summit & Expo, 1916
PWSA (USA) Conference, 1917
PXE International, 8901
The Pyramids, 8339

Q

Quad Canes, 623
Quad City Deaf & Hard of Hearing Youth Group: Tomorrow's Leaders for our Community, 8270
Quad Commander, 499
Quadtro Cushion, 242
Quality Care Newsletter, 8872
Quality First, 7774
Quality Improvement Organizations, 7615
Quality of Life for Persons with Disabilities, 5254
Quantum Books, 5279
Quantum Technologies, 5540
Quarterly Update, 9323
Queen Anne Health Care, 7200, 7200
Queen of Angels/Hollywood Presbyterian Medical Center, 6259
Queen of the Valley Hospital, 6260
Quest Books, 45
Quest Camp, 1040, 7932
Quest Magazine, 2301
Quest, Inc., 5986, 6769, 1079
Quest, Inc. - Tampa Area, 5987, 6770
Questar Corporation Contributions Program, 3313
Questions and Answers: The ADA and Persons with HIV/AIDS, 8802
Queue, 1695
Queue Inc, 1702
Queue Incorporated, 1736
Quick Reading Test, Phonics Based Reading, Reading SOS (Strategies for Older Students), 1842
Quick Talk, 1843
Quickie 2, 557
Quincy Rehabilitation Institute of Holy Cross Hospital, 7176

R

R82, Inc., 137, 325
RA Bloch Cancer Foundation, 3078
Race the Clock, 1844
Ragtime Industries, 6895
RAIL, 4380
The Rainbow Club, 1071
Rainier Vista Care Center, 7201
Raised Dot Computing, 1604
Raised Line Drawing Kit, 529
Raising Deaf Kids, 930
Raleigh Rehabilitation and Healthcare Cent er, 7348
Ralph H Johnson VA Medical Center, 5823
Ralph M Parsons Foundation, 2858
Ramapo for Children, 1282, 2749, 7907
Ramapo Training, 2749
Ramplette Telescoping Ramp, 384
Rampvan, 115
Rancho Adult Day Care Center, 6649
Rancho Los Amigos Medical Center, 6649
Rancho Los Amigos National Rehabilitation Center, 6261
Rand-Scot, 624
Rand-Scot, Inc., 163, 228, 353, 624
Random House, 8403, 8774
Random House Publishing, 8699, 8706
Ranger All Seasons Corporation, 562, 566
Rapahope Children's Retreat Foundation, 979, 2797, 8645
Rapaport Publishing, Inc., 8858, 8861
Rascal 3-Wheeler, 558
Rascal Convertable, 559
Rasmuson Foundation, 2799
Rasmussen's Syndrome and Hemispherectomy Support Network Newsletter, 8873
Raven Rock Lutheran Camp, 7933
Ray Graham Association for People with Disabilities, 6855
Raynaud's Phenomenon, 8803
Raytheon Company Contributions Program, 3035
RB King Counseling Center, 6850
RC Baker Foundation, 2857
RD Equipment, Inc., 146, 161
REACH, 8070
REACH of Dallas Resource Center on Independent Living, 4576
REACH of Dallas Resource on Independent Living, 5255
REACH of Denton Resource Center on Independent Living, 4577
REACH of Fort Worth Resource Center on Ind ependent Living, 4578
REACH Rehabilitation and Catastrophic Long-Term Care, 7042
Reach Rehabilitation Program: Americana Healthcare, 6856
REACH Rehabilitation Program: Leader Nursing and Rehabilitation Center, 7041
REACH/Resource Centers on Independent Livi ng, 4669
REACHing Out Newsletter, 5255
Reaching the Autistic Child: A Parent Trai ning Program, 8804
Reaching the Child with Autism Through Art, 61
Reaching, Crawling, Walking... Let's Get Moving, 9235
Read How You Want Large Print Books, 5272
Read: Out Loud, 1845
Reader Rabbit, 1846
Reader's Digest Foundation, 3167
Readers Digest Association, 3167
Reading and Deafness, 2571
Reading Comprehension Series, 1847
Reading for Content, 2041
Reading from Scratch, 2042
Reading in the Workplace, 1867
Reading Is for Everyone, 9236
Reading Rehabilitation Hospital, 4996
Reading with Low Vision, 9237
Reading, Writing and Speech Problems in Children, 8029, 8986
Readings on Research in Stuttering, 2572
Readings: A Journal of Reviews and Commentary in Mental Health, 2302
Readjusment Counciling Service Western Mountain Re, 5752
REAL Design, 212, 216, 217
Real Design Inc., 500
Reality of Dyslexia, 8030
Rear Closure Shirts, 1537
Rear Closure T-Shirt, 1538
Rebound: Northeast Methodist Hospital, 6456
Rebsamen Rehabilitation Center, 6235
Receptive-Expressive Emergent-REEL-2 Language Test, 2nd Edition, 2707
Recipe for Reading, 2043
Reclaiming Independence: Staying in the Dr ivers Seat When You Are no Longer Drive., 7812
Recognizing Children with Special Needs, 5455

Recording for the Blind & Dyslexic, 9238, 9313, 9322
Recreation Activities for the Elderly, 2573
Recreation Unlimited Foundation, 1338, 1339, 1340, 1341
Recreation Unlimited: Day Camp, 1338
Recreation Unlimited: Residential Camp, 1339
Recreation Unlimited: Respite Weekend Camp, 1340
Recreation Unlimited: Specialty Camp, 1341
Red Notebook, 4889
Red Rock Center for Independence, 4590
Redman Apache, 687
Redman Crow Line, 688
Redman Powerchair, 223, 687, 688, 714, 719
Reduced Effort Steering, 116
Reference and Information Services From NLS, 9239
Reference Manual for Communicative Sciences and Disorders, 2574
Reference Service Press, 2832, 3353, 3355, 3359, 3360, 3361, 3362, 3363, 3364, 3373, 3374, 3375
Regal Research & Manufacturing Company, 567
Regent, 560
Regenta Park, 6747
Regents' Center for Learning Disorders, 2708
Regional Access & Mobilization Project, 4181
Regional Access & Mobilization Project: Be lvidere, 4182
Regional Access & Mobilization Project: De Kalb, 4183
Regional Access & Mobilization Project: Fr eeport, 4184
Regional ADA Technical Assistance Center, 3724
Regional Center for Independent Living, 4461
Regional Center for Rehabilitation, 6650
Regional Early Childhood Director Center, 3754
Regional Library, 4798
Regional Rehabilitation Center Pitt County Memorial Hospital, 7076
Regional Resource Centers Program, 5541
Registry of Interpreters for the Deaf, 8169, 8253
Rehab Care, 6931, 7113
Rehab Engineering & Assistive Tech. North America, 1919
Rehab Home Care, 7077
Rehab Institute at Florence Nightingale He alth Center, 7341
Rehab Pro, 2303
REHAB Products and Services, 6851
RehabCare, 6932
Rehabiliation Engineering Research Center on Accessible Public Transportation, 5598
Rehabilitation & Nursing Center at Greater Pittsburgh, The, 7138
Rehabilitation Achievement Center, 6857
Rehabilitation and Healthcare Center of Mo nroe, 7349
Rehabilitation and Healthcare Center of Ta mpa, 7247
Rehabilitation and Research Center Virginia Commonwealth University, 7398
Rehabilitation Associates, Inc., 6704
Rehabilitation Center at McFarland Hospital, 6437
Rehabilitation Center at Thibodeaux Regional, 6931
Rehabilitation Center Baptist Hospital, 6436
Rehabilitation Center for Children and Adults, 6771
Rehabilitation Center of Lake Charles Memorial Hospital, 6344
Rehabilitation Center of Palm Beach, 7246
Rehabilitation Division, 6111
Rehabilitation Engineering and Assistive Technology Society of North America (RESNA), 453, 1645
Rehabilitation Enterprises of North Easter n Wyoming: Newcastle, 4649
Rehabilitation Enterprises of Washington, 7202
Rehabilitation Hospital of Indiana, 7282
Rehabilitation Hospital of the Pacific, 6801
Rehabilitation Institute of Chicago, 6852, 6853, 8447
Rehabilitation Institute of Chicago's Virginia Wadsworth Sports Program, 8883
Rehabilitation Institute of Chicago: Alexian Brothers Medical Center, 6858
Rehabilitation Institute of Ohio at Miami Valley Hospital, 6396
Rehabilitation Institute of Santa Barbara, 6651
Rehabilitation Institute of Sarasota, 6288
Rehabilitation Institute of Southern California, 6652
Rehabilitation International, 931, 7712
Rehabilitation International World Congress, 1920
Rehabilitation Interventions for the Institutionalized Elderly, 2575
Rehabilitation Nursing for the Neurological Patient, 2576
Rehabilitation Opportunities, 6949
Rehabilitation Research and Development Center, 5656
Rehabilitation Research Library, 4968
Rehabilitation Resource Manual: VISION, 2577
Rehabilitation Resource University, 2480
Rehabilitation Service of North Central Oh io, 4494
Rehabilitation Services, 7089
Rehabilitation Services Administration, 3405, 5969, 6529
Rehabilitation Specialists, 7043
Rehabilitation Technology, 2578
Reinberger Foundation, 3212
Reizen Braille Labeler, 530
Relationship Development Intervention with Young Children, 8031, 8987
Relaxation Techniques for People with Special Needs, 5456
Relaxation: A Comprehensive Manual for Adults and Children with Special Needs, 5257
Reliance House, 6705
Religious Signing: A Comprehensive Guide for All Faiths, 8271
Remedial and Special Education, 2304
Remedy, 7739
Removing the Barriers: Accessibility Guidelines and Specifications, 1954
Renaissance at 87th Street, 7270
Renaissance at Hillside, 7271
Renaissance at Midway, 7272
Renaissance at South Shore, 7273
Renaissance Center, 6772
Renaissance Clubhouse, 4308
RENEW: Gillette, 4647
RENEW: Rehabilitation Enterprises of North Eastern Wyoming, 4648
Reno Regional Office, 5758
Report Writing in Assessment and Evaluation, 2579
Research & Training Center on Mental Health for Hard of Hearing Persons, 4774
Research and Practice for Persons with Sev ere Disabilities, 7659
Research and Training Center, 5256
Research on Aging, 7740
Research Press, 2172, 2536, 5257, 5433, 5456
Research Press Company, 2173
Research to Prevent Blindness, 3168, 9170
Research!America, 5542
Research, Advocacy, and Practice for Compl ex and Chronic Conditions, 7660
RESNA, 7677
RESNA Annual Conference, 1919
Resource Center for Accessible Living, 4462
Resource Center for Independent Living, 4232, 4463
Resource Center for Independent Living, In c. (RCIL), 4233
Resource Center for Independent Living: Emporia, 4234
Resource Center for Independent Living: Minot, 4485
Resource Center for Independent Living: Ar kansas City, 4235
Resource Center for Independent Living: Bu rlington, 4236
Resource Center for Independent Living: Co ffeyville, 4237
Resource Center for Independent Living: El Dorado, 4238
Resource Center for Independent Living: Ft Scott, 4239
Resource Center for Independent Living: Ot tawa, 4240
Resource Center for Independent Living: Ov erland Park, 4241
Resource Center for Independent Living: To peka, 4242
Resource List for Persons with Low Vision, 9240
Resource Room, The, 2580
Resources for Independence, 4291
Resources for Independent Living, 4055, 4618
Resources for Independent Living: Baton Rouge, 4274
Resources for Independent Living: Metairie, 4275
Resources for People with Disabilities and Chronic Conditions, 5258
Resources for Rehabilitation, 2581, 2577, 5226, 5258, 9220, 9287
Resources in Special Education, 2339
RespectAbility, 932
Respiratory Disorders Sourcebook, 8805
Respironics, 262
Responding to Crime Victims with Disabilit ies, 2139
Restructuring for Caring and Effective Education: Administrative Guide, 2583
Restructuring High Schools for All Students: Taking Inclusion to the Next Level, 2582
Rethinking Attention Deficit Disorder, 8032
Retirement Research Foundation, 2976
Rettsyndrome.org, 8071
Rewarding Speech, 2044
Rex Bionics, Ltd., 501
Rhode Island Arc, 3260
Rhode Island Department Health, 3828
Rhode Island Department of Education: Office of Special Needs, 2232
Rhode Island Department of Elderly Affairs, 3829
Rhode Island Department of Mental Health, 3830
Rhode Island Developmental Disabilities Council, 3831
Rhode Island Disability Law Center, 3832
Rhode Island Foundation, 3261
Rhode Island Governor's Commission on Disabilities, 3833
Rhode Island Lions Sight Foundation, Inc., 1398
Rhode Island Parent Information Network, 3834
Rhode Island Services for the Blind and Visually Impaired, 3835, 6184
RIC Northshore, 6852
RIC Prosthetics and Orthotics Center, 6853
RIC Windermere House, 6854
Rich Foundation, 2937
Richard L Roudebush VA Medical Center, 5699
Richard W Higgins Charitable Foundation, 2994
Richmond Research Training Center (RRTC), 6212
Rickshaw Exerciser, 385
Ricon, 112, 347, 369, 386
Ricon Classic, 386
Ricon Corporation, 387
Riddle of Autism: A Psychological Analysis, 8033, 8988
Rifton Equipment, 220
Right Angle Hand Controls, 117
Right at Home, 5457
Right Hand Gas and Brake Control, 118
Right Turn, 1704
Riley Child Development Center, 6332
Riley Hospital For Children, Indiana Univ. Health, 1128
Riley's Children Foundation, 1136
Rimland Services for Autistic Citizens, 1123, 7934
Rio Grande Community Development Corporation, 1265
Rio Vista Rehabilitation Hospital, 6457
Ripley Healthcare and Rehabilitation Cente r, 7387
RISE, 6894
RISE-Resource: Information, Support and Empowerment, 4579
Rising Treetops at Oakhurst, 1262, 8382
Rita J and Stanley H Kaplan Foundation, 3169
River's Edge Rehabilitation and Healthcare, 7263
Riverdeep Incorporated, 1803
Riverside Community Hospital, 7224

Riverside Medical Center, 6859
Riverview School, 2200
Road Ahead: Transition to Adult Life for Persons with Disabilities (3rd Edition), 5085
Roadster 20, 561
Roanoke City Public Library System, 5025
Roanoke Memorial Hospital, 7184
Roanoke Regional Office, 5847
Robert Campeau Family Foundation, 3213
Robert Ellis Simon Foundation, 2859
Robert J Dole VA Medical Center, 5710
Robert Sterling Clark Foundation, 3170
Robert Wood Johnson Foundation, 3103
Robert Young Mental Health Center Division of Trinity Regional Haelth System, 6860
Robey W Estes Family Foundation, 3322
Robey W Estes Jr, 3322
RoboMath, 1705
Rochester Area Foundation, 3068
Rochester Institute Of Technology, 4972
Rock-King Wheelchair Kit, 689
Rocker Balance Square, 502
Rocky Mountain Resource & Training Institute, 6231
Rodale Inc, 7732, 7738
Rodale Press, 5183
Rodeo, 1779
Roger Randall Center, 6939
ROHO Group, 230, 233, 239, 240, 241, 242
Role Portrayal and Stereotyping on Television, 5259
Roll Chair, 221
Rollators, 625
Rollin M Gerstacker Foundation, 3056
Rolling Along with Goldilocks and the Thre e Bears, 5058
Rolling Hills Country Day Camp, 7935
Rolling Start, 4056
Rolling Start: Victorville, 4057
Rolls 2000 Series, 690
Rome Subregional Library for the Blind and Physically Handicapped, 4825
Ronald McDonald House Charities (RMHC), 933
Room Valet Visual-Tactile Alerting System, 503
Rosalind Russell Medical Research Center for Arthritis, 4775
Rose-Colored Glasses, 9241
Roseburg VA Medical Center, 5806
Rosen Publishing, 8705, 8740
Rosen Publishing Group, 7982
Rosewood Center, 6950
Rosomoff Comprehensive Pain Center, The, 6773
Rotary Camp, 1342
Rotary Club of Akron, 1342
Rotary International, 2784
Rotary Youth Exchange, 2784
Round Lake Camp, 1263
Roundup River Ranch, 1061, 8646
Routledge (Taylor & Francis Group), 2405, 2545, 5050, 5069, 5088, 5361, 5386, 7624, 7625, 7626, 7627, 7629, 7635, 7639, 7641, 7645, 7651, 7970, 7972, 8959, 8961, 9124
ROW Adventures, 5617
Rowan Community, 7230
Rowan Vocational Opportunities, Inc. (RVO), 6162
Royal C Johnson Veterans Memorial Medical Center, 5825
RP Foundation Fighting Blindness, 9183
RP Messenger, 9324
RSA Union Building, 3413
RTC Connection, 5256
Ruben Center for Independent Living, 4203
Rubicon Programs, 6653
RULES: Revised, 2706
Rural Center for Independent Living, 4405
Rush Copley Medical Center-Rehab Neuro Physical Unit, 6314
Rusk Institute of Rehabilitation Medicine, 6385
Rutherford Vocational Workshop, 6163
Rutland Mental Health Services, 7178
Rx Remedies, 7739
Ryan White HIV/AIDS Program, 934
Ryland Group, 3011

S

S W Georgia Regional Library, 4815
S. Karger Publishers, Inc., 7685, 7703
S.C. Vocational Rehabilitation Department, 6187
SACC Assistive Technology Center, 1646
Sacramento Medical Center, 5657
Sacremento State, 1626
Safari Scooter, 562
Safari Tilt, 222
Safe Path Products, 454, 454
Safety Deck II, 647
Sagamore Publishing, 39
Sage Journals, 7666, 7735, 7748
SAGE Publications, 2609
Sage Publications, 2174, 40, 1997, 2037, 2269, 2276, 2281, 2282, 2292, 2304, 2341, 2375, 2389, 2404, 2412, 2413, 2424, 2462, 2520, 2546, 2563, 2567, 2569, 2571, 2612, 2617, 2624, 2639, 2640, 2642, 2656, 2666, 2674, 2685, 2695, 2707, 2717, 2719, 2720, 2721, 2722, 5112, 5167, 7652, 7715, 7740, 7955, 7999, 8018, 8034, , 8265, 8757, 8978, 9150, 9269
SAILS, 4580
Saint Joseph Regional Medical Center- South Bend, 6880
Saint Jude Medical Center, 7225
Salem VA Medical Center, 5848
Salvation Army, 1196
SAMHSA News, 2336
Sampson-Katz Center, 6861
Samuel W Bell Home for Sightless, 4495
San Antonio Area Foundation, 3305
San Antonio Warm Springs Rehabilitation Hospital, 6458
San Bernardino Valley Lighthouse for the Blind, 6654
San Diego VA Regional Office, 5658
San Francisco Foundation, 2860
San Francisco Public Library for the Blind and Print Handicapped, 4776
San Joaquin General Hospital, 6587
San Joaquin Valley Rehabilitation Hospital, 6262
San Jose State University Library, 4777
San Juan Center for Independence, 4430
San Luis Medical and Rehabilitation Center, 7424
Sandcastle Day Camp, 8203
Sandhills School, 2750
Sandusky: Blue Water Center for Independen t Living, 4337
Sanilac County Community Mental Health, 6999
Santa Barbara Bank & Trust, 2839
Santa Barbara Foundation, 2861, 5107
Santa Clara Valley Blind Center, Inc., 6655
Santa Clara Valley Medical Center, 6263
Santa Fe Community Foundation, 3108
Sarasota Memorial Hospital/Comprehensive Rehabilitation Unit, 6774
Sarkeys Foundation, 3221
Savannah Association for the Blind, 6797
Savannah Rehabilitation and Nursing Center, 7254
Say it with Sign, 9242
Say What Clothing Identifier, 258
SAYdee Posters, 2045
SB Waterman & E Blade Charitable Foundation, 3350
SC Department of Health and Environmental Control, 1402
Scandinavian Exchange, 2785
Scanning WSKE, 1672
SCARC, Inc., 5988
SCATBI: Scales Of Cognitive Ability for Traumatic Brain Injury, 8034
SCCIL at Titusville, 4120
SCENE, 9325
Schaefer Enterprises, 6691
Schepens Eye Research Institute, 4904, 9330
Scheuer Associates Foundation, 2894
Schmieding Developmental Center, 2709
Schnurmacher Center for Rehabilitation and Nursing, 7342
Scholastic, 8717
School Of Medicine, Rheumatology Division, 4850
School Specialty, 1964, 1965, 1974, 1984, 1989, 1993, 1998, 1999, 2010, 2011, 2016, 2040, 2041, 2043, 2051, 2054, 2055, 2056, 2057, 2069
Schools And Services For Children With Autism Spectrum Disorders., 3755
Schroth School & Technical Education Center, 7037
Schwab Rehabilitation Hospital, 7274
SCI Life, 8852
SCI Psychosocial Process, 8428, 8874
SCILIFE, 8429
Scoffolding Student Learning, 2584
Scoota Bug, 563
Scooter & Wheelchair Battery Fuel Gauges and Motor Speed Controllers, 648
Scottish Rite Center for Childhood Language Disorders, 8935
Scottsdale Administrative Office, 6517
Scottsdale Healthcare, 6239
Screening in Chronic Disease, 5260
Scripps Memorial Hospital at La Jolla, 6264
Scripps Memorial Hospital: Pain Center, 6656
Sea Pines Rehabilitation Hospital, 6289, 6752
Seacrest Village Nursing Center, 7328
Seagull Industries for the Disabled, 5989
Seany Foundation, 2862
The Seany Foundation, 1017, 8597
Sears-Roebuck Foundation, 2977
Seat-A-Robics, 5458
Seattle Medical and Rehabilitation Center, 7203
Seattle Regional Office, 5851
Sebasticook Farms-Great Bay Foundation, 6940
Secret Agent Walking Stick, 626
Secretary State Office, 4939
Secure Retirement, The Newsmagazine for Mature Americans, 7742
Sedgwick Press/Grey House Publishing, 2127, 2128
See A Bone, 9243
See for Yourself, 9350
See What I Feel, 9244
See What I'm Saying, 9349
The Seeing Eye, 9282, 9327
Seeing Eye Guide, 9327
Seeing Eye, The, 9095
Seeing Voices, 8272
Seersucker Shower Robe, 1539
Seizures and Epilepsy in Childhood: A Guid e, 8807
Selecting a Program, 9245
Selective Nontreatment of Handicapped, 2585
Selective Placement Program Coordinator Di rectory, 2140
SELF Magazine, 7741
Self Reliance, 4121
Self-Therapy for the Stutterer, 8989
Sellersburg Health and Rehabilitation Cent re, 7283
Semiotics and Dis/ability: Interogating Categories of Difference, 2586
SEMO Alliance for Disability Independence, 4381
Senior Focus, 7775
Senior Health Care Management, 7245
Senior Program for Teens and Young Adults with Special Needs, 2751
Senior Resource LLC, 7616
Senior Service America, 7617
Senior Times Magazine, 7743, 7743
Sensation Products, 2046
Sensory University Toy Company, The, 2047
Sequanota Lutheran Conference Center and Camp, 1394, 8948
Sequential Spelling: 1-7 with 7 Student Re sponse Books, 2048
Serenity, 7744
Series Adapter, 504
SeriousFun Children's Network, 1069
SeriousFun Support Center Office, 1069
Sertoma Camp Endeavor, 1087, 8204, 8204
Sertoma Centre, 6021
Servcies for Students with Disabilities (S SD), 2117
Service Coordination for Early Intervention: Parents and Friends, 2587
Service Source, 5964

Services Center For Independent Living, 4058
Services for Independent Living, 4382, 4496, 5121
Services for Students with Disabilities, 2209
Services for the Blind, 4927
Services for the Blind and Visually Impaired, 3836
Services for the Blind Branch, 6000
Services for the Seriously Mentally Ill: A Survey of Mental Health Centers, 2588
Services Maximizing Independent Living and Empowerment (SMILE), 3991
ServiceSource Disability Resource Center, 6213
Setebaid Services, Inc., 1383, 8602
Seven Fifty-Five FS, 706
7 Steps for Success, 2344
Sex Education: Issues for the Person with Autism, 8035, 8990
Sexual Adjustment, 5261
Sexuality and Disabilities: A Guide for Human Service Practitioners, 5262
Sexuality and Disability, 2589
Sexuality and the Developmentally Handicapped, 5321
Sexuality and the Person with Spina Bifida, 8808
Shady Oaks Camp, 1124, 8648
SHALOM Denver, 6689
Shalom House, 4283
Shambhala Publications, 5142, 5191
Shands Rehab Hospital, 7248
Shannon Medical Center: RehabCare Unit, 6459
Shape Up 'n Sign, 9351
Share, Inc, 8589
Shared Visions, 9328
Sharing Solutions: A Newsletter for Support Groups, 9329
Sharing the Burden, 7649
Sharp Calculator with Illuminated Numbers, 531
Sharp Coronado Hospital, 6657
Shasta County Opportunity Center, 5934
Shattered Dreams-Lonely Choices: Birth Parents of Babies with Disabilities, 5322
Shaughnessy-Kaplan Rehabilitation Hospital, 6978
Shawmut Bank, 2895
SHC, The Arc of Medina County, 1330
Shelby County Community Services, 6862
Shelby Pines Rehabilitation and Healthcare Center, 7388
Shell Oil Company Foundation, 3306
Shenandoah Valley Workforce Investment Board, 4619
Shenango Valley Foundation, 3243
Shepherd Center for Treatment of Spinal Injuries, 6798
Sheridan Press,, 9276
Sheridan VA Medical Center, 5865
Sherman Lake YMCA Outdoor Center, 7937, 8649
Sherman Lake YMCA Summer Camp, 8649
The Shield Institute, 60
Shilo Inns & Resorts, 5599
Shining Bright: Head Start Inclusion, 5459
Shirley Ryan AbilityLab, 935
Shoe Horn and Sock Remover, 259
Shop Talk, 2590
Shop Til You Drop, 1780
Shore Community Services, 6022
Shore Training Center, 6022
Shore Village Rehabilitation & Nursing Center, 7302
Show Me How: A Manual for Parents of Preschool Blind Children, 9246
Shower and Commode Chair, 155
Shower Bathtub Mat, 154
Shreveport VA Medical Center, 5716
Shriner's Hospitals for Children Newslette r, 5059
Shriners Burn Institute: Cincinnati Unit, 6397
Shriners Burn Institute: Galveston Unit, 6460
Shriners Burns Hospital: Boston, 6355
Shriners Hospital for Children-Shreveport, 6345
Shriners Hospital for Children: Honolulu, 6306
Shriners Hospital Springfield Unit Springfield Unit for Crippled Children, 6356
Shriners Hospitals, 6482
Shriners Hospitals for Children St. Louis, 7017
Shriners Hospitals for Children Cincinnati, 6397
Shriners Hospitals for Children, Greenville, 6429
Shriners Hospitals for Children, Philadelphia, 6424
Shriners Hospitals for Children, Erie, 6425
Shriners Hospitals for Children, Houston, 6461
Shriners Hospitals for Children, Lexington, 6341
Shriners Hospitals For Children-Northern California, 6658
Shriners Hospitals for Children: Intermountain, 6472
Shriners Hospitals for Children: Los Angel es, 6659
Shriners Hospitals for Children: Portland, 6408
Shriners Hospitals for Children: Spokane, 6482
Shriners Hospitals for Children: Tampa, 6290
Shriners Hospitals for Children: Twin Cities, 7007
Shriners Hospitals, Philadelphia Unit, for Crippled Children, 6426
Shrinners Hospitals for Children, 6424
Sibling Forum: A FRA Newsletter, 5060
Sibling Information Network Newsletter, 2337
The Sibling Slam Book: What It's Really Li ke To Have a Brother or Sister with Special Needs, 5064
Sibling Support Project, 5064, 5065, 5066, 5308
Sibling Supporting Project, 5061
The Sibling Survival Guide, 5065
Siboney Learning Group, 1701
Sibpage, 2338
Sibshops: Workshops for Siblings of Children with Special Needs, 5061
Sickened: The Memoir of a Muchausen by Pro xy Childhood, 5263
Sickle Cell Disease Association of Illinois, 8546
Side Velcro Slacks, 1540
Side-Zip Sweat Pants, 1541
Sidney Stern Memorial Trust, 2863
Sierra 3000/4000, 564
Sierra Health Foundation, 2864
Sierra Pain Institute, 7025
Sight & Hearing Association, 8170
Sight by Touch, 9352
Sightings Newsletter, 9330
Sign Language Interpreting and Interpreter Education, 8273
Sign Language Studies, 8296
Sign Media, 8252
Sign of the Times, 9247
Signaling Wake-Up Devices, 505
Signature and Address Self-Inking Stamps, 532
Signature Group Inc., 7749
Signed English Schoolbook, 2591
Signed English Starter, The, 8274
Signing Family: What Every Parent Should Know About Sign Communication, The, 8275
Signing for Reading Success, 8276
Signing Naturally Curriculum, 2049
Signing: How to Speak with Your Hands, 8277
Signs Across America, 8278
Signs for Me: Basic Sign Vocabulary for Children, Parents & Teachers, 8279
Signs for Sexuality: A Resource Manual, 8280
Signs of the Times, 8281
SILC Department of Vocational Rehabilitation, 4270
SILC, Indiana Council on Independent Livin g (ICOIL), 4204
Silent Call Communications, 195
Silent Garden, The, 8282
Silicon Valley Community Foundation, 2865
Silicon Valley Independent Living Center, 4059
Silicon Valley Independent Living Center: South County Branch, 4060
Silicone Padding, 243
Silver Towers Camp, 1464
Silvercrest Center for Nursing & Rehabilitation, 6386
Simon & Schuster, 5117, 8049
Simon & Schuster/Touchstone Publishing, 7988
Simon Foundation, 8864
Simon Foundation for Continence, 8373
The Simon Foundation for Continence, 7706
Simon SIO, 1848
Simonton Cancer Center, 8526
Simplicity, 1580
Sinai Hospital of Detroit: Dept. of Opthalmology, 4909
Since Owen, A Parent-to-Parent Guide for Care of the Disabled Child, 5323
Sing Praise Hymnal for the Deaf, 8283
Singeria/Metropolitan Parent Center, 3756
Single Switch Games, 5577
Single Switch Latch and Timer, 5578
Sinus Survival: A Self-help Guide, 8809
Sioux Falls Regional Office, 5826
Siouxland Community Foundation, 2991
Siragusa Foundation, 2978
Siskin Hospital For Physical Rehabilitation, 7148
Siskin Hospital for Physical Rehabilitation, 7389
Sisler McFawn Foundation, 3214
Sister Cities International, 2786
Sivantos Group, 279
Sivantos US, Inc., 279
Six County, Inc., 7107
Sizewise, 685
Sjogren's Syndrome Foundation, 3022, 8865
SJR Rehabilitation Hospital, 7046
Skadden Fellowship Foundation, 3171
Skills Unlimited, 7067
SkiSoft Publishing Corporation, 1872
Skokie Accessible Library Services, 4843
Skokie Public Library, 4843
Skyway, 691
Skyway Machine, 691
SL Start Washington, 6220
Sleep Better! A Guide to Improving Sleep for Children with Special Needs, 5324
SleepSafe Beds, 170
Slicing Aid, 325
SLIDER Bathing System, 153
Slim Armstrong Mounting System, 1581
Slingerland Institute for Literacy, 7204
Slingerland Screening Tests, 2710
Slosburg Family Charitable Trust, 3083
Slosson Educational Publications, 2606
Slosson Educational Publications Inc., 1996, 7960
Small Appliance Receiver, 326
Small Differences, 5460
Small Wonder, 2050
Smart Kitchen/How to Design a Comfortable, Safe & Friendly Workplace, 1955
Smart Leg, 388
SmartScoot Lightweight Travel Scooter, 565
Smile-A-Mile Place, 968, 969, 970, 971, 972, 973, 974, 975, 8603
SMILES, 4350
SMILES: Mankato, 4351
Smith Kettlewell Rehabilitation Engineering Research Center, 9331
Smoke Detector with Strobe, 506
Smooth Mover, 389
SOAR, 1496
SOAR Summer Adventures, 1313, 7936
Social and Emotional Development of Exceptional Students: Handicapped, 2594
Social Development and the Person with Spi na Bifida, 8810
Social Learning Center, 6941
Social Security, 3467, 3518, 3519, 3545, 3595, 3596, 3837, 3896, 3931, 3941, 3958
Social Security Administration, 3406, 3517, 3647, 3725, 3777, 3402, 3520, 3581
Social Security Admission, 3445
Social Security Bulletin, 7776
Social Security Library, 4890
Social Security Online, 5543
Social Security, Medicare, and Government Pensions, 7650
Social Security: Albany Disability Determination, 3757
Social Security: Arkansas Disability Determination Services, 3455
Social Security: Atlanta Disability Determination, 3531
Social Security: Austin Disability Determination, 3879
Social Security: Baltimore Disability Determination, 3621
Social Security: Baton Rouge Disability Determination, 3603

Social Security: Bismarck Disability Determination, 3784
Social Security: Boston Disability Determination, 3628
Social Security: California Disability Determination Services, 3466
Social Security: Carson City Disability Determination, 3701
Social Security: Charleston Disability Determination, 3941
Social Security: Cheyenne Disability Determination, 3958
Social Security: Columbus Disability Determination, 3798
Social Security: Concord Disability Determination, 3714
Social Security: Decatur Disability Determination, 3532
Social Security: Des Moines Disability Determination, 3581
Social Security: Frankfort Disability Determination, 3595
Social Security: Fresno Disability Determination Services, 3467
Social Security: Harrisburg Disability Determination, 3825
Social Security: Hartford Area Office, 3484
Social Security: Helena Disability Determination, 3683
Social Security: Honolulu Disability Determination, 3545
Social Security: Jefferson City Disability Determination, 3672
Social Security: Lincoln Disability Determination, 3692
Social Security: Louisville Disability Determination, 3596
Social Security: Madison Field Office, 3951
Social Security: Maine Disability Determination, 3612
Social Security: Miami Disability Determination, 3518
Social Security: Mobile Disability Determination Services, 3423
Social Security: Oakland Disability Determination Services, 3468
Social Security: Olympia Disability Determination, 3931
Social Security: Orlando Disability Determination, 3519
Social Security: Phoenix Disability Determination Services, 3445
Social Security: Providence Disability Determination, 3837
Social Security: Sacramento Disability Determination Services, 3469
Social Security: Salem Disability Determination, 3812
Social Security: Salt Lake City Disability Determination, 3896
Social Security: San Diego Disability Determination Services, 3470
Social Security: Santa Fe Disability Determination, 3734
Social Security: Springfield Disability Determination, 3565
Social Security: St. Paul Disability Determination, 3660
Social Security: Tampa Disability Determination, 3520
Social Security: Tucson Disability Determination Services, 3446
Social Security: Vermont Disability Determination Services, 3908
Social Security: West Columbia Disability Determination, 3840
Social Security: Wilmington Disability Determination, 3493
Social Skills for Students With Autism Spe ctrum Disorders and Other Developmental Disorders, 2592
Social Studies: Detecting and Correcting Special Needs, 2593
Social Vocational Services, 5935
Socialization Games for Persons with Disabilities, 5264, 5579
Society for Cognitive Rehabilitation, 7887
Society for Disability Studies, 2118
Society for Equal Access: Independent Living Center, 4497
Society for Neuroscience, 7618, 7713, 7755
Society for Post-Acute and Long-Term Care Medicine (AMDA), 936
Society for Progressive Supranuclear Palsy, 8374, 8419, 8846
Society for Rehabilitation, 7108
Society for the Blind, 6660, 9096
Society of Nuclear Medicine and Molecular Imaging, 7745, 7721, 7722
Society's Assets: Elkhorn, 4644
Society's Assets: Kenosha, 4645
Society's Assets: Racine, 4646
Sociopolitical Aspects of Disabilities (2nd Edition), 5382
Sofia University, 937
Soft Touch, 1582, 1583, 1587, 1588, 1589, 1718, 1719, 1720, 1728, 1729, 1740, 1741, 1748, 1749, 1764, 1768, 1770, 1776, 1777, 1778, 1779, 1780, 1781, 1789, 1797, 1798, 1802, 1804
Soft Touch Inc, 1561, 1564, 1565, 1568, 1575
Soft Touch Incorporated, 1775
Soft-Touch Convertible Flotation Mattress, 244
Soft-Touch Gel Flotation Cushion, 245
Softfoot Ergomatta, 649
SoftTouch, 1586, 1791, 1792, 1793, 1794, 1795, 1796
SoftTouch Inc., 1584
SoftTouch Incorporated, 1585
SOLO Literacy Suite, 1822
Solo Scooter, 566
SoloRider Industries, 567
Solutions at Santa Barbara: Transitional Living Center, 6661
Solving Language Difficulties, 2051
Solving the Puzzle of Chronic Fatigue, 8811
Someday's Child, 5461
Somerset Community Action Program, Inc., 6142
Somerset Valley Rehabilitation and Nursing Center, 7044
Something's Wrong with My Child!, 5325
Sometimes I Get All Scribbly, 5326
Sometimes You Just Want to Feel Like a Human Being, 5265
Son Rise: The Miracle Continues, 8812
Son-Rise Program, 6979, 8905
Son-Rise: The Miracle Continues, 5327, 8036, 8991
Songs I Sing at Preschool, 1781
Songs I Sing at Preschool IntelliKeys Over lay, 1582
Sonic Alert, 196
Sonic Alert Bed Shaker, 171
Sonora Area Foundation, 2866
Sonoran Rehabilitation and Care Center, 7216
Sonova USA Inc., 300
Soon Will Come the Light, 8037
Sophie Russell Testamentary Trust Bank Of Hawaii, 2944
Sound & Fury, 5462
Sound Connections for the Adolescent, 8992
Sound Sentences, 1849
Soundings Newsletter, 8316
SourceAmerica, 6214
Sources for Community IL Services, 3997
South Arlington Medical Center: Rehab Care Unit, 6462
South Bay Vocational Center, 5936
South Carolina Assistive Technology Program (SCATP), 2233
South Carolina Assistive Technology Project, 3841
South Carolina Assistive Technology Progra m, 5266
South Carolina Client Assistance Program, 3842
South Carolina Commission for the Blind (SCCB), 3843, 6185
South Carolina Department of Children with Disabilities, 3844
South Carolina Department of Education: Office of Exceptional Children, 2234
South Carolina Department of Employment and Workforce (DEW), 6186
South Carolina Department of Mental Health, 3845
South Carolina Developmental Disabilities Council, 3846
South Carolina Governor's Committee on Employment of the Handicapped, 6187
South Carolina Independent Living Council, 4545
South Carolina State Library, 5000
South Carolina State University, 9211
South Carolina Vocational Rehabilitation Department (SCVRD), 6188
South Central Alabama Mental Health, 5870, 5871
South Central Alabama Mental Health (SCAMHC), 3424
South Central Iowa Center for Independent Living, 4213
South Central Kansas Library System, 4862
South Central Pennsylvania Center for Inde pendence Living, 4530
South Central Technical College (SCTC), 2210
South Central Wisconsin Directory of Servi ces for Older Adults, 2141
South Central Wyoming Healthcare and Rehabilitation, 7427
South Coast Medical Center, 6265, 7226
South Dakota Advocacy Services, 3851
South Dakota Assistive Technology Project: DakotaLink, 4554
South Dakota Department of Aging, 3852
South Dakota Department of Education & Cultural Affairs: Office of Special Education, 2235
South Dakota Department of Health, 3850
South Dakota Department of Human Services: Computer Technology Services, 1647
South Dakota Department of Human Services, 3853, 6189
South Dakota Department of Human Services: Div. of Service to the Blind & Visually Impaired, 6190
South Dakota Department of Labor, 3849
South Dakota Department of Social Services Division of Behavioral Health, 3854
South Dakota Division of Rehabilitation, 3855
South Dakota State Library, 5001
South Dakota State Vocational Rehabilitati on, 6191
South Dakota Workforce Investment Act Training Programs, 6192
South Georgia Regional Library-Valdosta Talking Book Center, 4826
South Louisiana Rehabilitation Hospital, 6346
South Miami Hospital, 6291
South Shore Healthcare, 7343
South Texas Charitable Foundation, 3307
South Texas Lighthouse for the Blind, 7171
South Texas Rehabilitation Hospital, 6463
South Texas Veterans Healthcare System, 5837
Southampton Fresh Air Home, 1298
Southeast Alaska Independent Living, 3981
Southeast Alaska Independent Living: Ketch ikan, 3982
Southeast Alaska Independent Living: Sitka, 3983
Southeast Center for Independent Living, 4309
Southeast Disability & Business Technical Assist., 3521
Southeast Kansas Independent Living (SKIL), 4243
Southeast Kansas Independent Living: Independence, 4244
Southeast Kansas Independent Living: Chanu te, 4245
Southeast Kansas Independent Living: Colum bus, 4246
Southeast Kansas Independent Living: Fredo nia, 4247
Southeast Kansas Independent Living: Hays, 4248
Southeast Kansas Independent Living: Pitts burg, 4249
Southeast Kansas Independent Living: Sedan, 4250
Southeast Kansas Independent Living: Yates Center, 4251

Southeast Ohio Sight Center, 7109
Southeast Wisconsin Directory of Services for Older Adults, 2142
Southeastern Blind Rehabilitation Center, 6507
Southeastern Diabetes Education Services, 966, 8601
Southeastern Michigan Commission for the Blind, 4338
Southeastern Minnesota Center for Independent Living: Red Wing, 4352
Southeastern Minnesota Center for Independent Living: Rochester, 4353
Southeastern Paralyzed Veterans of America, 5688
Southern Adirondack Independent Living, 4464
Southern Adirondack Independent Living Cen ter, 4465
Southern Arizona Association For The Visually Impaired, 6530
Southern Arizona VA Healthcare System, 5646
Southern California Chapter, 8378
Southern California Rehabilitation Service s, 4061
Southern Indiana Center for Independent Living, 4205
Southern Indiana Resource Solutions, 6042
Southern Maryland Center for LIFE, 4292
Southern Nevada Center for Independent Living: North Las Vegas, 4406
Southern Nevada Center for Independent Living: Las Vegas, 4407
Southern New England Rehab Center, 7376
Southern Oregon Rehabilitation Center & Cl inics, 5807
Southern Tier Independence Center, 4466
Southern Worcester County Rehabilitation Inc. D/B/A Life-Skills, Inc., 6980
Southside Virginia Training Center, 7185
Southwest Branch of the International Dyslexia Association, 3735
Southwest Center for Independence, 4078
Southwest Center for Independence: Cortez, 4079
Southwest Center for Independent Living (S CIL), 4383
Southwest Communication Resource, 7047
Southwest Conference On Disability, 1921
Southwest District Independent Living Program, 4133
Southwest Louisiana Independence Center: L ake Charles, 4276
Southwest Louisians Independence Center: Lafayette, 4277
Southwest Medical Center, 6404
Southwestern Center for Independent Living, 4354
Southwestern Commission Area Agency on Agi ng, 7786
Southwestern Idaho Housing Authority, 4154
Southwestern Independent Living Center, 4467
Soyland Access to Independent Living (SAIL), 4185
Soyland Access to Independent Living: Char leston, 4186
Soyland Access to Independent Living: Shel byville, 4187
Soyland Access to Independent Living: Sull ivan, 4188
Spa Area Independent Living Services, 3998
Space Coast Center for Independent Living, 4122, 5267
Space Coast CIL News, 5267
Space-Saver, 390
Spalding Rehab Hospital West Unit, 6692
Spalding Rehabilitation Hospital at Memorial Hospital of Laramie, 6488
Span-America Medical Systems, 232
Spartan Stuttering Laboratory, 938
Spatial Tilt Custom Chair, 223
Spaulding University, 4867
Spec-L Clothing Solutions, 1542
Special Camp For Special Kids, 1041
Special Care Dentistry Association, 8527
Special Care in Dentistry, 8875
Special Children, 8906
Special Children/Special Solutions, 5463
Special Clothes, 405, 407, 408, 416, 1498, 1499, 1500, 1501, 1502, 1503, 1504, 1505, 1507, 1509, 1526, 1543, 1544
Special Clothes Adult Catalogue, 1543
Special Clothes for Children, 5544
Special Clothes for Special Children, 1544
Special Edge, 2339
Special EDitions, 4727
Special Education and Rehab Services, 8919
Special Education for Today, 2596
Special Education Report, 2340, 5062
Special Education Today, 2595
Special Format Books for Children and Youth Ages 3-19, 5063
Special Hockey International (SHI), 8884
Special Kids Need Special Parents: A Resou rce for Parents of Children With Special Needs, 5328
Special Needs Advocacy Resource Book, 2711
Special Needs Center/Phoenix Public Library, 4755
Special Needs Project, 2175, 414, 2000, 2175, 2369, 2422, 2483, 5301, 5323, 6249, 7630
Special Needs Trust Handbook, 5268
Special Olympics, 8457
Special Olympics International, 8458, 8412
Special Parent, Special Child, 5329
Special Services Division: Indiana State Library, 4852
Special Services Summer Day Camp, 1299
Special Siblings: Growing Up With Someone with A Disability, 5269
Special Technologies Alternative Resources, 9248, 9326
Special Tree Rehabilitation System, 7000
Special U, 4930
Specialty Care Shoppe, 1545
Specialty Hospital, 6305, 7255
SpectraLift, 391
Spectrum Aquatics, 392, 393
Spectrum Products, 392
Spectrum Products Catalog, 393
Speech Adjust-A-Tone Basic, 197
Speech and the Hearing-Impaired Child, 2597
Speech Bin, 2052, 2712, 2044, 2045, 2690, 2706, 5581, 8042, 8969, 8992, 8996
Speech Bin-Abilitations, 8977, 8985, 8993
Speech Pathways, 9025
Speech-Language Delights, 2053
Speech-Language Pathology and Audiology: An Introduction, 2598
Spell of Words, 2054
Spellbound, 2055
Spelling Dictionary, 2056
Spelling Rules, 1850
Spenco Medical Group, 246, 243, 246
Spider Network Systems, 120
SPIN Early Childhood Care & Education Cntr, 6690
Spina Bifida and Hydrocephalus Association of Canada, 8529
Spina Bifida Association, 8528
Spina Bifida Association of America, 5281, 5312, 5574, 8713, 8718, 8726, 8733, 8738, 8739, 8744, 8773, 8777, 8779, 8796, 8799, 8801, 8806, 8808, 8810, 8813, 8818, 8819, 8830, 8834, 8878
Spina Bifida Program of Children's Nationa l Medical Center, 6723
SPINabilities: A Young Person's Guide to Spina Bifida, 8806
Spinal Cord Dysfunction, 2599
Spinal Cord Injury Center, 2752
Spinal Network: The Total Wheelchair Reso urce Book, 507
Spine, 8853
Spinner Knobs, 121
Spirit Magazine, 8412
Spirit of Change Magazine, 7746, 7746
The Spiritual Art of Raising Children with Disabilities, 5363
Spiritually Able: A Parents Guide to Teach ing Faith To Children with Special Needs, 5362
Spokane Center for Independent Living, 4627
Spokane VA Medical Center, 5852
SPOKES Unlimited, 4508, 9197
Sport Science Review: Adapted Physical Activity, 8402
Sportaid, 455
Sports n' Spokes Magazine, 5585
Sportster 10, 568
Spring Dell Center, 8171, 8317
Spring Dell Center Newsletter, 8317
Springboard Consulting, 1906
Springer Publishing, 2365, 2411, 2494, 2570, 2589, 7966, 8955
Springer Publishing Company, 2366, 2372, 2419, 2455, 2551, 2559, 2573, 2576, 2631, 2641, 5119, 5225, 5251, 5252, 5253, 5304, 7637, 7684, 7691, 7711, 7714, 7719, 7720, 8023, 8028, 8982
Springfield Center for Independent Living, 4189
Sproul Ranch, Inc., 8197
Square D Foundation, 2979
Squirrel Hollow Summer Camp, 1101, 7938
SS-Access Single Switch Interface for PC's with MS-DOS, 1579
St Frances Cabrini Hospital, 6347
St George's Society of New York, 3172
St Lukes Roosevelt, 4448
St Martin's Griffin, 8975
St. Anne's Nursing Center, 6292
St. Anthony Hospital, 6406
St. Anthony Hospital: Rehabilitation Unit, 6406
St. Anthony Memorial Hospital: Rehab Unit, 6333
St. Anthony's Hospital, 6293, 7249
St. Anthony's Rehabilitation Hospital, 6294
St. Augustine Rainbow Camp, 1343
St. Camillus Health and Rehabilitation Cen ter, 7344
St. Catherine's Hospital, 6486
St. Catherine's Rehabilitation Hospital and Villa Maria Nursing Center, 6295
St. Clair County Library Special Technologies Alternative Resources (S.T.A.R.), 4920
St. Cloud VA Medical Center, 5739
St. Coletta's of Illinois, Inc., 6015
St. David s Medical Center, 6464
St. David's Rehabilitation Center, 6464
St. Frances Cabrini Hospital: Rehab Unit, 6347
St. Francis Camp On The Lake, 1198
St. Francis Health Care Centre, 6398
St. Francis Rehabilitation Hospital, 7110
St. George Care and Rehabilitation Center, 7394
St. John Hospital: North Shore, 6361
St. John of God Community Services Vocational Rehabilitation, 6143
St. John Valley Associates, 7888
St. John's Nursing Center, 6296
St. John's Pleasant Valley Hospital Neuro Care Unit, 6662
St. John's Regional Medica Center- Industrial Therapy Center, 6663
St. Joseph Health System, 6266
St. Joseph Hospital, 6487
St. Joseph Hospital and Medical Center, 6240
St. Joseph Hospital Rehabilitation, 6373
St. Joseph Hospital Rehabilitation Center, 4853
St. Joseph Rehabilitation Center, 6266
St. Joseph Rehabilitation Hospital and Outpatient Center, 6382
St. Joseph's Professional Center, 8341
St. Jude Brain Injury Network, 6267
St. Jude Hospital, 6267
St. Jude Medical Center, 6268
St. Lawrence Rehabilitation Center, 7329
St. Louis Regional Office, 5747
St. Louis Society for the Blind and Visually Impaired, 7018
St. Louis VA Medical Center, 5748
St. Mark's Hospital, 7395
St. Martin's Griffin (Macmillan Publishers), 5290
St. Mary Medical Center, 6269
St. Mary's Medical Center: RehabCare Center, 6438
St. Mary's Regional Rehabilitation Center, 6365
St. Mary's RehabCare Center, 7149
St. Patrick Hospital: Rehab Unit, 6348
St. Patrick RehabCare Unit, 6932
St. Paul Abilities Network, 939
St. Paul Press, 5291
St. Paul Regional Office, 5740
St. Petersburg Regional Office, 5682

St. Rita's Medical Center Rehabilitation Services, 6399
St. Vincent Hospital and Health Center, 6367
Stae Agency, 3927
StairClimber, 627
StairLIFT SC & SL, 394
Stamford Hospital, 7234
Stand-Up Wheelchairs, 692
Standard 3-in-1 Commode, 280
Standard Wheelchair, 693
Standing Aid Frame with Rear Entry, 628
Standing on My Own Two Feet, 9249
Stanford Health Care, 2753
Stanley W Metcalf Foundation, 3173
STAR, 9326, 3650
Star Bright Books, 7973
Star Center, 1648
Starbridge, 940
Stark Community Foundation, 3215
Starkey Hearing Foundation, 301, 8172
Start-to-Finish Library, 1851
Start-to-Finish Literacy Starters, 1852
Starting and Sustaining Genetic Support Gr oups, 5383
Starting Over, 2057
Starting Points, 9250
State Agency for the Blind and Visually Impaired, 3758
State Department of Wyoming, 3962
State Division of Vocational Rehabilitation, 6334
State Education Agency Rural Representative, 3759
State Library of Kansas, 4863
State Library of Louisiana: Services for the Blind and Physically Handicapped, 4873
State Library of Ohio: Talking Book Program, 4985
State Mental Health Representative for Children and Youth, 3760
State of Alabama Independent Living/Homebo und Service (SAIL), 3971
State of Alaska, 2179, 4748
State of Connecticut Agency, 2184
State of Illinois Center, 3560
State Of Iowa, 3577, 4855, 4857
State of Maine, 3610
State of Massachusetts, 6079
State of Michigan, 3040
State of Michigan Workers' Compensation Agency, 3648
State of Nebraska, 3691
State of Nevada Client Assistance Program, 3702
State of Washington, 3938
State of West Virginia, 3939
State Office Building, 3616
State Office of Wisconsin, 3954
State Planning Council on Developmental Disabilities, 3546
State University of New York, 2787
State University of New York Health Sciences Center, 4969
State University of New York Press, 2428, 2580, 2586
State Workforce Board, 6066
Staten Island Center for Independent Living, Inc., 4468
Statesman Health and Rehabilitation Center, 7370
Statewide Independent Living Council of Ge orgia, 4134
Statewide Information at Texas School for the Deaf, 3880
Staunton Farm Foundation, 3244
Staunton Public Library Talking Book Center, 5026
Steady Write, 533
Steel Food Bumper, 327
Steelcase Foundation, 3057
Steele, 508
SteeleVest, 508
Steering Device, 122
Steering Wheel Devices, 123
Stella B Gross Charitable Trust C/O Bank of The West Trust Department, 2867
Step-by-Step Communicator, 198
Step-By-Step Guide to Personal Management for Blind Persons, 9251
Stepping Stones Inc. - Allyn Campus, 1344
Stepping Stones Inc. - Given Campus, 1332
Stepping Stones: Camp Allyn, 1344
Steps to Independence: Teaching Everyday S kills to Children with Special Needs, 8813
Steps to Success: Scope & Sequence for Ski ll Development, 2600
Sterling Ranch, 3992
Sterling Ranch: Residence for Special Women, 3992
Sterling-Turner Foundation, 3308
Stern Center for Language and Learning, 8936
The Steve Fund, 948
Stevens Publishing Corporation, 2259
Stewardship Foundation, 3332
Stewart Huston Charitable Trust, 3245
Stewart Rehabilitation Center: McKay Dee Hospital, 6473
Stick Canes, 629
Stickybear Early Learning Activities, 1782
Stickybear Kindergarden Activities, 1783
Stickybear Math I Deluxe, 1706
Stickybear Math II Deluxe, 1707
Stickybear Math Splash, 1708
Stickybear Math Word Problems, 1709
Stickybear Money, 1710
Stickybear Numbers Deluxe, 1711
Stickybear Reading Comprehension, 1853
Stickybear Reading Fun Park, 1854
Stickybear Reading Room Deluxe, 1855
Stickybear Science Fair Light, 1784
Stickybear Spelling, 1856
Stickybear Town Builder, 1785
Stickybear Typing, 1786, 1868
Still Me, 8403
STIX Diabetes Programs, 1482, 8647
Stocker Foundation, 3216
Stone-Hayes Center for Independent Living, 4190
Stonewall Community Foundation, 3174
Stop-Leak Gel Flotation Mattress, 247
Store @ HDSC Product Catalog, 456
Storybook Maker Deluxe, 1787
Stout Vocational Rehab Institute, 2476, 2579, 2643
Stove Knob Turner, 328
Straits Area Services, Inc., 6093
Strategies for Teaching Learners with Special Needs, 2601
Strategies for Teaching Students with Learning and Behavior Problems, 2602
Strategies for Working with Families of Young Children with Disabilities, 5330
Strawberry Lane Nursing & Rehabilitation Center, 7425
Streator Unlimited, 6863
Strength for the Journey, 1365, 8650
Stretch-View Wide-View Rectangular Illuminated Magnifier, 604
Strides Magazine, 8413
Strive Physical Therapy Centers, 6775
Strobe Light Signalers, 509
Stroke Connection Magazine, 8118, 8414
Stroke Smart Magazine, 8122
Stroke Sourcebook, 8814
Stroke Sourcebook, 2nd Edition, 8815
Structural Integration: The Journal of the Rolf Institute, 2305
Stryker, 248, 677
Student Advocate, 9332
Student Disability Services (SDS), 941
Student Guide, 3378
Student Independent Living Experience Massachusetts Hospital School, 4310
Student Teaching Guide for Blind and Visually Impaired College Students, 9252
Students with Acquired Brain Injury: The School's Response, 2603
Students with Disabilities Office, 1649
Students with Mild Disabilities in the Secondary School, 2604
Studio 49 Catalog, 2058
Study Power Workbook: Exercises in Study - Skills to Improve Your Learning and Your Grades, 5354
Stuttering, 8816
Stuttering & Your Child: Help For Parents, 9013
Stuttering Foundation Newsletter, 9014
Stuttering Foundation of America, 8937, 8989, 9013, 9014
Stuttering Severity Instrument for Children and Adults, 2713
Sub-Acute Saratoga Hospital, 6664
Substance Abuse and Mental Health Services Administration (SAMHSA), 3407
Succeeding With Interventions For Asperger Syndrome Adolescents, 8817
Successful Job Accommodation Strategies, 6297
Successful Job Search Strategies for the D isabled: Understanding the ADA, 8038
Successful Models of Community Long Term Care Services for the Elderly, 7651
Suffolk Cooperative Library System: Long Island Talking Book Library, 4970
Suffolk Independent Living Organization (SILO), 4469
Summaries of Legal Precedents & Law Review, 4728
Summer Camp for Children with Muscular Dystrophy, 8651
Summer Office, 1248
Summer@Carroll, 1181, 7939
Summit Camp, 1300, 7940
Summit Independent Living Center: Kalipsell, 4392
Summit Independent Living Center: Hamilton, 4393
Summit Independent Living Center: Missoula, 4394
Summit Independent Living Center: Ronan, 4395
Summit Ridge Center, 7045
Summit Ridge Center Genesis Eldercare, 7330
Sumner Regional Medical Center, 6439
Sun Trust Bank Atlanta, 2930, 2933, 2938
Sun-Mate Seat Cushions, 249
Sunbridge Care and Rehabilitation, 6776
Sunburst Projects, 8530
Sunburst Projects United States Headquarters, 1020, 8530, 8604
Suncoast Center for Independent Living, Inc., 4123
Sundial Special Vacations, 5618
Sunnyhill Adventures, 1226, 7941
Sunnyhill, Inc., 4384
Sunnyside Nursing Center, 6270
Sunrise Medical, 557, 660, 680
Sunset View Castle Nursing Homes Castle Nursing Homes, 7365
Sunshine Campus, 1301
Sunshine Services, 6896
SunTrust Bank, Atlanta Foundation, 2938
SUNY Buffalo, School of Architecture & Planning, 5598
Super Challenger, 1788
Super Grade IV Hand Controls, 124
Super Stretch Socks, 1546
Superarm Lift for Vans, 395
Superintendent of Public Instruction: Special Education Section, 2243
Superior Alliance for Independent Living (SAIL), 4339
Support Plus, 1547
Support Works, 8907
A Supported Employment Workbook: Individua l Profiling and Job Matching, 5080
Supporting and Strengthening Families, 2605
Supporting Success for Children with Heari ng Loss, 2176
Surdna Foundation, 3175
Suregrip Bathtub Rail, 156
SureHands Lift & Care Systems, 396
Surf Chair, 694
Survey of Direct Labor Workers Who Are Blind & Employed by NIB, 9253
Survivors Art Foundation, 62
Suttle Lake Camp, 1366, 8652

SVC Corporation, 1674
SWAB Steering Wheel, 119
Swedish Covenant Hospital Rehabilitation Services, 6864
Swindells Charitable Foundation Trust, 2895
Switch Basics, 1789
Switch Basics IntelliKeys Overlay, 1583
Switch Interface Pro 5.0, 1790
Sycamore Rehabilitation Services, 6043
Symptomatic Chiari Malformation, 8818
Synapse Adaptive, 406
Synergos Neurological Center: Hayward, 6665
Synergos Neurological Center: Mission Hills, 6666
Syracuse Community-Referenced Curriculum Guide for Students with Disabilties, 2059
Syracuse University, 788, 4955
Syracuse University, School of Education, 5179
Syracuse VA Medical Center, 5781
System 2000/Versa, 1673
Systems 2000, 569
Systems Unlimited/LIFE Skills, 5469

T

T AF KI D, 5782
T HI Brentwood, 6815
T J Publishers, 2015, 4674
T J Publishers, Distributor, 1966
TAC Enterprises, 7111
Tacoma Area Coalition of Individuals with Disabilities, 4628
Taconic Resources for Independence, 4470
Tactile Braille Signs, 511
Tactile Checkers Set, 5580
Tactile Thermostat, 512
Take a Chance, 5581
Taking Charge, 8819
Taking Charge of ADHD Complete Authoritative Guide for Parents, 8039
Taking Control of Your Diabetes (TCOYD), 8531
Taking Part: Introducing Social Skills to Young Children, 2715
Talisman Summer Camp, 1314, 7942, 8949
Talk to Me, 9254
Talk to Me II, 9255
Talkable Tales, 8993
Talking Bathroom Scale, 157
Talking Book & Braille Services Oregon State Library, 4991
Talking Book and Braille Service, 4943, 5535
Talking Book Center Brunswick-Glynn County Regional Library, 4827
Talking Book Department, Parkersburg and Wood County Public Library, 5039
Talking Book Library at Worcester Public Library, 4905
Talking Book Program, 5009
Talking Book Program/Texas State Library, 5009
Talking Book Service: Mantatee County Central Library, 4807
Talking Books & Reading Disabilities, 9256
Talking Books for People with Physical Dis abilities, 9257
Talking Books Library for the Blind and Physically Handicapped, 4808
Talking Books Plus, 4998
Talking Books Service Evansville Vanderburgh County Public Library, 4854
Talking Books Topics, 9334
Talking Books/Homebound Services, 4809
Talking Calculators, 201
Talking Digital Thermometer, 281
Talking Electronic Organizers, 534
Talking Food Cans, 329
Talking Screen, 1687
Talking Thermometers, 282
Talking Watches, 202
TalkTrac Wearable Communicator, 200
Tampa Bay Academy, 6777
Tampa General Rehabilitation Center, 6298, 6778
Tampa Lighthouse for the Blind, 6779
Tanager Place, 1145, 8619, 8632
TapGear, 125
Taping for the Blind, 9353
Tarjan Center at UCLA, 47
TASH, 942, 1896, 4729, 7659
TASH Connections, 4729
TASK Team of Advocates for Special Kids, 1650
Taylor & Francis, 15, 16, 2445, 2489, 2553, 7695, 7697, 7965, 8954
Taylor & Francis Group, 2364, 8987
Taylor & Francis Group, LLC, 7658
Taylor & Francis Online, 5374
Taylor Publishing Company, 7957
Tazewell County Resource Center, 6866
TBC Focus, 9333
TCRC Sight Center, 6865
TDI National Directory & Resource Guide: Blue Book, 8284
TEACCH, 8070
TEACCH Autism Program, 7889
Teach Me Phonemics Blends Overlay CD, 1584
Teach Me Phonemics Medial Overlay CD, 1585
Teach Me Phonemics Overlay Series Bundle, 1586
Teach Me Phonemics Series Bundle, 1791
Teach Me Phonemics Super Bundle, 1792
Teach Me Phonemics: Blends, 1793
Teach Me Phonemics: Final, 1794
Teach Me Phonemics: Initial, 1795
Teach Me Phonemics: Medial, 1796
Teach Me to Talk, 1797
Teach Me to Talk Overlay CD, 1587
Teach Me to Talk: USB-Overlay CD, 1588
Teacher Education Division (TED), 2119
Teacher of Students with Visual Impairment s, 2754
Teacher's Guide to Including Students with Disabilities in Regular Physical Education, 2607
A Teacher's Guide to Isovaleric Acidemia, 2346
A Teacher's Guide to Methylmalonic Acidemia, 2347
A Teacher's Guide to PKU, 2348
Teachers Institute for Special Education, 1757
Teachers College Press, 2420, 2429, 2430, 2512, 2517, 2566, 2637, 7994, 9194
Teachers Institute for Special Education, 1755, 1756
Teachers Working Together, 2608
Teachig Students with Special Needs in Inclusive Classrooms, 2609
Teaching Adults with Learning Disabilities, 2610
Teaching and Mainstreaming Autistic Children, 8041, 8995
Teaching Asperger's Students Social Skills Through Acting, 63
Teaching Basic Guitar Skills to Special Learners, 64
Teaching Children With Autism in the General Classroom, 2611
Teaching Children with Autism: Strategies for Initiating Positive Interactions, 8040, 8994
Teaching Children with Down Syndrome about Their Bodies, Boundaries, and Sexuality, 5346
Teaching Disturbed and Disturbing Students: An Integrative Approach, 2612
Teaching Every Child Every Day: Integrated Learning in Diverse Classrooms, 2613
Teaching Exceptional Children (TEC), 2306
Teaching Individuals with Physical and Multiple Disabilities, 2060
Teaching Infants and Preschoolers with Handicaps, 2614
Teaching Language-Disabled Children: A Communication/Games Intervention, 2615
Teaching Learners with Mild Disabilities: Integrating Research and Practice, 2616
Teaching Mathematics to Students with Learning Disabilities, 2617
Teaching Mildly and Moderately Handicapped Students, 2618
Teaching of Reading: A Continuum from Kindergarten through College, The, 2716
Teaching Orientation and Mobility in the Schools: An Instructor's Companion, 9258
Teaching Reading to Children with Down Syndrome: A Guide for Parents and Teachers, 2619
Teaching Reading to Disabled and Handicapped Learners, 2620
Teaching Reading to Handicapped Children, 2621
Teaching Self-Determination to Students with Disabilities, 2622
Teaching Special Students in Mainstream, 2143
Teaching Students Ways to Remember, 2061
Teaching Students with Learning and Behavi or Problems, 2624
Teaching Students with Learning Problems, 2623
Teaching Students with Mild and Moderate Learning Problems, 2625
Teaching Students with Moderate/Severe Disabilities, Including Autism, 2626
Teaching Students with Special Needs in Inclusive Settings, 2627
Teaching Test-Taking Skills: Helping Students Show What They Know, 2062
Teaching the Bilingual Special Education Student, 2629
Teaching the Learning Disabled Adolescent: Strategies and Methods, 2630
Teaching Visually Impaired Children, 9259
Teaching Young Children to Read, 2628
Tech Connection, 1651
Tech-Able, 1652
Techniques for Aphasia Rehab: (TARGET) Generating Effective Treatment, 8042, 8996
Technologists, Inc., 413
Technology Access Center of Tucson, 1653
Technology and Handicapped People, 2631
Technology Assistance for Special Consumers, 1654, 4747
Technology for the Disabled, 5464
Teen Tunes Plus, 1798
Teen Tunes Plus IntelliKeys Overlay, 1589
Teenagers with ADD, 8043
Teens & Asthma, 8877
Teichert Foundation, 2868
Telecommunications for the Deaf, 8243, 8284
Telecommunications for the Deaf (TDI), 8236
Telecommunications for the Deaf and Hard o f Hearing, 8173
Teleflex Foundation, 3246
Television Remote Controls with Large Numbers, 535
Temple Community Hospital, 6667
Temple University, 1644, 4525
Temple University Institute on Disabilities, 5537
Temporary Assistance for Needy Families (TANF), 5902
Ten Things I Learned from Bill Porter, 8820
Tenco Industries, 6897
Tenet South Florida, 6287
Tennessee Assistive Technology Projects, 3859
Tennessee Client Assistance Program, 3860
Tennessee Commission on Aging and Disability, 3861
Tennessee Council on Developmental Disabilities, 3862
Tennessee Council on Developmental Disabilities, 8859
Tennessee Department Human Services: Vocational Rehabilitation Services, 6193
Tennessee Department of Children with Disabilities, 3863
Tennessee Department of Education, 2236
Tennessee Department of Labor and Workforc e Development, 6194
Tennessee Department of Mental Health, 3864
Tennessee Division of Rehabilitation, 3865
Tennessee Hospital Association, 7619
Tennessee Human Rights Commission, 6195
Tennessee Jaycees and Tennessee Jaycee Foundation, 1415
Tennessee Library for the Blind and Physically Handicapped, 5002
Tennessee Protection and Advocacy, 3860
Tennessee State Library Archives, 5002
Tennessee Technology Access Program (TTAP), 4560
TERI, 5270
TERRA-JET USA, 570
Terra-Jet: Utility Vehicle, 570
Terrier Tricycle, 571

Terry-Wash Mitt: Medium Size, 158
Test Critiques: Volumes I-X, 2717
Test of Early Reading Ability Deaf or Hard of Hearing, 2718
Test of Language Development: Primary, 2719
Test of Mathematical Abilities, 2nd Editio n, 2720
Test of Nonverbal Intelligence, 3rd Editio n, 2721
Test of Phonological Awareness, 2722
Test of Written Spelling, 3rd Edition, 2723
TESTS, 2606
Tethering Cord, 8878
Texas Advocates Supporting Kids with Disabilities, 3881
Texas Association of Retinitis Pigmentosa, 9324
Texas Bleeding Disorders Camp Foundation, 1424
Texas Commission for the Blind, 3882
Texas Commission for the Deaf and Hard of Hearing, 3883
Texas Council for Developmental Disabilities, 3884
Texas Department of Assistive and Rehabili tative Services, 4581
Texas Department of Human Services, 3885
Texas Department on Aging, 3886
Texas Education Agency, 2237
Texas Education Agency: Special Education Unit, 2238
Texas Federation of Families for Children's Mental Health, 3887
Texas Governor's Committee on People with Disabilities, 3888
Texas Health and Human Services (HHS), 3889
Texas League City Campus, 7159
Texas Lions Camp, 1451, 8205, 8654, 9120
Texas NeuroRehab Center, 6465
Texas Respite Resource Network, 3890
Texas School of the Deaf, 2239
Texas Scottish Rite Hospital for Children, 2724
Texas Specialty Hospital at Dallas, 6466, 7172
Texas Speech-Language-Hearing Association, 8938, 9009
Texas Technology Access Project, 3891
Texas UAP for Developmental Disabilities, 3892
Texas Victoria Campus, 7158
Texas Workers Compensation Commission, 3893
Texas Workforce Commission (TWC), 6198
Texas Workforce Commission: Vocational Rehabilitation Services, 6199
Textbook Catalog, 9260
Textbooks and the Student Who Can't Read Them: A Guide for Teaching Content, 2632
That All May Worship: An Interfaith Welcom e to People with Disabilities, 5271
That's My Child, 5331
Theatre Without Limits, 66
Theoretical Issues in Sign Language Research, 8285
Therapeutic Activities with Persons Disabled by Alzheimer's Disease, 7652
Therapeutic Nursery Program, 2677
Therapeutic Touch International Association (TTIA), 949
Therapro, Inc., 148, 158, 252, 254, 255, 257, 277, 314, 318, 321, 322, 330, 331, 334, 464, 474, 491, 492, 496, 513, 526, 585, 2019
Therapy Putty, 513
Therapy Shoppe, 2063
There are Tyrannosaurs Trying on Pants in My Bedroom, 1799
There's a Hearing Impaired Child in My Class, 2636
They Don't Come with Manuals, 5333
They're Just Kids, 5334
Thibodaux Regional Medical Center, 6349
Thick-n-Easy, 330
Thigh-Hi Nylon Stockings, 1549
Thinking Differently: An Inspiring Guide for Parents of Children with Learning Disabilities, 5347
Thinklabs One Stethoscope, 283
Third Line Press, 5235
Thoele Manufacturing, 494
Thomas Nelson, 7661
Thoms Rehabilitation Hospital, 7078, 7078, 7996
Three Billy Goats Gruff, 1800
Three Little Pigs, 1801
Three R's for Special Education: Rights, Resources, Results, 5465
Three Rivers Center for Independent Living: New Castle, 4531
Three Rivers Center for Independent Livi ng: Washington, 4532
Three Rivers Center for Independent Living, 4214, 4533
Three Rivers Health Care, 6366
Three Rivers Independent Living Center, 4252
Three Rivers Independent Living Center: Clay, 4253
Three Rivers Independent Living Center: Ma nhattan, 4254
Three Rivers Independent Living Center: Se neca, 4255
Three Rivers Independent Living Center: To peka, 4256
Three Rivers News, 9261
Three Rivers Press, 7976
Three Rivers Press/Crown Publishing-Random House, 9
Threshold Center For Autism, 6736
Thresholds, 950, 6024
Through the Looking Glass, 4062, 4728, 5207, 5303, 5311, 5319, 5338, 5344, 5400, 5401, 7986, 8234, 9135, 9136, 9173
Thumb Industries, 7001
Thumbs Up Cup, 331
Thyroid Disorders Sourcebook, 8821
Thyssen Krupp Access Solutions, 397, 397
Tic Tac Toe, 5582
Tidewater Center for Technology Access Special Education Annex, 1655
TIDI Products, LLC, 630
Tilt-N-Table, 650
Tim's Trim, 126
Timber Pointe Outdoor Center, 1125
Timber Ridge Ranch NeuroRestorative Services, 6539
Timberland Opportunities Association, 7205
Timbertop Camp for Youth with Learning Dis abilities, 1491, 7943
Timex Easy Reader, 605
Tinnitus Today, 8301
Tisch Foundation, 3177
Title II & III Regulation Amendment Regarding Detectable Warnings, 4730
Title II Complaint Form, 4731
Title II Highlights, 4732
Title III Technical Assistance Manual and Supplement, 4733
TJ Publishers, 2023, 2474, 8208, 8210, 8215, 8216, 8235, 8242, 8271, 8277, 8279, 9137
TJX Companies, 3036
TJX Foundation, 3036
TLC Speech-Language/Occupational Therapy Camps, 2714, 6078, 6951
TLL Temple Foundation, 3309
TMX Tricycle, 707
To a Different Drumbeat, 5335
To Live with Grace and Dignity, 5273
To Love this Life: Quotations by Helen Keller, 9262
To Teach a Dyslexic, 2064
Tobii Dynavox, 179
Togus VA Medical Center, 5718
Tohatchi Area of Opportunity & Services, 6152
Toledo Community Foundation, 3217
Toll-Free Information Line, 8908
Tom Snyder Productions, 1716, 1825
Tomah VA Medical Center, 5860
Tomorrow's Promise: Language Arts, 1857
Tomorrow's Promise: Mathematics, 1712
Tomorrow's Promise: Reading, 1858
Tomorrow's Promise: Spelling, 1859
Tompkins County Office for the Aging, 7787
Tools for Students, 5466
Tools for Transition, 2065
Topeka & Shawnee County Public Library Talking Books Service, 4864
Topeka Independent Living Resource Center, 4257
Topics in Early Childhood Special Education, 2341
Topics in Spinal Cord Injury Rehabilitatio n, 8406
Torah Alliance of Families of Kids with Disabilities, 5782
Total Living Center, 4424
Touch of Nature Environmental Center, 1115
Touch the Baby: Blind & Visually Impaired Children As Patients, 9263
Touch-Dots, 536
Touch/Ability Connects People with Disabilities & Alternative Health Care Pract., 5274
TouchCorders, 1802
Touchdown Keytop/Keyfront Kits, 1605
Touchstone Neurorecovery Center, 6467
TouchWindow Touch Screen, 1803
Tourette Association of America, 7893
Tourette Association of America National E ducation Conference, 1922
Tourette Syndrome Association, 8876
Tourette Syndrome Association Children's Newsletter, 8879
Tourette Syndrome Association of Connecticut (TSA), 8653
Tourette Syndrome: The Facts, 8822
Tourette's Syndrome: Finding Answers and Getting Help, 8823
Tourette's Syndrome: Tics, Obsessions, Com pulsions: Developmental Psychopathology, 8824
Touro Rehabilitation Center - LCMC (Louisiana Children's Medical Center), 6935
TOVA, 1823
Toward Effective Public School Program for Deaf Students, 2637
Toward Independence, 4734
Toyei Industries, 6531
Trace Research and Development Center, 4891
Trail's Edge Camp, 1199
Training Resource Network, 5390
Training, Resource & Assistive-Technology, 6936
Trans Health Incorporated, 6388
Transaction Publishers, 7669
Transfer Bench, 284
Transfer Bench with Back, 224
Transfer Tub Bench, 159
Transition Activity Calendar for Students with Visual Impairments, 9264
Transition to College for Students with Visual Impairments: Report, 9265
Transitional Hospitals Corporation, 6799
Transitional Learning Center at Gavelston and Lubbock, 7173
Transportation Equipment for People with Disabilities, 127
Transylvania Vocational Services (TVS), 6164
Travelers Aid International, 5600
Treating Adults with Physical Disabilities : Access and Communication, 2638
Treating Cerebral Palsy for Clinicians by Clinicians, 2639
Treating Disordered Speech Motor Control, 2640
Treating Epilepsy Naturally: A Guide to Al ternative and Adjunct Therapies, 8825
Treating Families of Brain Injury Survivors, 2641
The Treatment and Learning Centers, 1167
Treatment Review, 2342
Tree of Life Publications, 8393
Treemont Nursing And Rehabilitation Center, 7174
Trekker 40, 572
Tri-County Center for Independent Living, 4385
Tri-County Independent Living Center, 4063, 4591, 5938
Tri-County Patriots for Independent Living, 4534
Tri-Grip Bathtub Rail, 160
Tri-Lo's, 573
Tri-State Resource and Advocacy Corporation, 4561
TRIAID, 571, 573, 700, 707
Triangle Community Foundation, 3189
Triangle J Council of Governments Area Agency on Aging, 7788
Triangle Y Ranch YMCA, 7944
Trinity Health Foundation, 6860
Trips Inc., 5620

Triumph 3000/4000, 574
Triumph Scooter, 575
TRU-Mold Shoes, 1548
True Friends, 1215, 1203, 1204, 1205, 8562, 8566
Truman Medical Center Low Vision Rehabilitation Program, 7019
Truman Neurological Center, 7020
Trumbull Park, 6867
Trunks, 1550
TS Micro Tech, 1660
TSA CT Kid's Summer Event, 8653
TSA Newsletter, 8876
TTYs: Telephone Device for the Deaf, 199
Tub Slide Shower Chair, 161
Tufts Medical Center, 6975
Tulsa City-County Library System: Outreach Services, 4988
Tulsa City: County Library System, 4988
Tunnell Center for Rehab, 6669
Tuomey Healthcare System, 7377
Turn Signal Cross-Over, 128
Turnkey Computer Systems for the Visually, Physically, and Hearing Impaired, 1688
Turtle Teasers, 1804
Tuscaloosa VA Medical Center, 5640
Tuscon Administrative Office, 6518
TV & VCR Remote, 510
Twin Lakes Camp, 8383, 8656
Twin-Rest Seat Cushion & Glamour Pillow, 250
Twitch and Shout, 5467
21st Century Scientific, Inc. - Bounder Power Wheelchair, 657

U

U CL A Medical Center, 6271
U S Department of Education/ NI DR R, 6315
U S Department of Education, 8887
U S Department of Health and Human Services, 3493
U S Department of Justice, 4730, 4733
U S Social Security Administration, 4890
U-Control III, 1590
U-Step Walking Stabilizer: Walker, 631
U.S. Department of Justice, 5087
U.S. Department of Justice, Civil Rights Division, 5090, 5091, 5093, 5476
U.S. Department of Veteran Affairs, 5637, 5643, 6507
UAB Eye Care, 6508
UAB Spain Rehabilitation Center, 2756, 7210
UCLA Medical Center: Department of Anesthesiology, Acute Pain Services, 6271
UCP Huntsville, 4747
UCP Washington Wire, 4735
Ukiah Valley Association for Habilitation, 6670
The Ultimate Guide to Sex and Disability, 5272
Ultrasonic Imaging, 7748
Ultratec, 302
Umpqua Valley Disabilities Network, 4509
UN Printing, 9267
Unbound, 7622
Uncommon Fathers, 5336
Undercounter Lid Opener, 332
Understanding & Controlling Stuttering: A Comprehensive New Approach Based on the Valsa Hyp, 8997
Understanding ADHD, 8089
Understanding and Accommodating Physical Disabilities: Desk Reference, 5276
Understanding and Teaching Emotionally Disturbed Children & Adolescents, 2642
Understanding Asthma, 8826
Understanding Asthma: The Blueprint for Breathing, 8827
Understanding Attention Deficit Disorder, 8090
Understanding Autism, 8091, 9020
Understanding Cystic Fibrosis, 8828
Understanding Down Syndrome: An Introduction for Parents, 8044
Understanding Multiple Sclerosis, 8829
Underwood Books, 7958
Underwood-Miller, 8048
Uni-Turner, 333
Unicorn Keyboards, 1671
Union Pacific Foundation, 3084
Unisex Low Vision Watch, 606
United Access, 129
United Art and Education, 2066
United Brachial Plexus Network, Inc., 8532
United Cerebral Palsy, 2122, 7894, 4735
United Cerebral Palsy Association, 3486
United Cerebral Palsy Association New York, 8580
United Cerebral Palsy Associations of New Jersey, 6145
United Cerebral Palsy Associations of New Jersey, 3724
United Cerebral Palsy Of Delaware, 1072
United Cerebral Palsy of Texas, 3894
United Disability Services, 33, 7726
United Foundation for Disabled Archers, 8460
United Methodist Camp Tekoa, 1312, 8195
United Methodist Church, 8183
United Methodist Church: Eastern Pennsylvania, 1390
United Methodist Publishing House, 7731
United Spinal Association, 1956, 4971, 8375
United States Access Board, 1936, 1937
United States Association of Blind Athletes, 9097
United States Blind Golf Association, 9360
United States Blind Golfers Association, 9098
United States Braille Chess Association, 9099
United States Deaf Ski & Snowboard Associa tion, 8175
United States Department of the Interior National Park Service, 5586
United States Disabled Golf Association (USDGA), 951
United States Golf Teachers Federation, 756
United States Olympic Committee, 8459
United States Trager Association, 952
United We Stand of New York, 3761
Unity Language System, 203
Univ. of Maryland, College of Information Studies, 4891
Universal Attention Disorders, 1823
Universal Hand Cuff, 334
Universal Institute Rehabilitation & Fitne ss Center, 6380
Universal Pediatrics, 953
Universal Switch Mounting System, 1591
University Afiliated Program/Rose F Kennedy Center, 3762
University Healthcare-Rehabilitation Center, 6474
University Legal Services AT Program, 4739
University Medical Center, 6369, 6437
University of Alabama, 3417
University Of Alabama at Birmingham, 6508
University of Arkansas at Little Rock, 9298
University of California Memory and Aging Center, 7789
University of Chicago Press, 8285
University of Cincinnati Hospital, 6400
University Of Cincinnati Uap, 4981
University of Colorado Health Sciences Center, 6272
University of Hawaii at Manoa, 7689
University of Idaho, 4830
University of Illinois, 1120, 8381
University of Illinois at Chicago, 4844
University of Illinois at Chicago: Lions of Illinois Eye Research Institute, 4844
University of Illinois Medical Center, 6868
University of Illinois Press, 8247
University Of Iowa, 7831, 7945, 8941, 8950, 9122
University of Iowa, 4856
University of Kansas, 3583
University of Maine at Augusta, 1633, 3605
University of Maryland Rehabilitation and Orthopaedic Institute, 2757
University of Miami, 6299
University of Miami: Bascom Palmer Eye Institute, 4810
University of Miami: Jackson Memorial Rehabilitation Center, 6299
University of Miami: Mailman Center for Child Development, 4811
University of Michigan, 2209
University of Michigan: Orthopaedic Research Laboratories, 4921
University of Minnesota, 4930
University of Minnesota at Crookston, 2788
University of Missouri, 4938
University of Missouri-Kansas City, 3668
University of Missouri: Columbia Arthritis Center, 4938
University of New Hampshire, 2219
University of New Mexico, 1921
University of North Carolina at Chapel Hill: Neuroscience Research Building, 4977
University of North Carolina at Chapel Hill, 8752
University of Oregon, 2789
University of Pennsylvania, 2776
University of Rochester Medical Center, 3763
University of South Carolina School of Medicine, 796, 3263
University of South Florida, 4803
University of Texas, 3892
University of Texas at Austin, 1649
University of Texas at Austin Library, 5011
University of Texas Southwestern Medical Center/Allergy & Immunology, 5010
University of Utah Health Care Burn Camp Programs, 1457
University of Virginia, 6477
University of Virginia Health System General Clinical Research Group, 5027
University of Virginia, Rehab Engineering Centers, 651
University of Washington, 2427
University Press of Mississippi, 8828, 8829
University Press of New England, 8795
Unseen Minority: A Social History of Blindness in the United States, 9266
UNUM Charitable Foundation, 3001
Unyeway, 5939
Up and Running, 1876
Upledger Institute International (UII), 954
UPMC Braddock, 7371
UPMC McKeesport, 7372
UPMC Passavant, 7373
Upper Coastal Plain Council of Governments Area Agency on Aging, 7790
Upper Peninsula Library for the Blind, 4922
Upper Valley Medical/Rehab Services, 6401
Uppertone, 514
Upstate Update, 9335
Upward Bound Camp, 1367
Urologic Care of the Child with Spina Bifida, 8830
US Administration on Aging, 7621
US Association of Blind Athletes, 9359
US Department of Education, 2902, 3378, 3403, 3405
US Department of Education: Office for Civil Rights, 3408
US Department of Health, 9024
US Department of Health and Human Services Office for Civil Rights, 4736
US Department of Health and Human Services, 2336, 3388, 3407, 5140
US Department of Housing & Urban Development, 3401, 5181
US Department of Justice, 3382, 3384, 4672, 4678, 4679, 4680, 4681, 4685, 4696, 4720, 4731, 4732, 5094, 5095, 5096, 5103, 5110, 5186, 5208, 8802, 9132
US Department of Labor, 4737, 3400, 3501
US Department of Labor Office of Federal Contract Compliance Programs, 4738
US Department of Labor: Office of Federal Contract Compliance Programs, 3409
US Department of Transportation, 3410
US Department of Veterans Affairs, 3411
US Department of Veterans Affairs National Headquarters, 5635
US Department Veterans Affairs Beckley Vet Center, 5858
US Office of Personnel Management, 3412
US Paralympics, 8459
US Role in International Disability Activities: A History, 5275
US Servas, 5601

US Social Security Administration, 7776
USA Deaf Sports Federation, 8334
Usher Syndrome, 8831
Using the Dictionary of Occupational Titles in Career Decision Making, 2643
USX Foundation, 3247
Utah Assistive Technology Program (UTAP) Utah State University, 4592
Utah Assistive Technology Projects, 3897
Utah Client Assistance Program, 3898
Utah Department of Aging and Adult Service s, 3899
Utah Department of Human Services, 3901
Utah Department of Human Services: Division of Services for People with Disabilities, 3900, 6200
Utah Division of Services for the Disabled, 3902
Utah Division Of Substance Abuse & Mental Health, 3901
Utah Division of Veterans Affairs, 5841, 5841
Utah Employment Services, 6201
Utah Governor's Committee on Employment for People with Disabilities (GCEPD), 6202
Utah Governor's Council for People with Disabilities, 3903
Utah Independent Living Center, 4593
Utah Independent Living Center: Minersville, 4594
Utah Independent Living Center: Tooele, 4595
Utah Labor Commission, 3904
Utah Protection & Advocacy Services for Persons with Disabilities, 3905
Utah State Library Division: Program for the Blind and Disabled, 5012
Utah State Office for Rehabilitation (USOR), 6203
Utah State Office of Education, 2240
Utah State Office of Education: At-Risk and Special Education Service Unit, 2240
Utah State Office of Rehabilitation, 6202
Utah State Office of Rehabilition: Vocational Rehabilitation, 6204
Utah State Office of Rehabilition: Service s for the Blind and Visually Impaired, 6205
Utah State University, 3897
UTHSC Center on Developmental Disabilities, 1412

V

V A Montana Healthcare System, 5750
V Foundation for Cancer Research, 5546
V OR T Corporation, 1744, 1811
V XI Corporation Incorporated, 1689
VA Ann Arbor Healthcare System, 5736
VA Boston Healthcare System: Brockton Division, 5728
VA Boston Healthcare System: Jamaica Plain Campus, 5729
VA Boston Healthcare System: West Roxbury Division, 5730
VA Central California Health Care System, 5659
VA Central Iowa Health Care System, 5706
VA Connecticut Healthcare System: Newington Division, 5669
VA Connecticut Healthcare System: West Haven, 5670
VA Greater Los Angeles Healthcare System, 5660
VA Hudson Valley Health Care System, 5783
VA Illiana Health Care System, 5697
VA Maryland Health Care System, 5724
VA Medical Center (116D), 5013
VA Medical Center, Washington DC, 5676
VA Montana Healthcare System, 5751
VA Nebraska-Western Iowa Health Care System, 5756
VA North Indiana Health Care System: Fort Wayne Campus, 5700
VA North Texas Health Veterans Affairs Car e System: Dallas VA Medical Center, 5838
VA Northern California Healthcare System, 5661
VA Northern Indiana Health Care System: Marion Campus, 5701
VA Pittsburgh Healthcare System, University Drive Division, 5817
VA Pittsburgh Healthcare System, Highland Drive Division, 5818
VA Puget Sound Health Care System, 5853
VA Salt Lake City Healthcare System, 5842
VA San Diego Healthcare System, 5662
VA Sierra Nevada Healthcare System, 5759
VA Southern Nevada Healthcare System, 5760
VA Western NY Healthcare System, Batavia, 5784
VA Western NY Healthcare System, Buffalo, 5785
VAK Tasks Workbook: Visual, Auditory and Kinesthetic, 2067
Valir Health, 6407
Valley Associates for Independent Living (VAIL), 4619
Valley Associates for Independent Living: Lexington, 4620
Valley Association for Independent Living (VAIL), 4583
Valley Association for Independent Living: Harlingen, 4584
Valley Center for the Blind, 6671
Valley Forge Specialized Educational Services, 2758
Valley Garden Health Care and Rehabilitati on Center, 7227
Valley Health Care and Rehabilitation Cent er, 7217
Valley Light Industries, 5940
Valley News Dispatch, 8045
Valley Regional Medical Center, 7391
Valley Regional Medical Center: RehabCare Unit, 6468
Valley View Regional Hospital-RehabCare Unit, 7116
Valpar International, 1869
ValueOptions, 5547
Van Ameringen Foundation, 3178
Van G Miller & Associates, 6885
Vancouver Health & Rhabilitation Center, 7411
Vancouver Health and Rehabilitation Center, 7206
Vanderbilt Kennedy Center, 1411
Vanderbilt Rehabilitation Center, 7140
Vangater, Vangater II, Mini-Vangater, 398
Vanguard School, The, 2758
VanMatre Rehabilitation Center, 6869
VANTAGE, 7749
Vantage Mobility International, 130
Variety Club Camp and Developmental Center, 1395
Vaughn-Blumberg Services, 6509
VBS Special Education Teaching Guide, 2644
Vector Mobility, 704
Vegetarian Voice, 7751
Veggie Life, 7752
Vehicle Access Remote Control, 131
Velcro Booties, 1551
Ventilator-Assisted Living, 8880
Ventura Enterprises, 632
Venture Publishing Inc., 5076
Ventures Travel, 5621
Verbal Behavior Approach: How to Teach Children with Autism & Related Disorders, 8046, 8998
Verbal View of the Web & Net, 7813
Verizon Foundation, 3179
Vermont Achievement Center, 6475
Vermont Assistive Technology Program, 4596
Vermont Assistive Technology Project: Department of Aging & Disabilities, 1656
Vermont Assistive Technology Projects, 3909
Vermont Assn for the Blind & Visually Impaired, 9337
Vermont Association for the Blind and Visually Impaired, 9100
Vermont Back Research Center, 8376
Vermont Center for Independent Living: Ben nington, 4597
Vermont Center for Independent Living: Chi ttenden, 4598
Vermont Center for Independent Living: Mon tpelier, 4599
Vermont Client Assistance Program, 3910
Vermont Community Foundation, 3314
Vermont Department of Aging, 3911
Vermont Department of Developmental and, 3912
Vermont Department of Disabilities, Aging and Independent Living (DAIL), 3913, 6207
Vermont Department Of Health, 3914
Vermont Department of Health: Children with Special Health Needs, 3914
Vermont Department of Labor, 6208
Vermont Department of Libraries - Special Services Unit, 5014
Vermont Department of Libraries -Special Services Unit, 5015
Vermont Developmental Disabilities Council, 3915
Vermont Division for the Blind & Visually Impaired, 3916
Vermont Division of Disability & Aging Services, 3917
Vermont Division of Vocational Rehabilitat ion, 6209
Vermont Interdependent Services Team Approach (VISTA), 2645
Vermont Overnight Camp, 1465
Vermont VA Regional Office Center, 5843
Vermont Veterans Centers, 5844
Versatrainer, 399
Vertek, 1866
VESID, 3764
Vestibular Board, 400
Vestibular Disorders Association, 5277, 8176, 5277, 8218, 8314, 8330, 8331, 8332, 8760
Vet Center, 5741, 5752
Vet Center Readjustment Counseling Service, 5737
Vet Health Administration U S Department of VA, 5790
Veteran Benefits Administration - Anchorage Regional Office, 5643
Veteran's Voices Writing Project, 5636
Veterans Benefits Administration, 5667, 5698, 5758, 5775, 5816, 5843, 5851
Veterans Benefits Administration U S Dept. of V A, 5655, 5664, 5671
Veterans Benefits Administration, U S Dept. of V A, 5650, 5653, 5658, 5682, 5684, 5690, 5692, 5703, 5709, 5713, 5717, 5719, 5725, 5735, 5740, 5743, 5747, 5754, 5761, 5767, 5779, 5791, 5793, 5796, 5799, 5804, 5814, 5820, 5822, 5826, 5830, 5839, 5847, 5854, 5862, 5866
Veterans Health Administration, 5666
Veterans Health Administration U S Department of V, 5657, 5695, 5797, 5824, 5859
Veterans Health Administration U S Department. of, 5669
Veterans Health Administration U S Deptartment of, 5660, 5726, 5772
Veterans Health Administration U.S. Dept. of VA, 5638
Veterans Health Administration, U S Department of, 5783, 5813
Veterans Health Administration, U S Dept. of V A, 5640, 5644, 5646, 5647, 5651, 5652, 5654, 5659, 5661, 5662, 5665, 5670, 5677, 5678, 5679, 5680, 5681, 5683, 5685, 5686, 5687, 5693, 5694, 5696, 5697, 5699, 5700, 5701, 5702, 5704, 5705, 5708, 5710, 5711, 5712, 5715, 5716, 5718, 5720, 5721, 5723, 5727, 5728, 5729, 5730, 5731, 5732, 5733, 5734, 5736, , 5738, 5739, 5742, 5744, 5745, 5746, 5748, 5751, 5753, 5755, 5756, 5759, 5760, 5762, 5766, 5770, 5773, 5774, 5776, 5777, 5778, 5780, 5781, 5784, 5785, 5786, 5788, 5789, 5792, 5794, 5795, 5798, 5801, 5801, 5805
Veterans Health Administration, U S Dept. of VA, 5825
Veterans Health Administration, U.S. Dept. of VA, 5639
Veterans Health Administration, US Dept. of VA, 5645, 5648, 5649, 5672, 5691, 5769, 5829, 5831
Veterans Support Center (VSC), 6206
VFW Auxiliary, 7750
Viability, 955, 6086
Vibra Health Care, 6276
Victor E Speas Foundation, 3079
Victoria Foundation, 3104
Victory Junction, 1315
Video Guide to Disability Awareness, 5468

Video Intensive Parenting, 5469
Video Learning Library, 8319
Views from Our Shoes, 5066
Viking Books, 9165
Villa Esperanza Services, 6672
Village Square Nursing And Rehabilitation Center, 6673
Vim & Vigor Magazine, 7753
Vinfen Corporation, 6981
Vinland Center Lake Independence, 4355
Vinsen Corporation, 6080
Vintage and Anchor Books, 8272
Vintage-Random House, 8022
VIP Newsletter, 2343
Virginia Autism Resource Center, 5028
Virginia Beach Foundation, 3323
Virginia Beach Public Library Special Services Library, 5029
Virginia Center on Aging, 7623
Virginia Chapter of the Arthtitis Foundation, 5030
Virginia Commonwealth University, 5022, 7623
Virginia Department for the Blind and Vision Impaired (DBVI), 3921, 6215
Virginia Department Of Education, 2242
Virginia Department of Education: Division of Pre & Early Adolescent Education, 2242
Virginia Department of Mental Health, 3922
Virginia Department of Veterans Services, 5849
Virginia Developmental Disability Council, 3923
Virginia Office for Protection & Advocacy, 3925
Virginia Office for Protection and Advocacy, 3926
Virginia Office Protection and Advocacy for People with Disabilities, 3924
Virginia State Library for the Visually and Physically Handicapped, 5031
Virginia's Developmental Disabilities Plan ning Council, 3927
The Viscardi Center, 728, 894, 6154
Visi-Pitch III, 1824
Vision Enhancement, 9267
Vision Forward Association, 9101
Vision Foundation, 3038
Vision Loss Resources, 7008
Vision Magazine, 8318
Vision Northwest, 7122
Vision World Wide, 9102
Visions & Values, 5278
VISIONS Center on Blindness, 1302, 9121
Visions Center on Blindness (VCB), 9103
VISIONS Vacation Camp for the Blind (VCB), 1302, 9121
Visiting Nurse Association of America, 8909
Visiting Nurse Association of North Shore, 6982
Vista Center for the Blind & Visually Impaired, 6674
Vista Center for the Blind & Visually Impaired, 9328
Vista Wheelchair, 695
Visual Aids and Informational Material, 9336
Visual Impairment: An Overview, 9268
Visual Impairments And Learning, 9269
Visually Impaired Center, 7002, 9301
Visually Impaired Persons of Southwest Florida, 6781
Visually Impaired Seniors as Senior Companions: A Reference Guide, 7653
Visually Impaired Veterans of America, 9104
Vital Signs: Crip Culture Talks Back, 5470
Vocabulary Development, 1860
Vocational and Rehabilitation Agency, 5995
Vocational and Rehabilitation Service - Decatur, 5891
Vocational Rehabilitation, 5903
Vocational Rehabilitation Agency: Oregon Commission for the Blind, 3813
Vocational Rehabilitation and Employment, 6387
Vocational Rehabilitation Program, 6061
Vocational Rehabilitation Service (VRS), 5875
Vocational Rehabilitation Service - Opelika, 5876
Vocational Rehabilitation Service - Dothan, 5877
Vocational Rehabilitation Service - Gadsde n, 5878
Vocational Rehabilitation Service - Homewo od, 5879
Vocational Rehabilitation Service - Huntsv ille, 5880
Vocational Rehabilitation Service - Jackso n, 5881
Vocational Rehabilitation Service - Jasper, 5882
Vocational Rehabilitation Service - Mobile, 5883
Vocational Rehabilitation Service - Muscle Shoals, 5884
Vocational Rehabilitation Service - Selma, 5885
Vocational Rehabilitation Service - Tallad ega, 5886
Vocational Rehabilitation Service - Troy, 5887
Vocational Rehabilitation Service - Tuscal oosa, 5888
Vocational Rehabilitation Services, 5908, 6025
Vocational Rehabilitation Services - Andal usia, 5889
Vocational Rehabilitation Services - Annis ton, 5890
Vocational Rehabilitation Services for the Blind, 6105
Voice, 9015, 9337
Voice Amplified Handsets, 204
Voice of the Diabetic, 8881
Voice of Vision, 9338
Voice-It, 1689
Voices for Independence, 4535
Voices of Vision Talking Book Center at DuPage Library System, 4845
VOLAR Center for Independent Living, 4582
Volta Review, 8297
Volunteer Transcribing Services, 2068
Volunteers of America (VOA), 956
Volunteers of America of Greater New Orlea ns, 4278
VSA - The International Organization on Ar ts and Disability, 67
VSA arts, 68
VSA Arts of New York City, 3765
VUE: Vision Use in Employment, 9366

W

W Troy Cole Independent Living Specialist, 4279
WA Department of Services for the Blind, 3932
Waban Projects, 958
Wabash Independent Living Center & Learning Center (WILL), 4206
Waco Regional Office, 5839
Wage and Hour Division of the Employment Standards Administration, 3501
Wagon Road Camp, 1303
Wakeman/Walworth, 3369
Walden Rehabilitation and Nursing Center, 7313
Walgreens Home Medical Center, 457
Walker Leg Support, 634
Walking Alone and Marching Together, 9270
Wallace Memorial Library, 4972
Walter Cronkite School of Journalism, AZ State U., 900
Walter Winchell Foundation, 5498
Walton Options for Independent Living, 4135
Walton Options for Independent Living: Nor th Augusta, 4546
Walton Rehabilitation Health System, 6800, 7256
Walton Way Medical, 458
War Memorial Hospital, 7412
Wardrobe Wagon: The Special Needs Clothing Store, 5548
Warner Books, 7947
Warner Robins Rehabilitation and Nursing C enter, 7257
Warren Achievement Center, 6870
Warren Grant Magnuson Clinical Center, 4892
Warren Memorial Hospital, 7399
Wasatch Valley Rehabilitation, 7396
Wasatch Vision Clinic, 7177
Washable Shoes, 1552
Washington Client Assistance Program, 3933
Washington Connection, 9367
Washington County Disability, Aging and Veteran Services, 3814
Washington County Vocational Workshop, 6026
Washington DC VA Medical Center, 5677
Washington Developmental Disability, 3934
Washington Ear, 9105
Washington Governor's Committee on Disability Issues & Employment, 3935
Washington Hearing and Speech Society, 3502
Washington Memorial Library, 4821
Washington Office of Superintendent of Public Instruction, 3936
Washington Square Health Foundation, 2981
Washington State Developmental Disabilities Council, 3937
Washington Talking Book and Braille Library, 5034
Washington University, 7546
Washtenaw County Library for the Blind & Physically Handicapped, 4923
Waterproof Bib, 1553
Waterville Public Library, 4880
Waupaca Elevator Company, 351
Waushers Industries, 7208
Wayfinder Family Services, 2870, 1001, 9107
Wayne County Regional Educational Service Agency, 1686
Wayne County Regional Library for the Blind, 4924
Wayne State University, 941
Wayne State University: CS Mott Center for Human Genetics and Development, 4925
WB Saunders Company, 8979
WCIB Heavy-Duty Folding Cane, 633
We Are PHAMALY, 69
We Can Do it Together!, 9354
We CAN Hear and Speak, 8286
We Can Speak for Ourselves: Self Advocacy by Mentally Handicapped People, 5337
We Magazine, 5549
We Media, 5550
We're Not Stupid, 8092
WebABLE, 5551
WebMD Magazine, 7754
WebMD, LLC, 7754
Webster Enterprises of Jackson County, Inc., 6165
Wediko Children's Services, New Hampshire Campus, 1247
Week the World Heard Gallaudet, The, 8287
Weekly Wisdom, 8072
Weiner's Herbal, 5279
Weitbrecht Communications, Inc. (WCI), 459
Welcome Homes Retirement Community for the Visually Impaired, 7003
Weldon Center for Rehabilitation, 6983
Well Mind Association of Greater Washington, 3503
Wellsouth Health Systems, 7292
Wendell Johnson Speech & Hearing Clinic, 8950
Wendell Johnson Speech And Hearing Clinic, 7831, 7945, 8941, 9122
Wes Test Engineering Corporation, 1871
West Central Illinois Center for Independent Living, 4191
West Central Illinois Center for Independe nt Living: Macomb, 4192
West Central Independent Living Solutions, 4386
West Florida Hospital: The Rehabilitation Institute, 6782
West Florida Regional Library, 4812
West Gables Health Care Center, 6783
West Hills Day Camp, 1304
West Michigan Learning Disabilities Foundation, 2743
West Palm Beach VA Medical Center, 5683
West Penn Burn Camp, 1396
West Suburban Hospital Medical Center, 6823
West Texas Lighthouse for the Blind, 7175
West Texas VA Healthcare System, 5840
West Virginia Advocates, 3942, 3943
West Virginia Autism Training Center, 5040
West Virginia Client Assistance Program, 3943
West Virginia Department of Aging, 3944
West Virginia Department of Children with Disabilities, 3945
West Virginia Department of Education: Office of Special Education, 2244
West Virginia Department of Health, 3946, 3952
West Virginia Developmental Disabilities Council, 3947

West Virginia Division of Rehabilitation Services (DRS), 3948, 6221
West Virginia Library Commission, 5041
West Virginia Research and Training Center, 2693
West Virginia School for the Blind Library, 5042
Westchester Disabled on the Move, 4471
Westchester Independent Living Center, 4472
Westchester Institute for Human Developmen t, 3766
Western Alliance Center for Independent Living, 4479
Western Alliance for Independent Living, 4480
Western Michigan University, 3630
Western New York Foundation, 3180
Western Psychological Services, 8088
Western Resources for dis-ABLED Independence, 4555
Western Washington University, 2790
WesTest Engineering Corporation, 1566
Westpark Rehabilitation Center, 7284
Westside Center for Independent Living, 4064
Westview Nursing and Rehabilitation Center, 7285
Weyerhaeuser Company Foundation, 3333
WG Hefner VA Medical Center - Salisbury, 5790
WGBH Educational Foundation, 6958, 8917
What About Me?, 5471
What About Me? Growing Up with a Developme ntally Disabled Sibling, 5067
What Do You Do When You See a Blind Person - and What Don't You Do?, 9271
What Everyone Needs to Know About Asthma, 8832
What is Auditory Processing?, 8288
What It's Like to be Me, 5068
What Museum Guides Need to Know: Access for the Blind and Visually Impaired, 9272
What Psychotherapists Should Know about Disabilty, 5385
What School Counselors Need to Know, 2646
What Was That!, 1805
Wheat Ridge Ministries, 2982
Wheel Life News, 651
Wheelchair Accessories, 652
Wheelchair Aide, 653
Wheelchair Back Pack and Tote Bag, 654
Wheelchair Bowling, 8436
Wheelchair Carrier, 401, 401
A Wheelchair for Petronilia, 8430
Wheelchair Getaways, 5628
Wheelchair Roller, 655
Wheelchair Sports, USA, 8461
Wheelchair with Shock Absorbers, 696
Wheelchair Work Table, 656
WheelchairNet, 5552
Wheelchairs and Transport Chairs, 697
Wheelers Accessible Van Rentals, 132, 5602, 5629, 5587
Wheelin Around e-Guide, 5587
When Billy Broke His Head...and Other, 5472
When I Grow Up, 5473
When Parents Can't Fix It, 5474
When the Brain Goes Wrong, 5280
When the Road Turns: Inspirational Stories About People with MS, 8833
When You Have a Visually Impaired Student in Your Classroom: A Guide for Teachers, 2647
When Your Student Has Arthritis, 8404
White Cane and Wheels, 5475
Whittier Trust, 2871
Whittier Trust Company, 2871
Whittier Union High School District, 5933
Whole Building Design Guide, 1957
Whole Person, The, 4387
Whole Person: Kansas City, 4388
Whole Person: Nortonville, 4258
Whole Person: Nortonville, The, 4259
Whole Person: Prairie Village, 4260
Whole Person: Prairie Village, The, 4261
Whole Person: Tonganoxie, 4262
Whoops, 1861
Why Won't My Child Pay Attention?, 8093
Wichita Public Library, 4865
Wichita Public Library/Talking Book Service, 4865
Wichita Public Library/Talking Book Servic e, 4866
Widex USA, Inc., 303
Wilderness Inquiry, 5603, 5622
Wiley, 5371, 5395
Wiley & Sons, 31, 43
Wiley Publishers, 7968, 8957
Wiley Publishing, 4670, 8038, 8965
Wiley-Blackwell, 5073
Wilkes-Barre VA Medical Center, 5819
Will Grundy Center for Independent Living, 4193
Willam G Gilmore Foundation, 2872
Willamette Valley Rehabilitation Center, 7123
William B Dietrich Foundation, 3248
William H Honor Rehabilitation Center Henry Ford Wyanclotte Hospital, 7004
William Hein & Company, 4689, 4697, 4700, 4701, 4713
William J and Dorothy K O'Neill Foundation, 3218
William Jennings Bryan Dorn VA Medical Center, 5824
William Morrow & Company, 8973
William Morrow Paperbacks (HarperCollins), 5347, 5360
William N Pennington Foundation, 3087
William S Hein & Co Inc, 4692
William S Hein & Company, 4740, 4719
William S Middleton Memorial VA Hospital Center, 5861
William Stamps Farish Fund, 3310
William T Grant Foundation, 3181
William Talbott Hillman Foundation, 3249
William V and Catherine A McKinney Charitable Foundation, 3250
Williams Lift Company, 402
Willough at Naples, 6784
Wilmer Ophthalmology Institute, 4881
Wilmington VA Medical Center, 5672
Wilmington Vet Center, 5673
Winchester Rehabilitation Center, 7400
Wind River Healthcare and Rehabilitation Center, 7428
Window-Ease, 515
Window-Eyes, 1690
Windsor Estates Health and Rehab Center, 7286
Windsor Rehabilitation and Healthcare Cent er, 7235
WINGS for Learning, 1697, 1703, 1704, 1767, 1774, 1835
Winkler Court, 7250
WinSCAN: The Single Switch Interface for PC's with Windows, 1592
Winston-Salem Industries for the Blind, 7079
Winston-Salem Regional Office, 5791
Winston-Salem Rehabilitation and Healthcar e Center, 7350
Winter Address, 1378
Winter Park Memorial Hospital, 6300, 7251
Winthrop Rockefeller Foundation, 2807
Winways at Orange County, 6675
Wiregrass Rehabilitation Center, Inc., 5892
Wisconsin Badger Camp, 1492
Wisconsin Board for People with Developmen tal Disabilities (WBPDD), 3953
Wisconsin Bureau of Aging, 3954
Wisconsin Coalition for Advocacy: Madison Office, 3955
Wisconsin Elks/Easterseals Respite Camp, 1493
Wisconsin Governor's Committee for People with Disabilities, 3956
Wisconsin Lions Camp, 1494, 8657
Wisconsin Lions Foundation, 1494, 8657
Wisconsin Regional Library for the Blind & Physically Handicapped, 5045
Wisconsin VA Regional Office, 5862
Wishing Wells Collection, 1554, 1525
Without Reason: A Family Copes with two Ge nerations of Autism, 8047, 8999
Wivik 3, 1806
WM Keck Foundation, 2869
Wolfner Talking Book & Braille Library, 4939
A Woman's Guide to Living with HIV Infecti on, 8666
Women to Women Healthcare, 959
Women with Attention Deficit Disorder: Embracing Disorganization at Home and Work, 8048
Women with Physical Disabilities: Achievin g & Maintaining Health & Well-Being, 5281
Women with Visible & Invisible Disabilitie es: Multiple Intersections, Issues, Therapies, 5386
Wonderland Camp, 1227
Woodbine House, 2177, 2450, 2619, 5058, 5336, 5343, 5346, 8005, 8043, 8223, 8698
Woodcock Reading Mastery Tests, 2725
The Woodlands Foundation, 1387
Woodrow Wilson Rehabilitation Center, 7186
Woodrow Wilson Rehabilitation Center Training Program, 4621
Woodside Day Program, 6716
Woodstock Health and Rehabilitation Center, 7209
Wordly Wise 3000, 2069
WordMaker, 1807
Words+, 1580, 1590, 1593, 1670, 1672, 1673, 1687, 1735, 1765, 1816, 1875
Words+ Inc, 1573
Words+ IST (Infrared, Sound, Touch), 1593
Work and Disability: Contexts, Issues & St rategies for Enhancing Employment Outcomes, 5396
Work in the Context of Disability Culture, 5282
Work Inc., 6087
Work Sight, 9273
Work Training Center, 5941, 5920
Work!, 2070
Work, Health and Income Among the Elderly, 7654
Work-Related Vocational Assessment Systems : Computer Based, 1869
Workers Compensation Board Alabama, 3425
Workers Compensation Board Illinois, 3566
Workers Compensation Board Iowa, 3582
Workers Compensation Board Louisiana, 3604
Workers Compensation Board Maryland, 3622
Workers Compensation Board Massachusetts, 3629
Workers Compensation Board Missouri, 3673
Workers Compensation Board Nevada, 3703
Workers Compensation Board New Hampshire, 3715
Workers Compensation Board New Mexico, 3736
Workers Compensation Board New York, 3767
Workers Compensation Board North Dakota, 3785
Workers Compensation Board Oklahoma, 3805
Workers Compensation Board Pennsylvania, 3826
Workers Compensation Board Rhode Island, 3838
Workers Compensation Board Vermont, 3918
Workers Compensation Board Washington, 3938
Workers Compensation Board Wisconsin, 3957
Workers Compensation Board Wyoming, 3960
Workers Compensation Board: District of Columbia, 3504
Workers Compensation Board: South Carolina, 3847
Workers Compensation Board: South Dakota, 3856
Workers Compensation Division, 3436
Workers Compensation Division Tennessee, 3866
Workforce and Technology Center, 6952
WorkForce West Virginia, 6222
Working Bibliography on Behavioral and Emotional Disorders, 2648
Working Together & Taking Part, 2071
Working Together with Children and Families: Case Studies, 2649
Working with Visually Impaired Young Students: A Curriculum Guide for 3 to 5 Year Olds, 2650
Workplace Skills: Learning How to Function on the Job, 1870
The Workshop, 6023
Workshops, Inc., 5893
WORLD, 957
World Association of Persons with Disabilities, 5553
A World Awaits You, 5089, 5583, 8415
World Chiropractic Alliance, 8112, 8377
World Experience Teenage Exchange Program, 2791
World Federation for Mental Health, 960

World Institute on Disability, 2355, 2507, 2638, 5205, 5248, 5275
World Institute on Disability (WID), 961
World of Options, 2792
World Research Foundation, 4756
World Service Office of Overeaters Anonymous, 8533
World Through Their Eyes, 9274
Worst Loss: How Families Heal from the Death of a Child, 5364
Worthmore Academy, 2759
WP and HB White Foundation, 2980
Write: Out Loud, 1808
Write: OutLoud, 1877
Writer's Showcase Press, 5172
WW Norton & Company, 5129, 8398
WY Department of Health: Mental Health and Substance Abuse Service Division, 3959
Wyman Center, 8622, 8633
Wyoming Client Assistance Program, 3961
Wyoming Department of Aging, 3962
Wyoming Department of Education, 2245, 5046
Wyoming Department of Workforce Services: Unemployment Insurance Division, 6225
Wyoming Developmental Disability Council, 3963
Wyoming Protection & Advocacy for Persons with Disabilities, 3964
Wyoming Services for Independent Living, 4650
Wyoming Services for the Visually Impaired, 5046
Wyoming State Rehabilitation Council (SRC), 6226
Wyoming's New Options in Technology (WYNOT) - University of Wyoming, 5047
Wyoming/Colorado VA Regional Office, 5866

X

Xavier Society for the Blind, 4973

Y

Y Camp, 8658
YAI: National Institute for People with Disabilities, 962
Yale New Haven Health System-Bridgeport Hospital, 6706
Yale University Press, 8797
Yale University: Vision Research Center, 4787
Yavapai Regional Medical Center-West, 5904
YMCA Camp Carter, 1430
YMCA Camp Chandler, 976, 8612
YMCA Camp Chingachgook on Lake George, 1305, 9123
YMCA Camp Fitch, 1397, 8206, 8384, 8659, 8951
YMCA Camp Ihduhapi, 8660
YMCA Camp jewell, 8663
YMCA Camp Kitaki, 8661
YMCA Camp Kon-O-Kwee, 1384
YMCA Camp of Maine, 8664
YMCA Camp Shady Brook, 8662
YMCA Camp Speers, 1388
YMCA Camping Services, 7905
YMCA of Greater Des Moines, 8658
YMCA of Greater Hartford, 8663
YMCA of Greater Oklahoma City, 8560
YMCA of Greater Pittsburgh, 1369
YMCA of Orange County, 1039, 7927, 8947
YMCA of Southern Arizona, 7944
YMCA of the Pikes Peak Region (PPYMCA), 8662
YMCA Outdoor Center Campbell Gard, 1345, 8665
YMCA Storer Camps, 1190
Yoga for Arthritis, 8437
Yoga for Fibromyalgia: Move, Breathe, and Relax to Improve Your Quality of Life, 8405
Yoga for MS and Related Conditions, 8438
You and Your ADD Child, 8050
You and Your Deaf Child: A Self-Help Guide for Parents of Deaf and Hard of Hearing Children, 8289
You May Be Able to Adopt, 5338
You Mean I'm Not Lazy, Stupid or Crazy?!: A Self-Help Book for Adults with ADD, 8049
You Seem Like a Regular Kid to Me, 9275
You Tell Me: Learning Basic Information, 1809
You Will Dream New Dreams, 5339
Young Children with Special Needs: A Developmentally Appropriate Approach, 2726
Young Onset Parkinson Conference, 1923
Young Person's Guide to Spina Bifida, 8834
Youngstown Foundation, 3219
Younker Rehabilitation Center of Iowa Methodist Medical Center, 6335
Your Child and Asthma, 8835
Your Child Has a Disability: A Complete So urcebook of Daily and Medical Care, 5340
Your Child in the Hospital: A Practical Guide for Parents (3rd Edition), 5348
Your Cleft Affected Child, 8836
Your Guide to Bowel Cancer, 8837
Your Role in Inclusion Theatre, 5283
Youth as Self Advocates (YASA), 964
Youth for Understanding International Exchange, 2793
Youth Leadership Camp, 8207
Youth MOVE National, 963
Youville Hospital & Rehab Center, 6984
Yuma Center for the Visually Impaired, 6532

Z

ZoomText, 1679
Zygo-Usa, 1674

Grey House Publishing

2021 Title List

Grey House Publishing

Visit www.GreyHouse.com for Product Information, Table of Contents, and Sample Pages.

Opinions Throughout History

Opinions Throughout History: The Death Penalty
Opinions Throughout History: Diseases & Epidemics
Opinions Throughout History: Drug Use & Abuse
Opinions Throughout History: The Environment
Opinions Throughout History: Gender: Roles & Rights
Opinions Throughout History: Globalization
Opinions Throughout History: Guns in America
Opinions Throughout History: Immigration
Opinions Throughout History: Law Enforcement in America
Opinions Throughout History: National Security vs. Civil & Privacy Rights
Opinions Throughout History: Presidential Authority
Opinions Throughout History: Robotics & Artificial Intelligence
Opinions Throughout History: Social Media Issues
Opinions Throughout History: Sports & Games
Opinions Throughout History: Voters' Rights

This is Who We Were

This is Who We Were: Colonial America (1492-1775)
This is Who We Were: 1880-1899
This is Who We Were: In the 1900s
This is Who We Were: In the 1910s
This is Who We Were: In the 1920s
This is Who We Were: A Companion to the 1940 Census
This is Who We Were: In the 1940s (1940-1949)
This is Who We Were: In the 1950s
This is Who We Were: In the 1960s
This is Who We Were: In the 1970s
This is Who We Were: In the 1980s
This is Who We Were: In the 1990s
This is Who We Were: In the 2000s
This is Who We Were: In the 2010s

Working Americans

Working Americans—Vol. 1: The Working Class
Working Americans—Vol. 2: The Middle Class
Working Americans—Vol. 3: The Upper Class
Working Americans—Vol. 4: Children
Working Americans—Vol. 5: At War
Working Americans—Vol. 6: Working Women
Working Americans—Vol. 7: Social Movements
Working Americans—Vol. 8: Immigrants
Working Americans—Vol. 9: Revolutionary War to the Civil War
Working Americans—Vol. 10: Sports & Recreation
Working Americans—Vol. 11: Inventors & Entrepreneurs
Working Americans—Vol. 12: Our History through Music
Working Americans—Vol. 13: Education & Educators
Working Americans—Vol. 14: African Americans
Working Americans—Vol. 15: Politics & Politicians
Working Americans—Vol. 16: Farming & Ranching
Working Americans—Vol. 17: Teens in America

Education

Complete Learning Disabilities Resource Guide
Educators Resource Guide
The Comparative Guide to Elem. & Secondary Schools
Charter School Movement
Special Education: A Reference Book for Policy & Curriculum Development

Grey House Health & Wellness Guides

Autoimmune Disorders Handbook & Resource Guide
Cancer Handbook & Resource Guide
Cardiovascular Disease Handbook & Resource Guide
Dementia Handbook & Resource Guide

Consumer Health

Autoimmune Disorders Handbook & Resource Guide
Cancer Handbook & Resource Guide
Cardiovascular Disease Handbook & Resource Guide
Comparative Guide to American Hospitals
Complete Mental Health Resource Guide
Complete Resource Guide for Pediatric Disorders
Complete Resource Guide for People with Chronic Illness
Complete Resource Guide for People with Disabilities
Older Americans Information Resource

General Reference

African Biographical Dictionary
American Environmental Leaders
America's College Museums
Constitutional Amendments
Encyclopedia of African-American Writing
Encyclopedia of Invasions & Conquests
Encyclopedia of Prisoners of War & Internment
Encyclopedia of Rural America
Encyclopedia of the Continental Congresses
Encyclopedia of the United States Cabinet
Encyclopedia of War Journalism
The Environmental Debate
The Evolution Wars: A Guide to the Debates
Financial Literacy Starter Kit
From Suffrage to the Senate
The Gun Debate: Gun Rights & Gun Control in the U.S.
History of Canada
Historical Warrior Peoples & Modern Fighting Groups
Human Rights and the United States
Political Corruption in America
Privacy Rights in the Digital Age
The Religious Right and American Politics
Speakers of the House of Representatives, 1789-2021
US Land & Natural Resources Policy
The Value of a Dollar 1600-1865 Colonial to Civil War
The Value of a Dollar 1860-2019
World Cultural Leaders of the 20th Century

Business Information

Business Information Resources
The Complete Broadcasting Industry Guide: Television, Radio, Cable & Streaming
Directory of Mail Order Catalogs
Environmental Resource Handbook
Food & Beverage Market Place
The Grey House Guide to Homeland Security Resources
The Grey House Performing Arts Industry Guide
Guide to Healthcare Group Purchasing Organizations
Guide to U.S. HMOs and PPOs
Guide to Venture Capital & Private Equity Firms
Hudson's Washington News Media Contacts Guide
New York State Directory
Sports Market Place

2021 Title List

Visit www.GreyHouse.com for Product Information, Table of Contents, and Sample Pages.

Statistics & Demographics

America's Top-Rated Cities
America's Top-Rated Smaller Cities
The Comparative Guide to American Suburbs
Profiles of America
Profiles of California
Profiles of Florida
Profiles of Illinois
Profiles of Indiana
Profiles of Massachusetts
Profiles of Michigan
Profiles of New Jersey
Profiles of New York
Profiles of North Carolina & South Carolina
Profiles of Ohio
Profiles of Pennsylvania
Profiles of Texas
Profiles of Virginia
Profiles of Wisconsin

Canadian Resources

Associations Canada
Canadian Almanac & Directory
Canadian Environmental Resource Guide
Canadian Parliamentary Guide
Canadian Venture Capital & Private Equity Firms
Canadian Who's Who
Cannabis Canada
Careers & Employment Canada
Financial Post: Directory of Directors
Financial Services Canada
FP Bonds: Corporate
FP Bonds: Government
FP Equities: Preferreds & Derivatives
FP Survey: Industrials
FP Survey: Mines & Energy
FP Survey: Predecessor & Defunct
Health Guide Canada
Libraries Canada
Major Canadian Cities: Compared & Ranked, First Edition

Weiss Financial Ratings

Financial Literacy Basics
Financial Literacy: How to Become an Investor
Financial Literacy: Planning for the Future
Weiss Ratings Consumer Guides
Weiss Ratings Guide to Banks
Weiss Ratings Guide to Credit Unions
Weiss Ratings Guide to Health Insurers
Weiss Ratings Guide to Life & Annuity Insurers
Weiss Ratings Guide to Property & Casualty Insurers
Weiss Ratings Investment Research Guide to Bond & Money Market Mutual Funds
Weiss Ratings Investment Research Guide to Exchange-Traded Funds
Weiss Ratings Investment Research Guide to Stock Mutual Funds
Weiss Ratings Investment Research Guide to Stocks

Books in Print Series

American Book Publishing Record® Annual
American Book Publishing Record® Monthly
Books In Print®
Books In Print® Supplement
Books Out Loud™
Bowker's Complete Video Directory™
Children's Books In Print®
El-Hi Textbooks & Serials In Print®
Forthcoming Books®
Law Books & Serials In Print™
Medical & Health Care Books In Print™
Publishers, Distributors & Wholesalers of the US™
Subject Guide to Books In Print®
Subject Guide to Children's Books In Print®

SALEM PRESS

2021 Title List

SALEM PRESS

Visit www.SalemPress.com for Product Information, Table of Contents, and Sample Pages.

LITERATURE

Critical Insights: Authors

Louisa May Alcott
Sherman Alexie
Isabel Allende
Maya Angelou
Isaac Asimov
Margaret Atwood
Jane Austen
James Baldwin
Saul Bellow
Roberto Bolano
Ray Bradbury
Gwendolyn Brooks
Albert Camus
Raymond Carver
Willa Cather
Geoffrey Chaucer
John Cheever
Joseph Conrad
Charles Dickens
Emily Dickinson
Frederick Douglass
T. S. Eliot
George Eliot
Harlan Ellison
Louise Erdrich
William Faulkner
F. Scott Fitzgerald
Gustave Flaubert
Horton Foote
Benjamin Franklin
Robert Frost
Neil Gaiman
Gabriel Garcia Marquez
Thomas Hardy
Nathaniel Hawthorne
Robert A. Heinlein
Lillian Hellman
Ernest Hemingway
Langston Hughes
Zora Neale Hurston
Henry James
Thomas Jefferson
James Joyce
Jamaica Kincaid
Stephen King
Martin Luther King, Jr.
Barbara Kingsolver
Abraham Lincoln
Mario Vargas Llosa
Jack London
James McBride
Cormac McCarthy
Herman Melville
Arthur Miller
Toni Morrison
Alice Munro
Tim O'Brien
Flannery O'Connor
Eugene O'Neill
George Orwell
Sylvia Plath
Philip Roth
Salman Rushdie
Mary Shelley
John Steinbeck
Amy Tan
Leo Tolstoy
Mark Twain
John Updike
Kurt Vonnegut
Alice Walker
David Foster Wallace
Edith Wharton
Walt Whitman
Oscar Wilde
Tennessee Williams
Richard Wright
Malcolm X

Critical Insights: Works

Absalom, Absalom!
Adventures of Huckleberry Finn
Aeneid
All Quiet on the Western Front
Animal Farm
Anna Karenina
The Awakening
The Bell Jar
Beloved
Billy Budd, Sailor
The Book Thief
Brave New World
The Canterbury Tales
Catch-22
The Catcher in the Rye
The Crucible
Death of a Salesman
The Diary of a Young Girl
Dracula
Fahrenheit 451
The Grapes of Wrath
Great Expectations
The Great Gatsby
Hamlet
The Handmaid's Tale
Harry Potter Series
Heart of Darkness
The Hobbit
The House on Mango Street
How the Garcia Girls Lost Their Accents
The Hunger Games Trilogy
I Know Why the Caged Bird Sings
In Cold Blood
The Inferno
Invisible Man
Jane Eyre
The Joy Luck Club
King Lear
The Kite Runner
Life of Pi
Little Women
Lolita
Lord of the Flies
Macbeth
The Metamorphosis
Midnight's Children
A Midsummer Night's Dream
Moby-Dick
Mrs. Dalloway
Nineteen Eighty-Four
The Odyssey
Of Mice and Men
One Flew Over the Cuckoo's Nest
One Hundred Years of Solitude
Othello
The Outsiders
Paradise Lost
The Pearl
The Poetry of Baudelaire
The Poetry of Edgar Allan Poe
A Portrait of the Artist as a Young Man
Pride and Prejudice
The Red Badge of Courage
Romeo and Juliet
The Scarlet Letter
Short Fiction of Flannery O'Connor
Slaughterhouse-Five
The Sound and the Fury
A Streetcar Named Desire
The Sun Also Rises
A Tale of Two Cities
The Tales of Edgar Allan Poe
Their Eyes Were Watching God
Things Fall Apart
To Kill a Mockingbird
War and Peace
The Woman Warrior

Critical Insights: Themes

The American Comic Book
American Creative Non-Fiction
The American Dream
American Multicultural Identity
American Road Literature
American Short Story
American Sports Fiction
The American Thriller
American Writers in Exile
Censored & Banned Literature
Civil Rights Literature, Past & Present
Coming of Age
Conspiracies
Contemporary Canadian Fiction
Contemporary Immigrant Short Fiction
Contemporary Latin American Fiction
Contemporary Speculative Fiction
Crime and Detective Fiction
Crisis of Faith
Cultural Encounters
Dystopia
Family
The Fantastic
Feminism

2021 Title List

SALEM PRESS

Flash Fiction
Gender, Sex and Sexuality
Good & Evil
The Graphic Novel
Greed
Harlem Renaissance
The Hero's Quest
Historical Fiction
Holocaust Literature
The Immigrant Experience
Inequality
LGBTQ Literature
Literature in Times of Crisis
Literature of Protest
Magical Realism
Midwestern Literature
Modern Japanese Literature
Nature & the Environment
Paranoia, Fear & Alienation
Patriotism
Political Fiction
Postcolonial Literature
Pulp Fiction of the '20s and '30s
Rebellion
Russia's Golden Age
Satire
The Slave Narrative
Social Justice and American Literature
Southern Gothic Literature
Southwestern Literature
Survival
Technology & Humanity
Violence in Literature
Virginia Woolf & 20th Century Women Writers
War

Critical Insights: Film

Bonnie & Clyde
Casablanca
Alfred Hitchcock
Stanley Kubrick

Critical Approaches to Literature

Critical Approaches to Literature: Feminist
Critical Approaches to Literature: Moral
Critical Approaches to Literature: Multicultural
Critical Approaches to Literature: Psychological

Critical Surveys of Literature

Critical Survey of American Literature
Critical Survey of Drama
Critical Survey of Graphic Novels: Heroes & Superheroes
Critical Survey of Graphic Novels: History, Theme, and Technique
Critical Survey of Graphic Novels: Independents and Underground Classics
Critical Survey of Graphic Novels: Manga
Critical Survey of Long Fiction
Critical Survey of Mystery and Detective Fiction
Critical Survey of Mythology & Folklore: Gods & Goddesses
Critical Survey of Mythology & Folklore: Heroes and Heroines
Critical Survey of Mythology & Folklore: Love, Sexuality, and Desire
Critical Survey of Mythology & Folklore: World Mythology
Critical Survey of Poetry
Critical Survey of Poetry: Contemporary Poets
Critical Survey of Science Fiction & Fantasy Literature
Critical Survey of Shakespeare's Plays
Critical Survey of Shakespeare's Sonnets
Critical Survey of Short Fiction
Critical Survey of World Literature
Critical Survey of Young Adult Literature

Cyclopedia of Literary Characters & Places

Cyclopedia of Literary Characters
Cyclopedia of Literary Places

Introduction to Literary Context

American Poetry of the 20th Century
American Post-Modernist Novels
American Short Fiction
English Literature
Plays
World Literature

Magill's Literary Annual

Magill's Literary Annual, 2021
Magill's Literary Annual, 2020
Magill's Literary Annual, 2019

Masterplots

Masterplots, Fourth Edition
Masterplots, 2010-2018 Supplement

Notable Writers

Notable African American Writers
Notable American Women Writers
Notable Mystery & Detective Fiction Writers
Notable Native American Writers & Writers of the American West
Novels into Film: Adaptations & Interpretation
Recommended Reading: 600 Classics Reviewed

SALEM PRESS

2021 Title List

SALEM PRESS

Visit www.SalemPress.com for Product Information, Table of Contents, and Sample Pages.

HISTORY

The Decades

The 1910s in America
The Twenties in America
The Thirties in America
The Forties in America
The Fifties in America
The Sixties in America
The Seventies in America
The Eighties in America
The Nineties in America
The 2000s in America
The 2010s in America

Defining Documents in American History

Defining Documents: The 1900s
Defining Documents: The 1910s
Defining Documents: The 1920s
Defining Documents: The 1930s
Defining Documents: The 1950s
Defining Documents: The 1960s
Defining Documents: The 1970s
Defining Documents: American Citizenship
Defining Documents: The American Economy
Defining Documents: The American Revolution
Defining Documents: The American West
Defining Documents: Business Ethics
Defining Documents: Capital Punishment
Defining Documents: Civil Rights
Defining Documents: Civil War
Defining Documents: The Cold War
Defining Documents: Dissent & Protest
Defining Documents: Drug Policy
Defining Documents: The Emergence of Modern America
Defining Documents: Environment & Conservation
Defining Documents: Espionage & Intrigue
Defining Documents: Exploration and Colonial America
Defining Documents: The Formation of the States
Defining Documents: The Free Press
Defining Documents: The Gun Debate
Defining Documents: Immigration & Immigrant Communities
Defining Documents: The Legacy of 9/11
Defining Documents: LGBTQ+
Defining Documents: Manifest Destiny and the New Nation
Defining Documents: Native Americans
Defining Documents: Political Campaigns, Candidates & Discourse
Defining Documents: Postwar 1940s
Defining Documents: Prison Reform
Defining Documents: Secrets, Leaks & Scandals
Defining Documents: Slavery
Defining Documents: Supreme Court Decisions
Defining Documents: Reconstruction Era
Defining Documents: The Vietnam War
Defining Documents: U.S. Involvement in the Middle East
Defining Documents: World War I
Defining Documents: World War II

Defining Documents in World History

Defining Documents: The 17th Century
Defining Documents: The 18th Century
Defining Documents: The 19th Century
Defining Documents: The 20th Century (1900-1950)
Defining Documents: The Ancient World
Defining Documents: Asia
Defining Documents: Genocide & the Holocaust
Defining Documents: Nationalism & Populism
Defining Documents: Pandemics, Plagues & Public Health
Defining Documents: Renaissance & Early Modern Era
Defining Documents: The Middle Ages
Defining Documents: The Middle East
Defining Documents: Women's Rights

Great Events from History

Great Events from History: The Ancient World
Great Events from History: The Middle Ages
Great Events from History: The Renaissance & Early Modern Era
Great Events from History: The 17th Century
Great Events from History: The 18th Century
Great Events from History: The 19th Century
Great Events from History: The 20th Century, 1901-1940
Great Events from History: The 20th Century, 1941-1970
Great Events from History: The 20th Century, 1971-2000
Great Events from History: Modern Scandals
Great Events from History: African American History
Great Events from History: The 21st Century, 2000-2016
Great Events from History: LGBTQ Events
Great Events from History: Human Rights

Great Lives from History

Computer Technology Innovators
Fashion Innovators
Great Athletes
Great Athletes of the Twenty-First Century
Great Lives from History: African Americans
Great Lives from History: American Heroes
Great Lives from History: American Women
Great Lives from History: Asian and Pacific Islander Americans
Great Lives from History: Inventors & Inventions
Great Lives from History: Jewish Americans
Great Lives from History: Latinos
Great Lives from History: Scientists and Science
Great Lives from History: The 17th Century
Great Lives from History: The 18th Century
Great Lives from History: The 19th Century
Great Lives from History: The 20th Century
Great Lives from History: The 21st Century, 2000-2017
Great Lives from History: The Ancient World
Great Lives from History: The Incredibly Wealthy
Great Lives from History: The Middle Ages
Great Lives from History: The Renaissance & Early Modern Era
Human Rights Innovators
Internet Innovators
Music Innovators
Musicians and Composers of the 20th Century
World Political Innovators

2021 Title List

SALEM PRESS

History & Government
American First Ladies
American Presidents
The 50 States
The Ancient World: Extraordinary People in Extraordinary Societies
The Bill of Rights
The Criminal Justice System
The U.S. Supreme Court

SOCIAL SCIENCES
Civil Rights Movements: Past & Present
Countries, Peoples and Cultures
Countries: Their Wars & Conflicts: A World Survey
Education Today: Issues, Policies & Practices
Encyclopedia of American Immigration
Ethics: Questions & Morality of Human Actions
Issues in U.S. Immigration
Principles of Sociology: Group Relationships & Behavior
Principles of Sociology: Personal Relationships & Behavior
Principles of Sociology: Societal Issues & Behavior
Racial & Ethnic Relations in America
World Geography

SCIENCE
Ancient Creatures
Applied Science
Applied Science: Engineering & Mathematics
Applied Science: Science & Medicine
Applied Science: Technology
Biomes and Ecosystems
Earth Science: Earth Materials and Resources
Earth Science: Earth's Surface and History
Earth Science: Earth's Weather, Water and Atmosphere
Earth Science: Physics and Chemistry of the Earth
Encyclopedia of Climate Change
Encyclopedia of Energy
Encyclopedia of Environmental Issues
Encyclopedia of Global Resources
Encyclopedia of Mathematics and Society
Forensic Science
Notable Natural Disasters
The Solar System
USA in Space

Principles of Science
Principles of Anatomy
Principles of Astronomy
Principles of Behavioral Science
Principles of Biology
Principles of Biotechnology
Principles of Botany
Principles of Chemistry
Principles of Climatology
Principles of Information Technology
Principles of Computer Science
Principles of Ecology
Principles of Energy
Principles of Geology
Principles of Marine Science
Principles of Mathematics
Principles of Modern Agriculture
Principles of Pharmacology
Principles of Physical Science
Principles of Physics
Principles of Programming & Coding
Principles of Robotics & Artificial Intelligence
Principles of Scientific Research
Principles of Sustainability
Principles of Zoology

HEALTH
Addictions, Substance Abuse & Alcoholism
Adolescent Health & Wellness
Aging
Cancer
Community & Family Health Issues
Integrative, Alternative & Complementary Medicine
Genetics and Inherited Conditions
Infectious Diseases and Conditions
Magill's Medical Guide
Nutrition
Psychology & Behavioral Health
Women's Health

Principles of Health
Principles of Health: Allergies & Immune Disorders
Principles of Health: Anxiety & Stress
Principles of Health: Depression
Principles of Health: Diabetes
Principles of Health: Nursing
Principles of Health: Obesity
Principles of Health: Pain Management
Principles of Health: Prescription Drug Abuse

SALEM PRESS

2021 Title List

SALEM PRESS

Visit www.SalemPress.com for Product Information, Table of Contents, and Sample Pages.

CAREERS

Careers: Paths to Entrepreneurship
Careers in the Arts: Fine, Performing & Visual
Careers in Building Construction
Careers in Business
Careers in Chemistry
Careers in Communications & Media
Careers in Education & Training
Careers in Environment & Conservation
Careers in Financial Services
Careers in Forensic Science
Careers in Gaming
Careers in Green Energy
Careers in Healthcare
Careers in Hospitality & Tourism
Careers in Human Services
Careers in Information Technology
Careers in Law, Criminal Justice & Emergency Services
Careers in the Music Industry
Careers in Manufacturing & Production
Careers in Nursing
Careers in Physics
Careers in Protective Services
Careers in Psychology & Behavioral Health
Careers in Public Administration
Careers in Sales, Insurance & Real Estate
Careers in Science & Engineering
Careers in Social Media
Careers in Sports & Fitness
Careers in Sports Medicine & Training
Careers in Technical Services & Equipment Repair
Careers in Transportation
Careers in Writing & Editing
Careers Outdoors
Careers Overseas
Careers Working with Infants & Children
Careers Working with Animals

BUSINESS

Principles of Business: Accounting
Principles of Business: Economics
Principles of Business: Entrepreneurship
Principles of Business: Finance
Principles of Business: Globalization
Principles of Business: Leadership
Principles of Business: Management
Principles of Business: Marketing